Primary Care Medicine

SECOND EDITION

ALLAN H. GOROLL, M.D.
Assistant Professor of Medicine
Harvard Medical School
Massachusetts General Hospital
Boston, Massachusetts

LAWRENCE A. MAY, M.D.
Assistant Clinical Professor of Medicine
University of California, Los Angeles
Los Angeles, California

ALBERT G. MULLEY, JR., M.D., M.P.P.
Assistant Professor of Medicine
Harvard Medical School
Chief, General Internal Medicine Unit
Massachusetts General Hospital
Boston, Massachusetts

With 56 contributors

Primary Care Medicine

Office Evaluation and Management of the Adult Patient

J.B. LIPPINCOTT COMPANY

PHILADELPHIA

London   *Mexico City*   *New York*   *St. Louis*   *São Paulo*   *Sydney*

Sponsoring Editor: Richard Winters
Manuscript Editor: Virginia Barishek
Indexer: Betty Herr Hallinger
Design Director: Tracy Baldwin
Design Coordinator: Susan Hess Blaker
Production Manager: Kathleen Dunn
Production Coordinator: George V. Gordon
Compositor: TAPSCO, Inc.
Printer/Binder: Murray Printing Company

Second Edition

6 5 4 3

Library of Congress Cataloging-in-Publication Data

Goroll, Allan H.
   Primary care medicine.

   Includes bibliographies and index.
   1. Family medicine. I. May, Lawrence A.   II. Mulley,
Albert G.   III. Title. [DNLM: 1. Physicians, Family.
2. Primary Health Care. W 84.6 G672p]
RC46.G56   1987   616   86-27341
ISBN 0-397-50717-8

*The authors and publisher have exerted every effort to ensure that
drug selection and dosage set forth in this text are in accord with
current recommendations and practice at the time of publication.
However, in view of ongoing research, changes in government regulations, and the constant flow of information relating to drug therapy
and drug reactions, the reader is urged to check the package insert
for each drug for any change in indications and dosage and for added
warnings and precautions. This is particularly important when the
recommended agent is a new or infrequently employed drug.*

To JOHN D. STOECKLE, M.D.

Contributors

Ann B. Barnes, M.D.[†]

Assistant Clinical Professor of Obstetrics and Gynecology
Harvard Medical School; and
Assistant Gynecologist
Massachusetts General Hospital
Boston, Massachusetts

Michael J. Barry, M.D.

Instructor in Medicine
Harvard Medical School; and
Assistant in Medicine
Massachusetts General Hospital
Boston, Massachusetts

Arthur J. Barsky, III, M.D.

Assistant Professor of Psychiatry
Harvard Medical School; and
Chief, Primary Care Psychiatry Unit
Massachusetts General Hospital
Boston, Massachusetts

Robert J. Boyd, M.D.

Clinical Associate Professor of Orthopaedics
Harvard Medical School; and
Visiting Orthopaedist
Massachusetts General Hospital
Boston, Massachusetts

David C. Brewster, M.D.

Associate Clinical Professor of Surgery
Harvard Medical School; and
Attending Surgeon
Massachusetts General Hospital
Boston, Massachusetts

† Deceased.

Lynn F. Butterly, M.D.

Clinical Research Fellow in Gastroenterology
Massachusetts General Hospital
Harvard Medical School
Boston, Massachusetts

Carolyn J. Crimmins, R.D., M.P.H., M.B.A.

Associate in Preventive Medicine
Harvard Medical School; and
Business Manager/Nutritionist
Cardiovascular Health Center
Massachusetts General Hospital
Boston, Massachusetts

Gregory D. Curfman, M.D.

Assistant Professor of Medicine and Preventive Medicine
Harvard Medical School
Boston, Massachusetts

Jules L. Dienstag, M.D.

Associate Professor of Medicine
Harvard Medical School; and
Assistant Physician
Massachusetts General Hospital
Boston, Massachusetts

Leslie S.-T. Fang, M.D., Ph.D.

Assistant Professor of Medicine
Harvard Medical School; and
Assistant Physician, Massachusetts General Hospital
Boston, Massachusetts

Lawrence S. Friedman, M.D.

Assistant Professor of Medicine
Jefferson Medical College
Thomas Jefferson University
Philadelphia, Pennsylvania

Jeffrey E. Galpin, M.D.

Director of International Medical Diagnostic, Inc.
Porton International; and
Associate Professor of Medicine
University of California, Los Angeles
Los Angeles, California

Ellie J.C. Goldstein, M.D.

Associate Clinical Professor of Medicine
University of California, Los Angeles
Los Angeles, California;
Director, R. M. Alden Research Laboratory; and
Senior Staff Physician
Santa Monica Hospital and Medical Center
Santa Monica, California

John D. Goodson, M.D.

Assistant Professor of Medicine
Harvard Medical School;
Assistant in Medicine and
Curriculum Director, Primary Care Program
Massachusetts General Hospital
Boston, Massachusetts

Allan H. Goroll, M.D.

Assistant Professor of Medicine
Harvard Medical School
Massachusetts General Hospital
Boston, Massachusetts

David A. Greenberg, O.D., M.P.H.

Professor of Optometry
Vice President for Academic Affairs/Dean
Illinois College of Optometry
Chicago, Illinois

Aina Julianna Gulya, M.D.

Assistant Professor of Surgery
Otology and Neurotologic Surgery
George Washington University Medical Center
Washington, D.C.

Eleanor Z. Hanna, Ph.D.

Instructor, Harvard Medical School; and
Director, Alcohol Clinic
Massachusetts General Hospital
Boston, Massachusetts

Mark S. Huberman, M.D.

Instructor, Harvard Medical School; and
Staff Oncologist
New England Deaconess Hospital
Boston, Massachusetts

Robert A. Hughes, M.D.

Instructor in Medicine
Harvard Medical School; and
Assistant in Medicine
Massachusetts General Hospital
Boston, Massachusetts

Steven E. Hyman, M.D.

Fellow in Genetics, Harvard Medical School; and
Fellow in Molecular Biology and Psychiatry
Massachusetts General Hospital
Boston, Massachusetts

Michael A. Jenike, M.D.

Assistant Professor of Psychiatry
Harvard Medical School; and
Director, Inpatient Psychiatric Unit
Massachusetts General Hospital
Boston, Massachusetts

Jesse B. Jupiter, M.D.

Associate Professor of Orthopaedic Surgery
Harvard Medical School; and
Assistant Orthopaedic Surgeon
Massachusetts General Hospital
Boston, Massachusetts

John P. Kelly, D.M.D., M.D.

Assistant Professor of Oral and Maxillofacial Surgery
Harvard School of Dental Medicine; and
Associate Visiting Oral and Maxillofacial Surgery
Massachusetts General Hospital
Boston, Massachusetts

Eric Kortz, M.D.

Clinical Fellow in Surgery
Harvard Medical School; and
Resident, General Surgery
Massachusetts General Hospital
Boston, Massachusetts

Steven R. Levisohn, M.D.

Instructor in Medicine
Harvard Medical School; and
Assistant in Medicine
Massachusetts General Hospital
Boston, Massachusetts

Richard R. Liberthson, M.D.

Associate Professor of Pediatrics
Associate Professor of Medicine
Harvard Medical School; and
Pediatrician, Associate Physician
Massachusetts General Hospital
Boston, Massachusetts

Jacob J. Lokich, M.D.

Chief of Medical Oncology, The Cancer Center
Medical Center of Boston;
Assistant Professor of Medicine
Harvard Medical School; and
Physician, New England Baptist and
  New England Deaconess Hospital
Boston, Massachusetts

Nicholas J. Lowe, M.D., F.R.C.P.

Professor of Medicine/Dermatology
Associate Chief, Division of Dermatology
Head, Psoriasis and Skin Treatment Center
School of Medicine
University of California, Los Angeles
Los Angeles, California

Michael N. Margolies, M.D.

Associate Professor of Surgery
Harvard Medical School; and
Associate Visiting Surgeon
Massachusetts General Hospital
Boston, Massachusetts

Lawrence A. May, M.D.

Assistant Clinical Professor of Medicine
School of Medicine
University of California, Los Angeles
Los Angeles, California

Charles J. McCabe, M.D.

Assistant Professor of Surgery
Harvard Medical School; and
Associate Director, Emergency Services
Associate Visiting Surgeon
Massachusetts General Hospital
Boston, Massachusetts

William E. Minichiello, Ed.D.

Instructor in Psychology
Harvard Medical School; and
Chief Psychologist
Psychosomatic Medicine Unit
Massachusetts General Hospital
Boston, Massachusetts

Albert G. Mulley, Jr., M.D., M.P.P.

Assistant Professor of Medicine
Harvard Medical School; and
Chief, General Internal Medicine Unit
Associate Physician
Massachusetts General Hospital
Boston, Massachusetts

Samuel R. Nussbaum, M.D.

Assistant Professor of Medicine
Harvard Medical School; and
Director, Endocrine Associates
Massachusetts General Hospital
Boston, Massachusetts

L. Christine Oliver, M.D., M.S.

Assistant Professor
Harvard Medical School; and
Assistant in Medicine
Massachusetts General Hospital
Boston, Massachusetts

Wayne L. Peters, M.D.

Assistant Clinical Professor of Medicine
University of Colorado School of Medicine; and
Medical Director
HealthMark Centers
Denver, Colorado

Amy A. Pruitt, M.D.

Assistant Professor of Neurology
Harvard Medical School; and
Associate Neurologist
Massachusetts General Hospital
Boston, Massachusetts

Marvin J. Rapaport, M.D.

Associate Clinical Professor of Medicine (Dermatology)
Division of Dermatology
School of Medicine
University of California, Los Angeles
Los Angeles, California

Ronald M. Reisner, M.D.

Professor-in-Chief
Division of Dermatology
School of Medicine
University of California, Los Angeles; and
Chief, Dermatology Service
Veterans Administration Wadsworth Medical Center
Los Angeles, California

Claudia U. Richter, M.D.

Clinical Instructor in Ophthalmology
Harvard Medical School; and
Assistant in Ophthalmology
Massachusetts Eye and Ear Infirmary
Boston, Massachusetts

James M. Richter, M.D.

Assistant Professor of Medicine
Harvard Medical School; and
Assistant Physician
Massachusetts General Hospital
Boston, Massachusetts

Nancy A. Rigotti, M.D.

Instructor in Medicine
Harvard Medical School;
Associate Director, Institute for the Study of Smoking
   Behavior and Policy
Harvard University; and
Assistant in Medicine
Massachusetts General Hospital
Boston, Massachusetts

Jerrold F. Rosenbaum, M.D.

Chief, Clinical Psychopharmacology Unit
Massachusetts General Hospital; and
Assistant Professor of Psychiatry
Harvard Medical School
Boston, Massachusetts

Robert T. Schooley, M.D.

Assistant Professor of Medicine
Harvard Medical School
Massachusetts General Hospital
Boston, Massachusetts

Linda C. Shafer, M.D.

Instructor in Psychiatry
Harvard Medical School; and
Assistant in Psychiatry
Massachusetts General Hospital
Boston, Massachusetts

William V.R. Shellow, M.D.

Associate Professor of Medicine (Dermatology)
School of Medicine
University of California, Los Angeles; and
Chief, Inpatient and Consultation Dermatology
Veterans Administration Wadsworth Medical Center
Los Angeles, California

Harvey B. Simon, M.D.

Assistant Professor of Medicine
Harvard Medical School; and
Associate Physician
Massachusetts General Hospital
Boston, Massachusetts

Daniel E. Singer, M.D.

Assistant Professor of Medicine
Harvard Medical School; and
Assistant in Medicine
Massachusetts General Hospital
Boston, Massachusetts

Alan Smith, M.D.

Clinical Assistant Professor in Medicine and
  Gastroenterology
University of Washington School of Medicine; and
Attending Staff Physician
Swedish Hospital Medical Center
Seattle, Washington

Arthur J. Sober, M.D.

Associate Professor of Dermatology
Harvard Medical School; and
Associate Dermatologist
Massachusetts General Hospital
Boston, Massachusetts

Roger F. Steinert, M.D.

Assistant Professor of Ophthalmology
Harvard Medical School; and
Assistant Surgeon in Ophthalmology
Massachusetts Eye and Ear Infirmary
Boston, Massachusetts

John D. Stoeckle, M.D.

Professor of Medicine
Harvard Medical School; and
Physician, Massachusetts General Hospital
Boston, Massachusetts

Katharine K. Treadway, M.D.

Instructor in Medicine
Harvard Medical School; and
Assistant Physician, Massachusetts General Hospital
Boston, Massachusetts

Jeffrey B. Weilburg, M.D.

Clinical Instructor in Psychiatry
Harvard Medical School; and
Director, Neuropsychiatry Section
Psychopharmacology Clinic
Massachusetts General Hospital
Boston, Massachusetts

William R. Wilson, M.D.

Professor of Surgery (Otolaryngology)
George Washington University Medical Center
Washington, D.C.

Foreword to the First Edition

Physicians have traditionally provided direct, initial, comprehensive care for patients as well as continuity of care. In the past two decades the growing proportion of specialist physicians has endangered this traditional role of the physician. The development of highly technologic, tertiary, inpatient medical care has preoccupied the attention of our teaching institutions. Coping with the increased armamentarium of diagnostic and therapeutic interventions has distracted some physicians from traditional roles in patient care. The primary care movement has been a national response to this situation aimed at providing more physicians skilled in dealing wisely and humanely with illness in their patients and providing the overall supervision and continuity of medical care that we expect of good generalists. It encourages these physicians to know their patients as human and social beings as well as bearers of organ pathology. Promotion of prevention as well as the practice of curing is an important part of primary care.

The concerns which have led to renewed attention of the medical profession to primary care medicine have had a very salutary effect on our teaching institutions. There has been a resurgence of training in the ambulatory setting. Medical students and residents have learned that many illnesses formerly thought to require hospitalization can be effectively managed in the ambulatory setting. As usual, this is not an original discovery; rather, it is a return to the emphasis that was very much a part of training programs in the earlier decades of this century.

Primary Care Medicine has grown out of the experiences of a group of young physicians who have pioneered in the rebirth of primary care medicine within the Harvard medical community. They have organized primary care practices which have served as training sites for other physicians and health workers. They have examined their own practices, as well as the published experience of others, in order to provide within this text a synthesis of the best available information for ambulatory management of adult medical patients. Their discussions are brief and practical rather than exhaustive, but the interested reader is provided with a key annotated bibliography which directs him to further sources of information. This book is not meant to compete with the traditional exhaustive textbook of Medicine. Rather, its brief, clear discussions and analyses of current knowledge are prepared for the busy practitioner who daily encounters many problems for which he needs to quickly know the best available answers.

To whom is the book addressed? To the primary care physician, of course. It will be his bible—a valuable source of guidance and of solace in innumerable management situations. But it is becoming increasingly evident that the medical subspecialist devotes a considerable portion of his practice time to the provision of first contact and continuous care of the medical needs of his patients. This book will, therefore, find a welcome place on the desk of both the medical subspecialist and the medical generalist and is addressed to everyone engaged in the clinical practice of adult Medicine.

Alexander Leaf, M.D.
Jackson Professor of Medicine
Harvard Medical School; and
Chief, Medical Services
Massachusetts General Hospital
Boston, Massachusetts
April 1981

Preface

Primary Care Medicine is designed to help those who provide primary care to adults. It attempts to delineate rational approaches to the screening, evaluation, management, and prevention of both the common and the "must-not-miss" clinical problems encountered in office practice. Good primary care requires not only accurate diagnosis and technically sound treatment, but also an understanding of the patient's perspective and his informational needs, an appreciation for costs and cost-effective measures, and an ability to make timely and appropriate referrals and hospital admissions. We have tried to address these essential components of primary care throughout the book.

This book is problem-oriented to facilitate its use in everyday practice. In each chapter, pertinent epidemiology, natural history, pathophysiology, clinical findings, and laboratory tests are considered in terms of their contribution to decision-making. When relevant data are not available, we alert the reader and suggest careful monitoring of the literature. Our aim is to present in a logical yet practical manner effective and efficient approaches to the problems encountered in the office.

The reception to the first edition has been gratifying. We have attempted to preserve its focus and style, while updating and enhancing its content. The knowledge base pertinent to primary care medicine has expanded at a sometimes frightening rate, which has made it necessary to rewrite almost every chapter (there are over 2000 new references in the annotated bibliographies). In doing so we have taken the opportunity to enrich the content and discuss some of the difficult clinical problems that plague even the experienced clinician (*e.g.*, asymptomatic complex ventricular irritability, diarrhea in the homosexual patient, appropriate degree of diabetic control, persistent low back pain, use of estrogens for menopause, chronic somatization).

To improve the utility of the book for office-based care, we have added chapters on office surgical procedures and sigmoidoscopy. Other new chapters are devoted to such important emerging problems as AIDS, Alzheimer's disease, and eating disorders. In many chapters there are new sections that deal with the special problems encountered by elderly, pregnant, and homosexual patients. In all, we address 230 clinical problems in this edition, with the ambitious goal of covering the breadth of primary care internal medicine for the student while providing sufficient depth in difficult areas to aid the experienced practitioner.

We are indebted to our families for their extraordinary patience and support, to our patients (who remain our most effective teachers), and to our mentors, colleagues, and students who have been a continuous source of stimulation and inspiration.

Finally, an extra special thank you to J. Stuart Freeman, Richard Winters, Virginia Barishek, the staff at J.B. Lippincott Company, and Jonathan Meyer for the devoted work and commitment to quality that were so essential to the publication of this book.

Allan H. Goroll, M.D.
Lawrence A. May, M.D.
Albert G. Mulley, Jr., M.D., M.P.P.

Contents

4. Respiratory Problems

5. Gastrointestinal Problems

6. Hematologic and Oncologic Problems

10. Musculoskeletal Problems

11. Neurologic Problems

1

Principles of Primary Care

1

Tasks of Primary Care
JOHN D. STOECKLE, M.D.

DEFINITION OF PRIMARY CARE

Primary care is coordinated, comprehensive, and personal care, available on both a first-contact and continuous basis. It incorporates several tasks: medical diagnosis and treatment, psychological assessment and management, personal support, communication of information about illness, prevention, and health maintenance.

This book addresses the clinical problems encountered by primary care physicians in office practice of adult medicine. In this setting, the physician's responsibilities and tasks extend beyond the narrow technological confines of medical diagnosis and treatment. Although a great deal of effort must be focused on accurate diagnosis and technically sound therapy, the other clinical tasks that complete the very definition of primary care also assume major importance.

Alongside this clinical definition of primary care stands a plethora of other definitions; these derive from organizational, functional, professional, and academic perspectives. For example, policy planners have defined primary care as a *level of medical services,* one that is provided outside the hospital. Presumably, primary care (community-based services) is, then, a less technical practice compared with secondary care (consultant or specialty services) and tertiary care (hospital services). This organizational definition provides a scheme for the allocation of public resources among these health services, each of which has a distinct professional, economic, institutional and political structure. For another definition, Alpert and Charney have looked at important *patient care functions* of doctors, namely, to provide access, continuity, and integration. Although this view is useful in describing the functions performed by practitioners for their patients within organized health services, it does not define the content of their clinical work. From the standpoint of professionalism, primary care has been defined as a *specialty* concentrating on humanistic medicine practiced outside the hospital, but devoid of the special procedures and technology that typically characterize medical specialization. This definition has been useful in organizing a segment of the profession, for example, family practice, and in providing a new curriculum for the education and training of doctors. From the university comes still another definition of primary care as an *academic discipline* concerned with the expansion of knowledge unique to primary practice and to personal care, a definition that contains the promise of a departmental position for primary care in the medical school.

Although each of these definitions presents a particular perspective about primary care and serves some special purpose, none explains the primary care physician's day-to-day work with patients.

By taking the perspective of the doctor's practice, primary care can be defined by several tasks: (1) medical diagnosis and treatment; (2) psychological diagnosis and treatment; (3) personal support of patients of all backgrounds, in all stages of illness; (4) communication of information about diagnosis, treatment, prevention, and prognosis; (5) maintenance of patients with chronic illness; (6) prevention of disability and disease through detection, education, persuasion, and preventive treatment. These tasks comprise the clinical work of doctors providing primary care. They not only restate medicine's central mandate of patient care, but also constitute a clinical definition of primary care to which the information in this text is applied.

THE TASKS AND THEIR RATIONALES

Except for medical diagnosis and treatment, the tasks that define primary care may seem merely vocational, that is, practical but not scientifically based. However, social science research has provided a logical and rational basis for the clinical work of primary care. The data derived from these studies concern the patients's illness rather than the doctor's definition of disease; they are contained in the cognitive, communicative and behavioral processes by which the patient defines being ill; and they are found in the clinical and social science literature on such topics as the patient's emotional reactions, personality, expectations, requests, attributions, views of treatment and social networks, to mention but a few. Knowledge concerning such aspects of care in conjunction with statistical thinking contributes a rational framework for the tasks of primary care.

Medical diagnosis and treatment remains a central task, although it is by no means the end point of care. As the patient's first contact with medical services, the primary doctor must not only be knowledgeable about disease, but must exercise critical judgment in determining the scope, site, and pace of the medical workup and management. In organizing diagnosis and management, the physician needs to know the clinical presentation and natural history of illness, the uses and limits of the laboratory, and the indications for and shortcomings of invasive tests and therapeutic measures. In continuing care, the issues are the same. The doctor's critical attitude toward the use of technology and the referral of patients for special therapies or diagnostic techniques remains essential. Chapter 2 considers methods developed in clinical epidemiology and decision analysis, which promise to help the clinician rationally choose among a sometimes bewildering array of diagnostic and therapeutic options.

Psychological diagnosis and treatment and personal support complement the medical components of care. Studies documenting the relationship between emotional reactions and illness, coupled with surveys showing a high frequency of such reactions in office practice, underscore their importance in patients seeking medical help. Recognition of anxiety, depression, sexual dysfunction, personality disturbance, and psychosis is necessary for the interpretation of bodily complaints, the communication of personal feelings, and the joint decision of doctor and patient on acceptable and effective treatment plans.

Recognition of emotional reactions alone is insufficient. The doctor's response to the normal patient's psychological defenses is essential to securing cooperation and relieving anxiety. Understanding the patient's defenses and personality style allows the clinician to provide meaningful support and to respond appropriately to the patient's emotional needs. The care rendered is then likely to be perceived as personal and psychologically acceptable. Much of this analysis of the psychological aspects of clinical practice derives from contributions by Kahana and Bibring, Lipsett, Balaint, and Zaborenko.

Information about the patient's expectations and requests is also important. *Expectations* often play a major part in seeking help, complying with treatment, and feeling satisfied with care. In their studies of illness behavior and patients' use of doctors, Zola and Mechanic viewed expectations as explanations of patients' decisions to go to see the doctor. If attention was not paid to the patient's reason for coming, the corollary was clear: the patient would not stay in treatment. In health centers in Israel, Shuval found specific expectations of visits to doctors: status enhancement in seeing socially important professionals; catharsis of grief, anger, and despair; sanctioning of failure to cope; and understanding and control of illness through medical "scientific" explanations. This brief list is by no means complete, for along with these so-called latent expectations are traditional or "real" medical ones—for example, that the doctor is a healer of disease and possesses techniques for its control, relief, or cure. Such expectations not only explain the decision to seek medical care but are, in fact, elements of the clinical tasks of personal support and communication of information about illness.

Newer clinical studies by Lazare and colleagues have separated *requests* from expectations. Requests are specific and concrete helping actions and behaviors identified by patients. These studies identified some 14 requests and demonstrated that their prompt recognition and negotiation benefited both patient and doctor. The doctor's interest in ascertaining what treatment the patient wants indicates a reciprocity that is associated with greater satisfaction and adherence to medical advice. These efforts are part of the task of personal support and management. Still other elements of the management task, such as decisions about continued care, referral, and discharge, are also realized through an understanding of requests; thus, physicians need both to elicit and to respond to them.

The communication of information about illness—the need to inform, explain, reassure, and advise patients—is essential to primary care. This task is often dependent on a knowledge of the patient's *attributions* (i.e., what the patient thinks is the cause of illness). If the patient's attributions differ from the doctor's and are not uncovered, his anxieties may not be relieved, nor will the doctor's explanation be accepted. Knowing how and what to tell the patient about his illness is often difficult, especially if the patient's interpretation of the illness has not been elicited.

Mechanic, for example, suggests that patients with bodily complaints may go to the primary care doctor not for relief of physical discomfort but rather to learn what causes their complaints and sometimes to obtain reassurance that their complaints have less serious causes than they thought. Such confirmation or correction of the patient's attributions is a kind of "attribution therapy." From a broader perspective, Kleinman assigns to attributions a major function in all medical care systems, namely, the control of illness through the explanation of its cause. In effect, the doctor's clinical or scientific explanations of illness provide labels, names, and models so that the patient feels his illness can be understood and controlled, regardless of its technical treatment. In essence, the patient's beliefs about illness need to be elicited so that they can be used in explanation, education, and reassurance. (See Appendix.)

Maintenance of the chronically ill requires continuous, long-term treatment and is a distinct task of primary care. Here, obtaining patient compliance is essential because most long-term treatment now takes place without daily medical supervision, and most of that treatment requires the self-administration of drugs. To improve adherence to therapy, it has become increasingly important to learn about the *patient's views of treatment* and actual self-treatment. So far the record on adherence to treatment has not been good. A wide discrepancy between what is prescribed and what is done typifies the literature of "following the doctor's orders," and the problem seems to be as much the doctor's as the patient's.

Knowledge about patients' views and behaviors can be used to design more effective therapeutic regimens and to alter therapeutic directions. Moreover, the act of eliciting information may improve communication between doctor and patient, thus strengthening their relationship and further promoting therapeutic efforts. More studies of patient views of treatment and of the dynamics of the doctor–patient relationship should provide new knowledge that can be used to enhance compliance.

Prevention of disease and disability, another modern component of primary care, emphasizes screening and reduction in risk factors to avoid the more elaborate technologies sometimes necessary for cure. The primary physician needs to know which conditions and risk factors are worth screening for and how best to detect and effectively manage them; thus, it is hoped that some potential causes of morbidity and mortality will be foreseen and prevented. (See Chapter 3.)

A less commonly considered but no less important aspect of prevention involves attention to the patient's *social network,* since illness is often precipitated by disruption of interpersonal relationships. For example, Parkes and others have noted an increased mortality and morbidity among recent widows, while Zola has reported that interpersonal crises were among the most frequent of five common circumstances that spurred the individual to come for medical attention. Knowledge of patients' social situations can help in prevention of illness and visits to the doctor by focusing attention on stresses that might be precipitants. Attention to social networks is important for personal treatment. If significant loss or separation occurs, a major part of treatment can involve helping the patient reestablish his social network, thus lessening dependence on professional help from the doctor, nurse, or social worker.

THE PROMISE OF PRIMARY CARE MEDICINE

So far the clinical tasks of primary care have been proposed as a perspective from which readers might view the information in this text. In addition, the tasks also promise changes in our ideas about standards of treatment, the doctor–patient relationship, professional relations, organization, prevention, clinical excellence, and clinical effectiveness.

Treatment. The ideal of personal treatment is revived and reemphasized. Though it is not entirely dead, the increasing size, specialization, and organization of practice often makes personal, patient-oriented treatment a luxury rather than a medical care necessity. Patient-centered treatment also means that specific therapeutic regimens must not only be technically correct, but designed to be acceptable to patients, especially since more patients than ever are being cared for on an outpatient basis.

Doctor–Patient Relationship. Patient-centered treatment in primary care practice implies a doctor–patient relationship in which the doctor acts out several behaviors that will enhance the patient's participation in care and treatment:

1. Making the relation more democratic by giving patients a part in decisions about the scope of diagnosis and alternatives of treatment.
2. Developing patient participation by transmitting appropriate information so that patients can make intelligent choices.
3. Attending to patients' feelings about illness and treatment with regard, genuine concern, and empathy.
4. Providing helping actions that are person-centered by eliciting, acknowledging, and responding to patients' own perspectives of their illness and care.
5. Responding by negotiation to the patients' choices, decisions, and requests; similarly, acknowledging and negotiating conflict even if in the relationship itself.
6. Promoting health education, self-help, and preventive behaviors by communicating information about diagnosis, treatment, and prevention.
7. Conveying respect for the person of the patient without regard to the patient's gender, race, ethnicity, or age.

Professional Relations. The primary physician's responsibility for accessible, integrated, and continuous care is enhanced and made central. One consequence is that decision making is now coordinated by the generalist; so often in the past it was not.

Organization. Because the goals of primary care include not only cure, but also prevention and health maintenance, the ambulatory site emerges as the major organizational setting for delivery of primary care services.

Prevention. The ideal of prevention in practice has been to deal with the individual patient seeking help. Primary care medicine also examines the epidemiology of the entire practice, and perhaps even its community base, to institute a program of effective preventive intervention.

Clinical Excellence. Skills in medical diagnosis and treatment have often been the only measure of clinical excellence. The ideal of excellence is now expanded to include skills in *all* clinical tasks of primary care. Moreover, the value of a carefully performed history and physical examination receives renewed emphasis as concerns about overuse of the laboratory and expensive high technology grow.

Clinical Effectiveness. The usual objective criteria for efficacy of diagnosis and treatment have been derived from the standards of clinical science. Consideration of subjective parameters such as patient acceptance and a sense of well-being is mandatory in the primary care setting and must be added to the assessment of clinical efficacy.

These themes on the clinical tasks and promises of primary care run through the chapters that follow, sometimes explicitly, sometimes latently; but they are always central to providing personalized care to patients.

ANNOTATED BIBLIOGRAPHY

Alpert JJ, Charney E: The Education of Physicians for Primary Care. DHEW Publication No 74–31B. US Government Printing Office, 1975 (*Functional definition of primary care.*)

Balaint M: The Doctor, the Patient and the Illness. New York, International Universities Press, 1957 (*A classic study of the British general practitioner's negotiations with patients about diagnosis and treatment.*)

Hicks D: Primary Health Care, a Review, Commissioned by the Department of Health and Social Security, London, Her Majesty's Stationery Office, 1976 (*Organizational definition of primary care.*)

Kahana RJ, Bibring GL: Personality types in medical management. In NE Zinberg (ed): Psychiatry and Medical Practice in a General Hospital, pp 108–123. New York; International Universities Press, 1965 (*Discusses the use of defense mechanisms derived from personality assessment in treatment.*)

Kasl SV, Cobb S: Health behavior, illness behavior and sick role behavior. I: Health and illness. Arch Environ Health 12:245, 1966 (*A thorough review of sociological and psychiatric studies on the factors that lead to a decision to seek help.*)

Kleinman AM: Toward a comparative study of medical systems: An integrated approach to the study of the relationship of medicine and culture Sci Med Man 1:55, 1973 (*A study that examines the specific and general significance of attributions.*)

Lazare A, Cohen F, Mignone R et al: The walk-in patient as a customer: A key dimension in evaluation and treatment. Am J Orthopsychiatry 42:872, 1972

Lazare A, Eisenthal S, Frank A et al: Studies on a negotiated approach to patienthood. The doctor–patient relation. In E Gallagher (ed): Fogarty International Center Series on the Teaching of Preventive Medicine, Vol 4. Washington DC, DHEW, 1977 (*Two studies that systematically examine requests of patients in a psychiatric clinic.*)

Lindemann E: Symptomatology and management of acute grief. Am J Psychiatry 101:141, 1944 (*A classic paper on the symptoms in medical patients.*)

Lipsett D: Medical and psychological characteristics of "crocks." Psychiatry Med 15:293, 1970 (*Describes the patient who needs to have bodily complaints and suggests a means of management that takes this need into account.*)

McDill MS: Structure of social systems determining attitudes, knowledge and behavior toward disease. In AJ Enelow, JB Henderson (eds): Applying Behavioral Sciences to Cardiovascular Risk. New York, American Heart Association, 1975 (*Reviews the potential use of networks in prevention of cardiovascular disease.*)

McKinlay JB: Social networks, lay consultation and help-seeking behavior. Social Forces 51:275, 1973 (*Uses networks to explain differences in help-seeking behavior.*)

McWhinney IR: General practice as an academic discipline. Lancet 1:419, 1966 (*Defines primary care from an academic perspective.*)

Mechanic D: Medical Sociology. New York, Free Press, 1968 (*A classic text detailing the interaction of social factors and illness.*)

Mechanic D: Social psychologic factors affecting the presentation of bodily complaints. N Engl J Med 286:1132, 1972 (*A sociological study that examines the factors influencing the patient's decision to seek medical help.*)

Parkes CM: Effects of bereavement on physical and mental health—A study of medical records of widows. Br Med J 2:274, 1964 (*One of a number of studies documenting increased morbidity and mortality among widows shortly after the death of their husbands.*)

Proger S: Doctor of primary medicine (editorial). JAMA 220:410, 1972 (*Defines primary care as a specialty rather than as a function.*)

Shuval JT, Antonovsky A, Davies AM: Social Function of Medical Practice: Doctor–patient Relationship in Israel. San Francisco, Jossey–Bass, 1970 (*An analysis of the rates and reasons for medical visits; provides a typology of the uses of medical visits.*)

Stoeckle JD, Zola IK, Davidson GE: On going to see the doctor. The contributions of the patient to the decision to seek medical aid. J Chronic Dis 16:975, 1963 (*An analysis of patients' expectations in medical practice.*)

Stoeckle JD, Zola IK, Davidson GE: The quality and significance of psychological distress in medical patients. J Chronic Dis 17:959, 1964 (*A review of the many studies of the psychological distress found in medical patients.*)

Waitzkin H, Stoeckle JD: The communication of information about illness: Clinical, sociological and methodological considerations. In ZJ Lipowski (ed): Advances in Psychosomatic Medicine: Psychosocial Aspects of Physical Illness, Vol 8, pp 180–216. Basel, S Karger, 1972 (*A review of the significance of and research on communication in medical practice.*)

Zaborenko RN, Zaborenko L, Hengea RA: The psychodynamics of physicianhood. Psychiatry 33:102, 1970 (*This study is illustrative of the importance of understanding patients' defenses and personalities and the uses this knowledge may have in the treatment relationship.*)

Zola IK: Studying the decision to see a doctor. In ZJ Lipowski (ed): Advances in Psychosomatic Medicine: Psychosocial Aspects of Physical Illness, Vol 8, pp 216–236. Basel, S Karger, 1972 (*The paper describes the typology of decisions and their dynamics.*)

Appendix: Approaches to Encouraging Compliance

That 20% to 80% of patients do not comply with medical advice is repeatedly quoted. Such dismal statistics are derived from a rigid definition of compliance as patients' all-or-nothing adherence to medical instructions, whereas their treatment behaviors are far more variable, ranging from the optimal cooperative response to the ritualistic, retreatist, and innovative. Regardless of the extent and variability of noncompliance, patients' adherence to medication regimens is critical in effectively treating medical disorders, as is their adoption and learning of appropriate behaviors (in eating, exercise, smoking, drinking, relaxation, and drug use) for preventing disease.

Explanations and theories of noncompliance have focused on patients' beliefs, attitudes, expectations, and feelings that interfere with their "taking pills" or "changing habits." Even if such factors do interfere, they can be changed. Compliance can be improved by practitioner–patient communication that responds to patient views and develops the patient's ability to adhere to medical advice through education and the learning of new behaviors. Fostering compliance is a major goal of patient education.

SPECIFIC STRATEGIES

The educational/communication strategies and techniques helpful in facilitating compliance begin with the doctor–patient relation. A positive, affiliative doctor–patient relationship is important for making the patient "ready" to receive patient education and to negotiate the goals and means of treatment. Moreover, the physician's explanations and educational efforts, in turn, contribute to that relationship. Specific strategies utilize persuasion, medical advice, feedback, and monitoring.

Persuasion, or Why Do It?
1. Describe immediate and long-term treatment benefits with health risk and cost. If possible, present treatment options and acknowledge if rationale differs from view of patient.
2. Assist patients in clarifying their priorities (requests) for treatment (*e.g.,* patients presenting with pain may request explanation rather than medication).
3. Use your expertise, experience, and relationship to assert your own expectations that the patient should comply, in supporting the patient's treatment choice and capacity to carry it out.

The Medical Advice, or What to Do
1. Adapt instruction to the patient's language and knowledge level, responding to any misconceptions about treatment.
2. Make directions explicit, simple, personalized, and operational (how many, what kind, and when to take "pills;"

organizing "pill taking" into the routine of the patient's everyday life).
3. Use multiple modes of communication, both verbal and written instructions and, where available, audiovisual materials that reinforce general knowledge about treatment. Enlist other members of the clinical team in providing instructions; also recruit family in the educational process.

Feedback, or What Advice Was Negotiated?
1. Have the patient repeat the medical advice given and the rationale for it.
2. Have the patient rehearse how medical advice will be carried out.
3. Jointly plan return visits, phone calls, and additional reviews with clinical team (nurse practitioners, physician assistants), if needed.

Monitoring Compliance, or What Have You Done?
1. At return visits review the patient's compliance by direct questioning, again eliciting the rationale along with the problems the patient experienced in treatment.
2. Use information to reexplain or redesign treatment, reinforce behaviors, and reward the patient.
3. Encourage and organize the patient's self-monitoring of treatment (*e.g.,* blood pressure measurements).

In general, these educational strategies and tactics are not systematically carried out in practitioner–patient communication. Their use in patient education should result in greater compliance with medical advice.

ANNOTATED BIBLIOGRAPHY

DiMatteo MR, Nicola DD: Achieving Patient Complaince. New York, Pergamon Press, 1982 (*Another thoughtful review with emphasis on what to do.*)

Harris L et al: Americans and their Doctors. New York, Pfizer Pharmaceuticals, 1985 (*More on the relationship.*)

Mumford E: The responses patients have to medical advice. In Understanding Human Behavior in Health and Illness. Baltimore, Williams & Wilkins, 1985 (*Responses range from the ritualistic to the innovative.*)

Sackett DL, Snow JC: The magnitude of compliance and non-compliance. In Haynes R, Sackett D (eds): Compliance in Health Care. Baltimore, Johns Hopkins University Press, 1979 (*One of many useful chapters in this book devoted to both academic and practical aspects of the compliance issue.*)

Stimson GV: Obeying the doctor's orders: A view from the other side. Soc Sci Med 8:97, 1974 (*A study that details what patients think after they have left the doctor's office.*)

Suarstad BL: Patient–practitioner relationships and compliance with prescribed medical regimens. In Aiken LH, Mechanic D (eds): Applications of Social Science to Clinical Medicine and Health Policy. New Brunswick, NJ: Rutgers University Press, 1986 (*Emphasis on the relationship to facilitate compliance.*)

2

The Selection and Interpretation
of Diagnostic Tests

Laboratory investigations are often essential to patient care. Although the history and physical examination remain the foundation of a clinical data base and sometimes suffice, the limits to what we can know about a patient are continually expanding with the addition of new diagnostic tests. These tests have many uses: to make a diagnosis in a patient known to be sick; to provide prognostic information for a patient with known disease; to identify an individual with subclinical disease or at risk for subsequent development of disease; and to monitor ongoing therapy. The ultimate objective is to reduce patient morbidity and mortality and improve satisfaction and sense of well-being. If the physician and patient are to reach these objectives, they must avoid some pitfalls along the way that may result from misuse or misinterpretation of laboratory tests.

Pitfalls are more likely to be avoided if the physician appreciates the inherent uncertainty and probabilistic nature of the diagnostic process and understands the relationship between characteristics of a diagnostic test and of the patient(s) being tested. Sometimes a diagnosis is evident when a patient presents with a pathognomonic constellation of signs and symptoms. In most cases, however, presenting signs or symptoms are not specific. Rather, they can be explained by a number of diagnoses, each with distinctly different implications for the patient's health. On completion of the history and physical examination, the clinician considers a list of conditions, referred to as the differential diagnosis, that might explain the findings. The diagnoses may then be ranked, reflecting an implicit assignment of probabilities to each. Such a ranking can be thought of as the physician's index of suspicion for each condition, based on knowledge and past experience with similar patients. The purpose of subsequent laboratory testing is to refine the initial probability estimates and, in the process, to revise the differential diagnosis. The probability of any particular disease on the revised list will depend on its probability of being present before testing and the validity of the information provided by test results.

THE VOCABULARY OF DIAGNOSTIC
TEST INTERPRETATION

Terminology is important in diagnostic test interpretation. Clinical pathologists often focus on a test's accuracy and precision. *Accuracy* is the degree of closeness of the measurement made to the true value, measured by some alternative "gold

standard" or definitive test. *Precision* is the test's ability to give nearly the same result in repeated determinations. Clinicians are more concerned with the ability of a test result to discriminate between persons with and persons without a given disease or condition; this discriminating ability can be characterized by a test's sensitivity and specificity. *Sensitivity* is the probability that a test will be positive when it is applied to a person who actually has the disease. *Specificity* is the probability that a test will be negative when it is applied to a person who actually does not have the disease. A perfectly sensitive test can rule out disease if the result is negative. A perfectly specific test can rule in disease if the result is positive. Because most tests are neither perfectly sensitive nor perfectly specific, the result must be interpreted probabilistically rather than categorically.

Although sensitivity and specificity are important considerations in selecting a test, the probabilities they measure are not in themselves what ordinarily concern the physician and the patient after the test result has returned. Both are concerned with the following questions: If the result is positive, what is the probabiity that disease is present? If the result is negative, what is the probability that the patient is indeed disease-free? These probabilities are known respectively as the *predictive value positive* and the *predictive value negative.* They are determined not only by the sensitivity and specificity of the test, but also by the probability of the disease being present before the test was ordered.

Relationships between sensitivity and specificity and positive and negative predictive values can be better understood by referring to a two-by-two table (Fig. 2-1). The two columns indicate the presence or absence of disease (note that a gold standard of diagnosis is assumed) and the two rows indicate positive or negative test results. Any given patient with a test result could be included in one of the four cells labeled *a*, *b*, *c*, or *d*. Definitions of sensitivity, specificity, predictive value positive, and predictive value negative can be restated using these labels. It is important to note that each of these four ratios has a complement. The complement of sensitivity (1 − sensitivity) is referred to as the *false-negative rate,* while the complement of specificity (1 − specificity) is referred to as the *false-positive rate.* These terms are often used ambiguously in the medical literature: the false-negative rate is confused with the complement of the predictive value negative which is termed the *false-reassurance rate;* the false-positive rate is confused with the complement of the predic-

Disease

		Present	Absent	
Test	Positive	a	b	a + b
	Negative	c	d	c + d
		a + c	b + d	a + b + c + d

Definitions

Sensitivity:	$\dfrac{a}{a+c}$	False negative rate:	$\dfrac{c}{a+c}$
Specificity:	$\dfrac{d}{b+d}$	False positive rate:	$\dfrac{b}{b+d}$
Predictive value positive:	$\dfrac{a}{a+b}$	False alarm rate:	$\dfrac{b}{a+b}$
Predictive value negative:	$\dfrac{d}{c+d}$	False reassurance rate:	$\dfrac{c}{c+d}$

Figure 2-1. The two-by-two table clarifies relationships between test characteristics (sensitivity and specificity) and predictive values of positive and negative test results. The clinician, interpreting a diagnostic test, can fill in the table if he is aware of the test's sensitivity and specificity and the patient's (population's) pretest probability (prevalence) of disease. Pretest probability is $(a + c)$ and $(1 -$ the pretest probability) is $(b + d)$. Multiplying $(a + c)$ by the sensitivity provides the value for a, and multiplying $(b + d)$ by the specificity provides the value for d. Values for cell c and cell b can be determined by simple subtraction. With the cells filled in, the predictive value of a negative or positive test can be calculated easily. It is worth noting that this calculation method is precisely equivalent to Bayes' theorem of conditional probability.

tive value positive, the *false-alarm rate.* The terms false-reassurance rate and false-alarm rate, have been designated to help avoid ambiguity.

INTERPRETING TESTS: REVISING DIAGNOSTIC PROBABILITIES

When the clinician interprets a test result, he usually processes the information informally. Rarely is a pad and pencil or calculator used to explicitly revise probability estimates. But sometimes the revision of diagnostic probabilities is counterintuitive; for instance, it has been shown that most clinicians rely too heavily on positive test results when the pretest probability or disease prevalence is low.

Attention to the two-by-two table indicates why predictive values are crucially dependent on disease prevalence. This is particularly true when one is using a test to screen for a rare disease. When a disease is rare, even a very small false-positive rate (remember, that is the complement of specificity) is multiplied by a very large relative number—that is, $(b + d) \gg (a + c)$. Therefore, b will be surprisingly large relative to a, and the predictive value positive will be counterintuitively low. Examples of this effect are evident in Table 2-1.

Consider the example of a noninvasive test to detect coronary disease applied to a 40-year-old man with a history of atypical chest pain. Based on test evaluations reported in the literature, the sensitivity and specificity of the test can be estimated at 80% and 90%, respectively. Based on symptoms and risk factors, the clinician estimates that the patient's pretest probability of coronary disease is 0.20. (This is the same as saying that the prevalence of coronary disease in a population of similar patients would be 20%.)

Referring to Figure 2-1, with a pretest probability of 0.20, $a + c = 0.20$ and $b + d = 0.80$. Multiplying 0.20×0.8 (the sensitivity) gives us a value of 0.16 for a (subtraction gives us a value of 0.04 for c). Multiplying 0.80×0.9 (the specificity) gives us a value of 0.72 for d (again, subtraction gives us 0.08 for b). The predictive value positive, then, is 0.16/0.24, or 0.66. The predictive value negative is 0.72/0.76, or 0.95.

The clinician can use another method to quickly revise probabilities to test his or her intuition. It requires an understanding of *odds* as well as probability. If P is the probability that a particular disease is present, the ratio of P to $(1 - P)$, or $P/(1 - P)$, is called the odds favoring that disease. The odds against that disease being present are represented by $(1 - P)/P$. Just as one can estimate the pretest probability of disease before diagnostic tests are performed, one can express that estimate as the pretest odds.

Pretest odds can be revised simply by multiplying a ratio called the *likelihood ratio,* which is the relative occurrence of the test result among persons with and without disease—that is, the probability of the result given the presence of

Table 2-1. Effect of Prior Probability (Prevalence)
on Predictive Value of Positive Test Results

PRIOR PROBABILITY (PREVALENCE), %	PREDICTIVE VALUE OF POSITIVE TEST, %		
	Sensitivity 90%/ Specificity 90%	*Sensitivity 95%/ Specificity 95%*	*Sensitivity 99%/ Specificity 99%*
0.1	0.9	1.9	9.0
1	8.3	16.1	50.0
2	15.5	27.9	66.9
5	32.1	50.0	83.9
50	90.0	95.0	99.0

disease divided by the probability of the result given the absence of disease. Note that the likelihood ratio is nothing more (or less) than the ratio of sensitivity to the false-positive rate (*i.e.,* 1 − specificity). It therefore includes all the information contained in estimates of sensitivity and specificity. When the pretest odds of a disease are multiplied by the likelihood ratio, the result—sometimes termed the post-test odds—represents the odds favoring disease given the test result.

Returning to the example, the patient with atypical chest pain could have his chances of having coronary disease expressed as odds rather than probability. A probability of 0.20 is equivalent to odds of 1/4 (0.20/0.80). The likelihood ratio for a test with a sensitivity of 0.8 and a specificity of 0.9 is 8 (0.8/[1 − 0.9]). The pretest odds can be converted to post-test odds simply by multiplying by the likelihood ratio: 1/4 × 8 = 2. Note that the post-test odds ratio of 2:1 is equivalent to the post-test probability of 0.66.

WHERE DOES THE INFORMATION COME FROM?

One of the reasons clinicians are reluctant to take a quantitative approach to diagnostic test interpretation is that such an approach suggests a precision that belies our uncertainty about pretest probabilities and about sensitivity and specificity of even commonly used tests. Estimation of pretest probability hinges on epidemiologic information about the incidence and prevalence of various diseases, modified on the basis of patient characteristics and presenting symptoms. This kind of information is all too rarely presented in the medical literature. Estimates are necessarily uncertain.

There is also uncertainty about the sensitivity and specificity of tests. Rarely are these values presented in medical texts, and test evaluations in the medical literature can sometimes be misleading. The clinician should be familiar with some of the reasons that a test rarely performs as well in general use as it does during the evaluation study that appears in the medical journal.

The False-Positive Rate and Pretest Probability: Overestimating Predictive Values

The importance of the pretest probability of disease in an individual patient (or the prevalence of disease in a population of such patients) for determining the predictive values of a test is often not fully appreciated and may lead to disappointment in the clinical performance of the test. Consider how, during its evaluation, the sensitivity and specificity of a test are estimated. Two groups of patients are assembled. One consists of patients known to have the disease in question as defined by some gold standard (represented by $a + c$ in Fig. 2-1). The other consists of persons without disease based on the same gold standard (represented by $b + d$). The test being evaluated is then applied to both populations. The proportion of those with disease who have a positive result ($a/a + c$) provides us with an estimate of the test's sensitivity. The proportion of those without the disease who have a neg-

ative test ($d/b + d$) gives us an estimate of the test's specificity. Our confidence that these estimates of sensitivity and specificity are accurate increases with the number of people in each group tested. The investigator can most efficiently maximize confidence in the estimates of both sensitivity and specificity by applying the test to disease and nondisease groups of equal size. It is not surprising, therefore, that tests are often evaluated by applying them to populations in which disease and nondisease occur with equal frequency, or nearly so.

If sensitivity, specificity, and predictive values are sufficiently high in such an evaluation study, the test is proposed for general use. What happens when the test is adopted and applied in a general population in which the disease is much less likely to occur than nondisease? The sensitivity and specificity should remain the same, but the predictive value positive will necessarily fall, and its complement, the false-alarm rate, will necessarily increase. This phenomenon is most important when the disease in question is rare, as is evident in Table 2-1.

Defining Disease for Diagnostic Test Evaluation: The Gold Standard Problem

To evaluate a diagnostic test, an investigator must be able to distinguish between persons with and without disease by some alternative method. Often this gold standard test is more invasive or more expensive than the newer, proposed test being evaluated. (The newer test would not be worth evaluating, if it did not confer some advantage for patient or clinician.) Sometimes a gold standard is not readily available. If the disease is one with a short, predictable natural history (*e.g.,* pancreatic cancer), an investigator may resort to follow-up, defining the absence of disease by morbidity-free survival over a specified period. But if the disease has a highly variable natural history (*e.g.,* coronary disease or most rheumatologic disorders), the follow-up approach becomes impractical. Instead, the investigator must rely on more arbitrary and often more subjective criteria to define disease, including combinations of tests, signs, or symptoms. Herein lies a potential pitfall that can affect the accuracy of the estimates of sensitivity and specificity. If the diagnostic criteria are not assessed independently of the test being evaluated, the sensitivity, specificity, or both will be overestimated.

The problem occurs in its most obvious form when a positive test result leads the investigator to a more extensive search for disease than was applied to those with a negative test. A related problem occurs when the test and the diagnostic criteria are very similar biologic measures. An example of this problem is the estimation of the sensitivity and specificity of isoenzymes for myocardial infarction. In the absence of a ready gold standard, investigators have used various criteria to define acute myocardial infarction. Some have included total enzyme levels among the criteria when evaluating the diagnostic value of isoenzymes. This will result in too optimistic estimates of sensitivity and specificity. To the extent that false-negative isoenzyme results are correlated with false-negative total enzyme results, the sensitivity of the isoenzyme test will be overestimated. To the extent that false-positive isoenzyme results are correlated with false-positive total enzyme results, the specificity of the new test will be overestimated.

The Narrow Spectrum Problem: Overestimating Sensitivity When the "Disease" Group Is Too Sick

When an investigator assembles a group known to have the disease in question by means of some gold standard, he may choose patients with unequivocal diagnostic (gold standard) findings. In doing so, the investigator may select a severely ill group that is not representative of the disease in the general population; that is, he will focus on too narrow a spectrum of disease.

Consider the investigator evaluating a noninvasive test for coronary artery disease such as an electrocardiographically monitored exercise tolerance test. To be sure that he is dealing with true coronary disease, he includes only people with unequivocal prior myocardial infarction or with classic angina symptoms. Using his chosen criteria for a positive test, he determines that the sensitivity of the test is 90%. What he (and the readers of his report) may not realize is that the test is more sensitive when coronary disease is extensive (two- or three-vessel rather than single vessel) or severe (99% stenosis rather than 80% stenosis) and that his gold standard criteria have selected for patients with extensive or severe disease. When the test is used to detect less extensive disease, producing more equivocal symptoms in the general population, its sensitivity will prove disappointing. Recognize that the sensitivity estimate provided by the evaluation is accurate for the narrow spectrum of disease severity found in the test population. The disappointment comes when that estimate is generalized inappropriately to include those with less severe disease.

An important historical example of the spectrum problem is the evaluation of carcinoembryonic antigen (CEA) as a test for colon cancer. Early studies, documenting very high sensitivity, were conducted in patients with extensive colon cancer. Enthusiasm for CEA as a screening test heightened (despite the low predictive value positive made inevitable by the disease's relatively low prevalence among asymptomatic persons). Later studies, however, proved the sensitivity of the test to be substantially lower among those with early limited disease, that is, among those most likely to benefit from early detection by a screening program.

The Comorbidity Problem: Overestimating Specificity When the "No-Disease" Group Is Too Well

In the same way that an investigator can assemble a "disease" group that is sicker than the population to which the test will eventually be applied, he can assemble a "no disease" group that is too healthy. Many tests will perform better when asked to discriminate between "disease A" and "no disease" than when asked to discriminate between disease A, on the one hand, and diseases B through Z, on the other. Consider the fledgling investigator who wishes to estimate the sensitivity and specificity of guaiac testing as a screening test for colonic cancer. He knows about the spectrum problem and has included in his "disease" group people with early cancers. For his "no disease" group, he has selected medical school students. It should be clear that this choice of controls will provide an estimate of specificity that is higher than could be expected when the test is generally applied to a population including older individuals more likely to have a nonmalignant source of occult bleeding. Obviously the controls should not have the target disease (*i.e.,* colon cancer). But if the investigator also excludes from the control population all comorbid conditions that the test might confuse with the disease (*e.g.,* peptic ulcer disease, diverticular disease, etc.), his estimate of specificity will be too optimistic.

Investigators can guard against such disappointments by drawing their "disease" and "no disease" populations from the target population in which the test will eventually be used. The spectrum of disease that should be detected in the target population should be represented in the "disease" group. Comorbid conditions that might be confused with that disease should be included in the "no disease" control group. Such an effectiveness evaluation of a diagnostic test might be preceded by a simpler study comparing very sick with completely well individuals. If it cannot discriminate between the very sick and the very well in such an efficacy study, the more difficult effectiveness trial need not be undertaken. The clinician can guard against being misled by reports of a test's efficacy by carefully considering the populations in which a test has been evaluated and not generalizing the results inappropriately to larger, more heterogenous groups.

How Does the Test Compare with Others?

A final reason for disappointment with the application of apparently promising tests is failure to consider adequately the test's potential role in the constellation of tests that are already available. Does the new test provide new information? Does it obviate the need for more invasive or more expensive tests? If the answer to these questions is no, the worth of the test and its evaluation are in obvious doubt.

WHICH TESTS SHOULD WE USE?

Perfect tests are rare. Clinicians must choose among tests with imperfect sensitivity and specificity. The physician frequently has some choice about the sensitivity and specificity of a test. Obviously, alternative tests—usually those that are more costly or invasive—may be more sensitive and more specific. A new technology or an improved skill in interpre-

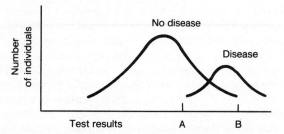

Figure 2-2. Hypothetical distributions of test results (*e.g.,* intraocular pressure measured by Schiotz tonometry) among patients with disease (*e.g.,* glaucoma) and without disease. Because the test is not perfect, the distributions overlap. If all patients with values to the right of *A* are said to have "positive" results, the test will be 100% sensitive but will have a low specificity. If all patients with values to the right of *B* are said to have "positive" results, the test will be 100% specific but will have a low sensitivity. The choice of a cutoff value between *A* and *B* depends on the relative importance of false-positive and false-negative results (see text).

tation may improve both measures. Often, however, the physician can increase sensitivity only by accepting a decrease in specificity. The most graphic examples of this principle involve tests that provide quantitative results, such as the measurement of intraocular pressure in glaucoma screening. Population studies indicate that a sensitivity of 70% and a specificity of 80% are reasonable estimates for Schiotz tonometry if the cutoff point for a positive test is 21.9 mmHg. Raising the discrimination value to 25.6 mmHg increases specificity to 95% but decreases sensitivity to 50%. The physician must trade one against the other. The general case is illustrated in Fig. 2-2. Note that the usual "normal" values for the test results are derived from frequency distributions of results among apparently well individuals; the potential trade-off between sensitivity and specificity is not considered.

Which is more important, sensitivity or specificity? In general, the answer depends on the cost—including patient inconvenience, morbidity, and mortality as well as dollars—of false-negative results compared with that of false-positive results, and the benefits of true negative and of true positive results. Sensitive tests or less stringent criteria for disease and the resulting low false-negative rate should be favored when effective treatment for the condition exists and the cost of lost opportunity is great. High specificity or more stringent criteria for disease and the resulting low false-positive rate

are most important when a positive diagnosis does not significantly influence therapy or outcome but may be a burden for the patient.

The clinician who is mindful of the purpose of making a particular diagnosis, who considers the natural history of disease as well as prognostic and therapeutic implications of the diagnosis, is likely to make efficient use of the laboratory while maximizing health benefits for his or her patients.

A.G.M.

ANNOTATED BIBLIOGRAPHY

Department of Clinical Epidemiology and Biostatistics, McMaster University Health Sciences Centre. How to read clinical journals: II. To learn about a diagnostic test. Can Med Assoc J 124:703–751, 1981 (*Part of a superb series that distills principles of clinical epidemiology for the practitioner.*)

Galen RS, Gambino SR: Beyond Normality: The Predictive Value and Efficiency of Medical Diagnosis. New York, John Wiley & Sons, 1975 (*Application of concepts of sensitivity, specificity, and predictive value to illustrate clinical problems.*)

Griner PF, Mayewski RJ, Mushlin AI et al: Selection and interpretation of diagnostic tests and procedures: Principles and applications. Ann Intern Med 94(4 Pt 2):557–600, 1981 (*A very well presented primer with many good examples.*)

Griner PF, Panzer RJ, Greenland P: Clinical Diagnosis and the Laboratory: Logical Strategies for Common Medical Problems. Chicago, Year Book Medical Publishers, 1986 (*A superb resource. Information about sensitivity or specificity of tests as well as recommended strategies.*)

McNeil BJ, Keeler E, Adelstein SJ: Primer on certain elements of medical decision-making. N Engl J Med 293:211, 1975 (*Concise review of applications of decision theory and information theory to the diagnostic process.*)

McNeil BJ, Abrams HL: Brigham and Women's Hospital Handbook of Diagnostic Imaging. Boston, Little, Brown, 1986 (*Sensitivities and specificities of tests as well as algorithms. Well referenced.*)

Ransohoff DF, Feinstein AR: Problems of spectrum and bias in evaluating the efficacy of diagnostic tests. N Engl J Med 299:926, 1975 (*Reviews problems in disease definition and population selection that may affect evaluations of diagnostic tests.*)

Sox HC, Jr: Probability theory in the use of diagnostic tests. Ann Intern Med 104:60, 1986 (*A succinct, clear presentation.*)

Vecchio TJ: Predictive value of a single diagnostic test in unselected populations. N Engl J Med 274:1171, 1966 (*Early paper pointing out the importance of prevalence to predictive value.*)

3
Health Maintenance and the Role of Screening

Public interest in health maintenance or, more positively, health enhancement has grown dramatically in recent years. Many Americans have demonstrated their interest in exercise, good dietary habits, maintenance of appropriate body weight, and stress reduction. Increased enthusiasm stems from growing awareness of associations between elements of lifestyle and health. Despite reliable evidence and public acceptance of these associations, however, many people continue to indulge in self-destructive habits such as smoking, overeating, and alcohol abuse. Efforts to alter such behavior are often frustratingly ineffective. Patients who seek reassurance from physician visits that include routine screening procedures often persist in behavior that greatly increases their risk of morbidity.

Physicians must acknowledge their primary role in prevention as that of educators. Accurate information regarding risk factors is most likely to reinforce health-enhancing behavior and alter self-destructive behavior. The physician must appreciate the potential for behavior modification and familiarize himself with local resources. Routine screening for specific diseases, the health maintenance activities most closely identified with the physician, should be performed selectively. The limits of screening tests as well as their potential health benefits should be clearly understood by every primary physician.

Specific risk factors and screening tests are discussed in subsequent chapters. This chapter will focus on the question, "What makes a disease or risk factor worth screening for?" The relationship between prevalence and predictive value of a test is particularly important in the screening situation (see Chapter 2). Because the physician is more interested in improving health outcomes for patients than simply in providing them with diagnoses, elements of the natural history of the disease and of the effectiveness of therapy are critically important.

CRITERIA FOR SCREENING

Whether or not a screening policy results in improved health outcomes depends on the characteristics of the disease(s), of the test(s), and of the patient population. These are summarized in Table 3-1.

NATURAL HISTORY OF THE DISEASE AND EFFECTIVENESS OF THERAPY

Screening tests are performed to identify asymptomatic disease. The alternative is to wait until the patient presents with symptoms and then make a diagnosis. The question then is, "What makes a disease worth diagnosing early?" The practical objective of screening is prevention of morbidity and mortality—not simply early diagnosis. There is little benefit to the patient, and perhaps considerable harm, in advancing the time of diagnosis of a disease for which earlier treatment does not influence outcome.

The importance of the natural history of the disease and effectiveness of therapy can be illustrated by considering Figure 3-1. As it shows schematically, some variable time after the biological onset of a disease, a diagnosis is possible using a screening test. This is followed by another variable time period during which the patient has no symptoms. Usually, a short time after symptoms appear, the clinical diagnosis is made. Eventually, after the course of therapy has been selected and completed, there is an identifiable clinical outcome that can range from cure and complete health to death.

Often, outcome depends somewhat on the point during the natural history of the disease at which therapy is initiated. This is most clear in the case of localized versus metastatic cancer. Many tumors can be readily excised, and the patient cured of the disease, during early stages. The opportunity for cure is often lost when tumor spread makes excision or other local therapy impractical. The "escape from cure" may not

Table 3-1.   Criteria for Screening

Characteristics of the Disease
Significant effect on the quality or length of life
Prevalence sufficiently high to justify costs
Acceptable methods of treatment available
Asymptomatic period during which detection and treatment
   significantly reduce morbidity and/or mortality
Treatment in the asymptomatic phase yields a better therapeutic
   result than treatment delayed until symptoms appear

Characteristics of the Test
Sufficiently sensitive to detect disease during the asymptomatic
   period
Sufficiently specific to provide acceptable predictive value
   positive
Acceptable to patients

Characteristics of the Population Screened
Sufficiently high disease prevalence
Accessibility
Compliance with subsequent diagnostic tests and necessary
   therapy

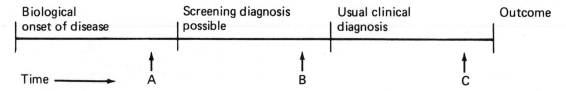

"Escape from cure" at point A: Screening may not affect outcome

"Escape from cure" at point B: High priority for screening

"Escape from cure" at point C: Education and improved access to
care may be more efficient than
screening tests

Figure 3-1. Relationships between screening and natural history of disease.

be as dramatic as the point of tumor metastasis; a disease may simply become more refractory to therapy, increasing the likelihood of morbid complications. The practical purpose of screening is to advance the time of the diagnosis to a point in the natural history of the disease when a relative or absolute "escape from cure" is less likely to have occurred.

While the natural history of any disease varies a great deal among individuals afflicted, some generalizations are worthwhile. If an "escape from cure" generally occurs at point A in Figure 3-1 or at any point before available screening tests can detect the disease in question, the value of screening must be questioned. The most common result will be bad news sooner for the patient but no difference in outcome. If "escape from cure" routinely occurs after symptoms appear (*e.g.,* at point C), screening may be valuable, but could likely be supplanted by patient and professional education programs aimed at ensuring early presentation and prompt diagnosis. Diseases in which "escape from cure" generally occurs after the disease is detectable but while it remains asymptomatic (*e.g.,* at point B) are the most appropriate targets of screening efforts.

Several points about the evaluation of screening programs can also be made with reference to Figure 3-1. Critics of indiscriminate screening point out that the benefits of a screening program can easily be overestimated if the relationship between time of diagnosis and natural history is not understood. One fallacy results from neglecting the importance of *lead time* when evaluating the effect of screening on subsequent survival. Because screening has the potential to advance the time of diagnosis from one point in the natural history to another and because survival is, by necessity, measured from the time of diagnosis rather than the time of onset, the survival of patients whose diseases are detected by screening should be expected to be longer than that of patients who present symptomatically. Extensive follow-up data on many

patients allow approximation of the average length of time by which the diagnosis is advanced by screening. This illusory gain in survival, the lead time, can then be subtracted from any measured difference in survival duration to learn the true benefits of the screening program.

The second fallacy that can lead to overestimation of screening benefits depends on the variability in natural history among individual cases of the same disease. Individuals who have less aggressive disease and thereby spend more time in a detectable but asymptomatic stage are, other things being equal, more likely to be detected by a screening test than are patients with more aggressive disease. If patients with indolent asymptomatic disease are more likely to have an indolent clinical course after diagnosis, patients diagnosed by screening should be expected to have longer survival rates than patients who present symptomatically. Arguments about the impact of such biological determinism rather than advancing the time of diagnosis have most frequently been raised with regard to breast cancer. They apply generally to questions of screening, however. This potential bias toward prolonged survival among patients detected by screening tests has been called *time-linked bias sampling.*

Neither of these arguments is meant to deny the value of screening for treatable disease. They simply advise caution in interpreting apparently favorable results based on unsophisticated measures of effectiveness.

VALIDITY OF AVAILABLE SCREENING TESTS AND POPULATIONS SCREENED

Diseases worth identifying usually have a relatively low prevalence in the asymptomatic population. As a result, the specificity of the diagnostic test used is the principal determinant of the predictive value positive of the test. Tests that may be very useful in diagnosis when the prior probability

Table 3-2. Recommendations of the American Cancer Society
for the Early Detection of Cancer in Asymptomatic Persons

TEST OR PROCEDURE	Sex	NEW RECOMMENDATION POPULATION Age	Frequency	PREVIOUS RECOMMENDATION
Chest x-ray		—Not recommended—		High risk persons, annually*
Sputum cytology		—Not recommended—		Not recommended
Sigmoidoscopy	M&F	Over 50	Every 3–5 years; after 2 negative exams 1 year apart	Persons over 40, annually
Stool guaiac slide test	M&F	Over 50	Every year	Persons over 40, annually
Digital rectal examination	M&F	Over 40	Every year	Same
Pap test	F	20–65; under 20 if sexually active	At least every 3 years; after 2 negative exams 1 year apart; more frequently in high-risk women§	Annual
Pelvic examination	F	20–40 over 40	Every 3 years Every year	Annual Same
Endometrial tissue sample	F	At menopause women at high risk†	At menopause	Same
Breast self-examination	F	Over 20	Every month	Same
Breast physical examination	F	20–40 over 40	Every 3 years Every year	Annual Same
Mammography	F	35–40 Under 50 Over 50	Baseline Consult personal physician Every year	No policy
Health counseling and cancer checkup‡	M&F M&F	Over 20 Over 40	Every 3 years Every year	"Periodic"

* Persons over 40 who smoke or are exposed to other lung carcinogens.
† History of infertility, obesity, failure of ovulation, abnormal uterine bleeding, or estrogen therapy.
‡ To include examination for cancers of the thyroid, testicles, prostate, ovaries, lymph nodes, oral region, and skin.
§ Early age at first intercourse, multiple sex partners.
(From the American Cancer Society: Report on the cancer-related health check-up. Cancer 30:194–240, 1980)

of disease is 10% or 20% may produce an unacceptable number of false-positive results when used in a screening situation. Such nonspecificity has been referred to as the *cost* of a screening test. The costs, including morbidity and patient concern, of diagnostic evaluations among patients with false-positive screens can far outweigh other costs of a screening program. The sensitivity and specificity of the screening test, costs, and patient acceptability are critical considerations in the decision to screen for disease.

The importance of disease prevalence in determining the predictive value positive is one basis for the use of risk factors in screening policy. By limiting screening to a high-risk population, the physician in effect increases the prevalence of the disease in the population tested (and alternatively increases the prior probability of the disease in any individual), thereby increasing the predictive value positive and decreasing the false-alarm rate and the number of false-positive results.

HEALTH MAINTENANCE—WHAT IS APPROPRIATE?

Periodic health evaluation has been recommended with varying degrees of enthusiasm throughout the 20th century. Many patients believe in its value; the majority of Americans feel that more health resources should be expended on preventive efforts. Recently, however, the value of periodic examinations and specific preventive measures has been questioned. Evidence regarding the effectiveness of periodic examinations, measured in terms of decreased morbidity and mortality, is fragmentary. Supporters argue that there are additional benefits of regular physician contact that result in a greater sense of well-being. Such contact provides opportunities for appropriate patient education.

Routine examinations should be tailored to the individual patient. The use of indiscriminate laboratory screening has been shown to increase consumption of health care resources

Age

16 17 18 19 20 21 22 23 24 25 26 27 28 29 30 31 32 33 34 35 36 37 38 39 40 41 42 43 44 45

History & Physical
MD Breast Exam
Pelvic Exam
Rectal Exam
*Hearing Assessment
**Tetanus-Diph-theria Booster
**Influenza Immunization
Blood Pressure
***Pap Smear
Cholesterol
*VDRL
*PPD
Stool for Occult Blood
Sigmoidoscopy
Mammography

F	B & S
ACS	CTF

F   Frame and Carlson
B & S   Breslow and Somers
ACS   American Cancer Society
CTF   Canadian Task Force on the Periodic
Health Examination

Figure 3-2.   Summary of recommendations of the four major studies.
*Canadian Task Force recommends that this be done on the basis of clinical judgment.
**At first visit, the physician should check the past immunization history according to the Centers for Disease Control recommendations for rubella, mumps, poliomyelitis, diphtheria/tetanus toxoids, pertussis.
***If sexually active. A blackened square indicates that a study has considered the maneuver and recommended it. Squares left empty do not necessarily indicate that the study considered but did not recommend the maneuver. (From Medical Practices Committee, American College of Physicians. Ann Intern Med 95:729, 1981)

without producing demonstrable benefit. Although the importance of characteristics of the patient, the diseases, and the test in determining appropriate prevention strategies must be recognized, summary recommendations can be useful. A number of reviews, each applying the criteria discussed in this chapter, have offered recommendations for preventive health care in *asymptomatic* persons *without* specific *risk factors*. The age-specific recommendations of Frame and Carlson, Breslow and Somer, the Canadian Taskforce on the Periodic Health Examination, and the American Cancer Society (ACS) are presented in Figure 3-2. The recommendations of the American Cancer Society represent a departure from earlier guidelines that included tests for lung cancer as well as earlier and more frequent tests for colon cancer and cancer

Age

46 47 48 49 50 51 52 53 54 55 56 57 58 59 60 61 62 63 64 65 66 67 68 69 70 71 72 73 74 75+

History & Physical
MD Breast Exam
Pelvic Exam
Rectal Exam
*Hearing Assessment
**Tetanus-Diphtheria Booster
**Influenza Immunization
Blood Pressure
***Pap Smear
Cholesterol
*VDRL
*PPD
Stool for Occult Blood
Sigmoidoscopy
Mammography

of the uterine cervix. Current ACS recommendations are summarized and contrasted with previous guidelines in Table 3-2.

The screening and health maintenance chapters that follow review evidence for and against a wide range of preventive measures that might be considered by the primary care provider. It should be noted that uncertainty about the natural history and effectiveness of therapy, the importance of specific risk factors, and the sensitivity and specificity of potential screening tests rarely, if ever, allow proof of the effectiveness of a screening procedure. Some conclusions and recommendations, necessarily based on speculative data, may be controversial.

A.G.M.

ANNOTATED BIBLIOGRAPHY

American Cancer Society: Report on the cancer-related health check-up. Cancer 30:194 240, 1980 (*A superb review of screening principles followed by detailed presentation and defense of current recommendations.*)

Breslow L, Somer AR: The lifetime health-monitoring program. N Engl J Med 296:60, 1977 (*Specific screening prescriptions by age group.*)

Canadian Taskforce on the Periodic Health Examination: The periodic health examination, 1984 update. Can Med Assoc J 130: 1278, 1984 (*An update of the very valuable 1979 report; provides recommendations for screening and health maintenance; based on very thorough study.*)

Feinleb M, Zelen M: Some pitfalls in the evaluation of screening programs. Arch Environ Health 19:412, 1969 (*Reviews problems with predictive value positive, lead time, and time-linked bias sampling.*)

Frame PS, Carlson SJ: A critical review of periodic health screening using specific screening criteria. J Fam Pract 2:29; 123; 189; 283; 1975 (*Considers 36 diseases. Screening recommended for only a few based on specific criteria.*)

Medical Practice Committee, American College of Physicians: Periodic health examination: A guide for designing individualized preventive health care in the asymptomatic patient. Ann Intern Med 95:729 732, 1981 (*Succinct summary of recommendations.*)

Screening for Disease. Lancet, October 5 to December 21, 1974 (18-part series). (*A review of screening with unenthusiastic conclusions.*)

Spitzer WO, Brown BP: Unanswered questions about the periodic health examination. Ann Intern Med 83:257, 1975 (*Reviews the issue in terms of impact on health and effect on the doctor–patient relationship.*)

4

Immunization

HARVEY B. SIMON, M.D.

Immunizations are an effective and important means of controlling many communicable diseases through primary prevention. The power of immunization programs is nowhere more evident than in the case of smallpox, which has been eradicated as a result of an aggressive worldwide vaccination program. But if smallpox vaccine has been rendered obsolete through its own effectiveness, the other immunizing agents have not. An appalling number of Americans have not received their recommended immunizations. In large part, this is a failure of public education and of access to health care delivery. But while the pediatrician has been traditionally effective in immunizing individual patients, the primary care internist too often overlooks the importance of immunization.

Except for travelers, patients rarely request immunizations. It is up to the physician, then, to initiate consideration of immunization. The first step is to take a detailed immunization history. In addition, a history of prior adverse reactions to vaccines and of egg allergy should be sought. Finally, it is important to be aware of the current prevalence of infectious diseases in the local community, and, in the case of the traveler, in other parts of the world.

GENERAL PRINCIPLES OF IMMUNIZATION

In general, live attenuated vaccines (Table 4-1) provide more complete and longer lasting immunity than inactivated agents. However, because live vaccines can produce serious disseminated disease in the immunosuppressed host, these preparations should be avoided in patients who are immunologically deficient (leukemia or lymphoma patients, steroid and cancer chemotherapy recipients, patients with agammaglobulinemia, etc.). Inactivated vaccines (Table 4-1) are safe in these patients.

Two inactivated vaccines can be given simultaneously at separate injection sites, as can an inactivated vaccine and a live vaccine. However, if significant local or systemic reactions are anticipated, as is often the case with cholera or typhoid vaccines, for example, it may be best to administer the vaccines on separate days. On theoretical grounds, it is desirable to separate vaccinations with live virus vaccines by at least 1 month. However, studies have shown that a combination of measles, mumps, and rubella vaccines can be given to children along with the trivalent oral polio vaccine without adverse reactions or loss of effectiveness.

In pregnancy, rubella vaccine is absolutely contraindicated because of its potential teratogenicity. In general, other live virus vaccines should be avoided in pregnancy unless the risk of exposure and illness clearly outweighs the possible risks of the vaccine itself. Inactivated vaccines are generally considered safe in pregnancy.

Passive immunity can interfere with active immunity but such interference is of little practical importance with inactivated vaccines, which can therefore be administered any time after the use of immune globulin. However, with live attenuated vaccines, it is best to defer immunizations until 3 months have elapsed following administration of immune globulin, blood, or plasma. If immune globulin becomes necessary after vaccination and the interval between the live, attenuated vaccine and the immune globulin is less than 14 days, the vaccine doses, should be repeated in about 3 months,

Table 4-1. Immunizing Agents

Live Attenuated Vaccines
1. Viral
   a. Polio
   b. Measles
   c. Rubella
   d. Mumps
   e. Yellow fever

Inactivated Agents
1. Viral
   a. Influenza
   b. Rabies
   c. Polio
   d. Hepatitis B
2. Bacterial
   a. Pneumococcus
   b. Meningococcus
   c. Hemophilus influenzae; type B
   d. Diphtheria (toxoid)
   e. Tetanus (toxoid)
   f. Pertussis
   g. Typhoid
   h. Cholera

Vaccines Prepared from Egg Media
1. Influenza
2. Rabies
3. Rocky Mountain spotted fever
4. Typhus
5. Yellow fever

Immunoglobulin Preparations for Passive Immunization
1. Human
   a. Immune globulin
   b. Tetanus immune globulin
   c. Measles immune globulin
   d. Hepatitis B immune globulin
   e. Rabies immune globulin
   f. Varicella-Zoster immune globulin
2. Equine
   a. Diphtheria antitoxin
   b. Botulism antitoxin

unless serologic testing demonstrates that antibody has been produced. Travelers requiring both vaccines and immune globulin should receive the immune globulin 2 weeks after completing the vaccinations, if possible.

Patients who have exhibited hypersensitivity reactions to a vaccine should not receive that product again. Individuals with egg allergies should not be given vaccines prepared in egg cultures (Table 4-1). If multiple-dose immunization schedules are delayed or interrupted, they should be resumed without administering additional doses, no matter how long the interval between doses. In general, immunization should be avoided during significant febrile illnesses. Mild upper respiratory infections, however, need not preclude immunizations.

The decision to immunize must include consideration of the frequency of the condition, chances of exposure, risks and benefits of immunization, and cost.

SPECIFIC IMMUNIZING AGENTS

Diphtheria and Tetanus Toxoid and Pertussis Vaccine

Although both diphtheria and tetanus are now uncommon in the United States, all individuals should receive the excellent protection afforded by the toxoids that are prepared by formaldehyde treatment of the bacterial toxins. Pertussis vaccine is indicated in all children below age 6 years, but older individuals are not nearly as susceptible to pertussis and should not receive the vaccine. Children between 6 weeks and 6 years of age should be given the combined diphtheria, pertussis, and tetanus (DPT) product. For patients first receiving immunization after age 6, three tetanus diphtheria (Td) injections should be administered, with the second dose given 1 to 2 months after the initial dose and the third dose 6 to 12 months later. A booster should be administered every 10 years.

Tetanus diphtheria immunization is the only immunization universally indicated in adults (Table 4-2), but is frequently overlooked. Immigrants and elderly individuals, particularly women and men who have not served in the military, are especially likely never to have been immunized.

If a patient has received a full primary tetanus series and boosters at regular 10-year intervals, additional boosters are not necessary at the time of injury. Other individuals should receive tetanus-diphtheria toxoids for minor wounds and both tetanus-diphtheria toxoids and tetanus immune globulin (TIG) for more serious wounds (Table 4-3).

Polio Vaccine

Although all children should receive polio vaccine, the very low incidence of poliomyelitis in the United States makes the routine immunization of adults unnecessary. Previously immunized travelers who are anticipating visits to rural areas of developing countries should receive a single booster dose of oral polio vaccine (TOPV), as should certain health care and laboratory workers who may be exposed to polio virus. An inactivated vaccine (IPV) is available for use in immunosuppressed patients. Previously *un*immunized adults who may be exposed to polio virus (through travel, occupation, etc.) should be given IPV because of the slight risk of vaccine-associated paralysis following OPV; three doses should be given at intervals of 1 to 2 months, with a fourth dose given 6 to 12 months later. Some authorities recommend two doses of IPV for unimmunized parents of infants who are to be given TOPV.

Measles, Mumps, and Rubella Vaccines

These three live attenuated virus vaccines are available in a combined preparation for use in children at age 15 months or older.

Table 4-2. Indications for Immunization in Adults

Primary Immunization or Booster in All Adults
Tetanus-diphtheria

Immunization in Selected, Vulnerable Individuals
Influenza (the elderly and debilitated)
Pneumococcus (sickle cell disease, splenectomy, elderly, and debilitated)
Rubella (women of childbearing age who are antibody negative; must avoid pregnancy for 3 months)
Meningococcus (splenectomy)
? Hemophilus influenzae, type B (splenectomy)

Immunizations in Certain Epidemiologic Situations
Hepatitis B vaccine (for certain high-risk individuals including selected medical and dental personnel, dialysis patients, recipients of frequent transfusions, residents and staff of institutions for the retarded, sexual contacts of HbsAg carriers, and male homosexuals)
Meningococcus (epidemics; possibly household contacts; only types A and C available)
Immune globulin (for household exposure to hepatitis A and possibly non-A-non-B hepatitis)
Hepatitis B immune globulin (hepatitis B negative patients who have acute intensive exposure to hepatitis B as in needle sticks)
BCG (selected tuberculin-negative individuals expecting intense exposure to tuberculosis)

Immunizations for International Travel (Depending on Area)
Typhoid (two injections plus booster)
Cholera (within 2 months of departure)
Yellow fever (Africa, South America)
Polio (Tropical or developing areas; booster or primary series if never immunized)
Plague (rural Vietnam, Cambodia, Laos)
Typhus (rarely necessary)
Immune globulin (for hepatitis A)

Passive Immunizations after Exposure
Rabies immune globulin (plus vaccine)
Tetanus immune globulin (plus toxoid)
Diphtheria antitoxin (plus toxoid)
Botulism antitoxoid
Immune globulin (for hepatitis A)
Hepatitis B immune globulin (for hepatitis B—acute intense exposure)
Vaccinia immune globulin (for complications of smallpox vaccination)
Varicella-Zoster immune globulin (for certain vulnerable individuals after exposure—available only from CDC)
Measles immune globulin (for certain vulnerable individuals after exposure)

Mumps vaccine is rarely indicated in adults. Nonimmune adult males are at risk of mumps orchitis. However, susceptibility is difficult to predict, since many adults with no history of clinical mumps are immune and the skin test is not a reliable predictor of immunity. Hence, routine mumps vaccination of adult males cannot be recommended. Immune globulin is not of proven value in postexposure prophylaxis.

Rubella vaccine is recommended for adolescent and adult women if serological tests for rubella antibody are negative, and if they are able to avoid pregnancy for 3 months following immunization. The most common side-effects of rubella vaccination are arthralgias. Rubella vaccine has not been demonstrated to cause congenital rubella syndrome or teratogenicity.

An inactivated measles vaccine was introduced in 1963, but was replaced by a much more effective live attenuated vaccine in 1967. Persons born before 1956 can be considered immune by virtue of natural infection. However, measles vaccine should be considered for persons born between 1957 and 1967 unless documentation of vaccination with atten-

uated vaccine after 1 year of age is available. Measles vaccination is particularly important for susceptible college students or health-care workers. Immunization of previously immune individuals is not harmful.

Smallpox

Universal smallpox immunization in the United States was abandoned in 1971 because of the disappearance of the disease. Vaccination is no longer recommended for travelers. The vaccine is now recommended only for laboratory personnel exposed to orthopox viruses. Smallpox vaccine is available to civilians in the United States only through the Centers for Disease Control (CDC).

Influenza Vaccine

Influenza remains a major worldwide problem because of frequent antigenic shifts in the virus. New vaccines are prepared in anticipation of the viral strains, which are expected to prevail during the winter flu season. Indications for

Table 4-3. Summary Guide to Tetanus Prophylaxis in Routine Wound Management—United States, 1985*

HISTORY OF ADSORBED TETANUS TOXOID (DOSES)	CLEAN, MINOR WOUNDS		ALL OTHER WOUNDS†	
	Td‡	TIG	Td‡	TIG
Unknown or < three	Yes	No	Yes	Yes
≥ three§	No‖	No	No#	No

* Important details are in the text.

† Such as, but not limited to, wounds contaminated with dirt, feces, soil, saliva, etc.; puncture wounds; avulsions; and wounds resulting from missiles, crushing, burns, and frostbite.

‡ For children under 7 years old; DTP (DT, if pertussis vaccine is contraindicated) is preferred to tetanus toxoid alone. For persons 7 years old and older, Td is preferred to tetanus toxoid alone.

§ If only three doses of *fluid* toxoid have been received, a fourth dose of toxoid, preferably an adsorbed toxoid, should be given.

‖ Yes, if more than 10 years since last dose.

Yes, if more than 5 years since last dose. (More frequent boosters are not needed and can accentuate side-effects.)

(Source: Morbidity and Mortality Weekly Reports 34:405, 1986)

vaccination vary from year to year, depending on vaccine availability, the likelihood of influenza epidemics, and vaccine toxicity. In general, the elderly and debilitated, particularly those with cardiopulmonary disease, should receive influenza vaccine in the autumn prior to the flu season. Other vulnerable individuals, including nursing home residents and those with renal disease, diabetes, sickle cell anemia, and immunosuppressed hosts, should also receive the vaccine. Health care workers who have extensive contact with high-risk patients should consider annual vaccination. Unlike other viral infections, a chemical agent, amantadine, is available to prevent clinical disease in patients exposed to influenza A_2. Amantadine is particularly useful in elderly patients directly exposed to the flu, as in nursing home outbreaks.

Meningococcus Vaccine

A quadravalent vaccine containing 50 mg each of cell wall polysaccharides from meningococcal types A, C, Y, and W-135 is now available. It is not recommended for general use, but is indicated for control of epidemics (as in the military) and for travelers to areas experiencing outbreaks of meningococcal meningitis. Meningococcal vaccine may be of some benefit in household contacts of patients with meningococcal disease. Meningococcal vaccine is immunogenic for splenectomized patients (except those who have received chemotherapy or radiotherapy for lymphoma); asplenic individuals should receive the vaccine.

Pneumococcus Vaccine

A multivalent vaccine prepared from pneumococcal capsular polysaccharides was licensed in this country from 1945 to 1947, but was withdrawn because of lack of use. Despite the use of penicillin and other antibiotics, however, pneumococcal pneumonia has remained a major cause of morbidity and mortality in the United States, with an estimated 500,000 cases annually and a case fatality rate of 5% to 10%. A vaccine released in 1977 contained 14 polysaccharide types, responsible for about 80% of pneumococcal disease. A new vaccine released in 1983 contains 23 polysaccharide types, responsible for about 90% of pneumococcal disease, and has replaced the 14-valent vaccine. The vaccine appears to be at least 70% effective in preventing pneumonia caused by these serotypes, and has been safe and well-tolerated thus far. Pneumococcal vaccine is indicated in individuals with increased susceptibility to pneumococcal infection, including splenectomized patients and those with sickle cell disease, nephrotic syndrome, cirrhosis, and chronic cardiopulmonary disease. Because mortality from pneumococcal pneumonia increases with age beyond age 50, the elderly can be expected to benefit from the vaccine as well; it is not clear, however, if age alone should be an indication for vaccination in the absence of underlying disease, or at what age such routine vaccination should be considered. Antibody response to pneumococcal vaccine has been poor below age 2.

Vaccination produces adequate antibody levels in patients with sickle cell anemia, nephrosis, uremia, diabetes, and asplenia, but vaccine failures have been reported in these groups as well as in normals. Because patients with Hodgkin's disease respond poorly after splenectomy plus chemotherapy and radiotherapy, it seems wise to administer vaccine to these patients as soon after diagnosis as possible. Although only 30% of myeloma patients respond serologically, vaccination seems reasonable in these high-risk patients.

Pneumococcal vaccine is safe. Side-effects consist mainly of pain and erythema at the injection site and occasional mild fever. Local side-effects appear to be increased following revaccination; protective levels of antibody persist for years, and revaccination is not recommended. Patients who have previously received the 14-valent vaccine in use from 1977 through 1983 should not receive the newer 23-valent vaccine, since the risk of local reactions does not seem to warrant the slight additional protection. The safety of pneumococcal vaccine for pregnant women has not been evaluated.

Pneumococcal vaccine and influenza vaccine can be administered simultaneously at separate sites without impairing efficacy or increasing toxicity.

Hemophilus Influenzae, Type B

H. influenzae, type B, is a major bacterial pathogen in childhood, causing meningitis, bacteremia, epiglottitis, pneumonia, and other invasive infections. Other strains of *H. influenzae,* however, are more likely to cause otitis media. In the United States, the risk of developing *H. influenzae,* type B invasive disease during the first 5 years of life is about 1 in 200. The risk is even higher in native Americans, blacks, individuals with asplenia, sickle cell disease, Hodgkin's disease, or antibody deficiencies, and in children who attend day care centers.

A vaccine prepared from *H. influenzae,* type B capsular polysaccharide was licensed in 1985. Vaccination is recommended for all children at 24 months of age. Whereas vaccination is less effective in younger children, it may be considered at 18 months in higher-risk children.

At present, there is not enough data to recommend the use of this vaccine in older individuals who may be vulnerable to *H. influenzae,* type B (splenectomy, etc.).

Rabies Vaccine and Rabies Immune Globulin

Although human rabies is rare in the United States (one to five cases per year), thousands of people are at risk because of animal bites and scratches. Approximately 25,000 persons receive prophylaxis in the United States each year. Rabies in domestic animals has become very uncommon, but wildlife (especially skunks, foxes, raccoons, and bats) still pose a risk. Fortunately, rabies prophylaxis has become much less toxic with the availability of the new human diploid cell rabies vaccine (HDCV) and human rabies immune globulin (RIG).

Preexposure rabies vaccination is recommended only for people with occupational exposure to rabies virus. Both active immunization with vaccine and passive immunization with rabies immune globulin, may be indicated after animal bites or scratches. Table 4-4 presents the U.S. Public Health Service guidelines for postexposure prophylaxis.

BCG Vaccine

Bacille Calmette-Guérin (BCG) vaccine is a live, attenuated strain of *Mycobacterium bovis,* which was introduced in 1922. Seniority notwithstanding, the efficacy of BCG is unknown. Earlier European trials showed up to 80% protection, but recent Indian trials showed little value. Because of the sharp decline in new cases of primary tuberculosis in the United States, BCG is recommended only in selected tuberculin-negative individuals with unavoidable intense exposure to tuberculosis, such as children of mothers with active tuberculosis. BCG may be useful in travelers anticipating close contact with people infected with tuberculosis, but an alternative approach is tuberculin skin-testing before and after travel, with administration of isoniazid in the event of skin-test conversion.

Table 4-4.   Guide to Postexposure Rabies Prophylaxis*

Animal Species	Condition of Animal at Time of Attack	Treatment of Exposed Human
Wild		
Skunk	Regard as rabid unless proven negative	RIG† + HDCV‡
Fox	by laboratory tests (the animal	
Coyote	should be killed and tested at once;	
Raccoon	observation not recommended)	
Bat		
Bobcat		
Other carnivores		
Domestic		
Cat or dog	Healthy and available for observation	None unless animal develops rabies§
	Unknown (escaped)	Consult public health officials; if treatment is indicated, give RIG + HDCV
Other	Rabid or suspected rabid	RIG + HDCV Consider individually‖

* These recommendations are only a guide. They should be applied in conjunction with knowledge of the animal species involved, circumstances of the bite or other exposure, vaccination status of the animal, and presence of rabies in the region. Public health officials should be consulted if questions arise.

† RIG (rabies immune globulin, human) is administered only once, at the beginning of therapy. The dosage is 20 IU/kg, one half intramuscularly in the buttocks and one half thoroughly infiltrated around the wound. Equine antirabies serum should be used only if RIG is not available. *All wounds should be thoroughly cleansed with soap and water.*

‡ HDCV (human diploid cell vaccine) is the vaccine of choice. One milliliter of vaccine should be given intramuscularly on days 0, 3, 7, 14, and 28. (The World Health Organization currently recommends a sixth dose 90 days after the first dose.) HDCV is so effective that serologic testing of recipients is no longer recommended.

§ RIG and HDCV should be started at the first sign of rabies in the biting dog or cat during a 10-day holding period.

‖ Bites of squirrels, hamsters, guinea pigs, gerbils, chipmunks, rats, mice, other rodents, rabbits, and hares almost never call for antirabies prophylaxis.

(Source: Modified from U.S. Department of Health and Human Services/Public Health Service/Center for Disease Control: Recommendation of the Immunization Practices Advisory Committee: Rabies Prevention—United States, 1984. MMWR 33:393, July 20, 1984)

Viral Hepatitis

Hepatitis A. Commercially available pooled human gamma globulin is of proven benefit in preventing or clinically modifying type A hepatitis (infectious hepatitis), particularly if it is given within 2 weeks of exposure to the virus. Individuals closely exposed to patients with hepatitis should be given gamma globulin, especially household contacts of patients. The recommended dosage is 0.02 ml per kilogram of body weight, or about 2 ml in adults. Immune globulin is also useful in preventing hepatitis A in travelers to underdeveloped areas where hepatitis is endemic; the dosage is 2 ml for brief travel, and 5 ml for travel of longer than 3 months, with repeat doses every 4 to 6 months if needed.

Hepatitis B. PASSIVE IMMUNIZATION. Two globulin products are currently available in the United States. Immune globulin (IG) is prepared from normal donors; although pre-1972 lots of IG had low anti-HBs titers, current lots have titers between 1:100 and 1:1000. Hepatitis B immune globulin (HBIG) is prepared from high titer donors and has titers of at least 1:100,000.

IG is of no *proven* efficacy in preventing hepatitis B but *may* have *some* value in chronic low-dose exposure (travelers, closed institutions, family contacts).

HBIG will prevent or modify some cases of hepatitis B following exposure. HBIG is indicated for hepatitis B antigen and antibody negative individuals with an *acute intense exposure* to hepatitis B (needle stick, sexual partner, oral ingestion). HBIG should be given in a dose of 0.06 ml/kg (5 ml for adults) as soon as possible. (See Tables 4-5 and 4-6.) HBIG is very expensive.

ACTIVE IMMUNIZATION. Plasma-derived vaccine. A vaccine has been developed from the plasma of healthy HBsAG carriers; 22-nm antigen particles are isolated from plasma, purified, inactivated by formalin, and absorbed to aluminum hydroxide. In human trials dating from 1975, the vaccine appears to be very safe and effective. It became available in 1982 and is recommended for high-risk individuals including certain medical, dental, and laboratory personnel, intimate contacts of hepatitis B patients, institution residents and staff, hemodialysis patients and their families, male homosexuals, and travelers to endemic areas. Two 20-μg doses of vaccine are administered one month apart, and a third dose is administered 6 months after the first. A dose of 40 μg is recommended for immunosuppressed patients and for those on hemodialysis.

Administration of HBIG with the first dose of hepatitis B vaccine does not interfere with immunization.

Because some of the plasma used to produce vaccine has been harvested from male homosexuals, concern has been raised about AIDS. Thus far vaccine appears safe—in fact, AIDs is *less* common in homosexuals who have received vaccine than in unvaccinated homosexual men.

Despite its excellent clinical record, the inactivated hepatitis B vaccine has been underutilized. For example, only 6% of susceptible hemodialysis patients and 32% of susceptible staff have received vaccine despite their high risk for infection. The major reason for this underutilization appears to be an unfounded fear of AIDS. Additional problems with the vaccine include suboptimal responses in certain recipients, including those with immunological abnormalities, probably because the extensive inactivation procedures used in manufacturing the vaccine reduce its immunogenicity.

Recombinant DNA vaccine. Because of the difficulties with inactivated hepatitis B vaccine produced from the plasma of chronic carriers, a new vaccine was developed utilizing recombinant DNA technology to produce hepatitis B surface antigen. No infectious particles are present in the preparation, but the hepatitis B surface antigen in the vaccine induces an immune response in vaccine recipients, with production of protective antibody. Clinical trials with the recombinant DNA vaccine have shown excellent antibody titers and safety.

The recombinant DNA hepatitis B vaccine was licensed for clinical use in the United States in 1986; the indications,

Table 4-5. Hepatitis B. Virus Postexposure Recommendations

| EXPOSURE | HBIG | | VACCINE* | |
	Dose	Recommended Timing	Dose	Recommended Timing
Perinatal	0.5 ml IM	Within 12 hr of birth	0.5 ml (10 Ug)IM	Within 7 days, repeat at 1 and 6 months
Percutaneous†				
Sexual	0.6 ml/kg IM or 5 ml for adults	Within 14 days of sexual contact	1.0 ml (20 Ug)IM§	Repeat at 1 and 6 months

* The first dose can be given at the same time as the HBIG dose but at a separate site.

† See Table 4-6.

§ Vaccine is recommended for homosexually active males and for regular sexual contacts of chronic HBV carriers, but optional for heterosexuals with a limited exposure.

(Source: U.S. Department of Health and Human Services/Public Health Service: Post-exposure prophylaxis of hepatitis B. MMWR 33:286, 1984)

Table 4-6. Recommendations for Hepatitis B Prophylaxis Following Percutaneous Exposure

| | EXPOSED PERSON | |
SOURCE	*Unvaccinated*	*Vaccinated*
HBsAg-positive	1. HBIG × 1 immediately* 2. Initiate HB vaccine† series	1. Test exposed person for anti-HBs‡ 2. If inadequate antibody,§ HBIG (×1) immediately plus HB vaccine booster dose
Known source High risk HBsAg-positive	1. Initiate HB vaccine series 2. Test source for HBsAg; if positive, HBIG × 1	1. Test source for HBsAg only if exposed is vaccine nonresponder; if source is HBsAg- positive, give HBIG × 1 immediately plus HB vaccine booster dose
Low risk HBsAg-positive	Initiate HB vaccine series.	Nothing required
Unknown source	Initiate HB vaccine series	Nothing required

* HPIG dose 0.06 mL/kg IM.

† HB vaccine dose 20 μg IM for adults; 10 μg IM for infants or children under 10 years of age. First dose within 1 week; second and third dose, 1 and 6 months later.

‡ See text for details.

§ Less than 10 SRU by RIA, negative by EIA.

(Source: MMWR 34:331, 1985)

dosage, and administration schedules for the two vaccines are identical, except that the recombinant DNA vaccine is not yet recommended for dialysis patients. The cost of the vaccines is similar. It is likely that as availability and experience increase, the recombinant DNA vaccine will replace the older vaccine.

Non A-Non B Hepatitis (NANB). IG is not of proven value but may be a reasonable precaution for intimately exposed individuals (needle stick, oral ingestion, sexual contact) in a dose of 0.06 ml/kg within 1 week of exposure.

The epidemiology and natural history of viral hepatitis, as well as its prevention, are discussed in Chapter 52.

Typhoid Fever Vaccine

Although typhoid vaccination is not required, it is recommended for people traveling to parts of Africa, Asia, and Central and South America where the disease is endemic. The immunization series consists of two subcutaneous injections separated by at least 1 month, with boosters every 3 years if needed for additional travel. Typhoid vaccine is only about 70% effective in preventing infection with *Salmonella typhi;* travelers should maintain vigilance with regard to food and water. Febrile reactions to the vaccine are relatively common.

Cholera Vaccine

Although cholera vaccine is incompletely effective, and the risk of cholera in Americans traveling abroad is low, cholera vaccination is required for travel to certain countries. One injection of vaccine prior to departure is sufficient for

travel certification; a full primary series for individuals traveling to areas in which the disease is endemic includes a second injection at least a week after the first, with a booster every 6 months if indicated.

Yellow Fever Vaccine

This live, attenuated viral vaccine is available only at designated yellow fever vaccination centers. Yellow fever is endemic in parts of tropical South America and Africa, and vaccination is required for travelers to these areas.

Typhus and Plague Vaccines

These vaccines are seldom indicated in American travelers, except for the occasional individual anticipating prolonged exposure in rural areas of Southeast Asia and other scattered remote regions.

Additional Prophylactic Measures
for International Travel

In addition to ascertaining and obtaining appropriate immunizations, the traveler faces a number of potential health problems. All travelers should be evaluated medically before a long or difficult trip and should be fully informed about their medical status. The patient with chronic illness may find it useful to take along medical summaries and copies of electrocardiograms. An adequate supply of medication is essential. Patients with potentially serious illnesses might best be advised to avoid medically unsophisticated areas of the world.

Malaria. Travelers to areas where malaria transmission might occur should be advised to take *malaria prophylaxis.* In most instances, the recommended drug is *chloroquine phosphate,* which is administered once weekly beginning at least 1 week prior to departure and continuing for 6 weeks after return. The drug is generally well-tolerated and serious toxicity on this schedule is rare, even if it is continued for prolonged periods. The dose of chloroquine is 5 mg per kilogram of body weight up to the full adult dose of 300 mg base (500 mg of chloroquine phosphate).

The prophylaxis of chloroquine-resistant *P. falciparum* malaria is a difficult problem. Chloroquine-resistant strains are found in parts of Southeast Asia, Central America (including Panama), northern South America, and Africa. Chloroquine-resistant *P. falciparum* malaria remains a difficult problem for travelers. In 1982, the CDC recommended the combined weekly use of chloroquine and *Fansidar* (pyrimethamine and sulfadoxine) as prophylaxis. Since then, however, 20 cases of severe mucocutaneous reactions, six of which were fatal, have been reported. Fansidar has been associated with Stevens–Johnson syndrome, toxic epidermal necrolysis, erythema multiforme, serum sickness, and hepatitis. Thus, new guidelines for travelers to areas with chloroquine-resistant malaria have been issued.

1. Travelers must be informed that malaria may occur up to 1 year after departure from an endemic area no matter which prophylactic regimen is used. The symptoms should be explained, and travelers should be prepared to seek medical care if symptoms arise.
2. Travelers should avoid contact with mosquitoes, especially between dusk and dawn, when most malaria transmission occurs. Screening and nets, clothing that covers most of the body, insect repellents (ideally containing N,N-diethyl-m-toulamide), and insect spray (containing pyrethrum) are all important measures.
3. Travelers to high-risk areas, particularly parts of Africa, should take regimens based on the length of stay. Those staying 3 weeks or less should take prophylactic chloroquine and carry a single three-tablet dose of Fansidar, to be taken as a self-treatment for malaria symptoms if medical care is not available. For those staying longer than 3 weeks, weekly use of Fansidar (one tablet, plus chloroquine) must be considered. Those who use Fansidar should discontinue its use at the first sign of mucocutaneous lesions. Alternative prophylactic agents include amodiaquine and doxycycline.
4. Fansidar should not be used by persons who are allergic to sulfonamides or pyrimethamine, or by pregnant women.

Traveler's Diarrhea. The prophylactic administration of doxycycline or trimethoprim-sulfamethoxazole or Pepto-Bismol may help prevent travelers' diarrhea. Travelers should be advised to seek medical attention if they develop severe or protracted diarrhea, especially if accompanied by passage of blood or mucus, or if high fever is present. However, medical care may be unavailable in some areas and "empirical" self-medication with trimethoprim-sulfamethoxazole (two tablets bid for 5 days) may be the only practical, if imperfect, alternative. Physicians faced with this problem should call the Center for Disease Control in Atlanta, Georgia, for the latest recommendations.

Travelers to tropical and underdeveloped areas should be cautioned to avoid potentially contaminated water and ice. Carbonated beverages, boiled water, and tea and coffee made with boiled water are generally safe. Chemical treatment of water with chlorine or iodine is also helpful, but while most pathogenic viruses and bacteria are killed, cysts capable of causing amebiasis or giardiasis may survive. Foods must also be selected with care. Most well-cooked hot food is safe, but raw fruits and vegetables should be avoided and dairy products should be consumed only if hygienic preparation and proper refrigeration are ensured.

Although traveler's diarrhea is an extremely common problem, guidelines for its management remain imperfect. Mild self-limited diarrhea should remain untreated, except for appropriate fluid replacement. Widely used obstipating agents such as diphenoxylate (Lomotil) may provide symptomatic relief, but can actually prolong the course of bacterial diarrheas. Many cases of traveler's diarrhea are caused by enteropathogenic strains of *Escherichia coli.*

FURTHER INFORMATION

An authoritative source of additional information on vaccinations and travel is the Center for Disease Control, 1600 Clifton Road, N.E., Atlanta, GA 30333. Useful publications include the *Morbidity and Mortality Weekly Reports,* which is available for a modest subscription fee from the *New England Journal of Medicine.* The annual *Health Information for International Travel* can be obtained from the superintendent of Documents, U.S. Government Printing Office, Washington DC 20402.

ANNOTATED BIBLIOGRAPHY

Bolan G, Broome CV, Facklam RR et al: Pneumococcal vaccine efficacy in selected populations in the United States. Ann Intern Med 104:1, 1986 (*Comparison of serotypes provides estimate of vaccine efficacy of 61% in persons over 65, but confidence limits were wide.*)

Eminia EA, Ellis RW, Miller WJ et al: Production and immunological analysis of recombinant hepatitis B vaccine. J Infect Dis 13:(suppl A)3, 1986 (*Reviews the development and properties of the vaccine.*)

Health and Public Policy Committee, American College of Physicians: Hepatitis B vaccine. Ann Intern Med 100:149, 1984 (*Recommendations from The Clinical Efficacy Assessment Project.*)

Immunizations and chemoprophylaxis for travelers. Med Lett 27: 33, 1985 (*A concise, authoritative summary.*)

Recommendations of the Immunization Practices Committee: Recommendations for protection against viral hepatitis. MMWR 34: 331, 1985 (*Recommendations for both passive and active immunization.*)

Recommendations of the Immunization Practices Advisory Committee: Update: Prevention of Hemophilus influenzae Type b Disease. MMWR 35:170, 1986 (*Recommendations for use of this new vaccine.*)

Sack DA, Kaminsky DC, Sack RB et al: Prophylactic doxycycline for traveler's diarrhea. Results of a prospective—blind study of Peace Corps volunteers in Kenya. N Engl J Med 298:758, 1978 (*A double-blind clinical trial demonstrating that prophylactic administration of doxycycline can reduce the incidence of "turista."*)

U.S. Department of Health and Human Services/Public Health Service: General recommendations on immunization. MMWR 32: 1, 1983. (*Recent CDC recommendations.*)

U.S. Department of Health and Human Services/Public Health Service: Prevention of malaria in travelers. MMWR 31(Suppl):1 1982. (*A detailed discussion of the chemoprophylaxis of malaria, including the difficult problem of chloroquine-resistant malaria. See also "Revise Recommendations for Malaria Chemoprophylaxis" MMWR 31:328.*)

2

Constitutional Problems

5
Evaluation of
Chronic Fatigue

Chronic fatigue is a frustrating problem to assess because it is so vague. Nevertheless, it is one of the most common complaints in the office setting; it is important because it is a sensitive though nonspecific indicator of underlying medical and/or emotional pathology. Regardless of cause, the patient typically reports a lack of energy, listlessness, and generalized disinterest in family, work, and leisure activities. Some patients inappropriately use the term *weakness* to describe their problem, though motor function remains intact. Many speculate that they have vitamin deficiencies, low iron, or anemia. Self-treatment with vitamin and iron supplements is common.

Many people bothered by fatigue come to the primary physician looking for an organic cause; few initially admit to an emotional problem, even though most studies of fatigue report psychological etiologies in the vast majority of cases. The primary physician has the task of determining whether the problem is mainly a physiological or an emotional one; sometimes both mechanisms coexist.

PATHOPHYSIOLOGY AND CLINICAL PRESENTATIONS

Almost all illnesses are capable of causing fatigue; however, a few are noteworthy for the prominence of the symptom in the clinical presentation. Fatigue is an important somatic symptom of *depression,* often coexisting with early morning awakening, appetite disturbances and multiple bodily complaints. Changes in central nervous system neurotransmitter metabolism are believed to play a major role in the pathogenesis of depression (see Chapter 223). *Chronic anxiety* may result in generalized fatigue, due in part to difficulty in obtaining adequate physical and psychological rest. Patients report trouble falling asleep and a host of associated bodily complaints. Many maintain their neck muscles in constantly tensed states, giving rise to occipital-nuchal headaches. Palpitations, difficulty breathing, chest tightness, and gastrointestinal troubles add to the clinical picture (see Chapter 222). Chronic insomnia from a variety of *sleep disorders* represents an important etiology of fatigue (see Chapter 228).

Some of the medications used to treat anxiety and depression have substantial sedating effects; when used in excess, they may actually worsen the patient's sense of fatigue rather than alleviate it. Of the *tricyclic antidepressants,* amitriptyline and *doxepin* are among the more sedating, which makes them useful when agitation is a problem, but they can cause some patients to feel "knocked out" (see Chapter 223). Chronic use of *hypnotics* may aggravate difficulty in falling asleep and contribute to fatigue (see Chapter 228). *Minor tranquilizers* such as diazepam (Valium) can cause tiredness when taken daily in frequent doses sufficient to result in accumulation of high serum levels of the drug and its active metabolites (see Chapter 222).

Antihypertensives that penetrate the central nervous system, such as *reserpine,* methyldopa, clonidine, and *propranolol,* may precipitate depression or fatigue. Reserpine has been found to cause depression when used in dosages exceeding 0.5 mg per day, especially in patients with a prior history of depression. Propranolol and other lipid-soluble beta-blocking agents can have a similar, though usually less severe, effect with fatigue being a more common complaint. In a series of 390 hypertensive patients taking propranolol, fatigue was the major reason for discontinuing the medication. Antihistamines used for allergic rhinitis are another common pharmacologic precipitant of fatigue.

Endocrine disturbances are treatable precipitants. Dysfunction of the thyroid, adrenal, pituitary, parathyroid, or endocrine pancreas can be subtle in onset, starting out inconspicuously as fatigue. For example, *hypothyroidism* may begin with fatigue, often in association with weight gain, dry skin, mild hoarseness, cold intolerance, and other signs (see Chapter 102). Patients with *Addison's disease* manifest insidious onset of fatigue in conjunction with weight loss, vague gastrointestinal upset, postural hypotension, and eventually, hyperpigmentation. *Panhypopituitarism* from postpartum hemorrhage or a tumor of the sellar region can cause fatigue. The patient with postpartum disease (Sheehan's syndrome) fails to lactate or menstruate; lassitude, decreased libido, and loss of axillary and pubic hair develop slowly. Later, symptoms of hypothyroidism may ensue.

Diabetes that is out of control with marked glycosuria is another endocrinologic etiology of fatigue. When glycosuria is severe enough to produce caloric wasting and fatigue, polyphagia, polyuria, and polydipsia usually exist (see Chapter 100). *Hyperparathyroidism* as well as other causes of hypercalcemia may present with fatigue and weakness. In an NIH series of 57 cases of primary hyperparathyroidism, fatigue was the most common symptom, occurring in 24%. *Apathetic hyperthyroidism* is an uncommon but important source of fatigue in the elderly. Presentation includes profound weight loss and unexplained atrial fibrillation, in addition to apathy and extreme fatigue (see Chapter 101).

Iron deficiency is often blamed for fatigue, although the correlation between iron deficiency anemia and fatigue is poor, especially when the anemia is mild (see Chapter 84). In a double-blind study of menstruating women with mild anemia due to iron deficiency, there was no significant difference between the effects of iron and placebo on fatigue. The relation between severe anemia (hematocrit <20) and fatigue is more direct. Lassitude prevails, at times in association with exertional dyspnea or with postural hypotension when blood loss is acute.

Chronic congestive heart failure and *chronic lung disease* are sometimes heralded by lassitude, but dyspnea is a prominent feature, along with other obvious signs of heart and lung disease (see Chapters 27, 36, and 44).

Most *chronic inflammatory, infectious,* and *neoplastic processes* are capable of precipitating fatigue; general malaise may even be the initial symptom. Fatigue may precede the joint symptoms of rheumatoid disease (see Chapter 153). Fever, night sweats, weight loss, or lymphadenopathy may contribute to the clinical picture. Marked fatigue and lymphadenopathy are the hallmarks of *acute infectious mononucleosis* (see Chapter 81) and may be seen with other viral illnesses such as *cytomegalovirus disease* and *viral hepatitis;* occasionally *acquired immunodeficiency syndrome* presents in this manner (see Chapter 142). Evidence of chronic Epstein–Barr virus infection has been found in some patients with a history of mononucleosis and a syndrome of chronic fatigue. The significance of the finding remains unclear, but may represent the cause of symptoms in some cases.

Chronic renal failure may present inconspicuously with fatigue and few localizing symptoms or signs aside from laboratory findings of azotemia, mild anemia, impaired renal concentrating ability, and an abnormal urinary sediment (see Chapter 139). *Hepatocellular failure* is an important source of lassitude. Jaundice, ascites, petechiae, asterixis, spider angiomata, and other signs of hepatic insufficiency usually contribute to the clinical picture. However, in chronic hepatitis, jaundice may be minimal while fatigue is prominent; the same holds for the prodromal phase of acute viral hepatitis (see Chapters 70 and 71).

DIFFERENTIAL DIAGNOSIS

Although the list of conditions that may present with fatigue is extensive, most cases have a strong overlay of anxiety and/or depression, even when the etiology is medical. Fatigue, of course, may accompany any illness, but those listed in Table 5-1 are notable for the prominence of lassitude in the clinical presentation. In a series of 300 cases of fatigue evaluated at the Lahey Clinic, 80% were due to an emotional problem, 4% to chronic infection, 3% to heart disease, 2% to anemia, and 1% to nephritis.

Table 5-1. Some Conditions Presenting as Chronic Fatigue

1. Psychologic
   a. Depression
   b. Anxiety
   c. Sleep disorders
2. Endocrine–Metabolic
   a. Hypothyroidism
   b. Diabetes mellitus
   c. Apathetic hyperthyroidism of the elderly
   d. Pituitary insufficiency
   e. Hyperparathyroidism or hypercalcemia of any origin
   f. Addison's disease
   g. Chronic renal failure
   h. Hepatocellular failure
3. Pharmacologic
   a. Hypnotics
   b. Antihypertensives
   c. Antidepressants
   d. Tranquilizers
   e. Drug abuse and drug withdrawal
4. Infectious
   a. Endocarditis
   b. Tuberculosis
   c. Mononucleosis
   d. Hepatitis
   e. Parasitic disease
   f. Chronic Epstein–Barr virus infection
   g. Cytomegalovirus
5. Neoplastic–Hematologic–Immunologic
   a. Occult malignancy
   b. Severe anemia
   c. Acquired immunodeficiency syndrome
6. Cardiopulmonary
   a. Chronic congestive heart failure
   b. Chronic obstructive pulmonary disease

WORKUP

In most instances, the evaluation of fatigue can be conveniently performed in the office. Two or three visits may be needed to establish the underlying etiology; at times the patient may insist that medical illness be ruled out before agreeing to discuss psychosocial matters.

History should begin with a thorough description of the fatigue to be sure that the patient is not confusing focal neuromuscular disease with generalized lassitude. Because depression underlies many cases of fatigue, it is essential to check for its somatic manifestations, such as early morning awakening, alteration of appetite, and multisystem functional complaints. It is also important to ask about significant losses, low self-esteem, and occurrence of crying spells and suicidal thoughts. Anxiety is suggested by unresolved conflict, persistent nervousness, recurrent bouts of excessive uneasiness, and trouble falling asleep. Any abuse of hypnotics or tranquilizers needs to be ascertained and considered as a cause of disturbed sleep and resultant fatigue. Fatigue in the elderly patient should not be ascribed to age; an underlying psychogenic or medical illness is likely.

A history of fever, sweats, weight loss, and adenopathy points toward smoldering infection and occult neoplasm. Symptoms suggesting a metabolic or endocrinologic cause include polyuria, polydipsia, changes in skin pigmentation and texture, hoarseness, cold intolerance, nausea, and abnormal menses. Symmetrical joint pain and morning stiffness are clues to underlying rheumatoid disease.

The past medical history should be noted for anemia, rheumatic fever, mononucleosis, heart murmur, recurrent urinary tract infection, proteinuria, liver disease, alcohol and drug abuse, and depression. Epidemiologic considerations ought to include exposure to tuberculosis, mononucleosis, and hepatitis; any risk factors for acquired immunodeficiency syndrome are important to note (see Chapter 142). Travel to areas where parasitic infections are endemic, work in meat-packing industries or on a farm, and sudden common source outbreak of illness are other potentially important epidemiologic clues.

A full listing of all the patient's medications should be obtained. Often overlooked are over-the-counter antihistamines that patients use for sleep, allergies, and colds. Most centrally acting antihypertensive agents are capable of causing fatigue and their use should be noted, as should that of all psychotropic agents.

Physical examination often provides important evidence and needs to be thorough. Vital signs should include postural pulse and blood pressure determinations, rectal temperature, and weight. If there is no fever on examination in the office, but it is suggested by history, then a 10 PM reading at home is indicated. Skin is assessed for change in pigmentation, purpura, dryness, rash, jaundice, and pallor. Endocarditis may

first be suggested by the finding of splinter hemorrhages or petechiae. Fundoscopic examination may reveal Roth's spots, diabetic retinopathy, or even, in rare instances, a tuberculoma. The sclerae are observed for icterus. If examination of the pharynx reveals petechiae at the junction of the hard and soft palate, mononucleosis ought to be considered.

Careful examination of all lymph nodes is essential; size, degree of tenderness, and distribution need to be noted. Diffuse adenopathy suggests malignancy and infection and is sometimes a sign of the acquired immunodeficiency syndrome (see Chapter 142). The thyroid is checked for goiter; the lungs for rales, consolidation, and effusion; and the heart for murmurs, rubs, gallops, and rhythm disturbances. Unexplained atrial fibrillation in the elderly may be a manifestation of apathetic hyperthyroidism.

The abdomen is palpated for organomegaly, masses, ascites, and hepatic tenderness. Rectal examination includes a look for masses, prostatic pathology, and occult blood. Genitalia should be checked for masses suggestive of malignancy and tenderness indicative of infection. Joints are assessed for signs of inflammation. A complete neurologic evaluation is necessary to be sure that the patient's fatigue is not really a manifestation of neuromuscular disease. Any tenderness, atrophy, focal weakness, or fasiculations in the muscles is noted. Deep tendon reflexes that have a slow relaxation phase are suggestive of hypothyroidism. Even visual field testing is important, for a pituitary lesion may produce a bitemporal hemianopsia.

Laboratory Studies. In the overtly depressed patient with an otherwise completely normal history and physical examination, there is no need to proceed with an extensive laboratory workup for occult medical illness. A complete blood count (CBC) and erythrocyte sedimentation rate (ESR) are often ordered for screening purposes, though the ESR is rather insensitive for detection of occult illness. A more difficult situation is the patient with no evidence of depression and an unrevealing history and physical. Here, a few extra studies are warranted to help rule out clinically subtle conditions that may present as fatigue. The list of such studies includes a serum calcium, BUN, creatinine, glucose, and transaminase. Thyroid function studies are often ordered in this situation but are rarely helpful in the absence of at least some clinical clue suggesting thyroid disease. However, the elderly patient with unexplained weight loss and atrial fibrillation is a strong candidate for apathetic hyperthyroidism and requires free thyroxine and total T_3 determinations.

The syndrome of chronic mononucleosis or chronic Epstein–Barr virus infection has received much attention in the lay press. Although there is some evidence it may be responsible for chronic fatigue in a limited number of patients (those with a history of mononucleosis who demonstrate periodic low-grade fever, lymphadenopathy, or persistent pharyngitis), the syndrome should not be used as an explanation for symptoms in the vast majority of chronically fatigued patients who have an otherwise unremarkable history and physical examination. Ordering *viral antibody titers* for EB virus in the occasional patient who has clinical evidence suggesting chronic infection is reasonable, but not in the much larger group of chronically fatigued individuals who have unremarkable histories and physical examinations.

PATIENT EDUCATION

It is often useful to provide patients with a substantive organic explanation for the way they are feeling, even if the etiology is psychogenic. Patients with underlying psychogenic disease need an especially thorough explanation of the grounds for the diagnosis and their symptoms; many come to the physician thinking they have a medical problem. For example, reviewing the diagnostic criteria for depression and describing the mechanism by which depression leads to fatigue (see Chapter 223) helps relieve some of the uncertainty and fear of underlying organic disease that accompanies symptoms. The attention given to "chronic mononucleosis" in the lay press often necessitates addressing the issue of its likelihood or lack thereof. Chronic mononucleosis has the potential for becoming the hypoglycemia of the 1980s, another "nondiagnosis" used to explain psychophysiologic symptoms.

SYMPTOMATIC RELIEF

When the cause of fatigue is endocrinologic, metabolic, or infectious, treatment needs to be specific and aimed at the underlying condition. Malignancy is often accompanied by a reactive depression that can be helped by development of a strong, supportive doctor–patient relationship (see Chapter 88). The fatigue of endogenous depression can be treated with support and tricyclic antidepressants; imipramine may be less sedating than amitriptyline (starting dose is 25 to 50 mg at bedtime, increased by 25 to 50 mg at a time). The sleep disorder caused by depression may respond well to small doses, with the fatigue dissipating as the patient gets a good night's sleep. Affective changes may not occur at low doses (see Chapter 223).

Anxiety-related fatigue can be difficult to treat. Prescribing antianxiety agents can lead to excessive use and worsening of symptoms (see Chapter 222); however, a brief and limited trial of benzodiazepine therapy at bedtime is worth an attempt; for example, 5 mg of chlordiazepoxide can help the patient to fall asleep and get much-needed rest. There is no evidence that any one benzodiazepine is superior to any other for sleep, although flurazepam is widely promoted and prescribed, often in conjunction with another benzodiazepine. (This can sometimes lead to excessive benzodiazepine intake.) Once symptomatic control of anxiety is accomplished, work can begin on helping the patient to deal with his problems.

A.H.G.

ANNOTATED BIBLIOGRAPHY

Abrams DI, Lewis BJ, Beckstead JH et al: Persistent diffuse lymphadenopathy in homosexual men. Ann Intern Med 100:801, 1984 (*A possible presentation of AIDS with adenopathy and fatigue being major clinical features.*)

Allan FN: Differential diagnosis of weakness and fatigue. N Engl J Med 231:414, 1944 (*A classic study of 300 patients presenting to the Lahey Clinic with fatigue; an emotional etiology was present in 80%.*)

Aurbach G, Mallette L, Patten B et al: Hyperparathyroidism: Recent studies. NIH conference. Ann Intern Med 79:566, 1973 (*Fatigue headed the list of symptoms reported in 57 cases of primary hyperparathyroidism; 24% reported the problem.*)

Croog SH, Levine S, Testa A et al: The effects of antihypertensive therapy on the quality of life. N Engl J Med 314:1657, 1986 (*Documents effects of methyldopa and propranolol on 626 men in a randomized double-blind study of antihypertensive therapies; both agents were associated with fatigue and lethargy in about 5% of patients.*)

Jerrett WA: Lethargy in General Practice. Practitioner 225:731, 1981 (*A review of 300 patients showed no advantage to laboratory testing in the absence of historical or physical clues.*)

Kales A, Bixler E, Tan T et al: Chronic hypnotic use: Ineffectiveness, drug withdrawal, insomnia, and hypnotic drug dependence. JAMA 227:513, 1974 (*Chronic hypnotic use may actually worsen the problem of sleeplessness and its attendant difficulties.*)

Severe depression caused by reserpine. Med Lett 18:17, 1976 (*Reviews the evidence linking reserpine with depression and advises against using doses in excess of 0.25 mg per day or prescribing to depressed patients.*)

Sox HC, Liang MH: The erythrocyte sedimentation rate. Ann Intern Med 104:515, 1986 (*A critical review arguing the test is not a useful screening procedure.*)

Straus SE, Tosato G, Armstrong G et al: Persisting illness and fatigue in adults with evidence of Epstein–Barr virus infection. Ann Intern Med 102:7, 1985 (*A report of 31 patients with chronic fatigue after infectious mononucleosis showing evidence of persisting infection in 23.*)

Thomas F, Mazzaferri E, Skillman T: Apathetic thyrotoxicosis: A distinctive clinical and laboratory entity. Ann Intern Med 72: 679, 1970 (*These patients are typically elderly, are depressed in appearance, and have marked weight loss. In this small series, 7 of 9 had atrial fibrillation and many presented with cardiac complaints.*)

Thompson K: Loss of Energy: Ageing or Disease? J Gen Pract (New Zealand) 1:34, 1984 (*A review suggesting that a loss of energy in the elderly is not normal and that fatigue present after a full night's sleep makes a psychological explanation more likely.*)

Wood M, Elwood P: Symptoms of iron deficiency anemia: A community survey. Br J Prev Soc Med 20:117, 1966 (*Correlation between hemoglobin concentration and symptoms was poor. Iron therapy produced no statistically significant improvement in symptoms.*)

Zacharias F: Patient acceptability of propranolol and occurrence of side effects. Postgrad Med J: 52(4):87, 1976 (*In a series of 390 hypertensives on propranolol, fatigue was reported as the most common side-effect, which limited dose; the incidence of the problem was less than 5%.*)

6
Evaluation of Fever
HARVEY B. SIMON, M.D.

Since antiquity, fever has been recognized as a cardinal manifestation of disease. Indeed, people identify fever as a sign of illness more readily than they recognize the importance of most other symptoms. In addition to causing concern, the presence of fever usually raises high therapeutic expectations. Even in the preantibiotic era, John Milton observed that "the feaver is to the Physitians, the eternal reproach" (1641); in the popular mind today, fever is equated with infection, and infections are expected to respond to the administration of "wonder drugs." As a result, the physician is faced with the challenge of defining the etiology of the fever, instituting appropriate therapy, and explaining the reasons for limiting antibiotic usage to bacterial infections.

PATHOPHYSIOLOGY AND CLINICAL PRESENTATION

Popular lore notwithstanding, 98.6°F (37°C) is *not* normal body temperature. In fact, there is no single normal value; like so many other biological functions, body temperature displays a circadian rhythmicity. In healthy individuals, mean rectal temperatures vary from a low of about 97°F (36.1°C) in early morning to a high of about 99.3°F (37.4°C) in late afternoon. In children, the normal range may be even greater. Moreover, physiologic factors such as exercise and the menstrual cycle can further alter body temperature. In practical terms, understanding the diurnal rhythm of body temperature is important for two reasons. First, many patients have been unnecessarily subjected to extensive workups and even psychologically invalided in the erroneous quest of a cause for deviation from the mythical "normal" of 98.6°F. Second, the fever of disease states is superimposed on the normal cycle, so that fevers are generally highest in the evenings and lowest in the mornings. As a result, frequent temperature recordings throughout the day are required to monitor fever in sick patients; the absence of fever in a single office visit does not exclude a febrile illness.

The presenting complaints of the febrile patient may be explained by the underlying disease process or by the fever itself. The signs and symptoms of fever vary tremendously. Some patients are asymptomatic; more often there is a sensation of warmth or flushing. Malaise and fatigue are common. The hypothalamus, acting through somatic efferent nerves, increases muscle tone in order to generate heat and raise body temperature; many febrile patients experience *myalgias* as a result.

These same factors account for one of the most dramatic manifestations of fever: the *shaking chill* or *rigor.* It is taught that rigor is a manifestation of bacteremia, but in fact any stimulus that raises the hypothalamic setpoint rapidly may produce a rigor. Patients experiencing a rigor exhibit uncontrolled violent shaking and trembling, and characteristically heap themselves with blankets even as their temperatures are shooting up. This phenomenon also has a physiologic basis. Despite the high central or core temperature, these patients subjectively feel cold because surface temperature is reduced. In order to generate fever in response to hypothalamic stimuli, cutaneous vasoconstriction occurs, skin temperature falls, and cold receptors in the skin sense this as cold. Quite the reverse occurs during defervescence; body temperature falls in response to cutaneous vasodilation, and drenching sweats typically terminate an episode of fever.

Other manifestations of temperature elevation include central nervous system symptoms ranging from a mild inability to concentrate to *confusion, delirium,* or even stupor, especially in the elderly or debilitated patient. High fevers (104°F–106°F) may produce *convulsions* in infants and young children without any primary neurologic disorder. Increased cardiac output is an invariable consequence of fever, and *tachycardia* typically accompanies fever. Tachycardia is so usual that its absence should lead one to suspect uncommon problems such as typhoid fever, in which relative bradycardia is typical (for unknown reasons), drug fever, and factitious fever. Patients with underlying heart disease may respond to the high output stress of fever with angina or heart failure.

Another sign of fever may be the so-called fever blister— *labial herpes simplex.* The problem is probably not precipitated by fever *per se,* for it is much more common in some infections, such as pneumococcal pneumonia and meningococcal meningitis, than in other febrile states.

Because fever accompanies infection so frequently, numerous investigators have tried to determine if fever has any protective or beneficial role. There are a few circumstances, such as central nervous system syphilis, in which elevations of body temperature may exceed the thermal tolerance of the infectious agent. In fact, induced fever was once a form of therapy for syphilis. In several animal models, fever enhances recovery from experimental infections; however, there is no such proven clinical benefit from fever in humans.

Is fever detrimental? Most otherwise healthy individuals can tolerate temperatures up to 105°F (40.5°C) without ill effects, although even in these individuals symptoms often warrant therapy. In children, high fevers should be suppressed because convulsions may occur. Patients with heart disease should also receive antipyretic therapy. Each 1°F of temperature increases the basal metabolic rate by 7%, resulting in increased demands on the heart, which may precipitate myocardial ischemia, failure, or even shock. In addition, extreme hyperthermia beyond 108°F (42.1°C) can cause direct cellular damage, probably by denaturing protein. Vascular endothelium seems particularly susceptible to such damage, and disseminated intravascular coagulation frequently accompanies extreme hyperthermia. Other structures that may be directly damaged are brain, muscle, and heart. Finally, metabolic derangements such as hypoxia, acidosis, and sometimes hyperkalemia can result from extreme pyrexia and, in turn, further contribute to coma, seizures, arrhythmias, or hypotension, which could be lethal. Nevertheless, patients have survived temperatures of up to 108°F without demonstrable organ damage, but mortality in this temperature range is appreciable. Body temperatures as high as 113°F have been demonstrated in humans, but these have been uniformly lethal.

DIFFERENTIAL DIAGNOSIS

Many inflammatory, infectious, neoplastic and hypersensitivity processes may produce fever. Most acute fevers are accompanied by obvious signs and symptoms of the underlying cause, such as upper respiratory infection, cystitis, and gastroenteritis. An untoward reaction to drug may produce fever, often in association with rash, arthritis, or edema. Among the drugs most commonly implicated are the antibiotics. However, unexplained persistent fever can be a major diagnostic challenge. Table 6-1 lists causes of "fevers of unknown origin," defined as those persisting for 3 weeks, exceeding temperatures of 101°F, and eluding 1 week of intensive diagnostic study.

WORKUP

The febrile patient presents a common but demanding problem in differential diagnosis. In most cases, a careful history and physical examination will provide important clues, so that laboratory studies can be used selectively. In addition, the initial office evaluation should help determine the proper pace of diagnostic tests and of therapeutic intervention. If the illness is insidious in onset and only slowly progressive, or if the patient is nontoxic and clinically stable, one may proceed with the workup in a deliberate manner on an ambulatory basis, utilizing serial clinical observations and time as key diagnostic tools. On the other hand, if the patient is a compromised host, or if he is acutely ill and toxic, several immediate diagnostic studies are mandatory, and treatment may even be required before all the results are available; hospitalization is usually necessary in such cases. Table 6-2 lists some factors that should prompt an aggressive approach to diagnosis and therapy.

Table 6-1.   Causes of Fever of Undetermined Origin

"The Big Three"
I. Infections: 40%
 A. Systemic
  1. Tuberculosis (miliary)
  2. Infective endocarditis (subacute)
  3. Miscellaneous infections: cytomegalovirus infection, toxoplasmosis, brucellosis, psittacosis, gonococcemia, chronic meningococcemia, disseminated mycoses
 B. Localized
  1. Hepatic infections (liver abscess, cholangitis)
  2. Other visceral infections (pancreatic, tubo-ovarian, and pericholecystic abscesses, and empyema of gallbladder)
  3. Intraperitoneal infections (subhepatic, subphrenic, paracolic, appendiceal, pelvic, and other abscesses)
  4. Urinary tract infections (pyelonephritis, renal carbuncle, perinephric abscess, prostatic abscess)
II. Neoplasms: 20%. Especially lymphomas, leukemias, renal cell carcinoma, atrial myomas, and cancers metastatic to bone or liver
III. Collagen–vascular disease: 15%. Including temporal arteritis and juvenile rheumatoid arthritis as well as systemic lupus erythematosus, rheumatoid arthritis, polyarteritis nodosa, Wegener's granulomatosis, and mixed connective tissue disease

Less Common Causes
 I. Noninfectious granulomatous diseases (especially sarcoidosis and granulomatous hepatitis)
 II. Inflammatory bowel disease
 III. Pulmonary embolization
 IV. Drug fever
 V. Factitious fever
 VI. Hepatic cirrhosis with active hepatocellular necrosis
 VII. Miscellaneous uncommon diseases (familial Mediterranean fever, Whipple's disease, etc.)
 VIII. Undiagnosed

(Modified from Jacoby GA, Swartz MN: Fever of unknown origin. N Engl J Med 289:1407, 1973)

Febrile illnesses are most commonly acute processes that are either readily diagnosed and treated (common bacterial infections) or self-limited despite the lack of a specific diagnosis (viral infections, allergic reactions). However, patients will occasionally present with undiagnosed fevers, fulfilling the classic criterion for "fever of unknown origin." In both situations, the key to diagnosis is often a meticulous history and physical examination.

History.   The infectious disease history should stress several items not routinely emphasized: (1) host factors, (2) epidemiology, (3) symptomatology, and (4) drug history. Regarding *host factors,* one should determine if the patient is basically healthy, or if he has an underlying disease that may render him unusually susceptible to infection. Patients with hematologic and other malignancies, acquired immunodeficiency syndrome (AIDS), diabetes mellitus, neutropenia, or sickle cell anemia may become infected with unusual opportunistic pathogens or may fail to respond normally to

Table 6-2. Febrile Patients Who Require
Special Attention

1. Vulnerable Hosts
   a. Age (very young or very old)
   b. Corticosteroid or immunosuppressive therapy
   c. Serious underlying diseases (neutropenia, sickle cell anemia, diabetes, cirrhosis, advanced COPD, renal failure, malignancies, AIDS)
   d. Implanted prosthetic devices (heart valves, joint prostheses, etc.)
2. Toxic Patients
   a. Rigors, prostration, extreme pyrexia
   b. Hypotension, oliguria
   c. CNS abnormalities
   d. Cardiorespiratory compromise
   e. New significant cardiac murmurs
   f. Petechial eruption
   g. Marked leukocytosis or leukopenia

common infectious agents. Patients taking corticosteroids or other immunosuppressive agents are especially vulnerable to infection. Individuals with implanted prosthetic devices such as artificial heart valves or hip prostheses are also at increased risk of serious infection. Finally, patients with past histories of certain infectious processes such as pyelonephritis may be prone to relapses or recurrences of similar problems.

Turning to *epidemiology,* it is helpful to ask if the patient has traveled to places where he may have been exposed to "exotic" infections such as typhoid fever or malaria. Less obvious factors such as exposure to animals may be of great importance. Vectors of infection may be found even among household pets, such as cats (cat-scratch disease and *Pasteurella multocida* cellulitis from bites or scratches, for example, and toxoplasmosis from fecal contamination), parakeets (psittacosis), and turtles (salmonellosis). A history of bites by stray dogs, skunks, or bats may suggest the possibility of rabies. More commonly, exposure to someone with a communicable disease such as tuberculosis or influenza can provide the central clue to diagnosis.

An inquiry into what is "going around" in the community may be helpful. A very localized outbreak of a flulike illness or atypical pneumonia may be a clue to *Legionella* infection (see Chapter 43). In areas with a large population of homosexuals, intravenous drug abusers, Haitians, or hemophiliacs, one needs to consider the possibility of AIDS and its complications (see Chapter 43). The patient's occupation is sometimes revealing as well; for example, abattoir workers may be exposed to brucellosis, leather workers to anthrax, and gardeners to sporotrichosis.

Attention to *symptomatology* may serve to pinpoint the site of infection. Localizing symptoms such as headache, alterations of consciousness, cough, dyspnea, flank pain, dysuria, or abdominal pain are particularly useful in focusing diagnostic studies. Finally, history should include a careful inquiry into any *drugs* used. Has the patient been taking antibiotics, which may alter his susceptibility to infection by favoring drug-resistant organisms or mask infection by rendering him culture negative? Does he have drug allergies or underlying problems such as renal failure, which may alter the choice of therapeutic agents? Is the patient taking any medications that may be responsible for fever as a manifestation of hypersensitivity?

Physical Examination. Unlike other conditions in which the physical examination is only confirmatory, essential clues may be uncovered by a detailed examination of the febrile patient. Vital signs should be determined in all cases. Fever is an important but nonspecific sign of infection; some patients with infections are afebrile whereas others may have a fever resulting from noninfectious causes such as hypersensitivity states and lymphoreticular malignancies. The shaking chill or rigor may suggest bacteremia but is also not specific. In the neonate or in occasional adults with overwhelming sepsis, hypothermia may be present. Respiratory distress may signal pulmonary infection or septic shock, and hypotension may be the presenting finding leading to a diagnosis of sepsis.

The skin and mucous membranes may provide crucial information. To cite a few examples: petechial eruptions suggest meningococcemia or Rocky Mountain spotted fever; pustular lesions, gonococcemia (see Chapter 116) or staphylococcal endocarditis; splinter hemorrhages and conjunctival petechiae, endocarditis; ecthyma gangrenosa, *Pseudomonas* septicemia; macular or vesicular eruptions, viral infections. Similarly, the optic fundi should be examined. Roth spots suggest endocarditis. Choroidal tubercles may be the only positive finding in miliary tuberculosis, and similar lesions may result from *Candida* septicemia.

The sinuses should be percussed for tenderness suggestive of sinusitis, and the tympanic membranes should be examined for effusion and erythema. The neck is checked for rigidity and focal tenderness. Careful examination of all the lymph nodes for enlargement may provide a very important clue to etiology (see Chapter 81); distribution needs to be noted. The breasts are examined for masses and tenderness. The chest is noted for rubs and signs of consolidation and effusion. A careful cardiac examination for murmurs and rubs is essential. The abdomen is checked for organomegaly, masses, tenderness, guarding, and rebound.

The genitorectal area is all too frequently overlooked, yet it is often a source of key information. The woman without an obvious source of fever must have a careful pelvic examination looking for cervical discharge, adnexal tenderness, and mass lesions (see Chapter 114). In men, the prostate and testicles need to be gently checked for tenderness and masses and the penis for discharge and rash (see Chapter 129). Rectal examination should include evaluation for discharge, tenderness, and masses (see Chapter 61); the stool is tested for occult blood.

Musculoskeletal examination may suggest inflammation or infection of the bone or joints if there is swelling, increased warmth, or tenderness. The neurologic evaluation should include a look for signs of meningeal irritation, the presence of focal deficits, and disturbances in mentation.

Laboratory Studies. If the history and physical examination provide strong indications of an infectious process, laboratory studies can be used selectively to confirm or refute the clinical diagnosis. For example, in the patient with an obvious viral upper respiratory infection, no studies are necessary. In patients with bronchitis, a sputum smear and culture may be all that is required, but if pneumonia is a possibility, a chest radiograph and complete blood count (CBC) are minimal additional requirements (see Chapter 43). In the patient with probable cystitis, a urinalysis and culture are sufficient, but if upper tract infection is suspected, especially as a complication of obstruction, then renal function tests, blood cultures, renal ultrasonography, and/or intravenous pyelography (IVP) deserve serious consideration (see Chapter 134).

In other patients, however, more extensive tests are needed to establish a diagnosis when the cause of fever remains unknown. Although such studies must be individualized, the approach to diagnosis of an obscure fever should include the following.

COMPLETE BLOOD COUNTS, DIFFERENTIAL, AND SEDIMENTATION RATE. Leukocytosis and a "shift to the left" suggest but do not prove bacterial infection. Toxic granulations, Döhle bodies, and vacuoles in polymorphonuclear leukocytes are suggestive of bacterial sepsis, but are not entirely specific. In most instances, the erythrocyte sedimentation rate (ESR) lacks the sensitivity and specificity needed for it to serve as an adequate means of detecting or ruling out such causes of fever as tumor, connective tissue disease, and infection. Although a very elevated ESR is an invitation to additional testing and may be a clue to a specific process such as temporal arteritis (see Chapter 156), many elevations are due to trivial conditions unrelated to the cause of fever. The ESR should be ordered and interpreted cautiously and not viewed as a screening test for "disease."

URINALYSIS. Pyuria strongly suggests urinary tract infection. Gram stain of the unspun urine specimen can be diagnostic (see Chapter 124).

RADIOGRAPHIC STUDIES. Chest radiographs may detect infiltrates, effusions, masses, or nodes even in the absence of abnormalities on physical examination, while KUB and upright abdominal films can disclose air–fluid levels in the bowel. Contrast studies and scans may be needed if there is suspicion of abscess, tumor, or other mass lesions (see below).

BLOOD CHEMISTRIES. The blood sugar determination is helpful in search of previously unsuspected diabetes mellitus. The test is also important in evaluating the significance of the sugar concentration in various body fluids. Liver function tests are useful in helping to define obscure sources of fever. For example, transaminase elevation suggests hepatitis, and

isolated rises in alkaline phosphatase point to infiltration of the liver.

EXAMINATION OF BODY FLUIDS. If there is any possibility of meningitis, a lumbar puncture is mandatory. Aspiration and study of pleural effusions, ascitic fluid, or joint effusions may be diagnostic. Such specimens should be examined directly by cell counts and stains (see below). Sugar and protein determinations help differentiate etiologies; in general, bacterial, mycobacterial, and fungal infections produce low sugar and high protein levels in body fluid.

CULTURES. If the patient has a heart murmur, or a prosthetic heart valve, or appears seriously ill, cultures of blood should be obtained. (Having at least two blood cultures from separate venipunctures is preferred.) Most patients should have cultures taken of urine (clean catch or catheterized specimen) and sputum. If other body fluids are obtainable, they should likewise be cultured. Special mycobacterial and fungal media are required if these agents are suspected, especially if the patient is a compromised host. Anaerobic cultures are important when one is dealing with a possible abscess or other infection of the pulmonary, gastrointestinal, or pelvic regions.

MICROSCOPIC EVALUATION. Any body fluid that can be obtained should be examined by the Gram stain technique. Sputum, urine, wound exudates, cerebrospinal fluid, pleural fluid, ascitic fluid and joint fluid often reveal the cause of infection on Gram stain. Even Gram stains of the stool may be helpful in certain specific situations, such as acute diarrhea with suspicion of staphylococcal enterocolitis. The presence of bacteria in a specimen of body fluid that is normally sterile is presumptive evidence of infection. This is particularly true when one is examining the spun sediment obtained from cerebrospinal fluid. Likewise, bacteria are not found in normal ascitic, joint, or pleural fluid. Bacteria in unspun urine correlates well with the presence of a significant urinary tract infection. However, Gram stains must be examined and interpreted with a certain amount of caution. For example, if one sees epithelial cells in a sputum specimen, one can be certain that the specimen contains mouth organisms and is not representative of conditions in the tracheobronchial tree. In such instances, one should obtain a better sputum sample. In the presence of bacterial pneumonia, the sputum usually contains many polymorphonuclear leukocytes and a large number of bacteria. Acid-fast stains are required to visualize mycobacteria (see Chapter 43), and specially stained wet mounts of body fluids can be useful in uncovering numerous types of fungal infections.

IMMUNOLOGIC STUDIES. Serologic tests (*e.g.,* Widal titers for salmonella, ASLO titers for streptococcal infections and acute rheumatic fever, the heterophil for infectious mononucleosis) and skin tests (especially the tuberculin test) can provide confirmatory evidence and need to be considered when clinical findings are suggestive. Testing for antinuclear antibody and rheumatoid factor may help in the diagnosis of a suspected vasculitis or rheumatoid disease. The presence of rheumatoid factor or immune complexes (Raji cell assay) can be clues to "culture-negative" endocarditis or underlying connective tissue disease (see Chapter 144). In the diagnosis of obscure fevers, it is often useful to freeze and save an "acute phase serum" for later comparison with a "convalescent serum."

The Undiagnosed Febrile Patient

Although an enormous number of studies are available for the evaluation of undiagnosed febrile illnesses, it is important to proceed with these in a logical, step-by-step fashion instead of subjecting the patient to a random series of expensive, time-consuming, uncomfortable, or even hazardous studies. The first step in the subsequent workup is to *document fever* by measuring rectal temperatures every 4 hours. If fever is documented, further testing should be directed to the most common causes of fever of unknown origin, as listed in Table 6-1. Obviously, the order of testing should be determined by clues present in the individual patient, beginning with the simplest, least expensive studies.

Radiographic and invasive studies may be revealing, but require careful selection. At times a contrast study or radionuclide scan will reveal a source of fever. *Abdominal ultrasonography* and *computed tomography* are used to identify abscess, tumor, or retroperitoneal adenopathy (see Chapters 53 and 81). *Bone marrow* or *liver biopsy* may detect a cancer. A lumbar puncture is unlikely to help unless nuchal rigidity or neurologic abnormalities are present. A blind *laparotomy* is not performed unless there are clear-cut clues to intra-abdominal abnormalities that cannot be evaluated with less invasive procedures.

Therapeutic trials. In the acutely ill patient it may be necessary to begin broad antibiotic coverage before the diagnosis is established. It is essential, though commonly forgotten, to obtain cultures of blood, urine, and other pertinent fluids prior to initiating treatment so that rational decisions can be made later concerning therapy. In the patient with a true "FUO," blind therapeutic trials are rarely helpful and are often confusing or even harmful. In this context it is useful to remember one definition of empiric therapy: that which the ignorant do to the helpless. In occasional patients with fever of unknown origin, therapeutic trials may be necessary, including intravenous antibiotics for suspected culture-negative endocarditis, combined chemotherapy for occult tuberculosis, or salicylates or steroids for noninfectious inflammatory disease. Such trials should always be conducted with a specific end point or time limit in mind, carefully planned observations, patient consent, and a mixture of humility and trepidation.

The second look. Despite the array of sophisticated technology available for the study of febrile illnesses, the history and physical examination remain the keys to diagnosis in most cases. Time can be a most valuable diagnostic tool. Unless the patient is progressively deteriorating, it may be advisable to interrupt the workup for a period of clinical observation, possibly with the aid of symptomatic therapy such as antipyretics. A second look, beginning with the history and physical examination, may then be fruitful.

SYMPTOMATIC THERAPY

The best therapy is obviously to treat the underlying cause. However, antipyretic therapy may provide comfort and prevent complications. The first issue, of course, is to determine if fever should be treated. Elevated temperature itself does not necessarily call for therapy. But if unpleasant symptoms are present, if the patient has limited cardiac reserve, or if the complications of fever are imminent, antipyretics should be administered.

Antipyretic therapy depends on the use of both chemical agents and physical methods. The most effective antipyretic drugs are the *salicylates* and *acetaminophen;* both appear to act on the hypothalamus to lower the thermal set point. Although parenteral salicylates are available, oral or rectal administration of either aspirin or acetaminophen is preferable. Doses of up to 1.2 g of either drug may be given to adults to initiate antipyretic therapy. In addition to intrinsic toxicities, it must be remembered that both aspirin and acetaminophen occasionally produce an overresponse, with hypothermia and even dangerous hypotension. Patients with typhoid fever or Hodgkin's disease, and the elderly and debilitated seem to be at somewhat greater risk for this uncommon complication. Other drugs that may be considered in special circumstances are the *phenothiazines,* which also act directly on the hypothalamus. However, phenothiazine therapy of fever has a substantial toxic potential and must be considered experimental.

Physical cooling is also extremely effective. At the simplest level, undressing the patient and exposing him to a cool ambient temperature will allow cooling by radiation; a bedside fan will promote cooling by convection, as well. Sponging with cool water or alcohol is also helpful, promoting evaporation. With extreme elevations (greater than 106°F), more drastic measures are necessary and hospitalization is urgent. *Immersion in an ice water bath* is the most efficient of these methods and may be indicated in hyperthermic emergencies such as heat stroke. All methods of physical cooling present the risk of hypothermic overresponse and should, therefore, be discontinued when the body temperature begins to fall below critical levels.

Hyperthermic emergencies are rare, but fever is common and most often presents as an unpleasant symptom rather than a medical crisis. It seems appropriate, therefore, to conclude with a comment about patient comfort. Although fever causes discomfort in most patients, use of physical cooling produces discomfort in virtually all individuals; often the treatment is remembered as far worse than the illness itself. As a result, these measures should be employed only when fever itself presents medical problems. The same is true to a lesser extent of aspirin and acetaminophen. In particular, many patients find rapid rises and falls of temperature very distressing; therefore, administering antipyretics every 4 hours for the first day or two of treatment may be preferable to waiting for the height of the fever spike.

INDICATIONS FOR ADMISSION

When temperature reaches 105°F, hospitalization needs to be considered. The very toxic or vulnerable patient (see Table 6-2) should be admitted promptly for aggressive study, monitoring, and control of temperature. With weight loss and debilitation, early hospitalization should also be considered. Moreover, when fever remains elevated beyond 101°F for weeks and ambulatory diagnostic efforts have been unsuccessful, it is often beneficial to bring the patient into the hospital for closer evaluation and documentation of fever; the advice of an infectious disease consultant can be helpful.

PATIENT EDUCATION

Whenever fever is suspected in the ambulatory setting, the patient should be instructed to keep a record of temperatures, preferably rectal, taken each evening, when elevations are most likely to occur. The patient needs to be assured that there is nothing abnormal about temperatures in the range of 97.0°F to 99.3°F.

ANNOTATED BIBLIOGRAPHY

Dinarello CA, Wolff SM: Molecular basis of fever. Am J Med 72: 799, 1982 (*An excellent basic science review of the mechanism of fever.*)

Dinarello CA: Interleukin-1 and the pathogenesis of the acute phase response. N Engl J Med 311:1413, 1984 (*A provocative review of some biologic mediators of fever.*)

Jacoby GA, Swartz MN: Fever of undetermined origin. N Engl J Med 289:1407, 1973 (*A concise clinical update on the etiologic considerations that should be undertaken in the patient with FUO.*)

Kumar KL, Reuler JB: Drug fever. West J Med 144:753, 1986 (*Superb review of drug fever, indicating that it most commonly accompanies systemic and cutaneous manifestation of a drug reaction but may be the sole feature in 3% to 4% of drug reactions.*)

Larson EB, Featherstone HJ, Petersdorf RG: Fever of undetermined origin: Diagnosis and follow-up of 105 cases. Medicine (Baltimore) 61:269, 1982 (*Cancer is now the leading cause of such fevers.*)

Petersdorf RG, Beeson PB: Fever of unexplained origin: Report on 100 cases. Medicine 40:1, 1961 (*A classic paper that defines the etiologies of FUO and details a logical diagnostic approach.*)

Simon HB: Extreme pyrexia. JAMA 236:2419, 1976 (*A study of the etiologies and consequences of temperatures of 106°F and above.*)

Sox HC, Liang MH: The erythrocyte sedimentation rate. Ann Intern Med 104:515, 1986 (*A critical review of the test, arguing that it is not a useful screening procedure.*)

Young EJ, Fainstein V, Musher DM: Drug-induced fever. Rev Infect Dis 4:69, 1982 (*Antibiotics were responsible for most cases.*)

7
Evaluation of Weight Loss

Involuntary weight loss is a very sensitive, though non-specific, symptom; it often suggests the presence of serious pathology, yet a substantial fraction of patients turn out to be free of organic illness. For example, in a series of patients with involuntary weight loss followed for 1 year, 50% either died or deteriorated over the course of the study; however, another 35% were well at the time of follow-up. In many cases of weight loss, accompanying symptoms readily suggest the cause, but when a marked fall in weight is the sole or predominant complaint, the assessment can be difficult. The primary physician needs to determine at the time of initial presentation who requires an extensive medical evaluation and who can be followed expectantly.

PATHOPHYSIOLOGY AND CLINICAL PRESENTATION

When the number of calories available for utilization falls below daily needs, weight is lost; 1 lb of fat is consumed for every 3500-calorie deficit. The principal mechanisms resulting in caloric deficits are reduced food intake, malabsorption, excess nutrient loss, and increased caloric requirements. Loss of fluid will also register as a fall in weight, with about 1 kg (2.2 lb) lost for every liter removed.

Although more than one mechanism may be operating in a given case, each mechanism has a few characteristic clinical features. Anorexia or disinterest in food typifies causes of *reduced intake.* Foul-smelling, bulky, greasy stools are seen in the later stages of *malabsorption;* subtle changes in stool consistency and frequency are noted earlier (see Chapter 58). Recurrent vomiting, profuse diarrhea, polyuria, or fistulous drainage can lead to *excessive loss.* Increased food intake, hyperactivity, or fever are prominent in cases of *increased demand.*

Many conditions associated with weight loss are clinically obvious and require little discussion, but others may be subtle in presentation, with few obvious manifestations beyond a substantial fall in weight. Anorexia nervosa, carcinoma of the pancreas, early malabsorption, apathetic hyperthyroidism of the elderly, and diabetes are examples of illnesses that sometimes fall into the latter category and deserve further elaboration.

The patient suffering from *anorexia nervosa* may deny any disturbance of appetite, yet persist in restricting food intake to the point of cachexia. The condition occurs predominantly among adolescent girls and young women. They decide to diet to an extreme degree, are preoccupied with a phobic concern about being fat, and are motivated by a relentless pursuit of thinness. Dieting persists because its psychological gratifications outweigh those derived from the intake of food. Paradoxically, the patient often reports feeling well and initially appears bright and undisturbed by the weight loss; anorexia is usually denied. At times, a few specific foods are the only ones consumed, for example, vegetable juices. Amenorrhea is invariable and appears shortly after weight loss begins. A variant of anorexia nervosa consists of surreptitiously induced vomiting following engorgement with food; hypokalemic alkalosis results (see Chapter 230).

Carcinoma of the pancreas is the archetypal neoplasm associated with dramatic weight loss. Mean age of onset is 55; males outnumber females 2 to 1. There are about 9.5 cases per 100,000 population. Weight loss is found in 79% to 90% at time of diagnosis and averages 15 to 20 lb. The degree of weight loss does not seem to correlate with size, location, or extent of disease. For example, in a series of 100 cases, eight patients had resectable tumors; of the eight, two had weight losses of 25 and 40 lb, respectively. Aversion to food is more typical of this malignancy than is true anorexia. In many instances, weight loss precedes all other symptoms; once jaundice and abdominal pain supervene, the tumor is usually far advanced. Many other gastrointestinal malignancies follow a similar clinical course.

In addition to occult malignancy, a host of other conditions may present predominantly with weight loss due to an appetite disturbance; these are described elsewhere: depression (see Chapter 223), alcoholism (see Chapter 224), the prodrome of viral hepatitis (see Chapter 70), hypercalcemia (see Chapter 96), uremia (see Chapter 139), hypokalemia, and digitalis excess (see Chapter 27).

Marked weight loss is a late sign of *malabsorption,* but modest reductions can occur in the early stages of illness when stools are noted to be a bit softer and more frequent than usual. Steatorrhea, abdominal discomfort, bloating, and pain accompany more dramatic falls in weight when disease is farther advanced. Early *Crohn's disease* in adolescents has been noted on occasion to begin inconspicuously with anorexia predominating. For example, in a small series of 11 adolescent girls labeled as having anorexia nervosa, 3 were shown to have Crohn's disease when barium studies were obtained. *Blind loop syndrome* and *giardiasis* may also have indolent presentations with weight loss and vague abdominal

discomfort; however, changes in stools are usually present as well, with patients reporting mushy, foul-smelling bowel movements (see Chapter 58).

Increased caloric demand due to hyperthyroidism is usually obvious; however, *apathetic hyperthyroidism* of the elderly may be mistaken for malignancy because weight loss is profound and the patient appears listless. The typical symptoms of excess thyroid hormone are absent, and unexplained atrial fibrillation is often present (see Chapter 101).

Although diabetes mellitus is commonly found in overweight adults, it may be the cause of weight loss when there is substantial wasting of calories due to a poorly controlled glycosuria. Young male insulin-dependent diabetics are sometimes plagued by diarrhea, which exacerbates fluid and nutrient losses; true malabsorption has been noted in a few (see Chapter 100).

Patients with an underlying medical cause for their weight loss usually present with symptoms and signs that strongly suggest organic illness. In a Veterans Administration (VA) medical center study of 91 patients with involuntary weight loss, the overwhelming majority were readily diagnosed on the basis of initial history and physical examination; only one patient had a truly occult malignancy. Clinical attributes from that study suggestive of a relatively benign etiology included fewer than 20 pack-years of smoking, no decrease in activities due to fatigue, no nausea or vomiting, normal physical examination, no recent change in appetite, and no history of cough that had recently changed.

DIFFERENTIAL DIAGNOSIS

The extensive number of causes of weight loss can be grouped pathophysiologically. Decreased intake, impaired absorption, increased loss, and excess demand are the principal mechanisms around which the differential can be organized (Table 7-1). Almost any illness can cause involuntary weight loss; the table emphasizes those conditions seen in the ambulatory setting that may present as unexplained loss of weight. Data are scarce on the frequency of etiologies. The VA study of 91 patients with weight loss included both hospitalized and ambulatory patients; cancer was the most common cause (19%); gastrointestinal disease ranked second (14%); psychiatric and cardiac problems, third (9%); nutritional/alcoholic, fourth (8%); followed by pulmonary, endocrine, and infectious causes. After a full medical evaluation and a year of follow-up, 26% were listed as having no apparent physical cause.

WORKUP

Because the workup of weight loss can be arduous, it is helpful when possible to first identify those patients likely to have a medical etiology and spare the remainder a major medical evaluation. The VA group developed a decision rule

Table 7-1.   Some Important Causes of Weight Loss

1. Decreased intake
   a. Anorexia nervosa
   b. Depression
   c. Anxiety
   d. Poor dentition
   e. Esophageal disease
   f. Gastrointestinal disease worsened by food
   g. Drugs (*e.g.*, digitalis excess, amphetamines, antitumor agents)
   h. Hypercalcemia
   i. Alcoholism
   j. Prodrome of viral hepatitis
   k. Hypokalemia
   l. Uremia
   m. Malignancy
   n. Chronic congestive heart failure
   o. Chronic inflammatory disease
2. Impaired absorption
   a. Cholestasis
   b. Pancreatic insufficiency
   c. Postgastrectomy
   d. Small bowel disease
   e. Parasitic infection (e.g., giardiasis)
   f. Blind loop syndrome
   g. Drugs (*e.g.*, cholestyramine, cathartics)
3. Increased nutrient loss
   a. Uncontrolled diabetes mellitus
   b. Persistent diarrhea
   c. Recurrent vomiting
   d. Drainage from a fistulous tract
4. Excess demand
   a. Hyperthyroidism
   b. Fever
   c. Malignancy
   d. Emotional states (*e.g.*, manic disease)
   e. Amphetamine abuse

using the data available from the initial history and physical to help select those patients for whom further investigation is warranted.

In their study they found that out of 123 clinical attributes tested, 6 proved to be independent diagnostic predictors of a physical cause for weight loss. These predictors included nausea or vomiting, a cough that had recently changed, and an abnormal physical examination (cachexia, abdominal mass, adenopathy, thyromegaly, etc.). Patients who remained fully active and smoked less than 29 pack-years were unlikely to have a physical etiology. Screening laboratory studies were only weak predictors. A discriminant rule was developed using these predictors. Its error rate was 12%; it misclassified 9 of 32 patients who proved not to have physical etiology and 2 of 59 with a physical cause of weight loss. Thus, on the basis of an initial history and physical examination, a good estimation of the probability of a serious underlying etiology was made. Whether the findings of this study can be generalized is as yet unproven; the work was carried out on a VA medical center population that was almost exclusively male, and many were inpatients. Nevertheless, the study suggests

that patients with no evidence of a physical etiology by history and physical examination are likely to have a good prognosis and might be more profitably evaluated for a psychiatric cause or poor caloric intake, rather than be subjected to extensive diagnostic testing in search of an occult malignancy or other serious medical etiology.

History. The first task is to document that weight loss has indeed occurred and to determine its extent. In the VA report, almost half of the patients considered for study were not shown to have weight loss when available records were checked. In the absence of recorded weights, meaningful historical data include change in clothing size, ability to give exact weight change, and confirmation of history by a family member.

History can be used to help identify the mechanism(s) responsible for the decline in weight by obtaining the details of daily food intake (including a calorie count), and inquiring into the presence of any appetite disturbance, steatorrhea, diarrhea, vomiting, polyuria, or symptoms of a hypermetabolic state.

When decreased intake is suspected, one needs to check for somatic symptoms of depression (see Chapter 223), excessive use of alcohol (see Chapter 224), poor dentition, fever, dysphagia, discomfort induced by eating, drug use, history of renal disease, symptoms of heart failure, melena, abdominal pain, anxiety, and exposure to hepatitis. If the patient is a young woman, anorexia nervosa should be considered, and inquiry into eating habits, self-image, and attitudes about weight is worthwhile. Family members should be questioned as well.

When impairment of absorption is suspected, inquiries are made into previous gastrointestinal surgery, the character of the stools, jaundice, history of pancreatitis, travel to an area known for giardiasis or other parasites, symptoms of inflammatory bowel disease (see Chapter 65), easy bruising, paresthesias, and sore tongue. Increased nutrient loss is assessed historically by ascertaining the quality and quantity of material lost, as well as the frequency and duration of the condition. Of major importance is checking for symptoms of diabetes such as polyuria and diarrhea. When excess demand is under consideration, the patient needs to be questioned about fever, malignancy, symptoms of hyperthyroidism and apathetic hyperthyroidism, amphetamine and thyroxine use, chronic anxiety (see Chapter 222), and manic states.

Physical examination should begin with an accurate weight determination. One then needs to check for wasting, apathetic appearance, fever, tachycardia, pallor, ecchymoses, jaundice, stigmata of hyperthyroidism, glossitis, poor dentition, goiter, adenopathy, signs of congestive heart failure, organomegaly, hyperactive bowel sounds, ascites, and abdominal and rectal masses. Stool should be obtained for gross and microscopic observation and guaiac testing. Position and vibration sense are tested for evidence of subacute combined degeneration and peripheral neuropathy.

Laboratory testing must be selective to avoid being wasteful and burdensome, for the number of potential investigations is enormous. History and physical examination will usually identify the basic mechanism(s) of weight loss and suggest specific causes that can be confirmed or ruled out by further investigation. Patients with a perfectly normal physical examination and a history devoid of any symptoms suggestive of underlying medical illness can probably be watched, and need not be subjected on the initial visit to a large battery of tests.

DECREASED INTAKE. The serum calcium, potassium, SGOT, BUN, and creatinine are worth ordering when the precise etiology of decreased intake remains obscure. A serum drug level should be obtained for any patient taking a digitalis preparation.

IMPAIRED ABSORPTION. A *qualitative stool fat examination* is the first step in the workup of suspected malabsorption. A 72-hour stool collection for *quantitative stool fat* provides further evidence. An upper GI series, d-xylose test, and Schilling test are also useful in helping to characterize the problem (see Chapter 52).

Should the d-xylose test be normal, there is a good chance the problem is one of pancreatic insufficiency rather than small bowel disease. A serum *amylase* may reveal pancreatitis (see Chapter 72), but a *secretin stimulation* test should be ordered to best assess exocrine function. If x-ray reveals blind loops, a C^{14} *glycyl choline test* will help document bacterial overgrowth, though usually the test is unnecessary.

For diagnosis of *giardiasis,* a stool sample suffices in many instances. Because parasites are passed intermittently, three or more stools on alternate days should be examined. Because the cysts are hardy, a fresh stool specimen is not required. Trophozoites are more likely to be found in acute cases. Examination of a duodenal aspirate or jejunal biopsy is resorted to when suspicion is high but stools are negative. Although these tests are more productive, they are cumbersome; some clinicians instead advocate a diagnostic trial of an antigiardial drug such as metronidazole.

INCREASED NUTRIENT LOSS. Laboratory assessment should include testing for significant glycosuria.

EXCESS DEMAND. Suspicion of hyperthyroidism necessitates free T_4 and total T_3 determinations, especially in the elderly apathetic patient with unexplained atrial fibrillation and weight loss. Some data suggest that a TRH stimulation test is a more sensitive means of detecting apathetic hyperthyroidism (see Chapter 101).

One of the most difficult diagnostic issues encountered in workup of weight loss concerns the possibility of *occult malignancy.* Deciding when to embark on a search for tumor requires an estimate not only of the likelihood of finding a malignancy, but also of the chances that it will be treatable. Unfortunately, by the time weight loss has occurred, most gastrointestinal malignancies are rather far advanced. When weight loss is the only symptom, pancreatic carcinoma may still be resectable if no other symptoms have appeared. There is hope that abdominal ultrasonography and computerized axial tomography will improve case detection and early identification of resectable tumors (see Chapter 53).

SYMPTOMATIC THERAPY

Most causes of weight loss require correction of the etiology and cannot be readily treated symptomatically. However, there are important exceptions to this generalization. Sometimes the severe anorexia associated with malignancy or use of antitumor agents can be overcome by use of phenothiazines or even tetrahydrocannabinol (see Chapter 74). The poor intake seen with hepatitis can be improved by providing small, frequent feedings, especially in the morning when nausea is less severe (see Chapter 70). Appetite disturbances associated with depression are often amenable to tricyclic therapy (see Chapter 223). Maldigestion due to pancreatic insufficiency can be compensated for by use of oral pancreatic enzyme preparations (see Chapter 72). The bacterial overgrowth of blind loop syndrome responds to oral broad-spectrum antibiotic therapy such as tetracycline 250 mg four times daily for multiple 10-day courses or for 3 or 4 days each week indefinitely. Caloric supplements in the form of medium-chain triglyceride and dextrose preparations can provide marked improvement when there is severe fat and carbohydrate maldigestion or malabsorption. Initially, 3 ounces are given with each meal; gradually this is increased to 6 ounces, including supplements between meals.

Fat-soluble vitamin supplements are also needed in cases of malabsorption to prevent malnutrition, even though caloric intake may be replenished. The fat-soluble vitamins A, D, and K are the most likely to be depleted. Dosage requirements in such cases are 25,000 units to 50,000 units per day for vitamin A, 30,000 units for vitamin D, and 4 mg to 12 mg for oral vitamin K. Monthly B_{12} injections of 1000 μg are needed for terminal ileal disease presenting with megaloblastic anemia (see Chapter 84). Control of excessive vomiting and diarrhea is discussed in Chapters 54 and 58, respectively.

INDICATIONS FOR REFERRAL AND ADMISSION

Anyone with marked weight loss suspected of having anorexia nervosa should be hospitalized and seen by a psychiatrist experienced in dealing with anorectics. When malabsorption is documented by 72-hour stool fat assessment, consultation with a gastroenterologist should coincide with proceeding to further assessment.

A.H.G.

ANNOTATED BIBLIOGRAPHY

Gullick H: Carcinoma of the pancreas. Medicine 38:47, 1959 (*A review of 100 cases. Weight loss occurred in 85.7%. Of eight patients with resectable neoplasms, weight loss was a notable and early symptom in two. There was no correlation between weight loss and site of disease.*)

Ihse I, Isaksson G: Pancreatic carcinoma. Clin Gastroenterol 13:961, 1984 (*A good review of diagnosis.*)

Kamath KR, Murugasu R: A comparative study of four methods of detecting *Giardia*. Gastroenterology 66:16, 1974 (*Mucosal biopsy was most sensitive, followed by duodenal aspiration and stool examination.*)

Marton KI, Sox HC, Krupp JR: Involuntary weight loss: Diagnostic and prognostic significance. Ann Intern Med 95:568, 1981 (*A prospective study attempting to identify predictors of serious pathology and poor prognosis.*)

Ryan ME, Olsen WA: A diagnostic approach to malabsorption syndromes. Clin Gastroenterol 12:533, 1983 (*A pathophysiologic approach.*)

Schwabe AD, Lippe BM, Chang RJ et al: Anorexia nervosa. Ann Intern Med 94:371, 1981 (*A comprehensive review.*)

Theologides A: Weight loss in cancer patients. CA 27:205, 1977 (*A consideration of this common complication.*)

Thomas FB, Massaferri EL, Skillman TG: Apathetic thyrotoxicosis: A destinctive clinical and laboratory entity. Ann Intern Med 72:679, 1970 (*Classic article describing this syndrome, which is characterized by marked weight loss, apathy, and atrial fibrillation in the elderly.*)

3

Cardiovascular Problems

8
Screening for Hypertension
KATHARINE K. TREADWAY, M.D.

Hypertension can justifiably be considered the most significant condition the practitioner concerned with health maintenance will meet in clinical practice. The size of the affected population is staggering—20% of adults in the United States have systolic pressures greater than 160 mm Hg or diastolic pressures greater than 95 mm Hg, including more than one third of people over age 70. Excess morbidity and mortality caused by hypertension have been well documented. The benefits of treatment for many, if not all, hypertensives have been proven. Nevertheless, despite improvement in hypertension management in recent years, many who should be treated remain either unaware of their elevated blood pressure, not treated, or not controlled.

Evaluation and management of the identified hypertensive patient are presented in Chapters 13 and 21. This chapter briefly reviews the epidemiology of high blood pressure, its importance as a risk factor, and the evidence for the effectiveness of therapy.

EPIDEMIOLOGY AND RISK FACTORS

Most estimates of the prevalence of hypertension derive from the Public Health Service National Health Examination Survey conducted during the early 1960s. Subsequent smaller surveys have substantiated both its prevalence (approximately 20% among all adults) and the importance of age, race, and sex as epidemiologic correlates.

Age. The prevalence rate of systolic hypertension rises steadily with age; diastolic pressures rise less steeply after the fifth or sixth decade. It is not clear whether this increase is limited to a subset of the population with a tendency toward hypertension or, more likely, whether a rise in blood pressure is part of aging. The prevalence of hypertension (using the rather stringent definition of systolic greater than or equal to 160 mm Hg or diastolic greater than or equal to 95 mm Hg) among persons aged 25 to 34 is approximately 5%. By age 55 to 64, it has risen to 35% to 40%.

Sex. Males in all age groups have a higher incidence of hypertension. In the third and fourth decades, it is more than twice as common among men than among women. The ratio decreases with advancing age, but a significant male predominance persists.

Race. A marked increase in prevalence has been documented among black men and women in all age groups. The overall prevalence ratio is 2:1, but it is higher in younger age groups and lower in older ones. Hypertension is also more severe among blacks. The relative rate of diastolic pressure greater than 115 mm Hg is nearly five times higher for blacks than whites.

Other Factors. Hypertension is more likely if there is a positive family history. There is a positive association between obesity and hypertension that appears to be independent of technical problems associated with sphygmomanometer cuff size. Increased salt intake has been incriminated; while crude linear relationships between average salt intake and hypertension prevalence have been described in populations, an individual's prior or current salt intake is not a predictor of blood pressure level. The role of psychological stress and resulting sympathetic stimulation appears to be variable. Blood pressure levels have been correlated with subjective estimates of increased stress in population studies. Cigarette smoking, an important risk factor in its own right, is not positively associated with increased blood pressure, but hypertensive smokers are at significantly greater risk to develop cardiovascular complications than are hypertensive nonsmokers. These and other forms of hypertension, including that associated with renal disease, are discussed in Chapter 13.

HYPERTENSION AS A RISK FACTOR FOR CARDIOVASCULAR MORBIDITY AND MORTALITY

Hypertension is the principal risk factor in the development of coronary artery disease as well as other forms of atherosclerotic disease. In addition, hypertension is the major cause of congestive heart failure, stroke, and renal failure. The combined results of epidemiologic studies indicate that middle-aged males with diastolic blood pressures of 95 to 104 mm Hg have a twofold increase in mortality due to coronary disease during a 10-year follow-up. If the diastolic level is 105 mm Hg or greater, the risk is threefold. Death rates from all causes were 60% and 200% greater in the respective hypertensive groups than among normotensive men. A 60% increase was also evident among men with diastolic blood pressures of 85 to 94 mm Hg compared with men with lower pressures.

Epidemiologic studies have clearly demonstrated the additive effects of multiple risk factors, namely, hypercholesterolemia, smoking, and diabetes, in predicting coronary artery disease.

Systolic hypertension has been shown to be the most powerful predictor of nonhemorrhagic and hemorrhagic stroke in males and females. Hypertensives have a fourfold risk of brain infarction compared with normotensives. The Framingham study has also shown hypertension to be the dominant predictor of congestive heart failure, with a sixfold increase in incidence among hypertensives.

NATURAL HISTORY OF HYPERTENSION AND EFFECTIVENESS OF THERAPY

With rare exceptions, hypertension is an asymptomatic disease. The natural history is one of insidious damage that is most often clinically silent for a decade or more. Consequently, it is a more ominous finding, and, in particular, a potent predictor of coronary disease, in younger age groups.

Arguments for the vigorous early treatment of moderately and severely elevated blood pressure rest on the convincing results of the Veterans Administration Cooperative Study. The data are summarized in Table 8-1. Among those treated, the rate of major nonfatal events and of cardiovascular death was reduced more than tenfold among severely hypertensive men and threefold among moderately hypertensive men. Treatment was most effective in reducing risks of stroke and congestive heart failure. There was no significant reduction in coronary events among patients with lowered levels of hypertension. A reduction in subsequent coronary events and death in patients with known coronary disease has been reported, but the available data are fragmentary. Middle-aged hypertensive men treated in a Swedish primary prevention trial have had lower incidences of fatal and nonfatal coronary events than their untreated counterparts.

Table 8-1. Results of Veterans Administration Cooperative Study

	DIASTOLIC 115–129 MM/Hg*		DIASTOLIC 90–114 MM/Hg†	
	Control (N = 70)	*Treated (N = 73)*	*Control (N = 194)*	*Treated (N = 186)*
Death	4	0	19	8
Other morbid events	23	2	57	14

* Veterans Administration Cooperative Study Group on Antihypertensive Agents, JAMA 202:1028, 1967 *(Average follow-up 18 months.)*
† ——, JAMA, 213:1143, 1970 *(Average follow-up 40 months.)*

The effectiveness of treating mild hypertension (diastolic blood pressure of 90 to 104 mm Hg) in patients without evidence of end-organ damage remains an area of controversy. Despite several recent studies designed to assess the benefit of therapy in this group, the results remain inconclusive. The Australian Therapeutic Trial in Mild Hypertension demonstrated lower cardiovascular morbidity and mortality among mild hypertensives (diastolic blood pressure 95 to 110 mm Hg) in the treated group than in the untreated group. However, most of the benefit was evident among those over 50 years of age and those whose diastolic blood pressure was greater than 100 mm Hg. Of particular interest is that during the 5 years of observation, almost half of the untreated group became spontaneously normotensive. Furthermore, the reduction in risk conferred by pharmacologic reduction of blood pressure was not as great as that associated with spontaneous normotension.

The Hypertension Detection and Follow-Up Program compared the treatment of hypertension by community physicians with that of special centers designed to provide aggressive, stepped care. Although overall cardiovascular mortality in the mildly hypertensive group was reduced by 26% after 5 years, the study failed to show benefit in those under age 50 or in white women. While this and other studies have not yet demonstrated a reduction in mortality in patients under 50, they have demonstrated that treatment achieves a reduction in hypertensive complications such as congestive heart failure and stroke.

It is clear that blood pressure levels alone cannot be the deciding factor in determining when hypertension should be treated. Age, race, sex, and the presence of other cardiovascular risk factors, as well as a family history of hypertensive complications, must all be considered when deciding whether or not to initiate pharmacologic treatment of hypertension. Particularly in the young patient with uncomplicated mild hypertension, the presumed benefits must be carefully weighed against the cost, inconvenience, and largely unknown risks of prolonged antihypertensive therapy.

SCREENING METHODS

The process of identifying patients with high blood pressure in the primary care setting is straightforward. Blood pressure determination should be a routine component of patient evaluation regardless of the presenting complaint. Reliable equipment is important. Aneroid manometers, if used, should be checked regularly. All personnel responsible for recording blood pressures should be aware of sources of measurement error, such as inappropriate cuff size.

Blood pressure is properly measured in both arms while the patient is seated comfortably. The cuff should be placed at heart level and as high as possible on the arm. The average of two successive measurements in each arm is recorded. Diastolic pressure is taken at the point at which sound disappears (Korotkoff 5) rather than when it changes in quality (Korotkoff 4). Cuff size must be adequate to avoid falsely elevated readings (cuff width greater than two-thirds the arm width, length of inflatable portion greater than two-thirds the arm circumference).

Using a standard size cuff in a muscular or obese adult will result in a reading that is as much as 10 mm Hg higher than the true blood pressure. To avoid this error, a large adult size cuff should be used in such patients.

Variability of blood pressure may be related to recent physical activity, emotional state, or body position. Although such factors must be kept in mind, the predictive value of the "casual" blood pressure determination has been validated. Nevertheless, the diagnosis of hypertension must never be made on the basis of a single reading, but rather should be based on multiple determinations.

CONCLUSIONS AND RECOMMENDATIONS

Hypertension is an extraordinarily common condition and the strongest predictor of subsequent cardiovascular and cerebrovascular morbidity and mortality. It is essentially asymptomatic, and end-organ damage is insidious. Benefits of antihypertensive therapy for a large segment of the population have been conclusively proven. The detection and appropriate management of hypertension is one of the foremost responsibilities of the practitioner. Specific recommendations regarding the evaluation and selection of patients for treatment are discussed in Chapters 13 and 21.

ANNOTATED BIBLIOGRAPHY

Berglund G, Sannerstedt R, Andersson O et al.: Coronary heart disease after treatment of hypertension. Lancet 1:1, 1978 (*Middle-aged hypertensive men treated with hypotensive drugs [usually starting with propranolol] had significantly lower incidences of fatal and nonfatal coronary events than untreated men. Data from the Goteborg primary prevention trial; controls were not randomized.*)

Burch GE, Shewey L: Sphygmomanometric cuff size and blood pressure recordings. JAMA 225:1215, 1973 (*Use of wrong size cuff can lead to erroneous reading.*)

Freis ED: Should mild hypertension be treated? N Engl J Med 307: 306, 1982 (*Reviews the evidence and recommends treatment for patients with borderline or mild hypertension and other risk factors, but withholding drug therapy from those without other risk factors.*)

Hypertension Detection Follow-Up Program Cooperative Group: The effect of treatment on mortality in "mild" hypertension. N Engl J Med 307:976, 1982 (*Twenty percent lower 5-year mortality was found in patients with diastolic blood pressures between 90 and 104 mm Hg who were treated intensively with stepped care compared with similar patients who were simply referred to their usual source of care for treatment.*)

Kannel WB, Wolf PA, McGee DL: Systolic blood pressure, arterial rigidity, and risk of stroke. JAMA 245:1225, 1981 (*Subjects with isolated systolic hypertension experienced two to four times as many strokes as did normotensive persons in the Framingham study.*)

Maxwell MH et al: Error in blood pressure measurement due to incorrect cuff size in obese patients. Lancet 2:8288, 1982 (*The standard adult size cuff results in readings of about 10 mm Hg in excess of the true pressure in obese patients. A large cuff is needed.*)

Paul O: Risks of mild hypertension: A ten-year report. Br Heart J 33:116, 1971. (*Reviews the data of six prospective studies in the United States. The increased risk of morbid and mortal cerebrovascular and cardiovascular events for men with diastolic pressures of 85 mm Hg to 90 mm Hg is evident.*)

Pickering TG, Harshfield GA, Kleinert HD et al.: Blood pressure during normal daily activities, sleep, and exercise. JAMA 247: 992, 1982. (*Average 24-hour pressures can be well predicted by measurements made in the physician's office in normal and hypertensive subjects but not in borderline hypertensives.*)

Veterans Administration Cooperative Study Group on Antihypertensive Agents: Effects of treatment on morbidity in hypertension. Results in patients with diastolic blood pressures averaging 115 through 129 mm. Hg. JAMA 202:1028, 1967

Veterans Administration Cooperative Study Group on Antihypertensive Agents: Effects of treatment on morbidity in hypertension II. Results in patients with diastolic blood pressure averaging 90 through 114 mm Hg. JAMA 213:1143, 1970

Veterans Administration Cooperative Study Group on Antihypertensive Agents: Effects of treatment on morbidity in hypertension III. Influence of age, diastolic pressure, and prior cardiovascular disease. Further analysis of side effects. Circulation 45:901, 1972 (*The studies described in these papers are the basis for the current approach to antihypertensive therapy. They are required reading for the primary care provider.*)

Weiss NS: Relation of high blood pressure to headache, epistaxis, and selected other symptoms. The United States Health Examination Survey of Adults. N Engl J Med 287:631, 1972 (*No clear relationship was shown between these symptoms and the level of blood pressure. They may be better indicators of retinopathy in both normotensive and hypertensive patients.*)

9
Screening for Hyperlipidemia
WAYNE L. PETERS, M.D.

Elevated serum levels of cholesterol and triglycerides are exceedingly common. Hyperlipidemia may be a manifestation of an underlying illness, but more often it reflects both genetic and dietary determinants. It is of significance because cholesterol is a major risk factor for atherosclerosis.

The total blood cholesterol is the sum of the cholesterol concentrations from the three major circulating lipoproteins—low-density lipoproteins (LDL), high-density lipoproteins (HDL), and very low-density lipoproteins (VLDL).

Total cholesterol = LDL cholesterol + HDL cholesterol + VLDL cholesterol. (Most laboratories use the fasting triglycerides divided by 5 to approximate VLDL cholesterol.)

In deciding whether and how to screen for hyperlipidemia, the primary physician must consider several questions: Which lipid elevations increase coronary risk? How practical is their detection? How effectively can these levels be lowered by diet and drugs? Will lowering these levels reduce the risk of a coronary event?

EPIDEMIOLOGY AND RISK FACTORS

Prevalence estimates of hyperlipidemia are based on rather arbitrary definitions of serum lipid elevations. More than 5% of American adults have total cholesterol levels greater than 275 mg/dl, and/or fasting triglyceride levels greater than 250 mg/dl. Although such levels may be considered upper limits of "normal" in the statistical sense, they should not be considered healthy. Coronary risk has been shown to increase curvilinearly with increasing total cholesterol levels, even within the American "normal" range. The two thirds of American adult males with total cholesterol levels greater than 200 mg/dl have an increased probability of developing heart disease, chiefly from the atherogenic LDL cholesterol component. Conversely, HDL cholesterol (especially the HDL_2 subfraction) is inversely and independently related to coronary risk, with its protective effect at least as strong as the atherogenic effect of LDL.

A review of the many factors that influence blood lipid levels (particularly serum cholesterol) provides a basis for identifying patients likely to benefit from lipid screening.

Genetic Factors. The genetic influence on serum lipid levels is important but has been clearly defined for only a fraction of patients with hyperlipidemia. Primary disorders inherited by means of a monogenic mechanism account for only a small fraction of patients with hyperlipidemia. Nevertheless, these disorders are among the most common of the inherited errors of metabolism. Polygenic inheritance is far more common. Polygenic hypercholesterolemia affects 5% of the general population.

Age. Cholesterol and triglyceride levels increase with age; total cholesterol increases, on the average, more than 2 mg/dl per year during early adulthood.

Sex. Men have higher total cholesterol levels than women until age 50. Women carry a higher proportion of cholesterol in the form of HDL (primarily the HDL_2 subfraction).

Diet. A diet high in *saturated fatty acids* raises total and LDL cholesterol levels, whereas *polyunsaturated fatty acids* lower them. Total and LDL cholesterol are also increased by *dietary cholesterol,* but the effect is smaller than that of saturated fatty acids. *Caloric excess* resulting in obesity is the most important dietary determinant of triglyceride levels. *Alcohol* has little effect on total cholesterol levels, but it can cause an acute rise in triglyceride level among people with hypertriglyeridemia. Moderate alcohol ingestion also causes a rise in HDL levels, but probably not in the "protective" HDL_2 subfraction.

Other Factors. Epidemiologic data suggest that regular aerobic physical *exercise* increases HDL cholesterol and HDL_2 mass level. Exogenous *estrogens* increase HDL_2 mass and can cause extreme increases in triglyceride levels among patients with hypertriglyceridemia. An independent relationship between *obesity* and low HDL cholesterol levels appears likely. Cross-sectional population studies have demonstrated a reduction in HDL cholesterol in *cigarette* smokers that is dose-dependent and independent of age, obesity, alcohol, hormone use, and exercise.

HYPERLIPIDEMIA AS A RISK FACTOR
FOR CORONARY HEART DISEASE

A number of large prospective studies, including those from Framingham and the Pooling Project (a study in which data from several American epidemiologic studies were pooled), have demonstrated the *total serum cholesterol* level to be a strongly positive, independent predictor of coronary heart disease risk below the age of 50. Over the usual range of total cholesterol values that many laboratories designate as "normal" (180 to 300 mg/dl), risk increases an average of fourfold to fivefold (Table 9-1). The addition of other coro-

Table 9-1. Probability of Developing Coronary Heart Disease in 6 Years Based on Age and Cholesterol Level in the Absence of Other Risk Factors (Expressed as Number of Cases per 100 Male Patients)

CHOLESTEROL LEVEL	AGE						
	35	40	45	50	55	60	65
185	0.4	0.9	1.8	3.0	4.5	5.7	6.4
210	0.5	1.2	2.2	3.6	5.1	6.2	6.6
235	0.8	1.6	2.9	4.4	5.8	6.8	6.9
260	1.1	2.2	3.6	5.3	6.7	7.4	7.1
285	1.6	2.9	4.6	6.4	7.6	8.0	7.4
310	2.2	3.8	5.8	7.6	8.7	8.7	7.6
335	3.1	5.1	7.3	9.1	9.9	9.5	7.9

(Based on data from the Framingham study as cited in Figure 9-1.)

nary heart disease risk factors such as glucose intolerance, smoking, and hypertension can markedly enhance this independent cholesterol-related risk (see Fig. 9-1). The positive relationship between total cholesterol and risk of coronary heart disease derives mainly from the *LDL cholesterol* component. Because LDL cholesterol accounts for about two thirds of the total cholesterol in the typical patient, the total cholesterol level is generally used as a proxy for LDL.

The ability to predict disease using the total cholesterol level can be enhanced by the addition of an *HDL cholesterol* determination. For every 10-mg/dl increment in HDL, there is a 50% decrease in coronary risk. Very high HDL levels (60 to 100 mg/dl) in vigorous, healthy patients may account for moderate elevations in total cholesterol (220 to 280 mg/dl), increases that do not represent enhanced risk of heart disease. The determination of a total cholesterol/HDL ratio helps to distinguish such low-risk individuals from others with elevated total cholesterol.

The Framingham study demonstrated that the *total cholesterol/HDL ratio* most efficiently predicts patients who are at increased risk. A ratio of 5 approximates the average or standard risk, with ratios of 10 and 20, respectively, denoting double and triple the risk. A ratio of 3.5 or less is considered optimal.

No American prospective study has found an independent contribution of *triglyceride level* to coronary risk, when other risk factors such as total cholesterol, HDL cholesterol, blood pressure, smoking, glucose intolerance, weight, ECG abnormalities, and personality are corrected for. Although hypertriglyceridemia is found in some cases of accelerated atherogenesis, its contribution to coronary risk remains to be proven. Moreover, premature cardiovascular disease is absent in some patients with familial hypertriglyceridemia or with chylomicronemia. Triglyceride levels above 500 mg/dl are associated with acute pancreatitis.

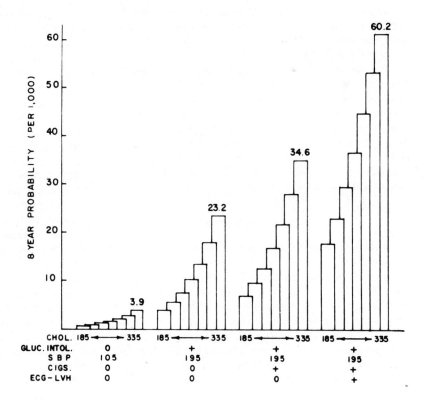

Figure 9-1. Risk of cardiovascular disease according to serum cholesterol at specified levels of other risk factors. ECG-LVH = electrocardiographic evidence of left ventricular hypertrophy; SBP = systolic blood pressure. [From the Framingham study, 18-year follow-up (Monograph No 28); 35-year-old men. Reprinted with permission of the Framingham study. Also in Ann Intern Med 90:86, 1971.]

EFFECTIVENESS OF TREATMENT

The validity of screening for hyperlipidemia depends, in part, on the ability of diet and drug therapy to lower lipid levels and the attendant cardiovascular morbidity. Decreased intake of cholesterol and saturated fat in a controlled setting results in serum cholesterol reductions of up to 30%. In more relevant studies of "free-living" patients, the reductions ranged from 6% to 15% and from 12% to 45% when drug therapy was added. Caloric and fat restrictions are usually effective in lowering triglyceride levels; prohibition of alcoholic beverages can enhance the dietary effects.

Diet and drug intervention trials have recently demonstrated a reduction in coronary morbidity and mortality with reduction of elevated total and LDL cholesterol levels. The Lipid Research Clinics' Coronary Primary Prevention Trial studied 3806 asymptomatic middle-aged men with primary hypercholesterolemia (type II hyperlipoproteinemia) for an average of 7.5 years, randomized in a double-blind fashion to either a treatment group receiving the bile acid sequestrant *cholestyramine resin,* or a control group receiving an indistinguishable placebo. All patients were asked to adhere to a cholesterol-lowering diet. The cholestyramine group experienced reductions in average total and LDL cholesterol that were 8.5% and 12.6% greater, respectively, than those obtained in the placebo group. The cholestyramine group experienced a 19% reduction in definite coronary heart disease death and/or definite nonfatal myocardial infarction, and significant ($p < 0.05$) reductions in the incidence of development of angina pectoris and new positive exercise test results. For each 1% reduction in total cholesterol, there was an approximate 2% decrease in risk.

The National Heart, Lung, and Blood Institute Type II Coronary Intervention Study examined the effects on the progression of coronary arteriosclerosis of therapy with cholestyramine versus those of a placebo for 5 years in 116 patients with angiographically documented coronary heart disease. This randomized double-blind study suggested that total and LDL cholesterol reductions retard the rate of progression of atherosclerosis. It follows that primary prevention, if undertaken, should be initiated early.

SCREENING METHODS

A random *total serum cholesterol level* is the most convenient screening test for the general population. Fasting is unnecessary because cholesterol is not acutely affected by diet. The initial search for hypercholesterolemia ideally should be done at or before the age of 20 years. Following an acute myocardial infarction (or other similar stress), total cholesterol levels will gradually fall by as much as 20%, but at the time of hospitalization the level may not be substantially different from baseline. A significant drop in total cholesterol and triglyceride levels has been demonstrated when a patient assumes a recumbent position; this occurs within 5 minutes and reaches a maximum of 10% to 12% within 20 to 30 minutes. Many automated *serum* cholesterol determinations give values 5% to 10% higher than the standard Abell–Kendall technique for *plasma* cholesterol used in Framingham and other studies because of the dilutional effect of cellular water in the plasma method.

If the initial total cholesterol in adults is above an optimal upper range of 180 to 200 mg/dl, a second confirmatory determination should be obtained. *Triglyceride determinations* are not recommended for screening purposes. Not long ago, *lipoprotein electrophoresis* was touted as a necessary test for the evaluation and treatment of hyperlipidemia. It has since been recognized that electrophoresis rarely contributes to clinical decision making (see Chapter 22).

At present, it is too early to recommend *HDL cholesterol* determinations for screening purposes, as test precision is inadequate in the majority of laboratories, especially in the range of 20 to 40 mg/dl, which is the high-risk zone for HDL cholesterol. If a laboratory with excellent quality control and an appropriate measurement technique for HDL is available, the ratio of total cholesterol/HDL cholesterol is more accurately predictive of risk than either measurement alone.

CONCLUSIONS AND RECOMMENDATIONS

- Epidemiologic studies have demonstrated that elevated total cholesterol (>200 mg/dl) and elevated LDL cholesterol (>125 mg/dl) levels are positive independent risk factors for the development of coronary heart disease in persons under the age of 65. The presence of other coronary heart disease risk factors dramatically accelerates this risk. Both genetic and dietary factors influence total and LDL cholesterol levels.
- Diet and drug therapy effectively reduce the total cholesterol and the atherogenic LDL cholesterol levels.
- Decreased coronary heart disease morbidity and mortality following the reduction of total and LDL cholesterol have been unequivocally demonstrated.
- HDL cholesterol is an independent negative predictor for the risk of developing coronary heart disease. One's ability to predict risk at any age, but especially over the age of 50, is enhanced by use of the total cholesterol/HDL ratio. A ratio of less than 3.5 is considered optimal.
- Regular aerobic physical exercise, weight loss in obese patients, and cessation of cigarette smoking elevate HDL cholesterol levels.
- Although hypertriglyceridemia is associated clinically with accelerated atherogenesis, its contribution to coronary risk has not been shown in epidemiologic study to be independent of total cholesterol level and other risk factors.
- A random total blood cholesterol measurement is recommended for all adults. Because of greater prognostic significance and increased likelihood of benefit from early in-

tervention, screening should be performed during early adulthood when possible. This is particularly important when there is a family history of hypercholesterolemia or premature coronary heart disease. If the level is greater than 200 mg/dl, then a repeat determination is indicated. If normal, a repeat check is recommended at least every 3 to 5 years.

- A fasting triglyceride level does not qualify as a useful screening test; however, it is useful in evaluating hypercholesterolemia (see Chapter 22).
- HDL cholesterol determinations are not currently recommended for screening purposes. Although an independent predictor of coronary risk, commercially available assays are too unreliable at the present time.

ANNOTATED BIBLIOGRAPHY

Brensike JF, Levy RI, Kelsey SF et al: Effects of therapy with cholestyramine on progression of coronary arteriosclerosis: Results of the NHLBI Type II Coronary Intervention Study. Circulation 69:313, 1984 (*Cholestyramine treatment retards the progression of coronary heart disease as assessed by angiography in patients with Type II hyperlipoproteinemia* [*primary hypercholesterolemia*].)

Grundy SM, Bilheimer D, Blackburn H et al: Rationale of the diet-heart statement of the American Heart Association: Report of the nutrition committee. Circulation 65:839A, 1982 (*A detailed review of the evidence for a diet–coronary heart disease relationship and the rationale for the American Heart Association dietary recommendations. An extensive and useful bibliography complements this article.*)

Kannel WB: High-density lipoproteins: Epidemiologic profile and risks of coronary artery disease. Am J Cardiol 52:9B, 1983 (*Specifically profiles the contribution of the individual values and ratios of total cholesterol, HDL cholesterol, and LDL cholesterol toward predicting cardiovascular risk.*)

Kannel WB, Castelli WP, Gordon T: Cholesterol in the prediction of atherosclerotic disease. Ann Intern Med 90:85, 1979 (*Reviews the associations between total cholesterol, LDL cholesterol, and HDL cholesterol and coronary risk.*)

Krauss RM: Regulation of high density lipoprotein levels. Med Clin North Am 66:403, 1982 (*Reviews the current concepts of the structure, metabolism, and factors influencing the levels of HDL in humans.*)

Lipid Research Clinics Program: The Lipid Research Clinics Coronary Primary Prevention Trial. JAMA 251:351, 1984 (*A significant reduction was observed in the incidence of coronary heart disease by lowering the total cholesterol and LDL cholesterol in asymptomatic middle-aged men with primary hypercholesterolemia.*)

Peters WL, Goroll AH: The evaluation of hypercholesterolemia in primary care practice. J Gen Intern Med 1:183, 1986 (*A comprehensive review; 74 references.*)

Pooling Project Research Group: Relationship of blood pressure, serum cholesterol, smoking, relative weight and ECG abnormalities to incidence of major coronary events. J Chronic Dis 31:201, 1978 (*A concerted epidemiologic evaluation of cardiac risk factors.*)

10

Exercise and Cardiovascular Disease

HARVEY B. SIMON, M.D.
STEVEN R. LEVISOHN, M.D.

In the past decade, exercise has become an American growth industry. An estimated 20 million to 40 million Americans jog regularly, making it the most popular participant sport. In addition, other active sports such as tennis and racquetball, cross-country skiing, and biking have grown in popularity. Unlike other recreational activities, these sports attract participants not only for their intrinsic pleasures but because they are widely believed to be beneficial to health. In the case of jogging, the public has been exposed to conflicting claims ranging from the hypothesis that marathon running helps prevent myocardial infarctions to warnings that long distance running is a health hazard. Because of these controversies, the primary care physician is increasingly called on to advise his patients about the effects of exercise on health and to prescribe an effective and safe exercise program.

PHYSIOLOGY AND CLINICAL IMPLICATIONS OF EXERCISE

Physical work may involve either aerobic or anaerobic metabolism, and may rely on either isotonic or isometric muscular activity. The concept of aerobic exercise provides the foundation for endurance training. The total amount of stored energy available to muscle groups in the form of preformed ATP and phosphocreatine is sufficient to sustain less than 10 seconds of maximal exertion. Clearly, energy must be generated continuously during exercise, and the majority of this energy comes from the metabolism of muscle glycogen. The availability of oxygen determines whether this metabolism will be aerobic or anaerobic. When oxygen supply is adequate, metabolism is aerobic and glycogen is completely metabolized to pyruvate and then to water and CO_2 through the Krebs cycle. With increasing exercise, the ability of the lungs to take up oxygen and of the heart and blood vessels to deliver it to muscle cells is exceeded, and metabolism becomes anaerobic. The costs of anaerobic metabolism are substantial. Anaerobic metabolism is inefficient; it generates only one third as much energy from each gram of glycogen, and increases production of lactic acid, resulting in muscle cramps, fatigue, and dyspnea. Lactic acid is buffered by bicarbonate, resulting in increased CO_2 production and hyperventilation. Clinically, an abrupt rise in respiratory rate indicates that the anaerobic threshold has been crossed. Endurance training can be expected to increase the anaerobic threshold, thus allowing more work to be performed under favorable aerobic conditions.

The goal of training is to improve cardiopulmonary function and muscular efficiency. The type of exercise is critical. While maximal exertion or anaerobic training may be of some benefit to certain competitive athletes, the cornerstone of training for fitness is endurance or *aerobic exercise* using large muscle groups in continuous rhythmic activity for prolonged periods. Jogging and brisk walking are ideal for this. Other good training activities include biking, swimming, cross-country skiing, rowing, and rope jumping. These activities provide *isotonic exercise* whereby skeletal muscle fibers change in length with little change in tension. Heart rate and cardiac output increase but peripheral vascular resistance falls. In contrast, sports depending on very brief bursts of intense activity such as weight lifting provide *isometric exercise* in which muscle tension increases with little change in fiber length. Such exercise produces a marked increase in peripheral vascular resistance and blood pressure with little increase in cardiac output. Aerobic power does not increase with isometric exercising, and the hypertensive response can be hazardous to patients with cardiovascular disease. Because arm work has a greater tendency to produce tachycardia and hypertension than does an equivalent degree of leg work, it is particularly important to limit the resistance level in arm exercises for patients with hypertension or heart disease. Sports that allow prolonged periods of inactivity such as baseball or golf are poor for cardiopulmonary conditioning. Similarly, while activities providing sustained but gentle muscular effort such as yoga can be important parts of a fitness program because they are excellent for promoting flexibility and strength, they are poor tools for attaining cardiopulmonary fitness.

The effects of regular exercise can be classified in terms of cardiovascular, musculoskeletal, metabolic, and psychological functions. The most thoroughly documented results of aerobic exercise concern changes in *cardiopulmonary performance*. Exercise requires an increase in the body's oxygen consumption, which is made possible by increased oxygen uptake by pulmonary ventilation, increased oxygen delivery by the heart and the peripheral circulation, and increased oxygen extraction by muscle. Endurance training enhances

the efficiency of these processes by both central and peripheral mechanisms. At rest and at submaximal work loads, the fit individual has a slower heart rate than does the untrained person. Stroke volume is increased so that cardiac output for a given work load is unchanged. While the achievable maximum heart rate is not increased by training, the maximum cardiac output and maximum oxygen consumption are greatly enhanced, so that the well-trained individual can both attain higher work loads and sustain them for prolonged periods before becoming exhausted.

Although there is little firm evidence that exercise increases myocardial oxygen supply or produces collateral vascularization in humans, myocardial oxygen demands for a given work load decrease. This diminution in myocardial oxygen consumption is made possible by the lower heart rate and lower systolic blood pressure that accompany exercise in the fit individual. This can be of particular benefit to the patient with angina, since this "double product" of HR × BP determines the angina threshold (see discussion of postmyocardial infarction rehabilitation in Chapter 26). In addition, animal studies have demonstrated increased coronary artery cross-sectional area, increased myocardial capillary density, and myocardial hypertrophy in rats and dogs forced to exercise.

The *peripheral effects* of exercise are of great importance in endurance training. Capillary blood flow to muscle is increased. Muscle fibers increase in volume, and muscle strength and endurance are enhanced. Muscle mitochondria increase in size and number, and respiratory enzymes increase. As a result, muscle oxygen extraction is improved. Training also improves neuromuscular coordination and musculoskeletal efficiency.

Another important cardiovascular effect of exercise is on the *blood pressure*. Systolic pressure normally rises during exercise, but this rise tends to be slightly less in the fit individual. More important, total peripheral resistance falls as a result of improved muscle blood flow and decreased circulating catecholamine levels. The net result in trained individuals is lower blood pressure, both during exercise and at rest. Because this effect is actually more prominent in hypertensive subjects, endurance training can be an important nonpharmacologic adjunct for the control of mild to moderate hypertension. Only small numbers of hypertensive patients have been studied, and although preliminary results are encouraging, additional trials will be needed before exercise can be firmly recommended in the treatment of hypertension.

Less well-established cardiovascular benefits of exercise training include a possible diminution of arrhythmias, perhaps because of lower catecholamine levels. In addition, exercise increases fibrolytic activity and decreases platelet adhesiveness; these hematologic effects may, to some degree, protect against atherogenesis. In these areas, too, the data are preliminary.

The *metabolic benefits* of exercise are well documented. *Weight control* is an important motivating factor for many runners. An average jogger can be expected to consume about 600 calories in an hour of running. Other endurance activities have similar effects (Table 10-1). While exercise alone will produce only a slow reduction in total body weight, the per-centage of body fat falls more rapidly, resulting in visible increases in muscle tone. Perhaps most important, runners become motivated to adhere to dietary patterns that will permit sustained weight control.

Another metabolic effect of great interest is that of regular exercise on the blood lipids. In many runners, serum *triglyceride* levels fall dramatically without changes in the dietary intake of fats or carbohydrates. The total *cholesterol* level changes less predictably, but *high-density-lipoprotein* levels tend to rise in runners, and these higher levels appear to be statistically linked to a lower risk for coronary artery disease (see Chapter 9).

The *psychological effects* of regular exercise are receiving a great deal of attention. Most individuals who engage in regular exercise develop an improved self-image. This can be of great importance in the rehabilitation of patients with ischemic heart disease (see Chapter 26), and can also be used to help motivate healthy individuals to modify other risk factors by following a prudent diet and discontinuing smoking. The recreational aspects of exercise tend to lessen anxiety and depression. Running is being studied as a tool for the treatment of depression, and early results in small groups of patients are encouraging. Nevertheless, the so-called runner's high proves elusive or illusionary for many joggers. Although exercise has many psychological benefits, it is hardly a panacea. Patients can be encouraged to exercise for both psychological and physical gains, but they must have realistic expectations.

In sum, regular endurance-type exercise improves cardiopulmonary performance and tends to lower blood pressure, body weight and fat, and serum triglycerides while elevating serum high-density lipoproteins. Physical fitness may also assist in the psychological response to stress. Because of the amelioration in all these risk factors, it would seem reasonable to expect regular exercise to lessen morbidity and mortality from cardiovascular disease. Many epidemiologic investigators have explored the effects of exercise on longevity. In evaluating these studies, it must be remembered that attention to inactivity as a risk factor is relatively recent, with most work being done in the last decade. In addition, there are many intrinsic difficulties in population studies of this type. Perhaps the greatest problem is that of potential bias introduced by self-selection: if healthier people tend to exercise more, then improved mortality in active people may relate to underlying factors rather than to exercise *per se.* Additional difficulties include problems in quantifying exercise and small sample sizes. Finally, there are numerous confounding variables such as psychosocial factors, diet, alcohol consumption, smoking, genetic background, body build, lipid levels, and blood pressure.

In light of these many problems, it is not surprising that there is some divergence in the results of studies, as well as some controversy about the interpretation of the results. Nevertheless, the majority of investigations suggest that reg-

Table 10-1. Approximate Metabolic Expenditures Associated with Selected Activities*

AVERAGE ENERGY OUTPUT	ACTIVITY
1 met	Rest
1½–2 mets 2–2½ kcal/min	Desk work Standing Strolling (1 mile/h)
2–3 mets 2½–4 kcal/min	Level walking (2 miles/h) Level biking (5 miles/h) Golf (power cart)
3–4 mets 4–5 kcal/min	Walking (3 miles/h) Biking (6 miles/h) Badminton Housework
4–5 mets 5–6 kcal/min	Golf (carrying clubs) Dancing Tennis (doubles) Raking leaves Calisthenics
5–6 mets 6–7 kcal/min	Walking (4 miles/h) Cycling (10 miles/h) Skating Shoveling garden soil Average sexual activity
6–7 mets 7–8 kcal/min	Brisk walking (5 miles/h) Tennis (singles) Snow shoveling Downhill skiing Water skiing
7–8 mets 8–10 kcal/min	Jogging (5 miles/h) Biking (12 miles/h) Basketball Canoeing Mountain climbing Ditch digging Touch football
8–9 mets 10–11 kcal/min	Jogging (6 miles/h) Cross-country skiing Squash or handball (recreational)
Over 10 mets Over 11 kcal/min	Squash or handball (competitive) Running 6 miles/h: 10 mets 8 miles/h: 13½ mets 10 miles/h: 17 mets

* Energy outputs are expressed in mets. One met is the energy expended at rest, and equals 3.5 ml O_2/kg body weight/minute. (Calorie consumption values are for a 70-kg person.)

(Modified from Fox SM, Naughty JP, Gorman DA: Physical activity and cardiovascular health. III. The exercise prescription; frequency and type of activity. Mod Concepts Cardiovasc Dis 41:6, 1972)

ular physical activity does indeed have a favorable effect on morbidity and mortality from cardiovascular disease. Perhaps the best known studies in this country are those of Paffenbarger and his co-workers. In a 22-year cohort analysis of 3686 San Francisco longshoremen who underwent multiphasic screening, it was found that high energy output at work reduced the risk of fatal myocardial infarction, especially in younger subjects. As expected, smoking and hypertension were independently associated with cardiac mortality. It was estimated that if low energy output, smoking, and hypertension could have been eliminated, this population might have had an 88% reduction in fatal myocardial infarctions over the 22 years of the study. In a retrospective study of 16,936 male Harvard graduates, the risk of first myocardial infarction was found to be inversely related to energy expenditure. Sedentary men were at 64% higher risk than were classmates who expended an extra 2000 kcal or more per week. Peak exertion in the form of strenuous sports enhanced the effect of total energy expenditure. Interestingly, varsity sports participation in college had no protective effect unless athletic activity was continued into subsequent adult years, implying that self-selection based on initial fitness or genetic endowment is not sufficient to explain these results. In this study the protective effects of adult exercise were found to be independent of other risk factors.

While these studies concentrate on the role of exercise in the prevention of cardiovascular disease, attention is also being directed to the role of physical training in the treatment of patients with established atherosclerotic heart disease. Data from these trials are statistically inconclusive because of problems with sample size and patient compliance, and because of the relative newness of these studies. Nevertheless, studies in this field demonstrate subjective improvement in exercising patients and indicate a trend toward a decrease in coronary events (see Chapter 26 on postmyocardial infarction rehabilitation).

MEDICAL SCREENING OF POTENTIAL EXERCISERS

The physician can and should play a central role in promoting physical fitness. An important goal is to provide patient motivation through education: a clear understanding of the benefits and techniques of endurance training enhances compliance. Medical screening of the prospective participant and prescription of an appropriate exercise program are essential for the person who has been inactive.

The first step in medical screening is obtaining a detailed personal and family history. Of particular importance in the family history is the presence of coronary heart disease, peripheral vascular disease, hypertension, stroke, diabetes, or sudden death. Each patient should be carefully questioned about symptoms that suggest cardiovascular disease, including chest pain, palpitations, dyspnea, undue fatigue, syncope, and claudication. It is very important to review health habits in detail, with special attention to previous exercise patterns, smoking, diet, and the use of oral contraceptive agents.

A complete physical examination is also vital to the medical screening of the prospective exerciser. Height and weight should be recorded and ideal lean body weight estimated. The blood pressure should be taken at rest with the patient supine and standing, and the heart rate and blood pressure recorded after mild exercise (stair climbing or situps are satisfactory for this purpose). The chest is examined for rales, wheezes, and rhonchi and the heart for cardiomegaly, gallops, murmurs, and rhythm disturbances. The peripheral pulses and abdomen need to be palpated to exclude the presence of peripheral vascular diseases or an aortic aneurysm. The musculoskeletal system should be evaluated both to exclude significant pathology and to determine if specific flexibility or strengthening exercises are required as part of the training program.

Several laboratory studies are helpful in the screening process. Most patients ought to have a CBC, urinalysis, and determinations of blood sugar, creatinine, and cholesterol. For patients over the age of 35 who have been sedentary, a resting electrocardiogram should be performed to look for evidence of ischemia, left ventricular hypertrophy, and disturbances of rhythm or conduction. A baseline chest roentgenogram will provide information on heart size, pulmonary parenchyma, and vasculature.

If any of these screening procedures discloses evidence of overt cardiopulmonary disease, *exercise stress testing* is mandatory before an exercise program is initiated. Even if preliminary screening is negative, stress testing may be helpful for high-risk individuals, including those with positive family histories, hypertension, diabetes, or hyperlipidemia. Obesity, cigarette smoking, and a previously sedentary life-style are further indications for stress testing. Because atherosclerotic heart disease is so prevalent in our society, stress testing is probably a prudent precursor to vigorous exercise programs in all males above age 40 and in all females above age 50, even if they are asymptomatic and apparently healthy. Although analyses of exercise stress testing in asymptomatic populations have cast doubt on the ability of the test to help identify underlying coronary disease in patients free of angina (see Chapter 31), the test is useful for uncovering exercise-induced arrhythmias and hypotension, evaluating the individual's exercise capacity, and establishing the maximal and target heart rate for use in the exercise prescription (see Chapter 26).

In special cases, additional studies may be desirable, such as an FEV1, vital capacity, and arterial blood gases in patients with subjective dyspnea or suspected pulmonary disease. Specialized ergometric testing can determine maximal oxygen consumption, total work capacity, and other physiologic parameters. Another powerful tool is 24-hour ambulatory monitoring for arrhythmias using the Holter monitor (see Chapter 24). Finally, telemetry can enable constant monitoring of heart rate and rhythm during actual jogging.

Medical screening and exercise testing should allow the physician to assign each patient to one of three categories: (1) Individuals with normal studies can undertake exercise programs without medical supervision. Even in these healthy individuals, however, individualized exercise prescriptions and guidance regarding training techniques and safety precautions will be of great value. (2) Patients with ischemic heart disease, moderate hypertension, or moderate chronic obstructive lung disease will benefit from graded exercise programs, but it is best that they be referred to specialized exercise rehabilitation programs that provide medical supervision and facilities for emergency treatment. People taking digitalis, nitrates, or beta blocking agents should be included in this supervised exercise group. However, if structured rehabilitation programs are not accessible, milder forms of exercise such as walking or stationary bicycling can still be recommended with appropriate precautions. (3) Physical exertion is contraindicated in the presence of congestive heart failure, ventricular irritability, unstable angina, uncontrolled hypertension, unstable diabetes, or uncontrolled epilepsy, although patients with these conditions can sometimes be enrolled in supervised programs if they respond to medical therapy. Patients with AV block, sick sinus syndrome, left ventricular or aortic aneurysms, and aortic valve disease should be excluded from exercise programs.

THE EXERCISE PRESCRIPTION

A fitness program depends on three elements: *frequency, intensity,* and *duration* of exercise. It is well established that at least three exercise sessions per week are required to develop and maintain fitness, and five sessions per week probably provide maximum benefit. Hence, the exercise prescription should call for at least three workouts each week. Many individuals prefer a routine of daily activity; this is certainly an excellent regimen but, especially during the first few months of training, it is advisable to schedule easier and harder workouts on alternate days to prevent injuries and allow the muscles to recover.

The intensity and duration of training are intimately related. Equal degrees of fitness can be attained through less intense exercise sustained over a long period or through more vigorous effort for shorter periods. Maximum cardiopulmonary fitness can be attained by 15 to 60 minutes of continuous aerobic exercises, strenuous enough to raise the heart rate to 60% to 80% of maximum or the oxygen uptake to 50% to 85% of maximum.

Obviously these optimal fitness goals must be attained very slowly and gradually, and the physician's exercise prescription should provide a practical means of attaining them. Both the starting point and the rate of progression depend on the health, age, and fitness of the participant. As a rule of thumb, the beginner should plan to jog for a daily duration of 10 to 12 minutes at a pace sufficient to increase his heart rate to 60% to 80% of maximum without producing breathlessness.

Each running session should include a 5- to 10-minute *warmup period.* At the beginning of exercise, even the well-conditioned athlete experiences some degree of dyspnea due to anaerobic metabolism, because it takes 45 to 90 seconds for cardiac output to increase enough to meet the new work load, thus providing the "second wind." A warmup period will minimize this initial anaerobic period and also allow muscles to loosen and stretch out, which prevents many injuries. For the runner, the warmup period should consist of stretching exercise, calisthenics, and a gradual progression from walking to slow jogging to running.

The actual *training period* should initially consist of a total of 10 to 12 minutes of exercise. At first, it is best to alternate periods of effort with periods of recovery. This is easily accomplished by alternately walking and jogging. For example, an unfit or older individual might alternate 1 minute of jogging with 1 minute of walking, repeating this cycle 10 to 12 times during each training day. When this can be accomplished with comfort, perhaps at the end of 10 to 12 times during each training day. When this can be accomplished with comfort, perhaps at the end of 10 to 20 sessions over 2 to 3 weeks, the schedule can be changed to 2 minutes of jogging alternating with 2 minutes of walking, with 6 cycles in each session. When this is mastered, the jogging ritual can be extended to 3 or 4 minutes with only 1 or 2 minutes of rest for 3 or 4 cycles, and then to two 6-minute runs with 1 or 2 minutes of walking in between. By the end of 1 to 2 months, most individuals should expect to be able to jog for 10 to 20 minutes continuously, and to cover 1 to 2 miles during this period.

Obviously, the young and athletic individual will progress more rapidly than the older or unfit one; but it is important to urge restraint on even the athletic individual—one of the most common causes of orthopedic injuries is attempting too much too quickly. Once a base of 10 to 20 minutes of jogging is well established, further progress should be encouraged. It is reasonable to increase running time or distance by a rate of about 10% per week; this can be accomplished by extending one or two sessions while preserving some short-distance days, or by gradually extending each session. At the end of 4 to 6 months, 3 to 4 miles of jogging 3 to 5 days per week will provide maximal conditioning. However, this level of activity must be maintained to sustain the cardiopulmonary benefits of running. Feelings of accomplishment and well-being usually provide motivation for sustained participation, often at even higher levels.

In addition to the duration of running, it is important to consider the intensity or *pace* of the exercise. The most precise guide available is the heart rate. Patients should jog at a pace sufficient to raise the pulse to 60% to 80% of maximum. When exercise testing has been performed, an observed maximal heart rate can be used for this calculation. In the absence of these data, the maximal heart rate can be predicted for healthy individuals by subtracting the age from 220. As a rough guide, the target of 60% to 80% of this maximum translates to 130 to 150 beats/minute for younger persons and to 110 to 125 beats/minute for older ones. The patient can be taught to take his carotid or radial pulse just before and immediately after exercise, and to adjust his pace to attain and maintain the target heart rate. It can be very helpful to have the patient keep a daily record of these figures together with the time and approximate distance covered. As training progresses, a more rapid pace will be required to achieve the target heart rate.

Many people find it difficult or unpleasant to take their pulses. In such cases, intensity of effort can be roughly gauged by the "talking pace"—the individual should go fast enough to feel that he is working hard while still being able to talk to a companion without a sensation of dyspnea. For most people, this will translate to a 10- to 12-minute mile at first with progression to 7- to 9-minute miles when fitness is attained.

The final element of the exercise prescription is the *cooldown period*. Following each training session, a period of 5 to 10 minutes of walking and stretching exercises is desirable. Very hot or very cold showers should be avoided.

PATIENT EDUCATION

It is clear that long-term prospective studies of large population groups will be needed to establish firmly the role of exercise in the prevention and treatment of cardiovascular disease. But primary care physicians need not await the results of these studies before advising their patients to exercise. Although smoking (see Chapter 32), hypertension (see Chapter 8), and hypercholesterolemia (see Chapter 9) are probably the most important treatable risk factors, physical inactivity appears to rank next. While patients should be told that exercise has not been proven conclusively to reduce mortality, initial studies are encouraging. Moreover, most people who exercise regularly will feel better, look better, and have enhanced capacities for work and recreation. These factors alone provide sufficient justification for the physician to encourage endurance-type exercise.

However, exercise is not without potential adverse effects, and patients should be educated about these factors as well. There is no question that exercise can precipitate cardiac arrhythmias or myocardial ischemia in individuals with coronary artery disease. Sudden death is a tragic if infrequent complication of exercise. Careful medical screening of po-

tential exercisers, an individualized exercise prescription, and meticulous supervision of high-risk patients can minimize complications. Closely controlled conditioning programs have even enabled survivors of myocardial infarctions to engage safely in marathon running (see Chapter 26). Some runners encounter exercise-induced asthma, particularly during periods of cold weather. Advising use of a face mask that warms inspired air often suffices, but sometimes a mild bronchodilator (see Chapter 45) is necessary. Extreme environmental conditions may also produce thermal stress ranging from frostbite to heat stroke. Here, too, prevention is the best treatment; the physician should be able to advise the runner about appropriate fluid intake, clothing, acclimatization, and safe duration of exposure. Similar advice can prevent dehydration and electrolyte imbalance.

Musculoskeletal injuries are very common and result from overuse, inflexibility, and muscle imbalance (see Chapters 149 and 151). Overuse is prevented by advising gradual increases in exercise; inflexibility and imbalance are avoided by stretching and strengthening exercises (see below). Providing advice about running shoes and running surfaces can also help lessen risk of injury.

PRACTICAL ADVICE FOR THE BEGINNING RUNNER

Food and fluid intake. It is best to avoid running within 2 hours of a substantial meal. Despite many claims to the contrary, no specific dietary programs are required for running. The obese runner should restrict calories to reduce, while the lean individual may require increased caloric intake to maintain weight. Competitive runners feel that increased carbohydrate intake during the 3 days prior to a race helps increase endurance, and there is some experimental evidence suggesting that such "carbohydrate loading" does increase muscle glycogen content. Adequate fluid intake is essential, particularly in warm weather. Although thirst will dictate the need for fluid replacement, it is best to begin drinking small amounts before thirst becomes overt, so that large volumes will not be needed at any one time. Water is excellent, though some runners prefer balanced electrolyte solutions or even carbonated beverages.

Climate. Thermal stress presents a great threat to the runner. When confronted with an abrupt change in climate, the runner should sharply reduce distance and speed for several days until acclimatization is achieved. In warm, humid weather, jogging should be confined to early morning or evening hours or shady locations, distances and speed should be reduced, fluids should be taken at frequent intervals during the run, and clothing should be light colored and lightweight. Environmental temperatures between 50°F and 60°F are ideal for running in shorts and T-shirts. Between 40°F and 50°F, a warmup suit is generally sufficient; below 40°F, gloves or mittens and a hat are important. Multiple layers of thin flexible clothing are better than a single bulky garment.

Woolen fabrics are ideal but a soft cotton layer should be next to the skin. An extra layer of thermal underwear is vital for temperatures below 30°F, and if winds are strong or temperatures drop below 15°F, an additional layer such as a turtleneck, extra shorts, and possibly a ski mask are required. Again, distances should be reduced in bitter cold, and it is particularly important to avoid wet conditions, which can lead to frostbite, especially of the feet.

Air pollutants may cause irritation of the upper and lower respiratory tract and carbon monoxide can impair oxygenation and precipitate angina. One should avoid running on heavily traveled roads, during rush hours, and on days when temperature inversions increase air pollution.

Safety is of utmost importance. The runner should run facing the flow of cars. Sidewalks are preferred when possible. Although country roads are ideal, it is desirable to run with a companion in isolated areas in case of injury. Daytime running is safer both because the runner is more visible to cars and because he can see road hazards more easily. Bright-colored clothing should be encouraged, and at night reflectorized vests are mandatory. Dogs are best avoided by means of an impromptu detour, but if this is not possible they can generally be intimidated by a firm command to "go home" or by the threat of a stick or stone.

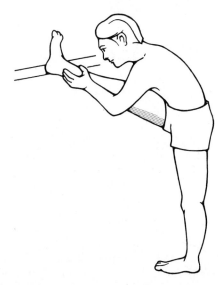

Figure 10-2. Hamstring stretch. Rest one leg on a sturdy table or desk. Keeping both legs straight, slowly bend forward at the waist so that you feel the hamstring stretch. Hold for 30 seconds Repeat with the other leg up.

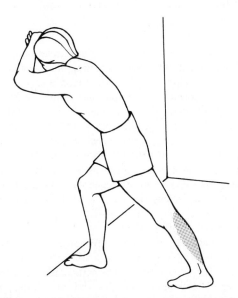

Figure 10-1. Calf, Achilles, and soleus stretch. Stand 3 feet from a wall with one foot forward, leaning forward to support your upper body by resting your forearms against the wall. Bend the forward leg at the knee. Keep the rear leg straight with the heel on the floor and slowly press your hips forward until you feel the calf stretch. Hold for 15 seconds. Relax and then repeat with the rear knee slightly bent so that you feel the Achilles stretch. Repeat with the other leg forward.

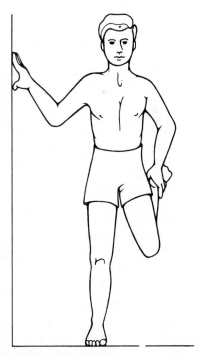

Figure 10-3. Quadriceps stretch. Stand at arm's length from a wall with your feet parallel to the wall. Rest your hand on the wall for support. Hold your ankle in your free hand and pull the foot back and up until the heel touches the buttocks, while leaning slightly forward from the waist. Repeat with the other leg.

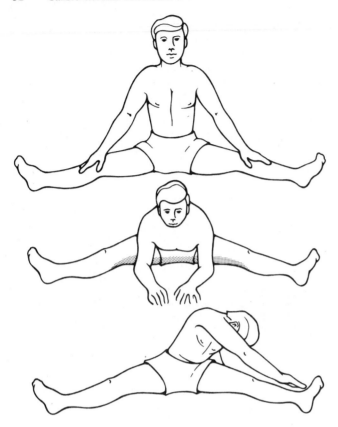

Figure 10-4. Hip and side stretch. Sit on the floor and spread your legs as far apart as possible. With your legs and back straight, bend forward from the waist until you feel a stretch at the inner thighs. Hold for 20 seconds. Relax, then twist at the waist and lean to touch your right hand to your left foot. Hold for 20 seconds. Repeat on the other side.

Equipment. One of the pleasures of running is that elaborate equipment is not required. However, good running shoes are essential. Many excellent shoes are available; the choice should be dictated by fit, comfort, and support rather than by endorsements or ratings. The toe box should provide enough room for dorsiflexion during takeoff, the sole should be flexible, and provide adequate cushioning, and the heel should be fairly snug without exerting pressure on the Achilles tendon. Most good running shoes are costly but can be expected to last for up to 1000 miles. Often, they can be resoled. Shoes are important, but other items ranging from stopwatches to designer sweat suits are optional to say the least. Good shoes will help prevent musculoskeletal injuries. In addition, a relatively soft running surface is helpful; grass and turf are best if they are smooth and level; asphalt is preferable to concrete.

Orthotics and other orthopedic devices are sometimes helpful for refractory problems. Patients with overuse injuries who fail to limit their activity may require a splint or cast to enforce inactivity, even if immobilization is not actually necessary for healing. The use of such devices requires referral to an orthopedist or podiatrist skilled in treating runners' musculoskeletal problems.

Stretching. Regular running produces asymmetric muscular development. The calf, hamstring, and Achilles can become overdeveloped and/or shortened and tight. Hill running and sprinting may produce similar effects on the quadriceps and hip flexors. A regular program of stretching exercises is essential to promote flexibility and balanced muscular development. These exercises are ideal for the warmup and cooldown periods before and after running.

Stretching routines are almost as numerous and varied as runners themselves. Four exercises are of particular value: the Achilles and soleus stretch (Fig. 10-1), the hamstring stretch (Fig. 10-2), the quadriceps stretch (Fig. 10-3), and the hip and side stretch (Fig. 10-4).

With increased running, more stretching will be necessary. In addition to flexibility, balanced muscular strength can be important. Bent knee situps are particularly valuable in strengthening abdominal muscles and preventing "side-stitches." Upper extremity strength is surprisingly important for runners. Pushups are the simplest upper extremity exercise, but advanced runners often include limited weight lifting or isometrics as well.

Running is not a panacea, but it has many cardiopulmonary, metabolic, and psychological benefits. The physician has a crucial role in the medical screening of potential runners, and he can prevent most problems with simple instructions. Periodic return visits may be necessary for dealing with various running-related problems. These visits afford the opportunity for the physician to counsel patience and persistence. Joggers who get through the difficult 2 or 3 months at the beginning of training are likely to develop running habits that are both enjoyable and healthful.

ANNOTATED BIBLIOGRAPHY

Reviews

(These four works provide comprehensive overviews of cardiovascular and metabolic aspects of exercise.)

Eichner ER: Exercise and heart disease. Epidemiology of the "exercise hypothesis." Am J Med 75:1008, 1983

Milvy P (ed): The marathon: Physiological, medical, epidemiological and psychological studies. Ann NY Acad Sci 301:1, 1977

Rigotti NA, Thomas GS, Leaf A: Exercise and coronary heart disease. Ann Rev Med 34:391, 1983

Wenger NK (ed): Exercise and the Heart. Philadelphia, FA Davis, 1978

Individual Papers

Cooper KH, Pollock, ML, Martin RP et al: Physical fitness levels vs. selected coronary risk factors. A cross-sectional study. JAMA 236: 116, 1976 (*A prevalence study of nearly 3000 men showing an inverse relationship between physical fitness and resting heart rate, blood pressure, body weight, percent body fat, and serum levels of cholesterol, triglycerides, and glucose.*)

Corfman GD, Thomas GS, Paffenbarger RS, Jr: Physical activity and primary prevention of cardiovascular disease. Cardiology Clinics 3:203, 1985 (*Part of a superb symposium on preventive cardiology.*)

Gibbons LW, Blair SN, Cooper KH et al: Association between coronary heart disease, risk factors and fitness in healthy adult women. Circulation 67:977, 1983 (*A study of 3000 subjects demonstrating an inverse relationship between risk factors and physical fitness in women.*)

Paffenbarger RS, Hale WE, Brand RJ et al: Work-energy level, personal characteristics, and fatal heart attack: A birth-cohort effect. Am J Epidemiol 105:200, 1977 (*A recent report on the 22-year cohort analysis of 3686 San Francisco longshoremen.*)

Paffenbarger RS, Hyde RT, Wing AL et al: Physical activity, all-cause mortality and longevity of college alumni. N Engl J Med 314:605, 1986 (*Documents prolonged survival among those who have increased physical activity.*)

Paffenbarger RS, Wing AL, Hyde RT: Physical activity as an index of heart attack risk in college alumni. Am J Epidemiol 108:161, 1978 (*A survey of the effects of exercise on coronary risk in 16,936 Harvard graduates.*)

Pickering TG: Jogging, marathon running and the heart. Am J Med 66:717, 1979 (*An excellent editorial and terse summary of the proven and as yet unproven effects of jogging on the heart and risk of cardiovascular disease.*)

Roman O, Camuzzi AL, Villalon E et al: Physical training program in arterial hypertension. Cardiol 67:230, 1981 (*Demonstrates achievement of a blood pressure reduction with exercise.*)

Scheuer J, Tipton CM: Cardiovascular adaptation to physical training. Annu Rev Physiol 39:221, 1975 (*A scholarly review on the cardiovascular effects of exercise in man and animals.*)

11
Bacterial Endocarditis Prophylaxis

Once universally fatal, bacterial endocarditis remains a serious disease, with a mortality rate of about 25%. Despite the now widespread availability of antibiotics; the incidence of this infection has not changed dramatically. Although controlled data are lacking, logic and pathogenesis of endocarditis argue that individual infections might be prevented by judicious use of prophylactic antibiotics. The primary care provider must be able to assess risks in individual patients. In addition, an understanding of the basis for prophylaxis recommendations is necessary if individuals likely to benefit from preventive measures are to be instructed effectively.

EPIDEMIOLOGY AND RISK FACTORS

Over the past several decades there has been a shift in the incidence of endocarditis to older age groups; the current mean age is about 50. Males predominate among patients over 50, but the sex ratio is more nearly equal among those under 50.

The risk of endocarditis in an individual patient is partially a function of the predisposing cardiac lesion and of the occurrence of procedures likely to induce bacteremia. However, as many as 30% to 40% of cases of endocarditis occur in the absence of underlying heart disease, and transient bacteremia is common. Additionally, the intensity of bacteremia, the characteristics of the bloodborne organisms, and host factors all play important roles. Since these additional determinants cannot be readily estimated, individual risk must be based on the diagnosis of predisposing lesions and the likelihood of bacteremia.

In the preantibiotic era, chronic rheumatic heart disease was the underlying lesion in 80% to 90% of cases of endocarditis. Currently, rheumatic heart disease is present in approximately 40% of patients with endocarditis. Congenital heart disease, undiagnosed murmurs, and atherosclerotic disease each account for 10% of underlying lesions. The remaining 30% to 40% of infections occur without known predisposing cardiac disease. In one series of 25 autopsies, 8 patients had no underlying heart disease.

Clearly, all individuals have some finite risk of developing endocarditis. Relative risks cannot be accurately estimated for specific heart lesions because of a lack of epidemiologic data. Because approximately 40% of endocarditis cases occur in the presence of *rheumatic heart disease* (which has a prevalence of slightly more than 1% in the adult population) and another 40% occur in the absence of heart disease, the risk of endocarditis is increased a hundredfold in the rheumatic heart as opposed to the normal heart.

Risk in *congenital heart disease* seems comparable. Patent ductus arteriosus, ventricular septal defect, and tetralogy of Fallot are the congenital lesions most commonly associated with endocarditis. Pulmonary and aortic stenoses constitute lesser risks. Atrial septal defect is very rarely responsible for endocarditis.

Idiopathic hypertrophic subaortic stenosis (IHSS) confers significant risk of endocarditis. In a series of 126 IHSS patients followed for varying periods up to 12 years, there were 3 definite cases and 3 suspected cases. Nine cases were reported in three other series, with a combined total of 158 patients with IHSS followed for varying periods.

Mitral valve prolapse is also associated with increased risk of endocarditis. One natural history study reported five cases of endocarditis in 855 patient-years of follow-up, an incidence higher than in patients free of valvular heart disease. A recent case-control study estimated that mitral valve prolapse confers an eightfold increase in endocarditis risk. Although this risk is substantially lower than that associated with rheumatic or other acquired valvular disease, the public health consequences are great because of the high prevalence of mitral valve prolapse. In one series of apparent failures of endocarditis prophylaxis, mitral valve prolapse was the most common underlying cardiac lesion.

Prosthetic valves involve special risks. Prosthetic valve endocarditis has been divided into two groups: (1) early, associated with surgery and most often involving nosocomial pathogens such as staphylococci, and (2) late, often following procedures that induce bacteremia and frequently associated with bacteria of low virulence. Late prosthetic valve endocarditis deserves special attention for two reasons: (1) organisms that are rarely able to infect damaged natural valves are more apt to infect prosthetic valves, and (2) when one deals with prosthetic valve endocarditis, the stakes are higher; treatment often involves valve replacement, and even with medical and surgical treatment overall mortality is significantly higher.

Another particularly high-risk group includes those who have previously had *endocarditis.* Recurrence rates as high as 10% have been cited, and third infections have been reported in some individuals. Table 11-1 summarizes known predisposing lesions in approximate order of risk. It must be kept in mind that the absolute risk of endocarditis, even for the patient at high risk, is extremely low, fewer than 1 case per 1000 tooth extractions.

The association of bacteremia with various events is shown in Table 11-2. Leading the list are dental procedures, rigid bronchoscopy, and genitourinary (GU) manipulations in the presence of urinary infection.

NATURAL HISTORY OF ENDOCARDITIS AND EFFECTIVENESS OF THERAPY

Untreated endocarditis is uniformly fatal. Current mortality rates are about 10% with natural valves and 25% to 65% with prosthetic valves. Death often follows congestive heart failure, arterial emboli, myocardial infarction, myocardial abscesses or other complications.

The efficacy of antibiotics used prophylactically has not been demonstrated. The large number of patients needed for such a study and the difficulties in identifying patients at risk and diagnosing episodes of potential bacteremia practically preclude such proof. Recommendations for prophylactic antibiotic regimens are based on experience with an experimental animal model.

RISK OF PROPHYLACTIC THERAPY

In the absence of previous sensitivity, the risk of serious reaction to penicillin prophylaxis is very small. No deaths were associated with the administration of benzathine penicillin G to over 300,000 Navy recruits for rheumatic fever prophylaxis. The largest studies have shown the incidence of all types of reactions to both intramuscularly and orally administered penicillin to be less than 1%. Approximately half of these reactions were considered serious. The risk of death due to serious penicillin reaction has been estimated at 1 to 2 per 100,000 patients receiving the drug.

Table 11-1. Cardiac Risk Factors for Endocarditis

1. High Risk
   a. Prosthetic heart valve(s)
   b. History of endocarditis
2. Moderate Risk
   a. Rheumatic or other acquired valvular disease
   b. Congenital heart disease (excluding atrial septal defect of the secundum type)
   c. Idiopathic hypertrophic subaortic stenosis
3. Probable Moderate Risk
   a. Mitral valve prolapse
   b. Undiagnosed murmurs

Table 11-2. Events Predisposing to Bacteremia

EVENT	PERCENTAGE OF INSTANCES IN WHICH BACTEREMIA OCCURS (%)
Dental extraction	75
Tooth brushing, flossing or irrigation	
Normal gingiva	20
Gingivitis	50
Bronchoscopy	
Fiberoptic	Less than 1
Rigid	15
Fiberoptic endoscopy	10
Sigmoidoscopy	5
Barium enema	10
Liver biopsy	5
Transurethral resection of prostate	
Sterile urine	10
Infected urine	50

Less information is available concerning risks associated with other prophylactic antibiotics. However, the rate of allergic reactions is probably significantly lower and, even with aminoglycosides, there is little toxicity when the drug is given for the brief period necessary for adequate prophylaxis.

IDENTIFYING PATIENTS AT RISK

As discussed previously, a rough estimate of risk can be made by identifying the underlying heart disease and estimating the likelihood that bacteremia will occur. Predisposing cardiac disease is detected by history and physical examination. A history of congenital or rheumatic heart disease and presence of a murmur indicate substantial risk. Documentation of IHSS or the presence of valve calcification can also be considered an indication for prophylaxis. All individuals with diastolic murmurs should be considered to be at risk.

Difficulty arises when the patient is *probably* at moderate risk. This is the case for most patients with mitral valve prolapse or with an isolated systolic murmur without a helpful history or other cardiac findings (see Chapter 15). Bacterial endocarditis prophylaxis for this group is controversial. The results of two independent risk–benefit analyses suggest that expected morbidity and mortality associated with penicillin therapy outweigh the benefits of prevention. Nevertheless, many clinicians continue to recommend prophylaxis. If prophylaxis is advised for patients in this group, it should be used only for high-risk procedures, which include dental work, rigid bronchoscopy, prostate surgery, and urinary catheter manipulation.

CONCLUSIONS AND RECOMMENDATIONS

- Clinical efficacy of endocarditis prophylaxis is difficult to demonstrate definitively. However, when the extreme degress of morbidity and mortality associated with the disease are weighed against the negligible risk associated with prophylaxis, vigorous preventive efforts are justified. It is estimated that about half of cases occur in patients with known predisposing heart disease following an anticipated episode of bacteremia, and thus may be preventable.
- Identifiable risk varies with the type of heart abnormality and the event responsible for bacteremia, as summarized in Tables 11-1 and 11-2.
- Because patients with prosthetic valves are especially susceptible, they should receive vigorous prophylaxis for any procedure—oral, genitourinary, or gastrointestinal—known to cause bacteremia. Similar vigorous therapy might also be applied to patients with a history of endocarditis. Specific recommendations for these *high-risk patients* are as follows.
  For dental procedures or surgery of the respiratory tract:
  1. Aqueous crystalline penicillin G (1,000,000 units IM) *mixed with* procaine penicillin G (600,000 units IM), *plus*
  2. Streptomycin (1 g IM)
  All of the above given 30 minutes before the procedure, followed by penicillin V (500 mg PO) given every 6 hours for eight doses.
  For patients allergic to penicillin:
  1. Vancomycin (1 g IV infused over 30 to 60 minutes), before the procedure, *followed by*
  2. Erythromycin (500 mg PO) given every 6 hours for eight doses.
  For GU or GI tract procedures:
  1. Aqueous crystalline penicillin G (2,000,000 units IM or IV) *or* ampicillin (1.0 g IM or IV), *plus*
  2. Gentamicin (1.5 mg/kg not to exceed 80 mg IM or IV) *or* streptomycin (1.0 g IM).
  Initial doses are to be given 30 to 60 minutes before the procedure. Ampicillin or penicillin doses are repeated every 6 hours for three to four doses. If gentamicin is used, the same dose is given every 8 hours for two additional doses. If streptomycin is used, the same dose is given every 12 hours for two additional doses. Additional doses may be necessary for prolonged procedures. On the other hand, a single dose may be sufficient for simple outpatient procedures. Longer intervals between doses may be appropriate in patients with significantly compromised renal function.
- Patients with congenital or acquired valvular disease or with undiagnosed murmurs thought to reflect an anatomic abnormality should receive prophylaxis for all dental and upper respiratory tract procedures. Genitourinary and gastrointestinal procedures associated with a high frequency

of bacteremia (including GU procedures in the presence of infected urine or prostate) should be done with antibiotic coverage. Endoscopy, barium enema, sigmoidoscopy, D & C, and intrauterine devices (IUD) insertion do not require antibiotic coverage.

Specific recommendations for these moderate-risk patients include the following:

1. Aqueous crystalline penicillin G (1,000,000 units IM) *mixed with* procaine penicillin G (600,000 units IM), both given 30 to 60 minutes before the procedure, *followed by* penicillin V (500 mg PO) every 6 hours for eight doses
2. Alternative when parenteral therapy is not feasible: penicillin V (2.0 g PO) 30 to 60 minutes before the procedure, *followed by* penicillin V (500 mg PO) every 6 hours for eight doses

For patients allergic to penicillin:

1. Vancomycin as recommended for high-risk patients with penicillin sensitivity, *or*
2. Erythromycin (1.0 g PO), 90 to 120 minutes prior to the procedure, *followed by* erythromycin (500 mg PO) every 6 hours for eight doses

This regimen may also be preferred to oral penicillin for patients taking penicillin continuously for rheumatic fever prophylaxis. Although endocarditis caused by penicillin-resistant organisms has not been a significant problem in such patients, it remains a theoretical concern.

• As in all preventive efforts, patient education is extremely important. All patients with identifiable risk should be urged to maintain a high level of oral health to minimize the potential for recurrent bacteremia. Patients receiving rheumatic fever prophylaxis must understand that their continuous therapy will *not* protect them from endocarditis.

A.G.M.

ANNOTATED BIBLIOGRAPHY

Allen HA, Leatham A et al: Significance and prognosis of an isolated late systolic murmur: A 9- to 22-year follow-up. Br Heart J 36: 525, 1974 (*Sixty-two patients with isolated late systolic murmur [33 also had a click] were followed for minimum of 9 years [mean 13.8]. Bacterial endocarditis occurred in 5 patients.*)

Bor DH, Himmelstein DU: Endocarditis prophylaxis in patients with mitral valve prolapse. Am J Med 76:711, 1984 (*An analytic review of the risks of endocarditis and drug prophylaxis concluding that no prophylaxis or prophylaxis with erythromycin is preferable to prophylaxis with a penicillin.*)

Clemens JD, Horwitz RI, Jaffe CC et al: A controlled evaluation of the risk of bacterial endocarditis in persons with mitral valve prolapse. N Engl J Med 307:776, 1982 (*A case-control study estimating a substantially higher risk—odds ratio of 8.2—of endocarditis for people with mitral valve prolapse than for those without it.*)

Clemens JD, Ransohoff DF: A quantitative assessment of pre-dental antibiotic prophylaxis for patients with mitral valve prolapse. J Chron Dis 37:531, 1984 (*A cost-effectiveness analysis concluding that the risk of postdental endocarditis in mitral valve prolapse may be outweighed by the risk of fatal reactions to parenteral penicillin prophylaxis.*)

Dismukes WE, Karchmer WE, Buckley M et al: Prosthetic valve endocarditis. Analysis of 38 cases. Circulation 48:365, 1973 (*Includes 19 cases of "late" endocarditis. Predisposing factors were identified in 12 cases, with dental or GU procedures incriminated in 7.*)

Doyle EF, Spagnuolo M, Taranta A et al: The risk of bacterial endocarditis during antirheumatic prophylaxis. JAMA 201:807, 1967 (*Sixteen cases of endocarditis were reported during 3615 patient-years of antirheumatic prophylaxis. No controls, but calculated incidence was not statistically different from that in historical control group. Four of the 16 organisms were penicillin-resistant.*)

Durack DT, Kaplan EL, Bisno AL: Apparent failures of endocarditis prophylaxis. JAMA 250:2318, 1983 (*Summary of 52 cases submitted to the National AHA Registry. Mitral valve prolapse was the most common underlying cardiac lesion; only 6 of 52 endocarditis patients received recommended antibiotic regimens.*)

Epstein EJ, Coulshed N: Bacterial endocarditis in idiopathic hypertrophic subaortic stenosis. Cardiologica 54:30, 1969 (*This paper reviews reported cases of endocarditis in a combined series of 158 patients with IHSS.*)

Everett ED, Hirschman JV: Transient bacteremia and endocarditis prophylaxis. A review. Medicine, 56:61, 1977 (*Incidence data for bacteremia associated with relevant clinical procedures gathered from the literature are reviewed.*)

Ivert TS, Dismukes WE, Cobbs CG et al: Prosthetic valve endocarditis. Circulation 69:223, 1984 (*Documents the high risk of both early and late endocarditis among people with prosthetic valves; the highest risk were for those with prior native valve endocarditis and mechanical rather than biological prostheses.*)

Kaplan EL, Anthony BF, Bisno A et al: Prevention of bacterial endocarditis. Circulation 56:39A, 1977 (*Summarizes the rationale and most recent AHA recommendations and recognizes the special risk of patients with prosthetic valves.*)

Lerner PI, Weinstein L: Infectious endocarditis in the antibiotic era. N Engl J Med 274:199, 1966 (*One hundred cases plus an extensive literature review.*)

Prophylaxis of bacterial endocarditis: Faith, hope and charitable interpretation (Editorial). Lancet 1:519, 1976 (*Argues the infeasibility of any clinical trial and the importance of experimental models.*)

Weinstein L, Rubin RH: Infectious endocarditis—1973. Prog Cardiovasc Dis 16:239, 1973 (*An update. Some information about susceptibility and predisposing events.*)

Wilson WR, Javmin DM, Danielson GK et al: Prosthetic valve endocarditis. Ann Intern Med 82:751, 1975 (*Gram-negative rods were found in 31% of late cases.*)

12
Rheumatic Fever Prophylaxis

Despite a decline in incidence that began before the availability of antibiotics, rheumatic fever and rheumatic heart disease remain significant causes of preventable morbidity. Primary prevention depends on appropriate diagnosis and effective treatment of Group A streptococcal pharyngitis, discussed in Chapter 218. Vaccination against streptococcal infection may be possible in the future, but current preventive measures depend on discriminating antibiotic use.

The prophylactic use of antibiotics has been shown to be effective for primary prevention during epidemics among closed populations. The major role of antibiotic prophylaxis, however, is in prevention of second attacks. The risk of recurrence following streptococcal infection is especially high in patients with evidence of carditis. Continuous streptococcal prophylaxis in patients with prior rheumatic fever is the major means of preventing the cardiac sequelae of rheumatic fever recurrences. It is the task of the primary physician to identify patients who would benefit from such prophylaxis and to provide the instruction necessary for long-term compliance.

EPIDEMIOLOGY AND RISK FACTORS

The epidemiology of rheumatic fever parallels that of streptococcal infection. Rare below age 5, it is most common in older children and adolescents. Incidence decreases after adolescence; cases after age 40 are very rare. There is no clear predilection for either sex.

Although a genetic predisposition has not been proven, an association between certain HLA antigens and rheumatic diseases has been identified, at least among white patients. Heterogeneity in the immune response to a specific streptococal cell-wall antigen, the Group A carbohydrate, has been demonstrated, but predictors of the hyperimmune response associated with the clinical sequelae of rheumatic fever have not been identified.

Racial differences in the incidence of rheumatic fever exist but disappear when socioeconomic status is considered; crowded living conditions is an important variable. Crowding may also explain the high incidence in cold climates and during winter months in temperate climates.

All demographic risk factors are heavily outweighed by a previous history of rheumatic fever. The likelihood of an attack following streptococcal infection is at least five times higher among individuals with previous rheumatic fever.

NATURAL HISTORY OF RHEUMATIC FEVER AND EFFECTIVENESS OF THERAPY

Rheumatic fever follows between 0.5% and 3.0% of ineffectively treated cases of Group A streptococcal upper respiratory infections. Diagnosis and appropriate antibiotic therapy will prevent rheumatic fever in the individual case, but such efforts cannot be expected to eliminate rheumatic disease because of the high proportion of streptococcal infections that are subclinical. Approximately one third of patients with primary rheumatic fever have no history of preceding respiratory infections. Another one third have symptoms but do not seek medical care. The remainder are ineffectively diagnosed or treated.

Among all patients with Group A streptococcal infection and a history of previous rheumatic fever, the recurrence rate is 15%. More specific rates can be estimated for subgroups depending on (1) the number of previous rheumatic attacks, (2) the interval since the last attack, and (3) whether or not there was evidence of carditis. Specific attack rates are summarized in Table 12-1.

Because of these high secondary attack rates and the ubiquity of the streptococcus, *continuous* antibiotic prophylaxis of streptococcal infection is the only feasible method of preventing rheumatic fever recurrences. Three antibiotic regimens have gained general acceptance:

Table 12-1. Risk of Recurrent Rheumatic Fever After Group A Streptococcal Infection

	PERCENTAGE RECURRENCES OF STREPTOCOCCAL INFECTION (%)
Interval Since Onset of Last Rheumatic Episode	
Up to 2 years	28
2–5 years	15
5 years and over	10
Number of Previous Attacks of Rheumatic Fever	
2 or more	27
1	14
Rheumatic Heart Disease	
Not present	13
Present	26

(Modified from Spagnuolo M, Pasternack B, Taranta A *et al:* Risk of rheumatic fever recurrences after streptococcal infections. N Engl J Med 285:641, 1971)

Table 12-2. Prophylaxis and Attack Rates of Streptococcal Infection and Rheumatic Fever Recurrences

	ORAL SULFADIAZINE (1 G DAILY)	ORAL PENICILLIN G (200,000 UNITS DAILY)	IM BENZATHINE PENICILLIN G (1.2 MILLION UNITS EVERY 4 WEEKS)
Number of patient-years	576	545	560
Number of streptococcal infections (rate/100 patient-years)	138 (24.0)	113 (20.7)	34 (6.1)
Number of rheumatic fever recurrences (rate/100 patient-years)	16 (2.8)	30 (5.5)	2 (0.4)

(Modified from Wood H, Feinstein AR, Tarant A et al: rheumatic fever in children and adolescent III. Comparative effectiveness of three prophylaxis regimens in preventing streptococcal infections and rheumatic recurrences. Ann Intern Med 60:31, 1964)

1. Benzathine penicillin G, 1,200,000 units IM every 4 weeks
2. Sulfadiazine, 1 g PO qd (500 mg for patients under 60 lb)
3. Penicillin G, 250,000 units PO bid

Although the effectiveness of erythromycin (250 mg PO bid) has not been studied, it is recommended for the rare patient allergic to both penicillin and sulfonamides. The classic study comparing the effectiveness of these three regimens in preventing streptococcal infection and rheumatic fever is summarized in Table 12-2.

There are no firm guidelines regarding the duration of continuous antibiotic prophylaxis following an episode of rheumatic fever. Factors that influence the likelihood of rheumatic recurrence following infection have already been reviewed. Within limits, the physician can estimate the risk of exposure of a particular patient to streptococcal infection. For example, parents of young children, teachers, and other school personnel, health care providers, and military personnel are at high risk.

RISKS OF ANTIBIOTIC PROPHYLAXIS

The risks of penicillin administration are discussed in Chapter 11 on endocarditis prophylaxis. It should be emphasized that, in a large series, reactions following parenteral administration were no more common than those following oral therapy.

CONCLUSIONS AND RECOMMENDATIONS

- Primary prevention of rheumatic fever depends on accurate diagnosis and treatment of symptomatic streptococcal upper respiratory infections. Prevention of rheumatic fever recurrences depends on continuous streptococcal prophylaxis of the patients at risk.
- Monthly injections of benzathine penicillin G (1,200,000 units IM) provide the most effective prophylaxis and are recommended in patients with a high risk of both strep-

tococcal exposure and a rheumatic recurrence after infection. Acceptable oral regimens in patients at lower risk include the following:

Sulfadiazine, 1 g PO qd, *or*

Penicillin G, 250,000 units PO bid, *or*

Erythromycin, 250 mg PO bid (in patients allergic to both penicillin and sulfa drugs)

- The duration of prophylaxis should be based on the risk incurred by the particular patient.
- All patients with rheumatic fever should be treated until age 25 or for 5 years following an episode (whichever is longer). In those with two or more previous attacks or with rheumatic heart disease, therapy should be continued until age 40 or for 10 years following the last episode. Prophylaxis in patients with rheumatic heart disease at high risk of streptococcal exposure should be continued indefinitely.

A.G.M.

ANNOTATED BIBLIOGRAPHY

Ayoub EM: The search for host determinants of susceptibility to rheumatic fever: The missing link. Circulation 69:197, 1984 (*Reviews evidence for genetic markers and immune hyperresponsiveness to streptococcal antigens among people predisposed to rheumatic fever.*)

Breese BB, Disney FA: Penicillin in the treatment of streptococcal infections. A comparison of effectiveness of five different oral and one parenteral form. N Engl J Med 259:57, 1958 (*No difference was found in reaction rates between IM and po use.*)

Holmberg SD, Faich GA: Streptococcal pharyngitis and acute rheumatic fever in Rhode Island. JAMA 250:2307, 1983 (*Of patients receiving throat cultures, nearly 90% were given antibiotic therapy before the culture results were known, and nearly 40% continued antibiotic therapy for 10 days regardless of results. Only three definite cases of rheumatic fever were identified during a 5 year period.*)

Kaplan EL, Bisno A, Derrick W et al: Prevention of rheumatic fever: AHA Committee Report. Circulation 55:1, 1977 (*Summary of argument for prophylaxis with recommendations.*)

Land MA, Bisno AL: Acute rheumatic fever: A vanishing disease in suburbia. JAMA 249:895, 1983 (*A retrospective analysis in Memphis–Shelby County detecting a 0.64 case per 100,000 population annual incidence of acute rheumatic fever. An accompanying editorial ponders explanations for the dramatic fall in acute rheumatic fever incidence in the United States.*)

McFarland RB: Reactions to benzathine penicillin. N Engl J Med 259:62, 1958 (*Reaction rate of 1.3% following single injection in 12,858 naval recruits.*)

Schwartz RH, Wientzen RL, Pedreira F et al: Penicillin V for group A pharyngeal tonsilitis. JAMA 246:1790, 1981 (*A randomized-control trial demonstrating a treatment failure rate of 31% for patients treated for 7 days compared with 18% for those treated for 10 days.*)

Sellers TF: An epidemiologic view of rheumatic fever. Prog Cardiovasc Dis 16:303, 1973 (*Reviews epidemiology.*)

Spagnuolo M, Pasternack B, Taranta A: Risk of rheumatic fever recurrences after streptococcal infections. N Engl J Med 285:641, 1971 (*Data are reviewed in Table 12-1.*)

Wood HF, Feinstein AR, Taranta A et al: Rheumatic fever in children and adolescents. III. Comparative effectiveness of three prophylaxis regimens in preventing streptococcal infections and rheumatic recurrences. Ann Intern Med 60:31, 1964 (*Data are reviewed in Table 12-2.*)

13
Evaluation of Hypertension
KATHARINE K. TREADWAY, M.D.

High blood pressure, if unrecognized or untreated, leads to the development of heart failure, renal failure, and stroke and is considered the most significant cardiovascular risk factor. In the majority of cases, the cause of hypertension is unknown. Moreover, the disease is usually asymptomatic prior to the advent of complications. The silent nature of hypertension, ignorance regarding its pathogenesis, and frustration caused by the long-term, empiric therapy required have fostered apathy in physician and patient alike. Blood pressure measurements are commonly omitted during routine physical examinations or emergency room visits. Follow-up for patients with high blood pressure is often limited or non-existent, and even when patients keep their appointments faithfully, they may not be taking their medications as prescribed.

Adequate therapy of high blood pressure has been shown to reduce morbidity and mortality. Even partial correction can reduce complications significantly. In light of the clearly demonstrated benefits of treatment, apathy toward high blood pressure cannot be justified.

DEFINITION

The definition of high blood pressure is arbitrary. Actuarial data have shown that morbidity and mortality related to complications of hypertension increase linearly with increasing levels of either systolic or diastolic blood pressure. Hence, no critical level of blood pressure exists beyond which risk becomes highly magnified. For the sake of definition, we identify as hypertensive those blood pressure levels associated with a greater than 50% increase in mortality: for men below age 45, 130/90 mm Hg; for men over age 45, 140/95 mm Hg; for women of all ages, 160/95 mm Hg.

Primary or *essential hypertension,* which accounts for over 90% of cases, is as yet without identifiable cause. Onset of disease is usually between ages 30 and 50, and a history of familial hypertension can often be elicited. *Secondary hypertension* has a definable etiology (Table 13-1), occurs within a wide age range, and is often abrupt in onset and severe in magnitude; family history is commonly negative. *Borderline hypertension* is blood pressure that intermittently rises above the normal levels for each given age group and sex. Established hypertension has been shown to develop more commonly in patients with borderline hypertension.

It is becoming increasingly apparent that the definition of hypertension must be individualized for each patient. The diagnosis derives not only from the absolute level of blood pressure, but also from the presence or absence of other *cardiovascular risk factors.* Factors identified by the Framingham study as significant contributors to cardiovascular risk are hypertension, cigarette smoking, elevated serum cholesterol levels, glucose intolerance, and electrocardiographic evidence of left ventricular hypertrophy with strain. Thus, the patient with borderline hypertension, a moderately elevated serum cholesterol level and a history of smoking has a fivefold higher risk of incurring cardiovascular disease than the patient with borderline hypertension alone. Clearly, the patient at higher risk should be considered a candidate for prompt reduction of blood pressure and risk factor modification. A probability profile based on these risk factors is available (see Kannel, 1976) and can be extremely useful in predicting whether or not therapeutic intervention is advisable.

PATHOGENESIS

Although the etiology of essential hypertension has not been defined, a large body of experimental evidence now has elucidated several mechanisms that undoubtedly play a role. Of these, the *renin–angiotensin–aldosterone system* is prob-

Table 13-1.   Primary versus Secondary Hypertension: Specific Screening Protocols

CAUSE (PREVALENCE, %)*	SCREEN	CONFIRMATION
Coarctation (NA)	Arm and leg BPs, chest x-ray	Angiography
Cushing's syndrome (0.1)	Cushingoid appearance; 1-mg dexamethasone suppression test	High-dose dexamethasone suppression test, etc.
Drug-induced hypertension (0.8)	History: amphetamines, oral contraceptives, estrogens, corticosteroids, licorice, thyroid hormone	
↑ Intracranial pressure (NA)	Neurologic evaluation	
Pheochromocytoma (0.2)	History of paroxysmal hypertension, headache, perspiration, palpitations *or* fixed diastolic ≥130 mm Hg; 24-hour urinary metanephrine or VMA	Catecholamine levels, angiography, CT scan
Primary aldosteronism (Conn's or idiopathic) (0.1)	Serum K^+, urine K^+, stimulated PRA	Aldosterone levels, venography with differential level, CT scan
Renal disease (2.4)	History of congenital disease, diabetes, proteinuria, pyelonephritis, obstruction; urinalysis; BUN or creatinine	Creatinine clearance, IVP, ultrasound, biopsy
Renovascular disease (1.0)	Suspect in young female or elderly patient with atherosclerosis, especially if abrupt in onset, negative family history, and abdominal bruit present	Digital subtraction or digital arterial angiography and differential renal vein renins

* (Danielson M, Dammstrom B: The prevalence of secondary and curable hypertension. Acta Med Scand 209:451, 1981)

elucidated several mechanisms that undoubtedly play a role. Of these, the *renin–angiotensin–aldosterone system* is probably the best understood. Renin is released by the kidneys and acts within the bloodstream to yield angiotensin II, a potent vasoconstrictor and primary stimulus for aldosterone release.

Renin production is inversely proportional to effective blood volume: anything that increases effective blood volume suppresses renin; anything that decreases effective blood volume stimulates renin. For example, in primary aldosteronism, autonomous production of the salt-retaining hormone aldosterone by an adrenal adenoma results in intravascular volume expansion and renin suppression. Conversely, in renal artery stenosis, decreased renal perfusion on the affected side is perceived by that kidney as decreased effective blood volume. Renin is secreted, and increases in angiotensin II and aldosterone result, thereby creating systemic hypertension and volume expansion. While renin initiates this form of hypertension, it is maintained in different patients by a varying ratio of elevated angiotensin II and aldosterone. Similarly, patients with essential hypertension can be placed in high, normal, or low renin groups. In contrast with patients with primary aldosteronism or renal artery stenosis, however, no pathogenetic lesion responsible for these different renin levels has yet been identified in these patients.

Dietary *sodium* has long been implicated in the pathogenesis of hypertension. Several lines of evidence support the importance of sodium intake in the development of hypertension. In cultures in which salt intake is low, hypertension is exceedingly rare. When members of those same cultures migrate into cultures in which salt intake is high, approximately 25% to 30% will develop hypertension. Sodium restriction has long been known to reduce blood pressure in a subset of hypertensives. In addition, there are many experimental animal models supporting the role of sodium in the development of hypertension.

The role of the *central nervous system* (CNS) and its afferent and efferent receptors is becoming increasingly appreciated. Neurohumeral and sensory inputs from the periphery profoundly affect the various vasoactive CNS centers. Their output is, in turn, modified by peripheral vascular reactivity, which is itself affected by the autonomic nervous system, Na^+ and Ca^{++} and other, as yet poorly defined humoral agents.

Studies on patients with borderline hypertension have allowed clear identification of subgroups in which a defect in autonomic nervous system controls exists, resulting in excessive sympathetic and reduced parasympathetic activity. Certainly pheochromocytoma provides a model for secondary hypertension based on excessive catecholamines.

Last, *cardiogenic factors* appear to be important in the development of hypertension. In certain strains of rats in which hypertension. In certain strains of rats in which hypertension develops spontaneously and is eventually fatal, cardiac hypertrophy occurs long before elevation of blood pressure.

The ways in which these various mechanisms interact with one another and the ability to determine which mechanism(s) play a dominant role in a given individual remain ill defined. Although we can make some approximate generalizations regarding the probable mechanisms responsible for the development of hypertension in certain groups (*i.e.,* sodium retention in blacks and excessive sympathetic tone in certain young white male populations), these remain too crude to apply to the individual and at present can serve only as a very rough guide to therapy.

CLINICAL PRESENTATION

Hypertension is usually asymptomatic until the development of substantial blood pressure elevation, in which case fatigue, headache, light-headedness, flushing, or epistaxis may be reported. The rare syndrome of *hypertensive encephalopathy*, seen when diastolic blood pressure rises rapidly above 130 mm Hg, is characterized by restlessness, confusion, somnolence, blurred vision, and nausea or vomiting; all these symptoms are related to increased intracranial pressure.

Certain forms of secondary hypertension may be characterized by specific symptoms. Thus, the patient with *coarctation* of the aorta may experience leg claudication as a result of lower extremity ischemia; the patient with *Cushing's syndrome* may complain of hirsutism or easy bruising; the patient with *pheochromocytoma* may experience excessive perspiration, severe paroxysmal headaches, or palpitations; and the patient with *primary aldosteronism* will be prone to symptoms of hypokalemia, that is, muscle cramps, weakness, and polyuria.

Once end-organ damage develops, symptoms will be related to congestive failure, renal failure, cerebrovascular insufficiency, peripheral vascular disease, or ischemic heart disease.

DIFFERENTIAL DIAGNOSIS

Over 90% of cases of hypertension are essential; secondary causes account for the remainder and are listed in Table 13-1.

WORKUP

History. Patient evaluation includes a careful interview with emphasis on family history of hypertension, diabetes, or cardiovascular disease; patient's age at onset of elevated blood pressure; diet, especially with regard to salt intake; presence of other cardiovascular risk factors (smoking, diabetes, lipid abnormalities); symptoms of cardiovascular disease (angina, dyspnea, claudication, etc.); use of agents that can cause hypertension (birth control pills, steroids, thyroid, amphetamines in diet pills or cold capsules, large quantities of licorice); symptoms of secondary hypertension as summarized above; and a history of renal disease or flank trauma.

Physical examination emphasizes weight measurement; funduscopy; thyroid examination; general cardiopulmonary examination; evaluation of peripheral vasculature including bilateral arm and leg pressure measurements, simultaneous radial and femoral pulse palpation, and auscultation for bruits; abdominal palpation and auscultation; observation for the stigmata of Cushing's syndrome, chronic renal failure, or neurofibromatosis; and complete neurologic evaluation.

Several commonly held beliefs regarding the diagnosis of high blood pressure have been challenged by epidemiologic data from the Framingham study. First, casual blood pressure determinations appear to be as reliable as basal levels in predicting long-term cardiovascular risk. This is not surprising if we understand that a person capable of anxiety-provoked hypertension in the setting of a physician's office may be equally apt to respond to the stresses of daily life with labile hypertension. Second, risk appears directly proportional to systolic or diastolic blood pressure, elevation of either equally predisposing to the complications of hypertension.

Blood pressure is properly measured in both arms while the patient is seated comfortably. The cuff should be placed at heart level and as high as possible on the arm. The average of two successive measurements in each arm is recorded. Diastolic pressure is taken at the point at which sound disappears (Korotkoff 5) rather than when it changes in quality (Korotkoff 4). Cuff size must be adequate to avoid falsely elevated readings (cuff width greater than two thirds of arm width, length of inflatable portion greater than two thirds of arm circumference).

Laboratory Studies. Recently, extensive laboratory evaluation of patients with high blood pressure has come under a great deal of criticism. The yield of curable cases of hypertension is small, and with increasing costs, extensive evaluation for all hypertensive patients would put undue stress on health resources.

Laboratory evaluation of high blood pressure has three purposes: (1) to ascertain the degree of end-organ damage resulting from hypertension, (2) to identify patients at high risk for the development of cardiovascular complications, and (3) to screen for secondary, possibly reversible forms of the disease. Despite the wide array of sophisticated diagnostic techniques now readily available, there is increasing evidence that the diagnosis of secondary hypertension can be made accurately and economically by the alert physician on the basis of a careful history, a physical examination, and only a few simple diagnostic tests.

Tests considered essential in the evaluation of high blood pressure include complete blood count, urinalysis, serum BUN or creatinine, serum K^+, fasting blood sugar, serum cholesterol, and electrocardiogram. The urinalysis provides evidence of primary renal disease. The extent of renal compromise due to renal disease or secondary to the hypertension itself is indicated by the BUN or creatinine. Fasting blood sugar, serum cholesterol, and ECG supply data regarding cardiovascular risk and ECG changes resulting from hypertension. Serum potassium is a valuable screening test for primary aldosteronism and should be known before diuretic therapy is instituted. Total cost of these determinations is reasonable. In most patients, evaluation should stop here.

Patients at somewhat higher risk for secondary hypertension include (1) those under 35, (2) those with rapid onset of elevated blood pressure and a negative family history, (3) those with severe hypertension, and (4) those who have failed to respond to empirical therapy despite compliance. Fortunately, in a majority of patients at high risk for secondary hypertension, a specific diagnosis will be suggested by history and physical examination. Thus, the patient with Cushing's syndrome should be easily identified by appearance; the patient with coarctation can be diagnosed by measurement of arm and leg blood pressure and simultaneous radial femoral pulse palpation; patients with pheochromocytoma or drug-induced hypertension (*e.g.,* due to use of oral contraceptives, decongestants, or diet pills) can often be identified in an interview; primary aldosteronism is almost always apparent from serum K^+; and renovascular disease is most common in young patients and in older ones in whom onset of hypertension is abrupt, especially if a flank bruit or diffuse vascular disease is detected.

When a specific form of hypertension is suspected, each possibility can be accurately screened as follows: Cushing's syndrome: 1 mg of dexamethasone suppression; coarctation: chest x-ray; pheochromocytoma: 24-hour urinary metanephrine or VMA; primary aldosteronism: stimulated plasma renin activity and urinary K^+: creatinine. An increase in VMA or metanephrines is very specific for pheochromocytoma; two normal levels obtained while the patient is hypertensive virtually rule out the diagnosis. Methyldopa can falsely elevate metanephrines. Should these tests return positive, diagnosis can then be confirmed by more extensive evaluation in patients considered good surgical candidates.

Considerable controversy remains regarding the best way to screen for renovascular hypertension. The available screening methods of plasma renin measurements, hypertensive IVP, and renal scan have been found lacking when applied in clinical practice. In patients in whom a high suspicion of renovascular hypertension exists (young female or elderly patient with atherosclerosis, especially if hypertension is abrupt in onset, negative family history and abdominal bruit present), a more definitive workup should be undertaken directly, using digital subtraction angiography (DSA) and bilateral renal vein renins. When clinical evidence of renovascular disease is less compelling, one may consider a hypertensive IVP in the evaluation, although its false-negative rate is as high as 40%. However, the more costly and invasive evaluation must be resorted to when the clinical presentation strongly suggests the diagnosis or when the hypertension is severe and difficult to control.

ANNOTATED BIBLIOGRAPHY

Ferguson RK: Cost and yield of the hypertensive evaluation: Experience of a community-based referral clinic. Ann Intern Med 82: 761, 1975 (*Emphasizes that secondary hypertension can be detected on the basis of a careful examination and only a few simple diagnostic tests.*)

Goldenberg K, Snyder DK: Screening for primary aldosteronism. J Gen Intern Med 1:368, 1986 (*An examination of the serum potassium's utility as a screening test for this condition.*)

Goldfine A: Pheochromocytoma. Clin Endocrinol Metab 10:607, 1981 (*Includes a critical review of available diagnostic studies.*)

Grim CE, Weinberger MH: Renal artery stenosis and hypertension. Semin Nephrol 3:52, 1983 (*Comprehensive discussion of evaluation and treatment.*)

The 1984 Report of the Joint National Committee on Detection, Evaluation, and Treatment of High Blood Pressure. Arch Intern Med 144:1045, 1984 (*Provides authoritative consensus panel view on workup.*)

14
Evaluation of Chest Pain

Chest pain is an important reason for unscheduled office visits. Concerns about heart and lung disease are uppermost in the minds of many who come for evaluation. Although many chest pains prove to be harmless, the primary physician must be skilled in accurately recognizing the signs of serious etiologies in the office, where one is limited to a careful history, physical examination, ECG, and perhaps chest x-ray. Particularly challenging are evaluating pleuritic chest pain and determining when atypical pain represents angina.

PATHOPHYSIOLOGY AND CLINICAL PRESENTATION

Most structures within, surrounding, or adjacent to the thorax are capable of producing chest pain. Pain originating from the *chest wall* is predominantly musculoskeletal in origin. It may last from a few seconds to several days and can be sharp, aching, or dull. The discomfort is characteristically aggravated by deep inspiration, cough, direct palpation, and movement. Sometimes the patient complains of chest tightness. Vigorous and unaccustomed exertion can lead to muscular and ligamentous strain. Common sites of involvement are the costochondral and chondrosternal junctions. *Precordial catch syndrome,* which is believed to result from muscle spasm, causes acute sharp pain worsened by breathing and terminated by stretching or taking a very deep breath. It occurs mostly in young adults. *Costochondritis (Tietze's syndrome)* causes localized swelling, erythema, warmth, and tenderness at the costochondral junction. *Rib fracture* is usually preceded by a history of trauma or evidence of underlying malignancy. Of interest is the observation that musculoskeletal pain appears to occur with increased frequency in patients with angina, leading to considerable diagnostic confusion.

Other components of the chest wall are sometimes responsible for pain. For example, nerve irritation from a flare-up of *herpes zoster* causes discomfort in a dermatomal distribution. The neurologic complaints range from hypoesthesia to dysesthesia and hyperesthesia. Pain may precede the appearance of the vesicular rash by 3 to 5 days and, especially in the elderly, persist long after the rash resolves (see Chapter 192). Nerve injury from root compression due to *cervical spine disease* or a *thoracic outlet syndrome* can lead to pain in the chest and upper arm, superficially resembling angina. In the outlet syndrome, a cervical rib may compress part of the brachial plexus, resulting in motor and sensory deficits that occur in the arm in an ulnar distribution; at the same time, there is discomfort in the chest and upper arm (see Chapter 161).

Inflammation or distention of the *pleura* also produces pain worsened by deep inspiration and cough, but movement and palpation have little or no effect. A host of etiologies can trigger the inflammatory process, including infection, pulmonary infarction, neoplasm, uremia, and connective tissue disease. The more florid the inflammation, the greater the pain; and infectious etiology is more likely to present with considerable pleuritic pain than is a low-grade serositis associated with connective tissue disease. Stretching of the pleura following a *spontaneous pneumothorax* results in the acute onset of pleuritic pain and dyspnea. The condition often accompanies emphysema, in which there can be rupture of a bleb being responsible. When the pneumothorax is large, deviation of the trachea may be noted as mediastinal shift occurs. *Pleurodynia* is a self-limited source of pleuritic pain. It is most common in children and young adults and associated with Coxsackie B infection. Usually there is a typical viral prodrome followed by acute onset of chest pain. Chest pain in the setting of a viral URI may also occur from cough-initiated injury to the chest wall or viral-induced bronchospasm.

Pericarditis may also be a source of pleuritic pain, resulting from spread of the inflammatory process from the relatively insensitive pericardium to the adjacent parietal pleura. The pain is sharp, aggravated by respiratory motion and sometimes precipitated by swallowing if the posterior aspect of the heart is involved. When the diaphragmatic surface of the pericardium is involved, pain will be referred to the tip of the shoulder. Change in position may alter the pain; patients often note lessening of the pain upon sitting up and leaning forward. Pericarditis can also produce a second type of pain that mimics angina. The most important physical finding associated with pericarditis is a two- or three-component rub.

Chest pain can be produced by disease of the *pulmonary parenchyma* if the process extends into the pleura or another pain-sensitive structure in the chest. Consequently, the pain is usually pleuritic in quality. Among the most important etiologies are *pneumococcal pneumonia* (see Chapter 43), *acute pulmonary tuberculosis* (see Chapter 47), and *pulmonary embolization with infarction.* Most pulmonary emboli do not cause pleuritic pain, because the major sources of pain—infarction and congestive atelectasis—occur only in the context of marked embolic obstruction to blood flow to the lung. It is estimated by some that fewer than 10% of embolic episodes are associated with pain. The most common manifestation of embolization is dyspnea, which is seen in virtually every case, though it may be transient. Tachypnea and tachycardia are the only consistently observed physical findings; they too may be evanescent. Pleural rub, effusion, fever, or hemoptysis suggests the presence of infarction.

Angina pectoris is the most important cardiac source of chest pain. Typically it is brought on by exertion, eating a large meal, or emotional stress and is relieved by rest or nitroglycerin. Sexual intercourse is a particularly common precipitant. Patients usually report a squeezing or pressure sensation and sometimes do not even refer to the discomfort as a pain. Descriptions of sharp pain are atypical. Radiation of the pain to the jaw, neck, shoulder, arm, back, or upper abdomen is common, and some patients experience pain in one of these locations without having any chest symptoms. At times the arm is reported to feel numb. The duration of symptoms ranges from 2 to 20 minutes. Pain lasting longer is suggestive of acute coronary insufficiency or myocardial infarction; fleeting pains of a few seconds duration are not anginal in origin. Prompt response to nitroglycerin is characteristic of mild angina; relief is usually obtained within 5 minutes.

Other forms of angina include *nocturnal angina* or angina decubitus, in which the patient experiences pain while lying down, often awakening with typical anginal pain in the middle of the night. It is postulated that this might be a manifestation of pump failure, with the heart unable to handle the increased return to the right side of the heart resulting from recumbency. Another suspicion is that the increased physiologic activity associated with REM sleep increases myocardial oxygen demand and triggers angina.

Variant angina as described originally by Prinzmetal is

characterized by anginal pain occurring exclusively at rest in conjunction with transient ST segment elevation on the electrocardiogram. Classically, this syndrome was associated with coronary artery spasm at the site of high-grade proximal fixed stenosis. Since the original description in 1959, however, a wider spectrum of clinical presentations and underlying pathology has been appreciated. Variant angina may occur with exertion as well as at rest. The pain syndrome may be chronic and stable rather than unstable. ST segment depression rather than elevation may be present on the electrocardiogram recorded during pain. Coronary artery spasm may produce these symptoms and signs with or without accompanying fixed coronary stenosis. Symptoms resulting from spasm are indistinguishable from those of classic angina due to fixed stenoses as well as atypical chest pain.

Atypical angina is a nonspecific term used to denote chest pain that differs in location or quality from the more typical form, yet is suggestive of angina in having similar precipitants, timing, or other features. As many as 50% of such patients prove to have coronary disease. Anginal pain is seen occasionally in *mitral valve prolapse;* however, most patients with prolapse and chest pain describe symptoms that are nonanginal in quality—that is, poorly correlated with exertion or emotion and unrelieved by nitroglycerin (see Chapter 15). The condition is common in young women.

A vexing clinical problem is the development of chest pain in the patient who has had coronary bypass surgery. The return of typical angina raises the spectre of graft occlusion. Pleuritic pain may be due to chest wall causes or pericardial inflammation, as occurs in the *postpericardiotomy syndrome.*

Aortic and esophageal problems are important etiologies of chest pain. *Acute aortic dissection* produces a tearing, severe, sudden pain that often radiates to the back between the shoulder blades. *Esophageal reflux* of gastric contents gives a retrosternal burning sensation brought on by consuming a large meal, lying down, or bending over; it is lessened by antacids. *Esophageal spasm* may simulate ischemic pain in that it is substernal, may radiate to the neck, shoulder, or arm, and is often relieved by nitroglycerin. It may occur with meals or acid reflux or come on spontaneously. Atypical pain due to *biliary tract disease* may also mimic angina, for it can present substernally and respond to nitroglycerin. On rare occasions, pancreatitis or peptic ulcer disease produces substernal chest pain. Occasionally, a patient with gaseous distention of the bowel in the area of the splenic flecture may present with discomfort in the left upper quadrant and precordium.

Anxiety, depression, cardiac neurosis, and malingering are the major psychogenic sources of chest pain. Patients with *anxiety* or *depression* describe a "heaviness" or "tightness" in the chest that lasts for hours to days. This sensation may be accompanied by a feeling of inability to take a deep breath. When there is associated hyperventilation, the re-

sulting hypocapnia leaves the patient lightheaded and tingling. *Cardiac neurosis* sometimes leads to reports of pain that are hard to distinguish from genuine angina; at other times the patient misinterprets a noncardiac chest pain. *Malingering* is characterized by a conscious effort to feign illness to obtain secondary gain. Although other forms of psychogenic chest pain may bring secondary benefits to the patient, there is no premeditated attempt to deceive.

DIFFERENTIAL DIAGNOSIS

The differential diagnosis of chest pain can be organized along anatomic lines, as outlined in Table 14-1.

WORKUP

A careful history remains a most effective means of determining the cause of the patient's chest complaint. For ex-

Table 14-1.   Differential Diagnosis of Chest Pain

I. Chest Wall
  A. Muscular disorders
    1. Muscle spasm (precordial catch syndrome)
    2. Pleurodynia
    3. Muscle strain
  B. Skeletal disorders
    1. Costochondritis (Tietze's syndrome)
    2. Rib fracture
    3. Metastatic disease of bone
    4. Cervical or thoracic spine disease
  C. Neurologic disorders
    1. Herpes zoster infection or postherpetic pain
    2. Nerve root compression
II. Cardiopulmonary
  A. Cardiac disorders
    1. Pericarditis
    2. Myocardial ischemia
    3. Prolapsed mitral valve
  B. Pleuropulmonary disorders
    1. Pleurisy of any etiology
    2. Pneumothorax
    3. Pulmonary embolization with infarction
    4. Pneumonitis
    5. Bronchospasm
III. Aortic
  A. Dissecting aortic aneurysm
IV. Gastrointestinal
  A. Esophageal disorders
    1. Reflux
    2. Spasm
  B. Others
    1. Cholecystitis
    2. Peptic ulcer disease
    3. Pancreatitis
    4. Splenic flecture gas
V. Psychogenic
  A. Anxiety (with or without hyperventilation)
  B. Cardiac neurosis
  C. Malingering
  D. Depression

ample, in a study detailing the prevalence of angiographically confirmed coronary artery disease in almost 5000 patients, the prevalence of disease in persons who gave a history of typical angina was 89%, whereas in people with nonanginal chest pain, the prevalence of coronary disease was 16%. Questioning should emphasize timing and precipitating and alleviating factors. Quality, location, and intensity of pain are notoriously misleading; for example, precordial pain radiating down the left arm is not a highly specific finding. A common pitfall is to provide classic descriptions to the patient who cannot give a crisp account of the complaint. All too often patients will agree to neat descriptions under the duress of a physician's interrogation. Their initial vagueness may have been more useful diagnostically.

A few of the more important pain patterns are worth mentioning in terms of the differential diagnosis each suggests and how one separates one cause from another. Pain brought on by exertion and relieved by rest is indicative of angina; but psychogenic chest pain may also behave in this fashion. With the latter, however, chest complaints are usually accompanied by a host of other noncardiac signs and symptoms (headache, lightheadedness, nervousness, hyperventilation, weakness, sighing, fatigue), and coronary risk factors are often absent. As with variant angina, episodes may come on at rest, but, unlike with angina, they are likely to last from hours to days. Prompt response (within 5 minutes) to sublingual nitroglycerin is not usually seen in psychogenic illness and can be a helpful distinguishing point.

Pain that worsens upon deep inspiration or cough suggests a pleural, pericardial, and chest wall source. Focal tenderness at the site of pain narrows the differential to chest wall disease. Tenderness and swelling at the costochondral or sternochondral junction are characteristic of costochondritis (Tietze's syndrome). Coexistent viral illness and clustering of cases argues for pleurodynia due to Coxsackie infection. In young adults, acute pleuritic pain that resolves upon stretching or taking a very deep breath is virtually diagnostic of the precordial catch syndrome.

Pleuritic pain relieved by leaning forward and occurring in the context of a recent transmural infarction, viral illness, uremia, tuberculosis, or collagen disease points to pericarditis. Pneumothorax should come to mind when pleuritic pain is sudden in onset and accompanied by dyspnea in a patient with emphysema or previous history of pneumothorax. Such pain also requires consideration of pulmonary embolization, especially in a patient at risk for thrombophlebitis (recent surgery, past history of embolization, unilateral leg edema, oral contraceptive use). Pleuritic pain with cough and sputum production may be an indication of pneumonitis with pleural involvement, as in tuberculosis or pneumococcal pneumonia.

Onset of a sudden, maximally severe, tearing chest pain in a patient with hypertension, history of blunt trauma, coarctation, Marfan's syndrome, extensive atherosclerosis, or known thoracic aneurysm should suggest dissecting aneu-

rysm. Pain may radiate to the back with descending aortic involvement. In such cases, a high index of suspicion may be lifesaving.

Chest pain brought on by eating may be due to angina, but esophageal, biliary, pancreatic, and peptic diseases should also enter into consideration. Response to nitroglycerin lessens the likelihood of pancreatic and peptic problems, but esophageal and cystic duct spasms as well as angina are relieved by nitroglycerin. Physical examination and contrast studies are often necessary to identify gastrointestinal causes of chest pain.

The age and sex of the patient are important in guiding workup. A young woman is very unlikely to have coronary disease, and therefore other explanations should be expected and vigorously sought. It is almost never worthwhile to subject a premenopausal female to an extensive evaluation to rule out coronary artery disease unless there are major risk factors present. Mitral valve prolapse is an important consideration in this age group. The patient should be informed of the low likelihood of coronary disease to minimize demand for unnecessary evaluation. The setting of chest pain can be exceedingly helpful. Chest pain following a URI is almost invariably due to cough-induced trauma or bronchospasm. Chest discomfort associated with fever and nonspecific viral symptoms is most likely due to pleurisy, pericarditis, or a viral pneumonia. Chest pain following unusual physical activity such as moving, a new athletic endeavor, or exercise suggests musculoskeletal etiologies. Pain that is exacerbated by movement of the arms or shoulders is almost definitely related to musculoskeletal abnormalities.

Physical examination deserves careful attention. General appearance can be telling. An anxious, sighing, hyperventilating individual should be readily noticeable, as should the person in respiratory distress or extreme pain. Vital signs should be checked for fever, tachypnea, and tachycardia. Pressure needs to be taken in both arms in a patient with a suspected aortic dissection. The skin should be noted for cyanosis, herpetic rash, pallor, jaundice, and xanthomas. Examination of the fundi may provide evidence of atherosclerotic, diabetic, or hypertensive disease. Carotid pulse is palpated for delay in upstroke, suggesting hemodynamically significant aortic stenosis, a treatable cause of angina (see Chapter 25).

The chest wall is examined for signs of herpes and trauma, as well as for focal tenderness and swelling. If pain is elicited, it is important to ascertain that the pain on palpation is identical to that complained of previously. One should listen for a pleural rub on inspiration and expiration and observe for signs of consolidation and effusion. Hyperresonance, absent breath sounds, and tracheal deviation from the midline point to a large pneumothorax that requires immediate attention.

In the cardiac examination, a three-component rub is indicative of pericarditis, but it is often evanescent. An S_4

and paradoxically split S_2 may accompany the chest pain of angina. A midsystolic click and late systolic murmur are evidence of a prolapsed mitral valve. Abdominal examination should focus on palpation of the right upper quadrant and epigastrium for tenderness and masses. Legs require careful examination for unilateral edema and other signs of phlebitis (see Chapter 30). Neurologic examination needs to include a careful look at the cervical and thoracic spine and extremities for focal tenderness and motor and sensory deficits.

Test selection should be based on the working differential diagnosis constructed from history and physical; routinely ordering a chest x-ray and an ECG on every patient with chest pain is wasteful and potentially misleading. However, if a patient insists on having an x-ray or ECG, the test is probably worth obtaining for the reassurance it may provide.

SUSPECTED ANGINA. It is important to keep in mind that the *resting ECG* and even the *exercise stress test* are often normal in patients with coronary disease (see Chapter 31). Moreover, there is a high incidence of false-positive stress tests among women who complain of chest pain; many have normal coronary vessels. The addition of *thallium scintigraphy* to the exercise stress test may be helpful. Exercise stress thallium imaging is highly sensitive and, when used discerningly in patients with equivocal or positive electrocardiographic findings during exercise, may also improve specificity of the combined procedures (see Chapter 31).

Other noninvasive tests have been used in the attempt to confirm or deny a cardiac etiology of chest pain. *Cardiac ultrasonography* is useful in suspected mitral valve prolapse, especially in a young woman with a click and atypical chest pain. ST-segment monitoring during continuous ambulatory electrocardiograms and estimation of left ventricular function during exercise radionuclide ventriculography have been shown to have high false-positive rates; their low specificity limits their clinical value.

Pain of gastrointestinal origin, due either to acid reflux into the esophagus, disordered esophageal motility including spasm, or both, is sometimes difficult to distinguish from cardiac pain. As many as 20% of patients with pain so characteristic of myocardial ischemia that it prompted coronary care unit admission have been shown to have esophageal disorders. A trial of antacid therapy can sometimes help identify an esophageal etiology. The *esophageal acid perfusion (Bernstein) test* and esophageal manometry, with or without attempts to provoke spasm, may be advisable as an alternative to coronary angiography when noninvasive tests to detect coronary disease have been unrevealing (see Chapter 56).

In the occasional instance when noninvasive testing and clinical data are inconclusive and coronary disease must be ruled out, it may be necessary to resort to *coronary angiography*. When coronary arteries are without significant occlusive disease, spasm must be considered. It may be advisable

for the angiographer to attempt to provoke spasm with small incremental doses of ergonovine. However, attempts to induce vasospasm are not without risk and should be performed only in the catheterization laboratory by those experienced in the technique.

PLEURITIC PAIN. Patients with pleuritic pain should have a *chest x-ray.* In a study of 97 young patients (ages 18 to 40) with pleuritic chest pain, the combination of history, physical examination, and chest film identified 95% of cases of proven embolization. The most frequent x-ray finding in cases of embolization was a unilateral effusion. When history and physical findings were used alone, the detection rate for embolization was 80%. When *lung scan* was added after the chest x-ray, there was only a 5% improvement in detection rate, but the scan did substantially reduce the number of false-positive diagnoses from 39% after history, physical and x-ray to 16% after scan. Other studies have shown that a normal scan virtually rules out the diagnosis of clinically significant embolism, but high false-positive rates have been reported, especially in those with preexisting lung disease and in the elderly. The addition of ventilation scanning has not resolved the problem. *Arterial blood gases* are insensitive and are often no help in identifying patients with pulmonary emboli.

Thus, history, physical examination, and chest x-ray can be used to identify patients who might have an embolism and require further assessment. If the patient is young and free of underlying lung disease, a scan can reduce the number of false-positive diagnoses. If the patient is elderly or has underlying lung disease, the scan is unlikely to be sufficiently specific; angiography without prior scanning is urged by some experts, especially if the considerable risk of anticoagulant therapy is high and a definitive diagnosis is needed before commencing treatment. The utility of an ECG in patients with suspected embolus is marginal. The electrocardiographic findings of acute right heart strain, $S_1Q_3T_3$, are helpful if present, but sensitivity is low and a normal ECG certainly does not rule out the diagnosis. Likewise, serum enzymes are insensitive and of little use.

The chest x-ray may also reveal pneumonitis. Pneumococcal pneumonia and tuberculosis often present with acute pleuritic chest pain and may be mistaken clinically for pulmonary embolism. Consequently, any patient with pleuritic pain and sputum production should have both *Gram* and *acid-fast stains* made. A pleural effusion may also be detected on chest film. Any nonloculated pleural effusion of unknown etiology should be tapped, Gram-stained, cultured, examined microscopically, and sent for cell count, glucose, lactic dehydrogenase (LDH), and protein determinations (see Chapter 39).

Suspicion of pneumothorax is an indication for a chest film, but if x-ray is not immediately available and the patient is in respiratory distress, decompression should not be delayed. Chest x-ray is also helpful in the diagnosis of aortic dissection; but if this condition is suspected, emergency admission and angiography are indicated; delaying admission to obtain a chest film is unwise.

When pericarditis is under consideration, an *ECG* is essential. However, the ECG changes of early repolarization, a harmless finding seen in young men, may closely resemble those of acute pericarditis. The presence of concave ST segment elevations in both limb and precordial leads and the presence of PR segment depressions in the precordial leads, if they occur in the limb leads, distinguish pericarditis from early repolarization. *Cardiac ultrasonography* may reveal a pericardial effusion. An ANA, BUN, and tuberculin skin test are indicated when the cause of pericariditis is not readily evident.

OTHER CONDITIONS. Only a few musculoskeletal disorders require chest x-ray: suspected rib fractures and cervical or thoracic spine disease. If a gastrointestinal etiology is suspected, a contrast study may be in order. The ECG may show T-wave depression in cholecystitis and pancreatitis and may mistakenly be interpreted as evidence of coronary disease.

The anxious patient with psychogenic pain may find a chest x-ray and/or electrocardiogram reassuring. In most instances, however, a thorough history and careful physical examination combined with a detailed explanation should suffice. Repeating tests "just to be sure" may begin to undermine the patient's confidence in the physician's explanation and even heighten anxiety, especially if there are repeat studies.

It is important to realize that as many as 10% to 15% of cases remain undiagnosed, even after careful and thorough evaluation. Nevertheless, in such instances it is still possible to rule out the presence of an acutely serious etiology. Most patients with chest pain that initially eludes diagnosis can be followed expectantly for the time being.

SYMPTOMATIC RELIEF

Relief of pain must be based on an etiologic diagnosis. To simply suppress the pain with analgesics or sedatives before a diagnosis is made may hide important clues. However, musculoskeletal forms of chest pain may require analgesia. When the diagnosis of costochondritis is certain, local injection with lidocaine into the point of maximal tenderness can provide dramatic relief. An antacid regimen and other antireflux and acid-reducing measures are helpful in patients with esophagitis (see Chapter 56). Nitrates and calcium channel blockers are sometimes of benefit to patients with esophageal spasm (see Chapter 57).

PATIENT EDUCATION

A careful and thorough explanation is essential to avoid precipitating a cardiac neurosis or unnecessary visits to several physicians for evaluation of chest pain. Patients making many visits usually harbor unexplored concerns that have not been adequately addressed in an open and detailed explanation. Discussion of concerns can be extremely reassuring and comforting to the patient and family; this must not be overlooked when workup reveals a benign etiology.

A.G.M. and A.H.G.

ANNOTATED BIBLIOGRAPHY

Armstrong WF, Morris SN: The ST segment during ambulatory electrocardiographic monitoring. Ann Intern Med 98:249, 1983 (*An editorial pointing out the many causes of ST-segment depression on Holter monitoring and the limited value of this test for the diagnosis of coronary disease.*)

Branch WT, McNeil BJ: Analysis of the differential diagnosis and assessment of pleuritic chest pain in young adults. Am J Med 75: 671, 1983 (*Analysis of previously published series of 97 patients with pleuritic chest pain with recommended diagnostic approach.*)

Davies HA, Jones DB, Rhodes J: Esophageal angina as the cause of chest pain. JAMA 248:2274, 1982 (*Of 77 patients presenting to the emergency room with anginal pain, 20% were demonstrated to have esophageal abnormalities as the explanation.*)

De Caestecker JS et al: The oesophagus as a cause for recurrent chest pain: Which patient should be investigated and which test should be used. Lancet 2:1143, 1985 (*Intensive study of 50 patients with recurrent chest pain and no cardiac involvement revealed oesophagus abnormalities in 60%.*) (*Endoscopy was useful for detecting esophagitis; ambulatory pH monitoring was the most sensitive test.*)

Diamond GA, Forrester JS: Analysis of probability as an aid in the clinical diagnosis of coronary artery disease. N Engl J Med 300: 1350, 1979 (*Provides data on probability of coronary disease by history and laboratory studies.*)

Epstein SE, Gerber LH, Borer JS: Chest wall syndrome. JAMA 241: 2793, 1979 (*A detailed description of 12 patients seen at the NIH, including a description of the physical maneuvers that might elicit the pain of chest wall syndrome.*)

Goldman L, Lee TH: Noninvasive tests for diagnosing the presence and extent of coronary artery disease. J Gen Intern Med 1:258, 1986 (*A rigorous analytic review of exercise electrocardiography, thallium scintigraphy, and radionuclide ventriculography.*)

Hoffman JR, Igarashi E: Influence of electrocardiographic findings on admission decisions in patients with acute chest pain. Am J Med 79:699, 1985 (*The electrocardiogram added nothing to the history and physical in determining which patient should be admitted from the emergency room.*)

Kayser HL: Tietze's syndrome—A literature review. Am J Med 21: 982, 1956 (*Points out the often epidemic nature of the illness;* best review.)

Kirshenbaum HD, Ockene IS, Alpert JS et al: The spectrum of coronary artery spasm. JAMA 246:354, 1981 (*Emphasizes the variability of clinical presentation of coronary artery spasm and the difficulty of diagnosis.*)

Ockene IS, Shay MJ, Alpert JS et al: Unexplained chest pain in patients with normal coronary arteriograms. N Engl J Med 303: 1249, 1980 (*Patients with chest pain and normal coronary arteries often remain symptomatically limited despite anatomic reassurance.*)

Robin ED: Overdiagnosis and overtreatment of pulmonary embolism. Ann Intern Med 87:775, 1977 (*A critical discussion of the shortcomings of methods of diagnosis of pulmonary embolism; argues that lung scan should be limited to ruling out embolism in young patients and that arterial blood gases are of no help.*)

Rozanski A, Diamond GA, Berman D et al: The declining specificity of exercise radionuclide ventriculography. N Engl J Med 309: 518, 1983 (*Documents the very low specificity, approximately 20%, which represents a dramatic decline from earlier estimates. This decline can be explained by pretest and post-test referral bias.*)

Spodnick DH: Differential characteristics of the electrocardiogram in early repolarization and acute pericarditis. N Engl J Med 295: 523, 1976 (*Presents data suggesting that one can differentiate between the two based on location and occurrence of ST and PR segment changes.*)

Wasserman AG, Katz RJ, Varghese PJ et al: Exercise radionuclide ventriculographic responses in hypertensive patients with chest pain. N Engl J Med 311:1276, 1984 (*Exercise radionuclide ventriculography proved to be neither sensitive nor specific for arteriographic coronary disease among patients with chest pain.*)

15
Evaluation of the Systolic Murmur

Systolic murmurs are frequently noted in otherwise asymptomatic patients. Most are harmless, but it is important to identify those that may represent hemodynamically significant lesions and thus require more extensive evaluation such as cardiac ultrasonography, fluoroscopy, and catheterization. In most cases, one should be able to make the initial assessment in the office by a careful history and cardiac examination supplemented by chest x-ray and ECG.

PATHOPHYSIOLOGY AND CLINICAL PRESENTATION

Systolic murmurs can be divided into two broad groups: *ejection murmurs,* midsystolic and crescendo–decrescendo in character and usually emanating from the aortic and pulmonic valve areas; and *regurgitation murmurs,* which are holosystolic or occur early or late in systole, and usually result from the backflow of blood through incompetent mitral or tricuspid valves. Ejection murmurs are common and do not always indicate underlying disease.

Ejection Murmurs

"Physiologic" murmurs occur when there is increased ejection velocity across a normal valve creating turbulence. Causes of increased velocity include fever, anemia, pregnancy, hyperthyroidism, exercise, and conditions associated with a large stroke volume (*e.g.,* aortic regurgitation, bradycardia, atrial septal defect). Dilation of the aorta, as in hypertension or aging, may also produce a flow murmur by causing turbulent flow in the dilated segment.

"Innocent" murmurs occur in normal hearts under resting conditions. The origin of such murmurs is a subject of debate, with recent evidence pointing to the aortic root. Since there is no obstruction in the outflow tract, the murmur reflects the normal ejection pattern of blood from the ventricles and is early systolic and crescendo–decrescendo. Because chamber pressures are normal, there is normal splitting of heart sounds. Valves are normal; there are no adventitious sounds or other murmurs.

Early *aortic* and *pulmonic valve disease* may produce murmurs identical to physiologic ones, except that the former are often accompanied by ejection clicks. If outflow tract obstruction increases, the murmur will usually become louder and more prolonged, and peak intensity will occur later in systole. In pulmonic stenosis, the murmur increases with inspiration, and the pulmonic component of the second sound is delayed as disease progresses.

Atrial septal defects (*ASD*) produce physiologic murmurs due to increased right ventricular stroke volume. However, unlike other physiologic murmurs, there is often wide and fixed splitting of the second sound due to left-to-right shunting of blood and a delay in right ventricular ejection.

Asymmetric septal hypertrophy (*ASH*) produces an ejection quality murmur that is affected by the size of the left ventricular cavity. Any maneuver that decreases blood flow to the left ventricle (*e.g.,* Valsalva) will increase the degree of obstruction and make the murmur louder. When there is marked obstruction, the murmur lasts through most of systole and its peak is delayed beyond midsystole.

Patients with physiologic or innocent murmurs are generally asymptomatic from a cardiac standpoint and usually have no previous history of heart disease. Patients with mild varieties of aortic or pulmonic stenosis, ASH, or a small ASD may be asymptomatic as well. Only in later stages of these illnesses do patients begin to complain of dyspnea on exertion, fatigue, etc. Symptoms may not develop until the problem is far advanced, as in aortic stenosis (see Chapter 28).

Regurgitant Murmurs

Regurgitant murmurs are associated with some abnormality of the mitral or tricuspid valves, but the underlying valvular incompetence may be mild or transient and of no clinical significance. Holosystolic murmurs and hemodynamically significant regurgitation are usually associated with *rheumatic heart disease,* dilated valve rings secondary to dilated *cardiomyopathy,* or dysfunction of the valve apparatus due to *myxomatous degeneration* of a chordae tendineae or *ischemia* and infarction of a papillary vessel. A *ventricular septal defect* may also explain a holosytolic murmur.

Far more common is *mitral valve prolapse* (MVP) with its late systolic murmur, most often preceded by a click; the redundant mitral valve leaflets prolapse into the atrium during late systole. Patients with the click and late murmur of mitral valve prolapse often have no other signs or symptoms of heart disease. Mitral valve prolapse appears to be more common among women than men; for one study 17% of healthy female volunteers had auscultatory findings, and 21% had echocardiographic findings of mitral valve prolapse (10% had both; 28% had one or the other). Other studies have suggested a prevalence of auscultatory findings of 5% to 10%. Asthenic builds in both men and women have been associated with MVP, as has small breast size in women. Nonspecific T-wave changes, particularly inferior lead T-wave inversion, have been described.

DIFFERENTIAL DIAGNOSIS

The differential diagnosis can be listed according to the underlying pathophysiology. Thus, systolic ejection murmurs can be classified as innocent, physiologic, aortic, and pulmonic. Regurgitant murmurs may be caused by incompetence of the mitral or tricuspid valves or a ventricular septal defect (Table 15-1).

WORKUP

The primary physician needs to separate cases that require extensive investigation from those that do not, on the basis of a careful history, physical examination, ECG, and chest x-ray. Patients suspected of having correctable, hemodynamically significant lesions often require further noninvasive study and cardiac consultation. In an occasional case, cardiac catheterization is indicated, for example, the asymptomatic athlete with suspected tight aortic stenosis.

The first step in evaluation is to distinguish the systolic ejection murmur from systolic regurgitant murmurs. Timing, quality, and location are the most helpful features. Ejection quality murmurs are crescendo–decrescendo, harsh, are best heard with the bell, are usually loudest at the base, and radiate into the neck and down to the apex. In some patients, the murmur may be higher-pitched and maximal at the apex, as

Table 15-1. Differential Diagnosis of Systolic Ejection Murmur

1. Innocent Murmurs
2. Physiologic Murmurs
   a. Exercise or emotion
   b. Fever
   c. Anemia
   d. Hyperthyroidism
   e. Conditions with large stroke volumes: atrial septal defect, aortic regurgitation, bradycardia
   f. Pregnancy
3. Aortic Murmurs
   a. Aortic stenosis
   b. Asymmetric septal hypertrophy
   c. Sub- and supravalvular fixed stenoses
4. Pulmonic Murmurs
   a. Pulmonic stenosis
5. Mitral Regurgitation Murmurs
   a. Rheumatic mitral insufficiency
   b. Mitral valve prolapse syndrome
   c. Congenital mitral valve disease
   d. Rupture of chordae tendinea
   e. Papillary muscle dysfunction
   f. Left atrial myxoma
   g. Dilated mitral valve ring
6. Tricuspid Regurgitation Murmurs
   a. Rheumatic tricuspid insufficiency
   b. Dilated tricuspid valve ring
7. Ventricular Septal Defect

in elderly people with aortic stenosis. The systolic murmurs of mitral and tricuspid regurgitation are characteristically high-pitched, well localized to the apex or left sternal border (unless very loud) and pansystolic or late systolic. A midsystolic click may precede the regurgitant murmur of mitral valve prolapse.

Perhaps the most valuable characteristic distinguishing ejection murmurs from regurgitant murmurs is the varying intensity of ejection murmurs with changes in cardiac cycle length. Although ejection murmurs increase markedly with cycle length, regurgitant murmurs change slightly, if at all.

Systolic Ejection Murmurs. Here, one must separate innocent and physiologic ejection murmurs from those due to significant aortic and pulmonic outflow tract obstructions and atrial septal defects. The former are usually midrange in frequency, less than 3/6 in intensity, peak in early systole, stop long before S_2, are heard best at the base, and can radiate to neck and apex. Valsalva maneuvers and standing decrease their intensity. The second sound is normally split; there are no clicks, heaves, S_3S_4, or other murmurs. The ECG and chest x-ray are normal. Signs of anemia, fever, hyperthyroidism, and anxiety should be sought.

The murmurs due to atrial septal defect and hemodynamically insignificant aortic and pulmonic stenoses may resemble physiologic murmurs. However, in most cases of ASD, there is widened and fixed splitting of S_2, and in over

90%, there is a conduction defect of the right bundle branch type producing a QRS and lead V_1 with an RSR' configuration. A normal ECG and normal splitting of S_2 make an ASD unlikely. When one is in doubt, an echocardiogram can be used to look for abnormal septal motion and right ventricular enlargement; a normal study rules out the diagnosis.

Mild aortic stenosis in the young patient may be impossible to distinguish from a physiologic murmur; the presence of an ejection click is an important clue to the former. As severity progresses, the murmur gets louder, a thrill becomes palpable, and the carotid upstroke is delayed. (In the elderly, the upstroke may be normal because of a loss of vessel compliance.) As stenosis progresses, the murmur tends to peak later in systole; however; this does not always occur. Left ventricular enlargement may begin to develop on chest film, and signs of hypertrophy appear on ECG. The absence of these findings does not rule out serious aortic stenosis (see Chapter 28). In older patients, the degree of valve calcification corresponds roughly to the severity of stenosis. Cardiac fluoroscopy and echocardiogram are useful for detection of valve calcification. Doppler study aids determination of gradient.

In asymmetric septal hypertrophy, the systolic ejection murmur peaks around midsystole, which helps distinguish it from an innocent murmur. Moreover, it is usually heard most clearly along the left sternal border, often increases with Valsalva maneuvers and standing, and decreases with squatting. The carotid upstroke is brisk and sometimes bisferiens in quality. The echocardiogram is diagnostic.

Hemodynamically significant pulmonic stenosis is suggested by wide splitting or absence of the pulmonic component of the second heart sound, an ejection click that decreases with inspiration, a prolonged and loud murmur (greater than 3/6 that may increase with inspiration, evidence of pulmonary artery dilation on chest film, and prominent R-wave in V_1 indicative of right ventricular hypertrophy. A normal ECG and an early systolic murmur rule out significant pulmonic stenosis. Mild hemodynamically insignificant pulmonic stenosis may be indistinguishable from an innocent murmur, but no therapy is indicated (other than the need for dental prophylaxis), and therefore misdiagnosis is of little consequence.

In summary, the key components of the initial evaluation of the systolic ejection murmur in the asymptomatic patient include attention to carotid upstroke, second sound, clicks, the quality, timing, intensity and location of the murmur, the effects of provocative maneuvers, ECG, and chest x-ray.

Regurgitant Murmurs. Here, duration and timing during systole are helpful distinguishing characteristics. Holosystolic murmurs are usually due to mitral insufficiency, tricuspid insufficiency, or a ventricular septal defect. The murmur of *mitral insufficiency* is first heard at the apex and radiates laterally into the axilla; it varies little with cycle length or with respiration. The murmur of *tricuspid insufficiency* is usually best heard at the lower left sternal border, but when

the right ventricle is very large, it may be heard at the apex. It does not radiate well to the axilla. Intensity is strongly influenced by respiration, increasing at the beginning of inspiration and fading during early expiration. The murmur of *ventricular septal defect* is best heard at the sternal border and does not radiate to the axilla. Intensity does not vary with respiration. It often has some midsystolic accentuation and may be confused with an ejection murmur.

Early systolic murmurs are relatively rare. The classic explanation is a ventricular septal defect small enough to close during systole with the decrease in ventricular size. Much more common is the late systolic murmur, often introduced by a midsystolic click, that signifies *mitral valve prolapse.*

When the auscultatory findings are considered in the context of the history, the remainder of the physical examination, ECG, and chest x-ray, the etiology and hemodynamic significance of the murmur may be apparent. Rheumatic heart disease or the dilated valve ring of dilated congestive cardiomyopathy should be evident. Hepatojugular reflux has been shown to be a highly specific sign of tricuspid regurgitation. A history of angina or MI, or the ECG findings of anteroseptal myocardial infarction may suggest papillary muscle dysfunction.

An *echocardiogram* can confirm the diagnosis of mitral valve prolapse with high sensitivity and specificity. Such confirmation should, however, be obtained discriminatingly. An echocardiogram is not necessary in the asymptomatic patient with auscultatory findings typical of click murmur syndrome. Echocardiographic documentation is advisable when atypical chest pain, palpitations, or other symptoms are associated with click murmur findings, particularly when therapy (other than endocarditis prophylaxis) is contemplated.

PATIENT EDUCATION

If the murmur is determined to be innocent, it is essential to provide careful explanation and reassurance. Anxiety may be precipitated by repeated auscultation and laboratory work that focuses on the heart. Excessive workup, if left unexplained, can lead to unnecessary concern and self-restriction of activity. Reassurance should include a discussion of the cause of the murmur and emphasize that other forms of heart disease have been ruled out. The patient with a harmless murmur should be specifically told that there is no need to restrict activity or undergo further evaluation at the present time.

Counseling is particularly important for the patient with *mitral valve prolapse.* Much uncertainty remains about the prognostic significance of MVP. Progression to hemodynamically significant mitral regurgitation, eventually requiring valve replacement, has been described but must be rare. An association with rhythm disturbances and sudden death has been described, but it is not clear that any increased risk of sudden death applies to the vast majority of asymptomatic people with MVP. Those with such worrisome findings as complex ventricular ectopic activity, prolonged QT intervals, ECG abnormalities, history of syncope, or family history of sudden death may be at increased risk. When these findings are present, specific therapy may be indicated (see Chapter 24). The patient with isolated MVP should be reassured. MVP has also been associated with transient cerebrovascular events and stroke, suggesting that the redundant mitral valve may be a source of emboli. Such events are, however, extremely rare. Anticoagulation is not currently advised for patients with MVP in the absence of other risk factors. MVP does confer some increased risk of infective endocarditis, and most clinicians agree that antibiotic prophylaxis is indicated for procedures likely to cause bacteremia (see Chapter 11).

A.G.M. and A.H.G.

ANNOTATED BIBLIOGRAPHY

Barnett HJM, Boughner DR, Taylor DW et al.: Further evidence relating mitral valve prolapse to cerebral ischemic events. N Engl J Med 302:139, 1980

Burde GD, DePasquale NP: Electrocardiography in the Diagnosis of Congenital Heart Disease. Philadelphia, Lea & Febringer, 1967 (*Describes right bundle branch pattern in patients with ASD.*)

Cheitlin MD, Byrd RC: The click murmur syndrome. JAMA 245: 1357, 1981 (*Reviews the epidemiology, etiology, and clinical significance; offers explicit management recommendations.*)

Devereaux RB, Brown WT, Kramer-Fox R et al: Inheritance of mitral valve prolapse. Ann Intern Med 97:826, 1982 (*Pedigrees of 45 probands with mitral valve prolapse suggest that the condition has autosomal dominant inheritance with age- and sex-dependent expression.*)

Epstein, SE et al: Asymmetric septal hypertrophy. Ann Intern Med 81:650, 1974 (*A detailed discussion of ASH, including clinical findings; 67 references.*)

Finegam RE, Gianelly RD, Harrison DC: Aortic stenosis in the elderly: Relevance of age to diagnosis and treatment. N Engl J Med 281:1261, 1969 (*Physical findings such as carotid upstroke and quality and location of the murmur may be misleading in assessing aortic stenosis in the elderly.*)

Maisel AS, Atwood JE, Goldberger AL: Hepatojugular reflux: Useful in the bedside diagnosis of tricuspid regurgitation. Ann Intern Med 101:781, 1984 (*Hepatojugular reflux had a specificity of 100% and a sensitivity of 66% in detecting tricuspid regurgitation. An increase in murmur intensity with deep inspiration was as specific and more sensitive.*)

Rosenberg CA, Derman GH, Grabb WC: Hypomastia and mitral-valve prolapse. N Engl J Med 309:1230, 1983 (*A report of an association between small breast size in women and mitral valve prolapse.*)

Stein PD, Sabbah H: Aortic origin of innocent murmur. Am J Cardiol 39:665, 1977 (*Presents extensive data for the aortic origin of innocent murmurs.*)

Tavel ME: The systolic murmur—innocent or guilty. Am J Cardiol 39:757, 1977 (*An editorial arguing that evaluation of the systolic murmur can be done without resorting to invasive procedures.*)

16
Evaluation of Leg Edema

Leg swelling can be a bothersome problem as well as an initial symptom of important underlying disease. Many suffer from chronic venous insufficiency, but occasionally the cause of the swelling is acute deep vein thrombophlebitis, nephrotic syndrome, or another serious condition. Accurate determination of etiology is essential if the clinician is to avoid such common mistakes as treating edema in elderly persons with digitalis when the actual cause is venous disease.

PATHOPHYSIOLOGY AND CLINICAL PRESENTATION

Edema is defined as an increase in extracellular volume. It develops if hydrostatic pressure exceeds colloid oncotic pressure, capillary permeability increases, or lymphatic drainage becomes impaired. Hydrostatic pressure is a function of intravascular volume, blood pressure, and venous outflow. Colloid oncotic pressure is dependent on the serum albumin concentration.

Decreased oncotic pressure is usually due to hypoalbuminemia, which can occur secondary to malnutrition, he-

patocellular failure, or excess renal or gastrointestinal loss of albumin. The resultant fall in intravascular volume from excessive transudation of fluid stimulates salt retention. This compensatory effort to maintain adequate intravascular volume leads to further edema formation because the underlying oncotic deficit remains. Edema sets in when the serum albumin concentration falls below 2.5 g per 100 ml. Leg swelling due to hypoalbuminemia is typically bilateral, pitting, and sometimes accompanied by edema of the face and eyelids (especially upon awakening).

Increased hydrostatic pressure may result from excessive fluid retention (such as is seen with congestive heart failure) or impairment of venous outflow. A localized increase in hydrostatic pressure develops in the legs during prolonged standing, especially if the valves in the leg veins are incompetent. Increased hydrostatic pressure due to fluid retention produces bilaterally symmetrical edema, whereas swelling due to venous insufficiency may be asymmetrical and accompanied by varicosities and other signs of venous disease (see Chapter 30). At times, the only sign of deep vein thrombophlebitis is an acutely swollen leg. Unilateral lower leg edema can also result from venous compression by, or rupture of, a popliteal (Baker's) cyst. A stroke that causes paresis in one leg may result in unilateral edema due to reductions in vascular tone and venous and lymphatic drainage; thrombophlebitis may ensue.

Increased capillary permeability can occur with immunologic injury, infection, inflammation, or trauma. A permeability defect is also believed to be responsible for *idiopathic edema,* a poorly understood but common problem seen almost exclusively in women. Although some patients report a periodicity to the problem that seems to parallel the menstrual cycle, careful studies have failed to find sufficient evidence to warrant the label "cyclic edema." The condition is especially aggravated by hot weather and standing, more so than occurs with venous insufficiency. Transient abdominal distention is common, and weight may fluctuate several pounds over the course of the day. The disorder is not progressive, but it can cause considerable discomfort. It is often accompanied by headache, fatigue, anxiety, and other functional symptoms. Some patients are bothered by nocturia.

Lymphatic obstruction hinders reabsorption of interstitial fluid. The swelling usually starts in the feet and progresses upward; often the problem is unilateral. The edema of lymphatic obstruction tends to have a brawny quality and evidences little pitting, except in its early stages. Recumbency provides only minor relief compared with edema from other causes.

DIFFERENTIAL DIAGNOSIS

The differential diagnosis of edema can be organized according to clinical presentations and pathophysiologic mechanisms (Table 16-1). Certain infiltrative conditions may be mistaken for edema, such as pretibial myxedema and lipedema (a familial, bilateral deposition of excess fat).

WORKUP

History. The distribution of the swelling should be ascertained from the patient. If edema is predominantly unilateral, the patient ought to be questioned about risk factors for thrombophlebitis such as use of oral contraceptives, recent surgery, previous phlebitis, and prolonged inactivity. Inquiry into recent injury, redness, tenderness, or fever may prove productive. If the edema is bilateral, it is important to check for a history of dyspnea on exertion, orthopnea, ascites, jaundice, proteinuria, chronic kidney disease, malnutrition, varicose veins, chronic diarrhea, rash and use of salt-retaining drugs such as corticosteroids, and estrogens. Antihypertensive drugs, including methyldopa and nifedipine, and nonsteroidal anti-inflammatory drugs, especially ibuprofen, have also been

Table 16-1.   Important Causes of Leg Edema

I. Unilateral or Asymmetric Swelling
  A. Increased hydrostatic pressure
    1. Deep vein thrombophlebitis
    2. Venous insufficiency
    3. Popliteal (Baker's) cyst
  B. Increased capillary permeability
    1. Cellulitis
    2. Trauma
  C. Lymphatic obstruction (local)
II. Bilateral Swelling
  A. Decreased oncotic pressure
    1. Malnutrition
    2. Hepatocellular failure
    3. Nephrotic syndrome
    4. Protein-losing enteropathy
  B. Increased hydrostatic pressure
    1. Congestive heart failure
    2. Renal failure
    3. Use of salt-retaining drugs (*e.g.,* corticosteroids, estrogens)
    4. Venous insufficiency
    5. Menstruation
    6. Pregnancy
  C. Increased capillary permeability
    1. Systemic vasculitis
    2. Idiopathic edema
    3. Allergic reactions
  D. Lymphatic obstruction (retroperitoneal or generalized)

associated with dependent edema. A report of acute facial swelling suggests an allergic reaction or hypoalbuminemia if the swelling is more chronic.

Physical examination should be used to detail the extent of the edema. Careful measurements of calf and thigh diameters can be very helpful. If the swelling is predominantly limited to one leg, the limb ought to be examined for tenderness, redness, increased warmth, varicosities, and a palpable thrombosed vein. Unfortunately, the utility of the physical examination for detection of deep vein thrombophlebitis is limited. The often mentioned signs of deep venous thrombosis—calf tenderness, palpable cord, positive Homan's sign—have not proved to be very sensitive or specific; unilateral edema may be the only clue aside from a suggestive history. It is important to check for pitting; if edema is prominent but pitting is only minimal, it suggests that lymphatic obstruction might be the cause.

The patient with bilateral leg edema should have the blood pressure measured for elevation, especially if there is a history of kidney problems; new onset of hypertension may be a sign of renal failure. The skin is checked for signs of hepatocellular failure (jaundice, spider angiomata, ecchymoses), the jugular veins for distention, the chest for rales and evidence of a pleural effusion, the heart for a third heart sound indicative of failure, the abdomen for masses, ascites, and other manifestations of portal hypertension, and the pelvis for masses. Any lymphadenopathy should be noted.

Laboratory Studies. The patient with unilateral edema may well have venous thrombosis and be at risk for life-threatening pulmonary embolus. Laboratory evaluation must be directed at excluding this condition. The definitive test for the detection of acute deep vein occlusion is the *venogram.* When performed by the experienced radiologist, it is nearly 100% sensitive and specific. A number of noninvasive methods have been developed. These include the iodine 125 (^{125}I) fibrinogen uptake test, measurement of blood velocity using a Doppler ultrasound probe, and impedance plethysmography. The *^{125}I fibrinogen uptake* test detects propagating clot in the calf and lower thigh but is expensive and not widely available. The *Doppler test* is very dependent on the experience of the observer. *Impedance plethysmography* is emerging as the most useful noninvasive approach to the patient with possible thrombophlebitis; it has a specificity of approximately 95% but limited sensitivity, especially for occlusions in the deep veins of the calf. Plethysmography is, therefore, very useful when it is positive. Unless there is a serious contraindication to anticoagulation, therapy in a patient with a positive test can be initiated without resorting to venogram. However, if clinical suspicion of thrombophlebitis is high, a negative result with impedance plethysmography should be followed either by a venogram or by serial plethysmography studies 2 and 4 days after the initial study. Strategies for the use of these tests are discussed further in Chapter 30.

A venogram may also detect the cause of lymphatic obstruction and should be obtained before lymphangiography is attempted in patients in whom lymphatic obstruction is suspected. Severe lymphatic obstruction may interfere with attaining a satisfactory lymphangiogram.

The patient with more generalized edema involving both legs should have a chest film in search of heart failure and pleural fluid, a urinalysis for detection of albuminuria, determinations of the serum creatinine and the BUN for evidence of renal insufficiency, and measurements of the prothrombin time and bilirubin for further documentation of hepatocellular failure. If the serum albumin is low and protein is detected in the urine, a 24-hour urine collection for albumin and creatinine is indicated (see Chapter 128).

PATIENT EDUCATION AND SYMPTOMATIC THERAPY

When edema is due to increased hydrostatic pressure or decreased oncotic pressure, a number of simple measures can provide the patient some symptomatic relief. The patient should be advised to restrict salt intake, avoid prolonged standing or prolonged sitting with the legs dependent, elevate the legs whenever possible, and avoid wearing garments that might restrict venous return (*e.g.,* garters and girdles). Proper support stockings might provide some added benefit. If possible, use of salt-retaining drugs should be discontinued or minimized. Severe edema may require diuretic therapy. (See Chapter 30 for details on therapy of venous insufficiency.) Lymphatic obstruction and increased capillary permeability do not respond well to these measures.

Patients with idiopathic edema are sometimes helped by salt restriction, support hose, elevation, and diuretic use in the early evening. In addition to diuretics, other drugs have been reported to be useful; these include propranolol and captopril. It is important to reassure the patient with this condition that the edema poses no threat to health. Furthermore, idiopathic edema often runs a self-limited course, subsiding spontaneously over a few months to several years.

Patients with chronic leg edema should be instructed to call the physician at the first sign of inflammation or unilateral increase in swelling.

A.G.M. and A.H.G.

ANNOTATED BIBLIOGRAPHY

Coggins CP: Edema. In RS Blackow (ed): Signs and Symptoms. Philadelphia, JB Lippincott, 1977 (*Excellent review of pathophysiology of edema.*)

Cranley JJ, Canos AJ, Sull WJ: The diagnosis of deep vein thrombosis, fallibility of clinical symptoms and signs. Arch Surg 111:34, 1976 (*Classic signs of deep vein thrombosis, muscle pain, tenderness, swelling, and the presence of Homans' sign occurred with approximately equal frequency in people with and without deep vein thrombosis.*)

Galloway JMD: The swollen leg. Practitioner 218:676, 1977 (*A clinically useful review that concentrates on the swollen limb resulting from local vascular problems.*)

Haeger K: Venous and Lymphatic Disorders of the Leg. Philadelphia, JB Lippincott, 1966 (*Detailed discussion of lymphatic obstruction.*)

Huisman MV, Buller HR, Tencate JW et al: Serial impedance plethysmography for suspected deep venous thrombosis in outpatients. N Engl J Med 314:823, 1986 (*Found to be nearly equal to venography for detection of deep venous thrombosis.*)

Ruschhaupt WF: Differential diagnosis of edema at the lower extremities. Cardiovasc Clin 13:307, 1983 (*A comprehensive review.*)

Streeten DHP: Idiopathic edema: Pathogenesis, clinical futures and treatment. Metabolism 27:353, 1978 (*Absolutely comprehensive review of the syndrome of idiopathic edema. All of the etiologic theories are studied with the conclusion that upright posture is an important contributor to excess transudation of fluid in more than 30% of the patients studied. Treatment is suggested, including reducing salt intake, reducing the duration of standing and sitting, and administering diuretic if done at 7 or 8 PM followed by recumbency for several hours; 84 references.*)

17

Evaluation of Arterial Insufficiency of the Lower Extremities

DAVID C. BREWSTER, M.D.

Vascular occlusive disease of the lower extremities is seen with greater frequency as patients continue to live longer and as atherosclerosis becomes more prevalent. Arteriosclerotic occlusive disease is by far the most common cause of arterial insufficiency, although lower extremity ischemia may also be caused by embolism, arterial dissection, trauma, thrombosis of an aneurysm, or other unusual conditions. It is more common in men, and increases in prevalence with age.

Proper clinical management requires the physician first to recognize the manifestation of ischemic disease and carefully evaluate its severity. Many patients with mild to moderate vascular insufficiency may be managed conservatively, whereas others with acute ischemia or more severe chronic ischemia that threatens to cause tissue necrosis require more intensive investigation and often surgery.

The primary physician must be able to differentiate between patients with arterial insufficiency and those with exertional limb pain due to other causes. Moreover, one needs to know the indications for and limitations of the newer non-invasive techniques for evaluating blood flow and the indications for arteriography and surgical referral.

PATHOPHYSIOLOGY AND CLINICAL PRESENTATION

Occlusive disease generally becomes symptomatic by gradual reduction of blood flow to the involved extremity or organ. Symptoms finally occur when a critical arterial stenosis is reached. Pressure and blood flow are not significantly diminished until at least 75% of the cross-sectional area of the vessel lumen is obliterated by the disease process. This is equivalent to approximately a 50% reduction in lumen diameter. More severe stenoses or even total occlusions may remain essentially asymptomatic as long as collateral circulation maintains sufficient blood flow around a lesion to satisfy the metabolic demands of the distal limb at rest and during exercise. Development of ischemic symptoms in the leg implies either inadequate collateral circulation or additional occlusive disease distal to the particular collateral bed. Thus, lesions in the aortoiliac segment may cause little difficulty unless, as is commonly the case, there is associated disease in the femoropopliteal arterial territory.

Arteriosclerotic plaques producing stenosis or occlusion of the arterial lumen are often segmentally distributed, with a predilection to arterial bifurcations. The infrarenal abdominal aorta and aortic bifurcation are common sites of disease, as are the iliac and femoral artery bifurcations. Diabetic patients seem prone to onset of arteriosclerosis at an earlier age, and often have a more distal distribution of occlusive arterial lesions.

The earliest manifestation of impaired arterial circulation is usually *intermittent claudication,* or muscular pain in the leg brought on by exercise and relieved within several minutes by rest. Blood flow is adequate for local metabolic demands at rest but cannot increase sufficiently to meet the increased oxygen demands of the muscle mass resulting from exercise, a situation quite analagous to the pain of angina pectoris. The relatively high resistance across collateral vessel beds limits the required threefold to fourfold increase of blood flow to the exercising leg.

As the severity of the occlusive process worsens, blood flow becomes inadequate for tissue needs even at rest, resulting in the manifestations of more severe arterial insufficiency: "ischemic rest" pain and tissue necrosis (gangrene or ischemic ulceration).

DIFFERENTIAL DIAGNOSIS

Lower extremity ischemia may also be caused by arterial embolism, dissection, trauma, thrombosis of an aneurysm, or thromboangiitis obliterans (Buerger's disease). Other non-vascular conditions may mimic the symptoms of claudication or ischemic rest pain. Pain in the hip, thigh, or knee region with walking is frequently a result of *degenerative disk disease, osteoarthritis* or the hip or knee, or *Paget's disease.* Sciatic or other radicular pain may cause confusion. Various other neurologic or musculoskeletal disorders may be at fault. *Cauda equina compression* by disk, tumor, or spinal canal stenosis produces a well-known "*pseudoclaudication*" syndrome. Such nonvascular causes of pain may be suspected when pain is not clearly related to a predictable amount of exercise and is not promptly relieved by cessation of activity.

Diabetic neuropathy can be difficult to differentiate from ischemic rest pain, particularly in a patient with diminished or absent pulses. In both conditions, a burning constant ache is often present in the forefoot and toes. The presence of paresthesias in addition to pain suggests a neurologic etiology.

True ischemic rest pain is usually worse with elevation, and frequently is relieved somewhat by dependency of the limb. Such features may be used in differentiation. In all such instances, noninvasive studies during exercise may be of substantial help in the differential diagnosis.

WORKUP

The diagnosis of peripheral vascular disease and an accurate assessment of its level and severity may be made by a careful history and physical examination to an extent not possible in many other disease states. The availability of effective treatment for peripheral vascular disease makes it mandatory that early and accurate diagnosis be established before end-stage problems develop, resulting in inevitable limb loss.

History. Intermittent claudication is the hallmark of vascular insufficiency, and a reliable history can be diagnostic. The pain of claudication is usually described as a cramp or ache in the calf or thigh muscles after walking a predictable distance. The location of the pain may help to localize the occlusive process. In some instances of proximal disease, the pain may be located principally in the hip or buttock region, causing confusion with other neuro-orthopedic conditions. The pain should be reproducible by walking a certain distance and should be relieved within minutes of stopping. If the walking distance required to produce the pain varies considerably from day to day, or if the patient must sit or lie down for more than several minutes to obtain relief, the physician should suspect other etiologies. Similarly, the pain should involve the same areas consistently and not different portions of the leg from day to day. Crampy pain occurring in the calf at rest, particularly at night, rarely signifies a vascular problem.

Complaints of *pain at rest* as well as with exercise suggests more advanced ischemia. A history of prior claudication is almost always obtained in such patients unless the distribution of the occlusive process is quite distal or in small vessels only. Ischemic rest pain typically involves the toes or forefoot, not the calf or thigh. It is usually improved with dependency of the limb and therefore is worse at night. Pain that is not confined to the distal foot, that is better with elevation, or that occurs in a patient without intermittent claudication should alert the physician to look for other possible causes, such as diabetic neuropathy or a neuro-orthopedic problem.

Symptoms of tissue necrosis will usually be quite apparent. Peripheral gangrene without prior symptoms should raise the possibility of embolic disease or small vessel occlusions due to conditions other than chronic arteriosclerosis. In patients with leg ulceration, historical clues suggesting a traumatic, dermatologic, or venous etiology should also be sought; many leg and foot ulcers are not ischemic in origin.

A complete history should include questioning for sexual difficulties; erectile impotence, long associated with severe aortoiliac occlusive disease, has been termed the *Leriche syndrome* after the French surgeon who first reported its significance in 1923. Finally, it is of utmost importance to note the existence of known risk factors for arteriosclerosis (family history, smoking, diabetes mellitus, hypertension, lipid disorders—see Chapter 9) as well as related problems in the coronary and cerebrovascular systems indicative of the systemic nature of arteriosclerosis. There is a high prevalence of coronary disease, stroke, and congestive failure in patients with peripheral arterial disease.

Physical Examination can help confirm, localize, and establish the severity of the arterial lesion. *Palpation of peripheral pulses* is the keystone of the examination. Palpation of the abdomen for the aortic pulsation, and of both extremities for femoral, popliteal, posterior tibial, and dorsalis pedis pulses should be routine in all patients. Reduced or absent pulses in the symptomatic region are characteristic of arterial insufficiency. Local factors such as edema or marked obesity may hinder palpation. Abnormally prominent pulsations suggest aneurysmal disease. *Auscultation* of the aortic and groin regions should also be performed, with the finding of *bruits* further supporting the possible existence of arterial occlusive disease. Simple exercise of the patient at the bedside may greatly intensify femoral bruits, and this is occasionally a useful maneuver. The absence of a bruit, however, has little meaning, since marked reduction of flow in a severely stenotic or occluded vessel will not produce a bruit.

Other useful findings are abnormal pallor on elevation of the legs, *rubor on dependency,* and *prolonged capillary filling time* (especially when one leg is compared with the other). Temperature differences and atrophic skin and nail changes are less reliable indicators of chronic arterial insufficiency. Careful spine, hip, knee, and neurologic examinations are important to rule out nonvascular causes of exertional lower extremity pain.

History and physical examination are usually sufficient to establish the diagnosis and provide a rough estimate of severity. In patients with mild to moderate disease and without limb-threatening ischemia or unacceptable activity limitations, no further investigation is necessary other than evaluation for potential risk factors such as smoking, diabetes, hypertension, and hyperlipidemia (see Chapters 32, 100, 8, and 9). Blood sugar determination may detect a previously undiagnosed diabetic, but there is still no firm evidence that tight control of the serum glucose level prevents or ameliorates vascular disease (see Chapter 100).

Noninvasive Vascular Laboratory Studies are indicated when the diagnosis or degree of impairment is uncertain, or when the disease is severe enough to warrant consideration of surgical correction. In recent years, a wide variety of noninvasive testing methods such as Doppler ultrasound have been developed to assess blood flow to the extremities. Many of these methods are widely available, simple to use, relatively inexpensive, and may be used repeatedly without risk or discomfort to the patient. Such tests may be extremely helpful in establishing a vascular etiology for complaints of pain in the leg and in quantifying clinical impressions, which are often somewhat imprecise. Because they can be used repeatedly, such tests are also particularly helpful in evaluating improvement or deterioration of the patient's condition over time and in assessing the benefit of various forms of treatment or operation.

Doppler ultrasound segmental limb pressures combined with *pulse volume recordings* are commonly used noninvasive studies. Sensitivity is improved when treadmill exercise is added to the examination. It should be emphasized that these methods are not meant to replace or lessen the value of a good history and physical examination but rather to supplement them and provide such additional information as site and severity of stenosis.

Arteriography has little place in the diagnostic evaluation of arterial insufficiency, and should rarely be used for such purposes. However, once a decision has been reached for surgical intervention (see Chapter 29), arteriography is indicated. The procedure is generally regarded as indispensible to the surgeon for precise localization of the disease process and proper selection of an operative procedure.

INDICATIONS FOR REFERRAL AND ADMISSION

Patients with rest pain or a nonhealing ischemic ulcer require consideration for surgery and ought to be referred to an experienced vascular surgeon. Patients with severe intermittent claudication that interferes with daily activity may also benefit from a surgical consultation, but often can be managed conservatively (see Chapter 29). Patients with gangrenous lesions of the lower extremities or an infected ischemic ulcer require prompt hospital admission, particularly if they are diabetic.

ANNOTATED BIBLIOGRAPHY

Fairbairn JF II: Clinical manifestations of peripheral vascular disease. In JL Juergens, JA Spittell Jr, JF Fairbairn II (eds): Peripheral Vascular Diseases, 5th ed, pp 3–49. Philadelphia, WB Saunders, 1980 (*A very thorough and complete textbook discussion of the manifestations of vascular disease, differential diagnoses, and methods of evaluation.*)

Goodreau JK, Creasy JK, Flanigan DP et al: Rational approach to the differentiation of vascular and neurogenic claudication. Surgery 84:749, 1978 (*Helpful discussion of diagnostic approach useful in differentiating vascular and nonvascular exercise-related pain.*)

Kempczinski RF: Clinical application of noninvasive testing in extremity arterial insufficiency. In RF Kempczinski, JST Yao (eds): Practical Noninvasive Vascular Diagnosis, pp 343–362. Chicago, Year Book Medical Publishers, 1982 (*A thoughtful discussion of utility and role of noninvasive laboratory studies in management of patients with lower extremity occlusive disease.*)

Pearce WH, Yao JST, Bergan JJ: Noninvasive vascular diagnostic testing. In Current Problems in Surgery. Chicago, Year Book Medical Publishers, August 1983. (*Excellent monograph describing methodology, advantages, and limitations of the wide variety of noninvasive techniques currently available.*)

Strandness DE Jr: Preoperative evaluation of vascular diseases. In H Hamiovici (ed): Vascular Surgery: Principles and Techniques, pp 17–38. New York, McGraw-Hill, 1976 (*Good discussion of the pathophysiology and hemodynamics of acute and chronic arterial occlusive disease, with good reference list.*)

18
Evaluation of Syncope

When confronted with a report of loss of consciousness, the primary physician needs to determine whether the patient has an underlying cardiovascular or seizure disorder that requires prompt attention or a less threatening condition that can be approached in a more leisurely fashion.

PATHOPHYSIOLOGY AND CLINICAL PRESENTATIONS

The pathophysiologic common denominator of circulatory syncope is inadequate cerebral perfusion that does not meet the brain's metabolic demands. Mechanisms that may be responsible include sudden decrease in peripheral vascular resistance, inadequate cardiac output, failure of vasoconstrictive reflexes, and functional or anatomic cerebral vascular occlusion; any number of these may be operative in a given case. Psychoneurologic mechanisms of syncope include hysteria and seizure activity. Metabolic disturbances usually do not result in syncope, though they may alter consciousness.

Vasodepressor syncope (the common faint) accounts for most episodes. Although vagal activity plays some role, and the episode is often labeled "vasovagal," the condition can be induced even when vagal activity is blocked by atropine. In response to an emotionally uncomfortable situation, fight or flight reactions are only partially mobilized. Marked peripheral arterial dilatation takes place, particularly in the muscular bed, resulting in reduced total peripheral vascular resistance. The fall in resistance is not accompanied by a compensatory increase in cardiac output. The failure of the heart to respond is believed to be a function of inadequate filling volume due to a shift of blood to the vascular bed in the muscles, which is outside the central venous reservoir. Perfusion pressure drops over the course of minutes and lightheadedness and syncope then ensue.

The patient experiences premonitory symptoms of sweating, epigastric queasiness, lightheadedness, and pallor. Dilation of the pupils, blurring of vision, yawning and sighing, or hyperventilation occur; the patient feels restless and unable to concentrate. The heart rate is rapid prior to loss of consciousness. By the onset of syncope, the pulse slows due to vagal influence. Shortly afterward, the person regains consciousness but feels weak, sweaty, and nauseated. Control of bladder and bowels is never lost.

Orthostatic hypotension is another cause of reduced cerebral perfusion pressure. Upon standing, reflex vasoconstriction and increase in heart rate fail to occur because of autonomic insufficiency. Hypotension progresses over seconds to a few minutes, until perfusion is inadequate for maintainence of consciousness. During the presyncopal period, there is no change in heart rate, nor do other signs of autonomic response, such as pallor, nausea, or sweating, occur. The period of syncope is brief, and consciousness returns promptly. Near syncope is common among these patients, as are impotence and bladder and bowel disturbances.

Carotid sinus hypersensitivity can cause marked reflex bradycardia and a fall in arterial resistance. Most patients with this condition are elderly and have underlying atherosclerotic heart disease manifested by ischemic changes on electrocardiogram. Massage of the carotid sinus often results in long asystolic pauses. Digitalis administration seems to aggravate the condition. Carotid sinus syncope may also cause a vasodepressor form of syncope in which heart rate remains unchanged. Minor events can trigger symptoms; wearing a tight collar, turning the head, or shaving may cause light headedness, sweating, pallor, and nausea, followed by fainting. When the predominant mechanism is asystole, the loss of consciousness can be precipitous.

Post-tussive syncope is characterized by loss of consciousness that follows a prolonged bout of forceful coughing. Men with chronic bronchitis are most often affected. The mechanism is believed to involve decreased cardiac output due to decreased venous return, increased cerebral vascular resistance secondary to hypocapnia, and compression of cerebral vessels by an increase in cerebrospinal fluid pressure. Prolonged Valsalva maneuvers have a similar effect; the increase in intrathoracic pressure impedes venous return and decreases cardiac output.

Postmicturition syncope takes place in the context of emptying a distended bladder. The typical setting involves a male who has gotten up at night to urinate after consuming considerable amounts of alcohol. Consciousness is lost without much warning. Drainage of ascitic fluid or a distended bladder may produce a similar effect. The mechanism is unknown. Valsalva maneuver and reflex vasodilatation have been implicated.

Cerebral vascular disease leads to syncope only when there is total or near-total occlusion of most major vessels supplying the brain. Lesser degrees of obstruction may contribute to minor lightheadedness upon standing. Patients with substantial cerebrovascular disease often have evidence of previous strokes manifested by focal neurologic deficits.

The subclavian steal syndrome results from occlusion of the proximal subclavian artery, leading to reversal of flow in the adjacent vertebral artery. When vascular resistance in the arm falls, for example, during exercise, flow is redirected away from the brain and ischemic symptoms may ensue.

Effort syncope suggests underlying cardiac disease. Exercise induces peripheral vasodilatation, but cardiac output cannot be increased adequately and syncope results. Severe aortic stenosis and marked asymmetric septal hypertrophy (ASH) obstruct the ventricular outflow tract to a degree sufficient to limit cardiac response to exercise. Total blockade of the mitral orifice from an atrial myxoma and pulmonary hypertension can have similar consequences. Loss of consciousness comes with little warning.

Cardiac arrhythmias and *heart block* may precipitate drop attacks that have none of the premonitory manifestations of vasodepressor syncope. Fewer than 5 seconds of consciousness remain once effective systoles have ceased. Palpitations are sometimes reported, and loss of consciousness can occur while person is supine. Important conditions associated with heart block and/or dysrhythmias include acute ischemia, sick sinus and preexcitation syndromes, prolapsed mitral valve, and digitalis toxicity. It seems that patients with chronic bifascicular and trifascicular block are more likely to have syncopal attacks, but those with syncope have not been found to have an increased risk of sudden death.

Vasovagal syncope refers specifically to instances in which the entire reflex is vagally mediated. Distention of a viscus (as occurs in esophagoscopy) is an example of a vasovagal etiology. Vagal influences also play roles in vasodepressor syncope and carotid sinus hypersensitivity by contributing to bradycardia and suppressing AV node conduction.

Metabolic factors (hypoxia, hyperventilation, hypoglycemia) are more likely to alter consciousness than to cause actual syncope. Restlessness, confusion and anxiety are prominent and precede loss of consciousness. When hyperventilation is responsible, the patient first complains of a smothering or suffocating feeling in conjunction with paresthesias in the limbs and circumorally (see Chapter 222). Syncope may take place while the patient is sitting or lying down. Hypoglycemia rarely causes loss of consciousness (see Chapter 97).

Hysteria produces syncope characterized by graceful fainting to the floor or couch, frequent presence of an audience, normal pulse, skin color and blood pressure, and an emotionally detached description of the episode.

Seizures differ from other causes of syncope in that aura, postictal symptoms, incontinence, and tonic–clonic movements often dominate the clinical picture. However, akinetic petit mal attacks have few of these features, though normal blood pressure and pulse help distinguish them from seizures having cardiovascular etiologies (see Chapter 164).

DIFFERENTIAL DIAGNOSIS

Important causes of syncope are listed in Table 18-1. The most important distinction to be made among possible etiologies is that between cardiac and noncardiac diagnoses. A number of recent studies provide clear evidence that the short-term prognosis for syncope due to underlying cardiac disease is much worse (1-year mortality rates of 18% to 33%) than for noncardiac or unexplained syncope (1-year mortality rates of 6% to 12%). In a series of 176 ambulatory patients evaluated for syncope, 9% had a cardiac etiology, 45% had vasomotor instability, 1% had seizures, 6% had other etiologies, and 3% were unexplained.

WORKUP

History, physical findings, and the resting 12-lead ECG are the most valuable elements of the evaluation of syncope. This limited data base suffices in 60% to 85% of cases in which a diagnosis is eventually made. The physician and patient should appreciate that even exhaustive evaluation often fails to identify an etiology for syncope. Fortunately, the prognosis for patients with a single unexplained episode of syncope is excellent.

History. One immediate objective is to determine whether a cardiac problem is responsible for the loss of con-

Table 18-1.   Important Causes of Syncope

1. Cardiac
   a. Arrhythmias (sick sinus syndrome, ventricular tachycardia, very rapid supraventricular tachycardia)
   b. Heart block (Stokes–Adams attacks)
   c. Aortic stenosis, severe
   d. Asymmetric septal hypertrophy, severe
   e. Primary pulmonary hypertension
   f. Atrial myxoma
   g. Prolapsed mitral valve
2. Vascular–Reflex
   a. Vasodepressor syncope (emotional upset)
   b. Orthostatic hypotension (ganglionic blocking agents, diabetes, old age, prolonged bed rest)
   c. Carotid sinus hypersensitivity
   d. Cerebral vascular disease, severe
   e. Subclavian steal syndrome
   f. Post-tussive syncope
   g. Valsalva syncope
   h. Postmicturition syncope (emptying distended bladder)
   i. Vasovagal syncope (distention of a viscus)
3. Psychological–Neurologic
   a. Seizures
   b. Hysteria
4. Metabolic
   a. Hyperventilation
   b. Hypoxia
   c. Hypoglycemia (rarely)

sciousness. The absence of premonitory symptoms in the presyncopal period suggests a sudden fall in cardiac output, whereas nausea, diaphoresis, pallor, and lightheadedness and more typical of reflex and vascular etiologies. Identification of precipitants requires asking about emotional upsets, crowded hot surroundings, sudden standing, prolonged and forceful coughing, Valsalva maneuvers, micturition, and vigorous exercise. Effort syncope is characteristic of hemodynamically significant obstruction in the ventricular outflow tract. Position just prior to syncope is worth noting because loss of consciousness while recumbent argues against a reflex or vascular mechanism. In considering heart disease, one needs to ask about a history of infarction, palpitations, chest pain, heart murmur, dyspnea on exertion, and use of digitalis and antiarrhythmic drugs, especially quinidine. A history of diabetes, stroke, use of antihypertensive agents, prolonged bed rest, impotence, and bladder and bowel incontinence should be checked for when the patient reports lightheadedness or syncope on standing.

It is important not to mistake other conditions for true loss of consciousness. Vertigo (see Chapter 160), neuroglycopenic symptoms (see Chapter 97), and the lightheadedness associated with an anxiety attack are sometimes confused with syncope.

A seizure disorder is usually not difficult to distinguish from circulatory syncope because of the preceding aura, motor activity, incontinence, and postictal symptoms of confusion, drowsiness, and paresis. However, when there are no motor manifestations, as in akinetic petit mal seizures, the differentiation may be impossible to make by history alone.

Reports from witnesses should be sought whenever possible. Activity, position, complaints, and appearance prior to syncope as well as duration of the episode, associated motor activity, and behavior upon regaining consciousness deserve attention. Some observers will even be able to report pulse and respirations.

Physical examination concentrates on the cardiovascular system. *Blood pressure* and *pulse* should be measured in both arms while the patient is supine and standing to detect postural effects and any occlusion of the subclavian artery. It may be necessary on occasion to wait as long as 5 minutes to obtain a postural fall in blood pressure. Torso and head, including the tongue, require scrutiny for signs of trauma sustained during a motor seizure.

Carotid pulses are auscultated for bruits and gently palpated for volume and carotid upstroke (see Chapter 15). If there is no evidence of carotid artery disease, one can massage the carotid and observe for reflex bradycardia and hypotension. The maneuver is indicated when a hypersensitive carotid sinus reflex is suspected. However, because it may also cut off blood supply and cause syncope when there is severe cerebral occlusive disease, it should not be attempted in such patients.

The neck veins are noted for distention and the chest for rales and rhonchi. The *heart* is palpated for heaves and thrills and is auscultated for clicks and murmurs with the patient in the supine, decubitus, and sitting positions. Systolic murmurs should be evaluated for evidence of aortic stenosis, ASH, and mitral valve prolapse (see Chapter 15). A variable diastolic murmur raises the question of atrial myxoma. Neurologic assessment includes a search for focal deficits indicative of prior stroke.

Provocative maneuvers are particularly helpful in identifying conditions that alter consciousness but do not cause syncope. Asking the patient to voluntarily hyperventilate or spin around may reproduce symptoms and confirm a clinical suspicion. Exercising the arm is worthwhile if subclavian steal syndrome is suspected.

Laboratory Studies. When the history suggests a common faint and the physical examination is normal, no laboratory studies are needed. Sudden loss of consciousness without warning is an indication for an *electrocardiogram* (ECG), looking not only for heart block and arrhythmias, but also for subtle clues such as a short PR interval, delta waves, or new onset of bundle branch block.

If the ECG is unrevealing but an arrhythmia or transient heartblock is suspected nonetheless, a *24-hour ambulatory ECG recording (Holter monitor)* should be ordered. However, the physician must appreciate how common rhythm disturbances are among asymptomatic patients, particularly the elderly. Paroxysmal supraventricular arrhythmias and complex ventricular arrhythmias have been demonstrated in as many as 13% and 50%, respectively, of healthy active asymptomatic persons over age 60. It is not surprising, therefore, that correlation between rhythm disturbances detected during Holter monitoring and symptoms is poor. In one study, more than 80% of patients with supraventricular tachycardia and more than 90% of patients with ventricular tachycardia were asymptomatic at the time of their arrhythmias. Although only 13% of all patients had symptoms correlated with arrhythmias, fully one third reported symptoms while their heart rate and rhythm were normal. In another study of more than 1500 patients referred for Holter studies because of syncope, arrhythmia-related symptoms occurred in only 2%. Syncope or (much more commonly) presyncope occurred without an associated arrhythmia in 15%.

An *exercise stress test* may detect arrhythmias not found during Holter monitoring. However, stress tests should not be performed in the evaluation of effort syncope unless and until tight aortic stenosis and other forms of outflow tract obstruction have been excluded.

Because of the limited specificity of Holter monitoring, *intracardiac electrophysiologic studies* have been advocated to detect cardiac causes of syncope. In some series, ventricular tachycardia inducible by programmed stimulation has been found in a majority of patients with recurrent unexplained syncope. In such cases, repeat electrophysiologic testing after selection of antiarrhythmic drugs provides a rational therapeutic endpoint. Such invasive testing is available only in specialized centers and is not without risk, particularly in the patient with underlying coronary disease. At present, electrophysiologic testing should be reserved for the patients with otherwise unexplained syncope that is recurrent or otherwise deemed life-threatening.

An *echocardiogram* may be valuable when a structural lesion, rather than a rhythm disturbance, is the suspected cardiac cause of syncope. Palpitations, inferior T-wave abnormalities, or a click and late systolic murmur may suggest mitral valve prolapse. The same test might identify an atrial myxoma. Effort syncope or a systolic ejection murmur may raise the question of aortic stenosis or asymptomatic septal hypertrophy (see Chapter 15).

The *electroencephalogram* (*EEG*) has repeatedly been shown to be of little use in evaluating syncope in the absence of either a history suggestive of seizure or neurologic deficits. Even when a seizure disorder is present, the routine EEG has a sensitivity of only 50%. Sleep studies and photic stimulation may improve sensitivity to 80% (see Chapter 164). Similarly, the *head computed tomography* (*CT*) *scan* should generally be reserved for patients with focal seizures or defects on neurologic examination; in one study, 7 of 20 patients with and none of 17 patients without such findings had abnormalities detected on CT scan.

Random blood sugar determinations are of little use in documenting hypoglycemia; a blood sugar at the time of symptoms is the best test (see Chapter 97).

SYMPTOMATIC THERAPY AND PATIENT EDUCATION

Vasodepressor syncope can be prevented by instructing the patient to lie down or at least put his head below his knees during the presyncopal period. The patient bothered by orthostatic hypotension needs to avoid abrupt postural changes by sitting on the edge of the bed in the morning before getting up. Girdles, garters, and other constricting garments should not be worn, but elastic stockings may be helpful in increasing venous return. One can advise the patient to avoid prolonged standing and to contract the calf muscles when standing to increase venous blood flow. It may be necessary to discontinue or alter dosages of drugs that contribute to postural hypotension, particularly diuretics, antihypertensive agents, and hypnotics. Loosening the collar is sometimes helpful for the person with a hypersensitive carotid sinus reflex. A demand pacemaker is indicated only when heart block or severe bradycardia has been proven responsible for syncope.

The patient whose syncope remains unexplained after discerning evaluation can be confidently reassured. The majority of patients presenting to the office-based practitioner have a vasodepressor-type reaction. A careful history, physical, and explanation helps to reassure such a patient of the benign nature of the syncopal event.

INDICATIONS FOR ADMISSION

Pending further study, it is safest to hospitalize patients with syncope suspected to be of cardiac origin or due to a seizure disorder of recent onset. If serious heart and neurologic diseases have been ruled out, further evaluation can safely proceed on an outpatient basis even though the etiology may remain undetermined. Family members should be instructed to make careful note of all events surrounding the syncopal period, including appearance, position, activity, complaints, and behavior. They might be taught to palpate the radial or femoral pulse to provide data on heart rate and rhythm during the episode. Admission to the hospital for observation of the obscure case is a difficult decision but is most useful when episodes are frequent.

A.G.M. and A.H.G.

ANNOTATED BIBLIOGRAPHY

Branch WT, Jr: Approach to syncope. J Gen Intern Med 1:49, 1986 (*A valuable review.*)

Day SC, Cook EF, Funkenstein H, et al: Evaluation of emergency room patients with transient loss of consciousness. Am J Med 73:15, 1982 (*Patients presenting to an emergency room with syncope are described; when a serious etiology is not readily found, prognosis is good.*)

Dimarco JP, Garan H, Harthorne JW et al: Intracardiac electrophysiologic techniques in recurrent syncope of unknown cause. Ann Intern Med 95:542, 1981 (*Among patients with three or more recurrences of syncope, electrophysiologic studies detected life-threatening arrhythmias in a majority, including 80% of those with coronary disease.*)

Eagle KA, Black HR, Cook EF et al: Evaluation of prognostic classification of patients with syncope. Am J Med 79:455, 1985 (*An outpatient study with 176 patients finding 8.5% with cardiac etiologies, 44.9% with vasomotor instability, 1.1% with seizures, 6% with others, and 39% unexplained.*)

Fleg JL, Kennedy HL: Cardiac arrhythmias in a healthy elderly population: Detection by 24-hour ambulatory electrocardiography. Chest 81:302, 1982 (*Among healthy, active persons aged 60 to 85, Holter monitoring disclosed paroxysmal atrial tachycardia in 13% and complex ventricular arrhythmias in 50%, including ventricular tachycardia in 4%.*)

Gibson TC, Heitzman MR: Diagnostic efficacy of 24-hour electrocardiographic monitoring for syncope. Am J Cardiol 53:1013, 1984 (*Of 1512 patients referred for Holter monitoring because of syncope, 15 had an episode of syncope, of which 7 were related to an arrythmia, and 241 reported presyncope, of which 24 were arrhythmia-related.*)

Kapoor WN, Karpf M, Wieand S, et al: A prospective evaluation follow-up of patients with syncope. N Engl J Med 309:197, 1983 (*A prospective study confirming the findings of Silverstein et al. that patients with a cardiovascular cause for syncope face much higher risk than those with noncardiovascular or unknown causes.*)

Kapoor W, Karpf M, Levey GS: Issues in evaluating patients with syncope. Ann Intern Med 100:755, 1984 (*An editorial describing emphasis on meticulous history, physical examination, and electrocardiogram with discriminating use of additional tests in an evaluation of patients with syncope.*)

Kwoh CK, Beck JR, Pauker SG: Repeated syncope with negative diagnostic evaluation. Med Decision Making 4:351, 1984 (*A sophisticated decision analysis approach to the question of whether or not to pace, including a well-structured review of the literature.*)

Lipsitz LA: Syncope in the elderly. Ann Intern Med 99:92, 1983 (*An extensive clinical review stressing the selective use of diagnostic tests in evaluating syncope as well as attention to drug effects and treatment of symptomatic abnormalities.*)

McAnulty JH, Rahimtoola SH, Murphy E et al: Natural history of high risk bundle branch block: A final report of a prospective study. N Engl J Med 307:137, 1982 (*A perspective study of 554 patients with chronic bifascicular and trifascicular block followed for 4 years. An incidence of complete heart block of only 1% per year was found. Moreover, heart block itself did not produce serious consequence.*)

Schatz IJ: Orthostatic hypertension. Arch Intern Med 144:773, 1984 (*A good review of the mechanisms and management.*)

Silverstein MD, Singer DE, Mulley AG et al: Patients with syncope admitted to medical intensive care units. JAMA 248:1185, 1982 (*Among this ICU population, those with cardiovascular syncope had a 19% 1-year mortality rate while those with noncardiovascular or unexplained syncope had a 6% rate. The authors conclude that patients discharged with unexplained syncope do not face increased risk of death during the subsequent year.*)

Weissler A, Warren J, Estes E et al: Vasodepressor syncope: Factors influencing cardiac output. Circulation 15:875, 1957 (*Vasodepressor syncope may occur even when vagal activity is blocked by atropine, thus arguing against a primary role for vagal effects in syncope associated with emotional upset. A classic paper.*)

Zeldis SM, Levine BJ, Michelson EL et al: Cardiovascular complaints: Correlation with cardiac arrhythmias on 24-hour electrocardiographic monitoring. Chest 78:456, 1980 (*The great majority of patients with arrhythmias were asymptomatic; only 13% had symptoms that correlated with arrhythmias and more than one third had symptoms without arrhythmias.*)

The following references document the association of syncope with various conditions and precipitants:

Engel GL: Psychologic stress, vasodepressor (vasovagal) syncope, and sudden death. Ann Intern Med 89:403, 1978

Ferrer M: Sick sinus syndrome. Circulation 47:635, 1973

Klotz PG: Syncope during prostatic examination. N Engl J Med 282:1046, 1970

Levin B, Posner JB: Swallow syncope: Report of a case and review of the literature. Neurology 22:1086, 1972

Mannick J, Suter C, Hume D: The subclavian steal syndrome: A further documentation. JAMA 182:254, 1962

McIntosh H, Estes E, Warren JV: Mechanisms of cough syncope. Am Heart J 52:70, 1956

Peters M, Hall R, Cooley D, et al: Clinical syndrome of atrial myxoma. JAMA 230:695, 1974

Proudfit WL, Forteza ME: Micturition syncope. N Engl J Med 260:328, 1959

Thames MD, Albert JS, Dalen JE: Syncope in patients with pulmonary embolism. JAMA 238:2509, 1977

Thomas JE: Hyperactive carotid sinus reflex and carotid sinus syncope. Mayo Clin Proc 44:127, 1969

19
Evaluation of Atrial Fibrillation in the Outpatient Setting

Atrial fibrillation (AF) is one of several dysrhythmias that can produce an irregularly irregular heart beat; it is often a manifestation of advanced heart disease, but sometimes is discovered incidentally on an office visit. Many patients tolerate the arrhythmia well and can be worked up thoroughly on an outpatient basis by means of noninvasive studies. Cases that present without other signs of underlying heart disease are particularly challenging; some are harmless while others are resistant to standard therapy and associated with potentially serious conditions that may elude diagnosis unless specifically sought. The primary care physician needs to know when it is safe to conduct the workup on an outpatient basis and how to carry out an efficient noninvasive evaluation.

PATHOPHYSIOLOGY

The postulated electrophysiologic mechanisms of AF include focal automaticity and a complex form of reentry. Factors that may precipitate and/or perpetuate AF include increased atrial size, increased atrial pressure, varying repolarization times of neighboring areas of atrial myocardium, and occurrence of atrial premature beats during the vulnerable period of an atrial cycle. Increases in circulating catecholamines may precipitate atrial premature beats. Ischemia and disease of the sinoatrial nodes also predispose to atrial dysrhythmias by suppressing the SA node and allowing other atrial foci to fire. Epidemiologic data from the Framingham study reveal that heart failure and rheumatic heart disease are the most powerful predictors of development of AF, suggesting that myocardial damage and left atrial dilatation are important precursors of the condition.

CLINICAL PRESENTATIONS

The hallmarks of AF are the characteristic electrocardiographic findings of an irregularly irregular ventricular rhythm and atrial fibrillatory waves. The fibrillatory waves range in appearance from fine irregular undulations of the baseline to very coarse waves. The QRS duration is usually normal but may widen with aberrant conduction and simulate ventricular tachyarrhythmias. The ST segments and T waves may be abnormal in appearance if there is rapid ventricular response, underlying heart disease, or use of digitalis.

AF can present as a paroxysmal or chronic dysrhythmia, both with and without evidence of underlying heart disease.

Its incidence in the Framingham study was 2% over 20 years. The overwhelming majority of AF patients in that study had evidence of underlying heart disease at the time of the arrhythmia's onset. AF was often a sign of advanced heart disease complicated by congestive failure; the onset was associated with a twofold increase in mortality.

Some patients with incidentally discovered AF are asymptomatic; however, if the AF is paroxysmal or the ventricular rate is very rapid, palpitations may be reported. If cardiac output falls precipitously, symptoms of heart failure may occur. Rapid rate may also lead to myocardial ischemia in patients with underlying coronary artery disease. Systemic embolization may be the first sign of AF and present as an acute neurologic or peripheral vascular event.

A number of acute noncardiac conditions can precipitate AF in the absence of clinically apparent heart disease; these include acute alcohol intoxication, decompensated chronic obstructive lung disease, pneumonia, and pulmonary embolization. However, AF does not always occur in the context of overt heart disease or an acute event such as sudden pulmonary decompensation. The entities associated with seemingly isolated bouts of AF deserve particular attention because detection is sometimes difficult and therapy is different from that for most other causes of AF (see Chapter 23).

Lone Atrial Fibrillation is a term used to denote AF in patients without underlying heart disease. Studies of military recruits found its prevalence to be about 1 in 10,000. Lone AF is a harmless condition in young people; they characteristically experience episodes precipitated by emotional stress, alcohol, use of stimulants, or smoking. There is no underlying heart disease, chamber enlargement, or risk of embolization. The prognosis is excellent. Some older patients are inappropriately diagnosed as "lone fibrillators" when the actual etiology may be one of the less clinically apparent etiologies such as early alcoholic cardiomyopathy, sick sinus syndrome, Wolff–Parkinson–White syndrome, or apathetic hyperthyroidism.

Alcoholic Cardiomyopathy. The early stages of alcoholic cardiomyopathy may present as paroxysms of AF triggered by binge drinking. The distinction between this condition and "lone fibrillation" triggered by alcohol may be difficult but is suggested by the finding of cardiomegaly even in the absence of heart failure. Abstinence can halt or even reverse the condition.

Sick Sinus Syndrome (bradycardia–tachycardia syndrome) is an important and sometimes subtle cause of AF. The condition accounts for about half of all cases requiring pacemaker implantation. Atrial tachyarrhythmias often alternate with symptomatic bradycardia and sinus arrest. Patients may experience episodes of palpitations, lightheadedness, or syncope. At times, the first manifestation of the condition may be paroxysms of AF. Identification is most important, because treatment directed only toward the AF may worsen the bradyarrhythmias. Paroxysmal AF due to sick sinus syndrome is associated with an increased risk of thromboembolism. The exact cause of this condition is unknown but seems to be related to diffuse degeneration of conducting system tissue.

Wolff-Parkinson-White Syndrome (WPW) is a preexcitation syndrome that can produce episodes of AF associated with very rapid ventricular response rates. In fact, a ventricular rate of greater than 200 beats/minute and no other known cause for AF should make one suspicious of WPW syndrome. The condition is believed to be at least partially congenital in nature and characterized by atrioventricular conduction through an anomalous accessory pathway. This anomalous conduction results in the characteristic baseline ECG findings of a shortened P–R interval (less than 0.12 second) and delta waves. Some WPW patients have normal baseline ECGs and show anomalous conduction only during tachyarrhythmias, making diagnosis difficult. The reported incidence of AF among patients with WPW ranges from 11% to 39%. WPW is an important cause of AF to recognize, because the AF may actually worsen with digitalis therapy (see Chapter 23), and has the potential to degenerate into ventricular tachycardia and fibrillation.

Apathetic Hyperthyroidism of the Elderly is another cause of AF that may appear to occur without evidence of underlying heart disease. These patients characteristically manifest marked apathy that may be mistaken for severe depression and impressive weight loss that may simulate occult malignancy (see Chapter 101). Sometimes, AF is the predominant manifestation of the condition. The usual signs and symptoms of thyrotoxicosis are absent. The AF is difficult to control with standard modes of therapy for AF but usually reverts to sinus rhythm with correction of the hyperthyroid state.

DIFFERENTIAL DIAGNOSIS

Atrial fibrillation is only one of a number of dysrhythmias that present as an irregularly irregular pulse. Frequent atrial premature beats, multifocal atrial tachycardia, paroxysmal atrial tachycardia or atrial flutter with variable block, sinus arrhythmia, and frequent ventricular premature beats all may produce an irregularly irregular rhythm.

The most common cause of AF in the community setting is hypertensive heart disease; however, only those hypertensive patients with evidence of left ventricular hypertrophy are likely to develop AF. The major causes of AF are listed in Table 19-1.

WORKUP

The diagnosis of AF is based on the characteristic *ECG findings* of an irregularly irregular ventricular response and atrial fibrillatory waves. These fibrillatory waves range from barely perceptible irregular undulations of the ECG baseline to very coarse waves. The standard lead best suited for detection of atrial activity is lead V_1, followed by leads II, III, and aV_F. Occasionally, the routine 12-lead ECG will show no atrial activity; in such instances, one can check lead V_{3R} for evidence of atrial activity or infer the diagnosis of AF based on the characteristic ventricular response pattern and a QRS of normal duration. Multifocal atrial tachycardia, paroxysmal atrial tachycardia, or atrial flutter with variable block, frequent atrial premature beats, and sinus arrhythmia all produce rhythms that can resemble AF, but the presence of P waves or flutter waves on ECG separate them from AF. If the ventricular response rate is too rapid to reveal atrial activity, vagal maneuvers and gentle carotid sinus message can be attempted (provided there is no evidence of carotid artery disease) to slow the rate and uncover any hidden fibrillatory or P waves.

Once the diagnosis of AF is established, one needs to determine if workup can proceed on an outpatient basis.

Table 19-1.   Important Causes of Atrial Fibrillation

Paroxysmal Atrial Fibrillation
"Lone fibrillation"
Acute ischemia
Alcohol intoxication and early alcoholic cardiomyopathy
Sick sinus syndrome
Wolff–Parkinson–White syndrome
Acute pulmonary embolization
Acute pericarditis
Acute pulmonary decompensation
Acute heart failure
Any cause of chronic AF

Sustained Atrial Fibrillation
Advanced rheumatic mitral valve disease
Chronic congestive heart failure
Advanced aortic valve disease
Advanced hypertensive heart disease
Coronary artery disease
Advanced cardiomyopathy
Congenital heart disease
Apathetic hyperthyroidism of the elderly
Sick sinus syndrome
"Lone" fibrillation
Constrictive pericarditis
Digitalis toxicity (rarely)

Prompt hospital admission is needed for the patient with evidence of acute congestive heart failure, ischemia, embolization, hypotension, or a very rapid ventricular response rate (>150 to 170 beats/minute). If there is no hemodynamic compromise, an outpatient workup can commence. A retrospective study of 97 patients with new onset AF who were admitted to the hospital as a routine procedure found that 98% had an uncomplicated course. The authors concluded that hospitalization is unnecessary for new onset of uncomplicated AF.

History. The young patient with a paroxysm of AF should be questioned about a prior history of such episodes, excess intake of stimulants and alcohol, emotional stress, fever, heart murmur, and chest pain. Older patients should be queried about preexisting heart disease, hypertension, chest pain, dyspnea, cough, calf pain, leg edema, fever, lightheadedness, near syncope, loss of consciousness, weight loss, depression, history of heart murmur or rheumatic fever, and any prior attacks of palpitations. A careful drug history should be taken with emphasis on alcohol abuse (see Chapter 224). Any use of digitalis should be noted; however, digitalis toxicity only rarely results in AF. A long-standing history of attacks dating from young adulthood suggests Wolff–Parkinson–White syndrome. The presence of marked weight loss and depression in an elderly patient with unexplained AF points to apathetic hyperthyroidism. The older patient with episodes of altered consciousness may suffer from sick sinus syndrome.

Physical Examination. In addition to noting heart rate, blood pressure, respiratory rate, jugular venous pulse, and other signs of hemodynamic status, the examination should be checked for apathetic appearance, evidence of marked weight loss, cyanosis, goiter, wheezes, friction rub, heart murmur, calf tenderness, asymmetrical leg edema, and signs of alcohol intoxication.

Laboratory Studies. The *electrocardiogram* often provides useful information beyond identification of the arrhythmia. A ventricular response rate greater than 200 beats/minute suggests WPW syndrome, as does a widened QRS due to aberrant conduction; delta waves may be seen within some of the aberrantly conducted beats. The appearance of the fibrillatory waves on ECG provides some hints of etiology. Coarse fibrillatory waves are most typical of AF due to rheumatic heart disease and other causes of marked left atrial enlargement, whereas fine fibrillatory waves are more common in cases due to atherosclerotic and hypertensive heart diseases. The ST and T wave segments should be checked for evidence of ischemia, strain, digitalis effect, and pericarditis (see Chapter 14). Advanced valvular and hypertensive forms of heart disease are suggested by finding ECG evidence of left ventricular hypertrophy.

A cardiogram taken after return to sinus rhythm should be checked for a shortened PR interval and delta waves diagnostic of Wolff–Parkinson–White syndrome. Occasionally, preexcitation is concealed on the resting ECG, so that the ECG of some WPW patients appears normal; in such instances the diagnosis of WPW syndrome can be difficult. Other clues to WPW syndrome include a ventricular response rate during AF of greater than 200 beats/minute and delta waves distorting the QRS complex.

A rhythm strip sometimes reveals sinus node disease, but often a 24-hour *Holter monitor* will be needed to detect the episodes of bradycardia and tachycardia that characterize the sick sinus syndrome. *Chest x-ray* is the best simple test for determining heart failure, cardiomegaly, and intrapulmonary pathology. Cardiomegaly may be the only evidence of underlying heart disease and an early sign of a cardiomyopathy. *Echocardiogram* provides an excellent noninvasive means of identifying valvular, congenital, cardiomyopathic, and pericardial forms of heart disease. The elderly, apathetic patient with unexplained AF requires measurement of *thyroid indices* to rule out hyperthyroidism. If the standard indices are normal, yet clinical suspicion remains high, a TRH stimulation test may provide a more sensitive test result. Although AF is a very uncommon manifestation of digitalis toxicity, a serum *digoxin level* is probably worth checking when no other etiology is apparent and the patient is known to be taking the drug.

In summary, the evaluation can be performed on an outpatient basis if the patient is tolerating the rhythm well and there is no evidence of failure, ischemia, or embolization. A careful history and physical examination supplemented by ECG, chext x-ray, and echocardiogram complete the evaluation in most patients. Patients with AF of unknown etiology should be studied further for evidence of sick sinus syndrome, apathetic hyperthyroidism, alcoholic cardiomyopathy, and WPW syndrome.

A.H.G.

ANNOTATED BIBLIOGRAPHY

Campbell RWF, Smith RA, Gallagher JJ et al: Atrial fibrillation in the preexcitation syndrome. Am J Cardiol 40:514, 1977 (*AF due to preexcitation syndromes can cause very rapid and aberrantly conducted ventricular responses; ventricular dysrhythmias can sometimes result.*)

Culler MR, Boone JA, Gazes PC: Fibrillatory wave size as a clue to etiologic diagnosis. Am Heart J 66:425, 1963 (*Coarse atrial fibrillatory waves found most frequently in patients with mitral valve disease and left atrial enlargement; also noted in "lone" AF and hyperthyroidism.*)

Ettinger PO, Wu DF, De La Cruz C Jr et al: Arrhythmias and the "holiday heart": Alcohol-associated cardiac rhythm disorders. Am Heart J 95:955, 1978 (*Paroxysmal AF may be a sign of early alcoholic cardiomyopathy and be induced by binge drinking.*)

Forfar JC, Miller HC, Toft AD: Occult thyrotoxicosis: A correctable cause of "idiopathic" atrial fibrillation. Am J Cardiol 44:9, 1979 (*Ten of 75 patients presenting with AF of unknown etiology were hyperthyroid by TRH stimulation testing. In a number of cases, the T$_4$ and total T$_3$ were normal.*)

Hanson HH et al: Auricular fibrillation in normal hearts. N Engl J Med 240:947, 1949 (*Classic paper describing the entity of "lone fibrillation."*)

Lowenstein SR et al: The role of alcohol in new onset of atrial fibrillation. Arch Intern Med 143:1882, 1983 (*Alcohol contributed to approximately two thirds of new cases of atrial fibrillation in this series.*)

Scarpa WJ: The sick sinus syndrome. Am Heart J 92:648, 1976 (*Good review of this condition and its many manifestations.*)

Shlofmitz RA, Hirsch BE, Meyer BR: New onset atrial fibrillation. J Gen Intern Med 1:139, 1986 (*A retrospective study showing that urgent hospitalization is rarely necessary.*)

20

Evaluation of Palpitations

Palpitations are disconcerting and often incite fear of serious heart disease, although the majority of cases seen in the office occur among the worried well. The patient with palpitations reports a disquieting awareness of his heartbeat, which may be described as a pounding, racing, skipping, flopping, or fluttering sensation. The primary physician must be able to diagnose and treat important dysrhythmias and provide convincing reassurance to the anxious persons with no underlying heart disease. The development of ambulatory monitoring (Holter monitoring) has improved detection of arrhythmias; its indications and limitations need to be understood.

PATHOPHYSIOLOGY AND CLINICAL PRESENTATION

Most healthy individuals are unaware of their resting heartbeat. Increase in stroke volume or contractility, sudden change in rate or rhythm, or unusual cardiac movement within the thorax may cause a perceptible beat. Isolated palpitations are noted when premature atrial or ventricular contractions are followed by a long pause; the prolonged filling time leads to an increase in stroke volume and the vigorous ejection of a large volume of blood on the next beat. A constant pounding is felt at rest by patients with hyperkinetic states (*e.g.,* fever, severe anemia, hyperthyroidism); the rate is rapid and the rhythm is regular. A regular rhythm is also noted in those with large stroke volumes due to aortic regurgitation and other forms of valvular heart disease.

Excess adrenergic stimulation results in increased contractility and sinus tachycardia, which may present as palpitations. Anxiety is a common cause of such catecholamine-induced palpitations. A heightened awareness of bodily sensations often compounds the problem. The normally perceptible heartbeat that occurs with exercise is not unpleasant unless one is preoccupied with worries about health. Hyperthyroidism may have a presentation similar to anxiety (see Chapter 101).

In rare instances, the source of adrenergic outpouring is a pheochromocytoma. Its incidence is less than 0.1%, with about half of cases presenting as paroxysms of palpitations, hypertension, perspiration, tremor, nervousness, and other signs of adrenergic stimulation. Episodes are often spontaneous in origin but may be triggered by emotion and thus mimic an anxiety attack. An insulin reaction can produce a similar clinical picture (see Chapter 100). Onset of palpitations from adrenergic stimulation can be abrupt; resolution is usually more gradual.

Any sudden change in rate or rhythm may be perceptible. Attacks of palpitations that are regular in rhythm and rapid in rate are not unique to catecholamine excess; paroxysms of supraventricular tachycardia (SVT), often referred to as paroxysmal atrial tachycardia (PAT), are an important cause. SVT occurs in a wide variety of patients, including those with normal hearts, sick sinus syndrome, mitral valve prolapse and other forms of valvular disease, coronary artery disease, cardiomyopathy, and the preexcitation syndromes (*e.g.,* Wolff–Parkinson–White syndrome). Onset of SVT is characteristically sudden and may be precipitated by excess coffee, alcohol consumption, emotional upset, or strenuous exertion. Often there is no obvious precipitant. Resolution is typically abrupt. A reentrant mechanism is postulated to account for SVT. Pathways that have been implicated involve the AV node, atria, and accessory conduction fibers. The dysrhythmia seems to be initiated by the occurrence of premature beats that alter conduction in the normal pathway. Paroxysms cease when the conducting properties of the reentrant circuit are disturbed by changes in vagal tone.

Some of the conditions associated with SVT are responsible for other dysrhythmias as well. For example, almost half of patients with sick sinus syndrome experience heart block or marked bradycardia in addition to bouts of SVT.

Sudden onset of palpitations with an irregular rhythm and rapid rate typifies paroxysmal atrial fibrillation (PAF) and may also be seen if there are runs of multifocal atrial tachycardia (MAT). PAF occurs in a host of settings (see Chapter 19) including alcohol excess, infection, and acute worsening of congestive heart failure; the condition is also found among otherwise healthy young people. MAT takes place in the context of severe pulmonary disease, particularly when there is an acute fall in PO_2 or pH. Frequent atrial or ventricular premature contractions can lead to a similarly irregular rhythm and rapid rate. Most chronic tachyarrhythmias do not produce palpitations.

Abnormal motion of the heart may be felt as a "turning over" or "flopping." The sensations are isolated and can occur with premature beats, the beat after a compensatory pause, or the beat after a blocked beat.

When there is serious underlying heart disease, palpitations are usually not the major or sole symptom. Syncope, near syncope, chest pain, or dyspnea suggests the presence of a significant cardiopulmonary illness.

DIFFERENTIAL DIAGNOSIS

The causes of palpitations can be listed in terms of their clinical presentation (Table 20-1).

WORKUP

History. The first priority is the detection of underlying heart disease. Inquiries into dyspnea, chest pain, and syncopal or near syncopal episodes are essential, as are questions about

Table 20-1. Important Causes of Palpitations

1. Isolated Single Palpitations
   a. Premature atrial or ventricular beats
   b. The beat following a blocked beat
   c. The beat after a compensatory pause
2. Paroxysmal Episodes with Abrupt Onset and Resolution (Rate Usually Rapid)
   a. Rhythm irregular
      1. Paroxysmal atrial fibrillation
      2. Paroxysmal atrial tachycardia with variable block
      3. Frequent atrial or ventricular premature beats
      4. Multifocal atrial tachycardia
   b. Rhythm regular
      1. Supraventricular tachycardias with constant block or 1:1 conduction
3. Paroxysmal Episodes with Less Abrupt Onset or Resolution (Rhythm Usually Regular, Rate Rapid)
   a. Exertion
   b. Emotion
   c. Drug side-effect (*e.g.,* sympathomimetics, theophylline compounds)
   d. Stimulant use (coffee, tea, tobacco)
   e. Insulin reaction
   f. Pheochromocytoma
4. Persistent Palpitations at Rest with Regular Rhythm (Rate Normal, Slow, or Rapid)
   a. Aortic or mitral regurgitation
   b. Large ventricular septal defect
   c. Bradycardia
   d. Severe anemia
   e. Hyperthyroidism (may also cause atrial fibrillation)
   f. Pregnancy
   g. Fever
   h. Marked volume depletion
   i. Anxiety neurosis

risk factors for coronary disease (see Chapters 8, 9, 10) and prior history of a heart murmur, rheumatic fever, myocardial infarction, and other forms of cardiac illness. A costly error is to mistake symptoms of anxiety, such as chest tightness and air hunger at rest, for evidence of organic heart disease. Use of all cardiotonic drugs should be detailed, including digitalis preparations, theophylline compounds, sympathomimetics, and anticholinergics. Use of tricyclic antidepressants is frequently associated with palpitations (see Chapter 223). Many over-the-counter cold remedies contain catecholamines or theophylline derivatives; their abuse may be responsible for symptoms.

A careful description of the palpitations in terms of onset, frequency, rate, rhythm, and pattern of resolution can sometimes be of help in diagnosis (see Table 20-1). Unfortunately, many patients are unable to give an accurate or detailed account of their symptoms. The relationship of the onset of symptoms to exertion can aid in separating the anxious individual, whose symptoms may occur at rest, and are usually not worsened by exertion from the patient with heart disease and impaired exercise tolerance. Identification of precipitants such as emotional upset, stimulant intake, fever, pregnancy, volume depletion, and severe anemia is essential, for their recognition can contribute to design of proper therapy. Inquiry into symptoms of an insulin reaction (see Chapter 100) and hyperthyroidism may also prove productive.

Physical Examination. At the beginning of the physical examination, one should look for evidence of excessive anxiety, such as tremor, sighing, and nervous mannerisms. Other important observations include determination of the blood pressure for elevation, marked postural change, and widened pulse pressure. The apical pulse is noted for rate and rhythm disturbances; relying on the peripheral pulse may be misleading when there is a pulse deficit, as occurs in atrial fibrillation or premature beats. The temperature should be recorded. The skin is examined for pallor and signs of hyperthyroidism, eyes for exophathalmos, neck for goiter, carotid pulse for upstroke, jugular venous pulse for distention and cannon waves, chest for rales, rhonchi, wheezes, and dullness, heart for heaves, thrills, clicks, murmurs, rubs, and S_3, and extremities for edema and calf tenderness. In addition to possibly providing important diagnostic information, the careful, unhurried physical examination can be of considerable use in reassuring the worried patient.

Laboratory Studies. Most patients with palpitations should have a resting *12-lead ECG*. Even if physical examination is completely normal and no disturbances of rate or rhythm are noted, one might detect evidence of conduction system disease (*e.g.,* bundle branch block or preexcitation) or signs of ischemia. In particular, the ECG needs to be studied for axis shifts, QRS widening, short PR intervals, and delta waves. If a dysrhythmia is noted on examination, it is worth obtaining a 2-minute rhythm strip to better characterize the problem. The anxiety-ladened person often insists on having an ECG and finds comfort in a normal result; unfortunately, in many cases the reassurance is only transient.

The development of continuous *ambulatory electrocardiographic monitoring* has proved to be an important addition to the diagnosis and understanding of dysrhythmias. When history, physical examination, and resting ECG have not provided a definitive diagnosis, it may be helpful to utilize ambulatory monitoring, particularly if the patient reports syncope or near syncope that seems to be cardiac in origin (see Chapter 18). Even when there is no syncopal history, patients with a preexcitation syndrome or bundle branch block on ECG, or evidence of mitral valve prolapse, cardiomyopathy, or coronary disease are candidates for monitoring, because they are at increased risk of having a clinically significant arrhythmia that requires treatment. The utility of the test in otherwise healthy patients who complain of palpitations is unclear at the present time, for it is known that healthy asymptomatic patients subjected to monitoring demonstrate a variety of dysrhythmias ranging from premature ventricular beats to very slow rhythms.

The high incidence of rhythm disturbances and the very poor correlation between the recorded "abnormalities" and reported symptoms is described in Chapter 18.

When palpitations are precipitated by exertion, *exercise stress testing* can contribute to assessment, especially in the patient with known or suspected coronary disease (see Chapter 31). In a study comparing the stress test to ambulatory monitoring, monitoring was found to be the more sensitive test for detecting most types of ventricular irritability in patients with coronary disease; however, there were instances in which ventricular tachycardia occurred on stress testing but did not appear on monitoring. Thus, the tests could be considered complementary.

Routine screening for endocrinologic causes of palpitations in the absence of clinical findings is of low yield. Patients with paroxysms of palpitations in conjunction with labile hypertension probably deserved to be screened for pheochromocytoma, although the condition is rare and screening tests have lacked the specificity and sensitivity required to minimize the rather high frequency of false-positive and false-negative results. The plasma catecholamine determination may be a more sensitive and specific test than the urinary VMA or metanephrines and, perhaps, better suited for diagnosis of pheochromocytoma. The test requires only a single venipuncture, rather than the 24-hour urine collection needed for VMA and metanephrine determinations; the patient needs to be supine for 30 minutes prior to the venipuncture. Metanephrines provide a more reliable index of pheochromocytoma than does the VMA.

SYMPTOMATIC RELIEF

When palpitations are a manifestation of neurotic concern, efforts should be addressed toward providing reassurance. Hasty words of comfort are worthless. A careful history and physical examination, combined with eliciting and responding to patient concerns, views, and requests, must take place before the patient can be told the palpitations are harmless. Such reassurance may be all that is needed, especially when combined with advice to increase physical activity and cut down on alcohol, coffee, smoking, and stress. Exercise stress testing may have a role in helping to reassure the anxious patient. If the palpitations persist and are bothersome, a trial of beta-blocker therapy may be beneficial. Often as little as 50 mg of atenolol or the equivalent per day decreases the frequency of symptoms to the point where they are tolerable. Use of minor tranquilizers is also worth incorporating into the program, but only in an episodic manner (see Chapter 222). All nonessential drugs capable of causing palpitations should be stopped.

Vagal maneuvers are often effective in halting SVT. Valsalva and carotid sinus massage (in the absence of carotid disease) can be taught to the patient and suggested as the first line of therapy after the onset of an attack. Digitalis and propranolol are effective in terminating SVT, but when SVT is due to a preexcitation syndrome, for example, Wolff–Parkinson–White syndrome, propranolol is preferred because digitalis may only prolong the problem by enhancing conduction in the accessory pathway. Prophylaxis of SVT attacks can be accomplished by avoiding known precipitants, such as alcohol and stimulants, and by using digitalis or propranolol; sometimes quinidine proves helpful by reducing the frequency of premature beats (the agent should usually be used in conjunction with digitalis, because of its vagolytic effects). Digitalis is the drug of choice for PAF. If SVT or PAF is accompanied by ischemia or failure, admission is urgent.

Treatment of MAT requires correction of the underlying pulmonary problem, rather than use of antiarrhythmic drugs. Improvement in oxygenation and pH status is essential. The approach to ventricular irritability depends on the setting in which it occurs (see Chapter 24). Correction of severe anemia, volume depletion, hyperthyroidism (see Chapter 101), fever (see Chapter 6), or congestive failure (see Chapter 27) is of prime importance to attaining symptomatic relief.

A.H.G.

ANNOTATED BIBLIOGRAPHY

Barnett PA, Peter CT, Swan HJC et al: The frequency and prognostic significance of electrocardiographic abnormalities in clinically normal individuals. Prog Cardiovasc Dis 23:299, 1981 (*An extensive review of this important and troublesome phenomenon.*)

Bravo EL, Tarazi RC, Gifford RW et al: Circulating and urinary catecholamines in pheochromocytoma. N Engl J Med 301:682, 1979 (*The serum catecholamine concentration proved to be the most sensitive and specific test for diagnosis, followed by the urinary metanephrines; the VMA determination was the least reliable.*)

Giffort RW Jr, Kvale WF, Maher FT et al: Clinical features, diagnosis and treatment of pheochromocytoma: A review of 76 cases. Mayo

Clin Proc 39:281, 1964 (*A classic article on the condition, emphasizing that it may mimic various common problems and requires biochemical confirmation for diagnosis.*)

Harrison DC, Fitzgerald MD, Winkle RA: Ambulatory electrocardiography for diagnosis and treatment of cardiac arrhythmias. N Engl J Med 294:373, 1976 (*Thorough review of the subject; 53 references.*)

Josephson ME, Kastor JA: Supraventricular tachycardia: Mechanisms and management. Ann Intern Med 87:346, 1977 (*Excellent discussion of pathophysiology and rational basis for therapy; 78 references.*)

Lowenstein SR, Gabow PA, Cramer J et al: The role of alcohol in new onset atrial fibrillation. Arch Intern Med 143:1882, 1983 (*Among 40 cases of new onset atrial fibrillation, alcohol caused or contributed to approximately two thirds; 90% of these converted spontaneously to sinus rhythm within 24 hours.*)

Narula OS: Wolff–Parkinson–White syndrome: A review. Circulation 47:872, 1973 (*A detailed description of the syndrome; 38 references.*)

Peters RW, Scheinman MM, Mondin G et al: Prophylactic permanent pacemakers for patients with chronic bundle branch block. Am J Med 66:978, 1979 (*Prophylactic permanent pacemaker insertion in 40 symptomatic patients with chronic bundle branch block and prolonged infranodal conduction times did not protect against sudden death. The incidence of sudden death appears to be related to the type and severity of underlying heart disease.*)

Rubenstein JJ, Schulman CL, Yurchak PM et al: Clinical spectrum of the sick sinus syndrome. Circulation 46:5, 1972 (*Classic article reporting on a series of 56 patients; over 60% of patients had bradycardia and SVT.*)

Ryan M, Lown, B, Horn H: Comparison of ventricular ectopic activity during 24-hour monitoring and exercise testing in patients with coronary heart disease. N Engl J Med 292:224, 1975 (*Monitoring proved better in exposing ventricular irritability, but there were instances when ectopic activity was detected only by stress testing.*)

Shand DG: Propranolol. N Engl J Med 293:280, 1975 (*A terse review of the drug; includes discussion of its use in anxiety to control palpitations; 20 references.*)

21

Management of Hypertension
KATHARINE K. TREADWAY, M.D.

Hypertension is one of the few conditions in medicine that can be readily detected and effectively treated in the asymptomatic period before irreparable harm is done. It ranks as the leading reason for office visits and prescription of medication. The frequency and importance of the problem demand that the primary physician be expert in its management.

PRINCIPLES OF THERAPY

When to Treat

The availability of effective medication with relatively few side-effects and the general belief that reducing blood pressure will protect against cardiovascular complications have led to increasingly early treatment, with many clinicians initiating therapy when the diastolic pressure reaches the range of 90 to 100 mm Hg (Table 21-1). However, no study to date has successfully determined exact guidelines for antihypertensive treatment in the general population.

Although controlled studies have shown that treatment of even very modest blood pressure elevation (diastolic pressures of 90 to 94 mm Hg) affords protection against stroke, congestive heart failure, and progression of hypertension, only half of available trials demonstrate that treatment of such mild hypertension protects against coronary artery disease. In one trial, there was a higher incidence of sudden death from coronary disease among the treatment group, believed linked to diuretic-induced arrhythmias. These results have led a national consensus panel to issue a note of caution in use of antihypertensive drugs, especially diuretics, in patients with diastolic pressures between 90 and 94 mm Hg.

Results in patients with greater elevations in diastolic pressure show more clear-cut cardiovascular benefit. Deciding when to begin treatment should be based not only on the average blood pressure, but also on the presence or absence of additional cardiovascular risk factors, end-organ damage, and age, sex, and race of the individual (see Chapter 8). For example, a young black male with a diastolic pressure of 95 mm Hg, a two pack-per-day smoking habit, arteriolar nicking on fundoscopic examination, and hypercholesterolemia requires earlier and more aggressive intervention than does a

Table 21-1. Algorithm for the Identification and Follow-up of High Blood Pressure

DIASTOLIC BP (mm Hg)	ACTION
120	Evaluate and treat immediately
105–119	Evaluate and treat
100–104	Evaluate and treat
95–99	Confirm on one separate occasion; initiate drug therapy, especially if there are additional risk factors for cardiovascular disease
90–94	Follow blood pressure at frequent intervals and initiate nonpharmacologic measures to lower BP. If BP fails to fall with nonpharmacologic treatment, institute drug therapy

white female with a similar blood pressure, an otherwise normal physical examination, and no additional cardiovascular risk factors.

The goal of therapy is reduction of diastolic blood pressure to below 90 mm Hg with a minimum of adverse side-effects.

Reports showing a significant reduction in deaths from cardiovascular complications attribute awareness and more effective control of blood pressure as primary factors.

Definition and indications for treatment of isolated *systolic hypertension* are less clear. Although epidemiologic data show an increased risk from systolic hypertension, no benefits of treatment have been demonstrated. Moreover, systolic hypertension is often very difficult to control. Therefore, treatment recommendations are conservative—to reduce systolic blood pressure by 10% in individuals under 35 years of age with systolic pressure greater than 140 mm Hg; in those 35 to 59 with systolic pressure greater than 150 mm Hg; and in those 60 or older with systolic pressure greater than 160 mm Hg. Systolic hypertension due to high output states such as aortic regurgitation or anemia should not be treated with antihypertensive medications.

Treatment Modalities

Nonpharmacologic Therapies. The mainstays of nonpharmacologic therapy are salt restriction, reduction of excess weight, and exercise (Fig. 21-1). All patients should be instructed in a *no-added salt diet* and encouraged to avoid processed foods that are high in sodium. Not only may salt restriction alone provide adequate control in some very mild cases, but it can profoundly affect the efficacy of pharmacologic therapy. One study demonstrated that in patients receiving diuretics who had an unrestricted salt intake, blood pressure was reduced by 4% compared with a 15% reduction for those on a low-sodium diet.

Weight reduction has been shown to achieve significant decreases in blood pressure, even when ideal weight has not been reached. The effect is independent of salt intake. All patients who are greater than 15% above their ideal body weight should be urged to lose weight. The relation between obesity and blood pressure is particularly strong among young to middle-aged adults.

Reduction in alcohol consumption. Epidemiologic data indicate a relationship between excess alcohol consumption and risk of hypertension. More than two drinks per day appears to significantly increase the risk of developing hypertension. Small-scale studies suggest that reducing alcohol intake of two or fewer drinks per day will result in a modest decrease in blood pressure in hypertensive drinkers.

Exercise of the aerobic variety helps to reduce weight, improves cardiovascular conditioning, and may help in patients with mild, uncomplicated hypertension. Patients with

Begin with nonpharmacologic measures (salt restriction, weight reduction, exercise, reduction in alcohol use)
↓
Initiate pharmacologic therapy with a thiazide diuretic (especially for elderly or black patients)
or
Initiate therapy with a beta-blocking agent (especially if young or with autonomic overactivity)*
↓
Substitute, rather than add, another first-line agent (thiazide or beta-blocker)
↓
Combine use of two first-line agents or add a second-line agent (*e.g.,* thiazide plus beta-blocker or methyldopa)
↓
Add a peripheral vasodilator (*e.g.,* hydralazine, prazosin) as a third agent
or
Use a converting enzyme inhibitor (captopril, enalapril) alone or with a diuretic; add a beta-blocker if necessary
or
Use clonidine, reserpine, or guanethidine with a diuretic
↓
Substitute minoxidil plus furosemide (especially for patients with renal insufficiency); add a beta-blocker if necessary
or
Substitute a calcium-channel blocker

Figure 21-1. Algorithm for treating hypertension.

* Converting enzyme inhibitors may also prove to be useful as first choice agents.

underlying heart disease should be evaluated medically (see Chapter 10) before engaging in any exercise program.

Behavioral therapies such as relaxation techniques and biofeedback programs have gained popularity in recent years, and some data suggest a modest benefit; however, these methods have yet to undergo rigorous clinical testing and should not be considered an alternative to more proven non-pharmacologic and pharmacologic treatments.

Pharmacologic Therapies. When nonpharmacologic therapies do not suffice or hypertension is moderate or severe, drug treatment should be initiated (see Table 21-2). Currently available pharmacologic agents useful in the treatment of hypertension may be classified into five major groups: diuretics, sympatholytics, vasodilators, calcium-channel blockers, and converting enzyme inhibitors.

DIURETICS remain the most commonly used agents for both initiation and maintenance of therapy. In most instances a *thiazide* is utilized. When used carefully in properly selected patients, thiazides are a safe, well-tolerated, and cost-effective means of treatment (see Table 21-2). Minimization of *hypokalemia,* the most important side-effect of thiazide use, can be achieved by concomitant limitation of salt intake and increased dietary potassium. At times, a potassium supplement or a potassium-sparing diuretic needs to be added to the patient's program, especially in patients with underlying coronary artery disease, who are at increased risk of arrhythmic complications. Worsening ventricular irritability has been demonstrated in the presence of ischemia and hypokalemia, and an increased risk of sudden death was noted in one large study among hypertensive patients having baseline electrocardiographic abnormalities who were treated with large doses of thiazides. Patients on thiazides who take a digitalis preparation are also very susceptible to developing dysrhythmias in the setting of hypokalemia. Regular monitoring of the serum potassium is essential when there is underlying heart disease. However, mild degrees of hypokalemia (3.0 to 3.5 mg/dl) in patients free of cardiac problems are probably harmless and need not be assiduously monitored or treated. More severe degrees of hypokalemia may cause muscle weakness.

Other side-effects of thiazide therapy include mild glucose intolerance, increase in serum lipids, and hyperuricemia. The degree of *glucose intolerance* in normal patients is usually insignificant, but those with diabetes may experience some worsening of control (see Chapter 100). Thiazides may *increase total cholesterol* and triglyceride levels, though the importance, if any, of these changes is not yet clear. Mild *hyperuricemia* occurs in as many as 60% of patients; however, only if the patient develops recurrent attacks of gouty arthritis or kidney stones is treatment of the hyperuricemia necessary (see Chapter 155). Nonsteroidal anti-inflammatory agents and estrogens may blunt the antihypertensive effects of thiazides.

Hypersensitivity reactions mandate immediate discontinuation of the thiazides and substitution of a loop, distal tubular, or phthalimidine derivative, although similar reactions may occur with each of these.

The *loop diuretics,* furosemide, ethacrynic acid, and bumetanide, should be reserved for patients with evidence of renal insufficiency (creatinine clearance less than 30% of normal) or with allergy to the thiazides.

The *distal tubular diuretics,* spironolactone, triamterene, and amiloride, provide no special advantage in initial management. Because of the tendency to develop gynecomastia with spironolactone, its use is limited to patients with Conn's Syndrome. The other potassium-sparing agents are used in patients with mineralocorticoid hypertension, thiazide hypersensitivity, or severe gout. In patients simultaneously receiving digitalis preparations or with ventricular irritability, in whom hypokalemia is a special risk, the potassium-retaining properties of these agents are advantageous whether used alone or in combination with thiazides. These drugs must be used with extreme caution in patients with a tendency to develop hyperkalemia—for example, patients with renal insufficiency, or insulin-requiring diabetics with renin deficiency.

It is well to avoid starting with a preparation that has a fixed combination of a thiazide and a distal tubular diuretic until the necessary dose of each is established. Fixed combinations may not provide proper doses and are usually more expensive. However, if the fixed dose is identical to the patient's optimal program, then a combination agent may facilitate compliance.

SYMPATHOLYTIC DRUGS include a variety of agents that may be further divided into those acting peripherally and those acting centrally. Included in the former group are the beta-blockers, prazosin, reserpine, and guanethidine.

Beta-blockers are highly effective in reducing high blood pressure. Several mechanisms have been proposed to explain their antihypertensive effect. There are now a variety of beta blockers available; all appear to be equally effective. In general, beta-blockers are well tolerated and may be used alone as initial therapy. The addition of diuretics, if needed, will enhance their effectiveness. These agents have a variety of side-effects including bradycardia, exacerbation of congestive heart failure, fatigue, impotence, decreased exercise tolerance, nightmares, and increased airway resistance. Acebutolol is associated with development of a lupus-like syndrome. In general, these agents should not be used in patients with asthma, heart failure, or significant COPD. *Metoprolol, atenolol,* and *acebutolol* are relatively cardioselective with a greater effect on beta$_1$ (cardiac) adrenoreceptors than on the beta$_2$ (vessel and bronchi) adrenoreceptors. In low doses, these drugs may be tolerated in some patients with COPD, but selectivity is lost at higher doses, including doses used for hypertension. *Pindolol* and acebutolol are beta-blockers with agonist as well

Table 21-2.   Antihypertensive Drugs

CLASS	DRUG	TRADE NAME	INITIAL/MAXIMUM DOSE (mg/day)	FREQUENCY OF DOSAGE	RELATIVE COST (dose in mg)
Diuretics	Thiazides				
	Chlorothiazide	Diuril	500/1500	bid	1.08 (1000)
	Hydrochlorothiazide	Hydrodiuril	50/150	bid	1.00 (100)
	Phthalimidine derivatives				
	Chlorthalidone	Hygroton	50/100	qd	0.81 (50)
	Metolazone	Zaroxolyn	2.5/5	qd	1.39 (5)
	Side-effects				
	$\downarrow$K$^+$, alkalosis, $\uparrow$uric acid, $\uparrow$blood sugar, $\uparrow$Ca^{2+}, ?$\uparrow$lipids, dermatitis, photosensitivity, $\downarrow$platelets, $\downarrow$WBC, $\downarrow$RBC, $\uparrow$PRA, may $\downarrow$glomerular filtration rate (GFR), GI or hepatic toxicity, pancreatitis, impotence				
	Distal tubular diuretics				
	Spironolactone	Aldactone	25/100	tid	4.87 (100)
	Triamterene	Dyrenium	100/300	qd	1.29 (100)
	Side-effects				
	$\uparrow$K$^+$, rash, hyperpigmentation, megaloblastic anemia (triamterene), $\uparrow$PRA, $\downarrow$GFR, nausea, vomiting, diarrhea, menstrual irregularities and gynecomastia (spironolactone), impotence, drowsiness, ataxia				
	Combination drugs				
	Spironolactone and hydrochlorothiazide	Aldactazide	1/4 tablets	bid	2.23 (2 tablets)
	Triamterene and hydrochlorothiazide	Dyazide	1/2 tablets	bid	8.0 (4 tablets)
		Maxide	1/2 tablets	qd	4.8 (1 tablet)
	Amiloride and hydrochlorothiazide	Moduretic	1/2 tablets	qd	5.6 (2 tablets)
	Side-effects				
	Same as for the constituent agents, except less $\uparrow$K$^+$ or $\downarrow$K$^+$				
Sympatholytics (centrally acting)	Methyldopa	Aldomet	250/3000	tid or qd	9.1 (1000)
	Side-effects				
	Drowsiness (usually transient), sedation, depression, impotence, fluid retention, orthostatic hypotension, positive direct Coombs' test (usually without clinical hemolysis), transaminase elevation, $\downarrow$PRA, GFR unchanged				
	Clonidine	Catapres	0.1/2.4	bid or qd	4.57 (0.6)
	Side-effects				
	Same as for methyldopa, plus weakly positive Coombs' test (without clinical hemolysis), sudden rebound hypertension with abrupt discontinuation of drug, bradycardia or heart block, impaired glucose tolerance				
	Guanabenz	Wytensin	8/64	bid	5.0 (8)
	Side-effects				
	Similar to clonidine				
Sympatholytics (beta-blocking agents)	Acebutolol	Sectral	400/800	qd	2.3 (400)
	Side-effects				
	Similar to propranolol, except lupus-like syndrome, less risk of bronchospasm, little orthostatic hypotension or bradycardia (beta$_1$ selective and alpha agonist)				
	Atenolol	Tenormin	25/100	qd	2.3 (50)
	Side-effects				
	Similar to propranolol, except less risk of bronchospasm and fewer CNS effects (beta$_1$ selective; low lipid solubility)				
	Labetalol	Trandate Normodyne	400/2400	bid	2.8 (400)
	Side-effects				
	Similar to propranolol except increased risks of orthostatic hypotension and impotence (nonselective beta blocker, selective alpha$_1$ blocker)				
	Metoprolol	Lopressor	100/400	qd or bid	2.2 (100)
	Side effects				
	Similar to propranolol except for less risk of bronchospasm (beta$_1$ selective)				

Table 21-2. Antihypertensive Drugs *(Continued)*

CLASS	DRUG	TRADE NAME	INITIAL/MAXIMUM DOSE (mg/day)	FREQUENCY OF DOSAGE	RELATIVE COST (dose in mg)
	Nadolol	Corgard	40/320	qd	3.2 (80)
	Side-effects Similar to propranolol (nonselective beta blocker)				
	Pindolol	Visken	20/80	bid	2.4 (10)
	Side-effects Similar to propranolol except less resting bradycardia (nonselective beta blocker; some agonist activity)				
	Propranolol	Inderal	40/2000	qid or bid	3.2 (120)
	Side-effects Bradycardia, congestive heart failure, bronchospasm, insomnia, depression, paresthesias, claudication, masking of hypoglycemia, impotence, sedation, possible preciptation of angina with abrupt discontinuation of drug, ↓PRA, ↓GFR, ↑K⁺, GI disturbances				
	Timolol	Blocadren	5/60	qd or bid	3.1 (20)
	Side-effects Similar to propranolol but less risk of CNS effects (nonselective beta blocker; low lipid solubility)				
Sympatholytics (peripherally acting)	Guanethidine	Ismelin	10/300	qd	1.78 (25)
	Side-effects Orthostatic hypotension (AM), weakness, bradycardia, diarrhea (dose related), nasal congestion, sedation (rare), impotence (retrograde ejaculation), ↑PRA				
	Reserpine	Raudixin Serpasil Sandril	100/300 0.1/0.5	qd	0.59 (0.25)
	Side-effects Drowsiness, nasal congestion, increased appetite, bradycardia, depression (can be severe), nightmares, ↑gastric acidity (may be ulcerogenic), parkinsonian rigidity, galactorrhea, postural hypotension (rare), impotence (rare), ?breast cancer (may promote development of preexisting disease)				
	Prazosin	Minipress	3.0/20	tid	3.96 (6)
	Side-effects Dizziness, drowsiness, headache, weakness, depression, palpitations, tachycardia, orthostatic hypotension, syncope (may occur suddenly after first dose), nausea, diarrhea, constipation, edema, dyspnea, rash, pruritus, dry mouth, blurred vision, impotence, urinary frequency, hallucinosis, ↓PRA				
Vasodilators	Hydralazine	Apresoline	40/400	qid or bid	1.22 (200)
	Side-effects Headache, tachycardia, palpitations, fever, weight gain, edema, lupus erythematosus-like syndrome (rare if dosage <200 mg/day), exacerbation of coronary insufficiency, ↑PRA, ↑ or −GFR				
	Minoxidil	Loniten	5/40	qd–qid	20 (20)
	Side-effects Sodium retention, peripheral edema, hirsutism, pericardial effusion; GFR unaffected				
Converting enzyme inhibitors	Captopril	Capoten	37.5/150	tid	9.9 (75)
	Enalapril	Vasotec	5/40	qd	10.7 (5)
	Side-effects Orthostatic hypotension, taste disturbance, leukopenia, agranulocytosis, pancytopenia, proteinuria, membranous glomerulopathy, acute renal failure in patients with bilateral renal artery stenosis or renal artery stenosis to solitary kidney				

as antagonist properties and hence less likely to cause bradycardia. *Labetalol* has alpha-blocking activities and hence acts similarly to the combination of a beta-blocker and vasodilator. It appears to be more likely to cause orthostatic hypotension and impotence. The beta-blockers with low lipid solubility (*e.g.,* atenolol, timolol) are less likely to penetrate the CNS and cause neuropsychiatric side-effects.

PERIPHERALLY-ACTING SYMPATHOLYTICS. *Prazosin* acts

peripherally to block alpha receptors causing arteriolar and venous dilatation. Because it affects both the venous and arterial systems, it causes less reflex tachycardia than pure arterial vasodilators. It may be used as an initial single agent in the treatment of mild hypertension, although it is more costly than diuretics, and many patients do not tolerate it well because of postural hypotension. Special note should be made of its tendency to cause profound orthostatic hypotension and syncope between 1 and 3 hours after the first dose. This can be avoided by giving a low dose (1 mg) at bedtime and instructing the patient to stay supine for at least 3 hours.

Guanethidine is a postganglionic blocker and is an effective antihypertension agent. However, its side-effects and the availability of much more easily tolerated medications should discourage its use unless and until other medications have failed. It causes significant postural hypotension, diarrhea, fatigue, impotence, and retrograde ejaculation. *Guanadrel* is a congener of guanethidine with a shorter duration of action but with the same array of side-effects and offers no advantage over guanethidine.

Reserpine is another postganglionic inhibitor. Its advantages are that its cost is low and it can be taken as a single daily dose. However, it has a number of significant side-effects including the development of severe depression, nightmares, drowsiness, nasal congestion, gastrointestinal disturbances, and bradycardia.

CENTRALLY ACTING SYMPATHOLYTICS. *Alphamethyldopa, clonidine,* and *guanabenz* are centrally acting sympatholytics that reduce blood pressure by stimulating central alpha receptors, which in turn reduce sympathetic outflow to the heart and vasculature. They should be considered second-line agents given to patients in whom diuretic therapy alone is inadequate and in whom beta-blockers have failed or are contraindicated. Because of their tendency to provoke secondary salt and water retention, in general, they should be used with a diuretic. Although all these agents frequently cause drowsiness, fatigue, and impotence, lower doses are often quite well tolerated, particularly in the older hypertensive population in whom beta-blockers may be less effective or poorly tolerated. Alphamethyldopa occasionally causes fever, acute or chronic hepatitis, and a Coombs' positive hemolytic anemia. Clonidine is more likely to cause sedation and dry mouth and is associated with the development of severe rebound hypertension following abrupt cessation of therapy. A slow-release transdermal patch is available and convenient, but very expensive. Skin irritation is common. Guanabenz is similar to clonidine in its action and side-effects.

ARTERIAL VASODILATORS. Hydralazine and minoxidil are arterial vasodilators that act directly to relax arterial smooth muscle, thus causing a reflex tachycardia and sodium and water retention. *Hydralazine* is typically used as a third-line agent in combination with a beta-blocker and a diuretic agent. In general, it requires dosing four times a day, which

often limits compliance. It typically causes headache, dizziness, and a lupuslike syndrome, especially in doses exceeding 200 mg/day. Because of its reflex tachycardia, it may exacerbate angina. *Minoxidil* is an extremely potent vasodilator that should be used only in patients with moderately severe hypertension uncontrolled by other medications. Both a beta-blocker and a loop diuretic must be used. Salt and water retention may be marked, requiring high doses of furosemide. Hypertrichosis is common. Minoxidil has been rarely associated with pericardial effusion and even more rarely with cardiac tamponade.

ANGIOTENSIN-CONVERTING ENZYME (ACE) INHIBITORS are represented by *captopril* and *enalapril*. This class of agents blocks the conversion of renin-activated angiotensin I to angiotensin II, an extremely potent vasoconstrictor that also stimulates the production of aldosterone. Although generally well tolerated, these agents can cause glomerular injury when used in high doses in patients with underlying renal disease. High-dose therapy with captopril has been linked to an occasionally fatal episode of agranulocytosis; skin rashes and taste disturbances also occur. When used in lower doses (*e.g.,* less than 150 mg of captopril per day) in patients with mild to moderate hypertension and no renal disease, the ACE inhibitors are effective and relatively free of side-effects. When compared in double-blind study to methyldopa and propranolol, captopril produced fewer side-effects and less impairment of the patient's sense of well-being.

The ACE inhibitors may be used alone or in combination with a diuretic or a beta-blocker. Because the ACE inhibitors block the production of aldosterone, they can lead to dangerous elevations in serum potassium when used in conjunction with a potassium-sparing diuretic or potassium supplementation; close monitoring of the serum potassium is indicated in such situations, but not when an ACE inhibitor is used alone. These agents should not be used in patients with unilateral or bilateral renal artery stenoses, because marked reduction in renal function may occur.

CALCIUM-CHANNEL BLOCKERS have proven useful as antihypertensive agents in patients with underlying coronary artery disease. *Nifedipine,* and, to a lesser extent, *diltiazem* have been found effective in lowering blood pressure in such patients. However, the need for frequent doses and the side-effects of nausea, anorexia, and peripheral edema limit their usefulness as antihypertensive agents.

TREATMENT RECOMMENDATIONS

- All patients should be put on a no-added salt diet, urged to lose weight if they are more than 15% above ideal weight, and advised to limit their alcohol intake to less than two drinks per day. Encouraging an exercise program (see Chapter 10) may also be of benefit.
- For patients with mild hypertension (diastolic pressures 90

to 100 mm Hg) and no associated cardiac risk factors, non-pharmacologic therapies can be initiated before resorting to drug treatment. However, if no improvement in blood pressure control is noted within several months, then pharmacologic treatment needs to be considered.

- For patients with mild to moderate hypertension (diastolic pressures 100 to 110 mm Hg), initial treatment should include all nonpharmacologic measures *plus* initiation of drug therapy with a single agent.
- For patients with moderate to severe hypertension (diastolic pressure greater than 110 mm Hg), initial treatment may require more than one agent from the outset.
- The agents of choice for initial therapy include thiazide diuretics, beta-blockers, and, perhaps, the ACE inhibitors.
- Thiazides are effective and very low in cost. Black patients, in particular, experience marked improvements in blood pressure control with thiazide use and sodium restriction. However, thiazide use in patients with cardiac disease may expose the patient to the risk of hypokalemia-induced dysrhythmias. Other potential disadvantages are their tendency to raise serum cholesterol and worsen glucose intolerance in diabetics.
- A beta-blocker is often preferred in the young hypertensive patient, because it is well tolerated and produces fewer metabolic derangements compared to the thiazides. Cost is greater, as is the frequency of such side-effects as fatigue and impotence. The less lipid-soluble preparations might cause fewer CNS side-effects.
- The ACE inhibitors are effective, better tolerated than the beta-blocking agents, and have no adverse effects on lipids; however, they are expensive. As experience with them grows and their safety becomes further established, they may emerge as the agents of choice for single-drug therapy of hypertension.
- Treatment should be initiated with a small dose of medication (*e.g.,* 25 to 50 mg/day of hydrochlorothiazide, 25 to 50 mg/day of atenolol, or 50 mg per day of captopril). In most patients, the goal is a gradual reduction in blood pressure to below 140/90; the guidelines are a bit more liberal for the elderly (see below). Rapid decreases blood pressure are unnecessary and likely to cause uncomfortable side-effects that compromise compliance. If a diuretic is not used, sodium restriction should be emphasized to avoid a return of hypertension from increased sodium reabsorption.
- If treatment with a single agent does not suffice, a second drug should be substituted for, rather than added to, the original regimen. This reduces side-effects, and by keeping the number of drugs to a minimum, enhances compliance. If the second drug does not work, switching to a third first-line agent may be tried before resorting to a two-drug regimen. When multi-drug therapy is required, the combination of a thiazide diuretic and a sympatholytic or beta-blocker is usually effective and a reasonable next step.

- Should hypertension persist despite use of a diuretic and a sympatholytic, hydralazine or prazosin is given as a third agent. This program will control 80% to 85% of all hypertensive patients, with minimal side-effects. An alternative to this three-drug program is to use an ACE inhibitor in combination with a diuretic; should that not suffice, a beta-blocker can be added. A third alternative is to prescribe a potent sympatholytic such as guanethidine in combination with a diuretic.
- Patients who are most difficult to control are candidates for the potent vasodilator minoxidil, usually in combination with a loop diuretic and a beta-blocker. Alternatively, a calcium-channel blocker may prove useful in this setting.

COMPLIANCE AND PATIENT EDUCATION

Unfortunately, most antihypertensive agents cause some uncomfortable side-effects. These factors naturally favor noncompliance with therapy. Attrition from treatment programs is high, and even when patients do keep their appointments faithfully, they may not be taking medications as prescribed. Nevertheless, recent evidence suggests that behavioral and educational efforts directed toward better compliance can be effective.

Home blood pressure determinations can successfully and inexpensively foster compliance. Provided the patient does not become obsessed or excessively alarmed, such determinations can provide useful information regarding blood pressure and its fluctuations in the home environment. Office visits can be minimized or promptly instituted if control is lost.

The increasing number of effective antihypertensive agents is allowing a greater degree of flexibility in treatment and *minimizing the number of pills* that need to be taken (an important cause of poor compliance). Thus, unpleasant side-effects can be circumvented by alternative therapeutic regimens. It is worthwhile mentioning in this regard the problem of impotence, which has been reported with the use of every available antihypertensive agent (although with particular frequency with certain sympatholytic agents). Both men and women should be questioned about sexual dysfunction shortly after initiation of antihypertensive therapy. Often the substitution of another drug or alteration in dosage will eliminate this problem.

Last, recent evidence suggests that patients who lose significant weight and modify their sodium intake while on antihypertensive medication may be able to tolerate either elimination of one or more antihypertensive agents or at least be controlled on lower doses. This potential for improved control by nonpharmacologic measures can be a powerful motivating factor and help achieve weight reduction and salt restriction.

SPECIAL TOPICS

Hypertension Associated with Estrogen-Containing Contraceptives. Elevation of systolic and diastolic blood pressure occurs in most patients receiving estrogen therapy over prolonged periods. Five percent of patients become hypertensive, and approximately one half of these remain hypertensive after hormonal therapy has been discontinued. Factors that predispose to the development of hypertension include family history or past history of high blood pressure, chronic renal disease, and hypertension with a previous pregnancy. A patient should be started on oral contraceptive or estrogen therapy only after a careful history has excluded these predisposing factors; once therapy is begun, continued blood pressure monitoring is required for the duration of treatment. The development of hypertension should prompt immediate cessation of therapy.

Hypertension Associated with Pregnancy. Hypertension that develops during pregnancy may represent either pre-eclampsia or exacerbation of preexisting hypertension. In the latter case, hypertension appears before 20 weeks of gestation, blood pressure is often quite high, and end-organ damage may already be evident. Patients with chronic hypertension are usually multigravidas. These patients are best managed by standard antihypertensive therapy as indicated, although, in general, the use of diuretics should be avoided unless control is not possible without them. Each of the commonly used agents appears safe and without adverse effects on the fetus, in particular, alpha-methyldopa, beta-blockers, and hydralazine. Clonidine, minoxidil, and ACE inhibitors are *not* established as safe during pregnancy and should be avoided.

Preeclampsia is characterized by a blood pressure of 140/90 mm Hg or higher, edema, and proteinuria, all of which appear in the third trimester. The typical patient is a very young primagravida. Multiple births, diabetes, or hydatidiform mole are common associated factors. It is now recognized that in early pregnancy blood pressure of normal women is low. This observation has led to clinical tests aimed at identifying patients at risk of the development of preeclampsia. Thus, a resting blood pressure above 110/75 mm Hg while the patient is sitting, or above 100/65 mm Hg while the patient is in the left lateral decubitus position, at 17 to 20 weeks of gestation, should alert one to the possibility of preeclampsia. Once diastolic blood pressure rises above 90 mm Hg, bed rest and, if necessary, hospitalization are indicated. Salt restriction and diuretic administration as therapies for preeclampsia are controversial; it is currently thought that they have the potential to aggravate this syndrome by stimulating the renin–angiotensin–aldosterone system.

Borderline Essential Hypertension. Borderline essential hypertension has become the focus of recent investigative interest. A subgroup of borderline hypertensive patients has been identified in whom excessive central nervous system sympathetic overactivity and parasympathetic underactivity result in a hyperdynamic, hyperkinetic state. These patients are characterized by increased cardiac output and heart rate. Although such patients respond well to therapeutic intervention with propranolol, the impact of treatment on disease progression and ultimate outcome has yet to be determined.

The Elderly Patient. Available epidemiologic and clinical trial data indicate that both systolic and diastolic hypertension in patients over age 65 carry increased cardiovascular morbidity and mortality and that treatment can lower the risk in patients with diastolic hypertension. Many elderly patients have isolated systolic hypertension (systolic pressure greater than 160 mm Hg and diastolics less than 90 mm Hg); as yet no evidence shows that reduction of isolated systolic hypertension reduces cardiovascular risk. The elderly do not tolerate volume depletion or sympathetic inhibition as well as young patients. Treatment of diastolic hypertension can proceed with small doses of a diuretic and avoidance of agents likely to cause postural hypotension. For those with isolated systolic hypertension, until more definitive data are available, it seems reasonable to begin with salt restriction and weight reduction. If the pressure does not come down to less than 160 mm Hg, then a cautious trial of diuretic therapy may be worth an attempt; the goal is a systolic pressure of less than 160 mm Hg.

The Diabetic Patient. Control of hypertension is particularly important in diabetics, because they are already very vulnerable to cardiovascular morbidity and mortality. Although thiazide diuretics may slightly worsen glucose intolerance, the effect is usually not of major clinical significance (see Chapter 100). Beta-blocking agents may mask the catecholamine-induced hypoglycemic response in patients taking excess doses of insulin, but this is rarely a problem, and usually the drugs are well tolerated in the well-tutored patient.

The Stroke Patient. Control of hypertension reduces the risk of recurrent stroke. The only pitfall is too rapid and too vigorous a reduction in blood pressure. Gradual reduction avoiding postural hypotension is the goal.

The Patient with Renal Failure. Hypertension can worsen renal function, and its control can slow progression of renal parenchymal disease. Sodium retention is usually a problem when the serum creatinine rises above 2.5 mg/dl and can lead to elevations in pressure. Furosemide, metolazone, and other potent diuretics may be needed to counter the sodium retention and reduce pressure. Beta-blocking agents, vasodilators, and ACE inhibitors are also effective, though captopril may worsen renal function. Minoxidil is used along with a diuretic in severe cases.

ANNOTATED BIBLIOGRAPHY

Croog SH, Levine S, Testa MA et al: The effects of antihypertensive therapy on the quality of life. N Engl J Med 314:1657, 1986 (*A multicenter randomized double-blind study of 626 men to determine the effects of captopril, methyldopa, and propranolol on their quality of life; captopril was the best tolerated.*)

Dustan HP: Nutrition and hypertension. Ann Intern Med 98:660, 1983 (*An editorial that takes a minimal view of the role of sodium, potassium, and calcium in the etiology of hypertension but acknowledges the importance of alcohol and obesity in the initiation and continuation of high blood pressure. This accompanies a 200-page symposium on nutrition and blood pressure control.*)

Freis ED et al: Veterans Administration cooperative study group on antihypertensive agents. I. Effects of treatment on morbidity in hypertension: Results in patients with diastolic blood pressures averaging 115 through 129 mm Hg. JAMA 202:1028, 1967. II. Results in patients with diastolic blood pressure averaging 90 through 114 mm Hg. JAMA 213:1143, 1970 (*The classic studies demonstrating that treatment of hypertension reduced morbidity and mortality from heart failure, renal failure, and stroke.*)

Freis, ED: Should mild hypertension be treated? N Engl J Med 307:306, 1982 (*Reviews the evidence and recommends treating patients with borderline or mild hypertension and other risk factors, but withholding drug therapy for those without other risk factors.*)

Helgeland A et al: Enalapril, atenolol and hydrochlorothiazide in mild to moderate hypertension: A comparative multicenter study in Norway. Lancet 1:872, 1986 (*In a study of 436 patients with mild to moderate hypertension, the three drugs that were compared showed similar efficacy with much greater patient tolerance of enalapril and hydrochlorothiazide and an important effect on potassium, uric acid, and blood sugar in patients on hydrochloroathiazide. They found a more favorable risk profile for the enalapril-treated group.*)

Holden RA, Ostfeld AM, Freeman DH et al: Dietary salt intake and blood pressure. JAMA 250:365, 1983 (*Dietary salt assessment and blood pressure therapy effectively lowered systolic blood pressure by reducing systemic vascular resistance.*)

Hypertension Detection and Follow-Up Program Cooperative Group: The five year findings of the Hypertension Detection Follow-Up Program. JAMA 242:2562, 1979 (*A randomized trial of stepped care versus referred care demonstrating a reduction in mortality with stepped care, including among those with mild hypertension.*)

Hypertension Detection Follow-Up Program Cooperative Group: The effect of treatment on mortality in "mild" hypertension. N Engl J Med 307:976, 1982 (*A 20% lower 5-year mortality was found in patients with diastolic blood pressures between 90 and 104 mm Hg who were treated intensively with stepped care compared with similar patients who were simply referred to their usual source of care for treatment.*)

Kannel WB, Wolf PA, McGee DL: Systolic blood pressure, arterial rigidity, and risk of stroke. JAMA 245:1225, 1981 (*Subjects with isolated systolic hypertension experienced two to four times as many strokes as did normotensive persons in the Framingham study.*)

Kaplan NM: Use of non-drug therapy in treating hypertension. Am J Med 96, 5 Oct 1984 (*Excellent review, documenting efficacies of nondrug treatments; 69 references.*)

Lindheimer MD, Katz AI: Hypertension and pregnancy. N Engl J Med 313:675, 1985 (*Includes a useful discussion of antihypertensive drug therapy in pregnancy.*)

MacMahon SW, Norton RN: Alcohol and hypertension. Ann Intern Med 105:124, 1986 (*An editorial summarizing the evidence linking the two conditions and recommending a limit of two drinks or less per day.*)

Medical Research Council Working Party: MRC trial of treatment of mild hypertension: Principal results. Br Med J 291:97, 1985 (*English trial of benefit of treating mild hypertension with either propranolol or a diuretic. Those treated had a reduction in stroke. There was no benefit in overall rates of coronary events. Diuretic therapy was more efective than sblocade in reducing the incidence of strokes. Propranolol reduced coronary events only in nonsmokers.*)

National Heart Foundation of Australia Study: Treatment of mild hypertension in the elderly. Med J Aust 2:398, 1981 (*Elderly patients with diastolic pressures greater than 95 mm Hg benefitted from therapy.*)

Patel C, Marmot MG, Terry DJ: Controlled trial of biofeedback-aided behavioral methods in reducing mild hypertension. Br Med J 282:2005, 1981 (*A modest but significant reduction in blood pressure was achieved and it persisted for the 1 year of follow-up.*)

Pettinger WA: Minoxidil and the treatment of severe hypertension. N Engl J Med 303:922, 1980 (*Reviews of the pharmacology and clinical use of this potent vasodilator.*)

Taguchi J, Freis ED: Partial reduction of blood pressure and prevention of complications in hypertension. N Engl J Med 291:329, 1974 (*This article makes the important point that even partial reduction of blood pressure reduces significantly the complications of hypertension.*)

Vardan S, Mookherjee S, Warner R et al: Systolic hypertension in the elderly. JAMA 250:2807, 1983 (*Thiazide therapy effectively lowered systolic blood pressure by reducing systemic vascular resistance.*)

Veterans Administration Cooperative Study on Antihypertensive Agents: Comparison of propranolol and hydrochlorothiazide for the initial treatment of hypertension. JAMA 248:1996, 1982 (*Propranolol and hydrochlorothiazide were equally efficacious among whites in the short term; hydrochlorothiazide was more effective during long-term therapy but induced more treatment withdrawal and biochemical abnormalities.*)

Vidt DG, Bravo EL, Fouad FM: Captopril. N Engl J Med 306:214, 1982 (*A brief review of pharmacology and clinical use including adverse effects.*)

Weinberger MH: Oral contraceptives and hypertension. Hosp Pract 10:65, 1975 (*Review summarizes current knowledge on oral contraceptives and hypertension.*)

Weinberger MH: Antihypertensive therapy and lipids. Arch Intern Med 145:1102, 1985 (*Mechanisms and implications of lipid changes associated with antihypertensive agents.*)

22
Approach to the Patient
with Hypercholesterolemia

WAYNE L. PETERS, M.D.

Hypercholesterolemia is a major risk factor for coronary artery disease (see Chapter 9). The importance of correcting this risk factor has been underscored by the Lipid Research Clinical Trials, which demonstrated reduced morbidity and mortality from coronary heart disease and slowed progression of atheromatous coronary lesions when total cholesterol and LDL cholesterol levels were reduced and HDL cholesterol was raised. Elevated levels of total serum cholesterol may be due to an inherited disorder of lipid metabolism, an underlying disease that causes lipid elevation, and/or dietary indiscretion. The primary treatment for most hyperlipidemias that result in hypercholesterolemia is diet; drug therapy is reserved for the diet-refractory case.

The primary care physician needs to know how to work up the patient who is found, on screening, to have an elevated serum total cholesterol, how to design an effective, yet practical dietary program, and how to carry out pharmacologic treatment when diet alone does not suffice.

PATHOPHYSIOLOGY

The heterogeneity of the hyperlipidemias can be a source of confusion in the approach to patients with elevated cholesterol levels. Consideration of the normal and pathologic physiology of lipids and their lipoproteins, and a review of the effect diet has on lipid metabolism facilitates an understanding of classification schemes, evaluation strategies, and treatment plans.

Lipoproteins

Lipids circulate in the blood attached to lipoproteins, which are involved in their delivery, storage, and clearance (Fig. 22-1). Lipoproteins (lipid + apoprotein) are composed of a central lipid core surrounded by a membranous coating of unesterified cholesterol, phospholipids, and apoproteins (Table 22-1). The principal lipoproteins are the chylomicrons, the very low-density lipoproteins (VLDL), the low-density lipoproteins (LDL), and the high-density lipoproteins (HDL).

Chylomicrons, the lowest density lipoprotein, carry predominantly triglycerides derived from dietary fat. The chylomicron particle is not considered to be atherogenic; the atherogenic potential of chylomicron remnants is a matter of dispute.

Very Low-Density Lipoproteins. The main function of VLDL is to transport triglycerides synthesized in the liver and intestines to capillary beds in adipose tissue and muscle, where they are hydrolyzed.

Normal VLDL is probably not atherogenic. The smaller and more cholesterol-rich VLDL remnants, which persist after hydrolysis, appear to have atherogenic potential. Persons with the genetic disorder familial dysbetalipoproteinemia (Type III or VLDL remnant hyperlipidemia) have accelerated atherogenesis. Animals that develop atherosclerosis secondary to cholesterol feeding have increased numbers of lipoproteins similar to human VLDL remnants. Although elevations of plasma triglycerides are common in patients with coronary heart disease (CHD), they are not uniformly independent predictors for CHD risk.

Low-Density Lipoproteins. LDL is the major carrier of cholesterol; it is responsible for supplying cholesterol to the tissues and regulating the serum cholesterol level. Two routes for LDL metabolism are available, a receptor-dependent mechanism and a scavenger (receptor-independent) pathway. Individuals with familial hypercholesterolemia can have absent, decreased, or defective receptors. When LDL levels in the plasma become excessive (as from dietary indiscretion), LDL is removed by the macrophages of the reticuloendothelial system by the scavenger pathway. Macrophages in the arterial wall eventually become overloaded with cholesterol esters and are converted to the "foam" cells that characterize early atherosclerosis.

Because the majority of plasma cholesterol (60% to 75%) is carried in the LDL particle, elevations of total cholesterol usually reflect increased LDL levels. The anatomic degree of coronary atherosclerosis has been directly linked to the concentration of LDL.

High-Density Lipoproteins. HDL (alpha lipoprotein) appears to be the primary component of a reverse cholesterol transport system carrying cholesterol from peripheral cells to the liver for catabolism. Nascent HDL particles are secreted by the liver and intestine and appear to have an affinity for free (unesterified) cholesterol from cell membranes or other lipoprotein particles (especially VLDL). Once free cholesterol is incorporated and esterified, the particle is designated HDL_2.

Strongly independent inverse correlations between HDL cholesterol and CHD have been reported from numerous

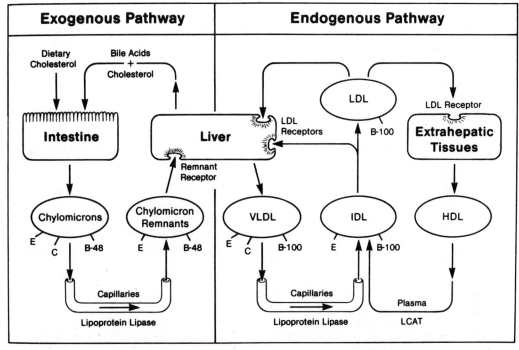

Figure 22-1.   Separate pathways for receptor-mediated metabolism of lipoproteins carrying endogenous and exogenous cholesterol. HDL = high-density lipoprotein; LCAT = lecithin:cholesterol acetyltransferase; LDL = low-density lipoprotein; IDL = intermediate-density lipoprotein; and VLDL = very-low-density lipoprotein. The distinction between exogenous and endogenous cholesterol applies to the immediate source of the cholesterol in plasma lipoproteins. After the exogenous cholesterol has been delivered to the liver and has been secreted in VLDL, it is considered endogenous cholesterol. The role of each lipoprotein is discussed in the text. HDL is shown as the lipoprotein that removes cholesterol from extrahepatic cells and delivers it to IDL through the action of plasma LCAT and a cholesterol ester–transport protein (From Goldstein JL, Kita T, Brown MS: N Engl J Med 309:288, 1983. Reprinted with permission.)

clinical and epidemiologic studies. HDL_2 seems to best reflect that relationship. Apoprotein A-I may be an even more useful discriminator for CHD than HDL. Obesity, tobacco use, lack of exercise, hypertriglyceridemia, maleness, and poorly defined genetic factors are associated with low HDL levels.

Because the addition of an HDL cholesterol level to a random total blood cholesterol leads to more precise prediction of CHD risk, some have suggested using the total cholesterol/HDL ratio or the LDL/HDL ratio as the best single

"number" for assessing CHD risk. A total cholesterol/HDL ratio of ≤4.5 implies reduced risk. The average ratio for individuals with CHD is 5.3 to 5.8, with values of 10 and 20 approximating double and triple the average risk.

Dietary Influences on Lipoproteins. Dietary fats have a major influence on plasma total cholesterol and LDL levels in persons consuming typical American diets. Although sensitivity to fats varies among individuals, the mean response

Table 22-1.   Composition of Plasma Lipoproteins

	PERCENT		PERCENT LIPID	
LIPOPROTEIN	*Protein*	*Cholesterol*	*Triglyceride*	*Phospholipid*
Chylomicrons	1–2	2–12	80–95	3–15
VLDL	10	9–24	50–80	10–25
LDL	25	57	13	30
HDL	50	30	10	60

to changes in dietary fatty acids (through feeding experiments) is approximated by the formula of Keys:

$$\Delta \text{ Total cholesterol} = 1.3(2\Delta S - \Delta P)$$

where ΔS and ΔP are the changes in the percentage of total calories contributed by saturated and polyunsaturated fats, respectively.

SATURATED FATTY ACIDS. Long-chain saturated fatty acids have no double bonds and are not essential for human growth and development. They predictably raise the total plasma cholesterol and LDL levels by causing increases in the rates of synthesis of LDL and/or LDL apoprotein B. The major sources of saturated fat in the American diet (see Table 22-2) are animal fats, that is, red meat (beef, pork, veal, lamb, ham) and whole milk products (milk, butter, ice cream, cream cheese, hard cheese, cottage cheese, yogurt). Chicken and turkey (prepared skinless) contain less saturated fat. The three plant sources of saturated fat are coconut oil, palm oil, and cocoa butter. Unfortunately for the consumer, coconut and palm oil are widespread additives in commercially prepared foods. Unless the consumer routinely reads product ingredient labels, these "invisible" fats can contribute a major share of dietary saturated fatty acids. Cocoa butter exerts a more modest hypercholesterolemic effect, perhaps because of its high concentration of stearic acid. Products made with hydrogenated vegetable oil or shortening contain artificially "saturated" fatty acids.

MONOUNSATURATED FATTY ACIDS. Monounsaturated fatty acids are present in all animal and vegetable fats. Oleic acid, a nonessential fatty acid with one double bond, is the most common dietary monounsaturate. These fatty acids cause either no change or lowering of LDL levels, depending on the fatty acid composition of the reference diet. Major dietary sources include olives, olive oil, peanuts, peanut butter, avocados, seeds, and nuts (almonds, filberts, pecans).

POLYUNSATURATED FATTY ACIDS. Polyunsaturated fatty acids (PUFA) are not synthesized by the body and therefore are essential fatty acids. They serve important functions in cellular membranes and as prostaglandin precursors. The two primary families of PUFA, n-6 and n-3, are named for the location of the first double bond counting from the methyl end of the fatty acid.

The most common n-6 PUFAs are linoleic acid (C18:2) and arachidonic acid (C20:4). Principal dietary sources of n-6 PUFA are the liquid vegetable oils (safflower, sunflower, soybean, corn) and products containing these oils (see Table 22-2). The n-3 PUFA, linolenic acid (C18:3), is found in certain vegetable oils (new rapeseed) and leafy vegetables. Eicosapentaenoic acid (C20:5) and docosahexaenoic acid (C22:6) are present in the oil of fish and shellfish.

Fish oils are being studied for the potentially antiatherosclerotic effects of PUFA. A low incidence of atherosclerosis was initially reported among Greenland Eskimos and subsequently confirmed among Japanese fishermen. Both groups ingest a marine-based diet, suggesting a potential dietary

Table 22-2.   Fatty Acid Composition of Commonly Consumed Foods
(as percentage of total fatty acids)

FOOD	SATURATED	MONOUNSATURATED	POLYUNSATURATED
Butter, cream, milk	65	30	5
Beef	46	48	6
Bacon and pork	38	50	12
Lard	42	45	13
Chicken	33	39	28
Fish	29	31	40
Coconut oil	92	6	2
Palm kernel oil	86	12	2
Cocoa butter	63	34	3
Olive oil	15	76	9
Peanut oil	20	48	32
Cottonseed oil	27	20	53
Soybean oil	16	24	60
Corn oil	13	26	61
Sunflower seed oil	11	22	67
Safflower seed oil	10	13	77

means of reducing atherosclerosis through ingestion of more fish and fish oils. Mortality from CHD was more than 50% lower in a group of Dutch men who consumed at least 30 g of fish per day than among those who did not eat fish. Both n-3 and n-6 PUFA cause decreased levels of total and LDL cholesterol, although eicosapentaenoic acid (EPA) may exert a greater LDL-lowering effect than linoleic acid on a gram-for-gram basis. In addition, EPA has shown a profound VLDL-lowering effect in early studies. The precise mechanisms for these lipoprotein effects are not presently understood. Polyunsaturated fatty acids may decrease the synthesis or increase the clearance of apoprotein B.

DIETARY CHOLESTEROL. Dietary cholesterol has a smaller effect than saturated fatty acids on raising plasma total and LDL cholesterol. Although standard formulas are available for precisely calculating this change, each 100 mg of dietary cholesterol raises plasma total and LDL cholesterol by approximately 7 mg/dl. Diet-derived cholesterol may be most hypercholesterolemic when consumed in diets with ratios of polyunsaturated to saturated fats (P/S) of less than 0.8. Possible mechanisms of action include increased LDL synthesis and/or decreased LDL catabolism.

Organ meats (brain, liver, kidney, heart, sweetbreads) and egg yolks are concentrated sources of dietary cholesterol (see Table 22-3). Although shrimp and crab contain moderate amounts of cholesterol, its effect in these foods may be offset by the concomitant presence of eicosapentaenoic acid. Cholesterol is absent in food derived from plant sources.

CARBOHYDRATES, PROTEIN, AND TOTAL CALORIC INTAKE. At present, there is no conclusive evidence that either dietary carbohydrate (simple sugar and complex carbohydrate) or protein (animal or vegetable) significantly affect LDL levels in humans. Increased total caloric intake associated with obesity *may* induce overproduction of VLDL triglycerides and synthesis of apoprotein B, both of which may raise LDL levels. HDL levels are depressed in overweight individuals.

FIBER. Oat bran, a water-soluble fiber, and legumes have a putative LDL-lowering effect. Modest decreases in LDL have also been reported for the gums guar and pectin, presumably by means of interference with bile acid reabsorption. Additional investigation is needed to establish with greater certainty the effects of the multiple constituents of fiber on blood cholesterol levels.

CLASSIFICATION AND WORKUP OF HYPERCHOLESTEROLEMIA

Hypercholesterolemia emerges as the common denominator for lipid and lipoprotein abnormalities associated with increased risk of coronary heart disease. A clinically useful classification system for these abnormalities specifies the underlying lipoprotein–cholesterol abnormality or abnormalities that contribute to the cholesterol elevation. A classification

Table 22-3. Cholesterol Content of Common Foods

FOOD	AMOUNT OF FOOD	CHOLESTEROL CONTENT (MG)
Brains	3.5 oz (100 g)	>2000
Liver, chicken	3.5 oz	555
Kidney	3.5 oz	375
Liver, beef	3.5 oz	300
Caviar	1 tbsp	>300
Egg yolk	1	252
Shrimp	3.5 oz	150
Crab	3.5 oz	100
Mackeral	3.5 oz	95
Lobster (cooked)	3.5 oz	85
Cheese, cheddar	3.5 oz	84
Veal	3.5 oz	70
Chicken, breast	3.5 oz	67
Beef	3.5 oz	65
Pork	3.5 oz	62
Clams	3.5 oz	50
Flounder	3.5 oz	50
Oysters	3.5 oz	50
Ice cream (regular)	1 cup	40
Butter	1 tbsp	35
Scallops	3.5 oz	35
Milk, whole	1 cup	14
Milk, 2%	1 cup	9
Milk, skim	1 cup	2
Margarine	1 tbsp	0

system for patients with hypercholesterolemia based on the quantitative lipoprotein–cholesterol abnormality permits stratification by risk of CHD (see Table 22-1), serves as an organizing scheme for differential diagnosis (see Table 22-2), and suggests specific dietary, behavioral, and/or drug interventions (see Table 22-3).

Classification and workup begin with making the diagnosis of hypercholesterolemia, which can be defined somewhat arbitrarily as a *total blood cholesterol* concentration of *greater than 200 mg/dl.* Above this level, the slope of the curve relating CHD risk to total blood cholesterol level begins increasing more steeply (see Chapter 9). Below this cholesterol concentration, the risk of CHD is usually modest and not a cause for concern. However, it must be recognized that there is no threshold level for CHD risk; the lower the total cholesterol, the lower the risk (with the exception of patients whose elevated total cholesterol is due solely to HDL elevation).

Hypercholesterolemia is best screened for by a *random total blood cholesterol* determination (see Chapter 9). A second determination is important to confirm the elevation. Two total cholesterol levels in excess of 200 mg/dl constitute a diagnosis of hypercholesterolemia. Once that diagnosis is established, the underlying lipoprotein–cholesterol abnormality producing the hypercholesterolemia needs to be identified.

Because total cholesterol can be expressed by the formula

Total cholesterol = LDL cholesterol

+ HDL cholesterol + VLDL cholesterol

one can readily calculate some of these terms if *triglyceride* and *HDL levels* are known from serum or plasma determinations. Lipoprotein electrophoresis, an expensive procedure, need not be done. HDL cholesterol determinations are now widely available and appropriate for workup of hypercholesterolemia, although some assays lack accuracy and reproducibility. The VLDL cholesterol can be estimated by the formula

VLDL cholesterol = Fasting triglyceride level ÷ 5

This determination requires a fasting sample because the triglyceride level is acutely affected by food intake. The estimate for VLDL cholesterol holds for fasting triglyceride levels up to about 400 to 500 mg/dl; beyond this range, the estimate becomes inaccurate. Knowing the total cholesterol, the HDL cholesterol, and the VLDL cholesterol, one can calculate LDL cholesterol from the formula

LDL cholesterol = Total cholesterol

− HDL cholesterol − VLDL cholesterol

In many laboratories, this LDL calculation has already been performed for the clinician. LDL cholesterol is directly measured by ultracentrifugation in only a few specialized lipid research laboratories.

With these determinations completed, the lipoprotein–cholesterol concentrations can be compared to reference levels and categorization of any lipoprotein–cholesterol abnormalities made, whether it is an elevated HDL cholesterol, an elevated LDL cholesterol, an elevated VLDL cholesterol, or a combination of elevations. Each of these subcategories of hypercholesterolemia has its own associated CHD risk (Table 22-4) and differential diagnosis (Table 22-5).

One *hypo*lipidemic state must be considered, especially in patients with symptomatic CHD and/or a family history of premature CHD (onset before age 55). A *depressed HDL cholesterol* level (HDL < 35 mg/dl with a total cholesterol/HDL ratio > 4.5) contributes to CHD risk as much as or more than a high LDL cholesterol level.

It is important to note that this classification system does not encompass all known lipid and lipoprotein disorders, but rather is limited to those most commonly associated with hypercholesterolemia and risk for CHD. The classification system of Fredrickson and Lees remains the standard for comprehensive classification, but it is cumbersome for guiding workup and management of most patients with hypercholesterolemia.

The possibility of a genetic disorder should be considered when extremes of any lipoprotein–cholesterol level are encountered and/or there is a history of premature CHD (onset of disease before age 55) in the patient or family members. Therapy in any instance will be the same—dietary and health-related behavioral intervention followed by drug therapy as necessary (see below). Screening of other family members for hypercholesterolemia is strongly recommended.

PRINCIPLES OF MANAGEMENT AND THERAPEUTIC RECOMMENDATIONS

The recent rigorously conducted Lipid Research Clinic Trials demonstrated reduced coronary heart disease morbidity and mortality and slowed progression of atheromatous coronary lesions when total cholesterol and LDL cholesterol levels were reduced. For every 1% reduction in cholesterol there was a 2% reduction in CHD risk. These results con-

Table 22-4.   CHD Risk Associated with Lipoprotein Cholesterol Abnormalities

LIPOPROTEIN–CHOLESTEROL	LEVEL (MG/DL)	ESTIMATED CHD RISK
LDL–cholesterol	125–185	Moderate
	>185	High
HDL–cholesterol	>65 (and total cholesterol/HDL ratio < 4.5)	Low
	<35 (and total cholesterol/HDL ratio > 4.5)	Moderate–high
VLDL–cholesterol	50–100 (or fasting triglycerides 250–500)	Low
	>100 (or fasting triglycerides > 500)	?

Table 22-5. Differential Diagnosis of Hypercholesterolemia

1. Moderate LDL Cholesterol Elevation: LDL = 125–185 mg/dl
   (In most individuals this is equivalent to a total cholesterol of 200–260 mg/dl)
   a. Dietary contribution (present in everyone to varying degrees)
   b. Genetic contribution (ill-defined for majority of people in this range)
   c. Secondary LDL increase (hypothyroidism, nephrotic syndrome, acute intermittent porphyria, Cushing's syndrome, dysproteinemia, obstructive liver disease)
2. Marked LDL Cholesterol Elevation: LDL > 185 mg/dl
   (In most individuals this translates into a total cholesterol >260 mg/dl)
   a. Dietary contribution (present in everyone to varying degrees)
   b. Genetic contribution (these known abnormalities account for a minority of cases)
      1. Polygenic hypercholesterolemia
      2. Familial combined hyperlipidemia
      3. Monogenic hypercholesterolemia (predominant LDL overproduction)
      4. Familial broad-beta (dysbeta) hyperlipoproteinemia
      5. Familial hypercholesterolemia (LDL receptor-mediated clearance defect)
   c. Secondary hypercholesterolemia (see above)
3. Elevated HDL Cholesterol: HDL > 65 mg/dl
   a. A high HDL explains the total cholesterol "elevation," with LDL levels < 125 mg/dl or the total cholesterol/HDL ratio ≤ 4.5; pattern predicts low risk for CHD and requires no treatment
4. Elevated VLDL Cholesterol: Fasting triglycerides > 250 mg/dl
   a. Dietary contribution—see also diet-related secondary cases below
      1. High carbohydrate diets may cause transient triglyceride increases
   b. Genetic contribution (triglycerides often >500 mg/dl)
      1. Familial combined hyperlipidemia
      2. Familial hypertriglyceridemia
      3. Familial broad-beta (dysbeta) hyperlipoproteinemia
      4. Genetic lipolysis defects
   c. Secondary (obesity, excessive alcohol intake, uncontrolled diabetes mellitus, uremia, nephrotic syndrome, dysproteinemia, oral contraceptives, thiazide diuretics, and beta-adrenergic blocking agents)
5. Depressed HDL Cholesterol: HDL < 35 mg/dl
   a. Genetic (poorly defined)—concomitant triglycerides often >250 mg/dl
   b. Behavioral (obesity, cigarette smoking, sedentary life-style)
   c. Drugs (progestins, anabolic steroids, androgens, some beta-adrenergic blocking agents, thiazide diuretics)
   d. Normal variant (if LDL correspondingly low, *i.e.,* <125 mg/dl)
6. Combination of the Above
   a. Many patients have more than one of these lipoprotein abnormalities contributing to their hypercholesterolemia and CHD risk. Although causation for each can be considered individually, therapies utilizing diet, behavior, and/or drugs often overlap

firmed the multiple strong epidemiologic associations of hypercholesterolemia with coronary heart disease and the vast array of supportive experimental animal and clinical hypolipidemic trials preceding them. Thus, a very sound scientific basis now exists for recommending efforts to reduce total blood cholesterol and LDL levels to achieve primary and secondary prevention of CHD. Precise data on just how much total and LDL blood cholesterol lowering is most effective and in whom it should be carried out are not currently available, but an estimate of CHD risk and need for treatment can be made on the basis of the patient's qualitative and quantitative lipoprotein–cholesterol abnormality or abnormalities (see Table 22-4). A rational treatment program can be designed in similar fashion (see below).

Diet

Dietary therapy represents the first line of therapy for both the treatment and prevention of clinically significant hypercholesterolemia (total serum cholesterol > 200 mg/dl) (Table 22-6). Reductions in total fat, saturated fat, and dietary cholesterol are recommended for all adults.

The National Institutes of Health has recommended that all Americans (except children under 2 years of age) (1) reduce total dietary fat intake from the current level of about 40% of total calories to 30% of total calories; (2) reduce saturated fat intake to less than 10% of total calories; (3) limit polyunsaturated fat intake to 8% to 10% of total calories; (4) reduce daily cholesterol intake to 250 to 300 mg; and (5) reduce total calories, if necessary, to correct obesity and maintain ideal body weight.

Available data suggest that modest amounts of PUFA (8% to 10% of total calories) should be present in the diet. At this level of intake, lipoproteins can be favorably affected while minimizing possible untoward effects (cholesterol gallstones, carcinogenesis, and/or unstable lipid fractions in cell membranes).

A phased approach maximizes adherence to recommended dietary changes. Total fat, saturated fat, and cholesterol intake are gradually reduced with partial replacement by polyunsaturated fat. Intake of complex carbohydrates (fruits, vegetables, cereals, pasta, grains, and legumes) is strongly encouraged. Table 22-7 outlines one such stepwise

Table 22-6.   Therapy for Hypercholesterolemia (Total Cholesterol > 200 mg/dl)

LIPOPROTEIN ABNORMALITY	TREATMENT WITH DIET/ HEALTH BEHAVIORS	TREATMENT WITH DRUGS
Elevated LDL cholesterol (>125 mg/dl)	Reduce total and saturated fat Reduce dietary cholesterol Increase PUFA (moderation) Lose weight if obese Increase water-soluble fiber	Cholestyramine Cholestipol Nicotinic acid Neomycin
Elevated VLDL cholesterol (fasting triglycerides >250 mg/dl)	Decrease total calories Lose weight if obese Exercise Decrease alcohol intake	Nicotinic acid Gemfibrozil Eicosapentaenoic acid
Elevated HDL cholesterol (>65 mg/dl and total cholesterol/HDL ratio < 4.5)	No therapy—low-risk profile	
Depressed HDL cholesterol (<35 mg/dl and total cholesterol/ HDL ratio > 4.5)	Lose weight if obese Regular aerobic exercise Stop cigarette smoking	?Gemfibrozil

approach to diet, the Massachusetts General Hospital phased diet, which uses a color-coded zone system. Each zone represents a particular level of expected total and LDL cholesterol lowering. Selection of a particular zone is based on the underlying lipoprotein abnormality and its attendant CHD risk. The early involvement of a registered dietitian facilitates patient understanding and adherence to the dietary regimens.

Moderate LDL Cholesterol Elevation (125 to 185 mg/ dl)—Moderate Risk. For this degree of elevation, the modest dietary changes of the yellow zone (phase I of the American Heart Association) should suffice and result in average total and LDL cholesterol reductions of 20 to 40 mg/dl. Individuals consuming a high-fat baseline diet are often more susceptible to diet-induced plasma cholesterol lowering. Most people with

moderate LDL elevation can approach the ideal range of LDL < 125 mg/dl and total cholesterol < 200 mg/dl without radically altering their diets. The weight loss that often accompanies a lower-fat diet may further contribute to lowering of LDL and an increase in HDL. Approaching and maintaining ideal body weight should remain a primary goal. Regular intake of fish rich in eicosapentaenoic acid and water-soluble fiber (oat bran, legumes) will further enhance decreases in LDL. Polyunsaturated fatty acids should constitute no more than 8% to 10% of total calories.

Marked LDL Cholesterol Elevation (>185 mg/dl)—High Risk. Attempts to dramatically reduce dietary saturated fat and cholesterol should be maximized in these patients. Motivated individuals can often avoid the consequences of life-

Table 22-7.   The Massachusetts General Hospital Phased Diet Guidelines

	AVERAGE U.S. DIET	ZONES		
		Yellow	*Blue*	*Green*
Total fat (as percentage of total calories)	40–45	30	25	20
Saturated	17	10	6	3
Monounsaturated	18	10	9	7
Polyunsaturated	7	10	10	10
Protein (%)	15–20	15	15	15
Carbohydrate (%)	40–45	55	60	65
Dietary cholesterol (mg)	500	300	200	100
P/S ratio	0.4	1	1.7	3.3
Range of average total/LDL cholesterol decrease (mg/dl)		20–40	40–60	60–80

long medication by strict adherence to blue- and green-zone guidelines (see Table 22-7). Four to 6 months should be allowed for implementation of these significant dietary life-style changes. The effect of any LDL cholesterol-lowering medication is enhanced by diets that restrict saturated fat and cholesterol intake. Concomitant therapy for any secondary cause of LDL cholesterol elevation (see Table 22-5) is indicated.

Depressed HDL Cholesterol (<35 mg/dl)—Moderate to High Risk. Although dietary fat restriction sometimes lowers HDL levels, the important change is the total cholesterol/ HDL ratio, which usually decreases; this change is associated with decreased risk of CHD. Weight loss, smoking cessation, and regular aerobic exercise may increase HDL by 5 to 15 mg/dl. Ethanol also elevates HDL levels, but consumption for this purpose is not advocated.

Elevated VLDL Cholesterol (Fasting Triglycerides > 250 mg/dl)—Low (?) Risk. Fasting triglycerides > 250 mg/dl are considered unlikely to be solely responsible for accelerated atherogenesis. Rather, they are often markers for other genetic lipoprotein disorders and/or numerous life-style or metabolic characteristics that are considered to be contributors to the atherogenic process. Low HDL, low apoprotein A-I, and high apoprotein B levels frequently accompany elevated triglycerides. Fasting triglycerides consistently above 500 mg/dl are associated with an increased risk for acute pancreatitis, and thus should be lowered. Weight loss and maintenance of desirable weight often decrease VLDL and triglycerides to normal levels. Avoidance of calorically dense foods (fat, alcohol, simple sugars) is crucial for success. Increased intake of complex carbohydrates may transiently raise VLDL synthesis and, therefore, triglyceride levels.

Drug Therapy

Although prudent modification of dietary intake remains the keystone for successful therapy of hypercholesterolemia, factors that should prompt consideration of drug therapy (Table 22-8) include (1) inadequate diet-induced LDL cholesterol lowering, (2) poor adherence to dietary recommen-dations, (3) high-risk hypercholesterolemia, and (4) potential for accelerated atherogenesis by the presence of other major CHD risk factors. The decision to begin potentially life-long medication should be made only after careful scrutiny, bal-ancing the expected benefits with the cost and side-effects of therapy, especially in low- to moderate-risk patients with un-complicated moderate elevations of LDL cholesterol or VLDL cholesterol. Selection of agent is a function of lipo-protein–cholesterol abnormality, drug mechanism of action, and patient tolerance of side-effects. The regimen should be tailored to the individual patient.

Marked LDL Elevation—High Risk. In many of these patients, strict adherence to a low-saturated-fat and low-cho-lesterol diet does not normalize the total cholesterol (<200 mg/dl) and LDL cholesterol (<125 mg/dl). The effectiveness of drug therapy has been demonstrated for primary and sec-ondary prevention of CHD from hypercholesterolemia due to LDL cholesterol elevation. Several drugs produce signifi-cant decreases in LDL cholesterol.

BILE ACID SEQUESTRANTS, cholestyramine (Questran) and colestipol (Colestid), are drugs of choice for initial therapy of hypercholesterolemia due to marked LDL elevations. These bile-acid-binding resins interrupt the normal entero-hepatic circulation of bile acids. The result is decreased return of bile acids to the liver, increased hepatocyte conversion of intracellular cholesterol into bile acids, and subsequent in-creases in the number of hepatic surface LDL receptors as the intracellular cholesterol concentration falls. These drugs are best tolerated when started in dosages of one or two pack-ets or scoopfuls daily and gradually increased to the usual four to six packets or scoopfuls per day. Constipation, the most common side-effect, can be prevented or alleviated by increased dietary fiber, bran cereal, stool bulk–producing agents, dried apricots, or prunes. Concomitant anionic drugs (*e.g.,* thiazides, thyroxine, digitalis, coumadin, tetracycline, vancomycin, and phenobarbital) should be taken 1 hour be-fore or 4 hours after the sequestrants to prevent their ad-sorption by the sequestrants. With high doses, steatorrhea and impaired absorption of the fat-soluble vitamins A, D, E, and K may occur, though this is rare. Vitamin supplemen-

Table 22-8. Drug Effects on Lipoproteins

DRUG	LDL	HDL	VLDL (TRIGLYCERIDES)
Bile acid sequestrants Cholestyramine (Questran) Colestipol (Colestid)	↓	↑ (slight)	← → (or) ↑
Nicotinic acid	↓	↑	↓
Neomycin	↓		
Probucol (Lorelco)	↓	↓	
Mevinolin (MK-803)	↓		
Gemfibrozil (Lopid)	Variable	↑	↓

tation would be advised in these cases. Bile acid sequestrants may cause modest increases in HDL and VLDL levels.

NICOTINIC ACID (NIACIN) is another first-choice agent for LDL cholesterol elevations. It inhibits the secretion of VLDL from the liver, which in turn decreases LDL production. An increase in HDL and the HDL_2 subfraction is frequently observed because of a decrease in the fractional catabolic rate for HDL. Nicotinic acid can be purchased without prescription in 100-mg and 500-mg tablets from some pharmacies and in most commercial vitamin/supplement outlets. Cutaneous flushing and pruritus occur in most individuals when the medication is started and when the dosage is increased. The flushing is mediated by prostaglandins and often mitigated by premedication with aspirin. Patient adherence is improved if these side-effects are explained prior to the initiation of therapy, but they often limit patient acceptance of the drug. To minimize episodes of flushing, nicotinic acid should be started at a dosage of 100 mg three times daily with meals. Gradual increments in dosage should be made as tolerated and should not exceed a total daily dose increase of 2.5 g a month. The dose for maximum LDL lowering is in the range of 3 g to 7.5 g per day. Liver enzymes (SGOT, SGPT, alkaline phosphatase), plasma glucose, and uric acid levels should be monitored periodically to detect early side-effects and ensure reversibility. Occasionally, the vasodilating effects augment postural hypotension caused by antihypertensive agents. The common development of dry skin responds to lanolin-containing lotions. The occasional acanthosis nigricans seen with the drug is reversible by discontinuing therapy. Mealtime doses decrease dyspepsia, nausea, and vomiting. Prior peptic ulcer disease constitutes a contraindication to nicotinic acid.

NEOMYCIN, a nonabsorbable aminoglycoside antibiotic, effectively lowers cholesterol when given in small oral doses. It appears to act by inhibiting intestinal cholesterol absorption with subsequent reductions in either VLDL synthesis or its conversion to LDL. In doses of 1 g twice daily, neomycin appears to be well tolerated and safe for prolonged administration in patients without preexisting renal, hepatic, or intestinal disease. No ototoxicity or nephrotoxicity has developed at this dose after 12 to 30 months of use for hypercholesterolemia. Mild nausea is usually avoided by mealtime dosages. Neomycin presently lacks FDA approval for use in hypercholesterolemia.

PROBUCOL (Lorelco) effectively lowers LDL cholesterol by uncertain mechanisms. Unfortunately, it usually lowers HDL cholesterol by a greater percentage than it does LDL cholesterol, which results in a higher, more atherogenic LDL/HDL ratio. This troublesome effect limits its use as a single agent, but probucol may be useful in combined therapy (see below). The usual dose is two 250-mg tablets twice daily. Diarrhea is the most common side-effect.

THE HMG-CoA REDUCTASE INHIBITORS, mevinolin (United States) and compactin (Japan), are currently undergoing clinical testing. They specifically inhibit 3-hydroxy-3-methylglutaryl coenzyme A reductase, the rate-limiting enzyme in cholesterol biosynthesis. Reductions of LDL cholesterol by 20% to 50% in normal and heterozygous hypercholesterolemic patients treated with mevinolin have been reported, and no troublesome side-effects have been reported. If continued testing produces no significant untoward effects, drugs of this class could revolutionize therapy for hypercholesterolemia due to elevated LDL cholesterol.

COMBINED DRUG REGIMENS utilizing the previously discussed medications have proven very effective in dramatically lowering LDL levels in individuals with marked hypercholesterolemia. Using two drugs with complementary sites of activity has produced normalization of LDL in many highly resistant cases. Colestipol and nicotinic acid have reduced LDL cholesterol by 40% in patients following coronary artery bypass surgery and by 55% in heterozygous familial hypercholesterolemia. Colestipol and probucol reduced LDL cholesterol by 29%, but the LDL/HDL cholesterol ratio was unchanged. Mevinolin plus colestipol and compactin plus cholestyramine have reduced LDL cholesterol in heterozygous familial hypercholesterolemia by 54% and 53%, respectively. Neomycin and niacin have lowered LDL cholesterol by 45% while raising HDL cholesterol by 36%. These studies imply that virtually any patient with hypercholesterolemia due to elevated LDL cholesterol can be treated effectively with various combinations of diet and drugs. Noncompliance secondary to unacceptable side-effects is usually the limiting factor for overall success.

Depressed HDL Cholesterol (HDL < 35 mg/dl)—Moderate to High Risk. No randomized clinical trial demonstrating a reduction in CHD mortality/morbidity by elevating HDL levels has been reported. Clinical trials to address this question are ongoing in Finland and the United States. Until the results are available, the routine use of gemfibrozil or nicotinic acid to raise HDL levels cannot be advised. Vigorous attempts to raise HDL cholesterol by regular aerobic exercise (see Chapter 10), cessation of smoking (see Chapter 49), and weight loss (in obese patients) (see Chapter 229) can be encouraged.

Elevated VLDL Cholesterol (Fasting Triglycerides > 250 mg/dl)—Low (?) Risk. No definitive clinical trial has been performed to determine whether drug therapy for any form of elevated triglycerides will decrease CHD morbidity and/or mortality. In the absence of an elevated LDL cholesterol, a depressed HDL cholesterol, premature heart disease in the individual or family members, and/or other risk factors for CHD (hypertension, cigarette smoking, obesity, diabetes mellitus), there is no evidence for increased cardiovascular risk from triglyceride levels between 250 and 500 mg/dl.

Drugs may be required to avoid abdominal pain and acute pancreatitis when chylomicronemia is present and/or fasting triglyceride levels are greater than 500 mg/dl. Vigorous attempts to incorporate triglyceride-lowering life-style changes—weight control, alcohol and fat restriction, and increased physical activity—should be continued during any drug therapy.

NICOTINIC ACID is very effective in lowering VLDL (triglyceride) levels (see previous section). Because of its favorable concomitant LDL-lowering and HDL-raising effects, it is particularly useful if these abnormalities are present.

GEMFIBROZIL (Lopid) lowers triglyceride levels by both reducing the synthesis of VLDL triglyceride and increasing its clearance by stimulating lipoprotein lipase activity. It also elevates HDL cholesterol, the HDL$_2$ subfraction, and apoprotein A-I, probably by increasing synthesis and lipoprotein lipase activity. The effects on LDL cholesterol are variable. The usual dose is one or two 300-mg capsules twice daily before meals. Contraindications include preexisting gallbladder disease, hepatic disease, or several renal dysfunction. Mild gastrointestinal symptoms are the most common side-effect.

CLOFIBRATE (Atromid-S) increases clearance of VLDL triglyceride by stimulating lipoprotein lipase activity. Its effects on raising HDL and the HDL$_2$ subfraction appear more modest than those of gemfibrozil. Clofibrate was associated with an increased incidence of gallstones in two large-scale trials and an increase in deaths from noncardiovascular causes compared with placebo patients in the World Health Organization study. Its use is, therefore, probably best restricted to patients with familial dysbetalipoproteinemia disease.

FISH OIL, EICOSAPENTAENOIC ACID (EPA), has remarkable VLDL and triglyceride-lowering effects. Four grams to 6 g of EPA daily lowers triglycerides 50% to 85% in normals and in patients with carbohydrate-induced and/or genetic hypertriglyceridemia. Clinical studies are ongoing to assess dose-response curves, to compare dietary and various supplement forms, and to determine possible adverse effects.

PATIENT EDUCATION

The importance of patient education in the management of hyperlipidemia, as with other cardiovascular risk factors, cannot be overemphasized, because treatment consists essentially of changing one's eating and exercise habits (see Chapters 229 and 10). The first step in therapy should be a careful review by the primary care physician of the importance of treating hypercholesterolemia. Detailed dietary instruction, weight loss (see Chapter 229) combined with a review of the patient's food preferences and budget will be needed to ensure compliance. Reinforcement can be provided by periodic visits to check weight, diet, and cholesterol level.

INDICATIONS FOR REFERRAL

Patients with high-risk lipoprotein–cholesterol disorders who do not respond to diet plus one or two first-line drugs should be referred for consultation with a physician familiar with drug treatment for lipid disorders.

The possibility of a genetic disorder and need for referral to a lipid unit should be considered when extremes of any lipoprotein cholesterol levels are encountered and/or there is a history of premature CHD (onset of disease before age 55) in the patient or family members. Lipid research laboratories can often categorize the specific genetic abnormalities in this setting by directly measuring LDL cholesterol with ultracentrifugation and precisely determining the apolipoproteins, HDL subfractions, and various enzyme or receptor systems. However, whatever more specialized testing is available, therapy in most instances is still the same—dietary and health-related behavioral intervention followed by drug therapy as necessary. Screening of other family members for hypercholesterolemia is recommended.

ANNOTATED BIBLIOGRAPHY

Arntzenius AC, Kromhout D, Barth JD et al: Diet, lipoproteins, and the progression of coronary atherosclerosis: The Leiden Intervention Trial. N Engl J Med 312:805, 1985 (*One of several recent large-scale clinical trials examining dietary intervention.*)

Brensike JF, Levy RI, Kelsey SF et al: Effects of therapy with cholestyramine on progression of coronary arteriosclerosis: Results of the National Heart, Lung and Blood Institute Type II Coronary Intervention Study. Circulation 69:313, 1984 (*A major clinical study documenting efficacy of therapy.*)

Castelli WP, Abbott RD, McNamara PM: Summary estimates of cholesterol used to predict coronary heart disease. Circulation 67:730, 1983 (*Includes discussion of cholesterol/HDL ratio.*)

Committee of Principle Investigators: A cooperative trial in the primary prevention of ischemic heart disease using clofibrate. Br Heart J 40:1069, 1978 (*There was an increased incidence of noncardiovascular deaths and gallstones; not a recommended drug.*)

Connor WE, Lin DS: The effect of shellfish in the diet upon the plasma lipid levels in humans. Metabolism 31:1046, 1982 (*Though high in cholesterol, their net effect may be neutral for CHD risk.*)

Dujovne CA, Krehbiel P, Decoursey S et al: Probucol with colestipol in the treatment of hypercholesterolemia. Ann Intern Med 100:477, 1984 (*An example of the usefulness of two-agent, combined drug therapy.*)

Ehnholm C, Huttunen JK, Pietinen P et al: Effect of diet on serum lipoproteins in a population with a high risk of coronary heart disease. N Engl J Med 307:850, 1982 (*Documents improvement by dietary intervention.*)

Fredrickson DS, Levy RI, Lees RS: Fat transport in lipoproteins—an integrated approach to mechanisms and disorders. N Engl J Med 276:34, 1967 (*A classic article, with their classification scheme.*)

Gordon T, Castelli WP, Hjortland MC et al: High density lipoprotein as a protective factor against coronary heart disease: The Framingham study. Am J Med 62:707, 1977 (*Some of the epidemiologic data on HDL as a protective factor.*)

Grundy SM, Bilheimer D, Blackburn H et al: Rationale of the diet-heart statement of the American Heart Association. Report of Nutrition Committee. Circulation 165(4):839A, 1982 (*Dietary recommendations from the American Heart Association; authoritative consensus view.*)

Hegsted DM, McGandy RB, Myers ML et al: Quantitative effects of dietary fat on serum cholesterol in man. Am J Clin Nutr 17:281, 1965 (*Detailed data on relation of dietary fat to lipid levels.*)

Hoeg JM, Gregg RE, Brewer HB, Jr: An approach to the management of hyperlipoproteinemia. JAMA 255:512, 1986 (*An accessible, authoritative review with algorithms for diagnosis and therapy.*)

Hoeg JM, Maher MB, Bou E et al: Normalization of plasma lipoprotein concentrations in patients with type II hyperlipoproteinemia by combined use of neomycin and niacin. Circulation 70:1004, 1984 (*Both agents decrease LDL levels.*)

Jenkins DJA, Leeds AR, Newton C et al: Effect of pectin, guar gum, and wheat fibre on serum-cholesterol. Lancet 1:1116, 1975 (*Results in modest decrease in LDL.*)

Kannel WB, Castelli WP, Gordon T: Cholesterol in the prediction of atherosclerotic disease. New perspectives based on the Framingham Study. Ann Intern Med 90:85, 1979 (*A review of epidemiologic data on risk factors; cholesterol, but not triglyceride, is an independent risk factor for CHD.*)

Kesaniemi YA, Grundy SM: Influence of gemfibrozil and clofibrate on metabolism of cholesterol and plasma triglycerides in man. JAMA 251:2241, 1984 (*Good review of these two agents.*)

Knapp HR, Reilly I, Alessandrini P et al: In vivo indices of platelet and vascular function during fish oil administration in patients with atherosclerosis. N Engl J Med 314:937, 1986 (*A report on the mechanisms of action of fish oil in protecting against atherosclerosis.*)

Kromhout D, Bosschieter EB, Coulander CDL: The inverse relation between fish consumption and 20-year mortality from coronary heart disease. N Engl J Med 312:1205, 1985 (*Intriguing data on PUFA in diet and decrease in risk of CHD.*)

Lipid Research Clinics Program: The Lipid Research Clinics Coronary Primary Prevention Trial results. JAMA 251:351, 1984 (*A landmark study demonstrating efficacy of dietary and drug interventions.*)

Mabuchi H, Haba T, Tatami R et al: Effect of an inhibitor of 3-hydroxy-3-methylglutaryl coenzyme A reductase on serum lipoproteins and ubiquinone 10-levels in patients with familial hypercholesterolemia. N Engl J Med 305:478, 1981 (*Reports the efficacy of this new type of lipid-lowering agent.*)

McManus BM, Wilson JE, Miller WE: "Normal" blood cholesterol levels. N Engl J Med 312:51, 1985 (*A critique of the notion of "normal."*)

Nessim SA, Chin HP, Alaupovic P et al: Combined therapy of niacin, colestipol, and fat-controlled diet in men with coronary bypass: Effect on blood lipids and apolipoproteins. Arteriosclerosis 3:568, 1983 (*A multifaceted approach to treatment in a high-risk group.*)

Peters WL, Goroll AH: The evaluation and treatment of hypercholesterolemia in primary care practice. J Gen Intern Med 1:183, 1986 (*An analytic, prescriptive review.*)

Schaefer EJ, Levy RI: Pathogenesis and management of lipoprotein disorders. N Engl J Med 312:1300, 1985 (*A comprehensive review of the confusing genetics of lipoprotein disorders.*)

Scott L, Caggiula AW, Farrand M et al: Counseling the patient with hyperlipidemia. Am Heart Assoc Publ No 70-061-A, 1984 (*A practical guide for patient education.*)

Shepherd J, Packard CJ, Bicker S et al: Cholestyramine promotes receptor-mediated low density lipoprotein catabolism. N Engl J Med 302:1219, 1980 (*An important effect of cholestyramine.*)

23

Management of Atrial Fibrillation and Other Supraventricular Tachycardias in the Outpatient Setting

Atrial fibrillation (AF) discovered in the office setting can usually be managed on an outpatient basis by the primary care physician, provided the ventricular response rate is not dangerously fast and there is no evidence of heart failure, ischemia, or embolization. The first therapeutic objective, regardless of etiology, is to control the ventricular response rate. A second priority is to assess the risk of embolization and determine the need for anticoagulation. Once the etiology is identified and the condition treated, candidacy for elective cardioversion can be considered if the AF does not resolve spontaneously.

CLINICAL COURSE AND NATURAL HISTORY

The paroxysms of atrial fibrillation that occur in young people who have *no underlying heart disease* are annoying but without consequence; although recurrent, they are not associated with embolization and have a good prognosis. Patients with paroxysms of AF due to the *sick sinus syndrome* have a worse prognosis. Their bouts of AF may be interspersed with episodes of severe bradycardia, leading to alterations in consciousness and even syncope. Systemic embolization also can occur.

Paroxysms of AF are also characteristic of *Wolff–Parkinson–White (WPW) syndrome;* recurrent attacks of AF and other tachyarrhythmias may be accompanied by very rapid ventricular response rates, which in some patients can degenerate into ventricular dysrhythmias causing serious hemodynamic compromise. The risk of serious ventricular dysrhythmias can be estimated by measuring the shortest R–R interval during an episode of AF. Any interval less than 180 milliseconds indicates high risk.

AF due to *alcoholic cardiomyopathy* begins with paroxysmal AF during binge drinking. If drinking continues, the cardiomyopathy progresses; however, the condition is potentially reversible with total abstinence.

AF from underlying *valvular or myocardial disease* may begin as paroxysms, but the episodes become more prolonged as left atrial pressure and size increase; eventually chronic fibrillation ensues. Before chronic fibrillation sets in, an episode of AF may be precipitated by such factors as acute heart failure, ischemia, fever, infection, hypoxia, or hypovolemia; correction of the precipitant often results in at least a temporary return to sinus rhythm. In the early stages of chronic AF, cardioversion may be successful in restoring normal sinus rhythm, but unless the underlying pathophysiology is corrected, the AF usually recurs and cardioversion becomes less effective.

Systemic embolization, and particularly *stroke,* are among the most serious complications of AF. Both prospective and retrospective studies have documented an increased risk of embolization in patients with AF. It used to be thought that such risk applied only to patients with AF due to rheumatic mitral valve disease; however, recent data from the Framingham study and elsewhere document significant increases in the rate of stroke for *all* patients with AF and underlying heart disease. Nevertheless, the risk of stroke in mitral disease is still 3 times that of other etiologies and as much as 17 times that of patients without atrial fibrillation. The risk from AF is statistically independent of other risk factors, such as heart failure and coronary artery disease.

Data from the Framingham study also reveal that risk of stroke is greatest at the onset of AF, with over 25% of AF-associated strokes occurring at the time of onset. In addition, the likelihood of having a recurrence of stroke within the first 6 months is twice as great in patients with AF compared with patients with stroke and no AF.

Chronic atrial fibrillation usually reflects serious cardiac pathology. In the Framingham study, onset of atrial fibrillation and heart failure were closely linked. The development of chronic atrial fibrillation was associated with a doubling of overall mortality and of mortality from cardiovascular disease.

PRINCIPLES OF MANAGEMENT

Rate Control

Heart rate is an important determinant of hemodynamic state. Regardless of the cause, the first priority is to control the ventricular response rate to less than 85 at rest and less than 110 after mild exercise (*e.g.,* 10 sit-ups or 10 stand-ups from a chair). The heart rate may appear well controlled at rest but rise markedly with mild effort; one needs to evaluate control both at rest and on exertion.

Digoxin is the drug of choice for control of the ventricular response rate in most conditions that cause AF. Digoxin functions by decreasing conduction through the AV node. The major exception to its use in AF is in cases of preexcitation (*e.g.,* Wolff–Parkinson–White syndrome) in which the drug may speed up the rate by favoring conduction through the bypass tract and shortening its refractory period. In the vast majority of cases, AF responds well to digoxin, which impedes conduction of atrial impulses arriving at the AV node. At times, AF reverts to sinus rhythm upon institution of digoxin therapy.

Most patients who present in the office setting with AF can be managed on an outpatient basis provided there is no evidence of ischemia or heart failure and the *ventricular rate* is not dangerously rapid (greater than *150–170* beats per minute). Initiating therapy with a maintenance dose of digoxin is reasonable if the ventricular rate is *less than 120* and well tolerated. About 5 days are required to achieve standard therapeutic serum levels, although the best measure of an adequate dosage is the heart rate. If the ventricular rate is *between 120 and 150* and well tolerated, outpatient management is still reasonable as long as the patient is reliable and the home situation is supportive. In such circumstances, more rapid digitalization is indicated. An oral loading dose of digoxin is given over the first 24 hours; the heart rate is monitored to assess the need for further immediate doses in the loading phase and to determine the appropriate maintenance doses. At the first sign of heart failure or ischemia, the patient requires hospital admission.

Patients who appear *refractory to digoxin* therapy for rate control require evaluation for factors that might be aggravating the rhythm disturbance. The rapid rate may be a physiologic response to heart failure, fever, hypovolemia, or hypoxia, or it may be a manifestation of the underlying etiology, such as hyperthyroidism, alcoholic cardiomyopathy, or Wolff–Parkinson–White syndrome. Treatment needs to be directed toward the precipitants and underlying etiologies (see below). Of particular importance is the need for abstinence from alcohol in patients suspected of having early *alcoholic cardiomyopathy* (see Chapter 27). Poor compliance is another possible cause of inadequate rate control; measurement of a serum digoxin level will help determine if this is the case.

Beta-blocking Agents and Calcium Channel Blockers.
At times, moderate doses of digoxin may not provide sufficient rate control, especially during exercise. Rather than escalate digoxin therapy to near toxic levels, one can add a beta-adrenergic blocking agent or verapamil to slow the rate. Controlled studies have shown both agents to be effective adjuncts to digoxin therapy. *Beta-blocking agents* work by increasing the refractoriness of the AV node and by blocking the beta-adrenergic effect of catecholamines on the heart rate. They are contraindicated in the presence of heart failure. *Verapamil,* a calcium-channel blocker, is also effective for control of chronic AF when used in conjunction with digoxin. It has a direct effect on the AV node, prolonging its refractory period and conduction time. The drug interferes with the clearance of digoxin and may result in increases in digoxin serum concentrations; adjustment downward of the digoxin dose is often necessary, as is careful monitoring of the digoxin dose. Verapamil has a negative inotropic effect and must be used with caution, if at all, in patients with heart failure.

Patients with AF due to *Wolff–Parkinson–White syndrome* require special mention. Patients with occasional bouts of AF that are well tolerated and self-limited require no treatment as long as the shortest R–R interval during an attack is greater than 180 milliseconds. No restrictions on activity are necessary. Patients with very rapid ventricular rates and hemodynamic deterioration during an attack of AF should be hospitalized and treated with urgent electrical cardioversion. Digitalis preparations should *not* be used. Outpatient management to prevent future episodes of AF from getting out of hand is accomplished on an empirical basis using quinidine, procainamide, disopyramide, or amiodarone. Inpatient electrophysiologic testing can help determine which agent is most likely to provide optimal control of ventricular rate during AF. Propranolol is sometimes helpful in protecting against episodes of AF but it should also be subjected to electrophysiologic study before it is used in patients with potentially serious attacks of AF.

Patients with the tachycardia–bradycardia form of *sick sinus syndrome* pose a therapeutic dilemma: although their AF usually responds well to digitalis preparations, the drug may worsen episodes of bradycardia. Consequently, pacemaker implantation is often necessary for patients with symptomatic bradycardia.

Treatment of AF due *hyperthyroidism* may require addition of a beta-blocking agent to achieve adequate rate control. Definitive treatment of the underlying thyroid disease (see Chapter 101) is essential to the successful prevention of future episodes of AF. At times, elective cardioversion (see below) is necessary to restore sinus rhythm after successful treatment of the hyperthyroidism.

AF patients with a slow ventricular response on no medications probably have underlying conduction system disease; digitalis may worsen the bradycardia and is indicated only if there is underlying heart failure. Patients with very slow rates on digoxin may have *digitalis toxicity,* especially if there are episodes of a junctional rhythm ("regularization of AF") or ventricular premature beats (see Chapter 27). In such instances, digoxin should be held and a serum level checked.

Anticoagulant Therapy—Prevention of Embolization

Prevention of systemic embolization and especially of stroke are the next most important therapeutic priorities after rate control. The recent epidemiologic data from the Framingham study suggest that the risk of stroke from AF is much greater than was previously thought and is not limited to patients with rheumatic mitral valve disease; it extends to all AF patients with underlying heart disease. Moreover, strokes appear to cluster around the onset of AF, suggesting that patients with recent onset of AF and those with paroxysms of the arrhythmia are at particularly high risk. This risk needs to be weighed against the risks of anticoagulant therapy.

Unfortunately, no controlled trials of anticoagulant therapy for stroke prevention in AF patients exist, so there are no definitive answers to date. (Prospective trials are in progress.) At present, the increasing safety of carefully monitored oral anticoagulant therapy (see Chapter 85) and its known efficacy in prevention of embolic stroke (see Chapter 165) appear to put the burden of proof on the physician who decides to withhold anticoagulant therapy. Because the chances of embolization are greatest at the onset of AF, the decision to anticoagulate should not be delayed.

The physician reluctant to anticoagulate solely on the basis of new onset AF and underlying heart disease should search for further clinical findings indicative of high risk. Such findings include prior embolic stroke, left atrial mural thrombus, tight mitral stenosis, left atrial enlargement, and poor cardiac output.

A related dilemma is whether or not to anticoagulate *prior to elective cardioversion.* The concern is that fresh atrial thrombus, which has not had sufficient time to organize, may be dislodged with resumption of vigorous and coordinated atrial contraction. Again, no definitive randomized prospective studies exist to resolve the issue. Pooling data from available retrospective studies produces a heterogeneous population of approximately 1650 AF patients who were not prophylactically anticoagulated prior to cardioversion. In this diverse group, the frequency of embolic events is calculated as 1.7%. The same pooled data show a rate of 0.7% for the 450 patients who were anticoagulated. Because the etiology and nature of the AF in many of these patients is not specified, the data cannot be used to identify high-risk subgroups. Although there is some suspicion that patients with rheumatic heart disease, cardiomegaly, left atrial enlargement, or a history of embolization are at increased risk of embolization from elective cardioversion, the available data are inadequate to substantiate this view. Prospective randomized studies are sorely needed.

If prophylactic anticoagulation is to be undertaken, it should be initiated at least 2 to 3 weeks before elective cardioversion (to allow existing thrombus to endothelialize) and continued for up to 1 week after cardioversion. Embolic episodes have been documented to occur as late as several days after cardioversion; this correlates with the time noted for resumption of full atrial mechanical function. It is important to note that if anticoagulant therapy is to be carried out, it must be done long enough in advance of elective cardioversion to permit organization of any preexisting left mural thrombus. Three to 4 weeks of warfarin therapy prior to cardioversion is the customary anticoagulant regimen.

Elective Cardioversion

Patients who cannot tolerate the fall in cardiac output or the increase in myocardial oxygen demand associated with AF are prime candidates for cardioversion. Urgent cardioversion is the treatment of choice for acute heart failure or myocardial ischemia. Indications for elective cardioversion include reduced exercise tolerance, symptomatic palpitations, persistence of AF after effective treatment of the underlying etiology, angina with onset of AF, and systemic embolization from left atrial stasis.

Cardioversion is contraindicated with digitalis toxicity (ventricular arrhythmias may ensue), a slow ventricular response rate in the absense of digitalis (this may lead to sinus arrest after cardioversion), and inability to tolerate quinidine and other agents used to maintain sinus rhythm after cardioversion.

Maintenance of sinus rhythm for more than 6 months after cardioversion is most likely in patients with recent onset of AF, coarse fibrillatory waves on ECG, and a left atrium that is within normal size limits. Conversely, those with chronic AF, left atrial enlargement, advanced mitral stenosis, or chronic congestive heart failure are least likely to attain long-term benefits from elective cardioversion; AF almost always returns within a short period of time.

Electrical cardioversion is the procedure of choice for converting AF to sinus rhythm. Pretreatment with quinidine and its continuation for 3 to 6 months after cardioversion enhance the probability of maintaining sinus rhythm. Digoxin is withheld for 2 days prior to cardioversion, because there is an increased risk of ventricular dysrhythmias when the heart is countershocked in the presence of high digoxin levels.

The risk of embolization is reported to range from 1% to 3% and can be reduced by prior anticoagulation (see above). *Pharmacological cardioversion* by quinidine is less optimal, since near-toxic doses of quinidine are required and inpatient monitoring is necessary to ensure safety.

PATIENT EDUCATION

The young patient with paroxysmal AF who is free of underlying heart disease needs to be fully reassured to prevent cardiac neurosis and the unnecessary restriction of activity. Such patients should be instructed to quit smoking, avoid sleep deprivation, and limit their use of alcohol and stimulants. They often benefit from use of relaxation techniques (see Chapter 222) at times of stress. WPW patients whose episodes of AF are brief, infrequent, and well tolerated can also be reassured and encouraged to remain fully active. Patients with AF secondary to alcohol abuse and evolving cardiomyopathy need to be informed of the risk of alcoholic cardiomyopathy and strongly urged to abstain from alcohol.

It is important to teach AF patients and family members to watch for signs of hemodynamic compromise, such as rapid heart rate, unexplained weight gain, worsening dyspnea on exertion, and decreased exercise tolerance. Patients often fear that long-term digoxin therapy will be habit-forming or injurious to the heart; reassurance and education about its use are often much appreciated. However, they need to be aware of the symptoms and signs of digitalis toxicity (see Chapter 27) so that correction of the problem is not delayed unnecessarily.

INDICATIONS FOR ADMISSION AND REFERRAL

Patients unable to tolerate their AF because of congestive heart failure or ischemia should be hospitalized immediately. The same is true if the ventricular response rate is extremely rapid. (>170 beats per minute). Electrical cardioversion may be urgent. Hospitalization is also indicated for patients refractory to medical therapy and those with new onset of embolization. Patients who are candidates for elective cardioversion need at least a temporary stay, even if only for the day.

Referral is indicated for patients with refractory AF, suspicion of Wolff–Parkinson–White syndrome, sick sinus syndrome, and AF resulting in hemodynamic compromise.

THERAPEUTIC RECOMMENDATIONS

• If there is no evidence of congestive failure, ischemia, or embolization, and the ventricular response rate is less than 150 beats per minute, outpatient management can be undertaken, provided the patient is reliable and the home environment is supportive.

- The first priority is to slow the ventricular rate. Digoxin is the drug of choice, although it is contraindicated in cases of AF due to preexcitation syndromes such as Wolff–Parkinson–White.
- If the heart rate is between 100 and 120 and is well tolerated, begin therapy with a maintenance dose of digoxin (0.25 to 0.375 mg per day). Control should be achieved within 5 days, the time it takes to reach a therapeutic serum level.
- If the rate is between 120 and 150 and well tolerated, begin therapy with an oral loading dose of digoxin (1.0 to 1.25 mg over 24 hours in divided doses) to achieve rate control more rapidly. The ventricular rate is monitored to determine the daily dose.
- The goal of rate control should be a heart rate of less than 85 at rest and less than 110 after modest exercise (*e.g.,* 10 stand-ups). The rate must be checked after exercise because it may rise markedly, even though it appears well controlled at rest.
- If rate control is difficult to achieve, check for failure, ischemia, fever, hypovolemia, hypoxia, recurrent pulmonary embolization, hyperthyroidism, and WPW syndrome. Treatment should be directed at the underlying condition. Hospitalize the patient if the AF is not well tolerated.
- Patients who are well controlled at rest but have rates that rise unacceptably with exertion (>120) might benefit from a cautious trial of adding a beta-blocking agent (*e.g.,* timolol 10 mg bid) or verapamil (80 mg tid) to the digoxin regimen. Do not use this regimen in patients with heart failure or preexcitation syndrome. Monitor the serum digoxin level regularly if verapamil is used, since it may rise.
- Young patients with brief and infrequent bouts of AF due to WPW need not be treated if episodes are well tolerated and the shortest R–R interval is greater than 180 ms. All others require prompt referral to a cardiologist. Do not treat them with digitalis.
- Patients with sick sinus syndrome may be very susceptible to bradycardia; use digoxin with care and only if there is no history of symptomatic bradycardia; obtain cardiac consultation if symptomatic bradycardia occurs.
- Although definitive studies are lacking, available epidemiologic evidence argues in favor of beginning oral anticoagulant therapy as early as possible in all AF patients with underlying heart disease, unless there is a serious contraindication to warfarin therapy (see Chapter 85). Patients with mitral valve disease, prior embolization, heart failure, left atrial thrombus, left atrial dilatation, and low cardiac output are at particularly high risk for systemic embolization, as are patients with paroxysmal AF due to underlying heart disease.
- Elective cardioversion is indicated for treatment of AF that persists after definitive treatment of its underlying etiology, rapid ventricular rate refractory to medical therapy, symp-

tomatic palpitations, and systemic embolization thought to arise from the left atrium. The need for prophylactic anticoagulation prior to elective cardioversion remains unproven. If this therapy is to be employed, it should be started 2 to 3 weeks before cardioversion and continued for 1 week after the procedure.
- Urgent cardioversion is needed for hemodynamic deterioration, ischemia, and extremely rapid rates (*e.g.,* >200).
- Synchronized electrical countershock is the preferred method of cardioversion. To maximize efficacy and minimize risk, it should be preceded by 3 to 4 weeks of oral anticoagulant therapy and by withholding digoxin and beginning quinidine sulfate (200 mg qid) 48 hours before cardioversion.
- Quinidine is continued for 6 months to prevent relapse. Patients least likely to hold in sinus rhythm after cardioversion are those with chronic AF, advanced mitral stenosis, chronic congestive heart failure, and other causes of marked left atrial dilatation.
- Patients with paroxysms of AF from whatever cause should be advised to use alcohol only in moderation and avoid bouts of acute intoxication, since such bouts increase vulnerability to AF.

MANAGEMENT OF PAROXYSMAL SUPRAVENTRICULAR TACHYCARDIAS

Paroxysmal supraventricular tachycardia describes a heterogeneous group of arrhythmias characterized electrocardiographically by a regular rhythm, rapid rate, and narrow QRS complex. Electrophysiologic studies have identified several mechanisms responsible for this class of arrhythmias. *Reentry* accounts for most cases and has been localized with greatest frequency to the AV node; less common sites of reentry are the AV nodal bypass tract (as in WPW syndrome), the sinus node, and the atria. The tachycardia is initiated by premature beats that dissociate refractoriness between conduction pathways and permit circulating electrical activity. The tachycardia ceases when conductivity in the reentrant circuit is altered. A separate form of supraventricular tachycardia, paroxysmal atrial tachycardia with block, is characteristic of digitalis intoxication, and results from *increased automaticity* in atrial tissues as well as block at the AV junction. These arrhythmias occur in young people with no apparent heart disease and in older patients with severe coronary, valvular, or myocardial disease.

There are some useful guidelines to help the clinician distinguish between reentry and increased automaticity. The rhythm disturbance is more likely to be reentrant if it is initiated by a premature beat, is perfectly regular (usually without defined P waves), and can be halted by vagal maneuvers such as Valsalva. Characteristics of increased automaticity include no initiating premature beat, a gradual increase in rate (the "warmup" phenomenon), and no response to vagal maneuvers.

In theory, selection of treatment modality can be based on the underlying pathophysiology. For reentrant cases, agents that can block the reentrant circuit should be more effective; these include digitalis, beta-blockers, and the calcium-channel blockers verapamil and diltiazem. Agents that stabilize the membrane (*e.g.,* quinidine, procainamide, disopyramide) are preferred for episodes due to increased automaticity.

In reality, there is much overlap and it is sometimes very difficult on clinical or even electrophysiologic grounds to predict which type of agent will work best. For example, the calcium-channel blocker verapamil has been found to be extremely effective in cases of multifocal atrial tachycardia, a condition characterized by increased automaticity. Although it is not useful to be dogmatic about drug selection, an attempt at determination of the underlying mechanism can help in the initial choice of therapy.

Both treatment of the acute tachyarrhythmia and prevention of recurrent episodes have been greatly enhanced by the advent of *calcium-channel blockers.* Verapamil prolongs AV nodal refractoriness, which helps terminate reciprocating AV tachycardias that involve the AV node. When used intravenously, verapamil is among the most effective drugs for terminating an acute attack. When used orally for chronic prophylaxis, it has proven to be safe and extremely beneficial, markedly reducing the frequency and severity of attacks without significant side-effects or complications. Studies using diltiazem have produced similar results. The effective verapamil dose for prophylaxis is 240 to 480 mg per day (usually given as 80 to 160 mg tid).

Need for *prophylactic therapy* is based on the frequency and severity of attacks as well as their effect on the patient's cardiac status. A young person may find the episodes annoying, but an elderly patient with coronary disease may develop myocardial compromise from the tachycardia. For patients with reentrant physiology who experience only one or two attacks per year and tolerate them without difficulty, it is best to teach them vagal maneuvers such as Valsalva and carotid sinus massage. These can be carried out at the onset of an attack. For patients with more frequent episodes and/or limited myocardial reserve, chronic therapy with a calcium-channel blocker, beta-blocker, or digitalis is worth a try. Patients with increased automaticity may benefit from one of the membrane-stabilizing antiarrhythmic agents, although verapamil has proven effective even in this setting.

A.H.G.

ANNOTATED BIBLIOGRAPHY

David D, Segni E, Klein HO et al: Inefficacy of digitalis in the control of heart rate in patients with chronic atrial fibrillation: Beneficial effect of an added beta adrenergic blocking agent. Am J Cardiol 44:1378, 1979 (*Digoxin often failed to control rate during exercise; increasing the digoxin dose to achieve maximum serum levels was of little benefit. Addition of timolol was effective and well tolerated.*)

Engel TR, Luck JC: Effect of whiskey on atrial vulnerability and "holiday heart." J Am Col Cardiol 1:816, 1983 (*Alcohol enhanced vulnerability to atrial fibrillation in patients without clinical evidence of cardiomyopathy or heart failure.*)

Graboys TB: The treatment of supraventricular tachycardias. N Engl J Med 312:43, 1985 (*An editorial summarizing current state of knowledge about these rhythm disorders and noting that our ability to treat is presently greater than our understanding of the problem.*)

Mauritson DR, Winniform MD, Walker WS et al: Oral verapamil for paroxysmal supraventricular tachycardia. Ann Intern Med 96:409, 1982 (*A long-term double-blind randomized trial demonstrating that verapamil is both safe and effective for prophylaxis of this arrhythmia.*)

Meyers DG, Gonzalez ER, Nelson WP: The role of prophylactic anticoagulation in cardioversion of atrial fibrillation. Cardiovasc Rev Reports 6:647, 1985 (*A critical review of the available evidence presented in pooled form, argues that few conclusions can be drawn from available data and that prospective randomized studies are needed.*)

Panidis JP, Morganroth J, Baessler C: Effectiveness and safety of oral verapamil to control exercise-induced tachycardia in patients with atrial fibrillation receiving digitalis. Am J Cardiol 52:1197, 1983 (*A double-blind controlled study demonstrating that oral verapamil plus digoxin is superior to digoxin alone and is safe. Digoxin serum levels increased with verapamil therapy.*)

Shlofmitz RA, Hirsch BE, Meyer BR: New onset atrial fibrillation: Is there a need for hospitalization? J Gen Intern Med 1:139, 1986 (*The authors present retrospective data that strongly suggest the answer is no.*)

Wolf PA, Kannel WB, McGee DL et al: Duration of atrial fibrillation and imminence of stroke: The Framingham study. Stroke 14: 664, 1983 (*A major contribution. Risk of embolic stroke in AF patients found to be maximal at onset of AF, independent of other risk factors for stroke, and substantial, even in AF patients without rheumatic mitral disease. Recurrence was twice as likely in patients with AF.*)

24

Management of Ventricular Irritability in the Outpatient Setting

The discovery of ventricular ectopy in the outpatient setting poses difficult questions for the primary care physician. At issue is whether the patient's ventricular irritability increases the risk of sudden death or merely represents an incidental finding. Treatment is often problematic, being fraught with considerable expense, morbidity, and in some instances even mortality. Investigators have sought to better identify patients at high risk for sudden cardiac death and to determine if suppression of ventricular ectopy improves survival. The primary care physician needs to know whom to treat, when to treat, how to select an antiarrhythmic agent, and how to monitor its efficacy.

CLINICAL PRESENTATION AND COURSE

Premature ventricular contractions (PVCs) are ubiquitous and commonly found among patients both with and without underlying heart disease. In studies of the general population, at least one PVC per routine electrocardiogram was found in 1% of Air Force recruits, 4% of life insurance applicants, 7% of men over the age of 34, and 40% to 75% of normal persons subjected to 24 to 48 hours of continuous ambulatory (Holter) monitoring. The incidence and prevalence of PVCs increase with age and with exercise.

In the ambulatory setting, ventricular irritability usually presents in one of several ways: (1) as an incidental finding on routine examination or ECG; (2) as an ECG finding in a patient being evaluated for palpitations, dizziness, or syncope; or (3) as a complication of underlying heart disease noted on resting ECG, exercise stress test, or Holter monitoring. In terms of assessing the prognostic significance of ventricular irritability, the crucial question is whether underlying heart disease is present or absent.

Benign Ventricular Arrhythmias

Initially, prospective studies of large populations of ambulatory men were thought to have shown a correlation between PVCs on routine ECG and subsequent sudden death; however, when these results were reexamined controlling for other cardiac risk factors, PVCs were not found to be an independent determinant of cardiac death in the general population. A recent long-term study of 73 *asymptomatic healthy subjects* with frequent and complex ventricular ectopy

(>60 beats/hour plus multiforms, repetitive forms, bigeminy, or R on T) showed no increased mortality after a mean follow-up of 6.5 years. Regardless of the presence and persistence of worrisome-looking ventricular irritability, these patients had a prognosis no different from that of other healthy people; there was no increased risk of cardiac death.

Other natural history surveys have also emphasized that in the absence of hypertension, angina, history of myocardial infarction, cardiomegaly on chest x-ray, or ECG signs of ischemia, left ventricular hypertrophy, or bundle branch block, people with PVCs are at no greater risk for cardiac death than the general population.

Potentially Malignant Ventricular Dysrhythmias

In comparison to patients free of underlying heart disease, the situation is more worrisome for patients with a variety of cardiac problems, such as those recovering from a *recent myocardial infarction.* In the Coronary Drug Project study of over 2000 survivors of myocardial infarction, the occurrence of even a single PVC on a routine ECG taken 3 months or more after the infarct was associated with a doubling of the mortality rate during the 3-year follow-up period. Numerous studies have revealed that the features most predictive of mortality are high frequency of PVCs (greater than 30 per hour over a 24-hour period) and presence of complex ventricular ectopy, especially repetitive beats three or more consecutive complexes). Prognosis is even worse in these patients when the ejection fraction is less than 0.4.

In patients with a history of *remote myocardial infarction,* the frequency and complexity of PVCs also influence prognosis. For example, in a 5-year study of 1739 male survivors of acute myocardial infarction, the absence of ventricular irritability on a 1-hour ECG recording performed 3 to 9 months postinfarction was associated with a 6% risk of sudden cardiac death over 5 years. The risk was 12% in patients with unifocal PVCs, and 25% in those with complex ventricular ectopy. Multivariate analysis showed that complex ventricular ectopy had the strongest influence on risk for sudden cardiac death.

The situation is similar for patients with other forms of heart disease that cause myocardial scarring and abnormal wall motion. Patients with hypertrophic or congestive cardiomyopathy, important valvular disease, mitral valve prolapse with myxomatous degeneration, congenital heart disease with ventricular hypertrophy, and revascularization or valve surgery have been found to be at increased risk of sudden death if experiencing frequent or complex PVCs, especially in the context of a reduced ejection fraction. The ventricular ectopy is not merely a manifestation of the underlying heart disease, but an independent predictor of prognosis.

Malignant Ventricular Arrhythmias

Nonsustained ventricular tachycardia is a worrisome dysrhythmia characterized by runs of ventricular tachycardia (VT) that spontaneously revert to sinus rhythm within several beats. In the context of chronic coronary artery disease and left ventricular dysfunction, it represents a very malignant form of electrical instability that is an independent risk factor for sudden death. A more benign form found in young patients with no demonstrable heart disease is characterized by resolution with exercise, no associated symptoms, and a regular, relatively slow rate (<150 beats/minute) with uniform cycle length and QRS morphology.

Recurrent sustained ventricular tachycardia is another malignant ventricular dysrhythmia. Its characteristic features are repeated episodes of ventricular tachycardia that can persist for several hours. Coronary artery disease and cardiomyopathy account for almost 90% of cases. About 1% of postinfarction patients experience this arrhythmia during the first year of follow-up. Without treatment, the 1-year mortality rate is about 40%. Response to treatment can be predicted by invasive electrophysiologic studies.

TORSADE DE POINTES is a rapid polymorphic ventricular tachycardia that often deteriorates into ventricular fibrillation. Its characteristics are a QRS axis that twists about the ECG baseline, going from positive to negative and back again, and an association with a prolonged QT interval. This is a very malignant ventricular dysrhythmia seen in patients with electrolyte abnormalities and drug toxicity (quinidine, tricyclic antidepressants).

In sum, the main determinants of prognosis in patients with ventricular ectopy are the presence of underlying heart disease and ventricular dysfunction, not simply the presence, frequency, or complexity of the PVCs. However, frequency and complexity of PVCs are independent predictors of sudden death in patients with a diseased myocardium. Patients with heart disease who manifest VT are at risk of sudden death.

As long as the asymptomatic patient with PVCs has no evidence of underlying heart disease, the prognosis appears fine, but what is the *probability of occult heart disease* in an otherwise apparently healthy patient presenting with PVCs? In a study of 25 such patients, presenting with frequent and complex PVCS and subjected to coronary catheterization and angiography, only 6 were found to have significant coronary artery disease (>50% luminal narrowing). The characteristics of the ventricular ectopy did not differentiate those with coronary disease from those without it. These asymptomatic patients were treated with modest doses of beta-blocking agents and have had no decrease in survival more than 5 years of follow-up.

PRINCIPLES OF MANAGEMENT

Management of patients with ventricular irritability discovered in the outpatient setting is one of the most difficult challenges in the office practice of medicine. Even with marked progress in identifying patients at risk, there are still important unanswered questions regarding the efficacy of antiarrhythmic therapy and appropriate therapeutic endpoint. Only a few small studies show that pharmacologic suppression of worrisome ventricular ectopy in patients with underlying heart disease will prevent ventricular tachycardia, ventricular fibrillation, and sudden cardiac death. The available studies have been limited to the most symptomatic of patients with the most malignant forms of ventricular irritability (such as those with syncope or survivors of resusitation who demonstrate recurrent VT). There are almost no data on the much larger group of patients who are asymptomatic yet have worrisome ectopy in the context of heart disease.

In addition, there are few objective guidelines for the conduct of antiarrhythmic therapy. With the exception of patients with VT monitored by programmed electrophysiologic study (see below), little is known about how much suppression is enough. Most researchers set arbitrary therapeutic endpoints (*e.g.,* total elimination of the most malignant forms of ectopy, 90% reduction in lesser forms, 50% reduction in all types of PVCs) and then await the results to assess the meaningfulness of the endpoint.

The setting of a meaningful treatment endpoint is complicated by difficulty documenting control; patients may show no further irritability on stress test or Holter monitoring, yet still suffer attacks of ventricular tachycardia. Moreover, there is up to a 10% chance of worsening the ventricular irritability with antiarrhythmic drugs; this adverse response is idiosyncratic, unpredictable, and associated with all classes of antiarrhythmics.

Thus, at the present time, treatment of patients with worrisome ventricular irritability remains, for the most part, problematic. Although programmed electrophysiologic study has helped rationalize the treatment of VT (see below), it requires cardiac catheterization and remains a limited resource currently available only at cardiac centers. In most instances, treatments of ventricular irritability (especially of PVCs) continues to be empirical.

Estimation of Risks

The decision to initiate treatment depends upon one's estimate of the risk of the arrhythmia and the expected benefit from antiarrhythmic therapy (which is often unknown); this needs to be balanced against the risk associated with treatment.

Patients with No Underlying Heart Disease. Asymptomatic patients with ventricular premature beats and no evidence of underlying heart disease require no treatment, because they have no increased risk of sudden death. However, before one concludes that the patient is free of heart disease, a thorough noninvasive evaluation is indicated, including ECG, chest x-ray, cardiac ultrasonography, and perhaps exercise stress testing. Even if the VPCs are complex or frequent, there is no need to initiate therapy, because such ventricular irritability has no influence on prognosis.

Patients with Underlying Heart Disease and Simple PVCs. Patients with underlying heart disease and infrequent, simple PVCs (<30 per hour and unifocal) are only at modestly increased risk, a risk which probably approaches the risk of the antiarrhythmic therapy itself. It is currently recommended that such patients who have no symptoms related to their arrhythmia be followed expectantly without instituting antiarrhythmic therapy. However, one might consider treatment of the underlying illness, such as beta-blockade for patients with coronary disease (see Chapter 25). Should symptoms develop or ejection fraction decline in conjunction with an increase in the frequency or complexity of the PVCs, then antiarrhythmic treatment ought to be considered.

Patients with Underlying Heart Disease and Complex PVCs. Patients with underlying heart disease and complex PVCs deserve consideration for antiarrhythmic therapy, especially if the patient has other indicators of poor prognosis such as a low ejection fraction (less than 0.40). Their ventricular irritability poses an independent risk of sudden death, a risk that probably outweighs the risk associated with antiarrhythmic therapy. However, treatment is problematic and empirical. No studies demonstrate that survival has been improved in such patients when treated with antiarrhythmic agents; it remains to be shown that suppression of PVCs by drugs will prevent cardiac sudden death. Moreover, there is no *a priori* means of selecting an effective therapeutic agent; trial and error remain the only guides (see below).

Patients with Underlying Heart Disease and Ventricular Tachycardia. Patients with heart disease and malignant forms of ventricular irritability (recurrent sustained ventricular tachycardia, torsade de pointes) are at great risk of sudden death, with annual mortality rates as high as 40%. They are the most important candidates for antiarrhythmic therapy; only in these patients has suppression of ventricular ectopy been shown to prolong survival. The situation is particularly serious in those who have already had an episode of resuscitation from near sudden death and those with poor left ventricular function. These patients require hospitalization for initiation of antiarrhythmic therapy.

Selection and Initiation of Therapy

There is no means of exactly predicting what effect a particular antiarrhythmic agent will have on a given patient. As noted above, selection of an agent is empirical and must be individualized; it is based on therapeutic response. Grouping agents by cellular electrophysiologic effects may be useful for classification, but available knowledge of the electrophysiology of most ventricular arrhythmias and drugs is still too fragmentary to allow matching an antiarrhythmic drug with a corresponding arrhythmia.

Therapy is initiated by chosing one of the commonly used antiarrhythmic agents and monitoring its effects on the targeted ventricular arrhythmia (see below). To be practical for chronic outpatient use, an antiarrhythmic must be available in an oral form and have an effective half-life of at least 6 hours. Choice of an agent is based on its reported efficacy, safety, duration of action, and the severity and frequency of side-effects (see Table 24-1).

The most commonly prescribed agents for outpatient treatment of ventricular irritability are quinidine, procainamide, and disopyramide. Mexiletine, flecainide, and tocainide appear promising and others such as amiodarone may have a role in more refractory cases. The beta-blocking agents have proven useful in selected situations.

QUINIDINE remains the first-line drug for outpatient treatment of chronic ventricular irritability, being among the most effective agents for suppression of a wide range of ventricular arrhythmias. Quinidine is available as a sulfate salt and in gluconated form; there are also sustained release preparations (see below). The 200-mg sulfate preparation has the same amount of quinidine base as the 324-mg gluconate tablet. Quinidine is almost fully absorbed from the gastrointestinal tract and has an elimination half-life of 7 to 10 hours, being metabolized by the liver and partially excreted unchanged by the kidneys. Renal failure does not increase serum levels appreciably. Peak serum levels are reached within 1 to 2 hours of taking quinidine sulfate and within 4 hours after taking a dose of quinidine gluconate. Quinidine reduces the clearance of digoxin and can double its serum concentration, necessitating reduction in digoxin dose when both are used simultaneously.

The most common side-effects of quinidine, and the ones most often responsible for discontinuation of the drug, are nausea, vomiting, and diarrhea. Sometimes switching from the sulfate to the gluconate form can lessen the gastrointestinal (GI) side-effects. Other common side-effects include tinnitus and vertigo. Hypersensitivity reactions are occasionally encountered; rash, thrombocytopenia, hepatitis, or hemolytic anemia may result. The most potentially serious side-effect is marked prolongation of the QT interval, usually a result of excessive dose but occasionally an idiosyncratic reaction to a single dose. Although some degree of QT prolongation is seen normally as therapeutic levels are achieved, marked

Table 24-1.   Some Agents for Outpatient Treatment of Ventricular Irritability

DRUG	DOSE (STARTING) (MG)	THERAPEUTIC SERUM CONCENTRATION (μM/ML)	ELIMINATION	ECG	ADVERSE EFFECTS
Quinidine	200 qid	2–6	Liver	↑QT, PR, QRS	GI, hypotension, heart block, syncope
Disopyramide	100 qid	2–8	Renal/liver	Same	GI, CHF, anticholinergic
Procainamide	375 q4h	4–10	Renal	Same	GI, lupus, CNS
Tocainide	400 q8h	3.5–10	Renal/liver	None	GI, CNS
Mexiletine	200 q8h	0.5–2	Liver	None	GI, CNS
Propranolol	10 qid	Not established	Liver	↑PR, QT	Heart block, CHF Bronchospasm
Amiodarone	200 qid	1–3.5	?	↑QT	Pulmonary fibrosis corneal deposits, neurologic, GI, drug–drug effects, thyroid
Flecainide	100 bid	Not established	Liver/renal	↑PR, QRS	Ventricular arrhythmias, heart block, CHF

prolongation is abnormal and increases the risk of VT and VF.

Several *long-acting quinidine preparations* are available (see Table 24-2) allowing administration as infrequently as q8h. The percentage of actual quinidine alkaloid in each preparation ranges from 60% to 82%, making dose adjustment important to ensure that a full dose of quinidine is provided when switching from quinidine sulfate (which is 83% quinidine) to a long-acting preparation. A common error is to forget to make the dose adjustment and inadvertently cut down on the patient's daily dose. Although long-acting preparations might help improve compliance and provide more even serum levels of the antiarrhythmic, they are considerably more expensive than generic quinidine sulfate (see Table 24-2).

DISOPYRAMIDE has many of the same electrophysiologic properties as quinidine and is also useful in the outpatient treatment of chronic ventricular irritability. It is well absorbed; about 60% is excreted unchanged by the kidney while the remainder is metabolized by the liver. The dose and frequency of administration need to be reduced in the setting of renal or hepatic failure. Serum half-life ranges from 5 to 9 hours, making q6h administration feasible. Disopyramide also comes in a sustained-release preparation that allows q12h administration and actually saves the patient money (see Table 24-2); however, generic disopyramide will soon be available and eliminate this cost advantage.

Unlike quinidine, disopyramide has a rather pronounced negative inotropic effect, limiting its usefulness in patients with heart failure and low ejection fraction. This negative inotropic effect is especially significant when the drug is used in conjunction with a beta-blocking agent. Although disopyramide does not cause the often troublesome gastrointestinal side-effects associated with quinidine, it does have sub-

Table 24-2.   Long-Acting Preparations of Common Antiarrhythmics

PARENT DRUG	QUINIDINE			PROCAINAMIDE	DISOPYRAMIDE
Preparation	Quinidex Extentabs	Duraquin/ Quinaglute	Cardioquin	Pronestyl SR Procan SR	Norpace CR
Compound	Sulfate	Gluconate	Polygalacturonate	HCl	Phosphate
Amount of active drug (%)	82	62	60		
Duration of action (h)	8	8	8	6–8	12
Incremental cost of using long-acting preparation (%)*	168	139	189	160	−23

* Costs are based on 1986 *Redbook* and they compare the wholesale price of a long-acting compound with the equivalent total daily dose of its generic preparation.

stantial anticholinergic activity that commonly produces urinary retention, constipation, blurred vision, and dry mouth.

PROCAINAMIDE is similar in its antiarrhythmic effect to quinidine and disopyramide. One major drawback to its use in the outpatient setting is its short serum half-life (3–4 hours), which necessitates frequent administration. Sustained-release preparations are on the market (see Table 24-1), making q6–8h administration possible and providing more steady plasma concentrations. The cost to the patient is increased considerably when switching from generic procainamide to a sustained-release preparation. The drug is well absorbed and excreted renally; in renal failure one needs to reduce the frequency of administration. Like quinidine and disopyramide, procainamide can cause AV block and should not be used in patients with high-grade heart block. Chronic use of procainamide is associated with appearance of antinuclear antibodies in about 80% of patients; 20% of these patients develop a drug-induced lupus syndrome. The rate of development of this syndrome is a function of acetylator phenotype; patients who slowly acetylate the drug are at greater risk.

MEXILETINE AND TOCAINIDE are new, orally effective analogues of xylocaine, that resemble the parent drug in activity against ventricular arrhythmias. Unlike quinidine, procainamide, and disopyramide, these agents do not prolong the PR, QRS, or QT intervals; thus, they hold promise as safe, effective agents in the treatment of ventricular irritability. Although they can suppress ventricular dysrhythmias refractory to previously available agents, their antiarrhythmic potency in crossover studies is about the same as quinidine and, like other agents, they occasionally worsen ventricular irritability. Response to parenteral xylocaine is a good predictor of response to these drugs. The relatively long half-lives of these agents (8–12 hours) makes possible dosage schedules that are practical for chronic outpatient use, that is, twice and three times a day. These agents can be used in conjunction with quinidine or other antiarrhythmics for added efficacy, and are even well tolerated in the presence of heart failure, having little negative inotropic effect. Of the two, mexiletine is the more negatively inotropic and also has a modest suppressive effect on AV nodal conduction.

Side-effects are mostly of the CNS and GI variety (tremor, ataxia, confusion, dizziness, nausea, anorexia); the GI upset can often be prevented by taking the medication with meals. Side-effects are dose-related and resolve with discontinuation of the drug. About 15% of patients are unable to tolerate these agents because of the CNS or GI side-effects. Because these agents are still new to the general medical community, they should not yet be considered the drugs of first choice for treatment of ventricular irritability, but the literature should be followed for future recommendations; these agents hold much promise.

FLECAINIDE is the first of a new class of local anesthetic-type antiarrhythmic agents that are capable of suppressing nonsustained ventricular arrhythmias. Unlike quinidine and procainamide, which are also local anesthetic derivatives, flecainide and its congeners do not prolong the QT interval, but do cause PR and QRS prolongation. The drug is well absorbed when taken orally; 50% is metabolized by the liver, 30% excreted unchanged by the kidneys. Flecainide has a half-life of 13 hours in healthy adults, making possible twice-a-day dosage; the half-life is prolonged in patients with heart failure, liver or kidney disease. The drug has proven superior to quinidine and disopyramide in suppression of complex ventricular irritability and unsustained ventricular tachycardia. However, it can aggravate existing ventricular irritability as well as precipitate ventricular dysrhythmias. Consequently, it is recommended that the patient be hospitalized and monitored during the initiation of flecainide therapy. Low-dose therapy is less likely to induce ventricular irritability. The agent can also cause heart block in patients with conduction disturbances and aggravate preexisting congestive heart failure. These properties make flecainide a potentially important and potent antiarrhythmic that should be reserved for serious cases of malignant ventricular irritability that do not respond to a first-line agent such as quinidine. It must be used with caution; consultation with a cardiologist may be helpful prior to initiating flecainide therapy.

AMIODARONE is a unique and potent antiarrhythmic drug that is effective for treatment of refractory life-threatening irritability, particularly recurrent ventricular tachycardia. Its effect on VT cannot be predicted from its response to programmed electrophysiologic study; Holter monitoring is used to judge the efficacy and adjust the dose. Pharmacokinetics are poorly understood; elimination half-life is estimated to be 30 to 60 days, making overdosage and toxicity potentially serious problems. However, the long half-life makes possible once-a-day dosage.

Amiodarone has several worrisome side-effects that are predominantly dose related. The most dangerous is pulmonary fibrosis preceded by a reversible patchy pneumonitis. Another complication is corneal deposits; these usually do not interfere with vision and disappear with discontinuation of the drug. GI upset is common, and clinical hepatitis occurs in 4% of patients. Ataxia and tremor also occur. The drug contains an iodinated segment that can interfere with thyroid metabolism. Amiodarone prolongs the QT interval and has a modest negative inotropic effect. Interactions with other drugs are substantial; amiodarone increases the serum levels of digoxin, quinidine, and procainamide and potentiates the effect of warfarin. Dose adjustments are necessary when amiodarone is used. In spite of all these side-effects, the drug is reasonably well tolerated when used carefully.

BETA BLOCKING AGENTS are useful for suppression of ventricular irritability related to digitalis toxicity, exercise, emotional stress, prolonged QT interval syndromes, and tricyclic antidepressants. Although these drugs are not particularly effective in directly suppressing ventricular irritability due to coronary artery disease, they are the only agents proven to prolong survival in patients with ischemic heart disease (see Chapter 25). The mechanism of this protective effect is unknown. Many of these agents have negative inotropic effects and can worsen heart block; they should be used with caution in patients with heart failure and conduction disturbances.

Determining a Therapeutic Endpoint and Monitoring Therapy

Since treatment of ventricular irritability is not without potentially serious risk, one needs to establish a measurable therapeutic endpoint for judging the efficacy of a treatment program. Antiarrhythmic therapy that fails to meet set criteria should be halted and another agent tried, because the risk of continued treatment probably outweighs any added benefit. Unfortunately, there are few physiologically or statistically meaningful guidelines for judging the adequacy of suppression of ventricular irritability. The field is marked by controversy. One group argues that suppression of VT induced by *programmed electrophysiologic study* is the only meaningful therapeutic endpoint; studies have shown that patients whose malignant ectopy can be controlled according to this criterion demonstrate prolonged survival (see below). Groups advocating the need for electrophysiologic study argue that noninvasive methods of determining adequacy of suppression are inadequate, because such suppression does not prevent induction of VT during electrophysiologic study and thus may not be truly protective.

On the other side of the argument are those who argue that noninvasive study can provide a meaningful and more easily determined therapeutic endpoint. They cite data from study of patients with symptomatic life-threatening ventricular arrhythmias; the goal of therapy was suppression of ectopy as determined by *Holter monitoring and exercise stress test.* Survival was markedly improved in the group who achieved complete suppression of VT and R-on-T, 90% suppression of multifocal PVCs, and greater than 50% suppression of all PVCs as measured noninvasively by Holter and stress tests.

At the present time, it remains unresolved whether noninvasive or invasive study is needed to determine adequate suppression of malignant ventricular arrhythmias. Differences in results are likely due to differences in the patient populations studied. Each means of judging a meaningful therapeutic endpoint may be justifiable for a given set of patients. Just which patients qualify for a particular method of determining a therapeutic endpoint is not yet known. The literature should be followed closely for new developments.

Although there is controversy concerning the appropriate therapeutic endpoint for patients with the most malignant forms of ventricular ectopy, at least some evidence now suggests that antiarrhythmic therapy can prolong survival in specific situations. It remains to be demonstrated that chronic suppression of less malignant but still worrisome PVCs prevents VT or decreases the risk of sudden death.

What should the clinician do when he feels compelled to act, even though consensus on determining the efficacy of therapy is lacking? One might utilize the continuous (Holter) ambulatory recording and exercise stress test when the patient has a ventricular arrhythmia that is frequent and spontaneous or stable and well tolerated; the goal of therapy and the criterion for selection of an agent would be suppression of the most malignant irritability, both at rest and with exercise. Patients with paroxysms of malignant ventricular irritability unrelated to exercise or daily activity, especially those with recurrent sustained VT, might be best evaluated by programmed electrophysiologic study, in which the arrhythmia can be provoked and the efficacy of therapy determined. Often Holter and stress tests are too insensitive for detection of these arrhythmias.

Even though treatment of ventricular irritability is still largely empirical and problematic, the primary physician can do much to ensure the safety of antiarrhythmic therapy and minimize iatrogenic complications. The most important measure is to individualize therapy and treat only with an agent that has proven effective by objective testing for the patient in question. Monitoring the *ECG* for evidence of excessive dose and idiosyncratic reactions is also essential. Quinidine, procainamide, and disopyramide can substantially *prolong the PR, QRS, and QT intervals* when serum levels are in the toxic range. Modest QT interval prolongation is to be expected and is a sign of therapeutic effect, but marked prolongation is an important sign of excessive dose and a need to withhold further medication. Marked prolongation of the QT interval can also occur idiosyncratically in some patients at the very onset of therapy; it should be watched for.

Measurement of *serum drug levels* is an important aid to the safe use of these antiarrhythmic agents (see Table 24-1). Proper interpretation of the data requires that levels be drawn long enough after the last dose so that one does not mistake a peak serum level for a steady-state one.

INDICATIONS FOR REFERRAL

Any patient found to have ventricular tachycardia in the setting of underlying heart disease should be referred to a cardiologist skilled in treatment of complex arrhythmias; programmed electrophysiologic study deserves consideration. Referral is also indicated for symptomatic patients with underlying heart disease and complex forms of PVCs that are refractory to quinidine and other first-line agents. The primary care physician would probably benefit from reviewing treatment plans with a cardiologist before initiating therapy of any patient with complex PVCs and underlying heart disease, even when formal referral is not pursued.

PATIENT EDUCATION

Patients with worrisome ventricular irritability pose a problem in patient education. On the one hand, the physician is reluctant to scare the patient who may be relatively asymptomatic; yet without full knowledge of the significance of the problem, compliance and monitoring of one's condition might suffer. Most patients and their families benefit from knowing the prognostic meaning of the ventricular arrhythmia and appreciate the frankness. Fear can be lessened by informing them of the efficacy of therapy for the most serious forms of ventricular irritability. Full disclosure improves compliance by reinforcing the importance of therapy; patients are also more willing to put up with annoying side-effects from the drugs.

Patient education is also crucial to patients with harmless forms of ventricular irritability. Knowing that the palpitations and abnormal ECG have no implications for long-term survival is tremendously reassuring and can prevent development of a cardiac neurosis and unnecessary restriction of activity.

CONCLUSIONS AND THERAPEUTIC RECOMMENDATIONS

- No antiarrhythmic treatment is needed for patients with infrequent (less than 30 beats/hour) unifocal PVCs, regardless of whether or not there is underlying heart disease. The risks of therapy outweigh any potential benefit.
- No antiarrhythmic treatment is indicated for patients with ventricular ectopy who are free of underlying heart disease, even though they may have frequent (greater than 30 beats/ hour) and/or complex PVCs (repetitive beats, R on T, bigeminy, multiform). These patients are at no increased risk of sudden cardiac death. However, a careful search for underlying heart disease should be made before concluding there is none.
- Patients with frequent and/or complex PVCs in association with underlying heart disease pose an unanswered question regarding need for treatment. Although they are at moderately increased risk of sudden death, *efficacy of therapy is yet to be proven.* If the patient is asymptomatic and the ectopy is readily detected by Holter and stress test, then the clinician who feels compelled to treat can probably try initiating therapy on an outpatient basis (see below). If the patient is symptomatic (near syncope, syncope), when admission is indicated to ensure maximally safe initiation of

therapy. The same holds for the asymptomatic patient who is of questionable reliability.

- If therapy is going to be started in the outpatient setting, it should be initiated only with a single agent. Choice of antiarrhythmic agent needs to be individualized. One must demonstrate the ability of the agent to suppress the target ectopy for the patient in question.
- Patients with underlying heart disease and asymptomatic PVCs might be started on an outpatient program consisting of quinidine sulfate 200 mg qid. Patients unable to tolerate the GI side-effects of quinidine sulfate can be tried on quinidine gluconate 324 mg q8h or disopyramide 100 mg qid. Alternatively, one can initiate therapy in patients known to respond well to xylocaine with tocainide 400 mg q8h. Consider a beta-blocking agent (*e.g.,* propranolol 20 mg qid) for patients with ectopy induced by exercise or emotional stress.
- Do not use loading doses when initiating antiarrhythmic therapy in the outpatient setting.
- Initiation of any antiarrhythmic agent (especially quinidine, procainamide, or disopyramide) on an outpatient basis should include administering the first dose in the office and having the patient stay for several hours to ensure there are no idiosyncratic reactions that might endanger the patient. This includes measuring the QT interval before and several hours after the first dose to be certain there is no excessive prolongation of the QT interval.
- Therapy can be advanced slowly until suppression of the malignant forms is achieved (as judged by stress test and Holter monitoring), serum drug levels reach the upper limit of the therapeutic range or side-effects become limiting. Study the patient for objective evidence of suppression of ectopy as soon as therapeutic drug levels are reached. *Do not continue indefinite use of an agent that does not objectively demonstrate efficacy.* If suppression cannot be demonstrated, then discontinue the agent promptly. Adverse effects of these agents are common, potentially dangerous, and unpredictable. Try a second drug. If still unsuccessful, obtain consultation; do not use agents you are unfamiliar with.
- Definition of therapeutic endpoint remains somewhat arbitrary, although complete suppression of the most malignant forms of ectopy should be sought.
- Once the appropriate agent and effective daily dose are established, one can consider switching to a long-acting preparation, provided that adjustment is made to ensure an equivalent dose of active ingredient and the patient's ability to afford the incremental cost of using a long-acting preparation.
- Patients with underlying heart disease and VT, especially those who are symptomatic, require prompt admission and referral. Antiarrhythmic therapy for these patients must be initiated in the inpatient setting. Consideration of pro-

grammed electrophysiologic study is indicated; the procedure may facilitate identification of an effective antiarrhythmic agent. Some argue that Holter and stress testing are sufficient to expose the malignant irritability and judge the efficacy of therapy.

• Monitor serum drug levels in all patients on chronic antiarrhythmic therapy; have a sample drawn a sufficient length of time ater the last oral dose (usually 4–6 hours) to avoid measurement of peak serum levels.

A.H.G.

ANNOTATED BIBLIOGRAPHY

Anderson JL, Mason JW: Testing the efficacy of antiarrhythmic drugs. N Engl J Med 315:391, 1986 (*Compares the efficacy of Holter monitoring versus electrophysiological study.*)

Bigger JT: Definition of benign versus malignant ventricular arrhythmias. Am J Cardiol 52(6):47C, 1983 (*An excellent review of the various forms of ventricular irritability and the risk associated with each of them.*)

Graboys TB, Lown B, Podrid P et al: Long-term survival of patients with malignant ventricular arrhythmia treated with antiarrhythmic drugs. Am J Cardiol 50:437, 1982 (*Risk of sudden death was dramatically reduced in survivors of resusitation when treated with antiarrhythmic agents, using as an endpoint suppression of ectopy found on Holter and stress tests.*)

Kennedy HL, Whitlock JA, Sprague MK: Long-term follow-up of asymptomatic healthy subjects with frequent and complex ventricular ectopy. N Engl J Med 312:1983, 1985. (*There was no increase in mortality among these healthy patients; mean duration of follow-up was 6.5 years.*)

Kennedy HL, Pescarmona J, Bouchard RJ et al: Coronary artery status of apparently healthy subjects with frequent and complex ventricular ectopy. Ann Intern Med 92:179, 1980. (*A subset being followed for complex and frequent ventricular ectopy volunteered for coronary angiography. One quarter were found to have significant coronary stenosis. No clinical features of their ventricular ectopy distinguished them.*)

Kupersmith J, Reder RF, Slater W: New antiarrhythmic drugs. Cardiov Rev Reports 6:35, 1985 (*Good review of newer agents. 75 references.*)

Lown B: Management of patients at high risk of sudden death. Am Heart J 103:689, 1982 (*Presents the view that stress testing and Holter monitoring adequately expose the malignant ventricular arrhythmias in 85% of patients at high risk of sudden death and that suppression of such ectopy is a sufficient therapeutic endpoint.*)

Meinertz T et al: Significance of ventricular arrhythmias in idiopathic dilated cardiomyopathy. Am J Cardiol 53:902, 1981 (*Ventricular irritability was a determinant of increased risk in these patients.*)

Roden DM, Woosley RL: Flecainide. N Engl J Med 315:36, 1986 (*A review of this potent new antiarrhythmic; a useful second tier drug for serious irritability.*)

Ruberman W et al: Ventricular premature complexes and sudden death after myocardial infarction. Circulation 64:297, 1981 (*Frequent and complex ventricular irritability in post-MI patients was associated with increased risk of sudden death.*)

Ruskin J: Ventricular extrasystoles in healthy subjects. N Engl J Med 312:238, 1985 (*An editorial summarizing current knowledge and pinpointing areas of continued uncertainty.*)

Ruskin JN, McGovern B, Garan H et al: Antiarrhythmic drugs: A possible cause of out-of-hospital cardiac arrest. N Engl J Med 309:1302, 1983 (*Provides evidence of sudden death due to drugs for treatment of ventricular irritability.*)

Ruskin J, DiMarco J, Garan H: Out-of-hospital cardiac arrest: Electrophysiologic observations and selection of long-term antiarrhythmic therapy. N Engl J Med 303:607, 1980 (*Documents the utility of programmed electrophysiologic study in the detection and treatment of malignant ventricular irritability.*)

Velbit V, Podrid M, Lown B et al: Aggravation and provocation of ventricular arrhythmias by antiarrhythmic drugs. Circulation 65:886, 1982 (*Ventricular irritability was worsened in about 10% of cases. It was not predictable and occurred with all classes of antiarrhythmics with about equal frequency.*)

25
Management of Chronic Stable Angina

The last 10 years have been a period of major progress in the treatment of symptomatic coronary artery disease. The long-acting nitrates, beta-blocking agents, calcium-channel blockers, coronary bypass surgery, and angioplasty provide an array of options for the treatment of angina. This medical and surgical armamentarium is complemented by dietary (see Chapter 22) and exercise programs (see Chapter 10), aimed at primary and secondary prevention.

The primary care physician must understand the indications and limitations of this sometimes bewildering list of therapeutic modalities to design the best possible treatment program for the individual patient.

PATHOPHYSIOLOGY

Angina is a manifestation of myocardial ischemia; it occurs when oxygen demand exceeds available vascular supply. Coronary artery stenosis due to atherosclerotic disease is by far the most common etiology. A greater appreciation for the importance of coronary vasospasm has developed, especially in patients with variant angina. Spasm has been documented in patients both with and without underlying atherosclerotic disease. Its prevalence was found to be 3% in patients undergoing coronary angiography with ergonovine stimulation, but the true prevalence is estimated to be far greater. Spasm is suspected of playing a role in acute myocardial infarction, as well as triggering anginal episodes. A wide range of precipitants have been described; these include neurogenic stimulation (*e.g.,* stress and cold), alpha-adrenergic stimulation in the setting of beta-blockade, abrupt nitrate withdrawal, ergonovine, and direct mechanical irritation from cardiac catheterization. There is some evidence that vasoactive peptides, platelets, and prostaglandins might play important roles. Other mechanisms are likely to be found in the near future.

Another important etiologic factor in the production of angina is hemodynamically significant aortic stenosis; it limits cardiac output and restricts flow to the coronary circulation. In addition, conditions that increase myocardial oxygen demand (*e.g.,* hyperthyroidism, fever) or decrease oxygen supply (severe anemia) can aggravate or precipitate angina in patients with underlying coronary artery disease, spasm, or aortic stenosis.

NATURAL HISTORY

The prognosis of patients with chronic stable angina due to coronary artery disease is a function of the location and severity of the stenoses. Combined data obtained prior to widespread use of bypass surgery reveal that patients with significant disease in one vessel have a mean annual mortality rate of 2.2%. This figure increases to 4.5% to 7.0% when the lesion involves the left main coronary artery. With stenosis of two vessels, the mean annual mortality rate is 6.8%; the rate rises to 11.4% for three-vessel disease. Other correlates of increased risk include evidence of left ventricular dysfunction such as cardiomegaly, symptoms of heart failure, and resting tachycardia. There is some data suggesting that survival is also a function of severity of symptoms. The development of unstable angina (rest pain, crescendo pattern, recent onset) is a bad prognostic sign. "Silent" ischemia (ischemic electrocardiographic changes in the absence of symptoms during continuous ECG monitoring) has been identified as a marker of an especially poor outcome in such patients.

The natural history of coronary artery spasm is highly variable, reflecting the diversity of this group of patients. An important variable is the presence or absence of underlying coronary disease. When spasm occurs in the absence of fixed stenoses, the prognosis is relatively good; in a series of 59 such patients followed for a mean of 5.9 years, 39% had spontaneous remissions and none died. Some investigators even suggest that spasm may be a temporary condition; however, myocardial infarction, heart block, and malignant arrhythmias have been documented in such patients, emphasizing that the condition is not a benign one. The prognosis of patients with spasm in the setting of underlying coronary stenosis is a function of the coronary anatomy; patients with multivessel disease are at greatest risk. Whether or not risk is significantly enhanced by the presence of spasm is as yet undetermined.

PRINCIPLES OF MANAGEMENT

Most medical therapies work by decreasing myocardial oxygen demand. Invasive procedures such as angioplasty and bypass surgery are designed to improve blood supply to the myocardium. Calcium-channel blockers act to do both. Oxygen demand can be lessened for a particular level of activity by reducing heart rate, contractility, heart size, or afterload. Agents useful for decreasing oxygen demand include nitrates, beta-blockers, and calcium-channel blockers. Exercise tolerance can be enhanced by improving peripheral oxygen extraction and promoting a sense of psychological well-being, as well as by decreasing oxygen demand and improving blood supply to the myocardium. Correction of any preexisting hypertension (see Chapter 21), heart failure (see Chapter 27), severe anemia (see Chapter 84), hyperthyroidism (see Chapter 101), or hypoxia is also essential to an optimal outcome.

Nitrates

Nitrates are smooth muscle relaxants that cause vascular dilatation, predominantly of the venous capacitance vessels, though they have a lesser effect on the arterial bed. Nitrates have no proven direct chronotropic or inotropic effects but are believed to decrease myocardial oxygen demand predominantly by reducing left ventricular filling pressure (preload) and end-diastolic volume; nitrates also have a modest effect on systemic blood pressure (afterload). A reflex tachycardia results from the reduction in systemic blood pressure. There is some suggestion that regional myocardial perfusion may be improved, but total coronary blood flow is not. Nitrates are moderately effective in lessening coronary vasospasm. Nitrates and beta-adrenergic blocking agents have complementary effects on myocardial oxygen demand and are often used together (see below).

Sublingual nitroglycerin (TNG) is effective for relief of anginal pain and can provide short-term (up to 30 minutes) improvement in exercise tolerance when taken prophylactically. Its advantages are low cost, rapid onset of action (30 seconds to 3 minutes), safety, and proven efficacy in providing symptomatic relief. Its main drawback is its short duration of action. TNG must be taken sublingually because oral doses are denitrified and inactivated on the first pass through the portal circulation. Since the drug is volatile, it must be kept in a stoppered, amber vial and stored in a cool place. Once a bottle of TNG is opened, the contents remain maximally effective for up to 6 months; after that it is best to assume that the TNG has lost some of its potency, and a fresh supply should be prescribed. Often the patient using old TNG will note that the side-effects of the drug, such as headache and burning under the tongue, are less pronounced, and there is less relief from angina.

An oral nitroglycerin spray is also available. It dispenses 200 metered doses of 0.4 mg each. The patient obtains the drug by spraying it onto or under the tongue. Onset and duration of action are identical to sublingual TNG tablets. Its main advantage is longer shelf life (3 years). Disadvantages include twice the expense of sublingual TNG and the need to carry around an inhaler. One potential advantage is better absorption in patients with dry mucous membranes.

Isosorbide dinitrate is the best studied of the oral nitrates that have been developed in efforts to improve on the short duration of action characteristic of TNG. Early studies failed to demonstrate any prolonged action for these so-called long-acting nitrates when used sublingually or in small doses orally when they were compared with TNG. It was not until larger single oral doses of isosorbide were utilized (20 to 40 mg) that controlled studies showed statistically significant improvements in hemodynamic parameters and exercise tolerance that persisted for up to 4 hours after a dose. A sustained release form (Tembids) is available but because of highly variable intestinal absorption, it is not recommended.

The onset of action of isosorbide taken orally is 15 to 30 minutes. A sublingual form has also been developed that has a more rapid onset of action, 5 to 15 minutes; its duration of action is about 2 hours. In addition, a chewable isosorbide preparation is marketed; its characteristics are similar to those of sublingual isosorbide. It remains unsettled whether the faster but shorter-acting forms of isosorbide are so superior to TNG for prophylaxis that they are worth the much greater cost. Long-acting prophylaxis appears to be best achieved by use of oral isosorbide and nitroglycerin ointment.

Nitroglycerin ointment has been rediscovered in recent years as an effectve method for providing long-acting prophylaxis. Improved exercise tolerance and hemodynamic effects have been found to persist for up to 6 hours after application. Because the ointment is messy and becomes irritating to the skin of some patients if applied to the same area around-the-clock, it is best suited for nocturnal use.

Transdermal nitroglycerin patches were developed with the hope that prolonged nitroglycerine administration could be achieved in a convenient-to-use form. Early reports suggested that the patches would provide 24-hour protection, because patches gave 24 hours of serum nitrate levels that approached the peak levels seen in patients using sublingual nitroglycerin. Moreover, initial studies of exercise tolerance showed that when patients begin using transdermal patches, they showed improved performance up to 24 hours after application of the patch. Unfortunately, the early reports were not confirmed. Studies done on patients after a week of continuous use of the patch failed to show any significant improvement in exercise tolerance beyond a few hours from time of application. Hemodynamic effects also were reduced after continuous patch use. Serum nitrate levels continued well above minimal therapeutic level, ruling out impaired absorption. The discrepancy between findings in patients tested acutely and after more prolonged therapy is believed due to the development of *nitrate tolerance.*

Tolerance is viewed as a consequence of the patch's ability to deliver a more steady serum nitrate concentration than that attainable with other long-acting nitrate preparations, which have half-lives of only 4 to 6 hours. Onset of tolerance is quite rapid, within 12 to 24 hours. Prevention of tolerance appears to require a regimen that provides for rapid increases and decreases in nitrate levels over the course of the day as well as a daily nitrate-free period. Until prospective studies provide more definitive data on proper use of transdermal patches, it is recommended that patients who are begun or continued on transdermal therapy might be best advised to limit patch wearing to no more than 12 hours per day. Moreover, physicians should continue use of the patch only in those patients who show definite clinical benefit; if there are none, then use of the patch should be terminated. In patients who have been using patches for months to years, termination is best conducted in a tapering fashion to avoid precipitating a nitrate withdrawal syndrome. The literature should be followed closely for further studies addressing the question of optimal transdermal nitroglycerin use.

Initiation of Nitrate Therapy. Determining the *proper dose* of a long-acting nitrate is achieved by monitoring the effect of the agent on heart rate, blood pressure, and exercise tolerance. Long-acting nitrate therapy should be introduced gradually; starting with too large a dose produces severe vascular headaches that force many patients to stop their medication. Beginning with a low-dose program (*e.g.,* 5 mg of isosorbide tid) and advancing it slowly over 1 to 2 weeks, one can achieve substantial nitrate doses without significant headache. Patients with migraine headaches may be very intolerant of nitrates; combining nitrate therapy with a beta-blocking agent often overcomes this difficulty, especially if the beta-blocker is started first.

The dosage can be increased until (1) customary activity can be undertaken without pain, (2) the heart rate at rest rises by 10 to 15 beats per minute, or (3) the blood pressure falls to the point of causing postural lightheadedness. The development of headache is not a reliable therapeutic endpoint, because this side-effect usually disappears with continuation of therapy.

There is little question as to the efficacy of nitrates for relief of anginal pain and improvement in exercise tolerance in patients with coronary artery disease. In addition, nitrates remain the drug of first choice in patients with variant angina due to coronary vasospasm. The effect of nitrates on prognosis is more difficult to determine, since most studies of survival involve multiple drug regimens combining nitrates with beta-blocking agents; such studies do document improved survival.

Beta-Adrenergic Blocking Agents

Beta-adrenergic blocking agents (see Table 25-1) reduce myocardial oxygen consumption by reducing contractility, blood pressure, and heart rate. The reduction in heart rate is also potentially beneficial in allowing more time for myocardial perfusion that occurs during diastole. Beta-blockers have demonstrated efficacy in prophylaxis of angina, improvement in exercise tolerance, and prolongation of survival in patients surviving myocardial infarction. In the landmark Norwegian Multicenter Study, postinfarction patients treated with timolol experienced a 45% reduction in sudden death. To date, no comparable trials have been conducted in patients with stable angina who have not experienced infarction.

The beta-blocking agents and nitrates nicely complement one another in the treatment of angina and are often used together. The beta-blockers can reduce the reflex tachycardia that may result from nitrate use; nitrates help minimize any increase in left ventricular end diastolic pressure that may ensue from the beta-blocker's negative inotropic properties.

The *adverse effects* of the beta-blockers include *heart failure* due to decreased contractility and *heart block* due to slowed conduction. Heart failure is a relative contraindication to use of most beta-blockers, as is heart block. Beta-blockade can cause symptomatic *bradycardia* in patients with underlying sinus node disease. In addition, beta-blockade can trigger *bronchospasm*. Even the relatively selective beta$_1$-blocking agents (see Table 25-1) can trigger bronchospasm in asthmatics when used in moderate doses. Beta-blockers also blunt the beta-adrenergic response to hypoglycemia; thus, these agents must be used with care in those taking insulin (see Chapter 101). A long-term study of anginal patients with functional class III or IV disease who took propranolol for 5 to 8 years showed that heart failure developed in 25%, but two thirds had a history of heart failure prior to therapy. All patients with a cardiothoracic ratio greater than 1:2 developed some degree of heart failure on propranolol. The incidence of asthma was 4%, was dose-related, and did not require complete discontinuation of the drug.

Depression and *fatigue* are frequently reported, especially with use of beta-blockers that are lipid soluble (see Table 25-1) and able to diffuse readily across the blood–brain barrier. Other CNS side-effects include *nightmares* and insomnia. The CNS side-effects are among the leading reasons for discontinuation of therapy.

Although *coronary vasospasm* has been documented in a few patients on beta-blocking agents in the setting of unopposed alpha-adrenergic stimulation, vasospasm resulting from use of beta-blockers is rarely a problem clinically, perhaps because these agents also decrease platelet aggregation, oxygen demand, and other factors that may contribute to vasospasm or angina. Beta-blockers have proven useful in patients with variant angina but are probably best used only in conjunction with agents that have vasodilating capacity, such as the nitrates or calcium-channel blockers. The newer beta-blockers with some intrinsic beta-adrenergic activity may prove useful. The literature should be followed closely for new developments in the use of beta-blockade in patients with coronary vasospasm.

Abrupt withdrawal of beta-blockade can precipitate an exacerbation of angina, acute coronary insufficiency, and even infarction. The issue of withdrawal is particularly common in anginal patients who are about to undergo cardiac surgery and will have most of their medications discontinued before surgery. Only a small proportion of anginal patients experi-

Table 25-1. The Beta-Blocking Agents

DRUG	HALF-LIFE (H)	LIPID SOLUBILITY	CARDIOSELECTIVITY	AGONIST ACTIVITY
Propranolol*	Up to 6	High	No	No
Metoprolol*	Up to 6	Moderate	Yes	No
Atenolol	Up to 24	Low	Yes	No
Nadolol	Up to 24	Low	No	No
Timolol	Up to 24	Low	No	No
Pindolol	Up to 12	Low	No	Yes
Acebutolol	Up to 12	Low	Yes	Yes
Labetalol	Up to 12	Low to moderate	No	No

* A sustained-release form of the drug is available.

ence a rebound in symptoms when beta-blockade is suddenly terminated. Those most likely to do so are patients on large doses who have achieved much benefit from beta-blockade. It has been hypothesized that the increase in beta-adrenergic receptors that results from long-term use may make these patients more sensitive to beta-adrenergic stimulation. Available reports indicate that beta-blockers can be withheld for up to 48 hours without risking any increase in angina. Patients who experience an exacerbation of angina usually do so between 2 and 6 days after abrupt discontinuation of therapy. Tapering therapy over the course of a week can prevent any precipitous reaction to withdrawal of beta-blockade.

Propranolol is the prototype beta-blocking agent. Although usually well tolerated, its disadvantages include relatively little cardioselectivity, a short serum half-life, and high lipid solubility that permits CNS penetration. In the last few years, several new beta-blockers have been developed in attempts to overcome some of the disadvantages associated with the parent compound.

Metoprolol differs from propranolol in that it is relatively cardioselective at low to moderate doses (selectivity is lost at high doses) and less likely to induce bronchospasm, making it a useful drug in angina patients who also suffer from chronic obstructive pulmonary disease. *Atenolol* is also cardioselective, but has the additional advantages of a longer half-life (up to 24 hours), allowing once-daily administration and low fat solubility that limits the CNS effects. *Acebutolol* is a third beta$_1$-selective drug, which, in addition, has some intrinsic sympathomimetic activity and does not slow heart rate as much as other beta-blockers. It has been linked to a lupus-like syndrome, the importance of which remains unclear. *Nadolol* also has a long half-like and low lipid solubility; however, it is not cardioselective. *Timolol* is a more potent beta-blocker with a very narrow therapeutic range. It can be administered on a twice-daily basis and does not penetrate the CNS readily; however, it is not cardioselective.

Pindolol was the first of the beta-blocking agents to possess some intrinsic sympathomimetic activity and produce less depression of contractility, conduction, and sinus node function. As a result, pindolol makes possible beta-blockade in anginal patients who might not otherwise tolerate such therapy because of marginal left ventricular function, bradycardia, or heart block. Experience with pindolol is still limited, and its use in such patients should be undertaken with extreme care. Pindolol's intrinsic beta effect gives it some vasodilating activity, which might make this agent the preferred beta-blocker for patients with vasospasm. The literature should be followed for reports on use of pindolol in these situations.

Labetalol differs from other beta-blockers in having an additional alpha-blocking effect. This quality gives the drug a more rapid onset of antihypertensive effect, but offers little advantage in the treatment of chronic stable angina. Adverse effects include greater degrees of postural hypotension and sexual dysfunction than seen with most other beta-blockers.

Proper *selection* of a beta-blocking agent depends on the clinical circumstances. For example, anginal patients with COPD or asthma whose symptoms cannot be adequately controlled with other drugs should be treated with a low dose of a relatively cardioselective agent (*e.g.,* atenolol or metoprolol). Those with modestly reduced left ventricular function, conduction system, or sinus node disease might best tolerate beta-blockade that combines some intrinsic adrenergic activity, as provided by pindolol or acebutolol. When fatigue or mild depression are present, a beta-blocker with minimal CNS penetration is best, such as atenolol or timolol. Compliance is facilitated by agents that can be administered on a once-daily basis (*e.g.,* atenolol). Propranolol was the first beta-blocker to be introduced and, although it lacks many of these potentially advantageous properties, many patients remain on it without difficulty and need not be switched to one of the newer (and usually more expensive) agents. Sustained-release preparations of propranolol and metoprolol have been developed for once-daily administration. Studies show these long-acting formulations to be as effective for control of angina as the standard formulations that must be given four times daily.

Initiation of beta-blocking therapy requires titration of dose against the resting and exercise heart rates. Lowering the resting heart rate to about 60 beats per minute at rest is usually considered evidence of sufficient beta-blockade; however, a subset of patients do not achieve adequate control of their angina at this level of beta-blockade. Further increases in dosage may be necessary to prevent chest pain; target heart rates as low as 40 to 50 beats per minute at rest and 100 with vigorous exercise have been suggested. The true measures of adequate therapy remain the supression of angina and improvement of exercise tolerance.

Calcium-Channel Blockers

Calcium-channel blockers (see Table 25-2) inhibit calcium transport through the "slow" calcium channel of the cellular membrane in myocardial, vascular, and other smooth muscle tissues. The net effects range from coronary and systemic vasodilatation to decreases in myocardial contractility and conductivity. Coronary vasodilation improves perfusion in patients prone to spasm, while arterial dilation and slowing of the heart rate reduce myocardial work and oxygen demand. These agents have proven particularly useful in combination with beta-blockers and nitrates for treatment of angina that has been otherwise refractory to medical therapy. No data exist as yet on the effect of calcium-channel blockers on survival. The first-generation calcium-channel blockers currently in wide use are nifedipine, diltiazem, and verapamil. They represent a spectrum of calcium-channel blocking activity.

Nifedipine is the most active peripheral vasodilator of the calcium-channel blockers, with its main effect being on the vascular smooth muscle of the peripheral arterial bed. Both coronary and peripheral arterial dilatation are produced,

Table 25-2. Properties of Calcium-Channel Blockers

DRUG	CORONARY DILATATION	PERIPHERAL ARTERIAL DILATATION	AV NODE DEPRESSION	SA NODE DEPRESSION	NET EFFECT ON LEFT VENTRICLE
Nifedipine	++	+++	0	0	+/0
Diltiazem	+	++	+	++	0
Verapamil	+	+	++	+	−

making this agent particularly useful for patients with the combination of coronary vasospasm and hypertension. Although nifedipine has some direct negative inotropic effects, the net effect on left ventricular function is minimal because the drug induces a strong beta-adrenergic reflex response to its arterial vasodilation. In some patients, a reflex tachycardia and hypotension occur; the tachycardia can be blunted by use of a beta-blocking agent. Unlike verapamil, nifedipine has no clinically significant suppressant effect on the sinoatrial (SA) or atrioventricular (AV) nodes and can be used safely in patients with underlying conduction system disease. Nifedipine has been shown to be effective in the treatment of chronic stable angina, unstable angina, and variant angina. Relative to other calcium-channel blockers, it is less potent but better tolerated in the treatment of chronic angina.

Verapamil is the calcium-channel blocker with the most pronounced net effects on myocardial contractility and conduction. It can precipitate heart failure in patients with underlying impairment of myocardial contractility and can slow conduction at the AV node to the extent that it is useful for treatment of supraventricular tachycardias (see Chapter 23). Compared to the other calcium-channel blockers, it has the greatest therapeutic efficacy, but also the highest frequency of adverse cardiac side-effects. *Diltiazem* more closely resembles verapamil than nifedipine. It causes greater slowing of the heart rate, but has less influence on the AV junction, contractility, and vascular tone than does verapamil.

Choice of calcium-channel blocker for use in chronic stable angina depends to a large extent on the state of the patient's myocardium and conduction system. Patients with sinus node dysfunction should not be started on diltiazem because of the risk of bradyarrhythmias; verapamil is relatively contraindicated in the presence of heart failure or conduction system disease. Nifedipine is the preferred calcium-channel blocker in situations in which cardiac side-effects would not be well tolerated, although it is less effective against angina than the other calcium-channel blockers. Moreover, nifedipine has marked effects on noncardiac smooth muscle, resulting in the highest incidence among calcium-channel blockers of extracardiac side-effects, such as peripheral edema, flushing, and postural hypotension.

Designing the Medical Regimen

There are three options for initial therapy. Traditionally, the *nitrates* were the agents of first choice, based on safety, modest cost, and efficacy in control of symptoms. *Beta-blocking agents* also achieve symptomatic relief, especially when angina is exercise-induced; moreover, they have shown ability to improve survival in patients with documented infarction. The efficacy of *calcium-channel blockers* and their unique mode of action suggests their use for at least some cases, such as those with rest pain and suspected spasm.

In the absence of comparative data, it is suggested that selection of *initial therapy for prophylaxis of angina* be individualized and based on the patient's clinical presentation. Patients who respond well to nitroglycerin are likely to have an excellent response to long-acting nitrates, whether they have exertional or rest angina. A beta-blocking agent provides excellent control for patients with exertional chest pain, and would be especially advantageous in patients who have a co-existing condition that would also benefit from beta-blockade (*e.g.,* hypertension or migraine). For patients with spasm, calcium-channel blockers have proven very effective. In studies comparing isosorbide to nifedipine, control of variant angina was equivalent for both agents. The efficacy of the other calcium-channel blockers compared with that of nitrates in patients with spasm remains to be determined. Diltiazem has a very low incidence of side-effects and might be considered for single-drug therapy if nitrates were poorly tolerated or did not control symptoms.

For patients with chronic stable angina who are not well controlled by use of long-acting nitrates alone, *addition of a beta-blocking agent* is the standard next step, being complementary in mode of action to nitrates. A new alternative suggested by some authorities is to *substitute a calcium-channel blocker* for a beta-blocking agent, especially a calcium-channel blocker that slows the heart rate (*e.g.,* diltiazem or verapamil) and can offset the reflex tachycardia of nitrates. Such two-drug therapy may be especially useful in patients who are poor candidates for beta-blockers (*e.g.,* those with depression or severe bronchospastic disease). Calcium-channel blockers have been shown in double-blind studies to be at least equal in efficacy to beta-blocking agents in patients with chronic stable angina. Patients responding better to calcium-channel blockers may have a component of coronary vasospasm and be served more optimally by an agent with coronary vasodilator activity.

Another new two-drug strategy is combined use of a *calcium-channel blocker and a beta-blocking agent.* Controlled, double-blind studies have demonstrated enhanced symptomatic relief with this strategy compared with the use of these agents alone. The improvement in control of angina is believed due to the additive diminution in heart rate and blood pressure that combination therapy achieves. The combination of *verapamil plus a beta-blocker* appears to be the most effective of the two-drug regimens for control of angina but is associated with the highest frequency of cardiac side-effects (*e.g.,* heart failure, heart block). *Nifedipine plus a beta-blocker* is well tolerated but relatively less effective. Results with diltiazem appear to parallel those with verapamil closely. Since beta-blocking agents are negatively inotropic and can slow the heart rate and conduction, combination therapy with verapamil or diltiazem is contraindicated in patients with heart failure, sinus node dysfunction, or conduction system disease.

Three-drug therapy using calcium-channel blockers in conjunction with beta-blocking agents and nitrates has been utilized for treatment of patients with severe chronic stable angina that is refractory to two-drug regimens. The addition of a calcium-channel blocker will often improve control and might even allow a decrease in nitrate and beta blocker doses, thus helping to reduce the troublesome side-effects that occur with using these drugs at maximal doses. Nifedipine is often the calcium-channel blocker first used in this context, because adverse cardiac side-effects are relatively minimal and its ability to decrease afterload may prove beneficial. However, nifedipine is also the least effective as a coronary vasodilator; trials of diltiazem and even verapamil may be necessary, provided there is no sinus node dysfunction, conduction system disease, or heart failure.

Some authorities have argued for substitution of a potent calcium-channel blocker for a beta-blocking agent before both are used simultaneously in a three-drug regimen; the rationale is the improved safety, simplicity of program, and lower cost.

Cautions. When combination therapy involving beta and calcium-channel blockers is undertaken, it is important to use reduced doses of both agents because of the potential for additive adverse effects on contractility, chronotropy, and conduction. Other cautions for use of combination therapy include avoidance of potent arterial vasodilators (captopril, prazosin, hydralazine) and agents with central alpha-adrenergic blocking effects (*e.g.,* clonidine, methyldopa). Care is also required when combination therapy is used in conjunction with digoxin therapy, because of the potential for further suppression of conduction through the AV node.

Antiplatelet Agents

Ever since platelets were found to participate in the formation of atherosclerotic plaque and release vasoactive substances, agents that suppress platelet function have been tried in patients with angina. Studies involving over 13,000 patients using aspirin, dipyridamole, or sulfinpyrazone have failed to demonstrate any statistically significant improvement in survival, with the exception of aspirin in patients with unstable angina. A long-term primary prevention trial with aspirin every other day is in progress.

Surgical Therapy

Although surgery clearly improves symptoms and functional status in patients who fail medical therapy, its ability to prevent infarction and prolong survival remains to be established. Several randomized multicenter studies of patients with stable angina have been conducted, and long-term follow-up data are becoming available.

The results suggest a benefit from surgery in those patients with the worst prognosis. At greatest risk are those with critical stenosis of the *left main coronary artery.* In the *Veterans Administration (VA) study* of 686 patients with stable angina, 95 patients had left main disease. Among those with left main disease randomized to surgery, survival was so dramatically improved that patients randomized to medical therapy were allowed to cross over and receive surgery. The average annual mortality in the surgical group was 3%. Direct comparison of long-term results with patients treated medically is impossible because almost half the medically treated group died and the other half were allowed to receive surgical therapy.

For patients without left main disease, there is controversy as to the benefit from elective bypass surgery. For example, it is known that patients with *three-vessel disease* also have a poor prognosis; do they benefit from surgery? In the VA study, 595 patients with stable angina who did not have left main disease were randomized and have been followed for 11 years; cumulative survival rates did not differ significantly among the medically and surgically treated groups. However, the study identified an important high-risk subgroup of patients with angiographic and clinical evidence suggestive of poor prognosis that showed a significant benefit from surgical therapy throughout all 11 years of follow-up. High angiographic risk was defined as three-vessel disease and impaired left ventricular function; high clinical risk included at least two of the following: resting ST depression, history of myocardial infarction, and history of hypertension. Only patients with combined high angiographic and clinical risk demonstrated improved survival from surgical therapy over the entire follow-up period. Patients in categories of lower risk did not benefit as much from surgery. Those having high risk in only one category (*e.g.,* three-vessel disease and impaired left ventricular function, but no clinical risk factors), showed some improved survival with surgery at 7 years of follow-up, but this benefit was no longer apparent by 11 years. (It has been suggested that late graft occlusion may be the cause for the deterioration in survival between years 7 and 11.) Patients with normal left ventricular function, low angiographic risk, and low clinical risk tended to do better throughout the 11 years of follow-up if treated medically, although their advantage was not statistically significant, except among patients with two-vessel disease.

In sum, the VA study suggests that surgery fails to improve overall survival, except among selected subgroups that have the very worst prognosis (*i.e.,* patients with left main disease; and patients with three-vessel disease, impaired left ventricular function, ST segment depression at rest, and history of hypertension or infarction).

Another multicenter randomized study was the Coronary Artery Surgery Study (CASS). This differed from the VA study in several respects: its patients had less serious illness (no left main disease or severe angina), and it examined the rate of infarction as well as mortality. There was neither prolongation of life nor prevention of myocardial infarction in patients treated surgically and followed up for 5 years compared with those randomized to medical therapy. Unlike the findings in the VA study, no subgroups showed a benefit from surgery. The subgroup most closely resembling the angiographically high-risk group of the VA study (three-vessel disease and an ejection fraction below 0.5) showed only a trend toward improved survival at 5 years; the trend was not statistically significant.

Thus, the emerging view is that bypass surgery may prolong survival, but only in patients with the very worst prognoses. Unforeseen developments such as late graft occlusion may limit the beneficial effects of surgical therapy that were noted enthusiastically in earlier reports. Hundreds of thousands of patients currently undergo bypass surgery annually, many with mild stable angina, in hope of achieving prolonged survival. It remains to be seen whether any beyond those with main left or clinically severe three-vessel disease derive lasting benefit from surgery. The most recent data suggests the majority of patients do not. Further reports from the VA and CASS studies should continue to illuminate this issue.

Detection of Patients Who Are Candidates for Surgery.
Patients with greater than 50% stenosis of the left main coronary artery are the prime candidates for bypass surgery and need to be identified. They represent 5% to 10% of patients with coronary artery disease. Unfortunately, no pattern of symptoms, signs, or resting electrocardiographic changes reliably identifies such patients. However, exercise stress testing has been found to be useful for detecting such patients. In *markedly symptomatic patients,* early ST segment changes during stage I or II of exercise, 2 mm or more of ST segment depression, downsloping ST segments, exercise-induced hypotension, and prolonged ST segment changes after the test (>8 minutes) have been reported to have some value in predicting left main coronary disease. The predictive accuracy (predictive value) of these criteria have been reported to range from 21% to 47%.

Most series relating exercise test results to coronary anatomy have been done in patients who are markedly symptomatic and have already undergone coronary arteriography. As a result, these studies are retrospective and contain a selection bias: the study populations are limited to previously catheterized patients. In addition, many studies were done without multiple lead recording, limiting their ability to detect global ischemia, a suspected manifestation of left main disease. When the above stress test diagnostic criteria were examined prospectively in 40 patients with suspected coronary disease but *few or no symptoms* and no previous catheterization, only the criterion of *global ischemia* (simultaneous anterior and inferior ST segment depressions) was found to significantly correlate with left main disease. The predictive accuracy was 57%.

There is some tentative evidence for the use of stress testing to identify a subset of minimally symptomatic patients with three-vessel disease who have a poor prognosis; such patients drop their ejection fractions with exercise. Whether or not this subgroup will benefit from surgery is untested at present.

These results suggest that anginal patients might benefit from exercise stress testing to screen for conditions such as main left disease that are associated with poor prognosis. Use of multiple electrocardiographic leads and measurement of ejection fraction might enhance the predictive value of testing; further confirmatory data are awaited. The severity of symptoms need not be the determining factor for who is tested.

Surgery for Patients with Coronary Spasm. Most studies of surgical therapy for patients with coronary spasm show disappointing results. The National Heart, Lung and Blood Institute's trial of surgical versus medical therapy in 79 patients with ST segment elevation during chest pain showed the surgical group with significantly higher rates of mortality and nonfatal infarction over the 36 months of follow-up. Surgical therapy should be considered only when medical therapy has failed and spasm has been documented in or about an area of fixed, critical stenosis and not in other vessels or distally.

Angioplasty. Percutaneous transluminal coronary angioplasty has been used predominantly to reestablish flow in symptomatic patients with single-vessel disease. The procedure requires coronary angiography and involves passing a balloon catheter into a stenosed vessel and inflating the balloon at the site of the stenosis to widen the lumen. Patients with high-grade proximal stenosis (>70%) of a single vessel have been considered the best candidates for the procedure, with many achieving at least short-term relief from symptoms and improvement in flow. However, high mortality has been reported in patients with proximal stenosis of the left main coronary artery undergoing angioplasty. Also, high rates of restenosis have been found in patients with variant angina subjected to angioplasty.

The long-term safety, efficacy, and cost-effectiveness of the procedure in comparison with medical therapy and bypass surgery remain to be established. The literature should be followed closely for developments in this area, especially as angioplasty is applied to treatment of multivessel disease. The need is acute for randomized controlled studies similar to those done for bypass surgery.

Treatment of Risk Factors and Aggravating Conditions

Heart Failure. When heart failure complicates angina, digitalis and/or a diuretic can provide some symptomatic relief (see Chapter 27). Digitalis may be needed to counter failure associated with the use of propranolol; nitrates cannot prevent the development of clinically significant congestive failure induced by beta-blockade. Although the positive inotropic effect of digitalis may increase myocardial oxygen demand, this increase can be offset by a reduction in heart size; a net decrease in oxygen requirements often results. Nocturnal episodes of angina that are triggered by failure will respond to treatment of the congestive failure. Sometimes symptoms of failure that occur at night are due to ischemia and labeled an "anginal equivalent"; reducing myocardial oxygen demands may alleviate the symptoms.

Stress. When acute anxiety or situational stress is known to precipitate chest pain, use of a minor tranquilizer such as a benzodiazepine (see Chapter 222) may be helpful in anticipation of an extremely stressful situation to prevent a severe bout of angina. Regular use of benzodiazepine tranquilizers, however, can lead to tolerance and even addiction and is no substitute for an adequate medical regimen. Beta-blocking agents are quite effective in limiting the adverse cardiac effects of anxiety by blocking the attendant adrenergic discharge.

High levels of life stress and social isolation have been found in carefully conducted prospective study to be important independent predictors of death from coronary disease. Although personality style, such as so-called *Type A behavior,* was initially thought to be an important risk factor, recent prospective studies have failed to confirm the earlier, widely publicized observations on personality style, which were based mostly on retrospective data.

The therapeutic implications of these findings include the importance of addressing the psychosocial stresses that the anginal patient encounters. An adequate evaluation includes a thorough psychosocial history with emphasis on those factors contributing to stress and social isolation. Less attention need be paid to altering the style of the hard-driving, impatient person; urging such patients to change their behavior may be less productive than helping them to deal with the stresses they encounter.

Obesity and Hypercholesterolemia. Weight reduction (see Chapter 229) is indicated in the patient who is more than 20% overweight. The goal is to reduce cardiac work and oxygen demand. Adherence to a low-saturated-fat, low-cholesterol diet (see Chapters 9 and 22) has been shown to lower the mortality from coronary disease and should be an essential part of the medical program for all patients with coronary disease. Whether or not regression of stenoses can be accomplished is currently under investigation. A halt in progression of plaque has been documented. Other dietary factors such as *coffee* and *alcohol* consumption do not appear to be of major significance, although a minor increase in HDL cholesterol has been noted with modest alcohol intake (see Chapter 22).

Smoking is a major aggravating factor for angina, not only because it contributes to the development of coronary disease, but also because the absorbed nicotine increases blood pressure and heart rate, thus increasing myocardial oxygen demands. Moreover, the rise in carboxyhemoglobin levels in the blood cuts down on the oxygen supply to the heart. Even passive smoking, that is, breathing the air in a smoke-filled room, has been shown to reduce exercise tolerance significantly in patients with chronic stable angina. Cessation of smoking is certainly not easy to achieve and may even produce some additional stress; nevertheless, the benefits in terms of symptomatic improvement may be impressive and may obviate the need to consider more aggressive antianginal therapy. Working with the patient to quit smoking is certainly worth a serious attempt and often succeeds when the physician takes a strong interest (see Chapter 49).

An Exercise Program can improve exercise tolerance. Uncontrolled data suggest that survival may be prolonged by exercise training; the issue remains controversial (see Chapters 10 and 26). Exercise programs may improve exercise tolerance by reducing peripheral oxygen demands (skeletal muscle efficiency improves), by decreasing the increment in heart rate and blood pressure that occurs with exercise, and by promoting a sense of psychological well-being.

Careful screening of patients who are potential candidates for exercise training is necessary to ensure safety. Patients should not take part in an exercise program if they have congestive heart failure, unstable angina, severe systemic hypertension, brittle insulin-dependent diabetes, severe lung disease, hemodynamically significant valvular heart disease, heart block, exertional hypotension, or poor motivation. Patients using ganglionic blocking agents are also advised against participating.

All patients who are enrolled should have an exercise stress test to determine the maximum heart rate at which they can safely exercise (see Chapter 26). Once this rate is established, the patient should be taught to measure his own pulse and instructed not to exceed the target rate. The optimal rate for achieving training benefit is 75% to 85% of the maximum for the patient's age, but the level may have to be set lower if angina, ischemic ST and T-wave changes, or arrhythmias occur at such rates.

The best exercises are isotonic ones that use the large muscles of the body (*e.g.,* walking, swimming, jogging, and cycling). Isometrics are to be avoided, because they are capable of inducing marked elevations in blood pressure and precipitating ventricular irritability. A 10- to 15-minute warmup period should start the session, followed by 20 to 30 minutes of more strenuous activity (see Chapter 10). To attain the optimal training benefit from exercise, there should be two to three periods of about 5 minutes each, during which the target heart rate is achieved. The session ends with time for cooling down. Conditioning requires at least three sessions per week.

Training should begin slowly, advance gradually, and not involve competitive activities until a full 3 months of activity at the target heart rate has been achieved and is well tolerated. Many patients report a new sense of confidence and well-being and a return to productive work; they avoid unnecessary restrictions of life-style, and depression often resolves.

PATIENT EDUCATION

Patient education is pivotal in the management of the person with angina, because the success of a medical regimen requires the intelligent use of drugs by the patient. If the patient lacks an understanding of the rationale behind therapy, he is apt to misuse the agents prescribed or to comply poorly. Counseling can prevent unnecessary restrictions in activity, excessive fear, and decline in life-style. Of particular concern to many patients is the safety of engaging in sexual intercourse. The issue should be addressed openly and directly, even if the patient does not raise the subject, for the worry and interference with marital life can worsen emotional stress and aggravate symptoms. Guidelines for engaging in sexual activity are similar to those for any other form of physical exertion. The oxygen demands of intercourse among married, middle-aged partners are about the same as those for climbing a flight of stairs. If intercourse takes place among unaccustomed partners, the physical and emotional stress may be greater and the oxygen requirements increased. When there is a question of how much activity the patient can safely tolerate, an exercise stress test can be of help; moreover, the test may have a reassuring effect on the overly cautious patient who has been needlessly limiting his activity.

The patient has an important role in helping the physician to gauge the effectiveness of therapy. Subjective reports of exercise tolerance have been found to correlate with objective ergometric findings. Thus, a careful history that reveals how well the patient is managing can provide a very practical means of judging the adequacy of the therapeutic program.

INDICATIONS FOR ADMISSION AND REFERRAL

Admission is required when the anginal pattern is increasing in frequency and/or severity and is becoming harder to control. Episodes that are starting to last more than 15 minutes and beginning to occur at rest as well as with exertion suggest the development of acute coronary insufficiency.

Hospitalization may also be of benefit to judge the adequacy of a medical regimen and to check on compliance when a patient reports insufficient relief of symptoms. Referral to a cardiologist for consideration of coronary angiography is indicated when maximum medical therapy has failed to control symptoms and when left main or severe three-vessel disease is suspected. The same is true if tight aortic stenosis is a consideration (see Chapter 28).

THERAPEUTIC RECOMMENDATIONS

- Help the patient to eliminate or reduce important risk factors such as smoking, excess intake of cholesterol and saturated fat, life stress and social isolation, and marked obesity.
- Treat any concurrent aggravating factors such as hypertension, heart failure, severe anemia, hyperthyroidism, hypoxia, or critical aortic stenosis.
- Employ nitroglycerin, 0.3 mg or 0.4 mg sublingually, for immediate symptomatic treatment of anginal episodes; instruct the patient to rest at the time of pain and to repeat the nitroglycerin if the pain does not resolve within 5 minutes. Advise the patient to maintain a fresh supply of nitroglycerin and to discard any bottle that has been open for more than 6 months or any tablets that fail to burn sublingually or cause throbbing headache.
- Instruct the patient to use sublingual nitroglycerin prophylatically if the anginal pattern is predictably related to events and short-term (<30 minutes) protection will suffice (*e.g.,* before carrying bundles, climbing a hill).
- If short-term prophylaxis is insufficient or the frequency and severity of episodes is too great for sublingual nitroglycerin alone, add a long-acting nitrate, a beta-blocking agent, or a calcium-channel blocker to the program. The choice of agent is determined by the clinical situation:
  1. *Nitrates.* For patients who respond well to nitroglycerin, begin an oral long-acting nitrate such as *isosorbide dinitrate.* The starting dose should be low to avoid severe headache (*e.g.,* 5 mg tid) and advanced slowly over 1 to 2 weeks in increments of 5 mg per dose; the interval between doses can be shortened from 8 to 6 to 4 hours if suppression of anginal episodes remains inadequate. Increase the dose until control is obtained, side-effects become intolerable, systolic blood pressure falls to 100 mm Hg, resting heart rate increases more than 10 beats per minute, or postural hypotension occurs. *Nitroglycerin paste* can be used as an adjunct to isosorbide therapy for nocturnal pain. Begin with 1 inch of the ointment applied to the precordium or any other part of the body before bed. Advance the dose of ½ inch at a time until a therapeutic endpoint is achieved. *Transdermal nitroglycerin patches* can be used as a nocturnal substitute for nitroglycerin paste. Begin with a 5 or 10-mg patch, applied before bed. Because of the risk of nitrate toler-

ance reported in patients using patches round-the-clock, consider removing the patch in the morning rather than using it as a 24-hour nitrate source.

2. *Beta-blocking agents.* For patients with exertional angina as well as those who do not respond well to nitroglycerin or have another condition that would also benefit from beta-adrenergic blockade (*e.g.,* hypertension or migraine headache), and have no serious contraindications to beta-blockade (heart failure, heart block, asthma, tight aortic stenosis, depression), begin a beta-blocking agent such as *atenolol* 50 mg qd. The dose can be increased every 3 to 4 days in 25 to 50-mg increments until control is achieved, the heart rate falls below 40 to 50 beats per minute, fatigue develops, or evidence of heart failure ensues.

   a. A beta-blocking agent can also be added to the regimen at the same time long-acting nitrates are begun; the effects of combined therapy are often synergistic, canceling out adverse cardiac side-effects and achieving good control with smaller doses of each agent.

   b. If you must terminate beta-blockade, do so only in a tapering fashion over several days and have the patient reduce activity during this time.

3. *Calcium-channel blockers.* This class of drugs can be used if coronary artery spasm is strongly suspected or if nitrates and beta-blocking agents do not adequately control symptoms. The choice of agent and number of drugs used depends on the clinical situation. For patients with severe angina complicated by heart failure, sinus node, or conduction system disease, add *nifedipine,* 10 mg qid, to the patient's ongoing program. Advance the dose in 10-mg increments until control is achieved or blood pressure falls below 100 mm Hg. For patients with no failure, sinus node, or conduction system disease, one might consider using an agent with greater antianginal effect such as *diltiazem,* starting with 30 mg tid, or *verapamil,* 80 mg tid. Monitor carefully for signs of heart failure, heart block, and bradycardia. Solo use of a calcium-channel blocker is worth considering in patients with variant angina not adequately controlled by nitrates. Two-drug therapy involving a calcium-channel blocker plus a long-acting nitrate or a beta-blocker may also be helpful in specific situations (see Principles of Therapy above).

- Consider use of exercise stress testing to screen noninvasively for conditions associated with poor prognosis, such as left main disease. Use of multiple leads and measurement of ejection fraction with exercise may increase the predictive value of test results.
- Begin an exercise program for the motivated patient; obtain a stress test first.
- Refer to a cardiologist for consideration of angiography and surgery if anginal pain remains refractory in spite of a max-

imal medical regimen or there is evidence suggestive of left main disease. Also refer any anginal patient with evidence of critical aortic stenosis.

- Admit patients with acute coronary insufficiency (unstable angina) and those with refractory pain who are suspected of poor compliance.
- Thoroughly review with the patient and family the rationale and proper use of medications; encourage the patient to help monitor the efficacy of therapy. Counsel him on allowable activity, encourage exercise as tolerated, and help him avoid self-imposed unnecessary limits on activity.

A.H.G.

ANNOTATED BIBLIOGRAPHY

Abrams J: Nitroglycerin and long-acting nitrates. N Engl J Med 302: 1234, 1980 (*Terse but good review, though slightly dated; 38 references.*)

Abrams J: Transdermal nitroglycerin and nitrate tolerance. Ann Intern Med 104:424, 1986 (*Reviews available data and suggests that transdermal preparations be used for no more than 12 hours per day to avoid development of tolerance.*)

Blumenthal DS, Weiss JL, Mellits ED et al: The predictive value of a strongly positive stress test in patients with minimal symptoms. Am J Med 70:1005, 1981 (*The finding of global ischemia during 12-lead monitoring of an exercise stress test correlated significantly with left main coronary stenosis; the finding had a predictive value of 57%.*)

Bonow RO, Kent KM, Rosing DR et al: Exercise-induced ischemia in mildly symptomatic patients with coronary artery disease and preserved left ventricular function: Identification of subgroups at risk of death during medical therapy. N Engl J Med 311:1339, 1984 (*Mildly symptomatic patients with three-vessel disease who had normal ejection fractions at rest but falls in ejection fraction with exercise had a poor prognosis.*)

Braunwald E: Mechanism of action of calcium-channel blocking agents. N Engl J Med 307:1618, 1982 (*Thorough review of mode of action as well good discussion of clinical uses of the various agents; 45 references.*)

CASS Principal Investigators: Myocardial infarction and mortality in the Coronary Artery Surgery Study (CASS) randomized trial. N Engl J Med 310:750, 1984 (*One of the landmark randomized studies on the efficacy and indications for bypass surgery. Neither prolongation of life nor prevention of infarction was demonstrated in this mildly symptomatic patient population.*)

Conti CR: Large vessel coronary vasospasm: Diagnosis, natural history and treatment. Am J Cardiol 55:41B, 1985 (*Comprehensive review of therapy as well as good summaries of natural history and diagnosis, 31 references.*)

Frishman WH: Beta adrenoceptor antagonists: New drugs and new indications. N Engl J Med 305:500, 1981 (*Reviews and contrasts the available agents in this important class of drugs.*)

Frishman WH: Atenolol and timolol, two new systemic beta adrenoceptor antagonists. N Engl J Med 306:1456, 1982 (*Reviews and compares the pharmacology and clinical effectiveness of these two newer agents.*)

Frishman WH et al: Comparative effects of abrupt withdrawal of propranolol and verapamil in angina pectoris. Am J Cardiol 50: 1191, 1982 (*No rebound effect was noted in those on verapamil; 2 of 20 patients had severe exacerbation of symptoms when propranolol was withdrawn.*)

Gottlieb SO, Weisfeldt ML, Ouyang P et al: Silent ischemia as a marker for early unfavorable outcomes in patients with unstable angina. N Engl J Med 314:1214, 1986 (*A poor prognostic sign; encountered in 50% in this study.*)

Graboys TB: Stress and the aching heart. N Engl J Med 311:594, 1984 (*An editorial summarizing the data on the relation between psychosocial stress and mortality from heart disease.*)

Kannel WG, Feinleib M: Natural history of angina pectoris in the Framingham study. Prognosis and survival. Am J Cardiol 29: 154, 1972 (*A community-based study showing an overall annual mortality rate of 4%.*)

Leon MB, Rosing DR, Bonow RO et al: Combination therapy with calcium channel blockers and beta blockers for chronic stable angina. Am J Cardiol 55:69B, 1985 (*Combined use in patients with refractory angina and preserved left ventricular function provides better results than either agent alone.*)

Luchi RJ, Chahine RA, Raizner AE: Coronary artery spasm. Ann Intern Med, 1979 (*Excellent review of pathophysiology and its clinical implications; 118 references.*)

Mock MB, Reeder GS, Schaff HV et al: Percutaneous transluminal coronary angioplasty versus coronary artery bypass. N Engl J Med 312:916, 1985 (*An editorial summarizing the current status of this technology and arguing that randomized controlled studies are needed to determine efficacy.*)

The Norwegian Multicenter Study Group: Timolol-induced reduction in mortality and reinfarction in patients surviving acute myocardial infarction. N Engl J Med 304:801, 1981 (*This landmark trial demonstrated a 45% reduction in sudden death among post-MI patients attributable to beta-blockade with timolol.*)

Parker JO: Efficacy of nitroglycerin patches: Fact or fancy? Ann Intern Med 102:548, 1985 (*An editorial reviewing the evidence for efficacy and raising the question of tolerance developing rapidly with patch use.*)

Parker JO: Propranolol in angina pectoris. Circulation 65:1351, 1982 (*Long-acting propranolol administered in a dose of 160 mg daily is as effective as 40 mg of standard propranolol given four times daily.*)

Reeves RJ, Oberman A, Jones UB et al: Natural history of angina pectoris. Am J Cardiol 33:434, 1974 (*A terse review of natural history studies and prognostic indicators. Concludes that the extent of coronary disease and performance of left ventricle are the best determinants of prognosis.*)

Reichek N, Sutton M: Long-acting nitrates. Ann Intern Med 97:774, 1982 (*An editorial critically reviewing the efficacy of nitrate preparations.*)

Ruberman W, Weinblatt E, Goldberg JD et al: Psychosocial influences on mortality after myocardial infarction. N Engl J Med 311:552, 1984 (*Degree of life stress and social isolation, but not personality style, were important predictors of mortality.*)

Veterans Administration Coronary Artery Bypass Surgery Cooperative Study Group: Eleven-year survival in the Veterans Administration randomized trial of coronary bypass surgery for stable angina. N Engl J Med 311:1333, 1984 (*Landmark study. Only those with a very high risk of dying [left main disease, very severe three-vessel disease] demonstrated a benefit from surgery after 11 years of follow-up; earlier benefits found at 7 years disappeared by year 11.*)

26
Cardiovascular Rehabilitation and Secondary Prevention of Coronary Artery Disease
GREGORY D. CURFMAN, M.D.

The major goals of a program in cardiovascular rehabilitation are to improve functional capacity in individuals with established heart disease and to develop and apply interventions aimed at halting the evolution and progression of the coronary atherosclerotic process. The first goal can be accomplished in a majority of patients, and recent information indicates that the second goal may also be very much within reach. Because the interventions sometimes require major changes in the patient's life-style, the influence of the primary physician is critically important. One needs to know what interventions are effective and how to tailor a rehabilitation program to the needs and capabilities of the individual patient.

STRUCTURE OF A CARDIAC REHABILITATION PROGRAM

Cardiovascular rehabilitation programs have traditionally been divided arbitrarily into four phases, which describe the temporal sequence of rehabilitative measures followed in patients with coronary artery disease.

Phase I is the *early rehabilitation* of the patient *during hospitalization* for an acute coronary event. The major goals of this phase include (1) prevention of physical deconditioning, (2) patient education regarding coronary risk factors, and (3) interventions aimed at preventing psychological disability resulting from the anxiety and depression that frequently follow an acute coronary event.

Physical deconditioning is avoided by initiating a program of low-level activity as soon as possible after clinical stability has been achieved. In practice, low-level activity can begin safely as soon as the third day after admission for an uncomplicated myocardial infarction, as soon as rest symptoms have been controlled in patients admitted for medical therapy of angina, and as soon as the patient who has undergone coronary artery bypass surgery is ambulatory.

Initial activity should consist of *slow walking* (60–80 steps per minute); the heart rate should not exceed 15 to 20 beats per minute above the resting level (or 10–15 beats per minute above the resting value in patients receiving beta-adrenergic blocking agents). An alternative low-level activity program can be initiated during hospitalization with a *stationary bicycle ergometer.* If no resistance is applied to the flywheel of a standard bicycle ergometer and the instrument is used in the "free-wheeling" mode, the systemic oxygen consumption achieved by the exercising patients is only 1.3 times resting oxygen consumption, that is, 1.3 mets (see Chapter 10). This low level of activity is comparable in intensity to slow walking and is quite safe for most patients. Either mode effectively prevents skeletal muscle deconditioning and atrophy. Low-level activity also improves morale; patients feel that they are contributing positively to the recovery process.

Prior to hospital discharge, most patients should be observed by their physician while *climbing a flight of stairs.* This will provide confidence that such tasks can be performed safely and will often uncover specific questions about what should and should not be done during the first weeks at home. *Submaximal exercise testing* before hospital discharge has been recommended and is performed routinely in some centers. A treadmill exercise test to a 5-MET level has been found to be safe even when performed within 10 days of an uncomplicated myocardial infarction.

The information obtained from stress testing has prognostic implications and may be useful in patient management. A negative submaximal test predicts an excellent prognosis during the subsequent year, whereas a test that is positive for ischemic electrocardiographic changes with or without anginal symptoms predicts a poorer outcome. In the latter instance, a more aggressive medical or surgical therapeutic approach may be indicated. Exercise testing can also be effective in exposing latent ventricular dysrhythmias and may help in selecting patients whose long-term prognosis may benefit from beta-adrenergic blocker therapy (see below). Successful completion of an exercise test before discharge from the hospital helps to restore patient confidence and suggests that the recovery process is proceeding smoothly.

Because discharge from the hospital after uncomplicated myocardial infarction is being recommended considerably earlier than in the past (often after only 1 week of hospital-

ization), exercise testing can be used to decide which patients can safely undergo early discharge. *Thallium scintigraphy,* in conjunction with submaximal exercise testing, may improve risk stratification after myocardial infarction. Thallium scanning after administration of the coronary vasodilator dipyridimole may also be helpful in stratifying patients into risk categories.

Phase II, the convalescence phase, begins at the time of hospital discharge and continues for 3 to 6 *weeks.* The goal of Phase II rehabilitation is to return the patient to the level of physical conditioning that existed prior to the cardiac event. Since evidence from experimental animal models suggests that high-level physical activity soon after myocardial infarction may promote infarct extension and possible ventricular aneurysm formation, the prescribed activity level remains relatively low during Phase II. *Exercise intensity* is regulated by monitoring peak heart rate, which should not exceed the level achieved during the predischarge submaximal exercise test. If the exercise test disclosed ischemic electrocardiographic changes, anginal symptoms, or ventricular dysrhythmia, the heart rate during exercise training sessions is maintained below the heart rate at which any of these pathologic events was observed. The exercise training modalities used during Phase II, as in Phase I, usually consist of *walking* and *stationary bicycling.* The process of educating the patient and the family about coronary risk factors is an important component of Phase II.

During *Phase III, the late convalescence–physical training phase,* the major goal is to increase the patient's level of physical conditioning. Based on a maximal exercise test performed 3 to 6 weeks after discharge, exercise prescription is rewritten to provide a greater physiologic training effect. This test allows the patient's heart rate and blood pressure responses to exercise to be quantitated and provides another screening test for latent myocardial ischemia and ventricular dysrhythmias. The exercise training modalities used during Phase II can be broadened during Phase III to establish a balanced exercise program that will have long-term patient appeal. Upper extremity conditioning may be added, especially in patients for whom upper extremity work is important on the job. During Phase III, efforts to modify risk factors continue. These include dietary interventions to lower the total serum cholesterol concentration to less than 200 mg/dl, raise HDL cholesterol concentration, and achieve ideal body weight (see Chapters 9 and 22). Hypertension control (see Chapter 21) and smoking cessation (see Chapter 49) are critically important. Stress management should be addressed (see Chapter 222), particularly as the patient faces a return to work. A well-balanced cardiac rehabilitation program needs to deal with all of these considerations, both in the patient and in the patient's family.

Phase IV is the *maintenance* or *follow-up phase* of cardiac rehabilitation. The goal is to encourage lifelong adherence to the health habits established during Phase III. Follow-up visits at 6- to 12-month intervals are important. Blood pressure and pulse measurement, serum lipid levels, and even repeat maximal exercise tolerance tests can provide useful feedback to the patient about his or her health practices and indicate areas that may require further life-style change to minimize coronary risk. Further research is needed to improve our understanding about the most effective methods of achieving permanent life-style modification.

THE EFFECTS OF EXERCISE TRAINING

Although it is a commonly held belief that exercise is beneficial for cardiovascular health, our understanding of how physical exercise influences the cardiovascular system and its diseases is far from complete. Nevertheless, substantial information is now available to support the use of exercise training to reduce the morbidity and mortality of cardiovascular disease. Moreover, there is increasing evidence that physical activity is protective against the development of first manifestations of coronary artery disease (primary prevention) (see Chapter 10).

A number of studies indicate the important role that exercise plays in the secondary prevention of coronary disease. The National Exercise and Heart Disease Program (NEHDP) was a large multicenter trial designed to investigate the effects of exercise conditioning on cardiovascular morbidity and mortality in patient who had survived a first myocardial infarction. In the study, 651 patients were assigned randomly to an exercise group or to a sedentary control group. During an average follow-up period of 3 years, the exercise intervention group demonstrated a 37% lower mortality rate than the sedentary control group, a 29% lower cardiovascular mortality rate, and an 87% lower rate of death due to recurrent myocardial infarction. Because of the relatively small number of patients involved, only the 87% reduction in death due to recurrent infarction was statistically significant. Nevertheless, the trends in mortality noted in this study suggest that exercise training may improve prognosis following myocardial infarction even over the relatively short time span of 3 years.

Regular physical exercise may benefit patients with coronary artery disease by a number of mechanisms. These include the physiologic "*training effect*"; because of the increase in peripheral oxygen extraction by working skeletal muscles and the increase in cardiac stroke volume that constitute the training effect, the cardiovascular system of the trained individual is able to deliver a given quantity of oxygenated blood to the peripheral tissues at a lower heart rate. Since systemic arterial pressure also tends to be somewhat lower during exercise in the trained state, the rate–pressure product (heart rate × systolic arterial pressure), which correlates closely with myocardial oxygen consumption under most physiologic conditions, is often substantially lower than in the untrained

state. The benefit to the individual with ischemic heart disease is obvious; it becomes possible for the trained individual to exercise to a higher level before reaching the critical rate–pressure product at which myocardial ischemia develops. Beta-adrenergic blockers benefit patients with angina pectoris in a similar fashion, by reducing heart rate and blood pressure during exertion. Unlike exercise training, however, beta-blocking agents also tend to reduce the maximal cardiac output that can be achieved during exertion, and thereby also decrease maximal oxygen consumption and exercise capacity.

Exercise training may benefit individuals with cardiovascular disease by other physiologic mechanisms as well. Aerobic exercise training results in *dilatation of large coronary arteries,* and this process may diminish the hemodynamic effect of existing coronary artery lesions. Some evidence also suggests that exercise training may improve collateral blood flow to ischemic zones. Coronary blood flow under conditions of maximal coronary vasodilatation may also be increased. Another beneficial effect of exercise conditioning is an *increase in HDL-cholesterol* concentration (see Chapter 9).

Other protective mechanisms of aerobic exercise that are of potential importance are an increase in fibrinolytic response to occlusive stimuli in the trained state. Exercise training has also been associated with an increase in ventricular fibrillation threshold in animal studies, suggesting that exercise conditioning may alter the electrophysiologic properties of the myocardium, rendering it less vulnerable to ventricular dysrhythmia.

ESTIMATING THE AMOUNT OF EXERCISE NEEDED

Although some information is available about *how much exercise is needed* to produce the beneficial physiologic effects discussed above, the issue remains unsettled. In the practice of cardiac rehabilitation, the generally accepted assumption is that one must achieve a physiologic training effect to obtain health benefits. Classic exercise physiology indicates that the training effect can usually be produced by any form of aerobic exercise (running, jogging, fast walking, cycling, rowing, cross country skiing, swimming) that is performed at least four times a week, for at least 30 minutes per exercise session, at an intensity resulting in a heart rate of 70% to 85% of a measured maximum. However, it is possible that less-intense aerobic activity may be effective in producing a training effect and the associated health benefits. Further investigations of this important question is clearly indicated.

The traditional and simplest method of determining an effective exercise intensity for patients undergoing exercise training in a cardiac rehabilitation program is to calculate 70% to 85% of a measured maximal heart rate. Some authorities suggest that the target heart rate should be determined by adding 60% to 70% of the difference between maximal and resting heart rates to the resting heart rate, whereas others argue that the most physiologic parameter to use as a training guide is the rate–pressure product, since this derived parameter is a more accurate measure of cardiac work than is heart rate alone. In practice, the traditional method of using 70% to 85% of a measured maximal heart rate as the target heart rate zone is generally the most efficient. This exercise intensity translates to approximately 60% to 80% of maximal oxygen consumption.

The relationship between heart rate and oxygen consumption (expressed as percentages of their respective maximum values) is not influenced by beta-adrenergic blockade. This point is of importance in cardiac rehabilitation because many patients receive beta-blocking agents as part of their therapeutic regimen (see below). In determining target heart rates for exercise training, the importance of measuring a true maximal heart rate during a formal graded exercise test is apparent, and this exercise test must be performed under the influence of beta-blockers if the patient will be receiving one of these agents during exercise training sessions. The mode of exercise used for exercise testing should be specific to the type of exercise planned for exercise training—that is, treadmill testing for walking/jogging programs and bicycle ergometer testing for cycling program. These two modes of exercise are used most commonly in cardiac rehabilitation programs.

OTHER INTERVENTIONS FOR SECONDARY PREVENTION

Exercise training is but one means of rehabilitation and secondary prevention in the patient with coronary disease. A balanced rehabilitation program should focus attention on other aspects of coronary risk as well, including hypertension (see Chapters 8, 13, and 21), hypercholesterolemia (see Chapters 9 and 22), cigarette smoking (see Chapters 32 and 49), obesity (see Chapter 229), and stress (see Chapter 222).

The long-term use of pharmacologic agents has been applied in an attempt to achieve secondary prevention of coronary disease. A number of randomized clinical trials have indicated that *beta-adrenergic blockade* reduces the total mortality rate, as well as the incidences of recurrent infarction and sudden death in patients following acute infarction. The most convincing studies leading to this conclusion were the Norwegian timolol study (39% reduction in total mortality, 28% reduction in reinfarction rate), and the American Beta-Blocker Heart Attack Trial (26% reduction in total mortality, 23% reduction in coronary incidence). The data derived from these studies are quantitatively similar to data from the NEHDP, although the many potential adverse side-effects of beta-blockers perhaps make this form of postinfarction therapy less appealing than a structured exercise program.

Other agents have been used for secondary prevention in patients with a history of myocardial infarction, but none has had as evident an effect as beta-adrenergic blockade. Both antiplatelet agents and anticoagulation therapy have been tried. A number of trials have suggested a modest reduction in death or reinfarction rates with long-term *aspirin* therapy or anticoagulation with warfarin. A recent randomized trial demonstrated no differences in mortality between groups of post-MI patients treated with aspirin or anticoagulation, but the absence of a placebo group leaves unanswered questions about effectiveness of either agent. Of interest is the observation that patients were less tolerant of long-term aspirin therapy than of anticoagulants. Recently, aspirin has been demonstrated to be efficacious in preventing myocardial infarction among male patients with unstable angina.

Even more controversial is the efficacy of *sulfinpyrazone.* Although a large-scale randomized trial reported a 32% reduction in 2-year cardiac mortality with sulfinpyrazone therapy, the findings have been rejected by many (including the Food and Drug Administration [FDA]) because of after-the-fact exclusion of some deaths during the analysis. Sulfinpyrazone has not been widely used for routine secondary prevention. Recently, the antiplatelet agents *dipyridamole* and aspirin together have been shown to be efficacious for a different but related purpose—the reduction of vein graft occlusion in the first year following coronary artery bypass surgery.

PATIENT EDUCATION

The patient who has suffered an acute coronary event is among those in greatest need of health education and individualized life-style counseling. Patient and family are apt to be depressed and frightened by the diagnosis of "coronary disease," believing the prognosis to be grim and fearing invalidism, especially if an infarction occurred. They need to be informed that in the vast majority of uncomplicated cases, a return to job and regular activity is the rule rather than the exception.

Prognosis is a major concern of the patient and family. Long-term survival rates after infarction have been the subject of prospective epidemiologic studies. Average annual mortality in the Framingham study was 5% for men and 7% for women. Patients at greatest risk for late cardiac death were found to have "malignant" ventricular irritability beyond the acute phase of illness, azotemia, previous infarction, persistent congestive failure, angina, or advanced age; once congestive failure ensued, 50% were dead within 5 years. Many of the complications of infarction are a function of the degree of myocardial damage; this is consistent with the observation that prognosis correlates with extensiveness of disease, a finding also supported by angiographic studies (see Chapter 25). Risk of postinfarction angina was 5.2% per annum; risk of a second infarction was 2.9% for men, 9.6% for women; risk of failure was 2.3%. Moreover, reduction of such rates has been achieved with beta-blockade and lowering of serum cholesterol. Specific statements to the patient and family concerning exercise capacity can be based on graded treadmill stress testing during the recovery period. There are some data suggesting that 1-year survival can also be estimated from a limited, treadmill exercise test done prior to discharge.

Counseling needs to begin in the predischarge period. Realistic concerns as well as excessive fears of incapacitation may dramatically alter self-image and diminish self-respect. The most effective way of dealing with such fears is to specifically elicit and address the patient's concerns, discuss the plan for recovery and rehabilitation, and provide an activity prescription. Knowing what one should and should not do during various stages of the recovery process can help eliminate some of the anxiety that accompanies having a serious illness.

General guidelines should be given. For example, unsupervised activities during the first month following an MI should require no more from 3 mets (see Table 10-1). By the time 6 to 8 weeks have passed, tasks requiring up to 5 mets will be safe for most individuals, provided a gradual increase in activity has not been interrupted by symptoms or complications. However, specific guidelines, tailored to the patient's personal occupational and recreational interests are essential.

Not all questions are raised by the patient. The timing of *sexual activity* should be routinely and openly discussed; myocardial infarction of sudden death during intercourse is an uncommon but widely feared event. Studies suggest that intercourse with a familiar partner requires 3 mets to 5 mets. Sexual activity can therefore be safely resumed by most patients as early as 4 weeks after myocardial infarction. The patient should be advised to avoid coital positions that require sustained isometric exercise, such as upper torso weight-bearing with the arms, during the early return to full sexual activity.

The period following an acute coronary event is also a time when patients are particularly susceptible to counseling about changes in life-style that reduce coronary risk. The primary physician is well positioned to take advantage of this opportunity. A balanced cardiac rehabilitation program offers the most positive approach. Often, the gratifying result some months later is a person who is healthier and more fit than he or she was before the acute coronary event.

ANNOTATED BIBLIOGRAPHY

The Anturane Reinfarction Trial Research Group: Sulfinpyrazone in the prevention of sudden death after myocardial infarction. N Engl J Med 302:250, 1980 (*A controversial randomized trial reporting a reduction in 2 year cardiac mortality of 32% among patients treated with sulfinpyrazone after their infarction.*)

Beta Blocker Heart Attack Trial Research Group: A randomized trial of propranolol in patients with acute myocardial infarction. JAMA 247:1707, 1982 (*This large-scale randomized trial among men and women with one prior myocardial infarction demon-strated a reduction in total mortality of 9.8% to 7.2% and in cardiovascular mortality from 8.5% to 6.2% among those treated with propranolol.*)

Chesebro JH, Fuster V, Elveback LR et al: Effect of dipyridamole and aspirin on late vein graft patency after coronary bypass operations. N Engl J Med 310:209, 1984 (*A randomized trial indicating significant reduction in vein graft occlusion during the first year following bypass surgery with dipyridamole and aspirin therapy.*)

Curfman GD: Cardiac rehabilitation and secondary prevention of coronary artery disease. Transition, June 1984 (*Portions of the current chapter appeared first in this review prepared by the author, and reproduced with permission of the editor.*)

EPSIM Research Group: A controlled comparison of aspirin and oral anticoagulants in prevention of death of myocardial infarction. N Engl J Med 307:701, 1982 (*No difference in mortality or reinfarction between groups given oral anticoagulants and aspirin following myocardial infarction.*)

Frishman WH, Furberg CD, Friederwald WT: B-adrenergic blockade for survivors of acute myocardial infarction. N Engl J Med 830:837, 1984 (*Reviews the clinical studies, potential mechanisms, and clinical use of beta-blockers after myocardial infarction.*)

Jones RJ: Aspirin and recurrent myocardial infarction. JAMA 244:667, 1980 (*An editorial reviewing the equivocal evidence provident by clinical trials.*)

Lewis HD, Davis JW, Archibald DG et al: Protective effects of aspirin against acute myocardial infarction and death in men with unstable angina. N Engl J Med 309:396, 1983 (*Men with unstable angina treated for 12 weeks with buffered aspirin at a 51% lower incidence of death of acute myocardial infarction than placebo-treated controls.*)

McNeer JF, Wagner GS, Ginsberg PB et al: Hospital discharge one week after acute myocardial infarction. N Engl J Med 28:229, 1978 (*A controlled study of early discharge in patients following uncomplicated myocardial infarction.*)

The Norwegian Multicenter Study Group: Timolol-induced reduction in mortality and reinfarction in patients surviving acute myocardial infarction. N Engl J Med 304:801, 1981 (*The landmark trial demonstrating a 45% reduction in sudden death among post-MI patients attributable to timolol therapy.*)

Paffenbarger RS, Hyde RT: Exercise in the prevention of coronary heart disease. Prev Med 13:3, 1984 (*A selective review of the effect of physical activity on primary and secondary prevention of coronary artery disease.*)

Pollock ML, Wilmore JH, Fox SM: Exercise in Health and Disease. Philadelphia, WB Saunders, 1984 (*A useful volume containing much practical information about the development of the exercise prescription.*)

Pryor DB, Hindman MC, Wagner GS et al: Early discharge after acute myocardial infarction. Ann Intern Med 99:528, 1983 (*Extensive review of studies of length-of-stay following myocardial infarction as well as attempts to identify low-risk patients for the posthospital course.*)

Rigotti NA, Thomas GS, Leaf A: Exercise and coronary heart disease. Annu Rev Med 34:391, 1983 (*An excellent review of the effects of exercise on the coronary atherosclerotic process and its clinical manifestations.*)

Shaw LW: Effects of a prescribed supervised exercise program on mortality and cardiovascular morbidity in patients after a myocardial infarction. Am J Cardiol 48:39, 1981 (*Results of the National Exercise and Heart Disease Project, which examined the effects of exercise on mortality and morbidity in patients after myocardial infarction.*)

Temple R, Pledger GW: The FDA's critique of the anturane reinfarction trial. N Engl J Med 303:1488, 1980 (*The rationale for rejecting the positive findings of an effect because of after-the-fact exclusion of certain deaths from analysis in the study.*)

Theroux P, Waters DD, Halphen C et al: Prognostic value of exercise testing soon after myocardial infarction. N Engl J Med 301:341, 1979 (*An important study that demonstrates both the safety and the usefulness of exercise testing early after myocardial infarction.*)

Van Camp SP, Peterson RA: Cardiovascular complications of outpatient cardiac rehabilitation programs. JAMA 256:1160, 1986 (*Documents the very low risk of cardiac events associated with supervised programs.*)

Wilhelmsen L, Sanne H, Elmfeldt D et al: A controlled trial of physical training after myocardial infarction. Prev Med 4:491, 1975 (*Results similar to those of the National Exercise and Heart Disease Project.*)

27
Management of Chronic Congestive Heart Failure

Chronic congestive heart failure (CHF) ranks among the most common of cardiac problems encountered in office practice. Although digitalis and diuretics remain the basic modes of therapy, vasodilators have proven to be important adjuncts, especially in patients with advanced heart failure refractory to other modes of treatment. Of particular importance is design of a drug regimen that is properly tailored to the patient's underlying pathophysiology. A thorough understanding of each agent's mode of action and indications for use is needed to prevent the iatrogenic complications that result from unwise use of drugs for CHF that have narrow therapeutic ranges, such as the digitalis preparations.

Successful management of CHF in the outpatient setting requires identification and correction of treatable underlying causes, elimination of precipitating factors, and judicious application of digitalis, diuretics, and vasodilators. Because multidrug regimens are often necessary, thorough instruction of patient and family is essential to limit the number of avoidable complications and prevent unnecessary hospitalizations that result from poor compliance or drug toxicity.

CLINICAL PRESENTATION AND COURSE

Regardless of etiology, the clinical manifestations of CHF are quite stereotyped and reflect the magnitude of the fall in cardiac output and the rise in pulmonary and systemic venous pressures. Initially and in mild cases, the patient may complain of fatigability, dyspnea on exertion, or unexplained weight gain; there may be few overt physical signs of failure, but chest x-ray often shows redistribution of pulmonary venous flow to the upper lung fields and/or an enlarged heart. Fatigue becomes increasingly prominent as cardiac output falls. As pulmonary congestion increases, dyspnea worsens, orthopnea is noted, and paroxysmal nocturnal dyspnea may be reported. At this stage, rates are frequently found on physical examination, but their absence does not rule out the presence of CHF. Sometimes failure-induced bronchospasm dominates the pulmonary examination. In severe cases, the chest film will show interstitial pulmonary edema. In chronic CHF, right-sided or bilateral pleural effusions are common. Ankle edema, jugular venous distention, and hepatojugular reflux are indicative of elevated systemic venous pressure; if CHF is predominantly left-sided, these findings may not be present. An S3 gallop is among the most specific physical signs of failure, but it is often difficult to hear. If left ventricular dilatation becomes very marked, a mitral regurgitant murmur may become evident. Pedal edema is one of the least specific signs of CHF; in the elderly, isolated pedal edema is more likely to be a result of venous insufficiency (see Chapter 16).

Since congestive failure is not a single disease, it does not have a uniform natural history. Clinical course and response to therapy depend on the nature of the underlying etiology and the state of the myocardium at the time of presentation. For example, the appearance of CHF in a patient with aortic stenosis is an ominous prognostic sign associated with a mean survival of no more than two to three years. However, if the valve is replaced before irreversible myocardial decompensation has occurred, the prognosis is altered dramatically (see Chapter 28). Cases of CHF caused by alcoholic cardiomyopathy, thiamine deficiency, hypertensive heart disease, and hyperthyroidism also have favorable outcomes if detected and treated early.

The Framingham study has provided interesting epidemiologic data concerning CHF in the community setting. The annual incidence rate for development of failure was 2.3 per 1000 for men and 1.4 per 1000 for women. The major causes were hypertension in one third of the patients, hypertension in combination with coronary disease in another one third, isolated coronary disease in about 10%, and valvular disease in another 10%. Sixty percent of patients had a serious noncardiac illness along with CHF. Five-year survival rates, regardless of cause, were only 50%.

Several factors have been examined for their correlation with prognosis. In an important study, plasma norepinephrine levels were found by multivariate analysis to correlate strongly with mortality risk and were superior to such catheterization data as pulmonary wedge pressure, cardiac index, mean arterial pressure, and heart rate. The higher the plasma norepinephrine level, the poorer the prognosis. Such observations, if confirmed, may provide useful and readily obtainable guides to prognosis in the future.

DIAGNOSIS OF HEART FAILURE

Heart failure is frequently a mistaken diagnosis. A common error is to attribute ankle edema or dyspnea to congestive heart failure. In a recent study of patients on digitalis for supposed CHF, 40% did not fulfill basic diagnostic criteria for the condition. *Right heart failure* is easier to document than left heart failure. It is defined as a right atrial pressure greater than 6 cm H_2O, manifested as a greater than 6 cm vertical distance from the level of the right atrium to the top of the jugular venous column. Ankle edema in the absence of jugular venous distention does not constitute a diagnosis of right heart failure.

Left heart failure is more difficult to diagnose solely on clinical grounds. The most specific findings, short of invasive measurement of the left atrial pressure, are found on chest x-ray and include upper zone flow redistribution, cardiomegaly, prominent interstitial markings, Kerley "B" lines, and perihilar haziness. Patients who develop CHF only with exercise may not show interstitial changes on a chest film done at rest. Historical and physical examination findings are neither very sensitive nor specific, but often provide important supportive evidence. Historical data of some diagnostic value are reports of paroxysmal nocturnal dyspnea and orthopnea. The finding of a third heart sound (S_3) is among the most sensitive and specific signs of a low ejection fraction (less the 40%), ventricular dilatation, and elevated atrial pressure. Basilar rales is another helpful sign. Left atrial enlargement (by the ECG criterion of terminal P-wave negativity in lead V_1 that exceeds 0.03 mm/sec) and cardiomegaly by chest film also have diagnostic value.

In the absence of florid radiologic evidence of pulmonary edema, the diagnosis of CHF is best supported by the finding of upper zone redistribution and one of the other historical, physical, or laboratory findings just noted. In the absence of even upper zone redistribution, the presence of any three other findings (*e.g.,* S_3, cardiomegaly, and basilar rales) constitutes reasonable evidence for the diagnosis.

PRINCIPLES OF MANAGEMENT

The first task is to search for and treat a reversible underlying etiology. All too often, many cases are encountered at the time irreversible myocardial damage has occurred, but when a treatable cause is present and detected early, there is an opportunity for definitive measures to bring about a successful outcome. Valvular disease (see Chapter 28), alcohol excess (see Chapter 224), hypertension (see Chapters 13 and 21), hyperthyroidism (see Chapter 101) and myxedema (see Chapter 102) are examples of conditions requiring etiologic therapy. A stereotyped approach with digitalis and diuretics that ignores etiology may lead to omission or delay of proper measures and result in loss of a unique therapeutic opportunity.

Correct selection and application of supportive treatment also requires identification of etiology. For example, digitalis usually proves helpful when there is an excess pressure load on the left ventricle, but if the specific cause of the pressure work is hypertrophic subaortic stenosis, addition of digitalis can increase contractility to the point of worsening outflow tract obstruction. The decision regarding initiation of therapy with digitalis or a diuretic is dependent on a clear formulation of the underlying pathophysiology.

Attention must be directed to the presence of precipitating factors. Severe anemia (see Chapter 78), high fever (see Chapter 6), tachycardia (see Chapters 19, 20, and 23), pulmonary infection (see Chapter 43), pulmonary embolization (see Chapter 14), excess salt intake, marked obesity (see Chapter 229) and excess exertion or emotional stress may worsen or precipitate failure in patients with decreased myocardial reserve. Use of beta-blockers (see Chapter 25) or other negatively inotropic agents may also bring on CHF. A careful search for these factors is essential.

The mainstay of supportive, symptomatic management is drug therapy. Digitalis, diuretics, and vasodilators have specific roles determined by their different hemodynamic effects. Digitalis is used mainly for its positive inotropic action, diuretics for their ability to reduce volume, and vasodilators to lessen preload and afterload.

Digitalis

Digitalis has been a cornerstone of treatment for congestive heart failure since the time of Withering, yet the precise indications for its use and documentation of its efficacy are just now emerging. Only two double-blind, placebo-controlled studies have been performed in patients with CHF and sinus rhythm. One, a nonrandomized study, examined elderly patients with stable CHF who were receiving chronic digitalis therapy. Most had New York Heart Association functional class II or class III disease; only one had a third heart sound. None of the 30 patients completing the study showed evidence of deterioration during the 3 months of placebo administration. However, there were some methodologic problems with the study, including a 25% attrition and no randomization. Despite these limitations, the study suggests it might be reasonable to cautiously withdraw digitalis in carefully selected, elderly CHF patients who manifest mild, stable CHF.

The other double-blind placebo-controlled study was randomized and showed that digitalis benefited only a subset of CHF patients, those with more chronic and severe CHF, characterized by greater left ventricular dilatation, greater reduction in ejection fraction, and an S_3. Multivariate analysis showed the presence of an S_3 to be the major correlate of response to digitalis. This suggests that it is not simply the severity and chronicity of the CHF that predicts response to digitalis, but more importantly the underlying pathophysiology. The pathophysiologic state necessary for production of an S_3 includes a severely reduced ejection fraction, marked left ventricular dilatation, and a high left atrial pressure. Patients in this study who had diuretic-induced reduction of left atrial pressure did not have an S_3 and did not improve further with digitalis therapy. Supporting evidence for the predictive value of an S_3 comes from a recent, uncontrolled, unblinded study of long-term digitalis therapy in nine patients with CHF. All showed objective improvement with digitalis; all had an S_3.

Indications for Therapy. The view that emerges from these studies is that digitalis is likely to benefit those chronic CHF patients who have a persistently elevated left atrial pressure, low ejection fraction, and left ventricular dilatation, manifested by the presence of a *third heart sound despite diuretic therapy.* Use of digitalis prior to initiation of diuretic therapy seems unwise, in view of the relative safety, of diuretic therapy, the narrow therapeutic range of digitalis, and the seriousness of digitalis toxicity. Available data indicate no excess mortality when digoxin is used for CHF in patients who have suffered recent infarction.

Digitalis remains the drug of choice for failure induced by *rapid atrial fibrillation* (see Chapter 23). The drug is also of use in patients with CHF resulting from *uncontrolled hypertension* or *severe aortic stenosis,* but is not a substitute for valve surgery when the aortic stenosis is critical (see Chapter 28). Digitalis has been shown to be ineffective in patients with heart failure resulting from hypertrophic cardiomyopathies, be they idiopathic or due to long-standing hypertension (a common etiology among outpatients, especially women). In fact, patients with hypertrophic subaortic stenosis may develop worsening outflow tract obstruction with use of digitalis. Digitalis is also of no proven benefit in cases of mitral stenosis, as long as the patient is in sinus rhythm, and is of no use in patients with episodes of CHF due to recurrent, transient ischemia. The efficacy of digitalis in *cor pulmonale* is in question; the drug is occasionally beneficial, but the results are not impressive and the risks of toxicity are increased in the setting of hypoxia.

Initiation of Therapy. Patients who are stable can be started on a maintenance oral dose without resorting to a loading dose. Full therapeutic serum levels can be achieved in 5 to 7 days with digoxin (see Digitalis Preparations, below). If the patient is less stable, but not so compromised as to require hospitalization, an oral loading dose can be given in divided amounts over 24 hours.

The decision to initiate digitalis therapy should not be made casually. The incidence of digitalis toxicity was found to be 23% in a prospective study of 900 consecutive admissions to the Boston City Hospital general medical service. Mortality from digitalis intoxication has averaged 22% in published series. Use of serum concentration measurements seems to have helped limit the incidence of toxicity. However, one cannot depend on serum levels alone for the diagnosis of digitalis toxicity, because there is considerable overlap in serum concentrations among those with and without evidence of toxicity.

Digitalis Preparations. Numerous digitalis preparations are available; the physician should become familiar with one or two, learn their pharmacokinetics, and use them predominantly. *Digoxin* is the most widely used. In the past, some variations in bioavailability had been noted among different brands; this seems to have been corrected. Half-life of digoxin is 36 hours; onset of action is 1 to 2 hours when taken orally; absorption from the GI tract ranges from 50% to 75% complete. Excretion is renal and decreases significantly with reduction in creatinine clearance. Therapeutic serum levels can be achieved in 5 to 7 days by prescribing a daily maintenance dose of 0.25 mg. When more rapid oral digitalization is desired, a loading dose of 1 to 1.25 mg. can be given in divided doses over 24 hours. Higher doses are not needed in obese patients; their nonlipid extracellular fluid volume is normal.

If a patient presents taking a digitalis preparation other than digoxin, it is best to leave him on the drug he is used to. The exception to this generalization concerns patients taking *digitalis leaf.* Because of its variable and unpredictable composition of digoxin and digitoxin, digitalis leaf should be discontinued, and one of the preparations containing only a single active ingredient used instead. *Digitoxin* may be beneficial when digitalis must be given to a patient with renal failure, because elimination of digitoxin is not dependent on renal function. However, a major disadvantage with digitoxin is its long half-life of 4 to 6 days, making for serious problems if toxic levels occur. Digoxin can be used safely in renal failure as long as renal function and serum levels are frequently checked and necessary dosage adjustments made.

Monitoring Therapy. Digitalis therapy requires careful monitoring. *Serum levels* should be measured at least three or four times per year, more frequently if there are changes in the patient's clinical status. It is hoped that this will help reduce the incidence of digitalis toxicity. A sample should be drawn at least 6 hours after the last dose, since there is a 4 to 6 hour rise in serum level after an oral dose. In most instances it is best to have the patient omit the day's dose when he comes to the office for a serum determination.

A number of factors can affect serum concentration, including renal function when digoxin is being used and hepatic function in digitoxin therapy. Absorption of digitalis from the gut remains adequate in CHF, but may fall in severe cases of malabsorption. Thyroid status can affect digitalis metabolism; hypothyroidism prolongs the half-life and hyperthyroidism shortens it. Treatment of thyroid disease needs to be accompanied by an adjustment of dose.

The serum level of digitalis is not in itself diagnostic of toxicity, because there is considerable overlap in serum concentrations among those with and without evidence of toxicity; but if the digoxin level is above 2.0 ng. per ml., the probability of encountering toxicity increases considerably. In one series, 80% of patients without evidence of toxicity had a digoxin level below 2.0 ng/ml; in 87% with toxicity, the level was above 2.0.

To avoid *digitalis toxicity,* even when the dose is closely followed, the physician needs to monitor factors that increase the "sensitivity" of the myocardium to the toxic effects of the drug. These include hypokalemia, elevations in serum calcium and magnesium, acute hypoxia, organic heart disease, and pulmonary disease with acute hypoxia.

Digitalis Toxicity. Symptoms of digitalis toxicity can be divided into noncardiac and cardiac manifestations. Anorexia, nausea, vomiting, diarrhea, visual disturbances including yellow halos around lights, and, in rare instances, delirium have been described since Withering's time. Arrhythmias are the predominant cardiac manifestation of toxicity. Digitalis can cause any type of rhythm and/or conduction disturbance because it affects automaticity of myocardial tissues as well as the conduction system. Ventricular irritability (especially bigeminy), paroxysmal atrial tachycardia with block, and junctional tachycardia are particularly characteristic of digitalis excess.

The unexplained onset of an arrhythmia in a patient on digitalis raises the possibility of drug-related toxicity. The drug should be withheld, a serum level obtained, a stat potassium level checked, and serious consideration given to immediate hospitalization for monitoring and parenteral antiarrhythmic therapy. The high incidence and mortality rate of this preventable and often treatable condition call for vigilance.

A few pitfalls in the use of digitalis must be pointed out: (1) digitalis should not be used unless there is genuine evidence of heart failure or atrial fibrillation. A most common error is to assume that ankle edema in the elderly is related to CHF and to begin digitalis for this reason. Most of the time the ankle edema is due to venous insufficiency. (2) Unless failure has a reversible cause that has been corrected, digitalis should not be discontinued. Patients who respond to digitalis need the drug chronically; they have been shown to deteriorate clinically and hemodynamically when the drug is withdrawn in experimental circumstances. (3) The ST-T wave changes on the ECG have no correlation with optimal or toxic dose levels and cannot be used for such determinations.

Diuretics

Diuretics are indicated when there is excessive fluid retention. Most patients with failure begin to retain sodium as cardiac output falls and renal perfusion diminishes. Initially, the increase in volume helps to produce a rise in diastolic filling pressure and maintain cardiac output by the Frank–Starling mechanism. However, the degree of fluid retention is often excessive, resulting in pulmonary congestion and/or peripheral edema. Abnormalities in release of atrial natriuretic peptide, prostaglandin metabolism, and neurohumeral regulation are believed involved in the process of volume overload. Precise roles remain to be delineated.

Selection of Agent and Initiation of Therapy. Therapy of CHF can be initiated with a diuretic when digitalis is not the drug of choice. If treatment has begun with digitalis, but volume overload persists, a diuretic can be added to the program; however, overzealous use of diuretics may worsen the situation by producing prerenal azotemia or a dangerous fall in filling pressure (as in critical aortic stenosis). Moreover, escalating diuretic therapy in mitral or aortic valve disease may inappropriately delay the timing of surgical therapy (see Chapter 28).

Diuretic therapy can be initiated with a *thiazide* when the symptoms of failure are mild or when the patient is asymptomatic but showing weight gain or x-ray findings indicative of early CHF. The degree of dyspnea on exertion and weight changes are the simplest clinical parameters to follow for gauging response to therapy in mild cases. For patients with renal impairment and mild CHF, *metolazone* can be useful. It is similar in potency to the thiazides, but more effective in the setting of azotemia.

Patients with more severe CHF, manifested by dyspnea at rest, orthopnea, or paroxysmal nocturnal dyspnea represent the other end of the spectrum. If it is judged reasonable to attempt outpatient management of such patients, a *loop diuretic* (i.e., furosemide or ethacrynic acid) is necessary. Small doses of loop diuretics may also benefit patients with mild to moderate failure that cannot be adequately controlled by thiazides. Caution is warranted when treating a patient for the first time with a loop diuretic, because a marked diuresis may be evoked, even from a small dose. If a thiazide had been used previously, it should be stopped rather than continued in conjunction with the loop diuretic, because the two agents are very potent when used together. The combination of a thiazide and loop diuretic is indicated in cases of failure refractory to large doses of the loop diuretic alone. The maximal effect of a loop diuretic can be achieved by using a single daily dose.

In decompensated CHF, absorption of oral furosemide declines, which accounts for the oft-noted reduction in efficacy during an exacerbation of heart failure. Parenteral administration of the drug or high-dose oral therapy is required to achieve diuresis. At times, supplementing oral therapy with an occasional intravenous administration of a loop diuretic in the office will suffice to counter worsening failure refractory to oral therapy.

The *potassium-sparing diuretics* are weak agents used mainly in conjunction with other diuretics to avoid the need to prescribe potassium preparations and to augment diuresis. Their onset of action is slow; full effect may take up to a week to become evident. The *mercurials* have dropped from use because of the need to administer them parenterally. They are more potent than the thiazides and can sometimes be used intramuscularly on an intermittent basis, as, for example, by the visiting nurse, to supplement oral diuretic therapy.

Monitoring Therapy. Monitoring postural signs, BUN, and creatinine are essential to avoid excess volume depletion and severe prerenal azotemia. When a potassium-wasting diuretic is being used in conjunction with digitalis therapy, it is critical to carefully monitor the serum potassium. The incidence of digitalis toxicity rises appreciably in the setting of hypokalemia. Use of a potassium-sparing drug necessitates watching for hyperkalemia.

Diuretic Preparations. The thiazides are sulfonamide derivatives, believed to inhibit sodium reabsorption in the cortical tubule. Although the number of thiazide preparations is large, they differ only in cost and duration of action. *Hydrochlorothiazide* is the least expensive and is available generically. Thiazides cause modest potassium depletion, which usually is not clinically important (see Appendix), unless there is concurrent ventricular irritability, ischemia, or use of digitalis. Under such circumstances, careful monitoring for hypokalemia and assiduous potassium supplementation are essential. Sometimes a potassium-sparing diuretic may be used instead of a KCl supplement (see below). Hyperglycemia and hyperuricemia are commonly encountered when thiazides are used. They are usually of little clinical significance (see Chapter 21). During the first 7 to 10 days of therapy, the serum calcium may rise, but it will stay elevated indefinitely only in patients with underlying hyperparathyroidism. Absorption from the gastrointestinal tract is rapid; onset of action is 1 hour, and half-life 12 to 24 hours.

Another sulfonamide diuretic is *metolazone,* an agent similar to the thiazides in site of action, but possessing a longer half-life and more effective for treatment of mild CHF in patients with impaired renal function. Metolazone has an effective half-life of 24 to 48 hours compared to 12 to 24 hours for the thiazides. Being a sulfonamide, it shares many of the same side-effects, such as hypokalemia, hyperglycemia, and hyperuricemia. The maximum daily dose is 10 to 20 mg. Metolazone can be combined with a loop diuretic for use in very refractory cases in which volume overload is a major problem.

The potent diuretics that act at the loop of Henle are *furosemide* and *ethacrynic acid.* Their absorption is rapid, and onset of diuretic action occurs within 30 to 60 minutes,

lasting 6 to 8 hours. Caution must be exercised, since serious volume depletion may occur with their use. Prerenal azotemia (manifested by a BUN–creatinine ratio of more than 20:1), postural hypotension, lightheadedness, and fatigue are clues to marked hypovolemia. Hypokalemia, hyperglycemia, and hyperuricemia may occur. Ethacrynic acid is potentially ototoxic, especially when used in combination with an aminoglycoside antibiotic such as kanamycin. Audiograms should be obtained if ethacrynic acid is to be given for a prolonged period.

Frequent urination is a common complaint in patients using these potent diuretics; evening doses should be avoided if possible. Starting dose of furosemide is 20 to 40 mg per day. If this amount does not produce the desired effect, the single dose should be increased rather than the frequency of doses. In many instances, one daily dose is sufficient, maximally effective, and well tolerated by the patient. Potassium loss can be countered by prescribing potassium supplements or adding a potassium-sparing diuretic (see further discussion).

Spironolactone, triamterene, and *amiloride* are the commonly used potassium-sparing diuretics. The former is an antagonist of aldosterone, the latter two are not, but clinically behave in a manner similar to spironolactone. All are weak diuretics when used alone and should never be used initially in CHF. Their role is to help preserve potassium and supplement diuresis. Serious hyperkalemia may occur, necessitating frequent serum potassium determinations and discontinuation of potassium supplements. These drugs should not be used in renal failure, since life-threatening hyperkalemia may ensue. Spironolactone has been known to cause gynecomastia; there is also a question of increased risk of carcinogenesis based on experiments in which high doses were given to rats.

Fixed combinations containing a potassium-sparing diuretic and a thiazide are heavily promoted and expensive (see Chapter 21), though they are convenient and facilitate compliance. Prior to prescribing such a preparation, the proper dose of each agent should be determined separately. The combination preparation is reasonable to use only if it can provide the exact dosages desired. Many combinations contain subtherapeutic thiazide doses.

Vasodilators

Advances in understanding the effects of preload and afterload on cardiac output in the failing heart have lead to the development of vasodilator therapy for chronic CHF. As heart failure worsens, a number of neurohumoral systems respond to maintain circulatory stability. The sympathetic nervous system and the renin-angiotension system are activated. The result is arterial and venous vasoconstriction. The arterial vasoconstriction raises systemic vascular resistance and blood pressure, increasing afterload and the work of the left ventricle. Under these circumstances, cardiac output drops in the failing heart. Venoconstriction increases venous return; normally the heart responds via the Frank–Starling mechanism to increase cardiac output, but not in the setting of heart failure. The result is increased pulmonary and systemic hypertension and no improvement in cardiac output. The progressive decrease in cardiac output and rise in venous pressure trigger further neurohumoral activity and a vicious cycle is established.

The goal of vasodilator therapy is to improve the preload and afterload environment of the failing heart. Agents that act on the arterial bed lower systemic resistance and reduce impedance to the ejection of blood from the left ventricle, thus augmenting cardiac output. Vasodilators that act on the venous bed decrease preload and reduce pulmonary and systemic venous congestion. Dyspnea and exercise tolerance improve. A multicenter Veterans Administration (VA) study found that vasodilator therapy significantly improved both survival and left ventricular function.

Selection of Agent. Most vasodilators have been found to improve circulatory dynamics when used acutely, but acute response does not predict efficacy of chronic therapy. Several double-blind, placebo-controlled trials ranging in duration from 2 to 6 months have now been completed to determine the efficacy of the most commonly prescribed vasodilators for chronic oral use in the outpatient setting. Patients were monitored for several months by serial clinical evaluations and exercise stress testing. Both *captopril* and *isosorbide dinitrate* have demonstrated significant and sustained improvements in cardiac function and exercise tolerance. Neither *prazosin* nor *hydralazine* proved significantly better than placebo; tolerance to their vasodilator effects has been reported with chronic use. The calcium channel blocker *nifedipine* has also been studied, but its effectiveness has not been established. Calcium channel blockers can depress left ventricular function (see Chapter 25) and their safety for long-term use in CHF is unknown. *Minoxidil,* a potent arterial vasodilator, was found in one controlled study to worsen heart failure and increase the death rate compared to placebo.

Isosorbide has proven especially useful in patients with CHF caused by ischemic heart disease. Isosorbide acts predominantly on capacitance vessels to reduce preload, though at the high doses required for use in CHF (up to 80 mg tid–qid), it also causes some arterial dilatation and modest decreases in systemic resistance. CHF patients with marked pulmonary and systemic venous congestion might benefit from use of isosorbide.

The *angiotensin converting enzyme (ACE) inhibitors* (captopril, enalapril) are very active on both the arterial and venous sides of the circulation, decreasing left ventricular filling pressure and increasing cardiac output. They not only block production of angiotensin II but also reduce peripheral sympathetic tone, inhibit bradykinin degradation, and stim-

ulate prostaglandin synthesis. The effect of ACE inhibitors on survival of patients with chronic CHF is the subject of ongoing investigation. Captopril in combination with furosemide has also been shown to decrease the hyponatremia that often complicates severe CHF. Adverse effects reported include hypotension, loss of taste, rashes (including necrotizing vasculitis), and neutropenia. Worsening renal function occurs in up to 25% of patients with underlying azotemia; there is little effect on kidney function in those with no preexisting renal impairment. Nevertheless, the BUN, creatinine, and urinalysis (for proteinuria) should be monitored. Since hypotension is common at the onset of therapy, it is recommended to start with small doses (*e.g.,* as little as 6.25 mg of captopril). The dose is then increased gradually (up to as much as 100 mg of captopril tid–qid).

Selection of the appropriate vasodilator for a given patient is still somewhat empirical, but consideration of the patient's pathophysiology and the vasodilator's predominant site of action can help guide drug selection. CHF patients with marked pulmonary congestion and peripheral edema might be candidates for isosorbide, whereas those with arterial hypertension or evidence of arterial vasoconstriction might obtain an increase in cardiac output by starting with captopril. Such crude guidelines may be helpful for selection of initial vasodilator therapy, but empiric observance of response to therapy remains the criterion for continuation of an agent or search for a new one. Combination therapy using isosorbide and hydralazine was effective in the VA study cited above.

Initiating Therapy. At present, it is recommended that vasodilator therapy be started only after the patient has failed to achieve an adequate response from diuretics and digitalis. It is important to inquire into exercise tolerance. Patients may note improvement at rest with use of digitalis and diuretics, but if exercise tolerance remains limited, then a trial of vasodilator therapy deserves consideration. Treatment need not be delayed until the end stages of CHF; both captopril and isosorbide have proven quite safe and well tolerated when used with care in CHF. Whether vasodilator therapy will be considered appropriate for initial therapy of CHF remains to be determined. The literature should be followed closely for new developments in this exciting and fast moving area.

New Agents and New Uses of Older Agents. Despite the development of vasodilator therapy, the search continues for agents that will improve contractility better and more safely than digitalis. The investigational bipyridine inotropic agent *milrinone* has shown promise for chronic oral use in severe CHF, producing sustained improvement in cardiac function and exercise tolerance without the worrisome side-effects noted with a related bipyridine, *amrinone.* (Although marketed for acute parenteral administration, amrinone has been withdrawn from trials for long-term outpatient use because of a 15% incidence of dose-related thrombocytopenia and fever, and marked gastrointestinal intolerance.) Milrinone has also been found to have some vasodilator effects. New uses for older vasodilators continue to be explored. Vasodilators that have proven ineffective as single agents for long-term therapy (*e.g.,* hydralazine, prazosin) may still have promise in vasodilator programs that utilize a combination of agents. For example, in the VA study noted earlier, the combination of isosorbide plus hydralazine proved efficacious; prazosin alone was not.

Anticoagulation Therapy

Although the presence of CHF is not *per se* an indication for warfarin anticoagulant therapy, it does increase the risk of thromboembolic disease in a patient with an underlying predisposition for an embolic event. For example, the CHF patient with venous disease who is put to bed for prolonged rest is at increased risk and deserves consideration for anticoagulation therapy. The same holds true for the patient in atrial fibrillation who develops CHF (see Chapter 23).

Concurrent Drug Use and Nonpharmacologic Measures

Use of medications that might depress left ventricular function or alter neurohumoral regulatory mechanisms should be undertaken with extreme care and only after the potential risk is weighed. For example, *beta blocking agents, disopyramide,* and such calcium channel blockers as *verapamil* are myocardial suppressants; they are relatively contraindicated for use in CHF. In a study of the role of prostaglandins in CHF, it was discovered that use of prostaglandin inhibitors, such as the *nonsteroidal anti-inflammatory agent* indomethacin, caused a worsening of CHF in patients with advanced disease complicated by hyponatremia; patients without hyponatremia were unaffected.

Fortunately, some important medications are not contraindicated in CHF. For example, the *tricyclic antidepressants* do not cause a reduction in left ventricular performance; they are relatively well tolerated, though they occasionally cause postural hypotension in CHF patients. A study of the effects of *acute intake of alcohol* on patients with functional class III or IV CHF found no deleterious effect on cardiac function; in fact, a modest reduction in afterload was noted, though the authors hastened to add that they were not recommending alcohol as a vasodilator.

Salt Restriction has traditionally occupied an important place in supportive therapy. It is probably most helpful in preventing unnecessary exacerbations of failure. Patients are placed on a no-added-salt diet, which provides about 4 g of sodium per day. The patient and family are instructed to prepare and serve meals without addition of salt and to avoid foods with large salt content, including canned ham (which is packed in salt water), bacon, catsup, and so on. Rarely is extreme salt restriction (*e.g.,* 1 to 2 g sodium diet) urged on the patient, since it is often unrealistic and unpalatable, leading to poor caloric intake and depression. Fluid restriction is reserved for severe cases that are complicated by hyponatremia.

The Activity Prescription has an important function in minimizing myocardial work demands while maintaining the patient's ability to live as fully as possible. The level of allowable activity needs to be tailored to the patient's medical status, life-style and responsibilities. Patients with symptoms of failure on moderate exertion (New York Heart Association class II disease) can continue to work as long as reasonable limits are placed on emotional and physical demands. It may be more stressful psychologically (and consequently physically) to have to quit one's job than to continue working in a somewhat more limited capacity. In most instances, the amount of allowable activity can be determined from an office visit by a careful history that elicits the degree of exertion that precipitates symptoms. At times, symptoms may be out of proportion to physical findings; taking a walk up a flight of stairs with the patient can provide helpful data regarding exercise tolerance. Treadmill testing is sometimes necessary to gauge exercise capacity, especially if the patient has coronary disease and it is unclear whether it is failure or ischemia that is limiting the patient. Regardless of etiology, a daily rest period and reduction of psychological stress are key means of lessening myocardial work in the patient with failure.

If weight is increasing, orthopnea worsening, and dyspnea on exertion more severe and brought on by less exertion, activity should be further restricted. A few days of bed rest are often beneficial and may obviate the need for hospitalization. The patient with failure who is put to bed should use a footboard or get out of bed periodically to avoid prolonged venous stasis and thrombus formation.

PATIENT EDUCATION

Because the medical program is often complex and the need for compliance is great, the physician must take the time to discuss with patient and family the rationale behind therapy and to set with them the guidelines for activity, diet, and use of medication. In this way they can become valuable partners in the treatment effort.

Patients should be instructed to weigh themselves each morning before breakfast and to keep a *weight record.* If their clinical status, weight, and medication program are stable, less frequent recordings are necessary. Patients are advised to call their physician when weight increases suddenly by more than 2 or 3 pounds, because this may be the earliest sign of increasing CHF and a forerunner of more severe symptoms. Reliable, intelligent patients may be instructed to adjust their diuretic doses according to weight. Debilitated or uncooperative individuals should have a family member of visiting nurse obtain weight recordings. Weight is among the most helpful parameters to follow in outpatient management of failure.

Patients and their families must know the identity of the medication being used. It is easy for the patient to become confused because multiple-drug regimens are common and many of the pills are similar in appearance. Medication booklets are invaluable. Each tablet is taped to the page alongside its generic and brand names, dose schedule, indication for use and warning signs of toxicity. For patients with poor eyesight, a family member or visiting nurse should put out and set aside the pills to be taken each day.

INDICATIONS FOR REFERRAL AND ADMISSION

Patients with refractory failure should be considered for hospital admission, because valuable observations can be made under controlled conditions that assure compliance with the medical regimen. Moreover, it may provide, an opportunity to search for a treatable underlying etiology that may not have been appreciated initially. If the patient is still refractory to therapy while in the hospital, it may be helpful to obtain a cardiac consultation regarding the use of oral vasodilator therapy. Starting such therapy in the hospital is the safest way to initiate a vasodilator program and allows close monitoring of response. Other indications for admission include worsening failure, evidence of digitalis toxicity, and inadequate support and supervision at home.

THERAPEUTIC RECOMMENDATIONS

- Identify the etiology of the CHF and any precipitating factors (*e.g.,* fever, anemia, atrial fibrillation, infection, salt excess); treat these specifically if they are amenable to therapy, rather than relying solely on symptomatic measures to ameliorate the CHF.
- Initiate a no-added-salt diet, but do not restrict water intake unless dilutional hyponatremia ensues.
- Begin diuretic therapy with a thiazide diuretic (*e.g.,* hydrochlorothiazide 50 mg bid) if the CHF is mild and there is evidence of volume overload or pulmonary venous congestion.
- Switch to or begin a "loop" diuretic (*e.g.,* furosemide 20–40 mg bid) if failure is moderately severe. Be careful of marked response to a loop diuretic in a patient who has never been treated with the agent before. Exert particular caution with use of potent diuretics in situations that require a high filling pressure (*e.g.,* tight aortic stenosis).
- In initial stages of loop diuretic use, divide daily dose to minimize the inconvenience of a large diuresis in the morning or evening that might interfere with activity. Avoid giving an evening dose if sleep is being interrupted by need to urinate frequently.
- If patient does not respond adequately to a loop diuretic that is being given in divided aliquots, try giving the entire daily dose at one time before escalating dose; an occasional intravenous dose of a loop diuretic in the office may also help in times of increased fluid retention. Addition of a thiazide or metolazone to loop diuretic therapy will often induce further diuresis in refractory patients; metolazone may be of particular help in the azotemic patient.
- In all forms of diuretic therapy monitor postural signs, serum potassium concentration, BUN, and creatinine. Cease any further increases in diuretic dose and consider a reduction if postural hypotension or severe prerenal azotemia develops.
- If after a full trial of diuretic therapy, the patient is not adequately improved, begin digitalis in those patients who manifest an S_3, which is indicative of a low ejection fraction, left ventricular dilatation, and elevated left atrial pressure.
- Begin digitalis before or in conjunction with diuretic therapy if the cause of the CHF is rapid atrial fibrillation, uncontrolled and severe hypertension, or tight aortic stenosis.
- Digitalis is contraindicated in hypertrophic cardiomyopathies and unstable or second-degree heart block. Digitalis is of no benefit to patients with mitral stenosis who remain in sinus rhythm or those with transient ischemia producing recurrent bouts of CHF.
- When CHF is mild, one can begin digitalis therapy with 0.25 mg per day of digoxin given orally; check serum level in 1 week and make any further dose adjustment on the basis of clinical response, serum level, BUN, and creatinine.
- If CHF is marked, but the patient does not require immediate hospitalization, one can start digitalis therapy with a loading dose of 1 to 1.25 mg of digoxin orally, given in divided doses over the first 24 hours. Then adjust dose as noted above.
- Monitor patients on digitalis by following the heart rate, rhythm, BUN, creatinine, potassium, and serum drug concentration. Patients on digoxin who experience a marked increase in BUN and creatinine should have a digoxin level checked and the drug held or dose reduced until a serum level is available to guide further administration. One can estimate the required dose from available nomograms or use the serum level as a guide. Serum digoxin level should be drawn at least 6 hours after the last dose, because there is a transient increase in serum level after an oral dose.
- Hypokalemia should be avoided, because it enhances sensitivity to toxic effects of digitalis, especially dysrhythmias. Admit to the hospital if paroxysmal atrial tachycardia with block, ventricular irritability, junctional tachycardia, or symptomatic bradyarrhythmias develop.
- Prevent potassium depletion with a dietary potassium supplementation (usually sufficient in thiazide therapy), an oral potassium preparation (often necessary when loop diuretics are used), or a potassium-sparing diuretic. If a potassium-sparing diuretic is prescribed, halt all other forms of potassium supplementation and continue to monitor the serum potassium.

- If an oral potassium preparation is employed, begin with an agent that provides chloride as well as potassium in order to avoid diuretic-induced hypokalemic alkalosis; however, if possible avoid KCl tablets, because of their risk of injury to the gastrointestinal mucosa (see Appendix).
- In patients refractory to digitalis and diuretics, consider vasodilator therapy especially if exercise tolerance remains poor. For patients whose pathophysiology is predominantly pulmonary and systemic venous hypertension, begin isosorbide dinitrate (10 mg qid) and increase dose as tolerated to a maximum of 80 mg qid. *Add* hydralazine 25 mg qid if additional vasodilator effect is needed, especially if there is an element of peripheral arterial hypertension.
- Alternatively, for patients with a mix of venous hypertension and arterial vasoconstriction, begin captopril (25 mg bid). Some patients experience marked hypotension with the first dose; a first dose of 6.25 mg is suggested in frail patients. Increase dose as tolerated to a maximum of 100 mg tid–qid. Monitor blood pressure, BUN, creatinine, and white blood cell count while on captopril therapy.
- Consider anticoagulant therapy for CHF patients if prolonged bed rest, atrial fibrillation, or congestive cardiomyopathy ensue.
- Avoid use of agents with negative inotropic effects; for example, most beta-blocking agents, disopyramide, and such calcium channel blockers as verapamil. Their use may worsen CHF.
- Provide patient and family with thorough instruction on purpose and proper use of medications prescribed for CHF. Advise patient to check his weight regularly, measuring it before breakfast and calling if there is an unexplained weight gain of more than 2–3 pounds over a week.
- Advise bed rest for exacerbations of CHF, but discourage major reorganizations of a patient's life-style unless symptoms are severe.
- Admit patients with refractory CHF, arrhythmias suggestive of digitalis toxicity, or inadequate support and supervision at home.
- Consider cardiac consultation if embarking on vasodilator therapy.

Appendix: Potassium Supplementation

Although there is considerable disagreement about the need for potassium supplementation in otherwise healthy patients receiving diuretics for hypertension, there is strong consensus regarding the importance of maintaining normokalemia in patients on digitalis. Diuretic-induced potassium depletion is particularly common in CHF due to the use of potent potassium-wasting agents. Hypokalemia exacerbates the risk of dysrhythmias due to ischemia and digitalis toxicity. Individual requirements for potassium replacement vary widely, necessitating regular monitoring of the serum potassium level, which is not an exact measure of total body potassium, but rather a rough guide to potassium requirements.

Supplements may be taken in the form of dietary additions or potassium-containing preparations. Amount needed is usually determined empirically, ranging from 0 to 60 mEq of supplement per day over and above normal dietary potassium intake. For patients on thiazides, dietary replacement often suffices. When furosemide or ethacrynic acid is used, a potassium preparation is usually a must (unless a potassium-sparing diuretic is used). *Dietary supplements* are the most palatable way to provide potassium. There are 15 mEq in a 10-oz glass of orange, pineapple, or grapefruit juice, a medium-sized banana, a baked potato, or two oranges. Tomato juice has almost twice the potassium content of orange juice but is high in sodium.

Salt substitutes contain KCl, but some are also 50% sodium chloride. Even those that are pure KCl do not provide adequate potassium.

Patients unable to sustain normokalemia by dietary means require a potassium supplement. There is plethora of potassium supplement preparations on the market. Oral potassium supplements combine potassium with any of a number of different anions. Only the chloride form is effective in correcting the hypokalemic alkalosis that results from diuretic use. However, any form will prevent potassium depletion unless sodium depletion is very severe. *Potassium chloride elixir* remains the safest and least expensive. It contains 20 mEq per 15 cc (one tablespoon). It is most easily taken in orange juice; unfortunately, about 50% of patients find it unpalatable, even when mixed in fruit juice. However, when faced with the cost of alternatives, many patients who complain of its taste are still quite willing to continue using it. Its safety, chloride content, and ability to deliver more milliequivalents of potassium per dose than most other preparations strongly recommend it.

Many types of potassium chloride tablets have been produced. The earliest preparations were found to lead to a high incidence of gastrointestinal ulceration, bleeding, obstruction, and perforation due to exposure of the intestinal mucosa to high local concentrations of potassium. To overcome this difficulty, a second generation of potassium chloride tablets were devised (Slow-K, Kaon-Cl, Klotrix, K-Tab) encoating the tablets in a *wax matrix,* which *slowed release* and reduced the frequency of GI complications, but did not eliminate the risk. Unfortunately, the complications continue to occur unpredictably with these agents. More recently, a *microencapsulated preparation* (Micro-K) has been promoted, containing KCl in the form of small crystals, each coated with a polymer permeable to water, theoretically helping to disperse the potassium and minimize locally high concentrations. Some uncontrolled endoscopic observations support this claim, but experience is still limited and this form of medication is very expensive, costing the patient almost ten times more than liquid potassium for an equivalent dose. Moreover, since each tablet contains only 8 mEq of potassium, multiple tablets are needed each day to provide the 15–45 mEq of potassium usually required.

Potassium gluconate and *bicarbonate* preparations are available. Some are in the form of liquids, others are effervescent tablets. Although they tend to be more palatable, their disadvantages include high cost (up to 50 cents per dose) and the absence of chloride to counter the alkalosis induced by diuretic use.

If all attempts at potassium supplementation fail, then a potassium-sparing diuretic is indicated. These agents are expensive and not without risk (*e.g.,* hyperkalemia). Therefore, they should not be used until other methods of potassium management have been tried.

A.H.G.

ANNOTATED BIBLIOGRAPHY

Arnold SB, Byrd RC, Meister W et al: Long-term digitalis therapy improves left ventricular function in heart failure. N Engl J Med 303:1443, 1980 (*An unblinded study of nine patients with documented CHF on chronic digitalis therapy; withdrawal of digitalis resulted in objective worsening of left ventricular function, which was restored after digitalis was resumed.*)

Braunwald E, Colucci WS: Vasodilator therapy of heart failure. N Engl J Med 310:459, 1984 (*An editorial that takes a very positive view of the role of vasodilators in treatment of CHF and briefly reviews approved and investigational agents.*)

Cohn JN: Unloading the heart in congestive heart failure. Am J Med 76(August 20, 1984):67, 1984 (*A terse review of the effects of preload and afterload reduction in patients with CHF; 26 references.*)

Cohn JN, Archibald DG, Ziesche S et al: Effect of vasodilator therapy on mortality in chronic congestive heart failure. N Engl J Med 314:1547, 1986 (*The multi-center VA study: combination of hydralazine and isosorbide improved both left ventricular function and survival.*)

Cohn JN, Levine B, Olivari MT et al: Plasma norepinephrine as a guide to prognosis in patients with chronic congestive heart failure. N Engl J Med 311:819, 1984 (*A single resting venous blood sample for plasma norepinephrine provided a better guide to prognosis than other commonly measured indices of cardiac performance.*)

Colucci WS, Wright RF, Braunwald E: New positive inotropic agents in the treatment of congestive heart failure. N Engl J Med 314:349, 1986 (*An authoritative review; includes discussion of amrinone and milrinone.*)

Dall JLC: Maintenance digoxin in elderly patients. Br Med J 2:705, 1970 (*When Digoxin was stopped in 80 elderly patients on chronic therapy, only one quarter showed signs of increasing failure. Most who had no change had little indication for being on the drug in the first place.*)

Dzau VJ, Hollenberg NK: Renal response to captopril in several heart failure: Role of furosemide in natriuresis and reversal of hyponatremia. Ann Intern Med 100:777, 1984 (*Captopril plus furosemide promoted correction of hyponatremia in patients with severe CHF; captopril enhances the effectiveness of furosemide.*)

Dzau VJ, Packer M, Lilly LS et al: Prostaglandins in severe congestive heart failure. N Engl J Med 310:347, 1984 (*Provides evidence for operation of both vasoconstrictor and vasodilator mechanisms in severe CHF complicated by hyponatremia; use of prostaglandin inhibitors may worsen CHF by interfering with prostaglandin-driven vasodilation.*)

Dzau VJ, Colucci WS, Williams GH et al: Sustained effectiveness of converting enzyme inhibition in patients with severe congestive heart failure. N Engl J Med 302:1373, 1980 (*Captopril therapy induced sustained improvements in clinical status and renal function among NYHA Functional Class IV patients.*)

Fleg JL, Gottlieb SH, Lakatta EG: Is digoxin really important in treatment of compensated heart failure? Am J Med 73:244, 1982 (*No deterioration noted upon withdrawal and 3 months of placebo therapy.*)

Francis GS: Sodium and water excretion in heart failure. Ann Intern Med 105:272, 1986 (*An editorial summarizing the significance of atrial natiuretic peptide and other factors influencing sodium and volume status in heart failure.*)

Glassman AH, Johnson LL, Giardina EV et al: The use of imipramine in depressed patients with congestive heart failure. JAMA, 250:1997, 1983 (*Imipramine did not cause a reduction in left ventricular performance in patients with pre-existing heart disease, but orthostatic hypertension was a frequent complication.*)

Green LH, Smith TW: Use of digitalis in patients with pulmonary disease. Ann Intern Med 87:459, 1977 (*A literature review that concludes that the efficacy of digitalis in corpulmonale is in question; there may be an associated increase in risk of digitalis toxicity.*)

Greenberg BH, Schutz R, Grunkemeirer GL et al: Acute effects of alcohol in patients with congestive heart failure. Ann Intern Med 97:171, 1982 (*Acute intake of a modest dose of alcohol caused mild vasodilation and no adverse effect on left ventricular function.*)

Lee DC, Johnson RA, Bingham JB et al: Heart failure in outpatients: A randomized trial of digoxin versus placebo. N Engl J Med 306:699, 1982 (*Only CHF patients with an S_3 that persists after diuretic therapy show benefit from long-term digoxin therapy.*)

Levine TB: Role of vasodilators in the treatment of congestive heart failure. Am J Cardiol 55:32A, 1985 (*An excellent review of available data on efficacy of vasodilators in CHF; 46 references.*)

McKee PA et al: Natural history of congestive heart failure: The Framingham study. N Engl J Med 285:1444, 1971 (*A community-based study of the epidemiology of CHF. Over two thirds of patients with CHF had hypertension alone or in combination with coronary artery disease.*)

Micro-K potassium supplement. The Medical Letter 24:71, 1982 (*This microencapsulated KCl preparation may be safer than previously available slow-release preparations, but controlled studies are lacking.*)

Muller JE, Turi PH, Rude RE et al: Digoxin therapy and mortality after myocardial infarction. N Engl J Med 314:265, 1986 (*No evidence of significant excess mortality was associated with digoxin use, when results were controlled for characteristics predictive of poor prognosis.*)

Mulrow CD, Feussner JR, Velex R: Reevaluation of digitalis efficacy. Ann Intern Med 101:113, 1984 (*A critical review of evidence on value of digitalis in CHF; rigorous analysis of available studies; 44 references.*)

Slow-release potassium. Medical Letter, 20:29, 1978 (*Reviews use of slow-release potassium tablets and concludes that small bowel ulceration continues to be reported in patients using these preparations.*)

Smith TW: Digitalis toxicity: Epidemiology and clinical use of serum concentration measurements. Am J Med 58:470, 1975 (*A review of the appropriate use of serum digitalis levels, arguing for cautious interpretation and use of results, since there is overlap between normals and those with evidence of toxicity.*)

Vasko MR, Brown-Cartwright D, Knochel JP et al: Furosemide absorption altered in decompensated congestive heart failure. Ann Intern Med 102:314, 1985 (*Absorption is reduced in severe CHF, accounting for the reduced efficacy of oral therapy.*)

Wilson JR, Reichek N, Dunkman WB et al: Effects of diuresis on the performance of the failing left ventricle in man. Am J Med 70:234, 1981 (*Diuresis improved ventricular function by reducing afterload; indicates that diuretics may help the failing heart by doing more than just reducing preload.*)

28

Management of Acquired Valvular Heart Disease

RICHARD R. LIBERTHSON, M.D.

As a result of increased physician awareness and improvements in noninvasive diagnostic techniques, the diagnosis of acquired valvular heart disease is being made earlier in the course of illness. Outpatient management has become commonplace because symptoms are frequently absent or mild at the time the condition is discovered. Although consultation with a cardiologist is often obtained, the responsibility for long-term care usually falls on the primary physician.

In order to properly manage the patient with valvular heart disease, the primary physician must be familiar with the condition's natural history, early warning signs of hemodynamic deterioration, and indications for and types of medical and surgical therapies. Of major importance is the proper timing of surgery.

NATURAL HISTORY

Mitral Stenosis

Most cases of mitral stenosis (MS) are rheumatic in origin, even though as many as 50% of patients cannot give a history of rheumatic fever. The symptom-free interval averages about 10 years (range is 3 to 25 years). In most instances, symptoms develop gradually over a decade, roughly paralleling the progression of stenosis; however, some people remain relatively free of complaints until stenosis becomes severe. Left atrial and pulmonary venous pressures increase substantially as valve area falls below 1.5 cm^2 and at this point, patients typically experience dyspnea on exertion. Any stimulus that rapidly increases blood flow or decreases the time available for diastolic filling can precipitate a sudden increase in pulmonary congestion and result in acute shortness of breath. Strenuous activity, fever, emotion, and onset of atrial fibrillation are often responsible for acute dyspnea.

Progressive narrowing of the valve orifice is accompanied by worsening exercise tolerance and increasing dyspnea. In patients with tight stenosis (valve area less than 1.0 cm^2) the period from onset of symptoms to incapacity averages 7 years, but the decline can be precipitous with the onset of atrial fibrillation or pneumonia. Persistence of chronic pulmonary hypertension, in which pulmonary vascular resistance rises out of proportion to the increase in wedge pressure. Cardiac output usually falls with onset of pulmonary hypertension, and fatigue may become a prominent symptom. The right ventricle hypertrophies in response to the rise in pulmonary artery pressure, and right heart failure and death ensue unless intervention occurs; deterioration may be rapid at this stage.

Atrial fibrillation complicates 40% to 50% of cases of symptomatic mitral stenosis. The correlation between development of atrial fibrillation and the severity of stenosis is slight and not due solely to the degree of left atrial enlargement. The loss of atrial systole and the increase in heart rate that characterize atrial fibrillation markedly reduce flow across the mitral valve and boost left atrial pressure. Premature atrial contractions and paroxysmal atrial fibrillation often precede sustained atrial fibrillation due to mitral stenosis.

Systemic embolization occurs in 10% to 20% of patients with MS. Age and presence of atrial fibrillation are the major determinants of risk; severity of stenosis is not a determinant, and, in fact, embolization may be a presenting symptom of MS.

In sum, there is typically a symptom-free period of about 10 years. Patients then begin to note dyspnea on exertion over the next 10 years, which progresses in many instances in the following decade. Once symptoms are present on minimal exertion, survival becomes markedly reduced. Patients with New York Heart Association class IV disease (symptoms at rest) have been found to have a 5-year mortality rate of 85%. Some patients have disease that does not progress and may remain stable indefinitely. In another subset of patients, symptoms do not develop until late in the illness.

Mitral Regurgitation

Patients with rheumatic mitral regurgitation (MR) can remain asymptomatic for many years, because the left ventricle dilates and adjusts well to the increase in volume load.

Onset of dyspnea and fatigue may not occur for decades. Symptoms take an average of 10 years to progress to the point of disability and need for surgery. It is not until very late in the course of the disease that myocardial reserve falters. Once the left ventricle fails, patients note progressive dyspnea and fatigue; symptoms become present at rest (functional class IV disease). If pulmonary hypertension develops, signs of right heart failure will ensue. Prognosis is poor at this stage.

Atrial fibrillation is found in upwards of 75% of cases, but the abrupt episodes of pulmonary congestion that typify mitral stenosis complicated by atrial fibrillation are less frequent in MR, although rupture of one of the chordae tendineae can result in sudden deterioration.

Nonrheumatic forms of chronic MR are commonly encountered in the outpatient setting. Etiologies include mitral valve prolapse, papillary muscle dysfunction, and calcified mitral valve annulus.

Mitral valve prolapse (MVP) usually does not produce hemodynamically significant regurgitation. Overall, prognosis is usually excellent. Palpitations and atypical chest pain are the most frequent symptoms; most are entirely asymptomatic. The amount of regurgitant flow has not been found to increase with time, and the need for mitral valve replacement is rare. There is a slight increase in risk of bacterial endocarditis; however, the cost–benefit prophylaxis is unresolved (see Chapter 11). The American Heart Association suggests prophylaxis for those with MVP who have evidence of mitral insufficiency. In the overwhelming majority of patients, mitral valve prolapse is of no clinical significance. A very small subset have ventricular irritability: rare patients have suffered ventricular fibrillation.

Papillary muscle dysfunction is responsible for as much as 10% of MR cases found clinically. Causes include ischemic injury, left ventricular dilatation, and cardiomyopathy. Ischemic heart disease is the most frequent etiology, with 40% of posterior infarcts and 20% of anterior infarcts accompanied by the development of papillary muscle dysfunction. The amount of regurgitant flow is highly variable. Severe MR and marked pulmonary congestion can occur, even in the context of only a minimal reduction in left ventricular ejection fraction. However, prognosis does depend on left ventricular systolic performance.

Calcification of the mitral annulus occurs in older people, often in conjunction with calcification of the aortic valve. The mitral lesion is usually not of hemodynamic significance, but heart block can develop if calcification extends into the ventricular septum.

Mixed Mitral Disease. Mortality is increased when significant stenosis and regurgitation occur simultaneously. In one large series of patients managed medically, the 10-year survival rate from the time of diagnosis was 33%.

Aortic Stenosis

Because of the marked ability of the left ventricle to hypertrophy and compensate for the pressure load, patients with aortic stenosis (AS) can remain symptom-free for many years, even with tight stenosis (valve area less than 0.7 cm^2). This is especially true in young patients; however, it must be remembered that sudden death can occur in asymptomatic individuals with critical AS. Onset of angina and effort syncope suggest a hemodynamically critical lesion that is limiting cardiac output, although in as many as 30% to 60% of AS patients with angina, there coexists significant occlusion of a coronary vessel. Survival averages about 3 years from the onset of angina or effort syncope. The development of congestive failure is an ominous sign, for it signals the inability of the myocardium to continue tolerating the enormous pressure load; survival averages about 2 years from the time failure is first noted. Over half of patients with AS die of congestive failure. Sudden death accounts for another 20%. The mean age of patients dying suddenly is 60; the mechanism of death in these cases is believed to be a dysrhythmia triggered by myocardial ischemia. The rate of stenosis is unpredictable and can progress rapidly over a few years, especially as the patient enters his 60s. Figures for survival are only averages; the range is wide, and many patients die soon after the onset of symptoms.

Age at clinical onset of AS is dependent in part on the underlying etiology. Significant AS appearing in a patient under the age of 30 is congenital in origin, due most often to a *bicuspid* valve. In approximately 15% of patients presenting for catheterization under the age of 30, obstruction is caused by a discrete subaortic membrane. Patients presenting between ages 30 and 70 have either a bicuspid valve or a valve damaged by *rheumatic fever.* Those who present with significant AS due to rheumatic fever are about 10 to 15 years older than patients who present with rheumatic mitral stenosis, due to the more gradual progression of the illness when it involves the aortic valve. Nevertheless, the course can be one of rapid deterioration. Many patients over 60 develop a systolic ejection murmur attributed to flow across thickened aortic valve leaflets; by age 80, half of the population has such a murmur. In a small percentage of *elderly patients,* hemodynamically significant stenosis develops due to heavy calcification of a tricuspid aortic valve.

Aortic Regurgitation

Rheumatic fever accounts for the largest number of cases of aortic regurgitation (AR). Most patients can live for decades with little incapacity, as the left ventricle dilates to accommodate the extra volume load. The latent period from occurrence of rheumatic fever to onset of clinical manifestations is about 10 years. During the following decade, symptoms appear and progress. The onset of symptoms is typically gradual, with palpitations being among the earliest changes noted by the patient, followed by dyspnea on exertion and fatigability. Appearance of LVH with strain and progressive cardiac dilatation are associated with a markedly increased risk of heart failure and death within 5 years. If exertional dyspnea worsens, other manifestations of congestive failure are likely to follow and signal the beginning of a rapidly declining phase of the disease due to left ventricular decompensation. At this stage, deterioration is rapid, with death occurring within 1 to 2 years of the onset of congestive failure. Angina is common, reported by almost 30% of patients; unlike the angina of aortic stenosis, it typically takes place at rest rather than upon exertion. Angina becomes more frequent when there is worsening heart failure. Sudden death may also occur in patients with severe aortic regurgitation.

Nonrheumatic causes of chronic AR include syphilis, myxomatous degeneration, and connective tissue disease. Aortic regurgitation secondary to untreated *syphilis* appears about 15 to 25 years after the initial infection and often has a more rapidly downhill course than AR due to rheumatic fever. *Myxomatous degeneration* has been found in 10% to 15% of cases of AR studied pathologically. The process is progressive and become clinically evident between the ages of 30 and 60. *Ankylosing spondylitis* is complicated by AR in about 3% of cases. The severity of the lesion is highly variable, and conduction defects are frequent. AR may appear before the onset of other symptoms, but in most instances it follows the appearance of arthritic symptoms by 10 to 20 years. The presence of severe AR shortens the otherwise normal life expectancy of patients with anklyosing spondylitis. *Reiter's syndrome* is associated with the development of AR in 5% of cases, typically in those with florid manifestations of the disease such as iritis, mucocutaneous changes, and extensive sacroiliac inflammation. Onset of AR occurs on an average of 15 years after the disease is first noted, often preceded by conduction disturbances. The severity and course of the AR are highly variable.

Mixed Aortic Valve Disease. Many patients with AS have some degree of AR, and vice versa. Whenever the gradient across the aortic valve is greater than 25 mm Hg in the context of significant regurgitation, there begins to develop a substantial pressure load as well as an increased volume load on the left ventricle. The clinical course is similar to that for isolated aortic stenosis of the same degree, although some clinicians believe there is an earlier onset of symptoms.

Combined Aortic and Mitral Disease. The etiology is mostly rheumatic; in fact, most cases of rheumatic fever produce some degree of multiple valve damage, though disease of one valve often dominates the clinical picture. The most common combination is aortic regurgitation in conjunction with mitral disease. Atrial fibrillation and systemic embolization are more frequent than in isolated AR, as is the severity of pulmonary symptoms. Less common is the coexistence of AS and MS. Symptoms and signs of AS are blunted by significant MS, such that pulmonary symptoms, atrial fibrillation, and systemic embolization may dominate the presentation, but there may be more angina and syncope than expected from isolated MS. Course is dictated by the severity of the individual lesions, but MS can delay the appearance of some of the manifestations of advanced AS.

ESTIMATING SEVERITY OF DISEASE

Mitral Stenosis

Symptoms provide crude indications of the severity of stenosis. Dyspnea correlates with increase in left atrial pressure and development of pulmonary venous congestion, but the relationship between degree of stenosis and elevation of left atrial pressure is variable. Fatigue occurs most often in the context of pulmonary hypertension, but the nonspecific nature of the symptom lessens its utility in estimating severity. Hemoptysis is related to pulmonary venous hypertension, but does not necessarily imply severe stenosis. Thus, history alone may fail to detect severe stenosis that is unaccompanied by marked pulmonary congestion; however, a worsening of dyspnea and a decline in exercise tolerance suggest hemodynamic deterioration and require further investigation.

On physical examination, the interval between the second heart sound and the opening snap, referred to as the *S_2-OS interval,* and the duration and timing of the diastolic murmur provide additional clues of severity. The S_2-OS interval is a function of the elevation in left atrial pressure. The greater the pressure, the shorter the interval. Unfortunately, the degree of MS is not the only determinant of left atrial pressure; the interval can be affected by factors other than valve area, such as heart rate and left ventricular pressure. Moreover, the valve must be mobile to snap; in advanced disease, the valve may calcify and the snap becomes inaudible. Nevertheless, the S_2-OS interval is useful because it can be determined at the bedside and does provide data that may help in judging severity when considered in the context of other findings. Perhaps the most precise use of the interval is in separating hemodynamically insignificant disease from moderate and severe MS. An interval of greater than 0.11 second at rest with a heart rate of 70 to 80 argues against a significant lesion (although there are exceptions). Patients with moderate to tight stenosis usually demonstrate intervals less than 0.08 second, which shorten with exercise. Proper estimation of the S_2-OS interval takes considerable practice.

The intensity of the *diastolic murmur* does not correlate with severity of stenosis, but its duration through diastole does. However, development of pulmonary hypertension may decrease cardiac output from the right side of the heart, result in a diminution of flow across the mitral valve, and consequently shorten the duration of the murmur.

Chest x-ray provides important evidence of severity. The earliest radiologic sign of MS is dilatation of the left atrium, which is best seen on a lateral view in conjunction with a barium swallow to outline the esophagus. The finding is not a very reliable manifestation of severity. A better sign is redistribution of pulmonary venous blood flow, producing dilatation of the upper zone pulmonary veins. Upper zone redistribution becomes prominent at a left atrial pressure of 25 mm Hg and parallels severity of stenosis. This change in pulmonary venous flow is very sensitive to changes in left atrial pressure, but not unique to mitral stenosis. Radiologic evidence of pulmonary hypertension (dilatation of the right pulmonary artery to 15 to 18 mm, rapid tapering of vessels, and right ventricular enlargement) strongly suggests advanced mitral stenosis, though again the findings are not specific for MS. Presence of Kerley B lines, perihilar haze, and other manifestations of interstitial edema are seen in patients with severe dyspnea due to MS; the absence of interstitial edema on chest film does not rule out tight MS, but a patient with dyspnea at rest should always show these changes on x-ray; otherwise, one must question the meaning of the shortness of breath. In sum, no single radiologic finding is specific for severe MS, but x-ray data can provide important supporting evidence.

The *electrocardiogram* is of limited utility for estimation of severity. The best ECG sign appears to be the QRS axis; a rightward shift to greater than +60° is associated with a valve area of less than 1.3 cm^2 in over 85% of cases. The absence of the rightward shift in axis means little. The greater the pulmonary artery pressure, the more likely right ventricular hypertrophy will appear on ECG.

Cardiac ultrasound study (echocardiography) is the most sensitive noninvasive method for evaluating mitral stenosis. One dimensional (M-mode) echocardiography readily identifies mitral valve thickening, calcification (when present), and the degree of limitation of valvular movement or excursion. Two-dimensional echocardiography (B-mode) provides even better information by allowing for direct visualization of the entire valve and its supporting apparatus, measurement of the valve orifice, left atrial and left ventricular chamber dimensions, and assessment of abnormality of other cardiac valves.

Cardiac doppler evaluation has become increasingly helpful in assessing the presence and magnitude of mitral stenosis, as well as detecting valvular incompetence. *Cardiac catheterization* is indicated when symptoms are progressive and cardiac surgery is being considered.

Mitral Regurgitation

A reasonable estimate of the severity of mitral insufficiency can be obtained by *history* and physical examination. Dyspnea on exertion and fatigability are early symptoms of hemodynamically significant regurgitation, though the absence of such symptoms does not rule out severe disease. On *physical examination,* severe MR produces left ventricular enlargement with a hyperdynamic, slightly diffuse, apical impulse displaced to the left but of normal timing and duration. In addition, there is a pansystolic murmur (its loudness does not correlate directly with severity), a loud S$_3$, often a mid-diastolic rumble from increased flow across the mitral valve, and at times wide splitting of the second sound due to shortening of left ventricular systole and early aortic valve closure. Cardiomegaly and left atrial enlargement are pronounced on *chest film.* A normal heart on chest x-ray and

absence of an apical pansystolic murmur rule out significant mitral regurgitation. The *ECG* reflects both left atrial and left ventricular enlargement, but is hardly specific for MR. The *two-dimensional echocardiogram* is useful for identifying the specific process causing the MR, be it rheumatic fever, prolapse, a ruptured chordae tendineae, or endocarditis. In addition, the severity can be ascertained by *doppler study* and by the magnitude of left atrial and left ventricular dilation.

Cardiac catheterization is indicated in patients with progressive symptoms and rapidly increasing heart size who are being considered for surgery. One needs to estimate degree of regurgitation, assess ventricular function, and check for the presence and severity of associated valvular and coronary disease.

Aortic Stenosis

There are numerous pitfalls in the clinical estimation of severity, especially in the elderly. Nevertheless, careful history and physical examination can provide important clues. Effort syncope, angina, and symptoms of congestive heart failure point to advanced disease with markedly reduced changes of 5-year survival. At times, it is impossible to tell clinically if these worrisome symptoms are due to AS. Because of the high prevalence of coexisting coronary disease, the presence of angina must be interpreted cautiously; cardiac catheterization and coronary angiography may be necessary.

Delay in carotid artery upstroke is one of the most helpful physical signs of significant AS. A normal upstroke in a patient under age 60 is strong evidence against important stenosis; however, upstroke may be normal in the elderly patient with severe stenosis and a stiff, noncompliant carotid artery. Particularly when there are prominent transmitted carotid thrills, the brachial arteries may better reflect the severity of aortic stenosis and should also be assessed by palpation. When coincidental aortic regurgitation is present, the upstroke may also be normalized in the presence of marked stenosis. A misleading delay in carotid upstroke can occur from the combination of systemic hypertension and congestive heart failure. Elevation of systolic blood pressure does not rule out hemodynamically significant disease, although a pressure greater than 200 and a pulse pressure in excess of 80 mm Hg are unusual when stenosis is marked.

In young patients, the intensity of the murmur usually correlates with severity; however, while it is generally true that critical aortic stenosis is unlikely in a young ambulating person who has less than a $^3/_6$ systolic ejection murmur, rare exceptions do occur. In patients with far advanced disease and a failing left ventricle, the murmur may decrease in intensity and appear insignificant as flow across the valve diminishes. In general, the longer the murmur takes to reach peak intensity, the greater the stenosis. Unfortunately, the timing of maximal intensity may not be delayed in some cases of severe stenosis, but if the murmur does peak after midsystole, the stenosis is usually significant. Because the murmur of AS in the elderly may lose its characteristic qualities, it is best to judge severity on the basis of symptoms and other findings.

A delay in the aortic component of the second heart sound is another sign of significant AS. S_2 may be single or paradoxically split. Calcification and increased rigidity of the valve will often diminish the intensity of the aortic closing sound; it may become inaudible. A forceful left ventricular impulse noted on palpation of the precordium is a reliable indication of secondary left ventricular hypertrophy due to significant outflow obstruction.

The *ECG* can contribute to the evaluation by showing signs of left ventricular hypertrophy (increased voltage and a strain pattern in the precordial leads V_{5-6}). The likelihood of finding a strain pattern (*i.e.,* ST and T wave depression in the apical and lateral leads), increases with the increase in gradient across the aortic valve. These ECG changes also identify patients at increased risk of sudden death, as fewer than 10% of patients succumbing to sudden death demonstrate a normal ECG. In children, the ECG is less helpful; even severe AS may not produce left ventricular hypertrophy and a strain pattern.

In the elderly, the degree of valvular calcification on *chest fluoroscopy* correlates with severity of stenosis. The absence of significant calcification in a patient over 60 greatly reduces the probability of important valvular stenosis. Poststenotic dilatation of the aorta suggests aortic valvular stenosis, but does not have quantitative meaning.

Echocardiography can help in the assessment of AS by identifying calcification, thickening, and decreased mobility of the aortic valve leaflets, findings that occur as AS progresses. Echocardiography is useful for delineating the etiology and morphology of stenosis, determining whether it is valvular or subvalvular, and if subvalvular, whether the stenosis is secondary to a discrete membrane, fibromuscular bar, or a hypertrophic myocardium as in IHSS. In the young patient with normal left ventricular function, the echocardiogram can provide an indirect estimate of the magnitude of the obstructive gradient. The echocardiogram also delineates the magnitude of left ventricular wall thickening and any associated valvular abnormality, particularly rheumatic valve disease. The *pulsed doppler* is useful adjunct to the echocardiogram for evaluating the severity of AS and any associated aortic insufficiency.

Cardiac catheterization is indicated in the young asymptomatic patient with evidence of severe stenosis, as well as in any patient with known aortic stenosis who begins to develop symptoms of angina, heart failure, or syncope. Elderly patients who are deemed healthy enough to be candidates for surgery should also have coronary angiography performed to identify significant occlusive disease that may be the source of symptoms or may limit chances of surviving surgery without correction at the time of valve replacement.

Aortic Regurgitation

Severity of AR can usually be well assessed clinically in cases of isolated valvular insufficiency. Marked regurgitation that is long-standing produces dyspnea, a loud diastolic murmur that extends beyond mid-diastole, an S_3, a bounding pulse, and a widened pulse pressure. The absence of a wide pulse pressure does not rule out hemodynamically significant AR, nor does the degree of widening necessarily correlate quantitatively with severity. Changes in peripheral resistance alone can cause large variations in pulse pressure. ECG and x-ray evidence of left ventricular hypertrophy and enlargement are indicative of long-standing significant regurgitation and suggest worsening left ventricular function if they progress.

The *echocardiogram* is useful for delineating the specific disease process in AR, be it rheumatic heart disease, annular dilation, or advanced luetic destruction. It is also of help in determining left ventricular size and evaluating left ventricular contraction. The *gated cardiac blood pool scan* contributes to the assessment by providing a measurement of ejection fraction and a view of contractility.

When aortic regurgitation occurs in the presence of coexisting aortic stenosis, mitral stenosis, or heart failure, the estimation of severity can be very difficult to judge on clinical grounds alone. Consultation with a cardiologist and catheterization are often needed.

PRINCIPLES OF MANAGEMENT

The major therapeutic objectives are to preserve exercise capacity, life-style, and life expectancy, and minimize the chances of endocarditis and systemic embolization. Proper timing of surgical intervention is essential to successful treatment. A common management error is to inappropriately delay surgery, allowing irreversible myocardial decompensation to develop; this increases the risk of operation and reduces the postoperative benefit. A physician can be lulled into a false sense of security by continuing to control symptoms through repetitive escalations of medical therapy. The need for progressive increases in medication suggests worsening myocardial function and the need for surgery. By ignoring the significance of such developments, the physician may miss the optimal opportunity for the best possible surgical outcome, long-term improvement and survival.

Early in the course of illness, symptoms of pulmonary congestion can be treated with digitalis and/or a mild diuretic regimen (see Chapter 27), but more advanced stages of disease require surgical intervention. Life expectancy and quality of life are clearly improved by properly timed valve surgery. Advances in design of prosthetic valves and improvements in operative technique have produced substantial reductions in surgical mortality. At present, mortality rates for patients undergoing valve surgery in major centers average less than 1% for mitral valvulotomy and less than 5% for mitral or aortic valve replacement. Operative mortality increases sharply when patients with advanced disease (*e.g.,* functional class IV) undergo surgery; nevertheless, imminent death is frequently inevitable unless surgery is undertaken. Consequently, patients with severe disease should not be denied an operation if there is reasonable evidence of sufficient myocardial reserve and thus a chance for meaningful improvement in life-style and survival postoperatively. The 5-year life expectancy rate for patients with class IV disease who live through valve replacement is usually less than 50%, but this figure is much better than the less than 5% rate for similar patients managed medically. Thus, even when surgery is inordinately delayed, it may still offer the patient some opportunity for prolonging survival.

Contraindications to valve surgery include serious coexisting noncardiac illness that would compromise survival and the existence of end-stage myocardial decompensation that would make surgery for naught.

Prior to surgery, medical therapy should be directed at control of heart failure (see Chapter 27), maintenance of a near normal life-style, and avoidance of potentially dangerous complications, such as arrhythmias (see Chapter 24), bacterial endocarditis (see Chapter 11), and embolization (see Chapter 23). Most people can be well managed on an outpatient basis for many years prior to the need for valve surgery, but escalation of medical therapy beyond the time when surgery is indicated must be avoided.

It is important to emphasize that patients who undergo valve surgery still have a "cardiac problem" after surgical correction, be it a prosthetic valve with a variable and still unknown late course, a need for anticoagulation and endocarditis prophylaxis, or an associated cardiac abnormality such as coronary, myocardial, or conduction system disease. All too often this is forgotten after the patient undergoes valve repair. Such patients need continued close follow-up and will always remain "cardiac patients."

Percutaneous balloon angioplasty is being utilized effectively and safely for relief of severe valvular aortic and mitral valvular stenoses. Specific indications remain to be defined, but the procedure has proven particularly useful for patients who are too ill to tolerate the risk of open heart surgery. Excellent palliation has been achieved. Duration of palliative effect is undetermined.

THERAPEUTIC RECOMMENDATIONS AND INDICATIONS FOR REFERRAL AND ADMISSION

- All patients with any form of valvular heart disease should receive prophylaxis for bacterial endocarditis (see Chapter 11).
- Patients under the age of 35 with previous rheumatic fever should be considered for rheumatic fever prophylaxis (see Chapter 12) particularly if they are frequent beta streptococcal infections or exposure to young children.

- Onset of atrial fibrillation with a rapid ventricular rate accompanied by acute hemodynamic deterioration is an indication for immediate hospital admission and treatment. Patients with slower rates who tolerate the atrial fibrillation can be digitalized on an outpatient basis (see Chapter 23).
- Occurrence of systemic embolization is an indication for urgent admission and intravenous anticoagulant therapy followed by long-term oral anticoagulant treatment (see Chapter 85). Some clinicians argue that valve surgery should be considered if embolization occurs; most concur that surgery is indicated if embolization happens repeatedly.

Mitral Stenosis

- Asymptomatic patients with mild to moderate stenosis need no restriction of activity. Those with evidence of tight stenosis and relatively few symptoms should be advised of the risk of precipitating symptoms by extreme exertion or pregnancy.
- Patients with mild dyspnea that occurs only on exertion can be started on a mild diuretic program (*e.g.,* 50 to 100 mg hydrochlorothiazide per day) and advised to follow a no-added-salt diet. Digitalis is of no benefit in isolated mitral stenosis unless there is atrial fibrillation. Extremely vigorous exertion and emotional upset should be avoided to prevent *precipitating* symptoms.
- Chronic coumadin anticoagulation is indicated for the patient with MS, particularly when there is atrial fibrillation (see Chapter 23).
- The development of signs of tight stenosis (see above), even if few symptoms are reported, is an indication for referral to a cardiologist for consideration of surgery. The same is true for worsening dyspnea that is inadequately controlled by a mild diuretic program and salt restriction.
- Young patients with evidence of isolated, tight MS with a pliable noncalcified valve should be considered for surgery early in the course of their illness, even before symptoms are disabling, because valvulotomy can be performed. The procedure provides symptomatic improvement that may last for 10 to 20 years, is less risky than valve replacement, and does not require chronic anticoagulant therapy.
- Older patients with fibrotic valves (absent opening snap, heavy valve calcification, and limited motion) must undergo valve replacement if surgery is needed. Since surgical mortality and complications are greater for valve replacement than for valvulotomy, surgery need not be advised until symptoms are more disabling. However, surgery should not be delayed until symptoms occur at rest or upon minimal exertion, because operative risk and long-term mortality increase substantially. A walk with your patient down a corridor or up a flight of stairs may be of great help in convincing both you and the patient that the time for surgery has arrived.
- Cardiac consultation for consideration of catheterization is indicated in the patient being considered for surgery when

there is a question of mixed mitral disease or involvement of multiple valves, or when symptoms are out of proportion to objective evidence of disease.

Mitral Regurgitation

- Asymptomatic young patients need no restriction of activity.
- Onset of fatigue and dyspnea can be treated with initiation of digitalis and diuretics, in conjunction with a no-added-salt diet. A modest diuretic program, such as 100 mg of hydrochlorothiazide, that adequately controls symptoms may suffice for years in patients with mild to moderate MR and is not an indication for surgery.
- The development of any increase in dyspnea that requires escalation of diuretic therapy is an indication for cardiac consultation concerning valve replacement. Progressive deterioration in clinical status and increasing heart size suggest presence of myocardial decompensation; prompt referral is indicated; medical therapy is no substitute for valve surgery.
- Use of vasodilators, particularly captopril (see Chapter 27), can benefit the inoperable patient.
- Refractory congestive failure due to MR is not a contraindication to surgery, though risk is increased. Prior to surgery, symptoms may be lessened by vasodilator therapy, which can diminish the proportion of regurgitant flow by decreasing afterload. Use of vasodilators can also benefit the inoperable patient.
- Patients with incapacitating dyspnea and pulmonary congestion felt to be due to *papillary muscle dysfunction* should be referred to the cardiologist for catheterization to determine if valve replacement will be of benefit. In one series, those with ejection fractions above 0.35 had the best surgical survival. If there is coexisting coronary disease, it should be treated (see Chapter 25).
- Patients with a *prolapsed mitral valve* rarely require treatment for ventricular irritability. Dyspnea is uncommon and digitalis, diuretics, and salt restriction are unnecessary, since the magnitude of the regurgitation is usually insignificant and rarely progressive. Occurrence of chest pain demands careful evaluation so that other etiologies are not mistakenly attributed to the valve disease (see Chapter 14).
- Patients with *calcification of the mitral valve annulus* should be followed for development of heart block. Regurgitant flow is usually small; consequently, dyspnea and pulmonary congestion are not major problems.
- Chronic anticoagulation is indicated in MR patients with atrial fibrillation, especially when accompanied by marked left atrial and left ventricular enlargement.

Aortic Stenosis

- Asymptomatic patients with mild AS do not require restriction of activity. However, young, asymptomatic patients with evidence of tight stenosis should be advised against physical exertion (e.g., competitive sports) and referred to a cardiologist for further evaluation and consideration of valvuloplasty or valve replacement. Cardiac catheterization is needed.
- Onset of angina, effort syncope, or congestive heart failure dictates serious consideration of valve surgery, because these are signs of critical stenosis and predict a poor prognosis unless definitive therapy is undertaken. Patients with these symptoms are at risk for sudden death. Medical therapy is no substitute.
- Congestive failure can be treated symptomatically on a temporary basis by prescribing digitalis and a diuretic program (see Chapter 27). Cautious use of furosemide (20 to 40 mg per day) may help reduce pulmonary congestion when fluid retention is marked, but the need for a high diastolic filling pressure must be kept in mind; overzealous diuretic therapy can cause a precipitous fall in cardiac output.
- Angina can be treated symptomatically with nitroglycerin pending surgery (see Chapter 25). Propranolol is contraindicated due to its negative inotropic effects. Coronary angiography is required at the time of cardiac catheterization to determine if there is coexisting significant coronary artery disease and the need for a bypass procedure at the time of valve replacement.
- Advanced age is not an absolute contraindication to valve replacement. Survival from surgery is predominantly a function of the patient's myocardial reserve. Consequently, patients in their 60s and 70s need not be denied surgery if they demonstrate good ejection fractions in the setting of severe AS.
- Because the lesion can progress rapidly over a few years, patients with AS should have careful longitudinal care and regular follow-up, even when disease appears hemodynamically insignificant and the patient is asymptomatic.

Aortic Regurgitation

- No activity restrictions are necessary in young asymptomatic patients with mild regurgitation.
- Patients with evidence of worsening left ventricular status (LVH with a strain pattern on ECG, increasing cardiomegaly on chest film) should be referred to a cardiologist for evaluation of surgery, even in the absence of disabling symptoms. Patients with these findings have been noted to have an increased 5-year mortality rate. Early identification of high-risk patients is suggested in the hope of correcting AR prior to the development of irreversible myocardial decompensation, which may occur rapidly at the time that symptoms of failure appear.
- Onset of early symptoms of pulmonary congestion (dyspnea on climbing more than one flight of stairs) in the absence of LVH with strain on ECG or marked cardiomegaly can

be treated medically with digitalization and a mild diuretic (50 to 100 mg hydrochlorothiazide). Progression of dyspnea to onset after climbing less than one flight of stairs or the appearance of LVH, strain, and an enlarging heart indicates the need for cardiac consultation and consideration of surgery.

Patients with dyspnea prompted by minimal exertion, orthopnea, or paroxysmal nocturnal dyspnea require prompt referral for surgery, because life expectancy is less than 1 year without surgery. Medical therapy with digitalis and diuretics may provide some symptomatic relief temporarily, but must not be used in place of valve surgery at this stage of illness.

PATIENT EDUCATION

By far, the most essential element of patient education is teaching the importance of endocarditis prophylaxis. The chances of compliance are certain to improve if time is taken to explain the rationale for prophylaxis and to inform the patient of the risks incurred if it is ignored. Proper procedure and situations requiring prophylaxis need thorough review (see Chapter 11). Patients who have had rheumatic fever require instruction prophylaxis against streptococcal infection (see Chapter 12).

Patients *and* their families should be fully briefed on allowable activity to avoid unnecessary restriction as well as the risk of sudden death (*e.g.*, the young asymptomatic patient with critical AS). If the safety of unlimited activity is in doubt, the patient should have a cardiac consultation. Patient confidence can be maintained by regular follow-up by the primary physician in conjunction with a consulting cardiologist when needed. It is helpful to inform the patient of the treatability of his condition and its excellent prognosis when therapy is properly timed and applied. Teaching the early warning signs of worsening disease to the patient who is mature and intelligent can help to enlist him in the monitoring effort. If the patient cannot be depended upon to relate symptoms accurately, perhaps a family member might be recruited to watch for early manifestations of progressive disease. Reviewing the proper use of digitalis and diuretics (see Chapter 27) is important for prevention of inappropriate and unauthorized escalation of the medical program when symptoms worsen. Instruction in anticoagulant therapy is also essential if it is to be used on a long-term basis (see Chapter 85).

ANNOTATED BIBLIOGRAPHY

Barnhorst DA, Oxman HA, Connolly DC et al: Long-term follow-up of isolated replacement of aortic or mitral valve with Starr-Edwards prosthesis. Am J Cardiol 35:228, 1975 (*Valve replacement improved life expectancy and symptoms.*)

Boucher CA, Wilson RA, Kanarek DJ et al: Exercise testing in asymptomatic or minimally symptomatic aortic regurgitation.

Circ 67:1091, 1983 (*Exercise gated blood pool scanning can help in management of aortic stenosis by providing information about the state of the left ventricle.*)

Brunnen PL, Finlayson JD, Short D: Serious mitral stenosis with slight symptoms. Br Med J 1:1958, 1964 (*Symptoms may be slight but young patients with tight stenosis are at risk for sudden deterioration; pregnancy was a major precipitant in this series of 20 patients.*)

Cheitlin MD, Gertz EW, Brundage BH et al: Rate of progression of severity of valvular aortic stenosis in the adult. Am Heart J 98: 689, 1979 (*Patients with aortic stenosis must be followed carefully and regularly, as this can be a progressive disease.*)

Chen JTT, Beliar VS, Morris JJ et al: Correlation of roentgen findings with hemodynamic data in pure mitral stenosis. Am J Roentgenol 102:280, 1968 (*When there is a prominent upper zone venous pattern and pulmonary artery dilation on chest film, the mitral stenosis is severe.*)

Cohn LH, Mudge GH, Pratter F et al: Five to eight year follow-up of patients undergoing porcine valve replacement. N Engl J Med 304:258, 1981 (*Documents rates of thromboemboli, endocarditis, and primary valve dysfunction in patients with porcine valves in the aortic and mitral valve positions.*)

Dalby AJ, Firth BG, Forman R: Preoperative factors affecting the outcome of isolated mitral valve replacement: A 10 year review. Am J Cardiol 47:826, 1981 (*Selection of the optimal time for mitral valve replacement remains a difficult problem, but there are helpful established guidelines.*)

Donner R, Carabello B, Black I et al: Left ventricular wall stress in compensated aortic stenosis in children. Am J Cardiol 51:946, 1983 (*When the myocardium is intact, as it usually is in the young, the echocardiogram can be helpful in quantifying the outflow gradient.*)

Frank S, Johnson A, Ross J, Jr: Natural history of valvular aortic stenosis. Br Heart J 35:41, 1973 (*In medically treated cases with significant stenosis, 50% were dead within 5 years and 90% within 10 years of diagnosis.*)

Friedman WF, Braunwald E: Accurate estimation of left atrial pressure without cardiac catheterization in mitral valve disease. Am J Cardiol 17:123, 1966 (*Dilatation of upper zone pulmonary veins is prominent when left atrial pressure reaches 25 mm Hg.*)

Fowler NO, Van Der Bel-Kahn JM: Indications for surgical replacement of the mitral valve. Am J Cardiol 44:148, 1979 (*A review which emphasizes timing of surgical therapy; 41 references are included.*)

Goldschlager N, Pfeifer J, Cohn K et al: Natural history of aortic regurgitation. Am J Med 54:577, 1973 (*Long asymptomatic period, but once symptoms occur, irreversible myocardial changes may have already taken place.*)

Graboys TB, Cohn PF: Prevalence of angina and abnormal coronary arteriograms in severe aortic stenosis. Am Heart J 93:683, 1977 (*Twenty % of patients had >75% luminal stenosis.*)

Greenberg BH: Aortic insufficiency: vasodilator therapy. Primary Cardiol 8:35, 1982 (*There is a role for afterload reduction in managing aortic insufficiency.*)

Greenberg BH, Massie BM, Botvinick EH et al: Beneficial effects of hydralazine in severe mitral regurgitation. Circ 58:273, 1978

(*Systemic afterload reduction has some beneficial role in the management of mitral regurgitation.*)

Grossman W: Aortic and mital regurgitation. JAMA 252:2447, 1984 (*Clinical review emphasizing the indications for and timing of surgical intervention in pure aortic and mitral regurgitation.*)

Hoagland PM, Cook EF, Wynne J et al: Value of noninvasive testing in adults with suspected aortic stenosis. Am J Med 80:1041, 1986 (*Enabled the designation of high- and low-risk groups.*)

Kaye D: Prophylaxis for infective endocarditis. Ann Intern Med 104: 419, 1986 (*A critical review of American Heart Association recommendations.*)

Morganroth J, Jones RH, Chen CC et al: Two-dimensional echocardiography in mitral, aortic and tricuspid valve disease. Am J Cardiol 46:1164, 1980 (*An authoritative review of ultrasound for the diagnosis of valvular heart disease.*)

Olsen KH, Biden H: Natural history of mitral stenosis. Br Heart J 24:349, 1962 (*Mortality for NYHA class III patients managed medically was 6% per annum and for class IV, 17% per annum.*)

Palacios IF, Lock JE, Keane JF et al: Percutaneous transvenous balloon valvotomy in a patient with severe calcific mitral stenosis. J Am Coll Cardiol 7:1416, 1986

Perloff JK: Acute severe aortic regurgitation. J Cardiovasc Med 8: 209, 1983 (*Authoritative review of the diagnosis and management of this condition.*)

Perloff JK: Evolving concepts of mitral valve prolapse. N Engl J Med 307:369, 1982 (*Makes the important point that patients with prolapse are a heterogeneous group with different presentations and prognoses; most have a harmless condition with an excellent prognosis.*)

Procacci PM, Savran SV, Schreiter SL et al: Prevalence of clinical mitral valve prolapse in 1,169 young women. N Engl J Med 294: 1086, 1976 (*Prolapse identified in approximately 10% of the normal population.*)

Radford M, Johnson RA, Buckley MJ et al: Survival following initial valve replacement for mitral regurgitation due to coronary artery disease. Circulation, 60:Suppl. II,39, 1979 (*Survival was a function of preoperative ejection fraction. Long-term survivors experienced reductions in heart failure.*)

Rappaport E: Natural history of aortic and mitral valve disease. Am J Cardiol 35:221, 1975 (*In large series of medically treated patients with mitral regurgitation, the 10-year survival was 60%.*)

Ross J: Left ventricular function and the timing of surgical treatment in valvular heart disease. Ann Intern Med 98:498, 1981 (*Reviews the problem of preservation of ventricular function relative to timing of mitral valve replacement for mitral insufficiency.*)

Rothenberg AJ, Clark JA, Carleton RA et al: Natural course of mitral stenosis. Clin Res 16:246, 1968 (*Symptoms correlated roughly with reduction in valve area. Few symptoms occurred when valve area was greater than 1.5 cm^2.*)

Spagnuolo M, Kloth H, Tianta A et al: Natural history of rheumatic aortic regurgitation. Circulation, 44:368, 1971 (*Young patients with marked LV enlargement, LVH on ECG and wide pulse pressure with diastolic less than 40 mm Hg are at high risk for failure or death.*)

Wood P: An appreciation of mitral stenosis. Br Med J 1:1051, 1954 (*Symptom-free interval from onset of rheumatic heart disease to onset of symptoms was 3 to 25 years with mean of 12 years. A classic study of mitral stenosis.*)

29

Management of Peripheral Arterial Disease

DAVID C. BREWSTER, M.D.

Although specific treatment to achieve regression of advanced arteriosclerosis does not yet exist (see Chapter 22), numerous therapeutic measures are available that can provide symptomatic improvement for patients with claudication and other manifestations of lower extremity arterial occlusive disease. In addition, great progress has been made in angioplasty and arterial reconstructive surgery for severe cases, resulting in the salvage of limbs which would otherwise require amputation.

The primary physician needs to know the natural history of the disease, as well as the indications for and effectiveness of both nonoperative and surgical management.

NATURAL HISTORY OF CLAUDICATION

A number of studies have examined the clinical course and prognosis of patients with intermittent claudication. In a series of 529 diabetic patients from the Mayo Clinic followed over 5 years prior to the advent of surgical reconstruction, only 3% came to amputation within 5 years if the only manifestation of their disease was claudication. Of the smokers who ceased smoking, none required amputation, but 11.4% who continued to smoke lost a limb.

A more recent study of 104 patients with claudication who underwent angiography also noted a relatively benign prognosis. Over a 6-month to 8-year follow-up (average 2.5 years), 79% remained stable or improved, and only 5.8% came to amputation. When patients were divided into mild, moderate, and severe disease groups on the basis of distance walked before onset of claudication, it was found that prognosis paralleled severity; the group with most severe disease accounted for five of the six amputations. Nevertheless, even in the most severe cases 69.4% stayed the same or improved, and only 15.1% came to amputation, underscoring the fact that progression to loss of limb is hardly inevitable.

In the Mayo Clinic series, the 5-year survival rate was 77.2% for patients with claudication, compared to 92.8% for a normal population matched for age and sex. The cause of death in over 75% of patients with claudication was believed to be coronary artery disease, underscoring the often systemic nature of atherosclerosis and its adverse effect on prognosis.

PRINCIPLES OF MANAGEMENT

Nonsurgical Measures

The basic tenet of nonoperative care is to control or limit disease progression while *stimulating collateral circulation.* As long as improvement in collateral flow outpaces the development of existing or new occlusive lesions, blood flow will be maintained and symptoms will remain stable or may actually improve. Perhaps the two most important methods of achieving these objectives are the *cessation of cigarette smoking* and regular daily exercise. Smoking appears to hasten progression of atherosclerosis and may also impair collateral flow by its vasoconstrictive effect. Significant occlusive disease is rare in nonsmokers. A possible stimulus for development of collateral circulation appears to be the demand created by *daily exercise,* although this is still unproven. Nevertheless, exercise programs significantly increase the claudication-free walking distance.

Careful attention to *foot care* (see below) is vital in prevention of limb loss. It has been estimated that up to 80% of amputations required in diabetics are attributable to poor foot care. Feet need to be inspected daily, especially when there is coexisting peripheral neuropathy that limits protective sensation.

Weight reduction can be helpful by lessening work load and reducing metabolic demands of the extremities. In addition, weight reduction may also help lower lipid levels. *Treatment of hypertension* (see Chapter 21) and *hyperlipidemia* (see Chapters 9 and 22) is advisable and may be of value in controlling progression of arteriosclerosis. Patients with extensive premature peripheral arterial disease (occurring before age 50) may suffer from heterozygosity for homocystinuria and should be tested for impaired homocysteine metabolism. Patients with the condition may respond to vitamin B_6 or folate. Proper *control of diabetes* is also important, although "tight" control does not seem to be of any additional help (see Chapter 100).

Pharmacologic treatment of arterial insufficiency remains controversial. *Vasodilators* are the most widely used class of drugs, but remain of unproven benefit. A wide variety of agents with differing mechanisms of action is available. Little convincing evidence exists to support their use in chronic obstructive vascular disease, particularly for claudication. We do not employ them. Although initial results with *prostaglandins* in occlusive disease were encouraging, later reports were less enthusiastic about their benefit, and further data are needed before their use can be recommended.

A new type of agent, *pentoxifylline,* is believed to improve capillary blood flow by increasing erythrocyte deformability. Randomized, double-blind multicenter study revealed at some centers a modest increase in patients' walking distance, but the increase was only 18% of that reported for exercise programs. *Antiplatelet agents* have been suggested, but there is no evidence suggesting benefit in lower extremity disease. *Anticoagulants* have no role in peripheral arterial disease.

Certain drugs may constrict peripheral arteries and *aggravate arterial insufficiency* and should therefore be avoided in occlusive arterial disease. *Ergot derivatives* are a classic example. Other commonly used drugs that may aggravate ischemic symptoms include beta-blocking agents and peripheral alpha-stimulating drugs. Both categories of drugs may worsen intermittent claudication and impede the healing of skin lesions.

Surgical Therapy

In patients with *claudication alone,* an operation should be considered only in those who are so significantly disabled by claudication that their ability to earn a living is compromised, or their desired life-style intolerably limited. The role of arterial reconstruction for claudication alone remains controversial. In general, the physician must attempt to determine the significance of ischemic symptoms in each patient. The patient's age, work requirements, social circumstances, and general state of health must all be considered. When doubt exists, referral for a surgical opinion is often useful.

Surgical referral is clearly indicated in patients with *advanced ischemia* resulting in *ischemic rest pain,* nonhealing *ischemic ulcerations,* or *gangrene.* Such limbs are clearly at risk, and arterial reconstruction is indicated, if feasible, to maximize chances of limb salvage. In such circumstances, patients should be referred for surgical investigation as soon as possible, before tissue necrosis or infection become too extensive. The morbidity and mortality of common revascularization procedures is in many instances less than that associated with major amputation. For poor risk patients, various "extra-anatomic" reconstructions are also available, which may be done with even more safety.

Many patients with significant arterial insufficiency that requires surgery also have underlying coronary disease that is hemodynamically critical. It may be clinically silent due to the exercise restrictions stemming from severe claudication. Such patients have high rates of perioperative morbidity and mortality. Dipyridamole–thallium stress testing before surgery helps to identify high-risk patients who may need coronary revascularization prior to peripheral vascular surgery.

Within the past decade, great progress has been made in the surgical management of arterial insufficiency. An experienced surgeon, with good anesthetic and postoperative management, may anticipate successful correction of aortoiliac occlusive disease with a mortality of only 1% to 2%, and excellent long-term patency of approximately 85% to 90% at 5 years. Femoropopliteal reconstruction may be done with even greater safety, although long-term patency is somewhat less, with approximately 70% to 75% of saphenous vein grafts still patent at 5 years. If the saphenous vein is unavailable for use, a number of suitable alternative prosthetic grafts have been developed within recent years. With improvement of direct reconstructive methods, lumbar sympathectomy is rarely considered a primary mode of treatment.

Percutaneous Transluminal Angioplasty is a promising therapeutic modality for peripheral arterial disease. It employs a balloon catheter that can be inserted percutaneously at a remote site, usually the femoral artery, and manipulated fluoroscopically within the diseased segment of artery. With balloon inflation to a pressure of 4 to 6 atmospheres, the arteriosclerotic plaque or occlusion is cracked and vessel lumen enhanced. The method is particularly applicable to localized proximal stenotic lesions or short segmental occlusions. In such circumstances, early results are generally good in experienced hands, and complication rates are low. Long-term follow-up results are not yet available, and are necessary to better define the role of balloon angioplasty in patients with peripheral occlusive disease. The technique is not suitable for the majority of patients with more widespread, diffuse occlusive disease. If feasible, angioplasty may be particularly helpful in patients who are poor risks for standard surgical correction; the procedure has a lower morbidity and mortality than standard surgery. In addition, it may be combined with surgery, for example, to correct a proximal iliac stenosis by balloon angioplasty and distal femoropopliteal bypass grafting.

Indications for angioplasty are the same as those for surgery: life-style-limiting claudication, ischemic rest pain, ulceration, or gangrene due to stenotic lesions of the iliac, femoral, or popliteal arteries.

PATIENT EDUCATION

Patient education is vital, as implementation of many of the measures just discussed required that the patient understand the nature of the problem as well as the factors that may aggravate the severity of symptoms. Patient compliance is essential in most nonoperative recommendations. Many patients come to the physician with great fear of limb loss. The favorable prognosis and likelihood of improvement are usually of great comfort and reassurance to the patient and family. The psychologic management of the patient is essential in preventing depression and invalidism. Emphasis should be on the positive prognosis and the patient's ability to improve his own condition by simple means. The patient with new claudication should be seen at 2- to 3-month intervals

for assessment of exercise tolerance and inspection of the feet for potential pressure points and ulcers. The need for foot care and immediate attention to the most trivial injury or lesion must be repeatedly emphasized.

INDICATIONS FOR REFERRAL AND ADMISSION

Refer only those patients for surgical consideration who have such severe disease (rest pain, nonhealing ulcers, early gangrene) that they are at risk for losing the limb and those with claudication whose life-style or livelihood are *intolerably* compromised by the inability to walk distances. Patients with signs of severe disease need prompt surgical attention. Urgent hospitalization is indicated for the patient with early gangrenous changes.

THERAPEUTIC RECOMMENDATIONS

- ***Cessation of smoking.*** The patient should be firmly told that he or she *must* stop smoking. The physician must be unequivocal about this, as patients often interpret half-hearted advice as only a suggestion (see Chapter 49).
- ***Continued exercise.*** In the patient with claudication, exercise is probably best achieved by daily walking. Patients are advised to walk to the point of discomfort, stop briefly, and then resume walking. It is important to emphasize to the patient that pain does not indicate harm or damage to the muscle, and that such a program will help rather than aggravate the condition. Any tendency to restrict activity, sometimes to the point of invalidism or confinement to the home, should be avoided, unless severe ischemia is present.

  Patients with more advanced ischemia and rest pain at night may benefit from raising the head of the bed on 6- to 8-inch blocks so that the feet and legs are made slightly dependent; gravity may aid blood flow enough to allow more comfortable sleep.
- ***Foot care.*** This aspect of preventive medicine is of extreme importance, particularly in the diabetic patient who often lacks protective sensation due to neuropathy and who may be more susceptible to infection. Because there is often a great deal of confusion about what is meant by "foot care," its components require elaboration:
  1. *Inspection.* The feet should be inspected daily for any scratches, cuts, fissures, blisters, or other lesions, particularly around the nail beds, between the toes, and on the heels.
  2. *Washing.* The feet should be washed daily with mild soap and lukewarm (never hot) water. Rinse thoroughly and dry gently but completely, particularly between the toes. Excessive soaking, leading to maceration, should be avoided.
  3. *Lanolin.* A moisturizing cream such as lanolin or Eucerin should be applied to the skin of the foot and heel but not between the toes. A light film, well rubbed in, will

prevent drying and cracking of the skin, often the genesis of a lesion, particularly on the heel. The cream should not be applied thickly or allowed to "cake" on the foot.

4. *Lambswool.* A small amount of lambswool or dry cotton or gauze may be placed between the toes to prevent lesions, which may occur if toes are allowed to rub together, particularly if orthopedic deformities of the toes are present.

5. *Powder.* An antifungal powder, such as Desenex, should be applied between the toes if excessive moisture or maceration is a problem.

6. *Proper footwear.* Properly fitting shoes with ample space in the forefoot are essential. Special shoes are rarely necessary.

7. *Podiatry.* Nails should be cut with extreme care, in good light, and only if vision is normal. They should be cut straight across and even with the end of the toe, never close to the skin or into the corner of the nailbed. Any abnormality of the nails as well as any corns or calluses should be treated by the physician or podiatrist.

8. *Avoidance of trauma.* Never use adhesive tape on the skin (paper tape is better), or any strong antiseptic solution. Avoid heating pads, hot packs, or heat lamps. Never walk barefoot.

It is the physician's responsibility to educate his patients in these points, and to urge them to contact him at the first sign of difficulty.

- *Weight reduction* (see Chapter 229).
- *Control of other risk factors* (e.g., hypertension [see Chapter 21], hyperlipidemia [see Chapter 22]). In patients with premature disease, test for homocystinuria and treat with vitamin B_6 and folic acid supplements if positive.
- *Surgical referral*
  1. *Patients with claudication alone.* An operation should be considered only in patients who are so significantly disabled by claudication that their livelihood or life-style is intolerably compromised by their inability to walk distances.
  2. *Patients with more severe disease.* People with rest pain, nonhealing ulcers, or early gangrene who have a limb which is in jeopardy should be considered for operation with some urgency.
  3. Consider preoperative dipyridamole–thallium stress testing to identify patients with high cardiac risk.

ANNOTATED BIBLIOGRAPHY

Boers GHJ, Smals AGH, Trijbels FJM et al: Heterozygosity for homocystinuria in premature peripheral arterial disease. N Engl J Med 313:709, 1985 (*A surprising percentage had the condition.*)

Boucher CA, Brewster DC, Darling C et al: Determination of cardiac risk by dipyridamole–thallium imaging before peripheral vascular surgery. N Engl J Med 312:299, 1985 (*An effective means of identifying high-risk patients preoperatively.*)

Coffman JD: Vasodilator drugs in peripheral vascular disease. N Engl J Med 300:713, 1979 (*A careful review of the available data and literature, suggesting that vasodilators are not effective in treatment of intermittent claudication or arterial insufficiency; 32 references.*)

Fairbairn JF II, Juergens JL: Principles of medical treatment. In Juergens JL, Spittell JA Jr, Fairbairn JF II (eds): Peripheral Vascular Diseases, p. 855. Philadelphia, WB Saunders, 1980 (*Comprehensive chapter on established and controversial aspects of medical management of arterial occlusive disease; 58 references.*)

Greenhalgh RM (ed): Smoking and Arterial Disease. Bath, England, Pitman Medical, 1981 (*Comprehensive survey of relationship of smoking and arterial occlusive disease.*)

Hallett JW Jr: Foot Care. In Hallett JW Jr, Brewster DC, Darling RC (eds): Manual of Patient Care in Vascular Surgery, p. 171. Boston, Little, Brown & Co, 1982 (*Good discussion of the key elements of proper foot care, with appropriate references.*)

Health and Public Policy Committee, American College of Physicians: Percutaneous transluminal angioplasty. Ann Intern Med 99:864, 1983 (*A position paper supporting the use of angioplasty for surgical candidates.*)

Hutchinson K, Oberle K, Crockford P et al: Effects of dietary manipulation on vascular status of patients with peripheral vascular disease. JAMA 249:3326, 1983 (*A double-blind randomized trial comparing American Heart Association Diet plus exercise with the Pritikin Maintenance Diet. Both groups had equal improvements in walking distance, but neither showed improvement in vascular parameters. Claims that the Pritikin diet causes regression of atherosclerosis were not substantiated.*)

Imparato AM, Kim GE, Davidson T et al: Intermittent claudication: Its natural course. Surgery 78:795, 1975 (*Study of 104 claudicators with angiographic control. Over a 6-month to 8-year follow-up, 79% remained stable or improved, and only 5.8% came to amputation; 25% eventually underwent arterial reconstruction.*)

Juergens JL, Barker NW, Hines EA: Arteriosclerosis obliterans; Review of 520 cases with special reference to pathogenic and prognostic factors. Circulation 21:188, 1960 (*General review of factors applying to natural history. Of patients who continued to smoke, 11.4% required amputation during the 5-year period, while none who stopped smoking had an amputation.*)

Larsen OA, Lassen NA: Effects of daily muscular exercise in patients with intermittent claudication. Lancet 2:1093, 1966 (*Controlled study showing benefit of exercise. No measurable increase in blood flow could be documented, however.*)

McAllister FF: The fate of patients with intermittent claudication managed nonoperatively. Am J Surg 132:593, 1976 (*A study of 100 patients with intermittent claudication followed for an average of 6 years; 78% either improved or remained stable. The study argues for restraint in bypass grafting.*)

Peabody CN, Kannel WB, McNamara PM: Intermittent claudication: Surgical significance. Arch Surg 109:693, 1974 (*Study of Framingham cohort with claudication followed an average of 8.3 years. Only 5% progressed to amputation, and 81% remained stable or improved. Effect of various risk factors on significant cardiovascular morbidity and mortality is emphasized.*)

Porter JM, Baur GM: Pharmacologic treatment of intermittent claudication. Surgery 92:966, 1982 (*Discussion of prior experience with vasodilating drugs and preliminary clinical experience with pentoxifylline, emphasizing a new concept in the pharmacologic treatment of claudication—namely drug modifications of hemorrheology, blood viscosity, and the microcirculation rather than vasodilatation.*)

Porter JM, Cutler BS, Lee BY: Pentoxifylline efficacy in the treatment of intermittent claudication. Am Heart J 104:66, 1982 (*A mul-*

ticenter, randomized, double-blind trial of pentoxifylline vs. placebo showing a modest increase in walking distance, but far less than that reported for exercise training.)

Waltman AC, Greenfield AJ, Novelline RA et al: Transluminal angioplasty of the iliac and femoropopliteal arteries. Arch Surg 117: 1218, 1982 (*Evaluation of the current indications for and results of balloon angioplasty in lower extremity occlusive disease.*)

30
Management of Venous Disease

DAVID C. BREWSTER, M.D.

Problems of the venous system (varicose veins, venous insufficiency, and phlebitis) are extremely prevalent among the elderly. Many physicians do little for the more mundane complaints referrable to the venous system because of lack of knowledge and confusion about pathophysiology and proper management. Such attitudes are unfortunate, because neglected venous problems can cause great disability and lead to occasional mortality. The primary management of venous diseases is still largely nonoperative, and great benefit is possible with well-conceived office care.

PATHOPHYSIOLOGY AND CLINICAL PRESENTATION

The high frequency of venous disorders of the lower extremities is unique to man and undoubtedly reflects the consequences of an upright posture and the effects of gravity. In order to return blood from the periphery to the right heart, the venous system in the legs must work against the force of gravity without the aid of organs specifically designed for this purpose. A number of factors work to lessen venous pressure in the leg and propel blood toward the heart; these include the "muscular pump" effect of the exercising calf musculature, the negative intrathoracic pressure created by the "bellows effect" of the chest wall with respiration, and the presence of multiple valves in both superficial and deep venous systems. The last prevents reflux of blood and serves to reduce pressure in the veins that would otherwise equal the weight of an uninterrupted column of blood from the heart to the foot (approximately 100 mm Hg).

A knowledge of basic anatomy of the venous system is vital to evaluation and management of lower extremity venous problems. The existence of two venous systems, superficial and deep, is well known. A third system linking the superficial and deep systems, the communicating or perforating veins, is less well recognized but of great importance. Valves also exist in the communicating veins, permitting flow from the superficial to the deep system but preventing retrograde flow.

When functioning properly, these three systems work in coordinated fashion. The deep system, composed of paired anterior and posterior tibial and peroneal veins, popliteal veins, and superficial and deep femoral veins handles approximately 80% to 90% of venous return, while the superficial network of greater and lesser saphenous systems is much less important in this respect.

Clinical disorders of the venous system usually stem from obstruction to venous return due to thrombosis of the vein lumen, or incompetent venous valves that allow reflux of blood and persistent elevation of venous pressure in the leg and foot.

Varicose Veins

Because the superficial veins lie in the subcutaneous tissue and lack the support afforded by muscle and fascial compartments, the superficial venous system is most prone to difficulty. Varicose veins are extremely common and probably affect some 10% to 20% of the adult population to some degree. They are more common in women, who also seem more likely to consult a physician for advice.

A family history of varicosities is present in the majority of patients and lends support to the concept of a hereditary or congenital etiology. It is unclear whether the primary problem is a congenital incompetence of valves or a weakness of the venous wall itself, which causes dilatation of the vein lumen and subsequent valve inadequacy. In any event, a self-perpetuating cycle ensues of venous reflux leading to further vein dilatation and valve failure. In time, the poorly supported superficial veins widen, elongate, and become tortuous. In a smaller percentage of patients the initial defect may be in the communicating veins, where poorly functioning valves allow abnormal flow toward the superficial system, causing eventual overdistension. In other patients, acquired factors such as old trauma or venous thrombosis may play a role. Factors that raise intraluminal vein pressure, such as repeated pregnancies, obesity, or wearing of tight garments that constrict the thigh, may be of importance. The final common pathway remains valvular incompetence.

Varicosities most commonly involve the veins of the greater saphenous system and its tributaries, and therefore occur principally in the medial and anterior thigh, calf, and ankle regions. The lesser saphenous system may also be involved, producing varicosities of the posterior calf and lateral ankle region. The exact distribution of involved branches is of real importance only when considering surgical correction.

The presenting symptoms of varicose veins are extremely variable, and often seem to bear little relationship to the apparent severity of the varicosities. It is well recognized that complaints are more frequent in women, particularly young women at the time of the menstrual period. Clearly, hormonal factors that favor fluid retention may aggravate venous distension, but in many such patients the main concern is over the cosmetic appearance of minor varicosities; other emotional factors are often superimposed.

Typically, patients complain of local aching or burning pain in the area of the varicosities, particularly at the end of the day after having been on their feet at work. "Tiredness," "heaviness," or a "bursting" sensation are commonly reported. Itchiness due to a stasis dermatitis may occur in the region of a severe and chronic varix, especially in the region of an incompetent perforating vein. Mild swelling of the ankle region may occur; however, this is relatively unusual with uncomplicated varicose veins. Similarly, ulceration due solely to varicose veins is rare. Severe swelling or recurrent ulceration almost always imply problems with the deep venous system (see below).

Large varices may be subject to trauma and bleeding. Much more commonly, however, the distended vein with sluggish blood flow may thrombose, leading to superficial phlebitis.

Chronic Venous Insufficiency

Chronic venous insufficiency, also called the *postphlebitic syndrome,* is a common chronic disorder that is particularly disabling if stubborn venous ulcers develop. Although the superficial venous system may be secondarily involved with varicose veins, the principal defect lies in the deep venous system.

A documented history of deep venous thrombosis can be obtained in fewer than one half of patients with chronic venous insufficiency, but is felt to be the etiology in most instances. Deep venous thrombosis may often be clinically silent, as documented by prospective ^{125}I-fibrinogen scanning studies in postoperative patients. Despite subsequent recanalization of deep venous occlusions, the phlebitic inflammatory process deforms or destroys venous valves in the deep system, and their incompetency results in reflux and increased venous pressure. Communicating veins undergo similar changes through valvular damage or simply by exposure to chronically elevated pressure from the deep venous system. Some authorities feel a congenital valvular incompetence may also play a role, similar to varicose veins of the superficial system. Regardless of cause, high venous pressure generated by muscular contraction forces blood through damaged valves in communicating veins toward the superficial system, resulting in "ambulatory venous hypertension." Such venous hypertension results in edema, usually most prominent in the calf and ankle region. Indeed, swelling is one of the hallmarks of chronic venous insufficiency, and usually differentiates the problem from simple varicose veins. Swelling of the thigh may occur, denoting valvular incompetence at the ileofemoral level as well. Generally, this is less severe and less troublesome than the edema of the lower leg.

Venous hypertension leads to not only interstitial fluid accumulation, but also to extravasation of plasma proteins and red blood cells into subcutaneous tissues. In time, this results in brawny induration of the skin and pigmentation of the thickened but fragile tissue. The presence of edema and continual high venous pressure result in reduced local capillary flow and relative hypoxia, which further increase the likelihood of tissue breakdown and subsequent healing difficulties. Eventually these processes and accompanying infection lead to damage of the lymphatics, aggravating swelling and local tissue breakdown.

The presenting complaints of patients with chronic venous insufficiency usually center around swelling or ulceration of the lower leg. Chronic recurrent swelling causes a sensation of tightness or bursting, as well as heaviness or aching of the limb. Naturally, this if often worst at the end of the day, and may largely disappear overnight.

Thrombophlebitis

The cause of acute thrombus formation in the venous system is often unclear, but in most instances factors contributing to the three basic elements of Virchow's triad (intimal damage, stasis, and hypercoaguability) can be identified. *Superficial thrombophlebitis* almost always occurs in varicose veins and is clearly a result of static blood flow in these channels. Trauma may occasionally be implicated. In the upper extremity, the cause is most often iatrogenic following intravenous cannulation. On examination, there will be pain and tenderness along the course of the vein, which may also be palpated as a tender cord or knot. There is often an inflammatory erythema locally.

Superficial thrombophlebitis that occurs in several locations over a short time span is sometimes called *migratory superficial phlebitis.* It can be an important clue to a more serious underlying problem such as occult malignancy, especially carcinoma of the pancreas. A hypercoaguable state seems to occur because of the tumor.

Deep venous thrombophlebitis (DVT) is notoriously more variable in its clinical presentation than superficial thrombophlebitis. Although most authorities have now abandoned emphasis upon the distinction between thrombophlebitis and phlebothrombosis, there may be a tremendous difference in presenting complaints and physical findings. Limbs with little or no pain, swelling, or tenderness may harbor extensive deep venous clot, while others with similar pathology may have marked clinical symptoms and signs. Classically, the patient complains of pain in the limb, worse with motion, walking, or dependency and better with rest or elevation of the extremity. There is frequently some swelling below the level of venous occlusion and tenderness to calf compression. Calf pain produced by dorsiflexion of the foot, a positive Homans' sign, is a classic but often absent finding. With extensive deep venous thrombosis, a dusky cyanosis may be present. Engorged or prominent superficial veins may be apparent and are very suggestive of deep venous obstruction. Unilateral edema of the leg may be the only finding.

EVALUATION

Varicose Veins

On physical examination one should note the extent and location of the varicosities, and more importantly, look for signs suggesting pathology in the deep venous system: thrombophlebitis, stasis changes, ulceration, swelling, and the like. Complaints of leg pain should be carefully evaluated to rule out other possibilities, such as arterial insufficiency, orthopedic or joint disorders, or neurologic problems. Severe varicosities occurring at a young age suggest a congenital arteriovenous malformation, while varicosities appearing after trauma should always raise the question of an arteriovenous fistula, which may produce a bruit.

Venous Insufficiency

Venous insufficiency needs to be distinguished from other causes of leg edema such as lymphatic obstruction and hypoalbuminemia (see Chapter 16). Moreover, leg ulcerations may be due to chronic arterial disease, which also needs to be ruled out. One inquires about claudication involving thigh or calf, rest pain that is relieved by dependency, and numbness or paresthesias. On examination, arterial disease is manifested by absent pulses, dependent rubor, and atrophic changes as well as ulceration. Bruits may be heard in the groin. Noninvasive studies can be helpful (see Chapter 17).

Superficial Thrombophlebitis

Physical examination should strive to exclude other diagnoses that may be confused with superficial thrombophlebitis, such as cellulitis or lymphangitis. In the latter two, one notes the absence of a palpable thrombosed vein, widespread distribution of erythema and swelling beyond the course of a vein, and identification of a possible focus of infection. Musculoskeletal causes of pain and tenderness should be sought, as well as possible neurologic disorders such as neuritis or radicular pain (see Chapter 161). Swelling of the extremity should also be carefully noted, as isolated superficial phlebitis should not contribute to generalized edema.

Deep Vein Thrombophlebitis

An accurate initial evaluation of patients with pain or swelling of one or both legs is of great importance, as deep venous thrombosis has potentially serious consequences. Differential diagnosis includes an extensive list of problems that may cause pain or swelling of the extremities (see Chapters 16, 149, and 161). Truly unilateral swelling, particularly extending above the knee, makes venous thrombosis more likely, but cellulitis or lymphedema must be considered. Pain alone is an unreliable symptom. The findings of calf tenderness and a "positive" Homans' sign are by no means conclusive. Numerous studies have demonstrated the relative inaccuracy of diagnosis by clinical examination, which is incorrect in up to 50% of cases.

The dilemma, then, is accurate diagnosis. *Contrast venography* is the single most reliable technique for detecting deep venous thrombosis, and is often referred to as the "gold standard" of diagnostic evaluation to which other methods are usually compared. Routine venography, however, has several disadvantages that make it impractical to use in all instances. The technique is relatively expensive and not always available, the necessary equipment is not portable, and the test is moderately uncomfortable for the patient. Moreover, there is a very small risk of thrombophlebitis associated with the procedure.

For these reasons, a wide variety of noninvasive methods have been developed for screening and diagnosis of patients, or at least identifying those truly requiring contrast venography or hospitalization. A detailed description and evaluation of each method is beyond the scope of this chapter, but some comments can be made about the weaknesses and advantages of different techniques.

The *Doppler method* has proven itself the most widely available and versatile noninvasive test. It can be used on nearly every patient under a wide variety of circumstances, the results are available immediately, and the examination can be repeated as necessary. The study is safe, painless, and rapid. Its sensitivity and specificity, as compared with venography, is over 90% for venous thrombi in the major ileofemoral veins above the knee, the most clinically important area. It is relatively insensitive to smaller thrombi in calf vessels below the knee; however, risk of embolization is much lower in disease below the knee. The same results and considerations apply to other modern methods of noninvasive testing such as *impedance plethysmography* (IPG), air plethysmography (PVR), or phleborrheography.

The most sensitive method for detecting calf thrombi is *radioactive fibrinogen scanning,* utilizing [125]I. This test is extremely sensitive and accurate for venous thrombi in smaller veins below the knee. However, results are not immediately available, as serial scans are necessary. The expense, time, high false-positive rate, and general unavailability of ^{125}I-tagged fibrinogen make it an impractical test for widespread screening of patients. It is most useful in prospective studies of patients, or when combined with other noninvasive modalities, in which case high sensitivity and specificity can be obtained.

Our own diagnostic approach utilizes Doppler examination of both lower extremities, with abnormalities best compared to the contralateral limb. In our study of 167 patients with Doppler techniques, comparing results to venography, diagnosis of above-knee thrombi was excellent (sensitivity 92.4%, specificity 90.7%). Doppler ultrasonography was also most useful in symptomatic outpatients, because of the lower incidence of calf thrombi in this group.

Several conclusions can be drawn from information provided by noninvasive evaluation in detecting DVT. Patients with strongly positive studies can be considered to have DVT involving veins above the knee and anticoagulated without venography. Conversely, patients with normal studies can be confidently observed without anticoagulants, with minimal risk. Repeat noninvasive studies are indicated if the patient's symptoms persist or worsen. When laboratory studies are equivocal, tests should be repeated in 48–72 hours. Finally, venography is indicated in postphlebitic patients, likely to have chronically abnormal and therefore unreliable noninvasive studies, and in those patients with a disparity between clinical and laboratory findings.

Noninvasive studies have made a great contribution in evaluating patients with possible DVT. The cost savings alone related to patients found to be free of DVT, in whom venography, anticoagulation, and hospitalization are avoided, is enormous. The necessity of firmly establishing the diagnosis by means other than history or physical examination cannot be overemphasized.

MANAGEMENT
Varicose Veins

Management of varicose veins can very often be satisfactorily accomplished by nonoperative means, based upon appreciation of the principal problem of valve incompetence and poor soft tissue support. Untreated, most varicose veins will slowly worsen, and may lead to increasing difficulty and disability. All patients will benefit from proper *elastic support* of medium weight, together with periodic *elevation* of the extremity at intervals during the day. Elastic support is best achieved by a properly fitted surgical stocking obtained from a hospital or commercial surgical company such as Jobst. The various stockings sold in department or drug stores are usually of too light weight and improper fit. Ace wraps are cumbersome and often applied improperly, creating a "tourniquet" effect at the knee level. In almost all instances it is our practice to use only a below-knee stocking, because proper compression is difficult to achieve in the thigh, above-the-knee stockings are difficult to keep up, and patient compliance is considerably less. Fortunately, varicosities in the thigh are much less often associated with symptoms or complications.

In addition, obese patients are urged to *lose weight,* and women are reminded to *avoid* the use of *tight garters* or panty girdles, which will constrict superficial venous return at the thigh level. *Prolonged standing* should be avoided as much as feasible.

Sclerotherapy has some enthusiasts but is not currently in wide use. A sclerosing solution such as 3% Sotradecol is injected into the vein lumen and a pressure dressing applied and maintained for several weeks. An inflammatory reaction causing eventual fibrosis and obliteration of the vein lumen is hoped for. Although we occasionally employ this for a small isolated varix, particularly a residual vein following surgical therapy, in our opinion, sclerotherapy is not indicated in the primary treatment of varicose veins.

Indications for surgical referral generally include persistently symptomatic varicose veins (particularly if a conservative program has been tried), cosmetic dissatisfaction, or recurrent episodes of superficial thrombophlebitis. The option of surgical therapy should probably be discussed initially, because some patients, particularly young women, will prefer this to chronic use of elastic support. In most instances of primary varicose veins, an excellent result can be expected from surgery with extremely low morbidity and a hospitalization of only 2 to 3 days. In experienced hands, the "recurrence" rate of varicose veins should be less than 10%.

Venous Insufficiency

Treatment of venous insufficiency is best initiated before the occurrence of venous ulceration, which will follow in many untreated cases. An understanding of the pathophysiology again emphasizes the importance of elastic support and periodic elevation of the extremity. *Patient education* is essential, because compliance is poor otherwise. A *knee-length heavyweight elastic stocking* is prescribed and must be worn religiously from the moment the patient gets out of bed until retiring at night. The leg is best elevated on a pillow or by raising the entire foot of the bed at night. *Periodic elevation* during the day is essential in most patients; it must be emphasized to the patient that the leg should be above the level of the heart for this to be effective. This must be done as often as necessary to prevent formation of edema. *Mild diuretic therapy (e.g.,* hydrochlorothiazide 50 mg qd) may be of some help in stubborn edema. The chronic and incurable nature of the problem must be made clear to the patient, while reassurance given that symptoms and problems are controllable and preventable by strict adherence to the above program.

Progression to the point of *ulceration* creates a much more troublesome problem. The ulcers may occur with even minor and unrecalled trauma due to atrophic, vulnerable skin and subcutaneous tissues. They usually occur in the lower medial leg just above the medial malleolus, usually overlying an incompetent communicating vein. These lesions will be refractory to all methods of care as long as venous hypertension from the incompetent deep system continues to be transmitted to the superficial tissues. Secondary infection (bacterial or fungal) is common, further impairing any chance for local tissue repair.

Management at this stage is much more difficult, time consuming, and often expensive. Preferred treatment is an extended period of *bed rest* with *elevation* of the involved extremity well above heart level at all times, combined with *wet to dry saline dressings* to the ulceration, applied three times daily. Hopefully such a program can be carried out at home by the family, perhaps with the help of a visiting nurse. Healing may be anticipated over a 2- to 4-week period. Hospitalization is generally not necessary unless dictated by social circumstances. Any infection should be cultured and treated appropriately with oral antibiotics; staphylococci and gram-negative rods are common. The patient should be urged to exercise the calf muscles repeatedly while in bed, ideally against a footboard, to minimize the occurrence of acute deep venous thrombosis.

Alternatively, particularly for patients who cannot afford extensive time off their feet, an *Unna paste venous boot* may be employed. Properly applied, this medicated bandage can supply good compression, does not require much patient cooperation, and allows the patient to remain ambulatory. Such boot dressings are best changed every 7 to 10 days. With some experience, many venous ulcers may be successfully handled in this fashion. Once healed, chronic use of a heavy-weight elastic stocking is resumed.

Surgical referral is advisable for recurrent or nonhealing ulcerations, because surgical interruption of incompetent communicating veins underlying these areas, together with stripping and ligation of associated superficial varicosities, may be indicated. In recent years, some surgeons have reported good results with direct repair of incompetent venous valves, or interposition of a competent valve from an arm vein into the deep venous system of the leg. Insufficient long-term experience exists, however, to ascertain the usefulness of such surgical therapy at this time.

Superficial Thrombophlebitis

Superficial thrombophlebitis in the lower leg is best managed by a combination of local heat, and compression with a good elastic stocking. Anti-inflammatory agents such as aspirin or one of the other nonsteroidal drugs may be useful. Antibiotics have no role. Women taking birth control pills should probably discontinue their use. The patient should avoid sitting or standing, but remain ambulatory to minimize the chance of developing any associated clot in the deep venous system. Pain and inflammation usually resolve within 1 to 2 weeks.

If superficial phlebitis extends above the knee, consideration of anticoagulation or ligation of the saphenous vein at the level of the saphenofemoral junction in the groin may be indicated, and surgical consultation should be considered. This is particularly true if the process has ascended while under treatment and observation. The rationale for such a policy is the increased risk of extension of thrombus into the deep system.

Deep Vein Thrombophlebitis

Deep vein thrombophlebitis above the knee is associated with a high risk of thromboembolization and requires immediate hospitalization for heparin therapy and subsequent initiation of oral anticoagulation. There are no definitive data on how long to continue oral anticoagulation, although it is customary to maintain therapy for 3 months after the first episode and for a longer period if there are recurrent bouts of thrombophlebitis. Data from randomized studies comparing high- and low-dose warfarin and warfarin versus "mini-dose" heparin for chronic therapy show that low-dose warfarin is the most cost effective.

ANNOTATED BIBLIOGRAPHY

Bergan JJ, Flinn WR, Yao JST: Clinical application of noninvasive testing in venous disease. In Kempczinski RF, Yao JST (eds): Practical Noninvasive Vascular Diagnosis, p. 389. Chicago, Year Book Medical Publishers, 1982 (*Useful review of current noninvasive testing methods available for venous disease, with proper perspective on their clinical role.*)

Cranley JJ, Canos AJ, Sull WJ: The diagnosis of deep venous thrombosis: Fallibility of clinical symptoms and signs. Arch Surg 111: 34, 1976 (*Documentation of the inaccuracy of clinical diagnosis.*)

Hanel KC, Abbott WM, Reidy NC et al: The role of two noninvasive tests in deep venous thrombosis. Ann Surg 194:725, 1981 (*A prospective study comparing accuracy and usefulness of Doppler ultrasonography and segmental air plethysmography, as compared with venography, in detection of DVT.*)

Hobb JJ: Surgery and sclerotherapy in the treatment of varicose veins. Arch Surg 109:793, 1974 (*Good review of treatment for this common problem, focusing on the advantages and proper indications for the use of each modality.*)

Huisman MV, Buller HR, tenCate JW et al: Serial impedance plethysmography for suspected deep venous thrombosis in outpatients. N Engl J Med 314:823, 1986 (*Found to be nearly equal to venography for detection of deep venous thrombosis.*)

Hull RD, Rascob GE, Hirsh J et al: A cost-effect analysis of alternative approaches for long term treatment of proximal venous thrombosis. JAMA 252:239, 1984 (*An analysis and review of data from randomized trials of alternative anticoagulant therapies, indicating that low dose oral therapy is the most cost-effective.*)

Juergens JL, Lofgren KA: Chronic venous insufficiency (postphlebitic syndrome, chronic venous stasis). In Juergens JL, Spittell JA Jr, Fairbairn JF II (eds): Peripheral Vascular Diseases, p. 809. Philadelphia, WB Saunders, 1980 (*Excellent discussion of the pathophysiology and clinical management of chronic venous insufficiency.*)

Linton RR: Post-thrombotic ulceration of the lower extremity: Its etiology and surgical management. Ann Surg 138:415, 1953 (*Classic article on the etiology and management of venous ulcerations.*)

Strandness DE, Langlois Y, Kramer M et al: Long term sequelae of acute venous thrombosis. JAMA 250:1289, 1983 (*Long-term sequelae including hyperpigmentation, pain, and swelling were not uncommon and were associated with occluded on incompetent distal deep veins.*)

31
Exercise Stress Testing
GREGORY D. CURFMAN, M.D.

The exercise stress test has become a widely employed method for detection of coronary artery disease. Assessments of exercise capacity, ventricular dysrhythmias, severity of coronary disease, and efficacy of antianginal therapy can also be accomplished by exercise testing. At present, the predominant method of exercise testing is continuous ECG monitoring of the patient during treadmill or stationary bicycle exercise. Thallium imaging techniques improve diagnostic accuracy in the detection of coronary disease, but also add substantially to the cost. The primary physician needs to know the sensitivity, specificity, and predictive value of the ECG exercise test and the factors that affect these parameters to appropriately order the study and properly interpret its results.

PHYSIOLOGICAL BASIS OF THE TEST

A complete assessment of the cardiovascular system often requires an evaluation of cardiovascular function under conditions of the enhanced metabolic demands of exercise. Evaluation of the heart in the resting state only reveals part of the story. The exercise stress test assesses the ability of the coronary circulation to supply sufficient blood to meet the increase in myocardial oxygen requirements generated by exercise. Since the rate of oxygen extraction by the heart is relatively fixed, increased oxygen supply is usually achieved by an increase in coronary blood flow. When stenosis limits adequate blood supply, ischemia may result, often manifested by anginal pain, ECG changes, or perfusion defects on a thallium scan. The demand placed upon the coronary circulation can be quantitated; the product of heart rate times systolic blood pressure closely parallels the measured myocardial oxygen consumption during isotonic exercise. Heart rate alone is almost as good an indicator of oxygen consumption. Since known quantities of work are being performed, the exercise stress test can provide a measure of exercise capacity as well as aid in detection of coronary disease.

APPROACHES TO EXERCISE TESTING

Exercise testing for detection of coronary disease generally utilizes dynamic (isotonic) rather than sustained-contraction (isometric) exercise. Isotonic exercise permits smoother increases in the rate–pressure product to be accomplished, allowing the patient's ischemic threshold to be approached gradually. Nevertheless, isometric exercise testing (*e.g.,* by sustained handgrip) can be of use in special situations, such as in assessing the safety of isometric activities in patients with known coronary disease.

Isotonic exercise testing protocols are divided into maximal and submaximal types, depending upon the level of exercise achieved during the test. A *maximal test* is defined as one in which systemic oxygen consumption reaches a plateau before exercise is terminated. Only by making serial measurements of oxygen consumption can one be certain that maximal exertion has been achieved. Because it is often not convenient to measure oxygen consumption during routine exercise testing, maximal effort is usually approximated by exercising the individual to his or her age-adjusted predicted maximal heart rate. Values for maximal predicted heart rate can be obtained from standardized tables or regression formulas, but the value 220 minus age in years for men and 210 minus age for women provide reasonable approximations of the true maximal heart rate. If a patient is receiving a beta-adrenergic blocking agent, the maximal predicted heart rate is not useful in judging when maximal effort has been accomplished. In this situation maximal effort can be approximated by having the patient exercise to exhaustion. The level of effort expended during the test can be assessed semiquantitatively using the scale of perceived exertion developed by Borg. If perceived effort is "very very hard" (19 or 20 on Borg's scale) at the termination of the test, it can be reasonably assumed that maximal exertion has been closely approximated.

A *submaximal exercise test* is by definition one in which maximal systemic oxygen consumption is not achieved. The test may be terminated prematurely by design (at a certain percentage of predicted maximal heart rate or at a given level of systemic oxygen consumption), or it may be terminated because of the appearance of angina, marked ischemic electrocardiographic changes, cardiac arrhythmias, severe hypertension, or hypotension. Tests terminated prematurely because a certain percentage of predicted maximal heart rate has been achieved are generally less useful than maximal exercise tests. Such submaximal tests provide little information about exercise capacity, and they often give less diagnostic information. In general it is best to continue the test to the predicted maximum heart rate, to maximal perceived effort, or until a pathologic event (angina, ischemia, arrhythmia, hypotension) occurs. One clinical situation in which submaximal testing has proved useful is in patients early *after myocardial infarction.* In this setting submaximal exercise testing to a 5 MET level (1 MET = 3.5 ml O_2 consumed/kg/min) has been useful in identifying patients at higher risk for subsequent coronary events and death.

Most maximal and submaximal tests are *multistage,* that is graded amounts of work are performed, with progressive increase in work load between stages. The objective of graded exercise is to obtain the greatest increase in heart rate before musculoskeletal fatigue limits the amount of exercise that the patient can perform. The previously used Master's exercise test was a single stage step test in which the intensity and amount of exercise were fixed; the test had a high rate of false-negative results because many patients did not sufficiently increase their heart rates during the performance of the test. Another disadvantage of Master's test was its inability to provide continuous ECG monitoring; ECGs were taken before and after exercise only, often reducing the amount of information available from the test.

Currently the *treadmill* and *bicycle ergometer* are the most popular devices used for exercise testing. Slightly higher values for maximal oxygen consumption can usually be obtained on the treadmill than on the bicycle ergometer, because a somewhat larger muscle mass is called upon during treadmill exercise. Many different exercise testing protocols are available for the treadmill and bicycle. Although the treadmill protocol developed by Bruce is very popular, it has the disadvantages of unequal changes in work load between stages, and a very abrupt increase in work load at stage IV, which is too vigorous for many cardiac patients. The protocols developed by Balke are characterized by a constant increment in work load from one stage to the next, and by a constant treadmill speed (walking pace), which is tolerated well by most patients.

Walking protocols are generally preferred over protocols that require running for diagnostic purposes in unfit populations. Bicycle ergometer protocols usually consist of 2- to 3-minute stages in which work load is increased by 10 to 30 W per stage, depending upon the level of physical conditioning of the subject. For both treadmill and bicycle tests, it is best to select a protocol that will allow the patient to reach maximal exertion within a 10- to 12-minute period. A longer test may be limited by an individual's endurance, and a shorter test usually increases the work load too rapidly.

Continuous *ECG monitoring* is employed during exercise testing. A modified V_5 lead (CM_5) is the one most commonly monitored. Test sensitivity can be increased by employing a three-lead system, since the CM_5 lead may not detect inferior ischemic changes. Further increases in sensitivity can be expected from recording 12-lead ECGs during exercise. In our own laboratory three leads are recorded each minute during exercise and 12 leads are recorded every 3 minutes. Because ischemic changes may not occur on the ECG until *after* exercise, monitoring is continued for at least 5 to 7 minutes into the recovery phase.

SENSITIVITY, SPECIFICITY, AND PREDICTIVE VALUE

ECG Testing

Myocardial ischemia may be manifested during the exercise stress test by ECG changes, by abnormal blood pressure and heart rate responses, or by angina. ECG changes, particularly alterations in ST segments that occur during exercise in the context of ischemia, have received the most attention and study. Sensitivity and specificity of ST segment changes in the diagnosis of coronary disease have been determined by correlating ECG findings with results of coronary angiography.

A number of factors affect sensitivity and specificity of the exercise test, including *severity of the underlying coronary disease* and the ECG criteria used for diagnosis of ischemia. For example, test sensitivity using the criterion of ST segment depression increased in one study from 40% to 76% as the extent of disease went from one-vessel to three-vessel stenosis. The *magnitude of ST segment depression* required for diagnosis affects sensitivity and specificity. One can achieve an increase in sensitivity by reducing the amount of ST depression required for the designation of ischemia, but at the cost of lowering specificity and obtaining more false-positive results. An analysis of pooled data showed that when the criterion for diagnosis of ischemia was 1 to 1.5 mm of ST depression, sensitivity was 23.3% and specificity 89%. When the amount of ST depression required was raised to 1.5 to 2 mm range, sensitivity fell to 8.8%, but specificity rose to 97.8%. This trade-off between sensitivity and specificity is characteristic of all tests having a quantitative standard for diagnosis (see Chapter 2).

Other aspects of *ST segment* change have been examined to improve sensitivity and specificity. Configuration of the ST segment has been subjected to careful study. A downsloping ST segment (Fig. 31–1) was found to have a specificity of 99%. Horizontal or plane depression of the ST had a specificity of 85%, and a slowly upsloping ST (greater than or equal to 1.5 mm ST depression at 0.08 second after the J point) had a specificity of 68%. Simple J-point depression without a slowly upsloping ST is a nonspecific finding and not diagnostic of ischemia. When the criterion for an ischemic response was at least 1 mm of downsloping or horizontal ST segment depression, the exercise test was found to have a sensitivity of 64% and a specificity of 93%. When a slowly upsloping ST was added to the list of acceptable criteria for ischemia, sensitivity increased to 76%, but at the expense of specificity, which fell to 82%.

A number of other factors alter the sensitivity and specificity of the ECG exercise test, including the *type of exercise protocol* used (submaximal tests appear to be less sensitive) and the *number of leads* used (a three-lead system improves sensitivity by about 10% over a single-lead system). The specificity of ST changes is limited by the fact that ST depression is not unique to coronary disease. Patients with valvular or

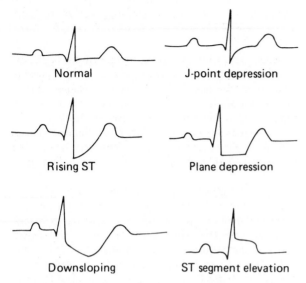

Figure 31-1. Exercise-induced ST segment changes.

hypertensive disease, nonischemic myocardial disease, and pre-excitation syndromes may demonstrate ST segment depression during exercise in the absence of ischemia. In addition, left ventricular hypertrophy, recent glucose ingestion, hypokalemia, and sedatives may produce *false-positive results*. Digitalis glycosides are notorious for their ability to cause deviations in ST segments. If possible, it is best to discontinue digitalis for at least 48 hours prior to testing. If this is not feasible, then exercise-associated ischemia should not be diagnosed until at least 2 minutes of ST segment depression is observed. Studies have also suggested that false-positive responses may be more common in women than in men by a factor as high as 3.

Investigators have searched for *other changes* that occur during the exercise test that might help to better identify patients with coronary disease. The changes in ST segments that occur with exercise do not provide a definite answer, but rather a probability statement of the likelihood of the patient having coronary disease. Among other variables studies have been *timing and duration of ST changes,* presence and severity of *ventricular dysrhythmias, heart rate* and *blood pressure changes,* and the coexistence of *exercise-induced angina.* In a recent series of 302 patients undergoing exercise testing and coronary angiography, the occurrence of *typical angina* during exercise had a sensitivity of 51% and specificity of 90%, compared with 76% sensitivity and 76% specificity for ST segment changes alone. In essence, exercise-induced angina had about the same diagnostic significance as did ST changes, especially when predictive values for these changes in the appropriate populations were compared.

A study that factored in all the possible exercise-induced variables that might help predict the presence of coronary

disease (ST configuration, depth of ST depression, timing of onset and duration of ST changes, occurrence of hypotension or inappropriately slow heart rate, and presence of malignant ventricular irritability) found only a 10% to 15% increase in test accuracy compared to that obtained by analyzing degree of ST segment depression alone. Some investigators are examining changes in R wave amplitude to see if these might contribute diagnostic information.

Knowledge of test sensitivity and specificity and attempts to improve them still do not provide the clinician with an estimate of the probability that coronary disease is present when a positive test result is encountered (*i.e.,* the predictive accuracy or predictive value positive of the test). Figures for the predictive accuracy of the exercise stress test have varied greatly from series to series, and between men and women, presumably because of wide differences in the prevalence of underlying coronary disease in the populations studied. The predictive accuracy of any diagnostic test is directly related to the prevalence of the disease in the population examined (see Chapter 2). As a result, a test will have a low predictive accuracy when disease prevalence is low, regardless of how sensitive and specific the test is.

Asymptomatic patients with few or no risk factors for coronary disease who are subjected to exercise testing and demonstrate "ischemic" changes are less likely to have underlying coronary disease and more likely to have a false-positive test. Therefore, asymptomatic individuals with an abnormal stress test should be screened carefully for possible causes of a false-positive response. In asymptomatic populations, abnormal ST segment responses should be viewed as a "risk factor" for coronary disease rather than as definite evidence of the disease. In these individuals, the incidence of coronary disease is about 6%, rising to 12% by the sixth decade.

Prevalence of coronary disease has been found to be 16% in patients with nonanginal chest pain, 50% in those with atypical pain, and 89% when typical angina is present. Consequently, the predictive value of a positive test is expected to be greatest in *patients with typical angina,* but in such instances the history of angina is almost as good as the test's predictive value (about 90%) in diagnosing coronary disease. The very high figures initially reported for the diagnostic utility and accuracy of the exercise test resulted from studies conducted on a referred population that had a high probability of coronary disease in the opinion of the referring physicians; these were the people in whom angiography was deemed most appropriate.

In essence, the exercise test adds little to the diagnosis of coronary disease in patients with typical angina, although exercise testing may be very useful in such patients to quantitate the amount of exertion required to induce ischemia, to obtain preliminary information about the extent of coronary disease (see Chapter 25), and to assess the efficacy of antianginal therapy. Also, exercise testing in asymptomatic individuals may produce false-positive responses, and care must be taken to avoid factors that may lead to a false-positive result. The test may be of help in diagnosis of *patients with atypical anginal pain* as long as the criteria for atypical pain are rather rigid (*e.g.*, two or three characteristics of classic angina must be present) though other features may be absent. In such settings, the predictive accuracy has been in the order to 40% to 50%. In general, exercise testing has its greatest diagnostic usefulness in individuals whose pretest likelihood of having coronary disease is moderate. An example would be a male over the age of 50 with an atypical chest pain syndrome and one or two coronary risk factors. In this situation a positive exercise test would substantially increase the post-test likelihood of underlying coronary disease, but a negative test would substantially reduce it.

Radionuclide Scan

Further attempts to improve the sensitivity and specificity of the exercise test have led to the development of radionuclide imaging techniques, such as the use of *Thallium 201,* which is taken up by myocardial cells via the sodium pump, similar to potassium ions. Thallium is distributed to the myocardium according to the regional coronary blood flow, and underperfused areas will take up less of the isotope and will appear as "cold" spots on the perfusion scan. When Thallium 201 is injected intravenously during exercise, myocardial uptake of the isotope is determined by regional differences in myocardial blood flow at the time of injection. Areas of myocardium that appear underperfused during exercise may "fill in" later during the 2 to 4 hours after exercise. Therefore, sequential scanning during and after exercise is required to diagnose hemodynamically significant coronary stenoses. Thallium scintigraphy has proved especially valuable in patients who have resting repolarization abnormalities on the ECG or left bundle branch block, both of which render interpretation of the standard exercise test difficult. Thallium scanning is also useful in patients whose standard exercise test results are suspected to be false positive or false negative. Thallium scans may demonstrate the size of the underperfused area of myocardium, information that can be useful in deciding whether coronary angiography should be performed for further evaluation of the patient.

Dipyridamole–thallium imaging represents a technique for noninvasively assessing coronary perfusion in patients unable to undergo exercise testing. Dipyridamole induces maximal coronary vasodilation; when used in conjunction with thallium myocardial imaging, the test has a sensitivity and specificity for detection of significant coronary disease comparable to that of exercise thallium imaging.

OTHER APPLICATIONS OF EXERCISE TESTING

1. Severity of Known Coronary Disease can be assessed by exercise stress testing. Factors correlating with severity and extensiveness of disease include depth of ST segment depression, early onset of ST changes, persistence of ST segment depression past 8 minutes into the recovery period, downward sloping ST configuration, hypotensive response at low workloads, and impairment of heart rate response to exercise (see Chapter 25). In addition, occurrence of both angina and ischemic changes during exercise have been reported to predict an increased likelihood of multivessel disease. Increase in R wave amplitude has been implicated as a sign of two- or three-vessel disease.

2. Assessment of Prognosis of Patients in the early postinfarction period may be aided by exercise testing. The greater the work load tolerated, the better the prognosis. Patients who developed angina on a limited exercise test conducted just before hospital discharge had twice the rate of postinfarction angina. Those with no ST segment changes had a 2.1% 1-year mortality, compared with a 27% mortality for those who did develop ST segment depression during exercise testing.

3. Determination of Exercise Capacity can be provided by the exercise stress test, since the patient is made to perform known quantities of work under direct observation and continuous ECG monitoring. This determination is essential for designing a safe cardiac rehabilitation program and may help to reassure the patient who is unnecessarily restricting activity out of fear of sudden death or infarction. The work level achieved during the test can be used to define the degree of incapacity (when it is in question) as well as provide guidelines for establishing safe levels of daily activity for the patient.

4. Detection of Ventricular Dysrhythmias can sometimes be facilitated by exercise testing, especially if the rhythm disturbance is believed to be exercise induced. However, except in a few cases of ventricular tachycardia, Holter monitoring (ambulatory ECG monitoring) was found in a careful study to be superior for detecting most types of ventricular irritability (see Chapers 20 and 24). Holter monitoring should be ordered in conjunction with an exercise test if the objective is optimal detection of dysrhythmias (see Chapter 20).

SAFETY AND CONTRAINDICATIONS

Reported mortality in a multicenter study involving 170,000 exercise tests was 0.01%. There was no relationship to the type of test or to exercise intensity. Morbidity requiring hospitalization was 0.2%. Safety is enhanced by a pre-examination history, a physical examination, and a resting ECG. Patients with unstable angina, uncompensated congestive failure, severe anemia, high-grade heart block, severe aortic stenosis, cor pulmonale, or severe hypertension should not undergo testing. A physician should be present throughout, and a defibrillator and other resuscitation equipment should be in the room. The test should be terminated if blood pressure or heart rate falls suddenly during exercise, or if exhaustion, angina, faintness, marked ST changes, severe hypertension, or serious arrhythmias occur (ventricular tachycardia, heart block, etc.). When performed by experienced personnel, exercise testing is very safe and is one of the most useful noninvasive tests for evaluating cardiovascular function and disease.

ANNOTATED BIBLIOGRAPHY

Bartel AG, Behar US, Peter US et al: Graded exercise stress tests in angiographically documented coronary artery disease. Circulation 49:348, 1974 (*Classic paper demonstrating that the depth of ST segment depression correlated with severity and extent of coronary disease.*)

Bruce RA: Methods of exercise testing. Am J Cardiol 33:715, 1974 (*A concise and thorough discussion of the differences in various methods of stress testing by one of the pioneers in the field.*)

Cohn K, Kamm B, Feteih N et al: Use of treadmill score to quantify ischemic response and predict extent of coronary disease. Circulation 59:286, 1979 (*Test accuracy using a multifactorial analysis was improved by only 10% to 15% over that achieved by use of ST criteria alone for evaluation of stress test results. Factors studied in the analysis included duration and onset of ST changes, blood pressure and heart rate responses, coexistence of exercise-induced chest pain, severity of ventricular irritability and magnitude and configuration of ST segment changes.*)

Council on Scientific Affairs, AMA: Indications and contraindications for exercise testing. JAMA 246:1015, 1981 (*Lists indications for exercise testing as well as absolute and relative contraindications.*)

Ellestad MH, Cooke BM, Greenberg PS: Stress testing: Clinical application and predictive capacity. Prog Cardiovasc Dis 21:431, 1979 (*A worthwhile review with emphasis on specificity, sensivity, and predictive value of the stress test. Also discusses recent work on utility of R wave changes in test interpretation. 144 references.*)

Epstein SE: Value and limitations of the electrocardiographic response to exercise in the assessment of patients with coronary artery disease. Am J Cardiol 42:667, 1978 (*Argues that the predictive value of the stress test is so low in asymptomatic patients that the test should not be used to screen for coronary disease. Agrees on its judicious use in symptomatic patients for providing information on prognosis and severity.*)

Epstein SE, Palmeri ST, Patterson RE: Evaluation of patients after acute myocardial infarction. N Engl J Med 307:1487, 1982 (*A somewhat controversial analysis of diagnostic tests available to select post-MI patients for coronary angiography.*)

Fortuin NJ, Weiss JA: Exercise stress testing. Circulation 56:699, 1977 (*Excellent, detailed review with 126 references.*)

Goldschlager N: Use of the treadmill test in the diagnosis of coronary artery disease in patients with chest pain. Ann Intern Med 97:383, 1982 (*An analytic review of the exercise stress test including an algorhythmic approach to atypical chest pain and a description of the role of thallium stress scintigraphy.*)

Leppo JA, Boucher CA, Okada RD et al: Serial thallium-201 myocardial imaging following dipyridamole infusion. Circulation 66:649, 1982 (*Diagnostic utility for detection of ischemic disease equalled that of exercise stress testing.*)

Martin CM, McConahay DR: Maximum treadmill exercise electrocardiography. Circulation 46:956, 1972 (*Provides data on the changes in sensitivity and specificity associated with different diagnostic criteria. When 0.5 mm ST depression is used, false-positive rate equals 43% and falls to 11% with 1.0 mm criteria.*)

Rifkin RD, Hood WB: Bayesian analysis of electrocardiographic exercise stress testing. N Engl J Med 297:681, 1977 (*Argues that the results of the stress test should be viewed as a probability statement, rather than as "positive" or "negative"; emphasizes the predictive value of various test results and the dependence of the predictive value on the prevalence of the disease in the population being studied.*)

Theroux PT, Waters DD, Halphen C et al: Prognostic value of exercise testing soon after myocardial infarction. N Engl J Med 301:341, 1979 (Performance of a limited treadmill test just prior to hospital discharge provided useful prognostic information.)

Weiner DA, Ryan TJ, McCabe CH et al: Exercise stress testing. N Engl J Med 301:230, 1979 (*A detailed study of data from the Coronary Artery Surgery Study examining the influence of the prevalence of coronary artery disease on the diagnostic accuracy of stress testing.*)

Weiner DA, McCabe C, Heuter DC et al: The predictive value of anginal chest pain as an indicator of coronary disease during exercise testing. Am Heart J 96:458, 1978 (*The occurrence of anginal pain during exercise was found to be as predictive of coronary disease as ischemic ECG changes alone.*)

4

Respiratory Problems

32
Health Consequences of Smoking
NANCY A. RIGOTTI, M.D.

Cigarette smoking is the major preventable cause of death in America, contributing to an estimated 350,000 deaths annually. Epidemiologic and experimental evidence has identified cigarette smoking as the primary cause of lung cancer and chronic obstructive pulmonary disease, and as a major risk factor for coronary heart disease. Smoking has been associated with other cancers, cerebrovascular and peripheral vascular diseases, and peptic ulcer disease. Smokers also suffer more acute respiratory illness. Maternal smoking during pregnancy increases risks to the fetus, and nonsmokers chronically exposed to tobacco smoke may suffer health consequences.

Although the epidemiologic case against cigarettes is convincing, the pathophysiology of the observed effects is not as well understood. Cigarette smoke, consisting of particles dispersed in a gas phase, is a complex mixture of thousands of compounds produced by the incomplete combustion of the tobacco leaf. Smoke constituents strongly implicated in causing disease are nicotine and tar in the particulate phase and carbon monoxide in the gas phase.

Strong evidence supports the benefits of smoking cessation, even for smokers with cardiopulmonary disease. Most smokers know that smoking has health risks and express the desire to quit, but find it difficult to do so. Some have turned to pipes, cigars, or cigarettes with reduced tar and nicotine yields in the belief that doing so reduces the danger of smoking. Smokers who become ill are more likely to stop smoking and are more susceptible to antismoking interventions. Changing the behavior of smokers should be a high priority for the primary care physician (see Chapter 49).

SMOKING AND PREMATURE MORTALITY

Smokers have a 70% higher mortality rate than nonsmokers. The risk of dying increases with the amount and duration of smoking and is higher in smokers who inhale. Coronary heart disease is the chief contributor to the excess mortality among cigarette smokers, followed by lung cancer and chronic obstructive pulmonary disease. Life expectancy is significantly shortened by smoking cigarettes.

SMOKING AND CANCER

The epithelium of the mouth, pharynx, larynx, and tracheobronchial tree is repetitively exposed to tobacco smoke containing many known carcinogens. These induce dysplastic changes in the epithelial cells, from which neoplasias are thought to arise. Smoke also dissolves in the saliva and is swallowed, exposing the upper gastrointestinal tract to carcinogens.

A strong association between smoking and *lung cancer* has been demonstrated in multiple prospective and retrospective epidemiologic studies, and corroborated by autopsy and animal experimental evidence. Lung cancer has been the leading cause of cancer death in men since the 1950s, and it surpassed breast cancer as the leading cause of cancer death in women in 1985. Male smokers have a tenfold higher risk of developing lung cancer, and the risk increases with the number of cigarettes smoked. Smokers exposed to asbestos or uranium are at especially high risk. The histologic types most clearly implicated are squamous cell and oat cell.

There is also strong evidence that smoking is a major cause of *cancers* of the *larynx, oral cavity,* and *esophagus.* The risk of these cancers increases with the intensity of exposure to cigarette smoke and is accelerated by alcohol consumption. Epidemiologic studies show an association between smoking and cancers of the bladder, pancreas, stomach, and uterine cervix. The evidence for causality is less strong for these cancers, and mechanisms of carcinogenesis are less clear.

SMOKING AND CARDIOVASCULAR DISEASE

Cigarette smoking is a major independent risk factor for *coronary artery disease.* Retrospective and prospective epidemiologic studies have demonstrated a strong relationship between smoking and coronary morbidity and mortality in both men and women. The coronary disease death rate in smokers is 70% higher than in nonsmokers, and the risk increases with the amount of cigarette exposure. The risk of sudden death is two to four times higher in smokers. Smoking is also a risk factor for recurrent cardiac arrest. In addition to increased coronary mortality, smokers have a higher risk of nonfatal myocardial infarction or unstable angina. Patients with angina lower their exercise tolerance if they smoke. Women who smoke and use oral contraceptives or postmenopausal estrogen replacement greatly increase their risk of myocardial infarction.

The *pathophysiologic mechanisms* are not all identified. Autopsy studies demonstrate more atheromatous changes in smokers than nonsmokers. Carbon monoxide in cigarette smoke decreases oxygen delivery to endothelial tissue, which may contribute to atherogenesis. In addition, smoking may trigger acute ischemia. Carbon monoxide decreases myocardial oxygen supply, while nicotine increases myocardial demand by releasing catecholamines that raise blood pressure, heart rate, and contractility. Carbon monoxide and nicotine also induce platelet aggregation that may cause occlusion of narrowed vessels.

Cigarette smoking is the most important risk factor for *peripheral vascular disease.* In patients with intermittent claudication, smoking lowers exercise tolerance and may shorten graft survival after vascular surgery. Smokers have more aortic atherosclerosis and an increased risk of dying from a ruptured aortic aneurysm. Smokers under age 65 have a higher risk of dying from cerebrovascular disease, and women who smoke have a greater risk of subarachnoid hemorrhage, especially if they also use oral contraceptives.

SMOKING AND PULMONARY DISEASE

Cigarette smoking is the primary cause of chronic bronchitis and emphysema. Smokers have a 5- to 25-fold increased risk of dying from chronic obstructive pulmonary disease, depending on the amount they smoke. Smoking activates leukocytes and alveolar macrophages to release proteases that can damage bronchioles and may contribute to the pathogenesis of chronic lung disease. Smokers have a higher prevalence of respiratory symptoms (cough, sputum, and dyspnea) than nonsmokers. Studies of pulmonary function indicate that impairment exists in asymptomatic as well as symptomatic smokers. Small airways dysfunction is the first pulmonary function abnormality to develop in smokers and may be a precursor of chronic lung disease. Smokers also have an increase in the normal age-related decline in FEV_1.

Smokers have a higher risk of acute as well as chronic pulmonary disease. Inhaling cigarette smoke impairs pulmonary clearance mechanisms by paralyzing ciliary transport. This may explain the susceptibility to viral respiratory infections, including influenza. Smokers who develop acute respiratory infections have longer and more severe courses, with a more prolonged cough.

OTHER HEALTH CONSEQUENCES

Smokers have a higher prevalence of *peptic ulcer disease* and a higher case–fatality rate. Duodenal ulcer patients who smoke are more likely to develop recurrent ulcers. Preliminary studies have reported a lower prevalence of ulcerative colitis in smokers. In case reports, smoking cessation has been associated with worsening of symptoms, and return to smoking with clinical improvement. This is a tentative association that may not be causal.

Smoking has been associated with increased *osteoporosis* in men and postmenopausal women. Female smokers weigh less than nonsmokers and have an earlier age of menopause; both of these factors are associated with osteoporosis and may contribute to the relationship between smoking and osteoporosis. Moreover, smoking depresses serum estrogen levels in postmenopausal women taking estrogen replacement therapy.

Maternal smoking during pregnancy contributes to fetal growth retardation. Infants born to mothers who smoke weigh an average of 200 g less but have no shorter gestations than infants of nonsmoking mothers. Carbon monoxide in smoke may decrease oxygen availability to the fetus and account for the growth retardation. Smoking during pregnancy has also been linked with higher rates of spontaneous abortion, fetal death, and neonatal death.

RELATED RISKS

Passive Smoking (Environmental Smoke Exposure)

Nonsmokers involuntarily inhale the smoke of nearby smokers, a phenomenon known as passive smoking. When smoking occurs in enclosed areas with poor ventilation, such as in buses, bars, and conference rooms, high levels of smoke exposure can occur. Acute exposure to smoke-contaminated air decreases exercise capacity in healthy nonsmokers and can worsen symptoms in individuals with angina, chronic obstructive pulmonary disease, or asthma.

Chronic exposure to smoky air occurs in the workplace and in the homes of smokers. Nonsmokers in smoky workplaces develop small-airways dysfunction similar to that observed in light smokers. Compared to the children of nonsmokers, children whose parents smoke have more respiratory infections throughout childhood, a higher risk of asthma, and alterations in pulmonary function tests. The long-term significance of physiologic changes in children and workers is not known. Because the evidence is not conclusive at present, a link between passive smoking and lung cancer is still controversial. In recent studies of nonsmoking women, those married to smokers had higher lung cancer rates than those married to nonsmokers. Chronic smoke exposure has not been associated with an increased incidence of cardiopulmonary disease in nonsmokers.

Pipe and Cigar Smoking

Because pipe and cigar smokers inhale less than cigarette smokers, smoke exposure is limited to the oropharynx, larynx, and esophagus. Their death rates for cancers at these sites are similar to the rates in cigarette smokers and much higher than nonsmokers. Overall mortality and rates of lung cancer, coronary artery disease, and chronic obstructive pulmonary disease are much lower in pipe and cigar smokers than in cigarette smokers and not much higher than in nonsmokers. However, cigarette smokers who transfer their habit of inhaling when they switch to pipes and cigars probably have higher health risks.

Low Tar and Nicotine Cigarettes

In 1980, the average cigarette delivered 14 mg of tar and 1 mg of nicotine, half as much as the average cigarette 25 years ago. Half the cigarettes now sold advertise reduced tar and nicotine yields. However, yields are determined by smoking machines and do not correlate with actual nicotine content. There is no evidence that smokers of reduced tar/nicotine cigarettes have less nicotine or carbon monoxide exposure, as measured by blood levels of metabolites. To compensate for the reduced nicotine delivered by these cigarettes, smokers may increase consumption or depth of inhalation. The cigarettes also contain new flavoring additives with unknown health consequences.

Lung cancer risk is reduced by 20% to 40% in smokers of filtered or low tar/nicotine cigarettes compared to higher tar/nicotine cigarettes, but the risk is still much higher than in nonsmokers. Laryngeal cancer risk may also be lessened. No data are available for cancers at other sites. For coronary artery disease, studies have detected no reduced risk for smokers of filtered or low tar/nicotine cigarettes.

HEALTH BENEFITS OF SMOKING CESSATION

Most health risks faced by smokers reverse upon smoking cessation, although years may be required for smokers to reduce risk to that of a lifetime nonsmoker. Prospective studies of former smokers demonstrate that their *overall mortality* and rates for *lung cancer* and *chronic obstructive pulmonary disease* decline toward the level of nonsmokers over 15 years. For *coronary heart disease,* half of the benefit is gained within

1 year of smoking cessation. This rapid reversal of risk suggests that smoking has a reversible, noncumulative effect on the cardiovascular system independent of atherogenesis. In *pregnant women,* the fetal growth retardation associated with smoking is reversible if smoking stops before the end of the second trimester.

Smokers who quit before developing chronic cardiovascular or pulmonary disease will have improved exercise tolerance, decreased frequency of cough, and improved pulmonary function. Small-airways dysfunction will improve, but may not return to normal, and the rate of decline of FEV_1 will slow. Smokers quitting after the development of chronic pulmonary or cardiovascular disease will have fewer *symptoms* of dyspnea, cough, sputum, or angina. There is less evidence that smoking cessation alters the *natural history* of these diseases once they have become symptomatic. Smokers who quit after a *myocardial infarction* reduce their subsequent mortality, compared to those who continue to smoke. Smokers undergoing *coronary or peripheral artery bypass graft* surgery may have longer graft survival if they stop smoking after surgery. In patients with *chronic obstructive lung disease,* the rate of decline in pulmonary function appears to slow after smoking cessation.

Summary and Conclusions

- Conclusive evidence indicates that smoking is the single most important cause of currently preventable morbidity and mortality.
- Smoking is associated with higher overall mortality and with higher morbidity and mortality due to coronary artery disease, chronic obstructive pulmonary disease, cerebrovascular and peripheral vascular disease, peptic ulcer disease, and cancers of the lung, oropharynx, larynx, and esophagus.
- Smokers with a chronic cardiopulmonary disease will have more symptoms (angina, claudication, dyspnea, wheezing, cough, and sputum) if they continue to smoke.
- Smokers without chronic disease suffer more frequent and more severe acute respiratory infections.
- Women who smoke during pregnancy increase fetal risks, and those who smoke and use oral contraceptives greatly increase their risk of thrombotic complications.
- Except for cancers of the oropharynx, larynx, and esophagus, pipe and cigar smokers who do not inhale have lower health risks than cigarette smokers.
- Smoking low tar/nicotine cigarettes does not reduce exposure to nicotine or carbon monoxide. These cigarettes do not lower cardiovascular risk and only partially reduce the smoker's risk of lung cancer.
- Smoking cessation reduces the smoker's risk of developing and dying of cancer or cardiopulmonary disease. Cessation is beneficial even in smokers who have developed a chronic disease.

ANNOTATED BIBLIOGRAPHY

Aronow WS: Effect of passive smoking on angina pectoris. N Engl J Med 299:21, 1978 (*Passive smoking lowers the exercise threshold at which angina develops.*)

Aronson MD, Weiss ST, Ben RL et al: Association between cigarette smoking and acute respiratory tract illness in young adults. JAMA 248:181, 1982 (*Women seeking medical care for the symptoms of a URI were more likely to be smokers. Smokers had more lower respiratory tract illness and a longer duration of cough.*)

Benowitz NL, Hall SM, Herning RI et al: Smokers of low-yield cigarettes do not consume less nicotine. N Engl J Med 309:139, 1983 (*Low-yield cigarettes do not contain less nicotine, and smokers of these cigarettes have no lower exposure to nicotine as measured by blood levels of a nicotine metabolite.*)

Castelli WB, Garrison RJ, Dawber TR et al: The filter cigarette and coronary heart disease: The Framingham study. Lancet 2:109, 1981 (*No reduction in coronary heart disease in smokers of filtered cigarettes.*)

Denfield J, Wright C, Krikler S et al: Cigarette smoking and the treatment of angina with propranolol, atenolol, and nifedipine. N Engl J Med 310:951, 1984 (*Cigarette smoking was demonstrated to interfere with the beneficial effects of all three antianginal drugs, but especially with nifedipine.*)

Fielding JE: Smoking: Health effects and control. N Engl J Med 313: 491, 555, 1985 (*A comprehensive, two-part review; 144 references.*)

Hallstrom AP, Cobb LA, Ray R: Smoking as a risk factor for recurrence of sudden cardiac arrest. N Engl J Med 314:271, 1986 (*Smoking was found to be the major risk factor for recurrence.*)

Jensen J, Christiansen C, Rodbro P: Cigarette smoking, serum estrogens and bone loss during hormone-replacement therapy early after menopause. N Engl J Med 313:973, 1985 (*Serum estrogen levels were lower in smokers than in nonsmokers, which may account for their greater rate and degree of osteoporosis, even with replacement therapy.*)

Kannel WB: Update on the role of cigarette smoking in coronary artery disease. Amer Heart J 101:319, 1981 (*A summary of the evidence linking smoking to risks of cardiovascular disease, with emphasis on data from the Framingham study.*)

Kark JD, Lebuish M, Rannon L: Cigarette smoking as a risk factor for epidemic A (H1N1) influenza in young men. N Engl J Med 307:1042, 1982 (*In a military unit, smokers had a higher risk of developing influenza (69% versus 47%) and more severe illness than nonsmokers.*)

McKinley SM, Bifano NL, McKinley JB: Smoking and age at menopause in women. Ann Intern Med 103:350, 1985 (*Women who smoke have an earlier onset of menopause.*)

Quimby GF, Bonnice CA, Burstein SH et al: Active smoking depresses prostaglandin synthesis in human gastric mucosa. Ann Intern Med 104:616, 1986 (*A possible mechanism for the link between smoking and ulcer disease.*)

Rogers RL, Meyer JS, Shaw TG: Cigarette smoking decreases cerebral blood flow suggesting increased risk for stroke. JAMA 250:2796, 1983 (*Cerebral blood flow measured by xenon inhalation seemed to be increased among smokers even when corrections were made for other stroke risk factors.*)

Ross AH, Smith MA, Anderson JR et al: Late mortality after surgery for peptic ulcer. N Engl J Med 307:519, 1982 (*Excess mortality among men following peptic ulcer treatment was attributable to smoking-associated disease.*)

Sontag S, Graham DY, Belsito A et al: Cimetidine, cigarette smoking, and recurrence of duodenal ulcer. N Engl J Med 311:689, 1984 (*Duodenal ulcers recur more frequently in smokers.*)

Sparrow D, Dawber RR, Colton T: The influence of cigarette smoking on prognosis after a first myocardial infarction. J Chronic Dis 31: 425, 1978 (*Analysis of Framingham data demonstrates lower mortality rates for smokers who quit after suffering a myocardial infarction.*)

Tager IB, Weiss ST, Munoz A et al: Longitudinal study of the effects of maternal smoking on pulmonary function in children. N Engl J Med 309:699, 1983 (*Measurements of FEV in children over a seven-year period suggest that maternal cigarette smoke may negatively affect the development of pulmonary function in children.*)

U.S. Department of Health, Education, and Welfare: Smoking and Health. Public Health Service Publication 1103, Washington, DC, 1964 (*The original Surgeon General's Report, which catalogued the evidence against smoking and first attracted wide public attention to the health risks of cigarettes.*)

U.S. Department of Health, Education, and Welfare: Smoking and Health: A Report of the Surgeon General, Public Health Service Publication 79-50066, Washington, DC, 1979 (*The first update of the 1964 report, extending the conclusions of the original report and reviewing new evidence on health risks. A comprehensive and readable reference.*)

U.S. Department of Health and Human Services: The Health Consequences of Smoking: Cancer 1982. US DHHS(PHS) Publication 82-50179, Washington, DC, 1982

U.S. Department of Health and Human Services: The Health Consequences of Smoking: Cardiovascular Disease. A Report of the Surgeon General. DHHS(PHS) Publication 84-50204, Washington, DC, 1983 (*Two in a series of yearly reports from the Surgeon General, each reviewing the evidence on a particular smoking-related topic.*)

White JR, Froeb HF: Small-airways dysfunction in nonsmokers chronically exposed to tobacco smoke. N Engl J Med 302:720, 1980 (*Nonsmokers chronically exposed to tobacco smoke at work have pulmonary function abnormalities comparable to light smokers.*)

Wilson PWF, Garrison RJ, Castelli WP: Postmenopausal estrogen use, cigarette smoking and cardiovascular morbidity in women over 50. N Engl J Med 313:1038, 1985 (*Risk was greatly exacerbated in smokers.*)

33
Screening for Lung Cancer

Lung cancer is the most common fatal malignancy among males. In recent years, it has claimed the lives of as many men as tumors of the colon and rectum, prostate, pancreas, and stomach combined. The incidence of lung tumors in males has been rising dramatically since 1930. More recently, a dramatic increase among women has been evident; lung cancer is now the leading cause of cancer deaths among women. More than 9% of American men and more than 4% of American women alive today will develop lung cancer during their lifetime; of these, 85% will die of the disease.

Most people are aware of the epidemic proportions of the lung cancer problem. Many have lost friends or relatives and know the grim prognosis of the disease. However, screening of asymptomatic individuals, whether or not it is restricted to those at high risk, can offer little reassurance. Efforts to improve the prognosis by early detection have been thwarted by the insensitivity of available tests, the characteristics of patients at high risk, and the aggressive natural history of most lung tumors. Without an understanding of these limitations, the primary care provider may expend resources that produce little more than exaggerated fear in some patients and inappropriate reassurance in others. Knowledge of the risk factors, the natural history, and the validity of available diagnostic tests provides a basis for the reasoned approach to many pulmonary symptoms (see Chapters 36 to 40).

EPIDEMIOLOGY AND RISK FACTORS

The epidemiology of lung cancer is dominated by its association with smoking. The dramatic increases in cancer death rates among men, and, more recently, among women can be attributed to increases in cigarette consumption. A dose-response relationship between duration and intensity of cigarette smoking and risk of lung cancer has been documented in men and women. When compared to nonsmokers, risks of lung cancer increase fivefold, tenfold, and twentyfold for men who smoke less than ½ pack, ½ to 1 pack, and 1 to 2 packs per day, respectively. A decrease in risk has been demonstrated in smokers who are able to stop and in those who smoke filter-tipped cigarettes. Cigar and pipe smokers incur much less risk, but again a dose–response relationship has been documented (see Chapter 32).

The association between smoking and cancer is strongest for the epidermoid (squamous cell) and small cell undifferentiated (oat cell) tumors. The relationship is less certain for adenocarcinoma (alveolar cell) and large cell undifferentiated (anaplastic) histologic types.

The observation that lung cancer occurs in males far more often than in females can be explained for the most part by differences in smoking patterns. In fact, lung cancer without a smoking history is more common among women. A slight apparent excess of lung cancer cases also occurs in urban areas and among low-income groups. The presence of polycyclic organic matter in urban pollution and in some occupational environments (see Chapter 35) may provide a partial explanation. On-the-job exposure to asbestos, chromate, nickel, and uranium has also been associated with significantly increased rates of lung cancer.

NATURAL HISTORY OF LUNG CANCER AND EFFECTIVENESS OF THERAPY

Lung cancer's rapidly progressive and usually inexorable course frustrates screening efforts. The 5-year survival rate is between 5% and 10%. At the time of symptomatic presentation, 75% of patients have lesions that are clearly unresectable. Of the remainder, 60% prove to be unresectable because of mediastinal involvement discovered by mediastinoscopy or thoracotomy. Five-year survival rates after resection in the relatively few remaining patients vary from about 9% for patients with oat cell tumors to 28% for patients with squamous cell tumors.

Reports of 5-year survival rates based on the symptoms present at the time of diagnosis are more relevant to the question of early detection. In a group of patients with overall 5-year survival of 7%, the 6% who were discovered while asymptomatic had an 18% survival rate, compared with 10% to 15% for patients with local symptoms and 6% for those with systemic symptoms. Nearly one third of the patients had symptoms of metastatic disease; none was alive 5 years later.

There are reports of higher survival rates after resection of *in-situ* lung cancer diagnosed by means of chest x-ray or sputum cytology followed by bronchoscopy, but this may represent little more than selection of slow growing or otherwise benign lesions. Some highly speculative estimates of growth rate suggest that squamous cell carcinoma and adenocarcinoma take as long as 10 and 25 years respectively to reach a size likely to be detected by x-ray. If such estimates are accurate and if there is wide variability in natural history, overestimation of benefits of early detection are likely due to the problems of lead time and time-linked-bias sampling (see Chapter 3).

SCREENING AND DIAGNOSTIC TESTS

Chest X-ray

A controlled British study of semiannual chest x-rays in over 29,000 men detected 101 lung tumors over a 3-year period. Seventy-six were detected in a control population of 25,000. The overall 5-year survival rates among cancer patients from the screened and control groups were 15% and 6%, respectively. Of the 101 cancers in the screened group, only 65 were detected by routine chest x-rays; the remainder presented symptomatically during screening intervals.

The value of chest x-ray screening was also addressed by the Philadelphia Pulmonary Neoplasm Project, which attempted to screen more than 6000 male volunteers over age 45 with semiannual x-rays. Lung cancer developed in 121 patients during a 10-year period, with an ultimate mortality rate of 92% at 5 years. The poor results were attributed to poor patient compliance with screening, patient and physician delay, advanced age or concomitant illness contraindicating surgical therapy, and inadequate sensitivity of the screening method.

The Kaiser Health Plan randomized trial of multiphasic health screening in approximately 5000 persons did not demonstrate any benefit from offering annual chest x-ray examinations. After 11 years of follow up, 25 lung cancer deaths had occurred among those randomized to the screening group, and 26 had occurred among controls. Three additional randomized trials of lung cancer screening are currently in progress.

Studies at the Mayo Clinic and at Memorial Sloan-Kettering Cancer Center have each randomized nearly 10,000 male smokers. In the Mayo study, those randomized to the close surveillance group are screened with both sputum cytology and chest x-ray examinations every 4 months, while control patients are asked, but not reminded, to have such studies annually. At Memorial Slona-Kettering, groups receive either annual chest x-ray and 4-monthly sputum cytologies or annual chest x-ray alone. A third study is underway at Johns Hopkins Hospital. Preliminary data from these studies indicate that screening may advance the time of diagnosis, with more cancers detected in an earlier stage; however, a reduction in cancer mortality has not been demonstrated.

It should be kept in mind that false-positive chest x-rays may engender considerable fear as well as the morbidity associated with confirmatory diagnostic tests. Although the specificity of radiographic screening has been shown to be 97%, it is still too low to give an acceptable predictive value. A Veterans Administration study of lung cancer screens found 438 false-positive x-rays compared with 97 true-positive readings for suspected neoplasm.

Cytologic Screening

The sensitivity of cytologic screening varies with the cell type and location of the tumor and the methods of specimen collection. It used to be thought that a single cytologic specimen would detect about 70% of squamous cell lesions and that three specimens would increase sensitivity to 90%. However, preliminary data from the large randomized trials conducted at the Mayo Clinic and Memorial Sloan-Kettering Cancer Center indicate that cytologic examination is much less sensitive. Only 10% of cancers in the Memorial Sloan-Kettering study and 16% of those in the Mayo study were detected initially by cytology alone. Presumably, these disappointing findings can be explained by the spectrum problem, that is, decreased sensitivity for early rather than late stage tumors (see Chapter 3). The specificity of sputum cytologic examination is about 98%, the same as that of chest x-rays.

It should be noted that, as diagnostic tests, x-ray and cytologic examination are complementary. In a Veterans Administration study, cytology alone had an overall screening sensitivity of 33% and a specificity of 98%. X-ray screening had a sensitivity of 42% and specificity of 98%. The sensitivity for combined x-ray and cytologic examination was 63%.

SUMMARY AND CONCLUSIONS

- Lung cancer is a major cause of morbidity and mortality, especially among men. The incidence is increasing among women.
- Smoking is the overwhelming risk factor for lung cancer. Occupational exposures are also relevant.
- Little is known about the presymptomatic natural history of lung cancer. It is presumed to be very variable. The 5-year survival despite all forms of therapy is 5% to 10%. Survival is slightly better when an asymptomatic lesion is detected.
- Cytologic examination of the sputum and chest x-ray are complementary diagnostic tests. However, neither is sensitive or specific enough to serve as a screening test.
- Large-scale early detection programs have demonstrated little benefit. Such efforts to improve prognosis have been thwarted by the usually rapid course of lung cancer, the characteristics of the patients at risk, and the relative insensitivity of available tests.

A.G.M.

ANNOTATED BIBLIOGRAPHY

(Additional references concerning the relationship of lung cancer to smoking follow Chapter 32.)

Boucot KR, Weiss W: Is curable lung cancer detected by semiannual screening? JAMA 224:1361, 1973 (*Reviews the data of the Philadelphia Pulmonary Neoplasm Project, in which 5-year survival in men offered semiannual x-ray screening was only 8%.*)

Dales LG, Friedman GD, Collen MF: Evaluating periodic multiphasic health check-ups: A controlled trial. J Chron Dis 32:385, 1979 (*The intervention included annual chest x-ray examination without demonstrable effect on lung cancer mortality.*)

Davies DF: A review of detection methods for the early diagnosis of lung cancer. J Chronic Dis 19:819, 1966 (*Somewhat dated but still useful review with 141 references.*)

Fontana RS: Early diagnosis of lung cancer. Am Rev Respir Dis 116: 399, 1977 (*Editorial optimistically interpreting results of combined screening program at Mayo Clinic.*)

Hubbell FA, Greenfield S, Tyler JL et al: The impact of routine admission chest x-ray films on patient care. N Engl J Med 312: 209, 1985 (*The impact of routine admission chest x-rays on the care of 742 consecutive patients admitted to a VA hospital was negligible; in only one case was a new pulmonary malignancy detected, but outcome was unaffected.*)

Kabat GC, Wynder EL: Lung cancer in nonsmokers. Cancer 53: 1214, 1984 (*A case-control study focusing on risk factors other than smoking; includes review of passive smoking risk studies.*)

Lilienfeld A et al: An evaluation of radiologic and cytologic screening for the early detection of lung cancer: A cooperative pilot study

of the American Cancer Society and the Veterans Administration. Cancer Res 26:2083, 1966

Schneiderman MA, Levin DL: Trends in lung cancer. Mortality, incidence, diagnosis, treatment, smoking and urbanization. Cancer 30:1320, 1972 (*Discusses increasing rates of smoking and lung cancer among women as well as cancer rates among urban dwellers and non-whites.*)

Seidenfeld JJ: Screening for bronchogenic carcinoma. Ann Intern Med 102:851, 1985 (*An editorial that summarizes available studies, including a large multi-center collaborative effort, and concludes that screening with chest x-ray and sputum cytology cannot be recommended as a cost-effective approach.*)

Tape TG, Mushlin AI: The utility of routine chest radiographs. Ann Intern Med 104:663, 1986 (*A comprehensive review of the issue.*)

Wynder EL, Goodman MT: Smoking and lung cancer: Some unresolved issues. Epidemiologic Reviews 5:177, 1983 (*An up-to-date review with special attention to passive smoke inhalation and the low yield cigarette.*)

34
Screening for and Prophylaxis of Tuberculosis

HARVEY B. SIMON, M.D.

Active tuberculosis is now a relatively rare occurrence in ambulatory practice; however, the possibility of the diagnosis is often brought to mind by the patient presenting with hemoptysis, chronic cough, or severe weight loss. Tuberculin reactivity remains prevalent. On a daily basis, the primary physician faces the question of whether or not to test for reactivity and how to respond when it is present.

EPIDEMIOLOGY AND RISK FACTORS

The decline in prevalence of tuberculosis in the United States during this century has been dramatic. At the turn of the century, a majority of Americans were infected before they reached adulthood, Today, only 25% of Americans over 50 and fewer than 5% of young adults react positively to tuberculin skin testing. Overall, about 7% of the population are positive reactors. Fewer than 5% of these have a history of clinical tuberculosis. Approximately 90% of new cases of clinical tuberculosis represent reactivation from the remaining pool of latent endogenous infection.

Not surprisingly, patients with tuberculosis tend to be clustered in certain population groups. The disease is more common in males, in the economically disadvantaged, in inner city residents, and in members of certain minority groups. The majority of patients with active disease are over 50 years of age, and the proportion of elderly patients appears

to be increasing. In a large study of nursing home residents, the prevalence of tuberculin skin test positivity was over 20% and the prevalence of active disease 2.4%. Other population groups with a disproportionately high incidence of tuberculosis include Hispanics, immigrants (especially from Southeast Asia), alcoholics, and patients with a history of gastrectomy, neoplasia, or other debilitating diseases.

NATURAL HISTORY OF TUBERCULOSIS AND EFFECTIVENESS OF THERAPY

Mycobacterium tuberculosis is transmitted by way of fresh droplet nuclei expelled by an individual with cavitary tuberculosis. It cannot be spread by hands, utensils, or other fomites, although organisms can be cultivated from room dust. While innoculation can occur via the gastrointestinal tract, the vast majority of infections in the United States begin in the lung (see Chapter 47). Rarely, primary infection results in early progressive disease; young children are at greatest risk for this complication. But in most cases, immunity develops over a period of several weeks, and hence the disease enters a latent stage.

Approximately 5% to 15% of new tuberculous infections eventually progress to serious disease. Risk is greatest during the years immediately following infection. Only 3% to 5% of patients without clinical disease 5 years after infection will suffer late reactivation.

Three strategies may be used in the prevention of clinical tuberculous infection. (1) biologic prophylaxis of uninfected individuals with BCG vaccine; (2) chemoprophylaxis of newly or recently infected individuals with isoniazid (INH); and (3) chemoprophylaxis of selected individuals with latent infections with INH.

Biologic prophylaxis in uninfected individuals is widely practiced in countries where tuberculosis is common. Bacillus Calmette-Guerin (BCG) vaccine is used for the prevention but not the therapy of tuberculosis. BCG vaccine is a live attenuated strain of *M. bovis,* which has little virulence in man. BCG vaccine has been in clinical use since 1922, but its role remains controversial. Early trials demonstrated that BCG could prevent tuberculosis in up to 80% of recipients, but recent trials on the Indian subcontinent have failed to demonstrate efficacy. Current preparations of BCG are well tolerated. BCG is not recommended for routine use in the United States. The vaccine produces a positive tuberculin test in recipients, and because of the low prevalence rate of new tuberculous infections in the United States (estimated at 0.03%), case-finding and INH prophylaxis are considered more effective. BCG vaccine should not be administered to PPD-positive individuals.

Chemoprophylaxis of newly or recently infected individuals, as identified by recent conversion to tuberculin reactivity, is an important method of preventing clinical disease. In patients who have not received chemotherapy, a positive skin test implies the presence of a few dormant but viable tubercle bacilli, which have the potential for reactivation. In a sense then, patients with positive tuberculin skin tests serve as their own reservoir for future clinical disease. It has been demonstrated that the administration of INH daily for 1 year reduces the risk of reactivation by up to 80%. Since the risk of progressive disease is greatest soon after infection, recent converters to tuberculin reactivity are most likely to benefit from such therapy. In general, individuals who have converted to tuberculin reactivity within 2 years should be considered for chemoprophylaxis. Close contacts of patients with active pulmonary tuberculosis deserve special attention. It has been recommended that children or adolescents who are exposed be treated with INH even if the tuberculin skin test is negative. If the test remains negative after 3 months of INH therapy, chemoprophylaxis can then be discontinued. Routine screening of all individuals below age 35 and INH treatment of positive reactors have also been recommended. Because the prevalence rate of positive reactions is less than 1% among children and adolescents, a positive reaction in a young patient may indicate recent exposure.

The chemoprophylaxis of selected patients with latent infections and long-standing positive tuberculin reactivity has also been advised. Patients who have recovered from clinical tuberculosis without the benefit of adequate chemotherapy should be considered for prophylaxis. It also seems reasonable to administer INH to those with positive tuberculin skin tests who are immunologically impaired hosts or who are positive for HTLV-III serology. Enthusiasm for INH prophylaxis must be tempered by the significant side effects of the drug. The major concern in the use of INH is its hepatotoxicity. This is quite rare in patients under age 20 and occurs in no more than 0.2% of those between ages 20 and 34. On the other hand, among patients over 50, more than 2% may develop INH-induced liver disease (see Chapter 47).

SCREENING AND DIAGNOSTIC TESTS

The tuberculin skin test, far more sensitive and specific than the chest x-ray, is the most useful test for the diagnosis of past or present tuberculous infection. The Mantoux test using the intradermal injection of Tween-80 stabilized purified protein derivative (PPD) is more reliable than multiple-puncture tests, such as the tine test. Three strengths of PPD are available: the first strength contains 1 tuberculin unit; the intermediate strength, 5 units; and the second strength, 250 units. Intermediate-strength PPD is the standard test material. The tuberculin skin test should be interpreted 48 to 72 hours after injection; the diameter of induration rather than erythema determines the interpretation: 0 to 4 mm is a negative reaction; 5 to 9 mm is doubtful; and 10 mm or more is positive. First-strength PPD should be reserved for patients in whom a very strong reaction is anticipated. Second-strength PPD should be reserved for individuals with negative reactions to a lower strength. A positive second-strength test in the face of a negative or doubtful intermediate-strength test is suggestive of infection with atypical mycobacteria and resultant cross-sensitization to PPD. Obviously, a positive tuberculin test does not by itself prove active disease. Repeated tuberculin skin tests can produce a booster effect; among hospital employees or other populations in which repeated skin testing may be necessary, a booster effect may be mistaken for tuberculin conversion. Confusion can be avoided by repeating negative or doubtful skin tests 1 week later: any increase in the diameter of induration can be attributed to the booster effect. In contrast, increased reactivity that occurs at 1 year, but not at 1 week, should be attributed to newly acquired infection.

False-negative reactions have been documented in up to 20% of patients with tuberculosis, particularly those individuals with overwhelming or advanced disease, malnutrition, or debility. Many of these patients are anergic, so that skin testing with *Candida* or streptokinase-streptodornase antigens can be useful in demonstrating overall immunologic impairment. Patients with clinical AIDS may have falsely negative PPD tests in the setting of active TB. The development of anergy is a poor prognostic sign.

In addition to the immunologic incompetence of the host, false-negative skin tests may result from mishandling of the antigen or from faulty injection technique. Tuberculin should never be transferred from one container to another, and skin tests should be given as soon as possible after the syringe is filled. Subcutaneous rather than intradermal injection may result in false-negative reactions. Since tuberculin sensitivity develops 2 to 10 weeks after initial infection, early skin tests may be negative in newly infected individuals.

Tuberculin skin testing is highly specific; however, cross-reactivity with atypical mycobacterial antigens may cause intermediate skin test reactions to occur in people who have not been exposed to *M. tuberculosis.* More often, individuals infected with atypical mycobacteria will have positive second-strength PPD reactions and weak or negative intermediate PPDs.

RECOMMENDATIONS AND CONCLUSIONS

- While active tuberculous disease has become uncommon in the United States, the prevalence of latent infection remains approximately 7%. Because the PPD test is useful in case-finding, BCG prophylaxis for PPD-negative patients is not recommended.
- For recent converters or positive reactors under age 35, INH should be given for 1 year while the patient is monitored carefully for development of hepatitis. INH should also be given to close contacts of patients with active pulmonary disease, particularly if the contact is a child or an adolescent; treatment can be discontinued if the patient remains PPD-negative for a 3-month period. Older patients who have recovered from clinical tuberculosis, have no evidence of active disease, but have never received chemotherapy should be considered for INH therapy. The decision to treat asymptomatic older patients needs to be tempered by the increased risk of INH-induced hepatitis in this age group.
- The tuberculin skin test can be useful in apparently healthy individuals. Because of its prognostic value and the importance of recent conversion, the PPD status of children and young adults should be determined. Individuals with a high risk of exposure to tuberculosis, such as those in the health professions, should have tuberculin tests on an annual basis so long as they remain PPD negative.
- PPD testing should be considered in asymptomatic patients who are confirmed to be HTLV-III positive. Prophylactic INH therapy may have important public health consequences, helping to prevent development and spread of clinical infection.

ANNOTATED BIBLIOGRAPHY

Barlow PB, Black M, Brummer DC et al: Preventive therapy of tuberculosis infection. Am Rev Respir Dis 110:371, 1974 (*A good review with specific recommendations for INH prophylaxis.*)

Boyd JC, Marr JJ: Decreasing reliability of acid-fast smear techniques for detection of tuberculosis. Ann Intern Med 82:849, 1975 (*Misleading title but very useful article pointing out high specificity [99%] of smears but low predictive value [45%] because of low prevalence. Sensitivity was 22%.*)

Clemens JD, Chuong JJH, Feinstein AR: The BCG controversy. A methodological and statistical reappraisal. JAMA 249:2362, 1983 (*A review of eight major controlled trials of BCG. Although the most recent trials failed to demonstrate efficacy, the three trials with superior methodology and statistics demonstrated 75% or greater protective efficacy. Further study of BCG will be necessary to resolve the controversy.*)

Comstock GW, Furculow ML, Greenberg RA: The tuberculin skin test. Am Rev Respir Dis 104:769, 1971 (*Standards for the administration and interpretation of the tuberculin skin test.*)

Holden M, Dubin MR, Diamond PH: Negative intermediate strength tuberculin sensitivity in active tuberculosis. N Engl J Med 285:1506, 1971 (*Emphasizes loss of potency due to adsorption of antigen. Tween-80 stabilized antigen had a sensitivity of 83%, superior to other preparations.*)

Hyde L: Clinical significance of the tuberculin test. Am Rev Respir Dis 105:453, 1972 (*Skin tests on 100 patients with active pulmonary TB provoked reactions greater than 5 mm in 90% and greater than 10 mm in 81%.*)

International Union Against Tuberculosis Committee on Prophylaxis: Efficacy of various durations of isoniazid preventive therapy for tuberculosis: Five year follow-up of the IUAT trial. Bull WHO 60:555, 1982 (*A cooperative European study of 27,830 tuberculin-positive adults with fibrotic pulmonary lesions. Fifty-two weeks of INH produced a 75% reduction in tuberculosis; 24 weeks of treatment provided a 65% reduction. Hepatitis occurred in 0.5% of the INH recipients, as compared with 0.1% in placebo recipients. For the 52-week regimen, the benefit/risk (tuberculosis averted/INH hepatitis) ratio was 2.1; for 24 weeks the ratio was 2.6.*)

Judson FN, Sbarbo JA, Tapy JM et al: Tuberculosis screening. Evaluation of a food handler's program. Chest 83:879, 1983. (*An evaluation of a skin test screening program of 6090 individuals. Screening was cost-effective, detecting 324 candidates for INH chemoprophylaxis at a cost of $45 each as well as four new cases of active tuberculosis.*)

Pitchenik AE, Cole C, Russell BW et al: Tuberculosis and acquired immunodeficiency syndrome among Haitians and non-Haitians in South Florida. Ann Intern Med 101:641, 1984 (*Documents the public health importance of testing and treating HTLV-III positive patients for tuberculosis.*)

Schacter EN: Tuberculin negative tuberculosis. Am Rev Respir Dis 106:587, 1972 (*Sixteen of 149 patients with clinical disease had negative tests. Ten with negative tests were infected with atypical organisms.*)

Stead WW, Lofgren JP, Warren E et al: Tuberculosis as an endemic and nosocomial infection among the elderly in nursing homes. N Engl J Med 312:1483, 1985 (*A study of 25,000 nursing home elderly showing a high prevalence of tuberculin reactivity and active disease; risk of new infection was great.*)

Thompson NJ, Glassrath JL, Snider DE Jr et al: The booster phenomenon in serial tuberculin testing. Am Rev Resp Dis 119:387, 1979 (*A good discussion of the booster phenomenon with guidelines for serial skin testing in high-risk population groups.*)

35

Prevention and Evaluation of Occupational Respiratory Disease

L. CHRISTINE OLIVER, M.D.
JOHN D. STOECKLE, M.D.

Occupational lung disease, one of the ten leading causes of work-related health problems in the United States, results from inhaled organic and inorganic dusts, irritant gases, and toxic fumes, which adversely affect both the upper and lower respiratory tracts. Although the true scope of occupational respiratory illness and disease is unknown, some estimates can be given. It has been estimated that approximately 65,000 males in the United States have clinically diagnosable asbestosis; moreover, by 2009 it is predicted that 19,000 cases of mesothelioma and 55,000 cases of lung cancer will occur in males with a history of occupational exposure to asbestos. Persons permanently disabled by respiratory disease due to previous exposure to cotton dust number about 30,000; active cotton mill workers partially disabled, about 85,000. Ten percent of active coal miners and 20% of retired miners have coal worker's pneumoconiosis (CWP). The U.S. Department of Labor has estimated that over one million workers are exposed to silica and that approximately 60,000 have silicosis.

Yet these figures underestimate the extent of occupational pulmonary disease. The reasons are several. First, since clinical findings of work-related respiratory disease resemble those of nonoccupational respiratory disease, diagnosis is often missed. Second, the latency period between exposure and the subsequent development of disease is often long, obscuring the causal relationship. Third, physicians often underdiagnose because they have inadequate training in occupational medicine. Fourth, occupational disease is underreported by health personnel. Moreover, the estimates do not include "paraoccupational" lung disease resulting from bystander exposure, from household contact with toxins carried home on work clothes, and from neighborhood exposures. Asbestos-related disease has been reported in family members of asbestos workers and in individuals living in close proximity to shipyards and asbestos-manufacturing plants. Chronic beryllium disease has resulted from residence in the neighborhood of beryllium plants and asthma from residence near grain elevators.

It is critical that the primary physician be familiar with occupational lung diseases and their diagnosis if unnecessary morbidity is to be avoided. Since acute respiratory symptoms due to toxic exposure are nonspecific, recognition of their relationship to the toxic agent is essential; continued exposure may result in needless, irreversible functional abnormalities. The diagnosis of established chronic occupational respiratory disease is also important. In such instances, the rate of functional deterioration or the risk of secondary disease such as neoplasia may be reduced by removal from the exposure, control of infection, and elimination of smoking.

PATHOPHYSIOLOGY AND CLINICAL PRESENTATION

Inhaled dusts, gases, and fumes exert their effect upon the respiratory tract in several ways. The first and most obvious is that of *direct irritation.* Excessive mucous secretion, cough, airway hyperreactivity, chest tightness or pain, dyspnea, pneumonitis, or pulmonary edema may develop. With such irritant gases as nitrogen dioxide (NO_2) and phosgene, a delay of 12 to 24 hours may precede the onset of pulmonary edema.

Second, dusts may be retained in the lungs, provoking a *fibrotic or granulomatous response.* In order to reach the lung, substances must have a particle size of 5 μm or less. Related to level of exposure, latency periods preceding the onset of clinical disease can be 15 to 20 years.

Third, *hypersensitivity* and abnormal function of the immune system may play a role in the development of occupational lung disease. Hypersensitivity is important etiologically in hypersensitivity pneumonitis and in certain types of occupational asthma. Increased circulating levels of immunoglobulins, rheumatoid factor (RF), antinuclear antibody (ANA), and alpha$_1$-antitrypsin have been observed in individuals with asbestosis. Reported peripheral blood T-lymphocyte abnormalities appear to be related to duration of asbestos exposure and to radiographic outcome. Elevated titers of circulating ANA and RF are seen in association with silicosis. Individuals with chronic beryllium disease are reported to have alterations in circulating T-lymphocytes and a high rate of blast transformation of lymphocytes compared to controls.

Fourth, *other host factors* are also important. Asbestos acts synergistically with cigarette smoke to increase the risk for lung cancer. The prevalence of bronchitis and airways obstruction is increased in smoking welders and coal miners compared to their nonsmoking coworkers. Finally, *social and economic factors* and work practices often determine the geographic proximity of home site to industrial sources of air pollution and affect the likelihood that family members will bring potentially toxic materials home on work clothes.

Occupational respiratory disease can be categorized clinically as follows (Table 35-1).

Industrial Bronchitis

Industrial bronchitis is characterized by cough and sputum. It may be associated with chronic airways obstruction. Acute bronchitis is self-limited. Chronic bronchitis is cough and sputum on most days, for 3 months or more per year, for 2 years or more. A nonspecific manifestation of airway irritation and inflammation, bronchitis may result from exposure to such agents as coal dust and silica, the irritant gases sulfur dioxide and chlorine dioxide, welding fumes, and vanadium pentoxide fumes.

Interstitial Lung Disease

Coal Worker's Pneumoconiosis (CWP) results from the deposition of coal dust in peribronchial tissues, with the formation of dust macules and the distention of terminal bronchioles. Occurrence and extent of disease depend both on the level of dust exposure and the rank of the coal, with anthracite being more fibrogenic than bituminous. CWP occurs in two forms: "simple pneumoconiosis," characterized by the presence of small dust nodules, usually less than 5 mm in diameter; and "complicated pneumoconiosis" or "progressive massive fibrosis" (PMF), characterized by large

Table 35-1. Classification of Occupational Respiratory Disease

Industrial Bronchitis
Causal agents: welding fumes, coal dust, sulfur dioxide, vanadium pentoxide

Pulmonary Fibrosis
Causal agents: asbestos, coal dust, silica, beryllium, talc, kaolin, and organic materials such as thermophilic actinomycetes, aspergillus, and animal proteins

Obstructive Airways Disease
Occupational asthma
Causal agents: toluene diisocyanate (TDI), phthalic anhydride, nickel, chromium, platinum salts, formaldehyde, *Bacillus subtilis* proteolytic enzyme, grains, animal products, epoxy resins, Western red cedar, mahogany, and oak
Byssinosis
Causal agents: cotton, flax, and hemp

Cancer
Causal agents: asbestos, arsenic trioxide, hexavalent chromium, nickel, bischloromethyl ether (BCME), chloromethylmethyl ether (CMME), vinyl chloride monomer, and radiation

Noncardiogenic Pulmonary Edema
Causal agents: nitrogen dioxide (NO_2), phosgene, chlorine, ammonia, and sulfuric acid

masses of dust and collagen tissue. The most prevalent respiratory symptom is chronic bronchitis, unrelated to radiographic appearance of the lungs and more common in smoking miners. Physiologic abnormalities on lung function testing are variable, and with the exception of single breath diffusing capacity for carbon monoxide ($DLCO_{SB}$), unrelated to radiographic appearance in simple CWP. Reduced $DLCO_{SB}$ is associated with category "p" opacities (<1.5 mm in diameter) of simple CWP and with advanced PMF. Airway obstruction may be seen in PMF and in association with chronic bronchitis.

Asbestosis is fibrosis of the lung parenchyma or pleura as a result of asbestos exposure. Pleural plaques may contain calcium. An early finding, usually occurring within 10 years of exposure, is the so-called "benign asbestos effusion." It may be unilateral or bilateral and often leaves behind residual pleural thickening at the costophrenic angle. Severity of asbestos-related pulmonary fibrosis is related both to total dose and to latency. Parenchymal asbestosis is more closely associated with dose and pleural asbestosis with latency in epidemiologic studies. Respiratory symptoms are nonspecific and depend on extent of disease. Physical examination may reveal characteristic dry end-inspiratory crackles at the lung bases and clubbing. Physiologic abnormalities include restrictive mechanics and impaired gas exchange. Small airways dysfunction, probably resulting from peribronchiolar fibrosis, may be an early finding. The posterior–anterior chest radiograph typically reveals irregular densities in the lower lung zones or the pleural plaques. Lateral views of the chest are useful in detecting *calcified hemidiaphragmatic plaques,* a hallmark of asbestos exposure. The value of oblique views in detecting pleural plaques is inversely related to risk for developing disease. Extensive pleural thickening has been associated with respiratory failure; the presence of pleural plaques has been associated with increased risk for subsequent development of lung cancer, mesothelioma, and parenchymal fibrosis. The effect of low-level exposure to asbestos in schools and other public buildings remains to be determined.

Silicosis results from exposure to silicon dioxide (SiO_2) or quartz, which is fibrogenic. Silica exposure occurs in a wide variety of occupational settings. Particularly important is bystander exposure. It is often the case that sandblasters are given respiratory protection, whereas workers around them are not. Like CWP, silicosis may occur in a simple nodular form or in a "complicated" form with PMF. Latency and severity of disease are directly related to level of dust exposure. Silicosis may occur after 1 to 2 years of high-level exposure. It may be complicated by mycobacterial or fungal infection. Radiographic abnormalities characteristically precede functional abnormalities and initially occur as small rounded opacities involving the upper lung zones. Hilar lymph nodes may become enlarged with "eggshell" calcifications. Physiologic abnormalities reflect the peribronchiolar location of the silicotic nodules and consist of small airways dysfunction and impaired gas exchange in the early stages. With PMF, obstruction, restriction, or a mixed pattern may develop.

Acute and Chronic Beryllium Disease results from the inhalation of beryllium. At risk are workers engaged in the manufacture of beryllium-containing products and in the electronics and aircraft industries. Acute disease follows inhalation of relatively high concentrations of beryllium. Its irritant effect upon the respiratory tract may produce nasopharyngitis, tracheobronchitis, or clinical pneumonitis. Chronic beryllium disease is a systemic granulomatous disorder often confused with sarcoidosis. Chest radiograph typically reveals a diffuse reticulonodular infiltrate, with hilar lymphadenopathy in about 40% of patients. Lung function tests may reveal obstruction or restriction and/or impaired gas exchange. The angiotensin$_1$-converting enzyme (ACE) is elevated in about 50% of individuals with active sarcoidosis, a finding that may be useful in distinguishing this entity from chronic beryllium disease. Elevated levels of beryllium in urine or tissue suggest the diagnosis and provide definitive evidence of exposure.

Hypersensitivity Pneumonitis (extrinsic allergic alveolitis) occurs following exposure to organic material. Causal agents include thermophilic actinomycetes, aspergillus, and serum and urine protein from animals and fish. Clinical disorders include farmer's lung, bird fancier's lung, bagassosis, humidifier fever, and animal handler's lung. Both acute and chronic reactions may occur. Chest radiograph may reveal miliary or larger discrete opacities in the middle and lower lung zones. Repeated exposure may result in recurrence of symptoms and ultimately in the development of chronic disease, with interstitial fibrosis on chest radiograph and impaired lung function on physiologic testing. The acute phase may be mild and pass relatively unnoticed. Antigen-specific precipitins appear in about 90% of cases.

So-called "benign pneumoconioses" occur following exposure to certain inert dusts. Chest radiograph reveals interstitial opacities. Lung function generally remains intact. These pneumoconioses follow exposure to iron oxide (siderosis), tin oxide (stannosis), barium (baritosis), and zirconium.

Obstructive Airways Disease

Occupational Asthma is reversible airway hyperreactivity caused by inhalation of substances in the workplace. It occurs in both nonatopic and atopic individuals. Symptoms include chest tightness, wheezing, dyspnea, and cough. Lung function tests may reveal small airways dysfunction and an obstructive defect that is partially reversible following administration of bronchodilators. Lung function may be observed to decline over the work shift or gradually over the work week. A fixed level of obstruction may ultimately develop.

Byssinosis is characterized by respiratory symptoms and obstructive airways disease and follows exposure to cotton, flax, and hemp dust. It is seen most commonly in the United States among cotton textile workers. Symptoms of chest tightness and dyspnea, with reduction in air flow rates, initially appear on the first day of the work week after a 2-day absence from work. These abnormalities may become persistent, resulting in chronic and irreversible disease with continued exposure. Diagnosis depends to a large extent on occupational history. The bract of the cotton plants is thought to contain the as-yet unidentified causal agent.

Cancer

Occupational exposures causally associated with cancer of the respiratory tract involve arsenic, chromium (hexavalent), nickel, vinyl chloride monomer, radiation, and possibly fumes from the welding of stainless steel. The chemicals bischloromethyl ether (BCME) and chloromethylmethyl ether (CMME) have been shown to cause small cell carcinoma of the oat cell type. Asbestos causes bronchogenic carcinoma, as well as mesothelioma, a tumor of the pleura and peritoneum. Asbestos and cigarette smoke act synergistically to increase the risk for lung cancer by 50 to 70 times, while asbestos alone increases the risk by a factor of three to five. Smoking does not affect the risk for malignant mesothelioma. Asbestos also increases the risk for cancers of the larynx and gastrointestinal tract.

NATURAL HISTORY OF DISEASE AND EFFECTIVENESS OF CONTROL

Although much remains to be learned about the natural history of most occupational lung diseases, practical control steps can be taken. It is worthwhile to distinguish agents that commonly cause acute symptoms and, with repeated exposures, may produce irreversible disease from other agents that produce disease evident only after a long asymptomatic latent period.

Byssinosis and bronchitis-pneumonia due to diisocyanate exposure are examples of acute reversible diseases that can progress to chronic, irreversible diseases with repeated exposure. Both are characterized by acute symptoms of coughing and wheezing that occur when the worker is re-exposed after a brief absence from work. Chronic obstructive changes can develop in those whose exposure continues despite symptoms. Some workers exposed to enzyme detergents have similar acute symptoms; progressive loss of elastic recoil is possible if exposure continues. Disorders due to organic dusts (farmer's lung) and toxic chemicals (beryllium) also produce both acute and chronic syndromes that are related to level and duration of exposure.

In contrast, diseases due to mineral dusts, such as coal worker's pneumoconiosis and asbestosis, become clinically manifest only after a long latent asymptomatic period. The clinical findings of coal worker's pneumoconiosis usually follow 10 years of exposure. Similarly, 10 to 20 years of low-level exposure is usually required to produce detectable pulmonary asbestosis. In the case of pleural asbestosis, exposure usually precedes the development of disease by 20 to 30 years. Silicosis also has a long latent period unless exposure is extremely intense. Despite improved dust control, termination of exposure has been advised for people with identifiable pulmonary disease. However, the extent to which progression of the disease can be influenced by cessation of exposure after the appearance of detectable abnormalities is not known.

DIAGNOSIS

Eliciting the *occupational history* is the most important step in the diagnosis of occupational respiratory disease. Although a chronologic lifetime work history is ideal, it is often unnecessary in the primary care setting. Three questions will usually suffice: (1) What is your current job? (2) What was your previous job? and (3) What is your usual job, that is, the one you have worked at the longest? It is important to obtain not only job title but also job description. Specific information about type, level, and duration of exposures is needed. It is important to characterize the temporal relationship of symptoms and disease to work, and to inquire about similar illness in coworkers and family members.

Lung function and other laboratory tests provide valuable diagnostic information. Reduction in the $DLCO_{SB}$ may be the only abnormality in developing pulmonary fibrosis. Small airways dysfunction may be an early sign of interstitial or obstructive lung disease. Pre- and post-shift spirometry is often useful in the diagnosis of occupational asthma or byssinosis. If history and clinical findings suggest the diagnosis of pneumoconiosis, chest radiograph should be interpreted according to the ILO System of Classification, developed by the International Labor Organization for standardization and more specific radiographic characterization and quantification of pneumoconiosis. Bronchial provocation by inhalation under carefully controlled conditions can be a useful tool in the diagnosis of occupational asthma.

Thorough documentation is essential not only for design of a treatment program, but also for disability and compensation determinations.

CONCLUSIONS AND RECOMMENDATIONS FOR PREVENTION

The role of the primary care physician in the prevention of occupational respiratory disease is as follows:

1. To appropriately recognize and diagnose work-related respiratory illness and disease.

2. To inform the patient of the diagnosis, making certain that he is aware of any occupational etiology. Ascertaining patient understanding is important because of statutes of limitation associated with legal remedies, such as worker compensation.

3. To inform the employee and/or a regulatory agency such as the Occupational Safety and Health Administration (OSHA) of any serious or potentially life-threatening hazards to the patient or coworkers in order to facilitate a workplace evaluation and eliminate the toxic exposure.

4. To encourage patients to abstain from habits such as smoking that are inherently toxic to the lungs and exacerbate the respiratory effects of occupational exposures.

5. To treat respiratory infections without delay. Unfortunately, there is often no specific treatment for occupational lung disease.

6. To institute appropriate surveillance for subsequent pulmonary disease.

Elimination of exposure through the use of rigorous engineering controls is the ultimate goal in prevention. Removal from the job should be a "court of last resort."

ANNOTATED BIBLIOGRAPHY

Barbee RA, Callies O, Dickie HA: The long term prognosis in farmer's lung. Am Rev Resp Dis 97:223, 1968 (*Fifty patients followed for an average of 6 years. Chronic disease occurred most commonly in those with a history of mild recurrent episodes each winter.*)

Beck GJ, Schachter EN, Maunder LR et al: A prospective study of chronic lung disease in cotton textile workers. Ann Intern Med 97:645, 1982 (*Retired cotton textile workers had progressive symptoms even after exposure to cotton dust had ended.*)

Becklake MR: Asbestos-related diseases of the lung and other organs: Their epidemiology and implications for clinical practice. Am Rev Resp Dis 114:55, 1976 (*Comprehensive review of epidemiology, pathogenesis, and clinical findings in asbestos-related disease.*)

Bouhuys A, Heapty LJ, Schilling RSF et al: Byssinosis in U.S. N Engl J Med 277:170, 1967 (*Chronic irreversible disease occurs mainly in reactors, those with acute reversible symptoms.*)

Carey TS, Hadler NM: The role of the primary physician in disability determination for Social Security and worker's compensation. Ann Intern Med 104:706, 1986 (*A useful guide to this practical issue.*)

Council on Scientific Affairs, AMA: A physician's guide to asbestos-related diseases. JAMA 252:2593, 1984 (*Answers to questions about the pathologic response to asbestos.*)

Craighead JE, Mossman BT: The pathogenesis of asbestos-associated diseases. N Engl J Med 306:1446, 1982 (*Extensive review of asbestos and related health problems.*)

Goodman LR: Radiology of asbestos disease. JAMA 249:644, 1983 (*Succinct, illustrated review.*)

Hammond EC, Selikoff IJ, Seidman H: Asbestos exposure, cigarette smoking and death rates. Ann NY Acad Sci 330:473, 1979 (*Study* of independent and interactive contributions of asbestos exposure and cigarette smoking to death from lung cancer in 17,800 asbestos insulation workers.)

McNeil BJ, Eddy DM: The costs and effects of screening for cancer among asbestos-exposed workers. J Chron Dis 35:351, 1982 (*A cost effectiveness analysis that favors colon cancer screening over lung cancer screening.*)

Parkes WR: Occupational Lung Disorders. Boston, Butterworths, 1982 (*Chapters 7, 8, 11, and 12 provide detailed discussion of silicosis, CWP, hypersensitivity pneumonitis, and occupational asthma with exceptional photographic illustration.*)

Program Plan of NIOSH by Program Areas for Fy 1983. DHHS (NIOSH) Publication 83-102, 1983 (*Sets forth the ten leading work-related health problems in the U.S. as determined by NIOSH on the basis of frequency, severity, and preventability.*)

Rom WN (ed): Environmental and Occupational Medicine, pp 481–489. Boston, Little, Brown & Co, 1983 (*Succinct review of acute and chronic beryllium disease, with discussion of pathogenesis, clinical findings, and differentiation from other granulomatous diseases.*)

Stoeckle JD, Hardy HL, Weber AL: Chronic beryllium disease, a report of 60 cases and selective review of the literature. Am J Med 46:545, 1969 (*Exposures occurred primarily during the manufacture of fluorescent lamps. Cor pulmonale was the usual cause of death.*)

Walker AM, Loughlin JE, Friedlander ER et al: Projections of asbestos-related disease 1980–2009. J Occ Med 25(5):409, 1983 (*Description of methods used to arrive at projections for current and future cases of asbestosis, lung cancer, and mesothelioma in U.S. males with occupational exposure to asbestos.*)

Wegman DH, Levenstein C, Greaves IA: Byssinosis: A role for public health in the face of scientific uncertainty. AJPH 73:188, 1983 (*Discussion of the scientific debate on the nature of byssinosis, its relationship to smoking, and the case for worker compensation in the absence of definitive data. References are given for the estimated prevalence of cotton dust–related disability.*)

Ziskind M, Jones RN, Weill H: Silicosis. Am Rev Resp Dis 113(5):643, 1976 (*Comprehensive review of silicosis, with discussion of history, sources and nature of exposures, pathogenesis, and clinical findings.*)

36
Evaluation of Chronic Dyspnea

Dyspnea is the subjective sensation of difficult or uncomfortable respirations. Patients commonly complain of "shortness of breath" to describe their respiratory difficulty. Acute dyspnea is most often a manifestation of anxiety (see Chapter 222), asthma (see Chapter 45), or sudden cardiopulmonary compromise; the patient usually comes to the emergency room for care. Patients with chronic dyspnea, even when severe, are more likely to present at the office. Long-standing dyspnea can usually be evaluated safely in the outpatient setting, provided the patient's condition is not rapidly deteriorating.

The major causes of chronic dyspnea are chronic obstructive lung disease and congestive heart failure; at times the differentiation can be difficult. Moreover, these etiologies often coexist; in such instances, the diagnostic task requires a determination of which cause is predominant. In evaluating the chronically dyspneic patient, one needs to check for precipitants and reversible components, in addition to determining cause. Also important are assessment of functional status, severity of deficits, and prognosis.

PATHOPHYSIOLOGY AND CLINICAL PRESENTATION

The pathophysiology of dyspnea involves disturbances of ventilation. Shortness of breath is experienced when ventilatory demand exceeds the actual or perceived capacity of the lungs to respond. The work of breathing may be increased because of altered chest wall mechanics, decreased lung compliance, airway obstruction, or exogenous factors such as obesity.

The location and workings of the system for detecting respiratory work are still incompletely understood. It has been hypothesized that an inappropriate relationship between length and tension of respiratory muscle fibers may be one triggering factor. The unmyelinated vagal nerve endings located between pulmonary capillaries and alveoli are believed to mediate the sensation of dyspnea in pulmonary edema.

There are several important clinical settings in which dyspnea occurs. *Congestive heart failure* (CHF) can cause dyspnea as pulmonary capillary pressure rises and fluid accumulates in the interstitium, leading to a fall in pulmonary compliance and a sense of difficulty breathing. The earliest symptom is often dyspnea on exertion. More severe failure is manifested by orthopnea and finally paroxysmal nocturnal dyspnea. Basilar crackles (rales) and a third heart sound are important signs of left heart failure and pulmonary venous hypertension; the third heart sound is one of the most specific signs of CHF (see Chapter 27). Peripheral edema and jugular venous distention are common manifestations of right heart failure, but these findings are very nonspecific, particularly leg edema (see Chapter 16). Contributing and precipitating factors include fever, acute ischemia, excessive dietary sodium intake, dysrhythmias, concurrent use of agents that are negatively inotropic (*e.g.,* beta blockers, disopyramide, verapamil), and poor compliance with medical regimen.

Besides CHF, there are a number of other causes of pulmonary venous hypertension that result in increased pulmonary capillary pressure and dyspnea; *mitral stenosis* is the most important etiology in this class of conditions.

Airway obstruction at any level of the respiratory tract can lead to difficulty breathing. *Tracheal stenosis* resulting from intrinsic disease or extrinsic compression is characterized by dyspnea in conjunction with stridor and inspiratory retraction of the supraclavicular space. *Chronic obstructive pulmonary disease* (COPD) (see Chapter 44) is the leading cause of airway obstruction. *Chronic bronchitis* is the subcategory of COPD that is defined as cough and sputum production that persists for 3 months or more in 2 consecutive years. Characteristically, these patients have a long-standing history of smoking, productive cough, and a slowly progressive decline in exercise capacity. In advanced stages, they may become plethoric, cyanotic, and cough incessantly; the term "blue bloater" has been applied to such patients. Tobacco-stained fingers, wheezes, coarse rales, rhonchi, and prolonged expiratory phase of respiration are often present on examination. Signs of cor pulmonale (right ventricular heave, jugular venous distention, leg edema) are late findings indicative of severe, advanced disease.

Another group of COPD patients are those with *emphysema*. Sputum production is minimal compared to that in patients with bronchitis, and there is less mismatching of ventilation and perfusion; consequently, hypoxia and cyanosis are less prominent. Gradual deterioration in exercise capacity takes place over many years. Patients with advanced emphysema appear thin and barrel-chested. They may purse their lips during expiration to keep their poorly supported airways from collapsing. The chest is hyperresonant, breath sounds are distant, and a few end-expiratory wheezes may be noted; expiration is prolonged.

COPD patients who suffer from *bronchiectasis* have a clinical presentation similar to those with chronic bronchitis, except their physical findings are more localized and their clinical course is more punctuated by recurrent episodes of pneumonia and purulent sputum production.

Asthma (see Chapter 45) is another of the obstructive airway diseases; it usually produces attacks of acute dyspnea, but airway obstruction may persist for a prolonged period after an acute episode and result in more chronic respiratory complaints, including exercise intolerance, cough, and sputum production. At times, sputum production may be the predominant early symptom and may be mistaken for infection. Diffuse wheezes are commonly noted on examination; in severe cases there is use of accessory muscles, retraction, and pulsus paradoxus. Exercise-induced asthma is common in young people and may contribute to recurrent dyspneic episodes.

Diffuse *interstitial lung disease* alters pulmonary compliance and may lead to a disturbance in the balance between ventilation and perfusion. The process is usually very gradual,

and often patients have few symptoms when pulmonary involvement is mild or even moderate; however, tachypnea and cyanosis ensue in severe cases. Diffuse, "dry," midexpiratory crackles are often heard on auscultation. As the interstitial process progresses, dyspnea and hypoxia worsen and exercise tolerance deteriorates.

Kyphoscoliosis is the major chest wall deformity capable of seriously impairing pulmonary musculoskeletal mechanics. Advanced cases can even terminate in cor pulmonale and respiratory failure. Among the extrapulmonary etiologies hindering lung mechanics are severe *obesity,* marked *ascites* (see Chapter 71) and large *pleural effusions* (see Chapter 39). Dyspnea is often the chief complaint in such patients.

Pulmonary vascular disease due to recurrent embolization or primary pulmonary hypertension can be the source of severe dyspnea; mortality is high. Patients with *recurrent emboli* often have a history of long-standing venous disease and episodes of deep-vein thrombophlebitis, though at times the source of emboli is hard to uncover. *Primary pulmonary hypertension* is a diagnosis of exclusion, found most commonly among women between ages 20 and 40. In both conditions, there is often a history of recurrent chest pain (see Chapter 14), dyspnea on exertion, and fatigue. Hyperventilation may result and be mistakenly attributed to anxiety. A history of Raynaud's phenomenon can be obtained in a substantial percentage of patients with primary pulmonary hypertension. *Secondary pulmonary hypertension* may also cause dyspnea; it results from long-standing pulmonary congestion, as seen in mitral stenosis (see Chapter 28). Regardless of etiology, signs of right heart failure develop over time (see Chapter 27).

Anxiety attacks are often confused with more serious etiologies, because the patient may appear to be in severe respiratory distress. The patient often reports chest tightness or claims that he cannot get in enough air. The florid, acute case is represented by the hyperventilation syndrome (see Chapter 222), but commonly there is a less dramatic, chronic feeling of dyspnea and fatigue that is affected little by exertion. Frequent sighing, multiple bodily complaints, nervousness, and a normal physical examination are typical of such patients.

DIFFERENTIAL DIAGNOSIS

The causes of chronic dyspnea encountered in the office setting are listed in Table 36-1.

WORKUP

History. The most difficult task in the evaluation of dyspnea is differentiating dyspnea due to cardiac disease from that resulting from pulmonary pathology. Both etiologies share a number of clinical features. For example, exertional dyspnea is common to both. A common misconception is

Table 36-1. Common Causes of Chronic Dyspnea

Cardiac
1. Congestive heart failure
2. Other causes of pulmonary venous congestion (mitral stenosis, mitral regurgitation)

Pulmonary
1. Chronic obstructive pulmonary disease
2. Pulmonary parenchymal disease (including interstitial diseases)
3. Pulmonary hypertension
4. Severe kyphoscoliosis
5. Exogenous mechanical factors (ascites, massive obesity, large pleural effusion)
6. Chronic asthma

Psychologic
1. Anxiety

that paroxysmal nocturnal dyspnea is chracteristic of heart failure. Unfortunately, this is not the case, because excessive secretions from COPD often pool at night, causing dyspnea due to airway obstruction and forcing the patient to sit up in order to clear his airway. The occurrence of wheezing is a nonspecific manifestation of large airway bronchospasm, whether due to asthma, bronchitis, or interstitial pulmonary edema.

In general, a past history dominated by chronic cough, sputum production, recurrent respiratory infections, occupational exposure, or heavy smoking points more to lung disease than to a cardiac origin. However, unless there is a strong history of previous lung disease or substantial sputum production, it may be very hard to distinguish a cardiac from a pulmonary source on the basis of history alone. Moreover, both may coexist concurrently. Physical findings and laboratory studies are often necessary for a better differentiation.

Dyspnea that is a manifestation of a chronic anxiety state may superficially mimic cardiopulmonary disease and cause some confusion. Onset at rest in conjunction with a sense of chest tightness, suffocation, or inability to take in air are characteristic features of the history. Also, there is little evidence of significant heart or lung disease, though there may be much fear of it. Multiple bodily complaints, history of emotional difficulties, absence of activity limitations, and lack of exacerbation upon exercising argue for a psychogenic cause. Unfortunately, patients with pulmonary hypertension may have episodes that can resemble anxiety-induced bouts of dyspnea; sometimes a young patient with primary pulmonary hypertension is incorrectly labeled "neurotic."

It is helpful to define as precisely as possible the degree of activity that precipitates the sensation of dyspnea, in order to estimate the severity of disease, determine the extent of disability, and detect changes over time. One means of achieving these objectives is to relate symptoms to the patient's daily activities and interpret the degree of restriction in terms of the expected endurance of a patient of similar age.

Factors that may contribute to the occurrence or worsening of dyspnea should be documented, including cigarette smoking, occupational exposure, excessive salt intake, weight gain, and increasing sputum production. The occupational history is particularly important, as the relationships between exposures and lung disease are becoming increasingly evident (see Chapter 35). The patient should be asked about hemoptysis; the symptom raises the possibilities of tumor, embolization with infarction, and pneumonia (see Chapter 38). Suspicion of embolization requires an inquiry into use of oral contraceptives, recent surgery, recurrent thrombophlebitis, and pregnancy (see Chapter 14).

Physical Examination should begin with a check for tachycardia, tachypnea, fever, and hypertension. Weight must not be forgotten, for it may be an early sign of worsening congestive failure (see Chapter 27). The patient's respiratory efforts need to be observed carefully to obtain an estimate of the amount of work expended in breathing; contractions of the accessory muscles of respiration suggest severe difficulty. Retraction of the supraclavicular fossa implies tracheal stenosis that has become critical. Pursed-lip breathing and a prolonged expiratory phase are signs of significant outflow obstruction. The best way to observe airflow obstruction is to have the patient take a deep breath and blow out at hard and fast as he can. The chest is examined for increased A–P diameter (suggestive of COPD) and deformity resulting from kyphoscoliosis or ankylosing spondylitis. Retraction of the intercostal muscles upon inspiration is characteristic of emphysema.

The chest should be percussed for dullness and hyperresonance and auscultated for wheezes, crackles, and quality of breath sounds. Crackles often represent fluid in the airway, as occurs with bronchitis, pneumonitis, and CHF. A normal pulmonary examination does not rule out respiratory pathology, but lessens its probability of being severe. Cardiac examination should focus on the presence of jugular venous distention, a third heart sound, murmurs of valvular heart disease, heaves, and carotid pulse abnormalities (see Chapters 27 and 28). It is important to recognize that many of the signs of right heart failure may be a consequence of long-standing pulmonary disease and therefore are not specific for a cardiac etiology. The abdomen is examined for ascites and hepatojugular reflux; the legs are checked for edema and other signs of phlebitis (see Chapters 16 and 30).

Laboratory Studies. The *chest x-ray* is essential to evaluation and should be studied for pulmonary venous redistribution, effusions, interstitial changes, hyperinflation, infiltrates, enlargement of the pulmonary arteries (indicative of pulmonary hypertension), cardiac chamber enlargement, and valve calcification. Upper zone redistribution of pulmonary blood flow is among the earliest x-ray findings of CHF (see Chapter 27); however, redistribution may also occur in COPD from destruction of vessels in the lower lung fields. The chest film is sometimes useful for detection of interstitial lung disease, because physical findings may be minimal. However, x-ray findings may also be unimpressive, necessitating further study (see below).

Simple *pulmonary function tests* can be reliably performed in the office on an inexpensive spirometer. The *FEV$_1$* and *vital capacity* are the most informative of these measurements for detecting obstructive and restrictive defects, and for determining severity. The ratio of FEV$_1$ to vital capacity is markedly reduced in clinically important obstructive disease. In restrictive disease, the ratio is close to 1.0, but the vital capacity is significantly reduced. An FEV$_1$ can also provide prognostic information; a reading of less than 1.0 liter per second is associated with a poor 5-year survival rate among patients with COPD (see Chapter 44). Patients suspected of having tracheal stenosis may require flow-volume studies to identify the lesion and determine its severity; referral is indicated.

Arterial blood gases (ABGs) are not routinely available in most office settings, but are worth obtaining when there is a question of deteriorating ventilation (*e.g.*, patient is observed to be breathing with accessory muscles); hospitalization should be considered when the PCO$_2$ is inappropriately elevated for the respiratory rate and repeat determinations reveal further pCO$_2$ increases. Drawing ABGs before and after exercise is helpful in assessing the severity of diffuse interstitial disease; a fall in pO$_2$ is evidence of a significant degree of interstitial disease. When use of accessory muscles is noted and the patient appears to be worsening, prompt hospital admission should be carried out, rather than taking time to obtain ABGs in the office.

A *single breath carbon monoxide diffusing capacity* may be the earliest sign of interstitial fibrosis. The test is particularly useful in evaluation of dyspnea associated with suspected occupational interstitial disease (see Chapter 35).

Sometimes the combination of history, physical examination, chest x-ray, and pulmonary function tests is not sufficient to determine the relative contributions of CHF and COPD to the patient's dyspnea. When findings are equivocal, it may be helpful to perform an old-fashioned but still useful test, the *circulation time;* in patients with CHF, the circulation time is prolonged by 4 or more seconds beyond the upper limit of normal (16 seconds). A *Gram's stain* of the sputum is often informative, especially when the patient is febrile, coughing more than usual, or reports a change in sputum.

The neurotic patient with anxiety-induced dyspnea often benefits from having a chest film and simple pulmonary function tests; the confirmation of a well-functioning respiratory system may provide some reassurance and lessen concern over bodily symptoms. At times, a walk with the patient up and down a few flights of stairs is just as convincing for both physician and patient. Climbing stairs with the patient complaining of dyspnea is also useful in those with suspected cardiopulmonary disease, for exercise tolerance can be quan-

titated in terms of flights climbed and the heart and respiratory rates attained.

SYMPTOMATIC MANAGEMENT AND PATIENT EDUCATION

Acute exacerbations of CHF (see Chapter 27), respiratory tract infections (see Chapter 43), large pleural effusions (see Chapter 39), and environmental irritants (see Chapter 35) can and should be dealt with promptly. Treatment of COPD (see Chapter 44), asthma (see Chapter 45), pulmonary venous congestion due to valvular heart disease (see Chapter 28), and anxiety (see Chapter 222) can also provide symptomatic relief. Regardless of cause, all patients with dyspnea should be advised to stop smoking; often the onset of even mild dyspnea is sufficient stimulus to quit, especially when combined with the physician's urging (see Chapter 49).

Many patients with chronic dyspnea request oxygen therapy at home. Such requests are reasonable if there is no evidence of carbon dioxide retention and the patient is bothered by chronic hypoxia; however, the majority of such patients have COPD and should not be given oxygen therapy until it is clear that they do not retain CO$_2$ (see Chapter 44).

The etiologies and precipitants of the patient's dyspnea should be discussed. Prognosis also requires elaboration, especially if it is different from the patient's perception. Some clinicians encourage selected patients with COPD or heart disease to engage in an exercise program; exercise tolerance is often improved, although the effect on survival remains unproven (see Chapters 10, 26, and 44). It is important that patients be reminded to note the level of activity that they can tolerate and report any decrease. Precipitants of worsening exercise tolerance should also be watched for. In this manner, patients can be enlisted in the diagnostic and monitoring efforts; their interest may help ensure compliance and facilitate management.

A.H.G.

ANNOTATED BIBLIOGRAPHY

Baumstark A, Swensson RG, Hessel SJ et al: Evaluating the radiographic assessment of pulmonary venous hypertension in chronic heart disease. Am J Radiol 142:877, 1984 (*Suggests the assessment can be quite accurate; sensitivity 0.75 and specificity 0.88.*)

Buehler JH, Gracey DR: Laboratory differentiation of cardiac and primary pulmonary dyspnea. Mod Concepts Cardiovasc Dis 43: 113, 1974 (*An excellent discussion of pathophysiology and the usefulness of pulmonary function tests in the evaluation of dyspnea.*)

Dodge R, Cline MG, Burrows B: Comparisons of asthma, emphysema, and chronic bronchitis diagnoses in a general population sample. Am Rev Respir Dis 133:981, 1986 (*There is a physician bias to label males as emphysematous; the study reinforces the fact that there is much overlap among these three diseases.*)

Editorial: The enigma of breathlessness. Lancet 1:891, 1986 (*A terse review of the difficult issues.*)

Lee DC, Johnson RA, Bingham JB et al: Heart failure in outpatients. N Engl J Med 306:699, 1982 (*Includes a discussion of clinical findings indicative of the diagnosis and predictive of response to therapy.*)

Jones NL: Exercise testing in pulmonary evaluation: Clinical application. N Engl J Med 293:647, 1975 (*Describes the use of exercise PFTs in evaluating dyspnea; preceded by article, N Engl J Med 293:341, 1975, detailing methods and physiology of exercise testing.*)

Nicklaus TM, Stowell DW, Christiansen WR et al: The accuracy of the roentgenologic diagnosis of chronic pulmonary emphysema. Am Rev Respir Dis 93:889, 1966 (*In patients with severe disease, the sensitivity of the CXR was 0.91 and specificity 0.96; these figures would be greatly reduced in patients with less severe disease.*)

Raffin TA: Indications for arterial blood gas analysis. Ann Intern Med 105:390, 1986 (*A critical review of uses for blood gas; 76 references.*)

37
Evaluation of Chronic Cough

A chronic cough poses a difficult evaluation problem because etiologies range from trivial conditions to life-threatening illnesses. Although many patients attribute their cough to cigarette-smoking, the primary physician must be aware of early signs suggesting a more worrisome cause (such as bronchogenic carcinoma) so that a prompt, efficient, and thorough evaluation can be undertaken without unnecessary testing and excessive delay.

PATHOPHYSIOLOGY AND CLINICAL PRESENTATION

The physiological function of cough is to remove foreign substances and mucus from the respiratory tract. It is a three-phased mechanical process that involves a deep inspiration, increasing lung volume, muscular contraction against a closed glottis, and sudden opening of the glottis. The maneuver produces and sustains a high linear air velocity to expel material from the respiratory tree.

Cough is a reflex response mediated by the medulla, but subject to voluntary control. The afferent limb may involve receptors in the larynx, respiratory tree, pleura, acoustic duct, nose, sinuses, pharynx, stomach, or diaphragm. The receptors respond to mechanical, inflammatory, or irritant stimuli. The trigeminal, glossopharyngeal, phrenic, and vagus nerves can carry the afferent signal. The efferent limb of the cough reflex involves the recurrent laryngeal, phrenic, and spinal motor nerves, which innervate the respiratory muscles.

The most common cause of recurrent cough is *cigarette smoking,* which may trigger the cough reflex by direct bronchial irritation or may induce inflammatory changes and mucus production, stimulating a self-propagating productive cough. Chronic cough and decreased flow rates have been observed in teenagers after only 3 to 5 years of smoking. Pipe and cigar smoking cause lesser degrees of difficulty.

Environmental irritants play a major role in production of cough in patients living in industrialized urban areas. Pollutants that are frequently involved are heavy smog, sulphur dioxide, nitrous oxide, and industrial gases such as ammonia.

In Britain, the relationship between air quality and production of cough has been documented. The dusts and particulate matter that are capable of producing pneumoconioses can contribute to the problem. The excessive drying of normal airway moisture that takes place in centrally heated homes (humidity may fall below 10% unless a humidifier is utilized) results in a persistent dry cough.

Carcinoma of the lung may present with cough in its early stages, particularly when an endobronchial lesion is present. Often the cigarette smoker notes a change in the pattern of his chronic "cigarette cough." Hemoptysis is noted in about 5% to 10% of early cases. Other clues are localized wheezing and purulent sputum suggestive of obstruction. In later stages, cough is present in conjunction with weight loss, anorexia, dyspnea, vomiting, and so on. In some instances, a systemic syndrome (e.g., inappropriate ADH secretion, hypertrophic pulmonary osteoarthropathy, dermatomyositis or peripheral neuropathy) may precede appearance of tumor.

Cough may be the predominant manifestation of *asthma.* Recent studies of asthmatics have emphasized that cough can occur in the absence of wheezing but in the presence of demonstrable airway obstruction. Marked mucus production is in part responsible for the cough (see Chapter 45).

Inflammation anywhere along the upper or lower respiratory tract is capable of producing cough, for receptors capable of transmitting impulses that stimulate cough are believed to be distributed throughout the respiratory system. The greater the inflammatory stimulus, the larger the white cell response and the more purulent the sputum. (The green coloration of very purulent sputum is due to the degeneration of white cells.) *Chronic bronchitis* is among the most common causes of chronic cough and sputum production. The condition is defined clinically as the presence of a productive cough that persists for at least 3 months for 2 consecutive years. A morning cough is often prominent, and bronchospasm a frequent accompaniment (see Chapter 44). *Bronchiectasis* is also characterized by cough and sputum production, but differs clinically from bronchitis in that there are more likely to be repeated bouts of hemoptysis and pneumonia. Copious amounts of purulent sputum are often produced. Chronic cough and sputum production commonly persist between episodes of pneumonia. Focal destruction of supporting lung tissue leads to dilatation of bronchi and focal findings of rhonchi and wheezes on physical examination. A history of suppurative pneumonia in childhood is sometimes elicited.

Nasal and *otic problems* are often overlooked as sources of chronic cough, but allergic rhinitis (see Chapter 220), sinusitis (see Chapter 217), impacted cerumen, or external otitis may be responsible. A persistent postnasal drip can be quite bothersome, and ranks as one of the leading causes that precipitates a visit to the physician. Otic problems cause a dry cough; nasal disease can lead to sputum production.

Interstitial lung disease and *extraluminal compression* may stimulate mechanical receptors and result in a nonproductive cough. Fibrotic diseases of the interstitium and pulmonary edema are examples of intrapulmonary etiologies, and hilar adenopathy, aortic aneurysm, and neoplasm are important extraluminal mass lesions. Chronic interstitial pulmonary edema produces nocturnal cough due to increased venous return at night, which worsens heart failure (see Chapter 27). When failure is severe, frothy pink or blood-tinged sputum may be noted.

Psychogenic cough is more prevalent in children but may occur in adults; characteristically, it is nonproductive, occurs at times of emotional stress, and ceases during the night.

Gastroesophageal reflux sometimes leads to aspiration of gastric juices, with resultant development of a chronic recurrent cough, often in conjunction with reflux on lying down.

DIFFERENTIAL DIAGNOSIS

The common causes of chronic cough are listed in Table 37-1. Rarer etiologies of cough include irritation of the pleura, diaphragm, pericardium, or stomach. Case reports of truly rare causes of cough include osteophytes of the cervical spine and pacemaker malfunction.

WORKUP

History. Because many etiologies of chronic cough are serious but potentially treatable illnesses, the prime objective of evaluation is to search for them; these include early lung cancer, heart failure, asthma, and tuberculosis. Moreover, identification of environmental precipitants is essential to successful therapy. Nonproductive cough should be distinguished from one that produces sputum or mucus. The color and nature of sputum and the timing of its production may be helpful in the diagnosis. Cough productive of purulent sputum indicates significant inflammation, while a scanty or nonproductive cough is usually noninflammatory. A cough described as "throat clearing" may be a manifestation of

Table 37-1.   Important Causes of Chronic or Persistent Cough

Environmental Irritants
1. Cigarette smoking (cigar and pipe smoking to a lesser degree)
2. Pollutants (sulfur dioxide, nitrous oxide, particulate matter)
3. Dusts (all agents capable of producing pneumoconioses)
4. Lack of humidity

Lower Respiratory Tract Problems
1. Lung cancer
2. Asthma
3. Chronic obstructive lung disease (especially bronchitis)
4. Interstitial lung disease
5. Congestive heart failure (chronic interstitial pulmonary edema)
6. Pneumonitis
7. Bronchiectasis

Upper Respiratory Tract Problems
1. Chronic rhinitis
2. Chronic sinusitis
3. Disease of the external auditory canal
4. Pharyngitis

Extrinsic Compressive Lesions
1. Adenopathy
2. Malignancy
3. Aortic aneurysm

Psychogenic Factors

Gastrointestinal Problems
1. Reflux esophagitis

postnasal drip. The history should also detail smoking habits, environmental and occupational exposures, previous allergies, asthma, sinusitis, chronic respiratory infections, and tuberculosis exposure. Associated symptoms of orthopnea, dyspnea on exertion, and paroxysmal nocturnal dyspnea strongly indicate heart failure; dyspnea may also reflect pneumonia or asthma. Hemoptysis suggests bronchitis, bronchiectasis, tumor, or tuberculosis, but also may be due to blood loss from the upper respiratory tract. Generalized wheezing is associated with obstruction from asthma or bronchitis, but localized wheezing may be a sign of tumor. Hoarseness is usually indicative of tracheobronchial disease with laryngeal involvement but may represent a tumor impinging on the recurrent laryngeal nerve. Associated heartburn and cough on lying down suggests reflux as the etiology.

Physical Examination should emphasize the upper and lower respiratory tracts, ears, neck, and cardiovascular system. The physician needs to examine the skin for cyanosis, the pharynx for postnasal discharge and tonsillar enlargement, the nose for polyps, discharge, and obstruction, and the ears for impacted cerumen or otitis. The trachea is palpated for position and the neck for masses and adenopathy. Auscultation and percussion of the lungs (including the apices) are done to detect wheezing, crackles, and signs of consolidation or effusion. During cardiac examination, the physician should evaluate the jugular venous pulse for distention and listen for an S_3 indicative of heart failure.

Laboratory Studies. Expensive testing can very often be held to a minimum when careful history and physical examination are combined with a few, simple, well-chosen studies. The chest film may be helpful when there is historical or physical evidence that raises the question of carcinoma, tuberculosis, heart failure, interstitial pneumonitis, bronchitis, or bronchiectasis. However, the test is overused. For example, many young, previously healthy nonsmokers with a cough that lingers during the winter for 3 to 4 weeks after a typical upper respiratory tract infection come to the office because they are afraid they have pneumonia. The decision to obtain a chest x-ray in a young patient is based on the clinical suspicion of pneumonia, or the patient's concern that he may have it. A study of 1819 patients revealed that the most significant findings predictive of pneumonia were sputum production, night sweats, fever, a respiratory rate greater than 25 per minute, rales, asymmetric respirations, and increased vocal fremitus. The presence of sore throat and rhinorrhea made pneumonia unlikely. The absence of suggestive symptoms and signs obviates the need for chest film, for the probability of encountering a process that requires antibiotic treatment is very small. Obviously, the chest film may be used to provide reassurance, but a careful history and physical should suffice for this purpose.

When a chest film is obtained and an infiltrate identified, a Gram's stain should be performed. In those at high risk for tuberculosis (*e.g.,* recent immigrants, immunocompromised hosts), an acid-fast stain for tubercle bacilli is needed.

Patients who give a history of producing purulent sputum in conjunction with cough but who cannot raise sputum at the time of examination should be instructed to drink a few glasses of water (which may facilitate sputum production), and be asked to remain a while until sputum can be raised. A common error in evaluating a productive cough is failure to obtain and examine the sputum. Culturing the sputum is also important, especially when tuberculosis is a possibility, because the acid-fast examination is not a very sensitive test and the diagnosis cannot be ruled out with certainty until three early morning sputum samples have failed to produce growth by 4 to 6 weeks (see Chapters 34 and 47).

When tumor is suspected (*e.g.,* heavy smoker with change in cough pattern) but the chest film is unremarkable, one should avoid hastily ordering expensive or invasive tests such as tomography and endoscopy. Cytologic testing of three early morning sputum samples can be a useful screening test for pulmonary neoplasm (see Chapter 33) and should be obtained when concern about carcinoma of the lung persists in spite of a normal chest film. Pulmonary histiocytes must be demonstrated on each specimen to prove that the sample of pul-

monary secretions is adequate. A "negative" test in the absence of histiocytes is the source of many false-negative results. Only if cytology is positive or clinical suspicion of cancer is extremely strong (new onset of hemoptysis in conjunction with cough) should the more invasive and expensive procedures be performed (see Chapter 38).

Evaluation of cough accompanied by shortness of breath should include a chest x-ray for signs of congestive failure (see Chapter 27) and a check of simple pulmonary function tests such as the FEV_1 and vital capacity in order to detect any significant bronchospasm that might be subject to treatment. A few whiffs of a bronchodilator can be given to measure the response to bronchodilators (see Chapters 44 and 45). Spirometry can be very useful in the puzzling case.

Patients with chronic bronchitis need not be subjected to repeated diagnostic studies whenever there is an increase or change in sputum production, because the most likely cause is an intercurrent tracheobronchitis due to pneumococci or *Haemophilus influenzae.*

Patients with reflux symptoms do not need radiologic study, but a diagnostic trial of antacids or histamine₂ antagonists may provide useful information.

SYMPTOMATIC THERAPY

The most effective therapy is to alleviate the underlying cause, although this is not always possible. Symptomatic management is directed at suppressing the cough and preventing complications that may result from coughing. Potential complications include musculoskeletal pain, rib fractures, pneumothorax, exhaustion, pneumomediastinum, post-tussive syncope (see Chapter 18), and rupture of subconjunctival or nasal veins. The occurrence of any of these complications may be a reason for occasionally suppressing a cough that has not been completely diagnosed.

The first priority and simplest manipulation is to remove or reduce irritants. Of paramount importance is cessation of smoking; this eliminated cough in 77% and reduced it in another 17% of patients within a month. Second, a properly humidified environment should be maintained. If a humidifier is used, it should be kept clean because it can become colonized with bacteria or fungi and cause infection or hypersensitivity pneumonitis. Third, adequate internal hydration should be encouraged, at least 1500 cc of fluid daily. These simple measures alone may abolish cough in many patients.

The patient with a chronic cough secondary to established underlying lung disease requires careful education. The patient must be informed that sputum should be expectorated when possible. Patients with chronic bronchitis or bronchiectasis can be taught how to cough with quiet, forceful expirations and how to perform postural drainage to promote removal of mucus from the bronchioles. Postural drainage is best timed before meals and at bedtime (see Chapter 44).

Patients with chronic cough often request and need temporary cough suppression to allow uninterrupted sleep or when complications of cough arise. A wide variety of agents have been used to treat cough. The most effective are the narcotic antitussives, which act centrally to suppress the medullary cough center. Other preparations are expectorants or mucolytic agents, which merely help to mobilize sputum; they can have a mild placebo effect as well, but it is not an impressive one. When cough significantly interferes with sleeping or eating, a narcotic cough suppressant should be used. Codeine is the drug of choice. It should be used in relatively small doses of 8 to 15 mg, at intervals of 2 to 4 hours, according to the patient's needs. Liquid and tablet preparations are equally effective. If a small dose does not suppress the cough, doses of up to 60 mg every 3 to 4 hours may be tried. It is worth noting that many patients expect to use a syrup for cough suppression; prescribing the drug in syrup form may provide some psychologic benefit. Patients for whom a narcotic antitussive is prescribed should be given small quantities and followed closely to ensure that the cough resolves and excessive use does not result. The obvious exception to this precaution is the patient with incurable lung cancer, who should receive the doses necessary to provide relief from the discomfort of persistent cough.

Nonnarcotic antitussives lack addiction potential but are not as effective as codeine. The most popular over-the-counter cough suppressant is dextromethorphan, which has a mild suppressant effect. Many over-the-counter preparations contain alcohol, sympathomimetics, and antihistamines. The mucolytic effects of alcohol are minimal; the sympathomimetics and antihistamines are of little use except in patients whose cough derives from chronic rhinitis (see Chapter 220). Some over-the-counter agents dull the peripheral sensory receptors; this is the rationale for putting mild topical anesthetics in sprays, syrups, and cough lozenges. They are of questionable utility.

Expectorants are heavily consumed. There are over 60 preparations containing guaifenesin; terpin hydrate is another popular expectorant. These agents are often combined with an effective cough suppressant and, as such, are associated with a beneficial effect, but by themselves they have no proven effect and represent an unnecessary expense. They are given when the patient insists on something for cough but lacks clear indications for cough suppression, or because the patient believes expectorants help him.

Patients with cough due to asthma respond to bronchodilators (see Chapter 45). An empiric trial of topical steroid therapy may help in suspected allergic rhinitis (see Chapter 220). Patients who respond to a short course of anti-reflux therapy should be considered for a more comprehensive program (see Chapter 56).

INDICATIONS FOR REFERRAL

Although endobronchial cancer is a feared etiology, it is not a common cause of chronic cough in the absence of other findings. However, the undiagnosed patient with risk factors for cancer (smoking, occupational exposure) deserves a consultation for consideration of bronchoscopy.

A.H.G. and A.G.M.

ANNOTATED BIBLIOGRAPHY

Bloustine S et al: Ear cough (Arnold's reflex). Otol Rhinol Laryngol 85:406, 1976 (*A clinical survey of 688 patients that revealed an incidence of the ear cough reflex of 1.74%, a reminder to examine the ear.*)

Brashear RE: Cough: Diagnostic considerations with normal chest roentgenograms. J Fam Pract 15:979, 1982 (*A concise review of both usual and unusual etiologies of acute and chronic cough.*)

Corrao W, Braman SS, Irwin RS: Chronic cough as the sole presenting manifestation of bronchial asthma. N Engl J Med 300:633, 1979 (*Six patients whose asthma presented as cough and had no prior history of wheezing.*)

Diehr P, Wood RW, Bushyhead J et al: Prediction of pneumonia in outpatients with acute cough—a statistical approach. J Chron Dis 37:215, 1984 (*A study of presenting symptoms in nearly 2,000 patients presenting with cough with and without radiographic evidence of pneumonia. A discriminate analysis scoring system is presented.*)

Irwin RS, Corrao WM, Pratter MR: Chronic persistent cough in the adult: The spectrum and frequency of causes and successful outcome of specific therapy. Am Rev Respir Dis 123:413, 1981 (*A series of 49 intensively studied patients revealing 12 with asthma, 14 with postnasal drip, 9 with asthma plus postnasal drip [usually following upper respiratory infection], 6 with bronchitis, 5 with esophagitis, and one each of malignant, cardiac, or interstitial origin.*)

Laudon RG: Smoking and cough frequency. Rev Respir Dis 114: 1033, 1976 (*A paper that confirms that smokers cough more frequently than nonsmokers.*)

McFadden FR Jr: Exertional dyspnea and cough as preludes to acute attacks of asthma. N Engl J Med 292:555, 1975 (*Wheezing may be absent as an early manifestation of an acute attack, and cough may dominate the clinical picture.*)

Stulbarg M: Evaluating and treating intractable cough. West J Med 143:223, 1985 (*An excellent review that focuses on a case where gastroesophageal reflux was the etiology of an intractable cough.*)

38
Evaluation of Hemoptysis

Because of its well-known associations with cancer and tuberculosis, hemoptysis is an alarming symptom for both patient and physician. Hemoptysis refers to coughing up of both blood-tinged and grossly bloody sputum. In the office, the primary physician is usually confronted with a patient who has noted sputum streaked with blood. Most patients prove to have inconsequential lesions, but a thorough evaluation is necessary because the seriousness of the etiology does not correlate with the amount of blood coughed up.

PATHOPHYSIOLOGY AND CLINICAL PRESENTATION

Inflammation of the tracheobronchial mucosa accounts for many cases of hemoptysis. Minor mucosal erosions can result from *upper respiratory infections* and *bronchitis;* blood-streaked sputum is often noted, especially if coughing has been vigorous and prolonged. Patients with *bronchiectasis* are more subject to recurrent episodes of grossly bloody sputum, because necrosis of the bronchial mucosa can be quite severe. Up to 50% of those with bronchiectasis experience hemoptysis. In the United States, hemoptysis occurring with *tuberculosis* is usually due to mucosal ulceration, although potentially fatal bleeding can occur when a blood vessel adjacent to a cavitary lesion ruptures. About 10% to 15% of patients with tuberculosis report some form of hemoptysis; most of these episodes are minor, involving sputum tinged with small amounts of blood. Endobronchial inflammatory injury from granuloma formation is the mechanism of hemoptysis associated with *sarcoidosis;* small amounts of blood-streaked sputum are occasionally noted.

Mucosal injury can also be a consequence of *bronchogenic carcinoma.* Disruption of endobronchial tissue may be minimal and cause little more than a trace of hemoptysis from time to time; hemorrhage is rare. Between 35% and 55% of patients with proven bronchogenic carcinoma report at least one episode of hemoptysis during the course of their illness; it is the presenting symptom in about 10% of cases. Carcinoma metastatic to the lung rarely results in hemoptysis. *Bronchial adenomas* are quite vascular, and commonly central and endobronchial in location; as a consequence, they frequently bleed, and recurrent episodes of hemoptysis are reported in about half of cases.

Injury to the pulmonary vasculature is an important source of hemoptysis. *Lung abscess* may result in damage to adjacent vessels and frequently presents with bloody as well as purulent sputum. *Necrotizing pneumonias,* such as those produced by *Klebsiella,* can cause substantial vascular disruption; 25% to 50% of patients cough up tenacious, bloody sputum referred to as "currant jelly." *Aspergillomas* are also capable of vascular injury; hemoptysis is the most common symptom of the condition. The patient with an aspergilloma is typically a compromised host with prior cavitary disease from tuberculosis, bronchiectasis, or the like. *Pulmonary infarction* secondary to embolization is characterized by sudden onset of pleuritic pain in conjunction with hemoptysis; embolization without infarction does not cause hemoptysis. Pulmonary contusion from blunt *chest trauma* may present with hemoptysis following a nonpenetrating blow to the thorax.

Marked elevations in pulmonary capillary pressure can cause vascular injury and extravasation of red cells. The pink, frothy sputum of *pulmonary edema* is a manifestation of this process. More grossly bloody sputum sometimes occurs in severe *mitral stenosis* when a dilated pulmonary-bronchial venous connection ruptures. Vasculitic injury is responsible for the hemoptysis found in *Wegener's granulomatosis* (see Chapter 220) and *Goodpasture's syndrome.* Hematuria often accompanies both conditions. Hereditary vascular malformations are subject to recurrent bleeding. *Arteriovenous malformations* may be accompanied by an audible bruit on auscultation of the lung. In *hereditary hemorrhagic telangiectasia,* there is often a family history of bleeding problems or prior episodes of bleeding from multiple sites; telangiectasias may be visible in the buccal cavity and on the skin. Bleeding into the interstitium characterizes *idiopathic pulmonary hemosiderosis.* This rare disease, uncommon in adults, is manifested by diffuse interstitial infiltrates, anemia, and hemoptysis.

Hemoptysis may be the first sign of a *bleeding disorder* or *excessive anticoagulant therapy;* however, there is usually an underlying bronchopulmonary lesion as well.

DIFFERENTIAL DIAGNOSIS

The most commonly reported etiologies of hemoptysis are chronic bronchitis and bronchiectasis, accounting for 50% to 70% of cases in many series. Bronchogenic carcinomas account for less than 5% of cases. Tuberculosis, pneumonia, and vascular lesions make up the remainder. Most prevalence figures are obtained from chest clinics and inpatient units serving preselected populations; therefore, they cannot be extrapolated to the primary care setting. The declining incidence of tuberculosis (see Chapter 34), more widespread use of fiberoptic bronchoscopy, and increases in cigarette smoking and lung cancer in women must be kept in mind when interpreting published clinical series. The more common and important etiologies of hemoptysis are listed in Table 38-1. In office practice, the nasal mucosa and oropharynx are more often the source of blood-tinged sputum than is the lower respiratory tract.

WORKUP

As noted earlier, most cases of blood-tinged sputum encountered in the primary care setting, especially those seen during the winter, are upper respiratory in origin. Such cases do not require further investigation. To avoid unnecessary workup for a pulmonary etiology, the history and physical examination should first focus on the nasal and oropharyngeal mucosa. Only in the absence of an upper respiratory bleeding source need further workup proceed in the manner detailed in the following paragraphs.

History. Evaluation of the patient with a suspected lower respiratory source of hemoptysis should begin with consideration of the epidemiology of the serious underlying causes. Concern about pulmonary neoplasm should be highest in the older male with a long history of heavy smoking or asbestos exposure. The elderly patient with evidence of old disease on chest x-ray should be presumed to have reactivated tuberculosis infection. The adolescent with hemoptysis may have a new infection due to recent tuberculosis exposure. The compromised host with previous cavitary disease is at risk for an aspergilloma.

Table 38-1.   Important Causes of Hemoptysis

Gross Hemoptysis
1. Tuberculosis (with cavitary disease)
2. Bronchiectasis
3. Bronchial adenoma
4. Bronchogenic carcinoma (uncommon)
5. Aspergilloma
6. Necrotizing pneumonia
7. Lung abscess
8. Pulmonary contusion
9. A-V malformation
10. Hereditary hemorrhagic telangiectasia
11. Bleeding disorder or excessive anticoagulant therapy
12. Mitral stenosis (with rupture of a bronchial vessel)

Blood-streaked Sputum
1. Any of the causes of gross hemoptysis
2. Upper respiratory tract infection
3. Chronic bronchitis
4. Sarcoidosis
5. Bronchogenic carcinoma
6. Tuberculosis
7. Pulmonary infarction
8. Pulmonary edema
9. Mitral stenosis
10. Idiopathic pulmonary hemosiderosis

The patient's description of the sputum associated with hemoptysis can be of some diagnostic help. Pink sputum is suggestive of pulmonary edema fluid; putrid sputum is indicative of a lung abscess; currant-jellylike material points to a necrotizing pneumonia; copious amounts of purulent sputum mixed with blood are consistent with bronchiectasis. The commonly described blood-streaked sputum is nonspecific.

History should also be examined for previous bleeding episodes, family history of hemoptysis, hematuria, concurrent pleuritic chest pain, known heart murmur or history of rheumatic fever, lymph node enlargement, blunt chest trauma, symptoms of heart failure (see Chapter 27), and use of anticoagulant drugs. Determining the amount of blood produced is not particularly helpful for diagnostic purposes beyond establishing whether the hemoptysis was gross or scant. As noted above, it is important to be certain that there is no history of a coexisting nasopharyngeal problem or source of gastrointestinal bleeding that the patient may be mistaking for true hemoptysis.

Physical Examination is directed at detecting nonpulmonary sources of bleeding as well as evidence of chest pathology and systemic disease. The vital signs should be checked for fever and tachypnea, the skin for ecchymoses and telangiectasias, and the nails for clubbing. Clubbing is associated with neoplasm, bronchiectasis, lung abscess, and other severe pulmonary disorders (see Chapter 41). Nodes are examined for enlargement, suggestive of sarcoidosis, tuberculosis, and malignancy (see Chapters 48 and 81). The neck is noted for jugular venous distention, consistent with heart failure, and severe mitral disease. Examination of the chest should include a search for bruits, signs of consolidation, wheezes, crackles, and chest wall contusion.

The history and physical findings can be used to determine the pace at which work-up should proceed, as well as the selection and sequence of laboratory tests. The patient with minimal hemoptysis may be followed at home, while evaluation takes place on an outpatient basis, as long as the patient is given explicit advice to return immediately if severe bleeding ensues. The patient with a suspected bleeding diathesis should not be sent home.

Laboratory Studies. The chest x-ray is essential to the assessment of most cases, for it may reveal a mass, abscess, infiltrate, interstitial changes, hilar adenopathy, signs of congestive failure (see Chapter 27), or evidence of significant mitral stenosis (see Chapter 28). Less common radiologic findings include peribronchial cuffing indicative of bronchiectasis and a crescentic radiolucency surrounding a coin lesion characteristic of an aspergilloma. Often the chest film is normal.

The sputum needs to be Gram stained if it appears grossly purulent or the patient is febrile. An acid-fast stain for tubercle bacilli is also essential, not only for diagnosis but for making a crude assessment of infectivity (see Chapter 47). The sensitivity of the acid-fast smear depends on the diligence with which the search for pathogenic organisms is made. In one series, only 20% of culture-positive samples were identified in advance by acid-fast smear. It should also be remembered that despite a very high specificity, the predictive value of a positive smear may be as low as 50% when the sputum specimens of low-risk patients are examined. A tuberculin skin test should be performed if the patient's PPD reactivity status is not known. It must be remembered, however, that approximately 7% of all adults (25% of adults over age 50) will have positive reactions. (See Chapters 34 and 47).

Sputum cytologies should be obtained in all patients in whom there is no clear diagnosis. The sensitivity of a single sputum cytology examination has been shown to be about 70% in the detection of squamous cell lesions, lower for other cell types. Three cytologic examinations increase sensitivity to 90%.

Additional diagnostic tests may be indicated in specific clinical settings; for example, tomography may further define a suspicious lesion seen on chest x-ray, and ventilation-perfusion scanning or angiography of the lung is indicated when the presentation suggests pulmonary embolization with infarction (see Chapter 14). Bleeding studies, such as a PT, PTT, platelet count, and bleeding time are needed if more than one site of bleeding is noted.

A difficult decision is when to refer the patient for bronchoscopy. The procedure often provides useful information when the diagnosis is still in doubt after chest x-ray and sputum examination. Moreover, the sensitivities of cytologic and bacteriologic studies are enhanced when specimens are obtained by bronchoscopy. Bronchoscopy is mandatory in all patients with massive hemoptysis who are being seriously considered for surgery, in order to localize the bleeding site. Rigid bronchoscopy is preferred in this situation.

The more common indication for bronchoscopy is to exclude the possibility of a tumor. It must be remembered, however, that the prevalence of cancer in an unselected population presenting with hemoptysis is low and that the risks of morbidity associated with bronchoscopy are not insignificant. Among patients presenting at a chest clinic complaining of hemoptysis, only 2% were subsequently found to have cancers. One could expect the prevalence among patients without suggestive chest x-ray findings and with negative sputum cytologies to be significantly lower. Patients with "positive" or "suspicious" cytology or a radiologic abnormality clearly are better candidates for endoscopy.

Serious complications are rare with fiberoptic bronchoscopy, but they do occur. In a review of 48,000 procedures, fewer than 100 life-threatening cardiovascular or respiratory complications were reported, most often in older individuals with COPD and coronary disease. Hypoxia occurs commonly following bronchoscopy. In the low-risk patient, fiberoptic bronchoscopy is indicated for unexplained, recurrent, mild hemoptysis and can be safely performed without hospitalization.

A.H.G., L.A.M., and A.G.M.

ANNOTATED BIBLIOGRAPHY

Boucot KR et al: Hemoptysis in older men. Geriatrics 14:67, 1959 (*A comprehensive statistical review of patients with hemoptysis from the Philadelphia Pulmonary Neoplasm Research Project. It found neoplasm in 80%, but hemoptysis was generally a late finding.*)

Fontana RS, Sanderson DR, Taylor WF et al: Early lung cancer detection. Am Rev Respir Dis 130:561, 1984 (*Results of screening with sputum cytology and x-ray examination.*)

Johnston RN, Lockhart W et al: Hemoptysis. Br Med J 1:592, 1960 (*A paper from a chest clinic that revealed 324 cases of hemoptysis representing 15% of the clinical population. Demonstrated that upper respiratory infection, bronchitis, and "no apparent diagnosis" were the leading causes of hemoptysis in an ambulatory population, done prior to advent of modern diagnostic techniques.*)

Selecky PA: Evaluation of hemoptysis through the bronchoscope. Chest 73:7415, 1978 (*Author takes the position that all patients with hemoptysis need bronchoscopy, unless they have malignant cells or acid-fast bacilli in the sputum.*)

Smiddy JF, Eliot RC: The evaluation of hemoptysis with fiberoptic bronchoscopy. Chest 64:158, 1973 (*An article that establishes the utility of transnasal fiberoptic bronchoscopy in a prospective study evaluating hemoptysis. The source of bleeding was located in 66 of 71 patients.*)

Surratt PM, Smiddy JF, Gruber B: Deaths and complications associated with fiberoptic bronchoscopy. Chest 69:747, 1976 (*Fifty-two severe respiratory complications and 27 severe cardiovascular complications in nearly 50,000 procedures.*)

Weaver LJ, Solliday N, Cugell DW: Selection of patients with hemoptysis for fibroptic bronchoscopy. Chest 76:719, 1979 (*Critical look at who needs bronchoscopy.*)

39
Evaluation of Pleural Effusions

Most pleural effusions encountered in the office are discovered as incidental findings and often pose a diagnostic challenge, for etiology is frequently unclear. Of major concern are the possibilities of tumor and infection. Outpatient evaluation of a pleural effusion requires skill in performance of a diagnostic thoracentesis in the office and the differentiation of a transudate from an exudate. The primary physician should be able to safely carry out the initial evaluation of a pleural effusion in the ambulatory setting, provided the patient's respiratory status is satisfactory and there is no evidence of serious acute illness.

PATHOPHYSIOLOGY AND CLINICAL PRESENTATION

The pleural cavity normally contains a small volume of serous fluid that serves as a lubricant. Fluid is formed by transudation from the parietal pleural surface and reabsorbed predominantly by the visceral pleura. Effusion results from excessive transudation of fluid or from an exudative process. Increased hydrostatic pressure and decreased colloid oncotic pressure produce transudates. Exudates result from inflammatory or infiltrative disease of the pleura and its adjacent structures; damage occurs to capillary membranes, and protein-rich material accumulates in the pleural space. Obstruction to lymphatic flow can also produce an exudative effusion.

Transudates

Since transudates are rarely associated with pleural inflammation, they are not usually accompanied by pleuritic pain, but may lead to shortness of breath if they are large enough to interfere with respiratory mechanics. They may be unilateral but are often bilateral. Physical examination of the lung reveals dullness and diminished breath sounds. If the effusion has produced some atelectasis, there may be bronchial breath sounds and increased vocal fremitus above the effusion. Most transudates have a protein concentration of less than 3.0 g per 100 ml, but chronic transudates may show higher concentrations. In a study of patients with longstanding effusions due to chronic congestive heart failure, a large percentage had pleural fluid protein concentrations in excess of 3.0 g per 100 ml.

Congestive heart failure is among the most common causes of transudative effusions. Left heart failure increases pulmonary capillary pressure (see Chapter 27), which forces excess fluid into the interstitium. Right ventricular failure contributes by raising central venous pressure, which elevates the hydrostatic force in the capillaries of the parietal pleura and diminishes fluid reabsorption. Most effusions due to congestive failure are bilateral, but at times there can be an isolated right-sided effusion; isolated left-sided effusions due to congestive failure are rare. The reason for the right-sided preference is unknown. Symptoms and signs of congestive failure (see Chapter 27) are usually evident. Over 85% of effusions resulting from heart failure have protein concentrations less than 3.0 g per 100 ml. The concentration may be greater if the effusion is chronic or the patient has recently been undergoing a brisk diuresis. The pleural fluid is usually clear, but it may be bloody and have red cell counts in excess of 5000 per ml.

Patients with an overexpanded extracellular volume due to severe *hypoalbuminemia* or *salt retention* develop edema in parts of the body where hydrostatic pressures are greatest, before showing evidence of pleural effusion. Cardiomegaly may be in evidence, but overt signs of congestive failure are usually absent. Edema is rare before the serum albumin falls below 2.0 to 2.5 g per 100 ml.

Intra-abdominal diseases are occasionally responsible for transudative effusions. Between 5% and 10% of patients with ascites due to cirrhosis develop a right-sided pleural effusion; the composition of the effusion resembles that of the ascitic fluid. In cases of pancreatitis or a subphrenic abscess, a "sympathetic effusion" with the characteristics of a transudate sometimes forms; it soon changes into an exudate.

Pleural effusions are common after cornary bypass graft surgery and do not imply serious pathology. The same holds for the postpartum patient.

Exudates

Since most exudates form as a consequence of pleural injury, they are often accompanied by pleuritic chest pain, especially in the acute phase when a friction rub may be heard before much fluid accumulates. The fluid is initially free-flowing, but may become walled-off and loculated when there is a marked inflammatory response. The protein content is usually greater than 3.0 g per 100 ml. The fluid is typically deep yellow or cloudy in appearance. The leukocyte count is often greater than 1000 cells per ml; a count greater than 10,000 is suggestive of an empyema, particularly if most of the cells are neutrophils.

Neoplasms are often responsible for the development of effusions. The majority of pleural fluid accumulations due to malignancies have the characteristics of exudates, though at times the protein concentration is less than 3.0 g per 100 ml. *Bronchogenic carcinoma* is the tumor most frequently associated with a pleural effusion. Fluid collects in most instances as a direct result of pleural invasion; unilateral effusions are the rule. Patients report dyspnea when the effusion is large and occasionally complain of pleuritic chest pain. The pleural fluid is usually clear and straw-colored, but it may be bloody and its glucose level may be very low. The white cell count is typically around 2500 per ml, with most cells being lymphocytes. Malignant cells are found in about 60% of instances. Unfortunately, the disease and its effusions are progressive; thoracentesis is followed by rapid reaccumulation.

Pleural effusions due to *metastatic carcinoma* are more likely to be bilateral than those due to bronchogenic carcinoma, for they occur as a consequence of lymphatic obstruction or diffuse seeding of the pleura. Carcinoma of the breast is the leading metastatic tumor producing pleural effusions. The characteristics of the pleural fluid are similar to those of effusions due to bronchogenic carcinoma. *Lymphoma* is another malignant cause of bilateral pleural effusions. The formation of a large effusion is a sign of advanced disease; there is often evidence of pleural, parenchymal, and lymph node involvement by the time a significant effusion appears. The pleural fluid may be a transudate or an exudate; most of the cells are lymphocytes. Cough and dyspnea accompany parenchymal involvement, but pleuritic pain is rare.

Mesotheliomas have become an increasingly important source of effusion as the incidence of asbestos exposure has increased. Only malignant mesotheliomas produce important pleural fluid accumulations. The latent period for mesothelioma formation ranges from 20 to 40 years after asbestos exposure; the degree of exposure may appear inconsequential (see Chapter 35). Chest pain, cough, and shortness of breath result from extensive pleural disease and large effusions. The fluid may be bloody and often contains malignant cells, which are sometimes hard to identify specifically as those of a mesothelioma. Since the tumor is only locally invasive, there are no signs of extrathoracic disease.

Impressive effusions can form as a consequence of *benign ovarian neoplasms (Meigs' syndrome).* The tumor produces ascites, and fluid tracks across the diaphragm and into the thorax. The effusion is typically on the right, but may be left-sided or even bilateral; it is exudative in quality, free of malignant cells, and similar in composition to the ascitic fluid from which it derives. Removal of the ovarian tumor results in prompt resolution of the effusion.

Infections are an important source of exudative pleural effusions. The effusion due to *postprimary tuberculosis* represents a delayed hypersensitivity reaction to spillage of organisms into the pleural space during early bacteremia or subclinical parenchymal disease (see Chapter 47). The effu-

sion is almost always unilateral. The patient may be relatively free of symptoms or complain of lethargy, fever, and weight loss; at times, the clinical picture is dominated by acute onset of pleuritic pain and fever. Cough and sputum are conspicuously absent. The chest x-ray may show little more than an isolated effusion, but the intermediate-strength tuberculin skin test is usually positive. The pleural fluid has the qualities of an exudate; the glucose concentration may be low. The white cell count averages 1000 to 2000 cells per ml; lymphocytes predominate; mesothelial cells are scarce (less than 2%). Neutrophils may be seen early in the course of the illness. Organisms are rarely found on acid-fast stain of the fluid and can be cultured from the fluid in only 25% of cases. Most of these effusions resolve spontaneously within a few months and leave little or no residual; however, symptomatic pulmonary parenchymal involvement eventually develops in over half of such patients (see Chapter 47).

Acute bacterial pneumonia may lead to the formation of a pleural effusion, but among the bacterial pneumonias encountered in ambulatory patients, effusions are uncommon. About 5% of patients with pneumococcal pneumonia develop an effusion; it is usually small and transient. Empyema is a rare but much more worrisome event, seen in less than 1%; most cases occur when proper antibiotic therapy is delayed. Cough, sputum production, fever, chills, and pleuritic pain are often prominent. Early on, the pleural fluid may be serous, but it quickly turns purulent with empyema formation. The fluid may be sterile if empyema does not develop; organisms can be isolated from most empyemas. In some instances, the pleural fluid offers the only opportunity for recovery of the causative organism. Characteristics of the pleural empyema fluid include a white cell count in excess of 5000 to 10,000 per ml, with neutrophils predominating. The concentration of glucose is typically less than 20 mg per 100 ml. Pleural scarring may be substantial if the empyema fluid is allowed to remain.

Viral pneumonitis and *mycoplasmal pneumonia* are sometimes associated with pleural effusions in the course of illness, but the effusions are small, transient, and of little consequence (see Chapter 43).

Pulmonary Embolization has been found to be accompanied by pleural effusion in up to 50% of cases. The effusions are usually small and not dependent on occurrence of pulmonary infarction. There is considerable variation in cell count, differential, and protein concentration. The effusions that result from infarction are more likely to be bloody. Bilateral effusions can be seen when emboli affect both lungs.

Systemic lupus erythematosus produces in many patients transient pleuropericardial inflammation during the course of the disease, usually after other signs and symptoms have appeared. There may be a brief period of pleuritic pain. On occasion, pleural involvement may be the disease's initial clinical presentation. In most instances, the pleural fluid has the characteristics of an effusion and may demonstrate low serum complement levels.

Rheumatoid Arthritis is much less likely to produce a pleural effusion than is lupus, but the fluid often persists. Less than 5% of patients experience pleuropericardial involvement; these individuals usually have a history of extra-articular manifestations and joint symptoms. Once in a while, the effusion is the first manifestation of rheumatoid disease. The effusion is an exudate, with a predominance of lymphocytes and a very low (less than 20 mg per 100 ml) glucose concentration. Although the fluid may contain rheumatoid factor, its presence is not unique to this disease.

Intra-abdominal Pathology occasionally results in the production of a pleural effusion. Patients with a recent history of abdominal surgery, intestinal perforation, or hepatobiliary disease are at risk for development of a *subdiaphragmatic abscess*. In addition to gastrointestinal symptoms, these patients may complain of pleuritic pain, fever, weight loss, and malaise. Often symptoms are nonspecific, causing considerable delay in the decision to seek medical help. The diaphragm on the involved side (which is the right in two thirds of cases) is elevated and moves poorly on fluoroscopy. A pathognomonic subdiaphragmatic air-fluid level may be present on chest film. The pleural fluid is usually sterile, though it may have a high leukocyte count. If the diaphragm has been perforated, an empyema can form. *Pancreatitis* may lead to a pleural effusion, particularly in the early phase of the disease. The effusions are most often on the left, but may be bilateral or right sided. The fluid characteristically has a high amylase concentration and is blood-tinged in one third of cases.

DIFFERENTIAL DIAGNOSIS

The etiologies of pleural effusions can be conveniently divided into those conditions that produce transudates and those that result in exudates (Table 39-1); nevertheless, some conditions can cause both. Chronic congestive heart failure is the etiology most frequently encountered in the ambulatory population. Neoplasms account for the majority of cases seen in referral populations. In a series reported from the Mayo Clinic, bronchogenic carcinoma was the leading cause of malignant pleural effusions, followed by breast cancer and lymphoma. Infection is the third most common etiology of fluid in the pleural space, with tuberculosis still accounting for a substantial proportion of effusions subjected to full evaluation. Bloody effusions are most often due to neoplasms, but are also seen with congestive heart failure, pulmonary embolization with infarction, tuberculosis, and pancreatitis. About 15% of effusions remain unexplained; most idiopathic effusions are exudates.

Table 39-1. Important Causes of Pleural Effusions

Transudates
Congestive heart failure
Hypoalbuminemia
Salt-retention syndromes
Ascites due to cirrhosis
Early phases of a sympathetic effusion
Neoplasm (on occasion)
Peritoneal dialysis
Postpartum
Cardiac bypass graft surgery

Exudates
Neoplasms
Bronchogenic carcinoma
Breast cancer
Lymphoma
Mesothelioma
Meig's syndrome
Infections
Tuberculosis
Bacterial pneumonia (including empyema)
Viral pneumonitis
Mycoplasmal pneumonia
Pulmonary embolization
Connective tissue disease
Rheumatoid arthritis
Systemic lupus erythematosus
Intra-abdominal disease
Subphrenic abscess
Pancreatitis
Idiopathic

WORKUP

History. Although definitive evaluation of a pleural effusion requires analysis of the pleural fluid, history can provide important clues and supporting evidence. The patient should be asked about the presence of fever, cough, sputum production, chest pain, dyspnea, edema, abdominal pain, prior history of malignant, hepatic, or renal disease, exposure to tuberculosis or asbestos, and symptoms of rheumatoid arthritis and systemic lupus (see Chapters 144 and 153). Cough, fever, and sputum production in conjunction with pleuritic chest pain suggests pneumonitis with pleural involvement. Pleuritic pain is also consistent with embolization (see Chapter 14), malignancy, and pleural inflammation with adjacent pericarditis due to connective tissue disease. Dyspnea may be induced by the effusion alone, but the symptom is indicative of congestive heart failure when accompanied by orthopnea and paroxysmal nocturnal dyspnea. A history of peripheral edema raises the possibilities of hypoalbuminemia, volume overload, and congestive failure. A history of alcohol abuse, recent abdominal surgery, or abdominal pain or distention points to a source below the diaphragm.

Physical Examination should determine the size of the effusion and the degree of respiratory compromise associated with it, as well as provide evidence for an underlying etiology.

The vital signs should be checked for fever, tachypnea, tachycardia, and weight change. The integument requires inspection for petechiae, purpura, spider angiomas, jaundice, clubbing (see Chapter 41), rheumatoid nodules, and rashes. The neck is noted for jugular venous distention and tracheal deviation; the lymph nodes, for enlargement. Findings of the effusion on examination of the lung include dullness to percussion and diminished breath sounds. If there is compression of adjacent lung, egophony and bronchial breath sounds may be heard above the effusion. A pleural friction rub may be audible, but is usually lacking when there is a considerable accumulation of fluid. The heart should be checked for an S_3, indicative of failure, and evidence of pericariditis, such as a three-component friction rub. The abdomen is examined for signs of ascites, organomegaly, and focal tenderness. The pelvic examination is done to rule out the presence of an ovarian mass, and the extremities are noted for edema, calf tenderness, and joint changes.

Laboratory Evaluation centers on chest film (for confirmation of the effusion's size and location) and on analysis of the pleural fluid. The chest x-ray should also be studied for pleural-based densities, infiltrates, signs of congestive heart failure (see Chapter 27), hilar adenopathy, coin lesions, and loculation of fluid (detection of which requires lateral decubitus views). Elevation of a hemidiaphragm and presence of a subdiaphragmatic air–fluid level are important radiologic signs of a subphrenic abscess. The location of the effusion may be helpful. Among transudative effusions due to cardiac failure, unilateral effusions tend to be right sided, and bilateral effusions usually are asymmetrical with more fluid on the right side. On the other hand, effusions associated with pericarditis, or with pancreatitis, tend to be left sided.

Although sampling of the pleural fluid is usually necessary for diagnosis, there are instances when thoracentesis need not be done on the first visit; these include the afebrile patient with clinical evidence of congestive heart failure, the postpartum woman who is otherwise well, the patient who has had bypass graft surgery, and the young patient with a small effusion in conjunction with a viral or mycoplasmal pneumonia. These individuals can be followed expectantly with repeat chest films; failure of the effusion to clear with resolution of the presumptive etiology is an indication for thoracentesis.

A *diagnostic thoracentesis* can be done safely and comfortably in the office on patients who have free-flowing effusions confirmed by lateral decubitus films. Ultrasound has been increasingly used to help guide thoracentesis, but in a careful study it has not been shown to enhance the safety or yield to the procedure except in situations of very small effusions. Thoracentesis for loculated effusions is more difficult and has a greater risk of pneumothorax; it is best not to tap such effusions in the office. There are a few pitfalls in thoracentesis technique that must be avoided. A common error is to enter the chest too far below the meniscus of the effusion,

risking penetrating the diaphragm or entering the diaphragmatic sulcus, which is likely to be sealed off from the effusion by lung tissue. To define the proper entry point, the lung fields should be percussed and auscultated to determine the upper border of the effusion. Because pleural fluid rises in a meniscus where it comes in contact with the parietal pleura, the needle should be passed into the chest one interspace *higher* than the upper border of the effusion as determined by examination. A few millimeters of penetration into the pleural space at the level of the meniscus will allow full drainage without the complications of a low entry. Injury to the neurovascular bundle along the inferior surface of the rib is avoided by aiming the needle just above the rib's *superior* margin, accomplished by "walking the needle" over the anesthetized surface of the rib. Pneumothorax is minimized by withdrawing or changing needle position as soon as air bubbles begin to appear or one feels the visceral pleura contacting the needle tip; the onset of coughing is common at this stage. The patient should be advised to resist the impulse to cough, for the act may impale the lung on the needle. Use of a large-bore Intracath (14 or 16 gauge) minimizes the risk of needle injury to the lung. A post-thoracentesis chest film should be obtained to be sure that a significant pneumothorax has not been produced.

The laboratory analysis of pleural fluid should begin with determination of *protein* and *LDH* concentrations; a simultaneous serum sample should also be sent for protein and LDH levels. The three most useful tests to identify a pleural exudate are pleural LDH level (>200 units), pleural-to-serum LDH ratio (>0.6), and pleural-to-serum protein ratio (>0.5). Used as a triad (any one of the separate tests positive), these tests have a sensitivity of 99% and a specificity of 98%. If this first step indicates that the effusion is a transudate, no further laboratory analysis of the fluid is indicated. In fact, because of the poor specificity of white and red blood cell counts, glucose level, amylase level, and even bacterial cultures (due to contamination), such tests performed on transudates may be misleading.

If any of the criteria for an exudate are met, the laboratory analysis should include differential cell count, bacterial culture (including cultures for anaerobes and mycobacteria), and *cytologic examination.* The cell count is rarely very helpful; a high white blood cell count may indicate infection but is nonspecific; a lymphocyte predominance may be suggestive of tuberculosis or malignancy but does not help in distinguishing between these two foremost explanations for exudative effusions without apparent cause. The sensitivity of cytologic examination depends on the mechanism of the malignant effusion and extent of disease; it may be as high as 95% in advanced disease but as low as 50% in early disease. A positive cytology, read by an experienced pathologist, is highly specific.

In certain circumstances, other tests may be useful. A low pleural fluid *glucose level* (<60 mg/dl) is a nonspecific finding associated with tuberculosis, other infection, or malignancy.

Very low glucose levels (<30 mg/dl) are most consistently associated with the effusion of rheumatoid arthritis. An elevated amylase level may point to pancreatitis as the cause of effusion, but it can also be seen in malignant effusion. Specific markers for malignancy such as carcinoembryonic antigen (CEA) level have not proved useful. Similarly, measurement of complement levels (CH50, C3, and C4) should be reserved for the rare instance when it is necessary to reduce the likelihood of an alternative co-morbid explanation for exudative effusion in the patient with rheumatoid arthritis or systemic lupus erythematosus. Pleural fluid ANA measurement may be useful in establishing the diagnosis of lupus pleuritis.

In about 15% of cases, the etiology of an exudative effusion is not evident after complete laboratory analysis of the pleural fluid. If the suspicion of tuberculosis or malignancy persists, pleural biopsy is indicated. Pleural biopsy alone may be less sensitive than cytologic examination of pleural fluid in detecting malignancy, but the two tests are complementary, with a sensitivity in excess of 90% when used together. Pleural biopsy is most useful in detecting tuberculosis with a sensitivity of 60% to 80%. Again, the biopsy information is complementary; fluid culture or pleural tissue (or both) will make the diagnosis of tuberculosis in up to 95% of those with the disease. Pleural tissue, as well as pleural fluid, should be submitted for mycobacterial culture.

When contemplating pleural biopsy, it should be anticipated that the majority of specimens will disclose only nonspecific inflammatory changes. Although as many as 20% of such patients will eventually have the diagnosis of malignant effusion made, the majority will have their effusion resolve spontaneously without serious sequelae.

INDICATIONS FOR ADMISSION AND REFERRAL

The acutely tachypneic patient in much discomfort obviously requires hospitalization, especially when embolization, severe congestive failure, or acute severe pneumonitis is likely. Few of these patients will present to the physician in the office, but the patient with a chronic and enlarging collection of pleural fluid is apt to be encountered. The person who appears to be tolerating the effusion without much discomfort can be evaluated and managed on an outpatient basis as long as there is no evidence suggestive of an empyema or a subphrenic abscess, conditions that require surgical attention. Referral is appropriate when malignancy or tuberculosis is suspected and pleural biopsy deemed necessary.

SYMPTOMATIC MANAGEMENT

The patient can be made comfortable prior to establishing a diagnosis. Pleuritic pain often responds to indomethacin;

the drug has the advantage over narcotics in that it does not have any suppressive effect on respiration. Removal of fluid is indicated when the effusion is compromising respiratory efforts. Usually no more than a liter should be removed at one time, in order to avoid intravascular volume depletion upon re-equilibration.

A.G.M.

ANNOTATED BIBLIOGRAPHY

Black LE: Pleural space and pleural fluid. Mayo Clin Proc 47:493, 1972 (*An excellent article reviewing pathophysiology.*)

Fine NL, Smith LR, Sheedy PF: Frequency of pleural effusions in mycoplasma and viral pneumonias. N Engl J Med 283:790, 1970 (*Small transient effusions are common in these conditions, but large effusions are rare.*)

Frist B, Kahan AV, Koss LG: Comparison of the diagnostic value of biopsies of the pleura and cytologic evaluation of pleural fluids. Ann Intern Med 7:507, 1972 (*Among 106 cases of malignant effusion, 97% had positive fluid cytology and 38% positive pleural biopsies; together, the tests had a sensitivity of 100%.*)

Hughson WG, Friedman PJ, Feigin DS et al: Postpartum pleural effusion: A common radiologic finding. Ann Intern Med 97:856, 1982 (*In a small prospective study, a majority of asymptomatic women had pleural effusions within 24 hours after delivery.*)

Hunder GG: Pleural fluid complement in systemic lupus erythematosus and rheumatoid arthritis. Ann Intern Med 76:356, 1972 (*Complement levels are low.*)

Light RW, Ball WC: Glucose and amylase in pleural effusion. JAMA 225:259, 1973 (*Tuberculosis and malignant effusions were not universally associated with low glucose values.*)

Light RW et al: Cells and pleural fluid. Arch Intern Med 132:854, 1973 (*Reviews the diagnostic significance of cell counts; concludes that the finding of many mesothelial cells is incompatible with tuberculosis; red cell counts greater than 100,000 suggested neoplasm, infarction, or trauma: predominant lymphocytes were consistent with tuberculosis or neoplasm.*)

Light RW et al: Pleural effusions: The diagnostic separation of transudate and exudate. Ann Intern Med 77:507, 1972 (*A classic article that details rigorous criteria for the separation of transudates from exudates.*)

Peterman TA, Speicher CE: Evaluating pleural effusions. JAMA 252:1051, 1984 (*Advocates a two-stage procedure identifying exudates with rapid determination of protein and LDH values, thereby eliminating need to order additional tests for transudates.*)

Poe RE, Israel RH, Vtell MJ et al: Sensitivity, specificity, and predictive values of closed pleural biopsy. Arch Intern Med 144:325, 1984 (*Sensitivity of 68% for malignant disease.*)

Weiss JM, Spodick DH: Association of left pleural effusion with pericardial disease. N Engl J Med 308:696, 1983 (*Patients with pericarditis tend to have unilateral pleural effusions that are left sided or bilateral effusions that are larger on the left; this is in contrast to the right-sided dominance in congestive heart failure.*)

40
Evaluation of the Solitary Pulmonary Nodule

The discovery of a solitary pulmonary nodule on chest x-ray is a worrisome finding, for it raises the possibility of malignancy. The patient is usually asymptomatic; solitary nodules are found at a rate of 1–2 per 1000 routine chest x-rays. Such a presentation identifies the subgroup of pulmonary malignancies with the greatest potential for cure; consequently, thorough assessment is of utmost importance. On the other hand, many of these lesions are not cancers, and to subject all patients to invasive studies can lead to unnecessary morbidity. The primary physician needs to determine the likelihood of malignancy on the basis of clinical and radiologic findings in order to identify the patient who requires referral for consideration of bronchoscopy, percutaneous needle biopsy, or thoracotomy. Workup can be initiated on an outpatient basis under the direction of the primary physician, pending the decision regarding the risk of cancer and the need for invasive study.

PATHOPHYSIOLOGY AND CLINICAL PRESENTATION

Solitary pulmonary nodules characteristically appear in the middle or lateral lung fields, surrounded by normal lung and unaccompanied by satellite lesions. They have smooth contours and are usually round ("coin" lesions) or oval. Neoplastic, granulomatous, vascular, and cystic processes are responsible for their formation. The nodule displaces normal aerated lung parenchyma and does not cause symptoms unless there is airway obstruction, pleural invasion, interference with respiratory mechanics, or involvement of blood vessels or nerves. Inflammatory lesions double in volume in less than 5 weeks; malignancies take between 1 and 18 months to double; benign nodules take longer. A solitary nodule that does not change in size over 2 years is benign. The older the patient, the greater the chances that the nodule is malignant; the probability is less than 2% below age 30 and increases by 10% to 15% with each succeeding decade.

DIFFERENTIAL DIAGNOSIS

By far, the most common causes of solitary pulmonary nodules are cancers and granulomas. The likelihood of malignancy in any individual case depends on the patient's age and other risk factors. But in most series, 40% to 50% of solitary nodules prove to be cancers. Of these, more than 75% are primary lung cancers, the remainder are metastatic lesions. Tumors of the breast, colon, and testicles are partic-

ularly prone to metastasize to the lung. Of the 50% to 60% of solitary pulmonary nodules that prove to be benign, 85% to 90% are granulomas; most are tuberculous but, in endemic areas, histoplasmosis and coccidioidomycosis are important considerations. Benign pulmonary tumors such as hamartomas explain about 5% of benign nodules. The remainder are bronchogenic cysts, hydatid cysts, pseudolymphomas, arteriovenous malformations, and bronchopulmonary sequestrations. Extrapulmonary lesions, such as skin lesions, moles, nipples, chest wall and rib lesions, and pleural plaques, may be confused with solitary lesions of lung parenchyma.

WORKUP

A most difficult diagnostic issue regards the need for resection of the unexplained solitary pulmonary nodule. Many surgeons argue that the risk of thoracotomy is small and potential benefit considerable, because resection of a nodule that proves to be an early primary lung cancer may provide the patient with a chance for cure. On the other hand, pulmonologists have argued that lesions that possess many of the criteria of benignity can be managed conservatively, and that definitive tissue diagnosis can be approached by bronchoscopy or needle biopsy without resorting to early thoracotomy (see Chapter 42). A review of the literature reveals passionate advocates on both sides; conclusive data taking into account morbidity and mortality of both approaches are lacking.

Identification of the patients most likely to have malignant lesions on the basis of noninvasive findings can help to select those who would be best suited to undergo a definitive, invasive diagnostic procedure. The patient's age, the doubling time of the lesion, and its x-ray appearance are among the most useful data for determining the chances of malignancy. The probability of cancer is 50% for patients in their sixties, but less than 2% for those under 30. Assessment of the doubling time, that is, the period during which the tumor doubles in volume, can be achieved efficaciously by review of previous chest films, if available. Before any further studies are undertaken, every effort should be made to locate old chest x-rays to determine the age and speed of growth of the nodule. A lesion that has been stable for 2 or more years is most likely benign; a nodule that has doubled in volume within 1 to 18 months is considered malignant until proven otherwise.

If previous films are unavailable, some useful information can be gleaned from the *radiologic appearance* of the nodule on the x-rays at hand. A most helpful sign is the presence of *calcification*. Laminated or concentric calcification is specific for granulomas. Central, diffuse, or homogeneous patterns of calcification are also associated with benign lesions, with rare exceptions. Radiographically visible calcium can occur in malignancies, however. A primary cancer may engulf a pre-existing calcified granuloma or scar; eccentricity of the calcium in the nodule should raise this possibility. Tomography may be helpful in more clearly defining the presence and distribution of calcification as well as the presence or absence of additional nodules or hilar adenopathy. Computed tomographic (CT) examination has often proved useful for evaluation. Initial reports of quantitative CT analysis utilized the attenuation coefficient on CT to distinguish benign from malignant nodules. However, reports that suggested that lower CT densitometry values predicted malignancy have not been uniformly successful when applied prospectively. Further study is currently in progress, and the possibility that magnetic resonance imaging (MRI) may prove more specific awaits further study and may help avoid some thoracotomies.

Location, size, and shape of the nodule, as it appears on chest x-ray are less valuable distinguishing signs. Both cancers and tuberculous granulomas are more common in the upper and middle lobes than in the lower lobes. Small lesions are more likely to be benign, but, if malignant, are still at a stage when detection and definitive diagnosis may have the greatest positive impact. Ill-defined borders suggest a primary malignancy, as does lobulation of the margin of the nodule. Cavitation occurs with nearly equal frequency in cancers and granulomas.

History is occasionally of help in elucidating the etiology of the nodule. Although symptoms are often absent, it is worth inquiring into a history of smoking, hemoptysis (see Chapter 38), known previous breast, bowel or testicular cancer, and systemic symptoms such as fever, night sweats, and weight loss. History of exposure to tuberculosis or residence in an area in which fungal disease is endemic raises the possibility of a granulomatous etiology.

Physical Examination is generally unrevealing, but a breast or testicular mass, occult blood in the stool, clubbing (see Chapter 41), cutaneous or mucosal telangiectasia, and an audible bruit over the chest wall (suggestive of a vascular etiology) should be excluded. Perhaps the most important part of the physical examination is careful palpation of lymph nodes, particularly those in the supraclavicular and axillary regions. If enlarged, such nodes can be biopsied, which may eliminate the need for thoracotomy or other invasive procedures.

Laboratory Studies. A number of other ancillary diagnostic studies may be of some help. An intermediate strength tuberculin test should be implanted (see Chapter 34); in endemic areas, fungal cultures and histoplasmin complement fixation titers may be of importance. Sputum cytologic examination is the least invasive means of confirming the presence of a malignancy. Three first morning samples should be obtained on consecutive days; yield is highest when the sample contains pulmonary histiocytes (a sign of a deep sample) and the lesion is in the upper lobes, centrally located, communicating with a bronchus, and large (see Chapter 33).

A conservative approach to further evaluation is reasonable in some circumstances. Criteria for withholding invasive study are (1) cytologic diagnosis of lung cancer with evidence of metastases, (2) lesions that have not enlarged in 5 years, and (3) in young patients, x-ray evidence that suggests benignity, such as solid or laminated calcium and sharp borders.

Invasive Studies. If the risk of malignancy is still not established after outpatient evaluation, one can progress to *bronchoscopy* and transbronchial brushings or biopsy for diagnosis of central lesions or *needle aspiration biopsy* under fluoroscopic control for diagnosis of peripheral lesions. *Thoracotomy* with resection is a third alternative (see Chapter 42).

Fiberoptic bronchoscopic examination with bronchial brushing and or biopsy may make a diagnosis in as many as 25% to 35% of peripheral lesions. But sensitivity is substantially lower when nodules are small and well circumscribed. *Needle aspiration* is a far more valuable approach to the diagnosis when the nodule is accessible to the transthoracic approach. A number of studies indicate that needle aspiration is highly sensitive (>95%) and highly specific for malignant lesions. Specific histologic types of malignant lesions can often be identified. Specific benign diagnoses are less often made on the basis of aspirated tissue. More extensive studies, such as mediastinoscopy and thoracotomy, are useful for planning therapy (see Chapter 42).

The choice of procedure depends on location of the lesion and available expertise. It is also important, when weighing the wisdom of an invasive procedure, to decide whether the patient could tolerate a resection. Patients with severe obstructive or restrictive disease should first undergo formal pulmonary function testing.

In sum, the evaluation of the patient with a solitary pulmonary nodule remains controversial. It appears at present that a conservative approach to evaluation is justified in patients judged to be at low risk for malignancy based on epidemiologic, historical, physical, and x-ray criteria. Patients at high risk for malignancy require a tissue diagnosis. A patient who falls between these two groups poses a dilemma, which should be shared with the patient so that a satisfactory plan can be devised. It may be reasonable to follow the patient with serial x-ray studies at 3-month intervals.

INDICATIONS FOR REFERRAL

Patients suspected on clinical and radiologic grounds of having a malignancy should be referred for tissue diagnosis.

Decisions regarding need for and type of invasive procedure should be made in conjunction with surgical and radiologic consultants. In situations where the probability of malignancy is unclear, the patient needs to be informed about the lack of diagnostic confidence based on noninvasive study, as well as the nature of further testing that would be undertaken. Patients who cannot emotionally tolerate the uncertainty should be advised to undergo a definitive procedure in order to end the constant worry about the possibility of malignancy. The patient who can live with such uncertainty and is reluctant to have a thoracotomy or biopsy could be followed at 3-month intervals with serial chest films for a period of 2 years.

A.G.M.
A.H.G.

ANNOTATED BIBLIOGRAPHY

Fulkerson WJ: Fiberoptic bronchoscopy. N Engl J Med 311:511, 1984 (*Reviews the indications, contraindications, and complications as well as diagnostic yield of fiberoptic bronchoscopy and endobronchial biopsy.*)

Godwin JD: The solitary pulmonary nodule. Radiol Clin North Am 21:709, 1983 (*A valuable clinical review including extensive discussion of the role of CT examination.*)

Lillington GA: The solitary pulmonary nodule/1974. Am Rev Respir Dis 110:699, 1974 (*A classic review of the problem.*)

Lillington GA, Stevens GM: The solitary nodule: The other side of the coin. Chest 70:322, 1976 (*An editorial that argues by example that early thoracotomy for every nodule, particularly in young people, would be uneconomic. It is suggested that needle biopsy or watchful waiting has a legitimate role in patients with low probability of malignancy.*)

Lillington GA: Pulmonary nodules: Solitary and multiple. Clin Chest Med 3:361, 1982 (*An update by one of the experts in the field; provides a thoughtful approach to the problem.*)

Nathan MH: Management of solitary pulmonary nodules: An organized approach based on growth rates and statistics. JAMA 227:1141, 1974 (*A very conservative approach advocated: observation of the nodule with serial x-rays for calculation of doubling time.*)

Toomes H et al: The coin lesion of the lung: A review of 955 resected coin lesions. Cancer 51:534, 1983 (*A useful series for statistics on types of lesions identified.*)

41
Evaluation of Clubbing

The term "clubbing" refers to enlargement and sponginess of the nail beds of the fingers and toes and reduction in the angle created by the nail and the dorsum of the distal phalanx. Clubbing is sometimes accompanied by a chronic subperiosteal osteitis, hypertrophic osteoarthropathy. Patients rarely complain of clubbed fingers; it is the physician who detects this abnormality as an incidental finding on physical examination. Since clubbing or hypertrophic osteoarthropathy may be the first clinical sign of a serious underlying condition, such as a pulmonary neoplasm, it is important for the primary physician to recognize these findings and investigate their possible causes.

PATHOPHYSIOLOGY AND CLINICAL PRESENTATION

Hypotheses explaining the pathogenesis of clubbing and osteoarthropathy implicate autonomic influences, AV shunting, and bloodborne substances. The precise pathophysiology remains uncertain, but it is known that intrathoracic vagotomy can abolish clubbing and osteoarthropathy, as can correction of an AV shunt or removal of a pulmonary tumor.

Pathologic examination of clubbed fingers reveals increased vascularity. In hypertrophic osteoarthropathy, the periosteum is found to be edematous, hyperemic, and infil-

trated by mononuclear cells. There is periosteal elevation, new bone formation, and endosteal resorption in the distal ends of long bones, metacarpals, and metatarsals. Soft tissue swelling in the distal ends of the fingers and toes may lead to clubbing.

Clubbing is usually asymptomatic. Patients with hypertrophic osteoarthropathy may complain of pain in the wrists, ankles, hands, and feet; erythema and effusions are sometimes noted. Hypertrophic osteoarthropathy may precede clubbing or occur without it, but most often the two appear together. Clubbing often takes place in the absence of osteoarthropathy. Either finding may develop prior to the clinical presentation of one of the conditions associated with it.

DIFFERENTIAL DIAGNOSIS

Clubbing and hypertrophic osteoarthropathy occur in as many as 5% to 10% of cases of bronchogenic carcinoma; metastatic lung tumors are rarely responsible for such changes. With the decline in the incidence of chronic pulmonary infectious diseases (such as tuberculosis, lung abscess, and bronchiectasis), carcinoma of the lung has emerged as the leading cause of hypertrophic osteoarthropathy. Clubbing and osteoarthropathy are seen in patients with cyanotic congenital heart disease with right-to-left shunts, subacute bacterial endocarditis, inflammatory bowel disease, and biliary cirrhosis. Clubbing is a classic sign of chronic hypoxemia in patients with chronic obstructive lung disease. There are hereditary forms of clubbing and hypertrophic osteoarthropathy that have no clinical significance. Unilateral clubbing is associated with impairment of the vascular supply to the arm that occurs with aortic, subclavian, or innominate artery lesions. Jackhammer operators may develop clubbing. Idiopathic hypertrophic osteoarthropathy, sometimes referred to as pachydermoperiostosis, is a benign condition that must be distinguished from hypertrophic osteoarthropathy secondary to systemic disease. These patients show periosteal new bone formation, swelling of the joints, and thickened and furred skin as well as clubbing. The benign syndrome can be differentiated from secondary hypertrophic osteoarthropathy by its development in adolescence, slow growth, paucity of joint symptoms, and absence of concurrent hepatic or pulmonary disease.

Clubbing must be differentiated from a number of other phalangeal conditions that resemble it. Many normal people, particularly blacks, have increased curvature of the nails. Infections of the terminal phalanges such as felons and chronic paronychia may be confused with clubbing, as may thyroid acropachy. Bilateral wrist and ankle complaints suggest a host of inflammatory joint diseases (see Chapter 144), in addition to hypertrophic osteoarthropathy.

WORKUP

The evaluation of clubbing should begin with confirmation of the characteristic physical findings: loss of the angle made by the nail and increase in the ballotability of the nail bed. Hypertrophic osteoarthropathy is identified by x-ray of the long bones; the typical changes are increase in periosteal thickness and new bone formation at distal ends. Once it is clear that clubbing or hypertrophic osteoarthropathy are present, an evaluation for an underlying etiology can commence.

History. Before an elaborate search for a serious illness is undertaken, it should be established whether clubbing has been lifelong and is present in other family members, indicative of the harmless familial variety. Symptoms such as cough, sputum production, hemoptysis, and dyspnea point to a respiratory problem and may have already triggered an evaluation of the lungs (see Chapters 36–38). The patient should be questioned about history of a heart murmur and exercise intolerance, as well as prior liver disease, crampy lower abdominal pain, diarrhea, bloody stools, and joint complaints. Smoking and other risk factors related to development of lung cancer (see Chapter 33) should be assessed. Exposure to tuberculosis also needs to be ascertained.

Physical Examination requires a check for fever, tachypnea, tachycardia, cyanosis, tobacco stains, jugular venous distention, barrel chest, wheezes, rhonchi, rales (crackles), signs of consolidation or effusion, heart murmur, skin lesions of hepatocellular disease and signs of cirrhosis (see Chapter 71). Lymph nodes should be palpated for enlargement and joints for hypertrophic changes.

Laboratory Studies. The only mandatory laboratory study is a chest x-ray, because an early pleural, pulmonary or mediastinal neoplasm may be asymptomatic. A CBC and stool examination for occult blood may be of help. Further evaluation of the liver, thyroid, heart, or bowel should be undertaken only if symptoms or physical findings suggest pathology in these areas. Patients with new onset of clubbing and a long smoking history should be followed for the development of pulmonary neoplasm; periodic examinations including sputum cytology and chest x-ray are appropriate.

The differentiation of osteoarthropathy from other conditions can be difficult. An extensive review of patients with clubbing and lung cancer showed that the symptoms of osteoarthropathy were often mistaken for arthritis and predated the diagnosis of neoplasm by a mean of 4.9 months. Frequent complaints of bilateral joint discomfort in the small joints, such as the wrists and hands, and an adequate response to aspirin or nonsteroidals tended to persuade physicians that they were dealing with rheumatologic disease. It was also noteworthy that they found acute elevations in acute phase reactants and a positive rheumatoid factor in 1 of 14 as well as antinuclear antibody in 5 of 12. The symmetrical involvement of small peripheral joints and the tendency to develop synovitis presents a significant diagnostic dilemma with some patients having a syndrome indistinguishable from that of an inflammatory arthritis.

SYMPTOMATIC MANAGEMENT AND PATIENT EDUCATION

There is no symptomatic therapy for clubbing. It is an innocuous cosmetic disturbance. Discomfort in the bones and joints secondary to hypertrophic osteoarthropathy can be treated with aspirin. Rarely, there are disabling joint symptoms; these may require extreme therapies such as corticosteroids or intrathoracic vagotomy. Such therapeutic options should be undertaken in consultation with a rheumatologist familiar with the condition.

Patient education is important in any condition where the physician discovers a potential sign of disease that is not obvious to the patient. It is likely that patients will be disturbed by the investigation and by the possibility of serious disease. The physician must take time to inform the patient that clubbing can be a harmless finding as well as a helpful guide to the early diagnosis of disease. The patient who smokes should be strongly advised to quit (see Chapter 49).

A.H.G.
L.A.M.

ANNOTATED BIBLIOGRAPHY

Schumacher HR Jr: Articular manifestations of hypertrophic pulmonary osteoarthropathy in bronchogenic carcinoma—A clinical and pathologic study. Arthritis Rheum 19:629, 1976 (*A detailed study and discussion.*)

Segal AN, Mackenzie AH: Hypertrophic osteoarthropathy: A ten year retrospective analysis. Semin Arthritis Rheum 12:220, 1985 (*An authoritative review with extensive study of 16 patients with hypertrophic osteoarthropathy; the differentiation from rheumatoid disease can sometimes be difficult.*)

Siegel RC: From clubbing to collagen. West J Med 134:352, 1981 (*A succinct review of pathophysiologic knowledge.*)

Stenseth JH, Clagett OT, Woolner LB: Hypertrophic pulmonary osteoarthropathy. Dis Chest 52:62, 1967 (*A review of 888 pulmonary neoplasms, revealing a 9.2% incidence of hypertrophic osteoarthropathy.*)

Trever RW: Hypertrophic pulmonary osteoarthropathy in association with congenital heart disease: Report of two cases. Ann Intern Med 48:660, 1958 (*Two case reports in a series of 3000 cases of cyanotic heart, revealing an incidence of 0.1%. Clubbing is far more frequent.*)

42

Approach to the Patient with Lung Cancer

JACOB J. LOKICH, M.D.
MARK S. HUBERMAN, M.D.

Carcinoma of the lung accounts for the highest number of annual cancer-related deaths (over 100,000 per year in the United States), and yet is among the most preventable of all cancers, in that a causative agent—smoking—has been identified. National incidence is 90 per 100,000 per year for men and 26 per 100,000 per year for women. Once established, most forms of lung cancer are minimally responsive to therapy, although there are important exceptions, for example, oat cell tumors. The reluctance of the American public to markedly alter its smoking habits has perpetuated the ever-increasing incidence of and death rate from lung cancer, which is currently rising as a consequence of increased smoking among women. The primary physician needs to be skilled in helping patients to quit smoking (see Chapter 49); alert to early signs of lung cancer; capable of conducting the workup, staging, and monitoring of the disease; and knowledgeable about recent advances in therapy and their effect on survival.

PATHOLOGY, CLINICAL PRESENTATION, AND COURSE

The common types of bronchogenic carcinoma are epidermoid, adenocarcinoma, small cell undifferentiated (oat cell), and large cell undifferentiated. Each has particular epidemiologic and clinical characteristics.

Epidermoid carcinoma is the most common lung cancer. It is predominantly a disease of men and accounts for more than 40% of all cases. Like most other bronchogenic carcinomas, there is a strong association with smoking. Most of these tumors occur centrally and can produce bronchial obstruction. They tend to ulcerate and may cause bleeding.

Adenocarcinomas are responsible for about 25% of lung cancers and many of those that present peripherally. They sometimes arise in areas of fibrosis secondary to prior pulmonary parenchymal damage. This cell type is less closely associated with smoking than others.

Undifferentiated small cell carcinoma (oat cell) is typically central in location and accounts for 25% of cases. These tumors derive from endocrine cells of the bronchial mucosa and can produce a variety of paraneoplastic syndromes (see Chapter 92). Most patients have advanced stages of disease at time of presentation, with 50% to 75% manifesting evidence of metastatic disease beyond the chest on routine staging.

Undifferentiated large cell carcinomas are, in most instances, probably a form of adenocarcinoma. Unlike well-differentiated adenocarcinomas, they are often centrally located and bronchoscopically visible as an endobronchial mass lesion. These cancers tend to metastasize hematogenously relatively early, leading to disease in the bones, liver, and brain.

Clinical presentation is partially a function of the tumor's location; central endobronchial lesions may produce symptoms early in the course of illness. Hemoptysis, cough, sputum production, and a localized wheeze are among complaints reported in *early phases;* however, the frequency with which these symptoms are noted in early disease is low. Hemoptysis occurs as a presenting symptom in only 7% to 10% of patients with lung cancer. On occasion, a systemic syndrome, such as hypertrophic osteoarthropathy (see Chapter 41), peripheral neuropathy, or inappropriate ADH secretion, may precede other evidence of disease.

Symptoms of *advanced disease* include anorexia, weight loss, nausea and vomiting, hoarseness (recurrent laryngeal nerve involvement), pleuritic chest pain, bone pain, and neurologic deficits. The *metastatic pattern* of lung cancer involves spread to the lymph nodes (25% to 45%), to the liver (30% to 45%), to the bone and bone marrow (20% to 40%), and to the central nervous system (20% to 35%). Variations in incidence figures for metastases are a function of the stage of disease and tissue type; for example, oat cell carcinoma more commonly spreads to the lymph nodes, marrow, and brain relative to other cell types.

The major *determinants of prognosis* in patients with lung cancer are *stage* at the time of diagnosis, histopathologic classification, and presence and duration of symptoms (Table 42-1). Lung cancer is staged according to extent of pulmonary parenchyma and lymph node involvement. Involvement of pulmonary parenchyma only is classified as *stage I;* spread to the draining hilar lymph nodes, *stage II;* and extension to the mediastinal lymph nodes *stage III.* About 25% of patients present with operable disease (stages I and II), but the majority present with stage III disease. The dismal prognosis for patients with lung cancer is related in part to the advanced stage of disease at the time of diagnosis. In those patients fortunate enough to have their disease confined to the lung (stage I), almost half may be cured by surgical approaches alone. With involvement of hilar lymph nodes, survival rates decrease dramatically, except those for epidermoid carcinoma.

Only 10% of patients developing lung cancer are cured, a statistic usually related to the advanced stage of disease at presentation. Of the patients presenting with metastasis or destined to develop metastasis, the most frequent sites include local or regional extension within the lung, and/or to bone, liver, and brain. Since the median survival for patients with lung cancer is less than 12 months, late metastasis is rare; the vast majority of the patients develop recurrence or distant metastasis within 12 months.

Oat cell carcinoma (undifferentiated small cell carcinoma) is unique in that prognosis appears to be independent of the anatomic distribution of the tumor at the time of diagnosis. Until recently, the 2-year survival for patients with oat cell disease, regardless of stage, had been approximately 6%; but, application of combined modality therapy (employing a multidrug regimen and radiation administered to the primary tumor and prophylactically to common sites of metastasis) has resulted in improvement of median survival from 1 to 2 months to 10 to 12 months (see below).

The poor survival figures for patients with lung cancer underscore the need for better methods of early detection of primary lung lesions. Unfortunately, local and regional disease is most often asymptomatic, and the sensitivity and specificity of available screening tests are limited (see Chapter 33). The new imaging techniques used in staging are not appropriate for screening and, in fact, have lead to an artifactual increase in survival data by detecting metastatic disease earlier.

WORKUP AND STAGING

Diagnosis and staging begin with noninvasive studies and proceed to increasingly invasive studies only as necessary. Many patients have concurrent chronic lung disease and may be seriously compromised by a complication of an invasive study. The histopathologic diagnosis may be obtained with a variety of procedures ranging from sputum cytology to thoracotomy (see Chapters 33 and 40, and Table 42-2). Staging is done to determine prognosis and treatment, and in particular to assess resectability of the tumor.

Table 42-1. Prognostic Determinants in Bronchogenic Carcinoma

STAGE	PROGNOSIS (2 YRS. DISEASE-FREE; %)	
Confined to lung	40–45	
Hilar node involvement	15*	
Mediastinum or chest wall involvement	10	
HISTOPATHOLOGY	**PREVALENCE (%)**	**MEDIAN SURVIVAL (MO)**
Epidermoid	50	6–9
Adenocarcinoma	25	6–8
Undifferentiated large	15	36
Undifferentiated small (oat)†	10	2
SYMPTOMS AND DURATION		**5-YEAR SURVIVAL (%)**
None		18
Local symptoms less than 6 months		16
Local symptoms greater than 6 months		9
Systemic symptoms with metastasis		6

* With epidermoid type, prognosis improves to 40%.

† With combination chemotherapy and radiation, the median survival is 10 to 12 months.

Table 42-2. Diagnostic and Staging Approaches
to Lung Cancer*

Sputum cytology
Scalene node biopsy
Mediastinoscopy
Bronchoscopy
Transbronchial biopsy
Transpulmonary biopsy
Thoracotomy (Chamberlain's procedure)

* In order of increasing invasiveness.

Diagnosis. *Chest x-ray* is the primary diagnostic modality, with the appearance of the lesion and its doubling time helpful in distinguishing benign from malignant disease (see Chapter 40). *Chest tomography* and, more recently, *computed tomography* add better definition of the lesion (*e.g.,* its pattern of calcification, if present) and help determine the presence of hilar and mediastinal involvement. *Sputum cytology* may be diagnostic and can even yield cell type in some instances; it must be obtained properly (deep, first morning sample with pulmonary histiocytes in evidence) to be of value in diagnosis. It is particularly helpful in diagnosis of central lesions, but a negative cytologic examination hardly rules out the diagnosis of cancer.

The scalene nodes should be carefully palpated. *Scalene node biopsy* is indicated when these nodes are enlarged; it can save the patient from a more invasive procedure for pathologic confirmation of the diagnosis.

The selection of invasive diagnostic procedures is determined in part by the location of the tumor. Peripheral lesions may be approached either with percutaneous needle biopsy or by a "minithoracotomy" (Chamberlain's procedure). In patients with clinically curable lesions (disease that appears localized to the parenchyma and draining hilar lymph nodes) the procedure of choice is a *thoracotomy with resection.* Surgical excision is particularly indicated for nodules with long doubling times or long disease-free intervals, especially if the nodules are solitary and unassociated with extrathoracic disease. Many thoracic surgeons believe that all patients should undergo *mediastinoscopy* for evaluation of the mediastinum and hilum prior to thoracotomy, since the presence of tumor in the mediastinum is a contraindication to resection. Early peripheral coin lesions are uncommonly associated with hilar or mediastinal extension, and *computed tomography* is often sufficient; however, computed tomography is not very sensitive and cannot be considered a substitute for mediastinoscopy in more advanced or central disease, in which the likelihood of microscopic nodal involvment is much higher. Reports of sensitivity in unselected cases are in the range of 50%.

For peripheral lesions, radiologically guided *transbronchial* or *percutaneous needle biopsy* deserves consideration. Reports on the diagnostic accuracy of these radiologically guided procedures quote sensitivity in excess of 90% and specificity over 95% when performed by skilled radiologists

using "fine needle" techniques that allow not only aspiration, but removal of a tiny core of material as well. However, sensitivity and specificity may be compromised by the inadequacy of the specimen sometimes obtained, which occasionally is an aspirate of cytologic material rather than a solid core of tissue; in such instances, the architectural relationships may be obscured or unavailable in cytologic specimens. A small pneumothorax usually results from these procedures, but it usually is of little clinical significance. For patients with limited pulmonary reserve who may be unable to tolerate any degree of pneumothorax, a controlled *thoracotomy* may also be preferable to needle aspiration.

Central lesions may be sampled by means of *endoscopic transbronchial biopsy, brushings, or washings.* Bronchoscopy is advocated by some as a routine procedure in the evaluation of all pulmonary lesions, but for peripheral pulmonary lesions, the accessibility by fiberoptic bronchoscopy may be limited.

Staging. The first priority of staging is to determine resectability, that is, to establish extent of hilar and mediastinal node involvement. The presence of a few involved ipsilateral nodes is no contraindication to resection. *Mediastinoscopy* performed through a cervical incision with biopsy of the mediastinal nodes is done to rule out microscopic involvement of contralateral nodes and establish candidacy for resection. Gross nodal involvement on chest x-ray or *computed tomography* obviates the need for mediastinoscopy, but as noted above, a negative CT scan does not rule out microscopic spread from central or late peripheral lesions.

The remainder of staging is determined by the tumor's cell type. For patients with *inoperable non-small cell carcinoma,* further staging is of little value, because the information would have minimal impact on decision making or estimation of prognosis. If there is no clinical evidence of metastatic disease, it is wasteful to routinely employ radionuclide scanning of the brain, bones, and liver (see Chapter 87). Similarly, although the use of tumor markers to identify and monitor occult sites of disease is under development, the current lack of effective systemic therapy precludes the usefulness of such measures for treatment decisions.

Staging is considerably different for patients with *small cell carcinoma.* Because the disease usually presents with evidence of bilateral nodal involvement, the issue is extent of disease rather than resectability. The goal is to distinguish between limited and extensive disease (the latter implies spread beyond the hemithorax of origin and regional nodes). Almost 25% of patients have marrow invasion, and marrow biopsy is done routinely. CT scanning of common sites of metastatic disease (*e.g.,* brain) may also be useful if the result will affect plans for therapy (see below).

PRINCIPLES OF MANAGEMENT

Surgery is the most effective mode of therapy for bronchogenic carcinoma and is associated with the lowest rate of morbidity. Unfortunately, only 45% of the patients who present with lung cancer can be explored with the possibility of successful resection. Of that group, only 60% (27% of all patients) have successful resections. Of this final group who undergo resection either by pneumonectomy or lobectomy, the 5-year survival or cure rate is approximately 25%. Thus, 7% of patients who present with lung cancer may be cured.

Less radical surgical procedures have become accepted for treating primary lung cancer. Pneumonectomy used to be performed in more than 70% of patients; it generally incorporated the hilar as well as mediastinal lymph nodes. A regional excision that employs wedge resection or lobectomy for peripheral lobe lesions is now being performed. The general surgical dictum is to employ the minimal degree of surgery necessary to remove all macroscopic evidence of tumor. The subsequent use of radiation therapy may augment local control, allowing for lesser surgery.

Radiation therapy for bronchogenic carcinoma has been used preoperatively to promote or convert inoperable tumors to technically resectable lesions (with curative intent following resection) and as definitive therapy for patients with stage III inoperable tumors without extrathoracic extension. As a postoperative adjunctive measure in bronchogenic carcinoma, radiation therapy has not significantly improved survival; however, it may reduce the extensiveness of local recurrence and consequently lower the incidence of severe pulmonary complications, such as superior vena cava syndrome or lobar collapse. Although there are reports of small improvements in long-term survival (less than 5%) associated with radiation doses up to 6000 rads for tumors confined to the hemithorax, the reports of improved survival are mostly anecdotal and not necessarily attributable to the administration of the radiation therapy.

Preoperative radiation therapy may promote the resectability of tumors and possibly extend survival rates. The *superior sulcus tumor* is one instance in which preoperative radiation therapy has improved the likelihood of cure in spite of contiguous extension of the tumor to bone or chest wall. In general, when surgery is used in combination with prior radiation, the resection almost always needs to be a pneumonectomy; in principle, surgery must incorporate all sites that were diseased prior to the radiation therapy.

Management of stage III disease deserves special comment. More than 70% of patients with bronchogenic carcinoma present with inoperable disease, either on the basis of extrathoracic extension of the tumor or intrathoracic extension to mediastinal lymph nodes, chest wall, or ribs. The latter group, with tumor limited to the chest at the time of presentation, is the most critical therapeutic challenge in bronchogenic carcinoma today. For patients with the superior sulcus variant, therapy that combines preoperative radiation with surgical resection has contributed to cures. With this singular exception, however, the majority of patients with stage III bronchogenic carcinoma develop distant metastases regardless of control of the primary tumor. Survival is a function of the rate and extent of systemic dissemination. The development of improved drugs or new combinations of chemotherapy must occur before hope can be offered to the patient with this stage of disease.

Treatment of small cell carcinoma has brought about impressive improvement in survival. Small cell disease is biologically unique among bronchogenic cancers, in that its cells are extremely sensitive to chemotherapy and radiation, probably due in part to their very rapid rate of proliferation. Surgical treatment is usually not possible, because 85% of patients have extensive disease at time of presentation.

The mainstay of treatment for small cell cancer is chemotherapy (see Table 42-3). Response is determined by stage of disease at time of presentation. Chemotherapy (with or without radiation), achieves a complete remission and a mean survival in excess of 1 year in over 50% of patients with *limited small cell disease.* Between 10% and 20% of this group may be free of relapse at 2 years, and disease-free survival in excess of 6 years is now being reported in a small fraction of patients (5%). There is active controversy about whether the addition of local radiation to the primary chest lesion improves the outcome for patients with limited disease.

Unfortunately, the results for *extensive small cell disease*

Table 42-3. Chemotherapy Programs for Small Cell and Non-Small Cell Lung Cancer

TUMOR CATEGORY	FREQUENCY (%)	REGIMENS	RESPONSE RATE (%)
Small cell	25	CAV	80
		C, MTX, CCNU	60–70
		C, E, A	70
Non-small cell*	65	CAP	40–50
		Vin, P	50
		VP-16, P	40
Other†	10	No established regimen	

C = cyclophosphamide; A = adriamycin; MTX = methotrexate; CCNU = nitrosourea; E = etoposide; Vin = vindesine; P = platinum.

* Includes epidermoid, adenocarcinoma, and large cell undifferentiated.

† Includes bronchoalveolar, giant cell, unclassified, and mixed types.

are not as good. Although the majority of patients demonstrate significant objective tumor regression with use of chemotherapy, complete response rates are less than 50%. Essentially all patients with extensive disease die within 2 years.

MONITORING

Monitoring patients with surgically resectable and potentially curable lung cancer is conditioned by the fact that there is little one can do for metastatic disease. Thus, monitoring is more specifically directed at searching for a new primary tumor in this high-risk population. Chest films are indicated at regular intervals, ranging from every 3 months during the first 2 years to every 4 to 12 months in later years. Routine monitoring for recurrent disease outside the chest is unnecessary in the absence of specific symptoms suggesting bone, liver, or brain metastasis.

Monitoring patients with extensive disease is directed at assessing the efficacy of therapy. One needs to select one or more objective measures of tumor burden (see Chapter 87) that can be followed conveniently to gauge response to treatment. Chest x-ray, CT scan, and bronchoscopy are commonly used.

MANAGEMENT OF COMPLICATIONS

Superior Vena Cava Syndrome. (See Chapter 92). Obstruction of the superior vena cava by lung tumor produces the classic clinical syndrome of facial edema, proptosis, suffusion of the conjunctivae, and dilation of the veins of the upper thorax and neck. Asymptomatic neck vein distention is an early manifestation. In late stages, the patient may complain of relentless headache. In patients with lung cancer, the syndrome is invariably caused by tumor extending into the right side of the mediastinum and compressing the venous system adjacent to the mediastinal lymph nodes. The secondary effects of compression are thrombosis and tumor invasion; if untreated, neurologic function may be compromised. The histopathologic types of lung cancer that lead to the syndrome are variable, but most commonly the culprit is undifferentiated small cell carcinoma.

The approach to evaluation and therapy has undergone some revision in recent years. Previously, it was believed that emergency radiation therapy was indicated regardless of whether or not a tissue diagnosis was available; the view was that the risk of an invasive procedure to obtain tissue outweighed its potential contribution to design of a treatment plan. More recent data indicate that the risk of evaluation in patients lacking a tissue diagnosis is low and that chemotherapy may be superior to radiation in some instances (*e.g.,* small cell cancer). Because superior vena cava syndrome may be the initial presentation of lung cancer, the issue of need for tissue diagnosis is frequently encountered in this setting. When the result will change the mode of therapy, tissue diagnosis should be attempted, taking care to minimize risk to the patient.

Even when a tissue diagnosis is not obtained, response to radiotherapy is rather good; in unselected series, more than 70% of patients demonstrate a response. Although patients with superior vena cava syndrome secondary to lung cancer have an inoperable tumor, the prognosis is no worse than for other patients with stage III lung cancer.

Malignant Pleural Effusion is another important complication. It occurs in 10% to 15% of patients with carcinoma of the lung and may be secondary to direct pleural implantation or a consequence of mediastinal obstruction to lymphatic drainage of the pleural surface. Only 20% to 30% of pleural effusions that develop as a consequence of bronchogenic carcinoma are cytologically confirmed, and many are transudates. Pleural biopsy is often required for definitive diagnosis.

The median survival for patients who develop a malignant pleural effusion is less than 3 months; therefore, the effusion should be monitored and treated only when it causes significant respiratory discomfort. The use of intrapleural chemotherapeutic agents (*e.g.,* bleomycin, fluorouracil) or chemical irritants, such as tetracycline, talcum powder, or quinacrine, may be effective in 50% to 60% of patients. The specific choice of agent for sealing the pleura is determined by morbidity of the treatment. The chemotherapeutic agents such as bleomycin and fluorouracil are relatively innocuous. On the other hand, nitrogen mustard and the "inert" irritants may result in a major secondary inflammatory response with reactive effusion and fever. Quinacrine (Atabrine) must be instilled repeatedly over a 5- to 7-day period to be maximally effective. Radiation therapy to the mediastinum or to the pleura has been of limited effectiveness. Surgical drainage with an intrathoracic tube for 2 to 3 days may result in a secondary inflammatory response adequate to seal the pleural space.

Tumor–Humoral Syndromes are associated with small cell carcinomas. Because the tumor is derived from endocrine cells of the bronchial mucosa, it is capable of producing ACTH, ADH, and even on occasion serotonin. The clinical pictures that may result are Cushing's syndrome, inappropriate ADH secretion, and carcinoid syndrome, respectively. In an autopsy series of 85 patients with small cell carcinoma, it was found that patients who manifested a paraneoplastic syndrome tended to have a more benign clinical course and longer survival; in addition, there was a significantly lower incidence of metastases to the central nervous system.

Complications of Surgical Therapy include prolonged air leakage due to a bronchopleural fistula, and postoperative intrapleural infection with empyema formation. Both are potentially serious and require prompt surgical attention. Pulmonary insufficiency is uncommon owing to careful preoperative pulmonary evaluation of candidates for resection; however, pneumonia in the remaining lung can lead to respiratory compromise.

Complications of Chemotherapy are those related to the use of such agents as cyclophosphamide, adriamycin, methotrexate, nitrosoureas, and cisplatin (see Chapter 89) in the treatment of lung cancer. Use of certain chemotherapeutic agents (*e.g.,* nitrosoureas, methotrexate) during the induction phase of radiation therapy in patients with small cell cancer is suspected of accounting for some of the late complications seen in long-term survivors.

Complications of Radiation Therapy include radiation pneumonitis, esophageal stricture, pericardial and myocardial fibrosis, rib fractures secondary to radiation-induced osteonecrosis, and radiation fibrosis.

PATIENT EDUCATION

Most laymen believe that lung cancer is fatal. Although prognosis and efficacy of treatment are indeed poor in most types of lung cancer, the patient with a newly discovered, suspicious pulmonary nodule needs to know that there are major differences in prognosis based on tissue type and stage of disease at time of presentation. Prior to completion of workup and staging, this background information can help sustain the patient and family through a worrisome period of uncertainty and provide a rationale for the procedures that need to be done. Once the diagnosis and extent of disease are known, the information can be shared and more precise estimates of prognosis and treatment plan can be given. Patients fortunate enough to have limited small cell disease or a resectable non-small cell tumor ought to be given the good news; those with less favorable disease should be told as much as they desire to know (see Chapter 88 on telling cancer patients about their diagnosis and prognosis).

The news of lung cancer in a loved one is very upsetting to family members, but the event can be used as an important opportunity to persuade smokers in the family to quit. Every effort should be made; prevention is still the best approach to lung cancer.

ANNOTATED BIBLIOGRAPHY

Ahmann FR: A reassessment of the clinical implications of the superior vena cava syndrome. J Clin Oncol 2:961, 1984 (*Argues that diagnostic workup is safe and useful for proper selection of treatment modality. Based on review of over 1800 cases.*)

Cohen MH, Matthews MJ: Small cell bronchogenic carcinoma: A distinct clinicopathologic entity. Semin Oncol 5:234, 1978 (*A synopsis of the important clinical features that make small cell (oat cell) lung cancer a unique entity.*)

Feinstein AR, Sosin DM, Wells CK: The Will Rogers phenomenon: Stage migration and new diagnostic techniques as a source of misleading statistics for survival in cancer. N Engl J Med 312: 1604, 1985 (*Describes an artifactual increase in survival of patients with lung cancer due to use of modern imaging techniques that pick up metastatic disease earlier.*)

Hoffman PC, Bitran JK, Golomb HM: Chemotherapy of metastatic non-small cell bronchogenic carcinoma. Semin Oncol 10:111, 1983 (*A comprehensive and updated introduction to the variety of combination chemotherapy regimens employed for each of the histopathologic types of non-small cell cancer, with a critical review of impact on survival. The critical role of cisplatin is emphasized; however, it is still controversial. The promise of many regimens provides an optimistic appraisal for lung cancer.*)

Johnson BE, Ihde DC, Bunn PA et al: Patients with small-cell cancer treated with combination chemotherapy with or without irradiation. Ann Intern Med 103:430, 1985 (*A series of 252 patients from the National Cancer Institute trials reports late results with documentation of prolonged survival in some.*)

Kessinger A, Foley JF, Lemon HM: Therapeutic management of small cell lung cancer: Fewer toxic reactions with lower chemotherapeutic drug dosages. JAMA 250:3188, 1983 (*The response rates and survival in this study are comparable to the high-dose regimens, with a substantial reduction in toxicity.*)

Livingston RB, Stephens RL, Bonnet JD et al: Long-term survival and toxicity in small cell lung cancer. Am J Med 77:415, 1984 (*Reports on a group of long-term survivors treated with combination of chemotherapy and radiation: 5% were alive at 6 years of follow-up. Points out the potential for disease-free survival in this condition.*)

de la Monte SM, Hutchins GM, Moore GW: Paraneoplastic syndromes and constitutional symptoms in prediction of metastatic behavior of small cell carcinoma of the lung. Am J Med 77:851, 1984 (*An autopsy series of 85 patients indicating that patients with paraneoplastic syndromes had a more benign clinical course and less CNS metastasis.*)

Payne CR, Stovin PG, Baker V et al: Diagnostic accuracy of cytology and biopsy in primary bronchial carcinoma. Thorax 34:294, 1979 (*Provides data on sensitivity and specificity of diagnostic measures.*)

Underwood GH, Hooper RG, Axelbaum SP et al: Computed tomographic scanning of the thorax in staging of bronchogenic carcinoma. N Engl J Med 300:777, 1979 (*A small series of 18 patients who underwent mediastinoscopy and CT. Sensitivity of CT was 40%; specificity 88%. CT is helpful if positive, but does not rule out the need for mediastinoscopy if negative.*)

43

Approach to the Patient with
Acute Bronchitis or Pneumonia in
the Ambulatory Setting

HARVEY B. SIMON, M.D.

Respiratory tract infections are among the most common acute problems seen in office practice; the majority are limited to the upper airway (see Chapters 46, 216–218). The cough, fever, chest discomfort, and dyspnea that may accompany lower respiratory infections provoke great concern in the patient, and the physician should respond with a careful evaluation designed to elucidate three basic issues: (1) Is the process limited to the trachea and bronchi, or is a frank pneumonia present? In general, patients with bronchitis respond well to ambulatory care, whereas patients with pneumonia should be considered for hospital admission. (2) Is the patient at increased risk for cardiopulmonary complications? The elderly patient with underlying cardiac or chronic lung disease may decompensate acutely from bronchitis alone, whereas otherwise healthy young individuals have a much greater tolerance for these infections. (3) What is the causative organism—is it bacterial or nonbacterial? Bacterial processes are usually more severe and require antibiotics, whereas viral infections are managed symptomatically.

PATHOPHYSIOLOGY AND CLINICAL PRESENTATION

The distinction between bronchitis and pneumonia is anatomic rather than etiologic; the same organisms can cause both syndromes, and patients may present with similar complaints, including fever, malaise, cough, and sputum production. Muscular-type chest wall discomfort produced from coughing occurs in both conditions, but individuals with pneumonia are more likely to have pleurisy or dyspnea as well as higher temperatures, chills, hypoxia, and a more "toxic" appearance. Similarly, although either type of infection can lead to sputum production, patients with bacterial pneumonia generally produce more sputum and are more likely to have hemoptysis.

The clinical distinction between bronchitis and pneumonia is based predominantly on physical examination and chest x-ray findings. Patients with bronchitis can have clear lungs or diffuse rhonchi and/or wheezes due to large airway secretions and bronchospasm, whereas individuals with pneumonia classically have rales, rhonchi, bronchial breath sounds and dullness to percussion over the involved areas of lung. Pleural effusions may accompany pneumonia. The chest x-ray in acute bronchitis usually reveals no infiltrate or signs of consolidation in contradistinction to the x-ray of the patient with pneumonia. But even this most clear-cut distinction between bronchitis and pneumonia can be misleading, for changes of chronic lung disease can simulate new infiltrates in some patients with bronchitis, while dehydration can minimize x-ray abnormalities in patients with pneumonia.

Patients with pneumonia are far more likely to experience complications such as hypoxia, cardiopulmonary failure, local suppuration (lung abscess or empyema), and spread of infection to other organs via the bloodstream. Clinical presentations are, in part, a function of the causative organism.

Gram-positive Organisms. *Streptococcus pneumoniae* is still the most common cause of bacterial bronchitis and pneumonia, accounting for up to 60% of all bacterial pneumonias. It is especially likely to be the agent infecting healthy young ambulatory patients, but it may affect all age groups. Classical clinical features include abrupt onset of fever with a single rigor, cough with rusty sputum, and pleuritic chest pain. Radiologic evidence of lobar consolidation is typical, but infiltrates can be patchy, especially in patients with chronic lung disease. The sputum Gram stain reveals abundant polymorphonuclear leukocytes and gram-positive diplococci (classically lancet-shaped) in pairs or short chains.

The most common complication of pneumococcal pneumonia is bacteremia, which occurs in about one third of patients. Bloodborne distant sepsis (septic arthritis, peritonitis, meningitis, etc.) is much less common. Sterile pleural effusions are common, while empyema is less frequent, and lung abscess is a rare complication. Delayed resolution of radiographic abnormalities is a relatively common occurrence and may take up to 6 to 8 weeks.

Staphylococcus aureus is the etiologic agent in up to 10% of bacterial pneumonias. Except in infancy, when it can be a primary infection, staphylococcal pneumonia most commonly follows a viral respiratory tract infection, particularly influenza. It may also occur as a nosocomial infection or as a result of bacteremic seeding of the lungs, especially in patients with staphylococcal endocarditis and/or intravenous drug abuse. Patients with staphylococcal pneumonia of respiratory or bloodstream origin are usually extremely ill. *S.*

aureus produces tissue necrosis, and the distinctive feature of staphylococcal pneumonia is the tendency to produce multiple small lung abscesses. Healing usually leaves some degree of residual fibrosis. Abundant polymorphonuclear leukocytes and gram-positive cocci in pairs, clumps, and clusters are found on the sputum Gram stain. Local suppurative complications, including lung abscess, empyema, and pneumothorax, are relatively common. Bacteremia with metastatic seeding of distant sites such as endocardium, bone, joints, liver, and meninges may occur.

Pneumonia caused by *Group A streptococci* is a rather uncommon infection, but has occurred in epidemics, especially in closed groups such as military units. Occasionally streptococcal pneumonia can occur following primary influenza pneumonia. Streptococcal pneumonia usually begins abruptly with fever, cough, and severe debility. Chest pain is prominent in most patients. The distinctive clinical and radiologic feature is rapid spread in the lung, with resultant early empyema formation. Initially, the empyema fluid may be quite thin, possibly due to the many enzymes elaborated by Group A streptococci, but later frank purulence occurs. Other complications such as lung abscess, bacteremia, metastatic infection, and poststreptococcal glomerulonephritis are uncommon. In patients with streptococcal pneumonia, the sputum Gram stain reveals numerous polymorphonuclear leukocytes and gram-positive cocci in pairs and short to long chains.

Gram-negative Organisms. While *H. influenzae* has long been recognized as a common cause of bronchitis in adults with chronic lung disease, there has recently been a greater recognition of frank pneumonias caused by this organism, sometimes with bacteremia. Most cases of bronchitis are caused by untypeable strains of *H. Influenzae,* but pneumonias are often caused by the more invasive encapsulated strains, especially type b. Radiographically, a bronchopneumonia pattern is typical. Abundant polymorphonuclear leukocytes and small pleomorphic gram-negative coccobacillary organisms are the characteristic findings in the sputum of patients with pneumonia or bronchitis due to *H. influenzae.* Complications of *H. influenzae* pneumonia in adults are uncommon, but in patients with underlying chronic lung disease, hypoxia and respiratory failure may develop.

Klebsiella pneumoniae typically produces pulmonary infection in debilitated patients, especially alcoholics, and is one of the only gram-negative bacillary pneumonias to occur with any frequency in ambulatory patients. It usually presents as an acute illness; rarely it may cause chronic pneumonitis. The organism has a high propensity to produce tissue necrosis, which accounts for the hemoptysis, dense lobar consolidation, and high incidence of abscess formation seen in this illness. Abundant polymorphonuclear leukocytes and large gram-negative bacilli, occasionally with thick capsules, are characteristically seen on sputum Gram stain. Lung abscess is a

common complication and is really part of the natural evolution of the disease. Empyema may occur.

Other gram-negative bacillary pneumonias were once rare, but have increased over the past 15 years and now account for up to 20% of bacterial pneumonias. They are principally hospital-acquired infections and remain quite rare in the ambulatory population. Patients with gram-negative bacillary pneumonia are typically debilitated from other illnesses and frequently have received antibiotic therapy, which alters their respiratory flora, thus accounting for the presence of these otherwise unusual pathogens. These pneumonias may result either from aspiration of gram-negative organisms present in the upper airway (often related to inhalation therapy), or from seeding of the lungs in the course of gram-negative bacteremia. *Bacteremic pneumonias* are characterized by multiple small areas of infection in both lungs. Abundant polymorphonuclear leukocytes and gram-negative bacilli are seen on sputum Gram stain. Complications including lung abscess, empyema, and bacteremia with metastatic spread of infection may occur.

Legionnaires' Disease. First identified in 182 patients in the 1976 Philadelphia outbreak, Legionnaires' disease is now recognized as an important cause of pneumonia around the world. The causative organism, *Legionella pneumophila,* is a filamentous, fastidious bacillus that survives in water and, to a lesser extent, soil. Human infection is acquired by inhalation of contaminated aerosols; person-to-person transmission is unknown. Legionnaires' disease may occur in sporadic cases or epidemics; hospital water supplies can be contaminated and nosocomial infections can occur. Middle-aged and elderly patients are most often affected, and immunosuppressed patients are particularly vulnerable. Nine serogroups of *L. pneumophila* have been recognized, and at least 7 other legionella species can cause human disease. The most important of these, *L. micdadei,* causes "Pittsburgh-agent" pneumonia in immunosuppressed patients.

The spectrum of clinical illness due to legionella infection ranges from mild upper respiratory disease (Pontiac fever) and self-limited atypical pneumonia to potentially fatal Legionnaires' disease and opportunistic infections in immunocompromised hosts. After a short prodrome, the full-blown form of Legionnaires' disease begins acutely with high fever, nonproductive cough, and dyspnea. *Pleuritic chest pain* occurs in about one third of cases. Extrapulmonary manifestations such as *diarrhea, confusion,* and *renal dysfunction* are common and can be clues to diagnosis. Although the typical patient is severely ill, milder cases have been recognized.

A pretibial rash and relative bradycardia occur in a few patients, but in most the physical examination is nonspecific. A modest leukocytosis and interstitial infiltrates or areas of patchy consolidation are characteristic laboratory abnormalities. The urinalysis, renal function tests, and liver function tests may be abnormal, and hypoxia can occur. Sputum is typically absent or scant. The sputum Gram stain fails to reveal pathogens, but *L. pneumophila* can sometimes be visualized in sputum or other specimens by direct immunofluorescent staining. The organisms can be cultured on charcoal yeast extract agar, and legionella antigens can be detected in the urine of some patients. In most instances, the diagnosis is made serologically (see later discussion).

Mixed Flora. *Aspiration pneumonias* result from aspiration of mouth secretions and bacteria into the lower respiratory tree. They are usually mixed infections caused by the aerobic and anaerobic streptococci, bacteroides, and fusobacteria, which are harmless normal flora of the upper airway, that cause pneumonia if they attain a foothold in lung parenchyma. Predisposing factors include alteration of consciousness (drugs, anesthesia, alcohol, head trauma) and diminution of gag reflex, permitting aspiration to occur. Patients usually are mildly to moderately ill but can be quite toxic, especially if lung abscess or empyema occurs. It must be stressed that hospitalized patients and ambulatory patients receiving antibiotics may have altered respiratory flora. Aspiration of mouth organism in such individuals may result in staphylococcal or gram-negative bacillary pneumonia, as discussed previously, rather than the pulmonary infection due to normal upper respiratory flora, as considered here. The sputum from patients with aspiration pneumonia may be malodorous, and characteristically shows abundant polymorphonuclear leukocytes and mixed flora, including gram-positive cocci in pairs and chains and pleomorphic gram-negative rods on Gram stain. Lung abscess and empyema are fairly common complications of aspiration pneumonia, especially if therapy is delayed.

Nonbacterial Organisms. *Mycoplasma pneumoniae* is one of the most common causes of nonbacterial pneumonia, and accounts for up to 20% of all pneumonias in some urban populations. It is the leading cause of the *atypical pneumonia syndrome* (fever, dry cough, nonspecific infiltrate on chest film) in otherwise healthy adults. The organism spreads via respiratory droplets and appears to have a long incubation period, so that slow spread among family members or other closed groups over a period of many weeks is characteristic. Although all ages can be affected, the greatest incidence of mycoplasmal pneumonia is in older children and young adults. The disease usually begins gradually. In addition to a nonproductive cough with fever and malaise, headache is a rather constant symptom. Physical examination discloses fine rales which are typically less extensive than the patchy alveolar densities (usually confined to one of the lower lobes) seen on chest x-ray. Occasionally examination of the tympanic membrane will also show a bullous myringitis. Laboratory studies reveal a normal white blood cell count and differential in most cases. The sputum is scant, with a predominance of mononuclear cells. Mycoplasma organisms are very small and lack cell walls; hence, they cannot be visualized with conventional microscopy. Mycoplasma pneumonia is usually a mild, self-limited illness, but can produce severe pneumonia in children with sickle cell anemia, in immunosuppressed hosts, and in the elderly. Uncommon complications include hemolytic anemia, encephalitis, Guillain–Barré syndrome, myopericarditis, and Stevens–Johnson syndrome.

VIRAL PNEUMONIA. Many viruses are capable of producing upper and lower respiratory tract infections, including adenoviruses, respiratory syncytial virus and parainfluenza virus. These infections are clinically indistinguishable except when part of a distinctive systemic viral illness such as rubeola in children or varicella in adults. Cytomegalovirus is a common cause of viral pneumonia in the immunocompromised host. The most important cause of viral pneumonia is influenza, which can be recognized by its epidemic spread and marked systemic symptoms such as fever and myalgias. Influenza pneumonia may be a mild or fulminant illness capable of causing lethal respiratory failure. Bacterial pneumonia, especially of the pneumococcal, staphylococcal, or streptococcal variety, is a frequent complication.

PSITTACOSIS. Psittacosis is caused by a member of the *Chlamydia* group of obligate intracellular parasites which are also responsible for lymphogranuloma venereum and trachoma. The disease is transmitted from parrots or other birds (including pigeons and turkeys) to man. The clinical features of psittacosis are indistinguishable from those of other nonbacterial pneumonias, with prominent headache, nonproductive cough, and fever. Occasionally a faint macular rash or splenomegaly develops.

Q FEVER. Caused by *Coxiella burnetii,* Q fever is unique among rickettsial infections in that pneumonia is prominent, there is no rash, and spread is through inhalation of infected dust particles rather than via the bite of an insect vector. The organisms reside principally in animals; human contact with cattle, sheep, goats, or with infected animal hides or hide products is the most important epidemiologic factor, and is often the only clue to diagnosis. The clinical features of Q fever are similar to those of the other nonbacterial pneumonias, except that hepatitis occurs in up to one third of patients.

OTHER ORGANISMS ranging from the tubercle bacillus (particularly during *primary tuberculosis,* see Chapter 47) to fungi (particularly *histoplasmosis* and *coccidiodomycosis*) and parasites (*Pneumocystis carinii* in the immunosuppressed host; see Chapter 142) can cause illnesses resembling the atypical pneumonias. In patients with COPD, *Branhamella catarrhalis* has been reported as a cause of pneumonia infiltrate.

DIFFERENTIAL DIAGNOSIS

In addition to the conditions listed in Table 43-1 and detailed above, noninfectious diseases can occasionally mimic

Table 43-1. Differential Diagnosis of Pneumonia

I. Bacterial Pneumonias
  A. Gram-positive
    1. *Pneumococcus*
    2. *Streptococcus*
    3. *Staphylococcus aureus*
  B. Gram-negative
    1. *H. influenzae*
    2. *Klebsiella*
    3. *Proteus, E. coli, Pseudomonas* and others
      (usually in hospitalized patients)
    4. Legionnaire's disease
  C. Mixed
    1. Aspiration pneumonia
  D. Mycobacterial
    1. Tuberculosis
II. Nonbacterial pneumonias
    1. *Mycoplasma*
    2. Viral
    3. Psittacosis
    4. Q fever
    5. *Pneumocystis carinii*
    6. Fungi

infectious processes. Bronchial asthma (see Chapter 45) and hypersensitivity pneumonitis are common examples. The radiologic findings associated with chronic pulmonary diseases, especially chronic bronchitis (see Chapter 44), and bronchiectasis (see Chapter 37), may be misleading if previous x-rays are not available. Atelectasis, pulmonary infarction, pulmonary edema (see Chapter 27), and lung tumors may also be confused with pneumonia.

WORKUP

History. A careful history should be taken, looking particularly for recent viral upper respiratory infection and any exposure to respiratory tract infection. Impaired cough and gag reflexes due to anesthesia, head trauma, intoxication, and neurologic disorders increase the risk of aspiration pneumonia. A history of recent travel may raise the question of unusual bacterial or fungal processes; and occupational exposures or animal (Q fever) and bird (psittacosis) contacts further broaden the differential diagnosis. It is particularly important to learn if the patient is a smoker and has underlying chronic lung disease or asthma (see Chapters 49, 44, and 45). The occurrence of such extrapulmonary symptoms as diarrhea and confusion suggests Legionnaires' disease.

It is important to distinguish between bacterial and nonbacterial diseases. Although this distinction can be difficult in individual patients, certain broad generalizations can be offered. Patients with bacterial pneumonias are more likely to have abrupt onset of illness and to be clinically sicker with higher temperatures, a higher incidence of chills, more copious sputum production, and a greater likelihood of developing significant pleural effusions. While both types of pneumonia can affect all ages, nonbacterial pneumonias are more common in older children and young adults. Such patients characteristically report a more gradual onset of symptoms with only moderate fever. Patients with viral and mycoplasmal pneumonias will often complain of a severe hacking cough, but substantial sputum production is unusual.

Physical Examination. The patient with bacterial pneumonia generally looks sicker, and chest examination usually reveals signs of consolidation, or at least localized rales and rhonchi. In contrast, the chest examination of patients with nonbacterial pneumonias typically shows only fine rales, and often the physical findings are less extensive than the radiologic abnormalities.

Physical examination is important not only to elicit signs of pneumonia itself, but to assess the overall status of the patient. High fever, marked tachycardia, hypotension, cyanosis, signs of hypercarbia (asterixis, confusion, papilledema), and alterations of mentation are indications for emergency hospitalization.

Laboratory Studies. When the patient is only mildly ill and has clear lungs, laboratory studies can be limited to a sputum Gram's stain, sputum culture, and a white blood cell count and differential. When pneumonia is suspected, PA and lateral chest x-rays are mandatory. If the patient appears quite ill, blood cultures should be obtained and thoracentesis considered, provided there is sufficient pleural fluid present. The fluid is sent for Gram's stain, culture, and protein, glucose, and LDH determinations (see Chapter 39).

Laboratory studies help distinguish between viral and bacterial causes. Patients with bacterial pneumonias are more likely to have a polymorphonuclear leukocytosis. If the chest x-ray reveals lobar or segmental consolidation, abscess formation or significant pleural effusions, bacterial pneumonia is more likely; a patchy infiltrate can occur in either type of process, but a true interstitial infiltrate suggests a nonbacterial etiology.

The key to diagnosis is *examination of sputum.* The sputum of the patient with bacterial pneumonia is typically thick and green to brownish in color. It may be blood-tinged. A good sputum specimen for microscopic examination and culture is crucial. If the patient cannot expectorate spontaneously, pulmonary physiotherapy, intermittent positive pressure breathing with humidified air, or nasotracheal suction may be used to obtain the specimen. If these fail, transtracheal aspiration should be considered. *Gram stain* of sputum from patients with bacterial pneumonia usually reveals abundant polymorphonuclear leukocytes and will often disclose the primary pathogen. Patients with nonbacterial pneumonias generally produce only scant quantities of thin sputum, though in the case of influenzal pneumonia it can be bloody; the Gram stain is noteworthy for an absence of bacteria and a scant cellular response. In patients with mycoplasmal pneumonia, mononuclear cells may predominate.

The value of the *sputum culture* is dependent upon obtaining a deep specimen. Often, sputum production is scant, as in cases of atypical pneumonia. Culturing an inadequate specimen is a waste of time. All cultures that are to be obtained should be sent before antibiotics are started. Some organisms are too fastidious to grow from sputum samples; other means of definitive diagnosis may be necessary. For example, pneumococci may fail to grow out from sputum samples, but can be isolated from blood cultures drawn during the early bacteremic phase of the illness.

Legionnaires' disease can be diagnosed by culture of the organism, antibody staining, or serologic study. In most instances, serologic study confirms the diagnosis. A single antibody titer of 1:256 is presumptive evidence, but confirmation requires demonstration of a fourfold rise in titer between acute and convalescent specimens, and a convalescent titer of at least 1:128. The organism can be isolated and cultured from sputum, lung, or pleural fluid, using charcoal yeast extract agar. Identification is sometimes made by fluorescent antibody staining of sputum.

Most *viral pneumonias* can be diagnosed on clinical grounds and epidemiologic evidence. Specific diagnosis depends on either serologic studies (which are retrospective) or viral cultures (which are not widely available). Recognition of influenza is important because contacts can be protected by prophylactic use of amantadine; diagnostic confirmation is worth seeking when influenza is suspected.

Mycoplasma can be grown in the laboratory only on specialized media. An important clue to diagnosis is the presence of cold agglutinins in the serum. Low titers (below 1:32 or 1:64) can occur in other disorders such as adenovirus and influenza infections, but high or rising titers are strongly suggestive of *M. pneumoniae* infection. Cold agglutinins may be absent, particularly in patients with mild disease, and specific serologic tests are then required. A new infiltrate in a patient with AIDS raises the question of *Pneumocystis* infection. Criteria for initiation of therapy range from dyspnea and hypoxia to recovery of the organism in sputum or bronchoscopy samples.

For *psittacosis,* a history of bird exposure is the key to diagnosis, and specific serologies are required for confirmation. The diagnosis of Q fever depends on specific serologies.

PRINCIPLES OF MANAGEMENT

Many patients with lower respiratory tract infections, especially those with acute bronchitis or mild pneumonia due to virus, *H. influenzae,* pneumococci, or mycoplasma, can be managed on an outpatient basis, provided that they are alert, reliable, have help available to them, and have no signs of serious compromise such as high fever, tachycardia, tachypnea, hypotension, cyanosis, or alterations of mentation. Oral antibiotic regimens can achieve therapeutic serum antibiotic levels. However, those with staphylococcal and gram-negative pneumonias must be treated with parenteral antibiotics and thus require hospitalization. The elderly and

individuals with poor home environments also deserve consideration for inpatient treatment.

There are certain general principles of management which apply, regardless of etiology. Adequate *hydration* is essential to help clear secretions; this can be achieved via attention to fluid intake and also through local airway humidification. *Expectorants* such as guaifenesin may be helpful to some patients in loosening the sputum, though there is no objective evidence that they make a significant difference in outcome. *Pulmonary physical therapy* can further help with secretions. (See Chapters 37, 44, 46.) In general, the cough reflex should not be suppressed in patients with bacterial infections, because coughing is an important mechanism for clearing secretions. However, if severe paroxysms of coughing produce respiratory fatigue or severe pain, temporary relief may be obtained with small doses of *codeine* (see Chapter 37). Chest pain should be treated with analgesics that do not suppress cough. Aspirin should be tried first, but for more severe pain, nonsteroidal anti-inflammatory agents or codeine may be needed. If narcotics are used, the patient must be carefully monitored for respiratory depression and excessive cough suppression. Fever can be controlled with aspirin or acetaminophen (see Chapter 6). If oxygen is administered prior to hospitalization, only very low FIO_2's (24% to 28%) should be utilized. Individuals with chronic lung disease who retain CO_2 depend on their hypoxic drive; excessive oxygen therapy may precipitate respiratory depression (see Chapter 44).

Specific therapy depends on the etiologic agent involved. While culture and sensitivity testing will require at least 24 to 48 hours to provide definitive information, the clinical setting, chest x-ray and sputum Gram's stain usually enable the physician to make a reasonable presumptive diagnosis and to initiate therapy promptly. Treatment can then be modified as necessary on the basis of culture results. For example, young, otherwise healthy patients with atypical pneumonia can be started on erythromycin, which will cover Mycoplasma and pneumococcal disease.

THERAPEUTIC RECOMMENDATIONS

Tables 43-2 and 43-3 summarize therapeutic recommendations for lower respiratory tract infections, acute bronchitis, and pneumonia.

Pneumococcal Disease

Penicillin is the drug of choice. Therapy should be continued until the patient has been afebrile for 3 to 5 days or for a total course of 10 to 14 days. A healthy young patient with disease confined to one lobe and a supportive home environment can be given an initial dose of intramuscular procaine penicillin and continued on oral penicillin at home with close follow-up. Most other patients should be considered for hospitalization initially and treated parenterally until substantial improvement occurs. Table 43-2 lists alternative

Table 43-2. Antibiotics of Choice for Outpatient Treatment of Lower Respiratory Tract Infections

ORGANISM*	DRUG OF CHOICE	ALTERNATE DRUGS
S. pneumoniae (pneumococcus)	Penicillin	Cephalosporins Erythromycin Lincomycin Clindamycin
Hemophilus influenzae	Ampicillin or Amoxicillin	Tetracycline Trimethoprim– sulfamethoxazole
Mycoplasma pneumoniae	Erythromycin or Tetracycline	
Q fever	Tetracycline	Chloramphenicol
Psittacosis	Tetracycline	

* Lower respiratory infections due to Group A streptococcus, *Staphylococcus aureus*, Legionnaire's disease bacillus *(Legionella pneumophilae)*, *Klebsiella pneumoniae*, *Pseudomonas aeruginosa*, *E. coli*, *Proteus mirabilis*, and other gram-negative bacilli require hospitalization for parenteral antibiotic therapy; the same is true for aspiration pneumonia due to mixed ''normal'' mouth flora.

antibiotics for the penicillin-allergic patient; tetracyclines should *not* be used because many pneumococci are now resistant to these agents.

An important development is the availability of a *vaccine* to prevent pneumococcal pneumonia. Although there are 83 capsular types of pneumococci, each with its own type-specific immunity, a relatively small number of serotypes account for most human infections. The vaccine incorporates 23 capsular types which together account for about 90% of pneumococcal pneumonias in the United States, and field trials suggest that it may be up to 80% effective in preventing pneumonia due to these 23 types. All patients who have undergone splenectomy or who have sickle cell disease should be vaccinated, because of their unique susceptibility to fulminating pneumococcal sepsis. In addition, immunosuppressed patients, the elderly, and individuals with chronic cardiopulmonary disease would seem to be good candidates for vaccination. Mild local pain and erythema are the only common adverse reactions to the vaccine, which is administered in a single 0.5-ml intramuscular or subcutaneous dose. Repeat doses of vaccine are not required. The vaccine can be given at the same time as influenza vaccine. Many patients received the original pneumococcal vaccine, which had 14 capsular antigens. It is uncertain whether patients who received the old vaccine should be revaccinated, but very high-risk patients probably should be.

Staphylococcus aureus

A parentally administered semisynthetic penicillin (or penicillin, if the organism is not a penicillinase producer) is the drug of choice, requiring hospitalization. Therapy should be continued until clinical and x-ray healing is apparent; this usually requires at least 2 to 4 weeks.

Table 43-3. Antibiotic Dosage Regimens for Ambulatory Therapy of Acute Bronchitis and Mild Cases of Pneumonia in Adults

DRUG	DOSE*	MAJOR TOXICITY†
Penicillin‡	250–500 mg every 6 h	Hypersensitivity
Ampicillin‡	250–500 mg every 6 h	Hypersensitivity GI intolerance
Amoxicillin‡	250–500 mg every 8 h	Hypersensitivity GI intolerance
Erythromycin	250–500 mg every 6 h	GI intolerance Hypersensitivity
Trimethoprim– sulfamethoxazole	2 tablets every 12 h or 1 double-strength tablet every 12 h	Hypersensitivity
Tetracycline	250–500 mg every 6 h	GI intolerance Hypersensitivity
Clindamycin	150–300 mg every 6 h	Enterocolitis Hypersensitivity
Cephalexin‡·§	250–500 mg every 6–8 h	Hypersensitivity

* All doses are for average-sized adults with normal renal and hepatic function. Consult manufacturer's recommendations for details.

† Only major toxicity is listed; see manufacturer's literature for additional adverse reactions. In addition, all antibiotics predispose to superinfection with resistant organisms and should be used with caution.

‡ Cross-sensitivity is shared among all of the penicillins. In addition, patients who are allergic to penicillins may be allergic to cephalosporins.

§ Other cephalosporins used orally include cephradine (similar to cephalexin), cefaclor (somewhat more active than cephalexin against H. influenzae), cefadoxril (can be given q 12 h).

Streptococcus pyogenes

Parenteral penicillin is the treatment of choice, requiring hospitalization. Therapy should be continued until clinical resolution, usually at least 2 weeks.

H. influenzae

Until very recently, ampicillin was the drug of choice for *H. influenzae* infections. In the past few years, an increasing number of ampicillin-resistant strains of this organism have been recognized. While ampicillin-resistant organisms still constitute a minority of strains, chloramphenicol or cefamandole should be used for initial therapy in the very sick patient, with a return to ampicillin if the organism proves sensitive. Cefamandole, a parenteral cephalosporin-like drug, is very effective against *H. influenzae,* including ampicillin-resistant strains. For patients with bronchitis, the oral tetracyclines and trimethoprim-sulfamethoxazole have been excellent alternatives to ampicillin. In general, patients with bronchitis should be treated for 7 to 10 days, and patients with pneumonia for 10 to 14 days.

Klebsiella and Other Enterobacteriaceae

Hospital admission for parenteral antibiotic therapy is required. Gentamicin is the drug of choice, pending results of susceptibility testing.

Legionnaires' Disease

Therapy during outbreaks is often initiated on clinical and epidemiologic grounds before the diagnosis is confirmed. Erythromycin is currently the drug of choice, 1 g intravenously four times daily. Treatment failures have been reported when seriously ill patients are given oral erythromycin; very mild cases may be managed on an outpatient basis with 500 mg erythromycin four times daily for 7 to 10 days. Close follow-up is mandatory.

Aspiration Pneumonia

A patient who aspirates cannot protect his airway and must be admitted. Penicillin is the drug of choice, and clindamycin is an excellent alternative.

Mycoplasma

Oral erythromycin or tetracycline is effective. The penicillins are inactive because mycoplasmas lack cell walls. Treatment should be continued for 1 to 2 weeks.

Viruses

Although there is no treatment for viral pneumonia, prophylaxis against influenza is extremely important. All elderly patients and those with underlying cardiopulmonary and chronic disease should be vaccinated annually with *polyvalent influenza vaccine* in the fall of each year. The vaccine is 70% to 80% protective, and it is prepared annually to correspond with the wild strains in circulation. The vaccine is made of purified, killed virus. There have been no reports of an increased incidence of Guillain–Barré with use of routine influenza vaccine; swine flu vaccine used only in 1976 was associated with an increased risk of neurologic complications. Serious reactions are rare, unless the patient is allergic to egg protein. Minor febrile responses and myalgias are sometimes noted.

Patients not immunized and at high risk of contracting influenza can be given oral *amantadine.* At a dose of 200 mg per day it can prevent or at least blunt clinical illness in 70% to 90% of patients exposed to influenza A (it has no activity against influenza B). Unfortunately, it must be taken daily during the period of risk to provide protection, and it causes neurologic side-effects (insomnia, dizziness, and confusion), particularly in the elderly. As such, it is best used during an epidemic to protect the frail unvaccinated population until an emergency vaccination program can be completed.

Atypical Pneumonia Syndrome

Most otherwise healthy ambulatory patients with fever, nonproductive cough, and nonspecific infiltrate have a self-limited disease that will resolve without treatment. However, since Mycoplasma is the most likely etiology in this patient population, an empirical course of erythromycin (see above) can be used to shorten duration of illness. Erythromycin is also likely to help in cases of Legionella infection presenting as mild atypical pneumonia; diagnosis and treatment may be based on epidemiologic grounds (*e.g.,* epidemic outbreak, common water source suspected). Epidemiologic data often form the basis for other treatment decisions, such as when there has been travel to an area endemic for histoplasmosis or coccidioidomycosis, or exposure to *Chlamydia psittaci* from handling of birds. Tetracycline is the drug of choice for Chlamydia infection. Patients with AIDS who come down with an atypical pneumonia require prompt consideration for *Pneumocystis carinii* infection. Trimethoprim–sulfa is usually the drug first administered and has proven effective when given parenterally. However, there is a high incidence of allergic reactions to the agent among AIDS patients, necessitating a switch to pentamidine.

Tuberculosis

See Chapter 47.

MONITORING THERAPY

Temperature, respiratory rate, chest examination, and white cell count will provide a reasonable estimate of recovery.

Repeating chest x-rays at frequent intervals is wasteful if the patient is progressing well clinically. It is important to recognize that clearing of radiologic findings often lags far behind clinical resolution; continued presence of a slowly resolving infiltrate is neither a sign of poor response to therapy nor indicative of serious prognosis. This is particularly true for pneumococcal disease, in which the patient feels much better although x-rays may still show an infiltrate up to 6 weeks later. However, x-ray examination is important for detection of complications such as lung abscess and empyema, and films should be obtained when the patient's condition is worsening or fever is not resolving.

INDICATIONS FOR ADMISSION

High fever, tachypnea, tachycardia, cyanosis, poor home environment, presence of an organism necessitating parenteral therapy, aspiration, lung abscess, empyema, and positive blood cultures mandate inpatient management. Elderly patients and those with preexisting cardiopulmonary disease should usually be admitted unless illness is very mild and close supervision is available at home. Most patients with AIDS ought to be hospitalized if pneumonitis develops.

PATIENT EDUCATION

Patients treated on an ambulatory basis need to be instructed to maintain a good fluid intake (approximately 2000 ml of liquid daily) in order to avoid inspissation of secretions and poor pulmonary toilet. Temperature should be taken and recorded each evening. Caution against overuse of any cough suppressant is important; emphasis should be on nighttime use only, allowing for sleep but permitting cough and mobilization of sputum during the day. Many patients think all coughing is bad; they need to understand its role in clearing the airways so they do not abuse their medication. If the patient is a smoker, he will probably have ceased smoking temporarily. This is an excellent opportunity to encourage the patient to quit, and, in fact, many do at this time (see Chapter 49). Patient and family should be instructed to watch for evidence of worsening (such as unremitting fever, drowsiness, dyspnea) and to call at first sign of difficulty.

ANNOTATED BIBLIOGRAPHY

Austrian R, Gold J: Pneumococcal bacteremia with special reference to bacteremic pneumococcal pneumonia. Ann Intern Med 60: 759, 1964 (*A classic study of clinical features and prognostic indicators in bacteremic pneumococcal pneumonia.*)

Denny FW, Clyde WA, Glezen WP: Mycoplasma pneumoniae disease: Clinical spectrum, pathophysiology, epidemiology, and control. J Infect Dis 123:74, 1971 (*An excellent description of clinical presentation.*)

Douglas RG Jr: Amantadine as an antiviral agent in influenza. N Engl J Med 307:617, 1982 (*Summarizes studies on amantadine and argues for its use during epidemics of influenza A.*)

Engleberg LA, Lerner CW, Tepper ML: Clinical features of Pneumocystis pneumonia in the acquired immune deficiency syndrome. Am Rev Respir Dis 130:689, 1984 (*Good description of its many forms.*)

Garibaldi RA: Epidemiology of community-acquired respiratory tract infections in adults. Am J Med 78(6B):32, 1985 (*Good update on epidemiology. Argues for careful etiologic diagnosis of community-acquired lower respiratory infections, given the wide array of pathogenic agents showing up in the community setting.*)

Health and Public Policy Committee, American College of Physicians: Pneumococcal vaccine. Ann Intern Med 104:118, 1986 (*Strongly recommends use of the vaccine; guidelines provided.*)

Jay SJ, Johannson WG, Pierce AK: The radiographic resolution of Streptococcus pneumoniae pneumonia. N Engl Med 293:798, 1975 (*A very helpful paper showing that delayed resolution of radiographic abnormalities is common in pneumococcal pneumonia, and that these x-ray findings in themselves need not raise concern about bronchial obstruction, neoplasia, or persistent infection.*)

La Force MA: Community-acquired lower respiratory tract infections: Prevention and cost-control strategies. Am J Med 78(6B):52, 1985 (*A provocative paper examining the utility of diagnostic, preventive, and treatment modalities.*)

Mayer RD: Legionella infections: A review of five years of research. Rev Inf Dis 5:258, 1983 (*An excellent overview of the epidemiology, pathogenesis, diagnosis, and management of this important infection.*)

Mostow SR: Pneumonias acquired outside the hospital. Med Clin North Am 58:555, 1974 (*A clinical overview of pneumonias in ambulatory patients.*)

Murray HW, Masur H, Senterfit LB et al: The protein manifestations of Mycoplasma pneumonia infection in adults. Am J Med 58: 229, 1975 (*The clinical spectrum of mycoplasmal pneumonia.*)

Musher DM, McKenzie SO: Infections due to Staphylococcus aureus. Medicine 56:383, 1977 (*A review of staphylococcal infections, including aerogenous and bacteremic pneumonias.*)

Nicotra B, River M, Luman JI et al: Branhamella catarrhalis is a lower respiratory tract pathogen in patients with chronic lung disease. Arch Intern Med 146:898, 1986 (B. Catarrhalis *in the sputum of chronic lung patients with pneumonic infiltrates should be suspected as pathogens. Treatment requires agents other than the penicillins.*)

Shapiro ED, Clemens JD: A controlled evaluation of the protective efficacy of pneumococcal vaccine for patients at high risk of serious pneumococcal infection. Ann Intern Med 101:325, 1984 (*A study using the case-control method which suggests that the vaccine is 70% effective for elderly patients. This paper also reviews previous trials and indications for vaccination.*)

Simon HB, Southwick FS, Moellering RC et al: Hemophilus influenzae in hospitalized adults: Current perspectives. Am J Med 69: 219, 1980 (*This study confirms the importance of nontypeable as well as typeable strains of* H. influenzae *in respiratory infections, and it points out that this organism can be a nosocomial pathogen and can participate in mixed infections.*)

44

Management of Chronic Obstructive Pulmonary Disease (COPD)

Chronic obstructive pulmonary disease (chronic bronchitis/emphysema) is a major cause of total disability, second only to coronary artery disease. Its prevalence approaches 30 per 1000. Because COPD is incurable and often irreversible, the prime goal of management is to preserve function and limit complications. In many instances, functional impairment can be minimized and exercise tolerance improved. Optimal management includes cessation of smoking (see Chapter 49), immunization against influenza and pneumococcal disease, control of bronchospasm, mobilization of secretions, improvement of exercise tolerance, and treatment of pneumonia and chronic hypoxia should they occur. The primary physician needs to know how and when to utilize bronchodilators, oxygen, pneumococcal and influenza vaccines, physical therapy measures, exercise training, and antibiotics in the management of patients with COPD. Physician attitude is also an important determinant of successful outcome.

PATHOPHYSIOLOGY, CLINICAL PRESENTATION, AND COURSE

The chronic obstructive pulmonary diseases are actually a diverse set of conditions sharing a pathophysiologic common denominator: slowing of the expiratory flow rate. The earliest manifestation of COPD appears to be an increase in small airway resistance.

The COPD patient may present clinically with any combination of cough, sputum production, wheezing, and shortness of breath. The presentation is a function of the severity of illness and the degrees of chronic bronchitis and emphysema to the clinical picture. Most patients have mixed disease, though one pathophysiology often predominates.

Emphysema. The primary pathophysiologic defect in emphysema is fragmentation of pulmonary elastic tissue, leading to destruction of alveolar architecture as well as of the capillary bed that lies within the alveolar wall. The loss of elastic tissue weakens the support structure that keeps noncartilaginous airways from collapsing during expiration; this leads to a fall in expiratory flow rates as the lung's normal elastic recoil is lost and poorly supported airways collapse during expiration. Recent studies suggest a reversible cholinergic component of airway obstruction responsive to atropine.

Inspiratory flow rates are normal because airway caliber is normal. Pulmonary compliance increases with the decline in elasticity. The size of the pulmonary capillary bed is reduced, causing carbon monoxide diffusing capacity to drop. The reduction in size of the vascular bed parallels the fall in alveolar surface area. Thus, ventilation still roughly matches perfusion, and significant hypoxemia does not ensue.

The *clinical picture* is dominated by dyspnea, particularly on exertion. Cough is only a minor complaint, and sputum production is scant. The patient with advanced disease is thin and tachypneic, often using accessory muscles of respiration and pursed-lip breathing. The latter helps keep noncartilagenous airways from collapsing during expiration. Cyanosis is uncommon, because pO_2 is only minimally reduced. The neck veins may seem distended, but only on expiration. The anterior–posterior diameter of the chest is increased; the percussion note is hyperresonant; and the breath sounds are distant. There are usually no signs of cor pulmonale, though the right ventricular impulse may be prominent due to displacement by hyperinflated lungs. As noted, hypoxemia is minimal and there is little if any carbon dioxide retention until the end stages of the disease.

Chronic Bronchitis. Inflammation of the cells lining the bronchial wall is the predominant pathophysiologic problem in chronic bronchitis. Smoking, air pollution, and prolonged exposure to other bronchial irritants are important etiologic factors; however, even after withdrawal of such irritants the inflammatory process often continues unabated. Edema, excess mucus production, and loss of ciliary transport result. Obstruction to airflow occurs with inspiration as well as with expiration. Widespread bronchial narrowing and mucus plugging produce hypoxemia due to mismatching of ventilation and perfusion. Hypercarbia results from impeded ventilation. Chronic hypoxia and hypercarbia increase pulmonary arterial resistance and may lead to development of cor pulmonale. Sudden worsening may precipitate acute right heart failure in severe chronic bronchitis. Compared to emphysema, chronic bronchitis causes much less parenchymal damage; diffusing capacity, lung volumes, and compliance are not greatly altered.

The role of infection in the genesis of acute exacerbations remains unsettled, though a recent double-blind, randomized, placebo-controlled trial found no difference in outcome between patients given tetracycline and those given a placebo.

The person with chronic bronchitis is often a smoker who presents with a history of chronic, productive cough. By definition, the cough must be present for at least 3 months each year, during 2 consecutive years. At first, the sputum production and cough occur just in the winter months, but soon the patient becomes symptomatic year round, with a history of frequent exacerbations. By the time dyspnea on exertion sets in, the disease is well advanced. Patients may report having to sit up at night to breathe; at times this may be a manifestation of congestive heart failure, which is not uncommon, but more careful questioning often reveals that the difficulty was precipitated by cough and relieved by raising sputum. Patients with severe chronic bronchitis are at increased risk of developing cor pulmonale, because they often become chronically hypoxic and develop an increase in pulmonary artery resistance that leads to right heart failure.

The chronic bronchitic patient is typically in his fifties at the time of presentation. He appears plethoric and cyanotic at the stage of severe disease, a time when many first come for help. Tobacco stains on the fingers and teeth are common, and there may be signs of cor pulmonale (distended neck veins, a right ventricular heave, a right ventricular gallop, and peripheral edema). The lungs sound noisy; crackles and wheezes are readily evident. The expiratory phase of respiration is prolonged. Because of the mismatching of ventilation with perfusion, hypoxia may be found on measurement of arterial blood gases. The pCO_2 rises as the patient's ability to effectively move air declines. Secondary polycythemia is common.

Clinical Course. The clinical course of COPD is generally progressive, though some individuals seem to reach a plateau clinically. Prior to the onset of symptoms, one can often detect an increase in the closing volume and a decrease in the maximum midexpiratory flow rate (sensitive measures of small airway disease); measures of large airway resistance are usually within normal limits during this phase of illness. The presymptomatic, small airway stage of COPD may represent a period of reversible disease; however, early fibrotic changes have been found in airways of such patients. It is unresolved whether intervention at the time of early small airway abnormalities will alter the course of disease and improve prognosis.

Longitudinal studies of symptomatic patients have shown a steady deterioration in pulmonary function with time. Using the forced expiratory volume at 1 second (FEV_1) as the measure of obstruction, an annual average decrease in flow rate of 50 to 60 ml per second has been noted. By the time the FEV_1 declines to 1 liter per second, the mean annual mortality approaches 10%. The onset of resting tachycardia and signs of cor pulmonale are other indicators of a poor prognosis.

A recent longitudinal 12-year study of 140 COPD patients provides confirmatory evidence for the importance of a number of predictors of survival and disability cited in several earlier studies. Although differences in entry criteria and methods make comparisons between studies difficult, several parameters are emerging as prognostically useful (see Table 44-1). Significant reductions in 12-year survival were found among patients with marked reduction in the ratio of FEV_1 to forced vital capacity (FVC), a substantial drop in FEV_1 or FVC, hypoxemia, hypercarbia, cor pulmonale, or decreased diffusing capacity.

The FEV_1 may be a more useful predictor of prognosis in advanced disease than the ratio of FEV_1 to FVC; in late disease, the FEV_1 often slows in its rate of decline and the FVC may fall more rapidly, thus preserving their ratio even in the setting of clinical deterioration. However, once the FEV_1 falls below 1 liter per second, it is less able to distinguish survivors from nonsurvivors. Other predictors of poor prognosis included heavy smoking and rate of decline of expiratory flow rates over time. Interestingly, the group with the lowest 12-year probability of survival still had a 40% chance of remaining alive.

Other investigators have found mixed venous oxygen concentration to be an important prognostic indicator; pulmonary hemodynamics were not predictive. Differences in patient populations make rigid extrapolation from studies of prognosis to individual patients unwise, but the parameters identified can be of qualitative use clinically. It remains very difficult to predict survival in individual patients.

Although prognosis for patients with COPD is not good, recent British and American studies have shown that stable, chronically hypoxemic patients (Po_2 <60) achieve prolonged survival when treated with continuous oxygen therapy. The exact mechanism of improved survival is not known, but pulmonary hypertension and secondary polycythemia decreased, and neuropsychiatric functioning improved.

WORKUP

Although the selection of treatment modalities is in part empirical, it is nevertheless helpful to identify the predominant pathophysiologic defects, their severity, effect on the patient's functional status, and any aggravating or precipitating factors. Clarification of these issues can help focus therapy and serve as a baseline for monitoring efficacy of treatment.

History. One should obtain a careful description of symptoms and activity limitations experienced in daily life,

Table 44-1. Predictors of Poor Prognosis in COPD

1. FEV1 < 40% of predicted; especially less than 1.0 liter/min
2. FEV1/FVC < 0.40
3. Arterial Po_2 < 55 mm Hg
4. Presence of cor pulmonale
5. CO_2 retention
6. FVC < 80% of predicted
7. Decreased single-breath diffusing capacity
8. Decreased mixed venous oxygen concentration

both at rest and with exercise. Smoking habits and environmental or work exposures to pulmonary irritants ought to be sought and specified. Quasiquantitative estimates of exercise capacity (*e.g.,* flights of stairs that can be climbed or distance that can be walked on level ground) are helpful, as is some indication of progression of symptoms over time.

Physical Examination. It is important to note any tachypnea, tachycardia, degree of prolongation of expiratory phase, cyanosis, clubbing, use of accessory respiratory muscles, wheezes, signs of consolidation, and evidence of cor pulmonale (jugular venous distention, peripheral edema, right ventricular heave, loud pulmonic closure sound, and right ventricular S_3).

Laboratory Studies are first directed at quantifying the degree of obstructive defect *and determining* the response to bronchodilators. Small airway disease can be detected during the asymptomatic phase of illness by ordering closing volume and maximal midexpiratory flow rate determinations. The degree of obstruction in larger airways can be assessed by measuring expiratory flow rates on an office spirometer; the most helpful measurement is the ratio of the forced expiratory volume at 1 second (FEV_1) to the vital capacity. Crude estimates of obstruction can be provided by the FEV_1 alone. Results are compared to predicted values. Patients with a 50% reduction in FEV_1 are often dyspneic on exertion; by the time the FEV_1 falls to 25% of predicted, they may complain of shortness of breath at rest. Determination of expiratory flow rates before and after inhalation of a bronchodilator (*e.g.,* isoproterenol) can provide a quick estimate of the benefit a patient may derive from bronchodilator therapy. The failure to obtain an improvement in flow rate from a few inhalations of a bronchodilator does not rule out the possibility of benefit, but it suggests the likelihood is not great.

A chest x-ray is helpful to detect complications of COPD, such as heart failure, pneumonia, or a pneumothorax. Arterial blood gases provide measures of oxygenation and ventilation. Hypoxemia and hypercarbia are manifestations of severe chronic bronchitis. Blood gases are particularly useful for documenting acute decompensation. In patients with severe chronic bronchitis, baseline studies of blood gases should be performed, so that gases obtained at times of marked subjective worsening can be compared to baseline determinations. Hematocrit and hemoglobin concentration provides a rough indication of the severity and chronicity of hypoxemia and the need for phlebotomy. The electrocardiographic abnormalities which appear in COPD generally reflect the severity of the lung disease and the presence of cor pulmonale. The ECG should be studied for sinus tachycardia, multifocal atrial tachycardia, peaked P waves (P pulmonale) and signs of right ventricular hypertrophy (*e.g.,* tall R wave in V_1 and deep S in lead V_6. Examination of the sputum is mandatory when acute pneumonitis is suspected.

PRINCIPLES OF MANAGEMENT

The prime goal of treatment is to improve the patient's functional status so that he can better carry out his daily activities. Elimination of precipitants and risk factors, prevention and treatment of infection, control of bronchospasm, mobilization of secretions, and avoidance of chronic hypoxia are the principal objectives of management. With the exception of chronic oxygen therapy in hypoxemic patients, treatment does not prolong survival, and therefore must be evaluated by the patient's subjective response. The success of treatment is strongly influenced by the physician's interest and the participation of patient and family in the program.

Avoidance of Precipitants and Risk Factors. Regardless of severity of disease or the types of deficits present, *all* COPD patients should be urged in the most emphatic way to *stop smoking.* A surprisingly large number of patients report little or no warning about smoking from their physicians; studies indicate that the physician's advice does lead some patients to cease smoking, especially those who are symptomatic (see Chapter 49). Halting the continuous insult to the airways produced by smoking may limit progression of the disease; survival rate is lower among patients who continue to smoke.

Reduction in exposure to other pulmonary irritants should be advised. Readily avoidable pulmonary irritants include aerosol deodorants, hairsprays, paint sprays, and insecticides. An occupational history should be reviewed (see Chapter 35) for important worksite irritants. Change in job or residence (for patients living in areas of severe air pollution) may be necessary, but should be urged only when the relationship between exposure and disease is strong; otherwise, the advice might cause more harm than good.

Prophylaxis Against Infection. Immunization against influenza is essential for all COPD patients. *Trivalent influenza vaccine* should be given each fall, at least 6 weeks before the onset of the influenza season. Serious reactions are rare unless the patient is allergic to egg protein. Mild fever and myalgias are sometimes noted. Due to ever-changing viral strains, vaccination must be done yearly. Should an outbreak of influenza occur, protection for patients who were not immunized can still be provided by prescribing oral *amantadine.* Amantadine is effective against known strains of influenza A. Recent studies demonstrated a protection rate of 78% against clinical disease. Its effects are additive to those of influenza vaccine and it can be given to very sick vaccinated patients who require maximum protection.

Pneumococcal vaccine is equally important for COPD patients. The latest preparation incorporates the capsular antigens of 23 species that are responsible for 90% of the pneumococcal pneumonia occurring in the United States. Mild erythema and pain at the injection site are the only common adverse reactions to the vaccine. The vaccine is administered as a single intramuscular injection of 0.5 ml. Repeat doses of the vaccine are not needed at the present time; antibody titers are remaining high in those vaccinated as long as 5 years ago.

There is no blunting of antibody response or increased frequency of adverse reactions when both the pneumococcal and influenza vaccines are given simultaneously. The only disadvantage is difficulty in determining the cause of hypersensitivity should a reaction occur.

There is conflicting evidence on the use of *prophylactic antibiotics*. Studies done on COPD patients in England suggested benefit from prophylactic use of antibiotics during the winter months, reducing the number of exacerbations and days lost from work. However, recent studies in the United States have failed to demonstrate evidence of reduced infection or significant benefit from the use of antibiotics, either prophylactically or at times of acute exacerbations. Nonetheless, when there is strong clinical evidence of infection (fever, change to purulent sputum loaded with white cells, new infiltrate), treatment with antibiotics is indicated. Because *pneumococci* and *H. influenzae* are the predominant organisms colonizing patients with COPD, *ampicillin* (or amoxicillin) is a reasonable first choice of antibiotic when there is evidence of infection. For patients allergic to penicillin, *tetracycline* and *trimethoprim–sulfamethoxazole* are reasonable alternatives, though they are not very effective against pneumococci. Cefaclor, an orally administered cephalosporin, is active against both pneumococci and H. flu; its major disadvantage is high cost.

Bronchodilators. Most bronchodilators act by increasing cyclic AMP (cAMP) levels, which, in turn, leads to relaxation of bronchial smooth muscle. The methylxanthines (theophylline and its derivatives) block phosphodiesterase, the enzyme that breaks down cAMP intracellularly. Beta-adrenergic agents increase synthesis of cAMP. The mechanism of action of the corticosteroids remains uncertain, but hypotheses include reduction in mucosal edema, inhibition of prostaglandins that cause bronchoconstriction, and increased responsiveness to beta-adrenergic agents.

The decision to employ bronchodilators and the choice of agent are somewhat empirical; trial and error are usually necessary to arrive at an optimal program. There is no evidence that bronchodilators alter prognosis. It is not always possible to predict who will respond to bronchodilators on the basis of response to a single exposure to isoproterenol, but those who show considerable improvement in FEV_1 are good candidates for a trial of therapy. All COPD patients with evidence of a severe obstructive defect should be considered for a trial of bronchodilators, even if they do not respond to a few inhalations of bronchodilator at the time of pulmonary function testing. In a study of ten such COPD patients with "irreversible" airflow obstruction (less than a 15% improvement in FEV_1 after inhaling a bronchodilator), a significant improvement in ventilatory function occurred

with both high- and low-dose theophylline therapy. However, patients did not report significant differences in degree of breathlessness at rest between placebo, low-, and high-dose therapy. Data from this study are limited to short-term effects. In a study of men with moderate to severe COPD using sustained-release theophylline, there was a significant improvement in dyspnea, but little change in objective parameters. In sum, a limited empirical trial is probably reasonable, but should not be continued unless there is clear-cut subjective or objective benefit.

Theophylline and its derivatives are effective and relatively inexpensive. They come in oral and rectal preparations, with the oral route preferred. Absorption of an oral dose approaches 90%; rectal administration is associated with erratic absorption and the potential for suddenly high serum concentrations that can cause dangerous side-effects. The disadvantage of a relatively short half-life (4 to 6 hours) for the theophylline compounds has been overcome with development of sustained-release preparations that provide therapeutic serum levels for up to 12 hours. Therapeutic serum levels range between 10 and 20 $\mu g/ml$. Wide variability in level for a given dose is due to differences in clearance, which is predominantly hepatic. Decreased clearance and increased serum levels occur with heart failure, hepatocellular disease, and such drugs as cimetidine and erythromycin; smoking and barbiturates increase clearance. Serious side-effects of theophylline and its derivatives include cardiac arrhythmias and seizures; nervousness, tremor, and gastrointestinal upset are the most common side-effects.

Fixed combination preparations containing subtherapeutic concentrations of theophylline in conjunction with adrenergic agents, expectorants, and barbiturates are to be avoided. Not only do they result in unnecessary cost to the patient, but the sympathomimetic ingredients may potentiate toxicity without improving therapeutic effect; moreover, the barbiturate hastens clearance of theophylline and may reduce respiratory drive in patients with CO_2 retention.

Beta-adrenergic agents constitute an increasingly important class of bronchodilators. Isoproterenol is the prototype beta agonist, but it is limited in usefulness by its very short half-life and lack of selectivity for bronchial smooth muscle. The advent of improved beta agonists with more pulmonary selectivity (so-called beta$_2$ agents) and longer duration of action represents an advance in bronchodilator therapy. Albuterol, metaproterenol, and terbutaline are currently the principal drugs in this class, available in both oral and inhaled preparations. The inhaled form is more rapidly acting and associated with fewer cardiac side-effects than the oral one, yet still acts for up to 6 hours. However, at high doses both the oral and inhaled forms lose their cardioselectivity. Oral terbutaline produces severe tremulousness in some patients when used at full doses; often it lessens with continued use, but it can persist. Use of both a theophylline preparation (*e.g.*, aminophylline) and a beta$_2$ agent (*e.g.*, terbutaline) can sometimes enhance bronchodilation and allow reduction in doses of each, helping to minimize side-effects and improve compliance.

The optimal *route of administration* for bronchodilators appears to be by inhalation. In a double-blind crossover study of 17 COPD patients with stable, chronic airflow obstruction, aerosol albuterol produced significantly greater improvements in FEV_1 than did a combination of oral terbutaline and aminophylline. Moreover, addition of the oral program to patients already on inhaled albuterol did not provide any additional bronchodilation, but did exacerbate side-effects. Data on long-term administration are not available, so these results must be interpreted cautiously.

The convenience and rapid onset of action of inhaled beta agonists sometimes lead to excessive use and the potential for tachyphylaxis. Reliance on inhalation therapy must be accompanied by thorough patient education regarding proper inhalation technique and frequency of administration.

The role of *intermittent positive-pressure breathing* (IPPB) therapy in COPD has been carefully studied and shown to be lacking in demonstrable benefit. A long-term (33 month), multicenter controlled study was conducted to settle the controversy surrounding the efficacy of this expensive treatment modality that is popular with many patients. There were no statistically significant differences in mortality, rate and duration of hospitalization, and change in lung function or quality of life among those taking bronchodilator by IPPB or compressor nebulizer. Moreover, there were no differences in response among any clinically relevant subgroups, such as those with more severe disease, copious sputum, or emphysema. There is no objective evidence for use of IPPB therapy in COPD.

Corticosteroids are the bronchodilator class of last resort. Prednisone has been shown to achieve 30% or greater improvement in FEV_1 over baseline measurements in patients refractory to all other bronchodilators. Side-effects limit the benefit of long-term steroid therapy (see Chapter 103). The significant morbidity may be reduced by rapidly tapering oral dosage as soon as control of bronchospasm is attained and switching to alternate-day therapy or use of an inhaled, nonabsorbable corticosteroid such as beclomethasone or flunisolide. Caution regarding underlying adrenal suppression must be exerted in switching from oral to inhaled steroids, especially in patients on prednisone at suppressive doses (>15 mg per day) for more than 4 weeks (see Chapter 103). Unfortunately, aerosol steroid preparations, although useful, have not proved as effective as oral prednisone. Nevertheless, only patients with totally refractory and incapacitating bronchospasm should be considered for chronic daily steroid therapy.

Anticholinergic Agents. A recent study in emphysema patients using an inhaled anticholinergic agent (atropine methonitrate) showed a degree of bronchodilation identical to that achieved with beta$_2$ agonists; this finding suggests a final common pathway for airway obstruction and a potentially new approach to treatment of bronchospasm in COPD.

Oxygen Therapy. Recent clinical trials have shown that survival is prolonged in COPD patients who are chronically hypoxemic (pO_2 less than 60 mm Hg) when they receive long-term *continuous oxygen therapy*. The more continuous the therapy, the better the effect; round-the-clock oxygen therapy is superior to nocturnal oxygen administration. There is a very small subset of patients who are hypoxemic only at night, and they alone may obtain optimal benefit from just nocturnal therapy. Most COPD patients with profound nocturnal hypoxemia also are hypoxic during the day and require continuous administration of oxygen. Concern about the potential for continuous oxygen therapy to worsen carbon dioxide retention has been proven unfounded. A study of the effect of supplemental oxygen on gas exchange in hypercarbic hypoxic patients with severe COPD found no clinically important increases in pCO_2 during sleep (when CO_2 retention is at its worst) and concluded that oxygen therapy can be used safely in such patients.

The need for *short-term supplemental oxygen* comes up during consideration of *air travel*. Prediction of need for oxygen and tolerance of the cabin environment can be accomplished by having the patient inhale a hypoxic gas mixture (17.2% O_2) that simulates the cabin environment of a jet aircraft at cruising altitude. To document the effect on pO_2, arterial blood gases can be obtained after inhaling this mixture for 20 minutes while at rest and with light exercise. Although there are no established guidelines for when oxygen supplementation is needed, a drop in pO_2 to below 50 mm Hg or the development of symptoms are reasonable indications for oxygen supplementation during flights longer than 2 hours. Airlines will provide an oxygen supply if notified at least 48 hours in advance of travel; their units provide flows of 2 to 4 liters per minute of 25% or 30% oxygen. Patients are usually not allowed to bring their own oxygen tanks into the cabin of domestic airlines.

Brief administrations of oxygen have been given to *improve exercise tolerance* in COPD patients. Studies on the effects of such oxygen use have been conflicting. When unblinded, exercise tolerance improves. When blinded and done in controlled fashion, little benefit can be demonstrated. Most hypoxemic COPD patients are chronically hypoxic and require continuous oxygen supplementation. The small subset of patients who are only hypoxemic and markedly dyspneic with exercise are the best candidates for a trial of short-term oxygen supplementation. A convenient means of identifying such patients is to measure their diffusing capacity during routine pulmonary function testing, rather than trying to obtain arterial blood gases just after or during exercise. A diffusing capacity above 55% has been shown to be 100% specific in excluding arterial hypoxemia during exercise; sensitivity was 68%. If oxygen is to be tried, it should be limited to those who have a reduced diffusing capacity and demonstrate consistently better performance on oxygen than on air when both are administered in single-blind fashion.

Control of Secretions. Patients bothered by heavy, tenacious sputum may obtain benefit by maintaining good *fluid intake,* assuring the adequate *humidification* of the indoor environment (particularly in centrally heated homes), and practicing *postural drainage* when clearance of secretions is difficult and cough is incapacitating. The simplest method of postural drainage is to have the patient lean over the side of the bed, rest the elbows on a pillow placed on the floor, and cough as a family member or visiting nurse gently pounds on the chest. For hydration, ultrasonic nebulizers are no better than the simple maintenance of good systemic hydration, though the moisture they deliver does reach deep into the tracheobronchial tree. Occasionally, bronchospasm can be triggered by a nebulizer, and its reservoir can become contaminated and serve as a source of airway infection. Nebulized detergents are of no proven use, but *mucolytic agents* such as acetylcysteine are capable of thinning secretions; they are usually reserved for patients on respirators and not commonly used in outpatient practice. Oral *expectorants* are very popular with some patients, but without proven clinical efficacy. These preparations need not be denied to the patient who feels that they are of benefit, but should not be the mainstay of the therapeutic program. Glyceryl guaiacolate and potassium iodide are the most frequently prescribed expectorants; many are available without a prescription.

Exercise Training. Among the simplest and most effective measures for improving exercise tolerance is an *exercise training* program. Walking has proven to be the best form of exercise for increasing the duration and intensity of activity in COPD patients. Three or four sessions per day are prescribed, ranging from 5 to 15 minutes each. The pace and duration of activity are matched to the patient's capabilities; most begin the program walking at a half-maximal pace and build gradually over a period of several weeks. At the end of the training period, heart and respiratory rates for a given level of activity are decreased; oxygen consumption also falls. Tests of ventilatory function are not significantly changed, but increases of 25% are attained in maximum duration and intensity of exercise. Many patients enjoy marked improvement in ability to carry out their daily activities.

Breathing exercises may have some beneficial effect, particularly in those patients who easily panic and hyperventilate when dyspneic. Teaching such individuals to take slow, deep, relaxed breaths and exhale against pursed lips can lessen the work of moving air and provide the patient who tends to panic with a sense of control over his breathing and a more relaxed respiratory pattern.

Management of Cor Pulmonale. Patients with chronic cor pulmonale can often be made more comfortable by careful attention to their volume status, degree of hypoxemia, and hematocrit. Reduction of excess intravascular volume can reduce edema; *diuretic therapy* (see Chapter 27) is an effective means of volume control. *Phlebotomy* is indicated when secondary erythrocytosis is severe enough to significantly reduce blood viscosity and impair oxygen delivery; this occurs when the hematocrit rises above 55.

Continuous *low-flow oxygen* therapy is indicated in cor pulmonale patients who are chronically hypoxic (see above). Survival is improved, although the precise mechanism of improvement is unknown; pulmonary vascular resistance and secondary polycythemia are only modestly decreased. Whether oxygen therapy prevents development or worsening of cor pulmonale is unsettled.

Focus is shifting to examination of cardiac output as a determinant of survival in patients with cor pulmonale. Augmented cardiac output is a normal response to a fall in pO_2. Many patients with cor pulmonale maintain a high cardiac index. It is suspected that a fall in cardiac output may be a determinant of poor prognosis. If this proves to be the case, then increased efforts at improving cardiac output may be indicated.

Previous attempts at inotropic therapy have produced equivocal results. *Digitalis* seems to help some patients, but not uniformly or predictably. The incidence of digitalis toxicity is high, aggravated by hypoxemia; clinical response is often equivocal. The drug is worth a try in patients with reduced cardiac output but should be continued only in those who show an objective as well as subjective response to therapy. Patients who do appear to improve with digitalis should be given a minimum maintenance dose and monitored closely for manifestations of digitalis toxicity (see Chapter 27). Future avenues of treatment include trials of pulmonary vasodilators, aimed at reducing right ventricular afterload and increasing cardiac output and oxygen delivery to the periphery. The newer inotropic agents are also likely to be tried.

Monitoring Therapy. Symptomatology remains one of the most important measures of efficacy. Semiquantitative reports from the patient on such parameters as number of stairs climbed or distance walked can be quite useful. Subjective assessment of bronchospasm has been found to correlate surprisingly well with FEV_1 measurement in asthmatics, and this probably is valid for COPD patients as well. Important aspects of the physical examination to be monitored include ratio of inspiration to expiration, respiratory rate, heart rate, jugular venous pressure, right ventricular impulse, and extremities (for edema). In patients with known CO_2 retention it is worth testing for asterixis, an indication of worsening ventilatory status with further carbon dioxide retention and encephalopathy. Serial determination of arterial blood gases, FEV_1, and FVC can help in objectively following the course of disease and detecting acute deteriorations.

INDICATIONS FOR ADMISSION AND REFERRAL

The patient who develops acute asterixis should be promptly admitted to the hospital; no oxygen should be administered on the way to the hospital for fear of further suppressing the respiratory drive. The same holds for the lethargic patient. Patients with refractory bronchospasm, severe cor pulmonale, or acute pneumonitis also require inpatient management. Consultation with a specialist in pulmonary medicine is indicated when considering chronic use systemic steroids for refractory bronchospasm, long-term continuous oxygen therapy for chronic hypoxemia, and inotropic agents for cor pulmonale.

PATIENT EDUCATION

The first priority is to stress the importance of cessation of smoking; this should be followed by design of specific program (see Chapter 49). Patients should be encouraged to maintain as much activity as possible and be provided with an exercise program if they can be motivated to comply. Patient, family, and physician should be involved in setting reasonable and realistic activity goals. Advice regarding adequate hydration and pulmonary toilet is basic to the care of chronic bronchitis patients. Patients likely to panic and hyperventilate when they become dyspneic often benefit from being taught slow, relaxed, deep breathing to institute in such circumstances.

Careful instructions regarding the indications and adverse effects of therapy can help the patient to carry out the prescribed program properly. Complex regimens should be written down and reviewed with both patient and family. It is essential to warn patients with CO_2 retention against unauthorized use of tranquilizers and sedatives, because of the risk of further suppressing their respiratory drive. Patients using inhalers should receive thorough instruction on their proper use (see Chapter 45); many treatment failures are due to poor technique. Such patients also require warning that excessive use of beta$_2$ agonists can lead to tachyphylaxis and cardiac side-effects; persistent overdoses of inhaled steroids (more than 20 puffs per day) can cause adrenal suppression.

Part of the patient education process should include instruction on self-monitoring and reporting of functional status. The involvement of the patient and the interest and concern of the physician have a considerable effect on the progress made by the COPD patient.

THERAPEUTIC RECOMMENDATIONS

- Insist on cessation of smoking and design a program for the patient (see Chapter 49).

- Advise the patient to reduce exposure to environmental irritants and known allergens and to maintain adequate humidity and hydration.

- Design, with patient participation, an exercise program; walking is probably the best exercise to utilize, though any aerobic exercise will suffice. Begin with an easily achieved level of activity (*e.g.,* half-maximal pace) and increase slowly in small increments. Frequency is 3 to 4 times daily, with duration ranging from 5 to 15 minutes.

- Administer trivalent influenza vaccine (0.5 ml IM) in the fall of each year to all COPD patients (except those having a known allergy to eggs) and at least 6 weeks before the usual winter onset of the flu season. Consider administering amantadine to unvaccinated COPD patients during an influenza epidemic.

- Administer pneumococcal vaccine to all COPD patients; dose is 0.5 ml IM and need be given only once; it can be given at the same time as the influenza vaccine.

- Advise patients bothered by heavy sputum production to keep well hydrated and to humidify the indoor environment (particularly those living in centrally heated homes). Nebulized detergents and oral expectorants are of no proven benefit. Teach postural drainage techniques to patients bothered by difficulty in raising sputum; teach slow, relaxed, deep breathing to patients likely to hyperventilate when dyspneic; a respiratory therapist may be of help in the teaching effort.

- For patients who have obvious bronchospasm or dyspnea on exertion and a substantial reduction in expiratory flow rate (*e.g.,* FEV_1 <1.5 to 2 liters per second or FEV_1/FVC <0.50), begin a trial of bronchodilator therapy. Start with an inhaled beta$_2$ adrenergic agent such as albuterol, metaproterenol, or terbutaline. Dose is two puffs from a measured-release, hand-held nebulizer q 6 h. Judge response on the basis of change in exercise tolerance and expiratory flow rates after about 1 week of therapy. Response to a single dose of inhaled bronchodilator does not predict response to continuous treatment. Be sure patient is instructed in and demonstrates proper inhaler technique. Warn about dangers from overuse of adrenergic agents.

- There is no evidence that delivery of inhaled bronchodilators by an intermittent positive-pressure breathing (IPPB) apparatus provides any benefit. The use of such expensive therapy is not recommended.

- If more bronchodilation is required, add an oral theophylline preparation, such as aminophylline 200 mg qid. Again, monitor for response after about 1 week of therapy before deciding to continue therapy indefinitely. If benefit is demonstrated, switch to a sustained-release theophylline preparation (*e.g.,* Theo-Dur or Slo-Phyllin) at a dose of 200 to 300 mg q 12 h. Check serum theophylline level (therapeutic range 10 to 20 $\mu g/ml$) to ensure proper dose.

- Patients in need of further bronchodilation can be given a trial of a poorly absorbed, inhaled corticosteroid such as beclomethasone or flunisolide, delivered by metered nebulizer. Dose is two puffs qid. Reserve systemic corticosteroids for refractory cases; hospitalization and consultation may be indicated.

- Initiate antibiotic therapy for patients with clinical infection (fever, purulent sputum, signs of consolidation). Initial drug of choice for outpatient therapy is amoxicillin 500 mg tid or ampicillin 500 mg qid. Tetracycline 500 mg qid and trimethoprim-sulfa double strength, one tablet bid, are alternatives for penicillin-allergic patients, especially if *H. influenzae* is the predominant organism.
- There is a controversy regarding the efficacy of antibiotic therapy for acute exacerbations of chronic bronchitis in the absence of obvious signs of infection. Most recent research has failed to detect significant benefit.
- For patients with cor pulmonale, begin a diuretic program (*e.g.,* furosemide 20 mg per day) when peripheral edema begins to occur; increase program as needed to control fluid accumulation caused by systemic venous hypertension. Phlebotomize the patient with secondary erythrocytosis when the hematocrit reaches the 55 to 60 range.
- Consider continuous low-flow oxygen therapy for patients with a PO_2 less than 60 mm Hg, particularly if PO_2 is in the 50 to 55 mm Hg range. Such patients are often beginning to manifest signs of cor pulmonale or require frequent phlebotomies to keep their hematocrit below 55.
- Consider a short-term trial of digitalis therapy in patients with severe right heart failure; treat for 2 weeks and check for objective signs of improvement (*e.g.,* decreased edema, lower jugular venous pressure, reduced heart size). Monitor carefully for evidence of digitalis toxicity (see Chapter 27).
- Review entire treatment program thoroughly with patient and family; encourage patient participation in setting goals and monitoring functional status.

A.H.G.

ANNOTATED BIBLIOGRAPHY

Anthonisen NR: Long-term oxygen therapy. Ann Intern Med 99: 519, 1983 (*A fine review of the recent evidence suggesting improvement in survival with chronic oxygen treatment: 60 references.*)

Anthonisen NR, Wright EC: IPPB trial group: Bronchodilator response in chronic obstructive pulmonary disease. Am Rev Respir Dis 133:814, 1986 (*The authors demonstrated that at some time or other, patients with COPD do manifest some bronchodilator responsiveness.*)

Anthonisen NR, Wright EC, Hodgkin JE: IPPB Trial Group: prognosis in chronic obstructive disease. Am Rev Respir Dis 133:14, 1986 (*Patient age and initial FEV_1 were the greatest determinants of mortality. Of the 985 patients with COPD but without hypoxemia, mortality was 23% in the 3 years of follow up.*)

Aubier M, DeTroyer A, Sampson M et al: Aminophylline improves diaphragmatic contractility. N Engl J Med 305:249, 1981 (*A finding that may justify a trial of aminophylline despite documented poor bronchodilator effect.*)

Baker JP: Intermittent positive pressure breathing or compressor nebulizer therapy. Ann Intern Med 99:715, 1983 (*Critically reviews the results of a multicenter study and agrees with the conclusion that IPPB therapy is without significant merit.*)

Bates JH: The role of infection during exacerbations of chronic bronchitis. Ann Intern Med 97:130, 1982 (*A summary of the controversy and some thoughts about why the issue remains unresolved.*)

Bolan G, Broome CV, Facklam RR et al: Pneumococcal vaccine in selected populations in the United States. Ann Intern Med 104: 1, 1986 (*Provides evidence for use in patients with COPD.*)

Eaton ML, Green BA, Church TR et al: Efficacy of theophylline in "irreversible" airflow obstruction. Ann Intern Med 92:758, 1980 (*A carefully documented study showing significant, dose-related improvement in ventilatory parameters; however, subjective response was less impressive.*)

Goldstein RS, Vivekanand R, Bowes G et al: Effect of supplemental nocturnal oxygen of gas exchange in patients with severe obstructive lung disease. New Engl J Med 310:425, 1984 (*Nocturnal oxygen therapy did not induce clinically important increases in PCO_2 during sleep in COPD patients with resting hypoxia and hypercarbia; argues for safety of continuous oxygen therapy in patients with CO_2 retention.*)

Green LH, Smith TW: Use of digitalis in patients with pulmonary disease. Ann Intern Med 87:459, 1977 (*Digitalis is of questionable benefit, and risk of toxicity is increased.*)

Gross NJ, Skorodin MS: Role of the parasympathetic system in airway obstruction due to emphysema. N Engl J Med 311:421, 1984 (*The inhaled anticholinergic agent atropine methonitrate was as effective as the $beta_2$ agonist salbutamol in achieving bronchodilation; data argues for a final common pathway in the reversible component of bronchospasm seen in emphysema and for a new direction in bronchodilator therapy.*)

Intermittent Positive Pressure Breathing Trial Group: Intermittent positive pressure breathing therapy of COPD: A clinical trial. Ann Intern Med 99:612, 1983 (*A multicenter controlled trial of 985 patients showing that IPPB was no better than nebulizer for administration of bronchodilator therapy.*)

Kanner RE, Renzetti AD, Stanish WM et al: Predictors of survival in subjects with chronic airflow limitation. Am J Med 74:249, 1983 (*A 12-year prospective study identifying important determinants of prognosis and confirming findings of earlier studies.*)

Kawakami Y, Kishi F, Yamamoto H et al: Relation of oxygen delivery, mixed venous oxygenation, and pulmonary hemodynamics to prognosis in chronic obstructive pulmonary disease. N Engl J Med 308:1045, 1983 (*A prospective study including right heart catheterization and follow-up 4 years later; found that mixed venous oxygen level was an important prognostic indicator; pulmonary and right ventricular hemodynamic measurements were not.*)

Lertzman MM, Cherniack RM: Rehabilitation of patients with chronic obstructive pulmonary disease. Am Rev Respir Dis 114: 1145, 1976 (*A superb review of therapeutic modalities in the management of chronic obstructive pulmonary disease.*)

Mahlerd A, Matthay RA, Snyder PE et al: Sustained-release theophylline reduces dyspnea in nonreversible obstructive airway disease.

Am Rev Resp Dis 131:22, 1985 (*A clinical trial in 12 ambulatory male patients with moderate to severe airway obstruction showed significant subjective improvement in symptoms.*)

Mendella LA, Manfreda J, Warren CPW et al: Steroid response in stable chronic obstructive pulmonary disease. Ann Intern Med 96:17, 1982 (*Six of forty-six patients with stable COPD had a clinically significant response to steroid therapy; there were no evident clinical predictors for steroid response.*)

Nicotra MB, Rivera M, Awe RJ: Antibiotic therapy of acute exacerbations of chronic bronchitis: A controlled study using tetracycline. Ann Intern Med 97:18, 1982 (*A double-blind, randomized, placebo-controlled trial in 40 moderately ill COPD patients; found no difference between patients on tetracycline and those taking placebo.*)

Owens GR, Rogers RM, Pennock BE et al: The diffusing capacity as a predictor of arterial oxygen desaturation during exercise in patients with COPD. N Engl J Med 310:1218, 1984 (*Diffusing capacity measured during routine pulmonary function testing at rest correlated well with degree of hypoxemia during exercise in patients with COPD; might prove a simple way to determine who would benefit from oxygen supplementation during exercise.*)

Pierson DJ: When to hospitalize the COPD patient. Chest, 73:126, 1978 (*Little objective evidence exists to help make this decision, but this well-conceived editorial provides intelligent guidance on treating people without hospitalization.*)

Sackner MA: Diaphragmatic breathing exercises. JAMA 231:295, 1975 (*A guide to applying this adjunctive therapy.*)

Sahn, SA: Corticosteroids in chronic bronchitis and pulmonary emphysema. Chest 73:389, 1978 (*A review of 17 published studies on the use of steroids concluding that benefit is restricted to individual patients; considers objectively monitored trials only.*)

Schwartz JS, Bencowitz HZ, Moser KM: Air travel hypoxemia with chronic obstructive pulmonary disease. Ann Intern Med 199:473, 1984 (*Measurement of arterial PO_2 on room air within 2 hours of flight or on breathing a hypoxic [17.2%] oxygen mixture for 15 minutes can be used to reliably preduct arterial PO_2 that will occur on flying in a commercial jet aircraft. Such testing can be used to determine who will need supplemental oxygen during flight. Accompanying editorial on p. 595 gives good summary of preflight medical evaluation.*)

Shim CS, Williams MH: Bronchodilator response to oral aminophyllline and terbutaline versus aerosol albuterol in patients with COPD. Am J Med 75:697, 1983 (*A randomized, double-blind crossover study indicating that the aerosol route is superior to the oral one for administration of bronchodilators in COPD.*)

Shim CS, Williams MH: Aerosol beclomethasone in patients with steroid-responsive COPD. Am J Med 78:655, 1985 (*A double-blind, randomized crossover trial comparing oral prednisone with inhaled beclomethasone. The beclomethasone did not prove to be an adequate substitute for oral corticosteroid therapy.*)

Sunderrajan EV, Byron WA, McKenzie WN et al: The effect of terbutaline on cardiac function in patients with stable chronic obstructive lung disease. JAMA 250:2151, 1983 (*Even small doses of terbutaline significantly increased right and left ventricular ejection fraction in patients with severe COPD.*)

Weitzenblum E, Sautegeau A, Ehrhart M et al: Long term oxygen therapy can reverse a progression of pulmonary hypertension in patients with chronic obstructive pulmonary disease. Am Rev Respir Dis 131:493, 1985 (*Sixteen patients with severe chronic obstructive pulmonary disease were treated with long-term oxygen therapy 15–18 hours a day, showing reversal of the progression of pulmonary hypertension in 12 of 16, but normalization was rarely observed.*)

45
Management of Asthma

Asthma is predominantly an outpatient condition, affecting about 2.5% of the population. It is characterized by airway hyperreactivity and sustained but reversible bronchial obstruction. Although there are no cures for asthma, effective means of control are available and include beta$_2$ adrenergic agents, theophylline, corticosteroids (both topical and systemic), and cromolyn. The primary physician needs to be skilled in the use of these agents and able to design a practical program that will minimize the frequency and severity of attacks. Many emergency room visits for treatment of asthma are avoidable.

PATHOPHYSIOLOGY, CLINICAL PRESENTATION, AND COURSE

The pathogenesis of asthma remains incompletely understood. The principal disturbances of pulmonary function are rapid development and persistence of reversible airway obstruction in response to stimuli that fail to affect normal persons. Among known *stimuli* are allergens, exercise, emotional stress, viral respiratory infection, and respiratory irritants. Both biochemical and neurogenic mechanisms have been postulated to account for the sustained but reversible bronchospasm that characterizes an acute asthmatic attack. Many of the substances likely to be involved in the genesis of bronchoconstriction, edema, and mucus production have been identified; however, precise roles and interrelationships remain to be elucidated. The list of *mediators* includes prostaglandin D$_2$, leukotrienes (slow-reacting substance of anaphylaxis), eosinophilic chemotactic factor, and histamine.

Allergen-induced asthma involves *immunologically triggered release* of bronchoconstricting substances from sensitized pulmonary mast cells. Sensitization occurs when IgE attaches to these cells and combines with the allergen, setting in motion a complex set of intracellular biochemical events that ends with degranulation of mast cells and release of biochemical mediators. An important component of this process is a fall in intracellular levels of cyclic AMP, which facilitates the degranulation process.

Elements of a *neurogenic pathway* have also been elucidated. Bronchial smooth muscle is responsive to autonomic influences; it is unsettled whether the effect is direct or via biochemical mediators. Vagal stimulation and cholinergic drugs cause bronchial constriction; beta-adrenergic stimulation appears capable of countering the cholinergic influences, either directly or by increasing adenyl cyclase activity, which raises intracellular cyclic AMP and blocks mediator release from mast cells. Bronchial irritants and emotional stress are thought to precipitate bronchospasm by way of triggering vagal reflexes.

In addition to the initial mediator-induced bronchospasm, many patients experience a second reaction occuring 6 to 12 hours later. This *late asthmatic reaction* is often more severe and less amenable to treatment than the initial one. Increases in neutrophil chemotactic factor correlate in time with the late reaction, suggesting a mast cell-mediated mechanism. Many patients with exercise-induced asthma also have late reactions with increases in neutrophil chemotactic factor.

Clinical Presentation. Be the pathway biochemical, neurogenic, or mixed, the net effect is bronchial edema, smooth muscle contraction, and excessive mucus production. Clinical manifestations include wheezing, dyspnea, cough, and sputum. Presentations range from pure bronchospasm with little cough and sputum, to a predominance of bronchorrhea and coughing that mimics bronchitis or an upper respiratory tract infection. In fact, cough and sputum production may be the initial symptoms of an asthmatic attack.

Cases are sometimes classified as "extrinsic" (triggered by a known allergen and often associated with elevated levels of IgE) or "intrinsic" (adult onset, no specific allergen evident). Patients with *extrinsic asthma* typically give a history of atopy and onset of symptoms during childhood or adolescence; however, the condition can occur at any age. Attacks may take place seasonally or year-round, precipitated by such common household allergens as the house-dust mite, animal dander, and fungal spores. IgE mediates the immediate reaction. Anxiety, inhalation of airway irritants, and exposure to perfumes and strong household odors can also precipitate asthmatic episodes in these patients. The course of attacks is usually self-limited, though some patients have severe bouts requiring hospitalization. Prognosis is relatively good, with 70% found to be symptom-free 20 years after onset.

Patients with *intrinsic asthma* usually begin having symptoms in the third or fourth decade. No identifiable allergen precipitates attacks in these patients. There can be much sputum production, sometimes making differentiation from chronic bronchitis difficult. Minor upper respiratory tract infections often precipitate attacks. Some patients present with exertional dyspnea or cough and no demonstrable wheezing, though expiratory flow rates are clearly reduced. Patients with intrinsic asthma are sometimes more refractory to treatment than those with extrinsic disease.

Other important clinical presentations include postexertional asthma, occupational asthma, and asthma associated with nasal polyps and aspirin sensitivity. *Postexertional asthma* is a form of airway hyperreactivity most common in children and adolescents. The stimulus is a reduction in the temperature of inhaled air, leading to mediator release in susceptible patients. Both initial and late phase reactions have been identified. Vigorous exercise on a cold dry day is particularly apt to trigger an attack; airway temperature can get quite low in such circumstances.

Occupational asthma has gained increasing recognition as an important cause of work-related disability. Exposure to irritant or toxic pollutants in the workplace and inhalation of allergens are the main sources of difficulty. Cold air, low concentrations of sulfur dioxide, fluorocarbons, and inert dusts are common irritants that stimulate reflex bronchospasm. Toxic gases such as high concentrations of sulfur dioxide, halogens, ammonia, acid fumes, and solvent vapors cause inflammatory bronchoconstriction. Important allergens include animal proteins, enzymes, grain and cereal dusts, seeds, vegetable gums, and legumes. Other substances have pharmacologic activity; there are histamine-releasing compounds in cotton dust, organic acids in wood dust, and numerous chemicals with anticholinesterase activity. Some agents provoke asthma through multiple mechanisms; toluene diisocyanate (TDI) has reflex, pharmacologic, betablocking, and IgE effects.

Patients with occupational asthma due to toxic or irritant substances characteristically report a direct relation between exposure and onset of symptoms. Those with allergen-induced disease note no symptoms at time of first exposure followed by occurrence of marked wheezing upon even minor repeat contact with the allergen (anamnestic response). Typically, patients with occupational asthma are symptom-free during days off from work, only to have a flare-up on returning.

The association between *nasal polyps and aspirin sensitivity* is a curious but important familial one. The bronchospasm may be marked.

Clinical Course. Regardless of the type of asthma, subclinical but significant bronchospasm remains for days to weeks after the wheezing of an acute attack subsides. The continuing obstruction is believed to represent residual small airway bronchoconstriction that resolves more slowly than large airway bronchospasm. The clinical recurrences that often develop shortly after the apparent resolution of an acute attack are most often not new episodes but relapses. No single clinical or laboratory parameter reliably predicts relapse (see below).

The long-term consequences of asthma are few. There is no evidence that it leads to such permanent pulmonary parenchymal damage as development of chronic bronchitis or emphysema. Overall mortality for all forms of asthma is 0.1% per year; the rate increases markedly to 3.3% for patients with episodes of status asthmaticus.

PRINCIPLES OF MANAGEMENT

The goals of therapy are to prevent attacks and control those that do occur. Before initiating therapy, it is important to verify that the patient's wheezing is not due to a nonasthmatic cause of bronchospasm, such as pulmonary edema, embolization, foreign body, or infection (see Chapters 27, 36, and 37).

Management of Acute Attacks and Chronic Active Disease

Most patients with acute asthmatic attacks can be managed on an outpatient basis, provided that proper therapy is promptly and fully instituted. The vast majority of patients seeking emergency room care do not need parenteral therapy. In a prospective study of 140 asthmatic patients who came for emergency room care, most presented because they either had no available medication, underutilized or improperly administered their medication, relied on over-the-counter preparations, or used fixed combination tablets or suppository forms that did not permit proper dosing. The asthmatic patient should be thoroughly instructed to initiate a full bronchodilator program at the first sign of a flare-up, and to report quickly to the primary physician if treatment does not seem to be working. Initiation of bronchodilator therapy at home can begin with a theophylline or beta-adrenergic preparation. Some patients with severe disease are likely to be on maintenance therapy at the time of an attack and require an increase in dose or addition of other agents.

Theophylline and its derivatives have been a mainstay of asthma therapy for decades, although it was not until 1974 that double-blind placebo-controlled crossover study definitively established that theophylline produces a significant decrease in the symptoms and signs of asthma. Success depended upon using higher doses than were previously utilized. Mechanism of action involves inhibition of phosphodiesterase, an enzyme important in the metabolism of cyclic AMP; recent data suggest that antagonism of adenosine may also be important. Theophylline is effective and relatively inexpensive; its major disadvantage is its narrow therapeutic range (10 to 20 mcg/ml). Below 10 μg/ml, bronchodilation falls off considerably.

ADVERSE EFFECTS. The serious adverse effects are clearly related to serum level. Serum levels in excess of 20 μg/ml are associated with a greatly increased risk of adverse side-effects. Conversely, when serum levels remain within therapeutic range, risk is minimized. For example, there has been concern about theophylline use in patients with *ventricular irritability*. Most studies have largely dispelled this view, finding that when serum levels remain in the therapeutic range, there is no significant increase in frequency or severity of ventricular ectopy. However, if levels exceed 35 μg/ml, life-threatening arrhythmias can occur. *Seizures* refractory to standard anticonvulsant therapy have occurred without warning when serum levels go above 40 μg/ml.

The minor gastrointestinal and neurologic side-effects are largely dose-related, but occur in some patients at normal or even subtherapeutic serum levels. *Nausea, vomiting, reflux, and diarrhea* are the common minor gastrointestinal effects. It was erroneously thought that the oral route of theophylline administration was responsible for the gastrointestinal upset; this theory lead to the use of subtherapeutic oral doses and manufacture of rectal suppository preparations. Suppositories should not be used; they have very erratic rates of drug release and absorption; serum levels are unpredictable. Common minor neurologic side-effects include *agitation, tremor, and insomnia*.

PHARMACOKINETICS. Oral theophylline is rapidly and thoroughly absorbed; onset of effect from an oral dose can be as early as 15 minutes with use of liquid hydroalcoholic preparations; by 1 to 2 hours almost 90% is absorbed. Half-life averages 6 hours but can range from 4 to 8 hours; there is much individual variation due to differences in clearance rates.

Rapidly absorbed theophylline preparations produce wide swings in serum levels; slow-release formulations give more stable serum concentrations and need be administered only every 8 to 12 hours. Clearance is achieved by hepatic biotransformation; only small amounts are excreted unchanged. Anything that alters hepatic microsomal activity will affect theophylline clearance. Clearance slows with liver disease, congestive heart failure, old age, infection, macrolide antibiotics (*e.g.,* erythromycin), cimetidine, high-dose allopurinol (600 mg/day), oral contraceptives, caffeine, and perhaps influenza vaccination; half-life may extend to as much as 8 hours in such circumstances. Clearance increases with smoking, eating of charcoal-broiled foods, phenytoin, and phenobarbital; half-life may shorten to 4 hours under such conditions.

PREPARATIONS. Liquid theophylline preparations (*i.e., elixir of theophylline*) contain alcohol, which is believed to speed absorption; although rapidly acting (onset within 15 minutes), it is more expensive, shorter in duration of action, and gives more erratic serum levels than other preparations. Its optimal use may be in oral treatment of acute exacerbations (see below). *Aminophylline* is a salt of theophylline, converted to the parent compound in vivo. It is the least expensive plain-tablet theophylline preparation and a mainstay of oral therapy for patients with slow clearance of the drug. Although usually given every 6 hours, it may be needed only every 8 hours in patients with prolonged clearance. As noted earlier, *aminophylline suppositories* are not recommended for use because of erratic absorption and unpredictable serum levels.

The *slow-release forms* of theophylline provide stable therapeutic serum concentrations with only 2 to 3 doses per day. Although many of the initial slow-release preparations were very erratic in performance, most have now been improved and certified by the Food and Drug Administration to produce therapeutic steady-state serum concentrations when given at the recommended doses and intervals. Patients who rapidly clear theophylline (*e.g.*, smokers) may require therapy every 8 hours with a slow-release preparation; patients who clear theophylline slowly may not need a slow-release formulation at all. On a cost-effectiveness basis, slow-release therapy is superior to use of plain tablets for most patients. The reliability of sustained-release forms, which need to be taken only once daily, remains unconfirmed. *Combination preparations* are to be avoided. They are expensive, often contain irrationally chosen ingredients (*e.g.*, barbiturates, useless expectorants), and do not permit adjustment of theophylline dose without increasing the intake of the other components that result in adverse side-effects (see below).

USE. Because of its narrow therapeutic range, theophylline is considered by some to be the drug of second choice for asthma, after the beta-adrenergic agents. Nevertheless, it occupies a central role in the treatment programs of many asthmatics. Use of theophylline in conjunction with a beta agonist for chronic asthma allows for enhanced bronchodilation at reduced doses of each and with fewer adverse side-effects. There is debate regarding efficacy of combined therapy in severe acute attacks. In the absence of an acute attack, initiation of outpatient theophylline therapy is best carried out gradually over the course of 1 week. A gradual approach helps to minimize adverse effects and achieve a therapeutic serum level safely. One starts with a total dose of 400 mg per day (using either plain or slow-release theophylline); after 3 days the dose is increased by 200 mg/day; 3 days later it is increased again by another 200 mg/day. Serum theophylline level is then checked 4 to 6 hours after the last dose, provided no dose has been missed for 3 days. Adjustment in dose is made according to serum level, which should fall in the 10 to 20 μg/ml range. Once a therapeutic level is attained, serum concentration need not be checked for several months, provided the patient's clinical situation, smoking status, and drug use do not change. Patients with levels that are too low are probably rapid metabolizers of the drug and should have their dose interval shortened. Obese patients need not be given extra high doses; area of drug distribution does not increase proportionally.

Adrenergic Agents. Catecholamines with beta activity and the selective noncatecholamine beta$_2$ agonists are potent bronchodilators, believed to act by increasing adenyl cyclase activity and production of cyclic AMP. There is a wide variety of adrenergic agents used for asthma, ranging from the very rapidly acting, short duration, nonselective isoproterenol to the long-acting, selective, beta$_2$ agonists. The advent of the selective beta$_2$ agonists provides bronchodilation that is rapid in onset, sustained, and relatively free of extrapulmonary side effects.

ISOPROTERENOL is the archtype catecholamine with predominantly beta-stimulating activity, used for decades by asthmatics to obtain rapid symptomatic relief of bronchospasm. Its major drawback is lack of selectivity, stimulating both bronchial (beta$_2$) and cardiac (beta$_1$) adrenergic receptors. The result is effective bronchodilation, but not without tachycardia and, in patients with underlying heart disease, risk of dysrhythmias and angina. Isoproterenol is ineffective by mouth because of gastric inactivation; consequently, it is available only in aerosol form for use in asthma. Tachyphylaxis develops with excessive use. Onset of action is within seconds; duration, less than 2 hours.

EPINEPHRINE is another time-honored catecholamine for treatment of asthma, especially severe acute attacks not halted by oral or inhaled medication. Its onset of action is rapid (within 1 to 2 minutes of subcutaneous injection); duration is short (about 30 minutes). Epinephrine stimulates alpha-adrenergic as well as beta-adrenergic receptors; the resulting vasoconstriction relieves mucosal edema and congestion but also raises blood pressure. The use of epinephrine in patients with coronary disease can trigger angina and arrhythmias.

SELECTIVE BETA$_2$ AGONISTS are the drug class of choice for initial therapy of asthma because of their relative selectivity for bronchial beta receptors, rapid onset (2 to 5 minutes) and prolonged duration of action (up to 6 hours) when taken by the aerosol route, and paucity of systemic side-effects. *Albuterol* (Proventil; Ventolin), *metaproterenol* (Alupent; Metaprel), *bitolterol* (Tornalate), and *terbutaline* (Brethine; Bricanyl) are the major drugs in this class for use in asthma. Most are available in both oral and inhaled forms; terbutaline can also be given as a subcutaneous injection for treatment of an acute attack. Bitolterol has a slightly longer duration of action than the other inhaled agents.

All beta$_2$ agents cause some *cardiotonic effects* when used in high doses. *Tremor* is common, particularly at the onset of oral therapy; it may be sufficiently disabling to cause termination of therapy, though it usually diminishes over time. Tremor has been particularly troublesome in patients taking terbutaline, though it has also been noted with metaproterenol use. Significant tachyphylaxis, manifested as failure to respond to parenteral epinephrine, has not been noted. Choice of a particular agent in this class is somewhat arbitrary, because all are quite similar in cost, action, and side-effects; a combination of patient preference, trial and error, and relative cost usually determine selection for long-term use.

ISOETHRANE (Bronkosol; Bronkometer) is a bronchoselective catecholamine that has been widely used for years, particularly as part of intermittent positive-pressure breathing (IPPB) therapy. It also comes in hand-held nebulizer form. Because it has a short duration of action and a potential for tachyphylaxis, its role has been supplanted by the newer non-catecholamine beta$_2$ agonists. Moreover, the efficacy of IPPB therapy has been called into serious question (see Chapter 44).

EPHEDRINE is an older noncatecholamine drug with nonselective beta-adrenergic effects that has been largely replaced by the newer beta$_2$ agonists. It is still available in irrational fixed-combination preparations (*e.g.,* Tedral; Marax). Its cardiac side-effects, short duration of action, and availability mostly in fixed-combination preparations argue against its continued use.

Corticosteroids. Oral and parenteral glucocorticoids (*e.g.,* prednisone, methylprednisolone, hydrocortisone) are reserved for patients with refractory bronchospasm. Their mechanism of action in asthma is not precisely known; the 6 to 8 hour delay noted between time of parenteral administration and onset of effect suggests that protein synthesis is required. Although highly effective, systemic glucocorticoids should not be used on a long-term basis if control can be achieved by other means; the side-effects of continued use are too destructive (osteoporotic fractures, adrenal suppression, skin changes, aseptic necrosis of bone, aggravation of diabetes mellitus; (see Chapter 103).

In an effort to achieve the advantages of chronic steroid therapy without the side-effects, *topical steroid aerosol preparations* have been developed. *Beclomethasone dipropionate* (Vanceril; Beclovent) is the best studied preparation; others include *flunisolide* (Aerobid) and *triamcinolone acetonide* (Azmacort). All are topically active, poorly soluble in water, and with little systemic effect at therapeutic doses.

PREDNISONE is the prototype oral glucocorticosteroid. Half-life is 12 to 24 hours. Administration of as little as 15 mg per day beyond 2 weeks will begin to suppress the adrenal–pituitary axis (see Chapter 103). It is optimal for short-term use to control an acute attack that is refractory to all other measures. A short course (*e.g.,* 7 to 10 days) administered on a rapidly tapering schedule is often very effective and will not result in adrenal suppression. A placebo-controlled, double-blind, randomized study of such prednisone use demonstrated that the group treated with steroids had significantly fewer symptoms and a lower rate of relapse.

Only those patients with chronic disabling bronchospasm refractory to all other forms of therapy should be considered for long-term, daily systemic steroid treatment. In most instances, use of a topical aerosol preparation in conjunction with theophylline and beta agonists will suffice, with short courses of high-dose systemic therapy reserved for severe exacerbations.

Cholinergic Blocking Agents. Atropine has been used to block the cholinergic pathway of mediator release. It is ad-

ministered in aerosol form to minimize systemic side-effects. The drug inhibits mucociliary function and is reserved for patients who have failed other forms of therapy, although some patients respond quite well to it.

Choice of Therapy

At present, the selective beta$_2$ adrenergic agents are the drug class of choice for patients with mild intermittent asthma. *Aerosol beta$_2$ therapy* is convenient, rapid in onset, prolonged in duration of action, and associated with a minimum of extrapulmonary side-effects. Its major shortcomings are limited effect on small airways when given as an aerosol and inability to reach areas of intense bronchospasm and mucus plugging. If ineffective, switching to an *oral beta agonist* preparation or adding *oral theophylline* is indicated.

When faced with a severe acute episode, *subcutaneous epinephrine* or *terbutaline* will terminate many attacks. Some suggest that *elixir of theophylline* can be used at home with similar efficacy and rapidity of onset, obviating the need for an office or emergency room visit. Patients totally unresponsive to nonsteroidal therapy require prompt admission to the hospital for parenteral therapy. Those with stubborn bronchospasm that lessens but does not fully resolve with nonsteroidal therapy may achieve control from a short, rapidly tapering course of *oral corticosteroids.*

Prophylaxis

Once an acute attack subsides, the goal of management shifts to prevention of future episodes. Identification of the responsible allergen is sometimes helpful, especially in industrial settings and in patients with extrinsic asthma, but in most instances extensive skin testing reveals a large number of allergens to which the patient is sensitive. Consequently, *desensitization treatment* is ineffective in most situations. Even in cases where a single known allergen has been identified, controlled studies have failed to demonstrate the efficacy of desensitization injections. Avoidance of the offending agent is good therapy where practical (*e.g.,* in industrial situations or when air pollution is heavy); unfortunately, this is not always feasible, and other methods of prophylaxis have to be used.

The inadequacies of immunotherapy and avoidance are not critical in view of the availability of effective pharmacologic agents for prophylaxis. It is felt that a daily *maintenance bronchodilator program* can help curb the frequency and severity of attacks. Beta agonists and theophylline are commonly used. Long-term controlled studies demonstrating the superiority of continuous therapy over intermittent use are lacking, but most authorities recommend a maintenance program when attacks have been frequent and severe. Cromolyn sodium, beclomethasone, and prednisone have been reserved for more refractory cases.

Cromolyn sodium is a unique and important prophylactic

agent that works by preventing degranulation of mast cells. It is most effective for prevention of episodes in children and those with exercise-induced bronchospasm. Because the drug possesses no direct bronchodilating or anti-inflammatory action, it plays no role in treating established asthmatic attacks. For children, adolescents, and those with exercise-induced asthma, cromolyn may precede use of other drugs. If such patients are already on maintenance bronchodilators and not adequately controlled, then adding cromolyn to the program may be beneficial. The drug is less likely to work in adults than it is in children, but should be considered before a patient is committed to more toxic therapy, such as long-term systemic prednisone. A 4- to 8-week trial is needed to assess efficacy.

Cromolyn is given as an inhaled powder; each dose comes packaged in a capsule that is inserted into an inhaler before use. The dose schedule for patients without exertional asthma is one capsule qid. For prophylaxis of exercise-induced asthma, the patient inhales the powder before engaging in exercise. Unfortunately, some patients experience a hypersensitivity reaction to the powder, thus limiting its general usefulness. Adverse effects are uncommon but include bronchospasm, cough, and irritation of the upper airway. Patients with exercise-induced asthma who cannot tolerate cromolyn can take a few inhalations of a *beta-adrenergic aerosol* before engaging in activity.

Patients who do not achieve adequate control from use of bronchodilators or cromolyn are candidates for a trial of *topical steroid therapy* (beclomethasone, flunisolide, triamcinolone). *Systemic steroids* are reserved for prevention of attacks in patients with a history of life-threatening asthma or recurrent disabling attacks that cannot be controlled by any other means.

Beclomethasone dipropionate is the best studied topical aerosol steroid preparation prescribed for treatment of asthma. Numerous controlled trials have demonstrated its efficacy in reducing the frequency and severity of attacks as well as making possible a reduction or discontinuation in systemic corticosteroid therapy. Benefit is achieved without clinically significant adrenal suppression or systemic steroid side-effects as long as the daily dose is less than 1 mg/day (approximately 20 inhalations/day). Onset of action is within 2 to 8 hours, but when therapy is begun, 24 to 48 hours may pass before symptomatic improvement is noted. Response is dose related and lasts about 6 to 8 hours.

Beclomethasone has dramatically reduced the number of patients requiring long-term systemic steroid therapy for control of asthma. In a study of 371 such patients followed for 1 year, 78% were well controlled without oral steroids or with only short-term prednisone therapy. In addition, beclomethasone appears to be superior to alternate-day prednisone, although cost and dose frequency are greater.

The most serious danger with topical steroid treatment is *adrenal insufficiency* at the time of switching from systemic

to nonabsorbable therapy. Patients previously maintained on long-term systemic corticosteroids have gone into shock and died when switched abruptly to topical therapy. Patients on long-term prednisone therapy in adrenally suppressive doses must be tapered slowly over several months when discontinuing systemic therapy (see Chapter 103). During periods of stress and flare-ups of asthma, topical therapy should be supplemented with large doses of systemic steroids; adrenal responsiveness may still be submaximal; moreover, topical medication may not penetrate obstructed airways where it is needed most.

The most frequent complication is mild *oropharyngeal candidiasis;* it responds well to nystatin mouthwash or clotrimazole troches and can be prevented by rinsing the mouth and pharynx with water after each dose. Some patients complain of hoarseness or throat irritation after inhaling beclomethasone; slight reduction in dose usually suffices. Some patients find that inhalation of beclomethasone triggers bronchospasm; use of an adrenergic agent beforehand will prevent it. As with any inhaler, proper technique is essential to obtaining a good therapeutic response (see below).

Although *adrenal–pituitary suppression* has been reported with long-term use of very high doses, this is a very uncommon complication, especially when daily dose is kept well below 1 mg/24 h (<20 inhalations/day). Physical changes of hyperadrenocorticism have never been reported with topical therapy.

Antibiotics have a very limited role in prophylaxis. Although viral upper respiratory infections frequently precipitate attacks (making *influenza vaccine* a must; see Chapter 44), bacterial infections do not. The occurrence of heavy sputum production has often been mistakenly attributed to infection when it was actually a manifestation of the asthma itself. However, in cases where bacterial infection is strongly suggested by sputum Gram's stain and confirmed by sputum culture, prompt treatment with an appropriate antibiotic (see Chapter 43) is important.

Choice of Therapy. Young patients and those with exercise-induced asthma might first be given a trial of *cromolyn* therapy before being started on a regular course of bronchodilators. Those with exercise-induced asthma who do not respond to cromolyn can try a few inhalations of a *beta-adrenergic aerosol* before engaging in activity. A maintenance dose of a beta agonist or *theophylline* often provides good prophylaxis in patients with frequent attacks. More refractory cases require steroids. A topically active *aerosolized corticosteroid* such as beclomethasone is added in patients coming off systemic steroid therapy, so that systemic steroids can be tapered or at least the daily dose of systemic steroid reduced.

Monitoring Therapy

Assessments of symptoms, signs, and expiratory flow rates remain the basic means of monitoring asthmatic patients and judging severity of illness. In a carefully conducted study of 96 asthmatic patients, *self-estimates of severity* and daily change in airway obstruction correlated better with peak expiratory flow rate measurements that did the clinical assessment of their physicians.

Certain physical findings, such as the ratio of inspiration to expiration, help to semiquantitatively judge the degree of bronchospasm. However, wheezes and related physical findings are not very sensitive indicators of airway obstruction. The absence of wheezes does not indicate resolution of bronchospasm (see below). *Pulsus paradoxus* and *sternocleidomastoid retraction* are signs of severe obstruction, suggesting an FEV_1 of less than 1 liter per second, but these findings are not inevitably present when expiratory flow rates are very low. Moreover, there is much variation between the degree of paradox and severity of bronchospasm.

Spirometry provides additional sensitivity. Careful studies correlating physical findings with spirometric readings have shown that the *forced expiratory volume* at 1 second (FEV_1) is still prolonged at the time wheezes disappear. Even after the FEV_1 has returned to normal, measures of small airway obstruction (*e.g., maximum midexpiratory flow rate*) continue to indicate bronchospasm.

The clearing of wheezes signifies little more than partial resolution of large airway bronchospasm; small airway bronchoconstriction may still be prominent and slower to resolve. Failure to continue therapy beyond resolution of audible wheezes is probably responsible for the high rate of relapse that accompanies acute episodes treated only while wheezes persist.

Sputum and blood eosinophil counts correlate with response to therapy in patients treated with steroids for an acute attack. Although blood eosinophilia is not an invariable feature of an acute exacerbation of asthma, it does decline with improvement of expiratory flow rate. The same holds true for sputum eosinophilia. The usefulness of the eosinophil count for predicting relapse and response to therapy is unsettled.

Arterial blood gases provide important information in severe cases, particularly adequacy of ventilation. A pCO_2 that is inappropriately high for the respiratory rate indicates ventilatory failure and urgent need for hospitalization. However, because arterial blood gases are not readily available in most office settings, decisions usually must be made without them. A *chest x-ray* rarely provides information of use in decision making.

Thus, some of the most easily obtained parameters (the patient's subjective assessment of severity, ratio of inspiration to expiration, pulsus paradoxus, sternocleidomastoid retraction, and FEV_1) are among the more meaningful guides to clinical status and severity of illness.

Pitfalls of Therapy

One of the most common reasons why outpatient treatment fails is *improper inhaler technique*. In a study of 30 asthmatic patients, 47% were found to be using improper technique and not getting an adequate dose of medication. Correct use of an inhaler is an essential skill for every asthmatic patient (see discussion of Patient Education).

Another important cause of treatment failure is *underutilization of medication*, often due to intolerance of side-effects. Systemic side-effects are most bothersome with oral therapy, particularly if the dose is not built up slowly. Starting off with full oral doses of beta₂ adrenergic agents is likely to cause uncomfortable tremulousness and tachycardia. Sudden high doses of theophylline will trigger nervousness and gastrointestinal upset. Patients come to regard therapeutic doses as too laden with side-effects. Therapy should be started at low doses and built up gradually unless there is a clinical urgency for doing otherwise.

Other common mistakes include reliance on *nonprescription agents,* such as low-dose epinephrine inhalers, and use of suboptimal prescription drugs, such as theophylline suppositories or fixed combination agents containing ephedrine. The epinephrine inhalers are too short acting to provide adequate relief from an attack. *Use of theophylline suppositories* is also ill-advised due to erratic absorption. The *fixed-combination agents* containing subtherapeutic doses of theophylline (120 mg/tablet) in combination with ephedrine (25 mg/tablet) provide too little theophylline and excess adrenergic stimulation if more than four tablets are taken in a 24-hour period. The result is poor bronchodilation and marked adrenergic side-effects. These preparations often contain barbiturates as well, which speed theophylline clearance and pose the added risks of ventilatory suppression and dependence.

Management of the Pregnant Patient

Fetal morbidity and mortality are increased if asthma goes uncontrolled during pregnancy. Most antiasthma drugs are safe to use both during pregnancy and when breast-feeding, although in some instances data are lacking due to the difficulty of performing controlled studies. Epinephrine increases the risk of fetal malformations, and the safety of the beta₂ agonists and cromolyn remain to be established; until safety is proven, they should be avoided if possible. Use of beclomethasone appears without serious consequence, and even systemic steroids can be prescribed if necessary. Theophylline is safe, as is penicillin. Erythromycin is a reasonable alternative in penicillin-allergic patients; tetracycline is contraindicated because it damages fetal liver, bone, and teeth. Some barbiturates have been linked to fetal malformations; many fixed-combination preparations contain barbiturates and should not be prescribed.

INDICATIONS FOR ADMISSION

One of the most difficult determinations is predicting the need for hospitalization at the time of initial presentation. Ability to make such predictions is particularly important for the care of patients with severe attacks who visit the office or emergency room. Some have argued that response to maximum nonsteroidal therapy is a good predictor of immediate outcome and need for admission. Most studies provide little evidence that any one parameter is predictive, although one group noted that patients who sat bolt upright on admission to the emergency room had a strong likelihood of requiring admission. Another group developed an index of multiple clinical parameters selected by multivariate discriminant analysis to predict need for hospitalization. Pulse rate greater than 120 per minute, respiratory rate greater than 30 per minute, pulsus paradoxus greater than 18 mm Hg, peak expiratory flow rate less than 120 liters per minute, moderate to severe dyspnea, accessory muscle use, and wheezing made up the presenting clinical parameters used in the index. Although in the investigators' setting the index was quite capable of distinguishing between those who needed admission and those who did not (sensitivity, 95%; specificity, 97%), it did not function nearly as well when applied prospectively by other investigators in their emergency room settings.

Lacking more definitive means of prediction, clinical status and response to therapy remain the most helpful guidelines for decision making. Consideration of hospital care is indicated for patients with an acute attack who manifest any one of the following:

1. subjective report of severe difficulty breathing
2. failure to respond to full nonsteroidal therapy, including subcutaneous epinephrine or terbutaline
3. use of accessory muscles of respiration (sternocleidomastoid retraction)
4. more than 10 mm Hg of pulsus paradoxus
5. FEV_1 <1.0 liter per second
6. arterial PCO_2 inappropriately high for respiratory rate
7. underlying cardiac condition
8. inadequate home situation or a history of poor compliance

PATIENT EDUCATION

Patients need to be made partners in management of their asthma, because good compliance and proper use of medication can minimize the severity and frequency of attacks. Because asthma is a condition that is characterized by periodic exacerbations, every patient who is capable of understanding his medications should be given instructions for initial self-treatment of an attack along with strong advice to call the physician if relief does not come quickly. Patients need to know that excessive delay may lead to refractory bronchospasm.

Addressing patient concerns and providing written information facilitates *compliance*. Many worry about becoming "dependent" on medication or "immune" to it. These fears need to be addressed openly. A medication booklet that lists prescribing information, side-effects, and indications for use alongside a picture of the medication can be very helpful

to patient and family. Often, patients mistakenly stop the wrong medication or cease therapy altogether because they were fearful or unfamiliar with the side-effects of their medications.

With the growing importance of aerosol therapy, *proper inhalation technique* is essential. Correct use involves coordinating inhalation with actuation of the canister nebulizer, a skill that takes some practice to master. Many patients make the mistake of inhaling first, then actuating the canister, holding their breath for 2 or 3 seconds more, and exhaling before taking the first inhalation. Others inhale through the nose. Because many patients cannot perform aerosol inhalation correctly after a demonstration, they need to practice under observation. Moreover, about half forget how to do it when tested on follow up. Repeat checks of technique are important.

Patients who develop bronchospasm from air pollution, pollens, or exercise need an *activity prescription*. Staying indoors, avoiding physical exertion, and using air-conditioning on particularly bad days are helpful. Those with exercise-induced asthma need not restrict themselves as long as prophylactic measures suffice; however, very cold dry days may be difficult.

Those with asthma due to occupational exposure or household factors need careful *counseling* when considering such difficult alternatives as leaving a job, giving up a favorite pet, or moving to a new location. Often less extreme measures are adequate. A number of patients with allergic asthma request advice about desensitization treatment. A trial of such therapy is reasonable if episodes are frequent and a single allergen is identified (see Chapter 220), but other prophylactic measures are more likely to control symptoms and do not require years of periodic injections.

Patients receiving steroids deserve an extra measure of instruction, particularly when switching over from systemic to aerosol therapy. Writing out the tapering schedule and emphasizing the importance of taking systemic steroids at the time of an exacerbation or major stress will help minimize the risk of adrenal insufficiency.

The pregnant patient with asthma will be reluctant to take medication. Detailed counseling about which medications can be used with safety and the importance of asthma control to the health of the fetus are needed to ensure compliance and alleviate concern.

THERAPEUTIC RECOMMENDATIONS

Prophylaxis

- Identify and advise avoidance of any known allergens or environmental irritants.
- Begin a trial of cromolyn therapy in children, adolescents, and those with exercise-induced asthma before initiating chronic bronchodilator therapy; an adequate trial is 4 to 8 weeks, inhaling one capsule qid or using cromolyn before vigorous activity. Alternatively, exercise-induced asthma

can be treated with a few inhalations of a beta-adrenergic agent before exertion.

- Start either slow-release theophylline (200 mg bid) or an inhaled beta$_2$ adrenergic agent (*e.g.,* aerosol albuterol 1 to 2 puffs q 6 to 8 h) for patients bothered by frequent flare-ups.
- Gradually increase dose of nonsteroidal bronchodilator until control is achieved or maximum dose reached.
- If a single agent does not suffice, reduce dose and use both theophylline and a beta-agonist.
- If nonsteroidal therapy does not reduce the frequency and severity of attacks, then begin beclomethasone inhaler (1 to 2 puffs qid).
- If maximum nonsteroidal therapy fails and the patient remains severely incapacitated, initiate systemic corticosteroid therapy for prophylaxis. No more than the minimum dose necessary to control symptoms should be prescribed; prednisone doses of 10 to 15 mg qod are often adequate and can be tried before escalating to daily prednisone therapy.
- For patients well controlled on oral glucocorticoids, attempt to substitute a topically active preparation for systemic therapy. Begin beclomethasone (2 puffs qid) and start tapering oral steroid therapy 1 week after initiating topical therapy (see Chapter 103 for details on tapering systemic steroids). Exert particular caution in tapering if the patient has been on daily systemic steroids for over a month. At times of stress and flare-ups, resume full dose of systemic steroid (*e.g.,* 60 mg prednisone/day) until episode passes.
- Administer trivalent influenza vaccine each fall at least 6 weeks before start of the flu season. Also administer pneumococcal vaccine, provided patient is not allergic to eggs (see Chapter 44).
- Prophylactic use of inhaler therapy early in the course of an upper respiratory infection may prevent an attack.

Acute Asthmatic Attacks

- If attacks are mild and infrequent, instruct the patient to use aerosol beta$_2$ adrenergic therapy (*e.g.,* albuterol inhaler) on an as-needed basis at the first sign of bronchospasm. Starting dose is 1 to 2 puffs q 4 to 6 h. Although risk of tachyphylaxis is small, the patient should be advised to use no more than 12 inhalations per 24 hours; systemic adrenergic side-effects ensue at greater doses. Maximum bronchodilation occurs with use of 2 to 3 inhalations spaced 10 to 20 minutes apart.
- If the beta agonist alone does not suffice or side-effects are bothersome, reduce dose by half and add oral theophylline to the program.
- If rapid onset of action is desired, start with 15 to 30 ml of elixir of theophylline (80 mg theophylline/15 ml in a base of 20% ethanol) followed a few hours later by a modest dose (200 mg bid) of a slow-release theophylline preparation. If rapid onset is not essential, begin with the slow-release theophylline and skip the elixir.
- If after 3 days symptoms are not well controlled, increase

theophylline dose by another 200 mg/day. Check serum theophylline level 4 hours after last dose. Therapeutic range is 10 to 20 μg/ml; adjust dose accordingly.

- When the clinical situation permits, begin treatment with beta agonists and theophylline at the low end of the dose range and advance gradually to minimize side-effects.
- If bronchodilation remains inadequate, use full doses of both agents, rather than extreme doses of a single drug.
- Whenever symptoms are difficult to control or side-effects are disabling, check serum theophylline level. Adjust dose accordingly.
- For intense acute attacks not promptly relieved by full doses of inhaled adrenergic therapy and oral theophylline, instruct the patient to come promptly to the office or emergency room. Give epinephrine 1:1000, 0.3 ml subcutaneously; repeat if necessary every 20 minutes, up to a total of three doses. An alternative to epinephrine is terbutaline 0.25 ml subcutaneously.
- Consider a brief trial of aerosol atropine if patient is unresponsive to adrenergic agents and theophylline.
- Advise the patient to keep well hydrated to prevent mucus plugging during a severe attack.
- Hospital admission for intravenous theophylline and systemic corticosteroids is indicated if there are signs of severe airway obstruction (pulsus paradoxus, FEV$_1$ <1 liter per second, use of accessory muscles of respiration, etc.).
- Selected patients with stubborn attacks that are uncomfortable and relatively refractory but unaccompanied by worrisome prognostic signs and not overly disabling can be given a cautious 7- to 10-day trial of outpatient prednisone, beginning with 60 mg per day and tapering to discontinuation over 7 to 10 days. Such a program should be reserved for extremely reliable patients who can be trusted to monitor themselves carefully; if there is any doubt, treat in the hospital.
- Once an acute attack has been brought under control, continue the full treatment program for at least 7 to 10 days after symptoms have resolved; then taper to a maintenance regimen.
- Avoid antianxiety agents, sedatives, fixed combination preparations, and rectal theophylline suppositories.
- Be sure patient is fully informed about his medications, their side-effects, and proper use. Demonstrate and check technique of inhaler use. Directly elicit and address any patient concerns.

A.H.G.

ANNOTATED BIBLIOGRAPHY

Adinoff AD, Hollister JR: Steroid-induced factures and bone loss in patients with asthma. N Engl J Med 309:265, 1983 (*Documents an increased prevalence of rib and vertebral fractures in asthma patients taking systemic steroids; found in 8 of 19, compared with 0 of 11 controls.*)

Aelony Y: "Noninvasive" oral treatment of asthma in the emergency room. Am J Med 78:929, 1985 (*Most patients who presented for emergency room care were fully controlled by instituting oral ther-*

apy at proper doses; argues that most emergency room visits are unnecessary.)

Baigelman W, Chodosh S, Pizzuato D et al: Sputum and blood eosinophils during corticosteroid treatment of acute exacerbations of asthma. Am J Med 75:929, 1983 (*Eosinophil counts correlated with objective measures of response.*)

Becker AB, Simons KJ, Gillespie CA et al: The bronchodilator effects and pharmacokinetics of caffeine and asthma. N Engl J Med 310:743, 1984 (*Caffeine was as effective a bronchodilator as theophylline in young asthmatic patients.*)

Bernstein IL: Occupational asthma: Coming of age. Ann Intern Med 97:125, 1982 (*An editorial providing an excellent and concise summary of progress in the field.*)

Bernstein IL, Johnson CL, Tse CS: Therapy with cromolyn sodium. Ann Intern Med 89:228, 1978 (*Thorough review of the use of this agent.*)

Brenner B, Abraham E, Simon RR: Position and diaphoresis in acute asthma. Am J Med 74:1005, 1983 (*Upright position and diaphoresis at time of emergency room presentation were surprisingly predictive of need for hospital admission.*)

Bukowsky JM, Nakatsu K, Munt P: Theophylline reassessed. Ann Intern Med 101:63, 1984. (*Detailed review, with emphasis on pharmacokinetic data, metabolism, and interactions with other drugs; 101 references.*)

Busse WW: The precipitation of asthma by upper respiratory infections. Chest 87:44S, 1985 (*A review of the mechanisms underlying viral-induced asthma.*)

Chan-Yeung M: Occupational asthma. Am Rev Respir Dis 133:686, 1986 (*A useful review of the occupations and compounds that may produce occupational asthma. A guide to eliminating environmental precipitants.*)

Fanta CH, Rossing TH, McFadden ER, Jr: Treatment of acute asthma: Is combination therapy with sympathomimetics and methylxanthines indicated? Am J Med 80:5, 1986 (*An emergency room study; found xanthines helpful when full doses of a beta agonist could not be used.*)

Fiel B, Swartz MA, Glanz K et al: Efficacy of short-term corticosteroid therapy in outpatient treatment of acute bronchial asthma. Am J Med 75:259, 1983 (*A double-blind, placebo-controlled study showing reductions in symptoms and rate of relapse.*)

Fischl MA, Pitchenik A, Gardner LB: An index predicting relapse and need for hospitalization in patients with acute bronchial asthma. N Engl J Med 305:783, 1981 (*An attempt using multivariate analysis to construct an index predicting prognosis; utilized eight clinical parameters; worked well in their setting.*)

Greenberger PA: Beclomethasone diproprionate for severe asthma during pregnancy. Ann Intern Med 98:478, 1983 (*Prevalence of congenital malformations was within the normal range among patients using the drug during pregnancy.*)

Mathison DA, Stevenson DD, Simon RA: Asthma and the home environment. Ann Intern Med 97:128, 1982 (*An editorial describing the allergens associated with house dust, household pets, ubiquitous fungi, and nonallergic irritants.*)

McFadden ER: Exertional dyspnea and cough as preludes to acute attacks of bronchial asthma. N Engl J Med 292:555, 1975 (*Presents evidence of intermittent episodes of cough and breathlessness that represent variants of asthmatic attacks.*)

McFadden ER, Jr: Clinical appraisal of the therapy of asthma: An idea whose time has come. Am Rev Respir Dis 133:723, 1986 (*A critical review of anticholinergics and the role of studies to evaluate optimal management of asthma.*)

McFadden ER, Kiser R, DeGroot WJ: Acute bronchial asthma: Relations between clinical and physiologic manifestations. N Engl J Med 288:221, 1973 (*Significant airway obstruction remains even after resolution of symptoms and signs. This residual bronchospasm may serve as the basis for repeated flares if therapy is discontinued too soon.*)

Nassif EG, Weinberger M, Thompson R et al: The value of maintenance theophylline in steroid-dependent asthma. N Engl J Med 304:71, 1981 (*Maintenance theophylline provided measurable clinical benefit in children with chronic steroid-dependent asthma.*)

Rose CC, Murphy JG, Schwartz JS: Performance of an index predicting the response of patients with acute bronchial asthma to intensive emergency department treatment. N Engl J Med 310:573, 1984 (*Could not reproduce the excellent predictive performance of the index developed by Fischl and co-workers.*)

Rossing TH, Fanta DH, McFadden ER: Effect of outpatient treatment of asthma with beta-agonists on the response to sympathomimetics in an emergency room. Am J Med 75:781, 1983 (*Prior use of sympathomimetics did not blunt response to their use in the emergency room setting; suggests that tachyphylaxis is not a clinically serious problem in most patients using adrenergic agents during an exacerbation.*)

Selner JC: Helping asthmatic patients control their environment. J Respir Dis 8:83, 1986 (*Useful practical advice.*)

Shim C, Williams MH: The adequacy of inhalation of aerosol from canister nebulizers. Am J Med 69:891, 1980 (*Almost half of patients studied were not using their inhalers properly and even after training, many still required further instruction and follow-up.*)

Shim C, Williams MH: Evaluation of the severity of asthma: Patients versus physicians. Am J Med 68:11, 1980 (*Patients were better at estimating the severity and change in their expiratory flow rates than were their physicians.*)

Shim C, Williams MH, Jr: Effects of odors in asthma. Am J Med 80:18, 1986 (*An experimental study that showed significant decline in FEV_1 and a survey that an overwhelming majority of asthmatics report worsening with exposure to one or more common odors.*)

Tashkin DP, Trevor E, Chopra SK, et al: Sites of airway dilatation in asthma following inhaled versus subcutaneous terbutaline. Am J Med 68:14, 1980 (*Inhaled terbutaline affected only large airways; oral therapy dilated both large and small airways.*)

Turner ES, Greenberger PA, Patterson R: Management of the pregnant asthmatic patient. Ann Intern Med 93:905, 1980 (*Detailed review of this special aspect of asthma management; 126 references.*)

Weinberger M, Hendeles L: Slow-release theophylline: Rationale and basis for product selection. N Engl J Med 308:760, 1983 (*Detailed review of these new preparations; 35 references.*)

Welsh PW, Reed CE, Conrad E: Timing of once-a-day theophylline dose to match peak blood level with diurnal variation in severity of asthma. Am J Med 80:1098, 1986 (*An example of the use of once-a-day therapy.*)

Williams MH: Beclomethasone dipropionate. Ann Intern Med 95:464, 1981 (*Five-year critical review of the topically active steroid.*)

46

Management of the Common Cold

HARVEY B. SIMON, M.D.

Upper respiratory tract infections are among the most frequent reasons for office visits; nevertheless, physicians see only a small fraction of patients with such problems, because most treat their symptoms at home with over-the-counter remedies or simply wait for the illness to pass by itself. Upper respiratory infections are the leading cause of absenteeism, accounting for an average of almost 7 days lost from work per person per year. Although a viral etiology accounts for the overwhelming proportion of cases, the physician must be alert for specifically treatable bacterial processes. In addition, familiarity with agents available for symptomatic relief is necessary because patients turn to their physicians when home remedies fail to help.

PATHOPHYSIOLOGY AND CLINICAL PRESENTATION

The upper respiratory tract is composed of two distinct types of epithelial surfaces. The oropharynx and nasopharynx are lined by a stratified squamous epithelium, and are normally teeming with a varied microbial flora. In addition, many potentially pathogenic bacteria can temporarily reside on these epithelial surfaces as "colonizers" without causing true infection. With a few exceptions, such as herpes simplex and E.B. virus, viruses are not usually long-term members of the normal flora of the respiratory tract.

Numerous host defense mechanisms protect the upper airway from infection. Mechanical defenses tend to prevent penetration of organisms from the nasopharynx and oral cavity into more vulnerable areas. These defenses include the cough, gag and sneeze reflexes, viscous mucous secretions entrap particulate material, and ciliary action propels such particles outward. In addition, local immunologic defenses attempt to deal with organisms that have breached the mechanical barriers. These defenses include lymphoid tissue, secretory IgA antibodies in respiratory secretions, and a rich vasculature capable of rapidly delivering phagocytic leukocytes.

The majority of upper respiratory infections are due to viral agents. Recent studies of pharyngitis suggest that about 30% of cases are Chlamydial in origin and another 5% to 10% each due to Mycoplasma and Group A streptococcus. Rhinoviruses are the most common viral agent associated with upper respiratory tract illness. Since there are over 110 antigenic serotypes, there is no cross immunity and reinfection with another serotype right after a recent cold is common.

Mechanisms of transmission include aerosolization of virus-laden respiratory secretions, and direct mucous membrane contact with virus from contaminated hands, other skin surfaces, and even table tops. Touching one's eyes or nose effects the inoculation. The timeless motherly warning that "you'll catch cold if you get wet or damp" has not been borne out by experimental study; at least such conditions are not sufficient in themselves to cause illness.

Numerous viral agents including rhinoviruses, respiratory syncytial virus, adenoviruses, influenza viruses, and parainfluenza viruses can cause an identical clinical picture. Incubation periods for viral URIs range from 1 to 5 days; virus shedding lasts up to 2 weeks. Typical symptoms include coryza, pharyngitis, laryngitis, headache, malaise, and fever, in various combinations. Ear and sinus discomfort is often present as well, but these symptoms are caused by mucosal edema, which impairs drainage, rather than by acute viral infection of these regions (see Chapters 216 and 217).

Whether known as the common cold, nasopharyngitis, or the "URI," these problems generally resolve spontaneously. Common viral upper respiratory infections rarely progress to pneumonia; most colds resolve spontaneously within 1 week, though symptoms may linger for several weeks.

PRINCIPLES OF MANAGEMENT

Once the virus has been contracted, there is no means of preventing cold symptoms. The enthusiasm that surrounded use of high-dose ascorbic acid for prophylaxis has waned as controlled studies have failed to demonstrate its efficacy. Therapeutic efforts are directed toward relieving nasal congestion, headache, and grippelike symptoms.

Millions of dollars are spent annually on over-the-counter cold remedies. Most contain a combination of ingredients, including antihistamines, sympathomimetic amines, and analgesics. Some even contain more than one antihistamine or sympathomimetic. Antitussives, caffeine, vitamin C, belladonna alkaloids, and expectorants are common additives as well. Antacids, laxatives, quinine, and papaverine are occasionally found.

Alpha-adrenergic agents are the most commonly used decongestants. They work by causing generalized vasoconstriction and thus reducing formation of secretions. Since they produce systemic vasoconstriction, sympathomimetics may raise blood pressure when used in doses sufficient to alleviate nasal congestion. There is no oral adrenergic agent that provides selective local vasoconstriction; nasal sprays are more effective for this purpose, but may be associated with rebound congestion after the drug effect subsides, leading to abuse of the spray. According to most authorities, nasal sprays are good for short-term therapy, while oral preparations are better when use is to continue longer than 10 days, since chronic spray applications interfere with ciliary action and irritate and dry the nasal mucosa, producing swelling.

Analgesics are quite useful for relief of the headache, fever, and achiness that often accompany a cold. Aspirin and acetaminophen have similar analgesic and antipyretic effects and are key ingredients in the combination cold remedies. Salicylate derivates such as salicylamide are sometimes used, though they are much less effective than aspirin. Plain aspirin is much cheaper than any combination of agents, and is preferred.

Expectorants are included in many preparations in the belief that they stimulate the flow of mucus. There is no evidence to support this view, even though these agents are widely prescribed and requested by patients. Warm steam from a vaporizer or cold mist from a humidifier are much more effective in loosening secretions. *Cough suppressants,* including narcotics such as codeine and non-narcotic agents such as dextromethorphan, are effective and useful symptomatically, especially in allowing the patient to sleep uninterrupted by cough. In many patients, a decongestant is even more effective in suppressing cough, since postnasal drip accounts for much of the cough stimulus. These agents are commonly available in combination with expectorants, though they may be prescribed alone, thereby saving the patient money.

Antihistamines have weak, atropine-type effects and may help to reduce secretions when used in therapeutic doses. Sleepiness is the major side-effect of most preparations. Combining multiple antihistamines in low amounts has no benefit over using one agent in a therapeutic dose.

Atropine, laxatives, caffeine, and antacids are present in subtherapeutic doses in combination preparations; they have little impact on symptoms and only increase costs. The vitamin C included has not been shown to have any effect, even when given in gram doses.

THERAPEUTIC RECOMMENDATIONS

Relief from the symptoms of a cold is best provided by rest, fluids, aspirin, and a vaporizer. A cough suppressant before bed (*e.g.,* 15 mg codeine sulfate) and a nasal decongestant spray (*e.g.,* phenylephrine; see Chapter 217) may aid in symptomatic management and are superior to expensive combination agents, which often contain irrational mixtures or subtherapeutic doses of active ingredients. Vitamin C has no proven role in prevention or alleviation of symptoms.

ANNOTATED BIBLIOGRAPHY

Coulehan JL, Eberhard S, Kapner L et al: Vitamin C and acute illness in Navajo schoolchildren. N Engl J Med 295:973, 1976 (*A double-blind trial of vitamin C and placebo in 868 schoolchildren. Vitamin C did not prove to be effective as either a prophylactic or a therapeutic agent.*)

Douglas RG, Lindgren KM, Couch RB: Exposure to cold environment and rhinovirus common cold. N Engl J Med 279:742, 1968 (*Your mother is wrong! Exposure to moisture and cold does not increase susceptibility to URIs, at least not in this study of volunteers experimentally infected with rhinovirus.*)

Garibaldi RA: Epidemiology of community-acquired respiratory tract infections in adults. Am J Med 78(6B):32, 1985 (*Good review of epidemiology and pathophysiology of URIs.*)

Simon HB: The immunology of exercise: A brief review. JAMA 252: 2735, 1984 (*Your mother is wrong again! There is no evidence that exercise lowers "resistance" to respiratory or other infection; nor is it protective.*)

Murphy S, Florman AF: Lung defenses against infection: A clinical correlation. Pediatrics 72:1, 1983 (*A comprehensive review of host defenses against pulmonary infection.*)

Oral cold remedies. Medical Letter 17:89, 1975 (*Critiques over-the-counter oral cold remedies and warns against their high cost, irrational combination of agents, and frequent use of subtherapeutic doses of active ingredients.*)

47
Management of Tuberculosis
HARVEY B. SIMON, M.D.

Tuberculosis may be encountered by the primary care physician as either of two very different clinical problems. By far the more common presentation is the patient with a positive tuberculin skin test but no active infection; up to 7% of the population in the United States today may be in this category. In contrast, only about 25,000 new cases of active tuberculosis are reported in the United States each year. One result of the declining incidence of tuberculosis is that its diagnosis and treatment have shifted from the sanatorium and the specialist to the community and the primary physician. If tuberculosis is less common today, it is still subtle because of a tremendous variety of clinical pictures. In a sense, the diagnosis of tuberculosis may actually be more difficult today because most physicians have had limited clinical experience with the disease, and are less likely to suspect its presence. In fact, it has been shown that diagnosis is delayed in many patients with tuberculosis admitted to university hospitals; some cases are recognized only at autopsy. In addition, the management of tuberculosis has undergone such tremendous changes in the chemotherapy era that studies have demonstrated suboptimal management by many general physicians in the United States. Clearly, diagnosis and treatment of tuberculosis remain a major challenge for the primary physician.

EPIDEMIOLOGY

With the elimination of bovine tuberculosis in the United States, virtually all cases are acquired through person-to-person aerosol transmission. People with active pulmonary infection shed infected droplets, which are then airborne into the environment. Because most infectious patients discharge relatively few organisms, casual contacts have a low risk of infection, and most secondary cases occur in household members, schoolmates, or other close contacts of the index case. Tuberculosis is more common in population groups where there is crowding and poverty (see Chapter 34). At present, only 10% of all "new" tuberculosis diagnosed in this country results from primary infection, the vast majority representing reactivation of latent endogenous infections.

Reactivation of tuberculosis occurs in less than 5% of all infected individuals, the remainder having positive skin tests but no clinical illness. Reactivation is most likely to occur within the first few years of the initial infection or at times of lowered host resistance, such as adolescence or the postpartum period. However, reactivation can occur many decades after initial infection and, in fact, is now most common in the elderly. As many as one fifth of patients with reactivated disease have histories of inadequately treated clinical tuberculosis. At times, a discrete insult to host defenses such as steroid therapy, alcoholism, malnutrition, neoplastic disease, or gastrectomy can be implicated, but more often it is impossible to identify the reason for reactivation.

Atypical mycobacterial infections are probably acquired from inhalation or ingestion of organisms from sources in nature; there is no evidence for person-to-person transmission.

CLINICAL PRESENTATION AND COURSE

Primary Infection. More than 90% of patients are entirely asymptomatic at the time of primary infection and can be identified only through conversion of the tuberculin skin test from negative to positive. The majority of these patients have normal chest x-rays, but fibrocalcific stigmata of infection are radiographically demonstrable in others. In the past, primary infection occurred almost entirely in childhood, but as the incidence of tuberculosis has declined, primary tuber-

culosis is also seen in adults. Recent reports have documented exogenous infection in elderly nursing home residents and suggest that nosocomial tuberculosis may be an important problem in nursing home settings.

Among symptomatic patients, four broad syndromes can be identified. Most common is an *atypical pneumonia* picture, with fever and nonproductive cough. Chest x-rays may show unilateral lower lobe patchy parenchymal infiltrates and/or paratracheal or hilar adenopathy. Although such patients should receive full antituberculous chemotherapy when diagnosed, the disease usually resolves, even without treatment. Another syndrome is *tuberculous pleurisy* and effusion. These patients have fever, cough, pleuritic chest pain, and sometimes dyspnea. Chest x-rays reveal unilateral pleural effusions, often without identifiable parenchymal lesions. The tuberculin test is almost always strongly positive. Diagnosis depends on examination and culture of the pleural fluid or on percutaneous needle biopsy of the pleura, since sputum cultures are positive in only 30% of such cases. Another syndrome is *direct progression* from primary disease to upper lobe involvement. Least common is early *systemic dissemination,* which used to be seen in children. In addition to these major manifestations, patients with primary tuberculosis may present with hypersensitivity reactions such as erythema nodosum.

Reactivation (Postprimary) Tuberculosis. This is the most common clinical form of tuberculosis and is seen most often in the elderly or debilitated patient. Symptoms usually begin insidiously and progress over a period of many weeks or months prior to diagnosis. Constitutional symptoms are often prominent, including anorexia, weight loss, and night sweats. Most patients have low-grade fever, but higher temperatures and even chills may be seen occasionally when the disease progresses more rapidly. In addition, most patients present with pulmonary symptoms, including cough and sputum production. Dyspnea is relatively uncommon in the absence of underlying chronic lung disease. A frequent complaint is hemoptysis, often in the form of bright red streaks of blood caused by bronchial irritation. Although physical examination is usually nondiagnostic, chest x-rays are highly suggestive of the diagnosis. Typical features include infiltration in the posterior apical pulmonary segments, which may be unilateral or bi-lateral, and which progresses to frank cavitation. Apical lordotic views and chest tomography may be helpful in documenting cavitary disease. Occasionally, postprimary tuberculosis may involve the lower lung fields, and in rare instances the chest x-ray may appear normal. The tuberculin skin test is positive in about 80% of patients with reactivation tuberculosis; patients with advanced disease are often malnourished and anergic.

Extrapulmonary Tuberculosis. Approximately 10% of all newly recognized cases of tuberculosis in the United States are extrapulmonary. While the frequency of pulmonary tuberculosis is declining, the incidence of extrapulmonary disease is remaining relatively constant. Although the clinical features of extrapulmonary tuberculosis vary widely, certain generalizations are possible. Past history is not a reliable guide to the diagnosis of extrapulmonary tuberculosis. Only 25% of patients have a past history of tuberculosis; of these, virtually all have been inadequately treated. There is typically a long latent period between the first episode of infection and the extrapulmonary presentation. Approximately 50% of patients with extrapulmonary tuberculosis have entirely normal chest x-rays; most of the others have stigmata of old inactive pulmonary disease, while a minority have coexisting active pulmonary infection. Although extrapulmonary disease can involve all organ systems, either singly or in various combinations, the most commonly affected areas are the genitourinary tract, the musculoskeletal system, and the lymph nodes.

The most common type of extrapulmonary tuberculosis is infection of an individual organ system. Such a patient is most often afebrile and can be entirely free of constitutional complaints. The illness typically pursues a very indolent course characterized by local organ dysfunction and eventual destruction rather than by progressive general decline. In fact, the differential diagnosis in these individuals more often suggests neoplastic disease than infection. The tuberculin skin test is almost always positive. Clinical syndromes in this category include genitourinary tuberculosis, tuberculous arthritis and osteomyelitis, tuberculous lymphadenitis, and many others.

Clinical infection with *atypical mycobacteria* is not seen very often in primary care practice. Representative syndromes caused by these organisms include cervical adenitis in children (scrofula), pulmonary infection, and cutaneous disease (swimming pool granuloma). Disseminated disease occasionally takes place in immunosuppressed individuals. For example, *M. avium intracellulare* has been a major problem causing disseminated infection in patients with AIDS.

DIAGNOSIS

The tuberculin *skin test* is the most sensitive test for diagnosis of infection with *Mycobacterium tuberculosis* (see Chapter 34); it is far more sensitive than the chest x-ray. A positive tuberculin test does not by itself prove there is active disease, but does indicate that infection has occurred. Negative tuberculin reactions have been documented in up to 20% of patients with tuberculosis, particularly those individuals with overwhelming or advanced disease, malnutrition, and debility. Many of these individuals are anergic, so that simultaneous skin testing with *Candida* or streptokinase-streptodornase antigens can be useful in demonstrating overall immunologic impairment.

When there is active pulmonary disease, the diagnosis of pulmonary tuberculosis can usually be confirmed by examination of the *sputum*. If patients are not able to produce sputum spontaneously, attempts should be made to induce sputum with the aid of hydration, pulmonary physiotherapy, IPPB, and mucolytic agents. Bronchoscopy may be necessary for obtaining appropriate specimens. Although cultures are necessary for a positive diagnosis and are more sensitive than smears, sputum specimens should be examined microscopically either by the traditional Ziehl–Neelsen (acid-fast) stain, or by the newer Truant fluorescent stain. Sputum or bronchoscopic washings should be examined both directly and after concentration by centrifugation and digestion. Carefully collected individual specimens are preferred to a 24-hour pool of sputum and saliva. Cultures of first morning fasting *gastric aspirates* are also helpful. Because gastric acid is toxic to mycobacteria, the collection bottles should contain a buffer such as sodium bicarbonate. Smears of gastric juice are misleading, because of the potential presence of saprophytic mycobacteria, and should not be performed.

Tissue biopsy is often required for diagnosis of tuberculous pleurisy or extrapulmonary disease, since sputum and gastric samples are usually negative for organisms in these situations.

PRINCIPLES OF TREATMENT

Prophylaxis in Uninfected Individuals. In many parts of the world where tuberculosis is common, Bacillus Calmette-Guerin (BCG) vaccine is used for the prevention of primary infection. It is intended only for prophylaxis and should not be given to patients with positive skin tests (see Chapter 34). Because the incidence of tuberculosis is relatively low in the United States, BCG is not routinely recommended in this country. Close contacts of patients with active pulmonary tuberculosis should be considered for isoniazid (INH) therapy, particularly if they are children, adolescents, or nursing home residents (see Chapter 34).

Prophylaxis in Tuberculin Converters and Those with Latent Disease. Prevention of active tuberculosis can be achieved with INH. However, the drug is not without toxicity; it can cause hepatocellular damage, particularly in older patients (see Appendix at the end of this chapter). An estimate of the risk of reactivation of tuberculosis needs to be weighed against the chances of drug-induced hepatitis in order to select patients for INH prophylaxis (see Chapter 34). In general, patients whose skin test has converted from negative to positive within the last 2 years should be considered for chemoprophylaxis. Older patients who have recovered from clinical tuberculosis but have never received chemotherapy should be evaluated to exclude active disease; if none is demonstrated, these individuals too may benefit from INH. Although firm data are lacking, it also seems reasonable to administer INH to immunologically impaired hosts with positive tuberculin skin tests, such as those with AIDS. Finally, it can be argued that all individuals below age 35 should be skin-tested at the time of routine medical evaluations, and that

INH should be administered to positive reactors (see Chapter 34). In contrast, patients over 35 with a positive skin test and no evidence or history of clinical tuberculosis should be followed and need not be treated, since at this age the risk of INH hepatotoxicity begins to outweigh the benefit of prophylaxis.

Patients with positive skin tests should be evaluated to exclude active infection. One needs to check for cough, fever, sputum production, pleuritic chest pain, lymphadenopathy, pleural effusion, pulmonary consolidation, and enlargement of the liver or spleen. A chest x-ray is essential, and complete blood count, differential, urinalysis, and liver function tests (particularly the alkaline phosphatase) may provide clues of active disease (*e.g.,* "sterile" pyuria or isolated alkaline phosphatase elevation). If no active infection is identified, the patient should be reassured, and the potential risks and benefits of INH therapy explained so that the patient can participate in therapeutic decision.

Treatment of Patients with Active Tuberculosis. Antituberculous drugs are the cornerstone of therapy. Since the patient will be noncontagious shortly after starting therapy, most treatment can be administered on an outpatient basis. The chemotherapy of tuberculosis is different from other antimicrobial programs and proceeds according to a unique set of principles:

1. The use of multiple drugs is necessary to prevent the emergence of drug-resistant organisms.
2. Single daily dosages are preferred.
3. Prolonged chemotherapy is necessary. Standard multiple-drug regimens require periods of 18 to 24 months. With combinations of newer agents, shorter regimens of 6 to 9 months have been found equally effective.
4. No matter what regimen is chosen, it is important to follow patients closely to insure compliance and to monitor for drug efficacy and toxicity. The currently available antituberculous regimens are so effective that prolonged surveillance is not necessary after completion of a full course of therapy.
5. Because chemotherapy will control the organisms, surgery is reserved for the treatment of complications such as restrictive pericardial scarring.
6. Elaborate programs of rest and diet have no place in modern treatment of tuberculosis.

Most patients with clinically active pulmonary tuberculosis should be hospitalized for the initial phases of therapy. As little as 2 weeks of multidrug therapy will greatly decrease the infectiousness of these patients, although a few mycobacteria may still be present on sputum smears or cultures. Hence, short-term admission to a general hospital is preferred, with early home care for patients who are reliable and clinically stable. Patients with extrapulmonary tuberculosis are much less infectious and can sometimes be managed entirely as outpatients.

CASE REPORTING AND PATIENT EDUCATION

All cases of tuberculosis should be reported promptly to public health authorities, so that contacts can be investigated and appropriate control measures instituted. However, it must be remembered that, particularly in elderly patients, the diagnosis of tuberculosis still carries social stigma and dire prognostic implications. Reassurance and education are therefore of great importance. It should be stressed that tuberculosis occurs in all social and economic classes, that modern chemotherapy is truly curative, that prolonged periods of hospitalization and isolation are no longer necessary.

Patients who are candidates for INH prophylaxis should understand the risks and benefits of INH therapy. If INH therapy is recommended and accepted, the patient should be instructed to discontinue the medication and report to the physician if adverse effects are noted, including skin rash, fever, fatigue, anorexia, abdominal distress, jaundice, or peripheral neuropathic symptoms. The importance of full compliance with the drug regimen, be it for prophylaxis or treatment of active disease, must be stressed.

THERAPEUTIC RECOMMENDATIONS

Prophylaxis

- In the United States, BCG prophylaxis is not recommended for prevention of infection (see Chapter 34).
- Recent conversion of a tuberculin skin test to positive is an indication for INH chemoprophylaxis. Average dose is 300 mg per day for 1 year. (Pyridoxine, 50 mg per day, is given with INH to prevent peripheral neuropathy.) Positive reactors who are under age 35 should also be considered for INH prophylaxis, as should close contacts of patients with active pulmonary disease, particularly if the exposed individual is a child or adolescent. In addition, older patients who have recovered from clinical tuberculosis but have never received chemotherapy should be considered for INH therapy if they have no evidence of active disease.
- The decision to use INH for prophylaxis involves weighing the risk of drug-induced hepatotoxicity (see Appendix at the end of this chapter) with the benefit of preventing active disease. The older the patient, the greater the risk of hepatitis. Risk begins to dominate beyond age 35.

Active Disease

- Patients with active disease require combination chemotherapy. Those with mild to moderate pulmonary or extrapulmonary disease can be treated with a two-drug regimen. INH plus rifampin or INH plus ethambutol are generally preferred in these circumstances (see Appendix). Patients with far advanced cavitary disease of the lung, meningitis, pericarditis, or miliary disease require triple-drug therapy, such as INH, rifampin, and ethambutol or streptomycin. Because of its superior tissue penetration, rifampin should always be included in triple-drug therapy of patients with tuberculous meningitis.

1. The usual dose of INH is 5 mg per kg body weight, which averages 300 mg per day for the adult. For initial therapy of life-threatening disease, doses of 10 to 15 mg per kg per day may be used. Ethambutol is available only in an oral preparation. Many authorities recommend initial therapy with 25 mg per kg body weight per day for the first 6 to 8 weeks of therapy, and then reduced doses of 15 mg per kg body weight per day for the remainder of the course. Good results have also been obtained with use of the lower dose throughout therapy. The average dose of rifampin in adults is 600 mg per day, administered in a single dose. Streptomycin must be given parenterally. The average adult dose is 1 g daily for the first 2 to 8 weeks of therapy, followed by 1 g twice a week.

2. Standard chemotherapeutic programs requiring the use of two antituberculosis drugs should be maintained for periods of 18 to 24 months, sometimes following an initial phase of three drugs for 2 to 3 months in the very sick patient.

3. *Short-course regimens,* using INH and rifampin together for periods for 6 to 9 months are a reasonable alternative when an 18- to 24-month regimen is impractical. On this program, failures do not exceed 5%. British studies have demonstrated excellent results with six months of INH, rifampin, and streptomycin or with nine months of INH and rifampin together with ethambutol or streptomycin for the first 2 months. More recent American studies have shown equally good results with just INH and rifampin for 9 months; following daily therapy for one month, these drugs can be administered twice weekly (INH 900 mg, rifampin 600 mg) for the remaining 8 months of treatment.

4. *Intermittent chemotherapy* is designed and should be reserved for unreliable outpatients who require supervised administration of drugs. After 3 months of standard daily treatment, these patients can be given 18 months of intermittent high-dose treatment in the format of INH 14 mg per kg and streptomycin 27 mg per kg, each taken twice a week. Streptomycin toxicity, however, can be expected in up to 10% of patients on this program; in such cases, high-dose ethambutol (50 mg per kg per dose) can be given instead.

5. *Drug resistance* is an increasing concern. In the United States, Asian and Hispanic patients are at greatest risk of harboring drug-resistant organisms. Whereas up to 10% of isolates from such patients may be resistant to INH or streptomycin, less than 1% are resistant to rifampin or ethambutol. When drug resistance is considered possible, initial therapy with INH, rifampin, and ethambutol is preferred. All isolates from patients previously treated for tuberculosis, as well as from Asians and Hispanics, should be tested for drug sensitivity.

6. Chemotherapy for tuberculosis is so efficacious that prolonged *follow-up* of successfully treated patients is not cost-effective. However, patients treated with newer short-course regimens should be followed for at least 1 year.

- Hospitalization should be considered in the initial stages of active pulmonary disease to minimize risk of spread. Two weeks of chemotherapy usually suffice to render the patient noninfectious.

- With the exception of *M. kansasii* and *M. marinum,* the majority of atypical mycobacteria are drug-resistant, making therapy difficult. So-called second-line antituberculous agents are sometimes necessary (see Appendix). Consultation with a specialist in mycobacterial disease is indicated.

Appendix: Antituberculous Chemotherapeutic Agents

Chemotherapeutic agents are separated into "first-line" and "second-line" drugs. The former include INH, ethambutol, rifampin, and streptomycin.

Isoniazid (INH). Introduced into clinical use in the early 1950s, INH remains the single most important antituberculous drug. Of importance is the excellent tissue penetration of this small, water-soluble molecule; the distribution of INH includes the central nervous system, tuberculous abscesses, and intracellular sites. The major metabolism of INH is by hepatic acetylation. Although metabolites are excreted by the kidneys, it is not necessary to modify INH doses except in advanced renal failure. INH is available both orally and parenterally; it is an inexpensive drug. The major toxicities of INH include:

1. Neurologic toxicity, ranging from peripheral neuropathy (which can be prevented by administration of 50 mg of pyridoxine daily) to much less common manifestations, including encephalopathy, seizures, optic neuritis, and personality changes.

2. Hypersensitivity reactions including fever, rash, and rheumatic syndromes with or without positive antinuclear antibodies.

3. Hepatitis, including serious clinical hepatitis in less than 2%, but a transient, clinically insignificant rise in SGOT

in 10% to 20%. Risk of clinically significant hepatitis increases with age.

The U.S. Public Health Service does not recommend routine SGOT determinations in individuals who are reliable and who are able to comply with directions for reporting symptoms of hepatitis. However, SGOT determinations can be helpful, particularly insofar as they give the physician an opportunity to briefly reinforce instructions and also because the surveillance is very reassuring to most patients. The problem with SGOT determinations is that between 10% and 20% of individuals receiving INH can be expected to show mild transient elevations in SGOT, which will return to normal even during continued therapy and are of no clinical significance.

Although precise data are lacking, a reasonable approach is to routinely determine the SGOT at monthly intervals for the first 3 months of therapy, since most SGOT abnormalities develop during this period. In symptomatic patients with elevated SGOTs, the drug should be discontinued and liver function tests monitored. In asymptomatic individuals with mild elevations of SGOT (perhaps up to 100 units), the drug can be continued, but the patient should be monitored weekly. If the SGOT fails to return to normal in 3 to 4 weeks, it seems prudent to discontinue the INH. On the other hand, even if a patient is asymptomatic, a single, more substantial elevation of SGOT, perhaps above 200 units, may be grounds to discontinue the agent. Again, it must be emphasized that these are "rules of thumb" rather than precise guidelines.

Rifampin is the newest of the major antituberculous drugs and rivals INH in its efficacy. Rifampin is a large, fat-soluble molecule that achieves excellent tissue penetration, including the central nervous system. The drug is excreted by the liver; modification of dosage is not required in renal failure but may be necessary in hepatic insufficiency. At the present time, only an oral preparation has been approved in the United States. Unlike INH and ethambutol, rifampin is actually a broad-spectrum antimicrobial, acting against some atypical mycobacteria, *M. leprae,* many bacteria (including staphylococci, meningococci, and various gram-negative bacilli), trachoma agent, and some viruses. Patients should be cautioned to expect orange discoloration of urine, sweat, tears, and saliva, which is of no clinical significance. Toxicities include hypersensitivity reactions (fever, rash, or eosinophilia), hematologic toxicities (thrombocytopenia, leukopenia, and hemolytic anemia), and a high incidence of hepatitis, including elevated SGOTs in up to 10%. Drug interactions occur; rifampin antagonizes the effect of warfarin, quinidine, oral contraceptives, and methadone. Rifampin should never be used in high-dose intermittent therapy because toxic reactions (including hemolytic anemia, thrombocytopenia, and hepatic failure) occur frequently. However, use of low-dose (600 mg) intermittent therapy given twice weekly appears well tolerated. Rifampin is an expensive drug.

Although rifampin is an extremely effective antituberculous drug, we prefer to reserve the agent for patients who cannot tolerate other first-line drugs, who are treatment failures, or who have overwhelming disease. Reasons for reserving this drug include its expense and its potential for hepatotoxicity, which can be particularly confusing in a patient simultaneously receiving INH. Finally, it is often helpful to have an excellent drug such as rifampin in reserve should problems develop during the course of treatment. However, most authorities recommend rifampin in the initial treatment of tuberculosis.

Ethambutol was introduced clinically in the United States in 1967 and represented a major advance in antituberculous chemotherapy. Ethambutol penetrates tissues well, including the central nervous system when the meninges are inflamed. The drug is excreted by the kidneys. Dose modification in renal failure should be based on serum ethambutol levels (available through the manufacturer) and monitored in patients with renal failure who require the drug. The major toxicities of ethambutol include hypersensitivity reactions, such as fever and rash, and optic neuritis, which is dose-related and usually manifested first by a loss of color vision. Less common side-effects include neuritis, GI intolerance, headache, and hyperuricemia. The cost of ethambutol is moderate.

Streptomycin, the first effective antituberculous drug, remains useful. Like other aminoglycosides, streptomycin has only a fair tissue distribution, being inactive at an alkaline *p*H in an anaerobic milieu, and penetrating the cerebrospinal fluid very poorly. Streptomycin is excreted by the kidneys, and dosage should be reduced in patients with renal failure. Major toxicities include hypersensitivity reactions and eighth nerve toxicity, especially to the vestibular division, resulting in vertigo. The cost of streptomycin is moderate. The drug is active against a variety of organisms in addition to *M. tuberculosis,* although many gram-negative bacilli have now become resistant due to widespread use over many years.

The "Second-line" Antituberculous Drugs tend to be both less effective and more toxic than the standard agents, but occasionally are of critical importance in patients with drug-resistant tuberculosis or atypical mycobacterial infection, and in those who cannot tolerate the standard therapies. Four agents are administered orally, including para-aminosalicylic acid (PAS), pyrazinamide, ethionamide, and cycloserine. For many years, PAS was considered a first-line drug, but its relatively weak tuberculostatic action and very high incidence of gastrointestinal intolerance has now relegated it to a secondary role. Two other drugs available parenterally—kanamycin, and capreomycin—are pharmacologically similar to streptomycin.

ANNOTATED BIBLIOGRAPHY

Barlow PB, Black M, Brummer DL et al: Preventive therapy of tuberculous infection. Morbidity and Mortality Weekly Report, 24: 71, 1975 (*The USPHS recommendations for the use of isoniazid in the "chemopropylaxis" of tuberculosis.*)

British Thoracic and Tuberculosis Association: Short-course chemotherapy in pulmonary tuberculosis: A controlled trial. Lancet 2:1102, 1976 (*A controlled study of 696 patients with culture-positive pulmonary tuberculosis. The authors recommend a regimen of INH and rifampin for 9 months supplemented by ethambutol for the first 2 months for treatment of pulmonary tuberculosis in Britain.*)

Daniel TM, Mahmoud AAF, Warren KS: Algorithms in the diagnosis and management of exotic diseases. J Infect Dis 134:417, 1976 (*Despite the obvious limitations of the algorithmic approach, this paper presents an accurate, practical, and concise overview of clinical tuberculosis and its management. It should be most helpful to physicians who see little tuberculosis and hence have come to regard it as an "exotic" disease.*)

Dutt AK, Jones L, Stead WW: Short-course chemotherapy with largely twice-weekly isoniazid-rifampin. Chest 75:441, 1979

Dutt AK, Moers D, Stead WW: Undesirable side effects of isoniazid and rifampin in largely twice-weekly short-course chemotherapy for tuberculosis. Am Rev Resp Dis 128:419, 1983 (*The initial and follow-up reports on the American trials of INH and rifampin for short-course chemotherapy.*)

East African/British Medical Research Councils: Controlled clinical trial of four short-course (6-month) regimens of chemotherapy for treatment of pulmonary tuberculosis. Lancet 2:237, 1974 (*An example of the British studies of short-course chemotherapy that have been conducted in Africa and also in the Orient. This study demonstrated excellent results with the use of INH, streptomycin, and rifampin for 6 months. Only 3% of 152 patients treated with this regimen relapsed. The cost effectiveness of this regimen has not been studied in the United States.*)

Guidelines for Short-Course Tuberculosis Chemotherapy. Morbidity and Mortality Weekly Reports 29:97, 1980 (*The USPHS recommendations for short-course chemotherapy, endorsing 9 months INH–rifampin as an acceptable alternative to standard 18–24 month regimens for pulmonary tuberculosis.*)

Hudson LD, Sharbaro JA: Twice weekly tuberculosis chemotherapy. JAMA 223:139, 1973 (*A study of 101 manifestly unreliable outpatients with active tuberculosis that demonstrates the usefulness of intermittent chemotherapy in this setting.*)

Johnston RF, Wildrick KH: "State of the art" review. The impact of chemotherapy on the care of patients with tuberculosis. Am Rev Resp Dis 109:636, 1974 (*A useful overview of the management of tuberculosis, which includes a discussion of skin testing, epidemiology, and BCG as well as chemotherapy.*)

Sharbaro JA: Tuberculosis: The new challenge to the practicing physician. Chest 68(Suppl):436, 1975 (*A very nice overview of tuberculosis today, with an emphasis on epidemiology.*)

Stead WW: Pathogenesis of the sporadic case of tuberculosis. N Engl J Med 277:1008, 1967 (*A lucid and important overview of the "unitary concept" of the pathogenesis of tuberculosis. This excellent paper clarifies relationship between primary infection, inactive disease, and reactivation tuberculosis.*)

Stead WW, Kerby GR, Schlueter DP et al: The clinical spectrum of primary tuberculosis in adults. Ann Intern Med 68:731, 1968 (*A clinical study of 27 adults with primary tuberculosis, which includes an excellent summary of the wide spectrum of events that may occur following initial infection by M. tuberculosis.*)

Stead WW et al: Tuberculosis as an endemic and nosocomial infection among the elderly in nursing homes. New Engl J Med 312:1483, 1985 (*This important paper shows that exogenous infection can occur in the elderly and that nosocomial tuberculosis may be an important problem in nursing homes. Despite the advanced age of these patients, INH prophylaxis was well tolerated and effective in tuberculin converters.*)

Wolinsky E: Nontuberculosis mycobacteria and associated diseases. Am Rev Resp Dis 119:107, 1979 (*A comprehensive and authoritative review of the "atypical mycobacteria". Although this paper is very long and contains more bacteriologic detail than will interest the primary care practitioner, it is nicely subdivided so that clinically useful information is readily accessible; 592 references.*)

Zakowsky P, Fligiel S, Berlin GW et al: Disseminated Mycobacterium avium-intracellulare infection in homosexual men dying of acquired immunodeficiency. JAMA 248:2980, 1982 (*An important atypical mycobacterial infection.*)

48
Management of Sarcoidosis
HARVEY B. SIMON, M.D.

Sarcoidosis is a disease characterized by formation of noncaseating granulomas, particularly in the lung but also occurring throughout the body. The precise etiology remains unknown, but activation of T-cell lymphocytes in the lung plays an important role in the pathogenesis of granuloma formation. In the United States, sarcoidosis is ten times more prevalent in blacks than whites; people of Scandinavian descent also have a high incidence of the disease. Females outnumber males. Onset is most often between ages 20 and 45.

Although a large percentage of patients with sarcoidosis are asymptomatic, diverse and clinically important syndromes do result; granuloma formation in the lung can be especially damaging, as can involvement in a number of other organ systems (*e.g.,* eye, gastrointestinal tract). Once diagnosis is established, the prime management decision regards need for corticosteroid therapy. Improved methods of monitoring disease activity have enhanced the clinician's ability to treat sarcoidosis effectively, while minimizing the risk of adverse effects from long-term steroids. The primary physician needs to know the most efficacious means of establishing the diagnosis, determining disease activity, and deciding upon the need for and duration of therapy with systemic steroids.

PATHOPHYSIOLOGY, CLINICAL PRESENTATION, AND COURSE

Pathophysiology. The cause of sarcoidosis is unknown. A variety of infectious and exogenous agents have been suggested as inciting factors, but whether one or several agents are involved remains conjectural. It is suspected that the granulomas and inflammatory reactions of sarcoidosis are due to an abnormal immunologic response to a provocative agent in susceptible hosts.

Although the etiology of sarcoidosis is unknown, the pathogenesis of its granulomatous inflammation is being clarified. Bronchoalveolar lavage studies reveal that the early stage of pulmonary sarcoid consists of an alveolitis, with an increased number of T-lymphocytes. Helper T-cells predominate, and there are an increased number of "activated" lymphocytes capable of secreting various soluble mediators or lymphokines, which may recruit monocytes and transform them into the macrophages of granulomas. The alveolites of early disease and the subsequent granulomatous inflammation are reversible, either spontaneously or with corticosteroid therapy, but the later fibrosis that characterizes advanced chronic sarcoidosis is irreversible.

In contrast to the increased numbers and activity of helper T-cells in the lungs, the peripheral blood of patients with sarcoidosis may show a decreased number of T-lymphocytes; this may account for the depressed cell-mediated immunity and cutaneous anergy observed in many such patients. However, the blood of patients with sarcoid often reflects increased activity of B-lymphocytes, accounting for the hypergammaglobulinemia and elevated antibody levels and circulating immune complexes that are often observed.

The granulomas of pulmonary sarcoidosis often resolve spontaneously, leaving the lung morphologically unscathed. However, in about 20% of patients, the process is more destructive, characterized by interstitial fibrosis, obliteration of capillaries, and destruction of pulmonary architecture. The end stage is formation of cystic spaces interspersed with bands of connective tissue. Once fibrotic changes occur, they are irreversible.

Clinical Manifestations of sarcoidosis reflect the sites of granulomatous inflammation. The most common presentation, especially in young adults, is bilateral hilar adenopathy, which occurs in 50% and is often detected on routine chest x-ray. About 25% present with bilateral hilar adenopathy and

pulmonary infiltrates, and 15% with infiltrates alone. Disease in the hilum is not associated with invasion or compression of bronchi or nodal calcification. Erythema nodosum or uveitis (manifested by red, watery eyes) may accompany hilar adenopathy. Some patients complain of cough, shortness of breath, wheezing, or chest discomfort as well as constitutional symptoms of fever, malaise, and fatigue.

Though pulmonary symptoms are the most frequent, sarcoidosis may present with extrathoracic disease, including hepatomegaly, splenomegaly, or uveitis. Other presenting manifestations include fever of unknown origin, granulomatous hepatitis, salivary and lacrimal gland enlargement, arthritis, peripheral adenopathy, and skin lesions. Hypercalcemia due to increased sensitivity to vitamin D is reported in 10% to 30%, but it is sustained in only 2% to 3%. Cardiac conduction abnormalities, such as heart block, and neurologic abnormalities (including facial palsies) are each seen in about 5% of cases. In addition, there are many case reports of unusual presentations.

Intrathoracic sarcoidosis can be divided into four stages. In stage 0 the chest x-ray is normal. In stage 1, bilateral hilar adenopathy is present; most patients are asymptomatic, and pulmonary function tests show normal mechanics, but the carbon monoxide diffusion capacity may be impaired. In stage 2, both hilar adenopathy and pulmonary infiltrates are present; pulmonary function tests show predominantly restrictive defects. In stage 3 disease, pulmonary infiltrates are present, but hilar adenopathy has resolved; restrictive and obstructive defects are present, and these patients may display clinical and radiographic findings or cor pulmonale. Whereas earlier stages of sarcoidosis are characterized by inflammatory changes that often resolve spontaneously, stage 3 reflects fibrosis and only 20% of patients experience spontaneous remission.

Diagnosis of sarcoidosis is sometimes a clinical challenge. It is increasingly accepted that asymptomatic, bilateral hilar adenopathy with or without uveitis or erythema nodosum is likely to be due to sarcoidosis. In a retrospective series of 100 patients with bilateral hilar adenopathy, conducted prior to the advent of AIDS, all 30 who were asymptomatic had sarcoid. Moreover, 50 of 52 with bilateral hilar adenopathy and negative physical examinations also had the disease. All eleven patients with neoplasm were symptomatic, and 9 had easily identifiable extrathoracic tumor upon physical examination. Among symptomatic patients, all with erythema nodosum or uveitis had sarcoid. Thus, the patient with bilateral hilar adenopathy who is asymptomatic, has a negative physical examination, or has erythema nodosum or uveitis does not necessarily require a biopsy to confirm the diagnosis of sarcoidosis. Nevertheless, some clinicians prefer to obtain a tissue diagnosis in all cases of sarcoidosis, including those with asymptomatic bilateral hilar adenopathy.

A decision to biopsy must be made by viewing the potential for discovering treatable conditions and balancing this probability against the risks associated with the procedure itself. For the diagnosis of hilar adenopathy, mediastinoscopy is the most direct approach and is usually well tolerated. For the documentation of pulmonary sarcoid, fiberoptic bronchoscopy with transbronchial biopsy is currently in favor. This procedure has a reported sensitivity of 60% to 80%. In addition, bronchoscopy allows direct visualization of the bronchial tree so that it can be helpful in ruling out tumor and obtaining samples of secretions for laboratory study. The major complication of transbronchial lung biopsy is pneumothorax; this is infrequent in experienced hands.

In patients with extrathoracic sarcoidosis, accessible sites for biopsy include skin lesions and enlarged peripheral lymph nodes. Biopsy of conjunctivae, salivary glands, and liver may reveal noncaseating granulomas, even when there is no clinical evidence of sarcoid in these tissues. Because of the low morbidity of salivary gland and conjunctival biopsies, these may be particularly useful. It must be remembered that the histologic appearance of sarcoid granulomas is not etiologically specific. Therefore, the other known causes of noncaseating granulomas must be ruled out, including tuberculosis, syphilis, berylliosis, brucellosis, Q fever, biliary cirrhosis, Wegener's granulomatosis, drug reactions, and local sarcoidal reactions in nodes draining solid tumors. Hodgkin's disease is particularly difficult to exclude with mediastinoscopy in patients presenting with unilateral or asymmetric hilar adenopathy.

The Kveim test has also been used in the diagnosis of sarcoidosis. The test requires the intracutaneous injection of heat-sterilized human sarcoid tissue, usually spleen. A positive reaction consists of the development of epithelioid granulomas detected on skin biopsy of the injection site at 4 to 6 weeks. The delay period, variability of the material available for injection, and the high incidence of false-positive and false-negative results (due to impure batches of antigen) have limited the usefulness of the Kveim reaction.

Other abnormalities that may be present in patients with sarcoidosis include cutaneous anergy, hyperglobulinemia, abnormal liver function tests, and elevated levels of lysozyme; none of these findings is specific, but together they are supportive of the diagnosis. Similarly, bone films of the hands may reveal changes suggestive of sarcoid.

Serum levels of angiotension converting enzyme (ACE) are elevated in many patients with sarcoidosis. ACE determinations lack both sensitivity and specificity for establishing a diagnosis of sarcoidosis, but ACE levels can be useful markers of disease activity and therapeutic responsiveness in individual patients (see below). The same is true of [67]gallium scanning; increased lung activity reflects active alveolitis, and scans can also detect disease activity in extrathoracic sites such as the lacrimal and parotid glands.

Natural History. Patients with clear lungs and asymptomatic hilar adenopathy have an excellent prognosis. In one large series of untreated cases, complete remission occurred in over 75% within 5 years. In 50% with untreated pulmonary parenchymal involvement, complete resolution was seen within 2 years. In one third of those in whom clearing did not occur, severe fibrosis developed. Overall, at 5 years, 87% were clinically well, 10% had died of respiratory failure, and 3% were disabled by pulmonary disease.

Most natural history data derive from referral centers. In a report from a nonreferral setting, 86 patients were followed for 10 years in a primary care practice; only 12 developed pulmonary fibrosis, and none experienced respiratory failure or cor pulmonale. This latter study suggests that the course of sarcoid may be more benign than has been reputed from referral centers, which are more likely to attract complicated cases.

Hepatic granulomas are present often, but clinically symptomatic hepatitis is much less common. In occasional patients, hepatic failure or portal hypertension occurs. Cranial and peripheral neuropathies tend to occur early in the disease and are usually transient; however, in some patients, significant neurologic damage is seen. Uveitis affects about 15%, comes on acutely and often resolves spontaneously. More worrisome is chronic iridocyclitis; it presents as pain and blurring of vision and may go on to produce cataracts, secondary glaucoma, and blindness. As noted above, hypercalcemia persists in about 2% to 3%, though it may be found transiently in up to 30%. Cardiac involvement with granulomata is found in 20% at autopsy, but only 5% have clinically significant disorders of conduction or impulse formation. Rarely, infiltration of the myocardium produces pump failure.

The course of patients with sarcoid may occasionally be complicated by infections such as tuberculosis, aspergillar fungus balls, candidiasis, and cryptococcosis, attributable in part to the disease and in part to the use of long-term steroid therapy.

PRINCIPLES OF MANAGEMENT, THERAPEUTIC RECOMMENDATIONS, AND MONITORING

The goals in the treatment of sarcoid include relief of symptoms and prevention of significant impairment of organ function. The natural history of sarcoid is variable, and hence the indications for therapy are often debatable. It is established that patients who present with asymptomatic bilateral hilar adenopathy or erythema-nodosum usually have a benign course, so that no treatment is indicated in the absence of symptoms.

The principal treatment for sarcoidosis is *systemic corticosteroid therapy.* The great variability in the disease's clinical course and the previous lack of sensitive indicators of disease activity have made it difficult to rigorously document the efficacy of steroid therapy. Older studies relied on such crude measures as symptoms, x-ray findings, and pulmonary function tests. Recent evaluations have examined the effect of corticosteroids on more direct indicators of the disease process (see below) and have found marked suppression of the alveolitis, but little influence on anatomic abnormalities present before initiation of steroid therapy.

The view that emerges from available studies is that glucocorticoids should be given to patients who are symptomatic and have clear evidence of active disease, such as an elevated angiotensin converting enzyme level or a very positive gallium scan. Most authorities recommend commencing with large doses of steroids (*e.g.,* 40–60 mg prednisone) given on a daily basis for anywhere from 6 weeks to 6 months, followed by tapering and/or switching to alternate day therapy if measures of disease activity indicate response. Steroid therapy is most effective if instituted early, because once the disease has progressed to fibrosis, the process cannot be reversed. However, there is no evidence that prophylactic treatment is worth the adverse effects of chronic steroid use (see Chapter 103).

Steroids consistently produce subjective improvement in dyspneic patients with early sarcoidosis and may even reduce pulmonary infiltrates when they are due to alveolitis or granulomatous changes. Lung volumes usually improve, but not necessarily the diffusing capacity, which may be permanently altered by destructive changes. Relapses upon cessation of therapy are frequent, necessitating close monitoring for at least 12 months after discontinuation of treatment. *Alternate-day steroid therapy* has proved successful as a maintenance program in some patients, controlling disease when given after an initial course of daily steroids; this approach minimizes the adverse effects of long-term steroid therapy.

Adrenal corticosteroids are also indicated for active ocular disease. Every sarcoid patient should have an ophthalmologic examination, especially if visual symptoms develop. Topical steroids may be used, but systemic therapy is usually added. Treatment is also indicated in the presence of significant or progressive involvement of any organ. Onset of hepatitis, facial nerve palsies, meningitis, myocardial conduction defects, hypercalcemia, or persistent constitutional symptoms (fever, fatigue) are other indications for treatment.

Whenever steroid therapy is carried out, objective documentation of response to treatment is essential. Because the predominant pathologic process in sarcoidosis is an alveolitis leading to granuloma formation, and corticosteroids work by suppressing the alveolitis, the optimal means of monitoring disease activity and response to therapy is to follow measures of the alveolitis. Previously employed means of objectively monitoring sarcoidosis (chest x-ray, lung volumes, diffusing capacity) have been unable to distinguish between extent of alveolitis and anatomic derangement. Although these parameters are useful for determining severity of disease, they are insensitive measures of disease activity and not very reliable for judging adequacy of therapy or need for continued treatment.

Monitoring. Bronchoalveolar lavage, gallium scanning, and angiotensin converting enzyme levels have proven to be more sensitive measures of disease activity. *Bronchoalveolar lavage* is used to sample inflammatory cells on the surface of the lower respiratory tract in an effort to gauge alveolar inflammatory activity. Cell type and state of activation are examined. Close correlations between lavage results and biopsy specimens have been documented. Results are usually expressed as the number and/or proportion of inflammatory and immune effector cells that are T-lymphocytes or IgG-secreting cells. Serial studies in sarcoid patients whose T-cell proportions remain low have shown little risk of deterioration in pulmonary function, whereas risk of further compromise is high in those with persistently high T-cell proportions. The number of cells decreases dramatically in patients who respond to corticosteroids. Lavage has been used extensively in some centers to monitor sarcoidosis, with little morbidity or discomfort noted. Concurrent bronchial inflammatory disease may distort the results.

Gallium scanning has proven very useful. Gallium concentrates in sites of acute and chronic inflammation. Increased uptake is a sensitive, but nonspecific marker of ongoing inflammation. Good correlations have been found between gallium scan findings and the severity, activity, and location of sarcoidosis as determined by lavage and biopsy; results also very closely parallel changes in clinical course. The test is noninvasive and exposes the patient to a minimal dose of radiation, thus allowing serial studies. Compared to other methods, gallium scanning has been found to be the most sensitive measure of disease activity. Its major disadvantage is its cost.

A less expensive alternative to gallium scanning is the serum *angiotensin converting enzyme* (ACE) level. Marked elevations in ACE among patients with sarcoid were found during investigations of how chronic lung diseases affect this important substance. ACE seems to be produced in large quantities by epithelioid cells within the sarcoid granuloma. Elevations are nonspecific and cannot be used for diagnosis of sarcoidosis, but do parallel the activity of the inflammatory process and provide a reasonably sensitive measure of disease activity. The sensitivity of ACE is slightly less than that of the gallium scan. If ACE is elevated from the outset, it makes for a very cost-effective means of monitoring disease activity and response to therapy. However, if the ACE level is not initially elevated, the gallium scan should be used to follow the course of the illness and adequacy of treatment.

Other nonspecific measures of inflammation, such as the *erythrocyte sedimentation rate* and *serum globulin level* have shown inadequate sensitivity to be useful for monitoring.

PATIENT EDUCATION

The diagnosis of sarcoidosis is far more common than are serious consequences of the disease. The nature of the disease should be carefully explained, with emphasis on its relatively benign, self-limited nature in the asymptomatic patient. Patients who are treated with steroids should be counseled about the side effects and risks inherent in such treatment (see Chapter 103). The need for careful follow-up must be emphasized in both the asymptomatic patient (to detect the development of functional abnormalities) and the patient with symptoms (to document objective benefits of treatment). Patients should be instructed about early signs of important complications, such as red eyes, blurred vision, eye pain, and dyspnea on exertion, so that therapy is not unnecessarily delayed.

ANNOTATED BIBLIOGRAPHY

Crystal RG, Roberts WC, Hunningham GW et al: Pulmonary sarcoidosis: A disease characterized and perpetuated by activated lung T-lymphocytes. Ann Intern Med 94:73, 1981 (*A comprehensive review of exciting new insights into the pathogenesis and immunology of sarcoidosis; 280 references.*)

Harkleroad LE, Young RL, Savage PJ et al: Pulmonary sarcoidosis: Long-term follow-up of the effects of steroid therapy. Chest 82: 84, 1982 (*Although only 25 patients were entered into this alternate-case steroid trial, a 15 year follow-up was available. There was no discernable benefit from early steroid therapy.*)

Israel HL, Fouts DU, Begys RA: A controlled trial of prednisone treatment of sarcoidosis. Am Rev Respir Dis 107:609, 1973 (*A prospective study of 90 patients. At 3 months, those on prednisone showed improvement in all pulmonary parameters measured, but over the long term there were no significant differences between groups on prednisone and those on placebo.*)

James DG: Kveim revisited, reassessed. N Engl J Med 292:859, 1975 (*An editorial arguing that previous reports of the lack of specificity of the test were due to preparation of impure batches of sarcoid splenic suspension and that the test is actually quite specific when proper antigen is used.*)

Johns CJ, Macgregor MI, Zachary JB et al: Extended experience in the long-term corticosteroid treatment of pulmonary sarcoidosis. Ann NY Acad Sci 278:722, 1976 (*A series of 192 cases of severe disease treated with prednisone. Clinical improvement resulted from treatment, and relapses were frequent when therapy was terminated. In cases where relapse occurs and recurs, long-term therapy with 10 to 15 mg of prednisone is required, often for years.*)

Koontz CH, Joyner LR, Nelson RA: Transbronchial lung biopsy via the fiber optic bronchoscope in sarcoidosis. Ann Intern Med 85: 64, 1976 (*A prospective study of 42 patients with suspected and later proven sarcoidosis. Test sensitivity was 63%. There was a higher probability of a positive biopsy in symptomatic patients.*)

Lawrence EC, Teague RB, Gottlieb MS et al: Serial changes in markers of disease activity with corticosteroid treatment in sarcoidosis. Am J Med 74:747, 1983 (*Serial evaluations of various disease activity markers with prednisone therapy. Gallium scan and ACE levels were the most sensitive measures of response.*)

Lieberman J, Schleissner LA, Nosal A et al: Clinical correlations of serum angiotensin-converting enzyme (ACE) in sarcoidosis. A longitudinal study of serum ACE, [67]gallium scans, chest roentgenograms and pulmonary function. Chest 84:522, 1983 (*One of many studies documenting the usefulness of longitudinal ACE determinations to follow disease activity. This careful study also measured other parameters and found [67]gallium scans particularly useful.*)

Reich JM, Johnson RE: Course and prognosis of sarcoidiosis in a nonreferral setting. Analyses of 86 patients observed for 10 years. Am J Med 78:61, 1985 (*A helpful natural history study suggesting that the course of sarcoid may be more benign than has been reputed from referral centers, which are more likely to attract complicated cases. Of the 12 patients in this study with pulmonary fibrosis, none have developed respiratory failure or cor pulmonale.*)

Siltzbach LE, James DG, Neville E et al: Course and prognosis of sarcoidosis around the world. Am J Med 57:847, 1974 (*A terse summary of clinical findings showing no differences of significance among different races and ethnic groups.*)

Winterbauer RH, Belic N, Moores KD: Clinical interpretation of bilateral hilar adenopathy. Ann Intern Med 78:65, 1973 (*A retrospective series of 100 cases. Authors argue asymptomatic patients with bilateral adenopathy only need not undergo biopsy for definitive diagnosis.*)

49

Smoking Cessation Techniques in Primary Care Practice

NANCY A. RIGOTTI, M.D.

Cigarette smoking is the major preventable cause of death in the United States. Strong evidence documents benefit from cessation of smoking, even for patients who have already developed chronic tobacco-related disease (see Chapter 32). Although the health risks of smoking are widely recognized, one third of adult Americans continue to smoke, and adolescents are taking up the habit in large numbers. Nevertheless, many people are eager to quit and often come to the primary physician for advice. Numerous studies have shown that physicians can change a patient's smoking habits. The primary care physician needs to be expert in motivating patients to quit and in advising them on the best means to accomplish their goal. This requires knowledge about available smoking cessation techniques and an appreciation of how and when to utilize them.

EPIDEMIOLOGY OF SMOKING AND QUITTING

Since 1964, when the Surgeon General's Report first publicized the health risks of smoking, there has been a decline in cigarette smoking by adults in the United States. This decrease is largely attributable to the increasing number of smokers who have quit, rather than to a fall in the number of smokers taking up the habit. Smoking in adolescence—the time when smoking usually begins—has fallen little since its peak in the 1970s. Adolescent girls are smoking in numbers comparable to boys; the historical gender difference continues to narrow. This is worrisome because women who smoke during the reproductive years incur special risks with pregnancy and oral contraceptive use. In 1980, 38% of men and 30% of women smoked regularly. Smoking is more common in populations that are nonwhite and have less education and lower incomes.

Nearly all smokers are aware of the health hazards of smoking and say they would like to quit, but most have difficulty doing so. In a recent national survey, only 30% of smokers who attempted to stop within the past year were abstinent for 6 months. Although the success rate for any single quitting attempt is low, smokers who repeatedly try to quit increase their likelihood of success. Lighter smokers are more successful than heavier smokers. Female smokers make more attempts to quit, but men are more likely to be successful. Smokers most likely to quit are those who expect their attempt to succeed, who have a strong belief in their personal control over events, feel competent and personally secure, and have a good social support system. The smoking habits of the spouse and, in some studies, friends, are important; those with nonsmoking spouses are more likely to succeed.

Health concerns are the most common reasons given by former smokers for quitting. However, the risks of lung cancer and heart disease are less often cited than are minor smoking-related ailments such as cough, dyspnea, and sore throat. Minor symptoms may successfully motivate a smoker to quit by making personally salient the more serious health risks of smoking. Illness in one smoker can influence other smokers to quit.

Other reasons for quitting cited by former smokers include a desire to exert self-control over one's life, aesthetic objections to the smoking habit, and fear of setting a bad example for others. The cost of cigarettes exerts little influence among adults.

The vast majority of exsmokers—95%—have quit on their own, without the aid of organized programs. Smokers who quit abruptly are more likely to be successful than those who attempt to gradually reduce the number of cigarettes smoked. Some reduction in cigarette consumption can be part of a smoker's preparation for quitting as long as a definite date for abrupt cessation is set.

WHY PEOPLE SMOKE

Smoking is a complex behavior that is initiated and maintained for different reasons. The influence of peers and parents appears to be most important in the initiation of smoking. Adolescents whose parents and friends smoke are more likely to begin smoking. Once the smoking habit is established, it is sustained by many factors.

Both pharmacologic and psychologic models have been proposed to explain what maintains smoking behavior. The *psychologic model* regards smoking as a learned behavior that continues because it is rewarding to the smoker. Certain situations, such as finishing a meal, become strongly associated with smoking and trigger the urge to smoke. Smokers also use cigarettes to handle environmental stress and regulate emotions, especially strong negative emotions like anger.

The *pharmacologic model* emphasizes physical addiction to nicotine. The smoker smokes to maintain a constant blood level of nicotine and thereby avert the *withdrawal syndrome,* characterized by falls in heart rate, blood pressure, basal metabolic rate, and changes in EEG rhythms and REM sleep patterns. Craving for nicotine is the most common subjective complaint of withdrawal, but other symptoms include irritability, inability to concentrate, daytime drowsiness and fatigue, sleep disturbances, headache, nausea, alteration in bowel habits, and increased appetite. Symptoms often begin within hours after cessation of smoking, but duration and severity are highly variable, representing different degrees of nicotine addiction among smokers. There is no simple test to measure nicotine addiction, but heavily addicted smokers tend to have their first cigarette shortly after arising, smoke more and stronger cigarettes, inhale deeply, and have difficulty not smoking for even a few hours.

The pharmacologic model can explain the difficulties with initial cessation but cannot explain why smokers have difficulty remaining abstinent after the first few days. In fact, the majority of smokers who stop temporarily resume smoking within a few months. Those few who remain abstinent for a year can be considered permanent exsmokers. Relapse usually occurs at times of interpersonal conflict, negative emotions, or social pressure to smoke. Alcohol is commonly involved. Cigarettes represent a familiar coping strategy resorted to at these times of high stress.

INTERVENTION TECHNIQUES

A wide variety of strategies exists to help people quit smoking, ranging from formal treatment programs administered in a group setting to self-help booklets designed for the individual smoker. There is currently no single superior smoking cessation technique. Little research has attempted to match individual characteristics of smokers with their responses to particular cessation programs. Strategies that combine behavioral and pharmacologic techniques appear to be most effective.

Most available techniques are more effective at helping smokers to quit than they are at maintaining long-term abstinence. Short-term cessation rates of 70% to 80% are common among programs. However, a predictable and rapid return to smoking follows initial cessation. A 1-year cessation rate of 30% to 35% is considered the standard for effective smoking cessation programs that involve self-selected, highly motivated patients.

Pharmacologic Methods. Pharmacologic methods aim to relieve symptoms of nicotine withdrawal. The use of *minor tranquilizers* to minimize withdrawal has not proved effective. *Lobeline* (Nikoban), a non-nicotine substitute whose autonomic effects mimic those of nicotine, is no more effective than placebo.

Nicotine chewing gum (Nicorette) allows the smoker to break the cigarette habit without enduring the symptoms of nicotine withdrawal. It also provides an oral substitute for cigarettes. Nicotine, released from the gum by chewing, is absorbed through the oral mucosa, resulting in blood levels comparable to those achieved by smoking. The rate of release is controlled by how fast the patient chews. Exposure to the other harmful constituents of cigarette smoke is avoided. Patients using the gum show less of a tendency to overeat upon cessation of smoking.

Nicotine gum is more effective than placebo when used in conjunction with a behavioral program for self-selected, motivated smokers attending a smoking withdrawal clinic; 1-year cessation rates of 30% to 50% have been reported, representing an advance over behavioral treatments alone. The gum may be especially useful in smokers heavily addicted to nicotine. When the gum is prescribed by physicians for less motivated patients, cessation rates are lower, and its effectiveness is less certain. In one randomized trial in Britain, nicotine gum added to a physician's advice to stop smoking led to more short-term smoking cessation than physician advice with or without a placebo gum, but there was no difference in cessation rates at 1 year, which were 10%. However, another study of British general practitioners found that adding gum to physician advice resulted in a significantly higher rate of long-term smoking cessation (9% at 1 year) than did physician advice alone (4%).

To use the gum, smokers are instructed to pick a target date when they will stop smoking. After that, they chew the gum whenever they have an urge to smoke, usually consuming a dozen pieces daily at the onset. Side-effects are mostly a consequence of overly vigorous chewing and release of excess nicotine—sore jaw, mouth irritation or ulcers, nervousness, dizziness, nausea, vomiting, hiccups, intestinal distress, headache, and excess salivation. To reduce these symptoms, smokers should chew the gum very slowly, just enough to detect a slight tingling taste in the mouth. Gum use continues in a tapering fashion until the craving for cigarettes ceases, usually by 3 to 12 weeks. Five percent to 10% of long-term users develop dependence and have difficulty stopping. Patients with recent myocardial infarction, unstable angina, or serious arrhythmias, and women who are pregnant or breast-feeding should avoid gum use. Best results are obtained when gum use is accompanied by a program to teach behavioral skills, either in a group or self-help format.

Behavioral Methods. The behavioral model of smoking has inspired a host of techniques to manipulate environmental cues that trigger or reward smoking. These techniques form the core of most smoking cessation programs in current use.

Stimulus-control strategies require the individual to identify and control environmental stimuli that trigger smoking. Cues are first identified by *self-monitoring.* The smoker carries a sheet wrapped around the cigarette pack on which he records the circumstances in which each cigarette is smoked. Environmental cues, identified from this daily log, are then progressively avoided or modified so that they no longer trigger smoking. The behavior is separated from its triggers by *progressive restriction* of the situations in which smoking is permitted. At a point in the relearning process, smoking stops altogether.

Controlled studies have not demonstrated impressive long-term cessation with this approach. Smokers may decrease their cigarette consumption but are less successful at total cessation, and those who stop have a high relapse rate. By itself, the technique is more effective in preparing the smoker to quit than in achieving long-term cessation.

Another stimulus-control strategy is *contingency contracting.* It requires the smoker to deposit money, which is returned if the maintenance of nonsmoking or program attendance is achieved.

Aversive conditioning techniques pair an unwanted act like smoking with an unpleasant stimulus to make the act less likely to occur. Smoking, real or imagined, has been paired with electric shock, an unpleasant imagined sensation like vomiting (*covert sensitization*) or a self-administered snap of a rubber band worn on the wrist. The most effective aversive stimulus is cigarette smoke, which is unpleasant even to a heavy smoker and has the advantage of being encountered by the smoker outside the laboratory. In the best-known technique, *rapid smoking,* the smoker is required to inhale every 6 seconds until unable to tolerate further smoking because of nausea, headache, or lightheadedness. A related technique is *satiation;* smokers purposely double or triple their base smoking rate for up to a day prior to cessation.

The rapid smoking technique effectively reduces the urge to smoke and produces high rates of short-term cessation, but relapse occurs rapidly unless other techniques are employed. The safety of rapid smoking has been a concern because of the smoker's intense exposure to nicotine and carbon monoxide. However, no serious medical complications have been reported with supervised use of rapid smoking among healthy people and those with mild cardiopulmonary disease.

Hypnosis. There is much interest in hypnosis; many hope it offers a painless way to stop smoking. Most studies evaluating hypnosis have been uncontrolled, with small samples and brief follow-up. Studies have reported abstinence rates of 20% to 25% at 1 year, comparable to the standard achieved by behavioral programs.

Acupuncture. The insertion of needles at acupuncture points, often around the ear, has been claimed to reduce the urge to smoke and lead to long-term cessation in several uncontrolled studies. However, randomized-control trial found no benefit; the cessation rate was less than 20%.

Organized Group Programs. Both nonprofit and commercial organizations offer group programs for smoking cessation. Most programs have a high drop-out rate and have not been adequately evaluated.

The oldest and best known is the Five-Day Plan developed in 1963 with sponsorship of the Seventh Day Adventist church. It consists of meetings on 5 consecutive nights and is low in cost. Techniques used are health education, encouragement to quit, and nonspecific support.

Adding behavior modification techniques to group programs has improved their effectiveness. SmokEnders is a costly commercial program consisting of 9 weekly meetings run by exsmokers. Cessation occurs after the fifth meeting, followed by group support. In one long-term study, 70% of smokers were not smoking at the end of the program and 39% remained abstinent 4 years later. However, on reanalysis, the long-term cessation rate was 24%, equivalent to the standard rates achieved by other behavioral programs. The American Cancer Society and the American Lung Association offer similar group programs at lower cost. More intensive group programs with extended follow-up offered in the medical setting have achieved better results.

Individual Aids. Booklets, audiovisual aids, telephone services, nonprescription filters, and chewing gum are available to help the smoker who wishes to quit on his own. Few have been evaluated. *Self-help manuals* range from booklets with practical tips on how to quit to longer books containing comprehensive programs of behavior modification. Many are available at minimal cost through nonprofit organizations like the American Cancer Society, the American Lung Association, and the National Cancer Institute (see Table 49-1). These groups also sponsor *telephone services* that provide education, encouragement, advice, and referrals. Use of the American Lung Association manuals has produced cessation rates of 12% at 1 month and 5% at 1 year.

A series of progressively stronger *filters,* which gradually restrict the tar and nicotine delivery from the smoker's own cigarettes, has not proved to be effective. A nonprescription *chewing gum* (Healthbreak) employs the principles of aversive conditioning. It releases silver salts into the mouth, which produce an unpleasant taste if a cigarette is subsequently smoked. Its effectiveness is dependent on patient compliance. The gum has reduced cigarette intake, but has not been shown to lead to long-term cessation.

THE PHYSICIAN'S ROLE

Health is the most common reason given by former smokers for quitting. Smokers who develop the symptoms of cardiopulmonary disease or become pregnant are more likely to quit smoking on their own and are more responsive to intervention efforts. Because physicians see smokers at these times, they can be especially influential in altering their patients' smoking habits.

The likelihood that a smoker will quit increases with the severity of the illness. Although fewer than 5% of smokers in the general population quit each year, 10% to 15% of men quit in the year after they are identified as being at high risk for coronary artery disease. One third of smokers in one study quit after the new diagnosis of angina, and many studies report that 30% to 50% of patients surviving a myocardial infarction stop smoking permanently. Increased rates of ces-

Table 49-1. Smoking Cessation Guides for Physicians and Patients

For the Physician

1. *The Physician's Guide; How to Help Your Hypertensive Patients Stop Smoking.* National Heart, Lung, and Blood Institute. NIH Publication 83-171, 1983.
   A well-designed guide detailing a practical, brief strategy and a more extended program, both applicable to all patients in office practice.
2. *Helping Smokers Quit Kit* (English and Spanish). National Cancer Institute
   A complete packet of materials for the physician's office, including a physician's guide and pamphlets to hand out to patients.

For the Patient

1. *Clearing the Air* (English or Spanish). National Cancer Institute.
2. *7-Day Plan to Help You Stop Smoking.* American Cancer Society
   Two free booklets providing a self-help program for smoking cessation.
3. *Quit for Good.* National Cancer Institute
   Two-booklet program for cesstion and maintenance available free to health professionals.
4. *I Quit Kit.* American Cancer Society
   A multimedia program, including booklets, a poster, a record, pins, and signs, providing a more extensive quitting program. Available at minimal cost.
5. *Freedom from Smoking in 20 Days* and *A Lifetime of Freedom from Smoking.* American Lung Association
   Two longer booklets available at minimal cost. The first provides an organized plan for quitting over 20 days; the second is a program to maintain abstinence.

sation are also reported in smokers with chronic obstructive pulmonary disease. During pregnancy, 20% of women smokers stop smoking, but the majority resume smoking after delivery. Many smokers quit temporarily when they have an acute respiratory illness.

Surveys indicate that physicians are not taking advantage of their opportunity to alter their patients' smoking habits. Fewer than one third of current smokers recall being told to quit by a physician. In fact, physician's advice can make a difference. The effectiveness of advice given by primary care physicians to stop smoking was demonstrated in a study of London general practitioners. Patients were randomized into three groups: one group routinely advised to stop smoking; another given the advice bolstered by a pamphlet and a warning to expect follow-up; and controls given no special advice. The groups receiving antismoking advice had significantly greater smoking cessation that was maintained for 1 year. The effect was enhanced with the leaflet and follow-up. The 5% cessation rate achieved was less than that reported by smoking cessation programs, but because many more smokers visit doctors than attend programs, brief physician's advice has a greater potential to alter smoking habits. A physician's advice appears to be more effective when the smoker is acutely ill or faces the new diagnosis of serious disease. In one study, smokers given brief antismoking advice during hospitalization for a myocardial infarction had a 63% 1-year cessation rate, compared to 27% of patients receiving no advice.

Physicians who devote more time to counseling smokers can expect to be even more effective. In one study, a regularly scheduled follow-up visit for smoking counseling was more effective than one-time advice. The physician can be most effective by advising all smokers to quit and providing more counseling to susceptible smokers—those with respiratory symptoms or the recent diagnosis of a serious smoking-related disease.

RECOMMENDATIONS

Smoking cessation strategy for office practice is summarized in Table 49-2.

1. *Assess smoking habits.* Smoking habits should be assessed as a part of every encounter in ambulatory practice. A smoking history should be taken from all smokers to assess the patient's current interest in quitting and to anticipate difficulties with cessation, such as a strong component of nicotine addiction or lack of social support. The smoker's prior cessation efforts and current medical and social situation can help guide treatment recommendations.

2. *Advise every smoker to stop smoking.* A firm statement to stop smoking should be made to all smokers at every visit. Total cessation is the goal.

3. *Motivate the smoker to attempt to quit.* This is the physician's primary role. The strategy should focus on health concerns, tailored to the individual's clinical situation. The

Table 49-2. Smoking Cessation Strategy for Office Practice

1. Assess smoking habits
   A. Smoking and quitting history
   B. Interest in cessation
   C. Likelihood of success
   D. Identify potential motivating factors
2. Advise every smoker to stop smoking
3. Motivate the smoker to attempt to quit
   A. Emphasize benefits of cessation
   B. Focus on short-term changes
   C. Tailor to the clinical situation
      1. Asymptomatic smoker
      2. Acute respiratory illness
      3. Chronic cardiopulmonary illness
      4. Pregnancy
   D. Address common fears
   E. Use physiologic feedback
4. Ask for a commitment to quit
5. Help the smoker to quit
   A. Physician counseling
   B. Self-help materials
   C. Nicotine gum
   D. Referrals to formal smoking withdrawal programs
   E. Anticipate problems
      1. Withdrawal symptoms
      2. Weight gain
6. Follow-up
   A. Put smoking on the problem list
   B. Follow-up visits or phone calls
   C. Continued monitoring at each visit

approach should be positive, emphasizing the benefits of cessation and including short-term benefits, such as increased exercise tolerance or improved taste and smell. The contribution of smoking to any of the patient's current symptoms should be emphasized.

The asymptomatic smoker may be the most difficult one to motivate. But most smokers do have minor smoking-related symptoms that would improve with cessation, such as morning cough or limited exercise tolerance. Smokers unable to quit for their own sake may do so for their children's health or a safe pregnancy.

Smokers with an *acute respiratory illness* commonly stop smoking for a few days on their own. The physician can suggest that the smoker take advantage of the period of reduced desire to stop smoking permanently. For the smoker with a *chronic disease* associated with smoking, the physician should point out the potential for reduced symptoms, improved function, and slowed progression of disease. Radiologic or pulmonary function tests can provide proof of smoking-related damage. However, these tests are not recommended for asymptomatic smokers because they do not detect early disease, and a normal result may give inadvertent reassurance to a smoker that his health is not being jeopardized.

Smokers reluctant to attempt cessation often harbor a specific concern, such as a fear of failure, weight gain, withdrawal symptoms, or loss of a pleasurable habit or a way to handle life stresses. Helping the smoker to clarify this concern and to develop his own counterarguments can be helpful. If the smoker remains unwilling to consider cessation, the physician should stop with a strong antismoking recommendation, but make a renewed effort at subsequent visits.

4. *Ask for a commitment to quit.* Encourage but do not force the smoker to set a date on which he will stop smoking, preferably within 4 weeks. Ideal quitting dates are landmarks like a birthday, anniversary, New Year's Day, or times when life stresses are minimized, such as the first day of a vacation. The physician should record the date in the medical record, as a reminder to follow the patient's progress.

5. *Help the smoker to quit.* The physician should be prepared to help smokers who express an interest in making a cessation attempt. The extent of this help will vary. The physician should express confidence in the patient's ability to quit, direct the smoker to sources of further help, and discuss anticipated withdrawal symptoms. Helpful behavioral hints should be offered (Table 49-3). Smokers concerned about weight gain should be advised to begin a concurrent exercise program and keep low-calorie snacks readily at hand; they may consider using nicotine gum if advised. Smokers who develop increased cough and sputum immediately after cessation should be reassured that this is temporary, common, and results from a return of ciliary clearance activities in the respiratory tract.

The majority of smokers will initially elect to stop on their own, and an individual attempt should be the physician's initial recommendation. These smokers will benefit from self-help material (see Table 49-1). Smokers heavily addicted to nicotine or with a history of severe withdrawal symptoms or large weight gains in prior quitting attempts may benefit from nicotine gum. It should be presented as an adjunct to a behavioral program that can minimize withdrawal symptoms but not make cessation painless.

Fewer than one third of smokers request an organized program. An individual or group program is appropriate for the smoker who is repeatedly unsuccessful in quitting on his own, expresses much doubt about his ability to quit, or has a low probability of success. The physician should be able to make appropriate referrals in the community.

6. *Follow-up.* Continued monitoring of the smoking habit is essential. Listing the problem on the patient's medical problem list will remind the physician to make its management part of the patient's continuing care. A return visit for follow-up smoking counseling is more effective than one-time advice. Smokers who quit should be congratulated but cautioned of the need to maintain vigilance against relapse. Exsmokers should be monitored carefully during the first year after cessation, when most relapses occur. For smokers whose attempts to quit were unsuccessful, the physician should focus on positive aspects, such as the duration of time the smoker was abstinent, and encourage another attempt.

Table 49-3. A Behavioral Program for Smoking Cessation

Rationale	Suggestions for the Smoker
Preparing to Quit	
1. Increase motivation	Write out a list of reasons to quit.
2. Make a commitment	Set a quit date. Sign a contract with family, friends.
3. Develop social supports	Enlist the support of nonsmoking friends, relatives, coworkers.
4. Self-monitoring to identify smoking cues	Keep a record of each cigarette smoked, noting circumstances, time, and how highly desired. Wrap this around cigarette pack with rubber band.
5. Progressive restriction	Eliminate least desired cigarettes; delay smoking first morning cigarette; smoke only at certain times or places.
6. Aversive conditioning	Fill a glass bottle with all your cigarette butts ("butt bottle").
7. Satiation	Oversmoke on the day before quitting.
Initial Cessation	
1. Avoid smoking cues	Eliminate all cigarettes, ashtrays, lighters from home and car. Spend the quitting day in places where smoking is not permitted.
2. Positive reinforcement	Reward self with a treat on quitting day.
3. Aversive conditioning	Look at "butt bottle" frequently. Wear rubber band on wrist and snap it when urge to smoke occurs.
4. Substitute oral stimuli	Chew on straws, toothpicks, carrot sticks, sugarless candy or gum.
5. Substitute activities for hands	Rubber bands, paper clips.
Relapse Prevention—Maintaining Nonsmoking	
1. Avoid smoking cues	Spend time in places where smoking is not permitted. Substitute situations associated with smoking (coffee, alcohol, end of meal) with other behaviors (tea, soft drink, brushing teeth, or taking a walk at end of meal).
2. Positive reinforcement	Treat self with money saved by not smoking.
3. Aversive conditioning	Wear rubber band on wrist and snap it when urge to smoke occurs.
4. Strategies to cope with urges to smoke	Take 10 slow deep breaths. Relaxation training. Incompatible activity (take a shower). Contact a nonsmoking friend.

ANNOTATED BIBLIOGRAPHY

Blum A: Nicotine chewing gum and the medicalization of smoking. Ann Intern Med 101:121, 1984 (*An editorial reviewing the evidence for and against the clinical utility of nicotine chewing gum and advocating greater involvement of physicians in more general smoking cessation efforts.*)

British Thoracic Society: Comparison of four methods of smoking withdrawal in patients with smoking related diseases. Br Med J

286:595, 1983 (*Multicenter randomized trial of patients attending chest clinics that demonstrated no long-term benefit when nicotine chewing gum was added to physician antismoking advice. Nicotine gum did increase short-term cessation rates.*)

Burt A et al: Stopping smoking after myocardial infarction. Lancet 1:305, 1974 (*Controlled prospective study of myocardial infarction survivors demonstrating the effectiveness of brief physician advice in-hospital, supplemented by nurse follow-up after discharge. At 1 year, 62% of those receiving the advice had stopped versus 27% in the control group.*)

Health and Public Policy Committee, American College of Physicians: Methods for stopping cigarette smoking. Ann Intern Med 105: 281, 1986 (*A critical review of methods. Emphasizes the importance of the physician's role.*)

Hjalmarson AIM: Effect of nicotine chewing gum in smoking cessation. JAMA 252:2835, 1984 (*A randomized trial demonstrating 1-year abstinence rates of 29% and 16% respectively for subjects with and without nicotine chewing gum. A critical review of nicotine gum efficacy trials appears on pages 2855–2858 of the same issue.*)

Hunt WA, Bespalec DA: An evaluation of current methods of modifying smoking behavior. J Clin Psychol 30:431, 1974 (*A classic review of 89 early studies, it described the characteristic relapse pattern among smokers who quit: 70% resume smoking within 3 to 6 months, after which relapse slows over 12 months.*)

Leventhal H, Cleary PD: The smoking problem: A review of the research and theory in behavioral risk modification. Psychol Bull 88:370, 1980 (*A comprehensive, review of why people smoke and the methods used to help them stop, it offers a synthesis of pharmacologic and psychologic models to explain smoking behavior.*)

Ockene JK, Hymowitz N, Sexton N et al: Comparison of patterns of smoking behavior change among smokers in the Multiple Risk Factor Intervention Trial (MRFIT). Prevent Med 11:621, 1982 (*Evaluation of the smoking component of a large study attempting to reduce risk factors in men at high coronary heart disease risk. Forty percent of men receiving an intensive behavioral intervention quit smoking for 4 years compared to 20% of those in the control group.*)

Pederson LL: Compliance with physician advice to quit smoking: A review of the literature. Prevent Med 11:71, 1982 (*Reviews the effectiveness of physician advice in different patient groups, concluding that the likelihood of smoking cessation correlates with the severity of the patient's disease.*)

Rose G, Hamilton PJS: A randomized controlled trial of the effect on middle-aged men of advice to stop smoking. J Epidemiol Comm Health 32:275, 1978 (*Physician counseling of British civil servants at high coronary disease risk led to 35% cessation rate at 3 years, compared to 14% in a control group, suggesting that patients made aware of their cardiac risk are susceptible to antismoking advice.*)

Russell MAH, Merriman R, Stapleton J et al: Effect of nicotine chewing gum as an adjunct to general practitioners' advice against smoking. Br Med J 287:1782, 1983 (*Randomized trial demonstrating the effectiveness of nicotine gum when prescribed by primary care physicians. At one year, 10% of smokers offered gum had stopped smoking.*)

Russell MAH, Wilson C, Taylor C et al: Effect of general practitioners' advice against smoking. Br Med J 2:231, 1979 (*A careful randomized controlled study in which routine advice to stop smoking resulted in a significant increase in cessation that was sustained over 1 year.*)

Sachs DPL, Hall RG, Hall SM: Effects of rapid smoking: Physiologic evaluation of a smoking cessation therapy. Ann Intern Med 88: 639, 1978 (*Rapid smoking elevates heart and respiratory rate and systolic blood pressure, and lowers P_{CO_2} but is not arrhythmogenic and is safe for healthy smokers.*)

U.S. Department of Health, Education, and Welfare: Smoking and Health: A Report of the Surgeon General, Washington, DC, Government Printing Office, 1979 (*The first update of the landmark 1964 report, this comprehensive book reviews the state of the art about the health effects of smoking and cessation techniques.*)

Wilson D, Wood G, Johnston N et al: Randomized clinical trial of supportive follow-up for cigarette smokers in a family practice. Can Med Assoc J 126:127, 1982 (*Patients scheduled for regular return visits to their family physician for continued smoking counseling were more likely to quit than those receiving one-time advice from their physician.*)

5

Gastrointestinal Problems

50
Screening for Gastric Cancer

For unknown reasons, the incidence of gastric cancer in the United States has been decreasing at a rate of 2% to 4% per year for the past several decades. During the 1930s, the death rate for gastric cancer was greater than 30 per 100,000; during the 1970s, the rate was approximately 10 per 100,000. At present, an American has an approximately 1% chance of developing gastric malignancy over his lifetime. Nevertheless, mortality remains high; approximately 75% of the 25,000 Americans who develop gastric cancer each year eventually die from the disease.

The usual insidious onset of the disease and the lack of suitable screening tests have thwarted preventive measures. Advances in endoscopic instrumentation, allowing more complete visualization of the stomach, have raised questions about unmet potential in prevention of gastric cancer deaths among high-risk populations. Some recommendations for routine endoscopic evaluation have sparked controversy. The primary care physician must understand the natural history of gastric cancer and the limitations of diagnostic tools in the detection of early disease.

EPIDEMIOLOGY AND RISK FACTORS

There is a marked international variation in the incidence of gastric cancer. Among the countries with the highest incidences are Chile, Japan, Finland, and Iceland. Incidence also varies, predictably, with age and sex. Men are twice as likely to develop gastric cancer in most countries. More than 60% of cases occur in people over age 65. Fewer than 10% of cases occur in people younger than age 30. The incidence among nonwhites and people in low socioeconomic groups in the United States is twice that among whites and the more well-to-do.

Genetic factors do not play a major role in determining risk for gastric cancer. It has been documented that migrants from areas of high risk (*e.g.,* Japan) eventually acquire the lower rates of their new home (*e.g.,* the United States). A genetically determined minor risk factor for gastric cancer is blood group; people with type A blood have a 10% increase in risk of developing gastric cancer.

A number of environmental factors have been suggested as explanations for the geographic variability of gastric cancer incidence. Phenol, present in all smoked foods, and the high salt concentration in salted fish and meat products have been linked to the high incidence of gastric cancer in Finland, Iceland, and Japan. Talc-treated rice has been implicated in Japan and Northern China. Provinces in Chile with high gastric cancer rates are agricultural, with high concentrations of nitrate present in the soil and drinking water. Nitrosamines, derived from nitrates and secondary amines, are suspected causes of gastric cancer in Chile and, to a lesser extent, in the United States where nitrates and nitrites are used as food additives in meat and fish.

A number of pathologic conditions, including gastric polyps and adenomas, have been associated with increased risk of stomach cancer. Gastric polyps are relatively infrequent; a prevalence of less than 0.5% has been documented in one autopsy series. The vast majority of polyps are hyperplastic and not associated with increased cancer risk. People with adenomas, particularly villous adenomas, have the same risk of cancer when the adenomas are found in the stomach as when they are in the colon. Some authorities have argued that peptic ulcer disease predisposes patients to gastric cancer. Carcinoma is found in approximately 3% of surgically resected gastric ulcers. It is likely, however, that ulceration follows carcinoma rather than *vice versa*. This association is the basis for the clinical practice of biopsying or resecting suspicious-appearing or persistent gastric ulcers.

A number of studies have demonstrated a statistical association between atrophic gastritis and gastric cancer. Achlorhydria and atrophic gastritis are common. Prevalence increases with age. An incidence of 1% per year of gastric cancer among patients with atrophic gastritis has been demonstrated in one study with yearly radiographic examination. The atrophic gastritis associated with pernicious anemia is also a risk factor for gastric cancer. Evidence indicates that patients with pernicious anemia have at least a fourfold increase in risk. Some studies have found even higher rates.

Prior gastric surgery for benign ulcer disease has long been considered a risk factor for subsequent gastric cancer. Increased risk was not evident early after surgery, but several Scandinavian studies suggested that those who lived more than 10 to 15 years following surgery faced a twofold to threefold increase in gastric cancer risk. Recommendations for annual endoscopic examination followed. More recently, a large population-based study conducted in Olmstead County, Minnesota, found gastric cancer to be no more common among patients with prior gastric surgery than among the population at large.

NATURAL HISTORY OF GASTRIC CANCER AND EFFECTIVENESS OF THERAPY

Gastric cancer typically has an insidious presentation. The most common initial symptom is epigastric discomfort. Later symptoms include early satiety, indigestion, weight loss, and other systemic symptoms. The percentage of patients who survive 5 years has not improved significantly in recent years; it remains at 20% of unselected cases. The patients who are operated on early in the course of their disease have a 60% to 90% 5-year survival rate.

Among highly selected patients with "early gastric cancer," defined as gastric cancer confined to the mucosa or submucosa but not extending to the muscularis propria, resection may be curative for as many as 95%. Intensive screening efforts in Japan have increased the proportion of gastric cancers detected in this early stage from approximately 5% to 30%. Efforts have not been as successful elsewhere, where fewer than 10% of cases meet criteria for early gastric cancer. The duration of the asymptomatic detectable period is unknown, but early gastric cancer has been found as long as 3 years after biopsies were originally misread as benign. The natural history of early gastric cancer appears to include protracted cycles of healing and ulceration.

SCREENING AND DIAGNOSTIC TESTS

None of the tests available for the diagnosis of gastric carcinoma are suitable for wide-scale screening efforts.

Gastric Cytology. Unlike cervical cytopathology, the collection and examination of specimens for gastric cytopathologic analysis is a laborious process. Samples must be obtained either by endoscopic scraping or by gastric lavage. Examination of the resulting slides usually takes 2 to 3 hours rather than the several minutes sufficient for the screening examination of cervical Pap smears. Many studies have demonstrated the sensitivity of gastric cytopathology studies to be approximately 90%. It is not known how much this figure is influenced by the spectrum of disease, that is, how sensitive cytology can be for the early, curable cancer. Specificity in a laboratory with experienced personnel should be approximately 97% to 98%. False-positives are often found in association with healing gastric ulcer and other gastric pathology. Although cytopathology is useful for further diagnosis in documented cases of abnormality of gastric mucosa, it cannot be recommended for indiscriminate screening.

Endoscopy. Similarly, endoscopy must be considered a diagnostic rather than a screening procedure. Sensitivity in making the diagnosis of gastric cancer is 90%. However, recent evidence suggests that endoscopic visualization is much less sensitive for early cancers, with a visual diagnosis being made in fewer than 50% of cases in some series. Multiple biopsies of any and all suspicious lesions can increase the sensitivity to 90%.

Diagnostic Radiology. The sensitivity of contrast studies in the diagnosis of gastric cancer has been reported to be as high as 95%. Obviously, however, it is least sensitive in cases of early disease and is too expensive and time-consuming to be considered a screening test in asymptomatic patients.

Stool analysis for occult blood (described in detail in Chap. 51) is an appropriate screening procedure for all gastrointestinal malignancies. Yearly guaiac testing has been recommended as part of the general screening for all adult patients. This is especially important for patients with identified increased risk of gastric cancer, such as those with a history of pernicious anemia or documented atrophic gastritis.

CONCLUSIONS AND RECOMMENDATIONS

- Despite a significant downward trend in incidence, gastric cancer remains a disease of high morbidity and mortality.
- The yearly analysis of stool for occult blood is indicated in all adult patients. This is especially important for those with a history of pernicious anemia, atrophic gastritis, or other gastric pathology.
- The value of gastric cytology, endoscopy, and contrast studies as routine procedures in high-risk patients is unproven. They are diagnostic procedures and should generally be reserved for symptomatic patients or patients with occult blood demonstrated by stool analysis.

A.G.M.

ANNOTATED BIBLIOGRAPHY

Ackerman NB: An evaluation of gastric cytology: Results of a nationwide survey. J Chron Dis 20:621, 1967 (*Survey of practices in U.S. hospitals indicating wide variation in validity of techniques. Not generally used for screening purposes but rather in response to symptoms or radiographic abnormalities.*)

Bedikian AY, Chen TT, Khankhanian N et al: The natural history of gastric cancer and prognostic factors influencing survival. J Clin Oncol 2:305, 1984 (*Useful review of natural history with an emphasis on clinical determinants of survival.*)

Green PHR, O'Toole K: Early gastric cancer. Ann Intern Med 97:272, 1982 (*An editorial reviewing endoscopic screening programs, which concludes that benefit remains unproven.*)

Hitchcock CR, MacLean LD, Sullivan WA: Secretory and clinical aspects of achlorhydria and gastric atrophy as precursors of gastric cancer. J Nat Cancer Inst 18:795, 1957 (*Review of data indicating increase of 4.5 and 21.9 times in risk among patients with achlorhydria and pernicious anemia. Recommends frequent radiographic studies.*)

Hoerr SO: Prognosis for carcinoma of the stomach. Surg Gynecol Obstet 137:205, 1973 (*Five-year survivals rates ranging from 83% to 11% depending on stage; overall 5-year survival rate of 18%.*)

Logan RFA, Langman MJS: Screening for gastric cancer after gastric surgery. Lancet 2:667, 1983 (*Accepts evidence for increased risk but, nevertheless, does not favor endoscopic screening.*)

MacDonald WC et al: Exfoliative cytology screening for gastric cancer. Cancer 17:163, 1964 (*Series of 500 patients with pernicious anemia or achlorhydria. Screening yielded three cases—none of which were asymptomatic, two of which were inoperable. The one false-positive finding resulted in an operative death.*)

Rubin P (ed): Cancer of the gastrointestinal tract: C. Gastric cancer diagnosis. JAMA 288:883, 1974 (*Collection of eight short articles that review the epidemiology, natural history, and diagnosis of gastric cancer.*)

Schafer LW, Larson DE, Melton LJ et al: The risk of gastric carcinoma after surgical treatment for benign ulcer disease. N Engl J Med 309:1210, 1983 (*No evident increase in the risk of gastric cancer following surgical treatment for benign peptic ulcer disease led the authors to conclude that there is no indication for endoscopic surveillance in this population.*)

51

Screening for Colorectal Cancer

MICHAEL J. BARRY, M.D.

Colorectal cancer is the most common malignancy found in both men and women, accounting for 13% of cancer deaths. Americans face a lifetime probability of developing a carcinoma of the colon or rectum of approximately 5%. This frequency, the long asymptomatic period of the disease, the availability of tests for early diagnosis, and the greater effectiveness of early therapy make screening for large bowel tumors a primary care priority.

EPIDEMIOLOGY AND RISK FACTORS

The incidence of colorectal cancer is greater in economically developed societies. The high-fat and low-fiber diet prevalent in Western societies has been implicated in the etiology of these cancers. Alterations in bile acid secretion produced by such a diet, and the subsequent bile acid metabolism by intestinal microflora, may produce carcinogens or cocarcinogens.

Advancing age is an important risk factor. The age-specific incidence increases into the eighth decade. The prevalence of asymptomatic colorectal cancer found incidentally at autopsy is about 1.5 per thousand in the sixth decade, 5 per thousand in the seventh decade, and 10 per thousand in the eighth decade.

Family history is also a risk factor; having a first-degree relative with colorectal cancer raises an individual's risk threefold. Familial polyposis is an autosomal dominant condition that confers virtual certainty of eventual malignancy. Total colectomy is usually performed at an early age. Patients with familial polyposis who have been treated with less than total colectomy need careful proctoscopic monitoring of the iliorectal anastomosis to remove polyps in residual rectal tissue.

Sporadic polyps are common lesions. Although the majority of small polyps are hyperplastic outcroppings unrelated to colorectal cancer, the prevalence of truly neoplastic polyps remains substantial; 15% of individuals in the seventh decade harbor adenomas greater than 0.5 cm, with one third of these being greater than 1.0 cm. Adenomas may actually contain malignancy, with the risk related to the size of the polyp. In one study, invasive cancer was found in only 0.5% of colonoscopically removed polyps from 0.5 to 0.9 cm in diameter, but in almost 15% of polyps greater than 3 cm in diameter. About 10% of neoplastic polyps have villous histology, tubular adenomas account for 70%, and the remainder have mixed histology. Villous histology confers greater risk, and these tumors tend to be larger and more sessile. Table 51-1 summarizes the relationship between invasive cancer and polyp size and histology. Clinical, pathologic, and epidemiologic evidence suggests many cancers begin as adenomatous polyps. Larger polyps, even if histologically benign, are best considered risk factors for eventual colorectal cancer. The degree

Table 51-1. Polypoid Lesions of the Colon and Rectum. Relation of Size to Cancer (1116 polypoid lesions, Massachusetts General Hospital, 1954–63)

DIAMETER (CM)	PERCENTAGE CANCEROUS
Less than 0.5	0.5
0.5–0.9	1
1.0–1.4	1.8
1.5–1.9	6
2–2.4	10
2.5–3.4	23
3.5 or larger	29

(Behringer GE: Changing concepts in the histopathologic diagnosis of polypoid lesions of the colon. Dis Colon Rectum 13:116–118, 1970)

of future risk from small (<1 cm) adenomas is still hotly debated.

Ulcerative colitis predisposes patients to a five to ten times greater risk of colorectal cancer; increasing risk with greater duration of disease and extent of involvement has been documented. Crohn's disease and ulcerative proctitis probably do not increase risk significantly.

Patients with resected colorectal cancers have a threefold greater risk of developing metachronous cancer in other locations of the colon. Recurrences of index cancers are usually extramural and not amenable to detection by screening.

The prevalence of synchronous colonic neoplasia is high and important to consider in the evaluation of the patient with a positive screening test. Synchronous adenomas occur in 40% to 50% of patients with an index polyp; 3% to 5% with a carcinoma will harbor a second one.

NATURAL HISTORY OF COLORECTAL CANCER AND EFFECTIVENESS OF THERAPY

Symptoms occur late in the course of colorectal cancer growth. It is likely that the mean duration of the asymptomatic detectable period is several years. When cancers are found after symptomatic presentation, 60% have already disseminated to regional nodes or distant organs.

Five-year survival rates vary dramatically with the stage of disease at the time of diagnosis. Older series with largely symptomatic tumors describe 65% survival for disease limited to submucosa (Duke's A), 45% for tumors invading through the muscularis but confined to the bowel (Duke's B), and 20% for tumors with positive regional nodes (Duke's C and D). Encouragingly, recent studies suggest that asymptomatic tumors have better prognoses even accounting for stage and occult interval; one study has described a 90% 15-year survival for asymptomatic Duke's A lesions discovered by proctosigmoidoscopy.

SCREENING TESTS

Digital Examination

In older series, 40% of colorectal cancers were within reach of the examining finger; it is now apparent that this is the case for fewer than 10% of tumors. However, the digital examination has almost no morbidity and the American Cancer Society recommends it annually after age 40.

Fecal Occult Blood Testing

Intermittent occult bleeding occurs with many asymptomatic colorectal cancers and large polyps. Individual guaiac impregnated filter paper slides (such as Hemoccult™) will regularly detect greater than 10 mg of hemoglobin per gram of stool. However, *in vivo* sensitivity for colonic neoplasia is greater than this figure would predict when serial samples of stool are tested to take advantage of the intermittent bleeding of these lesions. The fact that colonic tumors selectively enrich the stool surface with blood contributes to this sensitivity. When a single positive guaiac reaction is considered a positive screening test result, the standard protocol of testing two samples from stools on three consecutive days is 50% to 70% sensitive for colorectal cancer and large (>2 cm) polyps. Smaller polyps produce guaiac positivity only on occasion, but their high prevalence makes them the most common lesions found during the evaluation of patients with occult bleeding. Increasing the number of samples or hydrating slides before developing will increase sensitivity, but this procedure produces an unacceptable loss of specificity. False-positive tests may be due to nonmalignant bleeding gastrointestinal lesions or to foods with high peroxidase activity. Those due to the latter may be reduced by test diets free of rare red meat, horseradish, cantaloupe, or uncooked vegetables (especially broccoli, turnips, radish, or cauliflower). Ascorbic acid may cause false-negative tests, whereas iron and nonsteroidal anti-inflammatory drugs such as aspirin may cause false positives. Storage of slides for more than 4 days before development decreases their sensitivity, and should be avoided.

Individuals with a positive fecal occult blood test require a thorough evaluation for colorectal neoplasia. Colonoscopy is probably the most sensitive single test; it allows biopsy of suspicious lesions or polypectomy at the time of evaluation. It has been a clinical axiom that barium enema alone, which may have a sensitivity as low as 50% for early colorectal cancer (if done with single contrast), is insufficient to rule out cancer following a positive occult blood test. If colonoscopy must generally be done for biopsy confirmation after positive barium enema, and must also be done following a negative contrast study, logic and a sense of cost-effectiveness favor proceeding directly to colonoscopy to evaluate a positive test, bypassing both sigmoidoscopy and barium enema. In fact, this strategy was recently recommended by an international symposium on colorectal cancer. Air contrast barium enema may occasionally find lesions missed by colonoscopy but could be reserved for individuals in whom colonoscopy is incomplete (about 10% of procedures) or who have persistent occult bleeding.

Two randomized controlled trials are underway to determine whether periodic fecal occult blood testing reduces mortality. Data from these trials suggest that with a standard protocol about 4% of screenees will be positive, with 10% predictive value positive for colorectal cancer and up to 50% for all neoplasia (cancer plus polyps).

Proctosigmoidoscopy

Although older series reported that 75% of cancers were within range of the rigid sigmoidoscope, recent data documenting a proximal shift in the distribution of cancers as well as an average proctoscopic depth of insertion of only 15 to 20 cm have resulted in a revision of this estimate to as low as 25%. Although the yield of cancer is low in asymptomatic patients (perhaps 1 in 500 to 1000 examinations), some investigators have suggested that the real benefit of this test is identification and removal of rectal polyps, found in 2% to 12% of proctoscopies, to prevent future cancers. If this benefit is indeed the primary consideration, less frequent testing makes good sense given general agreement on the slow progression of the polyp–cancer sequence. The American Cancer Society now recommends proctosigmoidoscopy every 3 to 5 years after two negative studies a year apart at age 50.

When polyps greater than 0.5 cm are found at proctosigmoidoscopy, referral for colonoscopy to search for synchronous disease as well as to remove the index polyp for histology is recommended. Small polyps (<0.5 cm) often have a hyperplastic histology. Recent evidence suggests these small lesions can be removed with a biopsy forceps without histologic examination or subsequent pancolonic evaluation, but this controversial point requires further study. Periodic rigid sigmoidoscopy has not enjoyed wide acceptance by physicians and patients. New flexible instruments reaching further into the left colon may increase both patient acceptance and the sensitivity of the screening examination.

Other Tests

Contrast x-ray studies and colonoscopy are not screening tests for average-risk individuals. For subgroups at higher risk, especially after removal of a polyp or carcinoma, these tests may have a role, but the optimal frequency of restudy remains to be determined. Evaluation of multiple biopsies and/or cytology by means of colonoscopy is becoming an established practice in following individuals with ulcerative pancolitis of greater than 8 years' duration. Tumor markers such as carcinoembryonic antigen (CEA) are not suitable general screening tests because of low specificity and, in the patient with early cancer, low sensitivity as well.

CONCLUSION AND RECOMMENDATIONS

- The relatively high prevalence of colorectal cancer and characteristics of its natural history make detection in an asymptomatic stage with reduction of morbidity and mortality highly feasible, though still not conclusively proven. A careful history should identify individuals at especially high risk.
- Annual digital rectal examinations and fecal occult blood testing should begin at age 50 in average-risk individuals. Occult blood testing should follow a specific methodology, and positive tests should be thoroughly evaluated. Colonoscopy is probably the single best test for this purpose.
- The yield of proctosigmoidoscopy is small but significant, especially when polyps are considered. Primary care physicians can refer patients who require biopsy or polypectomy for colonoscopy since synchronous lesions are common. Proctosigmoidoscopy can be performed every 3 to 5 years after age 50 in patients willing to accept some short-term discomfort to reduce cancer risk.
- Individuals with a positive family history should begin a screening program at age 40, with the interval between proctoscopic examinations kept at every 3 years. Individuals with ulcerative pancolitis longer than 8 years or familial polyposis require periodic colonoscopy by a gastroenterologist. Patients who have had a cancer or a large (>1 cm) polyp removed may also be candidates for periodic endoscopy, but this point is debatable. Annual fecal occult blood testing and sigmoidoscopy should be done every 3 years at the minimum.
- Colonic polyps greater than 1.0 cm may contain invasive cancers or be precursors of future tumors and should generally be removed. When discovered by endoscopy, few additional resources are consumed and little extra morbidity is engendered by lowering the threshold for removal. Polyps smaller than 0.5 cm can be safely removed without histologic examination.
- Neither proctoscopy nor occult blood tests are sensitive enough to preclude the necessity for further evaluation of patients with gastrointestinal symptoms that are suggestive of colorectal cancer. Patients should be encouraged to report symptoms such as altered stool habit or hematochezia.

ANNOTATED BIBLIOGRAPHY

Burkitt DP: Etiology and prevention of colorectal cancer. Hosp Pract 16:67, 1984 (*Discusses theories of colorectal cancer etiology especially the high fat–low fiber hypothesis.*)

Crespi M et al: The role of proctosigmoidoscopy in screening for colorectal neoplasia. CA 34:158, 1984 (*Reviews multiple studies of the yield of sigmoidoscopy and examines the rigid versus flexible sigmoidoscopy controversy.*)

Crowley ML et al: Sensitivity of guaiac-impregnated cards for the detection of colorectal neoplasia. J Clin Gastroenterol 5:127, 1983 (*A 52% sensitivity for colorectal cancer is the lowest reported in* vivo *study and serves as a reminder that a negative occult blood series does not "rule out" cancer.*)

Fath RB, Winawer SJ: Early diagnosis of colorectal cancer. Annu Rev Med 34:501, 1983 (*Good concise review of risk factors, screening, and diagnostic tests.*)

Feczko PJ, Halbert RD: Reassessing the role of radiology in Hemoccult screening. Am J Radiol 146:697, 1986 (*Argues that double-contrast barium enema is a good initial test for evaluating Hemoccult-positive patients.*)

Gilbertsen VA et al: Colon cancer control study: An interim report. In Winawer S, Schottenfeld D, Sherlock P (eds): Colorectal Cancer: Prevention, Epidemiology, and Screening, 1980, p 261. New York, Raven Press (*Results of one of the two randomized trials of fecal occult blood testing for colorectal cancer.*)

Gnauck R, Macrae FA, Fleisher M: How to perform the fecal occult blood test. CA 34:134, 1984 (*Good review of methodology including test diets, storage delay, and interferring medications.*)

Lambert R, Sobin LH, Waye JD et al: The management of patients with colorectal adenomas. CA 34:167, 1984 (*Although good data are lacking, the algorithmic approach outlined makes academic sense.*)

Macrae FA, St John DJB: Relationship between patterns of bleeding and hemoccult sensitivity in patients with colorectal cancers or adenomas. Gastroenterology 82:891, 1982 (*Best in vivo study of sensitivity of occult blood test, examines the influence of the number of samples and the effect of hydration.*)

Macrae FA et al: Optimal dietary conditions for hemoccult testing. Gastroenterology 82:899, 1982 (*Examines the effect of diet on specificity, though unfortunately in young individuals only.*)

Morson BC: Polyps and cancer of the large bowel. In Hardley J, Morson BC (eds): The Gastrointestinal Tract: (International) Academy of Pathology Monograph, p 101. Baltimore, Williams & Wilkins, 1977 (*Reviews evidence for the polyp–cancer sequence.*)

Pollack ES, Nomura AM, Heilbrun LK et al: Prospective study of alcohol consumption in cancer. N Engl J Med 310:617, 1984 (*Men who were heavy consumers of beer had a threefold risk of colorectal cancer in this prospective study.*)

Sherlock P, Winawer SJ: Are there markers for the risk of colon cancer? N Engl J Med 311:118, 1984 (*Reviews genetic risks and the polyp controversy as well as prospects for a biochemical marker for colon cancer risk.*)

Shinya H, Wolff WI: Morphology, anatomic distribution and cancer potential of colonic polyps. Ann Surg 6:679, 1979 (*Colonoscopic experience with 7000 polyps, especially distribution, histology, and risk of cancer.*)

Spencer RJ, Melton LJ, Ready RL et al: Treatment of small colorectal polyps: A population-based study of the risk of subsequent carcinoma. Mayo Clin Proc 59:305, 1984 (*Suggests risk of subsequent cancer not increased if small polyps are removed without biopsy, or intensive follow-up.*)

Stroehlein JR, Goulston K, Hunt RH: Diagnostic approach to evaluating the cause of a positive fecal occult blood test. CA 34:148, 1984 (*Emphasizes the importance of colonoscopy.*)

Winawer SJ, Andrews M, Flehinger B et al: Progress report on controlled trial of fecal occult blood testing for the detection of colorectal neoplasia. Cancer 45:2959, 1980 (*Report on the other controlled trial of occult blood testing emphasizing predictive value of positive tests.*)

52
Prevention of Viral Hepatitis
JULES L. DIENSTAG, M.D.

Viral hepatitis is a contagious disease that afflicts more than 500,000 people in the United States each year. Although the majority of those infected with hepatitis viruses have no symptoms at all or a mild illness, severe, even fulminant, hepatitis develops in some patients; several thousand deaths per year are related to viral hepatitis. After acute hepatitis B, approximately 10% of patients become chronic virus carriers, and a proportion of these have chronic hepatitis. Of patients with transfusion-associated non-A, non-B hepatitis, chronic hepatitis develops in as many as 50%. In general, outbreaks of hepatitis are often traced to a source of hepatitis A virus; occasionally, clusters of hepatitis B follow exposure of several persons to contaminated needles, blood products, and the like. Among urban adult patients presenting to a primary care physician with sporadic cases of hepatitis, hepatitis B accounts for approximately one half, non-A, non-B hepatitis for 15% to 30%, and hepatitis A for the remainder. Currently, more than 90% of post-transfusion cases are attributable to

non-A, non-B hepatitis infection; the frequency of post-transfusion hepatitis B has been reduced dramatically by the introduction of blood donor screening for hepatitis B surface antigen (HBsAg).

Prevention of infection and prophylaxis against clinical disease are prime objectives in the management of viral hepatitis. The primary physician has major responsibility for these tasks, because patients and their contacts often present at a time when infectivity is high. Prevention of viral hepatitis requires a knowledge of the common modes of viral transmission, the periods of maximal communicability, and the efficacy of globulin preparations and vaccines.

EPIDEMIOLOGY AND RISK FACTORS

Hepatitis A Virus is shed in the feces, and transmission occurs predominantly by the fecal–oral route. Prior exposure to hepatitis A is manifested by the presence of antibody to the A virus (anti-HAV), which confers lifelong immunity. More than 80% of patients over age 60 are positive for anti-HAV; acute infection is rare in this age group. Because children and adolescents are least likely to have had previous exposure to the virus, they are the most susceptible to infection. Spread of infection is greatest when poor sanitary conditions and crowding exist. In a New York City study, 75% of low-income people had evidence of prior infection, compared with 20% to 30% of residents in middle- to upper-income neighborhoods. There is no carrier state.

Hepatitis B used to be considered a disease that resulted from parenteral exposure, but recent evidence suggests that nonpercutaneous transmission is a common mode of spread. Perinatal transmission from mother to offspring is common in developing nations. Patients with hepatitis B infection have been found to harbor hepatitis B surface antigen in saliva, semen, vaginal secretions, and breast milk, as well as in the serum. Spouses of patients with acute hepatitis and people with a large number of sexual partners (*e.g.,* male homosexuals) are maximally subjected to sources of nonpercutaneous transmission and have a markedly increased risk of contracting infection. About 0.1% of healthy blood donors are positive for HBsAg, as are 5% of drug addicts and an even larger proportion of patients in some dialysis units. Surgeons, laboratory technicians, oral surgeons, and other medical personnel exposed to blood and body fluids are at increased risk of contracting hepatitis B. Spread of infection from health personnel who are HBsAg carriers of antigen is a rare event, usually resulting from inadvertent patient exposure to their blood from cuts or abrasions. The development and application of sensitive screening methods for detection of HBsAg has greatly reduced the incidence of post-transfusion hepatitis type B. Currently, less than 10% of all post-transfusion hepatitis in the United States is due to B virus. Reliance on blood obtained from volunteer donors, less likely to contain the virus, has also reduced the frequency of post-transfusion hepatitis.

Hepatitis D Or Delta Hepatitis is a recently discovered type of hepatitis caused by a defective RNA virus that requires coinfection with hepatitis B (a DNA virus) to support its replication. Infection with this agent occurs either simultaneously with acute hepatitis B infection or is superimposed on chronic hepatitis B. Like hepatitis B, hepatitis D is transmitted by percutaneous inoculation and intimate contact. In nonendemic areas, such as the United States and western Europe, hepatitis D has been confined primarily to populations with frequent percutaneous exposures, such as drug addicts and hemophiliacs; in endemic areas, such as the Mediterranean countries, hepatitis D is transmitted primarily through intimate contact.

Non-A, Non-B Hepatitis was first recognized in transfusion recipients, 7% to 10% of whom have subclinical or clinically apparent hepatitis within 1 to 6 months following transfusion. Much more likely to occur after transfusion with blood from commercial donors, non-A, non-B hepatitis remains a complication of transfusion even when all-volunteer blood is used. More than 90% of all cases of transfusion-related hepatitis are classified by exclusion of hepatitis A and B as non-A, non-B hepatitis. Unfortunately, valid antigenic markers of this type of hepatitis remain elusive, and the diagnosis remains one of exclusion. Therefore, there are no virus-specific tests with which to screen donor blood. Non-A, non-B hepatitis is not confined to transfusion settings; it appears to be spread by the same modes as those spreading hepatitis B—that is, those associated with percutaneous or transmucosal exposure and intimate contact.

NATURAL HISTORY

Hepatitis A has an average incubation period of 30 days (range, 15–45 days) from the time of exposure to the onset of symptoms. An early manifestation of disease is elevation of the serum transaminase level, which occurs about a week before onset of flulike symptoms; however, fecal shedding of hepatitis A virus (HAV) has been found to occur even before the rise in transaminases and up to 2 weeks prior to the development of symptoms. HAV disappears from stool within 2 to 3 weeks, usually coinciding with the onset of jaundice and resolution of prodromal symptoms. A fall in viral titer parallels a rise in antibody titer, which persists indefinitely. Initially, the anti-HAV is of the IgM class; during convalescence anti-HAV of the IgG class becomes predominant. Therefore, a diagnosis of acute hepatitis A can be made by demonstrating IgM anti-HAV in a single serum sample. No episodes of chronic hepatitis or a carrier state have been found to result from hepatitis A infection. Fatalities are rare; fewer than 5% of cases of fulminant hepatitis are due to type A virus infection.

Hepatitis B infection is a much more variable disease. The incubation period averages 12 weeks, with a range of 4 weeks to 6 months. About 2 to 4 weeks prior to the onset of symptoms, HBsAg appears in the serum, followed by a rise in transaminase levels and symptoms. Antigen usually is cleared from the serum by 4 to 6 months; persistence of antigenemia beyond 6 months is considered chronic infection. Symptoms of acute hepatitis B typically last 4 to 6 weeks, but there is much variation, ranging from clinically inapparent disease to fulminant hepatocellular failure and death. Age, immunologic competence, degree of exposure, and virulence of the virus are postulated to be among the determinants of disease severity. About 10% of patients with syptomatic disease become chronic carriers of HBsAg; 1% to 2% progress to chronic active hepatitis; 1% die. Antibody to HBsAg appears at variable times after exposure, but 90% eventually develop anti-HBs, which persist indefinitely.

Antibody to the nucleocapsid core of HBV (anti-HBc) appears in the circulation within a week or so after HBsAg becomes detectable and persists indefinitely. Occasionally, during late acute infection, an interval occurs in which HBsAg has already disappeared, and anti-HBs has not yet become detectable. This so-called window period can be identified by the presence of anti-HBc; however, in routine practice and with the improved sensitivity of contemporary diagnostic tests, this window period is rarely identified. Most instances in which anti-HBc occurs in the absence of HBsAg and anti-HBs represent hepatitis B infection in the remote past. A test for anti-HBc of the IgM class (IgM anti-HBc) recently introduced can distinguish between acute or relatively recent acute hepatitis B (IgM positive) and remote infection or chronic carriage (IgM negative, anti-HBc of the IgG class). In a small proportion of cases of acute hepatitis B, HBsAg does not reach the threshhold for detection; in such cases, a diagnosis of acute hepatitis B can be established by detecting IgM anti-HBc.

The *e antigen* (HBeAg) has drawn attention as a predictor of infectivity. Needlestick exposure to blood from an HBsAg-positive person that is positive for HBeAg is associated with a high risk of infection. There was speculation that finding HBeAg early in the course of illness meant an increase in the probability of developing chronic hepatitis, but this has not been borne out. HBeAg appears transiently in the early phase of all hepatitis B infections, but only in a few does it persist and signify high infectivity.

Hepatitis D (Delta Hepatitis) is being recognized with increasing frequency in the United States. Its incubation period is similar to that for hepatitis B, and when both hepatitis B and hepatitis D infections are acquired simultaneously, a single clinically apparent episode of hepatitis may ensue. There is a slight increase in the risk of fulminant hepatitis when the two infections occur simultaneously, but, in general, the outcome of simultaneous acute hepatitis B and D is no different from the outcome of hepatitis B alone. In contrast, among patients with chronic hepatitis B infection, superimposed hepatitis D may lead to severe, fulminant hepatitis, convert a mild or asymptomatic chronic hepatitis B infection into a severe form of chronic hepatitis (chronic active hepatitis), or accelerate the course of chronic active hepatitis. A diagnosis of delta hepatitis is made by demonstrating the appearance of antibody to hepatitis D, anti-HD.

Non-A, Non-B Hepatitis was discovered when sera from patients with post-transfusion hepatitis were found to be negative for hepatitis A or B virus markers, as well as for markers of Epstein-Barr virus and cytomegalovirus. Better identification of this variant will have to await the availability of specific serologic tests. The mean incubation period is 7 weeks; as in hepatitis B, the range is wide—3 to 15 weeks—with 80% occurring within 5 to 10 weeks after transfusion. Only a quarter of patients become icteric, compared with two thirds of patients with post-transfusion hepatitis B, but one third to one half progress to chronic active hepatitis. In sporadic, nonpercutaneous cases, the chronicity rate is less than 10%.

PRINCIPLES OF PROPHYLAXIS

The principal means of prophylaxis are minimizing exposure to hepatitis virus and use of globulin preparations and vaccines. In many instances, globulin prophylaxis does not prevent infection, but it may reduce the chances of developing clinical hepatitis. Precautions against contact with the hepatitis patient are most appropriate during the prodromal stage of illness, when the patient sheds virus most heavily and/or when there is often little clinical evidence of hepatitis, making avoidance of contact with the virus difficult. Consequently, immunotherapy emerges as the mainstay of prophylaxis.

Hepatitis A. Prophylaxis for hepatitis A can be accomplished by use of standard *immune globulin* (IG). This globulin preparation contains high titers of anti-HAV and is about 80% effective in preventing clinical disease. The mechanism by which IG protects the exposed patient was believed to be passive–active immunization, in which passively administered antibody acts to minimize clinical illness but does not prevent infection. Newer analyses suggest that IG more often prevents infection entirely. IG must be administered within 1 to 2 weeks of exposure to be most effective. Patients with a prior history of serologically documented hepatitis A need not receive IG, for they are already protected by their own anti-HAV. Household contacts and small groups experiencing a common source outbreak (*e.g.,* an athletic team) should be given IG prophylaxis, if the outbreak is identified early enough. During the early phase of clinical hepatitis, when jaundice first appears, there may still be some shedding of virus; precautions such as avoiding intimate contact and careful washing of hands after contact are probably reasonable for a week or two longer. The patient should not serve food to others and may minimize transmission of virus by using disposable dishes and utensils. Because HAV has been cultivated *in vitro,* a vaccine is being developed and should be available within a few years.

Hepatitis B. The approach to prophylaxis of hepatitis B—based on providing the susceptible person with protective antibody, anti-HBs—has changed several times during the last decade. Before active immunization with a vaccine became available, the only alternative was passive immunoprophylaxis with globulins. Standard IG with negligible levels of anti-HBs and a high-anti-HBs-titer globulin—*hepatitis B immune globulin* (HBIG)—prepared from the plasma of persons with high-titer anti-HBs and containing anti-HBs at a titer in the range of 1:100,000 or higher, were compared in health workers sustaining a contaminated needlestick exposure, in sexual contacts of patients with acute hepatitis B, and in hemodialysis units. The results of all these studies were not always in agreement, and the studies were criticized for lack of appropriate controls and other faults in study design. A consensus emerged, however, that IG was as good as

HBIG in situations, such as in dialysis units, in which there was low-level continuous exposure, whereas HBIG was superior for prophylaxis in cases of temporally limited but intense exposure, such as a needlestick, a sexual exposure to someone with acute hepatitis B, or neonatal exposure at birth to an HBsAg-positive mother.

In some of these studies, the immune response after IG was found to resemble that expected after active immunization, with slowly evolving but long-lasting anti-HBs; subsequent analysis showed that these globulin lots, devoid of detectable anti-HBs, actually contained HBsAg complexed to anti-HBs. Thus, the HBsAg in these preparations provided vaccinelike active immunization. Contemporary lots of IG, prepared from plasma screened to eliminate HBsAg, no longer contain HBsAg and are unlikely to be as effective as the HBsAg-containing lots used in these studies. Even HBIG, which originally was thought to provide complete protection, was later found to attenuate clinical illness rather than to prevent infection and to protect by providing passive–active immunization (with long-lasting protection resulting from subclinical infection). HBIG continues to be recommended for needlestick or comparable transmucosal exposures to hepatitis B, for sexual contacts of patients with acute hepatitis B, and for babies born to HBsAg-positive mothers.

The advent of *hepatitis B vaccine* has made possible for the first time active immunization against hepatitis B infection. There are two vaccine preparations: one is made by monoclonal methods; the other is prepared from the plasma of chronic HBsAg carriers. The vaccine consists of the antigenic but noninfectious 22-nm particulate forms of HBV. The vaccine produced in the United States from HBsAg carriers undergoes a three-step inactivation process in which the HBsAg particles are subjected to treatment with pepsin, urea, and formalin, which cumulatively destroy the infectivity of all known viruses (including AIDS virus). Both preparations are safe, immunogenic, and effective in preventing HBV infection and illness. Currently, the vaccine is recommended for those with continuous exposure to hepatitis B or to blood (health and laboratory workers exposed to blood, dialysis staff and patients, family members of chronic HBsAg carriers, residents and staff of institutions for the mentally retarded, promiscuous homosexual men as well as heterosexuals, patients requiring frequent and multiple blood products or clotting factors, drug addicts, etc.). In addition, for those who require HBIG for acute, high-intensity HBV exposure, a course of hepatitis B vaccine may be substituted for follow-up doses of HBIG. Simultaneous administration of HBIG and vaccine in these situations provides the immediate high levels of passively acquired anti-HBs expected after HBIG is given alone and the long-lasting anti-HBs resulting from active immunization with vaccine alone. Several studies have shown that the two preparations do not interfere with each other.

An important goal in providing prophylaxis after accidental inoculation is to administer HBIG as soon as possible after the exposure—the earlier the better. Although studies of the efficacy of HBIG after needlestick allowed globulin administration up to 7 days after exposure, and although 7 days is usually selected as an arbitrary cutoff for prophylaxis in these situations, little protection can be expected after 48 hours of needlestick or exposure by birth to an HBsAg-positive mother. Thus, after an HBsAg-positive needlestick, if the anti-HBs status of the "stickee" is not known, early administration of HBIG is paramount, without delay to wait for the results of antibody testing. For babies born to HBsAg-positive mothers, optimally, HBIG should be given in the delivery room. After sexual contact, which is less direct than a percutaneous inoculation, longer delays can be permitted to assess the immune status of the exposed partner. Although determination of the HBeAg status of the contact case or inoculum source may provide information about relative infectivity, HBeAg status should not be a criterion for providing prophylaxis to contacts. First, the delay necessitated by waiting for HBeAg testing may invalidate efforts at prophylaxis, and second, infectivity can occur in the absence of HBeAg, although the likelihood is reduced.

Nonintimate household contacts do not require prophylaxis, nor do casual contacts at work. Such generalizations must be qualified by the infectivity and virulence of the virus at hand as well as the consequences of infection to the exposed person. All suspected sources of hepatitis B should be tested for HBsAg, and exposed persons can be checked for the presence of anti-HBs to see how susceptible to infection they are.

Reducing the spread of hepatitis B has been aided by screening blood donors for HBsAg. The person discovered to be an asymptomatic carrier requires attention. If the person is a health care worker who is free of symptoms and has normal liver function tests, he need not be removed from work unless proven to be a source of infection. Liver function and HBsAg status should be evaluated every 4 to 6 months to monitor for active disease. If such a person becomes symptomatic or shows signs of hepatitis, he should be advised to cease working temporarily until evidence of illness clears. Food handlers have not been implicated in the transmission of hepatitis B and, when HBsAg-positive, they need not be restricted. During acute hepatitis with symptoms, for their own comfort, they should be advised to refrain from work like anyone else with acute hepatitis B.

Risk of exposure to HBsAg ceases when antigen disappears from the bloodstream; this is usually within 6 to 8 weeks of infection. Repeat serum determinations of HBsAg can help define when precautions may be relaxed.

Hepatitis D (Delta Hepatitis). Prevention of delta hepatitis in persons susceptible to HBV infection can be achieved by administering hepatitis B vaccine. Once immune to HBV, a person is immune to hepatitis D as well. For HBsAg carriers, there is no effective immunoprophylaxis against infection with the delta agent. For them, prevention of delta hepatitis requires limitation of percutaneous and intimate contacts with patients known to be infected with hepatitis D.

Non-A, Non-B Hepatitis. The principal means of reducing the incidence of this type of viral hepatitis is to use volunteer blood in preference to commercial blood. The development of means to detect antigenic markers for the non-A, non-B variants will greatly facilitate prevention of the disease. IG and HBIG are of no proven benefit as prophylactic measures for post-transfusion non-A, non-B hepatitis; however, many authorities recommend IG for needlestick, sexual, or perinatal exposure to non-A, non-B hepatitis.

RECOMMENDATIONS AND PATIENT EDUCATION

Hepatitis A Precautions (to Be Continued Until a Week After the Onset of Jaundice)

- Advise the patient to wash hands thoroughly after use of the toilet.
- The patient need not be confined to home, but intimate contact should be avoided.
- Prohibit the patient from handling and serving food to others.
- Advise others to avoid contact with the patient's fecal material and to wash hands thoroughly if contact is made.

Hepatitis A Prophylaxis

- Administer IG to household contacts within 2 weeks of exposure: the dosage is 0.2 ml per kilogram; average adult dosage is 2 ml intramuscularly.
- Administer IG for contacts in an epidemic and for travelers to areas in which hepatitis A is endemic; the dose is the same as for household contacts, unless travel is prolonged; then the dose should be 0.05 ml per kilogram every 4 to 6 months.

Hepatitis B Precautions (to Be Continued Until HBsAg Clears from the Serum)

- All blood donors should be screened for HBsAg.
- Use volunteer blood, rather than blood from commercial donors.
- Preferentially use disposable syringes and needles.
- Have patient use separate razor, toothbrush, and other personal items.
- Have any materials containing HBsAg handled carefully, particularly blood samples and other bodily fluids; use of gloves is advisable.
- Recommend avoidance of intimate contact, but confinement to home is unnecessary.
- If the patient has acute disease and is sneezing or coughing productively, he should use a mask to minimize the risk of contact with saliva.
- Hands should be washed thoroughly after direct contact with the patient or with the patient's blood or body fluids.

Hepatitis B Prophylaxis

Preexposure. • Administer three 1-ml (0.5-ml for those under age 10) intramuscular injections of hepatitis B vaccine at 0, 1, and 6 months to persons in high-risk groups. These include health workers exposed to blood, residents and staff of custodial institutions for the developmentally handicapped, household and sexual contacts of chronic HBsAg carriers, promiscuous male homosexuals and promiscuous heterosexuals, patients with hereditary hemoglobinopathies and clotting disorders who require long-term therapy with blood products, and hemodialysis patients.

Postexposure • Administer HBIG intramuscularly, 0.06 ml per kilogram of body weight (approximately 5 ml), to those who sustain an accidental percutaneous or transmucosal exposure with HBsAg-positive blood or body secretions or needles/instruments contaminated with HBsAg-positive material. This globulin injection should be administered as soon after exposure as possible; although globulin injections are recommended up to 7 days after inoculation, their efficacy is nil beyond 2 days. Passive immunoprophylaxis with HBIG should be followed by a complete three-injection course of hepatitis B vaccine; these injections can be started at the same time as HBIG or within the first few days to a week after exposure.

- Administer HBIG, at the dose cited above, to sexual contacts of patients with *acute* hepatitis B as soon after exposure as is practical. Because recognition of hepatitis in a sexual contact is often delayed, early prophylaxis is usually impossible. In one study, prophylaxis within 30 days of recognized exposure was effective, but current recommendations call for prophylaxis within 14 days of exposure. Some authorities recommend a second HBIG injection 3 months after the first, if the sexual partner remains HBsAg-positive after initial detection; others recommend that the first HBIG dose be followed by a complete three-injection course of hepatitis B vaccine in all sexual contacts of patients with acute hepatitis B, regardless of the duration of the HBV infection.
- Administer 0.5 ml of HBIG intramuscularly to newborns of HBsAg-positive mothers immediately after birth, preferably in the delivery room. This should be followed by a complete three-injection course of hepatitis B vaccine, 0.5 ml per dose, preferably to be started within 7 days of birth.
- No prophylaxis is necessary for casual contacts or nonintimate household contacts.

Non-A, Non-B Hepatitis Precautions and Prophylaxis

- Precautions are the same as those for hepatitis B—that is, limitation of exposure to infected patients' blood and body fluids.
- There are no valid tests for use in screening blood to prevent non-A, non-B hepatitis.
- The best means of limiting transfusion-associated non-A, non-B hepatitis is to rely exclusively on volunteer rather than commercial blood donors.
- Although immune globulin has not been shown to be effective in preventing transfusion-related non-A, non-B hepatitis, some authorities recommend that IG be administered for exposures in which the inoculum size is much smaller than in transfusion settings, that is, to those who sustain a needlestick, to sexual contacts of acute cases of non-A, non-B hepatitis, and to babies born to mothers with non-A, non-B hepatitis. A single 5-ml dose (0.5-ml for newborns) has been suggested.

ANNOTATED BIBLIOGRAPHY

Alter HJ: The evolution, implications, and application of hepatitis B vaccine. JAMA 247:2272, 1982 (*Reviews the development of hepatitis B vaccine, studies done to prove its efficacy and safety, and recommendations for its use.*)

Alter H, Chalmer T, Freeman B: Health care workers positive for hepatitis B surface antigen: Are their contacts at risk? N Engl J Med 292:454, 1975 (*A prospective controlled study that showed no evidence of spread of hepatitis to 282 patients exposed to staff positive for HBsAg. Supports view that risk is low.*)

Alter H et al: Type B hepatitis: Infectivity of blood positive for e antigen. N Engl J Med 295:090, 1976 (*Presence of e antigen was found to be an important indicator of relative infectivity of HBsAg-positive serum, particularly after small-volume parenteral exposure.*)

Centers for Disease Control: Postexposure prophylaxis of hepatitis B: Recommendations of the Immunization Practices Advisory Committee. Ann Intern Med 101:351, 1984 (*The official CDC recommendations for use of HBIG and hepatitis B vaccine for postexposure prophylaxis are outlined; includes prophylaxis for needlestick exposure, sexual contacts of patients with acute hepatitis B, and newborns of HBsAg-positive mothers.*)

Dienstag JL: Non-A, non-B hepatitis. I. Recognition, epidemiology, and clinical features; II. Experimental transmission, putative virus agents and markers, and prevention. Gastroenterology 85:439, 743, 1983 (*A two-part extensive review of non-A, non-B hepatitis.*)

Dienstag JL, Feinstone SM, Kapikian AZ et al: Fecal shedding of hepatitis-A antigen. Lancet 1:765, 1975 (*Most shedding occurs prior to onset of jaundice.*)

Dienstag JL, Szmuness W, Stevens CE et al: Hepatitis A virus infection: New insights from seroepidemiological studies. J Infect Dis 137:328, 1978 (*A review of seroepidemiology studies which define the prevalence of hepatitis A infection and modes of transmission. Hepatitis A is transmitted by the fecal–oral route and not by percutaneous means.*)

Francis DP, Feorino PM, McDougal S et al: The safety of the hepatitis B vaccine. JAMA 256:869, 1986 (*Each of three inactivation steps in manufacture of the vaccine independently inactivates the AIDS virus.*)

Hoofnagle JH, Seeff LB, Bales ZB et al: Passive-active immunity from hepatitis B immune globulin. Ann Intern Med 91:813, 1979 (*A study of the mechanisms of immune globulin action in prophylaxis. Argues that infection is not prevented by HBIG, but clinical illness is. Suggests that ISG may cause active immunization in some instances.*)

Immunization Practices Advisory Committee: Inactivated hepatitis B virus vaccine. MMWR 31:317, 1982 (*Recommendations for the use of hepatitis B vaccine for populations at high risk of exposure to hepatitis B.*)

Krugman S: The newly licensed hepatitis B vaccine: Characteristics and indications for use. JAMA 247:2012, 1982 (*A brief but authoritative review that describes the vaccine and provides recommendations for its application.*)

Krugman S, Giles J: Viral hepatitis: New light on an old disease. JAMA 212:1019, 1970 (*Classic paper on natural history of hepatitis A and B and documentation of efficacy of gamma-globulin for prevention of hepatitis A.*)

Krugman S et al: Viral hepatitis, type B: Studies on natural history and prevention re-examined. N Engl J Med 300:101, 1979 (*Describes the serologic events in viral hepatitis as defined by contemporary tests for hepatitis B antigens and antibodies.*)

Mulley AG, Silverstein MD, Dienstag JL: Indications for use of hepatitis B vaccine, based on cost-effectiveness analysis. N Engl J Med 307:644, 1982 (*Hepatitis B vaccine, despite its high cost, actually saves medical care costs if administered to population groups with a sufficiently high risk of infection.*)

Redeker AD et al: Hepatitis B immune globulin as a prophylactic measure for spouses exposed to acute type B hepatitis. N Engl J Med 293:1055, 1975 (*Demonstrated high risk of hepatitis in spouses and efficacy of HBIG for prevention of clinical illness.*)

Rizzetto M: The delta agent. Hepatology 3:729, 1983 (*Dr. Rizzetto, the discoverer of the delta agent outlines the virology, serology, epidemiology, and clinical features of hepatitis D.*)

Seeff L et al: Type B hepatitis after needle-stick exposure: Prevention with hepatitis B immune globulin. Ann Intern Med 88:285, 1978 (*HBIG and IG without antibody were compared in a randomized, double-blind multicenter study. HBIG was significantly more effective in preventing hepatitis. The efficacy of IG compared with that of placebo was not studied.*)

Seeff LB, Hoofnagle JH: Immunoprophylaxis of viral hepatitis. Gastroenterology 77:161, 1979 (*A detailed review of the studies on which immunoprophylaxis is based; also provides an excellent approach to and rationale for decisions about preventive interventions.*)

Seeff LB, Koff RS: Passive and active immunoprophylaxis of hepatitis B. Gastroenterology 86:958, 1984 (*An updated review of the use of globulins and vaccine to prevent hepatitis B.*)

Szmuness W, Stevens CE, Harley EJ et al: Hepatitis B vaccine: Demonstration of efficacy in a controlled clinical trial in a high-risk population in the United States. N Engl J Med 303:833, 1980 (*A classic paper describing the landmark controlled trial of hepatitis B vaccine in homosexual men, establishing the safety and efficacy of the vaccine in preventing clinical and subclinical cases of hepatitis B.*)

53
Evaluation of Abdominal Pain

JAMES M. RICHTER, M.D.
LYNN F. BUTTERLY, M.D.

One of the most challenging problems faced by the primary physician is the outpatient assessment of abdominal pain. When the pain is acute in onset, triage decisions have to be made regarding the need for hospital admission and surgical intervention. If the pain is chronic or recurrent, the physician must design a safe, cost-effective plan for workup that will efficiently distinguish among a myriad of possible etiologies. In many instances, the exact cause of pain is not immediately evident. Nevertheless, a few basic determinations may help elucidate the underlying pathophysiology, which, in turn, can guide further assessment and decision making. Of particular importance is the need to decide on the proper speed and extent of evaluation.

PATHOPHYSIOLOGY AND CLINICAL PRESENTATION

The major mechanisms of abdominal pain include obstruction of a hollow viscus, peritoneal irritation, vascular insufficiency, mucosal ulceration, altered bowel motility, capsular distention or inflammation, metabolic imbalance, nerve injury, abdominal wall injury, referral from an extra-abdominal site, and emotional stress.

Clinical presentations of abdominal pain due to organ pathology or functional disturbances are determined, in part, by site of involvement. Although generalizations concerning the location of pain are at best crude, a few are clinically useful. Lower esophageal pain is usually subxyphoid or substernal but may be referred to the back. Gastric and duodenal disease produces epigastric discomfort, which sometimes radiates into the back. Pain from the small bowel is usually periumbilical but likely to occur in the right lower quadrant when the terminal ileum is involved. Most colonic pain is felt in the lower abdomen, particularly the left lower quadrant; with rectosigmoid problems, referral may be to the sacrum. Disease of the transverse colon may give upper abdominal discomfort. Gallbladder and common bile duct obstruction result in epigastric or right upper quadrant complaints, with characteristic radiation to the scapular region. Pancreatic pain is usually midline or with radiation into the back. Diffuse pain is seen with generalized peritonitis, metabolic disturbances, and psychogenic illness, though all may produce focal complaints.

Obstruction. Pain receptors in the bowel, biliary tree, and ureters respond to distention. The severity of the pain is a function of the speed of onset as well as the degree of distention. Obstruction that develops slowly over weeks to months may be relatively subtle in presentation, compared to the more dramatic picture produced by acute obstruction. In acute obstruction, the pain is severe, poorly localized, and "colicky" or wavelike in nature; it makes the patient restless. The pain of acute *small bowel* obstruction is greatest when the obstruction is proximal. The patient is often comfortable between bouts of pain. Severity decreases with time as bowel motility diminishes. Complete strangulation of small bowel is associated with steady pain from secondary vascular insufficiency or peritoneal irritation. Vomiting is common, particularly in proximal obstruction; when the problem is distal, vomiting is less frequent. Flatus and passage of small amounts of stool may occur at the outset, but they soon cease if the obstruction is complete. Diarrhea is noted in some cases of partial obstruction. On examination, the patient appears restless during bouts of pain. The temperature is typically normal or only mildly elevated. The abdomen may be distended, especially when the obstruction is distal. High-pitched, hyperactive bowel sounds are characteristic, but not always present. Tenderness to palpation is not impressive, unless leakage of bowel contents has occurred, causing peritoneal soilage. The stool is usually guaiac negative.

Large bowel obstruction is, in most instances, less painful and associated with less vomiting than is obstruction of the small intestine. Constipation or change in bowel habits often precedes complete obstruction. Diarrhea may occur with partial obstruction. Distention is greater than that seen in small bowel obstruction. Stools are frequently positive for occult blood, because malignancy and diverticular disease are common etiologies.

In cases of bowel obstruction, the white blood cell count may be normal, even in association with a strangulating obstruction—that is, with compromise of the intestinal blood supply in addition to blockage of the lumen. A plain radiograph of the abdomen (KUB and upright) in patients with small bowel obstruction often shows distention of loops of small bowel with air–fluid levels. This, together with an absence of gas in the large bowel (distal to the obstruction) is characteristic of small bowel obstruction. The radiographic appearance of colonic obstruction varies with the competency (or incompetency) of the ileocecal valve. If the valve is competent, less small bowel dilatation ensues.

Sudden *obstruction* of the *common bile duct* or *cystic duct* by a stone produces acute pain, sometimes referred to as biliary "colic." Obstruction and dilatation that occur gradually are often painless. Unlike the cramping pain of acute intestinal obstruction, the pain of acute biliary tract obstruction is mostly steady, lasting hours after sudden onset. In *acute cholecystitis,* the typical pain is maximal in the right upper quadrant or epigastrium, radiating to the scapular region, accompanied by nausea, vomiting, and fever without jaundice; at times there is only mild epigastric discomfort (see Chapter 69). In *common duct obstruction,* the pain is more likely to be epigastric and jaundice is noted soon after onset. Emesis may be prominent. Physical examination reveals a tender right upper quadrant. *Murphy's sign* (inspiratory arrest in response to right upper quadrant palpation) may be seen, and right upper quadrant tenderness to percussion or pressure over the gall bladder is also a suggestive finding. Laboratory investigation usually reveals a leukocytosis; mild hyperbilirubinemia may occur, usually after the initial onset of symptoms.

Obstruction within the *urinary tract* can present as abdominal pain. Acute ureteral blockade by a stone is extremely uncomfortable; the pain is cramping, beginning in the back and flank and radiating into the lower abdomen and groin. If acute pyelonephritis develops, upper abdominal pain, fever, and chills may ensue. Acute bladder outflow obstruction presents as lower abdominal distention and suprapubic pain. Symptoms of prostatism (see Chapter 133) may precede the episode.

Peritoneal Irritation may cause severe pain, because of the rich innervation of the parietal peritoneum. Focal injury results in well-localized discomfort that is described as sharp, aching, or burning. Spread of the irritant process leads to more generalized abdominal pain. Severity is related to the nature of the irritant and the speed at which the noxious exposure occurs. There can be reflex spasm of the overlying abdominal wall musculature, producing involuntary guarding. Rebound tenderness is prominent on physical examination. Most important, the pain is accentuated by pressure changes in the peritoneum, thus, palpation, coughing, or movement may increase the pain, leading the patient to lie still, in contrast to the restlessness of patients with "colicky" pain. Bowel sounds are often reduced or absent, especially when the irritation is generalized. The origin of the peritoneal irritant need not be intra-abdominal.

Vascular Disorders such as acute *arterial insufficiency* (due to atherosclerosis or embolus) may present with severe abdominal pain, although mild, constant pain may be the only symptom for several days. The pain of mesenteric arterial insufficiency may occur in the absence of tenderness and rigidity, and the diagnosis is not necessarily considered until signs of peritoneal soiling and shock ensue. *Dissection* or rupture of an abdominal aortic aneurysm produces severe acute abdominal pain that often radiates to the back or gen-

italia. *Mesenteric venous thrombosis* is a less common cause of intestinal ischemia than arterial occlusion; it may present similarly although it often has a more slowly progressive course. Both aortic dissection and mesenteric thrombosis typically result in pain complaints that are in excess of those elicited by physical examination.

Chronic arterial insufficiency may precede an acute episode of infarction, especially in cases of progressive atherosclerotic narrowing. The patient complains of episodes of cramping or dull midabdominal pain that come on 15 to 30 minutes after a meal and can last up to 2 or 3 hours. This so-called *abdominal angina* is greatest at times of maximal demand for blood supply to the bowel (*e.g.,* after a large meal). Some lose considerable amounts of weight because of the fear that eating will induce pain. Ischemic, abdominal pain also results from vascular occlusive crises of sickle cell anemia.

Mucosal Ulceration of the upper gastrointestinal tract is often accompanied by pain. Although the exact mechanism of pain in ulcer disease remains incompletely understood, it is believed that acid plays a major role. This hypothesis is supported by the observation that neutralization of acid often provides immediate relief. Pain pattern of duodenal ulcer disease usually parallels the acid-peptic cycle (see Chapter 64). Unless there is perforation or penetration into the pancreas, the pain is mostly confined to the epigastrium. Patients use such terms as "gnawing," "aching," and "burning" to describe their discomfort. Radiation of pain into the back in patients with duodenal ulcer suggests perforation into the pancreas.

Alteration In Bowel Motility may occur with functional disturbances, of which the *irritable bowel syndrome* is the best example. Spasmodic, nonpropulsive segmental contractions of large bowel result in development of high intraluminal pressures and cramping lower abdominal pain. Constipation alternating with diarrhea is a characteristic presentation (see Chapter 66). *Diverticular disease* is also associated with altered motility and pain (see Chapter 67). *Inflammation* often produces disturbances of motility and absorption, such as acute gastroenteritis and acute flares of inflammatory bowel disease (see Chapter 65). In most instances, the pain is diffuse, but occasionally it is focal and can simulate appendicitis or other surgical conditions. Fever, nausea, and vomiting are often prominent in the early stages of gastroenteritis; bowel sounds are usually hyperactive.

Intestinal Pseudoobstruction refers to a syndrome in which the clinical features of intestinal obstruction are found in the absence of a lesion, causing mechanical obstruction of the lumen. It may be chronic, with recurrence or persistence of symptoms, or may occur acutely (so-called *acute ileus*). Any part of the intestinal tract from the esophagus to the colon may be involved; there is a defect in propulsive forces in the involved segment. This results in the radiologic appearance of a partial obstruction. As in mechanical obstruction, the prominent clinical symptoms vary with the location of the pseudoobstruction, and may include vomiting (especially in proximal obstruction) or abdominal distention (most prominent in colonic obstruction); diarrhea or constipation can also be seen. It is noteworthy that the syndrome of chronic pseudoobstruction may precede the recognition of associated systemic diseases by many years (see below).

The causes of acute ileus include peritonitis (resulting from a variety of causes), systemic infections, ischemic bowel injury, abdominal operations (a common etiology), abdominal trauma, pharmacologic agents (associated with the administration of anticholinergic or narcotic drugs), and metabolic disturbances (such as electrolyte imbalance, especially hypokalemia). A few important causes of chronic intestinal pseudoobstruction are idiopathic, scleroderma, Parkinson's disease, opiates, phenothiazines, tricyclic antidepressants, antiparkinsonian medications, hypercalcemia, diabetes, myxedema, amyloid, radiation enteritis, and chronic laxative abuse.

Capsular Distention. Distention of the well-innervated capsule surrounding an organ can be another source of constant, *aching* abdominal pain. *Hepatic* capsular distention may result from hepatic swelling secondary to hepatitis, congestive heart failure, fatty infiltration, or subcapsular hematoma and may result in right upper quadrant pain. The pain of *splenic* capsular distention, as may occur secondary to blunt trauma, from an auto accident, is located in the left upper quadrant. With diaphragmatic irritation, the patient sometimes experiences pain radiating to the ipsilateral shoulder. With splenic trauma, there can be a deceptive period of many hours before peritoneal signs develop if a subcapsular hematoma temporarily retards the spilling of blood into the peritoneum.

Metabolic Disturbances may mimic intra-abdominal etiologies. *Porphyria* and *lead poisoning* sometimes simulate bowel obstruction, for they can cause cramping abdominal pain and hyperperistalsis. *Acute intermittent porphyria* (AIP) presents with moderate to severe colicky abdominal pain, which may be localized or generalized. Abdominal symptoms may be the result of intestinal dysmotility; vomiting and diarrhea are also common complaints. Fever and leukocytosis may be present but on examination the abdomen is found to be soft. Proximal muscle pain and a range of neuropsychiatric symptoms accompany the abdominal pain. The clinical features of *hereditary coproporphyria* and *variegate porphyria* are similar to those described for AIP; skin lesions may be prominent. A Watson–Schwartz test for urinary porphobilinogen may suggest the diagnosis of an acute attack in all three of these entities.

Lead poisoning may also present with abdominal pain. Such pain is typically wandering, poorly localized, colicky, and accompanied by a rigid abdomen. Encephalopathy, peripheral neuropathy, and anemia are associated features. The *urine coproporphyrin* is a more reliable test for this entity than is a serum lead level, which can be normal.

Ketoacidosis has been found to present with severe abdominal pain in 8% of instances and may be accompanied by emesis and an elevated white cell count. These symptoms are due at least in part to gastroparesis, which may occur in ketoacidosis. However, it should be remembered that acute intra-abdominal events such as cholecystitis may be the precipitants of ketoacidosis.

C'1 esterase inhibitor deficiency may result in episodic *angioneurotic edema* and severe abdominal pain. If this diagnosis is suspected, it is useful to check the serum level of C4, which is low in C'1 esterase inhibitor deficiency.

Nerve Injury from encroachment or irritation is an important mechanism of abdominal pain. The source of pain may be intra-abdominal, as occurs when a pancreatic cancer invades adjacent splanchnic nerves, or it may be extra-abdominal, as in herpes zoster irritating a nerve root that supplies an abdominal wall dermatome. Abdominal pain occurs in about 75% of patients with *cancer of the pancreas;* it is usually epigastric and most common in patients with tumor involving the body or tail of the pancreas. Sometimes the pain radiates to the back or is confined to it. Pancreatic malignancy also causes pain by other mechanisms, including obstruction of the common or pancreatic duct. Nerve root irritation from *herpes zoster* may be mistaken for an intra-abdominal process, especially before the rash appears. Often, the patient complains of a severe lancinating pain resembling an intra-abdominal source. There may be associated rectus muscle spasm simulating peritonitis, but unlike in peritoneal irriation, there is no effect on bowel function and palpation may actually aleviate the rectus muscle spasm. The pain of herpes infection often precedes the rash by several days and may persist after the skin clears, particularly in the elderly (see Chapter 192).

Abdominal Wall Pathology can also be mistaken for disease inside the abdominal cavity. Traumatic injury to the musculature of the wall produces pain that is constant, aching, and exacerbated by movement or pressure on the abdomen. The muscles may be in spasm, simulating the involuntary guarding of peritonitis. When a generalized myositis is responsible for the muscle pain, discomfort occurs in the limbs as well as in the abdomen. Occasionally, a tender mass in the wall, such as a rectus sheath hematoma, is found to be the source of difficulty.

Referred Pain from a process originating in the chest is sometimes an etiology of abdominal complaints. Pulmonary infarction and pneumonia of the lower lobes are among the chest problems that may present as pain in the upper abdomen; at times reflex muscle spasm even accompanies the pain. Upper abdominal pain, nausea, and vomiting may be the principal manifestations of an acute inferior myocardial infarction. Fortunately, most intrathoracic sources of abdominal pain are accompanied by symptoms and signs of cardiac or pulmonary disease.

Familial Mediterranean Fever (FMF) presents as episodic abdominal pain. Patients with this disorder often complain of abdominal swelling; an elevated erythrocyte sedimentation rate (ESR) may be noted during acute attacks. The etiology of FMF is still unknown, however, in some cases colchicine produces dramatic relief.

Psychogenic Pain. In most cases of psychogenic pain, the cause is an underlying irritable bowel syndrome, amplified in complex fashion by anxiety, depression, or other conditions which lead to exaggerated, unrealistic concerns about normal bodily functions. Many patients with psychiatric illness present to physicians with symptoms of irritable bowel syndrome. In a study of 29 patients with irritable bowel syndrome presenting to a university referral unit, 25 were found on evaluation to have an underlying psychiatric illness believed responsible for triggering their symptoms. Other patients with psychogenic pain have a pain pattern that shows little relationship to physiologic stimuli or anatomy.

In *neurotic patients,* a detailed history often reveals longstanding concerns about gastrointestinal symptoms that have been waxing and waning for years, but not worsening with time. There may also be a vague and complicated history of many undiagnosed symptoms involving multiple organ systems, again suggesting a heightened concern about bodily sensations. *Depressed patients* also manifest excessive worry and preoccupation with their bodies. Characteristically, their many bodily complaints occur in conjunction with early morning awakening, change in appetite, diminished libido, fatigue, and low self-esteem; there may be a history of an important personal loss or a family history of depression.

In patients with *hysteria,* the pain may have symbolic meaning and is often accompanied by recurrent nausea, vomiting, and diarrhea. Studies of such patients show an increased incidence of hospitalizations, operations, and medications for their pain compared with nonhysteric controls. The clinical presentation may be very confusing and the diagnosis is often missed. Diagnostic criteria include physical symptoms of several years' duration beginning before age 30, alteration of living pattern as a result of the symptoms, sickly appearance, history of conversion symptoms (dysphasia, loss of voice, double vision, fainting, memory loss, transient numbness, or paresis), and a potpourri of gastrointestinal, gynecologic, psychosexual, cardiopulmonary, and chronic pain complaints.

On physical examination, findings in patients with psychogenic abdominal pain are often neither very impressive nor in proportion to the amount of discomfort conveyed in the history. Even if severe discomfort is elicited, it may diminish with distraction.

Such features are characteristic of psychogenic abdominal pain but by no means universal. Although the clinical features vary greatly, what best characterizes psychogenic abdominal pain is not the constellation of symptoms, but the patient's disproportionate response to them.

DIFFERENTIAL DIAGNOSIS

Because the number of possible causes of abdominal pain is large, it is helpful to consider the differential diagnosis in terms of pathophysiologic mechanisms (see Table 53-1). Etiologies causing obstruction, peritoneal irritation, and vascular insufficiency are among the most dangerous. About 70% of mechanical small bowel obstruction is due to adhesions or external hernias; 90% of large bowel obstruction is attributable to diverticular disease and carcinoma. Acute arterial insufficiency results most often from systemic embolization due to atrial fibrillation, severe atherosclerotic occlusive disease, and hypoperfusional states. Pelvic pathology is a common extra-abdominal source of peritoneal irritation.

Other pathophysiologic mechanisms, such as nerve injury, metabolic imbalance, abdominal wall disease, and disordered motility may produce symptoms that superficially mimic a more worrisome etiology; but usually conditions associated with these mechanisms are more annoying than dangerous (an important exception is diabetic ketoacidosis). Pain re-

Table 53-1. Principal Mechanisms of Abdominal Pain

Obstruction	**Altered Motility**
1. Gastric outlet	1. Gastroenteritis
2. Small bowel	2. Inflammatory bowel disease
3. Large bowel	3. Irritable bowel syndrome
4. Biliary tract	4. Diverticular disease
5. Urinary tract	**Metabolic Disturbance**
Peritoneal Irritation	1. Diabetic ketoacidosis
1. Infection	2. Porphyria
2. Chemical irritation (blood, bile, gastric acid)	3. Lead poisoning
3. Systemic inflammatory process	**Nerve Injury**
4. Spread from a local inflammatory process	1. Herpes zoster
	2. Root compression
	3. Nerve invasion
Vascular Insufficiency	**Muscle Wall Disease**
1. Embolization	1. Trauma
2. Atherosclerotic narrowing	2. Myositis
3. Hypotension	3. Hematoma
4. Aortic aneurysm dissection	**Referred Pain**
Mucosal Ulceration	1. Pneumonia (lower lobes)
1. Peptic ulcer disease	2. Inferior myocardial infarction
2. Gastric cancer	3. Pulmonary infarction
	Psychopathology
	1. Depression
	2. Anxiety
	3. Neuroses

ferred from an extra-abdominal site is more of a problem; significant cardiac disease (*e.g.,* inferior myocardial infarction) or pulmonary pathology (*e.g.,* lower lobe pneumonia) may present as abdominal pain.

WORKUP

The first priority in the office evaluation of the patient with abdominal pain is to determine the likelihood of serious pathophysiology and the pace and extent of workup. Patients with acute pain need to be examined promptly for evidence of obstruction, peritoneal irritation, vascular compromise, and cardiopulmonary disease. The evaluation of chronic pain can be assessed at a more gradual pace, allowing time to get to know the patient and his problem before rushing into extensive testing.

History should include a complete description of the pain including localization, characterization, area of referral, time course of onset and resolution, and precipitating and alleviating factors. The chronological sequence of symptom occurrence should be clearly outlined.

In addition to carefully obtaining a complete description of the patient's pain, checking for specific items is needed: prior abdominal surgery, previous episodes of obstruction, known gallbladder or kidney stones, presence and nature of vomitus, passage of flatus, time of last bowel movement, occurrence of diarrhea, constipation or change in bowel habits, effect of movement on pain, presence of fever and rigors, development of distention, difficulties in urination, and presence of any cardiac or pulmonary symptoms. Inquiry into symptoms of pelvic pathology, such as dyspareunia, abnormal vaginal discharge, and irregular menstrual bleeding, should be included in the assessment of every woman with abdominal pain.

Frequently confounding variables in the assessment are the patient's perception of and response to the pain. Patients display widely varying tolerances to pain, yet the physician must learn to interpret accurately the "true" quality and quantity of the patient's experience. Psychological and ethnic factors alter expression and response to pain and must be taken into consideration, especially in cases of chronic abdominal pain. A thorough psychosocial history is essential. Substantial variation in pain perception, as well as communication, may be due to factors other than the pain itself. Exploring patient fears and concerns is often surprisingly productive.

On Physical Examination, particular attention ought to be paid to the patient's general appearance. The patient who appears reluctant to change position and keeps still is likely to have peritoneal irritation, whereas the patient with obstruction is often restless. It is important to check the vital signs for postural changes in blood pressure or heart rate,

because obstruction, peritonitis, and bowel infarction can produce large losses of intravascular volume. Any hypotension, atrial fibrillation, or fever should be noted; however, absence of fever does not rule out serious pathology, especially in the elderly or chronically ill patient. The skin is examined for jaundice, other stigmata of chronic liver disease, clubbing or spooning of the fingernails, signs of trauma, excoriations, prior surgical scars, evidence of dehydration or edema, rash (which may be dermatomal), and xanthomata. In addition, the sclerae are noted for icterus, the chest for splinting, a pleural friction rub, and signs of consolidation (particularly in the lower lobes), and the heart for murmurs, chamber enlargement, and signs of heart failure.

The abdominal examination should be performed with care to avoid unnecessary discomfort. A sharp increase in pain with coughing demonstrates rebound tenderness without the need for palpation and release. Examination of the abdomen includes checking for the presence of distention, altered bowel sounds (increase or absence), a hepatic rub or a vascular bruit, tenderness, guarding, rebound, hepatosplenomegaly, and masses (including a dilated aorta, loops of bowel, stool, or a distended bladder or uterus). An increased abdominal venous pattern suggests portal hypertension; periumbilical adenopathy suggests pancreatic cancer.

Pelvic and rectal examinations are essential parts of the evaluation, checking for masses and tenderness. These exams will certainly be more revealing if done gently. The fecal occult blood test is also mandatory.

If psychogenic pain or a major degree of psychocultural overlay is suspected, deep palpation ought to be done while the patient is distracted. Distracting an anxious patient while gently performing deep palpation may be the best way to demonstrate a lack of tenderness. One method used is to push deeply while auscultating with a stethoscope in a patient who is anxious about palpation.

In an elderly person with no history of somatizing, the presence of significant abdominal pain out of proportion to tenderness subsequently elicited by physical examination, suggests vascular compromise. The elderly person with an acute intra-abdominal process may at first show few signs of serious illness. Peritoneal signs may be absent or minimal. The only early clues may be unexplained mild fever, tachycardia, and vague abdominal discomfort. A high index of suspicion is needed.

Examining for nerve and muscle wall injury is often overlooked in the urgency of searching for more worrisome pathology. Two important signs of nerve involvement are pain in a dermatomal distribution and hyperesthesia. Both occur with nerve injury due to herpes zoster or nerve root impingement; however, hyperesthesia is also seen with focal peritoneal irritation. Testing is performed by gentle stroking of the skin overlying the area of pain. The rash of herpes may not appear until the time of the follow-up assessment. Abdominal wall pathology may be discovered by careful palpation of the wall for masses and muscle tenderness and by exacerbation of pain on contracting the muscles, as occurs with sitting up. Any pain on sitting up should not be confused with that due to involuntary muscle spasm from peritoneal irritation. The limbs should also be checked for muscle tenderness, which is suggestive of a generalized muscle disorder.

Laboratory Tests. Relatively few are needed at the time of initial assessment. Studies are aimed at determining the likelihood of obstruction, peritonitis, acute vascular insufficiency, metabolic disruption, and cardiac or pulmonary disease. The *complete blood count* (CBC) and *differential* are often helpful in confirming the presence of an acute inflammatory process. Though very nonspecific, the CBC and differential are reasonably sensitive in patients able to mount a normal acute inflammatory response. Unfortunately, the CBC may show little change in the elderly or chronically ill patient, even in an acute intra-abdominal emergency. The differential ought to be ordered even if the white cell count is "normal," because a shift to immature forms sometimes occurs without a significant elevation in the white count. At times a relatively benign condition such as viral gastroenteritis may produce an impressive elevation in the white cell count (as high as 20,000 cells/cc) accompanied by a marked shift to immature forms, simulating the peripheral blood picture of a patient with more worrisome disease. The CBC and differential must be carefully interpreted in the context of the entire clinical picture and not used alone to decide whether or not to admit the patient.

Supine and upright *plain films of the abdomen* are essential if one suspects bowel obstruction or perforation. Multiple (*i.e.,* ≥3) air–fluid levels, distention of the small bowel, and absence of gas in the large bowel are characteristic of complete small bowel obstruction; unfortunately, such findings are present in fewer than 50% of cases of bowel strangulation, especially in the early stages of obstruction. Partial mechanical obstruction may produce some loops of bowel with air–fluid levels, but there is also gas in the colon; the same findings are found in patients with adynamic ileus. In colonic obstruction with a competent ileocecal valve, only the large bowel appears distended, but if the valve is not competent, both large and small bowel demonstrate distention and gas, mimicking the findings of adynamic ileus. Distinguishing partial small bowel obstruction from ileus requires repeat films or a barium study. Suspected obstruction of the large bowel is an indication for a barium enema and usually a contraindication to performing an upper gastrointestinal series.

On the plain film (KUB), free air under the diaphragm indicates perforation of a viscus; absent psoas shadows suggest retroperitoneal bleeding, abscess, or mass; and displaced stomach or bowel (determined by gas patterns) may be caused by compression from a tumor. Plain films are also helpful in finding a biliary or renal stone, abdominal aortic calcification suggesting an aneurysm, or pancreatic calcification due to

pancreatitis. Calcification has been found on plain film of the abdomen in over 60% of abdominal aneurysms. A cross-table lateral view best demonstrates the lesion.

Although useful, plain films of the abdomen are commonly overutilized in evaluating abdominal pain. Limiting this study to patients with moderate to severe tenderness or high clinical suspicion of bowel obstruction, urinary tract calculi, trauma, ischemia, or gallbladder disease (regardless of degree of tenderness) was found in a retrospective study to be capable of reducing utilization by more than 50% without any significant reduction in the rate of detecting clinically important pathology. Plain films were not useful for detecting unsuspected pathology, especially in patients with mild tenderness on examination.

Using plain films to "rule out" serious pathology is possible only for bowel obstruction and perforation, in which the sensitivity of the plain film approaches 100%. Sensitivity for detection of other conditions is much lower.

Other simple tests can aid the initial evaluation. A *urinalysis* should be checked for pyuria, hematuria, bacteria, sugar, and ketones. Mild to moderate ketonuria is common when the patient has not eaten and is unrelated to diabetes; the diagnosis of ketoacidosis requires urine ketones in large concentrations (see Chapter 100). Red cells in the urine of a patient with flank pain suggest a stone in the ureter (see Chapter 134). The *BUN, glucose electrolytes,* and *amylase* levels can often be obtained on a stat basis. Elevation of the serum amylase occurs not only in pancreatitis, but also in intestinal obstruction, perforated ulcer, and biliary tract disease; additional information is needed to identify the source of the elevation (see Chapter 72). Although not especially specific, the serum amylase is quite sensitive.

Serum electrolytes can be helpful in cases of vomiting, diarrhea, or adynamic ileus; tests of renal and liver function, and blood sugar should also be determined when clinical findings are suggestive.

The initial investigation of acute upper abdominal pain should also include a *chest film* and *electrocardiogram,* looking for pleuropulmonary disease in the lower lobes and acute ischemic changes in the inferior myocardium. In patients with diarrhea, a microscopic *examination of the stool* for polymorphonuclear leukocytes is indicated (see Chapter 58).

In patients with ascites or those who have sustained abdominal trauma, an abdominal *paracentesis* with a small needle can add valuable information (see Chapter 71). This procedure should be performed in the lower abdomen where there is less chance of perforating a viscus or a large blood vessel. Nontympanitic areas of the right lower quadrant, left lower quadrant, or the linea alba (midline) are the usual sites.

The patient with acute colicky pain but no signs of obstruction or inflammation may have lead poisoning and should have urine samples checked for coproporphyrin. Serum lead levels are unreliable. The person with acute intermittent porphyria may also present with colicky pain. Often such individuals are thought to be psychiatrically disturbed because of abnormal behavior during an attack. The diagnosis is suggested by periodic attacks of cramping pain, constipation, nausea and vomiting, and neuromuscular symptoms in conjunction with the altered psychological state. The *Watson–Schwartz test* for urinary porphobilinogen is a reliable screening test for acute intermittent porphyria in patients who are symptomatic.

Once it is determined that acute obstruction, peritonitis, bowel ischemia, and worrisome metabolic and cardiopulmonary diseases are unlikely, further evaluation can be carried out on an outpatient basis, at a more gradual pace. Among the most productive diagnostic measures is repetition of the history and physical examination. An inconsistent history raises the question of psychogenic pain; however, constancy certainly does not rule out an emotional etiology. Many serious etiologies may lead to a worsening of the clinical picture in a few days; this is particularly true for bowel ischemia, which initially may have an indolent presentation. Any patient sent home with undiagnosed acute pain requires careful follow-up and reexamination.

Selection of radiologic *contrast studies* ought to be judicious and based on the need to confirm or rule out specific diagnoses. Blind searches that involve "running the bowel" in the absence of suggestive clinical evidence are wasteful, potentially misleading, and uncomfortable for the patient. Recurrent epigastric or right upper quadrant pain in conjunction with an elevated alkaline phosphatase is an indication for *ultrasonography* of the gallbladder (see Chapter 69).

Epigastric pain that parallels the acid–peptic cycle or responds to food or antacids suggests acid-peptic disease. There is little need for an *upper GI series* or *endoscopy* if the patient is under the age of 40 and the risk of gastric or esophageal malignancy is judged to be very low. Such patients can be safely treated for presumed ulcer disease without documenting the lesion. However, failure to respond to therapy or the presence of worrisome symptoms (melena, hematemesis, weight loss) necessitates a full evaluation, as does the occurrence of ulcer symptoms in older patients, who are at increased risk of gastric cancer (see Chapter 50).

All patients with lower abdominal pain and evidence of bleeding (be it gross or occult) should be evaluated by *colonoscopy* or the combination of *barium enema* and *sigmoidoscopy* to identify the source (see Chapter 60). However, the very young patient with constipation and obvious hemorrhoidal bleeding need undergo only a sigmoidoscopy to rule out associated rectosigmoid pathology. Sufferers of lower abdominal pain who have no bleeding, weight loss, or change in bowel habits are less likely to benefit from radiologic or endoscopic evaluation unless their symptoms are particularly severe or chronic.

At times, there is little clinical indication for a contrast study, but the patient insists on having an upper GI series or barium enema done to rule out a particular concern. The contribution of a normal test result to the peace of mind of the patient has to be taken into account when deciding which tests to obtain.

Sigmoidoscopy is a simple procedure with which much information about rectosigmoid masses or mucosal abnormalities can be obtained; it complements the barium enema (see Chapter 75). *Colonoscopy* may be useful especially when polyps, colitis, or cancer is a consideration. This study allows for biopsy of suspected cancer, polypectomy, and assessment of the extent of disease in patients with inflammatory bowel disease.

The patient with flank pain, hematuria, or pyuria may have a renal source for their abdominal pain. An *intravenous pyelogram* may help in looking for disease in the kidneys or ureters or for displacement of a ureter by an abdominal or retroperitoneal mass. *Renal ultrasonography* can reveal a stone or ureteral dilatation. *Pelvic ultrasonography* is indicated when a uterine or ovarian mass is noted on bimanual examination.

Abdominal ultrasonography and computerized body tomography have come to play important roles in the evaluation of abdominal pain, making major contributions toward the noninvasive detection of pancreatic malignancy and other upper abdominal tumors. *Ultrasonography* has become the test of choice for diagnosis of gallstones (see Chapter 69) and useful for detection of biliary and ureteral obstructions (see Chapters 62 and 134, respectively). It can help identify ascites and sometimes localize intra-abdominal abscesses. Ultrasonography has been instrumental in the detection of pancreatic tumors. The test's sensitivity for diagnosis of pancreatic carcinoma is reported to range from 65% to 85%. It is less specific, but specificity can be markedly improved by ultrasound-guided needle biopsy. Large amounts of bowel gas and fat limit the sensitivity of the ultrasonogram and result in a fraction of studies that are technically inadequate or indeterminate; however, its relatively low cost, its noninvasive nature, and the absence of radiation exposure make it an excellent screening test for detecting pancreatic disease.

Computed body tomography (CBT) has shown sensitivity and specificity similar to those of ultrasonography for detection of pancreatic cancer, but a much lower rate of indeterminate readings (in one study, 4% versus 23%). CBT is less dependent on the skill of the operator to yield a high-quality image than is ultrasonography, but it is more expensive and involves radiation exposure. In addition to imaging the pancreas, it provides excellent views of the liver, retroperitoneum, and spine. Both ultrasonography and CBT visualize the common bile duct, portal vein, and hepatic artery and detect any displacment, encroachment, or encasement of the major intra-abdominal vessels and organs.

Endoscopic retrograde cholangiopancreatography (ERCP) is more sensitive for detecting pancreatic cancer than ultrasonography and more specific, but success is very dependent on the skill of the endoscopist.

In sum, patients suspected of harboring a pancreatic malignancy should be screened with an ultrasound study for detection of a pancreatic mass. If the study is not technically adequate because of the presence of gas or fat, then CBT or ERCP should be ordered when a solid mass is identified; needle aspiration biopsy is usually needed to confirm a diagnosis of malignancy. Although much progress has been made in identifying a pancreatic mass in symptomatic patients, early detection in the asymptomatic period remains an elusive goal.

Evaluation Of Undiagnosed Pain. A most taxing problem arises when extensive medical evaluation is unrevealing and the physician is left with a suspicion of psychogenic pain, but little direct evidence to support the hypothesis. There may be pressure from patient and family to look harder for an "organic" cause and a tendency, out of frustration, to order progressively more invasive studies in search of such an etiology. The underlying psychological problems may be masked by pain complaints and hinder further inquiry into this area.

Fortunately, a number of important clues that might have emerged in the medical evaluation suggest a psychogenic etiology; these include an exaggerated response to the pain, a history of multiple undiagnosed bodily complaints, a nonprogressive clinical course that may span many years, lack of relation between symptoms and physiologic stimuli, inconsistent or distractable physical findings, and presence of somatic symptoms suggestive of depression (early morning awakening, fatigue, decreased libido, altered appetite).

When such suggestive evidence for a psychogenic etiology exists, further inquiry into psychosocial matters is essential, but it is important not to deny the reality of the patient's symptoms or suffering. To convey the message that "there is nothing really wrong" or that it is "all in your head" will only send the patient off in search of another medical evaluation, especially if the patient feels he has not been fully worked up for a medical etiology. An effective, nonalienating means of pursuing the psychosocial investigation is to engage the patient in discussing how the pain has affected his life and those around him. In addition, exploring the patient's fears, concerns, views, and expectations about the pain and its evaluation can help uncover important psychological information without resorting to a frontal assault that may compromise one's relation with the patient.

The timing of a detailed look into psychosocial issues deserves comment. Inquiry into the effect of the pain on the patient's life should be done at the outset of the evaluation, for it is an essential part of the data base on any patient. However, to suggest at the outset that the problem is probably psychogenic before completing a careful medical workup is to invite resistance and hostility. It is usually much easier to explore areas of stress, conflict, and loss once a thorough medical assessment has been concluded, serious organic illness ruled out, and specific patient concerns addressed.

Psychiatric consultation is indicated when there is evidence of serious depression (see Chapter 223) or hysteria. In those with neurotic complaints presenting with irritable bowel syndrome, thorough reassurance (which includes addressing patient concerns) delivered in sympathetic fashion can be most effective, especially when combined with a trial of increased dietary fiber. If a low-grade depression is suspected, a course of tricyclic antidepressant therapy (see Chapter 213) may be warranted. Where constipation is a problem, one should use a tricyclic agent with minimal anticholineric effects. Such empirical approaches to patients with psychogenic abdominal pain will often effect symptomatic relief without resorting initially to formal psychotherapy.

The patient with chronic or recurrent abdominal pain that defies explanation poses one of the most difficult problems in clinical medicine. In a study of 30 such patients presenting to a general internist, most had epigastric pain, distention, belching, and nausea without vomiting or weight loss. Symptoms often began at the time of a personal loss or other emotional stress. Depression was commonly found. When treatment was directed at depression, the pain disappeared in many instances. In a study of 64 patients with abdominal pain of unknown etiology, two thirds of the patients were women. The younger the age and shorter the duration of the symptoms, the better the chances were for improvement. Older women with pain for more than 3 months were least likely to improve or to be diagnosed. Of those subjected to laparotomy, a diagnosis was obtained in only 10%; the rate of improvement was the same as for those who did not undergo exploration. In 15% of the total study population, a cause for the patient's abdominal pain was found, but in only 6% did the condition requires surgery. Thus, very few patients with abdominal pain of unknown etiology are endangered by continued observation, as long as signs of serious pathophysiology are absent. The morbidity of exploratory laparotomy in such patients greatly exceeds the benefit. Unexplained pain that is present for less than 2 weeks is likely to resolve spontaneously, but such improvement is unlikely when pain has persisted for more than 3 months.

INDICATIONS FOR ADMISSION AND REFERRAL

Any evidence suggestive of peritoneal irritation, obstruction, or acute vascular compromise is an indication for immediate hospitalization and surgical consultation. Sometimes further observations made in the hospital can save the patient a surgical procedure, but no patient with the possibility of a condition that might require urgent surgery should be sent home from the office. Elderly patients are especially likely to have subtle presentations.

The patient with unexplained pain that has defied outpatient diagnostic attempts may benefit from further assessment in the hospital, especially if a need for large amounts of pain medication has developed. Admission provides an opportunity for 24-hour observation, specialty consultation, and assessment of the need for further study.

Where the diagnosis is unclear but admission does not seem warranted, assiduous, close follow-up is mandatory; repeated histories and examinations may subsequently yield the diagnosis and hence allow proper treatment. Such factors as the degree of distress manifested by the patient, the degree of temperature elevation, white blood count elevation or other laboratory abnormalities, and the ability of the patient to eat and drink all need to be assessed. Judgment also must be made as to whether or not a patient with undiagnosed abdominal pain should undergo more invasive testing. In general, patients with unexplained abdominal pain in conjunction with recurrent nausea and vomiting, jaundice, fever, weight loss of greater than 10% of body weight, or the presence of blood in the stool will require more extensive evaluation; consultations with the gastroenterologist, surgeon, and radiologist may provide valuable assistance. Further evaluation in these cases may include endoscopy, endoscopic retrograde cholangiopancreatography, abdominal computerized body tomography, or laparoscopy. Conversely, the internist may decide to follow a patient who appears well, and who has no systemic symptoms or laboratory abnormalities. If, however, the abdominal symptoms continue and the diagnosis remains unclear, it would seem prudent to refer the patient for further evaluation by a gastroenterologist.

SYMPTOMATIC THERAPY

Patients with acute abdominal pain of unknown etiology should not be given analgesics, because these may obscure important findings. Although the patient with undiagnosed chronic pain often requests pain medication, regular use of narcotics ought to be avoided, because the risk of addiction is extremely high; many such patients have underlying psychopathology and a strong potential for narcotic abuse. The patient with terminal cancer must not be denied the relief afforded by narcotics, even if the cause of pain is not fully defined (see Chapter 91).

As noted above, *therapeutic trials* for diagnostic purposes are sometimes informative and may bring relief from troublesome symptoms. Patients with suspected peptic ulcer disease can be given a course of antacid or histamine$_2$ blocker therapy (see Chapter 64); those with probable irritable bowel syndrome might be tried on a high-fiber diet (see Chapter 66); tricyclic therapy may prove beneficial to the depressed patient with abdominal pain of unclear etiology (see Chapter 223), though constipation may ensue and worsen the problem, if it is not due to depression.

ANNOTATED BIBLIOGRAPHY

Alpers DH: Functional gastrointestinal disorders. Hosp Pract 4:139, 1983 (*A review of the psychiatric conditions that present as functional gastrointestinal disorders; practical approach to diagnosis and treatment.*)

Anuras S, Shirazi S: Chronic pseudoobstruction. Am J Gastroenterol 79:525, 1984 (*The syndromes of acute and chronic colonic pseudoobstruction are differentiated; 99 references are included in this 1984 paper.*)

Cope A: Early Diagnosis of the Acute Abdomen, 14th ed. London, Oxford University Press, 1972 (*A concise, systematic approach to diagnosis of acute abdominal problems. Emphasis is on history and physical findings; required reading for the primary physician.*)

Drossman DA: Diagnosis of irritable bowel syndrome. Gastroenterology 87:224, 1984 (*An editorial discussing the difficulty in making the diagnosis.*)

Eisenberg RL, Heineken P, Hedgcock et al: Evaluation of plain abdominal radiographs in the diagnosis of abdominal pain. Ann Intern Med 97:257, 1982 (*An effort to develop criteria for the ordering of abdominal films in patients with abdominal pain.*)

Greenlee HB: Acute large bowel obstruction: An update. Surg Annu 14:253, 1982 (*A comprehensive paper covering the pathophysiology, clinical presentation, workup, and treatment of large bowel obstruction including a discussion of the surgical options for each of the common causes of obstruction.*)

Hill OW, Blendis L: Physical and psychological evaluation of "nonorganic" abdominal pain. Gut 8:221, 1967 (*This study of 31 consecutive patients with undiagnosed abdominal pain showed a high frequency of epigastric discomfort, distention, nausea, and belching without vomiting or weight loss. Bereavement or emotional upheaval often initiated symptoms.*)

Moosa AR: Diagnostic tests and procedures in acute pancreatitis. N Engl J Med 311:639, 1984 (*Reviews critically the host of tests available.*)

Ottinger LW: Mesenteric ischemia. N Engl J Med 307:535, 1982 (*Terse review of clinical presentations, diagnosis, and treatment.*)

Richter JM, Christensen MR, Simeone JH et al: Chronic cholecystitis: An analysis of diagnostic strategies. Invest Radiol (in press). (*An analysis of clinical utility of ultrasonography and other studies in the evaluation of abdominal pain.*)

Sarfeh IJ: Abdominal pain of unknown etiology. Am J Surg 132:22, 1976 (*Over two thirds of cases were in women. Improvement was most likely in younger patients with symptoms of less than 2 weeks' duration. Laparotomy did not influence the rate of improvement, and it established diagnosis in only 1 of 23 patients explored.*)

Scott PJ et al: Benefits and hazards of laparotomy for medical patients. Lancet 2:941, 1970 (*Exploration established a diagnosis in 69 of 81 patients with extensive medical workups and no firm diagnosis. A remediable cause was found in 40%, but the incidence of morbidity was 45%, and perioperative mortality was 15%.*)

Shatila AH et al: Current status of diagnosis and management of strangulation obstruction of the small bowel. Am J Surg 132:299, 1976 (*This retrospective study compares the etiologies as well as clinical and laboratory findings of simple obstruction and strangulation of the small bowel. Differentiation on the basis of clinical and laboratory findings is not found to be reliable, making early surgery necessary.*)

Spiro HM: Which tests for irritable bowel? Diagnosis (May 1984), p 110. (*An easy-to-read discussion of the clinical presentation and workup for irritable bowel syndrome by one of the field's leading authorities.*)

54
Evaluation of Nausea and Vomiting

Nausea and vomiting are extremely common presenting complaints, ranking in one study of primary care practice second only to symptoms of upper respiratory tract infection. Although in most instances the symptoms are due to self-limited disease, they may be a manifestation of a more serious underlying illness. The primary care physician needs to recognize the more worrisome causes of nausea and vomiting, provide relief from these debilitating symptoms, and correct any important fluid and electrolyte disturbances.

PATHOPHYSIOLOGY AND CLINICAL PRESENTATION

Two major central nervous system centers are involved in the vomiting reflex—the vomiting center and the chemoreceptor trigger zone. Irritation of vagal and sympathetic afferents in the pharynx, heart, peritoneum, mesentary, bile ducts, stomach, and bowel triggers impulses to the vomiting center in the medullary reticular formation. Gastric irritation, distention of a hollow viscus, myocardial ischemia, increased intracranial pressure, metabolic disturbances, drugs, pharyngeal stimulation, and emotional upset are important noxious stimuli that act through this pathway. Vestibular disturbances, centrally acting drugs, and metabolic derangements stimulate the chemoreceptor trigger zone in the floor of the fourth ventricle, which, in turn, activates the vomiting center. A cortical pathway to the vomiting center has been postulated to account for some forms of psychogenic vomiting.

The act of vomiting is a stereotyped response that varies little regardless of cause. Even so-called projectile vomiting (which is characterized by forceful emesis without prior nausea or retching), supposedly limited to cases of increased intracranial pressure, occurs in other conditions. Moreover, nausea, retching, and nonprojectile vomiting are seen with increased intracranial pressure.

Nausea and vomiting may be only one part of a symptom complex or dominate the clinical picture (as in psychogenic vomiting, early pregnancy, digitalis toxicity, and metabolic disturbances). Although there is considerable overlap among clinical presentations, some causes of nausea and vomiting are more likely to occur independent of meals, while others are characteristically associated with food intake. For example, early morning nausea and vomiting is quite typical of *metabolic etiologies.* Up to 75% of cases of diabetic ketoacidosis are accompanied by nausea and vomiting. Emesis and nausea are found among as many as 90% of patients in Addisonian crisis. Uremia may be heralded by similar symptoms; nausea often improves with correction of any associated hyponatremia, but can be refractory. Binge drinkers experience early morning nausea and dry heaves from excessive alcohol intake.

Early pregnancy is associated with mild early morning nausea and vomiting in over 50% of instances. The problem is severe in fewer than 1% of cases, leading to electrolyte abnormalities, dehydration, and weight loss. Most cases are mild; symptoms begin after the first missed period and terminate by the fourth month. Women with severe cases often have a history of vomiting in response to psychosocial stress. The diagnosis of pregnancy is sometimes overlooked.

In contrast to the causes of early morning vomiting, symptoms can be triggered shortly after eating by psychoneurotic illness, bile reflux, peptic ulcer disease, and gastritis. *Psychogenic vomiting* is characterized by years of recurrent emesis. It can often be traced back to childhood and is more common when there is a family history of vomiting. Patients report that symptoms appear just after eating and can be sufficiently controlled voluntarily to avoid vomiting in public. Some admit to inducing emesis; most are surprisingly untroubled by the problem. Nausea accompanies almost all episodes. A study of 20 patients with psychogenic vomiting revealed a marked predominance of women who were engaged in hostile relationships; abdominal pain and depression were uncommon.

Bulimia is a form of psychogenic emesis in which self-induced vomiting occurs, often after a period of binge eating. Preoccupation with being thin and preponderance among young women with poor self-images are characteristic. Laxative abuse frequently complicates the clinical picture (see Chapter 230).

A *pyloric channel ulcer* or *acute gastritis* may be associated with marked postprandial emesis. The vomiting in ulcer disease is believed due in part to irritation, edema, and spasm of the pyloric sphincter mechanism. Concurrent bleeding can lead to vomiting of coffee-groundlike material. Patients who undergo surgery for peptic ulcer may be troubled by recurrent *bilious vomiting,* which is believed due to reflux of bile into the stomach or gastric remnant. Patients vomit bile within 15 minutes of eating; little food is present. Nausea and a bad taste in the mouth are present on awakening in the morning.

Gastric retention results in vomiting of food eaten more than 6 hours previously. A succussion splash is detectable on examination, and food is seen in the stomach on upper GI series. In chronic cases there may be gastric outflow obstruction or atony secondary to diabetic neuropathy, anticholinergic use, or gastric malignancy. Transient gastric dilatation is a frequent concomitant of pancreatitis, peritonitis, gallbladder disease, and hypokalemia.

Acute episodes of vomiting accompany a host of conditions, ranging from the self-limited to the life-threatening. The most common is *viral gastroenteritis.* After many years of attributing this illness to viral infection, investigators have finally isolated and identified the responsible viruses. Explosive bouts of nausea and vomiting in conjunction with watery diarrhea, cramping abdominal pain, myalgias, headache, and fever are typical. Recovery is rapid in most instances, but symptoms may linger for 7 to 10 days.

Acute gastroenteritis that results from *food poisoning* due to *Salmonella* or *Shigella* infection has a similar clinical presentation and course; onset is 24 to 48 hours after exposure to the contaminated food. Domestic fowl represent the largest single reservoir of salmonella infection. Inadequate cooking is often responsible for human infection. Intake of pastries and similar items containing *staphylococcal enterotoxin* causes symptoms indistinguishable from viral gastroenteritis, except that onset is within 1 to 6 hours after eating the spoiled food, fever is rare, and complete clearing takes place by 24 to 48 hours. Clostridial food poisoning rarely produces prominent nausea and vomiting.

A number of intra-abdominal emergencies may precipitate acute emesis, such as peritoneal irritation and acute obstruction of a hollow viscus. Often they are *accompanied by severe abdominal pain* (see Chapter 53). *Intestinal obstruction,* especially of the proximal small bowel, produces marked nausea and vomiting of bilious material. Distention may be lacking, but intermittent cramping abdominal pain is characteristic. Feculent emesis is found in distal small bowel obstruction. In *acute pancreatitis,* emesis is seen in 85% of patients; however, upper abdominal pain radiating into the back is the cardinal symptom, occurring in 95% (see Chapter 72). Anorexia, nausea, and vomiting are early symptoms in more than 90% of patients with *acute appendicitis;* usually emesis clears early. As with pancreatitis, pain typically precedes other symptoms. *Acute pyelonephritis* may mimic a gastrointestinal etiology, by causing nausea, vomiting, and abdominal pain. *Acute cholecystitis* sometimes triggers acute emesis, but less regularly than does *acute cholangitis* due to sudden obstruction of the common duct.

Myocardial infarction may activate vagal afferents and produce nausea, vomiting, and epigastric discomfort simulating intra-abdominal disease. A prospective series of 62 patients with acute infarction revealed nausea and vomiting at the outset in 69% of those with inferior infarctions and 27% of those with anterior infarctions.

Neurologic emergencies can provoke severe bouts of acute emesis. In *midline cerebellar hemorrhage,* nausea and vomiting are profuse, in association with severe gait ataxia; meningeal signs and headache are seen as well. Within a few hours the patient may become comatose and die unless promptly diagnosed and treated (see Chapter 159). One third of patients with *increased intracranial pressure* experience vomiting. When it is sudden, forceful, and not preceded by nausea it is termed "projectile," but this presentation is not specific. Concurrent bifrontal or bioccipital headache is the rule. *Migraine headaches* and *vestibular disease* are less worrisome neurologic causes of acute emesis (see Chapters 159 and 160). The former is suggested by photophobia and throbbing unilateral headache, the latter by vertigo.

Of the many *drugs* that induce vomiting, *digitalis* intoxication is among the most serious. Anorexia is an early sign, followed by nausea and vomiting due to stimulation of the chemoreceptor trigger zone. Visual disturbances such as colored haloes are suggestive of the diagnosis (see Chapter 27). Hypokalemia and dehydration induced by vomiting may precipitate or worsen digitalis toxicity. Unfortunately, most *cancer chemotherapeutic agents* produce substantial nausea and vomiting (see Chapter 74).

Drug withdrawal as well as drug excess may trigger emesis. Nausea, dry heaves, and retching beginning at about 36 hours are characteristic features of the opiate withdrawal syndrome. Sweats, chills, and restlessness precede other symptoms; the vomiting peaks by 72 hours and subsides.

Anorexia, nausea, and vomiting often dominate the prodromal stage of *acute viral hepatitis* (see Chapter 70).

DIFFERENTIAL DIAGNOSIS

Table 54-1 lists some of the more common and important conditions associated with prominent nausea and vomiting. Causes of simple regurgitation are omitted from the list because they are usually manifestations of esophageal difficulties (see Chapter 57) and unaccompanied by emesis. The etiologies are listed for convenience according to clinical presentation; however, it is important to keep in mind that there can be considerable overlap and variation in the clinical picture. For example, some causes listed as being accompanied by abdominal pain may present with just isolated emesis.

WORKUP

History and physical examination supplemented by a few well-chosen laboratory studies are sufficient for diagnosis in most cases.

History should focus on such details as timing of symptoms, their relation to meals, characteristics of the vomitus, and associated complaints. Early-morning onset points to metabolic disturbances, alcoholic binge, and early pregnancy. Emesis precipitated by meals suggests psychogenic vomiting, pyloric channel ulcer, and gastritis. Onset a few hours after eating raises the possibility of gastric-outflow tract obstruction, gastric atony, or bowel obstruction. Emesis of food that was ingested more than 12 hours earlier strongly suggests gastric

Table 54-1.   Some Important Causes of Nausea
and Vomiting

NAUSEA/VOMITING AS PREDOMINANT OR INITIAL SYMPTOMS

Acute
1. Digitalis toxicity
2. Ketoacidosis*
3. Opiate use
4. Cancer chemotherapeutic agents
5. Early pregnancy
6. Inferior myocardial infarction*
7. Drug withdrawal
8. Binge drinking
9. Hepatitis

Recurrent or Chronic
1. Psychogenic vomiting
2. Metabolic disturbancies (uremia, adrenal insufficiency)
3. Gastric retention
4. Bile reflux postgastric surgery
5. Pregnancy

NAUSEA/VOMITING IN ASSOCIATION WITH ABDOMINAL PAIN†

1. Viral gastroenteritis
2. Acute gastritis
3. Food poisoning
4. Peptic ulcer disease
5. Acute pancreatitis
6. Small bowel obstruction and pseudoobstruction
7. Acute appendicitis
8. Acute cholecystitis
9. Acute cholangitis
10. Acute pyelonephritis
11. Inferior myocardial

NAUSEA/VOMITING IN ASSOCIATION WITH NEUROLOGIC SYMPTOMS

1. Increased intracranial pressure
2. Midline cerebellar hemorrhage
3. Vestibular disturbances
4. Migraine headaches
5. Autonomic dysfunction

* Abdominal pain is sometimes present.

† Abdominal pain is sometimes absent.

stasis and an organic etiology, as does vomiting of large volumes (>1500 cc/day). However, absence of such features hardly rules out organic disease.

Vomiting blood or coffee-ground material is indicative of gastritis and ulcer disease. Bilious vomitus means that the pyloric channel is open. When the material vomited is pure gastric juice, peptic ulcer disease and Zollinger–Ellison syndrome are suggested. Lack of acid suggests gastric cancer. Feculent material is a sign of distal small-bowel obstruction and blind-loop syndrome.

The history needs to include inquiry into abdominal pain, fever, jaundice, weight loss, abdominal surgery, external hernias, contaminated food source, family history of emesis, symptoms of diabetes, prior renal disease, ischemic heart disease, drug use (*e.g.,* digitalis, narcotics), visual disturbances, headache, ataxia, vertigo, last menstrual period, and concurrent emotional stresses and conflicts. Gentle questioning

about self-image, binge eating, and self-induced emesis is indicated when the patient is a young woman suspected of bulimia.

Physical Examination requires a check for postural hypotension, malignant hypertension, irregularities of rate and rhythm, Kussmaul breathing, pallor, hyperpigmentation, jaundice, papilledema, retinopathy, nystagmus, stiff neck, abdominal distention, visible peristalsis, abnormal bowel sounds, succussion splash, peritoneal signs, focal tenderness, organomegaly, masses, flank tenderness, muscle weakness, ataxia of gait, and asterixis. If there is a history of vertigo in conjunction with nausea, then the Barany maneuver (see Chapter 160) might reproduce symptoms and confirm the diagnosis of a vestibular etiology.

Patients suspected of having a "functional" disorder should be checked carefully for signs of autonomic insufficiency. Finding postural hypotension, lack of sweat, or blunted pulse and blood pressure responses to Valsalva suggests autonomic dysfunction and a bowel motility problem as the underlying etiology of the nausea and vomiting.

Laboratory Studies. In patients with emesis accompanied by acute abdominal pain, the first priority is to rule out an acute surgical etiology such as bowel obstruction, peritonitis, or blockage of a hollow viscus. *Plane and upright films of the abdomen* are indicated when such etiologies are suspected (see Chapter 53). Acute nausea and vomiting without associated abdominal pain may also be a clue to serious illness. If the patient is a known diabetic, ketoacidosis should be suspected and *serum ketones* checked. In a patient with strong risk factors for coronary artery disease an *electrocardiogram* should be obtained; inferior ischemia may present as gastrointestinal upset (see Chapter 14). Hepatitis might present like acute gastroenteritis, with anorexia, nausea, and vomiting; a *transaminase* determination can be diagnostic. The onset of pancreatitis may be dominated by emesis; a serum *amylase* is indicated. Acute onset of nausea and vomiting in conjunction with ataxia of gait and a stiff neck is very suggestive of a midline cerebellar hemorrhage; an emergency computed tomographic (*CT*) scan of the posterior fossa is needed.

Acute vomiting of unclear etiology without focal signs should also be pursued by carefully checking medications and *serum levels.* If a digitalis preparation is being taken, the drug should be withheld, an electrocardiogram obtained, a serum level ordered, and a potassium supplement prescribed if the potassium level is below 4.0 mg per 100 ml (see Chapter 27).

Recurrent vomiting of unknown etiology raises the question of a psychogenic cause. The patient with psychogenic vomiting may be recognized by the characteristic history of chronic emesis, with vomiting around mealtime, partial suppressibility, and a conflict-ridden social situation. The need for additional studies in such cases is best individualized, since some patients may insist on further testing while others may be comforted by knowing that extensive studies are not necessary. Any woman of childbearing age whose vomiting is suspected to have a psychogenic cause should always have a pregnancy test (see Chapter 109) before it concludes that emesis is emotional in origin.

Elimination of pregnancy and psychogenic causes leaves metabolic disorders and gastric pathology among possible antecedents of recurrent emesis. Metabolic disease is suggested by vomiting that occurs in the early morning. A urinalysis and determinations of the serum BUN, creatinine, electrolytes, and glucose should be obtained. An upper GI series can confirm gastric outlet obstruction or retention. Sometimes endoscopy is necessary for assessment of the stomach (see Chapter 64). The suspicion of hepatitis can be confirmed by obtaining a transaminase level (see Chapter 70).

Therapeutic Trials. Before a patient with unexplained vomiting is referred for psychiatric or motility studies, a therapeutic trial may have diagnostic utility and provide symptomatic relief. When there is suspicion of a motility disorder, a short course of a prokinetic agent such as *metoclopramide* can be useful. A therapeutic response is very suggestive of a motility disturbance. Patients suspected of having an underlying affective disorder sometimes respond to a 4- to 8-week trial of *antidepressant medication;* an agent with minimal anticholinerigic activity (*e.g.,* trazodone or desipramine) is preferred to minimize chances of gastrointestinal side-effects.

INDICATIONS FOR REFERRAL AND ADMISSION

Patients who remain undiagnosed after extensive evaluation, unresponsive to therapeutic trials, and without evidence or suspicion of an underlying psychiatric disturbance deserve consideration for gastric emptying and motility studies. These studies are done at only a few specialty centers; referral should be made in consultation with a gastroenterologist. Patients suspect of psychogenic vomiting need psychiatric consultation. Such patients may be seriously disturbed; suicidal attempts are not uncommon among bulimics and others with psychogenic emesis. Referral to a mental health professional skilled and experienced in the treatment of patients with eating disorders is optimal for those suffering from bulimia (see Chapter 230).

SYMPTOMATIC RELIEF

When a cause is identified, but treatment of the underlying condition does not adequately control the symptoms, antiemetic drug therapy may help provide symptomatic relief. The available agents work by suppressing the vomiting center, the chemoreceptor trigger zone, or peripheral receptors. Symptomatic therapy must not be used in lieu of making a diagnosis.

The phenothiazines are indicated for initial symptomatic treatment of vomiting caused by drugs and gastrointestinal disorders. They suppress the chemoreceptor trigger zone and probably the vomiting center and peripheral receptors as well. *Prochlorperazine* (*Compazine*) is the phenothiazine used most often for vomiting; it can be given in doses of 5 to 10 mg orally, every 6 hours, or 25 mg rectally, twice daily. This class of drugs is not effective for motion sickness or vestibular disease.

The antihistamine *meclizine* (*Antivert*) acts on the vestibular system and the chemoreceptor trigger zone. It is best for prevention and control of motion sickness and nausea and vomiting caused by vestibular disturbances. Other antihistamines with quicker onset and shorter duration of action such as *dimenhydrinate* (*Dramamine*) enjoy considerable popularity for motion sickness. The average dosage of meclizine is 25 mg, three times daily, for vestibular disease and 25 to 50 mg, at least 1 hour before a trip for motion sickness. Meclizine is teratogenic in animals and is not indicated for vomiting due to pregnancy. Moreover, it can cause drowsiness and should not be used prior to driving or use of machinery. *Transdermal scopolamine* is also effective for prevention of motion sickness. The major side-effects are dry mouth and lightheadedness. A single patch lasts up to 72 hours.

A few specific problems require elaboration:

Vomiting due to *cancer chemotherapy* is a major problem for patients being treated by drugs for malignancy. Phenothiazines usually suffice; but tetrahydrocannabinol has also demonstrated the ability to suppress chemotherapy-induced nausea and vomiting (see Chapter 74).

Morning sickness is best treated with small morning feedings and support; the goal is to try to avoid use of antiemetics. If an occasional episode is particularly severe, a long-established antihistamine such as dimenhydrinate may help. The prolonged, severe form of nausea and vomiting due to pregnancy does not respond to drugs but may remit with hypnosis and/or supportive psychotherapy.

Psychogenic vomiting is best approached by attention to the conflicts troubling the patient. No controlled studies have been done on the effectiveness of antiemetics; fortunately, patients often do not request medication for symptomatic relief.

Hepatitis. Phenothiazines are metabolized by the liver and in rare instances can cause jaundice; their use in controlling nausea and vomiting due to hepatitis requires close supervision. (See Chapter 70.)

A.H.G.

ANNOTATED BIBLIOGRAPHY

Ahmed S, Gupta R, Brancato R: Significance of nausea and vomiting during acute myocardial infarction. Am Heart J 95:671, 1977 (*Nausea and vomiting occurred in 69% of patients with inferior infarctions, compared with 27% of those with anterior infarctions.*)

Biggs J: Vomiting and pregnancy. Drugs 9:299, 1975 (*A terse review of clinical presentation and therapy.*)

Bordfield P: A controlled double-blind study of trimethobenzamide, prochlorperazine and placebo. JAMA 196:116, 1966 (*Prochlorperazine was the most effective.*)

Bothe F, Beardwood J: Evaluation of abdominal symptoms in the diabetic. Ann Surg 105:516, 1937 (*A classic study in which 75% of patients in ketoacidosis had nausea and vomiting; 8% had severe abdominal pain and elevated white counts simulating an acute abdomen. Also makes the point that intra-abdominal disease can precipitate ketoacidosis.*)

Drugs for relief of nausea and vomiting. Med Lett 16:46, 1974 (*An authoritative critique of available agents.*)

Hill OW: Psychogenic vomiting. Gut 9:348, 1968 (*A study comparing 20 patients with psychogenic vomiting to 22 patients with psychogenic abdominal pain. A high frequency of hostile living situations and symptoms coming on at mealtime characterized patients with vomiting.*)

Malagelda JR, Camillieri M: Unexplained vomiting: A diagnostic challenge. Ann Intern Med 101:211, 1984 (*A useful review of approaches to this difficult situation. Details neuromuscular disorders that may present as unexplained emesis; 61 references.*)

Rimer D: Gastric retention without mechanical obstruction. Arch Intern Med 117:287, 1966 (*A good review of the problem, detailing the causes of this condition; 73 references.*)

Sallen SE, Cronin C, Zelen M et al: Antiemetics in patients receiving chemotherapy for cancer. A randomized comparison of delta-a-tetrahydro-cannabinol and prochlorperazine. N Engl J Med 302:135, 1980 (*THC proved superior to prochlorperazine in this double-blind randomized crossover trial.*)

55
Evaluation of Indigestion

"Indigestion" is used to denote gastrointestinal discomfort coincident with the intake and digestion of food; the English use the word "dyspepsia." Symptoms subsumed under the heading of indigestion include upper abdominal discomfort, distention, eructation, nausea, heartburn, and even emesis. Almost everyone experiences such symptoms at one time or another, but recurrent or persistent complaints may reflect an underlying gastrointestinal, hepatobiliary, or psychogenic disorder. In addition, indigestion may be the presenting complaint of patients with cardiac, neurologic, or metabolic disease.

Patients bothered by indigestion often resort to home remedies or over-the-counter preparations. Remedies for "acid indigestion, heartburn, and gas" are sold by the millions each year. The prevalence of indigestion is estimated to be as high as 250 per 1000 population, with a peak in the 25- to 44-year-old age group with men outnumbering women by almost 2 to 1.

Indigestion's frequency, associated discomfort, and potential for serious underlying disease make a thorough yet efficient evaluation essential. It is estimated that more than 25% of patients with indigestion have more than one cause for their symptoms. The challenge confronting the primary care physician is to evaluate the patient cost-effectively and provide reassurance and symptomatic relief to the vast majority who have little more than a functional gastrointestinal disturbance.

PATHOPHYSIOLOGY AND CLINICAL PRESENTATION

The broad definition of indigestion encompasses a wide spectrum of etiologies and mechanisms, ranging from dysmotility and gastroesophageal reflux, at one end of the GI tract, to irritable bowel at the other end. The seriousness of illness is similarly broad, from functional disease to gastric and pancreatic malignancies. Symptoms listed under the rubric of indigestion or dyspepsia include heartburn, dysphagia, eructation, bloating, abdominal pain or discomfort, nausea and vomiting, and food intolerance.

Heartburn is a specific symptom that refers to the retrosternal burning sensation that occurs with esophageal reflux (see Chapter 56). It occasionally occurs in conjunction with esophageal spasm. Gastroesophageal reflux ensues from either reduced resting lower esophageal sphincter pressure or transient inappropriate relaxation of the sphincter, which allows reflux of stomach contents into the esophagus. Reductions in lower esophageal pressures have been recorded in response to meals high in carbohydrate and fat, coffee drinking, and cigarette smoking.

Dysphagia, or difficulty swallowing, is also a specific symptom of esophageal disease (see Chapter 57). It may result from neuromuscular disorders (*e.g.,* myasthenia gravis, multiple sclerosis, idiopathic pseudoobstruction, or cerebrovascular accident), primary esophageal dysmotility (*e.g.,* achalasia or diffuse esophageal spasm), or anatomic abnormalities (*e.g.,* peptic and malignant strictures). Neuromuscular or primary motility disorders cause difficulty swallowing both liquids and solid foods. In contrast, anatomic strictures characteristically present with selective dysphagia for solids; in advanced cases, there may be progression to difficulty swallowing liquids as well.

Eructation is a common feature of indigestion due to functional causes. Patients troubled by chronic belching have been observed to swallow air just prior to belching, thus unconsciously worsening the problem. Twenty percent to 60% of intraluminal gas represents swallowed air. The reason for the air swallowing (aerophagia) is unclear, although some investigators have observed that eructation seems to provide transient relief of abdominal discomfort. Anxiety and drinking of carbonated beverages can lead to aerophagia. Food gulping, gum chewing, smoking, and loose dentures have also been implicated but not proven to be causes of excessive air intake.

Bloating and flatulence often accompany eructation. Controlled studies have shown that in symptomatic patients there is an exaggerated pain response to normal degrees of intestinal distention without evidence of increased gas volume or production. Washout studies in patients complaining of "excess gas" have revealed no difference in total gas content compared with that in normal controls. In symptomatic patients, however, transit of gas through the bowel is delayed, with increased reflux of gas from jejunum to stomach, suggesting that altered motility may underlie the complaint of excess gas in such patients.

Carbohydrate malabsorption can cause flatulence. Certain foods contain high amounts of nonabsorbable sugars, which when eaten in substantial amounts, are fermented by colonic bacteria into excessive amounts of methane, H_2, and CO_2; flatulence ensues. The most common example of such carbohydrate malabsorption is lactose malabsorption in persons deficient in the small bowel mucosal enzyme lactase. An analogous situation may occur in normal individuals after ingestion of certain vegetables, particularly legumes, which contain the oligosaccharides raffinose and stachyose for which we lack the necessary disaccharidases. This is the mechanism by which beans cause excess flatulence. Neutralization of stomach acid by bicarbonate in the duodenum also results in generation of large amounts of CO_2, which may be especially high after fatty meals. Fatty foods may also delay gastric emptying, resulting in a bloated feeling; hence, symptoms associated with fatty foods are not limited to patients with gallbladder disease.

Abdominal pain or discomfort is a frequent component of indigestion. Biliary, gastric, or esophageal inflammation, peptic ulceration, functional motility disturbances and tumor have all been implicated. These etiologies result in visceral pain that is typically midline, poorly localized, and described as "aching," "gnawing," "burning," or "cramping." Unfortunately, the pain pattern is rarely specific for a particular etiology (see Chapter 53). Patients with underlying psychiatric illness do not manifest a particular form of abdominal discomfort, but rather respond in exaggerated fashion to minor functional symptoms (see Chapter 53).

Nausea and vomiting may be manifestations of psychogenic illness or a disorder of the stomach, duodenum, gallbladder, liver, or pancreas (see Chapter 54).

Food intolerance is another common complaint patients report when they speak of indigestion. *Fatty foods* are frequently implicated. Delayed gastric emptying, excessive CO_2 production, pancreatic insufficiency, and gallbladder disease

constitute the major mechanisms of fat intolerance. *Lactase deficiency* is common among non-Caucasians and leads to GI upset on intake of lactose-rich foods. Most milk products cause symptoms in such patients, although some yogurts are better tolerated because the bacteria used in processing often provide enough lactase to enable digestion. True *food allergies* rarely occur in adults. Gluten is known to be toxic to patients with celiac sprue, but the more common occurrence of indigestion associated with specific food items such as certain fruits, vegetables, or spicy foods remains unexplained.

DIFFERENTIAL DIAGNOSIS

Common causes of indigestion include peptic ulcer (both gastric and duodenal), gallbladder disease, functional illness, and esophageal reflux. Gastric carcinoma is occasionally responsible for the symptoms; angina, gastritis, and pancreatitis may be sources of acute "indigestion." In a British general practice study, 50 consecutive patients with indigestion were evaluated by upper GI series, oral cholecystogram, and endoscopy, revealing 50% with ulcer, 32% with functional problems, 12% with gallbladder disease, and single cases of gastric carcinoma and esophageal stricture.

Data from a Scandinavian series of 197 consecutive outpatients with upper abdominal discomfort evaluated by history, physical examination, barium studies, and endoscopy provided similar results. More than half of the patients had unrevealing evaluations and were labeled as having "functional" illness. In separate studies of patients chronically complaining of functional symptoms, a high prevalence of underlying psychiatric pathology has been found; in one study the rate was as high as 80%. Depression, anxiety disorders, and hysteria were particularly common in this group.

Indigestion is sometimes a manifestation of disease originating outside the gastrointestinal tract. Important etiologies include myocardial ischemia (see Chapter 14), neuromuscular disease, and diabetes (see Chapter 100).

WORKUP

The main objective is to distinguish patients with potentially important pathology from those with minor functional complaints. Data obtained from the history and physical examination are not entirely discriminating but may be sufficient to allow a reasonable approximation of the diagnosis. No single laboratory or radiologic test is diagnostic; each must be interpreted in light of the overall clinical picture. Putting every patient through a battery of radiologic studies is wasteful.

History. The first task is to elicit a detailed description of what the patient is experiencing, because the term "indigestion" may mean different things to the patient and the physician. Of particular importance is the presence of associated symptoms that augur a potentially serious underlying illness, such as unexplained weight loss, melena, jaundice, chest pain, fever, neuromuscular difficulty, postural light-headedness, back pain, or change in bowel habits. Inquiry into symptoms of diabetes, coronary disease, and psychiatric problems may also provide important contributory information.

Although the history must include a careful description of the patient's symptoms and particularly the pattern of any abdominal pain, it is essential not to overestimate the meaning of such information.

A group of English investigators prospectively examined the presentations of 360 patients complaining of indigestion to identify the clinical findings that best distinguish the more common, yet easily confused, causes of indigestion—namely, functional disease, cholecystitis, gastric ulcer, gastric cancer, and duodenal ulcer. Some features of the clinical presentation proved helpful in identifying underlying etiology. *Pain location* limited to the right upper quadrant was almost always due to gallbladder disease, although half of the patients with this condition reported only epigastric pain, as did most with functional illness, ulcer, and malignancy. *Chronicity* of complaints varied among etiologies. Pain of less than 3 months' duration showed a strong chance of being due to gastric cancer; duration of 6 to 12 months was characteristic of gastric ulcer; duration of 1 to 3 years was typical of gallbladder disease and functional illness; and duration of 5 to 10 years or more was typical of duodenal ulcer.

Pain radiation was often nonspecific. It was referred to the back in 25% to 30% of patients with ulcer and functional problems and 59% of patients with gallbladder disease. Radiation to the shoulder was rather specific for cholecystitis, but occurred in only 18% of patients. *Alleviating factors* were of some discriminative value. A beneficial response to food was characteristic of patients with duodenal ulcer and rare in those with other conditions. Milk provided temporary relief in 15% to 20% of patients with ulcer disease and in 8% with functional problems, pointing out its lack of specific meaning. Antacid response was nonspecific, occurring in 37% of patients with ulcers and in 26% of those with functional disease. Even a small fraction of those with gastric cancer (9%) and gallbladder disease (6%) obtained relief with antacids. Surprisingly, more than 50% of all patients in the study reported that pain was not aggravated by food intake; this feature was reported by 80% of those with cholecystitis, 60% with functional illness, and 50% with ulcer or tumor. If the pain was worsened by eating, the probability of duodenal ulcer was low (10%) and the probability of x-ray negative dyspepsia was high (70%). A relationship of symptoms to fatty food intake was not unique to patients with gallbladder disease (see Chapter 69).

Pain pattern was studied. The majority of patients with continuous pain were shown to have gastric cancer. When there were pain-free periods of 1 month or more, the cause

usually proved to be duodenal ulcer or functional illness. Although more than 80% of patients with gallbladder disease had acute attacks of pain, so did 50% with functional disease, 64% with gastric ulcer, and 72% with gastric cancer. Pain that awoke the patient from a sound sleep was seen most often with duodenal ulcer (70%), but was also reported by one third of patients with each of the other underlying etiologies.

Age proved helpful. Gastric cancer was rare under age 50. Gastric ulcer peaked in the 50- to 59-year age group; duodenal ulcer was rare after age 60, but cholecystitis peaked in the 60- to 69-year age range. Most patients aged 20 to 29 had functional problems or duodenal ulcer disease.

Associated symptoms were of variable use in identifying cause. Anorexia, nausea, and vomiting were found equally among the different groups, including those who proved to have functional illnesses as well as those with an organic lesion. Jaundice and pale stools pointed to biliary tract disease but also occurred in a few patients with gastric cancer, secondary to obstruction of the common duct. Most had normal bowel habits. Diarrhea and constipation were equally infrequent among the different groups. Weight loss of greater than 7 pounds was most common in cancer patients (85%) and gastric ulcer (61%), but was also seen in 25% to 45% of those with functional, gallbladder, and duodenal-ulcer problems.

This important study illustrates that many traditional notions about indigestion contain numerous misconceptions. For example, fatty-food intolerance is not unique to cholecystitis, nor is pain relief by antacids specific for ulcer disease. The location, severity, and quality of pain are nondiagnostic except for the right upper quadrant localization seen in half of those with gallbladder disease. Radiation into the back is common and of little help in discriminating among causes. Although pain radiation into the shoulder points to cholecystitis, it is found only in a fraction of such cases. Weight loss, anorexia, nausea, and vomiting are also frequent nonspecific accompaniments of any etiology. In spite of these potential pitfalls, a carefully taken history improved a diagnostic accuracy by 20% to 30%.

Physical Examination is often unrevealing. Epigastric tenderness correlates poorly with the presence of ulcer disease. Many patients experience some discomfort on deep palpation in the epigastrium, but the finding is of little diagnostic value. Particular attention should be paid to checking for the presence of jaundice (suggesting liver or biliary disease), adenopathy (suggesting infection or tumor), tenderness, a succussion splash (suggesting gastric outlet obstruction), an abdominal mass, and a positive stool guaiac test.

Laboratory Studies. When the history points strongly to a specific etiology, further laboratory study is indicated. For example, the patient reporting pain very suggestive of biliary colic (see Chapter 53) should be further evaluated by *ultrasonography* of the gallbladder. Sensitivity is 90% to 95% for detection of stones, although the finding of stones does not per se prove the link between symptoms and gallbladder disease; the diagnosis remains predominantly a clinical one. When reflux is a prominent part of the clinical picture in a patient over the age of 50, especially if associated with dysphagia, a *barium swallow* is indicated to check for stricture and malignancy (see Chapter 57).

In most patients presenting with indigestion, the history is too vague to allow a precise diagnosis, but it is also usually devoid of worrisome features. Nevertheless, traditional teaching is that all dyspeptic patients should undergo *upper GI series* and/or *endoscopy* early in their evaluation. Such an unselective approach to evaluation is proving to be both wasteful and misleading if the pretest probability of serious underlying disease is low (see Chapter 2). In some instances, a *diagnostic trial of empiric therapy* may be a more useful first step before resorting to radiologic or endoscopic investigation. In a study of 100 dyspeptic patients under age 50, a course of empiric therapy was prescribed for most at the time of initial presentation prior to upper GI series and endoscopy. Patients were told to take antacids, have frequent small meals, and stop smoking. For purposes of the study, all the subjects underwent radiologic and endoscopic evaluation. In a minority (24%), an abnormality was detected; in only a small fraction (11%) of cases was the detected abnormality of sufficient importance to affect decision making. Significant findings most often occurred in patients who were refractory to empiric therapy or strongly suspected on other grounds of harboring a malignancy. The investigators argued that unless symptoms were refractory to empiric therapy, cancer was strongly suspected or aggressive medical therapy was being contemplated (*i.e.,* use of histamine₂-blockers), the physician could dispense with barium studies and endoscopy in dyspeptic patients under age 50.

Other investigators have also attempted to define criteria for selection of dyspeptic patients in need of radiologic study. In a series of 483 ambulatory patients with indigestion subjected to upper GI series, abnormalities were discovered in only 20%. Four attributes were identified as 95% predictive of an abnormal study: a prior history of peptic ulcer, age greater than 50 years, relief of pain with antacid or food, and abdominal pain that occurs within an hour of eating. The authors concluded that routinely ordering upper GI x-ray films in patients with indigestion was wasteful and that with greater selectivity the number of studies ordered could be markedly reduced without any adverse impact on patient management.

The most worrisome *must-not-miss* cause of indigestion is an underlying *gastrointestinal malignancy*. The prevalence (and therefore the risk) of malignancy increases substantially in dyspeptic patients *over* the age of 50. In this age group, contrast studies and/or endoscopy should be considered especially when the history is suggestive of serious pathology. In a cost-effectiveness analysis comparing symptomatic em-

piric therapy (low-dose antacids or anticholinergics) with empiric ulcer therapy (high-dose antacids or H₂-blockers) and radiologic/endoscopic evaluation prior to therapy, mortality was minimized if radiologic evaluation preceded selection of therapy and if endoscopy was done when a gastric ulcer was found on upper GI series. However, the cost per additional life saved by this strategy was $2 million (estimates subject to assumptions regarding incidence of gastric cancer and relative benefit of early diagnosis).

In sum, an empiric course of therapy appears safe and reasonable as a first step in patients under the age of 50, who have a low risk of upper gastrointestinal malignancy or another worrisome etiology. In patients over age 50, it may be more appropriate to begin with an upper gastrointestinal contrast study, because of the increased risk of malignancy. Upper gastrointestinal endoscopy has been shown to be more sensitive and specific than contrast study for detection of pathology (see Chapter 64); however, the role of endoscopy in the evaluation of indigestion has not yet been clearly defined. Until it is, endoscopy should be used reservedly because the prognosis for x-ray negative dyspepsia is quite favorable. For example, a prospective English general practice study of 75 dyspeptic patients who were radiologically negative showed that 75% were symptom-free within 6 years; only 3% eventually manifested an ulcer or other important pathology. X-ray negative patients need not be restudied or undergo endoscopy unless there is a persistently strong suspicion of cancer, symptoms worsen, or their pattern changes, suggesting a new diagnosis.

X-ray negative patients are usually labelled as having "functional disease." It is important to keep in mind the high frequency of underlying *psychiatric illness* among such patients who chronically and persistently complain of indigestion yet show little evidence of important gastrointestinal or extra-abdominal pathology. Their characteristic presentation is an exaggerated response to their symptoms, although there is nothing diagnostic about the symptoms themselves, which span the entire range of dyspeptic complaints. Often the primary physician finds himself compelled to study such patients radiologically and endoscopically in order to "clear the air" and provide a modicum of reassurance. Once patient concerns have been addressed, it is important to inquire gently into psychosocial issues (see Chapter 53). In many instances there is little data to support a psychiatric diagnosis, and labelling a patient as having such a condition without confirmatory evidence is inappropriate. However, in those who do provide supportive information, the process of inquiry will help the patient refocus attention onto the problems underlying his gastrointestinal complaints and begin dealing with them.

Before one concludes that a patient has "functional" disease, consideration of underlying cardiac, metabolic, and neuromuscular problems is in order. Patients with "indigestion" brought on by exertion or having a history of cardiac problems or risk factors should have an evaluation for ischemic disease, beginning with an *electrocardiogram* at the time symptoms occur. Patients troubled by excessive bloating, gas, and loose stools may benefit from a *lactose tolerance test* or, more simply, a trial of a *lactose-restricted diet* (see Chapter 58) to rule out lactase deficiency. *Motility studies* are sometimes resorted to in patients who elude diagnosis and remain unresponsive to empirical therapy, yet are believed to suffer from a motility disturbance due to underlying autonomic dysfunction. Clues to autonomic dysfunction include postural hypotension, abnormal responses to Valsalva maneuver, and absence of sweating (see Chapter 18). Motility testing is an elaborate and expensive procedure; it should not be undertaken without the consultation of a gastroenterologist.

SYMPTOMATIC THERAPY

When the precise cause of symptoms remains unidentified after serious disease has been ruled out, an empiric trial of *antacid* or *H_2-receptor antagonist* therapy is often recommended. In one randomized, placebo-controlled study of such empirical therapy in nonulcer dyspepsia, no therapeutic benefit over placebo was demonstrated for either cimetidine or antacids; both treatment and placebo groups showed significant and nearly identical reductions in abdominal discomfort. In another, cimetidine produced a modest benefit. In most instances, primary physicians resort to such therapy for patients complaining of dyspeptic symptoms.

Cessation of alcohol intake and *smoking* will lessen chances of peptic ulceration and gastritis. Before resorting to *histamine$_2$ blockers* (see Chapter 64), for symptomatic treatment especially in older patients at risk for gastric cancer, one should attempt to identify a specific anatomic abnormality. Many dyspeptic patients are now on chronic cimetidine or ranitidine programs without a clear-cut indication.

For patients with excessive belching and gas, advice includes cessation of the repetitive aerophagia (used to induce belching) and limiting carbonated beverages, gum chewing, and cigarette smoking. Such patients will find that eating slowly (*i.e.,* not gulping their food) and not reclining after meals (which makes release of the gastric air bubble difficult) can help. *Simethicone* is widely touted in commercials for relief of "gas"; there is no evidence, however, that it works. One study, though, reported some success with *activated charcoal tablets* taken with meals. A trial of avoiding foods high in nonabsorbable carbohydrates such as beans and some whole grains and fruits might be recommended in patients who remain bothered by gaseousness. One frequently overlooked offender is sorbitol, an ingredient of many "sugar-free" gums and mints.

Other measures worthy of consideration in patients with indigestion include an empiric trial of a *lactose-free diet* and changing to frequent small meals. Recognizing that some patients with "indigestion" may suffer from a motility dis-

order, an attempt to augment intestinal motility may be worthwhile. *Metoclopramide* taken before meals speeds gastric emptying and often relieves symptoms of nausea and bloating. Because there is a high frequency of irritable bowel syndrome in patients with indigestion, a *high-fiber diet* may be remarkably helpful. *Anticholinergic medications,* often in combination with a tranquilizer (*e.g.,* Donnotal, Librax), have been widely prescribed over the years for symptomatic relief, but are of no proven benefit. Prolonged use of such preparations should be avoided because of the risk of developing tranquilizer dependence. *Benzodiazepines* are rarely, if ever, indicated. They have no proven "bowel-relaxant" effect. *Antidepressants* may be helpful in some dyspeptic patients who evidence signs and symptoms of depression (see Chapter 223).

PATIENT EDUCATION

The role of counseling and reassurance in managing patients with indigestion cannot be overemphasized. Many come with fears of cancer, ulcers, or other forms of major pathology. Most patients with functional symptomatology are able to cope with their symptoms, even when triggered by psychological stress, provided a thorough evaluation has been conducted and their concerns have been directly addressed. For the majority of patients with indigestion, the pace of symptoms and the degree of disability allow time for the primary physician to get to know the patient, initiate simple therapeutic measures, and address patient concerns. A trusting patient–doctor relationship is among the most efficacious means of dealing with dyspeptic patients. Unhurried explanation should minimize the patient's need to obtain further workup and multiple "second opinions."

INDICATIONS FOR REFERRAL

There are relatively few indications for referral. In most instances, diagnosis will be possible if time is taken to obtain a detailed history and become familiar with the patient. The major reason for referral is for performance of endoscopy to rule out the possibility of a gastric malignancy (see Chapter 64). The gastroenterologist can also be of help in deciding if an autonomic motility disorder is a serious consideration. Psychiatric consultation is needed when there is strong suspicion of significant psychiatric illness (severe depression, hysteria, incapacitating anxiety neuroses). Considerable discussion with the patient is beneficial before making the psychiatric referral so that the patient does not feel abandoned or rejected.

A.H.G.

ANNOTATED BIBLIOGRAPHY

Alpers DH: Functional gastrointestinal disorders. Hosp Pract 4:139, 1983 (*Argues that an overwhelming majority of "functional" illness* is accompanied by an underlying psychiatric disorder. Provides guidelines for evaluation and management.)

Crean GP et al: Ulcer-like dyspepsia. Scand J Gastroenterol 17:9, 1982 (*Careful history is essential in dyspepsia; better data base accumulation can improve diagnostic accuracy.*)

Goodson JD, Richter JM, Lane RS et al: Empiric antacids and reassurance for acute dyspepsia. J Gen Intern Med 1:90, 1986 (*Symptoms improved and requests for diagnostic tests decreased.*)

Gregory DW et al: Natural history of patients with x-ray negative dyspepsia. Br Med J 2:519, 1972 (*Shows that this can be a helpful diagnosis and carries a good prognosis—76% of patients were symptom-free at 6 years; only 3% developed ulcers.*)

Hoirocks JC, DeDombal FT: Clinical presentation of patients with dyspepsia. Gut 19:19, 1978 (*Prospective evaluation of 360 patients with emphasis on clinical presentation of five major disease categories.*)

Hyams JS: Sorbitol intolerance: An unappreciated cause of functional gastrointestinal complaints. Gastroenterology 84:30, 1983 (*Sorbitol may produce gas, bloating, cramps, and diarrhea particularly with higher doses.*)

Jain NK, Patel VP, Pitchumoni CS: Activated charcoal, simethicone, and intestinal gas: A double blind study. Ann Intern Med 101:61, 1986 (*Activated charcoal achieves superior results to simethicone, which was only effective for upper gastrointestinal gaseous distress.*)

Kolars JC et al: Yogurt—An autodigesting source of lactase. N Engl J Med 310:1, 1984 (*Bacterial lactase in yogurt allows lactase-deficient persons to tolerate yogurt as a source of milk.*)

Lennard-Jones JE: Functional gastrointestinal disorders. N Engl J Med 308:431, 1983 (*A wise overview of the problem, including an approach to workup and treatment.*)

Lesser PB, Bond JH, Levitt MD: Role of intestinal gas in functional abdominal pain. N Engl J Med 293:524, 1975 (*Symptomatic patients' bowels contain normal amounts of gas; symptoms seem to be due to abnormal sensitivity to distension and disordered motility.*)

Levitt MD: Excessive gas: Patient perception versus reality. Hosp Pract 7:143, 1985 (*A thorough review with an emphasis on the patient's view of the problem; practical in orientation.*)

Marton KI et al: Clinical value of upper GI x-ray series. Arch Intern Med 140:191, 1980 (*Examines utility of UGI x-rays in 483 ambulatory patients; significant abnormalities were found in 20%. They identify patient characteristics to improve utilization of UGI series.*)

Mead GM et al: Uses of barium meal examination in dyspeptic patients under 50. Br Med J 4:1460, 1977 (*This group also finds UGI series overused in younger patients.*)

Mollman KM et al: A diagnostic study of patients with upper abdominal pain. Scand J Gastroenterol 10:805, 1975 (*Of 197 consecutive nonacute medical patients evaluated with standard investigation, x-ray negative dyspepsia was found in half. Pain related to eating meals was helpful in this group.*)

Nyren O, Hans-Olov A, Bates S et al: Absence of therapeutic benefit from antacids or cimetidine in non-ulcer dyspepsia. N Engl J Med 314:339, 1986 (*A double-blind randomized study showing equally significant reductions in abdominal discomfort in placebo, antacid, and cimetidine-treated groups; there was no difference in response among the groups.*)

Read L, Pass TM, Kamaroff AL: Diagnosis and treatment of dyspepsia—A cost-effectiveness analysis. Med Decis Making 2:415, 1982 (*Uses a model to compare empiric therapy with UGI series with or without endoscopy prior to selecting therapy.*)

Talley NJ, McNeil AH, Piper DW: Randomized, double blind, placebo controlled cross over trial: Cimetidine and pirenzepine and nonulcerative dyspepsia. Gastroenterology 91:149, 1986 (*An interesting paper that addresses whether cimetidine is useful in the heterogeneous syndrome of patients without definable disease. Cimetidine was superior to placebo in decreasing the number and severity of upper abdomen pain episodes, but the absolute improvement was small.*)

56

Evaluation of Heartburn and Gastroesophageal Reflux

ALAN SMITH, M.D.
JAMES M. RICHTER, M.D.

Heartburn is a universally experienced gastrointestinal complaint indicative of gastroesophageal reflux. The term describes a retrosternal burning sensation, radiating upward, usually because of reflux of stomach acid into the esophagus. It is exacerbated by large meals, by supine posture, or occasionally by bending over. Heartburn ranges in severity from an occasional episode of postprandial discomfort without sequelae to a syndrome of severe esophageal inflammation, stricture, bleeding, and even esophageal carcinoma. The burning or hot sensation is usually alleviated, at least temporarily, by antacids. In one survey of presumably normal hospital staff, a 7% prevalence of daily heartburn was found; 36% of these same persons experienced heartburn once each month.

The evaluation and treatment of gastroesophageal reflux disease is best conducted in stepwise fashion.

PATHOPHYSIOLOGY AND CLINICAL PRESENTATION

The modern concept of reflux esophagitis emerged in 1935 with the proposal that esophagitis was caused by "the irritant action on the mucosa of free hydrochloric acid and pepsin." Through the 1940s and 1950s gastroesophageal reflux was believed to be related primarily to anatomic factors, specifically to the presence of a *hiatus hernia*. Today many patients complain of "hiatus hernia" when referring to their heartburn. Although there may be some modest predisposition to reflux disease among patients with hiatus hernia, careful studies refute a close association between hiatus hernia and gastroesophageal reflux.

Esophageal manometry studies in the 1960s showed that the physiologic action of the *lower esophageal sphincter* is critical to maintaining a pressure barrier between the stomach and the esophagus. Subsequent studies suggested that the pathogenesis of reflux disease is multifactorial, depending on more than just a decrease in the resting tone of the lower esophageal sphincter. Transient inappropriate relaxations of the lower esophageal sphincter, decreased secondary peristalsis, and defective mucosal resistance have all been implicated.

The lower esophageal sphincter is a complicated region of smooth muscle modulated by the interaction of hormonal, neural, and dietary factors. The hormone gastrin increases resting lower esophageal sphincter tone, while estrogens, progesterone, glucagon, secretin, and cholecystokinin all decrease lower esophageal sphincter pressure. Vagus nerve input helps maintain resting tone, as does alpha-adrenergic stimulation. Pharmacologic agents that increase sphincter tone include bethanechol, metoclopramide, pentobarbital, histamine, edrophonium, and antacids. Anticholinergics, theophylline, meperidine, and the calcium-channel blockers all decrease the resting tone. Tobacco, ethanol, chocolate, and foods with high concentrations of fat or carbohydrate all decrease lower esophageal sphincter pressure and increase heartburn. Citrus fruits and fruit juices often exacerbate symptoms; the mechanism by which they cause heartburn is not clear. Although pregnancy may cause reflux because of increased intra-abdominal pressure, the primary reason for heartburn in pregnancy is reduced lower esophageal sphincter pressure due to increased circulating levels of progesterone and estrogen.

Much emphasis has been placed on measurement of *lower esophageal sphincter pressures,* but there is enormous variation and overlap between patients with symptomatic gastroesophageal reflux and normal subjects. Normal lower esophageal sphincter pressure ranges from 12 to 30 mm Hg. Though single value determinations for lower esophageal sphincter pressure are fraught with inaccuracies, it is reasonable to assume that lower esophageal sphincter pressures of less than 6 mm Hg are apt to allow reflux, and lower esophageal sphincter pressures greater than 20 mm Hg should prevent gastroesophageal reflux. Pressures between 6 and 20 mm Hg are found in both patients and controls. Recent studies using 24-hour intraesophageal pH monitoring suggest that in many patients reflux occurs as a result of transient inappropriate lower esophageal sphincter relaxations rather than low basal tone.

Other factors involved in reflux disease include alterations in esophageal mucosal resistance to caustic liquids, impaired esophageal clearance (secondary peristalsis), and prolonged rates of gastric emptying. Saliva may be an important protective mechanism, inducing peristalsis as well as aiding in washout, dilution, and neutralization of acid refluxed into the esophagus.

Heartburn predictably accompanies gastroesophageal reflux. The patient characteristically complains of retrosternal ache or burning within 30 to 60 minutes of eating, especially after large meals. Symptoms are made worse by lying down or bending over; many patients learn to avoid lying down after meals. Heartburn can mimic cardiac ischemia, and some patients describe a chest heaviness or pressure, which may radiate to the neck, jaw, or shoulders. In some cases *regurgitation* of fluid or food particles may occur, particularly at night. The patient may describe soiling of the pillow with gastric contents or may awake because of coughing or a strangling sensation. *Nocturnal aspiration* is occasionally associated with gastroesophageal reflux and can cause recurrent pneumonias and bronchospasm. A *reflex salivary hypersecretion,* or "*water brash*" is sometimes described by patients with reflux. Water brash is especially common in children, but direct questioning is often required to determine its occurrence.

Pain or difficulty swallowing usually suggests long-standing reflux disease with *either* active inflammation, stricture, or both. Solid food may stick in the distal esophagus (with or without stricture formation), although food usually passes into the stomach after repeated swallows or drinking liquids. Chronic gastroesophageal reflux may result in alteration of the distal esophageal mucosa, from the usual stratified squamous epithelium to a columnar epithelium. This mucosal change is called *Barrett's esophagus* and is associated with esophageal ulcers, strictures, hemorrhage, and increased risk of adenocarcinoma. Classic radiologic presentation is a midesophageal ulcer or stricture. *Bleeding* may accompany reflux esophagitis, and be either slow and chronic, resulting in iron-deficiency anemia, or brisk, resulting in hematemesis.

DIFFERENTIAL DIAGNOSIS

The diagnosis of gastroesophageal reflux disease is secure when the patient describes heartburn and experiences regurgitation of stomach contents. However, many patients report only a dull substernal discomfort or ache, and in such circumstances the physician must consider myocardial ischemia, esophageal spasm, high-amplitude esophageal peristalsis, cholelithiasis, and mediastinal inflammation. Gastroesophageal reflux may accompany peptic ulcer disease (particularly in gastric hypersecretory conditions), functional dyspepsia (see Chapter 55), and cancer of the gastroesophageal junction. Esophageal infections with opportunistic organisms such as cytomegalovirus, herpes virus, and *Candida albicans* can cause heartburn in the immunocompromised host. Reflux esophagitis may also accompany intestinal dysmotility syndromes, including idiopathic intestinal pseudoobstruction, or secondary pseudoobstruction due to scleroderma. Diabetic gastroparesis may predispose to reflux and heartburn, because of retarded emptying of gastric contents.

WORKUP

History. The characteristic history of a retrosternal burning sensation radiating upward, associated with large meals and supine posture, is virtually diagnostic of reflux disease. An attempt should be made to identify any aggravating factors such as intake of fatty foods, concentrated sweets, alcohol, peppermint, coffee, tea, anticholinergics, calcium-channel blockers, and theophylline compounds. Inquiry should be made regarding response to antacids. Surgery near the gastroesophageal junction, for example, prior antireflux surgery or vagotomy, may predispose to reflux disease. A history of Raynaud's phenomenon raises the possibility of scleroderma. Consideration of achalasia, malignancy, esophagitis, and stricture is indicated if dysphagia is part of the clinical presentation (see Chapter 57).

Physical Examination. The physical examination is generally unrevealing, but several points are worth special attention. Sclerodactyly, calcinosis, and telangiectasia suggest underlying scleroderma (see Chapter 144). The epigastrium should be carefully examined for the presence of a mass lesion, and the stool should be examined for presence of occult blood.

Laboratory Studies. No single test is accepted as the standard for the diagnosis of reflux disease. Fortunately, a careful history is sufficient for the diagnosis in the majority of patients, and laboratory tests are needed only in atypical or severe cases. Initial therapy can be instituted on the basis of history alone. If there is dysphagia, painful swallowing, significant weight loss, or occult blood loss, the patient should undergo a barium swallow and upper GI series or endoscopy to rule out a neoplasm or a complication of acid–peptic disease. Suspected damage to esophageal mucosa due to reflux disease can be assessed by *endoscopy* in conjunction with *biopsy* (suction biopsy yields more tissue than endoscopic punch biopsies and give more meaningful information). The *barium swallow* may show inflammation, ulceration, or stricture, but is normal in most cases. It remains the most widely used test for reflux, but its sensitivity may be as low as 25% and it is far less accurate than a careful history. Its

main utility is in searching for stricture and tumor. In atypical cases, the *Bernstein acid perfusion test* is often employed to see if symptoms are due to reflux; however, the Bernstein test is rarely needed when the patient gives a classic description of heartburn, and the test requires careful interpretation since false-positives are common. The most sensitive and specific test is the 24-hour esophageal pH monitor, but it is very expensive, not universally available, and usually unnecessary. However, it does allow correlation of activity to symptoms and reflux of acid. Nevertheless, history still remains the mainstay of diagnosis.

Symptomatic Management. Therapy for reflux disease is best approached in a stepwise fashion beginning with simple interventions (see step 1 below), then adding medications (steps 2 and 3), and ultimately, in refractory cases, employing antireflux surgery (step 4). For many patients with a classic history and no evidence of complications, it is appropriate to begin with step 1 therapy; no laboratory studies are necessary. In many cases this empiric trial will be all that is required to relieve the patient's symptoms. Further testing and more aggressive treatment become necessary only in those cases with poor response to step 1 therapy, in cases where the history is unclear, and in patients with heartburn plus dysphagia or weight loss.

Step 1
a. Dietary manipulations—avoidance of foods high in fat or carbohydrate.
b. Weight reduction if obese.
c. Avoidance of large evening meals near bedtime.
d. Elevation of the head of the bed with 6-inch blocks under the bedposts (pillows are not adequate).
e. Avoidance if possible of medications that decrease sphincter tone, including theophylline compounds, calcium-channel blockers, meperidine, and anticholinergics.
f. Avoidance of cigarettes, alcohol, and coffee.
g. Antacids after meals and at bedtime.

Step 2. Add:
   Cimetidine or ranitidine to suppress gastric acid production (See Chapter 64 for regimens).

Step 3. Add:
a. Bethanechol (a cholinergic agent that raises lower esophageal sphincter pressure and improves acid clearance by the esophagus—the usual dose is 25 mg four times per day), *or*
b. Metoclopramide (a dopamine antagonist that augments gastric emptying and raises lower esophageal sphincter tone). However, as many as one third of patients may not tolerate the latter drug because of CNS side-effects.

Step 4. Consider:
a. Antireflux surgery (this is rarely indicated); it should be reserved for patients with stricture, bleeding, pulmonary aspiration, or very refractory symptoms. The choice, and

ultimate success, of a fundoplication procedure depends on the experience of the surgeon.

b. A major complication from surgery is difficulty with gastric emptying, which can lead to chronic bloating. Before subjecting a patient to surgery, it is important to be sure gastric emptying is relatively normal.

PATIENT EDUCATION

Successful management depends on the patient's compliance with medications, diet, and postural measures. A thorough explanation of the mechanisms of reflux and its aggravating factors helps provide a rational basis for the patient's action. Patients need to realize that no single measure will alleviate the discomfort of reflux, but when all are performed together, relief is extremely likely. The lack of connection between hiatus hernia and reflux also deserves mention because it is a common misunderstanding and often leads to a belief that surgery is required for treatment.

ANNOTATED BIBLIOGRAPHY

Albibi R, McCallum RW: Metoclopramide: Pharmacology and clinical application. Ann Inter Med 98:86, 1983 (*Detailed review of this drug that is useful in some cases of esophageal spasm.*)

Behar J, Brand DL, Brown FC et al: Cimetidine in the treatment of symptomatic gastroesophageal reflux. Gastroenterology 74:441, 1978 (*A five-center U.S. double-blind study documenting efficacy of cimetidine therapy in treating reflux disease.*)

Cohen S: Pathogenesis of coffee-induced gastrointestinal symptoms. N Engl J Med 303:122, 1980 (*Suggests that LES dysfunction and gastroesopageal reflux are the cause of coffee-induced heartburn in susceptible individuals.*)

Costell DO: Medical therapy of reflux esophagitis. Ann Intern Med 93:926, 1980 (*Editorial to the Thamik et al. Reference below— a good, concise outline of therapeutic options in reflux disease.*)

Dodds WJ, Hogan WJ, Helm JF, Dent J: Pathogenesis of reflux esophagitis. Gastroenterology 81:376, 1981 (*The most complete scientific review available on this topic. Emphasizes the importance of transient LES relaxation; 231 references.*)

Fink SM, McCallum RW: The role of prolonged esophageal pH monitoring in the diagnosis of esophageal reflux. JAMA 252:1160, 1984 (*Designates indications for use.*)

Helm JF, Dodds WJ, Pelc LR et al: Effect of esophageal emptying and saliva on clearance of acid from the esophagus. N Engl J Med 310:284, 1984 (*Documents the importance of proper emptying and saliva on mucosal integrity.*)

Jonsell G, DeMeester P: Comparison of diagnostic methods for selections of patients for antireflux operations. Surgery 95:2, 1984 (*A review of what should be done before subjecting patients to surgery.*)

Pope CE II: In Sleisenger MH, Fordtran JS (eds): Gastroesophageal reflux disease. In Gastrointestinal Disease, 3rd ed, Chapter 27, pp 449–476. Philadelphia, WB Saunders, 1983 (*Excellent summary by one of the experts in this field, including a discussion of surgical therapy; 164 references.*)

Richter JE, Castell DO: Drugs, foods, and other substances in the cause and treatment of reflux esophagitis. Med Clin North Am 65:1223, 1981

Richter JE, Castell DO: Gastroesophageal reflux. Ann Intern Med 97:93, 1982 (*The best current, concise review of this entity, with emphasis on diagnostic studies and stepwise therapy.*)

Richter JE: A critical review of current medical therapy for gastrointestinal reflux. J Clin Gastroenterol 8(suppl I):72, 1986 (*An absolutely superb review of all of the important studies relating to the efficacy of therapy; 69 references.*)

Silverstein BD, Pope CE: Role of diagnostic tests in esophageal function. Am J Surg 139:744, 1980 (*A summary of available studies and their indications.*)

Sjogren RW, Johnson LF: Barrett's esophagus: A review. Am J Med 74:313, 1983 (*Concise clinical review of the conditions, etiology, epidemiology, diagnosis, and treatment; 120 references.*)

Spechler SJ, Goyal RK: Barrett's esophagus. N Engl J Med 315:362, 1986 (*Comprehensive review with discussion of cancer risk, diagnosis, and management; 104 references.*)

Thamik KD, Chey WY, Shah AN, Gutierrez JG: Reflux esophagitis: Effect of bethanechol on symptoms and endoscopic findings. Ann Intern Med 93:805, 1980 (*Shows efficacy of cholinergic therapy for reflux disease.*)

Winnan GR, Meyer CT, McCallum RW: Interpretation of the Bernstein test. A reappraisal of criteria. Ann Intern Med 96:320, 1982 (*Reviews technique of this useful test, emphasizing that pain with acid infusion may persist during subsequent infusion of saline and that esophageal peristalsis is important in restoring intraesophageal pH to normal.*)

57
Evaluation of Dysphagia

Dysphagia is the unpleasant sensation of difficulty swallowing. The patient reports that food seems to get caught before reaching the stomach. The discomfort is experienced shortly after swallowing. Because true dysphagia is an important manifestation of esophageal disease, it should be fully assessed and not misinterpreted and dismissed as psychogenic or functional in origin.

PATHOPHYSIOLOGY AND CLINICAL PRESENTATION

Dysphagia implies an abnormality in swallowing and arises from either a loss of coordinated motor activity or from mechanical obstruction, be it intrinsic narrowing or extrinsic compression. *Transfer dysphagia* (oropharyngeal dysphagia) most often occurs as a consequence of neurologic disease and presents as difficulty initiating the act of swallowing. In most instances, other neurologic symptoms (nasal speech, dysphonia, and dysarthria) dominate the clinical picture, but at times, difficulty swallowing is the major complaint. Aspiration takes place with swallowing, and fluid regurgitates into the nose. Cough following deglutition may be a manifestation of abnormal upper esophageal sphincter function. Mechanical obstruction of the pharynx or upper esophagus may also produce oropharyngeal dysphagia.

Achalasia, the most common cause of motor dysphagia, is a slowly progressive disorder with a chronic course. There is aperistalsis, partial or incomplete relaxation of the lower esophageal sphincter (LES), and increased resting LES pressure. Vigorous tertiary esophageal contractions are seen early in the disease in young patients and may result in chest pain, but pain is not an invariable accompaniment. Lesions in the dorsal vagal nucleus, vagal trunks, and myenteric ganglia have been found; there is speculation that this perhaps represents damage caused by a neurotropic virus. As a consequence of neuron loss, the esophagus demonstrates exquisite sensitivity to gastrin and cholinergic agents. Swallowing liquids and solids are equally difficult, yet by eating slowly and drinking small amounts, the patient may be able to consume a full meal. Pain is reported by 70% to 80% of patients, especially if they eat or drink rapidly. Very cold liquids or emotion may provoke symptoms. Patients find that repeated swallowing or performing a rapid Valsalva maneuver can help pass material into the stomach. Regurgitation is common and can be provoked by changes in position or by physical exercise; pulmonary aspiration sometimes results. Patients may demonstrate foul breath because of retained esophageal material.

Squamous cell carcinoma of the esophagus is sometimes a complication of achalasia; it occurs in 5% to 10% of patients.

Carcinoma-induced achalasia is seen with tumors at the gastroesophageal junction. Adenocarcinoma of the stomach is the most common of these neoplasms. The mechanism by which tumor induces achalasia is unclear, but manometric findings are identical to those of primary achalasia. Patients are typically over 50 years of age and complain of marked weight loss and symptoms of dysphagia that are less than a year in duration.

Esophageal spasm, an important motor disorder, is characterized clinically by dysphagia and substernal chest pain, and manometrically by demonstration of simultaneous contractions throughout the esophagus in more than 10% of wet swallows. It differs from achalasia in that it is intermixed with normal peristaltic activity. A related form of motor dysfunction, picturesquely labelled *"nutcracker esophagus"* has a similar clinical presentation. Its manometric profile consists of peristaltic contractions that are of exceptionally high amplitude and long duration; there are no simultaneous contractions. LES pressure and relaxation are abnormal in many of these patients. Reflux occasionally precipitates the contractile abnormalities. About 3% to 5% of patients develop achalasia, and degenerative changes are noted in ganglia and nerves, suggesting that these may be early or mild forms of achalasia. Supersensitivity to gastrin and cholinergic agent can be demonstrated. Dysphagia results when the esophageal contractions interfere with bolus transit. Chest pain seems to be a consequence of prolonged contractile waves.

Together, these esophageal motor disorders account for many cases of noncardiac substernal chest pain, the "nutcracker" variety being the more common. The disorders simulate angina pectoris by presenting substernally, dissipating with nitroglycerin, and even radiating in angina-like fashion. The chest pain and dysphagia often occur separately; heartburn may be reported as a preceding symptom. The pain is frequently nocturnal, awakening the patient from sleep. Chest discomfort need not occur in relation to swallowing, but sometimes is triggered by drinking very hot or very cold liquids. Dysphagia is noted with both liquids and solids. Some asymptomatic patients manifest the radiologic and manometric criteria for esophageal spasm but rarely experience discomfort.

Scleroderma can result in a decrease in lower esophageal sphincter tone as well as a lack of propulsive motor activity. Reflux is more of a problem than is dysphagia, but as many as 20% of patients may suffer some difficulty in swallowing. About 75% of patients with scleroderma have esophageal involvement (see Chapter 56).

Mechanical obstruction differs clinically from motor dysfunction in that the patient has more difficulty with solids than with liquids. The duration of symptoms is shorter (less than 1 year) for patients with malignancy than it is for those with benign causes of obstruction; progression is often rapid. Most patients with tumor are over age 50 and report marked weight loss. The location of discomfort does not necessarily represent the site of obstruction, for the pain may be referred. Spontaneous pain is not a common feature of neoplasm involving the esophagus. Patients with stricture due to severe esophagitis usually have a long-standing history of reflux.

Inflammatory lesions of the pharynx or esophagus may cause pain on swallowing; there is no disturbance of esophageal motility, but swallowing is made difficult by the pain. Even saliva may be irritating.

Tablet ingestion may produce esophageal irritation. The most commonly implicated drugs are tetracycline, quinidine, potassium tablets, nonsteroidal anti-inflammatories, and iron preparations. The elderly are at greatest risk because they are likely to consume more tablets, use less water, and have age-related decreased saliva production. The discomfort will often be associated with the tablets and will generally decrease over a period of a few days. Infectious esophagitis caused by *Candida, Herpes simplex,* or *Cytomegalovirus* is being increasingly recognized in patients on long-term broad-spectrum antibiotics, and in the growing number of patients immunocompromised with AIDS. Viral or fungal esophagitis rarely occurs in immunologically intact individuals; when it does, it is usually short-lived and self-limited.

Sometimes *globus hystericus* is confused with dysphagia. The patient complains of a constant "lump in the throat." There is no actual difficulty swallowing food, even though there is a perception of something in the throat or esophagus. Symptoms are unrelated to swallowing, and esophageal function is normal.

DIFFERENTIAL DIAGNOSIS

The causes of dysphagia can be divided into motor and obstructive categories and are often subdivided according to whether they affect the upper or lower esophagus. Pharyngeal–upper-esophageal motor dysfunction is usually a consequence of a neurologic disease, such as pseudobulbar palsy, myasthenia gravis, multiple sclerosis, amyotrophic lateral sclerosis, or Parkinson's disease. The important esophageal motor disorders are achalasia, diffuse esophageal spasm, and scleroderma.

Upper esophageal mechanical obstruction may be due to tumor, Zenker's diverticulum, sideropenic webs, or an enlarged thyroid. Etiologies of obstruction in the lower portion of the esophagus include carcinoma, stricture, webs, and rings.

Most esophageal cancers are of the squamous cell variety, though half of those in the distal half of the esophagus are adenocarcinomas, suggesting that they arise in the cardia of the stomach. Stricture occurs from chronic reflux, corrosive agents, and prolonged nasogastric intubation. Causes of extrinsic esophageal compression include mediastinal tumors and aortic aneurysm. Acute dysphagia should cause one to consider infection, tablet-induced irritation, and food impaction.

True dysphagia must be distinguished from conditions that may produce esophageal pain without interfering with the mechanics of swallowing, as occurs with most forms of esophagitis. The patient with globus hystericus reports a constant sensation of something in the throat, but swallows normally.

No detailed population studies have been done on the prevalence of dysphagia and the relative frequencies of its etiologies.

WORKUP

History. A tentative diagnosis can often be made by history. A British study found that history alone could provide an accurate diagnosis in about 80% of cases. The most important historical features include the duration and progression of symptoms, relation of symptoms to solids and liquids, effect of cold on swallowing, and response to swallowing a bolus. Inquiry into these aspects of the problem help in the important task of differentiating a motor disorder from mechanical obstruction. Motor disease is suggested by gradual onset, slow progression, chronic course, equal difficulty with liquids and solids, aggravation of symptoms on swallowing cold substances, and passage of a bolus by repeated swallowing, forceful drinking, Valsalva maneuver, or throwing back the head and shoulders. Mechanical obstruction is characterized by more rapid onset and progressive course, more difficulty with solids than with liquids, no aggravation with cold foods, and regurgitation upon trying to swallow a bolus. The location of discomfort helps to locate the lesion only if it is very high or very low in the esophagus; a distal lesion may cause pain referred to the neck. Hiccups point to difficulty in the terminal portion of the esophagus. Intermittent dysphagia for solid food only, is indicative of a lower esophageal (Schatzki) ring.

Other historical features also have some discriminative value, including presence of pain, reflux, and neurologic defects. Pain in conjunction with dysphagia suggests spasm or achalasia, though pain may occur in these conditions without concurrent difficulty in swallowing. Pain on swallowing saliva alone is characteristic of mucosal inflammation. A history of heartburn in conjunction with difficulty swallowing solids argues strongly for a stricture secondary to chronic reflux esophagitis, especially if the problem is chronic. Scleroderma also is suggested when symptoms of reflux occur with dysphagia. Dysphagia that comes on only after activity, in association with motor aphasia, diplopia, or dysphonia, is indicative of myasthenia. Tremor or difficulty in initiating movement suggests Parkinson's disease (see Chapter 162). Other historical facts to note are recent use of topical upper respiratory or inhaled steroid aerosols, broad spectrum antibiotics, and concurrent immunodeficiency (*e.g.,* AIDS).

The pace of illness is important to note. Very acute dysphagia suggests infection, irritation, or food impaction. Rapid progression is due to tumor until proven otherwise, whereas slow progression is most consistent with a motor disorder. Weight loss may occur with any etiology and has little value in differentiating one etiology from another. The same is true for regurgitation.

Physical Examination. The skin is noted for pallor, signs of scleroderma (sclerodactyly, telangiectasias, calcinosis), and hyperkeratotic palms and soles (a rare finding suggestive of esophageal carcinoma). The mouth should be examined carefully for inflammatory lesions, ill-fitting dentures, and pharyngeal masses. Lymph nodes are palpated in the neck and elsewhere for any enlargement suggestive of neoplasm (see Chapter 81), and the thyroid for a large goiter. The abdomen is checked for masses, tenderness, organomegaly, and occult blood in the stool (suggestive of neoplasm and esophagitis). Neurologic examination should include testing for tremor, rigidity, and fatigability as well as cranial nerve deficits.

Laboratory Assessment consists of barium swallow to rule out an obstructive lesion, followed by endoscopy and/or manometry depending on the clinical and x-ray findings. Mechanically obstructing lesions will be identified by *barium swallow,* but some cases of gastric carcinoma may show little more than intrinsic narrowing and require endoscopy and biopsy if the history is suspicious of malignancy (rapid progression, marked weight loss). Radiologic diagnosis of motor disorders can be difficult, for early achalasia and esophageal spasm may produce few findings on barium swallow. The characteristic radiologic features of achalasia include dilatation, segmental contractions, and termination of the distal esophagus into a narrowed segment (often referred to as a "break"). When the patient is upright, an air–fluid level may be present on the barium esophagram. If diffuse esophageal spasm occurs during barium examination, it produces multiple tertiary contractions and differs from achalasia in that there is no break. Functional assessment of dysphagia is facilitated by performing all barium studies with the patient in the supine position to cancel the effect of gravity, and by dipping a piece of bread into barium to better trace the movement of solid food. Ciné studies sometimes help in diagnosis of oropharyngeal dysphagia.

Failure of the barium swallow to reveal a probable etiology leaves the primary physician with the difficult decision of whether or not to proceed with ordering endoscopy and/or

manometry. Suspicion of a motor disorder is best pursued by *manometry,* especially in confusing cases in which there are therapeutic implications. Although potentially diagnostic, manometry often gives indeterminate data. Many patients suspected of achalasia or esophageal spasm fail to show typical manometric findings of these conditions. They end up being placed in a category of nonspecific motility disease. Nevertheless, many authorities insist on manometric data before concluding a patient has esophageal spasm or a related motor disorder. The need to rule out tumor or another type of obstructing lesion is an indication for *esophagoscopy.* However, endoscopy for x-ray negative dysphagia is generally low in yield. Consultation with a gastroenterologist skilled in evaluation of esophageal disease is useful at this point. Finding an obstructing lesion on barium examination usually requires endoscopic assessment for direct visualization, cytology, and biopsy. The high frequency of esophageal pathology in patients with genuine dysphagia is a strong argument for thorough evaluation of every patient.

SYMPTOMATIC RELIEF

Regardless of etiology and pending definitive diagnosis, all patients with dysphagia require an adequate caloric intake that can be swallowed with a minimum of discomfort. The patient suspected of having mechanical obstruction should be advised to take predominantly liquids or soft solids.

A conservative approach sometimes suffices in patients with mild motor disease. The person with achalasia is often able to manage reasonably well by eating slowly, drinking small quantities at a time, and avoiding cold foods. A trial of nitroglycerin before eating may provide some help to the patient with possible esophageal spasm and serve as a crude diagnostic test as well; anticholinergic agents are of no proven benefit. Longer-acting nitrates and calcium channel blockers (*e.g.,* nifedipine) have smooth muscle relaxant qualities that may be helpful for relief of spasm. Antacids sometimes provide relief and are worth a try, especially if reflux seems to trigger symptoms. Patients with severe achalasia get little relief from dietary or drug manipulations; esophageal dilatation or myotomy is needed. Myotomy is more effective but requires major surgery and often produces severe reflux. Consequently, esophageal dilatation is usually the first invasive procedure for treatment of severe motor disease.

Patients with mechanical obstruction often require dilatation or surgery, but there are many exceptions. The person with a lower esophageal ring is best treated by advising slow intake of small amounts; dilatation does not work very well. Restoration of adequate iron intake will reverse the pathologic changes of sideropenic dysphagia, unless a carcinoma has ensued in the pharynx. Carcinoma of the upper or middle third of the esophagus is often unresectable and best treated by radiation therapy; considerable palliation is sometimes achieved. Treatment of oropharyngeal dysphagia due to obstruction is approached surgically (*e.g., removal of a Zenker's diverticulum or large goiter*), whereas attention to the underlying neurologic deficit is necessary in cases due to motor dysfunction, though myotomy may help as well. The patient with globus hystericus can be given thorough reassurance, although symptoms are not likely to resolve easily.

The patient who is referred for further evaluation and therapy should continue to be followed closely by the primary physician to be certain that the patient's nutrition is not overlooked during therapy of the underlying disease and to keep the patient informed of the overall diagnostic and therapeutic plan.

A.H.G.

ANNOTATED BIBLIOGRAPHY

Castell DO, Knuff TE, Brown FC et al: Dysphagia. Gastroenterology 76:1015, 1979 (*Reviews dysphagia as a complication of conditions causing reflux.*)

Castell DO: Medical therapy for reflux esophagitis. Ann Intern Med 104:112, 1986 (*An editorial reviewing current therapy.*)

Clouse RE, Lustman PJ: Psychiatric illness and contraction abnormalities of the esophagus. N Engl J Med 309:1337, 1983 (*Creates an association between psychiatric illness including depression and symptomatic esophageal motility disorders, many presenting as chest pain.*)

Cohen S: Motor disorders of the esophagus. N Engl J Med 301:184, 1979 (*Authoritative review by one of the field's leading investigators; 120 references.*)

Dipalma JA, Prechter GC, Bradie CE: X-ray negative dysphagia: Is endoscopy necessary? J Clin Gastroenterol 6:409, 1984 (*Endoscopy in x-ray dysphagia is generally of low yield.*)

Edwards DAW: Discriminative information in the diagnosis of dysphagia. J R Coll Physicians London 9:257, 1975 (*Critical discussion of important historical data; diagnostic accuracy by history alone is close to 80%.*)

Goyal RK et al: Lower esophageal ring. N Engl J Med 282:1298, 1970 (*An uncommon but important cause of obstructions.*)

Hollis JB, Castell DO: Esophageal function in elderly men: A new look at presbyesophagus. Ann Intern Med 80:371, 1974 (*A careful study that finds esophageal function is rather normal in elderly people, suggesting that disordered motility is most likely caused by disease and should not be attributed to aging.*)

Hurwitz AL, Duranceau A: Upper esophageal sphincter dysfunction: Pathogenesis and treatment. Am J Dig Dis 23:275, 1978 (*A review of the causes of oropharyngeal dysphagia and a presentation of the results of cricopharyngeal myotomy as a method of relieving symptoms; 48 references.*)

Jordan PH: Dysphagia and esophageal diverticula. Postgrad Med 61:155, 1977 (*An excellent review of diverticula and the etiology of the symptom dysphagia.*)

Kikendall JW, Freedman AC, Oyewole MA et al: Pill-induced esophageal injury: Case reports and review of the medical literature. Dig Dis Sci 28:174, 1983 (*A review of an often overlooked etiology.*)

Kilman WJ, Goyal RK: Disorders of pharyngeal and upper esophageal sphincter motor function. Arch Intern Med 136:592, 1976 (*Thorough discussion of oropharyngeal motor diseases.*)

Mukhopadhyay AK, Graham DY: Esophageal motor dysfunction in systemic diseases. Arch Intern Med 136:583, 1976 (*Connective tissue disease, metabolic problems, and neuromuscular disorders are reviewed.*)

Orlando RC, Bozymski EM: Clinical and manometric effects of nitroglycerin in diffuse esophageal spasm. N Engl J Med 289:23, 1973 (*Nitroglycerin can provide relief, though the study is uncontrolled.*)

Patterson DJ, Graham DY, Smith JL et al: Natural history of benign esophageal stricture treated by dilatation. Gastroenterology 85:346, 1983 (*The natural history of 154 patients with esophageal stricture treated with bougienage. Improvement occurred in 84.5% and 36% required no further dilatation during a 4-year follow up. Many patients, however, require repeat dilatations.*)

Richter JE, Castell DO: Diffuse esophageal spasm: A reappraisal. Ann Intern Med 100:242, 1984 (*Argues for a manometric diagnosis of spasm; critical review of diagnostic criteria.*)

Spechler SJ, Goyal RK: Barrett's esophagus. N Engl J Med 315:362, 1986 (*Comprehensive review; 104 references. Emphasizes risk of adenocarcinoma.*)

Tavitian A, Raufman JP, Rosenthal L: Oral candidiasis as a marker for esophageal candidiasis in the acquired immunodeficiency syndrome. Ann Intern Med 104:54, 1986 (*A useful clinical marker.*)

Vantrappen G, Hellemans J: Treatment of achalasia and related motor disorders. Gastroenterology 79:144, 1980 (*A review of surgical and nonsurgical approaches to symptomatic therapy.*)

58

Evaluation and Management of Diarrhea

JAMES M. RICHTER, M.D.

Diarrhea is an affliction familiar to everyone. It is clinically characterized as the frequent passage of unformed stools. Most episodes are brief, self-limited, and well tolerated without need for medical attention. However, when diarrhea becomes severe or chronic, a thoughtful evaluation is needed to ensure proper management. As the physician of first contact, the primary physician needs to be skilled in the care of patients suffering from diarrhea. Major tasks include making an expeditious clinical diagnosis of acute diarrheas, deciding when to use antibiotic therapy, preventing and treating traveler's diarrhea, efficiently evaluating patients with chronic diarrhea, and providing symptomatic relief while evaluation is in progress.

PATHOPHYSIOLOGY AND CLINICAL PRESENTATIONS

Diarrhea is a change in a patient's bowel habits, manifested by increased stool volume, looseness, and frequency. The pathophysiologic common denominator is an increased water content of stools, which may be due to increased fluid secretion, decreased water absorption, or altered bowel motility. At times several mechanisms are operative. *Increased fluid secretion* can be triggered by inflammation, hormones, or enterotoxins. The resulting secretory diarrhea has the characteristics of a stool volume that remains in excess of 500 ml/24 hours in spite of fasting, a low stool osmolality, and a normal stool electrolyte concentration. *Decreased reabsorption of fluid* occurs with abnormalities of the bowel mucosa, loss of reabsorptive surface, or the presence of unabsorbable osmotically active materials in the bowel lumen, such as lactose in patients with lactose deficiency. Patients with diarrhea due to decreased reabsorption typically respond to fasting with a decrease in stool volume to less than 500 ml/24 hours; stool osmolality is increased and its sodium and potassium concentrations are low. *Altered bowel motility* decreases the contact time with the bowel mucosa, limiting fluid reabsorption; it can ensue after vagotomy or may be hormonally triggered, as in hypergastrinemia.

Clinical presentation depends, in part, on the site of involvement. *Small bowel diarrheas* tend to result in passage of large, loose stools in conjunction with periumbilical or right lower quadrant pain. There may be diarrhea after meals or after eating certain foods, but this is also seen with patients suffering from malabsorption, osmotic diarrhea, a fistula, or the dumping syndrome. *Large bowel diarrheas,* especially those due to disease of the left colon and rectosigmoid, are manifested by passage of frequent, small, loose stools in conjunction with crampy, left lower quadrant pain or tenesmus.

Acute Diarrheas

A diarrhea is categorized as "acute" if its duration is less than 2 weeks. Infectious etiologies dominate and include viral, bacterial, and parasitic agents. Bacteria cause diarrhea by producing a toxin in contaminated food or after ingestion, or by invading the bowel mucosa. Parasites tend to invade the bowel wall, although some cause diarrhea by coating the absorptive surface.

Viral gastroenteritis is the most common cause of acute diarrhea, yet the organisms have only recently been isolated and identified. Epidemics of viral gastroenteritis are particularly common. More than 40% of outbreaks of nonbacterial gastroenteritis investigated by the Centers for Disease Control during a 5-year period were linked to the Norwalk virus. Outbreaks have been found to occur during all seasons and include waterborne, foodborne, and person-to-person modes of transmission. They last about a week. Vomiting is the prominent symptom in children, diarrhea in adults. After an incubation period of 48 to 72 hours, symptoms usually begin abruptly with diarrhea, nausea, vomiting, headache, low-grade fever, abdominal cramps, and malaise; they resolve spontaneously within 24 to 96 hours. The diarrhea tends to be predominantly of the small bowel variety and secretory in quality. Abdominal examination reveals diffuse tenderness (without guarding) and hyperactive bowel sounds. The white count is usually normal but may be elevated. Stools are usually free of leukocytes, but occasionally white cells are found, mimicking an invasive etiology.

Staphylococcus aureus is a common contaminant of custard-filled pastries and processed meats. The organism produces an enterotoxin that causes nausea, vomiting, abdominal cramps, and diarrhea within 2 to 8 hours of eating the contaminated food. Symptoms usually last less than 12 hours. A common-source pattern and lack of fever are typical.

Clostridium perfringens is another common food contaminant, especially of foods that have been warmed on steam tables. The organism releases an enterotoxin after sporulation in the intestine. Consequently, the incubation period of 8 to

24 hours is a bit longer than that for staphylococcal food poisoning. Symptoms include diarrhea, abdominal cramps, and occasionally some vomiting. It too has a common-source epidemiology, and there is no fever.

Bacillus cereus is a toxin-producing bacterial contaminant of rice and bean sprouts. One form of toxin-induced illness leads to vomiting but no diarrhea; in another, there is severe abdominal cramping and diarrhea. Incubation is 8 to 16 hours after ingestion of contaminated food. The symptoms are self-limited.

Salmonella species cause diarrhea by invading the bowel wall. Patients who lack gastric acidity are at increased risk of infection; stomach acid is an effective deterrent. The most common form of *Salmonella* infection is a self-limited diarrheal illness resulting from ingestion of contaminated food (eggs and poultry are often the source). Children are at greatest risk; late summer and fall are the times of peak incidence. Although most episodes of salmonellosis are mild, debilitated patients are at risk for serious bacteremia. In the typical outpatient case, symptoms begin 12 to 36 hours after ingestion and resolve within 5 days, although they may persist for up to 2 weeks. The initial presentation is rather nonspecific though indicative of a small bowel process: watery diarrhea, cramps, nausea, vomiting, and fever. In addition to colonization, an enterotoxin is released that stimulates the secretory diarrhea. In later stages, invasion spreads to the large bowel and leukocytes may be noted in the stool. A distinguishing feature of salmonellosis is that the leukocytes are often mononuclear cells. In severe cases, dysentery can develop.

Typhoid fever, a rare but "must-not-miss" form of salmonella disease, is caused by infection with *S. typhi.* About 500 cases occur in the United States each year, mostly among young people. Infections are both waterborne and foodborne. Although only a small percentage of patients with typhoid fever develop diarrhea, it does occur. The classic and most severe form is a "pea-soup" diarrhea developing in the third week of illness. Early symptoms suggestive of the condition are progressive fever, relative bradycardia, evanescent rash on the trunk ("rose spots"), splenomegaly, cough, headache, and right lower quadrant abdominal pain.

Shigella infection produces an invasive diarrheal illness. Transmission is by the fecal–oral route, and stubborn reservoirs include day care centers, Indian reservations, urban ghettos, and rural villages in developing countries. Young children are at greatest risk and often the source of infection within a family. The illness proceeds in two stages. First, there is colonization in the small bowel, resulting in a watery diarrhea and periumbilical pain, followed in a few days by invasion of the large bowel producing small frequent stools, tenesmus, and polymorphonuclear leukocytes on smear. In florid cases, the patient has fever, toxicity, bloody diarrhea, nausea, vomiting, and cramps. Most often the disease is more subtle and may be difficult to distinguish from other diarrheal illnesses accompanied by fever.

Campylobacter jejuni infection is now responsible for more cases of diarrhea in the United States than either *Salmonella* or *Shigella.* Infection derives most often from animal sources such as poultry and household pets; fecal transmission between people also occurs. The incubation period is 2 to 7 days. Clinically, the illness resembles that caused by *Salmonella* or *Shigella;* however, symptoms may persist longer. The relapse rate is as high as 20%, although the illness is usually self-limited and resolves within a week. In half of all cases, a Gram stain of the stool shows characteristic curved gram-negative rods arranged in "seagull wing" fashion. The organism grows best on a special medium incubated at 42°C; it will not grow on plates customarily used for isolation of *Salmonella* and *Shigella.*

Yersinia enterocolitica also causes an illness that resembles salmonellosis. Patients become infected by eating contaminated meat or dairy products. The incubation period is 12 hours to 3 days. An intense regional lymphoid reaction may arise in the terminal ileum (the portal of entry for the organism) and result in a clinical picture of fever, right lower quadrant abdominal pain, and diarrhea that can simulate the onset of Crohn's disease. From 10% to 40% of patients develop fever, arthralgias, polyarthritis, or erythema nodosum. The illness is usually self-limited.

Vibrio parahemolyticus and *non-toxin-producing V. cholera* are pathogenic *Vibrio* species that have caused outbreaks of diarrheal disease among people eating raw seafood, particularly oysters and sushi-style red snapper and salmon. The incubation period is measured in hours to several days. The illness that ensues is usually mild and self-limited, though an occasional patient may present with fever, nausea, vomiting, and crampy diarrhea.

Cryptosporidiosis is a protozoan infection being recognized with increasing frequency, especially among *immunocompromised patients,* such as those with *AIDS.* In these patients, the infection can produce a profuse watery diarrhea with stool volumes that may exceed 3 liters per day. Although the illness is usually self-limited, it may persist in immunocompromised hosts. Otherwise healthy, immunocompetent patients develop a mild illness; they become infected from occupational contact with animal dung; symptoms resolve spontaneously within 5 to 21 days.

Diarrhea in homosexual men may additionally ensue from infection with *Neisseria, Giardia, Entamoeba histolytica, Campylobacter, Chlamydia, Shigella,* or *Salmonella.* In a study of 194 homosexual men, a polymicrobial origin was identified in a major proportion of those presenting with diarrhea, tenesmus, and rectal pain.

Drug-induced diarrheas may occur as a result of excessive fluid secretion (alcohol, phenolphthalein, and castor oil), reduction of fluid absorption (magnesium-containing antacids), or stimulation of bowel motility (caffeine-containing beverages and herbal teas). Broad-spectrum antibiotics can cause diarrhea by allowing overgrowth of potentially pathogenic species such as *C. difficile* (see below). Almost any drug can cause gastrointestinal upset and diarrhea (see Table 58-1 later in the chapter).

Traveler's Diarrheas

Patients traveling from industrialized to developing nations are at considerable risk for developing diarrhea. Etiologic agents include *Escherichia coli, Salmonella, Shigella, Entamoeba histolytica, Giardia lamblia, S. typhi,* and *Vibrio cholera.*

E. coli are responsible for a large proportion of cases labeled as "traveler's diarrhea" or "turista." The problem originates from poor food handling practices. The clinical presentation depends on whether the infecting strain is simply a toxin producer or is also capable of bowel wall invasion. With enterotoxin production, a watery diarrhea ensues because of the toxin's promotion of fluid secretion in the small bowel. With bowel wall invasion, a dysenteric presentation is possible, with hemorrhagic colitis and fever. A cytotoxin has been isolated from invasive strains. A third mechanism of *E. coli* diarrhea is adherence to the upper small bowel, effectively coating the absorptive surface; impaired absorption and diarrhea without systemic signs result.

Entamoeba histolytica usually exists in a commensual relationship with the host, and most patients harboring the protozoan are asymptomatic carriers. Occasionally, this relationship breaks down and the ameba invades the colonic wall, resulting in an acute bloody diarrhea. The clinical presentation ranges from mild to fulminant illness. Occasionally the illness is mistaken for inflammatory bowel disease (see Chapter 65, and may have a protracted course with exacerbations and remissions. Asymptomatic carriers such as returning tourists and immigrants are often the source of infection in developed countries. Because amebiasis does not have a soil phase, it is not restricted to warmer climates. Well-documented outbreaks have occurred in the United States and Europe, in addition to those that originate in developing countries. Amebiasis can be spread by sexual contact and is prevalent among promiscuous homosexuals.

Giardia lamblia ranks as a leading parasitic cause of diarrhea, especially overseas, but also in the United States. Infection with the flagellated protozoan is particularly common where water supplies are contaminated by human sewage, but the organism is also endemic to such areas as the Rocky Mountains and Leningrad. The exact means by which *Giardia* causes diarrhea remains unsettled, although heavy infestations can lead to malabsorption by coating large areas of the small bowel, particularly the lower duodenum and upper jejunum. The majority of patients with giardiasis are asymptomatic, but the organism is being recognized ever more frequently as an important cause of acute, intermittent, and chronic diarrheas in the United States. The ensuing loose stools may be watery or greasy; mucus is often present, but

blood is rare. The patient may complain of epigastric or periumbilical discomfort. Mild steatorrhea and malabsorption occur with heavy parasite burdens.

Cholera is the prototypical secretory diarrheal disease. It results from drinking water contaminated with *Vibrio cholerae.* Most outbreaks are pandemic in the Indian subcontinent, Southeast Asia, Africa, and the Middle East. Isolated outbreaks have been reported in Mediterranean countries. In the United States, rare outbreaks sometimes occur along the Gulf Coast. The disease ranges in severity from a mild illness to fulminant, life-threatening diarrhea with copious production of gray, watery, mucoid ("rice water") stool. In severe cases, fluid losses may reach over 1 liter per hour, accompanied by vomiting, muscle cramps, and severe thirst. Being a noninvasive diarrhea involving the small bowel, cholera causes no tenesmus and the stool contains no leukocytes. Dehydration, serious volume depletion, and a metabolic acidosis may ensue. In mild cases, the patient reports painless, nonbloody diarrhea of abrupt onset.

Chronic and Recurrent Diarrheas

Although the number of etiologies is vast, consideration of a few exemplary conditions provides a good sense of the range and types of presentations.

Irritable bowel syndrome (see Chapter 66) is the most common of the motility disorders responsible for chronic diarrhea. It can present as diarrhea alternating with constipation, or as chronic, recurrent diarrhea. Some studies report a high frequency of associated psychiatric disease. In addition to diarrhea and constipation, patients may complain of distention, cramping, and mucus-laden stools. The condition waxes and wanes over many years. Many patients with this condition exhibit preoccupation with their bowels. Neither fever nor fecal leukocytes are present.

The *inflammatory bowel diseases* (see Chapter 65) are typical of the diarrheas that result from inflammatory destruction of the bowel wall. Abdominal pain, bloody stools, purulent discharge, and fever are seen in patients with active disease affecting the large bowel. Extraintestinal manifestations occur and may involve the skin, joints, liver, and heart. Microscopic examination of the stool reveals red cells and leukocytes.

Pseudomembranous colitis develops when normal bowel flora are suppressed by use of broad-spectrum antibiotics allowing *C. difficile* (a cytotoxin-producing gram-negative rod found in 6% of normal adults) to proliferate. The antibiotics most often responsible are *ampicillin* and *clindamycin,* but other broad-spectrum agents have also been implicated. Immunocompromised patients, the elderly, and those with underlying bowel disease are most susceptible. Fever, abdominal pain, profuse watery stools, and fecal leukocytes are typical clinical features; the illness may range from mild to severe. Symptoms usually start after the initiation of a course of antibiotic therapy, but onset can be delayed for as much as 4 weeks; symptoms sometimes persist for months, mimicking inflammatory bowel disease. The sigmoidoscopic finding of nodular, inflammatory ulcers or yellow-white mucosal plaques is characteristic.

Diabetic enteropathy is a hypomotility disorder that results from diabetes-induced autonomic neuropathy. When the small bowel is involved, the ensuing stasis allows bacterial overgrowth, which causes fat malabsorption resulting from bacterial deconjugation of bile acids. With involvement of the large bowel, the patient experiences distressing nocturnal diarrhea. Postural hypotension, impotence, and other symptoms and signs of autonomic insufficiency may accompany the diarrhea and suggest the diagnosis.

The *dumping syndrome* is another motility disorder, seen most commonly in patients who have undergone gastrectomy and gastroenterostomy. Patients complain of sweating, postural lightheadedness, tachycardia, and diarrhea following meals; foods and liquids rich in carbohydrates are most likely to trigger symptoms. Lying down minimizes symptoms, as does avoidance of concentrated sweets. Symptoms begin shortly after surgery and often subside within 12 months; they sometimes persist. Besides altered motility, other mechanisms, such as osmotic factors, are believed to be operative in this syndrome, although their precise contributions remain to be elucidated.

Villous adenoma causes a secretory, noninflammatory chronic diarrhea. Watery diarrhea, independent of food and fluid intake, is typical; severe potassium depletion can result. In some patients with this tumor, excessive secretion of mucus occurs, with loss of sufficient protein to produce hypoalbuminemia and a protein-losing enteropathy syndrome.

Malabsorption of fat or carbohydrate can lead to an osmotic diarrhea. Some of the osmotically active substances may also stimulate increased bowel secretion of fluids and electrolytes. *Malabsorption of fat* characteristically presents as foul, bulky, greasy stools. Patients may note that the stools seem to be "sticky" and difficult to flush down the toilet. Steatorrheic stools "float" not because of their fat content but because of an increase in trapped gas. Associated symptoms are a function of the severity of the caloric and vitamin deficiencies that ensue and may include weight loss, ecchymoses, bone pain, glossitis, muscle tenderness, and peripheral neuropathy. Cramping lower abdominal pain typically precedes bowel movements.

Malabsorption of lactose due to *lactase deficiency* is the prototype of carbohydrate malabsorption diseases leading to an osmotic diarrhea. It is particularly common among blacks, Indians, Orientals and Jews; onset is typically in adulthood. A secondary form of the disease may develop in patients suffering from extensive disease of the small bowel. Patients report nausea, bloating, cramps, and diarrhea after ingesting more than their customary intake of milk products. Weight loss and steatorrhea are absent or mild; appetite remains good.

Avoidance of milk products (except for yogurts containing live cultures, which provide lactase) terminates symptoms. Diagnosis is confirmed by an abnormal lactose tolerance test or a hydrogen breath test (detects excessive hydrogen production from bacterial metabolism of undigested lactose).

Chronic laxative abuse is an important and often occult etiology of chronic diarrhea. Patients suffering from bulimia (see Chapter 230) tend to use laxatives chronically and surreptitiously in a relentless attempt to lose weight. Depending on the type of agent used, either a secretory or osmotic diarrhea may develop. Agents associated with secretory diarrheas include castor oil and phenolphthalein preparations. Osmotic diarrheas occur when the patient takes a preparation that contains magnesium (*e.g.,* milk of magnesia) or another poorly absorbable substance. These substances appear in the stool and can be tested for if laxative abuse is suspected. Patients who abuse laxatives may present with unexplained dehydration, electrolyte depletion, or preoccupation with weight loss.

Incontinence

A number of patients who complain of "diarrhea" actually suffer from incontinence. Typically, their stool volumes are normal (less than 250 ml/day), though their stools may be soft. Poor sphincter tone and evidence of stool incontinence are found on physical examination.

DIFFERENTIAL DIAGNOSIS

Acute Diarrhea. The differential diagnosis for acute diarrhea is dominated by infectious agents (Table 58-1). Viruses are the single most important, frequent cause. Staphylococcal toxin, clostridial toxin, and ingestion of *Campylobacter, Salmonella, Shigella,* and enteropathogenic *E. coli* are common bacterial etiologies. *Giardia* and amebae are less frequent sources of acute diarrhea in the United States. Drugs are important and common causes of diarrhea, especially antibiotics, laxatives, magnesium-containing antacids, and other agents such as quinidine and guanethidine. Alcohol and caffeine-containing beverages should be considered. Most causes of chronic diarrhea are also capable of acute presentations.

Chronic Diarrhea. The differential diagnosis is even more extensive for chronic diarrhea. The infectious agents and drugs discussed under acute diarrheal disease may be responsible, but the likelihood of parasites such as amebae or *Giardia* increases. Inflammatory bowel diseases must also be considered. Absorption defects resulting from sprue, bile-salt deficiency, lactase deficiency, intestinal lymphoma, Whipple's disease, and pancreatic insufficiency may cause chronic diarrhea. The patient who has had gastrointestinal surgery may develop diarrhea on the basis of postgastrectomy dumping syndrome, fistulas, blind loops, loss of parasympathetic innervation, or extensive bowel resection. Diarrhea may be

Table 58-1. A Differential Diagnosis of Diarrhea

ACUTE DIARRHEA	CHRONIC OR RECURRENT DIARRHEA
Viruses	**Protozoa**
	Giardia lamblia
Bacterial Toxins	*Entamoeba histolytica*
Staphylococcus	*Cryptosporidiosis*
Clostridium	
	Inflammation
Bacteria	Ulcerative colitis
Salmonella	Crohn's disease
Shigella	Ischemic colitis
Escherichia coli	Pseudomembranous colitis
Campylobacter	
Yersinia	**Drugs**
B. Cereus	Laxatives
Vibrio parahaemolyticus	Antibiotics
Vibrio cholerae	Quinidine
	Guanethidine; other
Protozoa	antihypertensive agents
Giardia lamblia	Caffeine
Entamoeba histolytica	Digitalis
Drugs	**Functional**
Laxatives	Irritable bowel syndrome
Antibiotics	Diverticulosis
Caffeine	
Alcohol	**Tumors**
	Bowel carcinoma
Functional	Villous adenoma
Anxiety	Islet-cell tumors
	Carcinoid syndrome
Acute Presentations of Chronic	Medullary carcinoma of
or Recurrent Diarrhea	thyroid
(See next column)	
	Malabsorption
	Sprue
	Intestinal lymphoma
	Bile-salt malabsorption
	Whipple's disease
	Pancreatic insufficiency
	Lactase deficiency
	Other disaccharidase
	deficiencies
	Alpha-beta lipoproteinemia
	Postsurgical
	Postgastrectomy dumping
	syndrome
	Enteroenteric fistulas
	Blind loops
	Parasympathetic denervation
	Short bowel syndrome
	Other
	Cirrhosis
	Diabetes mellitus
	Heavy-metal intoxication
	Other neurogenic diarrheas
	Hyperthyroidism
	Addison's disease
	Pellagra
	Scleroderma
	Amyloidosis

caused directly by neoplasms, particularly villous adenoma. Diarrhea alternating with constipation raises the possibility of colonic carcinoma, irritable bowel syndrome, or diverti-cular disease of the bowel. A variety of extraintestinal conditions may be responsible, including cirrhosis, alcoholism, pellagra, and heavy-metal intoxications from lead, mercury, or arsenic. Occasionally, chronic diarrhea may develop with endocrinopathies such as Addison's disease, hyperthyroidism, and diabetes mellitus.

WORKUP

The first task is to confirm that the problem is indeed diarrhea and not simply an occasional loose stool or frequent defecation of formed stools. The term "diarrhea" specifically denotes the frequent passage of unformed stools. Once diarrhea is confirmed, one should seek an etiologic diagnosis to guide therapy, especially in severe or persistent cases.

Acute and Traveler's Diarrheas

History. The *nature of the bowel movements* should be determined, including their frequency, consistency, volume, and the presence of gross blood, pus, or mucus (see Tables 58-2 and 58-3). *Associated symptoms* such as fever, abdominal pain, and rash also deserve attention. Fever, blood, or pus suggests an invasive process, though blood may also result from anal pathology or irritation unrelated to the etiology of the diarrhea. Mucus free of leukocytes is a hallmark of irritable bowel syndrome. The macular "rose spot" rash on the trunk is an important clue for typhoid, a rare, but "must-not-miss" diagnosis. Patients with periumbilical or right lower quadrant pain and copious volumes of watery stool are likely to have a small bowel etiology. Those with left lower quadrant discomfort or tenesmus and frequent, small volumes of stool are probably suffering from an etiology that involves the large bowel.

Epidemiologic information is critical to making an etiologic diagnosis of acute diarrhea, because the clinical presentation is often nonspecific. Travel, food intake, and personal contacts require careful review. In more than 50% of cases, "*traveler's diarrhea*" results from exposure to enterotoxigenic *E. coli; Salmonella, Shigella, Giardia,* and *Campylobacter* account for the remainder. Although most cases occur with travel to developing nations, this is not always true (*e.g.,* risk of giardiasis with travel to Leningrad or the Rocky Mountains).

Onset of diarrhea within hours of ingesting a potentially contaminated food is suggestive of *food poisoning;* this is confirmed by checking if others were similarly affected. Foodborne illness with a short incubation period and no fever indicates ingestion of a preformed enterotoxin. Presence of fever and a slightly longer incubation period are characteristics of an infectious etiology (see Table 58-3). Custard-filled pastries, processed meats, foods warmed on steam tables, eggs, poultry, raw seafood, raw milk, rice, and bean sprouts are among the foods often implicated in food poisoning.

Table 58-2.   Important Features of Some Acute Diarrheas

ETIOLOGY	NATURE OF THE DIARRHEA			ASSOCIATED SYMPTOMS AND SIGNS	EPIDEMIOLOGIC DATA	LABORATORY RESULTS
	W/S	OB	GB			
Viral	+/+	−	−	n, v, fever, myalgias abdominal cramps, headache	Occurs in short-lived epidemics	WBC: nl or elevated Stool: usually no WBC
S. aureus	−/+	−	−	n, v, no fever	Custards; incubation: 2–8 h	WBC: nl Stool: no WBC
Clostridium perfringens	+/+	−	−	n, v, no fever	Steam tables incubation: 8–24 h	WBC nl Stool: no WBC
B. cereus	+/+	−	−	n, v, no fever	Rice, sprouts	WBC: nl Stool: no WBC
Salmonella	+/−	+	+	n, v, fever, in some cases dysentery	Eggs, turtles, poultry	Stool: WBC + Culture +
S. typhi	+/+ "Pea soup"	+	−	Rose spots, HA, splenomegaly, bradycardia, fever, toxic	Water, food	Stool: monos, culture +
Shigella	+/− Dysentery	+	−	n, v, fever, toxic in severe cases	Ghettos; day care centers; Indian reservations	Stool: WBC + Stool: WBC + Culture +
Campylobacter	+/− Dysentery	+	+	n, v, fever	Poultry, pets	Stool: WBC + Culture +
Yersinia	+/+	+	−	Simulates Crohn's disease and appendicitis; joint complaints	Dairy products, meat	Stool: WBC + Culture +
Vibrio sp.	+/+	−	−	n, v, cramps, occasionally fever	Raw seafood; 2-day course	Stool culture +
Cryptosporidia	+/−	−	−	occasionally n, v, cramps, dehydration	AIDS patients, immunosuppressed	Stool for o & p +
Giardia	See Table 58-3					
E. histolytica	See Table 58-3					

W/S = watery/soft
OB = occult blood
GB = gross blood
n = nausea
v = vomiting
o & p = ova and parasites
+ = present
− = absent
nl = normal
WBC = white blood cells

Person-to-person spread is an important source of infection that needs to be explored. Among *male homosexuals,* diarrhea often has a polymicrobial etiology; *Neisseria, Chlamydia, Entamoeba histolytica, Lymphogranuloma venereum, Giardia,* and *Campylobacter* are additional pathogens to consider. *Children* who attend day care centers may contract rotavirus, *Giardia, Shigella, Cryptosporidiosis,* or *Campylobacter.*

A good *drug history* is essential; any drug may cause diarrhea. It is particularly important to question for use of laxatives, magnesium-containing antacids, excess alcohol, caffeine-containing beverages, herbal teas, antibioties, digitalis, quinidine, loop diuretics (furosemide, ethacrynic acid), and antihypertensive agents.

Physical Examination. Vital signs must be checked for postural changes, a reflection of significant volume depletion. Any elevation in temperature or loss of weight needs to be noted. The skin is examined for rashes, the lymph nodes for enlargement, and the abdomen for tenderness, guarding, rebound, abnormal bowel sounds, organomegaly, and masses. A rectal examination and fecal occult blood test complete the physical.

Laboratory Studies. The laboratory workup should be individualized. The patient who feels well except for frequent loose stools requires no immediate laboratory testing. On the other hand, the patient who is ill with fever, nausea, abdominal cramps, or other systemic symptoms requires more ex-

Table 58-3.   Important Features of Traveler's Diarrheas

ETIOLOGY	NATURE OF THE DIARRHEA			ASSOCIATED SYMPTOMS AND SIGNS	EPIDEMIOLOGIC DATA	LABORATORY RESULTS
	W/S	OB	GB			
E. coli	+/−	−	−	Usually no fever; though occasionally toxicity	Contamination of water, food	Stool: WBC −; can also be +
Entamoeba histolytica	+/+ dysentery	+/−	+/−	Can simulate inflammatory bowel disease, asymptomatic carriers	Returning tourists; immigrants	Stool + for o & p; + serology
Giardia	−/+	−	−	Upper abdominal pain	Contamination of water supply	Stool + for o & p
V. cholera	+/− "rice water"	−	−	Marked dehydration, cramps, vomiting	Contamination of water supply	Stool: WBC −
Shigella	See Table 58-2					
Salmonella	See Table 58-2					

tensive evaluation, beginning with a *methylene blue stain* of *stool or mucus.* A drop of the sample is placed on a microscope slide and mixed thoroughly with two drops of methylene blue solution. After a cover slip is placed over the mixture, it is ready for viewing under the microscope. If methylene blue is not available, a *Wright's stain* or Gram stain will suffice to demonstrate the presence of leukocytes. Finding large numbers of white cells suggests an inflammatory or invasive diarrhea, such as occurs with *Shigella, Salmonella, Campylobacter,* invasive *E. Coli,* and *Entamoeba.* The presence of mononuclear cells is characteristic of salmonellosis. An occasional white cell is of no pathologic significance. Leukocytes may be absent from the stool in the early phases of shigellosis and pseudomembranous colitis.

In selected instances a *Gram stain* of the stool will give etiologic information. For example, in about half the cases due to *Campylobacter,* the Gram stain will demonstrate gram-negative rods arranged in characteristic gull-wing configuration. If either occult blood or leukocytes are present in the stool, appropriate *bacterial cultures* should be obtained. Detection of *Campylobacter* or *Yersinia* requires plating on specific medium at 42°C; the usual medium for *Salmonella* and *Shigella* will not suffice.

Patients with large numbers of leukocytes in the stool and severe illness should undergo *sigmoidoscopy* to examine the appearance of the colonic mucosa; samples of the mucus and cultures can also be obtained (see evaluation of chronic diarrhea for details). Preparatory enemas and cathartics should be avoided so as not to distort the appearance of the bowel wall (see Chapter 75).

If the diarrhea persists for 2 weeks or more, a secondary evaluation is indicated. Stools should once again be examined for blood and leukocytes. A second stool should be sent for bacterial culture and a fresh specimen examined for *ova and parasites.* Ova and parasite examinations are fraught with limitations that must be kept in mind. If *giardiasis* is a consideration, at least three stool samples are necessary, because excretion of the organism is intermittent. Aspiration of jejunal contents or passage of a string into the upper jejunum may be necessary to demonstrate trophozoites; such efforts usually produce positive results in infected patients. Identifying *E. histolytica* trophozoites by stool examination can be difficult; their visualization is easily impaired by the presence of barium, bismuth, and kaolin compounds. False-negative stool examinations also result from preparatory enemas (which lyse the organism) and antibiotics (tetracycline and sulfonamides reduce shedding of trophozoites into the stool).

If symptoms persist and the diagnosis remains uncertain, the patient requires further assessment for a chronic or recurrent diarrheal syndrome (see below). The patient who becomes markedly dehydrated or toxic is a candidate for hospital admission, or at least several hours of intravenous fluid replacement in an emergency room.

Chronic or Recurrent Diarrhea

History. If an acute episode of diarrhea has not resolved within 2 weeks or a pattern of recurrent diarrhea develops, several additional etiologies must be considered (see Table 58-1). The history is reviewed for new findings as well as for a *characterization of the diarrhea* and any *associated symptoms* (Table 58-4). Rectosigmoid pathology is suggested by frequent passage of small, loose stools in association with crampy, left lower quadrant abdominal pain or tenesmus. Small bowel disease is a consideration when there are large, loose bowel movements in conjunction with periumbilical or right lower quadrant pain, or when diarrhea occurs shortly after a meal or ingestion of certain foods. *Diarrhea following meals* should lead to a search for malabsorption, an osmotic etiology, the dumping syndrome, or a fistula. The presence of foul, bulky, *greasy stools* further supports the diagnosis of fat malabsorption. *Bloody stools* require investigation for neoplasm, invasive infection, and inflammatory bowel disease. The presence of *fever* has similar diagnostic implications.

Table 58-4.   Features of Representative Chronic Diarrheas

| ETIOLOGY | NATURE OF THE DIARRHEA | | | ASSOCIATED SYMPTOMS AND SIGNS | LABORATORY RESULTS |
	W/S	OB	GB		
Irritable bowel syndrome	−/+ Mucus prominent	−	−	Bloating, intermittent alternating constipation	Stools: − for WBC/RBC
Ulcerative colitis	+/+	+	+	Fever, abdominal pain, extraintestinal disease, bowel ulcers/inflammation	Stools: + for WBC/RBC Endoscopy: +
Crohn's disease	−/+	+/−	+/−	Abdominal pain, obstruction, skip areas	Proctoscopy +/− WBC +; O & P −
Pseudomembranous colitis	+/+	+/−	+/−	Simulates inflammatory bowel disease clinically; bowel ulcers/plaques	Stools: + for *C. difficile* toxin/WBC/RBC
Diabetic enteropathy	+/+	−	−	Signs of autonomic insufficiency; occasionally malabsorption	Stools: + for fat (in small bowel type)
Dumping syndrome	+/+	−	−	Gastric surgery; occurs with meals; sweats, tachycardia	Normal
Malabsorption of fat	−/+ Steatorrhea	−	−	Weight loss, vitamin deficiency, sprue, pancreatic disease	Stools: + for fat
Lactase deficiency	+/+	−	−	Associated with milk products, cramping, bloating	Abnormal lactose tolerance test
Laxative abuse	+/+	−	−	Wasting, bulimia, dehydration	Stool + for laxatives
Villous adenoma	+/− Secretory, mucus	+	−	Protein wasting, no relation to meals	Hypokalemia, low albumin
Colon cancer	+/+	+	+	Change in bowel habits	Iron deficiency

CHO = carbohydrate
O & P = ova and parasites
+ = positive
− = negative
w/s = watery/soft
OB = occult blood
GB = gross blood

Frothy stools and *excessive flatus* are signs of fermentation of unabsorbed carbohydrates. *Alternating diarrhea and constipation* point to irritable bowel syndrome, as does *mucus* in the stool. The absence of intermittent constipation in a patient complaining of chronic diarrhea does not rule out the diagnosis.

Recent *travel* in conjunction with diarrhea that persists for more than 2 weeks raises the possibilities of giardiasis and amebiasis; pseudomembranous colitis is a consideration if the traveler has a recent intake of antibiotics. The slow resolution of traveler's diarrhea suggests postdysentery lactase deficiency and postdysentery irritable bowel syndrome.

A thorough review of drug intake is mandatory. A history of surreptitious *laxative abuse* may be hard to elicit, but inquiring gently and nonjudgmentally into feelings of low self-esteem and body image may provide suggestive information when a young, intense woman presents with chronic diarrhea and wasting. Previous abdominal surgery should be specified, looking for procedures that may have produced blind loops and allowed for bacterial overgrowth. *Sexual history* is relevant; promiscuous male homosexuals have an increased risk of polymicrobial enteritis (see above). A *psychosocial history*

is needed to check for factors that may contribute to an irritable bowel syndrome.

Physical Examination. A complete physical examination is mandatory and may confirm suspected causes as well as establish the severity of the disease. Any fever, dehydration, postural hypotension, or cachexia should be noted. The skin should be inspected for jaundice, pallor, and rash. The abdomen is examined for distention, ascites, hepatomegaly, tenderness, rebound, and masses. Rectal examination may reveal fecal impaction, perirectal fistula, or a patulous anal sphincter. Stool is tested for occult blood.

Laboratory. Blood tests are helpful but rarely diagnostic. They should include a *complete blood count* for evidence of anemia and leukocytosis, *serum electrolytes* for detection of serious losses and imbalances, *amylase* for pancreatic disease, *liver function tests* and *prothrombin time* for hepatobiliary disease, and *serum calcium* and *glucose* for metabolic conditions that can lead to diarrhea. Eosinophil counts are normal in most parasitic infections that cause diarrhea; worms, not protozoan, stimulate peripheral eosinophilia. Previously ordered, but not very sensitive or specific markers of malabsorption, are the serum carotene and serum B$_{12}$ levels.

Sigmoidoscopy performed without cleansing enemas is a potentially definitive procedure. It should always be done when there is blood or pus in the stool or other evidence of rectosigmoid pathology. The presence of mucosal ulceration, plaques, friability, and bleeding should be noted and *smears of the mucus* carefully examined for inflammatory cells. The finding of mucus without leukocytes helps confirm the diagnosis of irritable bowel syndrome, while the presence of pus directs the evaluation toward infection and inflammation. Nodular inflammatory ulcers and yellow-white mucosal plaques are characteristic of pseudomembranous colitis. Ulceration is also noted with inflammatory bowel disease and amebic colitis.

Amebic disease and pseudomembranous colitis are often mistaken for inflammatory bowel disease. Patients with recent antibiotic exposure and an inflammatory exudate require evaluation for pseudomembranous colitis. Their *stool* should be assayed for *C. difficile toxin,* although it must be understood that some patients without disease harbor the organism and might show detectible amounts of toxin in the stool.

If there is ulceration of the rectosigmoid mucosa and suspicion of *amebic disease* on the basis of epidemiologic data, *fresh mucosal smears* should be made. Proper technique for identification of trophozoites involves sampling the periphery of the ulcers with a glass rod or metal spatula; cotton swabs are inadequate, because the organisms adhere too firmly and do not readily transfer to a slide. Multiple *stool examinations for ova and parasites* can also be ordered. False-negative examinations for trophozoites are common and result from use of preparatory enemas, recent exposure to antibiotics, and concurrent use of barium, bismuth, or kaolin.

When there is serious clinical and epidemiologic suspicion of amebic disease and yet ova and parasite examinations are negative, *serologic testing* is indicated. The standard test is an indirect hemagglutination (IHA) assay. A positive titer is in excess of 1:128. It takes 2 to 4 weeks for seroconversion to occur. By the time most patients with amebic disease present with diarrhea, they are seropositive. Serologic testing is 85% sensitive in the setting of intestinal disease and 95% sensitive with extraintestinal spread. Serologic testing is useful in nonendemic areas where most people are seronegative, but less meaningful among patients from endemic areas where there may be a high frequency of seropositivity from carrier states and chronic exposure. An ELISA test for *E. histolytica* antigen in the stool is under development.

Other patients who ought to have *stools* searched for *ova and parasites* include those who have traveled to areas endemic for *Giardia,* homosexuals (who have an increased incidence of giardiasis), and immunocompromised hosts, including those with AIDS (who are at risk for cryptosporidiosis). Fresh loose stools are needed for identification of trophozoites; less fresh specimens can be used for detection of ova. Several stool examinations may be necessary. Some times small bowel aspiration or even biopsy is necessary establish the diagnosis of giardiasis or cryptosporidiosis.

Three other stool tests deserve note. A simple and quick test in patients suspected of laxative abuse is to *alkalinize the stool;* if it contains phenolphthalein (a common ingredient of many over-the-counter laxatives) it will turn pink. Patients suspected of fat malabsorption should have a stool sample subjected to *Sudan stain* for qualitative detection of fat. Those with a positive qualitative study are candidates for a *72-hour quantititative stool fat determination.* Normally, stool fat should not exceed 6% of daily fat intake. Stool fat in excess of 6 g per day while on a test diet of 100 g of fat per 24 hours indicates fat malabsorption. Other studies of help in defining the location and nature of a suspected malabsorption problem include a *d-xylose test* for detection of small bowel disease and a *secretin-stimulation* test or a *Chymex* test (an indirect measure of chymotrypsin) for pancreatic insufficiency. For suspected lactase deficiency, a *lactose-tolerance test* can be obtained, though more practical is a diagnostic trial of restricting milk products for several days.

Barium enema and *upper GI series* best demonstrate anatomic abnormalities (blind loops, fistulas, and tumors). A barium enema is useful when inflammatory bowel disease and malignancy are being considered. However, the radiologic appearance of the bowel is not always definitive (*e.g.,* amebiasis can simulate the picture of inflammatory bowel disease). It is important to remember that barium obscures identification of ova and parasites, necessitating completion of stool collections prior to obtaining a barium study. *Sigmoidoscopy* or *endoscopy* is indicated for elusive cases and suspected inflammatory bowel disease; the procedure allows for direct visualization, mucosal smears, and biopsy (See Chapter 75).

Therapeutic Trials sometimes obviate the need for more elaborate studies. As noted above, cessation of diarrhea in response to *restriction of milk products* strongly supports the diagnosis of lactose intolerance. Other recognized empiric trials include a course of *antibiotic therapy* in patients suspected of blind-loop syndrome, a trial of *metronidazole* for patients with a travel history and clinical picture consistent with giardiasis, and use of *pancreatic enzymes* in patients believed to be suffering from pancreatic insufficiency.

Chronic Diarrhea of Unknown Etiology

Patients who remain undiagnosed after an extensive evaluation often turn out to have irritable bowel syndrome or surreptitious laxative abuse. The latter is most prevalent among young, professional women preoccupied with their weight, and having low self-esteem and a poor body image (see Chapter 230). An otherwise unexplained hypokalemia is also suggestive of laxative abuse.

If a diagnosis has not been made, it may be worthwhile to further characterize the type of diarrhea by determining *stool volume, osmolality,* and *electrolyte content.* A stool volume of less than 200 ml per day is strongly suggestive of irritable bowel syndrome. Osmotic diarrheas show increased stool osmolality and low sodium and potassium concentrations. The differential diagnosis of osmotic diarrhea includes ingestion of nonabsorbable solutes (magnesium, bran), maldigestion of food, and malabsorption of osmotically active substances (*e.g.,* carbohydrates).

Stool volumes in excess of 1 liter per day indicate a secretory diarrhea. Occult etiologies include surreptitious laxative abuse, villous adenoma, carcinoid syndrome, pancreatic cholera (from secretion of vasoactive intestinal peptide), and other similarly rare conditions.

PRINCIPLES OF MANAGEMENT

Acute Diarrheas

The vast majority of acute diarrheal illness should be managed by *maintaining hydration* and waiting for the spontaneous resolution of symptoms. Often, hydration can be maintained by use of oral fluids, even in cases of profuse diarrhea. Solutions rich in electrolytes and sugar facilitate absorption of water. An 8-oz glass of fruit juice to which is added a pinch of table salt and a half-teaspoon of honey or a teaspoon of table sugar makes a well-tolerated replacement solution. Nondiet cola drinks that have been allowed to stand and lose their carbonation are a reasonable substitute. Either can be taken along with a similar-size glass of water containing ¼-teaspoon of baking soda to replenish losses in stool electrolytes, which in acute infectious diarrhea are Na:125 mEq/liter, K:20 mEq/liter, HCO_3:45 mEq/liter, and Cl:90 mEq/liter.

Absorbent preparations are commonly used for symptomatic therapy of simple acute diarrhea. Solutions of *kaolin* and *pectin* have no proven benefit but seem to be harmless; however, they should not be relied on in the treatment of severe diarrhea. Doses of *bismuth subsalicylate (Pepto-Bismol)* in excess of those recommended on the bottle (*e.g.,* 2–3 tablespoons every 3 hours) are sometimes effective (see below). *Opiates* such as *diphenoxylate* (dispensed as a combination with small amounts of atropine [Lomotil] to discourage abuse) and *loperamide* are effective in the symptomatic treatment of diarrhea by directly inhibiting the motility of the intestinal smooth muscle. Diphenoxylate and loperamide are derived from meperidine but have less effect on the central nervous system. They should be used cautiously, if at all, in conditions in which toxic megacolon is possible (*e.g.,* inflammatory bowel disease). Their use should also be restricted in certain bacterial diarrheas, such as shigellosis, to avoid prolonging the clinical course. The usual dose of diphenoxylate is 2.5 to 5 mg, every 4 hours, up to 20 mg per day. Loperamide is given as 2 or 4 mg, every 4 hours, up to 16 mg daily. Lower maintenance dosages will often be sufficient after initial control is achieved. Other opiates are potent antidiarrheal agents but carry a higher risk of addiction; they

are useful when their coincident analgesic activity is needed. Deodorized tincture of opium (0.5–1 ml), paregoric (4 ml), or codeine (30–60 mg) can be given orally every 4 hours. *Anticholinergics* are useful only for the irritable bowel syndrome (see Chapter 66).

Antibiotics should *not* be used routinely for acute bacterial diarrheas, since most are self-limited. Antibiotics have minimal effect on the course of illness and may prolong the asymptomatic bacterial carrier state. Moreover, one risks triggering an antibiotic-induced diarrhea. Exceptions include typhoid fever and severe cases of shigellosis, pseudomembranous colitis, *Campylobacter,* and *Yersinia.* In addition, elderly debilitated patients and others who would be endangered by a *Salmonella* bacteremia (persons with prosthetic heart valves or sickle cell anemia) should receive a course of antibiotics to limit distant complications. *Salmonella bacteremia* and *typhoid fever* can be treated with parenteral *ampicillin* or oral *chloramphenicol;* in milder cases, oral *trimethoprim-sulfamethoxazole* (one double-strength tablet bid for 2 weeks) suffices.

Patients suffering severe dysentery caused by *shigellosis* can be treated with oral *ampicillin* (500 mg qid for 3–5 days), but antibiotic sensitivity testing is needed because ampicillin-resistant strains are common. *Trimethoprim–sulfamethoxazole* (one double-strength tablet bid for 3–5 days) is an excellent alternative. Pending stool culture results, a few days of empiric therapy for shigellosis is reasonable if the epidemiologic history is suggestive and the patient is experiencing severe bloody diarrhea. Antiperistaltic drugs are contraindicated. *Campylobacter* is sensitive to oral *erythromycin* (500 mg qid for 7 days). Most patients with *Yersinia* infection have a self-limited illness, but toxic patients are candidates for oral *chloramphenicol* (50 mg/kg/day in four divided doses for 7–10 days) or parenteral therapy.

Pseudomembranous colitis usually resolves without antibiotic treatment, but oral *vancomycin* liquid suspension (as little as 125 mg qid for 7–10 days) and *metronidazole* (750 mg tid for 5–10 days) have both proven capable of controlling the disease, though relapses are common and retreatment is often necessary. *Cholestyramine* (one packet in water tid) is used in conjunction with antibiotics to help bind the enterotoxin; it has proven useful in difficult cases.

Symptomatic patients suffering from diarrhea due to parasitic infection also benefit from definitive antimicrobial therapy. *Entamoeba histolytica* responds to *metronidazole* (750 mg tid for 5–10 days) for treatment of trophozoites and *diiodohydroxyquin* (650 mg tid for 21 days) for elimination of cysts. *Giardiasis* is treated with quinacrine (100 mg tid for 7 days) or metronidazole (250 mg tid for 7–10 days). Retreatment is often necessary.

Traveler's Diarrhea

The objectives of treatment of traveler's diarrhea include prevention of illness and provision of symptomatic relief.

Because the majority of "turista" cases are caused by enterotoxigenic *E. coli,* prophylaxis has been aimed at combatting this organism. *Doxycycline,* a tetracycline derivative, taken on the day of travel (200 mg) and daily (100 mg) while away has proven useful, though as many as 40% of toxigenic *E. coli* strains are resistant to the drug. Moreover, the drug itself often causes GI upset. An alternative antibiotic approach is daily use of *trimethoprim–sulfa* (one double-strength tablet per day), either prophylactically or for symptomatic therapy; use after the onset of diarrhea has proven quite effective. Prophylactic use of antibiotics has been in vogue, but the growing awareness of antibiotic-induced diarrhea, the high frequency of bacterial resistance to some agents, and the efficacy of bismuth-containing agents is leading to less reliance on antimicrobials.

Bismuth subsalicylate (*Pepto-Bismol*) has proven very effective in both prophylaxis for and treatment of traveler's diarrhea when used in large doses (60 cc qid). Unlike antibiotics, it has the advantage of not altering the normal bowel flora. Its mechanism of action is believed to involve inhibiting bacterial colonization by toxigenic bacterial strains. Bismuth turns the stools black; it is useful to warn patients of this side-effect so its occurrence does not cause alarm.

Many find taking *diphenoxylate* more convenient for symptomatic relief of traveler's diarrhea; in most instances, it can be used for brief periods with safety, except when *Shigella* or *Salmonella* infection is a serious consideration (*i.e.,* when there is fever or rectal bleeding).

Although much attention has been given to pharmacologic agents for prophylaxis, care in what one eats and drinks remains the single most important means of preventing traveler's diarrhea. Avoid use of local water supplies when they are in question. This includes foregoing fresh vegetables, which may have been washed in such water, and even use of ice cubes. Drinking bottled water is preferable.

Chronic Diarrhea

To be effective, therapy for chronic diarrhea needs to be etiologic. For example, steroids and sulfasalazine are needed to control diarrhea caused by exacerbations of inflammatory bowel disease (see Chapter 65). Malabsorption due to pancreatic insufficiency necessitates use of enzyme supplements (see Chapter 72). Lactase deficiency requires limitation of milk products or use of exogenous lactase. The dumping syndrome responds to small feedings. Persistent pseudomembranous colitis is an indication for antibiotic therapy (see above). Cessation of surreptitious laxative use cures the diarrhea that accompanies it (see Chapter 230). In the setting of irritable bowel syndrome, a high-fiber diet is indicated (see Chapter 66). Unlike treatment of acute diarrhea where many causes are self-limited and nonspecific measures aimed at symptomatic relief are appropriate, effective management of chronic diarrhea requires an etiologic diagnosis and specific therapy. Simply suppressing symptoms without identifying

a cause may delay identification of a serious underlying condition (*e.g.,* colon cancer).

Chronic Diarrhea Of Unknown Etiology. For patients who remain undiagnosed after an extensive workup, yet appear otherwise well, a trial of therapy for irritable bowel syndrome (see Chapter 66) is reasonable. Many such patients with unexplained diarrhea turn out to have a bowel motility disorder and associated psychosocial stresses. Clues to the diagnosis include absence of weight loss, normal laboratory studies, and a suggestive psychosocial history. Failure to respond after 4 weeks of therapy should lead to gastroenterologic consultation. One should not resort to nonspecific antidiarrheal agents for treatment of undiagnosed patients.

INDICATIONS FOR ADMISSION AND REFERRAL

Most patients with diarrhea can be managed on an outpatient basis. However, those who are unable to maintain their hydration orally and become significantly volume depleted (posturally hypotensive) require serious consideration for hospital admission and parenteral fluid replacement. Sometimes, several hours of intravenous fluids given in the emergency room will suffice and obviate an admission. Infants, elderly persons, and those with chronic or debilitating illnesses are particularly vulnerable to the complications of volume depletion and deserve closest watching. Patients with inflammatory diarrheas manifested by bloody, purulent diarrhea and fever are also candidates for possible admission.

Referral to a gastroenterologist is indicated for patients with complicated inflammatory bowel disease, undiagnosed chronic diarrhea, or a requirement for colonoscopy or intestinal biopsy. One particularly difficult issue worthy of consultation is the need for small bowel sampling in patients with suspected parasitic disease who have repeatedly negative stool examinations for ova and parasites.

PATIENT EDUCATION

Because most acute diarrheas are self-limited, the patient with no evidence of serious underlying pathology can be reassured and advised to concentrate on maintaining hydration. The sugar and electrolyte preparations described in this chapter are easy to take and should be encouraged. Many people think that taking fluids will seriously worsen their diarrhea, and they request opiates or antibiotics; the proper role for such agents needs to be reviewed and their unrestricted use limited. Many ask if kaolin-pectin preparations are helpful; there is no evidence that they alter symptoms or the course of the illness, but neither are they harmful. Although antibiotics have been in vogue for prophylaxis of traveler's diarrhea, patients should be informed of the emergence of resistant strains, the potential complications of antibiotic use, and the efficacy of bismuth preparations. A few bottles of a bismuth preparation (*e.g.,* Pepto-Bismol), a few tablets of diphenoxylate for "emergencies," and advice to use bottled water and avoid foods likely to be contaminated (*e.g.,* raw vegetables washed with local water) represent reasonable alternatives to antibiotic prophylaxis. Patients with chronic undiagnosed diarrhea need to be prepared for a potentially extensive evaluation. In the meantime, advice on perianal care is much appreciated and ought not to be overlooked while investigation proceeds.

Perianal Hygiene. Much can be done to relieve the perianal discomfort that accompanies severe unrelenting diarrhea. *Sitz baths* for about 10 minutes two or three times a day can be very soothing, followed by gentle drying with absorbent cotton (not toilet paper or towels). Washing with warm water on *absorbent cotton* after each bowel movement is also helpful in lieu of using toilet paper, which can be quite irritating. Also important is avoidance of soap. A short course of *hydrocortisone cream* may be useful when there is considerable anal inflammation. Some patients report that cleaning gently with cotton pads soaked with *witch hazel* (Tucks) provides considerable relief. Ointments containing topical anesthetics should be avoided; they can be irritating in themselves.

Recovery Phase. Following resolution of diarrhea, it is best to avoid milk and dairy products for approximately another 7 to 10 days, since mild lactose intolerance commonly accompanies many cases. The best foods to begin eating are easily digested, high-carbohydrate substances such as bananas, rice, baked potato, and applesauce. Continued repletion of fluid is important.

ANNOTATED BIBLIOGRAPHY

Bartlett JG et al.: Role of *Clostridium difficile* in antibiotic-associated pseudomembranous colitis. Gastroenterology 75:778, 1978 (*Study demonstrates that most pseudomembranous colitis is associated with cytotoxin produced by* Clostridium difficile.)

Bayless TM et al.: Lactose and milk intolerance: Clinical implications. N Engl J Med 292:1156, 1975 (*A study of the prevalence, characteristics, and diagnosis of lactose intolerance in adults.*)

Blacklow NR, Cukor G: Viral gastroenteritis. N Engl J Med 304:397, 1981 (*Reviews the epidemiology and clinical characteristics of Norwalk virus and rotavirus as well as other miscellaneous diarrhea-inducing agents.*)

Blaser MJ et al: Campylobacter enteritis in the United States: A multicenter study. Ann Intern Med 98:360, 1983 (*Campylobacter was more frequently isolated than both* Salmonella *and* Shigella *combined.*)

DuPont HL: Cryptosporidiosis and the healthy host. N Engl J Med 312:1319, 1985 (*A summary of current knowledge.*)

DuPont HL et al: Treatment of traveler's diarrhea with trimethoprim-sulfamethoxazole and with trimethoprim alone. N Engl J Med 307:841, 1982 (*Either agent when used after the onset of diarrhea terminated most cases within 24 hours: an alternative to prophylactic treatment.*)

DuPont HL, Ericsson CD, Johnson PC: Chemotherapy and chemoprophylaxis of traveller's diarrhea. Ann Intern Med 102:260, 1985 (*A good summary on the current state of knowledge and recommendations to avoid risky foods and to replace fluids and use loperamide or bismuth subsalicylate if diarrhea occurs. Trimethoprim sulfa may be used in patients with moderate to severe diarrhea.*)

DuPont HL, Hornick RB: Adverse effect of Lomotil therapy in shigellosis. JAMA 260:1525, 1973 (*Lomotil therapy may cause fever and toxicity may be prolonged in patients with shigellosis.*)

Eastham EJ, Douglas AP, Watson AJ: Diagnosis of *Giardia lamblia* infection as a cause of diarrhea. Lancet 2:950, 1976 (*Retrospective review of 31 patients found that* Giardia *is not considered often or early enough.*)

Fekety R: Recent advances in management of bacterial diarrhea. Rev Infect Dis 5:246, 1983 (*Comprehensive summary of pathophysiology, diagnosis, and treatment.*)

Gebhard RL, Gerding DN, Olson MM et al: Clinical and endoscopic findings in patients early in the course of *Clostridium difficile*-associated pseudomembranous colitis. Am J Med 78:45, 1985 (*Useful paper on the early features of this condition, including fever, leukocytosis, abdominal pain, diarrhea, and even an ileus; also illustrates early sigmoidoscopic appearance of the bowel mucosa.*)

Gorbach SL et al: Traveler's diarrhea and toxigenic *Escherichia coli.* N Engl J Med 292:933, 1975 (*Classic report documenting that traveler's diarrhea is often due to enterotoxigenic* Escherichia coli.)

Graham DY, Estes NK, Gentry LO: Double blind comparison of bismuth subsalicylate and placebo in the prevention and treatment of enterotoxigenic E. coli-induced diarrhea in volunteers. Gastroenterology 85:1017, 1983 (*A study of 32 volunteers confirming the effectiveness of bismuth subsalicylate in preventing diarrhea.*)

Harris JC, DuPont HL, Hornick RB: Fecal leukocytes in diarrheal illness. Ann Intern Med 76:697, 1972 (*A classic article that established that fecal leukocytes indicate inflammatory causes of diarrhea, such as shigellosis, salmonellosis, typhoid fever, invasive* E. coli, *and inflammatory bowel disease.*)

Ho DD et al: Campylobacter enteritis: Early diagnosis with Gram's stain. Arch Intern Med 142:1858, 1982 (*Gram stain had a sensitivity of 43% and a specificity of 99%.*)

Kaplan JE, Gary W, Baron RC et al: Epidemiology of Norwalk gastroenteritis and the role of Norwalk virus in outbreaks of acute gastroenteritis. Ann Intern Med 96:756, 1982 (*Only recently have the agents responsible for viral gastroenteritis been identified. This paper is an epidemiologic and clinical review of this important type of viral gastroenteritis.*)

Kolars JC, Levitt MD, Aouji M et al: Yogurt, an autodigesting source of lactose. N Engl J Med 310:1, 1984 (*Yogurt is well tolerated by lactase-deficient patients; yogurts containing live cultures release lactase and permit digestion of lactose.*)

Nolan CM, Johnson KE, Coyle MB et al: Campylobacter enteritis: Efficacy of antimicrobial and antimotility drugs. Am J Gastroenterol 78:621, 1983 (*Treatment with tetracycline or erythromycin shortened the course of illness, but antimotility drugs prolonged it.*)

Palmer DL et al: Comparison of sucrose and glucose in the oral electrolyte therapy of cholera and other severe diarrhea. N Engl

J Med 292:1107, 1977 (*A discussion of the uses and limitations of oral fluid and electrolyte therapy in severe diarrhea.*)

Palmer KR, Corbett CL, Holdsworth CD: Double blind crossover study comparing loperamide, codeine and diphenoxylate in the treatment of chronic diarrhea. Gastroenterology, 79:1272, 1980 (*Loperamide was more effective than diphenoxylate, as effective as codeine, and had fewer side-effects than either agent.*)

Quinn TC, Goodell SE, Fennell C et al: The polymicrobial origin of intestinal infections in homosexual men. N Engl J Med 309:576, 1983 (*An important finding.*)

Read NW et al: Chronic diarrhea of unknown etiology. Gastroenterology 78:264, 1980 (*The clinical features, evaluation, and follow-up of 27 patients with undiagnosed diarrhea are reported and a checklist for evaluation is presented.*)

Sazie ESM, Titus AE: Rapid diagnosis of campylobacter enteritis. Ann Intern Med 96:62, 1982 (*Describes the gram stain "gull wing" sign, which had a sensitivity of 65% and specificity of 95% in this study.*)

Silva J et al: Treatment of *Clostridium difficile* colitis and diarrhea with vancomycin. Am J Med 71:815, 1981 (*Oral vancomycin proved extremely effective and terminated symptoms within 7 days in all patients tested.*)

Wolfson JS et al: Cryptosporidiosis in immunocompetent: A characterization of 43 cases. N Engl J Med 312:1278, 1985 (*Produces a self-limited diarrhea.*)

59

Approach to the Patient with Constipation

Constipation is a universal affliction of Western civilization, resulting in part from a diet low in crude fiber. It is among the most frequent reasons for self-medication and is particularly troublesome in the elderly. More than $200 million are spent annually in the United States on laxatives; a survey of Londoners revealed 30% admitting to recent laxative use.

There is no uniform definition of constipation. To some, it means movements that are too infrequent or stools that are too hard. Others complain of incomplete or difficult evacuation. Among normal people, bowel habits widely vary, and there are diverse perceptions of what constitutes normal function. Population studies show that most normal people have more than three bowel movements per week, with men likely to have at least five. Stools less than 35 g per day are well below the lower limit of normal.

The primary physician must be able to uncover any underlying pathology as well as to provide symptomatic relief to those without a structural lesion. The prevalences of excessive laxative use and inadequate dietary fiber make it imperative that the physician be knowledgeable about the actions and adverse effects of available laxative preparations as well as dietary alternatives to their use.

PATHOPHYSIOLOGY AND CLINICAL PRESENTATION

The process of elimination of fecal waste requires two processes: filling of the rectum by colonic transport and reflex defecation of stool. Constipation may arise secondary to interference with either of these processes. The time it takes food to reach the anus is partially a function of the amount of fiber in the diet. Normal people placed on a diet containing 15 g of bran fiber per day have twice the number of movements per week of those on an uncontrolled diet. Patients with constipation solely on the basis of low dietary fiber usually have intermittent complaints that fully resolve with alteration of diet alone.

Exercise has an important effect on propulsion of bowel contents. Colonic transit has been observed to be significantly greater in physically active people than in those who get little exercise. Previously active persons often become constipated when put to bed on account of illness. Less dramatic, but probably no less important, is the leading of a *sedentary lifestyle;* constipation is common in inactive people.

Metabolic and endocrine disturbances can slow colonic transport. Hypokalemia, hypercalcemia, hypothyroidism, and diabetes are the most important of these in terms of frequency or potential reversibility. *Hypokalemia* can produce a generalized ileus and in most often seen in patients who take diuretics. Chronic laxative abuse may also produce hypokalemia; characteristically, there is surreptitious use of laxatives and diuretics, self-induced vomiting, pathologic desire to lose weight, and a personality disorder. Such patients present with fatigue and electrolyte disturbances. When constipation is caused by *hypothyroidism,* other manifestations of the disease are usually present, though sluggish bowel movements may be the presenting complaint. Constipation is a bothersome problem in some patients with *diabetes:* 20% of those with neuropathy report severe difficulty. Significant *hypercalcemia* (serum calcium greater than 12 mg/100 ml) can slow bowel motility.

Habitual use of *laxatives* is associated with impaired motor activity. The typical clinical picture is a long history of chronic constipation or a desire to feel "well cleaned out," followed by increasing laxative dependence, decreasing response, and ultimately a sluggish, poorly contracting bowel. Whether there is a prior underlying motor disorder or actual damage from laxative use is unsettled.

Mechanical *obstruction* from tumor, stricture, or volvulus may be responsible for the new onset of constipation. Cramping abdominal pain and distention in conjunction with a marked change in bowel habits are characteristic (see Chapter 53). Constipation occurs in more than 50% of patients with colonorectal cancers; it is usually a symptom of advanced disease but may be the presenting complaint.

New onset of constipation may also be precipitated by drug use. *Opiates* and agents with anticholinergic activity such as *antidepressants* are frequently implicated. An underlying depression is often contributory, and bowel complaints may be one of many somatic symptoms (see Chapter 223). The exact mechanisms by which emotional difficulties lead to constipation remain unclear, but the fact that they play an important role is widely recognized. Experiments in patients with the irritable colon syndrome, in which constipation can be an important difficulty, provide some clues regarding pathophysiology (see Chapter 66).

A lesion in the *innervation* of the bowel can result in constipation. Spinal cord pathology, transection of pelvic nerves, and ganglion abnormalities can all induce failure of normal bowel function. In most instances, other neurologic deficits are present. Disease limited to loss of neurones in the bowel wall typically presents as chronic, refractory constipation; it may date from childhood or be associated with long-standing laxative use.

A permanently damaged neuromotor apparatus is a consequence of *scleroderma*, whereas functional disturbances in motor activity are noted in *irritable colon syndrome* (see Chapter 66) and *diverticular disease* (see Chapter 67). Constipation results when there is an excessive degree of nonpropulsive contractions and segmentation of bowel contents. Diarrhea may quickly supervene if distal contractions cease while proximal hyperactivity continues.

Inhibition of the rectal defecation reflex has been documented in cases of local anal pathology, neurogenic disease, chronic use of laxatives, and voluntary suppression. Patients with this problem are found to have stool packed into the rectal ampulla. *Voluntary suppression* of the urge to defecate is usually a concomitant of a hectic life-style or deep-seated neurotic inhibitions. The resulting intermittent constipation may lead to excessive use of laxatives and enemas and damage to the reflex emptying mechanism.

Some authorities believe that substantial fluid intake is essential to normal bowel movements, though this is not well established. Water is known to be an effective means of distending the stomach and stimulating intestinal activity. The consistency of stool is a function of how much water it contains, which is a result, in part, of how much is taken into it.

DIFFERENTIAL DIAGNOSIS

The causes of constipation can be grouped according to pathophysiology. *Impaired motility* can be seen with inadequate dietary fiber, inactivity, laxative abuse, irritable colon syndrome, tumor, stricture, inflammatory bowel disease, diverticulitis, hypothyroidism, hypokalemia, diabetes, hypercalcemia, pregnancy, and scleroderma. Opiates, anticholinergics (including the tricyclic antidepressants), ganglionic blockers, calcium- and aluminum-containing antacids, disopyramide, calcium channel blockers, and antihistamines slow colonic motility. *Obstruction* may be secondary to tumor, stricture, or volvulus. *Neurologic disorders* that may hinder transport include multiple sclerosis and cord lesions. *Local anorectal pathology* such as hemorrhoids and fissures, strictures, abscesses or proctitis, and voluntary suppression retard rectal emptying. Chronic laxative abuse and rectocele formation reduce the muscle strength available for defecation. Last, but not uncommon, constipation is associated with *emotional difficulties* such as depression and neurotically excessive concern with one's bowels.

WORKUP

History. Evaluation begins with definition of the size, character, and frequency of bowel movements, followed by a determination of the problem's chronicity. Acute constipation is more often associated with organic disease than is a long-standing problem. Chronic complaints that wax and wane over months and years point to a functional disturbance, often compounded by habitual laxative use. Inquiry is needed into symptoms that suggest an underlying gastrointestinal problem, such as abdominal pain, nausea, cramping, vomiting, weight loss, melena, rectal bleeding, rectal pain, and fever. Anorexia, bloating, belching, flatus, mucus in the stool, headache, depression, and anxiety should also be recorded; these symptoms may be associated with constipation of any etiology but often accompany functional disorders.

It is helpful at the first visit to take a history of working, eating, and bowel habits. Inquiry into dietary fiber intake and physical activity is essential. Laxative use and drug intake, including antacids, need to be reviewed carefully. The patient's concerns and views should be sympathetically elicited.

Physical Examination should assess the patient's weight and nutritional status. Skin is noted for pallor and signs of hypothyroidism (see Chapter 102). The abdomen is examined for masses, distention, tenderness, and high-pitched or absent bowel sounds. Rectal examination includes careful inspection and palpation for masses, fissures, inflammation, and hard stool in the ampulla. The last finding rules out significant obstruction and poor colonic motility and suggests that the problem is inadequate rectal emptying. The stool is noted for color and consistency and tested for occult blood. Anal sensitivity and reflexes are noted. Disordered innervation of the anus is indicated by finding that the anal canal opens wide when the puborectalis muscle is pulled posteriorly. Anoscopy is needed to identify internal hemorrhoids, fissures, tumors, and other local pathology. Neurologic examination should be performed to search for focal deficits and delayed relaxation phase of the ankle jerks, suggestive of hypothyroidism.

Laboratory Studies. Radiologic investigation is of limited use unless evidence from history and physical examination suggests a specific etiology, such as obstruction. Acute onset of constipation requires ruling out obstruction and ileus, especially when accompanied by abdominal discomfort; supine and upright films of the abdomen, plus measurements of serum potassium and calcium levels are indicated. Suspicion of colonic obstruction requires a barium enema or colonoscopy. The finding on colonoscopy of pigmented colonic mucosa is common in patients who abuse anthraquinone laxatives such as castor oil or senna. Any hint of diabetes or hypothyroidism can be verified by urinalysis, serum glucose and thyroid-stimulating hormone determination (see Chapters 92 and 102).

An important diagnostic concern in the elderly is the possibility of constipation being due to a colonic neoplasm. Blood in the stool, weight loss, or iron-deficiency anemia mandates sigmoidoscopy followed by barium enema. More than 25% of patients with colorectal carcinomas present with constipation. However, the elderly person with no evidence of obstruction, anemia, or occult blood loss can probably be followed for a few weeks on a conservative program that includes more dietary fiber, increased exercise, and monitoring of stool guaiacs, before it is decided to subject the patient to the discomfort of colonoscopy or barium enema. If symptoms resolve and stools are negative for occult blood, the probability of malignancy or obstruction is low, and the patient need not undergo further testing at that time. A return visit for repeat assessment ought to be scheduled within 4 to 8 weeks.

When the cause of constipation is obscure, it is helpful to stop all nonessential medications. The codeine in a cough suppressant, the calcium in an over-the-counter antacid, or the iron in a multiple vitamin may be responsible for an otherwise puzzling diagnostic problem.

SYMPTOMATIC MANAGEMENT AND PATIENT EDUCATION

Symptomatic management is appropriate for the patient with a functional etiology. The first intervention is careful patient education about diet and use of laxatives. Explanation is needed to reassure the patient that a daily bowel movement is not essential to good health and that comfortable patterns of elimination depend on good living and eating habits. The patient should *stop taking laxatives,* enemas, and nonessential

drugs that may suppress colonic motility. The *fiber* content of the diet should be increased by adding bran, fruits, green vegetables, and whole-grain cereals and breads. Most studies show that 15 g of fiber per day is needed for the best effects, but the amount can be individualized. A large breakfast including bran cereal, juice, milk or coffee, and whole-grain bread is helpful. *Daily exercise* should be prescribed and based on the patient's physical capacity. It is important to inform the patient with chronic constipation that normal function may take many weeks to return. Often immediate results are expected; when they do not appear, the patient becomes despondent, stops the program, and returns to laxative and enema use.

Some patients refuse to eat bran because it makes them feel bloated and gassy. The patient can be reassured that these side-effects usually resolve within a month of continued use. If dietary and exercise efforts fail or the patient insists on medication, a nondigestible fiber residue such as ground *psyllium* seed (Metamucil) can be beneficial. It acts to increase bulk by means of its hydrophilic properties, but it must be taken with plenty of fluids to prevent formation of an obstructing bolus; the usual dose is one teaspoon in 8 oz of liquid, three times a day. The one existing controlled study of psyllium's efficacy showed significant improvement in symptoms with its use. However, the placebo group showed an equally large improvement, suggesting that explanation, reassurance, and increased attention are also important to improved bowel function.

When fecal impaction is present, a *hypertonic enema (e.g.,* Fleet's) will often relieve the situation. In addition, the patient can be instructed to squat over the toilet by standing on a chair in front of the bowl, providing a more favorable position for evacuating the rectum. Only rarely does one need to resort to disimpaction.

Trying to establish a convenient, uninterrupted *time for defecation* each day may be useful; 15 to 20 minutes following breakfast provides a good opportunity, for spontaneous colonic motility is greatest during that period. Continuing this routine each day regardless of travel or situational stress ought to be encouraged. Although there are no controlled studies proving the efficacy of this approach, it seems to help some people, though days or weeks can pass before success is noted.

Prevention of constipation during an illness that requires bed rest can be achieved by use of a high-fiber diet, bulk agents, and a commode, in preference to a bedpan. Correction of any coincident hypokalemia is important (see Chapter 27). There is no evidence that prophylactic use of laxatives or stool softeners is effective. A randomized controlled study of dioctyl sodium sulfosuccinate (Colace), a popular and expensive stool softener, failed to demonstrate any effect on the quality or frequency of stools. Use of minor tranquilizers in overly anxious patients has little direct effect on constipation. When severe depression requires use of antidepressants, the least constipating agent, that is, one with minimal anticholinergic activity, should be selected. All tricyclics have some anticholinergic activity, but desipramine and trazodone seem to have the least (see Chapter 223).

The importance of taking time to explain and answer questions cannot be overstated. Successful management of functional constipation is based on excellent patient cooperation. A patient who has used a particular agent for decades needs to be told why it is being removed from the program; otherwise, chances of compliance are small. Chronic laxative users should be warned that it may take 4 to 6 weeks before spontaneous movements return. Patience and sympathetic support can be rewarding, but expectations of quick results must not be raised.

(See Chapters 61, 66, 67, 68 for management of specific etiologies.)

A.H.G.

ANNOTATED BIBLIOGRAPHY

Burkitt D, Walker A, Paintner N: Effect of dietary fibre on stools and transit times and its role in causation of disease. Lancet 2: 1408, 1972 (*Classic paper on fiber and its link to constipation and other bowel problems.*)

Connell A, Hilton C, Irvine R et al: Variation of bowel habits in two population samples. Br Med J 2:1095, 1965 (*A population study helping to define the range of normal for bowel activity and the prevalence of constipation.*)

Darlington RC: Over-the-counter laxatives. J Am Pharm Assoc 6: 470, 494, 1966 (*Provides figures on spending for over-the-counter preparations; dated but enlightening and still valid.*)

Goodman J, Pang J, Bessman A: Dioctyl sodium sulfosuccinate: An ineffective prophylactic laxative. J Chronic Dis 29:59, 1976 (*A randomized prospective study of patients admitted to the hospital. The drug made no difference in quality or frequency of stools.*)

Graham DY, Moser SE, Estes MK: The effect of bran on bowel function and constipation. Am J Gastroenterol 77:599, 1982 (*Twenty grams of wheat or corn bran reduced transit time by 50% and improved constipation clinically in 6 of 10 constipated women.*)

Holdstock D et al: Propulsion in the human colon and its relationship to meals and somatic activity. Gut 11:91, 1970 (*Physical activity was found to stimulate mass movements, and inactivity reduced them.*)

Hull C, Greco RS, Brooks DL: Alleviation of constipation in the elderly by dietary fiber supplementation. J Am Geriatr Soc 28: 410, 1980 (*In an institutional geriatric population, adding bran prevented constipation and reduced laxative use.*)

Katz L, Spiro H: Gastrointestinal manifestations of diabetes. N Engl J Med 275:1350, 1966 (*Constipation is a frequent gastrointestinal complaint of diabetics.*)

Kirwn WO, Smith AN: Colonic propulsion in diverticular disease, idiopathic constipation and the irritable bowel syndrome. Scand J Gastroenterol 12:331, 1974 (*Transit time is prolonged in all three diseases and can be significantly reduced by bran.*)

Longstreth GF, Fox DD, Youkeles MS et al: Psyllium in irritable bowel syndrome: A double-blind study. Ann Intern Med 95:53, 1981 (*Both treatment and control groups showed equally impressive degrees of improvement, suggesting that other factors are also operative, such as attention, explanation, and reassurance.*)

Oster JR, Materson BJ, Rogers AI: Laxative abuse syndrome. Am J Gastroenterol 74:451, 1980 (*A review article outlining this important cause of chronic constipation.*)

Roth HP, Fein SB, Shurman JF: The mechanisms responsible for the urge to defecate. Gastroenterology 32:717, 1957 (*Describes normal process of defecation and provides physiologic basis for understanding disease states.*)

Rutter K, Maxwell D: Constipation and laxative abuse. Br Med J 2: 997, 1976 (*Good description of laxative abuse.*)

60
Evaluation of Gastrointestinal Bleeding
JAMES M. RICHTER, M.D.

Ambulatory patients frequently report gastrointestinal bleeding to the primary physician. The report might be of a tarry stool, some bright red blood passed by the rectum, or vomiting that produced fresh or changed blood. Sometimes, the only manifestation is a screening stool test positive for occult blood. Patients who do not feel ill may not present immediately for evaluation, and their symptoms often resolve without specific therapy. The primary physician must decide how extensively and aggressively to pursue a diagnosis in such patients. Proper decision making requires a knowledge of the probability of a serious underlying lesion and the sensitivity and specificity of barium studies and endoscopy.

PATHOPHYSIOLOGY AND CLINICAL PRESENTATION

Hematemesis usually represents bleeding proximal to the ligament of Treitz, although the site of blood loss may, on rare occasions, be in the jejunum. The absence of hematemesis does not, however, exclude the possibility of active upper gastrointestinal bleeding. Melena is usually seen with blood loss proximal to the ileocecal valve, where hemoglobin is converted into hematin, which gives the stool its tarry quality. Right colonic bleeding may also cause melena when transit is slow. Bright red blood most often originates in the left colon or anorectal region, though very brisk movement of blood from more proximal sites can lead to a similar presentation.

Manifestations of blood loss are a function of the rate of bleeding. Postural signs are important evidence of acute or significant volume loss. When the patient stands up from a supine position, and the heart rate rises by 10 or more beats per minute and/or the blood pressure falls by at least 10 mm Hg, one must assume that serious hemorrhage exists. Patient descriptions of the volume of bleeding are frequently unreliable.

DIFFERENTIAL DIAGNOSIS

The chief causes of gastrointestinal bleeding can be conveniently grouped by site of blood loss. Important esophageal etiologies are esophagitis, ulcer, neoplasm (occult blood loss), varices, and Mallory–Weiss lacerations. Gastric lesions that frequently bleed include ulcers, gastritis, and cancer. Duodenitis and ulceration are responsible for most bleeding from the duodenum. Sources in the small bowel and large bowel include Meckel's diverticulum, inflammatory bowel disease, benign and malignant neoplasms, diverticulosis, hemorrhoids, and anal fissures. Vascular lesions, such as hereditary hemorrhagic telangiectasia, may occur anywhere throughout the digestive tract, though angiodysplasia is generally limited to the colon and distal small bowel.

The prevalence of specific disorders varies with the population studied, diagnostic methods employed, and time of investigation in relation to bleeding. A recent British series of 277 patients with melena or hematemesis provides representative prevalence figures in a population composed of both outpatients and patients seen in emergency rooms. More than 85% of the patients in this study underwent endoscopy; diagnosis was also made by upper GI series or at surgery: 20% had duodenal ulcers, 15% had gastric ulcers, 12% had Mallory–Weiss tears, 11% had esophageal varices, 5% had gastritis, and 1% had gastric cancer. In 21%, no cause was found (half of these patients did not undergo endoscopy), and in 5% multiple lesions were detected.

In a study of 311 patients who complained of anorectal bleeding and were evaluated by careful physical examination, sigmoidoscopy, and barium enema, 79% had lesions of the anal canal, 15% had rectal and colonic disease, and 7% had perianal skin problems. Leading causes were hemorrhoids in 54%, fissure in ano in 18%, neoplasm in 6.5%, and inflammatory bowel diseases in 5%. In 8% no cause was found at the time of the examination. Most of the neoplasms were more than 10 cm above the anus.

In a series of 239 patients with undiagnosed rectal bleeding subjected to colonoscopy, 40% had significant lesions; 16% were found to have polyps; 10% had inflammatory bowel disease; 9% had carcinomas missed by barium enema; and 3% had diverticular disease, hemangiomas, or other causes. In a large percentage of these patients, no cause was found. In a study of anemic competitive runners, an increase in fecal hemoglobin was detected.

Patients with gastrointestinal bleeding while on anticoagulant therapy are likely to have an underlying lesion. In a study examining 3800 courses of anticoagulant therapy, gastrointestinal bleeding occurred in 45 patients. In 32, a source was determined: 13 had hemorrhoids, 9 had peptic ulcers, 7 had neoplasms, and 3 had other lesions.

Nosebleeds and respiratory-tract bleeding must be considered in the differential diagnosis of melena and guaiac positive stools. A false-positive stool-guaiac test result can be produced by use of glycerol guaiacolate, the popular expectorant, or a meal of rare red meat. Black stools may result from bismuth (Pepto-Bismol), iron, charcoal, or spinach intake; red stools can occur from eating large quantities of beets.

WORKUP

History and physical examination may provide information regarding the location and severity of bleeding, but additional investigations are usually necessary to determine the exact cause. In the previously mentioned series of 311 cases of anorectal bleeding, history and physical examination alone yielded a definite diagnosis in 28%. Nevertheless, history and physical examination have important roles that may obviate the need for more invasive testing or help in selecting an optimal procedure.

History. Before proceeding with an extensive workup, the physician ought to be certain that the report of blood loss is accurate; dark stools must not be mistaken for genuine melena. One should check for intake of preparations that will turn stool black, such as Pepto-Bismol, iron, or charcoal; eating beets will turn it red. A recent meal of red meat will produce a false-positive stool Hemoccult test result (see Chapter 51). The claim that HemoQuant testing reduces the false positive rate remains unsubstantiated.

An approximate bleeding site can be determined by the nature of the blood loss, that is, whether it is melena, hematemesis, or bright red blood from the rectum. A crude estimate of rate and severity can be obtained by asking about postural lightheadedness. The actual volume lost is not reliably obtained from the history, although very large amounts should be taken seriously.

When the patient complains of voluminous blood loss or lightheadedness, a careful check for postural change in vital signs is indicated before proceeding with a complete ambulatory assessment. Immediate hospital admission should be arranged if blood pressure falls more than 10 mm Hg to

15 mm Hg, or the heart rate increases by more than 10 to 15 beats per minute when the patient stands up from a supine position. Measurement of the hematocrit in the acute phase of blood loss may show deceptively little decline if there has not been sufficient time for reequilibration of intravascular volume.

Once it is clear that the degree of blood loss does not pose an immediate hazard, office evaluation can proceed. When hematemesis is reported, sources of esophageal, gastric, and duodenal bleeding must be sought. History of cirrhosis, chronic liver disease, or alcoholism point to esophageal varices. Use of aspirin, alcohol, and anti-inflammatory agents suggest bleeding due to ulceration or gastritis. History of peptic ulcer or the presence of epigastric pain responsive to antacids or related to food intake raises the possibility of bleeding from a gastric or duodenal ulcer. It is worth noting, however, that another explanation for bleeding may be present in patients with a history typical of ulcer disease.

When no hematemesis is noted, the source may still be from above the ligament of Treitz; however, small bowel and colonic lesions must be considered as well. Diarrhea, urgency, tenesmus, and lower abdominal cramping suggest inflammatory bowel disease (see Chapter 65). With ulcerative colitis, diverticulosis, and other forms of rectosigmoid disease, there is often some frank rectal bleeding. Weight loss or change in bowel habits raises suspicion of colonic cancer. A history of diverticular disease may be a clue to the cause of blood loss, but a coincident carcinoma must be ruled out. Many patients with rectal bleeding admit to past or present hemorrhoidal problems, but in almost half of the cases another lesion is found to be the cause of blood loss. Although note should be taken of oral anticoagulant use, most patinets who experience GI bleeding on warfarin have underlying pathology.

Physical Examination. The skin is inspected for pallor, ecchymoses, petechiae, telangiectasias, jaundice, and spider angiomata. The nose and pharynx are examined for sources of bleeding. Lymph nodes are palpated for enlargement and the abdomen for organomegaly, ascites, masses, or rectal lesions. Supraclavicular adenopathy or a rectal shelf mass points to a bowel malignancy. The stool is checked for color and occult blood (see Chapter 51). Careful external observation and anoscopic examination (see Chapter 75) of the anorectal tissues are essential.

If the patient describes convincing hematemesis, one may assume that the bleeding is from the upper tract, but if there is evidence of recent significant bleeding of uncertain origin, a nasogastric tube should be passed to aspirate gastric contents and test for the presence of blood. The guaiac test may be insensitive for heme unless the acidic aspirate is neutralized with a few drops of NaOH.

Laboratory Studies should be obtained to determine the chronicity and magnitude of blood loss as well as the presence of coincident disease. Hemoglobin concentration should be measured in all patients; however, if blood loss is acute, the hemoglobin concentration may not yet accurately reflect the severity of blood loss. Studies of coagulation such as platelet count, prothrombin time, and partial thromboplastin time are often useful in checking for acute precipitants to bleeding, as are tests of liver and renal function.

Rectal bleeding. The main concern is the likelihood of colon cancer; risk increases with age. Less than 5% of such cancers occur in patients under age 40 and less than 1% in those under age 30. Thus, if the physical examination or anoscopy reveals a bleeding hemorrhoid or other cause of local anal pathology in a young patient, it may be unnecessary to proceed with further tests. The finding on sigmoidoscopy of guaiac-negative stool from above the bleeding point also provides reassurance. On the other hand, 80% of colorectal malignancies are found in patients over 50. When a person over 50 presents with rectal bleeding, a thorough search for tumor is required even if a local lesion such as a hemorrhoid is discovered. Twenty-seven percent of patients with carcinoma of the rectum and 10% of those with carcinoma of the sigmoid have been noted to have coincidental hemorrhoids.

There are increasing data describing yields of diagnostic procedures. In the series of 311 patients with bright red rectal bleeding subjected to history, physical examination, sigmoidoscopy, and barium enema, the history diagnosed 5%, the physical examination raised the figure to 28%, and the addition of *sigmoidoscopy* provided an explanation in 90%. Barium enema raised the yield in this series only another 3%, probably because of the unusually large number of lesions in this study that were within reach of the sigmoidoscope. Cumulative data suggest that only 30% of colonic malignancies can be viewed by sigmoidoscopy (see Chapter 51). Consequently, persons with rectal bleeding in the age group at high risk for large bowel malignancy should undergo additional study. *Barium enema* has a sensitivity of 70% to 90% for detecting carcinoma and 70% for polyps greater than 5 mm in diameter. Cancers most often missed are in the cecum or rectosigmoid or are obscured by concurrent diverticulosis or ulcerative colitis. Air-contrast techniques improve the results.

The advent of *colonoscopy* has improved the identification of bleeding sources. About 40% of cases of frank rectal bleeding or occult blood loss with normal sigmoidoscopy and normal routine barium enema shown previously undetected lesions when studied by colonoscopy. About 10% have cancers, another 10% have polyps, 10% have inflammatory bowel disease, and 5% have telangiectasia. Furthermore, carcinomas and polyps were detected in 20% of patients when only diverticula were seen with barium enema. Although the role for colonoscopy is not yet entirely settled, most patients with bleeding over the age of 50 should have colonoscopy either primarily, if they have a normal barium enema and normal sigmoidoscopy, or if they show only diverticula on barium study.

Upper gastrointestinal bleeding. Endoscopy has proven superior to barium studies for the evaluation. The sensitivity of the *UGI series* is around 60%, compared to 95% for *endoscopy*. Esophagitis, Mallory–Weiss tears, and gastritis are readily seen by endoscopy and undetectable radiologically. Moreover, barium obscures mucosal detail and interferes with endoscopy for 24 to 48 hours. Thus, for suspected acute brisk upper gastrointestinal bleeding, endoscopy is the procedure of first choice, with barium study reserved as a supplementary procedure for patients with inactive bleeding, unexplained chronic blood loss, or suspected small bowel disease. However, the improvement in detection has neither increased survival nor decreased transfusion requirements. Improved patient outcome will require advances in treatment of upper gastrointestinal bleeding.

Should everyone with suspected upper gastrointestinal hemorrhage be subjected to urgent endoscopy? The question is hotly debated. Available data suggest that only high-risk subgroups need undergo urgent endoscopy. Those with chronic alcoholic liver disease appear to be at particularly high risk for dangerous bleeding, given their propensity for varices, ulcers, and erosive gastritis. A randomized controlled trial of 206 patients assigned to routine early endoscopy or no initial endoscopy showed no difference in outcome, except for patients who continued to bleed in spite of medical therapy. Thus, history of alcoholic liver disease or evidence of persistent bleeding on medical therapy emerge as the most compelling reasons for proceeding to urgent endoscopy. The finding of a visible vessel has serious prognostic implications (*i.e.*, risk of uncontrolled or recurrent bleeding).

INDICATIONS FOR ADMISSION AND REFERRAL

The patient with brisk, gross bleeding requires emergency ward evaluation, as does the person with less dramatic evidence of blood loss but whose hematocrit has fallen sharply or whose vital signs show hemodynamic instability. Workup of the patient with mild or slow blood loss can proceed safely on an ambulatory basis if the patient does not have serious cardiopulmonary disease and is responsible enough to recognize and promptly report signs of worsening blood loss or volume depletion. The patient with acute hematemesis or lower gastrointestinal bleeding who has normal barium studies and sigmoidoscopy ought to be seen by the gastroenterologist for consideration of endoscopy.

SYMPTOMATIC MANAGEMENT

Modest falls in hematocrit that accompany chronic low-grade gastrointestinal blood loss can be treated with oral iron ($FeSO_4$, 300 mg tid) to make up for the resulting iron deficiency (see Chapter 84). Marked, but gradual, decreases in hematocrit are usually well tolerated unless the patient has cardiopulmonary disease. Most patients do not need trans-fusion unless they are symptomatic. Oral iron usually produces a prompt reticulocytosis and at least partial correction of the anemia. Patients with presumed anal bleeding can be given fiber supplements or stool softeners to decrease mechanical trauma to the lesion (see Chapter 68).

ANNOTATED BIBLIOGRAPHY

Ahlquist DA, McGill DB, Schwartz S et al: Fecal blood levels in health and disease: A study using HemoQuant. N Engl J Med 312:1422, 1985 (*A report of a new technique for stool testing to detect occult blood loss. Claims increased sensitivity and specificity for detection of blood loss and occult malignancy. However, an accompanying editorial cites methodologic problems with this study, urges caution regarding its conclusions, and suggests continued use of the much less expensive Hemoccult test for now.*)

Conn HO: To scope or not to scope. N Engl J Med 304:967, 1981 (*A thoughtful editorial addressing this difficult question. Good summary of available data.*)

Coon U, Willis P: Hemorrhagic complications of anticoagulant therapy. Ann Intern Med 133:386, 1974 (*More than half of patients who bled on anticoagulant therapy had an identifiable underlying gastrointestinal lesion.*)

Dooley CP, Larson AW, Stacen H et al: Double-contrast barium meal and upper gastrointestinal endoscopy. Ann Intern Med 101: 538, 1984 (*Extensively reviews the literature comparing the sensitivity and specificity of these modalities as well as a study indicating that endoscopy was substantially more sensitive—92% versus 54%—and more specific—100% versus 91%—than double contrast barium swallow. An accompanying editorial points out the gold standard problem of this study and argues the merits of the radiologic approach.*)

Eastwood DL: Does endoscopy benefit the patient with acute upper gastrointestinal bleeding? Gastroenterology 72:737, 1977 (*Neither an improvement in patient survival nor a decrease in transfusion requirements could be demonstrated.*)

Foster DN, Miloszewski K, Losowsky M: Stigmata of recent hemorrhage in diagnosis and prognosis of upper gastrointestinal bleeding. Br Med J 1:1173, 1976 (*A series of 277 consecutive cases of hematemesis, melena, and upper GI bleeding seen in emergency and outpatient settings. Duodenal ulcer, gastric ulcer, Mallory Weiss lesions, and esophageal varices led the list of causes.*)

Goulston KJ et al: Evaluation of rectal bleeding. Lancet 2:261, 1986 (*Retrospective study of 145 consecutive patients over the age of 40 with rectal bleeding finding colorectal malignancies would have been missed on clinical basis alone. The authors suggest colonoscopy or good air contrast barium enema combined with flexible sigmoidoscopy be carried out in patients over age 40 with rectal bleeding.*)

Graham DY: Aspirin and the stomach. Ann Intern Med 104:390, 1986 (*Comprehensive review. Notes that degree of mucosal injury seen by endoscopy does not predict risk or degree of bleeding.*)

Layne EA, Mellow MH, Lipman TO: Insensitivity of guaiac slide for detection of blood in gastric juice. Ann Intern Med 94:774, 1981 (*Sensitivity of the guaiac test was low and greatly enhanced by neutralizing the acid with a few drops of NaOH.*)

Peterson WL, Barnett CC, Smith HJ et al: Routine early endoscopy in upper gastrointestinal tract bleeding. N Engl J Med 304:925, 1981 (*A randomized controlled trial in which no advantage was found for early endoscopy, though analysis of subgroups shows those with alcoholic liver disease and those who continue to bleed in spite of therapy require endoscopy.*)

Peterson WL, Fordtran JS: Quantitating the occult. N Engl J Med 312:1448, 1985 (*An editorial commenting on the report of HemoQuant published in the same issue. Urges caution in interpreting the results because of methodologic problems with the study. Also a good review of the utility and shortcomings of the stool-guaiac test.*)

Shapiro RH: The visible vessel: curse or blessing. N Engl J Med 300: 1438, 1979 (*An editorial reviewing the utility of endoscopy, with emphasis on defining a high-risk group of patients with upper gastrointestinal bleeding.*)

Steer ML, Silen W: Diagnostic procedures in gastrointestinal hemorrhage. N Engl J Med 309:646, 1983 (*Concise but very useful review of the operating characteristics of endoscopy, radionuclide imaging, angiography, barium contrast studies, and exploratory surgery in the diagnosis of both upper and lower gastrointestinal hemorrhage.*)

Stewart JG, Ahlquist DA, McGill DB et al: Gastrointestinal blood loss and anemia in runners. Ann Intern Med 100:843, 1984 (*Documents an increase in fecal hemoglobin level associated with competitive running, which may explain anemia and iron deficiency among long-distance runners.*)

Suchman AL, Griner PF: Diagnostic uses of the activated partial thromboplastic time and prothrombin time. Ann Intern Med 104: 810, 1986 (*An excellent review that states screening PTs and PTTs add no information to patients without a history of increased bleeding. A further note that the PT and PTT are sufficiently sensitive that if both are normal there is no indication for further investigation of a clotting factor abnormality.*)

Tedesco F et al: Colonoscopic evaluation of rectal bleeding. Ann Intern Med 89:907, 1978 (*Colonoscopy discovered cancers in 10% of patients with normal sigmoidoscopies and normal barium enemas and in another 10% with diverticula alone on barium enema. As in a similar British study, almost 40% had a detectable cause of blood loss.*)

Williams JT, Thompson JPS: Anorectal bleeding: Study of causes and investigative results. Practitioner 219:327, 1977 (*Diagnosis was made in 90% of cases by history, physical examinations, and sigmoidoscopy. A barium enema improved the yield by only 3% of cases. In 75% the cause was local and pathologic, but most tumors were 10 cm above the anus.*)

61
Evaluation of Anorectal Complaints

Anorectal complaints often go incompletely evaluated. Although they are usually a result of minor conditions, etiologies range beyond the trivial to inflammatory bowel disease, cancer, and infection. In addition, anorectal problems generate a substantial amount of worry and discomfort. As a result, they deserve careful and thorough evaluation by the primary care physician. An increasingly frequent diagnostic challenge is the evaluation of anorectal problems in male homosexuals.

PATHOPHYSIOLOGY AND CLINICAL PRESENTATION

Anorectal complaints result from traumatic, vascular, infectious, inflammatory, neurologic, and malignant etiologies. Symptoms include pain, discharge, itching, mass, and fecal incontinence. *Pain* is most often a manifestation of anal pathology; anal and perianal skin are richly innervated with pain-sensitive nerve fibers; rectal tissue is relatively insensitive to pain. A fissure, distention by abscess or hemorrhoid, invasion by tumor, or marked inflammation can lead to considerable discomfort. Secondary anal sphincter spasm may ensue, prolonging and intensifying the pain. *Discharge* ensues

from inflammation of the rectal mucosa or drainage of an abscess. Cancer, abscess, and thrombosed hemorrhoids can produce an anorectal *mass;* condylomata acuminata may also cause anal skin nodularity. *Itching* represents a minor form of skin irritation seen with a variety of mechanical and inflammatory lesions; it is intensified by moisture in the perianal area. Chronic itching leads to excoriation, edema, thickening, fissuring, and lichenification of the perianal skin. *Bleeding* is a common and important manifestation of anorectal pathology; its causes range from hemorrhoids and fissures to carcinoma and inflammatory bowel disease (see Chapter 60).

Hemorrhoids are the most common anorectal problem, affecting about half of patients over the age of 50. They represent dilatations of the anorectal vascular network. Although the traditional view is that hemorrhoids are venous varicosities resulting from straining at stool, they do not always present in a fashion consistent with this postulate. For example, hemorrhoids develop in early pregnancy in many young women, long before there is significant intra-abdominal pressure from a large fetus. Moreover, hemorrhoidal bleeding is characteristically arterial in quality (bright red) rather than the dark variety that would be expected from a strictly venous source. External hemorrhoids are covered by pain-sensitive anal skin and arise from the inferior hemorrhoidal plexus. Internal hemorrhoids are covered by the much less pain-sensitive rectal mucosa and represent dilations of the superior hemorrhoidal plexus. Many patients with hemorrhoids have been found to have increased resting anal sphincter pressures; the pathogenetic significance of this pressure increase remains unclear.

Clinical presentation depends in part on the location of the hemmorhoid and the presence of complications. External hemorrhoids that have thrombosed present as tender bluish swellings. Internal hemorrhoids often bleed, but only when they prolapse do they present as a mass; when irreducible, they are subject to thrombosis. Recurrent bleeding may be seen with either type; sudden rupture may cause rather dramatic, though relatively harmless, bright red bleeding.

Fistula-in-ano is a communication between the anal canal and the perianal skin. It is usually nontender. The external opening may be single or multiple, with a granulation tissue bud and chronic seropurulent drainage. Occasionally, an indurated cord of tissue may be palpable, extending from the external fistulous opening toward the anal canal. The fistula may result from rupture or surgical drainage of a perirectal abscess; other etiologies include Crohn's disease, carcinoma, tuberculosis, radiation therapy, lymphogranuloma venereum, and anal fissures. Patients complain of persistent and irritating drainage of blood, pus, or mucus.

Perirectal abscess and fistula-in-ano are two stages of the same disease process, beginning as infection in the anal glands that empty into the anal crypts at the mucocutaneous junction, and subsequently spreading into the adjacent tissue. The abscess thus formed often drains through the perianal skin. Symptoms and signs are a function of the size and location of the abscess. The first manifestation is rectal pain, which may occur before any mass becomes palpable. Patients characteristically complain of constant, throbbing pain in the perianal region or in the rectum. A mass may be identified externally on examining the anus or internally on palpating the rectum. Perirectal abscess formation is a particularly important problem in patients with Crohn's disease, immunodeficiency states, and hematologic disorders.

An *infected pilonidal cyst or sinus* is most common in males between ages 16 and 30. These are midline, in the area of the natal cleft. Multiple sinuses may be present. Recurrent secondary infections are frequent.

Carcinoma of the perianal skin or anorectal tract typically does not cause pain until relatively late in its clinical course, often in the setting of a large ulcerated bleeding lesion. Earlier lesions present as painless nodules or plaques. Pruritus, mucoid drainage, and change in bowel habits are more subtle manifestations that sometimes occur.

Proctalgia fugax, as the term implies, is fleeting, but severe rectal pain believed to be related to spasm of the levator ani and coccygeal muscles. Although usually brief, symptoms can last for more than 30 minutes. Suspected precipitants include chronic trauma from poor posture; psychogenic factors may also be operative. There are no associated physical findings, except for muscle tenderness on digital examination.

Proctitis, inflammatory disease of the rectum, has a wide variety of etiologies ranging from infection and trauma to radiation and inflammatory bowel disease. Regardless of the cause, the presentation is usually one of mucopurulent discharge, rectal bleeding, and, in severe cases, rectal pain and tenesmus. Patients with *ulcerative proctitis* demonstrate on sigmoidoscopy an inflamed rectal mucosa and a clearly demarcated upper border, above which the mucosa is normal. Systemic symptoms and extraintestinal manifestations are rare when the disease is limited to the rectum. The risk of carcinoma is small, and fewer than 10% to 15% of patients develop diffuse colitis.

Infectious proctitis occurs mostly among promiscuous *male homosexuals* who engage in frequent rectal intercourse with multiple partners. Gonorrhea, amebic disease, chlamydia, and herpes simplex infections are prominent in this population (see below). *Gonococcal proctitis* is especially common. The rate of asymptomatic carriage of gonorrhea among promiscuous male homosexuals is reportedly as high as 60% to 70%. Symptomatic gonococcal proctitis presents with discharge and rectal discomfort (see below). Diarrhea is the hallmark of symptomatic *amebic infection, shigellosis,* and *Campylobacter* infection (see Chapter 58). *Herpes simplex* proctitis can be a very painful condition, accompanied by tenesmus, constipation, rectal ulceration, and discharge. Involvement of the sacral nerve roots can lead to bladder and erectile difficulties, paresthesias, and pain in the thighs and buttocks.

Solitary rectal ulcer is a rare condition of unknown etiology associated with rectal discharge, bleeding, and occasionally, dull pain. The characteristic finding on sigmoidoscopy is a single shallow ulcer 7 to 10 cm from the anus; its borders may be heaped or nodular. Chronicity is the rule; complications are rare. These must be distinguished from cancer and lymphogranuloma venereum by biopsy.

Pruritus ani (chronic perianal itching) is not a diagnosis but rather a syndrome that results from a variety of mechanical and inflammatory lesions. Anatomic lesions that produce chronic discharge (such as *fistulas, fissures,* and *hemorrhoids* with intermittent mucosal eversion) can result in pruritus ani. There are a variety of infectious etiologies. *Anogenital warts (condylomata acuminata)* are viral in origin and generally transmitted by sexual contact. They may be confined to the perianal region or also involve the penis, vulva, and anal canal. Multiple, soft, filiform excrescences characterize these lesions, which may enlarge, become confluent, and even bleed. *Gonococcal proctitis* can lead to anal soreness, burning, and purulent discharge. Infestations with *pinworm (Enterobius vermicularis)* typically cause nocturnal anal itchiness, especially among children but sometimes spread to involve adult family members. Nocturnal symptoms are due to the daily evening migration of the female pinworm downward to deposit eggs on the perianal skin. Anal involvement is characteristic of some systemic dermatologic diseases, such as *psoriasis* and scabies. *Contact dermatitis* or *eczema* resulting from use of a topical agent is common and can complicate the diagnosis of the original cause of pruritus. Applied initially as a remedy for itching, the agent may only aggravate the problem by causing skin sensitization. Itching is intensified by moisture in the perianal area and often aggravated by use of topical agents applied in an attempt to quell symptoms. Passage of *alkaline stools* (as occurs in severe diarrhea) can have an irritant effect on the anal skin. Persistent anal itching may be a form of *neurodermatitis;* such patients characteristically present with multiple excoriations. *Candidal infection* is found among diabetics, homosexuals, and those recently taking broad-spectrum antibiotics; perianal erythema and itching are presenting manifestations.

Fecal impaction ranks as one of the major sources of anorectal discomfort among the elderly and bedridden. Chronic, incomplete evacuation leads to formation of an obstructing bolus of desiccated hard stool in the rectum. Symptoms of anal discomfort and constipation are typical, but anorexia, malaise, or nonspecific lower abdominal fullness may be all that is reported. Paradoxically, diarrhea rather than constipation is sometimes the only complaint, because of the collection of liquid stool distending the proximal colon and passing around the obstructing bolus. Unless this is corrected by disimpaction, complications such as intestinal obstruction, rectal prolapse, and even bowel perforation may ensue.

Fecal incontinence follows damage to the normal anal sphincter mechanism. Perianal disease, anal surgery, and neurologic disease can have devastating psychosocial consequences when they compromise the anal sphincter. Some patients lose the ability to sense rectal distention as well as to constrict the external sphincter. In others with only a weakened sphincter, the prognosis is less grim; biofeedback methods can be employed to help them regain continence.

Anorectal problems in homosexuals and others engaging in receptive anal intercourse deserve further comment, because they can be quite complex in etiology and presentation. In a major study, more than 80% of homosexual men presenting to a venereal disease clinic with anorectal or intestinal symptoms were infected with one or more sexually transmissible anorectal or enteric pathogens. Three principal syndromes were noted: a *proctitis* characterized by anorectal pain, lesions, and discharge, but no evidence of disease above the rectum; a *proctocolitis* that, in addition to proctitic manifestations, included diarrhea, tenesmus, and inflammation extending into the sigmoid mucosa; and an *enteritis* (see Chapter 58) that consisted of diarrhea and abdominal pain, but no anorectal symptoms or signs.

As noted above, gonococcal, herpetic, chlamydial, and syphilitic forms of proctitis occur with increased frequency among these patients. In the carefully documented venereal disease clinic study of 119 symptomatic patients and 75 randomly selected asymptomatic homosexual men mentioned earlier, the prevalence of anorectal *gonorrhea* was reported to be 31% among those with symptoms. In the same series, *herpes simplex* virus was cultured from 19% of symptomatic men; all isolates were type 2. Rectal mucosal ulcerations were present in the majority and yielded herpes virus. *Syphilis* was also common in this series; 3% of symptomatic individuals were found to have anal chancres, another 3% had evidence of secondary anorectal syphilitic disease (erythematous nodular or indurated rectal mucosal lesions that were biopsy positive).

A clinical and sigmoidoscopic picture of *proctocolitis* occurred in about 15% of cases. Such patients complained of anorectal discomfort, tenesmus, diarrhea, constipation, and abdominal cramps. On sigmoidoscopy, inflammatory changes started at the rectum and entended beyond 15 cm into the sigmoid colon. *Campylobacter, Entamoeba histolytica, Chlamydia,* and *C. difficile* were significantly correlated with the enterocolitis; often more than one organism was recovered. Polymicrobial infection is commonplace among symptomatic male homosexuals with many sexual partners.

Although much of the proctitis in this population is infectious in origin, *culture-negative proctitis* occurs with some frequency and has been linked to exposure to the *coloring agents* and scents found in some of the lubricants used for anal intercourse. Several etiologies may present simultaneously. The patient complaining of hemorrhoidal pain may actually have concurrent gonorrhea, allergic proctitis, and chlamydial infection. Traumatic complications of rectal intercourse include prolapsed hemorrhoids, anal fistulas and fissures, perirectal abscesses, rectal ulcers, and anal tears. Foreign bodies are sometimes recovered.

DIFFERENTIAL DIAGNOSIS

The differential diagnosis of anorectal problems can best be considered in anatomical terms, depending on whether symptoms and signs are predominantly anal, anorectal, or rectocolitic (see Table 61-1). This is particularly true when considering the causes of anorectal disease in male homosexuals (see Table 61-2).

WORKUP

History. Although a careful physical examination is the single most important part of the evaluation, history can provide important epidemiologic and etiologic information. Determining whether the condition is predominantly anal (local pain only), anorectal (local anal pain plus rectal discomfort, tenesmus, rectal discharge, constipation), or rectocolonic (rectal discomfort, tenesmus, rectal discharge, plus diarrhea, abdominal pain, bloating, nausea) helps to focus the evaluation.

Patients with anal complaints ought to be questioned about masses, nodules, focal tenderness, history of hemorrhoids, psoriasis, passage of hard stool, bleeding, discharge, generalized itching, nocturnal pattern, and recent trauma. Detailed inquiry into the use of topical medications (many of which are sensitizing), involvement of other household members or sexual partners, and hygienic practices should also be made.

For those with anorectal involvement, check into symptoms of inflammatory bowel disease (see Chapter 65), obtain a careful and detailed sexual history focusing on numbers of partners and practice of receptive rectal intercourse, and note any reports of inguinal adenopathy (seen with herpes and lymphogranuloma), sacral root paresthesias, and difficulty with micturition (other telltale symptoms of herpes simplex infection). Those with rectocolonic symptoms are likely to have either inflammatory bowel disease or a polymicrobial infection from rectal intercourse; consideration of associated symptoms and risk factors is indicated.

Physical Examination. Thorough and gentle inspection of the anus and perianal region is the *sine qua non* of suc-

Table 61-1.   Differential Diagnosis
of Anorectal Problems

PROBLEM	DIFFERENTIAL DIAGNOSIS
Anal discomfort	Hemorrhoids Fissure-in-ano (hard bowel movement, cancer, venereal disease) Fistula-in-ano (perirectal abscess, Crohn's disease, carcinoma, radiation, TB, lymphogranuloma venereum) Perirectal abscess (Crohn's disease, immunodeficiency, hematologic disorders) Infected pilonidal cyst Carcinoma of the anal epidermis Infections (syphilis, candidiasis, condylomata accuminata)
Rectal discomfort	Proctitis (ulcerative, gonococcal, amebic, herpetic) often accompanied by discharge and bleeding Perirectal abscess Impaction Proctalgia fugax Solitary rectal ulcer
Pruritus ani	Excess moisture (poor hygiene), pinworms, eczema, scabies, diabetes, liver failure, irritants (topical agents, alkaline stools), fissure, early cancer, neurodermatitis, anal infections (see above)
Incontinence	Rectal surgery, neurologic disease, perianal disease

Table 61-2.   Differential Diagnosis of Anorectal
Problems in Male Homosexuals

SYNDROME	ETIOLOGY
Proctitis	*N. gonorrhea* Herpes simplex *Chlamydia* (nonlymphogranuloma strains) Syphylis Condylomata acuminata Trauma Chemical irritants
Proctocolitis	*Campylobacter* *Shigella* *Entamoeba histolytica* *Chlamydia* (lymphogranuloma strains)
Enteritis	*Giardia lamblia*

cessful diagnosis of anorectal problems. One examines the anal skin for erythema, eczema, psoriatic patches, ulcerations, vesicles, fistulas, fissures, condylomata, nodules, hemorrhoids, and inflammatory changes. The presence of perianal or rectal ulcers in association with proctitis in a male homosexual is indicative of syphilis or herpes simplex. If the lesions appear as scaling plaques, a look at the skin of the extensor surfaces of the extremities might provide additional evidence for a diagnosis of psoriasis. In a very anxious patient with multiple excoriations over other parts of the body, suspect neurodermatitis as the cause of pruritus ani. If an inflamed anorectal mucosa is encountered, gonorrhea needs to be considered and inquiry into rectal intercourse pursued.

Stretching the perianal skin will reveal fissures, which come into view at the anal verge, most often in the posterior midline but occasionally in the anterior midline. With chronic fissures, there is scarring and induration as well as an associated hypertrophied anal papilla at the pectinate line; a skin tag marks the external limit. Crohn's disease is likely in those with multiple fissures, recurrent fistulas, or perirectal abscesses. A painless hard nodule or plaque in the anal region may represent carcinoma. When the lesion is ulcerated, the diagnosis is more obvious and the disease more advanced.

Digital rectal examination is almost always an essential component of the examination. However, in the presence of a painful fissure, it can be an extremely painful procedure that is likely to alienate the patient and cause such pain as to make adequate examination impossible. The same applies to use of anoscopy in such patients. On the other hand, rectal examination should never be deferred in patients who are not acutely and severely uncomfortable. One needs to check for masses (both fluctuant and firm), discharges, ulcerations, and other mucosal changes as well as test the stool for occult blood. Ascribing anorectal symptoms to hemorrhoids without performing as complete an examination as possible is a common reason for delay in diagnosis of carcinoma.

Palpation for enlarged lymph nodes should not be overlooked. Prominent inguinal adenopathy is characteristic of herpetic and chlamydial infections (lymphogranuloma venereum species).

Diagnostic Studies. Unless the patient has a very painful lesion, *anoscopy* needs to be performed (see Chapter 75) to visualize the canal and mucosa adequately and obtain samples of any discharge. One inspects for mucosal inflammation, fissure, fistula, mass, plaque, ulcer, and discharge. Patients with rectal inflammation, fistula formation, nonhealing fissures, bleeding, or diarrhea are candidates for *sigmoidoscopy*. Involvement of the sigmoid mucosa suggests inflammatory bowel disease (see Chapter 65, and infectious forms of colitis (see Chapter 58). Patients with atypical fissures, especially those that fail to heal, painless hard anorectal nodules, and mucosal ulcerations are candidates for *biopsy* to rule out malignancy, inflammatory bowel disease, and chronic infection (syphilis, tuberculosis). Children complaining of nocturnal pruritus ani can be evaluated for pinworm infestation by taking a cellophone tape impression of the anus and microscopically examining it under low power for the characteristic eggs.

Male homosexuals engaging in receptive anal intercourse with many sexual partners should undergo *anoscopy* to determine the nature of rectal involvement and to obtain samples of mucus for *Gram stain* and *culture on Thayer–Martin plates.* A positive Gram stain is excellent presumptive evidence of gonorrhea, although a negative smear does not rule out the diagnosis. Any chancrelike lesions should be subjected to *darkfield* examination for spirochetes. A *serologic test for syphilis* is also obtained.

Homosexual patients with evidence of rectal pathology on anoscopy require *sigmoidoscopy;* establishing the extent of mucosal involvement helps narrow the list of possible etiologies. Those with a *proctocolitis* picture of mucosal involvement extending above 15 cm or symptoms of colitis (diarrhea, nausea, abdominal cramping) should be *cultured for Campylobacter, Chlamydia* (lymphogranuloma strains), and *Shigella* and have their stools examined for the *ova and trophozoites* of *Entamoeba histolytica.* Those with *proctitis* only (no mucosal disease above 15 cm) are more likely to have gonorrhea, herpes simplex, or chlamydial infection (nonlymphogranuloma strains) and can be cultured accordingly. Viral cultures are not necessary, because the diagnosis of herpes simplex proctitis can usually be made on the basis of its characteristic clinical presentation (severe anorectal pain, multiple perianal ulcers, rectal ulceration, inguinal adenopathy, difficult micturation, impotence, and paresthesias in the S_4 and S_5 distributions).

SYMPTOMATIC MANAGEMENT AND INDICATIONS FOR REFERRAL

Patients with anal pain due to *fissure* should initially be treated symptomatically. Lubricants, such as mineral oil, and agents providing a soft, bulky stool, such as methylcellulose, will decrease trauma and counteract the attendant sphincter spasm. Frequent warm sitz baths provide intermittent relief of pain and spasm. Topical analgesics are of limited use and may result in skin sensitization. Systemic analgesics are sometimes necessary, but if narcotics are used, increased constipation may occur. If the pain has not improved by conservative measures in several days to weeks, the patient should be referred for surgical treatment, which has a high success rate. In general, chronic or recurrent fissures will require surgery more often than acute or superficial fissures. In patients in whom the pain of fissure precludes digital or instrumental examination at the first visit, these may be done at the time of surgical treatment under adequate anesthesia.

Established *perirectal abscess* will not resolve on antibiotics alone; the proper treatment is surgical drainage. Antibiotic therapy should be reserved for patients with extensive cellulitis, signs of systemic infection, immunosuppression, valvular heart disease, or intravascular prostheses. Incision and drainage of a perirectal abscess usually requires anesthesia and is not often an office procedure. Similarly, the treatment for an infected pilonidal sinus is surgical drainage, which is accomplished satisfactorily under local anesthesia.

The only successful treatment for *fistula-in-ano* is surgical. However, patients with inflammatory bowel disease should not undergo surgery for fistula because this will usually fail as long as there is any active proximal disease. Surgery is reserved for palliation of complications of fistula, that is, drainage of recurrent perirectal abscess.

For management of *hemorrhoids,* see Chapter 68. Suspicion of carcinoma and need for biopsy require surgical consultation.

Specific therapy for *pruritus ani* is related to identification of a specific etiology—for example diabetes in the patient with candidiasis. Identification of the cause may be a challenging exercise to the primary physician. Pruritus resulting from anatomic lesions will generally remit with correction of the underlying cause. *Anogenital warts* are effectively treated with topical application of 25% podophyllin in tincture of benzoin repeated every 1 to 2 weeks. The patient is instructed to bathe between 6 and 12 hours after the application. Care should be taken to avoid applying the compound to intact skin. If anoscopy reveals intra-anal warts at the initial examination, curettage and electrocoagulation under anesthesia will be necessary.

All family members should be treated simultaneously for *pinworms.* Pyrantel pamoate (Antiminth) is the drug of choice; a one-time oral dose of 11 mg per kilogram of body weight usually suffices. Preventive measures are difficult to enforce, except for handwashing before meals and after bowel movements. The best prevention is simultaneous treatment of all members of the household.

Often, however, no specific cause is found, and pruritus appears to be a form of neurodermatitis affecting the perianal skin. However, the symptoms are often relieved by careful attention to *perianal hygiene* following bowel movements, keeping the perianal skin dry with application of witch hazel, and using topical steroid ointments (0.25% hydrocortisone ointment) for several weeks to break the cycle of itching and skin changes caused by scratching. When contact dermatitis is thought to be caused by topical agents, the offending medication should be discontinued.

For treatment of *gonorrheal proctitis,* see Chapter 116.

While awaiting culture results, *homosexuals* with a non-specific *proctitis* (inflammation limited to the lower 15 cm of the bowel and no ulcers) should be treated empirically by covering for gonorrhea (with 4.8 million units of procaine *penicillin* intramuscularly preceded by 1 g of oral probenecid) and *Chlamydia* (with *tetracycline* 500 mg qid for 7 days). Both infections may be present simultaneously. Tetracycline (9.5 g over 4 days) is an alternative to penicillin in penicillin-allergic patients, but the failure rate of tetracycline therapy for gonococcal proctitis is three times that of intramuscular penicillin (see Chapter 116). The presence of ulceration suggests syphilis and herpes simplex, but does not rule out concurrent gonorrhea and chlamydial infection; polymicrobial infection is found in about 25% of patients.

Patients with *fecal incontinence* have achieved some benefit from *biofeedback* technique. However, only those who retain some degree of rectal sensation are candidates for biofeedback. The technique requires responding to the feeling of rectal fullness.

PATIENT EDUCATION

When poor or excessive personal hygiene, application of irritating agents, or neurotic behavior are responsible for symptoms, the relationship between rectal discomfort and precipitants should be explained so that the patient can take appropriate corrective action. Patients who obtain temporary relief of symptoms by applying a topical sensitizing agent may be reluctant to halt their medication if no other therapy is advised. Daily sitz baths can be prescribed in their place. Prevention through counseling is an important component of therapy in male homosexuals. Patients need to know that receptive anal sex with multiple partners carries a very high risk of intestinal infection and that they should certainly refrain from sexual activity if they become symptomatic.

A.H.G.

ANNOTATED BIBLIOGRAPHY

Alexander-Williams J: Causes and managements of anal irritation. Br Med J 287:1528, 1983 (*A good review with the British clinical approach.*)

Goodell SE, Quinn TC, Mkrtichian PA et al: Herpes simplex virus proctitis in homosexual men. N Engl J Med 308:868, 1983 (*Documents the high frequency and distinctive clinical presentation of this infection.*)

Jensen SL et al: Management of acute anal fissure. Br Med J 292:1167, 1986 (*Sitz baths and bran worked best.*)

Lebedeff DA, Hochman EB: Rectal gonorrhea in men: Diagnosis and treatment. Ann Intern Med 92:463, 1980 (*A prospective study of 1200 men detailing the clinical presentation, utility of Gram stain and culture, and response to therapy.*)

Lieberman DA: Common anorectal disorders. Ann Intern Med 101:837, 1984 (*A superb review with 107 references.*)

Owen WF: Sexually transmitted disease and traumatic problems in homosexual men. Ann Intern Med 92:805, 1980 (*A good review of the multitude of problems faced by homosexual men practicing receptive anal intercourse; 60 references.*)

Quinn TC, Goodell SC, Mkrtichian E: Chlamydia trachomatis proctitis. N Engl J Med 305:195, 1981 (*C. trachomatis of LGV immunotypes is associated with severe acute proctitis that mimics Crohn's disease.*)

Quinn TC, Stamm WE, Goodell SE et al: The polymicrobial origin of intestinal infections in homosexual men. N Engl J Med 309:576, 1983 (*An important paper documenting the polymicrobial nature of intestinal infection in this population. The authors detail three major types of clinical presentations and suggest a diagnostic and therapeutic approach to each.*)

Quinn TC, Goodell SE, Fennell C et al: Infections with Campylobacter jejuni and Campylobacter-like organisms in homosexual men. Ann Intern Med 101:187, 1984 (*Describes the clinical presentation of infection with this class of organisms; about 25% of symptomatic patients were infected with the organism.*)

Ramanujmps PRA, Sad ML, Abcarian H et al: Perianal abscesses and fistulas: A study of 10,023 patients. Dis Colon Rectum 27:595, 1984 (*Largest available series.*)

Smith LE, Henrich SD, McCullah RD: Etiology and treatment of pruritus ani. Dis Colon Rectum 25:358, 1982 (*Practical article on mundane but important issue.*)

Wald A: Biofeedback therapy for fecal incontinence. Ann Intern Med 95:146, 1981 (*The technique proved helpful in those who retain some degree of rectal sensation.*)

62

Evaluation of Jaundice

JAMES M. RICHTER, M.D.

The onset of jaundice usually prompts the patient or his family to seek medical attention. When associated symptoms are minimal, the patient is likely to present on an ambulatory basis, concerned about hepatitis or cancer. The primary physician needs to distinguish between jaundice due to hepatocellular dysfunction and that resulting from biliary tract obstruction; the former can be managed medically, but the latter requires direct intervention to relieve the obstruction. More specific determination of etiology is a secondary task that is less important to initial decision making. Effective clinical assessment necessitates familiarity with the mechanisms and clinical presentations of jaundice as well as the indications for and limitations of the noninvasive diagnostic studies available in the outpatient setting.

PATHOPHYSIOLOGY AND CLINICAL PRESENTATION

The mechanisms responsible for jaundice include excess bilirubin production, decreased hepatic uptake, impaired conjugation, intrahepatic cholestasis, extrahepatic obstruction, and hepatocellular injury. Clinically, jaundice becomes noticeable when the serum bilirubin reaches 2.0 to 2.5 mg per 100 ml. The yellow hue may be mimicked by carotenemia, but in the latter there is no scleral icterus. Deeply jaundiced patients often demonstrate a greenish tinge resulting from the oxidation of bilirubin to biliverdin.

Excess bilirubin production results from accelerated red cell destruction. Occasionally, markedly ineffective erythropoiesis may be responsible. The excessive amounts of hemoglobin and resultant bilirubin released into the bloodstream overwhelm the normal liver's capacity for uptake, and an unconjugated hyperbilirubinemia ensues. Total bilirubin rises as a result of the increased indirect fraction. All tests of hepatocellular function are normal (as are urine and stool appearances). Symptoms, signs, and laboratory tests point to hemolysis or ineffective erythropoiesis (see Chapter 78).

Decreased uptake and conjugation are other mechanisms of unconjugated hyperbilirubinemia. The only evidence of hepatocellular dysfunction is an increase in unconjugated bilirubin. Frequently there is a concurrent, acquired illness such as an infection, cardiac disease, or cancer. Hereditary conditions, such as Gilbert's and Crigler–Najjar syndromes are often responsible. *Gilbert's syndrome* is the most common cause. It is a benign disorder that produces recurrent self-limited episodes of mild jaundice. Typically, the unconjugated

fraction rises to no more than 1.5 to 3.0 mg per 100 ml. In Gilbert's syndrome, fasting and minor illness can precipitate jaundice.

Intrahepatic cholestasis may occur at a number of levels: intracellularly (*e.g.,* hepatitis), at the canalicular level (when estrogen-induced), at the ductule (phenothiazine exposure), at the septal ducts (primary biliary cirrhosis), and at the intralobular ducts (cholangiocarcinoma). Regardless of site, there are similarities in presentation. Jaundice comes on gradually, the patient feels well, and weight loss is slow; pruritus is common. The liver is large, smooth, and nontender; it may be firm but not rocky hard. Splenomegaly is unlikely except in primary biliary cirrhosis. Stools are pale and steatorrhea is present in severe cases. There is a hyperbilirubinemia, predominantly of the conjugated fraction, with marked alkaline phosphatase elevation, mild transaminase rise, and normal serum albumin. Urine is dark and positive for bilirubin. Prothrombin time may be prolonged due to malabsorption but is reversible by vitamin K injection.

Extrahepatic obstruction occurs when stone, stricture, or tumor block the flow of bile within the extrahepatic biliary tree. A history of gallstones, biliary tract surgery, or prior malignancy may be elicited. The gallbladder is sometimes palpable, especially when there is gradual development of obstruction allowing time for painless dilatation of the biliary tree. Sudden onset with pain results from passage of a stone that becomes wedged into the common duct; fever and sepsis may follow shortly thereafter, indicating cholangitis. Weight loss is a nonspecific finding, but when marked and accompanied by jaundice, it suggests carcinoma of the head of the pancreas or metastatic disease obstructing the common duct. Extrahepatic obstruction and intrahepatic cholestasis may be identical in presentation. The liver is usually enlarged; tenderness is minimal unless cholangitis or rapid distention occurs. A rock-hard mass strongly points to malignancy. As in intrehepatic cholestasis, conjugated bilirubin exhibits the greatest rise in association with a high serum alkaline phosphatase and a mild to moderate increase in the transaminase level. Any prolongation of prothrombin time is at least partially reversible with parenteral vitamin K. Urine is dark because of the conjugated bilirubinuria. Stools are pale from absence of bile.

Hepatocellular disease is typified by hepatitis, with prodromal symptoms of anorexia, nausea, abdominal pain, and malaise preceding jaundice (see Chapters 52 and 70). Hepatic tenderness and some hepatomegaly are common, but there is usually less liver enlargement than with obstruction. There may be ecchymoses. Transaminases may reach dramatic levels, except in cases of non-A, non-B and alcoholic hepatitis, in which the rise is no more than five times normal. The alkaline phosphatase rises modestly to two to four times above the baseline. Urine is dark, stools are pale. There may be evidence of decreased protein synthesis. The prothrombin time is the first measure of synthetic function to become abnormal, because the half-lives of the clotting factors made in the liver are less than 7 days. If synthetic function remains depressed beyond 2 weeks, the serum albumin begins to fall. Chronic hepatocellular disease may lead to fibrosis and cirrhosis with portal hypertension, peripheral edema, ascites, gynecomastia, testicular atrophy, bleeding, and encephalopathy (see Chapter 71).

DIFFERENTIAL DIAGNOSIS

The causes of jaundice are extensive but can be grouped according to major pathophysiologic mechanisms and type of hyperbilirubinemia (conjugated or unconjugated) (Table 62-1). It is important to recognize that more than one mechanism can be operating in a given case. The vast majority of cases are due to obstruction, intrahepatic cholestasis, or hepatocellular injury. In young patients, hepatitis predominates. In the elderly, stones and tumor are often responsible. Drugs account for many cases of intrahepatic cholestasis, and often mimic extrahepatic etiologies.

WORKUP

History and *physical examination* often provide a diagnosis or at least indicate whether the underlying pathophysiology is hepatocellular injury or biliary obstruction. In a study of 61 cases of jaundice documented by liver biopsy, history and physical examination alone correctly identified 70% of viral hepatitis cases, 80% of cirrhosis cases, and 77% of those with obstructive jaundice. *Key historical items* found useful in this study for descriminating among etiologies included presence of abdominal pain (indicative of obstruction) and history of alcoholism, exposure to hepatitis, and flulike onset (all suggestive of a hepatocellular etiology). Of little

Table 62-1. Differential Diagnosis of Jaundice
by Pathophysiologic Mechanisms

A. Unconjugated Hyperbilirubinemias (urine negative for bilirubin)
  1. Increased bilirubin production
  2. Decreased hepatic uptake of bilirubin
  3. Decreased conjugation
B. Conjugated Hyperbilirubinemias (urine positive for bilirubin)
  1. Hepatocellular disease
  2. Intrahepatic cholestasis
  3. Extrahepatic obstruction

descriminant value were history of weight loss, pruritus, nausea, vomiting, and distaste for tobacco. Dark urine and pale stools confirm a conjugated hyperbilirubinemia, but do not distinguish between hepatic and obstructive disease. Absence of abdominal pain does not rule out obstruction, especially that which develops slowly from tumor growth or primary biliary cirrhosis. History should also be checked for other hepatocellular disease risk factors (*e.g.,* travel to an area endemic for hepatitis, raw shellfish consumption, intravenous drug abuse, taking of potentially hepatotoxic drugs, etc.). History of gallstones, previous biliary tract surgery, and high fever point toward an obstructive cause. Family history of episodic jaundice in the setting of an intercurrent illness is consistent with Gilbert's disease. Intrahepatic cholestasis is a consideration if the patient reports use of estrogens, phenothiazines, and other drugs that can cause cholestasis.

Physical Examination. Findings that favor a diagnosis of hepatocellular disease include a small liver, signs of portal hypertension (ascites, splenomegaly, prominent abdominal venous pattern), asterixis, peripheral edema (from hypoalbuminemia), spider angiomata, gynecomastia, and palmar erythema. Mild to moderate hepatic enlargement and mild tenderness to punch are also consistent with hepatocellular disease, especially that due to acute hepatitis. A palpable gallbladder (Courvosier's sign) suggests malignant obstruction of the common bile duct. Marked hepatic enlargement (6 cm or more below the inferior costal margin) occurs with both extrahepatic obstruction and metastatic cancer to the liver. If obstruction is acute in onset, there may be some associated guarding, rebound tenderness, and fever. The finding of ecchymoses is consistent with both obstructive and hepatocellular mechanisms. The same is true for detection of pale stools and dark urine.

Laboratory Investigation can be utilized to identify the predominant pathophysiology and to assess severity, especially when history and physical findings are nondiagnostic. Testing begins with a check of the *urine for bilirubin.* Since only conjugated bilirubin appears in the urine, its presence indicates a conjugated hyperbilirubinemia and the possibility of cholestasis, obstruction, or hepatocellular injury; its absence argues for excess bilirubin production, decreased uptake, and impaired conjugation. Determinations of *direct* and *indirect serum bilirubin* levels quantitatively confirm urinary findings and indicate disease severity.

An elevation predominantly of the unconjugated bilirubin fraction and a negative urinary bilirubin should initiate a search for hemolysis (see Chapter 77), ineffective erythropoiesis, hereditary causes of jaundice, and concurrent systemic illness. Standard "liver function tests" add little to the assessment of unconjugated hyperbilirubinemia; they are normal or very mildly and nonspecifically elevated.

Conjugated hyperbilirubinemia and a positive urine necessitate a check of the *transaminase, alkaline phosphatase, prothrombin time,* and *serum albumin.* Mechanical obstruction and intrahepatic cholestasis are characterized by marked rises in *alkaline phosphatase* (greater than four to five times normal) and modest elevations in *transaminases* (two to three times normal). Hepatocellular disease characteristically causes a proportionately far greater rise in serum transaminase levels than in alkaline phosphatase concentrations. Two exceptions are non-A, non-B hepatitis and alcoholic hepatitis; transaminases are often only mildly elevated (no more than two to three times the upper limits of normal).

Unfortunately, not all conditions in which the alkaline phosphatase is markedly elevated have an obstructive pathophysiology. A cholestatic picture occasionally occurs in some cases of hepatocellular injury, such as with viral, alcoholic, and drug-induced forms of hepatitis. However, a low-alkaline phosphatase (under 50 international units per 100 ml) is rarely seen in the presence of extrahepatic obstruction.

Further separation of hepatocellular disease from cholestatic and obstructive conditions can be attempted by studying measures of liver synthetic function. A prolonged *prothrombin time* unresponsive to parenteral vitamin K is strongly suggestive of hepatocellular failure. Cholestasis and obstruction may also produce prolongation of the protime, but it can be reversed by vitamin K. *Serum albumin* levels fall when substantial hepatocellular injury has occurred and synthetic capacity has been suppressed for a few weeks. Interpretation of the albumin level requires consideration of dietary intake and sources of possible protein loss.

In most instances, hepatocellular disease can be distinguished from cholestasis and extrahepatic obstruction on the basis of clinical data, liver function tests, and response to vitamin K.* On the other hand, cholestasis and obstruction may be indistinguishable without further testing. The distinction is critical to management, because mechanical obstruction requires direct surgical, endoscopic, or radiologic intervention to restore bile flow.

Clinical evaluation and liver function tests have a sensitivity of 90% for detection of obstruction, but a predictive value of only 75%; 25% of patients suspected on clinical grounds to have obstruction turn out to have hepatocellular disease with a cholestatic picture. Thus, the clinical impression of obstruction must be confirmed by imaging techniques. When the clinical likelihood of obstruction is low, imaging studies are generally unnecessary.

Study of the biliary tree is necessary to differentiate intrahepatic cholestasis from extrahepatic obstruction and can be achieved by ultrasonography, computed tomography (CT), percutaneous transhepatic cholangiography, and endoscopic retrograde cannulation. Intravenous cholangiography has

been replaced by ultrasonography and CT as the primary noninvasive means of detecting biliary tree obstruction; its disadvantages included a high rate of false negatives and many allergic reactions to the iodinated dye that was used. Moreover, it fails to visualize the biliary tree once the bilirubin rises above 3 mg%.

Ultrasonography has emerged as the noninvasive study of choice in the evaluation of jaundice. Specificity is better than 90%. Sensitivity ranges from 47% to 90%, depending on the duration and degree of bile duct obstruction. Cases of early, acute, or intermittent obstruction may be missed unless ultrasound study is repeated after the ducts have had a few days to dilate. False positives may occur from ductal dilatation that persists after cholecystectomy or relief of obstruction. In about half of cases, ultrasonography cannot indicate the level of obstruction, nor is it particularly good at detecting the cause of the obstruction, unless it is due to a mass in the head of the pancreas. Stones in the common duct are frequently missed.

Computed tomography is similar to ultrasonography in sensitivity, specificity, and predictive value for diagnosis of obstructive jaundice. It has many of the same shortcomings and also the added disadvantages of greater expense and radiation exposure. As such, it is a second-choice test after ultrasonography, with a better ability to detect the level of obstruction. However, if surgical intervention is being considered, more definitive anatomic information, as provided by cholangiography, is often necessary.

If obstruction is strongly suspected on clinical grounds (even if the ultrasonography or CT is negative) or if additional anatomic detail is required for planning treatment, *percutaneous transhepatic cholangiography* or *retrograde cannulation* of the common bile duct is indicated. Both procedures are relatively safe, have similar complication rates, have similar rates of visualization, and provide equally diagnostic information. The predictive value for demonstration of obstruction is 99% and grounds for direct intervention. A negative study all but rules out obstruction, although there are exceptions. Some authorities suggest that proceeding directly to one of these procedures and skipping noninvasive study is indicated when there is very strong clinical suspicion of obstruction.

Transhepatic cholangiography is technically simple in patients with dilated intrahepatic ducts; however, 3% to 10% of patients experience cholangitis, hemorrhage, or bile leakage. Retrograde cholangiography is more difficult but allows examination of the ampulla and pancreas and has a slightly lower incidence of serious complications. For patients who may have a retained common duct stone after cholecystectomy, the opportunity to perform an endoscopic papillotomy makes the retrograde cholangiogram advantageous. Techniques have been developed for draining an obstructed biliary tract either endoscopically or transhepatically. Overall, both procedures are valuable diagnostically and have therapeutic

---

* Instances of anaphylaxis have been reported with intravenous use of vitamin K. Intramuscular or subcutaneous administration is preferable.

uses as well; final selection is based on the clinical circumstance as well as on local availability and expertise. Selection should be made in consultation with a surgeon, radiologist, or gastroenterologist experienced in evaluating obstructive jaundice.

Other studies deserve comment, more for their limited usefulness than because they are indicated in evaluation of jaundice. *Plain films* of the abdomen and *upper GI series* rarely provide diagnostic information. *Hepatobiliary scintigraphy* is better suited for diagnosis of cholecystitis; it provides poor anatomic resolution and often cannot distinguish between intrahepatic cholestasis and extrahepatic obstruction. *Liver biopsy* is sometimes important for determining the cause of hepatocellular injury (see Chapter 70), but is unwise in the setting of possible obstructive jaundice because it can lead to bile peritonitis. Once obstruction is ruled out or relieved, biopsy might be a consideration if there still is concern about hepatocellular disease (*e.g.,* biliary cirrhosis).

INDICATIONS FOR ADMISSION, CONSULTATION, AND REFERRAL

Most patients with jaundice will turn out to have acute viral hepatitis and can be managed on an ambulatory basis, unless they are unable to maintain their hydration or begin to show evidence of severe hepatocellular failure (see Chapter 71). Admission is mandatory when jaundice is complicated by fever and peritoneal signs indicative of cholangitis. Intravenous antibiotics and prompt surgical consultation are required.

As noted earlier, when there is clinical suspicion of extrahepatic obstruction, consultation with a gastroenterologist, surgeon, or radiologist experienced in the evaluation of jaundice can be very useful, especially when there is difficulty differentiating between intrahepatic cholestasis and extrahepatic obstruction.

When hepatocellular disease is suspect, and there is evidence of hepatic failure, portal hypertension or encephalopathy, or when jaundice persists longer than 3 months, liver biopsy may be indicated for definitive diagnosis. Consultation should be sought with a gastroenterologist familiar with liver disease and needle biopsy techniques.

SYMPTOMATIC RELIEF

Mild jaundice in itself is innocuous, but more marked elevations in bilirubin may produce considerable pruritus. Presumably the mechanism involves bile salt deposition in the skin, although recent evidence refutes this view. Cholestyramine has been used successfully to treat pruritus and is worth a try in patients who are quite uncomfortable. One 9-g packet of the powder containing 4 g of cholestyramine resin is mixed in orange juice or applesauce and taken three times a day. Absorption of fat-soluble vitamins may be impaired by cholestyramine, and oral or parenteral supplements of vitamins A, D, and K can be prescribed. Absorption of drugs may also be interfered with; drugs should be taken at least 1 hour before cholestyramine. Constipation or diarrhea are minor common side-effects.

ANNOTATED BIBLIOGRAPHY

Datta D, Sherlock S: Cholestyramine for long term relief of the pruritus complicating intrahepatic cholestasis. Gastroenterology 50: 323, 1966 (*Cholestyramine is effective; 4 to 7 days of therapy are required before relief is obtained.*)

Felsher B, Rickard D, Redeker A: The reciprocal relation between caloric intake and the degree of hyperbilirubinemia in Gilbert's syndrome. N Engl J Med 283:170, 1970 (*An increase in unconjugated bilirubin occurred with fasting or low caloric intake—approximately 400 calories.*)

Mueller PR, van Sonnenberg E, Simenone JF: Fine needle transhepatic cholangiography. Ann Intern Med 97:567, 1982 (*The radiologist's view of this technique and its central role in the evaluation of biliary obstruction.*)

Lapis J, Orlando R, Mittelstaedt C et al: Ultrasonography in the diagnosis of obstructive jaundice. Ann Intern Med 89:61, 1978 (*In a study of 47 cases of with cholestatic jaundice, there were no false positives. The false-negative rate was 6% when bilirubin greater than 20 mg% and 53% when bilirubin less than 10 mg%.*)

Levine R, Klatskin G: Unconjugated hyperbilirubinemia in the absence of overt hemolysis. Am J Med 36:541, 1964 (*A series of 366 patients with a high proportion traceable to a concurrent illness rather than a hereditary condition. Cardiac disease, infection, cancer, and inflammatory bowel disease accounted for more than 50%.*)

O'Connor KW, Snodgrass PJ, Swonder JE et al: A blinded prospective study comparing four current noninvasive approaches in the differential diagnosis of medical versus surgical jaundice. Gastroenterology 84:1498, 1983 (*A comparison of clinical evaluation, ultrasonography, computed tomography, and biliary scanning in the evaluation of jaundice demonstrating the importance and accuracy of clinical evaluation.*)

Richter JM, Silverstein MD, Schapiro RH: Suspected obstructive jaundice: A decision analysis of diagnostic strategies. Ann Intern Med 99:46, 1983 (*A comparison of comprehensive diagnostic strategies for the investigation of suspected obstructive jaundice.*)

Scharschmidt BF, Goldberg HI, Schmid R: Approach to the patient with cholestatic jaundice. N Engl J Med 308:1515, 1983 (*Good review of tests available for workup of obstructive jaundice.*)

Schenker S, Balint J, Schiff L: Differential diagnosis of jaundice: Report of a prospective study of 61 proved cases. Am J Dig Dis 7: 449, 1962 (*A study of the merits of clinical features and laboratory tests in the differential diagnosis of jaundice.*)

63

Approach to the Patient
with an External Hernia

MICHAEL N. MARGOLIES, M.D.

Abdominal hernias are exceedingly common, often causing occupational disabilities and posing the risk of incarceration and strangulation of bowel. Fortunately, adequate evaluation can usually be performed in the office by means of history and physical examination. The primary physician must distinguish between patients who require surgical referral and those who may be managed expectantly.

PATHOPHYSIOLOGY AND CLINICAL PRESENTATION

A hernia is a defect in the normal musculofascial continuity of the abdominal wall that permits the egress of structures not normally passing through the parietes. In general, the significant feature of hernia is not the size of the protrusion or the sac, but the size and rigidity of the defect in the abdominal wall. Fixation and rigidity of the hernial ring are the features that lead to incarceration and strangulation. The distinction between congenital and acquired hernia is not often clear, as many hernias that appear following trauma or straining represent a congenital predisposition, such as indirect inguinal hernia in the adult. This distinction has little bearing on management, although it may make considerable difference to the patient who may be compensated if the hernia can be attributed to trauma at work. Some of these hernias are incidental to, and antedate, the perceived injury.

Disorders resulting in increased intra-abdominal pressure may contribute to the appearance of a hernia and affect the postoperative management as well. For example, chronic cough due to cigarette smoking or bronchitis can precipitate or worsen herniation; the same is true of symptomatic prostatism.

The symptoms of an uncomplicated or reducible external hernia are related not to its size but to the degree of pressure on its contents. Patients with large scrotal hernias containing much intestine may have few symptoms other than a dragging sensation. A mass appears upon standing, which reduces when the patient is supine. Pain may be intermittent, disappearing when the hernia is reduced. Patients with small hernias containing an entrapped knuckle of bowel may have rather severe pain and nausea. Many patients with femoral, umbilical, or epigastric hernias may be entirely unaware of their existence.

An *irreducible* or *incarcerated hernia* is one in which the contents cannot be replaced into the abdomen. Here the mass remains palpable with the patient relaxed and in the supine position. A *strangulated hernia* is an irreducible one in which the blood supply to the entrapped bowel loop has been compromised, resulting in small bowel obstruction and infarction. These patients complain of colicky abdominal pain, nausea, and vomiting and show signs of small bowel obstruction with distention, tympany, and hyperperistalsis. In addition, careful examination demonstrates a tender, irreducible groin or ventral hernia.

Indirect inguinal hernias, which account for one half of all hernias in adults, pass through the internal abdominal inguinal ring along the spermatic cord through the inguinal canal, and exit through the external inguinal ring. In the male, these can descend into the scrotum. *Direct inguinal hernias* pass through the posterior inguinal wall medial to the inferior epigastric vessels, through Hesselbach's triangle. *Femoral hernias* pass through the femoral canal inferior to the inguinal ligament and become subcutaneous in the fossa ovalis. It is often difficult to distinguish between these three forms, especially when there is incarceration and the sac is large.

Indirect inguinal hernias are eight to ten times more common in men than in women, whereas femoral hernias are three to five times more common in women than in men. Nevertheless, the most common hernia in women is the indirect inguinal type. The diagnosis is less often made in women because physical examination of the external inguinal ring is more difficult. Direct hernias increase in incidence with advancing age and are the least likely of the external hernias to incarcerate or strangulate. Strangulation is common in femoral hernias.

The majority of patients with strangulated inguinal hernias are aware of the hernia prior to strangulation. In contrast, nearly half of those with strangulated femoral hernias are unaware of the hernia prior to strangulation. In addition, groin pain and tenderness are absent in a significant percentage of cases of strangulated femoral hernia.

The commonly encountered ventral hernias include umbilical, epigastric, and incisional varieties. Ventral hernias are often more obvious with the patient standing. *Umbilical hernias* pass through the umbilical ring and represent failure of the ring to obliterate after birth. In the infant, these often close spontaneously within the first 2 years of life. In the adult, they are more common in women and are associated with obesity, multiparity, and cirrhosis with ascites. Umbilical hernias are often missed because they are obscured by subcutaneous fat. There is a high risk of incarceration and strangulation and a greater mortality than with inguinal hernia because large bowel is frequently entrapped.

Incisional hernias are those that develop in the scar of a previous laparotomy or in a drain site. They are associated with a previous postoperative wound infection, dehiscence, malnutrition, obesity, and smoking. They are more common in vertical than in transverse scars. Incisional hernias often have multiple defects and several rings. They are frequently irreducible or only partially reducible because of adhesions within the sac. Patients with very large incisional hernias may be remarkably free from symptoms of intestinal obstruction, although incarceration is common; strangulation is relatively uncommon because of the usually large size of the defects.

Epigastric hernias occur through the linea alba between the xiphoid process and the umbilicus. They may be quite difficult to detect in the obese patient and must be looked for in patients with epigastric pain. Incarcerated epigastric hernia may produce symptoms that mimic peptic ulcer disease or biliary colic.

DIFFERENTIAL DIAGNOSIS

Recognizing a hernia usually presents little difficulty, although distinguishing one type of inguinal hernia from another can sometimes be complicated. Differential diagnosis of an entrapped femoral hernia includes not only inguinal hernia but femoral lymphadenopathy, saphenous varix, psoas abscess, and hydrocele. On occasion it is impossible to differentiate an incarcerated femoral hernia from a single enlarged femoral lymph node (the lymph node of Cloquet).

EVALUATION

Diagnosis and evaluation of external hernias require no more than a brief history and careful physical examination; laboratory and radiologic studies are unnecessary unless major complications have resulted.

History. The patient is questioned about groin pain, swelling, ability to reduce the hernia, circumstances of onset, and aggravating and alleviating factors, such as exacerbation on standing, straining, or coughing. Acute onset of colicky abdominal pain, nausea, and vomiting suggest entrapment and strangulation in a patient with a known hernia.

Physical examination is directed toward distinguishing among (1) hernias that are uncomplicated and require no therapy, (2) those that can be repaired electively, and (3) those in which emergency surgery is the safest course. The physical examination is also important in distinguishing the anatomic type of hernia, because prognosis and likelihood of incarceration and strangulation differ among the various types. The patient with a reducible hernia should be examined in both the supine and standing positions. Inspection is often as important as palpation for detection. Examination should

include a Valsalva maneuver to increase intra-abdominal pressure. In the male, small inguinal hernias are looked for by invaginating the scrotal skin while the patient is standing. To detect ventral hernias, the patient should be supine and then asked to lift the head from the examining table and to bear down to tense the abdominal wall.

If a hernia is irreducible, the physician should look for local tenderness, discoloration, edema, fever, and signs of small bowel obstruction. It is often difficult to distinguish a simple incarceration from early strangulation; for this reason these two lesions are managed identically by immediate referral to a surgeon. Surgical exploration is the only way to be certain that no compromised bowel is trapped in the hernia sac. Conversely, when signs of small bowel obstruction are present, it is essential to examine thoroughly for a strangulated femoral hernia because groin pain and tenderness may be absent.

A few conditions are believed to have more than a chance association with hernias, and some argue that they should be screened for. Whether or not the adult patient with a recent hernia is more likely to have an occult carcinoma of the colon remains a source of controversy. It had been suggested that patients undergo routine sigmoidoscopic examination and barium enema. However, if the patient reports no change in bowel habits and the stools are repeatedly guaiac-negative, it is probably unnecessary to submit him to more extensive investigation for occult malignancy. Symptoms and signs of prostatism are frequently present in the elderly male with hernia and may require relief prior to herniorrhaphy. The entire abdomen ought to be examined for masses, hepatomegaly, and ascites, which are sometimes associated with hernia formation.

PRINCIPLES OF MANAGEMENT AND INDICATIONS FOR REFERRAL

Patients with *symptomatic reducible inguinal hernias* should undergo elective repair for relief of symptoms and prevention of strangulation. Reduction by means of a truss is unsatisfactory even in patients with relative medical contraindications to surgery. Moreover, surgical repair can be done under local anesthesia in the high-risk patient.

In patients with a *nontender incarcerated inguinal hernia* of recent onset, but without signs of inflammation or bowel obstruction, it may be safe to attempt gentle reduction ("taxis"). This is best accomplished with the patient supine and the hips and knees flexed. If gentle pressure over the hernial sac fails to reduce the mass further, efforts should be abandoned and the patient referred for surgery forthwith. Often the patient has more experience in reducing his own hernia than the physician. Patients with evidence of strangulated groin hernias should be subjected to immediate operation regardless of medical contraindications; if untreated, death will result from bowel necrosis.

Patients with *reducible femoral hernias* should undergo prompt elective repair because of the high incidence of strangulation. Whenever there is a question of an incarcerated femoral hernia, it is safest to proceed immediately with surgical exploration.

In *umbilical hernias,* surgery is unnecessary if on physical examination there is a small asymptomatic fascial defect without protrusion. When herniation is detected, however, umbilical defects should be repaired, as there is a high risk of incarceration and strangulation. The danger of strangulation is compounded by the greater likelihood of colonic entrapment with a resultant higher mortality rate than in hernias in which small intestine is strangulated. Therefore, all incarcerated umbilical hernias should be managed as if they were strangulated. Elective umbilical herniorrhaphy should be avoided in patients with ascites; instead, efforts should be directed toward reducing the ascites (see Chapter 71). The problem in patients with cirrhosis and ascites is made more difficult when the skin overlying the sac thins out and poses the risk of rupture.

Patients with small neck *incisional hernias* or tender incarceration should undergo repair on an urgent basis. Patients who have trophic changes or ulceration in the skin overlying incisional hernias are also candidates for urgent surgery. In some instances, cellulitis of the skin overlying the hernia sac occurs and is difficult to distinguish from strangulation of the contents of the sac. Management of large incarcerated incisional hernias that occur in the abdomen in very obese patients is a particular problem. Major efforts should be directed toward weight reduction before repair if it is possible to procrastinate. If there is doubt, however, as to the presence of intestinal obstruction or viability of the contents of the sac, the advice of a surgeon should be sought promptly.

Factors contributing to hernia formation should be corrected if possible. Prostatectomy is occasionally required following repair of hernia, and the patient with symptoms of prostatic obstruction should be advised of this possibility. Patients with chronic bronchitis and emphysema, or with chronic cough due to cigarette smoking, should be urged to stop smoking promptly to diminish symptoms caused by the hernia and to decrease the possibility of postoperative complications.

PATIENT EDUCATION

Patients who are to be managed conservatively must be taught to watch for signs of complications. It is the responsibility of the physician to instruct the patient in the symptoms of incarceration and strangulation and in the urgency of seeking help should they occur. If the patient is deemed incompetent to make such observations and to obtain help promptly, a strong case can be made for proceeding with surgery. Patients scheduled for elective surgery also require instruction, because incarceration occasionally occurs prior to the planned operation.

Many patients with asymptomatic or mildly symtomatic reducible hernias will be reluctant to undergo surgery because their symptoms are minimal. If they fall into the high-risk group, for example, femoral or small neck incisional hernias, they should be informed of the strong likelihood of strangulation and the minuscule morbidity and mortality associated with surgery.

ANNOTATED BIBLIOGRAPHY

Anson B, McVay CB: *Surgical Anatomy,* 5th ed. vol I, pp 461. Philadelphia, WB Saunders, 1971 (*Extensive description of the anatomy of the inguinal and femoral regions.*)

Brendel TH, Kirsh I: Lack of association between inguinal hernia and carcinoma of the colon. N Engl J Med 284:369, 1971 (*One view of the relationship of hernia to colon carcinoma.*)

Clain A: Hamilton Bailey's Physical Signs in Clinical Surgery, 15th ed. Chicago: Year Book Medical Publishers, 1973 (*Details the differential diagnosis of hernia based on physical signs.*)

Dunphy JE, Botsford TW: Physical Examination of the Surgical Patient: An Introduction to Clinical Surgery, 4th ed, p 117. Philadelphia, WB Saunders, 1975 (*A concise, well-illustrated approach to physical examination of patients with hernia.*)

64
Management of Peptic Ulcer Disease

Peptic ulcer disease continues to be a major source of morbidity and a health problem of substantial importance. Prevalence estimates for active disease range from 1.5% to 2.0%. About 350,000 new cases are diagnosed annually. Five percent to 10% of the population will experience peptic ulcer disease in their lifetime. Males outnumber females by 2 to 1. Duodenal ulcers account for 80% of cases. In men, peak prevalence of duodenal ulcer occurs between the ages of 45 and 54; for gastric ulcer, peak occurs between the ages of 55 and 64. For unexplained reasons, the frequency of peptic ulcer disease is declining.

Developments in pharmacologic therapy have augmented the medical treatment of ulcer disease. The need for surgery has decreased markedly. Of particular significance are the more potent antacids, the histamine H_2-receptor antagonists, and surface-active agents such as sucralfate. The goals of management are to alleviate pain, promote healing, limit complications, and prevent recurrences while minimizing the costs and side-effects of treatment. The primary care physician must be well versed in the medical management of peptic ulcer disease, capable of designing an effective ulcer regimen and identifying patients who require referral for endoscopy or surgery.

PATHOPHYSIOLOGY AND CLINICAL PRESENTATION

Most peptic ulcers arise in the stomach and duodenum, areas exposed to gastric acid and pepsin. Although the precise mechanisms of ulcer formation remain incompletely understood, the process appears to involve the interplay of acid production, pepsin secretion, and mucosal defense mechanisms.

Excess acid production is the hallmark of duodenal ulcer disease, with significant increases noted in basal and peak acid outputs, parietal and chief cell masses, and responses to food and hormonal stimulation. Some patients demonstrate *rapid gastric emptying,* which raises the acid exposure of the proximal duodenum. *Pepsin* secretion is also elevated in duodenal ulcer disease. Gastric acid production is relatively normal in patients with gastric ulcers.

An appreciation for the importance of *mucosal defense mechanisms* is emerging. Major determinants of mucosal integrity include mucus secretion, bicarbonate production, mucosal blood flow, and cellular repair mechanisms. *Prostaglandins* have been found closely linked to mucus production, bicarbonate secretion, and repair. By helping to maintain a neutral *p*H and aqueous environment at the surface of the gastric epithelium, mucus and bicarbonate protect the mucosa from acid, pepsin, and other potentially injurious agents. *Compromise of the mucus barrier* may result from increased mucus degradation, decreased secretion or production of defective mucus. Bile acids, pepsin, pancreatic enzymes, and mechanical forces contribute to mucus degradation.

A host of psychological, dietary, pharmacologic, and hereditary factors have been implicated in causation or aggravation of ulcer disease. *Stress* has long been considered a key precipitant, a view supported by a higher incidence of chronic stress in ulcer patients than in controls, increased acid production in response to stress, and a more prolonged course and poorer prognosis in those with chronic severe anxiety. In addition, psychological studies have found that patients who develop ulcers view life stresses more negatively than do controls. Acid hypersecretion and ulcer formation have been observed in small-scale studies of patients undergoing severe emotional stress; with subsidence of stress, acid secretion falls and ulcers heal. Confirmation of these small-scale observations will strengthen the association between stress and ulcer disease.

Alcohol and *coffee* have also been implicated, but never definitively proven to be causative factors. Coffee, including decaffeinated forms, stimulates acid secretion, as do other caffeine-containing beverages. Beer is almost as potent a stimulant of acid secretion as gastrin. Epidemiologic evidence links *smoking* with ulcer disease. For example, cigarette smokers are twice as likely to develop ulcers as nonsmokers. Risk of gastric ulcer correlates with the number of cigarettes smoked, and those with ulcers show increased rates of smoking. Rates of recurrence are dramatically increased in those who smoke; healing is markedly slowed. Impaired prostaglandin production has been demonstrated in the gastric mucosa of smokers.

The contribution of *glucocorticosteroids* to ulcer formation has been debated ever since these agents first became available. Multiple randomized controlled trials have produced conflicting results, as have two major meta-analyses examining pooled data from such trials. The first analysis concluded that steroids did not cause ulcers unless they were administered for more than 30 days or in a total dose exceeding the equivalent of 1000 mg of prednisone. The second analysis, which was done 7 years later, included additional studies but excluded others; it found that the incidence of ulcers varied directly with steroid dosage and was significantly increased, even in patients treated for less than a month or receiving less than 1000 mg. Although the increase in risk was double that of patients not taking steroids, it remained low at about 2%. The debate continues. However, even if steroids do increase the chances of ulcer formation, the risk remains small.

Aspirin and other *nonsteroidal anti-inflammatory agents* cause superficial gastric erosions, though only unbuffered aspirin has been unequivocally proven to cause gastric erosions leading to ulceration. Whether or not the others cause chronic ulceration is unknown, but epidemiologic evidence points to a relationship between the use of these agents and gastric ulcers. Moreover, endoscopic study has shown significant mucosal injury from both plain and tablet forms of buffered aspirin, though not with enteric coated preparations, unless there is delayed gastric emptying. Injury is believed to be related, in part, to inhibition of prostaglandin synthesis.

Heredity plays some role. Parents, siblings, and children of ulcer patients have increased incidences of ulcer, and studies of twins show greater concordance (*i.e.,* both twins affected) among identical than among fraternal twins. Increased meal-stimulated gastrin release and pepsin secretion have been found to be hereditary traits among ulcer patients and their families.

Clinical Presentation. Peptic ulcers usually occur at or near mucosal transition zones, areas thought to be particularly vulnerable to the effects of acid, pepsin, bile, and pancreatic enzymes. Gastric ulcers are found in the atrium at the lesser curvature, near the junction of the acid-secreting parietal cells, and the antral mucosa. Duodenal ulcers arise mostly at the junction of the antrum and duodenum.

The clinical presentations of gastric and duodenal peptic ulcers are somewhat similar but rather nonspecific. Patients may present with pain, bleeding, or obstruction, or they may be symptom-free. Epigastric pain, relieved by antacids and occurring in clusters of daily symptoms for a few weeks separated by pain-free periods of months, is characteristic of peptic disease. Duodenal ulcer pain is classically relieved by food, absent before breakfast, and responsible for awakening the patient at night; it starts 2 to 3 hours after a meal. However, careful studies of patients with documented duodenal ulcers have shown that in some individuals pain is often worsened by meals, present before breakfast, and continuous rather than periodic. Gastric ulcer pain is more likely to be precipitated by food and often radiates from the epigastrium to the back or substernal region. It, too, can awaken the patient and be relieved by food. In both conditions, the pain may be dull, aching, gnawing, or burning in quality, consistent with its visceral quality.

Clinical Course. Since most patients receive some form of treatment, available data pertain to clinical course rather than true natural history. Studies done before aggressive use of antacids or histamine H2-receptor antagonists showed that most ulcers healed completely by 4 weeks, though large ones in the stomach could take up to 12 weeks. The majority of patients became pain-free within the first 4 weeks; however, there was little correlation between cessation of pain and healing of the ulcer. Recurrences were frequent. The 5-year recurrence rates ranged from 30% to 90%. Although it was rare for a patient to have more than two or three repeat gastric ulcers, multiple recurrences were not unusual for those with duodenal ulcers. There was no correlation between recurrence rate and ulcer size, duration of symptoms, or location. Recurrent ulcers healed just as rapidly and completely as original lesions. The rate of developing a major complication, such as hemorrhage, perforation, or obstruction was less than 1% per year. Bleeding was slightly more common from duodenal than from gastric ulcers and two to three times more common than perforation.

With the advent of newer medical therapies, the clinical course of peptic ulcer disease has improved. High-dose antacids, cimetidine, ranitidine, and sucralfate all speed the rate of healing for duodenal ulcers; cimetidine and ranitidine reduce the rate of recurrences. Antacids, cimetidine, and ranitidine hasten healing of gastric ulcers; ranitidine and cimetidine help to prevent recurrences. The effect of sucralfate on the clinical course of gastric ulcers is less well defined.

To date, there is no evidence that medical therapy prevents hemorrhage, perforation, or obstruction. Moreover, in controlled studies, medical treatments show little advantage over placebo for pain relief, in part because of a very strong placebo effect. Although prevention of ulcer recurrence has been demonstrated for the histamine H2-receptor antagonists, risk returns to its previous level once they are discontinued.

Surgical therapy has also affected the clinical course. Antrectomy lowers recurrence rates for duodenal ulcer to 5% per year; selective proximal gastric vagotomy also substantially lowers recurrences, although to a lesser extent (see below).

WORKUP

A presumptive diagnosis of acid-peptic disease can often be made on clinical grounds alone (see Chapter 53). As long as the risk of underlying gastric cancer is inconsequential (those less than 40 years of age) and there are no associated complications (*e.g.,* bleeding, perforation, or obstruction), a clinical suspicion of ulcer disease need not be confirmed by barium study or endoscopy to initiate therapy. Patients over the age of 40 are at greater risk of gastric cancer and should undergo either upper GI series or endoscopy to document the nature and location of the lesion when there is strong clinical suspicion of ulcer disease.

The *choice of diagnostic procedure* remains a subject of debate. Endoscopists correctly argue that gastroscopy is superior to barium study for detection of gastric ulcer and malignancy, especially since brushings and biopsy can be performed at the same time. Radiologists counter that by using air contrast techniques, they can approach the sensitivity of endoscopy with a procedure that is one third the cost, safer, and more comfortable for the patient. The issue remains unsettled.

A related diagnostic dilemma is what to do when barium study reveals a benign-appearing gastric ulcer. About 4% of all gastric ulcers prove to be malignant, with many manifesting radiologic signs of cancer. Radiologic criteria for malignancy include irregular shape, nodular base, absense of radiating gastric folds, folds that are blunted or stop before the ulcer, and rigidity of adjacent stomach. Ulcers in the fundus are at increased risk of being malignant; those within 1 cm of the pylorus are almost always benign. Using these criteria, sensitivity of barium study for detection of gastric malignancy is reported to be in the range of 80% to 85%, compared with 95% for endoscopy with biopsy and brushing. However, if all gastric ulcer patients are routinely subjected to endoscopy, it would cost tens of thousands of dollars to find a single case of cancer. Because the prognosis is not particularly good for patients with a malignant gastric ulcer (the 5-year survival is 25%–35%), the potential for benefit by adding endoscopy to every gastric ulcer patient's workup does not appear very great. A less costly alternative is to refer for endoscopy and biopsy only those patients with radiologically suspicious gastric ulcers and those with ulcers that fail to heal fully (see below). The literature should be followed for further cost-benefit studies.

PRINCIPLES OF THERAPY

The major objectives of therapy are to speed healing, reduce pain, and prevent complications and recurrences while minimizing the costs and side-effects of therapy. Although peptic ulcer disease represents a heterogeneous set of disorders, the overall approach to medical therapy centers on reducing gastric acidity and protecting the mucosal barrier. Antacids are employed to neutralize acid and histamine H_2-receptor antagonists to inhibit its secretion. Sucralfate is believed to form a protective coating over the injured mucosa, absorb pepsin, and inactivate bile acids. Under study are a host of additional therapies, ranging from prostaglandin analogues to colloidal bismuth preparations. Avoidance of substances and stresses that are potentially injurious to the gastric mucosa complement the therapeutic effort. Surgery remains an option for treatment of refractory disease and complications.

Duodenal Ulcer. The *choice of agent* is a matter of physician and patient preference. Antacids, histamine H_2-receptor antagonists (cimetidine and ranitidine), and sucralfate all speed the healing of duodenal ulcers. Antacids have the advantage of safety, since little is absorbed; however, compliance becomes a problem because of the need for frequent large doses. Costs are greatest for a ranitidine program, but the drug is well tolerated, convenient to use, and free of major adverse effects or important drug–drug interactions. Cimetidine remains a drug of proven efficacy with an excellent safety record; its main disadvantage is its effect on hepatic drug metabolism. Like antacids, sucralfate acts locally, but must be taken frequently. Many patients are treated with antacids plus an H_2-receptor antagonist; such combination therapy may be of benefit in severe cases.

The *duration of treatment* should be at least a full 4 weeks, the time needed for complete healing of duodenal ulcers in about 90% of patients. Resolution of pain cannot be used as a therapeutic endpoint; cessation of pain correlates poorly with completion of healing. Premature termination of therapy commonly occurs and increases the risk of symptomatic relapse. Patients who remain symptomatic after 4 weeks of therapy are likely to still have an unhealed ulcer; their treatment program should be extended for another 2 to 4 weeks. There is no need to change the program.

Failure to achieve pain relief after 8 weeks is an indication for documenting the ulcer's status and considering a *switch to another agent.* Some patients treated with cimetidine have benefitted from changing to ranitidine. Increasing the dosage of an agent is less effective than switching. *Adding a second agent* to the regimen may help. Antacids plus a histamine H_2-receptor antagonist may achieve better results than either alone; the combination of an H_2-receptor antagonist and sucralfate is worth a try if other combinations fail.

Although some authorities advocate endoscopic or radiologic *documentation of healing,* there are no studies showing this to be cost-effective in uncomplicated cases in which symptoms resolve within 4 weeks and do not recur. The need for documentation should be based on how it will affect clinical decision making. Persistence or recurrence of pain, symptoms of gastric outlet obstruction, and evidence of bleeding are among the indications for study.

Maintenance therapy is indicated for those with documented recurrences within 1 year, bleeding, or a concurrent condition necessitating use of anticoagulants (see Chapter 85). Maintenance programs with documented prophylactic efficacy include a single 150 mg dose of ranitidine given before bed and 300 mg of cimetidine given twice daily or 400 mg at bedtime. The efficacy of antacids for maintenance is unknown. Most authorities recommend continuing maintenance treatment for 1 year; the optimal duration of therapy remains unknown, as do the consequences of prolonged suppression of gastric acid production (see below). Although the relapse rate for medical maintenance therapy is ten times that of surgical therapy, most patients can be spared an operation. An alternative to daily maintenance therapy is empirical treatment of pain recurrences. The efficacy of this approach is yet to be determined, but it is used widely by patients.

Debate continues about the safety of chronically suppressing gastric acid production. There is concern that absense of acid will permit bacterial overgrowth, which in turn may lead to formation of the carcinogen nitrosamine. A once-daily ranitidine regimen allows sufficient acid secretion during a part of the day to suppress bacterial overgrowth.

Recurrences are closely linked to continuation of smoking and poor compliance with a maintenance regimen. Cessation of smoking is the first priority. If the patient has been on low-dose maintenance therapy when a recurrence develops, full-dose therapy should be initiated. Whether or not such patients benefit from switching to or adding a second agent is not known for sure, but this is worth trying. Refractory cases ought to be evaluated for *Zollinger–Ellison syndrome,* especially when there are multiple ulcers, occurrences in unusual places, marked abdominal pain, or a secretory diarrhea (due to hypergastrinemia). Such patients often manifest evidence of multiple endocrine adenomatosis (concurrent hyperparathyroidism, pituitary tumors, etc.) A fasting serum gastrin level in excess of 500 pg/ml in the presence of acid hypersecretion is diagnostic.

Gastric Ulcer. The principles guiding treatment are similar to those for duodenal ulcer. Antacids, H_2-receptor antagonists, and sucralfate all speed the rate of healing. The necessary antacid dose is about half that required in duodenal ulcer disease. Duration of therapy also differs, because healing often takes longer and is a function of ulcer size. Larger ulcers can take up to 12 weeks; only 50% heal by 4 weeks. Ulcers that fail to heal completely need to be evaluated endoscopically, with brushings and biopsy performed to rule out cancer. Maintenance therapy with a histamine H_2-receptor antagonist helps to prevent recurrence, though total suppression of acid production is unnecessary and probably undesirable, since it encourages bacterial overgrowth.

Nonpharmacologic Therapies

Diet. Contrary to common belief, there is no evidence that any particular dietary manipulation promotes healing or reduces acidity. The one exception is that avoidance of eating before bedtime probably reduces nocturnal acid levels by removing the postprandial stimulus to acid secretion. Otherwise, bland diets, frequent feedings, small feedings, and avoidance of spices, fruit juices, and acidic foods have never been shown to affect the course of ulcer disease. Milk is also without specific benefit; in fact, its high content of protein and calcium stimulates gastric acid secretion. Some patients claim that certain foods "disagree" with them; these can be avoided, but not for the sake of altering acid production. Intake of *coffee* (including decaffeinated forms) and other caffeinated beverages ought to be limited, but need not be eliminated entirely; their link with ulcer disease is not especially strong.

Avoidance of Agents Injurious to the Mucosal Barrier. A program to limit recurrences and speed healing should address chronic use of agents injurious to the mucosal barrier. However, as noted above, of the many agents implicated in ulcer disease, only *unbuffered aspirin* has been unequivocally proven to cause gastric erosions leading to ulceration. *Ethanol* also damages the mucosal barrier and can cause gastritis, but its use has never been definitively tied to ulcer formation. Indomethacin, phenylbutazone, and most other *nonsteroidal anti-inflammatory agents* can cause mucosal erosion and bleeding from an existing ulcer, but they do not result in back diffusion of hydrogen ions, and do not increase the risk of developing ulcer disease. As noted above, *glucocorticosteroids* exacerbate the chance of developing an ulcer, but the risk remains low and concurrent use of a prophylactic regimen is not required unless other risk factors are present.

Alleviating Emotional Stress. Those with difficult home or work situations may benefit from counseling by the primary physician. Treatment begins with a careful history eliciting pertinent psychosocial information. The very act of discussing these issues and the opportunity to ventilate one's feelings to a supportive listener may in itself lessen tension and help point the way to solutions. A short course of minor tranquilizer therapy is sometimes helpful to augment supportive psychotherapy and help the patient cope with the combination of stress and illness (see Chapter 222). Before the days of cost-containment, very stressed patients were hospitalized to facilitate ulcer healing; however, only stays in excess of 4 weeks were shown to be effective, making this form of therapy impractical today.

Smoking impedes the healing of peptic ulcers and might interfere with the action of H_2-receptor antagonists. Cessation should be urged during recovery from an ulcer. Although the role of smoking as a causative factor in ulcer disease is less well established, there is ample medical justification to advise its discontinuation (see Chapters 32 and 49).

Pharmacologic Therapies

Antacids remain a mainstay of therapy, because they are effective, relatively inexpensive, and safe. When used in a dose sufficient to buffer gastric acid (*e.g.,* 140 mEq, 1 hour after a meal), they have been shown endoscopically to be more effective than placebo in promoting healing of duodenal ulcers. Lower doses have been demonstrated by endoscopy to promote healing of gastric ulcers. These agents are no more effective than placebo for relieving pain due to duodenal ulcer, although they are better than placebo in gastric ulcers. This effect on gastric ulcer pain has stimulated speculation as to other mechanisms of action, including formation of a protective coating, inactivation of irritant bile acids, and stimulation of prostaglandin synthesis.

The *buffering capacities* of liquid antacid preparations vary considerably, ranging from 6 to 128 mEq per 15 ml. Liquids are superior to tablets in buffering capacity (see Tables 64-1 and 64-2). Calcium carbonate preparations are among the most potent in neutralizing capacity, but their usefulness is limited by the fact that they stimulate rebound acid secretion. The most effective liquid antacids contain magnesium and aluminum hydroxides. When the aluminum hydroxide mixes with acid, nonabsorbable aluminum salts are formed, which by themselves are constipating. The magnesium salts formed are also poorly absorbed, but frequently cause diarrhea, an effect that may not be completely canceled by the constipating action of the aluminum. If diarrhea becomes a problem, one can alternately use an antacid containing only aluminum hydroxide. Many of the liquid antacids contain considerable amounts of sodium. A low-sodium preparation is sometimes needed to avoid sodium excess in patients who must restrict salt intake. Tables 64-1 and 64-2 list relative strengths of common liquid and tablet antacids and their sodium content.

Studies correlating healing with acid neutralizing capacities indicate that substantial doses of antacids are needed in

Table 64-1. Characteristics of Major Liquid Antacids

PREPARATION	NEUTRALIZING CAPACITY (mEq/ml)	VOLUME FOR 140 mEq (ml)	SODIUM CONTENT (mg/5 ml)	RELATIVE COST*	BUFFERS
Maalox TC	4.2	33	<1.0	1.0	Al/MgOH$_2$
Titralac	4.2	33	11.0	0.7	CaCO$_3$
Delcid	4.1	34	1.5	1.0	Al/MgOH$_2$
Mylanta II	3.6	39	1.0	1.5	Al/MgOH$_2$
Camalox	3.2	44	2.5	1.2	Al/MgOH$_2$ CaCO$_3$
Gelusil II	3.0	47	1.3	1.7	Al/MgOH$_2$
Basaljel ES	2.9	48	23.0	2.4	AlCO$_3$
Riopan	2.7	50	<1.0	1.5	Magaldrate
Mylanta	2.5	55	<1.0	1.7	Al/MgOH$_2$
Alternagel	2.4	60	2.0	1.9	AlOH$_2$
Maalox Plus	2.3	61	1.0	1.7	Al/MgOH$_2$
Maalox	2.3	61	1.0	1.5	Al/MgOH$_2$
Gelusil	2.2	64	<1.0	1.9	Al/MgOH$_2$
Riopan Plus	1.8	78	0.7	1.5	Al/MgOH$_2$
Di-Gel	1.8	80	15.0	2.2	Al/MgOH$_2$
Amphogel	4	100	7.0	2.9	AlOH$_2$

* Reference cost is that of a 140 mEq dose of Maalox TC liquid. (Source: Green Book, 1986)

the treatment of duodenal ulcer; however, as little as 120 mEq per day has proven effective in healing gastric ulcers. Previous failures to demonstrate the effectiveness of antacids may have been due to inadequate doses. About 140 mEq at a time is necessary to bring the gastric pH into the 3.5 to 5.0 range. Typical 30-ml doses of many popular antacids provide

Table 64-2. Characteristics of Major Antacid Tablets

PREPARATION	NEUTRALIZING CAPACITY (mEq/tablet)	DOSE FOR 140 mEq (tablets)	SODIUM CONTENT (mg/tablet)	RELATIVE COST*	BUFFERS
Camalox	16.7	8	1.5	1.2	Al/MgOH$_2$
Basaljel	15.4	9	2.0	1.5	AlCO$_3$
Mylanta II	11.0	13	1.3	2.0	Al/MgOH$_2$
Tums	10.5	13	2.7	1.2	CaCO$_3$
Alka II	10.5	13	2.0	1.2	CaCO$_3$
Riopan Plus	10.0	14	0.3	1.7	Al/MgOH$_2$
Titralac	9.5	15	0.3	1.2	CaCO$_3$
Gelusil II	8.2	17	2.1	2.5	Al/MgOH$_2$
Rolaids	6.9	20	53.0	2.0	AlCO$_3$
Maalox Plus	5.7	25	1.4	2.5	Al/MgOH$_2$
Digel	4.7	30	10.6	2.5	Al/MgOH$_2$ MgCO$_3$
Amphogel	2.0	70	7.0	8.5	AlOH$_2$

* Reference cost is that of a 140 mEq dose of Maalox TC liquid. (Source: Green Book, 1986)

only 60 mEq. Even though contents listed on labels of weak and strong antacid preparations are similar, the relative amounts and solubilities of ingredients do vary, accounting for differences in potency.

The *timing* of the antacid dose affects the degree of acid neutralization. If given with a meal, the antacid is wasted, because food is a perfectly adequate buffer. When antacid is given 1 hour after eating, gastric acidity is minimized for another 1½ to 2 hours, countering the food-induced stimulation of acid secretion. A second dose 3 hours after a meal provides another hour of acid neutralization and tides the patient over to the next meal.

Problems associated with antacid use are relatively few, but important to recognize. Diarrhea is common as a result of the cathartic effect of insoluble magnesium salts. Treatment is to alternate therapy with an antacid containing only aluminum hydroxide. Antacids enhance the absorption of dicumarol and L-dopa and decrease absorption of cimetidine, phenothiazines, sulfonamides, INH, and penicillin. Potent antacids can cause premature release of aspirin from enteric coated tablets when both are taken simultaneously. Phosphate depletion is possible in patients using an aluminum-containing antacid—insoluble aluminum phosphate forms. Excess sodium absorption has already been mentioned. Magnesium-containing antacids should be avoided in renal failure; the small amounts of magnesium absorbed cannot be eliminated. Calcium can be absorbed and precipitate hypercalcemia if renal function is depressed. Calcium also triggers rebound acid secretion, making such antacids irrational choices.

A *cost-effective* antacid regimen employs an agent with a high degree of neutralizing capacity and low cost per therapeutic dose. Several liquid preparations have such qualities and stand out as the best buys; moreover, they are also among the lowest in sodium (see Tables 64-1 and 64-2). Compared with tablets, liquid antacid preparations are less expensive but not as convenient to use; tablets are particularly well suited for use at work. Although antacids are safe and effective, their cost and inconvenience can mount when they must be taken seven times a day. A full antacid program may approach the cost of H_2-receptor antagonist therapy. Trying to achieve adequate acid neutralization with antacid tablets alone can become difficult; at least eight tablets must be taken just to obtain 140 mEq of acid neutralizing capacity.

The ability of antacids to *prevent recurrences* remains unproven. Some patients report benefit from continuing to take a dose of antacid before bed, but the efficacy of such therapy is still unconfirmed. Antacid use prn is also extremely common but difficult to study; there are no definitive data on its role in preventing ulcer disease.

Histamine H_2-Receptor Antagonists. The development of agents capable of inhibiting parietal cell acid production represented a major advance in the medical therapy of peptic ulcer disease. Cimetidine and ranitidine are the two leading examples of this class of drugs. They act not only to block histamine-stimulated acid secretion, but also that triggered by pentagastrin, food, and physiologic vagal reflexes. Reports on the magnitude of reductions in acid secretion range from 50% to 95%. As noted earlier, both agents speed the healing of duodenal and gastric ulcers and prevent recurrences when used chronically at maintenance doses.

Cimetidine is the prototype histamine H_2-receptor antagonist and still ranks worldwide as among the most frequently prescribed drugs. When given four times daily in 300-mg doses, it is equal to high-dose antacids, randitine and sucralfate in its ability to accelerate the healing of *duodenal ulcers.* Similar results have been obtained with doses ranging from 0.8 g to 2.0 g per day; within this range, there seems to be little difference in efficacy. The latest regimen is a single 800 mg dose; its efficacy in preliminary studies is good. More data are needed before it can be recommended. A course of cimetidine therapy does not change the risk of recurrence. Regardless of duration of treatment, recurrence rates after completion of therapy range from 45% to 70% at 3 months and from 75% to 90% at 1 year. However, a low-dose maintenance program (300 mg bid) has been shown to substantially reduce the frequency of recurrences to about 15% per year. A similar effect is obtained with a single 400 mg dose at bedtime.

Cimetidine also facilitates healing of *gastric ulcers.* Although early studies failed to demonstrate any benefit, probably because of concomitant use of antacids in the placebo group. Latter trials prohibiting antacid use in the control group showed significant improvement in the rate of healing over that achieved with a placebo. When cimetidine was compared with high-dose antacids (seven doses/day), both were equally efficacious. Compared with low-dose antacids (15 cc of Maalox TC 1 hour after meals and before bed) and placebo, cimetidine proved superior to the placebo and slightly better than the antacids in both speed of healing and the proportion of patients who improved. Gastric ulcer patients who continue to smoke or take aspirin have blunted responses to cimetidine; however, with the addition of antacid therapy to a cimetidine program, even patients who must use aspirin or other nonsteroidal agents (*e.g.,* those with severe rheumatoid disease) heal their gastric ulcers.

PHARMACOKINETICS. Cimetidine is rapidly and completely absorbed after oral administration. Peak blood levels occur 45 to 90 minutes after a 300-mg dose. Significant inhibition of acid production persists for at least 4 hours. As noted above, there is preliminary evidence suggesting that a single 800 mg dose at bedtime is nearly as effective as 300 mg four times a day, but more data are needed. Absorption is significantly inhibited by concurrent intake of antacids containing magnesium or aluminum; the two should not be taken closer than 1 hour apart. Most of the drug is excreted unchanged in the urine; 15% is metabolized by the liver. Patients in renal failure require reduction in frequency of administration (*e.g.,* q12h when the serum creatinine rises above 3.0 mg/dl).

Side-effects and *adverse reactions* are relatively minor and occur infrequently (in fewer than 5% of patients). In controlled studies, the frequency of side-effects was indistinguishable from that for placebo; however, in long-term studies, the frequency of adverse reactions exceeds that for placebo. The most commonly experienced adverse reactions include diarrhea, nausea, vomiting, rash, dizziness, and headache. The incidence of each is less than 1%. The *CNS effects* are most prominent in the elderly, the very young, those with renal or liver disease, and those receiving high doses. Lethargy, confusion, slurred speech, agitation, and visual hallucinations have been reported; the drug crosses the blood–brain barrier in humans. *Gynecomastia* ranks among the most troubling of side-effects, and is especially prevalent among patients taking the drug at high dosages for treatment of Zollinger–Ellison syndrome. The cause is believed to involve the drug's weak antiandrogenic effect, which also results in a small reduction in sperm count. Isolated cases of *granulocytopenia* have been reported in the setting of severe underlying illness and multiple drug use. Small, clinically insignificant increases in serum creatinine and liver enzymes are noted occasionally.

A *question of carcinogenicity* has been raised, in relation to chronic suppression of gastric acidity leading to increased formation of nitrosamine (a potent carcinogen) from bacterial overgrowth. At present, there are conflicting laboratory study results on nitrosamine production and no documented evidence of increased rates of gastric cancer; however, the advisability of long-term, total suppression of acid production comes into question.

Cimetidine impairs hepatic drug metabolism by *inhibiting liver microsomal enzymes.* Hepatic clearance is slowed; the serum half-lives of hepatically metabolized drugs such as *warfarin, diazepam, chlordiazepoxide, phenytoin,* and *theophylline compounds* are extended. The net effect is a potentiation of drug effect when cimetidine is taken; dose reductions are essential, as is monitoring of serum levels. The effect of cimetidine on hepatic microsomal enzymes lasts for about 2 weeks after the drug is stopped. Cimetidine also reduces *propranolol* clearance, in part because of a slowing of hepatic blood flow.

Ranitidine is five to ten times more potent on a weight basis than cimetidine, and thus is given in lower dosages. Its ability to inhibit acid secretion is equal or superior to that of cimetidine and the effect lasts 12 hours. Ranitidine has promoted healing in a proportion of patients with refractory gastric ulcer, duodenal ulcer, or Zollinger–Ellison syndrome

who did not respond to cimetidine. A single dose at night has been found to be as effective as cimetidine in preventing recurrence of duodenal ulcer, reducing recurrence rate to less than 25%. Oral doses are well absorbed, though only 50% is bioavailable because of first-pass inactivation by the liver. About 25% of an oral dose is excreted unchanged in the urine.

Adverse effects are fewer and less serious than those of cimetidine; however, experience with ranitidine is less extensive. Unlike cimetidine, ranitidine has no antiandrogenic effect; other side-effects are similar: diarrhea, dyspepsia, loss of libido, dizziness, and mental confusion. Ranitidine also differs from cimetidine in *not decreasing hepatic drug metabolism,* or at least not impairing it to the same degree. However, the drug does decrease hepatic blood flow. Minor liver function abnormalities occasionally occur; they are reversible.

Sucralfate is a complex of aluminum hydroxide and sulfated sucrose that is believed to act by forming a barrier on the ulcer base, inhibiting pepsin activity and binding bile salts. It has no acid-neutralizing activity, and little is absorbed. In controlled trials, the drug is comparable to cimetidine and ranitidine in effectiveness in healing peptic ulcers. The agent also reduces the recurrence rate for gastric ulcers. It is most effective when taken 1 hour before meals and at bedtime, although twice daily administration of double-strength doses has proven adequate for treatment of duodenal ulcer. Some data suggest an added benefit when sucralfate is used with an H_2-receptor antagonist to promote healing of gastric ulcers. The main side-effect is constipation. The drug binds phosphate and has been reported to cause hypophosphatemia in patients with abnormal renal function. Sucralfate may interfere with the gastrointestinal absorption of tetracycline, digoxin, phenytoin, and cimetidine. The cost of daily sucralfate therapy is intermediate between that of cimetidine and ranitidine.

Anticholinergic Agents can suppress the parasympathetic muscarinic activity that triggers gastric acid secretion, especially the nocturnal surge. These agents are not as potent as H_2-receptor antagonists in suppressing acid production, but occasionally they are used to supplement the H_2-receptor antagonists in patients with refractory disease. The frequency and severity of anticholinergic side-effects make therapy intolerable for many patients. Because more effective, better tolerated agents are available, anticholinergics have only limited usefulness.

Prostaglandin Analogues are currently undergoing clinical testing. They may represent an attempt to exploit prostaglandin-mediated maintenance and repair of gastric mucosa. The literature should be followed for reports of their use.

Surgery

The *proximal gastric vagotomy* effectively limits recurrences without producing the disabling side-effects associated with earlier forms of surgery for duodenal ulcer disease. The operation involves selective severing of the nerve supply to the acid-secreting fundus; the nerves to the antrum are left intact, preserving control of gastric emptying. The incidence of ulcer recurrences is slightly higher (10%) than with vagotomy and antrectomy (5%) but similar to vagotomy and pyloroplasty (12%). Surgical mortality is lower and such potentially disabling postsurgical side-effects as the dumping syndrome and diarrhea are much less common. The operation is technically demanding and should be considered only by surgeons specifically trained to perform it. The procedure should not be done in patients with delayed gastric emptying. Distal gastrectomy with excision of the ulcer remains the procedure of choice for gastric ulcer.

The most serious *indications for surgery* include brisk bleeding of 6 units to 8 units of blood in 24 hours (see Chapter 60), recurrent bleeding episodes, perforation, gastric outlet obstruction refractory to medical therapy, and failure of a benign gastric ulcer to heal after 15 weeks. Operations are most often done in patients who fail to respond to medical therapy and have disabling symptoms that interfere with their lives.

PATIENT EDUCATION

Enlisting the patient's active involvement and overcoming much of the mythology surrounding ulcer disease are prime objectives of the patient education effort. Before they go to the physician, many patients put themselves on bland diets, increase their intake of milk products, and purchase calcium carbonate antacid tablets in efforts at self treatment. Some even take aspirin for pain relief. Even when a medical program has been designed, common errors made by patients are stopping medication as soon as the pain disappears, taking antacids with meals (which wastes the antacid), taking cimetidine at the same time as antacids (which impairs cimetidine absorption), and stopping antacids when diarrhea develops. Careful explanation and attention to detail are central to a successful program.

Use of coffee, alcohol, and tobacco need to be reviewed. Many physicians insist that coffee-drinking be stopped, though this may cause more difficulty than is warranted by its role in pathogenesis. Cessation of smoking is indicated, however, because smoking retards ulcer healing. Alcohol intake should also be discouraged.

Counselling the patient with situational stress is often beneficial, but any suggestion to change jobs or family situations because an ulcer has developed is probably unwarranted and potentially counterproductive. There is no evidence that such extreme solutions contribute to healing, and they may actually heighten stress. One useful supplement to counseling is teaching simple relaxation techniques; these are especially useful for patients bothered by multiple somatic manifestations of stress (see Chapter 222).

The patient needs to be taught to watch for complications of ulcer disease. In particular, the manifestations of gastrointestinal bleeding should be well understood so that there is no delay in seeking help. If the question of elective surgery arises, the patient should be made a full partner in the decision, since there are few definite guidelines for operation. A value judgment is necessary, and the costs and benefits of surgery versus continued medical therapy need to be discussed.

MONITORING THERAPY AND INDICATIONS FOR REFERRAL AND ADMISSION

Gastric Ulcer. If the lesion was detected initially by x-ray film, has all the hallmarks of a benign lesion (see above), and heals fully on follow-up barium study, then endoscopy can probably be forgone. Small ulcers should be reevaluated for healing at 6 weeks and large ones at 12 weeks. If, however, full healing has not occurred, then endoscopic evaluation and biopsy are needed, especially in patients over age 40, who are at increased risk of gastric cancer. It must be remembered that even malignant ulcers may shrink in size in response to therapy. Delay or failure to heal requires consultation with the gastroenterologist to review the medical program and the chances of cancer.

Because *duodenal ulcer* is far less likely to represent malignancy, monitoring by x-ray film and endoscopy is reserved for documenting a suspected complication such as bleeding. Periodic repetition of studies is unnecessary and expensive, even when typical symptoms recur, unless a different course of therapy such as surgery is contemplated. Following stool guaiacs and blood counts can help detect bleeding, as can careful questioning of the patient.

Refractoriness to therapy is an indication for referral to the gastroenterologist. Admission is mandatory when symptoms of hemorrhage, penetration, perforation, or gastric outlet obstruction are present; both surgeon and gastroenterologist need to be consulted.

A most difficult issue is when and whom to select for *elective surgery.* Much has to do with the patient's preferences; gross generalizations are meaningless. Clearly those with recurrent major bleeds, gastric outlet obstruction, or evidence of malignancy need to be seen by the surgeon. Seventy-five percent of patients with intractable pain obtain relief when treated surgically, but subgroups with alcohol abuse, character disorders, or severe neuroses do poorly when operated on. The decision to resort to elective surgery for recurrent disease should be made in conjunction with the patient, weighing the small risk of operative mortality and the morbidity of postgastrectomy syndrome against the morbidity and cost of recurrent pain, time lost from work, and need for chronic drug therapy.

THERAPEUTIC RECOMMENDATIONS

- Avoid, or at least limit to the extent medically possible, the use of agents potentially injurious to the gastric mucosa, including plain and buffered aspirin, nonsteroidal anti-inflammatory agents, and steroids.
- Advise cessation of smoking and a decrease in use of coffee (including decaffeinated forms) and other caffeine-containing beverages; complete cessation of coffee intake is unnecessary.
- Do not restrict any foods or insist on a bland or milk-laden diet. Frequent small feedings are unnecessary, and a bedtime snack may stimulate nocturnal acid secretion. The patient should avoid only foods that cause discomfort.
- Begin an antacid, H_2-receptor antagonist, or sucralfate, basing selection on patient preference, capacity for compliance, affordability, and potential for interaction with other medications the patient may be taking.
- Begin ranitidine when trying to maximize compliance or minimize drug–drug interactions and side-effects; if expense is a major concern, consider another agent. The starting dose is 150 mg bid, taken with meals.
- Begin a magnesium–aluminum hydroxide liquid antacid with high acid neutralizing capacity and low sodium content (*e.g.,* Maalox TC) if the patient is reliable and one needs to minimize systemic effects and drug–drug interactions. Prescribe sufficient amounts to provide 140 mEq/dose for treatment of duodenal ulcer and 70 mEq/dose for gastric ulcer (see Table 64-1). Give the doses 1 and 3 hours after meals and before bed. If diarrhea develops, alternate this with an aluminum hydroxide antacid (see Table 64-1).
- Begin cimetidine if previously used by the patient and well tolerated; cimetidine is less expensive than randitine, but it involves greater frequency of doses and more side-effects and drug–drug interactions. The dosage is 300 mg qid, taken with meals and before bed. Exert caution if patient is taking propranolol, warfarin, benzodiazepines, phenytoin, theophylline compounds, or other drugs metabolized by hepatic microsomes; cimetidine potentiates their effect. Avoid taking this drug at the same time as antacids; separate them by at least 1 hour.
- Begin sucralfate if the patient has been unable to tolerate antacids or H_2-receptor antagonists, but avoid it if compliance or constipation is a problem. The dosage is 1 g qid, taken 1 hour before meals and before bed. Avoid taking it simultaneously with digoxin, tetracycline, phenytoin, or cimetidine; sucralfate inhibits their absorption.

- For duodenal ulcer, continue therapy for a full 4 weeks or until symptoms resolve, whichever is longer. For gastric ulcer, continue treatment until healing has been demonstrated. Do not stop therapy simply because symptoms resolve.
- For patients refractory to single-agent therapy, add an agent from another drug class or switch to another drug in the same class.
- Thoroughly instruct the patient on how to carry out the therapeutic program and review common misconceptions.
- Attend to stress-related issues, but avoid recommending a major job or geographic change.
- Document full healing of a gastric ulcer by endoscopy or upper GI series at 6 weeks for small ulcers and at 12 weeks for large ones. No follow-up examinations are needed for uncomplicated duodenal ulcers.
- Obtain endoscopy with brushings and biopsy of gastric ulcers that appear suspicious on upper GI series or fail to heal completely.
- Advise patients with refractory cases to cease smoking entirely and omit all nonenteric-coated salicylates and nonsteroidal anti-inflammatory agents; if using enteric-coated aspirin, do not take them at the same time as antacids.
- Treat recurrences in a fashion similar to the initial episode.
- If two episodes of ulcer disease occur within 1 year, initiate prophylactic maintenance therapy with ranitidine (150 mg qhs) or cimetidine (300 mg bid or 400 mg qhs). Continue this treatment for 1 year.
- Refer the patient with refractory pain, multiple ulcers, frequent recurrences, or associated secretory diarrhea to the gastroenterologist for consideration of Zollinger–Ellison syndrome, as well as for review of the medical program and need for endoscopy.
- Admit patients with evidence of bleeding, gastric outlet obstruction, or perforation and obtain surgical consultation.

ANNOTATED BIBLIOGRAPHY

Barr GD, Kang JY, Canalese J et al: A two year perspective control study of maintenance cimetidine in gastric ulcers. Gastroenterology 85:100, 1983 (*Cimetidine in doses of 400 bid prevented gastric recurrence over 1 year but did not appear to provide significant benefit over the 2-year period.*)

Buchman E, Kaung DT, Dolank D et al: Unrestricted diet in treatment of duodenal ulcer. Gastroenterology 56:1016, 1969 (*Dietary restrictions made little or no difference.*)

Conn Ho, Blitzer BL: Nonassociation of adrenocorticosteroid therapy and peptic ulcer. N Engl J Med 294:473, 1976 (*The first of two studies examining pooled data; concludes there is little association between steroids and risk of ulcer.*)

Curatolo PW, Robertson D: The health consequences of caffeine. Ann Intern Med 98:641, 1983 (*Thorough review; examines the evidence linking caffeine with ulcer disease and acid secretion; 281 references.*)

Danilewitz M, Tim LO, Hirschowitz B: Ranitidine suppression of gastric hypersecretion resistent to cimetidine. N Engl J Med 306: 20, 1982 (*One of many reports showing the efficacy of switching to ranitidine when cimetidine does not work.*)

Dooley CP, Larson AW, Stace NH et al: Double-contrast barium meal and upper gastrointestinal endoscopy. Ann Intern Med 101: 538, 1984 (*A randomized study that indicate superior sensitivity and specificity for endoscopy but admits that cost-benefit is not established.*)

Drake D, Hollander D: Neutralizing capacity and cost effectiveness of antacids. Ann Intern Med 94:215, 1981 (*Excellent reference data on comparative characteristics of available antacids.*)

Freston JW: Cimetidine. Ann Intern Med 97:573,728, 1982 (*An exhaustive two-part review of the accumulated experience with the drug; 161 references.*)

Friedman DG, Siegelaub AB, Seltzer C: Cigarettes, alcohol, coffee and peptic ulcer. N Engl J Med 290:469, 1974 (*An epidemiologic study from the Kaiser-Permanente organization showing an increased prevalence of ulcer disease in smokers. Coffee consumption and alcohol were correlated with cigarette smoking, but were not independent determinants of prevalence of ulcer disease.*)

Gelfand DW, Ott DJ, Munitz HA, Yu M: Radiology and endoscopy: A radiologic perspective. Ann Intern Med 101:550, 1984 (*An editorial arguing that radiologic evaluation of ulcer disease is more cost-effective than endoscopy.*)

Goldberg MA: Medical treatment of peptic ulcer disease: Is it truly efficacious? Am J Med 77:589, 1984 (*A critical look at the state of medical therapy, arguing that we have a long way to go.*)

Greenblatt DJ, Abernethy DR, Morse DS et al: Clinical importance of the interaction of diazepam and cimetidine. N Engl J Med 310:1639, 1984 (*Shows that the interaction is not clinically important when diazepam is used in modest doses; warns against extrapolating to large doses or use in the elderly.*)

Greenfield S, Kaplan S, Ware JE: Expanding patient involvement in care. Ann Intern Med 102:520, 1985 (*Demonstrates that involvement leads to improvements in outcome.*)

Grossman MI, Kurata JH, Rotter JI et al: Peptic ulcer: New therapies, new diseases. Ann Intern Med 95:609, 1981 (*Review of research into mechanisms of disease and treatment; 168 references.*)

Hirschowitz BI: Natural history of duodenal ulcer. Gastroenterology 85:967, 1983 (*An excellent review of the natural history of duodenal ulcer addressing the critical issue of what to do about the typical lifelong relapse rate of 70% to 80% of peptic ulcer and a lifetime risk of potentially serious complications of 20%.*)

Ippolit A, Elashoff J, Valenzuela J et al: Recurrent ulcer after successful treatment with cimetidine or antacid. Gastroenterology 85:875, 1983 (*Recurrence rates after antacid therapy were 29% at 3 months and 56% at 6 months, compared with 36% and 55% after cimetidine.*)

Isenberg JI, Peterson WL, Elashoff JD et al: Healing of benign gastric ulcer with low-dose antacid or cimetidine. N Engl J Med 308: 1319, 1983 (*Demonstrates efficacy for both cimetidine and low-dose antacids, although cimetidine was superior.*)

Jensen RT, Gardner JD, Raufman JP et al: Zollinger-Ellison syn-

drome: Current concepts and management. Ann Intern Med 98: 59, 1983 (*A good review; 94 references.*)

Lanza FL, Royer GL, Nelson RS: Endoscopic evaluation of the effects of aspirin, buffered aspirin, and enteric-coated aspirin on gastric mucosa. N Engl J Med 303:136, 1980 (*Plain and buffered aspirin caused mucosal injury; enteric-coated aspirin did not.*)

Levant JA, Walsh JH, Isenberg J: Stimulation of gastric secretion and gastrin release by single oral doses of calcium carbonate. N Engl J Med 289:555, 1973 (*Calcium carbonate causes rebound acid hypersecretion, even though it is a good neutralizing agent.*)

Mahl GF: Anxiety, HCl secretion and peptic ulcer etiology. Psychosom Med 12:158, 1950 (*Acute anxiety raises acid secretion.*)

Messer J, Reitman D, Sacks HS et al: Association of adrenocorticosteroid therapy and peptic ulcer disease. N Engl J Med 309:21, 1983 (*The second analysis of pooled data; finds that there is an increase in risk of ulcer disease, although the absolute risk is small.*)

Peterson WL, Sturdevant RA, Frankl HD et al: Healing of duodenal ulcer with an antacid regimen. N Engl J Med 297:341, 1977 (*Documents the efficacy of high-dose [1000 MEQ: per day] antacid therapy in healing duodenal ulcers compared with that of a placebo. Also shows a surprisingly high rate of pain relief by placebo and delay in healing in cigarette smokers.*)

Richardson CT: Sucralfate. Ann Intern Med 97:269, 1982 (*Terse but useful editorial on the place of sucralfate in treatment of ulcer disease.*)

Richardson CT: Pathogenic factors in peptic ulcer disease. Am J Med 79(Suppl 2C):1, 1985 (*Excellent summary of pathophysiology.*)

Rutter M: Psychological factors in short-term prognosis of physical disease. 1. Peptic ulcer. J Psychosom Res 7:45, 1963 (*Severe anxiety prolongs recovery and makes relapse more likely.*)

Sedman AJ: Cimetidine-drug interactions. Am J Med 76:109, 1984 (*A short review of the clinically important interactions; 90 references.*)

Sogtag S, Graham DY, Belisto A et al: Cimetidine, cigarette smoking, and recurrence of duodenal ulcer. N Engl J Med 311:689, 1984 (*Finds that smoking is a major factor in recurrence of duodenal ulcer.*)

Spiro HM: Is the steroid a myth? N Engl J Med 309:45, 1983 (*An editorial that examines the contradictory data on this topic.*)

Spiro HM: Moynihan's Disease? The diagnosis of duodenal ulcer. N Engl J Med 291:567, 1974 (*Argues for attending more to the patient than to the ulcer itself with repeat endoscopies and barium studies.*)

Steinberg WM, Lewis JH, Katz DM: Antacids inhibit absorption of cimetidine. N Engl J Med 307:400, 1982 (*The original U.S. report of this important interaction.*)

Thompson JC: The role of surgery in peptic ulcer disease. N Engl J Med 307:550, 1982 (*An editorial that nicely summarizes the indications for surgery and the procedures currently available.*)

Van Deventer GM, Schneidman D, Walsh JH: Sucralfate and cimetidine as single agents and in combination for treatment of active duodenal ulcers. Am J Med 79(Suppl 2C):39, 1985 (*Both were well tolerated and equally effective; combination therapy produced the most rapid rate of healing.*)

65
Management of Inflammatory Bowel Disease

JAMES M. RICHTER, M.D.

Ulcerative colitis and Crohn's disease account for most of the inflammatory bowel disease seen in primary care practice. Abdominal pain, diarrhea, and bleeding are among the presenting manifestations. The first priority is to distinguish inflammatory bowel disease from other causes of diarrhea (see Chapter 58). The chronicity, potentially disabling symptoms, risk of malignancy (in the case of ulcerative colitis), and occasional refractoriness to medical therapy make management a major challenge. The primary care physician needs to know how to treat exacerbations, maintain remissions, and psychologically sustain these patients through difficult times. Competent care is based on a thorough understanding of the roles for sulfasalazine, corticosteroids, surgery, and psychological support. Although patients with severe or refractory disease may need to be referred to the gastroenterologist, most others can be well managed by the primary care physician.

PATHOPHYSIOLOGY, CLINICAL PRESENTATION, AND COURSE

Ulcerative Colitis is an idiopathic, diffuse inflammatory disease of the *bowel mucosa.* The disease typically begins in adolescence or young adulthood, but may occur at almost any age. Caucasians are affected more often than blacks. Prevalence is highest among Jews. The cardinal symptoms are bloody diarrhea and abdominal pain; in severe cases, fever, anorexia, and weight loss are present as well. The variability of presentations is remarkable, ranging from malaise and no symptoms referable to the colon, to fever, prostration, abdominal distention, and passage of large volumes of liquid stool.

The disease need not be confined to the bowel; extracolonic manifestations include arthritis, uveitis, jaundice, and skin lesions. The course is characteristically chronic, recurrent, and unpredictable. An insidious presentation does not predict a benign course, and a fulminant onset may be followed by long, relatively asymptomatic periods.

Ulcerative colitis almost always involves the *distal colon and rectum,* making diagnosis possible by sigmoidoscopy. The mucosa becomes edematous, obscuring the fine network of submucosal vessels. The moist, glistening mucosal surface is lost, and a granular appearance develops. The bowel wall is friable, bleeding spontaneously or when touched with a swab. In advanced cases, *pseudopolyps* and discrete *ulcers* may be seen. Smears of mucus from the bowel wall show polymorphonuclear leukocytes. Barium enema documents the extent of disease. Radiologic findings range from mucosal denudation to frank ulceration, with loss of haustral markings and a tubular appearance. There are *no skip areas.*

Liver involvement occurs in the form of *pericholangitis and fatty infiltration;* these are common histologic findings in ulcerative colitis but are seldom symptomatic. Much less frequently, chronic active hepatitis, cirrhosis, or sclerosing cholangitis is seen. A migratory, *monoarticular arthritis* affecting the large joints develops in 10% of patients. This arthritis often coincides with an exacerbation of colitis and resolves with control of the underlying disease. *Ankylosing spondylitis* also occurs, but runs a course independent of the colitis. *Uveitis* or episcleritis may be seen at any time during the course of the disease. *Erythema nodosum,* pyoderma gangrenosum, and oral aphthous ulcerations are found in about 5% of patients, usually during active colitis.

The *prognosis* for patients with ulcerative colitis seen in the primary care setting is far better than that for patients studied in referral centers, who are likely to have more severe disease. A recent community-based study done over 10 years found that 87% went into complete remission after the first attack and only 8% developed chronic persistent disease. In 30% no further attacks occurred over 5 years, and in 74% disease was limited to the distal bowel (rectum or rectosigmoid). The overall mortality rate was no different from that of the general population, although it was increased in patients with severe first attacks or extensive disease.

The *risk of cancer* is enhanced and a function of the extent and duration of disease. Risk begins to increase substantially after 8 years of illness. In a long-term community-based study, the risk of cancer in those with pancolitis was 12% at 26 years. This figure is considerably lower than the oft-quoted risk of 1% to 2% per year that derives from referral center studies; still, it is an increased risk and little cause for complacency.

Ulcerative Proctitis. Typically, the patient with ulcerative proctitis is a young adult who presents with rectal bleeding and tenesmus. The bleeding is usually not severe; it is sometimes mistakenly attributed to hemorrhoids. Diarrhea or constipation may accompany the bleeding, but often there are only small frequent bowel movements associated with a small amount of mucus. On sigmoidoscopy, an edematous, friable rectal mucosa is observed; the bowel above the rectosigmoid is uninvolved. On barium enema or colonoscopy, the remainder of the large bowel is normal. The clinical presentation of ulcerative proctitis is not pathognomonic; the condition must be distinguished from infectious forms of proctocolitis (see Chapter 61).

Ulcerative proctitis is a variant of ulcerative colitis, distinguished by the limited extent of inflammation, its good prognosis, and paucity of serious complications. However, relapses are common. Fewer than 15% progress to generalized ulcerative colitis. The distant complications of ulcerative colitis are rare, and carcinoma of the rectum develops no more often than in unaffected individuals.

Crohn's Disease. This condition is a chronic, relapsing inflammatory disorder of the alimentary tract, with a peak incidence in the second and third decades. The inflammation is characteristically discontinuous, with diseased segments of bowel separated by normal areas. Crohn's disease has a tendency to cause strictures, fistulas, and abscesses, because the granulomatous inflammatory process may extend through all layers of the bowel wall. The condition often affects the distal ileum and right colon, but frequently it involves only the small bowel or colon. It may occur in any portion of the alimentary tract, from the buccal mucosa to the anus.

Extraintestinal involvement occurs in 15% to 20% of cases, with arthritis, ankylosing spondylitis, uveitis, erythema nodosum, aphthous oral ulcers, and pyoderma gangrenosum being the predominant manifestations of disease outside the bowel. In addition, cholelithiasis and nephrolithiasis have a higher incidence in these patients that in the general population.

Symptoms vary, depending on the location and extent of disease. Diarrhea and abdominal pain (particularly in the right lower quadrant) are cardinal symptoms, occurring in almost 80% of patients. Weight loss, vomiting, fever, perianal discomfort, and bleeding are also common complaints. Constipation may be an early manifestation of obstruction. Symptoms can develop quite subtly or present in fulminant fashion with the patient systemically toxic.

Physical examination may reveal a discrete abdominal mass, especially in the right lower quadrant, but usually a normal abdomen or doughy loops of bowel are found. Abdominal or perianal fistulous tracts are noted on examination in up to 10% of patients. Extraintestinal findings include inflamed joints, spinal deformities, erythema nodosum, pyoderma, uveitis, and aphthous ulcers.

Sigmoidoscopy is abnormal in fewer than 20% of cases; fistulous tracts and discrete inflammatory ulcers are sometimes encountered in the rectosigmoid. *Barium enema and upper GI series* often show segmental involvement of large and small bowel, often with strictures, fistulas, and ulcers.

The primary abnormality in Crohn's disease is submucosal, causing radiologic studies to sometimes appear normal. In such cases, *colonoscopy* aids diagnosis by demonstrating segmental disease and ulceration that may be missed on barium enema.

Prognosis. Though it is difficult to extrapolate from referral center data to patients seen in primary care settings, a pattern emerges of disease activity that waxes and wanes over many years. Disease-free intervals may last as long as several years or even decades, but recurrences are the rule. Several years of relief from symptoms may be afforded by surgical resection, but there is no evidence that any medical and surgical therapy alters the ultimate course of the illness. In referral center series, as many as 70% of patients ultimately require surgical resection.

WORKUP

Proper management requires confirming the diagnosis and determining the extent of disease. One proviso should be kept in mind: because these illnesses often occur in women of childbearing age, attempts should be made to minimize their x-ray exposure and carefully select only the most necessary radiologic studies.

Ulcerative Colitis. The diagnosis is usually based on the clinical presentation, sigmoidoscopic demonstration of inflammation, and the exclusion of bacterial and parasitic infections by culture and examination for ova and parasites (see Chapter 58). Because the disease almost invariably affects the distal colon and rectum, *sigmoidoscopy* is an essential component of the workup. The procedure is best performed without cleansing preparations, so as not to distort the appearance of the bowel mucosa (see Chapter 75). In acute phases of the illness, the mucosa appears *friable* and inflamed; there is loss of the normal vascular pattern. As the disease progresses, a *purulent exudate* and discrete small *ulcers* may form. With severe colitis, there may be pus and spontaneous bleeding as well as large ulcers. Chronic phases of the disease are characterized by a *granular mucosa* and inflammatory *pseudopolyps* (tags of damaged mucosa and granulation tissue).

When the sigmoidoscopic picture is nonspecific, one should *culture and examine the stool* for *C. difficile, Entamoeba histolytica, Campylobacter, Shigella, Salmonella,* and *N. gonorrhea* (see Chapters 58 and 61). *Rectal biopsy* is usually unnecessary but indicated when one needs to confirm the diagnosis and exclude conditions such as Crohn's disease of the rectosigmoid, amebic colitis, and pseudomembranous colitis. *Barium enema* or *colonoscopy* is used to provide supportive evidence and document the extent of disease; it should be postponed until disease activity begins to subside, because there is a small risk of perforation when the procedure is performed on an acutely inflamed bowel.

Crohn's Disease of the colon may mimic ulcerative colitis clinically. Differentiating features include "skip areas" in the colon, significant small bowel involvement, fistulas, and granulomas on biopsy. The diagnosis is suggested by a history in a young person of recurrent postprandial lower abdominal pain and altered bowel habits; it is reinforced by finding on physical examination a mass or tenderness in the right lower quadrant. Radiologic contrast studies are needed for a more definitive assessment. The *small bowel phase of an upper GI series* shows segmental narrowing, areas with loss of the normal mucosal pattern interspersed with areas of normal mucosa, fistula formation, and the "*string sign*" (a narrow band of barium flowing through an inflamed or scarred area) in the terminal ileum.

Colonic disease may be documented by *air contrast barium enema,* with asymmetic segmental changes distinguishing Crohn's disease of the large bowel from ulcerative colitis. Disease of the terminal ileum can often be detected on barium enema; however, radiologic involvement of the terminal ileum is not unique to Crohn's disease. Some ulcerative colitis patients also demonstrate inflammatory changes in the terminal ileum ("backwash ileitis"), but they lack the skip pattern characteristic of Crohn's disease.

Sigmoidoscopy demonstrates rectosigmoid inflammation in the 20% to 50% of patients with disease in this area; however, the findings are often nonspecific (mild erythema). *Colonoscopy* is needed in difficult cases and helps in judging the extent and severity of disease. *Biopsy* can be diagnostic but is usually unnecessary unless the diagnosis remains unsubstantiated; it should be avoided when acute inflammation is present.

PRINCIPLES OF MANAGEMENT

Comprehensive management requires attending to the patient's medical, psychological, and nutritional needs. For the most part, treatment is empirical and directed at providing symptomatic relief. However, surgery does offer the possibility of cure for patients with ulcerative colitis, and studies have shown prophylatic benefit from sulfasalazine. The inflammatory bowel diseases are chronic illnesses that require long-term management and support for the patient and the family.

Ulcerative Colitis

Because the disease typically follows a relapsing course with acute exacerbations and intervals of remission, the approach to treatment depends on the patient's current clinical status. During remission, treatment is prophylactic; during flare-ups, the goal is control of the inflammatory process. For refractory and widespread disease, surgery requires consideration.

Dietary and Nutritional Measures. No specific diet improves or exacerbates ulcerative colitis. However, reduction in dietary *fiber* may be of some benefit during periods of active disease. In patients with inactive disease, 1 or 2 teaspoons of *psyllium* hydrophylic colloid (Metamucil) in water daily often helps to bind the stool. There is an increased incidence of lactase deficiency in these patients; an empirical trial of a *milk-free diet* is reasonable when diarrhea persists despite other evidence of clinical remission. Those who are anemic from blood loss need oral or parenteral *iron* supplementation (see Chapter 84). Oral iron may be poorly tolerated, necessitating parenteral administration. Anemia may also be due to folic acid deficiency. *Folic acid* supplementation is indicated when intake of leafy vegetables and fresh fruits is poor or when sulfasalazine is being taken (see below). Anemia may also be due to chronic disease and not respond to dietary and nutritional measures.

Sulfasalazine. The drug is recommended as initial treatment for mild to moderate disease and for prevention of relapses. After oral administration, about 70% reaches the colon, where it is metabolized by intestinal bacteria, resulting in the local release of sulfapyridine and the salicylate analogue 5-aminosalicylate, which seems to be the active moiety. Sulfasalazine's precise mechanism of action remains speculative; hypotheses include effects on prostaglandin synthesis and metabolism and inhibition of migration of polymorphonuclear leukocytes.

Randomized controlled studies have shown the drug to be effective as *initial treatment* for patients with mild to moderate symptoms when given in doses of 4 g per day for 2 to 4 weeks. About 80% of patients respond. Because sulfasalazine is less effective than corticosteroid therapy, it is reserved for relatively mild cases; however, combined use with steroids has been suggested for early treatment of severe disease.

Controlled studies have also documented the drug's efficacy for *prophylaxis* and maintaining remissions. In one major study, more than 65% of patients given maintenance doses of 2 g per day remained symptom-free for at least 1 year compared with 25% of patients given placebo. The prophylactic effect of maintenance therapy persists when the drug is continued beyond 1 year. The optimum dose is 2 g per day (4 g/day provides even better protection, but the frequency of side-effects is markedly increased).

Sulfasalazine is usually well tolerated, although minor *side-effects* occur in about one third of patients. *Rash and fever* are common hypersensitivity reactions to the sulfa moiety, whereas *nausea, vomiting, headache, and hemolysis* are common dose-related side-effects. Patients unable to tolerate full doses of sulfasalazine because of gastrointestinal upset often do better when reintroduced to the drug more gradually. Taking it with meals also helps. Potential *hematopoetic effects* include anemia (from folic acid deficiency, hemolysis, or marrow suppression), granulocytopenia, and thrombocytopenia. *Low sperm counts* and qualitative sperm abnormalities have been noted in men taking the drug, usually after about 2 months of therapy; these conditions reverse when the medication is stopped. *Hepatitis* and *nephritis* have also been reported.

Desensitization has been successful in patients with minor allergic reactions (rash, fever). Such patients are started on doses of a fraction of a tablet (1–30 mg per day were used in studies) and slowly advanced over 2 to 4 weeks until therapeutic doses are achieved. The drug has been used with safety in pregnant and nursing patients. Work on sulfa-free preparations is ongoing, including the development of a *5-aminosalicylate* retention enema for treatment of disease limited to the distal colon.

Drug interactions associated with sulfasalazine use include inhibition of folic acid absorption and a 25% reduction in *digoxin* bioavailability. Sulfasalazine's metabolism is slowed when *cholestyramine* or *broad-spectrum antibiotics* are used concurrently, an effect of uncertain clinical significance. *Ferrous sulfate* appears to have a similar effect on sulfasalazine, although iron absorption is not appreciably hindered; these drugs should not be taken at the same time.

Glucocorticosteroids. Steroids suppress the inflammatory process of ulcerative colitis. *Systemic preparations* are used in markedly symptomatic patients with *extensive disease.* Those without systemic toxicity can be well cared for at home by starting with the equivalent of 60 mg prednisone per day. Patients too ill for oral therapy (those with vomiting, high fever, or signs of bowel distention) should be admitted to the hospital. Once symptoms lessen, the dosage is gradually tapered over 4 to 8 weeks to the lowest dosage that maintains control. Usually, daily steroid therapy is necessary; *alternate-day therapy* rarely suffices to control acute episodes but may help to maintain a remission.

Patients with mild to moderate acute colitis limited to the distal colon can be treated with *rectally administered steroids.* Topical forms include hydrocortisone suppositories given one to three times daily or a retention enema given at night. These programs are capable of inducing remissions in patients with distal disease. The hydrocortisone will always reach the sigmoid; more proximal spread is variable. About one third is absorbed systemically, but adrenal suppression is not a major problem. Steroid suppositories and foams in conjunction with sulfasalazine work well to control disease limited to the rectum (ulcerative proctitis).

When uveitis and colitis flare simultaneously, oral steroids are often effective for both. In the absence of active colitis, the uveitis may be treated with topical steroids and mydriatics. The best means of treating other systemic manifestations (erythema nodosum, pyoderma gangrenosum, and oral aphthous ulcerations) is to control the underlying disease.

Opiates are useful for providing symptomatic relief of diarrhea during acute phases of illness and chronic active colitis. They must be used with *caution* in acutely ill patients

because of the risk of precipitating *toxic dilatation.* Diphenoxylate, codeine, tincture of opium, paregoric, and loperamide all limit the number of bowel movements. They are given before meals and at bedtime. Loperamide is among the most effective and least addicting, but is considerably more expensive. Codeine is excellent for short-term use and superior to diphenoxylate in efficacy. Tincture of belladonna and other anticholinergics help to control cramps.

Psychological Support. The suspicion that psychiatric problems precipitated development of ulcerative colitis, has not been borne out by subsequent study. Consequently, formal psychotherapy directed at uncovering intrapsychic conflict is unnecessary. However, forming a close, supportive, and empathetic patient–doctor relationship is invaluable to psychologically sustaining the patient through his illness (see below).

Screening for Cancer. All patients with clinical or radiologic evidence of *pancolitis* of *7 or more years* should be screened for cancer; at this point the incidence of cancer begins to rise substantially. Since the bowel cancer is often multicentric, the best method of screening is *colonoscopy* with multiple biopsies. There is no agreement on the frequency of screening; recommendations range from yearly to once every 3 years. Worrisome findings include *stricture* and *dysplasia.* Mild dysplasia is an indication for repeat study in 3 months. Severe dysplasia and stricture formation require consideration of colectomy; the risk of cancer is very high in the presence of such findings.

Surgery. A most difficult issue is determining the necessity and timing of surgery. Indications for *elective surgery* include *suspicion of cancer* and *failure of long-term medical management.* For patients who prove refractory to medical therapy, total colectomy offers complete cure of bowel disease and remission of most peripheral manifestations. Many patients actually welcome an ileostomy after years of painful, bloody diarrhea. Patients with severe, persistent disease requiring continuous, high-dose corticosteroids that cannot be tapered after 6 to 12 months deserve serious consideration for surgery, as do those with frequent, severe relapses or complications from prolonged exposure to systemic steroids (see Chapter 103). In each case, the morbidity of active disease and the threat of cancer must be weighed against the risks of major surgery and the inconvenience of a permanent ileostomy. The mortality of elective colectomy is 1% to 3%, with the majority of patients having no postoperative complications. Stoma revision is necessary in 10% to 20% of cases.

Crohn's Disease

Most patients can be treated on an outpatient basis by judicious use of medications and careful follow-up. A strong working alliance between the patient and primary physician is essential, because the disease is chronic and incurable.

Diet. Adequate nutrition is critical to the promotion of healing. Sufficient protein and calories must be provided, but in a manner that limits the stress put on an inflamed and often strictured bowel. Patients with cramps and diarrhea should have the *fiber* content of their diet *reduced;* those with steatorrhea will benefit from a *decrease* in *fat* intake to less than 80 g per day. An empiric trial of *restricting milk products* may terminate diarrhea due to lactase deficiency, which often accompanies the illness. More severely ill patients require partial *bowel rest,* which removes the stimulus that food has on bowel motility and secretion. Although there is no special advantage to commercially prepared *elemental dietary preparations (e.g.,* Magnacal, Ensure, Sustacal, Isocal), they are convenient and usually well-tolerated sources of the extra nutrition needed during exacerbations.

Vitamin and mineral deficiencies are common and must be corrected for proper healing and avoidance of such complications as anemia and bone disease. *Folic acid* supplementation is particularly important in patients taking sulfasalazine, which impairs its absorption. Patients who have had ileal surgery may need extra *vitamin B_{12}. Vitamin D* levels are likely to be low when intake is poor or steatorrhea is a problem. An oral supplement of 4000 IU or more usually suffices. Most vitamin and mineral deficiencies can be overcome by taking a multiple vitamin containing about five times the normal daily vitamin requirements and such minerals as iron, calcium, magnesium, and zinc.

Antidiarrheal Agents. The use of these agents in Crohn's disease is similar to that in ulcerative colitis (see above). The risks include addiction and exacerbation of obstructive symptoms.

Sulfasalazine. The National Cooperative Crohn's Disease Study demonstrated limited efficacy of sulfasalazine in patients with disease of the colon. The drug did not benefit patients with disease limited to the small bowel. Doses of 2 to 4 g per day are used to treat acute exacerbations of abdominal pain and diarrhea in patients with colonic involvement. Improvement typically occurs within 4 to 8 weeks. Chronic use of sulfasalazine does not maintain remissions. The drug in combination with corticosteroids is not better than steroids alone and has not been shown to have a steroid-sparing effect or allow more rapid tapering of steroids once a remission has been induced.

Glucocorticosteroids. When a patient is acutely ill or has not responded to sulfasalazine, systemic steroids are indicated. Patients with small bowel involvement are especially responsive. *High doses (e.g.,* the equivalent of 60 mg prednisone per day) should be used initially. As disease activity subsides, the dose can be empirically tapered to the minimum necessary to control symptoms. As much as 4 months of steroid therapy may be necessary to treat an exacerbation. Sometimes, *alternate-day regimens* will suffice to control disease activity;

they have the advantage of minimizing the steroid side-effects (see Chapter 103). Unfortunately, as noted before, sulfasalazine has not been shown to have a steroid-sparing effect.

Although steroids occupy a central place in the treatment of Crohn's disease, they are *ineffective for maintaining remissions* or preventing exacerbations. Prophylactic steroids are not indicated in Crohn's disease. Moreover, some extraintestinal manifestations and perianal disease do not respond very well to glucocorticoids.

Other Agents. Antibiotics and immunosuppressive agents have been tried, based on the possibility of an infectious or immunologic component to the disease. Relatively high doses of *metronidazole* (750–2000 mg/day) taken for prolonged periods are clearly helpful for patients with perianal disease. Preliminary data suggest the drug may be as effective as sulfasalazine for treatment of enteric disease, but this role is not yet clearly established. Patient acceptability is often limited by gastrointestinal upset, metallic taste, and paresthesias.

The immunosuppressive agents *azathioprine* and its metabolite *6-mercaptopurine* (6-MP) have been subjected to controlled study with variable results. Azathioprine tried at modest dosages to minimize the risk of marrow suppression proved no better than placebo. Higher-dosage studies using 6-MP demonstrated a *steroid-sparing effect, healing of fistulas,* and amelioration of other signs and symptoms. Although the agent is effective, onset of action is slow. Also, at higher dosages, the risk of *marrow suppression* rises substantially; prolonged therapy has been linked to *carcinogenesis,* adding to the reluctance to use such agents in young patients. Initiation of immunosuppressive therapy should not be done without gastroenterologic consultation.

Surgery. Eventually, as many as 70% of patients will require surgery because of *debilitating disease, persistent fistulas, obstruction, abscess,* or *severe bleeding.* The objective of surgical therapy is to remove grossly involved bowel and spare as much normal-appearing bowel as possible. Most patients will have many productive years after surgery; however, the recurrence rate is 30% to 50% per decade. The most common operation is removal of a diseased portion of the terminal ileum with an *ileocolonic anastamosis.* For patients with colonic involvement, *colectomy* with an internal anastamosis connecting the ileum to the sigmoid colon may provide several years of relief without resorting to ileostomy. Ileostomy is necessary in those with marked rectosigmoid disease. Twenty percent to 40% of ileostomies have to be revised within 5 years because of recurrence of disease in the stomal area.

No known medical regimen is capable of preventing postsurgical recurrences. Surgical treatment is undertaken with reluctance and only in the setting of severely disabling disease or serious complications, because, unlike its role in ulcerative colitis, it is not a cure. Reoperation is often necessary; the result is a steadily decreasing remnant of functional bowel. All attempts should be made to preserve as much of the right colon as is possible; its loss often leads to disabling postsurgical diarrhea.

PATIENT EDUCATION

The education and support of the patient and the family are essential. Fears abound when patients are told they have ulcerative colitis or Crohn's disease. These diagnoses conjure up images of colostomy, recurrent hospitalizations, invalidism, and social isolation. It is important to emphasize that the vast majority of patients lead fully functional lives and many obtain satisfactory control of their disease through medical therapy.

Since these are chronic diseases that affect young adults, the questions of *conception, pregnancy, and childbearing* will arise. Although there is some familial pattern to the occurrences of the inflammatory bowel diseases, transmission is not purely genetic and there is ample evidence that while the disease is in remission, fertility is essentially normal and healthy full-term infants can be delivered. However, conception might be a problem when the male patient is taking sulfasalazine (see above). Women with ulcerative colitis are prone to suffer new attacks or exacerbations during the first trimester of pregnancy and have a spontaneous abortion, rate of about 10%. Pregnancy seems to inhibit relapses during later trimesters. Women with active ulcerative colitis should be counseled to postpone getting pregnant until they have been in remission for about a year.

The issue of *cancer risk* in patients with long-standing and extensive ulcerative colitis can be addressed directly and clearly, reassuring those with minimal disease that their risk is nil. The primary physician can do much to prepare the patient who requires *colectomy* and subsequent *ileostomy* with frank but sensitive discussion. Many patients have fears and anxieties that they will not discuss unless they are broached by the physician. Another helpful approach is to have a person of the same age and sex who has had an ileostomy discuss the procedure and its consequences with the patient. Seeing that one can go on to lead a fully active life is very comforting. Where available, a local association of ostomates is a valuable resource.

Many patients can be taught to *adjust their medication* within a prearranged set of guidelines and limits. Dosages of sulfasalazine to be used for mild exacerbations can be specified and extra supplies of medication provided, allowing the patient to play an active role in his care and ensuring prompt treatment of a flare-up. Antidiarrheal agents can also be provided for prn use, but only to very reliable patients who are not likely to abuse them. Patients should be *instructed to call* if fever develops, diarrhea worsens, bleeding occurs, or abdominal pain becomes marked.

The need for a steady exchange of information with the patient and careful explanation of procedures and therapies cannot be overemphasized, nor the importance of close follow-up and availability. Attentiveness and responsiveness help alleviate much of the fear and worry that accompany inflammatory bowel disease and support the development of an effective therapeutic alliance. Additional information and support is available to the patient from the local chapter of the National Ileitis and Colitis Foundation.

INDICATIONS FOR REFERRAL AND ADMISSION

Referral for gastroenterologic consultation is indicated when full dosages of sulfasalazine and oral corticosteroids fail to control a flare-up inflammatory bowel disease. In addition, patients with disabling, chronic, refractory disease ought to see the surgeon and gastroenterologist for consideration of surgery. The pancolitis patient with long-standing disease needs referral for periodic colonoscopy and biopsy. Patients with extraintestinal disease should undergo an ophthalmologic consultation that includes a slit lamp examination to check for uveitis.

Prompt hospitalization for parenteral management is indicated for patients who are toxic, bleeding heavily, in severe pain, or too sick to obtain adequate nutrition orally. Bowel rest, nasogastric feeding of elemental diets, and parenteral steroids are prescribed and surgical consultation obtained, especially if there is severe bleeding, toxicity, distention, or evidence of peritoneal irritation. Home nasoenteric feeding has been demonstrated for carefully selected patients with malabsorption and weight loss refractory to conventional outpatient therapy. Nocturnal tube feedings of a low-fat elemental diet can correct such nutritional problems, but the program requires patients who can insert their own feeding tubes at night.

MANAGEMENT RECOMMENDATIONS

Ulcerative Colitis

General Measures
- Document mucosal inflammation with sigmoidoscopy.
- Reduce dietary fiber during an exacerbation.
- Advise adequate rest and sleep.
- Prescribe a folic acid supplement (1 mg per day) when leafy vegetables are restricted or sulfasalazine is being used.
- Add oral iron supplementation (300 mg ferrous sulfate tid) when there is considerable rectal bleeding and documented iron-deficiency anemia.
- Schedule visits frequently in the early phases of the illness to provide psychological support and close monitoring. Phone checks are helpful.
- Prescribe a short course of opiate therapy (*e.g.,* loperamide 2–4 mg or codeine 15 mg before meals and at bedtime) for temporary symptomatic control of troublesome diarrhea in patients with mild to moderate disease; avoid prolonged

use and use in patients with severe disease (high risk of toxic dilatation).

- If mild diarrhea persists during remissions, initiate a trial of psyllium hydrophyllic colloid (1 teaspoon in 8 oz of water once or twice daily); if this is still unsuccessful, try restricting milk products.
- Refer for periodic colonoscopy and biopsy patients who have pancolitis lasting more than 7 years.

Mild to Moderate Disease

- Begin *sulfasalazine,* 500 mg qid with meals, and increase the dosage as tolerated over several days to 4 g per day. Continue this dosage for 2 to 4 weeks until symptoms abate, then decrease it to the smallest dosage that maintains control of symptoms (usually 2 g per day, though sometimes 4 g per day are required).
- If sulfasalazine fails to achieve control within 3 weeks, add oral *prednisone;* begin with a dose of 40 mg per day. Initially give in divided doses for patients who are having symptoms round-the-clock, but change to a qAM program as soon as possible to limit the degree of adrenal suppression. Continue this dosage for 7 to 10 days.
- If control is achieved, begin tapering prednisone by 5 to 10 mg every 2 weeks to the lowest dosage necessary to suppress disease activity. An alternate-day program (using the same total weekly dose that maintains control) may be tried to minimize chronic steroid therapy side-effects (see Chapter 103).
- Once steroids are tapered off and disease activity ceases, decrease sulfasalazine to a maintenance dose of 2 g per day and continue for at least 1 year to maintain remission.

Moderate to Severe Disease

- Start with *prednisone,* 60 mg per day in divided doses, and *sulfasalazine* at 4 g per day. Once the symptoms come under control, give the entire prednisone dose in the morning and begin tapering empirically by 5 mg per week. Continue the sulfasalazine at 1 g qid indefinitely.
- If food intake is inadequate over time because of nausea or abdominal pain, consider supplementing the diet with a nutritionally balanced, *low-residue liquid dietary preparation (e.g.,* Magnacal, Ensure, Sustacal, Isocal).
- Monitor carefully for marked blood loss, volume depletion, severe abdominal pain, distention, and peritoneal signs; any of these is an indication for prompt hospital admission, parenteral therapy, and urgent surgical consultation.
- Refer for consideration of elective surgery, patients refractory to maximal medical therapy, those requiring daily steroids for prolonged periods (>6 months), and those found on cancer screening to have a stricture or dysplasia.

Ulcerative Proctocolitis

- If disease is limited to the rectosigmoid, begin treatment with oral sulfasalazine (as noted above) or topical hydrocortisone. Administer hydrocortisone rectally, using a 100-mg *retention enema* taken once nightly, a 25-mg *suppository* once or twice daily, or a 90-mg *foam* preparation once or twice daily. Selection of preparation can be based on patient preference and empirical results. Continue hydrocortisone until symptoms clear; continue sulfasalazine for prophylaxis.

Crohn's Disease

General Measures

- Document the extent of disease by barium studies or colonoscopy. Postpone barium enema and colonoscopy until disease activity subsides.
- Limit the fiber content of the diet in patients with cramps and diarrhea.
- Decrease the fat intake to less than 80 mg per day when there is steatorrhea.
- Conduct a trial of restricting milk products from the diet of patients with diarrhea; if the diarrhea promptly improves, continue with a lactose-restricted diet.
- Supplement the diet with a multivitamin preparation that contains five times the normal daily vitamin requirements plus iron, calcium, magnesium, and zinc.
- Consider short-course opiate therapy (*e.g.,* loperamide mg or codeine 15 mg with meals and before bed) for symptomatic relief of diarrhea; use caution, obstruction may be aggrevated and prolonged use can lead to narcotic dependence.
- Advise partial bowel rest and use of elemental, low-residue dietary preparations when cramps and diarrhea are severe.
- Admit for refractory disease, severe bleeding, toxicity, abdominal pain, abscess formation, or evidence of obstruction. Such patients need surgical consultation.

Colonic Disease

- Begin *sulfasalazine* 500 mg qid and quickly increase the dosage to 1 g qid over several days; continue for 4 to 8 weeks.
- If there is no response to sulfasalazine, *switch to prednisone* 60 mg per day; qid dosages may be required at the outset for round-the-clock control.
- As disease activity subsides, give the entire dosage in the morning and begin tapering it to the lowest dosage that controls the symptoms. Continue this dosage until all evidence of disease activity ceases (as long as 4 months); an alternate-day schedule may suffice.

Perianal Disease

- Prescribe *metronidazole* (750–2000 mg per day) for refractory perianal disease; a prolonged course of treatment may be necessary.

Ileal Disease

- The effectiveness of sulfasalazine for ileal disease is not well established, although some patients with mild disease may benefit. Begin with *prednisone* (60 mg per day) and use in the same fashion as for colonic involvement (see above).

• Consider use of *6-mercaptopurine* for patients with fistulas, refractory symptoms, or requirements for very high steroid dosages. Since the prolonged high-dose therapy required can cause marrow suppression and carcinogenesis, obtain gastroenterologic consultation before initiating therapy.

ANNOTATED BIBLIOGRAPHY

Bernstein LH, Frank MS, Brandt LJ, Boley SJ: Healing of perineal Crohn's disease with metronidazole. Gastroenterology 79:375, 1980 (*Documents the drug's usefulness in therapy of chronic perianal abscesses and fistulas.*)

Block GE: Surgical management of Crohn's colitis. N Engl J Med 302:1068, 1980 (*Terse and useful review of available surgical approaches, including discussion of criteria for patient selection.*)

Disanayake AS, Truelove SC: A controlled therapeutic trial of long-term maintenance treatment of ulcerative colitis with sulfasalazine. Gut 14:923, 1973 (*This study documents the efficacy of sulfasalazine for prophylaxis; recurrence rate was one fourth that of the control group.*)

Donaldson RM: Management of medical problems in pregnancy: Inflammatory bowel disease. N Engl J Med 312:1616, 1985 (*Good practical review of this difficult management issue.*)

Dworken HJ: Ulcerative colitis: A clearer picture. Ann Intern Med 99:717, 1983 (*Reviews data on prognosis derived from community-based studies and argues for a more optimistic view of the illness.*)

Farmer RG, Whelan G, Fazio VW: Long-term follow up of patients with Crohn's disease. Gastroenterology 88:818, 1985 (*Relationship between clinical pattern and prognosis.*)

Foley JH: Ulcerative proctitis. N Engl J Med 282:1362, 1970 (*A classic article describing the condition, its course, and therapy.*)

Glotzer DJ, et al: Comparative features and course of ulcerative and granulomatous colitis. N Engl J Med 282:582, 1970 (*A classic review comparing and contrasting the two conditions.*)

Halstead CH, Gandhi G, Tamura T: Sulfasalazine inhibits the absorption of folates in ulcerative colitis. N Engl J Med 305:1513, 1981 (*A report documenting this important side-effect of sulfasalazine.*)

Hawkey CJ: Salicylates for the sulfa-sensitive patient with ulcerative colitis. Gastroenterology 90:1082, 1986 (*A review of studies on use of nonsulfa-containing salicylates for inflammatory bowel disease.*)

Heymsfield SB, Smith-Andrews JL, Hersh T: Home nasoenteric feeding for malabsorption and weight loss refractory to conventional therapy. Ann Intern Med 98:168, 1983 (*An interesting approach that allows properly selected patients with severe disease to remain at home.*)

Jick H, Walker AM: Cigarette smoking and ulcerative Colitis. N Engl J Med 308:261, 1983 (*A provoking report of an inverse statistical relationship between smoking and ulcerative colitis; the accompanying editorial puts the finding into proper perspective.*)

Kirsner JB, Shorter RG: Recent developments in nonspecific inflammatory bowel disease. N Engl J Med 306:775, 837, 1982 (*A recent review of progress in therapy and understanding of pathogenesis; 391 references.*)

Klotz UK, Maier K, Fischer C et al: Therapeutic efficacy of sulfasalazine and its metabolites in patients with ulcerative colitis and Crohn's disease. N Engl J Med 303:1499, 1980 (*Finds that 5-aminosalicylate is the active moiety of sulfasalazine and may be an alternative for patients who cannot take sulfa-containing drugs.*)

Lennard-Jones JE et al: Cancer in colitis: Assessment of the individual risk by clinical and histological criteria. Gastroenterology 73:1280, 1977 (*Cancer risk is correlated with duration of disease and mucosal dysplasia. A protocol for detection is proposed.*)

National Cooperative Crohn's Disease Study. Gastroenterology 77:825, 1979 (*A multicenter controlled study demonstrating the efficacy of sulfasalazine in acute disease of the colon. No improvement was observed in patients whose disease was confined to the small bowel.*)

Peppercorn MA: Sulfasalazine: Pharmacology, clinical use, toxicity and related new drug development. Ann Intern Med 101:377, 1984 (*Authoritative and clinically useful review of the drug; 140 references.*)

Present DH, Korelitz BI, Wisch N et al.: Treatment of Crohn's disease with 6-mercaptopurine. N Engl J Med 302:981, 1980 (*A long-term randomized double-blind study showing that 6-MP is effective in the management of refractory Crohn's disease. The accompanying editorial by Sleisenger puts the study's results into context.*)

Purdy BH, Philips DM, Summers RW: Desensitization for sulfasalazine skin rash. Ann Intern Med 100:512, 1984 (*Presents a practical means of desensitization; patients with more serious allergic reactions are not candidates for this procedure.*)

Sacher DB: Cancer in ulcerative colitis: Good news and bad news. Ann Intern Med 95:642, 1981 (*A terse look at new data on risk and means of detection.*)

Singleton JW: Corticosteroids for Crohn's disease. Ann Intern Med 90:983, 1979 (*A excellent editorial summarizing the use of corticosteroids in Crohn's disease; argues for its selective use.*)

Sleisenger MH: How should we treat Crohn's disease? N Engl J Med 302:1024, 1980 (*Discusses the role of immunosuppressive therapy and analyzes available studies that give conflicting results.*)

Ursing B, Almy T et al: A comparative study of metronidazole and sulfasalazine for active Crohn's disease. A Cooperative Crohn's Disease Study in Sweden. II. Results. Gastroenterology 83:550, 1982 (*This study of 78 patients showed metronidazole able to produce results comparable to those of sulfasalazine; moreover, the drug worked in some patients who failed to respond to sulfasalazine.*)

Whelan G, Farmer RG, Fazio VW: Recurrence after surgery in Crohn's disease, relationship to location and disease. Clinical pattern and surgical indication. Gastroenterology 88:1826, 1985 (*Six hundred and fifteen patients followed by the Cleveland Clinic from 1966 to the present show a high index of recurrence after operation.*)

Whittington PF, Barnes HV, Bayless TM: Medical management of Crohn's disease in adolescence. Gastroenterology 72:1338, 1977 (*A useful guide for therapy. A major consideration is restricted use of steroids to avoid arresting growth.*)

66
Management of the Irritable Bowel Syndrome

The irritable bowel syndrome is a prevalent disease in modern society, reportedly accounting for half of gastrointestinal complaints seen by physicians and ranking as a major cause of industrial absenteeism. The condition has been referred to by many names, including "irritable colon syndrome," "mucous colitis," and "spastic colon." It can be defined as a functional disturbance of intestinal motility, strongly influenced by emotional factors. Patients seek help because of gastrointestinal symptoms, fear of serious illness, and psychological problems. Irritable bowel can mimic organic disease, often goes unrecognized, and results in extensive workups and frustrating attempts at therapy. The primary physician must become expert in the diagnosis and management of this very common condition to avoid unnecessary investigations and to initiate effective symptomatic therapy.

PATHOPHYSIOLOGY AND CLINICAL PRESENTATION

Irritable bowel syndrome is a disturbance of bowel motor activity. Nonpropulsive colonic contractions and slow-wave myoelectric patterns at 2 to 3 cycles per minute constitute about 40% of electrical and contractile activity at rest in patients with irritable bowel syndrome, compared with 10% in normals. These contractions are felt to impede propulsion of stool, and when excessive, they account for the constipation and discomfort so prevalent in this condition. The diarrhea often seen in the syndrome is believed to occur as a result of increased contraction in the small bowel and proximal colon and diminished activity in the distal large bowel, creating a pressure gradient and causing accelerated movement of intestinal contents. Meals cause an increase in colonic contractions, but controlled study has shown that patients with irritable colon syndrome have a significantly exaggerated increase in response to food from that of normals.

Emotional stress has long been considered an important contributing factor. Hypermotility in response to stress has been documented, and a high prevalence of psychiatric illness has been uncovered. A psychological study of 29 patients with irritable bowel syndrome and 33 controls found that 72% of the former had a psychiatric illness, compared with only 15% of the controls. Psychiatric symptoms usually preceded bowel complaints. Hysteria and depression were the most common emotional disorders. A hospital-based epidemiologic study of 102 patients with irritable colon syndrome revealed a significantly higher frequency of life stresses in this group than among 735 individuals in the control group.

Laboratory experiments correlating response to a stress interview with sigmoid motility and symptoms have shown that when patients expressed coping behavior, they had heightened sigmoid contractions and were most often troubled by constipation and abdominal pain; when exhibiting depressive behavior, they had diminished sigmoid activity and diarrhea.

The commonly encountered syndrome of diarrhea alternating with constipation may reflect the different responses to stress that an individual may manifest. Moreover, laboratory study of normal individuals subjected to experimentally induced stress showed similar bowel responses, suggesting that irritable colon physiology is a normal reaction to severe stress. What seems to characterize the patient persistently bothered by irritable colon symptoms is the greater prevalence of serious situational stresses, psychopathology, and perhaps learned visceral responses to threatening situations. This psychophysiologic response to stress may be altered by agents affecting gut motility, such as anticholinergics.

Clinical presentation is illustrated by a series of 50 patients treated in an outpatient unit. Most of the patients (62%) experienced onset of symptoms before age 40; 50% were under 30 at time of onset; and one quarter were under 20. *Chronicity* was the rule, with little change in symptoms over time, except for waxing and waning. Duration was in years. Only 14% actively carried a diagnosis of irritable bowel syndrome. *Abdominal pain* was present in 90%, *mucous* stools in 36%, *pelletlike stools* in 38%, *diarrhea* alone in 10%, *excessive flatus* in 36%. Fifty percent considered their symptoms related to stress; 34% denied this; 66% manifested symptoms of anxiety or depression. The abdominal pain was most often in the left lower quadrant or lower abdomen (62%), but in 28% there were multiple sites of pain. Upper abdominal involvement occurred in 38%. The pain was typically achy rather than crampy, often relieved by a bowel movement or passage of flatus. It was unusual for the pain to awaken the patient. Radiation was variable, and even extended into the left chest and arm when gas was trapped in the splenic flexure.

Small, hard, infrequent stools and an empty rectal ampulla characterize the constipation. Prolonged retention of stool allows for full absorption of intestinal water content. The diarrhea is typically small in volume, associated with visible amounts of mucus, and may follow a hard movement by a few hours. There may be urgency. Dyspepsia and excessive gaseousness are also reported (see Chapter 55). Weight loss is rare; symptoms usually parallel situational stresses.

CLINICAL COURSE

Irritable bowel syndrome is a chronic, relapsing condition with no evidence of significant morbidity or mortality. A prospective British study providing follow-up at 2-month intervals over 3 years found that severity waxed and waned, but the constellation of symptoms remained remarkably constant. At 1 year, 50% were unchanged, 36% improved, 12% were symptom-free and 20% were worse. The symptom-free period was usually less than a few months. One third of employed patients lost time from work. There was no correlation between time lost and number of visits to the doctor; 40% made five or fewer visits, and 46% made none at all. At 2 years, a similar pattern was found. Only one patient remained symptom-free from the first year.

Studies on clinical course identified groups of patients with different prognoses. The group with symptoms triggered by a major life stress enjoyed long symptom-free periods after the acute problem abated, whereas those with continuous intestinal complaints in response to daily living rarely became asymptomatic.

PRINCIPLES OF MANAGEMENT

Patient education, support, diet, and drugs are the basic therapeutic approaches available for dealing with irritable bowel syndrome. No single modality has proven successful in randomized, placebo-controlled studies. A sequential approach that begins with patient education and support minimizes the need to resort to drugs for provision of symptomatic relief.

The first rule in caring for these patients is to *take their symptoms seriously* and not dismiss them as inconsequential or imaginary. One cannot overemphasize the therapeutic benefit of a careful and *thorough history and physical examination,* combined with a few simple laboratory studies (perhaps even a limited sigmoidoscopy in patients very worried about "colitis"). Eliciting the *patient's concerns* (*e.g.,* cancer, inflammatory bowel disease) and then directly checking for and addressing them are essential to any reassurance effort and a *sine qua non* of effective care.

The physician needs to go beyond allaying fears to *providing a specific diagnosis;* these patients strongly believe there is something awry and will not accept a conclusion that "there's nothing wrong with your bowels." By the end of the initial office visit, the diagnosis of irritable bowel syndrome is usually evident. The diagnosis and its pathophysiology should be discussed along with the prediction that tests being ordered for the sake of thoroughness are going to be normal. In this way, the patient does not leave frustrated, feeling the "doctor cannot find what is wrong." *Explanation* (perhaps aided by diagrams) of how psychological stresses can lead to functional alterations in bowel motility helps patients with a psychophysiologic basis for their illness to better understand it. Patients without evident psychopathology and those unable to face the issue can at least be educated about the relationship between bowel motility disturbances and their symptoms.

A distinguishing characteristic of patients who suffer from irritable bowel syndrome is their exaggerated emotional response to their bowel symptoms. Sometimes, the best intervention is withdrawing all previously prescribed medications and simply listening empathetically to the patient's problems, helping him cope with his life situation. The establishment of a supportive *doctor–patient relationship* in conjunction with providing reassurance, explanation, and advice can have an important impact on outcome. When such care was given to patients in the prospective British study cited earlier, most reported feeling better, less concerned about their bowels, and more able to cope with their symptoms and the stresses of daily life. Even though there were frequent relapses, these seemed to be less important when they occurred in the context of close medical support.

Since the prevalence of underlying psychopathology is very high in patients with irritable bowel syndrome, definitive therapy often requires *identifying and addressing* the patient's *psychological difficulties.* In the context of conducting a thorough workup, the clinician needs to sensitively elicit details of the patient's life situation, aspirations, accomplishments, frustrations, and losses. Concerns, fears, expectations, and responses to previous life stresses can also be very informative, as can the mental status of the patient on examination. Anxiety disorders are commonly identified, but depression (see Chapter 223) and hysteria (see Chapter 222) often go unrecognized.

When specific underlying psychopathology is identified, treatment should be directed toward it. Success rates are high in such circumstances. In a study of 67 patients with irritable bowel syndrome, 56 were felt to suffer from *depression* and received a *tricyclic* agent. More than 50% become symptom-free, 33% improved, and 20% showed no benefit. *Amitriptyline* in low doses (25–50 mg qhs) has been found to be particularly effective, because its anticholinergic activity helps relieve diarrhea. One must be careful not to give benzodiazepines (*e.g.,* diazepam) to depressed patients who manifest anxiety; these agents will only worsen the depression (see Chapter 223). An antidepressant with anxiolytic properties (*e.g., doxepin*) is more appropriate.

Treatment of patients with *hysteria* and other somatization disorders first requires withdrawing the vast array of medications prescribed by the multitude of physicians they have visited over the years, and then setting up regularly scheduled visits for them to talk about their symptoms and personal problems. Such supportive therapy by the primary physician often suffices to alleviate much of their complaining and need for medication.

When bowel symptoms are not due to a well-defined psychiatric illness, use of psychotropic agents is less effective. A double-blind controlled study of 52 patients manifesting nonspecific anxiety showed that *diazepam* had no effect on bowel complaints compared with placebo. *Relaxation techniques* can be taught to such patients, often with surprisingly good results. The efficacy of *biofeedback* is undetermined; the method has not been subjected to controlled study.

Although a major part of the therapeutic effort in irritable bowel syndrome involves redirecting the patient's attention away from his bowels, it is often necessary to provide some patients with symptomatic relief before they are willing to turn their attention to the factors precipitating their symptoms. *Dietary manipulations* are sometimes helpful. Both low-residue and high-fiber diets have been tried. There is no evidence that low-residue diets are of any use. Results of studies examining *bran and high-fiber diets* are variable. In a double-blind trial of 50 patients eating a standardized bran biscuit or placebo, there was no difference in effect. Both groups reported subjective improvement in more than 50% of the subjects. A more recent controlled, but unblinded British study of 26 patients showed significant improvement in symptoms and colonic motor activity in the bran-fed group compared with controls. Certainly there is no harm in prescribing a high-fiber diet, and it may have other health benefits such as reducing the risk of colon cancer (see Chapter 51).

Use of *bulking agents,* such as the hydrophyllic colloid *psyllium* (Metamucil), is another frequently employed approach. In a double-blind controlled study of 77 patients, both placebo and control groups demonstrated significant improvement in symptoms. Personality factors and physician attention were important predictors of outcome. These results and those involving use of bran reinforce the importance of a multifaceted approach to treatment.

Many patients insist they have "*food allergies*" as the cause of their symptoms. True food allergies are rare and typically cause acute hypersensitivity reactions, not chronic gastrointestinal complaints. No changes in colonic motor activity have been found to occur in such patients on intake of the offending food. However, *food intolerances* are often noted in patients with irritable bowel syndrome. Coffee, citrus fruits, and caffeine are among the long list of substances purported to trigger symptoms. Sorbitol, a common sweetener in candies, is capable of causing bloating and diarrhea if taken in large amounts (see Chapter 58). Some food intolerances are mislabelled as irritable bowel syndrome. For example, patients with *gluten* intolerance (adult celiac disease, nontropical sprue) may present with abdominal discomfort and diarrhea. Persistent diarrhea, bloating, cramping, and excessive flatus may be manifestations of underlying *lactose* intolerance (see Chapter 58). A 1- to 2-week trial of restricting a suspected offending food or substance is reasonable when clinical suspicion is high.

Drug therapy efforts should proceed only in the context of a balanced program that includes patient education and support. Precipitously or prematurely resorting to pharmacologic measures in a hasty attempt to completely suppress symptoms can lead to frustration and excessive, even dangerous, escalations of drug intake. In fact, at the outset of therapy, it is often useful to *stop all nonessential medicines* that may affect bowel function, especially irritant laxatives.

Nevertheless, there is a role for carefully selected, short-term applications of medication when some symptomatic relief is deemed necessary. Patients suffering from *disabling diarrhea* may benefit from short courses of an *opiate* derivate (*e.g.,* diphenoxylate or loperamide). Caution needs to be exercised because of the *risk of abuse* in these patients. Patients bothered by *abdominal pain and distention* sometimes benefit from use of an *anticholinergic* agent (*e.g.,* dicyclomine). Although these agents have been shown to inhibit the postprandial increase in nonpropulsive colonic contractions, their clinical effectiveness is unproven; however, the consensus is that they are worth a try in cases in which nonpharmacologic measures have failed. Use only for short periods. They can worsen constipation. *Combination preparations* containing tranquilizers and anticholinergics should be avoided; they are heavily promoted, yet of no proven benefit (many contain barbiturates).

PATIENT EDUCATION

Because irritable bowel syndrome is a condition characterized by an exaggerated response to symptoms, patient education is central to effective management. As noted earlier the basic elements of the patient education effort include addressing patient fears, providing a specific diagnosis, and explaining the psychophysiologic basis of symptoms. In addition, when important situational stress or psychopathology is uncovered, it needs to be discussed openly so that the patient can begin to focus on the underlying issues rather than on his bowel symptoms. Sometimes, having the patient keep a diary of his symptoms, stresses, and feelings can help reveal connections that have otherwise eluded him. The major lesson to be mastered by patients with irritable bowel syndrome is the relationship between their psychological state and symptoms, a message that often takes patience, sensitivity, and skill to communicate effectively. Once this is understood and a supportive relationship is established, patients begin to cope better and spend less time obsessing about their bowels or searching for the elusive medication that will cure them.

INDICATIONS FOR REFERRAL AND ADMISSION

This is a condition in which a continuous relationship is essential, and any perceived need for referral should be acted on only after thorough discussion with the patient. In general, referral is helpful when there are refractory disabling symptoms, such as uncontrollable diarrhea, or when serious psychopathology is encountered. A hospital admission may, in rare circumstances, be appropriate and very beneficial in helping the patient to learn new means of coping with stress and providing a respite from an intolerable living situation.

MANAGEMENT RECOMMENDATIONS

- Take the patient's bowel complaints seriously; do not minimize their importance or deny their "reality."
- Elicit a full psychosocial data base as well as a complete history of the patient's bodily symptoms.
- Identify, discuss, and treat specifically any underlying depression (see Chapter 223), anxiety disorder (see Chapter 222), or other psychiatric condition.
- Provide a thorough explanation of the diagnosis and directly address the patient's concerns and fears.
- Establish a supportive relationship and begin supportive psychotherapy for patients with underlying situational or psychosocial stresses.
- Stop all nonessential medicines that may affect bowel function, especially irritant laxatives.
- For the patient bothered predominantly by constipation, increase dietary fiber and recommend regular exercise.
- Add a bulking agent such as psyllium (Metamucil), 1 rounded teaspoon in 8 oz of water, tid, if constipation is still troublesome.
- Resort to a trial of anticholinergic therapy (*e.g.,* dicyclomine 20 mg qid) only if other measures have failed and the patient finds abdominal pain and distention intolerable; may also be useful for diarrhea. Use only for short period of time.
- For the patient with diarrhea, recommend an increase in dietary fiber. If short-term symptomatic relief is essential, prescribe a 2- to 5-day supply of diphenoxylate with atropine (Lomotil) or loperamide, 1 tablet bid prn. Exert caution with opiate use because of its addiction potential in this chronic condition.
- Dietary restrictions are usually unnecessary. However, if there is a strongly suggestive history of intolerance to a food or substance, consider a 1- or 2-week trial of restricting its intake.
- Avoid use of sedatives, tranquilizers, and combination preparations.
- Help redirect the patient's attention from his bowel symptoms and the search for a cure to the factors responsible for the condition.
- See patient at regular intervals and be available for help at times of increased stress.

A.H.G.

ANNOTATED BIBLIOGRAPHY

Almy T: Experimental studies on the irritable colon. Am J Med 10: 60, 1951 (*Classic experiments on relation of stress to bowel activity.*)

Cann PA, Read NW, Holdsworth CD: What is the benefit of coarse wheat bran in patients with irritable bowel syndrome. Gut 25: 168, 1984 (*A study of 38 patients showed that bran did help pain, constipation, diarrhea, and urgency, as did placebo, except for constipation, which responded better with bran.*)

Deutsch E: Relief of anxiety and related emotions in patients with gastrointestinal disorders. Am J Dig Dis 16:1091, 1971 (*Diazepam relieved anxiety but did not improve bowel symptoms any better than did placebo.*)

Drossman DA, Powell DW, Sessions JT Jr: The irritable bowel syndrome. Gastroenterology 73:811, 1977 (*A superb review emphasizing motility factors, diagnosis, treatment, and prognosis of this difficult syndrome; 86 references.*)

Esler M, Goulston K: Levels of anxiety in colonic disorders. N Engl J Med 288:16, 1973 (*Patients with predominant diarrhea were significantly more anxious and more neurotic by psychometric testing than normals or those with constipation and pain.*)

Hislop I: Psychological significance of the irritable colon syndrome. Gut 12:452, 1971 (*Fifty-six of 67 patients with irritable colon syndrome were treated with tricyclic antidepressants. More than 80% reported significant improvement.*)

Ivey KJ: Are anticholinergics of use in the irritable colon syndrome? Gastroenterology 68:1300, 1975 (*A careful review of the use of anticholinergic drugs that concludes that although the evidence is dubious, they appear to be of some benefit in patients with pain or constipation as their major syndrome. Use is advised when patients fail to respond to routine measures; 53 references.*)

Jones AV, McLaughlan P, Shorthouse M et al: Food intolerance: A major factor in the pathogenesis of the irritable bowel syndrome. Lancet 2:115, 1982 (*Patients with irritable bowel may be intolerant to wheat, corn, dairy products, coffee, tea, or citrus fruits.*)

Kruis W, Thieme C, Weinzierl M et al: A diagnostic score for the irritable bowel syndrome, its value in the exclusion of organic disease. Gastroenterology 87:1, 1984 (*An elaborate regression study of irritable bowel syndrome characteristics providing a weighted score with high specificity and sensitivity.*)

Lennard-Jones JE: Functional gastrointestinal disorders. N Engl J Med 308:431, 1983 (*A succinct review of the epidemiology, clinical presentation, management, and treatment of functional gastrointestinal disease.*)

Longstreth GF, Fox DD, Youkeles MS et al: Psyllium therapy in the irritable bowel syndrome. Ann Intern Med 95:53, 1981 (*A randomized double-blind, controlled study showing that both treatment and controlled groups improved significantly; points out the strong psychological overlay of symptoms and efficacy of supportive measures.*)

Manning A, Heaton K, Harvey R et al: Wheat fibre and irritable bowel syndrome. Lancet 2:417, 1977 (*A controlled but unblinded study of 26 patients showing significant improvement in symptoms and colonic motor activity in the bran-treated group only.*)

Marzuk PM: Biofeedback for gastrointestinal disorders: A review of the literature. Ann Intern Med 103:240, 1985 (*Biofeedback has not been adequately studied to draw any conclusions about its efficacy in irritable bowel syndrome.*)

Newcomer AD, McGill DB: Clinical importance of lactose deficiency. N Engl J Med 310:42, 1984 (*An editorial on the role of lactose deficiency in clinical syndromes including irritable bowel syndrome.*)

Sullivan M, Cohen S, Snape W: Colonic myoelectric activity in irritable bowel syndrome. N Engl J Med 298:878, 1978 (*Patients with irritable bowel syndrome and abnormally prolonged increase in postprandial motor activity, which was reduced by an anticholinergic agent.*)

Treacher DF et al: Irritable bowel syndrome: Is barium enema necessary? Clin Radiol 37:87, 1986 (*A retrospective analysis of 114 patients, which found that the barium enema rarely revealed useful information in patients who had normal hematologic and biochemical screening, especially in those under age 50.*)

Waller S, Misiewicz J: Prognosis in the irritable bowel syndrome. Lancet 2:754, 1969 (*Symptoms wax and wane with little permanent resolution, but supportive therapy helps patients to cope.*)

Wangel A, Deller D: Intestinal motility in man. III. Mechanisms of constipation and diarrhea with particular reference to the irritable colon syndrome. Gastroenterology 48:69, 1965 (*A motility study of the large bowel, demonstrating increased proximal and distal activity aggravated by food and emotion in patients with constipation and pain, and diminished distal activity in those with diarrhea.*)

Whitehead WE, Engel BT, Schuster MM: Irritable bowel syndrome: Physiological and psychological differences between diarrhea-predominant and constipation-predominant patients. Dig Dis Sci 24:277, 1979 (*Suggests there is a relationship between clinical presentation and underlying psychological state.*)

Young S, Alper D, Norland C et al: Psychiatric illness and the irritable bowel syndrome. Gastroenterology 70:162, 1970 (*Seventy-two percent of patients with irritable bowel syndrome in a general group practice have an underlying psychiatric illness; only 28% were properly recognized and diagnosed.*)

67

Management of Diverticular Disease

Diverticula, abnormal herniations of colonic mucosa through the muscularis, are extremely common and increase with age. Autopsy studies estimate their presence in 20% of people over 40 and in 70% of those over 70. About 15% of people with the condition develop attacks of diverticulitis. It is possible that the recent emphasis on increasing the fiber content of the diet will reduce the incidence of diverticulosis in Western countries. The primary physician encounters many elderly patients with gastrointestinal complaints referable to diverticular disease. The physician must effectively and economically recognize and treat mild manifestations of disease, reduce the chances of complications, and decide when admission and surgical intervention are necessary.

PATHOPHYSIOLOGY, CLINICAL PRESENTATION, AND COMPLICATIONS

Increased intracolonic pressure causes herniation of colonic mucosa. Consequently, diverticula occur most frequently in the sigmoid where the colon is narrowest and pressure highest. Diverticula show a predilection for points of relative weakness in the muscularis where branches of the marginal artery penetrate the colonic wall. Current research indicates that the *low fiber content* of modern diets has a causal role, producing less bulky stool and increased intracolonic pressure. Conditions associated with abnormal co-

lonic activity and segmentation, such as irritable colon syndrome, may contribute to the pathogenesis of diverticula; this remains speculative. The possibility of muscular degeneration has been suggested but remains unproven.

The diverticular sac can become inflamed when undigested food residues and bacteria get trapped in the thin-walled sac; blood supply is mechanically compromised and bacterial invasion ensues. Microperforations can occur, producing peridiverticular and pericolonic inflammation.

Most diverticula are asymptomatic and discovered incidentally on barium enema. However, colonic motor activity is sometimes disturbed, and intermittent left lower quadrant pain results. Constipation is common, as is constipation alternating with diarrhea, and occasionally there is tenderness. *Diverticulitis* is characterized by left lower quadrant pain, tenderness, fever, and leukocytosis in a patient with known diverticulosis. Frequently a tender mass is noted. The diagnosis is made clinically during an acute attack and confirmed later by barium enema, once the risk of perforation subsides. At times, the radiologic findings resemble those of cancer or Crohn's disease, and colonoscopy is needed for more definitive evaluation.

The major complications of diverticular disease are perforation, obstruction, and bleeding. Perforations may lead to abscess formation. The abscesses may spontaneously drain into the bowel or erode into an adjacent organ, such as the ureter, bladder, or vagina, forming fistulas. Perforations that fail to become walled off may cause peritonitis. Those that enter the vagina result in vaginal gas or feces; those that erode into the urinary tract lead to dysuria or pneumaturia. Chronic inflammation can thicken the bowel wall and cause obstruction. Erosion into a blood vessel may result in brisk rectal hemorrhage. The incidence of hemorrhage, obstruction, or perforation was 15% in a 15-year study from the Lahey Clinic.

PRINCIPLES OF MANAGEMENT

The goals of therapy are prevention of symptoms, relief of pain, and avoidance of complications. Since diverticular disease is felt to be, in part, a manifestation of a low-fiber diet, *bran* has been tried in therapy. Prospective British studies of bran use have shown reversal of abnormal bowel physiology and reduction in symptoms in over 90% of cases. The average amount of bran needed to achieve an effect is 15 g per day. Some individuals are bothered by flatulence and bloating during the first 2 to 3 weeks of bran use, but this usually resolves.

Patients unable to tolerate bran may be treated with bulk agents such as *psyllium* (Metamucil). Irritant laxatives should be avoided. The efficacy of *anticholinergics* is controversial; painful spasm may be lessened, but the risk of constipation is increased, raising the likelihood of inspissation of fecal material. Indigestible materials (*e.g.,* seeds) that may block the mouth of a diverticulum should be omitted from the diet.

Diverticulitis can be treated at home when symptoms are mild and there is no evidence of peritonitis. The aim of therapy is to markedly reduce bowel activity to lessen the chance of perforation. *Rest* and clear *liquids* usually suffice. Strong analgesics and antipyretics should not be prescribed because they may mask signs of worsening inflammation. Broad-spectrum oral *antibiotics* such as amoxicillin or cephalexin are customarily used, especially when fever exceeds 101°F, though their efficacy is unproven.

An important decision in the therapy of diverticulitis is whether to treat the patient medically or opt for elective *surgical resection* of the involved bowel after initial resolution of symptoms. Proponents of surgical therapy argue that the frequency of complications warrants prophylactic operation once a patient experiences an attack of diverticulitis. The courses of 132 patients at Yale–New Haven Hospital with documented uncomplicated diverticulitis were analyzed. Of the 99 treated medically and 33 treated surgically, the rates of recurrence were almost identical. Moreover, three quarters never had more than one attack. The increased length of hospitalization and postoperative morbidity were not balanced by a marked reduction in rate of recurrence or complications. However, the presence of abscess, perforation, or obstruction is an indication for surgery. Although controlled data are lacking, most authorities recommend treatment with a high-fiber diet after acute symptoms have ceased.

INDICATIONS FOR ADMISSION AND REFERRAL

The development of a temperature greater than 101°F, persistence of pain for more than 3 days, and increasing pain indicate need for admission. A markedly elevated white count may be the only clue to a deteriorating situation; many patients with diverticulitis are elderly and may not demonstrate much fever, abdominal pain, or peritoneal signs. The management of a patient with bleeding, abscess, or perforation requires surgical consultation; operative intervention may be urgent.

THERAPEUTIC RECOMMENDATIONS AND PATIENT EDUCATION

For the patient with known diverticula and occasional pain or constipation the following recommendations should be observed:

- Increase the fiber content of the diet. The best sources are bran, root vegetables (particularly raw carrots), and fruits with skin. Bulk laxatives such as psyllium hydrophilic mucilloid (Metamucil) can be used in patients who cannot tolerate bran, but are relatively expensive.
- Inform patients that any bloating or flatulence due to bran intake usually resolves with continued use.
- Advise patients to avoid foods with seeds or indigestible material that may block the neck of a diverticulum, such as nuts, corn, popcorn, cucumbers, tomatoes, figs, strawberries, and caraway seeds.
- Have patients avoid laxatives, enemas, and opiates because they are potent constipating agents.
- Anticholinergics should be reserved for refractory cases.
- Instruct patients to report fever, tenderness, or bleeding without delay.

For patients with mild diverticulitis (temperature less than 101°F, white cell count below 13,000 to 15,000) the following recommendations should be observed:

- Prescribe bed rest and a clear liquid diet.
- Use mild nonopiate analgesics for pain.
- Monitor temperature, pain, abdominal examination for signs of peritonitis, and white count for elevation.
- Consider a broad spectrum antibiotic (*e.g.,* amoxicillin 500 mg tid) if the patient is slow to improve.

A.H.G.

ANNOTATED BIBLIOGRAPHY

Almy T, Howell DA: Diverticular disease of the colon. N Engl J Med 302:324, 1980. (*An authoritative review; 119 references.*)

Boles R, Jordan S: Clinical significance of diverticulosis. Gastroenterology 35:579, 1958 (*An analysis of 294 patients with diverticulosis; mean duration of follow-up was 15 years. Frequency of hemorrhage, obstruction, or perforation was 15%.*)

Boulos PB, Karamanolis DG, Salmon PR et al: Is colonoscopy necessary in diverticular disease? Lancet 1:95, 1984 (*Authors argue that air contrast barium enemas yield inaccurate results in about one third of cases; colonoscopy detected neoplasms in 31% of patients with diverticulosis.*)

Horner JL: Natural history of diverticulosis of the colon. Am J Dig Dis 3:343, 1958 (*A study of 503 patients followed in the ambulatory setting for 1 to 18 years [mean 8 years]. Incidence of diverticulitis was about 15%.*)

Larson D, Masters S, Spiro H: Medical and surgical therapy in diverticular disease. Gastroenterology 71:734, 1976 (*A report of 132 patients followed for a mean of 9.8 years [range 6 to 12 years] after medical or surgical therapy for acute diverticulitis. There was no significant difference in outcome; in about 75% of instances no further problems occurred among those in either group.*)

Painter N, Almeida A, Colebourne K: Unprocessed bran in treatment of diverticular disease of the colon. Br Med J 2:137, 1972 (*Seventy patients treated with bran in a prospective but uncontrolled study. More than 90% showed marked improvement in symptoms.*)

Taylor I, Duthie H: Bran tablets and diverticular disease. Br Med J 2:988, 1976 (*A cross-over trial of bran tablets, high roughage diet, and a bulk agent with an antispasmodic with 20 patients. All the agents improved measurements of bowel function, but bran was the most effective in relieving symptoms and normalizing colonic motor activity.*)

68
Management of Hemorrhoids

Hemorrhoids are a source of much misery though they are of no consequence unless they thrombose, prolapse, or bleed. Therapy is directed toward relief of symptoms, and should be accomplished with a minimum of discomfort, cost, and time lost from work. Simple approaches to pain relief and sensible modification in bowel habits to prevent progression constitute the essentials of medical therapy. The primary physician must be certain that symptoms are attributable to hemorrhoids, alleviate any anxiety about neoplasm, provide conservative medical therapy, and decide on the need and timing of surgery.

PATHOPHYSIOLOGY AND CLINICAL PRESENTATION

Theories explaining the etiology of hemorrhoids invoke a number of mechanisms, including increased venous pressure secondary to upright posture and straining at stool, arteriovenous communications in rectal tissue, and prolapsed cushions of tissue secondary to loss of support. Clinically, hemorrhoids are associated with pregnancy, portal hypertension, and constipation. The relative absence of hemorrhoids in African populations that have high-residue diets has led to the suggestion that an increase in dietary fiber might prevent the development of hemorrhoids.

Hemorrhoids may be classified by presentation as first degree when they merely bleed, second degree if they prolapse on high pressure but return spontaneously, and third degree when the anal suspensory ligament is stretched to the point of permanent prolapse. Hemorrhoids are considered to be *internal* when derived from the superior hemorrhoidal plexus above the dentate line, and *external* when located below the dentate line and covered by squamous epithelium.

Pain, incomplete defecation, constipation, excessive moisture, rectal itching, bleeding, or detection of a prolapsed mass are the common presentations. Hemorrhoids are regularly encountered as incidental findings on physical examination. Skin tags are evidence of previous hemorrhoids that have thrombosed, leaving connective tissue. The complications of hemorrhoids include bleeding, prolapse, and thrombosis.

PRINCIPLES OF MANAGEMENT

In most cases it is not necessary to remove hemorrhoids to treat them effectively. Symptomatic relief and a halt to progression can usually be achieved by use of simple local measures and minor changes in diet. For a painful attack, a *cold pack* applied for the first few hours offers considerable relief. Hot *sitz baths* (with a little salt added to the water to make it a more isotonic solution) are very soothing and effective when used at least once or twice daily for about 20 to 30 minutes. Softening the stool helps minimize straining and can be accomplished by increasing *dietary fiber* and making short-term use of *stool softeners* (*e.g.,* dioctyl sodium sulfosuccinate). Irritant laxatives should be avoided. Patients should set aside a regular time each day to have an unhurried bowel movement and avoid vigorous wiping. Stubborn itching and inflammation respond well to *topical corticosteroids;* hydrocortisone cream and suppositories are quite adequate and relatively inexpensive.

A host of *over-the-counter preparations* are heavily promoted. Many contain a topical anesthetic, such as benzocaine or pramoxine. *Benzocaine* may produce some temporary pain relief, but it is quite sensitizing; the resultant allergic response may actually worsen symptoms. *Pramoxine* is another topical anesthetic found in popular OTC preparations (Anusol,

Tronolane Cream, etc.). It is similar in efficacy to benzocaine, acting within 3 to 5 minutes of application and lasting several hours, but is less sensitizing. However, the cream formulation can still be irritating because of the presence of paraben preservatives. *Preparation H* is among the best-selling and most widely advertized of OTC hemorrhoidal therapies. It contains shark liver oil, live yeast cell derivatives, and phenyl mercuric nitrate; none of these agents, singly or in combination, has been shown to have any beneficial effect on hemorrhoids, though they are promoted as being able to shrink hemorrhoids and reduce inflammation.

Hemorrhoids that bleed repeatedly, prolapse, produce intractable pain, or thrombose deserve surgical evaluation. Internal hemorrhoids that have been bleeding persistently or prolapsed can be removed in the surgeon's office by utilizing *rubber-band ligation.* A rubber band is placed at the base of the hemorrhoid; within a week the lesion sloughs. Sometimes multiple attempts are necessary. *Injection of sclerosing agents* (*e.g.,* 5% phenol in oil) into the upper pole of an internal hemorrhoid is another means of dealing with internal hemorrhoids; the procedure has fallen out of favor because of its association with scarring of the anal canal. *Cryosurgery* is relatively painless and does not require anesthesia, but it produces a foul-smelling discharge for about a week and, occasionally, stricture is a late occurrence. Excruciatingly painful external hemorrhoids that have thrombosed can be excised under local anesthesia and the *clot removed.*

Definitive *hemorrhoidectomy* is the treatment of last resort. In contrast with the other surgical therapies mentioned, it requires hospitalization, and the recovery period can extend over several weeks. Moreover, there is a risk of compromising the competence of the anal sphincter. Nevertheless, it does represent a serious treatment option for patients with disabling, refractory disease.

THERAPEUTIC RECOMMENDATIONS

- Advise frequent hot sitz baths for relief of pain. At the initial recognition of pain, the patient can apply a cold pack for the first few hours, then take hot baths three or four times a day.
- If inflammation and itching are present, prescribe a suppository preparation containing a steroid, for example, hydrocortisone.
- Topical anesthetics may be useful for the acute relief of severe pain. If this form of therapy is to be used, an agent that is minimally sensitizing (*e.g.,* pramoxine) should be chosen.
- Treat constipation by having the patient increase dietary fiber and use a stool softener, such as dioctyl sodium sulfosuccinate, 100 mg tid. Following resolution of acute symptoms, the high-fiber diet should be continued.

- For thrombosed hemorrhoids:
  1. Instruct the patient to lie prone with ice applied to the thrombosed hemorrhoid.
  2. Prescribe oral analgesics; codeine may be required.
  3. Prescribe stool softeners.
  4. Conservative therapy should be successful in 3 to 5 days; otherwise refer the patient for surgical removal of the clot, which will relieve the pain promptly.
- Intractable symptoms require surgical therapy. The specific method chosen depends on the surgical expertise available in the community.

PATIENT EDUCATION AND PREVENTION

Instruction in proper diet and bowel habits is extremely helpful.
- Advise the patient to increase the intake of dietary fiber; suggest bran, carrots, green vegetables, and fruits with skin. Some people find foods such as chili, onions, and alcohol irritating. If this applies to your patient, suggest avoidance of them.
- Emphasize the importance of providing a regular time to have bowel movements. After bowel movements, the patient should avoid vigorous wiping; patting ought to suffice, and it minimizes irritation.
- Instruct the patient not to linger on the toilet or strain at stool. Long periods of standing should be avoided.
- Caution the patient against use of irritant laxatives.
- At the first sign of recurrent symptoms, institute frequent hot sitz baths.
- Instruct the patient to pat dry rather than wipe or rub.

A.H.G.

ANNOTATED BIBLIOGRAPHY

Anscombe AR et al: A clinical trial of the treatment of hemorrhoids by operation and Lord procedure. Lancet 2:250, 1974 (*A prospective study of two groups of 100 patients comparing hemorrhoidectomy and dilatation. The success rates were 98% and 84%, respectively, with dilatation producing fewer days of disability.*)

FDA Advisory Review Panel on OTC Hemorrhoidal Drug Products. Fed Register 45:35576, 1980 (*Concludes it is unclear whether topical anesthetics are effective for treatment of hemorrhoids.*)

Lieberman DA: Common anorectal disorders. Ann Intern Med 101: 837, 1984 (*Extensive review of the anatomy and physiology of the anus and rectum with special attention to hemorrhoids, fissure-in-ano, pruritus ani, and fecal incontinence; required reading for all primary physicians.*)

Murie JA, Sim AJ, MacKenzie I: Rubber band ligation versus haemorrhoidectomy for prolapsing haemorrhoids. Br J Surg 69:536, 1982 (*A long-term prospective clinical trial showing that ligation is effective, except for permanently prolapsed painful lesions.*)

Outpatient treatment of hemorrhoids (editorial). Br Med J 2:651, 1975 (*An editorial emphasizing that it is unnecessary to completely remove hemorrhoids to relieve symptoms. The excellent results and cost-saving of "ambulatory proctology" are noted.*)

Prasad GC et al: Studies on etiopathogenesis of hemorrhoids. Am J Proctol 27(3):33, 1976 (*An excellent review of the pathogenesis of hemorrhoids.*)

Taggart REB: Hemorrhoids and palpable anorectal problems. Practitioner 212:221, 1974 (*A succinct, complete review of the current alternatives in treating hemorrhoids. Other anal lesions, infection, fissure, fistula, pruritus, and prolapse are discussed.*)

To tie; to stab; to stretch, perchance to freeze (editorial). Lancet 2: 645, 1975 (*Concludes that hemorrhoidectomy should be reserved for failure of other methods.*)

Treatment of hemorrhoids. Med Lett 17:7, 1975 (*A one-page summary of new methods, calling attention to the possibility of non-surgical therapy.*)

What are hemorrhoids? (Editorial). Br Med J 4:365, 1975 (*A review of the theories concerning pathogenesis of hemorrhoids.*)

69

Management of Asymptomatic Gallstones and Chronic Cholecystitis

Gallbladder disease affects over 15 million Americans, and more than 350,000 cholecystectomies are performed each year. Many patients with stones are asymptomatic, while others suffer from chronic cholecystitis, with recurrent bouts of abdominal discomfort. The occurrence of asymptomatic gallstones or chronic cholecystitis requires that the primary physician determine who is a candidate for cholecystectomy and who can be managed conservatively.

CLINICAL PRESENTATION AND COURSE

Gallbladder disease may be asymptomatic or manifested by recurrent pain. Characteristically, *biliary colic* is rather sudden in onset, builds to a maximum within 1 hour, is steady, localized to the right upper quadrant or epigastrium, lasts 2 to 4 hours, and occasionally radiates to the left or right scapula. There is often nausea and vomiting. *Dyspeptic symptoms,* fatty food intolerance, belching, and bloating have also been attributed to chronic gallbladder disease, but the association has not been proven. Prospective studies have shown that such symptoms are just as common in middle-aged women without gallstones as in those with them. When patients with these symptoms are operated on, the dyspepsia often persists after cholecystectomy. Reflux of bile into the stomach has been noted in such individuals.

The rare patient with biliary colic, who has a normal gallbladder study on routine oral cholecystogram and ultrasound, may have acalculous gallbladder disease, an uncommon condition, or multiple small stones undetectable by conventional methods. These subtle forms of gallbladder disease may be discovered by observing delayed gallbladder emptying in response to a fatty meal or cholecystokinin.

The *clinical course* of untreated gallbladder disease is not known precisely. Two prospective studies, totaling 1300 patients who had at least one bout of pain, showed that over a follow-up period of 5 to 20 years, 30% had *recurrent pain,* and 20% experienced *complications* such as jaundice, cholangitis, or pancreatitis; half remained asymptomatic. Because all patients in these studies had pain requiring a hospital admission, this patient population probably represented a group with a greater likelihood of complications than one with a predominance of asymptomatic stones. In a more representative retrospective cohort study of 123 people with silent gallstones, there was no mortality from the condition and a 15-year accumulative probability of biliary pain of only 18%.

Although there is no certainty that the onset of complications will be preceded by episodes of biliary pain, a study of 600 patients found that more than 90% of patients who suffered a complication of gallbladder disease had prior warning symptoms of biliary colic, though these were often mild and ignored. Most patients with pain on presentation had similar patterns of pain on follow-up. When 112 patients with asymptomatic stones were followed without surgery for 10 to 20 years, 27% eventually complained of dyspepsia, 19% had biliary colic, and 4.5% experienced transient jaundice. No deaths resulted from delay of surgery.

In sum, the asymptomatic patient seems to have a relatively favorable prognosis. Individuals with recurrent pain have twice the rate of complications. Increased risk is also associated with stones larger than 2.5 cm, age over 60, and diabetes.

Some authorities believe there is a cause-and-effect relationship between gallstones and carcinoma of the gallbladder. The cancer occurs mostly in older women. The association with stone formation is based on circumstantial autopsy data and is not universally accepted. If the risk is real, it is likely to be small.

PRINCIPLES OF THERAPY

The available therapies include surgery and gallstone dissolution. In some instances no therapy is indicated. Lithotriptic methods are being evaluated.

Surgery. Symptomatic patients with recurrent biliary colic and a nonvisualizing oral cholecystogram or a gallbladder ultrasound examination that shows stones should undergo *elective cholecystectomy.* The risk of complications is far greater than the risk of surgery. This is especially true for diabetics. However, there is no evidence that the vast numbers of patients with asymptomatic gallstones would benefit from surgery. Even though surgical mortality is only 0.5%, the risk of conservative management is not much different and involves far less expense, morbidity, and time lost from work.

The decision to operate on elderly patients and those with serious underlying illness has to be individualized. Surgical mortality rises above 4% in patients over the age of 60, as does the risk of complications from gallbladder disease. Operating on all women over 65 with stones to prevent carcinoma of the gallbladder would result in more deaths from surgery than lives saved.

Chenodiol. The search for an effective medical therapy to dissolve gallstones has led to investigations of *chenodiol* (formerly called chenodeoxycholic acid). The agent desaturates the cholesterol content of the bile by suppressing hepatic cholesterol synthesis and decreasing biliary cholesterol secretion. It is given to patients with functioning gallbladders and *symptomatic radiolucent cholesterol gallstones.*

The efficacy and safety of chenodiol was evaluated in the National Cooperative Gallstone Study (NCGS), involving 916 patients. In the group treated with 750 mg of chenodiol a day for 2 years, stones dissolved completely in 13.5% and partially in another 27%. In the group of patients treated with a low-dose regimen of 375 mg per day, only 5.2% experienced complete dissolution. Stone disappearance among controls was 0.8%. When patients with partial stone dissolution were treated for another 1 or 2 years with 750 mg or 375 mg per day, complete disappearance of stones occurred in 23% and 16%, respectively. Other studies show that doses in excess of 750 mg per day can achieve greater rates of stone dissolution.

The best results are obtained in patients with small floating cholesterol stones. The effects of therapy can be well documented by periodic oral cholecystogram or gallbladder ultrasound. Therapy is contraindicated in patients with inflammatory bowel disease or peptic ulcer, because the drug increases bile acids, which may be harmful to colonic and gastric mucosa.

Unfortunately, stones recur in about half of patients within 5 years, with most reappearing within 1 year after therapy is stopped. This high recurrence rate suggests a role for chronic *suppressive therapy,* but in the only controlled study testing the prophylactic efficacy of chenodiol, a maintenance dose of 375 mg per day was unable to prevent recurrences of gallstones in patients who initially achieved stone dissolution.

Chenodiol is not without its *adverse effects.* In the NCGS, transaminase elevations occurred in 30% of patients treated with 750 mg per day. The *hepatotoxicity* was reversible, but it raises the question of more serious liver injury with higher doses or more prolonged courses of therapy. Other adverse effects include a *rise in low-density lipoprotein cholesterol levels* and *diarrhea.* Finally, chenodiol is very expensive, costing the patient well over $2 per day; this expense can be prohibitive if several years of therapy are contemplated.

A less toxic gallstone-dissolving agent, *ursodeoxycholic* acid, is available commercially in Europe but not in the United States. Reports suggest it is considerably safer, causing little hepatotoxicity or diarrhea.

In summary, medical therapy is an alternative for symptomatic patients with cholesterol gallstones who are too sick or unwilling to undergo elective cholecystectomy. However, the need for prolonged treatment, hepatotoxicity, and reformation of stones after termination of therapy make this approach suboptimal. Moreover, it is very expensive.

Lithotripsy. Extracorporeal shock wave techniques, which have proved very useful for renal stone disease (see Chapter 134), have been applied to patients with symptomatic gallstones. Adjuvant therapy with chenodiol is needed to help dissolve the remaining fragments. About 10% of patients experience choledocholithiasis, which can be treated successfully by endoscopic extraction. Further experience with this technique is required before its applicability to gallstone disease can be ascertained.

Other Measures. Gallstone formation has been noted with use of oral contraceptives and clofibrate. Patients taking these agents should be monitored for gallstones and taken off the drugs if any evidence of stone formation or cholecystitis develops. There is no evidence that dietary measures such as a low-fat diet or avoidance of particular foods are of any benefit. Dyspepsia responds to antacids in 25% to 50% of cases (see Chapter 55), and even surgery sometimes relieves such symptoms, though not with any consistency.

THERAPEUTIC RECOMMENDATIONS

- Patients who are completely asymptomatic should be followed and need not undergo cholecystectomy unless they are in the high-risk group, for example, are diabetic or have a stone larger than 2.5 cm. The decision regarding elective surgery in the elderly has to be individualized.
- Patients with recurrent biliary colic and radiologic evidence of gallbladder disease should undergo elective cholecystectomy, provided they can tolerate surgery.
- Symptomatic patients with radiolucent cholesterol gallstones, who are too frail or unwilling to undergo elective cholecystectomy, can be given a trial of chenodiol, 250 mg bid for the first 2 weeks and then 375 mg bid thereafter. The dosage is reduced if diarrhea ensues, and therapy is stopped if transaminase elevations develop. Therapy may

need to be continued for more than 2 years to achieve gallstone dissolution. The effects of therapy should be monitored with an oral cholecystogram or gallbladder ultrasound every 6 months.

- Clofibrate and oral contraceptives should be stopped, or dosages decreased, in patients with stone formation.
- There is no need to alter the diet or restrict fats in the treatment of biliary colic; anticholinergics are of no benefit.
- Dyspeptic symptoms should be treated with antacids. Avoidance of foods that precipitate symptoms may be worth a try. Severe refractory dyspepsia occasionally responds to surgery when gallstones or a nonopacifying gallbladder is present.

PATIENT EDUCATION

The asymptomatic patient needs to be reassured of the benign nature of his illness and should not be pushed into surgery or unnecessary dietary restriction. Dyspepsia may respond to antacids, and, thus, careful instruction in their use is indicated. The reluctant person at high-risk for complications of gallbladder disease requires a thorough explanation of the chances of complications and of the relatively low risk of elective surgery. However, the choice of elective surgery is the patient's, and initial refusal should be respected. In such instances, a trial of medical therapy and/or approaching the patient at a later date about surgery may produce better results than simply discharging the patient because he refuses elective operation. On the other hand, the very anxious patient with asymptomatic gallstones who steadfastly insists on surgery out of concern for future complications might be allowed to undergo elective cholecystectomy to provide peace of mind, provided there are no medical contraindications to undergoing surgery.

A.H.G.

ANNOTATED BIBLIOGRAPHY

Bennion LJ, Grundy SM: Risk factors for development of cholelithiasis in man. N Engl J Med 299:1161, 1978 (*Authoritative review, of current knowledge.*)

Carveth SW, Priestley JT, Gage R: Size and number of gallstones in acute and chronic cholecystitis. Mayo Clin Proc 34:371, 1959 (*Stones larger than 2.5 cm are more likely to precipitate attacks of cholecystitis than are smaller stones.*)

Cole WH: The false normal oral cholecystogram. Surgery 81:121, 1977 (*Stones and gallbladder disease are missed in 2% to 4% of studies because of the small size of the stones or the presence of acalculous disease. Thus, the false-negative rate is 2% to 4% for oral cholecystograms.*)

Comfort MW, Gray HK, Wilson JM: The silent gallstone: A ten- to twenty-year follow-up study of 112 cases. Ann Surg 128:931, 1948 (*There were no deaths in this group attributable to delay of surgery, and only 19% had episodes of colic during the period of follow-up.*)

Cooperberg PL, Burhenne HJ: Real time ultrasonography in calculus gallbladder disease. N Engl J Med 302:1277, 1980 (*Sensitivity of 98% and a specificity of approximately 95% were reported. Comparison with oral cholecystography in a subsample showed greater sensitivity and the same specificity for ultrasound.*)

Dolgin SM, Schwartz JS, Kressel HY et al: Identification of patients with cholesterol or pigment gallstones by discriminant analysis of radiographic features. N Engl J Med 304:808, 1981 (*Describes oral cholecystogram findings that help identify patients with cholesterol stones; buoyancy was highly predictive of cholesterol composition; a discriminant function was used to facilitate categorization.*)

Dunn FH et al: Cholecystokinin cholecystography. JAMA 228:997, 1974 (*Controlled evaluation in the diagnosis of patients with acalculous disease.*)

Gracie WA, Ransohoff DF: The natural history of silent gallstones. N Engl J Med 307:798, 1982 (*A retrospective cohort study of 123 people identified no mortality associated with asymptomatic gallstones and a 15-year accumulative probability of biliary pain of only 18%.*)

Isselbacher KJ: Chenodiol for gallstones: Dissolution or disillusion. Ann Intern Med 95:377, 1981 (*An editorial taking a "jaundiced" view of chenodiol therapy.*)

Marks JW, Shu-Ping L et al: Low-dose chenodiol to prevent gallstone recurrence after dissolution therapy. Ann Intern Med 100:376, 1984 (*The cumulative recurrence rate was 27% at 3.5 years. Low-dose therapy was ineffective in preventing recurrences.*)

Marks JW, Baum RA, Hanson RF et al: Additional chenodiol therapy after partial dissolution of gallstones with two years of treatment. Ann Intern Med 100:382, 1984 (*Complete dissolution occurred after 1 or 2 years of further therapy in as many as 23% of those who showed partial results during the first 2 years of therapy.*)

Mujahad Z, Evans JA, Whalen JP: The nonpacified gallbladder on oral cholecystogram. Radiology 112:1, 1974 (*Persistent nonvisualization of the gallbladder after the second dose has a sensitivity of more than 95% for detecting diseased gallbladders.*)

Mulley AG: Shock-wave lithotripsy. N Engl J Med 314:845, 1986 (*An editorial suggesting caution regarding applicability of lithotripsy to therapy of gallstones.*)

Newman HF, Northrup JD, Rosenblum M et al: Complications of cholelithiasis. Am J Gastroenterol 50:476, 1968 (*More than 90% of those who experienced complications had one or more prior episodes of colic.*)

Palmer RH: More on chenodiol: Continued treatment and prevention of recurrences. Ann Intern Med 100:450, 1984 (*An editorial reviewing the lessons learned from the NCGS.*)

Price WH: Gallbladder dyspepsia. Br Med J 3:138, 1963 (*Frequency and severity of dyspeptic complaints are unrelated to presence or absence of gallstones.*)

Ransohoff DF, Gracie WA, Wolfenson LB et al: Prophylactic cholecystectomy or expectant management for silent gallstones. Ann Intern Med 99:199, 1983 (*A decision analysis suggesting a very small survival benefit for prophylactic cholecystectomy that may well be offset by monetary costs, morbidity, and time preferences.*)

Rhine JA, Watson L: Gallstone dyspepsia. Br Med J 1:32, 1968 (*Of 32 patients undergoing cholecystectomy for dyspepsia, 13 still had similar symptoms after surgery.*)

Rosenberg L, Shapiro S, Slone D: Thiazides in acute cholecystitis. N Engl J Med 303:546, 1980 (*The relative risk of acute cholecystitis among patients who used thiazide during the month prior to hospital admission was 2; for those who used thiazides for 5 or more years, the relative risk was 2.9.*)

Sauerbruch T, Delius M, Paumgartner G et al: Fragmentation of gallstones by extracorporeal shock waves. N Engl J Med 314:818, 1986 (*A cautiously optimistic report.*)

Schein CJ: Acute cholecystitis in the diabetic. Am J Gastroenterol 51:511, 1969 (*Cholecystitis can be a lethal disease in the diabetic; documents increased risk in this subpopulation.*)

Schoenfield LJ, Lachin JM et al: Chenodiol (chenodeoxycholic acid) for dissolution of gallstones: The National Cooperative Gallstone Study. Ann Intern Med 95:257, 1981 (*A randomized, double-blind controlled study of the efficacy of chenodiol in treatment of cholesterol stones; the best data available.*)

Thistle JL, Cleary PA, Lachin JM et al: The natural history of cholelithiasis: The National Cooperative Gallstone Study. Ann Intern Med 101:171, 1984 (*Among 305 patients receiving placebo therapy, the most important predictor of biliary tract pain was a history of pain.*)

Wenckert A, Robertson B: The natural course of gallstone disease. Gastroenterology 50:376, 1966 (*About 30% of patients managed medically and followed for 5 to 20 years had attacks of colic, and another 20% had complications. These high figures are due in part to the fact that all were hospitalized initially, and well over half had nonvisualizing gallbladders, a sign of more advanced disease.*)

70

Management of Viral Hepatitis

JULES L. DIENSTAG, M.D.

More than 50,000 cases of viral hepatitis in the United States are reported to the Centers for Disease Control each year; the actual number is estimated to be ten times as high. Hepatitis B accounts for about 50% of all cases, and non-A, non-B hepatitis is responsible for over 90% of episodes that are transfusion-related. Mortality from all types of viral hepatitis is well below 1%, except for the recently recognized delta hepatitis (hepatitis D), in which the mortality rate may reach 5%. In addition, a proportion of patients with acute types B, non-A, non-B, and D hepatitis progress to chronic infection. Some become asymptomatic carriers; in others, the course progresses to chronic hepatitis, which is associated with an increased risk of cirrhosis and death.

The primary physician needs to be skilled in the management of viral hepatitis, an illness encountered frequently in the outpatient setting. Because no practical, specific therapy is available for acute or chronic viral hepatitis, the goals of management are limited to providing symptomatic relief and medical support, preventing the spread of infection to contacts, and minimizing and treating the consequences of chronic hepatitis. Effective outpatient management requires knowledge of the natural history of viral hepatitis, the methods for serologic diagnosis (see Chapter 62) and monitoring of the disease course, the indications for prophylaxis (see Chapter 52), and the means for recognizing the outcomes of severe acute and chronic diseases.

CLINICAL PRESENTATION AND NATURAL HISTORY

Acute Viral Hepatitis. In most instances, acute viral hepatitis is a self-limited illness; on the order of 85% of hospitalized patients and over 95% of outpatients recover completely and uneventfully within 3 months. A majority of persons with acute viral hepatitis never become jaundiced; their illness is mistakenly labeled as a nonspecific viral syndrome unless liver biochemical tests, such as aminotransferase levels, are ordered. A large proportion of patients remain asymptomatic, especially children. In elderly or immunologically compromised patients, the prognosis is more guarded, with increased risk of severe and protracted disease.

Prodromal symptoms occur after an *incubation period* of 2 to 4 (rarely 6) weeks for hepatitis A, 4 to 24 weeks for hepatitis B (with or without simultaneous acute delta hepatitis infection), and 3 to 15 weeks (80% within 5 to 10 weeks) for post-transfusion non-A, non-B hepatitis (shorter incubation periods of 1 to 4 weeks are common in factor-VIII-infusion-associated non-A, non-B hepatitis among hemophiliacs). Characteristically, *prodromal symptoms* consist of 1 to 2 weeks of malaise, anorexia, nausea, vomiting, change in senses of taste and smell, low-grade fever, right upper quadrant or midepigastric abdominal discomfort, and fatigue. Aminotransferase elevations may precede or coincide with the onset of prodromal symptoms.

If jaundice develops, it usually does so as prodromal complaints begin to subside, although persistence of prodromal symptoms is observed in more severe cases. By the time 6 to 8 weeks have elapsed, most patients are well on their way to full recovery. Occasionally, an isolated, mild aminotransferase elevation persists after clinical recovery. If it resolves within 3 to 6 months, the mild elevation has no prognostic significance.

There are a number of variations on the classic clinical presentation of viral hepatitis. The most ominous is the development of *fulminant hepatitis,* with overwhelming liver cell necrosis and signs of liver failure—encephalopathy, ascites, and coagulopathy. Mortality, despite the best medical care, approaches 80%. This complication is seen more often in cases of hepatitis B (especially when there is simultaneous delta hepatitis infection) than in those of hepatitis A or non-A, non-B.

In 5% to 10% of cases of acute type B hepatitis, the prodromal phase of illness may be characterized as a *serum-sickness-like syndrome,* with urticaria, arthralgias, fever, and polyarticular arthritis. Some patients with acute viral hepatitis have a *cholestatic* illness, with marked jaundice, elevation of serum alkaline phosphatase activity, and pruritus lasting 1 month to several months.

Approximately 5% to 10% of patients with viral hepatitis appear to suffer mild *relapses* during convalescence. Some of these apparent relapses actually represent instances of *second infections* with another hepatitis virus. Still, clinical and biochemical relapses have been documented in cases of hepatitis A and B. (Some relapses of hepatitis B may represent the clinical expression of simultaneous delta hepatitis infection.) Relapses, often multiple, are quite common after non-A, non-B hepatitis. In general, these relapses are not associated with the development of chronic hepatitis.

Progression to Chronic Hepatitis. The risk of progression varies among the several types of viral hepatitis. Although an occasional case of *hepatitis A* may be slow to resolve and last more than 6 months, chronic hepatitis associated with hepatitis A has not been documented. On the other hand, chronic hepatitis develops in 1% to 2% of patients with acute clinically apparent *hepatitis B,* and 5% to 10% become chronic hepatitis B surface antigen (HBsAg) carriers. Although most carriers are asymptomatic and have a nonprogressive course, a small proportion may actually have subtle and insidious progression to chronic liver disease. Rarely, acute hepatitislike exacerbations can occur in these chronic hepatitis B carriers; these events may represent superimposed infection with another hepatitis virus (A, non-A, non-B, or delta hepatitis) or reactivation of hepatitis B. The likelihood of chronic hepatitis is not increased in patients with simultaneous acute hepatitis B and D (delta hepatitis).

In *transfusion-associated non-A, non-B hepatitis,* as many as 50% of patients experience elevations in aminotransferase that persist for more than a year after acute infection; histologic evidence of chronic hepatitis can be detected in liver-biopsy tissue. Current observations suggest that, among patients with transfusion-associated chronic non-A, non-B hepatitis, cirrhosis develops within 5 to 10 years after the onset of acute hepatitis. The frequency of chronic hepatitis is lower and its severity is less after non-A, non-B hepatitis acquired in the absence of percutaneous inoculation.

Progression to chronic hepatitis is often manifested by little more than persistence of *mild symptoms and biochemical abnormalities* for 6 or more months; many patients remain anicteric. In patients with hepatitis B, *persistence of hepatitis B surface antigenemia* is associated with an increased

risk of chronic hepatitis; however, there are no reliable early predictors of chronicity. Reports suggesting that early detection of HBeAg in acute hepatitis B is associated with an increased risk of chronic hepatitis have not been borne out. On the other hand, *late persistence of HBeAg* is likely to be associated with chronicity.

Chronic Hepatitis. There are two general categories of chronic hepatitis, nonprogressive "chronic persistent hepatitis" and progressive "chronic active hepatitis." Because clinical differences between these two categories may be quite subtle, a distinction between them requires liver biopsy. *Chronic active hepatitis* is identified by the presence of a mononuclear-cell portal infiltrate that not only expands portal zones but also extends beyond the portal tract into the adjacent periportal lobular area with erosion of the limiting plate of periportal hepatocytes ("*piecemeal necrosis*"). Fibrous septae extending into the lobule are also characteristic, and a proportion of patients with chronic active hepatitis, up to 50% in some reported series, have cirrhosis on their initial liver biopsies. A more severe form of this lesion includes "*bridging necrosis,*" in which confluent necrosis and cell dropout span lobules (portal–portal and portal–central bridges.)

In contrast, *chronic persistent hepatitis* represents mononuclear-cell inflammation confined to the portal tract; the limiting plate of periportal hepatocytes is not eroded, and hepatocellular necrosis and inflammation do not extend into the lobule. Some authorities distinguish yet another category of chronic hepatitis, "*chronic lobular hepatitis,*" in which the inflammatory process and hepatocellular necrosis involve the lobule but in which other features of chronic active hepatitis are absent. This morphologic pattern can be considered intermediate between chronic active and persistent hepatitis and resembles slowly resolving acute hepatitis.

Differentiation between chronic active hepatitis on the one hand and chronic persistent and lobular hepatitis on the other is important for prognostic purposes. Chronic persistent hepatitis is a nonprogressive liver disorder with an excellent prognosis; progression to cirrhosis is extraordinarily unlikely. The same is true for chronic lobular hepatitis. In contrast, chronic active hepatitis tends to be a progressive disease, associated with an increased risk of cirrhosis and death.

Progression to Cirrhosis. Although progression to cirrhosis and eventual death are distinct possibilities in patients with untreated chronic active hepatitis, these outcomes are not inevitable in all cases; different categories of severity can be distinguished. Patients with marked, *disabling symptoms, sustained aminotransferase elevations* of greater than *ten times normal, gamma globulin* levels *twice normal,* or *bridging* or *multilobular collapse* on biopsy are at increased risk of progressive disease. Patients fulfilling these clinical and biochemical criteria of severe disease were found to have a

40% 6-month fatality rate. In those with bridging or multi-lobular necrosis, cirrhosis developed in 40% and death occurred in 20% after 5 years. In contrast, patients with piecemeal necrosis alone in the absence of bridging or multilobular necrosis and patients with minimal symptoms are not at risk for death, and progression to cirrhosis is rare (3%–10%). In a substantial proportion of patients with histologically confirmed chronic active hepatitis, symptoms may be minimal or absent, and the disease may be clinically quiescent for long periods.

On the other side of the coin, the benignity of chronic persistent hepatitis is not absolutely uniform; this lesion has been documented to deteriorate to chronic active hepatitis and to progress to cirrhosis in three situations: (1) in patients with an initial histologic diagnosis of chronic active hepatitis whose liver *biopsies improve with therapy,* allowing them to be classified as chronic persistent hepatitis; (2) in *immunosuppressed* patients with a histologic diagnosis of chronic persistent hepatitis; and (3) in patients with chronic persistent hepatitis B who become *superinfected with the delta agent.*

These histologic distinctions are very important in patients with nonviral chronic hepatitis; chronic active hepatitis usually responds to immunosuppressive therapy, while chronic persistent hepatitis requires no therapeutic intervention. The natural history and responsiveness to such therapy of viral chronic active hepatitis appear to be different. In patients with chronic active hepatitis associated with hepatitis B virus infection, the course may be quite benign. In these patients with mild chronic active hepatitis, progression is slow, and survival is prolonged even in the absence of therapeutic intervention. On the other hand, if chronic active hepatitis B is severe, progression may be relentless.

A Stanford University study of the natural history of chronic hepatitis B showed that the 5-year survival of chronic persistent hepatitis B was 97%, that of chronic active hepatitis B was 86%, and that of cirrhosis associated with hepatitis B was 55%. In patients with chronic hepatitis B, conversion from HBeAg to anti-HBe may signal an improvement in liver histology, whereas superinfection with the delta agent is usually associated with a deterioration in histology and an acceleration of the disease process. Life-long infection with hepatitis B virus, such as occurs primarily among those infected at or shortly after birth, is associated with an increased risk of hepatocellular carcinoma, whether cirrhosis is present or not.

In patients with chronic non-A, non-B hepatitis after transfusion, the predominant histologic finding is chronic active hepatitis. Generally, however, these patients rarely fulfill clinical or histologic criteria for severe chronic active hepatitis, and often, spontaneous improvement over time can be demonstrated. Still, despite this apparent relative benignity, long-term follow-up studies have shown that, even with mild elevations in aminotransferase activity and absence of symptoms, chronic non-A, non-B hepatitis may progress insidiously; as noted above, cirrhosis develops in 20% of these patients within 5 to 10 years.

PRINCIPLES OF MANAGEMENT

Acute Viral Hepatitis. Generally a benign and self-limited illness, acute viral hepatitis can be managed in most cases on an outpatient basis. Hospitalization should be reserved for high-risk patients (the elderly, immunocompromised persons, patients with difficult-to-manage underlying chronic diseases, etc.) and those with marked prothrombin time prolongation, encephalopathy, ascites and edema, inability to maintain oral intake, hypoglycemia, and/or hypoalbuminemia. There is *no specific therapy* for acute viral hepatitis that will accelerate convalescence or prevent sequelae. The goals of care are to maintain *adequate nutrition* and *patient comfort,* to *avoid* additional *hepatocellular insults* from hepatotoxic medications and alcohol, and to *prevent the spread* of infection to others.

Neither specific dietary manipulations, corticosteroid therapy, nor strict bed rest has any beneficial effect on the course or prognosis of acute, uncomplicated or acute, severe viral hepatitis. *Oral contraceptives* need not necessarily be stopped, but *alcohol* intake should be omitted and use of other drugs known to cause liver injury discontinued or monitored carefully. *Exercise* does not interfere with recovery; patients should be encouraged to engage in as much physical activity as they can tolerate without discomfort or undue fatigue.

The symptoms may be quite incapacitating. Nausea and vomiting can be controlled by cautious use of antiemetics; however, because phenothiazines cause cholestatic hepatitis in approximately 1% of patients, *nonphenothiazine antiemetics,* such as *trimethobenzamine,* should be used. Small, *frequent feedings,* especially in the morning when nausea is at a low ebb, can ensure adequate calorie intake. No specific foods need be restricted. In patients with cholestasis and pruritus, *cholestyramine* usually provides relief. Certainly, the identification of a patient with acute viral hepatitis should prompt consideration of prophylactic measures to limit the spread of infection to contacts (see Chapter 52).

In cases of fulminant hepatitis, neither corticosteroids nor any other specific intervention has been shown to be of any benefit. The most effective approach involves vigorous medical management with meticulous attention to details of the multisystem dysfunction that accompanies acute liver failure. Ideally, such patients should be treated in an intensive care unit.

Chronic Hepatitis. Treatment of chronic hepatitis depends on the type and severity of the disease. The goals of therapy are to relieve symptoms, prevent cirrhosis, and reduce the chances of mortality. Because *chronic persistent hepatitis* has an excellent prognosis, *no treatment,* beyond simple symptomatic relief and preventive measures, is indicated. The same is true for chronic lobular hepatitis.

Chronic active hepatitis tends to be a more serious and progressive condition. As noted above, *severe* chronic active hepatitis manifested by bridging or multilobular necrosis or the combination of aminotransferase levels greater than ten times normal, globulin levels twice normal, and marked symptoms has a poor prognosis. Controlled prospective trials, such as a major study conducted at the Mayo Clinic, have demonstrated clinical, biochemical, and histologic resolution of severe chronic active hepatitis in 80% of cases treated with prednisone or a combination of *prednisone* and *azathioprine.* Remission of histologic features to those of chronic persistent hepatitis or to normal were observed within 6 to 36 months. Moreover, therapeutic intervention in cases with severe symptoms and advanced pathologic changes on liver biopsy was associated with a significant reduction in mortality.

Only 15% to 20% of patients with a diagnosis of chronic active hepatitis fulfill criteria of severe disease. The need for and efficacy of *immunosuppressive therapy* (corticosteroids with or without azathioprine) in the majority of patients with chronic active hepatitis, especially those with *B virus disease,* remains *unknown.* The controlled Mayo Clinic studies cited above included only a few patients with chronic active hepatitis B; they were less responsive than patients with non-B disease. The few available studies on the utility of immunosuppressive therapy in HBsAg-positive patients give conflicting results. In a prospective, controlled trial of prednisolone in Chinese patients with HBsAg-positive chronic active hepatitis, therapy was not helpful and even tended to be harmful. The study has been criticized for its small size, low-dose regimen, limitation to patients with mild-to-moderate disease, and inapplicability of results obtained in Chinese patients (who acquire their infections in childhood) to Westerners (who become infected during adulthood). However, other data indicate that immunosuppressive agents increase the level of virus replication and suggest on theoretical grounds that it might be unwise to treat antigen-positive patients with such therapy.

Nevertheless, some patients with chronic active hepatitis B do respond, at least clinically and biochemically, to immunosuppressive therapy, as demonstrated in a controlled Taiwanese study. Moreover, the fact that immunosuppressive therapy increases the level of virus replication has never been extended to show that such an increase in virus replication translates into a deleterious effect on liver histology. Others have pointed out that for patients with severe, disabling, life-threatening chronic active hepatitis B, no alternative effective therapy exists, many trials of antiviral therapy notwithstanding. Therefore, some authorities do advocate immunosuppressive therapy in the more desperate cases, hoping for an anti-inflammatory effect that outweighs the adverse impact on virus replication.

Still, immunosuppressive therapy in patients with HBsAg-positive chronic active hepatitis, as well as with non-A, non-B chronic active hepatitis, should be considered with reluctance. Some authorities have abandoned immunosuppressive therapy altogether for patients with HBsAg-positive or other types of virally induced chronic active hepatitis. Others refer their patients with severe chronic active hepatitis B to special centers where experimental trials of antiviral therapy are being conducted; some reserve immunosuppressive therapy for those in whom HBeAg is undetectable. And still others resort occasionally to immunosuppressive therapy, at least to a 3- to 6-month trial, in patients with severe HBsAg-positive chronic active hepatitis who are totally disabled by their disease.

Because the decision to treat a patient with chronic active viral hepatitis is a very difficult one, embarking on such a course will rarely be done by a primary care physician without the consultation of someone very experienced in treating this type of patient. On the other hand, primary care physicians will have opportunities to provide long-term management and follow-up for these patients. In addition, many patients with presumed chronic viral hepatitis will turn out to have nonviral liver disease, and the primary care physician should be familiar with the therapeutic approach to this category of patients with chronic liver disease.

In patients with nonviral or viral *mild* or *asymptomatic chronic active hepatitis, immunosuppressive therapy* is *not indicated.* In such patients, the probability of morbidity and mortality is low, and the efficacy of therapy has not been demonstrated. Therefore, therapy of undocumented benefit must be weighed against the very high likelihood of complications. Long-term corticosteroid therapy is associated with serious complications in a high proportion of patients (see Chapter 103). Two thirds of patients treated with prednisone alone in the Mayo Clinic study of chronic active hepatitis experienced at least one serious adverse effect attributable to the corticosteroid. This approach is likely to remain in effect unless and until the efficacy of immunosuppressive therapy in such patients is demonstrated in a controlled trial.

The Immunosuppressive Program. For patients who are deemed appropriate candidates for immunosuppressive therapy, the regimen popularized by the Mayo Clinic has been utilized. The immunosuppressive program consists of *high-dose prednisone* or *reduced-dose prednisone* in combination with *azathioprine.* Treatment is initiated with 60 mg of prednisone, and the dose is reduced over the course of a month to a maintenance level of 20 mg. An alternative is a combination regimen in which therapy is initiated with 30 mg of prednisone combined with 50 mg of azathioprine; the azathioprine dose remains constant, while the prednisone dose is reduced over the course of the first month to a maintenance level of 10 mg. During a controlled study of the two regimens, 67% of patients treated with the high-dose steroid-alone program, but only 10% of those treated with the combination low-dose steroid/azathioprine program, experienced severe steroid complications after 18 months of therapy. Azathioprine-induced bone marrow suppression may occur in patients receiving the combination-therapy regimen, and they must be monitored closely. Neither azathioprine alone nor alternate-day prednisone therapy have been found to be effective alternative regimens. In European trials, lower-dose corticosteroid regimens, without an initiating high-dose phase, have also been found effective.

Therapy is continued until there is objective evidence of remission, that is, a fall in aminotransferase activity to a level under twice normal and resolution of morphologic features of chronic active hepatitis. Occasionally unacceptable drug toxicity (azathioprine hepatotoxicity or marrow toxicity, intolerable gastrointestinal upset, compression fractures) or failure to respond necessitate premature cessation of therapy. In responsive cases, symptoms improve within 6 months, aminotransferase levels within 12 months, and histology within 24 months. Rarely, more than 36 months are necessary to achieve remission. After 4 years the likelihood of drug-induced complications becomes greater than the likelihood of beneficial drug effect; nevertheless, some patients cannot be weaned from maintenance treatment and require indefinite continuation of therapy.

Once remission is achieved, therapy is discontinued by gradual tapering of prednisone over 6 weeks. Patients are monitored closely for signs of relapse, which occur in 50% of patients; relapse is especially common in patients with cirrhosis, often necessitating prolonged therapy for many years or multiple courses of treatment. Approximately 20% of patients fail to respond to conventional doses but may respond to higher doses. Relapses usually occur early; if remission lasts more than 6 months after cessation of therapy, relapse is less likely. Most cases of relapse are accompanied by symptoms and biochemical abnormalities, but in 10% of cases, the only sign of relapse is a change in histology. After relapse, 80% of patients respond again to reinitiation of therapy; after cessation of therapy, again, the relapse rate is 50%.

As noted earlier, the information reviewed here on therapy and its outcome in patients with chronic active hepatitis refers primarily to a population of patients with severe HBsAg-negative disease (nonviral for the most part). Unfortunately, when HBsAg-positive patients (or patients with chronic non-A, non-B hepatitis) are treated in this way, the outcome and the likelihood of success are less predictable.

For patients with *HBsAg-positive chronic active hepatitis,* especially for those with high levels of virus replication (HBeAg-positive, DNA polymerase-positive, and/or HBV DNA-positive), *antiviral therapy* may become the indicated approach in the future. Trials of the efficacy of *interferon* and adenine arabinoside have been in progress for more than a decade; however, neither of these drugs alone or in combination has been shown to have a significant long-term beneficial impact on hepatitis B viral infection or on the accompanying inflammatory liver disease. In addition, adverse effects are not insubstantial. Currently, such antiviral therapy remains *experimental* and is not available routinely. In the future, different regimens (*e.g.,* low-dose, long-term therapy or high-dose corticosteroid therapy and withdrawal followed by antiviral chemotherapy), different combinations, and new antiviral agents may prove more effective.

MONITORING COURSE AND RESPONSE TO THERAPY AND INDICATIONS FOR REFERRAL AND ADMISSION

Acute Viral Hepatitis. The patient can be followed by observing symptoms and monitoring hepatocellular function. An aminotransferase level once monthly is useful to judge the presence of ongoing disease, though the absolute level is not a particularly sensitive determinant of disease severity in the acute phase of illness. Prothrombin time is a good measure of hepatocellular synthetic function and should be checked when the patient first presents and when there is suspicion of worsening. Serum bilirubin also correlates with severity. A fall in serum albumin indicates hepatocellular failure, but because its half-life is 28 days, this change will not become apparent until late in the acute illness.

An office visit 2 weeks after the first presentation is often helpful to be sure there is no worsening and that the patient is managing satisfactorily. Thereafter, follow-up depends on how well the patient feels. At 3 months, a repeat aminotransferase, bilirubin, albumin, prothrombin time, and, in cases of hepatitis B, hepatitis B surface antigen should be performed to ascertain disease activity, severity, and antigen status.

If symptoms and laboratory evidence of activity persist after 3 months, repeat evaluations at monthly intervals are indicated. Referral for liver biopsy is not necessarily indicated if the illness has not resolved by 6 months. Many patients will continue to improve gradually after 6 months, and in many cases, because therapy for chronic viral hepatitis is limited, liver biopsy will not alter therapy. Biopsy should be reserved for the most severe cases, either for prognostic information or as confirmation of disease severity before immunosuppressive (or antiviral) therapy is initiated. It is particularly important to obtain help from a hepatologist, gastroenterologist, or pathologist experienced in interpreting biopsy material obtained from patients with chronic hepatitis; diagnosis depends on histologic appearance and can be difficult.

Chronic Hepatitis. Patients with mild *chronic persistent hepatitis* may be followed casually, but those who are symptomatic deserve careful monitoring and periodic reassessment to be sure there are no signs of progression. When *chronic active hepatitis* has been identified, very close follow-up is vital. If prednisone and azathioprine are used, weekly and later biweekly platelet and white cell counts are required. Aminotransferase, bilirubin, and gamma globulin levels ought to be obtained at 2 weeks, then every 1 to 3 months to monitor response and identify treatment failure. A complete evaluation should be performed every 6 months, including a liver biopsy if clinical and biochemical remission has occurred.

The need for and value of repeat liver biopsies at regular follow-up intervals is controversial. After the initial biopsy, which is necessary to initiate therapy, many authorities make subsequent decisions about duration and direction of therapy based on clinical and biochemical responses, without reliance on liver histology. Admission to the hospital is indicated for worsening mental status, bleeding, refractory ascites, or poor home environment. Patients with mild chronic active disease who do not receive therapy should be monitored in similar fashion and biopsied again if symptoms or biochemical parameters worsen.

PATIENT EDUCATION

Hepatitis often affects previously vigorous people accustomed to full activity. The prolonged course and magnitude of malaise commonly precipitate a reactive depression. Thorough explanation of the disease's course, design of a sensible treatment program that actively involves the patient and family, and close follow-up can maximize compliance and minimize depression.

Instruction concerning diet and activity is central to a comprehensive treatment program. In particular, it is important to prevent unnecessary restriction of activity and to ensure adequate nutrition. Patients can be told to do as much as they feel like doing, as long as they avoid overtiring themselves. Small, frequent meals, especially in the morning, are tolerated best. No foods need be restricted, but carbohydrates seem to be the best-tolerated food when nausea is pronounced.

THERAPEUTIC RECOMMENDATIONS*

Acute Viral Hepatitis

- Maintain adequate caloric intake and a balanced diet. Small feedings are tolerated best, especially in the morning. No foods need be restricted.
- Ensure adequate rest, but activity need not be unduly restricted if the patient feels capable of it.
- Omit potentially hepatotoxic agents, especially alcohol.
- Treat severe pruritus with cholestyramine.
- Treat severe nausea and vomiting with a nonphenothiazine antiemetic, such as trimethobenzamide (Tigan) suppositories.
- Admit the patient to the hospital if signs of marked worsening of hepatocellular function occur, for example, encephalopathy, bleeding, prolongation of prothrombin time.

* See Chapter 52 for prophylactic measures.

Also consider admission for maintaining adequate caloric and fluid intake when symptoms are severe.
- Check aminotransferase, prothrombin time, bilirubin, albumin/globulin, and HBsAg at onset and at 2 and 12 weeks. Any patient with evidence of persistent symptoms or laboratory abnormalities should be retested every 4 weeks. Referral for liver biopsy is reserved for a combination of failure to resolve infection and inflammation by 6 to 12 months and persistence of disabling symptoms.

Chronic Hepatitis

- Follow patients with chronic persistent hepatitis at regular intervals and rebiopsy if there are signs of marked worsening. Otherwise treat symptomatically. Steroids are not indicated.
- Immunosuppressive therapy should be avoided in patients with HBsAg-positive (or other viral) chronic active hepatitis. Some authorities do recommend such therapy for severe, disabling, life-threatening cases.
- In nonviral types of chronic active hepatitis (or in the very rare patient with viral chronic liver disease for whom no other options exist), begin high-dose prednisone (60 mg daily) or combination prednisone (30 mg) plus azathioprine (50 mg), also given daily, in patients with severe disease manifested by multilobular or bridging necrosis, disabling symptoms, and marked aminotransferase and globulin elevations. Combination therapy is preferred for the elderly, diabetics, and others who cannot tolerate long-term high-dose steroids.
- Taper prednisone by 5 to 10 mg at a time over the course of a month until a maintenance dose of 10 mg (with 50 mg of azathioprine) or 20 mg is established.
- Monitor aminotransferase, bilirubin, and globulins at 2 weeks, then every 1 to 3 months. If the patient is taking azathioprine, obtain platelet and white cell counts weekly for 3 months and biweekly to triweekly thereafter.
- Continue maintenance therapy for at least 24 to 36 months; then consider attempting discontinuation of therapy with a 6-week period of phasing out medication.
- Failure to achieve clinical improvement within 2 to 8 months of initiating therapy is an indication for consultation and consideration of high-dose treatment.
- Treat relapses in the same manner as new cases.
- Perform a full evaluation every 6 months, including liver biopsy when there is evidence of clinical improvement or worsening.
- Patients who are HBsAg-positive but asymptomatic probably need not be treated. The same applies to those with minimal clinical disease, antigen negativity, and necrosis limited to the periportal region. These individuals should be seen regularly and rebiopsied if symptoms and chemistries worsen.
- Admit the patient to the hospital when there is evidence of marked worsening of hepatocellular function.

ANNOTATED BIBLIOGRAPHY

Berk PD et al: Corticosteroid therapy for chronic active hepatitis. Ann Intern Med 85:523, 1975 (*An editorial that argues that not all forms of chronic active hepatitis have the same prognosis and that selectivity should be exercised in treating, because therapy is associated with a high morbidity.*)

Boyer JL: Chronic hepatitis—A perspective on classification and determinants of prognosis. Gastroenterology, 70:1161, 1976 (*Correlates histology with prognosis; a critical review with 66 references.*)

Czaja AJ, Summerskill WHJ: Chronic hepatitis: To treat or not to treat? Med Clin North Am 62:71, 1978 (*A discussion of the factors influencing the decision to treat. Severity of disease is the most important factor.*)

DeCock KM, Govindaragan S, Chin KB: Delta hepatitis in the Los Angeles area: A report of 126 cases. Ann Intern Med 105:108, 1986 (*A review of delta hepatitis found that it causes fulminant hepatitis with a 23% fatality rate and a high incidence in intravenous drug users and male homosexuals.*)

Dienstag JL: Non-A, non-B hepatitis. I. Recognition, epidemiology, and clinical features. II. Experimental transmission, putative virus agents and markers, and prevention. Gastroenterology 85:439, 1983 (*An in-depth review of non-A, non-B hepatitis with more than 400 references. Includes a detailed discussion of clinical features and outcome.*)

Dienstag JL, Isselbacher KJ: Therapy of acute and chronic hepatitis. Arch Intern Med 141:1419, 1981 (*A review of therapeutic options and management of viral and nonviral acute and chronic hepatitis.*)

Gregory PB, Knauer CM, Kempson RL et al: Steroid therapy in severe viral hepatitis: A double-blind, randomized trial of methylprednisolone versus placebo. N Engl J Med 294:681, 1976. (*An important prospective controlled trial of corticosteroid therapy for acute, severe hepatitis, primarily viral. Showed that such therapy was not beneficial and suggested that it was even deleterious. Very influential in altering physician practice; as a result, corticosteroids are not used for such cases.*)

Hoffnagle JH, Davis GL, Pappas SC et al: A short course of prednisolone in chronic type B hepatitis. Ann Intern Med 104:12, 1986 (*A randomized, double-blind, placebo-controlled study showing prednisolone was of no value and potentially harmful.*)

Koretz R, Suffin S, Gitnick G: Posttransfusion chronic liver disease. Gastroenterology 71:797, 1976 (*A prospective study of 47 patients with post-transfusion hepatitis. Chronic hepatitis, manifested by transaminase elevations for 20 weeks, developed in over 50%. About half of these individuals had the chronic active variety. Age, sex, number of units transfused, presence or absence of symptoms, and underlying illness were unrelated to risk of chronic hepatitis. Many had non-A, non-B disease.*)

Krugman S et al: Viral hepatitis type B: Studies on natural history and prevention re-examined. N Engl J Med 300:101, 1979 (*An updated and detailed evaluation of natural history, utilizing advances in immunologic techniques to reexamine sera collected in classic natural history studies.*)

Lam KC et al: Deleterious effect of prednisolone in HBsAg-positive chronic active hepatitis. N Engl J Med 304:380, 1981 (*A prospective, placebo-controlled, pair-randomized trial of low-dose prednisolone in Chinese patients with mild-to-moderate HBsAg-positive chronic active hepatitis. The treated group experienced no benefit and actually had an increased rate of delayed remission, relapse, complications, and death. This study is part of the data cited in withholding immunosuppressive therapy from patients with HBsAg-positive chronic active hepatitis. It has been criticized for its small size, its pair randomization, its low-dose treatment protocol, and its inclusion of primarily mild-to-moderate, rather than severe, disease.*)

Nefzger M, Chalmers T: The treatment of acute infectious hepatitis: Ten year follow-up study of the effects of diet and rest. Am J Med 35:299, 1963 (*A classic prospective study on the impact of diet and rest in 460 servicemen; no particular diet or activity program made any difference in long-term outcome.*)

Rizzetto M et al: Chronic hepatitis in carriers of hepatitis B surface antigen, with intrahepatic expression of delta antigen: An active and progressive disease unresponsive to immunosuppressive treatment. Ann Intern Med 98:437, 1983 (*Demonstration that liver histology in patients with chronic hepatitis B and delta hepatitis was severe—all but a few had chronic active hepatitis or cirrhosis—and that progression of disease was rapid and unrelenting. Development of cirrhosis and mortality were observed in follow-up studies, and the rate of such progression was higher than expected in patients with chronic hepatitis B alone. Unfortunately, immunosuppressive therapy had no beneficial impact.*)

Sagnelli E et al: Serum levels of hepatitis B surface and core antigens during immunosuppressive treatment of HBsAg-positive chronic active hepatitis. Lancet 2:395, 1980 (*One of several studies showing that immunosuppressive therapy in HBsAg-positive chronic active hepatitis increases the level of hepatitis B virus replication; one of the bases for withholding such therapy in HBsAg-positive cases of chronic active hepatitis.*)

Schalm SW, Summerskill WHJ, Gitnick GL et al: Contrasting features and responses to treatment of severe chronic active liver disease with and without hepatitis Bs antigen. Gut 17:781, 1976 (*Retrospective analysis of the Mayo Clinic controlled trial of immunosuppressive therapy in severe chronic active hepatitis; showed that HBsAg-positive patients responded less well and had a higher mortality than HBsAg-negative patients.*)

Summerskill WHJ, Korman MG, Ammon HV et al: Prednisone for chronic active liver disease: Dose titration, standard dose, and combination with azathioprine compared. Gut 16:876, 1975 (*Results of the Mayo Clinic prospective double-blind randomized trial showing that prednisone or prednisone plus azathioprine was superior to placebo and azathioprine alone in treating severe chronic active hepatitis.*)

Weissberg JI et al: Survival in chronic hepatitis B: An analysis of 379 patients. Ann Intern Med 101:613, 1984 (*Five-year survival curves were derived for the outcome of the various types of chronic liver disease associated with hepatitis B. Five-year survival rates were 97% for patients with chronic persistent hepatitis, 86% for those with chronic active hepatitis, and 55% for those with chronic active hepatitis and cirrhosis. Age over 40, bilirubin elevation, ascites, and spider nevi were identified by multivariate analysis as factors associated with a poor prognosis and high risk of death.*)

Wright EC et al: Treatment of chronic active hepatitis: An analysis of 3 controlled trials. Gastroenterology 73:1422, 1977 (*A critique of the major studies. Concludes that they do demonstrate a reduction in cirrhosis and mortality for patients with severe antigen-negative disease who are treated with steroids.*)

71

Management of Cirrhosis and Chronic Liver Failure

LAWRENCE S. FRIEDMAN, M.D.

Cirrhosis represents an irreversible state of chronic liver injury. However, the cirrhotic patient may be kept comfortable, active, and independent if precipitants of hepatocellular injury can be eliminated and complications prevented. The responsibility for long-term management of patients with cirrhosis and chronic liver failure often rests with the primary care physician, who needs to be capable of dealing with such potential difficulties as ascites, peripheral edema, encephalopathy, infection, bleeding, and electrolyte imbalances.

CLINICAL PRESENTATION AND COURSE

The *initial presentation* of a patient with cirrhosis may be rather dramatic when ascites, encephalopathy, or brisk variceal bleeding brings the patient to medical attention. More subtle manifestations include splenomegaly, a firm liver edge, or such signs of hepatocellular failure as jaundice, palmar erythema, Dupuytren's contractures, spider angiomata, parotid and lacrimal gland hypertrophy, gynecomastia, testicular atrophy, loss of axillary and pubic hair, and clubbing. An isolated elevation of the alkaline phosphatase may be the only finding in early primary biliary cirrhosis; a bronze appearance to the skin is characteristic of hemochromatosis. Routine liver function tests usually do not define the specific cause of liver disease, but the serum albumin concentration and degree of prothrombin time prolongation provide useful measures of hepatocellular function and severity of liver failure (see Chapter 62).

The *clinical course* depends in part on the nature, severity, and activity of the underlying hepatic disease. In patients with alcoholic cirrhosis, survival is inversely related to continued alcohol ingestion. In one study, patients with biopsy-proven alcoholic cirrhosis who abstained from alcohol had a 5-year survival rate of 60%, compared with a rate of 40% for those who continued to drink. The 5-year survival was only 30% for patients in whom jaundice or ascites developed. In a recent study of patients with symptomatic *primary biliary cirrhosis,* the average length of survival from the onset of symptoms was about 12 years, whereas the survival of asymptomatic patients did not differ from that of a control population matched for age and sex. The prognosis of patients with postnecrotic cirrhosis is difficult to assess because it is hard to date its onset; the cirrhosis develops insidiously over years from subclinical chronic active hepatitis.

Portal hypertension, fluid retention, and encephalopathy are the major sequelae of cirrhosis; they lead to varices, ascites, hypersplenism, edema, and coma. Variceal bleeding occurs in 20% to 30% of all cirrhotic patients, one third of whom die during the initial hospitalization, one third rebleed within 6 weeks, and one third survive 1 year or more. The principal causes of death in patients with cirrhosis are variceal bleeding, encephalopathy, and infection. In addition, patients with cirrhosis, especially those with chronic hepatitis B infection, are at increased risk for hepatocellular carcinoma.

PRINCIPLES OF MANAGEMENT

Cirrhosis and Its Underlying Etiologies

Alcoholic cirrhosis requires complete *abstinence* from further alcohol intake. Attention to good nutrition, daily multiple vitamin supplements (including 1 mg of folic acid), and correction of any iron deficiency or electrolyte deficits are important supportive measures. The search continues for agents that might halt hepatic fibrosis and promote hepatocyte regeneration. Glucocorticosteroids, propylthiouracil, colchicine, and insulin in conjunction with glucagon have been under investigation. The results have been variable with some agents and promising with others. None of these can be recommended at present, but the literature should be followed for further study results.

Primary biliary cirrhosis can cause severe pruritus, which may be relieved by *cholestyramine* in a dose of 4 g orally with meals. Because of decreased fat absorption from low intestinal bile-salt concentrations, these patients are particularly prone to develop deficiencies of the *fat-soluble vitamins.* They may require supplemental vitamin K (10 mg subcutanously every 4 weeks), vitamin D (50,000 U orally two to three times a week or 100,000 U intramuscularly every 4 weeks) with oral calcium (1 g daily), and vitamin A (25,000 U orally per day). Night blindness unresponsive to vitamin A may be due to zinc deficiency, which is treated with oral *zinc sulfate* (220 mg/day). For patients with steatorrhea, *medium-chain triglyceride* preparations often help. Corticosteroids do not alter the course of illness, but there is suggestive evidence for such an effect with D-penicillamine. Further controlled trials are needed before the drug can be recommended for noninvestigational use.

Secondary biliary cirrhosis can be halted by relieving or bypassing the obstruction to bile flow.

Hemochromatosis is treated with weekly *phlebotomies* of 500 ml until the serum iron and ferritin levels fall to normal; then they are performed as needed.

Wilson's disease responds to *D-penicillamine* therapy, which should be carried out in conjunction with a hepatologist experienced in using the drug.

Some forms of **chronic active hepatitis** benefit from *corticosteroid* therapy (see Chapter 70).

Complications

Ascites and edema result from increased portal pressure, hypoalbuminemia, secondary hyperaldosteronism, and impaired free water clearance. Although ascites, in itself, is not a hazard, gross ascites can cause abdominal discomfort and respiratory compromise; under such circumstances it ought to be treated. Before treatment is initiated, a *diagnostic paracentesis* is indicated in patients with new onset of ascites, worsening hepatic function, fever, or increasing encephalopathy to exclude infection and malignancy.

The cornerstone of ascites management is *restriction of salt intake* to 1 g of NaCl (400 mg sodium) per day. In the absence of encephalopathy, a daily protein intake of at least 50 g is recommended. *Water intake* should be curtailed to 1500 ml daily if marked hyponatremia (reflecting retention of free water) is present. An effective program of salt and water restriction requires a cooperative patient and a conscientious family. A dietitian can provide invaluable assistance. The patient should be instructed to check his weight daily; measuring abdominal girth is an unreliable index of fluid loss because of variations due to gaseous distention of the gastrointestinal tract.

The maximum amount of ascites that can be mobilized in 24 hours is limited to 700 to 900 ml, although peripheral edema can be mobilized at a faster rate. Therefore, the goals of therapy are loss of no more than 0.5 kg of body weight a day in patients with ascites only and of no more than 1 kg a day in those with both ascites and peripheral edema. Fluid losses exceeding these amounts may result in intravascular volume depletion, hepatorenal syndrome, and encephalopathy.

If diuresis has not ensued after 1 week of rigid salt restriction, diuretic therapy may be initiated. *Spironolactone* is the agent of first choice, because its diuretic action is mild and unlikely to cause rapid intravascular volume depletion. Moreover, it is a specific aldosterone antagonist that can counter the hypokalemic alkalosis commonly seen in cirrhotic patients with ascites. The initial dosage of spironolactone is 100 mg a day orally in divided doses. If diuresis does not follow within 1 week, the daily dosage may be increased by 100 mg every 4 or 5 days to a maximum of 600 mg daily. It is useful to monitor urinary electrolyte concentrations, because diuresis should follow a significant rise in urinary sodium and a fall in urinary potassium. If natriuresis and diuresis do not occur on a maximal dosage of spironolactone, *furosedmide* (starting at 20 mg daily) or *hydrochlorothiazide* (starting at 50 mg daily) may be added. However, potent diuretics must be used with extreme care to avoid precipitating azotemia, hypokalemia, and encephalopathy.

Failure to maintain diuresis suggests intravascular volume depletion, as do the onset of tachycardia and an orthostatic fall in blood pressure. An oral or intravenous fluid challenge of several hundred milliliters of isotonic fluid can confirm the presence of hypovolemia by inducing a temporary increase in urine output.

A minority of patients are truly refractory and fail to respond to diuretic therapy. Therapeutic *paracentesis* then becomes a consideration. Paracentesis of 1 to 2 liters is generally not recommended except to prevent imminent rupture of an umbilical hernia, to relieve severe abdominal pain, or to lessen disabling respiratory embarrassment. The beneficial effects are short-lived, and there is the risk of inducing a serious depletion in intravascular volume as ascitic fluid rapidly reaccumulates. Only patients with incapacitating and truly refractory ascites should be referred for consideration of *peritoneovenous (LeVeen) shunt* placement; results with this device have been variable and shunt insertion is associated with a high incidence of complications, especially infection and coagulopathy.

Hepatic encephalopathy is thought to be produced by one or more intestinally derived toxic substances that escape hepatic detoxification as a result of portasystemic shunting and hepatocellular dysfunction. Elevations of arterial and venous ammonia levels usually, but not always, correlate with the presence of hepatic encephalopathy. Venous levels may be falsely elevated when a tourniquet is left on too long at the time of blood drawing. Ammonia levels are useful in following the clinical state of individual patients. Important precipitating factors include gastrointestinal bleeding, excessive dietary protein intake, hypokalemic alkalosis, infection, constipation, use of sedative or hypnotic drugs, surgical procedures, and volume depletion resulting from diuresis or paracentesis. Precipitants are identified in about 50% of patients; the prognosis is usually better in those with an identifiable contributory factor than in those in whom the onset of encephalopathy is associated only with worsening hepatic function.

Mild encephalopathy may be managed on an ambulatory basis. Aside from excluding gastrointestinal bleeding, avoiding and correcting fluid and electrolyte disturbances, and discontinuing tranquilizers and sedatives, the mainstay of therapy is *restriction of dietary protein* intake to 30 to 40 g per day, while maintaining a daily caloric intake of 1500 kcal. In addition, simple gut cleansing with enemas or cathartics is effective when bleeding, constipation, or a large dietary protein intake has led to encephalopathy. Patients should be monitored with routine mental status examinations that include five-point star and signature testing and examination for asterixis.

Specific therapy for encephalopathy begins with *lactulose,* a synthetic, nonabsorbable disaccharide, which is metabolized to organic acids by enteric bacteria, causing an osmotic catharsis. In addition, lactulose suppresses the growth of ammonia-forming bacteria in favor of lactose-fermenting organisms. The initial dosage for patients with mild encephalopathy is 15 ml to 30 ml orally every 4 to 6 hours, with adjustments thereafter to produce two to three loose stools a day. Side-effects of oral lactulose include diarrhea and abdominal distress, which usually resolve after a reduction in dosage.

Lacutlose is as effective as *neomycin,* a poorly absorbed, broad-spectrum aminoglycoside antibiotic, which preceded lactulose as the drug of choice for treatment of encephalopathy. Neomycin acts by decreasing the intestinal concentration of ammonia-forming bacteria. Prolonged use in doses of 4 g per day or more results in significant serum drug levels and risk of serious ototoxicity and nephrotoxicity, especially in patients with underlying renal insufficiency. The drug also causes malabsorption. The recommended maximum oral dose is 1 g twice daily. Delivery of neomycin to the colon can be enhanced by administration with sorbitol, either orally or as an enema. In rare patients who fail to respond to either lactulose or neomycin, the two may be given together; in some patients the effect appears to be additive.

Oral and intravenous *amino acid formulations,* containing high concentrations of branched-chain amino acids and low levels of aromatic amino acids may be beneficial in controlling encephalopathy while maintaining positive nitrogen balance. Substituting vegetable for animal protein may be similarly effective. Further studies are required before such protein formulations can be recommended as sole therapy for encephalopathy.

Coagulopathy in patients with cirrhosis results from reductions in vitamin K-dependent clotting factors (II, VII, IX, and X) secondary to decreased hepatic protein synthesis and increased plasma proteolytic activity. In addition, bile-salt deficiency, neomycin therapy, and malnutrition may contribute to malabsorption of vitamin K, and hypersplenism may account for thrombocytopenia. If a patient with cirrhosis is discovered to have a prolonged prothrombin time, a trial of *vitamin K* 10 mg subcutaneously daily for 3 days will correct hypoprothrombinemia caused by bile-salt deficiency, neomycin, or malnutrition but not hypoprothrombinemia related only to hepatocellular disease. Otherwise, in the absence of bleeding, measures to correct abnormal coagulation parameters are generally not indicated.

Variceal bleeding in a cirrhotic patient requires hospitalization, and consultation with a gastroenterologist or surgeon skilled in managing this complication. Nevertheless, the primary physician must be familiar with current modes of therapy to judge how well the proposed treatment fits in with the overall plan of care for the patient. Emergent management of patients with bleeding esophageal varices begins with intravenous administration of *vasopressin* (0.1–0.6 U/minute) to decrease portal venous pressure and constrict splanchnic vessels. Insertion of a *Blakemore–Sengstaken* tube to compress varices directly may be used to stabilize patients who continue to bleed. Some studies suggest that administration of *nitroglycerin* with vasopressin may have the advantage of preserving coronary and renal blood flow without inhibiting the portal pressure-lowering and splanchnic vasoconstrictive effects of vasopressin.

Injection sclerotherapy, a technique in which varices are visualized at endoscopy and thrombosed by direct injection of sclerosing agents, has gained widespread popularity. Sclerotherapy appears to be useful in controlling acute variceal bleeding and, when repeated several times over 2 to 3 months, in preventing recurrent bleeding after acute variceal bleeding is controlled. Whether or not this therapy improves survival in cirrhotic patients with variceal hemorrhage is still unsettled, and it is possible that, like portasystemic shunt surgery, sclerotherapy may only substitute death from hepatic failure for death from variceal bleeding. Nevertheless, because its acute complication and mortality rates are low, sclerotherapy has become the treatment of choice for managing cirrhotic patients who bleed from varices. It has replaced portasystemic shunt surgery, which is now reserved for those who bleed despite repeated sclerotherapies.

Another recent development in the management of varices has been the long-term oral administration of *propranolol.* When prescribed in dosages that produce β-blockade, propranolol lowers portal venous pressure and decreases the frequency of recurrent variceal bleeding. Initial success with this therapy has been reported in patients with well-compensated cirrhosis. However, preliminary studies to determine the role of propranolol in the prevention of recurrent variceal bleeding in patients with decompensated cirrhosis (*i.e.,* those with ascites, hypoprothrombinemia, and encephalopathy) have been less encouraging.

Portasystemic shunt surgery remains the final and perhaps definitive procedure for patients with recurrent variceal hemorrhage due to portal hypertension. Extensive experience and a number of prospective studies have yielded the following observations: (1) the likelihood of recurrent variceal bleeding is significantly reduced after portasystemic shunting; (2) a significant improvement in long-term survival following portasystemic shunting has *not* been demonstrated, both because operative mortality rates are high and because underlying hepatic function, the principal determinant of survival, is unaffected by surgery; (3) portasystemic shunt surgery is not indicated in patients with varices that have never bled; (4) by preserving portal blood flow, selective shunt procedures such as the distal splenorenal shunt may be preferable in patients with demonstrable preoperative portal perfusion of the liver; they appear to be associated with a lower incidence of postoperative encephalopathy than conventional portacaval shunts are; and (5) side-to-side portacaval or proximal splenorenal shunts are the most effective operations for relieving ascites, because they decompress hepatic sinusoids, but they still have some attendant risk of precipitating encephalopathy.

THERAPEUTIC RECOMMENDATIONS AND MONITORING

- The patient should maintain a caloric intake of at least 2000 to 3000 kcal per day.
- Use of alcohol or other hepatotoxic agents must be prohibited.
- The patient should avoid tranquilizers and sedatives.
- Monitor prothrombin time, serum albumin, and bilirubin to assess the severity and progression of hepatocellular dysfunction.
- Check stools at each visit for evidence of occult bleeding.
- Check for asterixis and other signs of encephalopathy at each visit.
- A diagnostic paracentesis should be performed in patients with the new onset of ascites or clinical deterioration in the setting of preexisting ascites.
- In patients with unexplained clinical deterioration, a serum alpha-fetoprotein level should be measured to screen for hepatoma.
- For the treatment of ascites, patients should be instructed to restrict daily salt intake to no more than 1 g (400 mg of sodium) and to consume at least 50 g of protein per day. Consulting with a dietitian and providing the patient and his family with specific menus and food lists are essential.
- Restriction of fluid intake to 1500 ml is necessary only for marked hyponatremia (serum sodium concentration less than 125 mEq/liter).
- If salt restriction does not result in diuresis, begin spironolactone 100 mg daily in divided doses. If natriuresis and diuresis do not occur after 1 week, the daily dose of spironolactone may be increased by 100 mg every 4 to 5 days to a maximum of 600 mg per day.
- If spironolactone alone is ineffective in causing diuresis, furosemide 20 mg or hydrochlorothiazide 50 mg may be added to the regimen and cautiously increased in dosage; extreme care must be taken, however, to avoid inducing intravascular volume depletion and irreversible hepatorenal syndrome. The goal of therapy should be to lose no more than 0.5 kg per day in patients with ascites only and 1 kg per day in those with both ascites and peripheral edema.
- During therapy for ascites, the patient should be monitored closely for signs of volume depletion, azotemia, and hypokalemia. Frequent checks of pulse, postural changes in blood pressure, and serum potassium, BUN, and creatinine should be made. Diuretics should be withheld at the first sign of intravascular volume depletion.
- Potassium supplementation with 20 to 40 mEq KCl elixir per day may be necessary for patients with hypokalemia but must be administered cautiously to patients on potassium-sparing diuretics, such as spironolactone.
- At the first sign of encephalopathy, restrict dietary protein intake to 20 to 30 g per day. Start clinical monitoring of mental status, asterixis, and five-point star or signature testing. Venous ammonia levels may be monitored, with the caution that levels correlate inexactly with clinical encephalopathy.
- When protein restriction alone fails to control encephalopathy, begin oral lactulose, 15 to 30 ml every 4 to 6 hours, with subsequent adjustments in the dosage to allow two to three soft stools a day. Alternatively, give oral neomycin 1 g twice daily.

INDICATIONS FOR REFERRAL AND ADMISSION

Prompt hospitalization is required for patients with gastrointestinal bleeding, worsening encephalopathy, and increasing azotemia. Intractable cases of marked ascites may respond to elective admission and strict sodium restriction. Decisions about the management of variceal bleeding and indications for elective portasystemic shunt surgery are best made in consultation with a gastroenterologist and surgeon.

PATIENT EDUCATION AND SUPPORT

It should be emphasized to the patient and family that prognosis can be improved and symptoms lessened by careful adherence to the prescribed medical program. In particular, dietary discipline and omission of alcohol are central to a successful outcome and should be stressed. Many of these patients are chronic alcoholics with low self-esteem. A nonjudgmental, sympathetic physician can be instrumental in providing support, raising self-esteem, and improving the chances of compliance. Depression is a frequent accompaniment of the later stages of chronic liver disease and is manifested by failure to comply with the medical regimen and outright expressions of wanting to die. Treatment is very difficult. Antidepressant drugs may cause oversedation and thus are risky. There are no simple measures, but the physician's concern and support can help enormously.

ANNOTATED BIBLIOGRAPHY

Borowsky SA, Strome S, Lott E: Continued heavy drinking and survival in alcoholic cirrhotics. Gastroenterology 80:1405, 1981 (*A Study of 54 patients discharged from the hospital after treatment for alcoholic cirrhosis and first-time ascites; 12 of 15 [80%] continued heavy drinkers died in a mean time of 7.2 months after discharge, whereas 22 of 23 abstainers were still alive after a mean follow-up of 14 months.*)

Campra JL, Reynolds TB: Effectiveness of high-dose spironolactone therapy in patients with chronic liver disease and relatively refractory ascites. Dig Dis Sci 23:1025, 1978 (*Spironolactone doses as high as 600 mg daily were shown to be effective in patients with ascites presumed to be "refractory" at lower doses.*)

Conn HO: The rational management of ascites. Prog Liver Dis 4: 269, 1972 (*Comprehensive discussion of pathophysiology and treatment of ascites.*)

Conn HO, Leevy CM, Vlahcevic ZR et al: Comparison of lactulose and neomycin in the treatment of chronic portal-systemic encephalopathy; a double-blind controlled trial. Gastroenterology 72:573, 1977 (*The drugs were found to be equally effective and free of significant toxicity.*)

Epstein M: Peritoneovenous shunt in the management of ascites and the hepatorenal syndrome. Gastroenterology 82:790, 1982 (*Authoritative discussion of the various types of peritoneovenous shunts, their physiologic consequences, their complications, and the role of shunts in clinical practice; argues that the peritoneovenous shunt should be reserved for patients whose major medical problems will be addressed by relief of ascites and in whom adequate conservative therapy has been ineffective.*)

Fraser CL, Arieff AI: Hepatic encephalopathy. N Engl J Med 313: 865, 1985 (*A comprehensive review; 147 references.*)

Graham DY, Smith JL: The course of patients after variceal hemorrhage. Gastroenterology 80:800, 1981 (*Of 85 consecutive variceal bleeders, one third died in the initial hospitalization, one third rebled within 6 weeks, and one third survived at least 1 year. Long-term survival after the initial 2 weeks following the bleeding episode was not different from that of unselected cirrhotics without bleeding.*)

Hoyumpa AM, Desmond PV, Avant GR et al: Hepatic encephalopathy. Gastroenterology 76:184, 1979 (*A thorough and practical review of clinical, pathophysiologic, and therapeutic aspects of encephalopathy.*)

Lebrec D, Poynard T, Hillon P, Benhamou J-P: Propranolol for prevention of recurrent gastrointestinal bleeding in patients with cirrhosis. N Engl J Med 305:1371, 1981 (*A double-blind placebo-controlled study showing a decrease in the incidence of variceal rebleeding from 96% to 50% at 1 year in patients receiving propranolol in dosages that reduced the heart rate by 25%; the study was restricted to patients with minimal or absent ascites, jaundice, and encephalopathy.*)

MacDougall BRD, Westaby D, Theodossi A et al: Increased long-term survival in variceal haemorrhage using injection sclerotherapy: Results of a controlled trial. Lancet 1:124, 1982 (*The incidence of recurrent variceal bleeding was 8% in patients in whom varices were obliterated compared with 75% in control patients not receiving sclerotherapy. In this study survival was shown to be significantly improved in the sclerotherapy group.*)

Powell WJ Jr, Klatskin G: Duration of survival in patients with Laennec's cirrhosis. Am J Med 44:406, 1968 (*Classic paper showing improved survival in cirrhotic patients who abstained from alcohol compared with those who continued to drink heavily.*)

Rector WG: Drug therapy for portal hypertension. Ann Intern Med 105:96, 1986 (*Critical review of vasopressin, propranolol, and somatostatin.*)

Rikkers LF: Operations for management of esophageal variceal hemorrhage. West J Med 136:107, 1982 (*Elegant and critical review of the various types of portasystemic shunt procedures and the indications for their use.*)

Roll J, Boyer JL, Barry D, Klatskin G: The prognostic importance of clinical and histologic features in asymptomatic and symptomatic primary biliary cirrhosis. N Engl J Med 308:1, 1983 (*Survival data on 280 patients. The average survival was 11.9 years in symptomatic patients; jaundice, hepatomegaly, and ascites were each associated with a poor prognosis.*)

Shear L, Ching S, Gabuzda GJ: Compartmentalization of ascites and edema in patients with hepatic cirrhosis. N Engl J Med 282:1391, 1970 (*Classic study demonstrating that the maximum rate at which ascites can be absorbed is 930 ml per 24 hours and concluding that the therapeutic aim in patients with ascites should be weight loss of no more than 0.5 kg daily.*)

Webber FL: Therapy of portal-systemic encephalopathy: The practical and the promising. Gastroenterology 81:174, 1981 (*Concise review of established and experimental approaches to the treatment of encephalopathy.*)

72

Management of Pancreatitis
JAMES M. RICHTER, M.D.

The primary physician may encounter pancreatitis in three forms that lend themselves to ambulatory management: (1) recovery phase of acute pancreatitis, (2) chronic, mild relapsing pancreatitis presenting as recurrent abdominal pain, and (3) pancreatic insufficiency, with diarrhea and weight loss.

In the United States, most cases of pancreatitis are a result of excess ethanol ingestion or biliary tract disease, chiefly among middle-aged alcoholic men and elderly women with gallstones, respectively. A penetrating duodenal ulcer, trauma, hypercalcemia, hypertriglyceridemia, vascular disease, tumor, heredity, ampullary stenosis, and drugs such as thiazide diuretics, glucocorticosteroids, azathioprine, and sulfasalazine are also associated with pancreatitis. Frequently, no etiology is found. The course, response to therapy, and prognosis are largely functions of the etiology.

The primary physician must be able to distinguish acute pancreatitis from other causes of acute upper abdominal pain (see Chapter 53), pancreatic insufficiency from other causes of steatorrhea (see Chapter 58), and chronic pancreatitis from pancreatic carcinoma. Objectives of management include relief of pain, removal of precipitants, and assurance of adequate nutrition.

DIAGNOSIS, CLINICAL PRESENTATION, AND COURSE

Acute Pancreatitis. The manifestations of acute pancreatitis disease are produced by inflammatory breakdown of pancreatic architecture, with release of digestive enzymes into the intersititium of the gland, leading to autolysis. Typically, acute pancreatitis produces constant epigastric, periumbilical, or left upper quadrant pain radiating to the back, often increased by food and decreased by upright posture. Vomiting can be quite persistent. Examination reveals abdominal tenderness and may include decreased bowel sounds, distention and fever.

The diagnosis of acute pancreatitis is supported by increases in the serum amylase and serum lipase, and an amylase-creatinine clearance ratio greater than 5. The *serum amylase* is elevated principally in pancreatic disease, but may also be high in renal insufficiency, salivary gland disease, biliary tract obstruction, and such other intra-abdominal conditions as perforated peptic ulcer, mesenteric infarction, and small bowel obstruction without detectable pancreatitis. The serum *lipase* is more specific but less sensitive; it is a good confirmatory test. The *amylase–creatinine clearance ratio* was thought to convey added specificity, but is a nonspecific consequence of decreased renal amylase clearance that often accompanies severe pancreatitis, as well as diabetic ketoacidosis and cutaneous burns. Recently, assays for *trypsinogen* and *amylase isoenzymes* have been developed; they are useful confirmatory tests, but the serum amylase remains the best initial diagnostic study. At times *ultrasonography* can be used for diagnostic purposes; it shows edema of the gland, as well as any biliary tract pathology. Radiologic *contrast study* of the stomach and duodenum help to rule out peptic ulcer disease when the clinical presentation is unclear.

The *course* of acute pancreatitis depends on the severity of the disease and the underlying etiology. In a patient recovering from acute pancreatitis, symptoms are reliable indicators of disease activity. Elevated enzymes in an otherwise asymptomatic patient are usually of no significance. The serum amylase routinely falls to normal within several days, but may remain elevated for weeks after an uncomplicated illness. In other instances, persistently elevated enzymes in an asymptomatic individual may be a clue to the presence of a silent pseudocyst. If a mass is palpable or pain recurs, a pseudocyst should be ruled out by ultrasonography of the upper abdomen. *Pseudocysts* arise in about half of patients with severe pancreatitis, mostly in those with alcohol-induced disease. Spontaneous resolution occurs over 3 months in about 50% of patients; those with lesions over 2 cm usually require surgical removal.

Chronic pancreatitis characteristically presents and proceeds as bouts of mild to severe recurrent epigastric pain, often occurring in *chronic alcoholics* after years of excessive drinking. Sometimes chronic pancreatitis is heralded by a severe attack of acute pancreatitis. At other times, there may be mild pain or simply the painless insidious onset of exocrine insufficiency and diabetes. The pain of chronic pancreatitis is not entirely constant and often varies in intensity over days to weeks. There may be exacerbations of pain, nausea, and vomiting after eating or drinking alcohol. Elevated serum amylase and amylase–creatinine clearance ratios are helpful, but the sensitivity of these tests is lower than in acute pancreatitis.

Individuals who present with chronic recurrent abdominal pain and a history of relapsing pancreatitis usually do not present difficult diagnostic problems, but the patient without such a history requires more extensive assessment. A *plain film of the abdomen* may reveal *pancreatic calcification,* a late finding in alcoholic pancreatitis. *Ultrasonography* may demonstrate a diffusely enlarged gland, local mass, or pseudocyst. If ultrasound evaluation is normal and pancreatic disease is strongly suspected on clinical grounds, *pancreatic function testing* or *computerized axial tomography* should be done. Two normal studies correctly predict a normal pancreas in 90% of cases. An abnormal finding in any one study warrants further evaluation to distinguish between chronic pancreatitis and pancreatic carcinoma. At institutions where the technology exists, *endoscopic retrograde pancreatography* has proven to be an effective diagnostic technique. Abdominal angiography may be helpful when retrograde pancreatography is unavailable or fails.

The course of chronic pancreatitis is variable and depends on removal of precipitating factors. Presently, it is not known how cholelithiasis causes pancreatitis, but successful and early surgical therapy almost always prevents recurrent or chronic pancreatitis. With recurrent disease, pancreatic insufficiency may gradually develop over years, manifested by weight loss and steatorrhea. Although mild glucose intolerance may occur early in the disease process, the onset of clinical diabetes is a late complication and a sign of advanced disease.

Pancreatic Insufficiency. Patients with pancreatic exocrine insufficiency complain of weight loss and frequent, greasy bowel movements. Weight loss is often striking but nonspecific in this population, which tends to substitute alcohol for other forms of nourishment. Steatorrhea is a late development, not seen until more than 80% of pancreatic exocrine function has been lost. Objective evidence of maldigestion may be obtained by a *qualitative examination for stool fat* with Sudan stain. Where this is not available, a 72-hour *quantitative stool fat* analysis can also be used to establish the presence of steatorrhea and a *d-xylose test* to exclude small bowel mucosal disease. The *bentiromide test* is a simple outpatient study for detecting pancreatic exocrine insufficiency. When bentiromide (500 mg) is given orally, it normally is acted upon by pancreatic chymotrypsin to produce paraaminobenzoic acid, which is absorbed by the small bowel and excreted in the urine. In normal persons, greater than 50% is excreted in 6 hours. This test appears to have a sensitivity of 80% and a specificity of 90% for exocrine insufficiency. When significant uncertainty persists, direct pancreatic function tests, such as secretin stimulation, may be needed to demonstrate exocrine insufficiency objectively. A small group of patients with pancreatic insufficiency do not give a prior history of recurrent abdominal pain; they should be evaluated for hemochromatosis and cystic fibrosis.

PRINCIPLES OF MANAGEMENT

Acute Pancreatitis. About 50% of patients have mild, self-limited disease and will recover spontaneously. Such patients with mild pain and no vomiting may be treated on an ambulatory basis with restriction of fat and protein and careful monitoring. Patients with more severe disease who require hospitalization generally tolerate a full diet before discharge from the hospital, although a *diet moderately restricted in fat* is often recommended to lessen the degree of pancreatic stimulation. *H₂-receptor antagonists, antacids,* and *anticholinergics* are frequently given with the hope of reducing the stimulus to pancreatic secretion, but are of no proven benefit. If a patient returns with severe pain and vomiting, he should be readmitted.

Identification and treatment or removal of precipitants, such as alcohol abuse, hypercalcemia, stones, and hypertriglyceridemia are essential to successful therapy. Of the conditions associated with pancreatitis, alcoholism is the most difficult to deal with. Even the pain of pancreatitis often does not dissuade the dedicated drinker from abusing alcohol. Nevertheless, the *treatment of alcoholism* should be undertaken with considerable effort (see Chapter 224), since there is much to gain by the cessation of drinking. A check for drugs associated with pancreatitis is indicated (thiazides, corticosteroids, estrogens, azathioprine).

All patients should undergo evaluation of the biliary tract by *ultrasonography* to rule out stone disease, a treatable cause of pancreatitis. The oral cholecystogram is less useful, because it may not visualize until 4 to 6 weeks after a bout of acute pancreatitis. After an acute episode, a *serum calcium* should be repeated, because *hypercalcemia* can be masked by the decrease in calcium that may result from an attack. Repeatedly elevated *fasting triglyceride determinations* suggest the diagnosis of another treatable etiology.

Chronic Pancreatitis. Patients with chronic pancreatitis may develop recurrent bouts of pain and vomiting indistinguishable from acute pancreatitis. Those with severe pain and inability to maintain hydration orally should be admitted. Others with less severe exacerbations may be managed on an outpatient basis. Many are bothered by chronic pain.

Initial treatment consists of eliminating causative factors (see above) and attempting to control the often disabling *pain.* Pancreatic enzymes, low-fat diets, anticholinergics, and antacids may decrease pancreatic secretion but do not reliably lessen the pain. Nonnarcotic analgesics (aspirin, acetaminophen) should be tried but are usually inadequate, necessitating use of more potent agents. *Methadone* is the narcotic best suited for long-term outpatient use. The establishment of a *supportive doctor–patient relationship* complements pharmacologic pain control efforts.

Numerous *surgical procedures* have been designed to alleviate the pain of chronic pancreatitis; none is totally effective. Patients with persistent pain in the absence of gallbladder disease or alcoholism should have an endoscopic *retrograde pancreatogram* to search for a surgically treatable anatomic abnormality, such as pancreas divisum. If a markedly dilated duct is found, suggesting obstruction, a modified *Puestow sphincteroplasty procedure* can be performed to improve drainage of pancreatic juices into the small bowel. The operation may provide reasonable pain relief without removal of pancreatic tissue. Pseudocysts should be drained internally; however, reduction in pain is not consistently achieved. Sometimes partial or even subtotal pancreatectomies are attempted for control of pain; at best, results are equivocal.

In patients with severe active disease, the pancreas is progressively destroyed, and eventually the pain subsides as the disease "burns" itself out. Then the management priority shifts to treatment of pancreatic insufficiency.

Pancreatic Insufficiency. Management of pancreatic insufficiency begins with a therapeutic trial of oral pancreatic enzymes to judge efficacy of therapy. The patient who benefits from use of exogenous enzymes will tolerate the unpleasant taste and mild discomfort they cause. *Pancreatic enzymes* are available as extracts of hog pancreas. *Pancreatin* contains trypsin, amylase, and some lipase, while *pancrealipase* contains trypsin, amylase, and extra amounts of lipase. The usual dose is 0.5 g to 2.5 g with each meal. Because enzyme preparations are partially inactivated by gastric acid or require increased alkalinity in the duodenum, they may work better when given with antacids, bicarbonate, or H₂-receptor antagonists. *Medium-chain triglycerides* are often helpful, for they can be absorbed in the absence of lipase. Therapy can be assessed by monitoring symptoms, weight, and qualitative stool fat determinations. Clinically significant fat-soluble vitamin deficiencies are uncommon, perhaps because intact bile secretion prevents complete fat malabsorption.

Most patients with chronic pancreatitis have abnormal

glucose tolerance tests. Mild glucose intolerance can be watched, but insulin dependence may occur. Hypoglycemia may be a problem, because loss of glucagon secretion leads to a "brittle" diabetic state, but ketoacidosis is rare. The vascular complications of diabetes seldom appear, perhaps because most patients do not survive long enough.

PATIENT EDUCATION

Most patients know little about the pancreas and its role in digestion. Moreover, few are aware of the connection between alcohol abuse and pancreatitis. Patient cooperation regarding diet, alcohol intake, and use of enzyme extracts may be facilitated by a better understanding of the function of the pancreas and the nature of pancreatitis. Also, patients with acute pancreatitis who are making good recoveries can be comforted by the fact that recurrence is not common when the underlying cause is treated.

The patient with intractable pain and narcotic dependence poses one of the most difficult problems encountered in clinical medicine. A major pitfall is the development of an adversarial relationship between patient and physician concerning the need for narcotics. Although there are no simple solutions, it is essential to elicit, understand, and respond to patient concerns, fears, and needs at the very outset. A well-informed patient who has confidence in his physician and in himself requires less pain medication than one who is scared, feels abandoned, and is in conflict with his doctor.

INDICATIONS FOR ADMISSION AND REFERRAL

Some patients present with rather mild symptoms, but later develop a fulminant illness. Patients over age 55 are at risk for a serious progression, as are those who manifest fever, tachycardia, hyperglycemia, serum calcium below 8.0 mg/dl, or amylase over 1000 mg/dl at the time of initial presentation. Such individuals deserve admission for careful monitoring, even if they do not appear seriously ill at the outset. Patients who cannot maintain oral hydration also require admission. Surgical consultation is indicated if an anatomic abnormality, pseudocyst, or obstructive lesion is detected on workup of the pancreas and biliary tract. Patients with refractory pain might benefit from evaluation by a gastroenterologist skilled in endoscopic retrograde pancreatography.

MANAGEMENT RECOMMENDATIONS

Recovery Phase of Acute Pancreatitis

- Begin feedings with foods rich in carbohydrates and low in protein and fat. Gradually increase the amount of protein in the diet as tolerated, followed by slow resumption of fat intake.
- Check for and treat any underlying alcohol abuse (see Chapter 224), hypertriglyceridemia (see Chapter 22), or hypercalcemia (see Chapter 96).

- Eliminate, if possible, use of drugs associated with pancreatitis (azathioprine, estrogens, thiazides, corticosteroids).
- Obtain ultrasound examination of the gallbladder and biliary tract; refer the patient for surgery if stones are found.

Chronic Pancreatitis

- Check for and treat any inciting cause, such as, alcoholism, biliary tract disease, hypercalcemia, hyperlipidemia (see above).
- Readmit the patient if severe recurrent acute pancreatitis develops.
- Temporarily limit fat intake during flare-ups.
- Begin with mild analgesics for pain control, such as aspirin or acetaminophen 600 mg every 4 hours.
- Pain unrelieved by mild analgesia is an indication for a course of narcotic analgesics, such as methadone 5 or 10 mg every 6 or 8 hours.
- Further evaluation is needed to rule out carcinoma, pseudocyst, and biliary tract disease. Begin with ultrasonography and proceed to CT scan if ultrasonography is technically unsatisfactory.
- Refer the patient for surgery if a treatable lesion is found.
- Aggressive surgical procedures other than sphincteroplasty aimed at relieving ductal obstruction do not reliably relieve pain.

Pancreatic Insufficiency

- Give oral pancreatic extract with each feeding in doses of 0.5 to 2.5 g (2 to 8 tablets) with full meals and 0.5 g with snacks. Lack of effect may require addition of an antacid (*e.g.,* 60 cc of Mylanta with each meal) or H_2-receptor antagonist (*e.g.,* ranitidine, 150 mg bid) to neutralize gastric acid and prevent enzymes from becoming inactivated.
- Provide a high-calorie diet, rich in carbohydrate and protein.
- Supplement the diet with a medium-chain triglyceride preparation. Restrict fat in symptomatic steatorrhea.
- Monitor glucose tolerance and treat clinical diabetes, if present, with insulin, cautiously; these patients often exhibit "brittle" disease.

ANNOTATED BIBLIOGRAPHY

Ammann RW, Akobintz A, Largiader F et al: Course and outcome of chronic pancreatitis: A longitudinal study of a mixed medical–surgical series of 245 patients. Gastroenterology 86:820, 1984 (*An excellent clinical course/natural history study.*)

Arvanitakis C, Cooke AR: Diagnostic tests of exocrine pancreatic function. Gastroenterology 74:932, 1978 (*Excellent review of the major methods used to test exocrine function.*)

Bank S, Marks IN, Vinik AI: Clinical and hormonal aspects of pancreatic diabetes. Am J Gastroenterol 64:13, 1975 (*A clinical description of pancreatic diabetes, its therapy, and its distinctive properties.*)

Di Magno EP et al: A prospective comparison of current diagnostic tests for pancreatic cancer. N Engl J Med 97:737, 1977 (*A prospective clinical study demonstrating the utility of ultrasonography, pancreatic function testing, and endoscopic retrograde pancreatography in the evaluation of the patient with chronic abdominal pain suggestive of pancreatic carcinoma or chronic pancreatitis.*)

Geokas MC, Baltaxe HA, Banks PA et al: Acute pancreatitis. Ann Intern Med 103:86, 1985 (*A review of recent developments in pathogenesis, diagnosis, and therapy: 166 references.*)

Karasawa E, Goldberg HI, Moss AA et al: CT pancreatogram in carcinoma of the pancreas and chronic pancreatitis. Radiology 148:489, 1983 (*Irregular calcified ducts are characteristic of chronic pancreatitis, whereas in pancreatic cancer, smooth or beaded dilatation is the most frequent finding.*)

Mallory A, Kern F, Jr: Drug-induced pancreatitis: A critical review. Gastroenterology 78:813, 1980 (*A good review of the drug causes of pancreatitis and how to separate presumptive from definite.*)

Moossa AR: Diagnostic tests and procedures in acute pancreatitis. N Engl J Med 311:639, 1984 (*Critically reviews tests and procedures for the diagnosis of acute pancreatitis, emphasizing those that are useful in assessing the severity of an attack.*)

Niederau C, Grendell JH: Diagnosis of chronic pancreatitis. Gastroenterology 88:1973, 1985 (*A superb, absolutely comprehensive review of biochemical and imaging approaches to the diagnosis of chronic pancreatitis; 247 references.*)

Richter JM, Schapiro RH, Mulley AG et al: Association of pancreatitis and its treatment by sphincteroplasty of the accessory ampulla. Gastroenterology 81:1104, 1981 (*Patients with pancreas divisum develop recurrent acute pancreatitis more frequently than people with normal anatomy.*)

Saunders JHB, Wormsley KG: Pancreatic extracts and the treatment of pancreatic exocrine insufficiency. Gut 16:157, 1975 (*Provides a detailed review of pancreatic extracts, pancreatic replacement therapy, and the assessment of the efficacy of pancreatic replacement.*)

Steinberg WM, Goldstein SS, Davis SS et al: Diagnostic assays in acute pancreatitis. Ann Intern Med 102:576, 1985 (*Compares sensitivity and specificity of amylase, lipase, trypsinogen, and amylase isoenzyme assays for diagnosis of acute pancreatitis. Recommends use of amylase as the initial study of choice, with any of the others useful for confirmation.*)

Toskes P: Bentiromide as a test of exocrine function in adults with pancreatic exocrine insufficiency. Determination of appropriate dose of urinary collection interval. Gastroenterology 85:565, 1983 (*The standardization of the bentiromide test as a simple outpatient test for pancreatic insufficiency.*)

Van Dyke JA, Stanley RJ, Berland LL: Pancreatic imaging. Ann Intern Med 102:212, 1985 (*A critical review of current imaging techniques. Argues that CT is the best initial study. Although ultrasonography can provide comparable information without radiation exposure, it is often compromised by technical factors impairing the adequacy of the study; 50 references.*)

Warshaw AL, Popp JW Jr, Schapiro RH: Long-term patency, pancreatic function, and relief after lateral pancreaticojejunostomy for chronic pancreatitis. Gastroenterology 79:289, 1980 (*The modified Puestow procedure offers pain relief with preservation of pancreatic tissue in patients with a dilated pancreatic duct.*)

73

Management of Gastrointestinal Cancers

JACOB J. LOKICH, M.D.

Recent developments in combining chemotherapy and radiation therapy with surgery for treatment of gastrointestinal cancer have added substantially to palliation and potential for cure, although mortality is still high (50% to 80%). Moreover, improvements in management of the gastrointestinal complications of cancer, such as obstruction, ascites, and cachexia, have improved the quality of life for these patients (see Chapter 74).

Gastrointestinal malignancies are among the most common tumors found in adults. The treatment of local disease is the province of the surgeon, but management of advanced disease is a responsibility coordinated by the primary physician. It is important to know the indications and limitations of available treatment modalities in order to make best use of therapies offered by the surgeon, radiation therapist, and oncologist.

ESOPHAGEAL CANCER

Carcinoma of the esophagus is difficult to diagnose and treat because symptoms usually do not occur until late in the course of illness. Of the 9000 new cases of esophageal cancer diagnosed annually, less than 5% survive 5 years. Risk factors include *smoking* and *alcohol consumption*, and the malignancy may occur in conjunction with other tumors commonly associated with smoking, such as those of the lung, bladder, head, and neck. Palliation remains the predominant therapeutic option, because the diagnosis often does not become apparent until the tumor has reached advanced stages. Symptoms at presentation include *dysphagia* and progressive *inanition,* manifestations of late disease. Early symptoms may go unnoticed because they can be very nonspecific, such as an isolated episode of choking on a bolus of meat or new onset of reflux.

Tumors of the esophagus may develop in the cervical, midthoracic, or lower third segment; most are of the squamous cell variety, although adenocarcinoma may appear in a Barrett's esophagus. Tumor may extend regionally into the trachea as well as vertically up and down the esophageal mucosa and submucosa. Distant metastases occur in the liver and intra-abdominal node-bearing areas. At the time of diagnosis, less than one-third of patients have cancer confined to the esophageal wall, a stage in which cure is possible with surgical resection. Although median survival is less than 1 year, newer approaches to chemotherapy raise potential for cure to as much as 20%.

The morbidity of esophageal carcinoma is due largely to the severe dysphagia and inanition that characterizes advanced disease. Many patients are unable to swallow their own saliva. Even partial obstruction leads to weight loss and cachexia. *Blenderized diets* and *liquid diet supplements* help maintain adequate nutrition. Hyperalimentation is employed as a temporary means of parenterally feeding a malnourished patient who has potential for meaningful survival.

There are few controlled studies available to help define the optimal approach to therapy. *Surgical resection* is possible in patients with disease confined to the distal esophagus as determined by CT scan of the abdomen and thorax. For patients with nonresectable disease, surgical palliation can be provided by *placement of a polyvinyl Celestin tube.* Peroral endoscopic tube placement is becoming more common and avoids the 10% mortality of palliative surgery. Gastrostomy provides no symptomatic relief from the disabling dysphagia.

Radiation has been used as a preoperative technique, though randomized studies show no benefit. Attempts at radical curative radiation therapy are reserved for patients with cancer confined to the cervical esophagus when surgical resection would require laryngectomy. Radiation has also been used as a palliative measure to relieve dysphagia in patients who are not candidates for a surgical procedure; results are not very satisfactory. The complication rate is high due to the tendency of a heavily irradiated esophagus to perforate and surrounding structures (mediastinum, trachea, spinal column) to experience radiation damage. Use of lower radiation doses in *combination with chemotherapy* ("photochemotherapy") has produced encouraging results. When 5-fluorouracil and mitomycin-C or platinum are given in conjunction with radiation, up to 75% of patients achieve major reductions in tumor size, making some tumors amenable to surgical resection. Half of patients who subsequently undergo surgical removal show no evidence of residual tumor.

Laser therapy is available for palliation in patients too ill to undergo surgery or radiation. Results are encouraging, adverse effects are few, and therapy can be performed on an outpatient basis after an initial 2 to 3 day hospitalization. Relief is achieved, but there is no change in survival rate.

Prevention and earlier detection remain the most effective means of dealing with this devastating cancer. Efforts to en-

courage cessation of smoking (see Chapter 49) and alcohol abuse (see Chapter 224) can lower risk. A better means of early detection is sorely needed.

GASTRIC CANCER

There are approximately 25,000 new cases of gastric cancer annually, representing just less than 3% of all cancers. The incidence has been decreasing slightly over the past decade, but mortality remains relatively unchanged, with over 50% dying of this disease. Nonspecific abdominal pain, gastric ulceration with or without bleeding, weight loss, and obstruction are the major patterns of clinical presentation, mostly manifestations of advanced disease. Predisposing factors include *previous gastric surgery* (usually Billroth II anastomosis) and *pernicious anemia* with *achlorhydria.* Nitrates have been implicated as a dietary risk factor. About 95% of these tumors are *adenocarcinomas,* with those that are well differentiated and circumscribed having a much better prognosis than those that are poorly differentiated and infiltrative.

Clinical presentation can be subtle, making early diagnosis difficult. *Gastric ulcer* is an important presentation, characterized by a suspicious appearance on barium study or a more benign-appearing radiologic defect that fails to heal after 6 weeks of full medical therapy (see Chapter 64). *Endoscopic evaluation* with brushings and biopsy is indicated. About 95% of patients are curable if the lesion is confined to the gastric mucosa; 85% if it has gone no farther than the submucosa, an extension that occurs rather early on.

The disease often progresses silently until signs of metastatic disease, such as enlargement of the *left supraclavicular lymph nodes* or *ascites,* become evident and cause the patient to seek medical attention. Spread occurs by direct extension as well as by seeding of the lymphatics, blood vessels, and peritoneal surface. Metastases develop locally as well as at distant sites, most frequently the *liver* (40%), *lung* (15%), and *bone* (15%). Among patients who come to surgery, approximately 80% are found to have *lymph node* metastases, while 40% have *peritoneal involvement* and 35% show spread to the liver or lung.

Surgery is the primary mode of treatment, both for cure and palliation. Median survival for patients managed by complete surgical resection is in excess of 3 years. Subtotal or total gastrectomy is optimal for management of bleeding or obstruction related to tumors at the gastroesophageal junction. *Linitis plastica* or total wall involvement of the stomach is incurable and not manageable by surgery. *Adjuvant chemotherapy* employing 5-fluorouracil in conjunction with a nitrosourea has improved survival and potential cure rate for surgically resected disease; approximately 20% achieve cure with combined therapy. *Chemotherapy* used alone in patients with metastatic disease has produced responses in almost 40% of patients, with duration of response averaging 9 months but having no impact on survival. Complete responses are rare. Adenocarcinomas of the stomach are *not radiosensitive* at tolerable doses.

Patient monitoring should be guided by symptoms and not by routine testing for potential metastatic sites, since only palliative therapeutic options exist for patients with advanced disease.

PANCREATIC CANCER

Carcinoma of the pancreas is the fourth leading cause of cancer death in the United States. Mortality is high (well over 90% at 5 years) due partially to difficulties in early detection, which stem from the tumor's retroperitoneal location. Pancreatic cancer has been increasing in frequency, with 25,000 new cases annually. Hypotheses regarding pathogenesis include concentration and excretion of carcinogens by acinar cells inducing neoplastic transformation among ductal cells. Established risk factors include heavy *alcohol consumption* and heavy *smoking*. Diabetes mellitus, chronic pancreatitis, and exposures to dry-cleaning chemicals and gasoline are also suspected contributing factors. The validity of a statistical association with coffee consumption remains controversial.

Clinical presentation is a function of the tumor's location. Carcinoma of the head of the pancreas is capable of obstructing the biliary tree, upper gastrointestinal tract, or pancreas (see Chapter 62). Disease of the body or tail is more subtle in presentation, with vague upper abdominal or back discomfort, unexplained weight loss, unexplained depression, and migratory thrombophlebitis among its initial manifestations. Pancreatic cancer is also an important cause of ectopic hormone production (insulin, glucagon, ACTH) and unexplained onset of diabetes.

The *natural history* of pancreatic carcinoma is dominated by regional extension into the retroperitoneum and liver. Median survival for patients with extrapancreatic tumor is 12 weeks from time of presentation, and 19 to 42 weeks for those with tumor confined to the pancreas. *Diagnosis* has been facilitated by utilizing *ultrasonography* and *computed tomography* to localize a pancreatic mass and direct needle aspiration, but there has been no significant improvement in early detection. *CA 19-9*, a tumor marker developed with monoclonal antibody technology, is being tested for its utility in detecting and monitoring pancreatic cancer. The literature should be followed for the results of ongoing studies of its utility.

Management is difficult. The chance for cure is very limited, because it depends on surgically removing the entire tumor, which is usually well advanced by the time it is detected. Only patients with small lesions at the head of the pancreas are candidates for *curative surgery.* The risks of surgery are great, the operations formidable, and postoperative complications serious. Operative mortality approaches or even exceeds the 5-year survival rate. The decision to subject a patient with pancreatic cancer to a major operation with a high degree of operative mortality and only modest chances for substantially improved survival must be made individually.

A small resectable tumor at the head of the pancreas, heralded early by obstructing the common bile duct and causing jaundice, can be removed utilizing the *Whipple procedure* (a radical pancreatoduodenectomy). The operation is a surgical tour de force and should be attempted only by surgeons able to perform it with less than 5% mortality. The Whipple procedure offers significant palliation, though few patients survive 5 years. *Total pancreatectomy* and radical partial pancreatectomy have been offered as alternatives to the Whipple procedure; debate continues as to which is best. Most surgery for pancreatic cancer is done for palliation because extrapancreatic extension has already occurred. Biliary and gastrointestinal *bypass procedures* are employed to alleviate obstructions caused by tumor.

Radiation therapy has had several applications in treating pancreatic cancer. Intraoperative radiation therapy appears to offer some promise. Postoperative radiation is sometimes used after a Whipple procedure to reduce the chances of local recurrence. The adjuvant application of radiation, combined with *5-fluorouracil* has slightly enhanced the potential for survival in patients with inoperable disease. Radiation therapy has also been used for control of intractable retroperitoneal pain; 4 to 6 months of relief have been reported.

Supportive measures are important in patients who have undergone pancreatectomy. Insulin and pancreatic enzyme preparations are needed (see Chapters 100 and 72). Insulin requirements are in the range of 20 to 30 units per day.

COLON CANCER

Cancer of the colon is the most common visceral neoplasm in the western hemisphere; 90,000 new cases occur annually in the United States. As many as 50,000 deaths annually are attributed to the malignancy. Suspected etiologic factors include bile acids and other chemical carcinogens present within the bowel lumen. Patients at high risk include those with long-standing *pancolitis* (see Chapter 65), *familial polyposis,* and *Gardner's syndrome* (polyps, osteomas, epidermoid cysts, soft tissue tumors). Some families with a strong predisposition to colonic cancer have demonstrated autosomal dominant inheritance for the condition. *High-fiber diets* are associated with lessened risk, perhaps because they speed transit time in the bowel. Very preliminary data suggest that diets high in *calcium* may slow epithelial cell proliferation in subjects at high risk for familial colonic cancer; whether such a diet is useful as a preventive measure in selected patients remains to be seen.

The clinical *manifestations* of colon cancer are related to the site of the tumor. Tumors of the ascending colon may be asymptomatic until late stages, producing little more than mild *iron deficiency* anemia or intermittently *guaiac-positive stools.* Tumors of the descending colon and sigmoid can cause symptoms earlier in the course of illness, presenting as *rectal bleeding,* melena, or *change in bowel habits* (diarrhea as well as constipation). At the time of surgery, 50% to 75% of patients demonstrate tumor that has penetrated the bowel wall; 60% of these show regional metastases.

Prognosis depends on extent of penetration and local spread. The *Dukes' classification* remains the standard staging system. Category A patients have tumor limited to the submucosa and a 5-year survival of 85% to 90%. Those with stage B disease, invasion of the bowel wall but no nodal involvement, have a 5-year survival of 60% to 65%. Once the serosal surface and lymph nodes are involved, stage C, survival falls to about 30%.

The most common *sites of metastasis* are the *liver* (60% overall and 30% of solitary metastases) due to portal blood flow draining the intestines, the *peritoneal surface* (30%), and the *lung* (20%). Brain, skin, and local recurrences occur in less than 5%.

Management begins with screening for early detection; colon cancers are curable if identified before transmural invasion ensues. The *stool guaiac* examination is central to this effort (see Chapter 51). For patients in whom a tumor is detected, a good quality barium enema or *colonoscopy* extending to the cecum is essential before surgery, because about 3% of patients have synchronous tumors.

Surgery is the primary modality of therapy, both for cure and for palliative purposes to prevent or relieve bowel obstruction. The recognition that adenomatous polyps, villoglandular polyps, and villous adenomas may harbor cancers or be premalignant has led to the recommendation of *polypectomy* when detected, aided greatly by fiberoptic colonoscopy. Cancer confined to the polyp is considered carcinoma *in situ;* detectable invasion of the stalk or muscularis necessitates *colectomy.*

Radiation therapy has no established role in colon cancer, in contrast to its important place in the treatment of rectal cancer (see below). *Chemotherapy,* either as an adjuvant to surgery or for metastatic disease, has not advanced substantially since the introduction of *5-FU* in 1956. The response to 5-FU is in the range of 20% to 25%; complete remission is rare and there is no established improvement in survival. Improved delivery by infusion therapy or regional delivery to the liver or in conjunction with biochemical modulation through ancillary drugs is being investigated. Adjuvant chemotherapy has been employed in a number of prospective randomized trials; to date, all such trials have failed to demonstrate any advantage. At one point claims were made for high-dose vitamin C. Randomized, double-blind control study has shown that such therapy is no better than placebo.

Monitoring and follow up are essential for detection of a second bowel cancer (occurring in up to 5% of patients) and appearance of new polyps. Regularly scheduled *colonoscopy* should begin 6 months after surgery and take place every 24 to 36 months if no polyps are found and every 6 months if

they are. Any encountered polyps are removed. If colonoscopy is unavailable or cannot reach the cecum, air-contrast *barium enema* is an adequate substitute. Early detection of recurrent or metastatic disease has been aided by sequential monitoring of the plasma *carcinoembryonic antigen (CEA).* Although not adequate as a means of screening for colon cancer, CEA monitoring can be of benefit for detecting recurrence. The utility of detecting metastatic disease is limited, for there are few therapeutic options and none, at present, that need to be employed if the patient is asymptomatic. The recommended interval for CEA determinations is every 6 months for the first 2 years, provided that the CEA fell to very low levels with surgery. Detection of recurrent or metastatic disease would lead to a therapeutic intervention in the patient.

RECTAL CANCER

Rectal cancer is one of the most common cancers, with over 40,000 new cases and 10,000 deaths each year in the United States. The condition is defined anatomically as a bowel malignancy below the peritoneal reflection or within 15 cm of the anal verge. It is distinct from carcinoma of the anus or perianal area, which is generally derived from squamous epithelium.

The cancer commonly presents with occult or frank rectal bleeding, with or without an alteration in bowel habits. Tenesmus is usually a late symptom representing extension of the tumor beyond the bowel wall. Rectal or perianal pain is a consequence of the invasion of the pararectal structures in the sacral plexus. Tumor often arises on the posterior wall, making it particularly important to examine the rectal ampulla on routine rectal examination.

The tumor tends to invade locally and to recur in the pelvis alone or in association with distant metastases to the liver or lung, bypassing the intra-abdominal cavity. The tendency to recur locally has resulted in the application of adjunctive therapies, particularly radiation in conjunction with surgery to maximize long-term local control.

Management consists of *surgical resection,* aided by adjuvant radiation therapy. When possible, an effort should be made to *preserve the anal sphincter.* Tumors of the upper two-thirds of the rectum can usually be resected in conjunction with construction of an anastomosis; those of the lower third require an *abdominoperineal resection* with a permanent sigmoid colostomy. Sometimes unwise attempts are made to limit the resection in order to preserve the sphincter; inadequate surgical margins are taken, leading to local recurrence and death. Alternatives to abdominoperineal resection include local excision, fulguration, and intrarectal radiation therapy. Only patients with small exophytic tumors in the lower third of the rectum should be considered for such alternative therapy.

Radiation complements surgical therapy. The development of the surgical stapler and application of adjuvant radiation therapy postoperatively has permitted an anterior resection with primary anastomosis in many patients who would otherwise require a colostomy. In patients with locally advanced disease, preoperative radiation may reduce tumor size and allow for subsequent resection. CT scan is useful for determining extent of disease. Radiation can reduce the local recurrence rate of tumors that penetrate the bowel wall.

The use of *chemotherapy* for rectal cancer is very limited and similar to that for advanced colon cancer (see above). In regional or local primary tumor, the adjuvant application of chemotherapy in conjunction with radiation may increase the disease-free survival rate.

Careful *follow-up* is important because several forms of recurrent and metastatic disease are amenable to treatment. Isolated recurrences in the pelvis, lung, or liver can be resected with excellent results and some chance of cure. For this reason, yearly chest films, careful pelvic examinations, and alkaline phosphatase determinations are recommended.

Patients who have undergone abdominoperineal resection with permanent or temporary colostomy need careful counselling preoperatively and after surgery to help them adapt to their situation. Becoming comfortable with the details of ostomy care as well as having an opportunity to discuss their fears and concerns (sexual function, odor, appearance, bag changes, recurrence of cancer) are essential components of the rehabilitation effort. Ostomy groups and stoma nurses are important resources for the patient, but there is no substitute for a supportive, understanding patient–physician relationship.

SYNCHRONOUS HEPATIC METASTASES

Not uncommonly, hepatic metastases are discovered at the same time or even prior to discovery of the primary tumor, as is often the case with cancer of the colon. *Synchronous metastases* may represent up to 15% of new cases of colon cancer. In the presence of symptoms that are specifically derived from the primary tumor, such as bleeding or obstruction, a primary surgical resection is often undertaken if the patient has a life expectancy (on the basis of the hepatic metastases) that exceeds 2 months. In the presence of an asymptomatic primary tumor in the bowel, however, therapeutic efforts are directed first at the metastatic disease; if successful, a surgical approach to the primary tumor may be undertaken. This approach assumes that the median survival for patients with hepatic metastases does not exceed 6 months; therefore, in patients not responding to chemotherapy, the likelihood of dying of distant disease far exceeds the likelihood of significant complications from the primary tumor site.

ANNOTATED BIBLIOGRAPHY

Esophageal Cancer

Cello JP, Gerstenberger PD, Wright T et al: Endoscopic neodymium-YAG laser palliation of nonresectable esophageal malignancy. Ann Intern Med 102:610, 1985 (*An initial report of laser use to alleviate luminal obstruction; a promising therapy for patients with inoperable disease.*)

Kelsen D, Hilaris B, Coonley C et al: Cisplatin, vindesine and bleomycin chemotherapy of local, regional and advanced esophageal carcinoma. Am J Med 75:645, 1983 (*Sixty-three percent of patients with esophageal cancer responded to chemotherapy alone (without radiation) and 82% with local or regional disease were resectable; 3 of 34 had no visible primary tumor.*)

Leichman L, Steiger Z, Seydel HG et al: Preoperative chemotherapy and radiation therapy for patients with cancer of the esophagus: A potentially curative approach. J Clin Oncol 2:75, 1984 (*A discussion of a combined-modality approach to esophageal cancer in which 50% of patients coming to resection had no detectable tumor.*)

Gastric Cancer

Cullinan SA, Moertel CG, Fleming TR et al: A comparison of three chemotherapeutic regimens in the treatment of advanced pancreatic and gastric carcinoma. JAMA 253:2061, 1985 (*Although higher response rates are reported for combinations of drugs, single agent 5-FU is comparable to the more complex and expensive regimens when measured by survival.*)

Gastrointestinal Tumor Study Group: Controlled trials of adjuvant chemotherapy following curative resection for gastric cancer. Cancer 49:1116, 1982 (*The only prospective controlled trial in which chemotherapy improved the cure rate of surgery for gastric cancer.*)

Green PHR, O'Toole R: Early gastric cancer. Ann Intern Med 97:272, 1982 (*Reviews methods for early detection of gastric cancer and argues that endoscopy and biopsy should be done on all radiologically detected lesions; admits that there is no proof as of yet that this will reduce the mortality rate for gastric cancer.*)

Health and Public Policy Committee, American College of Physicians: Endoscopy in the evaluation of dyspepsia. Ann Intern Med 102:266, 1985 (*Recommends endoscopy in patients with 6 to 8 weeks of dyspepsia that remains refractory to therapy.*)

O'Brien MJ, Burakoff R, Robbins EA et al: Early gastric cancer. Clinicopathological study. Am J Med 78:195, 1985 (*Early gastric cancer now comprises a greatly increased portion of lesions leading to gastric resection, presumably due to use of endoscopic biopsy for benign-appearing gastric ulcers that fail to heal.*)

Pancreatic Cancer

Brooks JR, Culebras JM: Cancer of the pancreas: Palliative operation, Whipple procedure or total pancreatectomy? Am J Surg 131:516, 1976 (*Reviews the arguments for and against both procedures.*)

Cullinan SA, Moertel CG, Fleming TR et al: A comparison of three chemotherapeutic regimens in the treatment of advanced pancreatic and gastric carcinoma. JAMA 253:2061, 1985 (*Although higher response rates are reported for combinations of drugs, single agent 5-FU is comparable to the more complex and expensive regimens when measured by survival.*)

Gudjonsson B, Livingstone EM, Spiro HM: Cancer of the pancreas: Diagnostic accuracy and survival statistics. Cancer 42:2494, 1978 (*The 5-year survival was 0.4%, calculated from 61 studies.*)

MacMahon B, Trichopoulos D, Warren K et al: Coffee and cancer of the pancreas. N Engl J Med 304:630, 1981 (*The controversial study showing an association between coffee consumption and pancreatic cancer; admits the association does not prove causality.*)

Van Dyke JA, Stanley RJ, Berland LL: Pancreatic imaging. Ann Intern Med 102:212, 1985 (*A critical review of current imaging techniques. Argues that CT is the best initial study because ultrasound studies are often technically unsatisfactory, though the latter can give very good information at lower cost and without radiation exposure.*)

Colonic Cancer

Bresalier RS, Kim YS: Diet and colon cancer. N Engl J Med 313:1413, 1985 (*Summarizes the data linking dietary factors and colon cancer.*)

Burt RW, Bishop T, Cannon LA et al: Dominant inheritance of adenomatous polyps and colorectal cancer. N Engl J Med 312:1540, 1985 (*Documents an autosomal dominant inheritance in a "cancer-prone" family.*)

DeCosse JJ: Are we doing better with large bowel cancer? N Engl J Med 310:782, 1984 (*Reviews progress in treating colon cancer.*)

Gastrointestinal Tumor Study Group: Adjuvant therapy of colon cancer—Results from a prospectively randomized trial. N Engl J Med 310:737, 1984 (*The importance of concurrent placebo controls is emphasized and reinforced by this study, in which no advantage for adjuvant chemotherapy was observed and an increased risk of leukemia was identified.*)

Lipkin M, Newmark H: Effect of added dietary calcium on colonic epithelial-cell proliferation in subjects at high risk for familial colonic cancer. N Engl J Med 313:1381, 1985 (*Shows a normalization of proliferation and raises the possibility of a role for added calcium in selected patients—very preliminary data, but interesting.*)

Moertel CT, Childs DS, Reitemier RJ et al: Combined 5-fluorouracil and supervoltage radiation therapy of locally unresectable gastrointestinal cancer. Lancet 2:875, 1969 (*The original prospective randomized trial that established improved survival as a conse-quence of adding chemotherapy to routine radiation therapy for extensive gastrointestinal cancer.*)

Rectal Cancer

Gastrointestinal Tumor Study Group: Holyoke ED, Stablien DM, Thomas PRM et al: Prolongation of disease-free survival in surgically treated rectal carcinoma. N Engl J Med 312:1465, 1985 (*This prospective randomized trial is the first and only such trial to demonstrate the advantage of adjuvant radiation plus chemotherapy for rectal cancer; a subsequent analysis indicated a survival advantage as well.*)

Gunderson LL, Sosin H: Areas of failure found at reoperation (second or symptomatic look) following "curative surgery" for adenocarcinoma of the rectum: Clinicopathologic correlation and implications for adjuvant therapy. Cancer 34:1278, 1974 (*This important retrospective study established that the biologic behavior of rectal cancer was characterized by local recurrence: provided the rationale for use of adjuvant local radiation therapy.*)

Klingerman MM: Preoperative radiation therapy in rectal cancer. Cancer 36:691, 1975 (*A still useful summary of the use of radiation therapy as a preoperative modality.*)

Creagan ET, Moertel CG, O'Fallon JR et al: Failure of high-dose vitamin C therapy to benefit patients with advanced cancer. N Engl J Med 301:1189, 1979 (*This careful study conclusively demonstrates that high-dose vitamin C is no more effective than placebo.*)

Sandler RS, Freund DA, Herbst CA et al: Cost effectiveness of preoperative carcinoembryonic antigen monitoring in colorectal cancer. Cancer 53:193, 1984 (*Although the cost of identifying a resectable tumor with CEA monitoring ranged from $10,000–$20,000, the actual cost might be less if more effective therapies were available.*)

Steele G, Ellenbery S, Ramming K et al: CEA monitoring among patients in multi-institutional adjuvant GI therapy protocols. Ann Surg 196:162, 1982 (*This study failed to establish optimal guidelines for monitoring CEA, but suggests that (1) rising CEA levels indicate recurrent disease, (2) abnormal CEA levels are common with rectal tumors, and (3) a rising trend rather than isolated elevation is important as a predictor.*)

74

Managing the Gastrointestinal Complications of Cancer and Cancer Therapy

JACOB J. LOKICH, M.D.

The gastrointestinal symptoms that accompany cancer and cancer therapy are among the most difficult for the patient to bear, often compromising nutritional status and quality of life. Problems may arise from primary disease, metastases, side effects of therapy, or metabolic disturbances. Successful primary care of the cancer patient necessitates attending to the anorexia, nausea, vomiting, pain, ascites, and other gastrointestinal problems that often worsen their lives.

ANOREXIA, NAUSEA, VOMITING, AND CACHEXIA

Weight loss, inanition, and protein depletion with marasmus are common systemic effects of primary as well as metastatic cancer. These are a consequence of anorexia, taste distortion, vomiting, maldigestion, malabsorption, and mal-utilization (see Table 74-1). Such factors combine to induce the self-perpetuating and debilitating cycle of food rejection secondary to tumor growth, which simultaneously weakens host immune mechanisms and promotes tumor growth. Moreover, host tolerance to radiation and chemotherapy is compromised, thus restricting the ability to tolerate thera-peutic doses of either form of treatment.

Malnutrition. The *mechanisms* responsible for cachexia are multiple, and many are poorly understood. Anorexia is thought to be due, in part, to a tumor-induced polypeptide that can affect the satiety center in the brain. Additionally, chemotherapeutic agents are capable of distorting taste and irritating the gastrointestinal tract, leading to vomiting, pain-ful stomatitis, and ulcerative enteritis. Disorders of digestion and absorption ensue from malnutrition, obstructive lesions, and surgical therapies, such as gastrectomy or intestinal bypass procedures. Abnormal caloric utilization is a consequence of tumor-related changes in the body's metabolism, with food intake and lean body mass being channeled to support the tumor's caloric demands.

Detection of mild to moderate malnutrition is important. Manifestations include a 10% weight loss, serum albumin less than 3.5 g/dl, total lymphocyte count less than 1500, and a serum creatinine that is low for the patient's size. More severe malnutrition is characterized by further weight loss, a serum albumin less than 3.0, and a lymphocyte count under 1000.

The *goals* and *methods* of nutritional therapy vary ac-cording to the patient's clinical situation. *Hyperalimentation* is indicated for temporary nutritional support of the patient during very toxic therapy. A preoperative course of intensive nutritional support can lower the risk of sepsis and surgical mortality. However, most controlled studies of hyperalimen-tation and other nutritional therapies have failed to dem-onstrate any significant improvement in response to che-motherapy or radiation, lessening of side-effects from these treatment modalities, prolongation of survival, or improved tolerance to greater doses or longer periods of treatment.

Central hyperalimentation lines can now be maintained at home, provided the patient and family are capable of mas-tering the procedures necessary to ensure the sterility of the line and integrity of the infusion apparatus. Availability of a visiting hyperalimentation nurse is also helpful. The access site can be maintained as a heparin lock, allowing the patient to disconnect easily from the infusion. About 12 to 14 hours per day are needed for infusions, administered in solutions containing 4.2% or 5.2% amino acids and 20% to 25% glucose. The infusion schedule provides the patient with 10 to 12 hours a day of independence and opportunity to ambulate. Careful monitoring of metabolic parameters, including glu-cose, calcium, phosphate, magnesium, BUN, and creatinine is essential, as is close coordination with a hyperalimentation consultant.

A malnourished patient with an obstructed or injured upper alimentary tract may benefit from the passing or sur-gical placement of a *feeding tube,* provided the remainder of the gastrointestinal tract is intact. Tube placement permits implementation of an *enteral hyperalimentation* program, leading to restoration of strength and, ultimately, lessened dependence. Enteral hyperalimentation is particularly suited to patients who have undergone radiation or surgery in the upper alimentary tract. Long (43-inch), flexible silicon nasal feeding tubes make possible administration of feedings di-rectly into the distal duodenum or proximal jejunum, re-ducing the risks of aspiration and reflux that occur with gas-

Table 74-1. Factors That Determine Weight Loss in Cancer Patients

FACTOR	MECHANISM	TREATMENT
Anorexia	Associated with hepatic metastases and possibly mediated by a paraneoplastic polypeptide suppressing appetite center	Appetite stimulant
Taste distortion	Dysguesia or irritant effect of drugs	None
Vomiting	Emesis secondary to therapy (drugs, radiation)	Intermittent chemotherapy schedule Prochlorperazine tetrahydrocannabinol
Oral stomatitis	Secondary to chemotherapy	Topical anesthesia
Maldigestion	Secondary to enzymatic insufficiency	Pancreatic enzyme
Malabsorption	Secondary to obstruction or alteration of mucosal surface	Antitumor measures
Malutilization	Metabolic derangement related to tumor secretion or a consequence of mechanisms that compensate for limited nutrient availability	Antitumor measures

trostomy feedings. When a feeding tube cannot be passed nasally, feedings can be administered through a jejunostomy.

Enteral hyperalimentation utilizes milk-based and soy-based formulas, as well as less viscous formulations, although sometimes a pump is needed. The formulas are quite hypertonic and must be started at less than full strength (usually ¼ strength) and increased over several days, as tolerated. Cramps, dumping syndrome symptoms (flushing, tachycardia, sweating), and diarrhea are the major manifestations of intolerance. The goal is 2000 to 3000 calories per day.

For patients with upper alimentary discomfort but retained ability to swallow liquids, a *nutritionally complete liquid preparation* may offer a more comfortable and palatable means of keeping well nourished. These preparations are available commercially and reasonably well tolerated. Most contain all necessary vitamins and minerals. Lactose-free formulations are available for those who might have acquired lactose intolerance. Blenderized meals are another alternative.

Anorexia, Nausea, and Vomiting. For the vast majority of cancer patients, the main gastrointestinal problems are anorexia and nausea. Treatment is difficult; multiple contributing factors are often operating simultaneously. Although the most effective means of overcoming anorexia is to achieve control of the underlying malignancy, patients need practical suggestions for immediate use. *Small frequent feedings* (about six per day) of foods high in protein and calories should be advised. *Liquid dietary supplements* in the form of milkshakes and commercial preparations are excellent if tolerated. If nausea is prominent, the patient should be advised to try foods that are *salty,* beverages that are *cool and clear,* and desserts such as *gelatin* and *popsicles.* Dry foods such as *toast* and *crackers* also help. Dieticians recommend that the food be served in a *relaxed* family or group setting, *attractively prepared* and readily available. When *altered taste* makes food unpalatable, meat should be avoided and dairy products substituted as the main source of protein. *Acidic foods* may stimulate appetite in situations where taste acuity seems to wane, as might use of *extra seasoning* and spicy foods. There are some reports of *zinc* being used to treat dysgeusia, but results are not very impressive.

Foods to *avoid* when nausea is prominent include those that are excessively *sweet, greasy,* or *high in fat.* Corticosteroids have sometimes been used to stimulate appetite, but their effect is transient and not worth the major side-effects associated with the high doses needed to achieve an increase in appetite. Tricyclic antidepressants (*e.g.,* imipramine) have an appetite-stimulating effect that is nonspecific but sometimes useful.

Chemotherapy-induced emesis can be a vexing problem. Often an effective antitumor program has to be halted because of intolerance to the GI side-effects. Design of an antiemetic program requires knowing the propensity of various agents to cause emesis and the timing of its onset in relation to drug administration. Cisplatin, nitrosoureas, and nitrogen mustard are especially potent inducers of gastrointestinal upset. The chemotherapy schedule ought to be set up so that there are no more than two to three applications per month. Most often the treatments produce self-limited nausea and vomiting episodes that are only of a few hours' duration, but the experience can be very demoralizing and even lead to psychogenic emesis in anticipation of therapy.

Prochlorperazine remains the first-line agent for treatment of drug-induced emesis. It is most effective when taken several hours before administration of chemotherapy and continued on a regularly scheduled basis for the next 24 hours (see Table 74-2). Route of administration has little influence on effectiveness. *Metoclopramide* has been useful for treating nausea and vomiting induced by cisplatin; it must be given intravenously, beginning ½ hour before chemotherapy. *Haloperidol* has played a useful antiemetic role, especially in patients undergoing combination chemotherapy. Psychogenic vomiting that occurs in anticipation of chemotherapy responds to intravenous *lorazepam* in conjunction with behavioral *desensitization* therapy.

One approach to management is to have the patient use a mild tranquilizer the day before chemotherapy. On the day of treatment, a prochlorperazine spansule or suppository is

Table 74-2.   Drugs for Management of Chemotherapy-Induced Emesis

DRUG	INDICATION	DOSE
Prochlorperazine	First-line agent	5–15 mg q4h PO or IM; begin 4–8 h before chemotherapy
Haloperidol	Combination chemotherapy program	3 mg IM q2h; begin 1 h before chemotherapy
Metoclopramide	Cisplatin therapy	1–2 mg/kg IV q2–3h for up to 6 doses; begin ½ h before chemotherapy
Lorazepam	Anticipatory vomiting	1–2 mg IM q6h prn
Tetrahydrocannabinol	Young patient refractory to other therapy	5–15 mg q4h PO; begin 4–8 h before chemotherapy

given 4 to 8 hours before treatment. Normal food intake before chemotherapy is encouraged because it minimizes retching on an empty stomach, which produces muscle cramps and pain. One hour before anticipated emesis, another dose of prochlorperazine is given, followed by doses every 4 hours as needed. *Tetrahydrocannabinol* has been found effective in studies of young patients with severe emesis uncontrolled by prochlorperazine. Disturbing side-effects made it ineffective in the elderly. The agent is rarely used.

Recent trials suggest that multidrug regimens utilizing prochlorperazine along with metoclopramide, phenobarbital, or other agents may provide enhanced antiemetic effect. The main drawback to phenothiazine therapy is precipitation of extrapyramidal symptoms, which are most likely to occur when daily doses exceed 50 mg per day (see Chapter 168) and necessitate discontinuation of therapy. Under such circumstances, the mild antiemetic *trimethobenzamide* (Tigan) is worth a try, though less effective than prochlorperazine.

A few treatable etiologies need to be considered when a patient presents with refractory emesis. Persistent vomiting can be a manifestation of bowel *obstruction* or severe *ileus,* etiologies that respond to decompression by *nasogastric suctioning. Hypercalcemia* and *hypokalemia* may be causes as well as consequences of vomiting; monitoring of electrolytes and correction of any imbalances can help lessen the anorexia, nausea, and vomiting that sometimes accompany them.

Stomatitis. The management of chemotherapy-induced stomatitis includes avoidance of very hot, cold, spicy, and salty foods; smoking; alcohol; and use of a *topical anesthetic paste.* Viscous xylocaine preparations are not very helpful because they wash away quickly and thus provide only very transient relief; paste preparations last considerably longer. Unfortunately, taste distortion can occur as a consequence of the topical anesthetic effect.

When radiation therapy to the head and neck results in *xerostomia* and *mucositis,* the dryness and thick secretions can be lessened by chewing gum or sucking on hard candy, acts that help stimulate salivation. Use of gravies and avoidance of dry foods helps deglutition in patients whose salivary glands are damaged by radiation. In refractory situations, artificial saliva preparations can be used.

DIARRHEA AND CONSTIPATION

Diarrhea is another gastrointestinal nemesis well known to cancer patients. When it ensues from radiation or chemotherapy-induced enteritis, the problem is usually self-limited, resolving within the 1–2 weeks that it takes for the mucosal surface to reconstitute itself. If persistent or troublesome, low doses of *diphenoxylate* (Lomotil) can be prescribed for symptomatic relief. *Steatorrhea* is experienced by patients who have undergone pancreatectomy or suffer from pancreatic insufficiency; intake of several *pancreatic enzyme* tab-

lets with each meal (see Chapter 72) usually clears up the diarrhea. The postgastrectomy patient is at risk for the symptoms of the *dumping syndrome* (see Chapter 58). Avoidance of *sweets* and large *fluid volumes* (especially those rich in sugar) helps prevent attacks, as does lying down after a meal.

Constipation can be a very troublesome, often unavoidable consequence of *narcotic use* for pain control. However, prophylactic institution of some simple measures can help prevent disabling symptoms and fecal impaction. These include a *high fiber diet,* good *fluid intake* (at least 2 liters per day), use of *stool softeners* (e.g., dioctyl sodium sulfosuccinate), and, if necessary, administration of a gentle *laxative* before bed (e.g., milk of magnesia 15 ml). Constipation may also be a sign of *obstruction* in the lower intestinal tract or ileus, etiologies that need to be ruled out before escalating laxative therapy. *Hypokalemia* and *hypercalcemia* are two other important causes that deserve attention.

PERITONEAL IMPLANTS, BOWEL OBSTRUCTION, AND FISTULAS

Peritoneal implants within the abdominal cavity may develop in either a diffuse miliary pattern or coalesce into large mass lesions capable of causing obstruction. A surgical *bypass* procedure or regional surgical resection ("*debulking*") is indicated under such circumstances for palliation when there is some hope of prolonging meaningful survival. For patients with an indolent malignancy, particularly those with a localized point of obstruction, an aggressive surgical approach is worthy of consideration. Implants centered in the pelvic area may lead to formation of fistulae communicating with the bladder or skin; local *surgical excision* or *radiation* therapy can help control the problem.

MALIGNANT ASCITES

Ascites may occur as a complication of diffuse peritoneal implantation or secondary to portal venous hypertension. Occasionally, ascites may be the most debilitating symptom as a consequence of abdominal distention and pain; but often a significant clinical effect is the marasmus that occurs as a consequence of sequestration of the protein-rich fluid in the abdomen.

A surgical *shunt procedure* that employs a one-way valve catheter that is placed in the peritoneal cavity and run subcutaneously into the jugular venous system (the so-called LeVeen or peritoneal–jugular venous shunt) has been employed in patients with nonmalignant ascites and more recently in patients with neoplastic effusions. Excellent control of the ascites due to malignancy has been achieved, as increased abdominal pressure and a negative intrathoracic pressure cause ascitic fluid to move across the one-way valve into the venous system. This system allows for the restitution of body stores of amino acids and proteins and improves nutritional status as well as decreases abdominal distention. One complication from use of these shunts has been the development of disseminated intravascular coagulation in some patients resulting from the presence of thromboplastinlike material in the ascitic fluid. Patients with prolonged prothrombin times are at particular risk for this complication; consequently, surgery candidates should be carefully screened and have a prothrombin time obtained beforehand. Because of complications, shunt procedures have not been widely utilized.

The use of surgical drainage for ascites is not as effective as it is for effusions of the pleural space. Similarly, intra-abdominal instillation of chemotherapeutic agents and radioisotopes has been relatively ineffective. Sclerosing drugs and irritants to seal the peritoneal space are not recommended, since an irritant effect on the bowel may result in necrosis, perforation, or secondary fibrosis and adhesions leading to obstruction.

OBSTRUCTIVE JAUNDICE

Surgery is the usual treatment, often not feasible in patients with extensive porta hepatis disease extending into the liver. Alternatively, one can consider *percutaneous placement of a stent*. The procedure involves transcutaneously introducing a catheter into the liver of the inoperable patient and lodging it in the dilated ductal system. If it is possible to thread the catheter through the obstruction and establish a channel into the small bowel, then a closed drainage system can be set up, making bile available for digestion; otherwise biliary flow has to be directed externally. The procedure should only be attempted by individuals skilled in placement of such stents. Major complications do occur, particularly

recurrent *cholangitis*. The routine prophylactic use of tri-methoprim–sulfamethoxazole has helped minimize the frequency and severity of such episodes. The procedure can be uncomfortable and the stents have a tendency to become dislodged. However, if successful, significant palliation and improvement in quality of life can result for the patient willing to undergo stent placement.

Radiation therapy has also been used to treat obstructive jaundice caused by tumor in the porta hepatis. It is particularly useful in patients with radiosensitive neoplasms (*e.g.,* breast, lymphoma).

ANNOTATED BIBLIOGRAPHY

Devereux DF, Greco RS: Biliary enteric bypass for malignant obstruction. Cancer 58:981, 1986 (*A retrospective analysis of percutaneous versus surgical methods for treating the obstruction; surgery seems superior.*)

Gralla RJ, Itri LM, Pisko SE et al: Antiemetic efficacy of high-dose metoclopramide. N Engl J Med 305:905, 1981 (*A randomized controlled study showing the drug to be effective in cisplatin-induced vomiting.*)

Kris MG, Grolla RJ, Clark RA et al: Consecutive dose-finding trials: Adding lorazepam to the combination of metoclopramide plus dexamethasone. Cancer Treat Rep 69:1257, 1985 (*The use of multiple agents directed at suppression of the vomiting center as well as blocking anticipatory vomiting and other mechanisms is illustrated by these sequential trials.*)

Morrow GR, Morrell C: Behavioral treatment for the anticipatory nausea and vomiting induced by cancer chemotherapy. N Engl J Med 307:1476, 1982 (*Describes the phenomenon and details behavioral approaches to treatment.*)

Penta JS, Poster DS, Bruno S et al: Clinical trials with antiemetic agents in cancer patients receiving chemotherapy. J Clin Pharmacol 21(suppl):11s, 1981 (*A good review of available therapies.*)

75

Sigmoidoscopy and Other Anorectal Examinations

LAWRENCE S. FRIEDMAN, M.D.

Sigmoidoscopy is a basic technique for evaluating patients with gastrointestinal complaints and screening asymptomatic individuals for colorectal cancer. Rigid sigmoidoscopy can be performed within the context of an office visit. The necessary equipment is inexpensive to purchase, easy to master, and simple to maintain; the scope section is disposable, facilitating cleanup. The development of the flexible fiberoptic sigmoidoscope makes possible visualization of bowel previously beyond reach. However, fiberoptic instruments are much more expensive to purchase and maintain, and harder

to master. The ultimate role for fiberoptic sigmoidoscopy in primary care practice remains unsettled. The primary care physician should be able to perform a rigid sigmoidoscopic examination.

INDICATIONS FOR SIGMOIDOSCOPY

Sigmoidoscopy provides for direct visualization of the colonic mucosa. As such, it is an essential part of the evaluation of patients presenting with a host of complaints or problems referable to the large bowel (see Table 75-1). Also, sigmoidoscopy can supplement barium studies by providing additional observations of abnormalities detected on barium enema, such as polyps and other suspected mass lesions. In patients with known inflammatory bowel disease, sigmoidoscopy is useful for monitoring disease activity and response to therapy.

In asymptomatic individuals, sigmoidoscopy can be an important screening procedure for early detection of colorectal cancer. About one third of colorectal cancers are within reach of the rigid sigmoidoscope. It appears that asymptomatic rectal cancers discovered by sigmoidoscopy are less advanced and survival rates better than in patients with symptomatic cancers. Whether mass screening by sigmoidoscopy is superior to stool guaiac testing for early detection of colorectal cancer is still a subject of debate, especially in terms of cost effectiveness (see Chapter 51). Some authorities recommend that for patients with an average risk of colorectal cancer, sigmoidoscopic examinations be performed at age 50, age 51, and then every 3 to 5 years. Studies are in progress regarding this issue, and the literature should be followed for their findings.

ANORECTAL EXAMINATION

An anorectal examination is indicated in all patients who are to undergo sigmoidoscopy and should be incorporated into all complete physical examinations in adults. No bowel preparation is necessary, but the physician must establish rapport with the patient by taking a history and performing

Table 75-1.   Indications for Sigmoidoscopy

Symptoms
Rectal pain
Rectal discharge
Bright red bleeding per rectum
Hematochezia
Persistent or recurrent diarrhea
Change in bowel habits
Chronic constipation
Unexplained weight loss

Signs
Abdominal or rectal mass
Enlarged sentinel lymph node
Guaiac-positive stool
Unexplained hepatic nodule or enlargement or other signs of
   metastatic cancer

Laboratory Abnormalities
Unexplained iron deficiency anemia
Mass or polyp on barium enema
Other laboratory manifestation of metastatic disease from
   unknown primary lesion

Screening
Patients at high risk for colorectal malignancy (ulcerative colitis,
   familial polyposis)
Patients at average risk of malignancy (controversial)

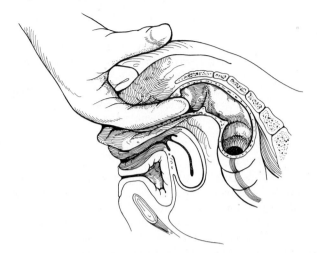

Figure 75-1.   Digital examination.

other parts of the physical examination first. Apprehension and embarrassment may be minimized by explaining each step, describing the anticipated sensations, and draping the patient to expose only the perineum.

Inspection. The patient may be examined in either the knee-chest or left lateral decubitus (Sims') positions. After retraction of the buttocks, the perianal skin and anal orifice are inspected for fecal material (reflecting poor hygiene, painful lesions that make cleansing difficult, or incontinence), drainage, dermatoses, scars, prolapsed hemorrhoids, fistulas, fissures, abscesses, hematomas, condylomata, and carcinomas. Lesions are described anatomically (*e.g.,* anterior, right-sided), not with reference to the face of a clock. Perineal, and sacrococcygeal tissues should be palpated with the gloved but unlubricated index finger for tenderness, induration, fluctuance, or masses.

Palpation. Digital examination of the rectum is then performed by placing the gloved, lubricated index finger at the anal orifice and gently inserting as the patient bears down. The small finger may be used in patients with painful or stenotic anal lesions. Anesthetic ointment may be helpful if a tender lesion is present. The anal sphincter tone and strength of contraction are noted, and the finger is swept circumferentially as it is advanced into the rectum. Abnormalities sought include fissures, fistulous tracts, abscesses, villous and pedunculated polyps, and cancers. Rarely, foreign bodies may be encountered. Internal hemorrhoids are not palpable unless they are thrombosed. In inflammatory bowel disease the mucosa may feel gritty. Stool in the rectum is deformable, distinguishing it from other rectal masses. The rectal ampulla should be checked carefully (see Fig. 75-1); it is often overlooked and may harbor a neoplasm.

The average effective depth of insertion of the index finger is 7.5 cm. In women, care must be taken not to mistake the cervix for a rectal "tumor" along the anterior rectal wall; the cervix is smooth and symmetric. In men the prostate and, if possible, the seminal vesicles should be examined. Finally, on withdrawal the examining finger should be inspected for the character of feces and the presence of blood, pus, or mucus. A test for occult blood should be performed, unless gross blood is evident.

Anoscopy

Anoscopy may be a useful adjunct to the anorectal examination, particularly in the evaluation of bright red rectal bleeding, perianal pain, or suspected hemorrhoids. Anoscopes are metal or disposable plastic tubes with a diameter of 2 cm at the tip and a length of 7 cm. A built-in light source may be present or an external light source may be required, depending on the make of anoscope. With the patient in the same position as for the anorectal examination, the lubricated anoscope is held in the right hand with the thumb pressing on the obturator as the instrument is introduced with slow gentle pressure. The instrument is first directed along the longitudinal axis of the anal canal toward the umbilicus and then pointed more posteriorly at the anorectal angle. It is inserted the full length and held in the left hand so that the flange rests against the anus. The obturator is removed and the anoscope is slowly withdrawn as the mucosa is examined.

The normal anal mucosa is pink with a visible delicate network of submucosal vessels. In patients with proctitis the vascular pattern is typically obliterated and the mucosa may be friable, that is, it may bleed easily on gentle swabbing. Anoscopy is particularly helpful in identifying hemorrhoids, which may appear as purple bulges into the lumen; occasionally blood may be seen to issue from a hemorrhoid. Fissures may be identified at the anal verge.

Rigid Sigmoidoscopy

Preparation. Satisfactory cleansing of the bowel can be achieved in most patients with a single tap water or phosphasoda (Fleet) enema administered 45 minutes before sigmoidoscopic examination. If the examination has been scheduled in advance, the patient can be instructed to self-administer one or two enemas at home on the morning of examination. Adequate preparation is particularly advisable in older individuals, who often have large amounts of retained stool in the rectal vault.

In patients with diarrhea or suspected inflammatory bowel disease, it is preferable to forego enema cleansing before sigmoidoscopy. These patients can usually achieve adequate preparation by having a bowel movement just before the examination. Moreover, because enemas may induce edema and erythema of the mucosa, prior enema administration may make it impossible for the observer to distinguish subtle mucosal changes caused by proctitis from those induced by the enema.

Because of the low risk of endocarditis associated with sigmoidoscopy in patients with valvular heart disease, antibiotic prophylaxis is not recommended except for patients with prosthetic valves (see Chapter 11). In these individuals the recommended regimen is aqueous penicillin G 2,000,000 U IM or IV, or ampicillin 1 gm IV plus gentamycin 1.5 mg/kg (not more than 80 mg) 30–60 min before the procedure; the gentamycin is repeated every 8 hours for two more doses. For penicillin-allergic individuals, vancomycin 1 gm IV is substituted for penicillin.

Sedation and analgesia are seldom necessary but may be used in patients with painful anal lesions.

Technique. The patient is examined in the same position as for the rectal and anoscopic examinations. The left lateral decubitus (Sims') position is better tolerated than the knee–chest position by older and debilitated patients and may be less embarrassing to patients in general. However, knee–chest permits greater range of scope motion. If available, a tilt-table designed for sigmoidoscopy minimizes the discomfort for the patient and eliminates the rather awkward position required of the examiner when Sims's position is used.

The sigmoidoscope is a rigid metal or disposable plastic tube, 25 cm long and approximately 1.5 cm in diameter. Newer rigid sigmoidoscopes have distal fiberoptic lighting, a proximal magnifying lens, and a connection for air insufflation. Additional standard equipment includes long cotton swabs, suctioning apparatus, and biopsy and grasping forceps.

The lubricated instrument is inserted with the right hand holding the obturator firmly in place and with gentle pressure against the anal sphincter as the patient bears down. Alternatively, if the rectal examination is performed with the left index finger, the sigmoidoscope may be guided over the withdrawing examining finger to avoid having to dilate the anal sphincter a second time. The sigmoidoscope is initially directed toward the umbilicus and then posteriorly at the anorectal junction (see Fig. 75-2).

Once past the anorectal ring, the obturator is withdrawn, and the sigmoidoscope is advanced with the lumen in view at all times. Unless stool is present, insertion is easy until the rectosigmoid junction is reached at about 12 to 15 cm from the anus. At this point the lumen bends forward sharply and to the left. The patient may experience painful spasm and should be reassured and instructed to breathe slowly and deeply to ensure relaxation of abdominal muscles as the instrument is slowly advanced. Air insufflation should be kept to a minimum to avoid painful colonic distention. When a tight bend in the lumen is encountered and the direction of the lumen is not obvious, it is best to withdraw the sigmoidoscope slightly until a smooth crescentic band of mucosa appears in the field of view. This band always represents the anterior aspect of the mucosa as it bends behind the band,

and the sigmoidoscope can be advanced again just beyond the band and deflected in the same direction, where the lumen should be expected to appear (see Fig. 75-3). It is important not to push the sigmoidoscope blindly and to desist when the mucosa blanches or the patient experiences severe pain.

Although it is desirable to pass the sigmoidoscope the entire 25 cm, complete insertion is often not possible. In fact, even in the hands of an experienced sigmoidoscopist, the average depth of insertion is 16 to 20 cm. Furthermore, it is important to note whether the sigmoidoscope is advancing, up the lumen or merely distending the rectal mucosa.

Examination of the mucosa is conducted on slow withdrawal of the instrument. The tip is swept circumferentially to visualize all areas of the wall, and air is injected in small amounts to flatten out folds and allow adequate inspection. As noted earlier, the normal mucosa is pale pink with a visible network of submucosal blood vessels. Occasionally some blood produced from enema tip trauma may be present. The mucosa should be examined and described; any lesions should be noted and the distance from the anal verge recorded. Occasionally blood may be found to come from a point above the reach of the instrument; this should be noted.

Biopsies of suspicious lesions and abnormal mucosa may be obtained with angled forceps. Mucosal biopsies should be shallow and taken from the posterior rectal wall, where the risk of perforation is small. Bleeding from biopsy sites usually stops with pressure from a swab or by application of silver nitrate sticks. Because of the risk of perforation, barium enema examination should be avoided for at least 5 days after a sigmoidoscopic biopsy.

The entire sigmoidoscopic examination should take from 2 to 5 minutes. However, the goal should never be speed, but rather thoroughness and assurance of patient comfort.

Complications. Perforations are rare, occurring in no more than one in 10,000 sigmoidoscopies, and are more likely if the examiner persists in pushing the sigmoidoscope forward in a bowel that is fixed at any point, as by tumor. Bleeding from biopsy sites is infrequent. Arrhythmias have been reported rarely.

Flexible Fiberoptic Sigmoidoscopy

The most widely used flexible fiberoptic sigmoidoscopes are 60 to 65 cm long with large-caliber suction and biopsy channels, full control of tip deflection by two-hand dials, and controls for air insufflation and water instillation. The diameter of the shaft is 11 mm, making the instrument narrower and longer than the rigid sigmoidoscope. The control dials and buttons are managed with the left hand as the examiner views the colon through the eyepiece; advancement of the instrument up the colon is accomplished with the right hand. Acute angulations of the colon are traversed by various combinations of tip deflection, shaft twisting, and repetitive back-and-forth motions; however, even accomplished sigmoido-

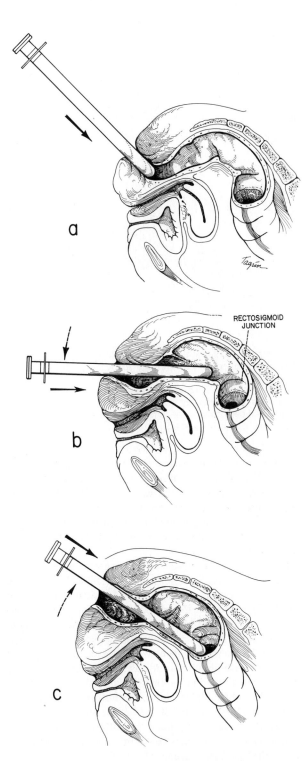

Figure 75-2. Overview of rigid sigmoidoscopic examination: (*A*) Tip of sigmoidoscope is inserted into anal canal in direction of umbilicus; (*B*) At anorectal junction (about 3 cm from anus) tip is deflected toward sacrum; (*C*) At rectosigmoid junction (about 12 to 15 cm from anus) tip is deflected anteriorly and to left.

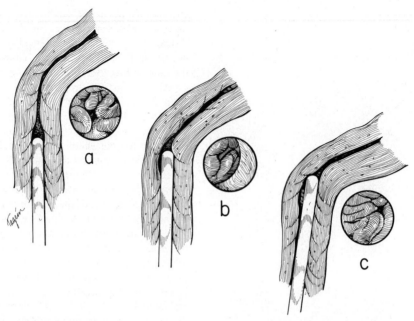

Figure 75-3. Maneuvering a rigid sigmoidoscope past an angulation in the sigmoid colon: (*A*) Advancement of sigmoidoscope through straight portion of colon; view through scope shows concentric lumen with radiating mucosal folds. (*B*) As bend in colon is reached, a crescentic band of mucosa is seen in front of the lumen as it bends. To maneuver past this angulation the scope is first withdrawn 1–2 cm as the tip is deflected *away* from the lumen. The scope is then readvanced slowly as the tip is deflected back toward the lumen *behind* the crescentic mucosal band. (*C*) Lumen reappears as the bend is transversed.

scopists may encounter difficulty in advancing the instrument through very sharp angles. The procedure can be done in the office or clinic, usually with no sedation or anesthesia, and with a preparation of only one or two phosphasoda enemas.

The advantage of the flexible sigmoidoscope over the rigid sigmoidoscope is its ability to examine a longer segment of colon. While the average depth of insertion of the rigid instrument is no more than 20 cm, the average depth of insertion for the flexible instrument in the hands of experienced endoscopists is about 50 cm. Consequently, the diagnostic yield of flexible sigmoidoscopy is greater than that of rigid sigmoidoscopy. For example, in comparative studies the flexible instrument identified two to six times more neoplasms and detected some abnormalities, such as diverticula, not generally within reach of the rigid sigmoidoscope. In addition, the flexible instrument is tolerated by the patient as well or better than the rigid instrument.

The apparent advantages of flexible sigmoidoscopy must be weighed against the observation that as a screening test, it detects no more than two-thirds of colorectal polyps and cancers. Moreover, patients undergoing either rigid or flexible sigmoidoscopy for gastrointestinal symptoms may still require additional tests, such as a barium enema or colonoscopy, to complete the evaluation. Thus, the decision to perform flexible rather than rigid sigmoidoscopy in a given instance may be more a matter of physician preference, cost, and convenience than of an apparent improvement in diagnostic yield. Currently, the most clear-cut advantage of flexible over rigid sigmoidoscopy would appear to be in the screening of asymptomatic patients for colorectal cancer, in which case a barium enema or colonoscopy would not be performed unless indicated.

Other factors to consider in deciding whether to use flexible instead of rigid sigmoidoscopes in a clinical practice are expense and convenience. Flexible fiberoptic instruments are much more expensive than disposable plastic rigid sigmoidoscopes and are more likely to be damaged and require occasional costly repairs. In addition, the flexible instrument must be cleaned thoroughly between patients, and the average duration of examination is at least 10 minutes, so that the time involved in using the instrument per patient is much greater for the flexible than the rigid instrument. Moreover, cleaning and proper care of the flexible sigmoidoscope requires an assistant. In a busy clinical practice, use of the flexible sigmoidoscope may be less practical and efficient than use of the rigid instrument.

Finally, the flexible sigmoidoscope has not yet been widely evaluated in a primary care setting staffed by physicians with no prior experience with fiberoptic instruments. Preliminary data suggest that nearly any physician can learn to use the flexible instrument, but only with supervised instruction. The diagnostic yield of the flexible sigmoidoscope in the hands of primary care physicians has not been evaluated, either in comparison with the rigid instrument or in comparison with experienced endoscopists. Recently, a shorter 30-cm flexible sigmoidoscope has been introduced and in preliminary studies appears to be quite easy to learn to use with minimal instruction. Whether the shorter instrument has sufficient advantage over the longer one to justify its commercial distribution has not yet been determined. Until experience with flexible sigmoidoscopy has been more thoroughly evaluated in the primary care setting, it would seem wise for primary physicians to master the technique of rigid sigmoidoscopy but to remain alert to the possibility that flexible sigmoidoscopy may prove advantageous in the future.

ANNOTATED BIBLIOGRAPHY

American Society for Gastrointestinal Endoscopy: Flexible Sigmoidoscopy: Guideline for Clinical Application, 1986 (*A booklet that summarizes the training requirements for primary care physicians to utilize a flexible scope. Most experts suggest 7 to 10 procedures to use the 35-cm scope and 15 to 30 procedures to master the 60-cm scope.*)

Bohlman TW, Katon RM, Lipshutz GR et al: Fiberoptic pansigmoidoscopy: An evaluation and comparison with rigid sigmoidoscopy. Gastroenterol 72:644, 1977 (*In a comparative study of flexible and rigid sigmoidoscopy in 120 patients, the flexible instrument was inserted nearly three times as far (55 cm vs 20 cm) and identified pathologic lesions three times as often (39% vs 13%) as the rigid instrument.*)

Coller JA: Technique of flexible fiberoptic sigmoidoscopy. Surg Clin North Am 60:465, 1980 (*Detailed and well-illustrated description of the technique of flexible sigmoidoscopy.*)

Lehman GA, Buchner DM, Lappas JC: Anatomical extent of fiberoptic sigmoidoscopy. Gastroenterol 84:803, 1983 (*A 60 cm examination, achieved in 50% of those examined, viewed the entire sigmoid colon 80% of the time.*)

Madigan MR, Halls JM: The extent of sigmoidoscopy on radiographs with special reference to the rectosigmoid junction. Gut 9:355, 1968 (*Failure to insert the rigid sigmoidoscope to 25 cm in a majority of patients was usually due to the acute angulation of the rectosigmoid junction.*)

Nelson RS: Proctoscopic examination: Step-by-step guide. Hosp Med 16:39, 1980 (*Clearly written and well-illustrated description of technique of rigid sigmoidoscopy.*)

Nivatvongs S, Fryd DS: How far does the proctosigmoidoscope reach?: A prospective study of 1000 patients. N Engl J Med 303:380, 1980. (*Average depth of insertion of rigid sigmoidoscope was 19.5 cm–20.3 cm in males and 18.6 cm in females.*)

Schrock TR: Examination of the anorectum, rigid sigmoidoscopy, and flexible fiberoptic sigmoidoscopy. In Sleisenger MH, Fordtran JS (eds): Gastrointestinal Disease, pp 1276–1280. Philadelphia, WB Saunders, 1983 (*Comprehensive discussion of indications for and techniques of both rigid and flexible sigmoidoscopy.*)

Winawer SJ, Cummins R, Baldwin MP et al: A new flexible sigmoidoscope for the generalist. Gastrointest Endosc 28:233, 1982 (*Initial experience of a primary physician with a new 30 cm flexible sigmoidoscope; depth of insertion >26 cm in 85% of cases.*)

6

Hematologic and Oncologic Problems

A

Hematology

76
Screening for Anemia

Anemia is a sign of illness rather than a diagnosis in itself. The incidental finding of a low hematocrit or hemoglobin level suggests a host of underlying conditions that range from the trivial to the life-threatening. Patients with fatigue or other subjective symptoms often ask about their "blood count;" the absence of anemia in such instances is reassuring. But is the otherwise well patient likely to benefit from either the identification or treatment of asymptomatic anemia? The answer to this question depends on the prevalence and nature of conditions most likely to cause asymptomatic anemia and the relationship between hemoglobin level and those symptoms attributed to its reduction.

EPIDEMIOLOGY AND RISK FACTORS

By far the most common cause for asymptomatic anemia is iron deficiency due to inadequate dietary replacement of iron lost from the body. Daily iron requirements for males and postmenopausal females are between 0.5 and 1 mg. Because additional iron is needed by menstruating and pregnant women, their daily requirements are 2 mg and 2.5 mg respectively. Since only 5% to 10% of the 10 to 20 mg of the iron contained in the average adult diet is absorbed, it is not surprising that iron deficiency is common in women of childbearing age. Population studies have found 10% to 20% of menstruating women to have abnormally low concentrations of hemoglobin (usually less than 12 g per 100 ml). Between 20% and 60% of pregnant women have hemoglobin levels below 11 g per 100 ml. Anemia is less likely to occur in women taking birth control pills and more likely to occur in women with intrauterine devices. Iron deficiency is rare in adult males; if present, it is a clear indication for diligent investigation of the gastrointestinal tract. Absorption of iron may be decreased after gastrectomy or in the presence of achlorhydria.

Sideroblastic and megaloblastic anemias are much less common. Pernicious anemia, the most common form of B_{12} deficiency, has a prevalence of 0.1% in individuals of Northern European extraction. It is much less common among other ethnic and racial groups. Folate deficiency is common during pregnancy and in patients with alcoholic liver disease, when it is often accompanied by sideroblastic anemia. Anticonvulsant drugs including phenytoin, primidone, and phenobarbital may interfere with folate absorption with resulting megaloblastic anemia. Thalassemia minor is a common cause of mild anemia in patients of Mediterranean or Far Eastern extraction. Sickle cell disease and trait, by far the most common hemoglobinopathy, is discussed in the following chapter.

NATURAL HISTORY OF ANEMIA AND EFFECTIVENESS OF THERAPY

Obviously, the natural history of anemia depends on the underlying cause. What symptoms can mild or moderate anemia itself be expected to cause? The hyperkinetic symptoms that follow compensatory increases in cardiac stroke volume and heart rate are rarely present before hemoglobin levels have fallen to 7.5 g per 100 ml. Other highly subjective symptoms including irritability, fatigue, and headache have been attributed to milder degrees of anemia. A British survey, however, found no relationship between the frequency of such symptoms and the level of hemoglobin (ranging from 8 to 12 g per 100 ml) among women found to have iron deficiency anemia during a screening program. There was indirect evidence that levels under 8 g per 100 ml were associated with symptoms severe enough to prompt presentation to a physician. Among the asymptomatic women identified by screening, no benefits from treatment were detected. Another report from Britain demonstrated a prevalence of anemia of 10% among screened women. There was a noteworthy absence of treatable underlying conditions other than iron deficiency and, again, no demonstrable benefits from treatment. It has been noted by some investigators that symptoms occur earlier, with higher hemoglobin concentrations, in megaloblastic anemia, but supporting evidence is fragmentary.

SCREENING AND DIAGNOSTIC TESTS

The laboratory measurements of hematocrit and hemoglobin concentrations are straightforward. Automated methods are reliable and reproducible when specimens are properly handled.

Mean hematocrit for adult men at sea level is 46%, with a range of 41% to 51%; for women the mean is 42% and the range 37% to 47%. Slight differences may be noted when automated techniques are used to measure the hematocrit. Normal mean hemoglobin concentration is approximately 16 g per 100 ml for men, with a range of 14 to 18 g per 100 ml; for women the mean is 14 g per 100 ml and the range is 12 to 16 g per 100 ml. In men over 65, the mean falls to 13.5 g per 100 ml; in women over 65, 13.1 g per 100 ml. It must be remembered, as with all continuous laboratory variables, that the choice of a reference value for defining normality is arbitrary. This is particularly true in light of the unclear relationship between significant symptoms and mild "anemia."

CONCLUSIONS AND RECOMMENDATIONS

- Anemia is a common condition. It may be secondary to serious underlying disease or simple dietary deficiency. Determination of hemoglobin concentration or hematocrit is recommended as part of the evaluation of many varied presenting complaints.
- Iron deficiency anemia is common among women of childbearing age, particularly those who are pregnant.
- There is no clear relationship between degrees of mild to moderate anemia and significant symptoms. No clearly measurable benefits following the treatment of mild anemia have been identified in screening studies.
- While determination of a complete blood count may provide clues to the presence of early treatable disease such as GI malignancy, more specific alternatives such as stool testing for occult blood are available. Routine screening for anemia in nonpregnant, asymptomatic patients is not recommended.

A.G.M.

ANNOTATED BIBLIOGRAPHY

Committee on Iron Deficiency: Iron defieicny in the United States. JAMA 203:407, 1968. (*Reviews prevalence studies of iron deficiency anemia.*)

Elwood PC, Shinton NK, Wilson IL et al: Haemoglobin, Vitamin B$_{12}$ and folate levels in the elderly. Br J Haematol 21:557, 1971 (*Ten percent of males with hemoglobin less than 13 g/100 ml; 10% of females less than 12.5 g/100 ml. No megaloblastic anemia found.*)

Elwood PC, Waters WE, Greene WJW et al: Symptoms and circulating haemoglobin level. J Chron Dis 21:615, 1969 (*Symptoms not correlated with hemoglobin level in those found anemic on screening.*)

Elwood PC, Waters WE, Greene WJ et al: Evaluation of a screening survey for anemia in adult nonpregnant women. Br Med J 4:714, 1967 (*Not very extensive follow-up but no serious underlying disease detected among anemic women.*)

Zadeh JA, Karabus CD, Fiedling J: Hemoglobin concentration and other values in women using an intrauterine device or taking corticosteroid contraceptive pills. Br Med J 4:708, 1967 (*Hemoglobin levels fall with IUD use. Increase with birth control pill use.*)

77

Screening for Sickle Cell Disease and Sickle Cell Trait

Sickle cell disease is the most common of the clinically significant hemoglobinopathies. In the United States, the disease and trait occur almost exclusively among blacks. During the late 1960s and early 1970s, sickle cell disease received a great deal of attention in the medical and lay press. The importance of screening for individuals with disease and trait was stressed. Some states legislated mandatory screening programs.

Sickle cell disease (the SS hemoglobin homozygous state) is usually identified during childhood. Patients whose anemia is not identified by screening are often diagnosed after presentation with impaired growth, increased susceptibility to infection, or painful crisis. Screening of adults is aimed at the identification of asymptomatic carriers of sickle trait (the AS hemoglobin heterozygous state). The principal objective is to reduce the prevalence of the homozygous condition by means of genetic counseling. Whether or not screening benefits the people screened has been debated. Screening performed without subsequent education and counseling can be harmful. An understanding of the natural history of sickle cell trait and disease, sensitivity to the concerns of affected patients, and selective use of available screening tests are all necessary if such harmful effects are to be avoided.

EPIDEMIOLOGY AND RISK FACTORS

Sickle cell disease has a prevalence of about 0.15% among black children in the United States. Double heterozygotes, including those with hemoglobin SC or S-beta-thal, are even less common. Prevalence of sickling disease is lower among adults, since the life span of SS homozygotes and double heterozygotes is decreased.

Screening surveys have documented a prevalence of sickle trait of 7.4% among black veterans and 8.7% in the black community of San Francisco. Some studies have shown regional differences in prevalence. Prevalence does not decrease with age. Sickle cell trait is present in low frequency in Southern Italy and higher frequency in parts of Greece. It remains a very rare finding in Americans of Mediterranean extraction.

NATURAL HISTORY OF SICKLE CELL DISEASE AND EFFECTIVENESS OF THERAPY

The natural history of sickle cell disease is variable. Most children exhibit failure to thrive and suffer frequent infections. Anemia is usually moderate but can become severe, often as a result of infection or folate deficiency. The course is punctuated by painful crises precipitated by infection, dehydration, or hypoxia. Organ infarction, congestive heart failure, cholelithiasis, and skin ulcers are some of the complications of chronic disease. Because supportive care has been improved, life expectancy for patients with sickle cell disease has increased. However, it remains significantly shortened.

In contrast, life expectancy is not affected by sickle cell trait. AS red blood cells sickle at much lower oxygen tension than SS cells. The only clinical abnormality that occurs with any frequency among patients with sickle cell trait is painless hematuria, presumably the result of small infarcts of the renal medulla where red cells are particularly susceptible to sickling.

The vastly different health implications of sickle cell trait and sickle cell disease have been lost on some screened individuals and, unfortunately, some physicians. Concern about risk of sudden death has been raised by four case reports of army recruits previously unknown to have sickle trait who

died during basic training at a moderately high altitude. Increased risk of sudden death among people with sickle cell trait has not been confirmed. On the contrary, extensive examinations of people with sickle cell trait have disclosed no differences in x-rays, ECG findings, spirometry, blood chemistries, and psychologic factors when compared to controls matched for age, sex, and race. Sickle cell trait is not significantly less frequent among black athletes, including professional football players, than it is among blacks in general.

If the principal reason for screening adults is to provide genetic counseling, it is important to consider the effectiveness of such counseling. Evidence suggests that identification and counseling of heterozygotes do not alter marriage and parenthood decisions. The individual who does not wish to make such decisions on the basis of carrier status is not likely to benefit from screening. Some families have been traumatized by questions of paternity raised by indiscriminate screening. Because of the confusion among patients and physicians about differences between sickle cell disease and trait, unnecessary anxiety may be the most common result. Surveys have demonstrated that many internists and general practitioners do not sufficiently understand the implications of screening test results to properly counsel patients.

SCREENING AND DIAGNOSTIC TESTS

Screening tests for sickle cell trait are inexpensive and reproducible. Tests for sickling, including the use of 2% metabisulfite solution and the more expensive commercial methods, are positive in the presence of hemoglobin S but do not distinguish between homozygotes, heterozygotes, and double heterozygotes (hemoglobin S combined with thalassemia or hemoglobin C). Hemoglobin electrophoresis can also be performed inexpensively.

A number of techniques have been developed to diagnose sickle cell disease during early gestation of fetuses at risk. Chorionic biopsy has been used to successfully identify sickle cell disease during the first 6 to 8 weeks of pregnancy. The availability of prenatal diagnosis should be explained prior to screening. Careful counseling must also precede the responsible application of any prenatal diagnostic method. Risks of the procedure to mother and fetus, risks of false positive and negative test results, and acceptability of therapeutic abortion should be discussed.

CONCLUSIONS AND RECOMMENDATIONS

- Sickle cell disease is a serious health hazard that usually presents during early childhood.
- Sickle cell trait is associated with minimal risk of morbidity. The principal reason for screening adults for the presence of sickle trait is to facilitate genetic counseling.
- Indiscriminate screening followed by inadequate counseling may be harmful and is not likely to provide benefits to

individuals who will not revise marriage and parenthood decisions on the basis of test results.

• Screening for sickle trait should be offered to black adults in reproductive age groups. Implications of test results should be fully explained before testing is performed.

A.G.M.

ANNOTATED BIBLIOGRAPHY

Farfel MR, Holtzman NA: Education, consent, and counseling in sickle cell screening programs: Report of a survey. AJPH 74:373, 1984 (*Of 52,000 persons screened in Maryland during a 1-year period, 25% were screened without informed consent.*)

Goossens M, Dumez Y, Kaplan L et al: Prenatal diagnosis of sickle-cell anemia in the first trimester of pregnancy. N Engl J Med 309: 831, 1983 (*Earlier diagnosis of sickle cell disease is possible through chorionic biopsy techniques.*)

Jones SR, Binder RA, Donowho EM: Sudden death in sickle-cell trait. N Engl J Med 282:323, 1970 (*Four cases of sudden death among 4000 black army recruits undergoing basic training at high altitude.*)

Kellon DB, Beutler E: Physician attitudes about sickle cell disease and sickle cell trait. JAMA 227:71, 1974 (*An editorial based on responses to a questionnaire that suggest misunderstanding of screening implications by a significant proportion of internists and family practitioners.*)

Motulsky AG: Frequency of sickling disorders in U.S. blacks. N Engl J Med 288:31, 1973 (*Estimates prevalence of double heterozygotes as well as SS disease at birth [1 in 625 with SS; 1 in 833 with SC; and 1 in 1667 with S-beta-thal] and in the population.*)

Murphy JR: Sickle cell hemoglobin in black football players. JAMA 225:981, 1973 (*The rate of Hb AS among black football players in the NFL was 6.7%.*)

Petrakis NL, Wiesenfeld SL, Sams BJ et al: Prevalence of sickle-cell trait and glucose-6-PD-deficiency. N Engl J Med 282:767, 1970 (*An 8.7% prevalence of sickle trait among over 4000 San Francisco blacks.*)

Sears DA: The morbidity of sickle cell trait. Am J Med 64:1021, 1978 (*Extensive review with 296 references concluding that while certain abnormalities do occur with increased frequency in sickle cell trait, survival is not impaired.*)

Whitten CF: Sickle-cell programming—An imperiled promise. N Engl J Med 288:319, 1973 (*Lists the arguments against indiscriminate screening.*)

78

Evaluation of Anemia

Anemia is a common problem in primary care practice. It is not a diagnosis but rather a sign of underlying disease, particularly in men and nonmenstruating, nonpregnant women, in whom readily detectable pathology is found in over 50% of cases.

Because anemia is defined as a reduction in hematocrit or hemoglobin concentration, its definition is necessarily quantitative and arbitrary. Mean hematocrit or hemoglobin concentrations vary widely, depending on age distribution, sex, and altitude of residence of the populations tested. However, World Health Organization criteria for anemia based on hemoglobin concentration have become widely accepted in recent years: adult males, below 13 g/dl; menstruating women, below 12 g/dl; pregnant women, below 11 g/dl. Such arbitrary cut-off values are essential for population-based studies, but the physician should recognize that they may have little meaning for the individual patient. Studies that have used response to therapy as a gold standard for the diagnosis (*e.g.*, a rise in hemoglobin concentration after administration of iron in populations without any other cause for anemia) have demonstrated a marked overlap in distributions of hemoglobin or hematocrit for "anemic" and "normal" populations. The physician must also keep in mind that anemia is defined in terms of concentration. If plasma

volume is expanded, a spurious diagnosis of anemia may be made when the total red cell mass and hemoglobin are normal. If plasma volume is contracted, a true anemia may be masked.

PATHOPHYSIOLOGY AND CLINICAL PRESENTATION

The pathogenesis of anemia is conceptually straightforward. There is either marked blood loss, inadequate production, or excessive destruction; often two or more mechanisms are operating simultaneously. Decreased production occurs when there are defects in stem cell proliferation or differentiation, DNA synthesis, hemoglobin synthesis, or a combination of these deficiencies. Excessive destruction can result from membrane disorders, abnormal hemoglobins, enzyme deficiencies, and a host of extrinsic problems such as mechanical or antibody-mediated disruption.

Clinical presentation of the patient with anemia depends on abruptness of onset, severity, age, and ability of the cardiopulmonary system to compensate for the decrease in blood volume and oxygen-carrying capacity. When onset is gradual, symptoms may be minimal due to adequate time for compensatory adjustments to decreased hemoglobin. Important responses to anemia include an increase in 2,3-DPG (facilitating oxygen delivery to tissues) and expansion of the plasma volume.

There are few symptoms when the hematocrit is above 30, the anemia gradual in onset, and the patient otherwise healthy. However, if the hematocrit falls further, dyspnea and mild fatigue may begin to appear upon strenuous exertion. Greater reductions in hematocrit result in cardiopulmonary symptoms that come with less activity. Age and cardiopulmonary reserve are also important determinants of symptoms. A potpourri of nonspecific complaints frequently accompanies anemia, including headache, tinnitus, poor concentration, palpitations, vague abdominal discomfort, anorexia, nausea, and diarrhea or constipation. Tachycardia and diminished peripheral resistance occur as the hemoglobin falls below 7.5 g per 100 ml; a systolic flow murmur due to high output is common. Pallor is an obvious finding best seen in the conjunctivae, but it is of little help in judging severity.

More specific clinical findings depend on the etiology, which can best be classified on the basis of red cell morphology (as determined by appearance on a Wright-stained peripheral smear or by autoanalyzer determinations of mean corpuscular volume and degree of anisocytosis).

Microcytic Anemias. *Iron deficiency* is characterized by slow development. In mild cases the relation between the anemia and symptoms is tenuous. Fatigue, headache, and irritability are frequently noted by women with iron deficiency, but a community study of 295 anemic patients showed no correlation between symptoms and hemoglobin concentration. The headache, paresthesias, and burning tongue sometimes occurring in this condition have been thought to be caused by low tissue levels of cellular iron. Double-blind studies examining the effect of iron vs. placebo in relieving symptoms are conflicting. Menorrhagia is another complaint attributed by some investigators to instances of iron deficiency, but this is disputed by others. Pica and dysphagia (due to an esophageal web) are classic, though rare, features today.

The physical findings that occur in iron deficiency are a bit more specific than are symptoms. Atrophic glossitis is commonly found, as is cheilitis. Koilonychia, with spooning, ridging, and thinning, are rare. Other physical findings and symptoms are manifestations of the underlying cause. The earliest laboratory changes are depletion of marrow iron stores and a corresponding fall in serum ferritin. These are followed by a decrease in serum iron and an increase in transferrin, producing in many cases a reduction in the percent saturation to below 16%. The first change in the peripheral blood is a drop in the hematocrit and hemoglobin. Only with increasing severity (hemoglobin below 9 g per 100 ml) do red cells become microcytic and eventually hypochromic.

Chronic blood loss is the most frequent cause of iron deficiency in adults. Malabsorption of iron and inadequate dietary intake are seldom major factors, though heavy antacid use and gastrectomy can inhibit iron uptake. Most menstruating women show depletion of iron stores, since the equivalent of 20 mg of iron is lost each month, and 500 mg iron is lost with each pregnancy, while daily normal iron intake provides only 1 mg. Long distance runners have been shown to lose enough blood in their GI tracts to produce iron deficiency anemia.

In the *anemia of chronic disease,* symptoms are those of the underlying illness. Chronic inflammatory diseases, chronic infections, and neoplasms are the most common etiologies. The anemia is usually moderate, with hemoglobins in the 7 to 11 g per 100 ml range. Both serum iron and iron-binding capacity are reduced; marrow iron stores and ferritin are normal or increased. The smear is most often normocytic, but can be hypochromic and even microcytic, mimicking iron deficiency. The serum iron falls before anemia sets in; percent saturation may be less than 16%, again simulating iron deficiency.

Thalassemia minor is typically asymptomatic and discovered during evaluation of a microcytic hypochromic anemia that does not respond to iron. Many persons with this hereditary condition are of Mediterranean ancestry. There are no characteristic physical findings. The red cell count is elevated, and the smear may reveal targeting and basophilic stippling in addition to some polychromatophilia, poikilocytosis and anisocytosis.

Sideroblastic anemias are a heterogeneous set of disorders, including a primary type which may be a preleukemic state, a pyridoxine-responsive variant, and other variants associated with rheumatoid arthritis, polyarteritis, malabsorption, chronic alcoholism, cancer, porphyria, lead poisoning, and true pyridoxine deficiency. In the primary type, patients are typically over age 60; liver and/or spleen are palpable in over 50%. The smear is dimorphic; since some cells are normochromic and others hypochromic, confusion with iron deficiency can result. Anisocytosis and poikilocytosis are pronounced. Serum iron is elevated, and iron binding capacity reduced. Marrow iron stains show many abnormal ringed sideroblasts.

Macrocytic Anemia. *Vitamin B_{12} deficiency* results most frequently from reduced gastric production of intrinsic factor, as occurs in pernicious anemia. The more than chance association with Hashimoto's thyroiditis and vitiligo has suggested an autoimmune mechanism. Blind loop syndrome, total gastrectomy, and terminal ileal disease are other causes. Dietary lack is very rare, since B_{12} is available in everyday foods and body stores contain a 3-year reserve. Onset is gradual; in pernicious anemia, symptoms usually become evident in the sixth decade. Sore tongue and numbness and tingling in the extremities are classic symptoms of B_{12} deficiency, but anorexia, diarrhea, and other gastrointestinal complaints may predominate. The neurologic manifestations also include disturbances of position and vibratory sense, due to lesions in the posterior columns of the spinal cord, and incoordination, spasticity, and up-going toes indicative of damage to the corticospinal tract. The neurologic syndrome is uncommon, but may present in the absence of anemia. Mild memory loss, depression, and irritability sometimes appear as well.

By the time the anemia is discovered, it may be quite severe. Hypersegmented polymorphonuclear leukocytes are an early finding specific for the megaloblastic anemias. Oval macrocytes are also characteristic, though poikilocytosis is considerable. The MCV rises above 100, and serum B_{12} falls below 100 pg/ml. In pernicious anemia, achlorhydria is found on histamine stimulation.

Folate deficiency is more likely to follow inadequate dietary intake than is B_{12} deficiency, because bodily stores are limited to a 3-month reserve. Chronic alcohol abuse is the classic setting. Increased demand for folate, as in pregnancy, hemolysis, malignancy, and severe psoriasis, is another precipitant. Malabsorption syndromes, such as sprue, and drugs that inhibit folate uptake, such as phenytoin and other anticonvulsants, also can precipitate the anemia. The same is true for folate antagonists such as methotrexate, trimethoprim, and triamterene. Hematologic features resemble those of B_{12} deficiency; there are no neurologic deficits.

Normochromic, Normocytic Anemias. Hemolytic anemias are a diverse group. Inherited forms are due to intrinsic red cell defects; acquired types depend primarily on extraerythrocytic mechanisms such as immunologic or mechanical injury. Clinical presentations vary according to rate of destruction, compensatory adaptations, and underlying etiology. Jaundice sets in when the liver's capacity to conjugate the excess bilirubin from hemoglobin breakdown is exceeded; the serum level of unconjugated bilirubin climbs. Splenomegaly evolves as trapping of damaged red cells progresses. Sudden fever, chills, headache, back and abdominal pain, and hemoglobinuria characterize severe acute hemolysis.

The peripheral smear is normochromic normocytic, but may be macrocytic due to release of immature forms during rapid red cell destruction and regeneration. Polychromatophilia is typical, and nucleated red cells, stippling, spherocytes, schistocytes and Howell-Jolly bodies are often noted. The reticulocyte count is elevated unless there is an accompanying marrow defect.

Sickle cell disease is the most prevalent hemolytic condition in the black population. *Sickle cell trait* is asymptomatic and anemia is absent, though mild hematuria due to sickling in the hypertonic renal medulla sometimes occurs. The peripheral smear is normal except for an occasional target cell. Hemoglobin electrophoresis reveals less than 50% of total hemoglobin to be of the S variety. *Sickle cell anemia* is a less benign problem. Painful aplastic crises, leg ulcers, hepatomegaly, hematuria, renal concentrating defects, and mild jaundice can occur; a cardiac flow murmur is common.

Painful crises are precipitated by stress and characterized by pain in the lower extremities, back, or abdomen. Fever and leukocytosis may be present as well. Attacks last up to a week and then resolve spontaneously. Aplastic crises are due to a concurrent illness that suppresses erythropoiesis, leading to marked worsening of anemia. The smear is normochromic; sickled cells may be noted as well as target forms. Hemoglobin electrophoresis reveals a predominance of hemoglobin S (see Chapter 77).

Drug-induced hemolysis is being recognized more frequently. Three mechanisms have been identified: (1) adsorption to the red cell of drug–antibody complexes, as occurs with quinidine; (2) drug adsorption to the red cell, followed by binding of antidrug antibody, as found with penicillin; (3) induction of a red cell "autoantibody," noted with long-term methyldopa use, but rarely causing significant hemolysis. The hallmark of most drug-related hemolytic episodes is a positive direct Coombs test.

Aplastic anemias are usually idiopathic, but they may be linked to a chemical agent or an idiosyncratic drug reaction. Onset is gradual, with fatigue and bleeding noted first; infection is a later problem. There is no organomegaly. The smear appears normochromic normocytic, but the number of platelets is diminished. There are no signs of increased red cell production. The reticulocyte count is zero, and a pancytopenia is present.

The *anemia of chronic renal failure* is due to reduction in both production and survival or red cells. Lack of erythropoietin and metabolic injury to erythrocytes are postulated mechanisms. The severity of the anemia parallels the degree of azotemia. The smear is normochromic normocytic; burr cells are sometimes prominent.

Hypothyroidism is associated with a number of anemic states. Iron deficiency may occur secondary to heavy menstrual bleeding. Also, a macrocytic picture that clears upon administration of exogenous thyroid hormone is not uncommon. A true megaloblastic anemia due to B_{12} deficiency occurs in about 10% of hypothyroid patients with a macrocytic smear; the relation between hypothyroidism and pernicious anemia is unresolved, but an autoimmune mechanism is postulated. More typical of hypothyroidism is a mild normochromic normocytic anemia.

Liver disease is responsible for a host of anemias, especially when accompanied by alcoholism and poor diet. Folate deficiency, marrow suppression, hypersplenism, bleeding and bile salt alteration of the red cell membrane all contribute. The smear shows considerable poikilocytosis with spiculated red cells and some macrocytes; if folate deficiency occurs, a megaloblastic picture is superimposed.

DIFFERENTIAL DIAGNOSIS

A practical method for organizing the many causes of anemia is to group them according to (1) the appearance of the Wright-stained smear of the peripheral blood and (2) the electronically determined red cell indices. This method allows for classification of etiologies into normochromic-normocytic, hypochromic-microcytic, and macrocytic categories (see Table 78-1) and facilitates workup.

The majority of patients who present with anemia have iron deficiency. In a London general practice, 95% of women and 50% of men with anemia had iron deficiency. In males and the elderly, this is very likely to be due to occult bleeding from an underlying lesion. In the London study, 95% of men with iron deficiency had blood loss from a gastrointestinal source. In a British study of anemia in the elderly, 110 patients over age 65 who presented with anemia were evaluated; 70% had iron deficiency and about half had evidence of gastrointestinal blood loss. In 40% of these cases, the etiology was listed as "undetermined," but many patients did not undergo full work-up because of advanced age. Prevalence of iron deficiency anemia among premenopausal women is conservatively estimated to be 15%, rising to over 30% during pregnancy.

In the London survey, anemia was attributed to chronic disease in 4% (probably an underestimate) and to B_{12} deficiency in 8%. The British study of elderly patients reported 14% had folate deficiency and 9% had a low B_{12} level.

Table 78-1. Differential Diagnosis of Anemia by Red Cell Morphology

Microcytic (MCV 50–82, MCHC 24–32)
1. Iron deficiency
    a. Chronic blood loss
    b. Inadequate intake
    c. Inadequate absorption
    d. Excess demand
2. Abnormal hemoglobins
3. Thalassemias
4. Sideroblastic anemia
5. Chronic disease

Normochromic-Normocytic (MCV 82–92, MCHC 32–36)
1. Hemorrhage
2. Hemolysis
3. Aplastic anemia, pure red cell aplasia
4. Marrow infiltration
5. Hypothyroidism
6. Chronic disease
7. Chronic renal failure
8. Cirrhosis
9. Early iron deficiency

Macrocytic (MCV >100, MCHC 32–36)
1. B_{12} deficiencies
2. Folic acid deficiencies
3. Antimetabolites
4. Accelerated erythropoiesis (acute hemolysis, hemorrhage)
5. Increased membrane surface area (liver disease)
6. Myxedema
7. Aplastic anemia

WORKUP

The diagnosis of anemia is based on measurement of the *hematocrit* and/or *hemoglobin concentration* of venous blood. Any abnormal test result needs to be repeated for confirmation before further evaluation is undertaken. Proper interpretation requires consideration of the patient's *intravascular volume status*. An overly expanded plasma volume will dilute the red cell mass and lead to a false-positive diagnosis. Conversely, dehydration can mask an underlying anemia. Examination of the Wright-stained *peripheral blood smear* and autoanalyzer-determined *red cell indices* (MCV, MCHC) are the time-tested means of classifying anemias and initiating evaluation.

The peripheral smear and red cell indices should be examined in conjunction with one another; they provide complementary information. Dependence on only one can lead to errors in diagnosis. For example, anemia due to both iron and B_{12} deficiencies often produces a dimorphic population of microcytic and macrocytic red cells readily observed on peripheral smear, yet the electronically determined mean corpuscular red cell volume will calculate the average size and erroneously suggest a normocytic type of anemia. The Wright-stained smear can also mislead when used alone; moreover, it often lacks sensitivity. Cells that easily flatten out (as in liver disease) may appear larger on smear than they actually are; the MCV will give a more correct determination of size. The sensitivity of the smear in detection of iron deficiency has been found to be as low as 49%.

Determination of red cell size on the peripheral smear is facilitated by utilizing the nucleus of the mature small lymphocyte as a good reference standard for normal red cell diameter. One can also make a control smear of known blood to help judge abnormalities. Use of the mean corpuscular volume and appearance on peripheral smear serves to classify the anemia morphologically and to facilitate evaluation.

Recent advances in flow cytometry have made possible an automated means of determining how much variability there is in the size of the patient's red cells. This measure of anisocytosis is referred to as the *red cell distribution width (RDW)*. Technically, the RDW is the coefficient of variation of cell volume; it serves as a means of detecting red cell heterogeneity, previously available only by examination of the peripheral smear. Although examination of the Wright-stained smear still provides information unobtainable from other sources (*e.g.,* appearance of other blood elements), the smear could be supplanted by the combined use of the MCV and RDW for initial classification of anemias (see Table 78-2).

Not all automatically determined cell indices have proven valuable. Recent studies suggest that the mean corpuscular hemoglobin concentration (MCHC) and the mean corpuscular hemoglobin (MCH) add little to the evaluation of ane-

Table 78-2. Classification of Anemias by Use of Data from Automated Cytometry

MCV < 80 MICROCYTOSIS	MCV 80–100 NORMOCYTOSIS	MCV > 100 MACROCYTOSIS
Low RDW		
Anemia of chronic disease	Hypoproliferation (*e.g.,* renal failure)	Aplastic anemias
Most thalassemias	Hereditary spherocytosis	Myelodysplastic syndromes
	Anemia of chronic disease	
High RDW		
Iron deficiency	Sickle cell disease	Megaloblastic anemias
Sideroblastic anemia	Early iron deficiency	Acute hemolysis or hemorrhage
Hemoglobin H	Marrow infiltration	Liver disease
	Chronic hemolysis	

mia, although the MCHC still is used as a means of quantifying degree of hypochromia.

Once a morphologic categorization is made, either by reference to red blood cell indices or by direct visualization of the peripheral smear, further evaluation can commence, often by carefully examining all blood elements on the peripheral smear.

Microcytic Hypochromic Anemias. The basis for classification is hypochromia and microcytosis as manifested by small red blood cells with an increase in the area of central pallor on smear, a mean corpuscular hemoglobin concentration below 32, and a mean corpuscular volume below 82. In early stages, not all features may be present. History should focus on any abnormal blood loss, change in bowel habits, melena, heavy aspirin use, family history of anemia (especially in those of Mediterranean descent), concurrent malignancy, symptoms of chronic infection or chronic inflammatory process, number of pregnancies, pica, dysphagia, history of lead exposure, dietary iron intake, quantity of menstrual blood loss, gastric resection, changes in nails, and soreness of the tongue. Physical examination includes checking for glossitis, cheilitis, koilonychia, splenomegaly, rectal mass, guaiac positivity, pelvic mass, and signs of chronic infectious, inflammatory, or neoplastic disorders.

There are a number of readily available tests that usually allow a confident etiologic diagnosis when the patient presents with microcytic anemia. Because iron deficiency is by far the most common cause, measurement of *serum iron* and *total iron binding capacity (TIBC)* is usually the first step. *Percent saturation* [(Fe/TIBC) $\times$ 100] is a sensitive measure of iron deficiency. In a study of 132 patients with documented iron deficiency, including 17 with normochromic normocytic smears, all had percent saturations of 16% or less. However,

the specificity of the test is limited by the finding that some patients with the anemia of chronic disease also have percent saturations that fall below 16%. The more typical pattern in anemia of chronic disease is a low iron and low TIBC in contrast to the low iron and increased TIBC characteristic of iron deficiency.

When it is unclear whether the cause of anemia is iron deficiency or chronic disease, a more direct measure of iron stores will settle the issue: iron stores are low or absent in iron deficiency and normal or increased in anemia of chronic disease. *Bone marrow aspiration* and examination comprise one measure of measuring iron stores, but it has been shown that absence of iron on aspirated specimens is not a specific finding unless there are generous amounts of marrow stroma in the aspirated sample; bone marrow biopsy is more specific.

Bone marrow examination is now used relatively infrequently because of the availability of *serum ferritin* radioimmunoassays. Serum ferritin is a soluble protein in which excess iron is stored. In normal subjects, serum ferritin level is directly proportional to body iron stores. Mean serum ferritin level in adult men is approximately three times higher than in menstruating women. In men and postmenopausal women, ferritin level increases gradually with advancing age. While the "normal" range for serum ferritin is, therefore, controversial, a level less than or equal to 12 μg/l has been shown to be highly specific (>97%) for iron deficiency. Sensitivity is also high in the absence of other diseases. However, infection, chronic disease, and liver disease will elevate serum ferritin levels, thereby masking the diagnosis of iron deficiency when it coexists with anemia of chronic disease. Most studies indicate that, under these circumstances, a serum ferritin level below 50 μg/l is consistent with iron deficiency, and a trial of iron therapy may be indicated. When the ferritin level is above 100 μg/l, it is not likely that iron deficiency is contributing to the anemia; when the level is between 50 and 100 μg/l the diagnosis is uncertain. One can resort either to marrow examination or a therapeutic trial.

A therapeutic trial of oral iron therapy can also be used in the uncomplicated case as a simple alternative to ferritin level or marrow examination. The reticulocyte count should be monitored over a 7- to 10-day period. A significant rise in the reticulocyte count is strong evidence for the diagnosis of iron deficiency. Microcytic anemia with lower serum iron that fails to respond can then be studied by ferritin or marrow examination.

In thalassemia, serum iron is normal or increased, and the iron-binding capacity and the percent saturation are normal. In hemoglobinopathies, the serum iron and iron-binding capacity are normal as well. In sideroblastic anemias, the serum iron is increased and the total iron-binding capacity decreased.

If serum iron and iron-binding capacity are *normal* and the patient is of Mediterranean extraction, a *hemoglobin A₂ determination* can help make the diagnosis of thalassemia trait. Similarly, *hemoglobin electrophoresis* can help detect an abnormal hemoglobin. If the serum iron is *increased,* a check of the hemoglobin A₂ level is needed to rule out thalassemia; a *marrow aspirate,* in which increased numbers of abnormal sideroblasts are sought, is also needed.

To summarize:

1. The important initial tests in the evaluation of microcytic hypochromic anemia are a determination of the serum iron, total iron-binding capacity, and percent saturation.
2. When percent saturation is below 16%, a diagnostic trial of iron therapy can be tried.
3. Alternatively, a serum ferritin determination and/or bone marrow aspiration can be ordered.
4. Hemoglobin electrophoresis, A₂ determination and, occasionally, bone marrow study supplement the work-up when serum iron is normal or increased.

Macrocytic Anemias. The criteria for inclusion in this group are a mean corpuscular volume greater than 100, a normal mean corpuscular hemoglobin concentration, and macrocytes on smear. (Often the latter are hard to detect in mild cases.) Marked macrocytosis identified electronically is clinically significant. For example, in a study of 100 patients with mean corpuscular volumes (MCV) greater than 115, over half had folate and/or B₁₂ deficiency; another 25% had liver disease or alcoholism accompanied by liver disease.

The first objective is to distinguish megaloblastic from nonmegaloblastic causes. The *peripheral smear* is the single most helpful test. Hypersegmented polymorphonuclear leukocytes are the earliest and most specific sign of a megaloblastic anemia, seen in over 65% of cases. Oval macrocytes are also characteristic. An increase in hypersegmented polys can be screened for by counting the number of neutrophils with five or more lobes in a routine 100-cell-differential.

Finding three neutrophils with five lobes or even one with six is strong presumptive evidence for megaloblastic anemia. *Bone marrow aspiration* may be needed in confusing situations, but in most instances a peripheral smear should do. It must be remembered that megaloblastic marrow changes can revert to normal within 12 to 24 hours of therapy, and thus treatment should be delayed if marrow examination is anticipated. However, neutrophil hypersegmentation may persist for up to 2 weeks after onset of vitamin replacement.

If the anemia has been identified as megaloblastic, the next step is to determine whether it is due to folate or B₁₂ deficiency. History and physical examination can give important clues. A history of gastric surgery or raw fish intake, or symptoms of terminal ileal disease, vitiligo, hypothyroidism, steatorrhea, glossitis, or subacute combined system disease suggest B₁₂ deficiency. Alcoholism, poor nutrition, pregnancy, blood dyscrasias, sprue, severe psoriasis, and anticonvulsant intake suggest folate lack. Antimetabolite therapy with folate antagonists such as methotrexate can cause a megaloblastic picture with normal serum folate levels.

Obviously, *serum folate* and B₁₂ determinations are helpful, but there are a number of pitfalls in interpreting the results. Many assays for B₁₂ levels are bioassays; recent antibiotic intake can interfere with them. Recent green vegetable intake can cause a false rise in the folate level. Also, B₁₂ levels may be low in patients with folate deficiency alone; thus, both folate and B₁₂ levels must always be measured together.

A *therapeutic trial* of folate or B₁₂ (they should never be given simultaneously) can be used when serum assays are unavailable or the results confusing. The hematocrit and reticulocyte counts are measured twice prior to administration, then followed every few days up to 10 days after a small but effective dose of B₁₂ (*e.g.,* 100 μg IM) or folate (1 mg IM) is given. The trial is positive if a significant rise in reticulocyte count occurs within 10 days. Large doses are not used because they can cause a nonspecific reticulocytosis in patients with megaloblastic anemias.

To distinguish B₁₂ deficiency due to malabsorption from that due to lack of intrinsic factor, an *oral Schilling test* with and without intrinsic factor is used. An unlabeled intramuscular dose of 1000 μg of B₁₂ is given to saturate binding sites prior to the oral radioactive dose. Both urine and plasma levels of labeled B₁₂ are measured to maximize accuracy. The difficulty with the test is that B₁₂ deficiency can itself cause malabsorption, confusing test interpretation. Thus, the test should be postponed until the deficiency is corrected. In malabsorptive states there will be no improvement with intrinsic factor, whereas there will be in pernicious anemia. Currently, there is no reliable test widely available for determining folate malabsorption.

Nonmegaloblastic macrocytic anemias can be divided into subgroups in which marrow activity is increased, normal, or decreased. To make this determination, a *reticulocyte count* is needed. The normal range is 0.8% to 2.5% in males and

0.8% to 4.1% in females. To correct for the degree of anemia, the reticulocyte count is multiplied by the hematocrit and divided by 0.45. Increased reticulocytes are due to hemorrhage or hemolysis. Normal or decreased levels occur in myxedema, liver disease, myelophthisic states, chronic disease, and hypoplastic anemia. The patient should be questioned and examined carefully for symptoms of any of these conditions, and the smear studied again. In myelophthisic processes, there may be a particularly large number of teardrops on peripheral smear; a *bone marrow biopsy* will confirm the diagnosis.

To summarize:

1. Peripheral smear is examined for hypersegmented polys and oval macrocytes.
2. If they are present, serum B_{12} and folate levels are ordered.
3. Alternatively, a diagnostic trial of a small dose of B_{12} or folate can be performed, monitoring reticulocyte count.
4. When B_{12} deficiency is detected, a Schilling test is helpful to differentiate between lack of intrinsic factor and malabsorption.
5. The reticulocyte count and peripheral smear examination are important to evaluation of nonmegaloblastic cases; bone marrow biopsy is indicated if a myelophthisic process is suspected.

Normochromic Normocytic Anemias. This category encompasses a diverse group of conditions that can be classified according to marrow response. A *reticulocyte count* is obtained. If increased, it suggests hemolysis or recent hemorrhage. If there is no history of recent hemorrhage, a careful drug history; an examination for splenomegaly; determinations of bilirubin, haptoglobin, and lactic dehydrogenase (LDH); and a Coombs test should be undertaken to assess the possibility of hemolysis. Common drugs implicated in the different types of drug-induced immune hemolytic anemias include quinidine, penicillin, methyldopa, and the cephalosporins. Bone marrow examination in cases of hemolysis is unnecessary.

If the reticulocyte count is not appropriately elevated, a search for metabolic causes of marrow suppression, such as renal failure, myxedema, Addison's disease, and alcoholic liver disease is in order. In addition, early iron deficiency may present as a normochromic, normocytic anemia, as can the anemia of chronic disease. Serum iron and total iron-binding capacity should be checked and a calculation of the percent saturation made. If the *peripheral smear* shows considerable numbers of teardrop forms and fragmented cells, suggesting a myelophthisic process, a *bone marrow biopsy* is indicated (an aspiration of the marrow may only yield a dry tap).

A very low or absent reticulocyte count is suggestive of an aplastic anemia, especially if accompanied by evidence of pancytopenia on peripheral smear and cell counts. History of drug use (*e.g.,* chloramphenicol, phenylbutazone, anti-

metabolites, gold), toxin exposure (benzene, insecticides), or recent viral illness may provide a clue to etiology. In the majority of instances, the history is unrevealing. Bone marrow biopsy is diagnostic.

To summarize:

1. The reticulocyte count is checked.
2. If the count is elevated, evidence for recent hemorrhage or hemolysis is sought.
3. If the reticulocyte count is not elevated, a search for underlying renal, endocrine, or liver disease should be undertaken, as well as an evaluation for early iron deficiency anemia, and anemia of chronic disease.
4. If the peripheral smear shows many teardrop forms and fragmented cells, a marrow biopsy is indicated.
5. If the reticulocyte count is practically zero and the peripheral blood count and smear show a pancytopenia, a marrow biopsy is necessary.

SYMPTOMATIC THERAPY

Few patients who present with an anemia of gradual onset require immediate correction of the anemia. The one exception is the patient with angina who may be compromised by the decrease in oxygen-carrying capacity. In almost all other instances, evaluation should proceed in an orderly manner and therapy withheld until a specific diagnosis can be made and a specific therapy implemented (see Chapter 84). The all too common practice of simultaneously prescribing multiple hematinics can obscure important findings. The elderly and others with symptoms and limited cardiopulmonary reserve should be admitted for inpatient evaluation and consideration of transfusion therapy.

PATIENT EDUCATION

Patients commonly think an anemia is due to vitamin or iron deficiencies. Many try self-treatment prior to seeing a physician; others request vitamin therapy. A common error among both patients and physicians is to attribute symptoms of depression, such as fatigue and listlessness, to an underlying anemia. Unless the hematocrit is well below 30, or the patient has very little cardiopulmonary reserve, this attribution is unjustified (see Chapter 5).

The patient needs to be told to what extent his anemia accounts for his symptoms, what the possible causes are, and what the appropriate work-up will involve. Attention to these details is likely to enlist patient cooperation, lessen anxiety, and foster a better working relationship between doctor and patient.

A.H.G. and A.G.M.

ANNOTATED BIBLIOGRAPHY

Bainton D, Finch O: The diagnosis of iron-deficiency anemia. Am J Med 37:62, 1964 (*A classic study examining the specificity and sensitivity of the serum iron, TIBC, and percent saturation.*)

Bessman JD, Gilmer PR Jr, Gardner FH: Improved classification of anemias by MCV and RDW. Am J Clin Pathol 80:322, 1983 (*A description of the utility of automated cytometry in evaluation of anemia.*)

Camitta BM, Storb R, Thomas ED: Aplastic anemia: Pathogenesis, diagnosis, treatment and prognosis. N Engl J Med 306:645, 712, 1982 (*A two-part comprehensive review.*)

Cartwright G: The anemia of chronic disorders. Semin Hematol 3: 351, 1966 (*Excellent review with 73 references.*)

Committee on Iron Deficiency: Iron deficiency in the United States. JAMA 203:407, 1968 (*Documents the absence of hypochromia in microcytosis early in the course of iron deficiency. The earliest findings are loss of stainable iron in the marrow and fall in the serum iron with rise in the total iron-binding capacity. Good review of epidemiology and workup.*)

Cook JD: Clinical evaluation of iron deficiency. Semin Hematol 19: 6, 1982 (*A detailed clinical review of the tests for iron deficiency, including serum ferritin and free erythrocyte protoporphyrin as well as older standbys.*)

Crosby WH: Reticulocyte count. Arch Intern Med 141:1747, 1981 (*A detailed discussion of this important laboratory study and its clinical significance.*)

Edwin E: The segmentation of polymorphonuclear neutrophils in hypovitaminosis B_{12}. Acta Med Scan 182:401, 1967 (*Sixty-four percent of patients with B_{12} deficiency exhibited hypersegmentation on smear. Good discussion of errors in counting lobes.*)

Entisham M, Cape R: Diagnosing and treating anemia. Geriatrics 32:99, 1977 (*Good summary of studies of anemia in the elderly.*)

Frank MM et al: Pathophysiology of immune hemolytic anemia. Ann Intern Med 87:210, 1977 (*A lucid review of types and their mechanisms.*)

Fry J: Clinical patterns and course of anemias in general practice. Br Med J 2:1732, 1961 (*Clinical epidemiology of anemia as seen in a London general practice.*)

Huebers HA, Finch CA: Transferrin: Physiologic behavior and clinical implications. Blood 64:763, 1984 (*The best recent review on transferrin, which includes discussion of clinically relevant issues.*)

Lindenbaum J: Small intestinal function in B_{12} deficiency. Ann Intern Med 80:326, 1974 (*Provides evidence for malabsorption due to, rather than as a cause of, B_{12} deficiency.*)

Linnell JC, Matthews DM: Cobalamin metabolism and its clinical aspects. Clin Sci 66:113, 1984 (*A review of B_{12} that covers both physiologic and clinical issues.*)

Lipschitz D, Cook J, Finch C: A clinical evaluation of serum ferritin as an index of iron stores. N Engl J Med 290:1213, 1974 (*A study correlating serum ferritin levels with iron stores; a level of less than 12 ng/ml was specific for iron deficiency.*)

McPhedran P et al: Interpretation of electronically determined macrocytosis. Ann Intern Med 78:677, 1973 (*The finding of an MCV greater than 115 was associated with folate or B_{12} deficiency in over 50% and with liver disease in another 25%.*)

Steinberg MH, Dreiling BJ: Microcytosis: Its significance and evaluation. JAMA 249:85, 1983 (*A brief review of causes and diagnostic test results.*)

Stewart JG, Ahlquist DA, McGill DB et al: Gastrointestinal blood loss and anemia in runners. Ann Intern Med 100:843, 1984 (*Documents significance of occult blood loss among long distance runners.*)

Taymor M, Sturgis S, Yahia C: The etiological role of chronic iron deficiency in production of menorrhagia. JAMA 187:323, 1974 (*A double-blind study documenting iron superior to placebo in improving menorrhagia.*)

Tudhope G, Wilson G: Anemia in hypothyroidism. Q J Med 29: 513, 1960 (*A detailed hematologic study of 116 cases of hypothyroidism, revealing anemia in over 30%; pernicious anemia occurred in 7%.*)

Van der Weyden M, Rother M, Firkin B: Metabolic significance of reduced B_{12} in folate deficiency. Blood 40:23, 1972 (*Low B_{12} levels can occur in folate deficiency; the reduction is usually moderate and improves with folic acid replacement.*)

Victor M, Lear A: Subacute combined degeneration of the spinal cord. Value of serum B_{12} determinations. Am J Med 20:896, 1956 (*The neurologic deficits may occur in the absence of anemia.*)

Wood M, Elwood P: Symptoms of iron deficiency anemia: A community survey. Br J Prev Soc Med 20:117, 1966 (*In 295 patients studied, there was little correlation between symptoms and serum hemoglobin concentration.*)

79
Evaluation of Polycythemia

An elevated red cell count, hemoglobin concentration, or hematocrit often occurs as an unexpected finding, noted coincidentally on obtaining an automated complete blood count. The upper limit of normal for a hematocrit is 52% for males, 47% for females. In the context of marked dehydration or severe lung disease, the elevation comes as no surprise; but in the absence of such concurrent disease, a search for an underlying cause is warranted. Possible etiologies include polycythemia vera, occult malignancy, right-to-left shunts, and hemoglobinopathies. The finding may even be spurious. In most instances, the primary physician should be able to distinguish among the variety of etiologies on clinical grounds, aided by a few simple laboratory studies.

PATHOPHYSIOLOGY AND CLINICAL PRESENTATION

True polycythemia, as opposed to relative or spurious polycythemia, is defined as an absolute increase in red cell mass. It may represent a stem cell defect, as in polycythemia vera, or be triggered by excess erythropoietin production, as in the secondary polycythemias.

Polycythemia Vera is a myeloproliferative disorder. The etiology is not completely understood, but the disease appears to occur secondary to an intrinsic cellular defect and is not dependent on erythropoietin. It is characterized by abnormal proliferation of all blood elements in the bone marrow and extramedullary sites, producing absolute erythrocytosis, leukocytosis, thrombocytosis, splenomegaly, a hypercellular bone marrow and, often, myeloid metaplasia and myelofibrosis. Polycythemia vera is an uncommon disease, with an incidence in the United States of 4 to 5 cases per million per year, or about 1000 new cases in the United States per year. However, the prevalence of the disease is relatively higher because of the long life span in the majority of patients. The peak age of onset is 50 to 60.

A small percentage of patients with polycythemia vera have a relatively benign course, with red cell volume controlled by occasional phlebotomy, and pruritus and hyperuricemia controlled by medication. Polycythemia vera can evolve into a malignant, disordered condition with the development of myeloid metaplasia, myelofibrosis, and acute leukemia.

It is not surprising that the presence of true polycythemia is often unsuspected, since symptoms develop gradually and are frequently vague and rather nonspecific. In early stages, the patient may be entirely asymptomatic, with an elevated hematocrit being the only manifestation. As the disease progresses, the white cell and platelet counts rise, and symptoms ensue as the red cell volume expands. Most are attributable to hyperviscosity, hypervolemia, and consequent sluggish blood flow, which take place when the hematocrit rises above 55. Headache, dizziness, vertigo, tinnitus, fullness of the head, and blurred vision are among the common neurologic symptoms. Patients may complain of angina pectoris or claudication when there is coexisting atherosclerotic disease. Generalized weakness, fatigue, sweating, and lassitude are frequently reported. Gastrointestinal complaints may predominate—for example, fullness, belching, epigastric discomfort. In polycythemia vera, a classic symptom is pruritus after bathing, believed due to abnormal histamine release. Also, gouty joint complaints occur in the context of marked secondary hyperuricemia caused by increased cell turnover. Left upper quadrant discomfort is a manifestation of the significant splenomegaly usually seen in polycythemia vera.

Hemostasis is disturbed in polycythemia vera due to hyperviscosity and defects in platelet function. Patients may present with bleeding in uncommon sites, such as hepatic, mesenteric, or retinal veins, or with bleeding in the form of epistaxis, menorrhagia, easy bruisability, or oozing from the gums.

On examination, the patient has a deep red appearance; peripheral cyanosis and ecchymosis may be noted. Blood pressure is usually normal. Hepatomegaly is present in 40% and splenomegaly in 70%.

In about 60% to 70% of cases, the white count rises above 12,000. Over half of patients experience increases in platelet count. The red cells appear normochromic and normocytic, unless iron deficiency develops. The erythrocyte sedimentation rate is frequently very low. Erythropoietin levels are below normal. Leukocyte alkaline phosphatase concentrations are increased in 80%, as are B_{12} levels due to an increase in B_{12}-binding proteins.

Secondary Polycythemia (erythrocytosis) represents the majority of cases of increased red cell mass. The increase is usually an appropriate physiological response to tissue hypoxia and occurs when the PaO_2 falls chronically below 55 mm Hg or, more precisely, when the arterial oxygen saturation (SaO_2) drops below 92%. Obvious mechanisms of hypoxia include residence at high altitudes and severe pulmonary disease, but cyanotic heart disease, increased carboxyhemoglobin from heavy cigarette smoking, and hemoglobinopathies with high affinities for oxygen can have a similar deleterious effect on tissue oxygenation.

Decreased tissue oxygenation is thought to be detected in the kidneys, causing release of erythrogenin, which acts enzymatically on a plasma protein substrate to form erythropoietin. There also seems to be a less sensitive nonrenal system for detecting tissue hypoxia and producing erythropoietin. Erythropoietin is a glycoprotein hormone that stimulates RNA synthesis, causing hematopoietic precursor cells to proliferate and differentiate into early erythroblasts. These cells mature at a faster than normal rate; early release of reticulocytes from the marrow and increased heme synthesis results. The increase in red cell mass improves tissue oxygenation, to the extent that hyperviscosity does not compromise it.

Pathologic Secondary Polycythemia results from inappropriate erythropoietin production, occurring autonomously in the absence of generalized tissue hypoxia. Renal diseases and a host of malignancies have been implicated. Inappropriate erythropoietin levels due to renal disorders and malignancies are very unusual occurrences, but it is important to be aware of them, since polycythemia may be an early clue to their existence. About 1% to 3% of renal cell carcinomas have erythrocytosis as a manifestation, occurring at a time when cure is possible. Hydronephrosis, renal artery stenosis, and renal cystic diseases are occasionally associated with elevations in erythropoietin; the mechanism is felt to be a reduction in blood flow to normal tissue. Huge uterine myomas, cerebellar hemangiomas, and hepatomas are also causes, although the mechanisms are unclear; up to 10% of hepatoma patients in one series had erythrocytosis.

Relative Polycythemia (also referred to as Gaisböck's syndrome, stress erythrocytosis, and spurious erythrocytosis) denotes a heterogeneous set of conditions, characterized by an increase in hematocrit without an increase in red cell mass. One subset of patients has a high-to-normal erythrocyte mass and a low-to-normal plasma volume. The other has a normal erythrocyte mass and a low plasma volume. Most patients with relative erythrocytosis are obese, middle-aged, hypertensive men. About one third of such patients experience thromboembolic complications. Those with a low plasma volume have the highest incidence of thromboembolization. The cause of relative polycythemia is unclear, but smoking appears to play a role. Loss of weight, cessation of smoking, control of hypertension, and implementation of exercise help alleviate the condition.

DIFFERENTIAL DIAGNOSIS

Patients with polycythemia can be separated on the basis of their underlying pathophysiology into three diagnostic categories: (1) polycythemia vera, (2) secondary polycythemia, and (3) relative polycythemia. Secondary polycythemia can be subdivided into physiologic and pathologic varieties (Table 79-1).

WORKUP

History. The first objective is to differentiate patients with polycythemia vera from those with secondary polycythemias. Important historical points suggesting a secondary polycythemia include high altitude residence, known congenital heart disease, history of heart murmur and cyanosis, smoking

Table 79-1. Differential Diagnosis of Polycythemia

A. Polycythemia Vera
B. Secondary Polycythemia
  1. Physiologic (due to systemic hypoxia)
    a. High altitude
    b. Right-to-left shunt
    c. Heavy smoking
    d. Severe pulmonary disease
    e. Abnormal hemoglobin with high O_2 affinity
  2. Pathologic (no systemic hypoxia)
    a. Renal cell carcinoma
    b. Uterine myoma
    c. Cerebellar hemangioma
    d. Hepatoma
    e. Hydronephrosis
    f. Cystic kidney disease
    g. Renal artery stenosis
C. Relative Polycythemia
  1. Marked volume depletion
    a. Protracted vomiting
    b. Persistent diarrhea
    c. Excessive diuretic use
  2. High-to-normal erythrocyte mass, low-to-normal volume
    a. Hypertensive, obese, middle-aged, male smoker

more than two packs per day, symptoms of chronic lung disease, familial occurrence, and history of renal cystic disease. Patients with polycythemia vera are free of such history and should be checked for symptoms of hyperviscosity or bleeding, such as lassitude, headache, pruritus, sweating, easy bruising, abdominal pain, menorrhagia, and epistaxis. History of diuretic use, vomiting, diarrhea, hypertension, and stress suggest relative or spurious polycythemias.

Physical Examination includes checking for hypertension, cyanosis, clubbing, ecchymoses, signs of chronic lung disease, heart murmurs, hepatic enlargement, splenomegaly, and abdominal and pelvic masses.

Laboratory Evaluation should begin with a *complete blood count, platelet count* and *peripheral blood smear examination.* Two-thirds of patients with polycythemia vera have an elevated WBC count, usually to 12,000–25,000/mm^3, and occasionally as high as 50,000–100,000/mm^3, with increased immature forms and basophils. Half of polycythemia vera patients have thrombocytosis, with platelet counts in the 450,000 to 1,000,000 per mm^3 range. Large, bizarre platelets and megakaryocytic fragments may be seen on the blood smear. In secondary and spurious polycythemia, the WBC, platelet count, and blood smear are normal. In polycythemia vera, red cell morphology becomes abnormal with progression of disease. With the development of myeloid metaplasia, anisocytosis and poikilocytosis with tear-drop forms, ovalocytes, elliptocytes, and nucleated red blood cells are seen.

An *arterial blood gas* with *oxygen saturation (SaO$_2$)* determination is important in the assessment of less obvious cases. A PaO$_2$ less than 55 mm Hg and a SaO$_2$ less than 92% indicate significant hypoxemia. In two-pack-per-day cigarette smokers, the SaO$_2$ determination that is calculated from the measured PaO$_2$ and a standard blood oxygen dissociation curve may be misleading. This method will given an erroneously high SaO$_2$ if carboxyhemoglobin levels are elevated; polycythemia due to increased carboxyhemoglobin will be missed. This problem can be avoided by ordering an SaO$_2$ determination that is measured directly rather than calculated from PaO$_2$.

The diagnostic criteria for polycythemia vera are an elevated total red cell volume, normal SaO$_2$, and splenomegaly. In the absence of splenomegaly, at least two of the following should be present: an elevation in platelet count (over 400,000/mm^3), white cell count (over 12,000/mm^3), *leukocyte alkaline phosphatase, serum B$_{12}$ level,* or unbound B$_{12}$-binding capacity.

If polycythemia vera and hypoxia-induced secondary polycythemia are ruled out, one should look for signs and symptoms of renal lesions and tumors, especially renal cell carcinoma. An *IVP* with *nephrotomograms* or *CT scan* of the abdomen may be diagnostic. When there is a strong family history of polycythemia, one should obtain a *hemoglobin electrophoresis* in search of a mutant hemoglobin with an abnormally high oxygen affinity. *Radioimmunoassay for erythropoietin* will confirm a secondary polycythemia and can be ordered if one needs further evidence to distinguish primary from secondary polycythemia. Usually this expensive test is unnecessary, because clinical data suffice to make the distinction.

Relative polycythemia should be suspected if the patient has signs of significant volume depletion or is an obese, middle-aged, hypertensive male smoker with a stressful lifestyle. Only when clinical evidence is insufficient to distinguish relative polycythemia from other forms, should a *determination of red cell mass* be ordered. The calculation of red cell mass is rather elaborate and requires a laboratory experienced in its measurement. A radioisotope label (chromium-51) is administered to tag the red cells and perform the calculation. Body habitus needs to be taken into account when interpreting the result. Tall muscular individuals will have a greater red cell mass than short fat ones, because blood volume is greater in muscle than in fat. A normal red cell mass is diagnostic of relative polycythemia.

SYMPTOMATIC THERAPY

When possible, treatment should be etiologic (*e.g.,* correction of a right-to-left shunt, removal of a erythropoietin-secreting tumor). Cessation of cigarette smoking (see Chapter 49) is an important goal; in patients with relative erythrocytosis or reactive polycythemia due to heavy smoking and high carboxyhemoglobin levels, the hematocrit will begin to fall within a week and return to normal 3 to 4 months after smoking is terminated. For selected patients with severe chronic obstructive pulmonary disease, chronic oxygen therapy may help normalize arterial oxygen saturation (see Chapter 44).

When polycythemia cannot be treated etiologically, red cell mass can be reduced safely and effectively by *phlebotomy.* Phlebotomy improves oxygen delivery, relieves hyperviscosity symptoms, and prevents the thromboembolic and hemorrhagic complications associated with polycythemia. The risk of such adverse effects begins to rise substantially as the hematocrit moves into the 55 to 60 range. The target hematocrit is in the low to mid 40s, the level at which tissue oxygenation is optimal in normovolemic patients.

Phlebotomy is especially useful in patients with polycythemia vera and pathologic secondary polycythemia. Even in cases where the polycythemia represents a physiologic accommodation to chronic hypoxemia, phlebotomy may be indicated if the polycythemic response becomes excessive (hematocrit > 60) and threatens oxygen delivery. Reducing the hematocrit below 55 improves exercise tolerance in polycythemic patients with severe chronic obstructive pulmonary disease.

Phlebotomy is conducted by removing up to 500 ml of blood as often as every 2 to 3 days to achieve a hematocrit below 55. For patients who do not tolerate such large losses of volume (*e.g.,* the elderly), phlebotomy is limited to no more than 250 ml once or twice a week. Iron deficiency may ensue and should be corrected because microcytic erythrocytes increase blood viscosity. The severely polycythemic patient who is to undergo surgery requires phlebotomy to prevent compromised hemostasis. Preoperative phlebotomy should be followed by administration of a volume expander to correct volume depletion.

Control of *polycythemia vera* with phlebotomy alone is usually possible in cases where platelet and WBC counts remain relatively normal. Phlebotomy has been shown to increase median survival from 2 to 12 years. Frequency of treatments is a function of the hematocrit and symptoms. Most symptoms can be alleviated by reducing the hematocrit to around 50; however, continued frequent phlebotomy is recommended until a normal hematocrit is achieved (mid 40s in men, low 40s in women). A maintenance schedule can then be set up based on monthly monitoring.

Myelosuppressive therapy deserves consideration when phlebotomy proves inadequate, thrombocytosis develops, or extramedullary hematopoiesis ensues. The optimal treatment is yet to be identified; a longitudinal investigation by the Polycythemia Vera Study Group has compared P_{32}, alkylating agents, and hydroxyurea. Although P_{32} and *alkylating agents* (*e.g.,* chlorambucil) are effective, they are also leukemogenic; as such, they are reserved for elderly patients. *Hydroxyurea* appears to be a reasonable alternative, free of leukemogenic effects, yet capable of suppressing the disease. Its disadvantages include frequency of administration, large number of pills that must be taken, and far less sustained remissions than P_{32}. Patients who fail hydroxyurea therapy can be given a treatment of P_{32}, especially if they are elderly; it will induce a 6- to 24-month remission and is less leukemogenic than alkylating agents.

Polycythemia vera patients bothered by *pruritus* may respond to *cyproheptadine* (12 to 16 mg/day) or *cimetidine* (300 mg bid to qid). Secondary *hyperuricemia* occurs in this disease and can lead to acute gout; *allopurinol* (300 mg/day) administered once daily prevents gouty attacks and should be considered when the uric acid rises above 9 to 10 mg/dl.

PATIENT EDUCATION AND INDICATIONS FOR REFERRAL

Patient education is essential to encourage smokers to give up cigarettes (see Chapter 49) and chronic obstructive pulmonary disease patients to follow a maximal program for improving oxygenation (see Chapter 44). The patient's understanding of the basis of his disease and its prognosis should help in achieving compliance (see Chapter 1). When polycythemia vera is diagnosed, patients should be referred to a hematologist for design of a treatment program. Referral is also appropriate when diagnosis is difficult and measurement of red cell mass or bone marrow biopsy is being considered.

A.H.G.

ANNOTATED BIBLIOGRAPHY

Adamson JW: Familial polycythemia. Semin Hematol 12:383, 1975 (*Molecular and physiological mechanisms of familial polycythemias.*)

Balcerzak SP, Bromberg PA: Secondary polycythemia. Semin Hematol 12:353, 1975 (*Excellent review of pulmonary physiology related to tissue hypoxia-induced polycythemia and other classes of secondary polycythemia.*)

Berk PD, Goldberg JD, Silverstein MN et al: Increased incidence of acute leukemia in polycythemia vera associated with chlorambucil therapy. N Engl J Med 304:441, 1981 (*Incidence of acute leukemia was 13 times that of patients treated with phlebotomy and 2.3 times that of those given P32; from the polycythemia vera study group.*)

Chetty KG, Brown SE, Light RW: Improved exercise tolerance of the polycythemic lung patient following phlebotomy. Am J Med 74:415, 1983 (*Patients with COPD show improved exercise tolerance when the hematocrit is lowered by phlebotomy to less than 55.*)

Berlin NI: Diagnosis and classification of the polycythemias. Semin Hematol 12:339, 1975 (*Reviews differential diagnosis and work-up of polycythemia.*)

Brown SM: Spurious (relative) polycythemia: A nonexistent disease. Am J Med 50:200, 1971 (*Patients with this condition were men with high normal red cell masses and low normal plasma volumes.*)

Golde DW, Hocking WG, Koeffler HP et al: Polycythemia: Mechanisms and management. Ann Intern Med 95:71, 1981 (*A comprehensive review of pathophysiology, evaluation, and therapy.*)

Milligan DW, MacNamee R, Roberts BE et al: The influence of iron-deficient indices on whole blood viscosity in polycythemia. Br J Haematol 50:467, 1982 (*Iron deficiency increases viscosity. This means that iron replacement is indicated during phlebotomy therapy.*)

Modan B: An epidemiological study of polycythemia vera. Blood 26:657, 1965 (*Incidence was 4 per million; median age was 60. Sex ratio was close to 1:1.*)

Smith JR, Landaw SA: Smokers' polycythemia. N Engl J Med 298:6, 1978 (*Occurs in heavy smokers and resolves when smoking is stopped.*)

Thomas DJ et al: Cerebral blood-flow in polycythemia. Lancet 2:161, 1977 (*Documents marked reduction in blood flow that returns to normal after repeated phlebotomies.*)

Wasserman IR: The treatment of polycythemia vera. Semin Hematol 13:57, 1975 (*The natural history of polycythemia vera and early findings of the polycythemia vera study group.*)

Weinreb NG, Shih CF: Spurious polycythemia. Semin Hematol 12:397, 1975 (*Review of the topic and results of study of 69 patients.*)

80
Evaluation of Bleeding Problems

The bleeding diatheses seen in the office setting range from abnormal screening studies obtained in preparation for major surgery, to complaints of easy bruising, petechial rashes, or recurrent episodes of unexplained frank blood loss. Sometimes, the only manifestation is a low platelet count, prolonged prothrombin time, or a delay in the bleeding time. When the volume of blood loss is small, rate of bleeding slow, and risk of serious hemorrhage low, evaluation may take place in the outpatient setting. The workup involves examination of the intrinsic and extrinsic clotting systems as well as checking blood vessels, platelet function, and platelet quantity to identify which part of the hemostatic apparatus is at fault. Often a careful history and physical examination, supplemented by a few simple laboratory studies, can yield a clinically meaningful answer and guide therapy. An important objective is to determine if the problem is inherited or acquired. At times, an anatomic lesion coexists with a bleeding diathesis; the clinician always needs to address this possibility, especially when the bleeding originates from the gastrointestinal tract (see Chapter 60), urinary tract (see Chapter 127), lung (see Chapter 38), or vagina (see Chapter 108).

PATHOPHYSIOLOGY AND CLINICAL PRESENTATION

Hemostasis is achieved by the interplay of the coagulation cascade, platelets, and vessel wall. The platelets provide the initial hemostatic plug in response to vascular injury, followed later by generation of fibrin at the site of damage. Blood coagulation is a carefully controlled process, limited by endogenous anticoagulants. Normal hemostasis represents a delicate balance between coagulant and anticoagulant factors. Any upset in this system of checks and balances may result in bleeding or thrombosis.

Qualitative Platelet Disorders

Platelet function defects can be classified according to the step in platelet activity that is affected: adhesion, aggregation, activation, secretion, or acceleration of coagulation. Patients with isolated qualitative platelet defects have a prolonged bleeding time in conjunction with normal-appearing platelets that are adequate in number.

Defective Adhesion. The most important form of impaired adhesion is *von Willebrand's disease,* a hereditary condition most commonly inherited in autosomally dominant fashion. There is decreased secretion or abnormal synthesis of a glycoprotein polymer needed for adherence of platelets to the site of vascular injury. There is also a deficiency of factor VIII procoagulant, giving rise to a prolongation in the partial thromboplastin time. Platelet agglutination fails to occur in the presence of the antibiotic ristocetin, a laboratory characteristic of this disease that is useful for its detection. Mucous membrane bleeding is a frequent manifestation. The severity of bleeding is variable and most severe among homozygous individuals, who may bleed from the gastrointestinal tract; hemarthrosis is rare. An acquired adhesion defect occurs when high doses of *semisynthetic penicillins* or *cephalosporins* are taken; these agents can coat the platelet surface and reduce binding to glycoprotein.

Defective Aggregation. Patients with *Glanzmann's thrombasthenia* are missing a bridging protein called glycoprotein IIb/IIIa. Their platelets cannot bind to fibrinogen and thus fail to aggregate via fibrinogen cross-links. *Clot retraction is abnormal;* the bleeding time is markedly prolonged. Serious bleeding can occur. Patients taking high doses of *semisynthetic penicillins* or *cephalosporins* also demonstrate reduced binding to fibrinogen.

Defective Activation and Secretion. Patients with activation problems have impaired production or impaired response to prostaglandin-dependent activators such as thromboxane A2, which attracts platelets and constricts vessels. *Nonsteroidal anti-inflammatory agents* affect platelet activation and secretion by inhibiting cyclooxygenase, which helps convert arachidonic acid to thromboxane. In addition, they inhibit release of ADP needed for platelet aggregation. The effect can be induced by as little as 600 mg of aspirin and persist for the life span of the platelets made during aspirin therapy. Severe bleeding does not result, but an underlying bleeding diathesis may be aggravated. In patients with *storage pool disease,* the ADP and serotonin contents of platelet granules are reduced or released prematurely, as occurs in patients who have undergone *cardiopulmonary bypass.* Bleeding is typically mild and the bleeding time only mildly prolonged.

Defective Acceleration of Coagulation. When platelets bind factors V and X on their surface, the rate of prothrombin conversion is greatly accelerated. Patients whose platelets cannot bind these clotting factors have a mildly prolonged prothrombin time, normal bleeding time, and normal tests of platelet aggregation.

Quantitative Platelet Defects

A normal platelet count ranges from 150,000 to 300,000 platelets per cubic centimeter. *Thrombocytosis* (by definition, counts in excess of 400,000) may lead to impairment of platelet function, occasionally causing mucous membrane bleeding or hemorrhage following trauma or surgery. Bleeding from thrombocytosis most often occurs from myeloproliferative disease.

Counts below 100,000 are classified as *thrombocytopenia,* but the risk of serious posttraumatic bleeding does not occur until the platelet count falls below 50,000. The risk of spontaneous bleeding rises as the count drops below 20,000. Petechial rash in dependent areas may be an initial manifestation. The lesions differ from those due to vasculitis in that they are not pruritic, not tender, flat, and without an erythematous blush. Hemorrhagic bullae in the buccal mucosa are very characteristic. Bleeding may initiate from the gastrointestinal or urinary tract. Thrombocytopenia develops when there is increased platelet destruction, decreased production, or abnormal pooling.

Increased Destruction is the most common cause of thrombocytopenia. The primary mechanism is immunologic, associated with drugs, viruses, lymphoproliferative disorders, and connective tissue diseases such as lupus. For example, certain drugs act as haptens, binding to serum proteins to form an antigenic substance that stimulates antibody production against it. The platelet is destroyed when it adsorbs the antigen-antibody complex.

Idiopathic Thrombocytopenic Purpura (ITP) ranks among the major causes of platelet destruction. Although a platelet-bound IgG antibody has been detected and found useful for diagnostic purposes, its pathophysiologic significance remains to be determined. The condition is most common in young adults, children, and women. In adults the condition is more chronic, characterized by a waxing and waning course. There are few spontaneous remissions. The spleen is usually not palpable, though it might be slightly enlarged. There is no lymphadenopathy, hepatomegaly, or sternal tenderness, helping to distinguish it from other causes of thrombocytopenia. Mild fever is sometimes noted.

Drug-induced thrombocytopenia is an idiosyncratic reaction, with quinidine among the most frequently involved agents. Rapid fall in platelet count to levels below 10,000 are not uncommon, and acute hemorrhage may ensue. Prompt return of the count to safe levels is typical as soon as the responsible drug is withheld.

The thrombocytopenias associated with *chronic lymphocytic leukemia* (CLL) and *systemic lupus erythematosus* (SLE) follow clinical patterns similar to ITP. In addition, lymphadenopathy and splenomegaly are found in the majority of patients with CLL, and 25% have hepatomegaly as well. In

SLE, arthritis and arthralgias are reported in 90%, skin rash in 70%, lymphadenopathy in 60% and renal disease in 50% (see Chapter 144). Platelet counts below 100,000 are not frequent, being reported in about 15% of cases.

Decreased Production implies bone marrow failure. The bone marrow may be suppressed by drugs, depressed after a viral infection, or replaced by tumor (see Chapter 78). Thrombocytopenias due to conditions causing *marrow failure* or a *myelophthisic process* usually occur in the context of a generalized pancytopenia. On occasion, individual drugs cause selective *inhibition of platelet production*. Chlorothiazide, tolbutamide, and ethanol are among the best documented. Megakaryocyte production suffers in *megaloblastic anemia* and quickly improves with replacement therapy. Transient thrombocytopenia may follow influenza, hepatitis, rubella, and other viral diseases.

Increased Pooling can be seen in disorders associated with an abnormally enlarged spleen. Splenomegaly results in excessive trapping and a fall in number of circulating platelets.

Regardless of etiology, there are a few characteristic features of the blood loss due to thrombocytopenia. Typical are the appearance of petechiae and slow oozing after trauma, rather than brisk bleeding. Mucosal bleeding is common, and menorrhagia or epistaxis may be presenting complaints.

Defects of the Intrinsic Pathway

These conditions prolong the partial thromboplastin time (PTT) by impairing the synthesis of clotting factors of the intrinsic pathway. Fortunately, many of the resultant clotting factor deficiencies do not cause serious bleeding, but the most common ones, the hemophilias, do.

Hemophilias A and *B* represent deficiencies of *factors VIII* and *IX* respectively. They account for over 80% of patients with inherited bleeding diatheses and, being *X*-linked, affect only males. The risk of bleeding depends upon the degree of factor deficiency. Patients with as little as 5% of normal concentrations experience little bleeding; those with 1% to 5% may bleed after minor trauma; those with less than 1% undergo spontaneous hemorrhage, typically into muscle and weight-bearing joints. Bleeding can also occur into the CNS, genitourinary tract, and retroperitoneum. Detection may be difficult if factor levels are in excess of 25%, because the PTT will be normal. Chromosomal mapping is being developed to help detect female carriers.

Factor XI deficiency occurs mostly among Ashkenazi Jews, inherited as an autosomal recessive disorder. A severe insult such as major trauma or surgery is needed to precipitate bleeding.

Deficiencies of the other intrinsic pathway factors may cause a prolongation of the PTT but do not lead to clinical bleeding problems, even in the setting of major surgery or serious trauma.

Defects of the Extrinsic Pathway

The major clotting factors of the extrinsic pathway (II, VII, X) are dependent for their synthesis and modification upon a healthy liver and an adequate dietary intake of vitamin K. Some vitamin K also derives from bacterial production by gut flora. Hereditary deficiencies of extrinsic pathway factors are very rare. Most bleeding traced to the extrinsic pathway is due to impaired vitamin K production or liver disease. Causes include *hepatocellular insufficiency, cholestasis* (impairing absorption of lipid-soluble vitamin K), *poor dietary intake,* and use of *broad-spectrum antibiotics* that kill normal gut flora. The characteristic laboratory finding is a prolongation of the *prothrombin time (PT)*. Prolongation of the PT is also an early manifestation of *coumarin* anticoagulant therapy. Coumarin derivatives inhibit vitamin K-dependent, postsynthetic modification of factors II, VII, IX, and X; this prevents them from being able to bind calcium and achieve biologic activity (see Chapter 84).

Vascular Defects

Vascular defects are characterized by purpuric bleeding into the skin and mucous membranes in the absence of a detectable clotting factor or platelet abnormality. Ecchymoses and/or petechiae are the predominant manifestations. The most common form occurs as a result of aging, so-called *senile purpura.* Atrophy of connective and fatty tissues makes the vessels fragile and subject to ecchymotic bleeding, especially in areas of chronic sun exposure (face, neck, dorsum of hands, forearms). The skin fragility and easy bruising seen with *Cushing's syndrome* are believed to have a similar basis, due to the catabolic effects of prolonged corticosteroid excess. *Scurvy* causes defective collagen synthesis; affected patients may present with gingival bleeding or hemorrhage into subcutaneous tissue and muscle. Perifollicular bleeding is characteristic. *Purpura simplex* is a mild condition seen in otherwise healthy women; they experience ecchymoses mostly in the lower extremities (sometimes colorfully referred to as "devil's pinches"), especially during menstrual periods. Most cases are believed to be acquired, and some have been linked to use of nonsteroidal anti-inflammatory agents.

Hereditary disorders of connective tissue (*e.g.,* Marfan's syndrome, Ehlers–Danlos syndrome) produce structural defects in supporting connective tissue and in major vessels. Bleeding ranges from easy bruising to serious hemorrhage. In *Rendu–Weber–Osler disease,* the developmental anomaly is telangiectasia formation due to lack of vessel support and contractility. Bleeding from these thin, convoluted networks of venules and capillaries might result from minor trauma or occur spontaneously. The telangiectatic lesions are violaceous, flat, usually no larger than a few millimeters, and range in shape from pinpoint to spiderlike. They occur on mucous membranes, face, trunk, palmar, and plantar surfaces. Unfortunately, the lesions also arise in major viscera, leading to risk of serious hemorrhage. The clinical course is often one of repeated hemorrhagic episodes.

A host of pharmacologic agents can induce purpuric bleeding in the absence of demonstrable platelet or clotting factor abnormalities. *Drug-induced vascular purpura* is thought to have an autoimmune mechanism, with antibodies directed at the endothelial surface, though the responsible antibodies have yet to be identified. Drugs in this category include *procaine penicillin, thiazides, quinine, iodides, sulfas, and coumarins.* The bleeding ceases when the drug is withdrawn.

Paraproteinemias (cryoglobulinemia, macroglobulinemia, myeloma) can lead to damage of the endothelial surface as immune complexes and paraproteins precipitate from the serum. The sludging and hyperviscosity commonly associated with these conditions also causes capillary anoxia. The bleeding that ensues is multifactorial in origin, resulting from impairment of clotting factor and platelet activity as well as endothelial damage.

Minor purpuric bleeding caused by *immune complex formation* sometimes occurs with *systemic lupus, rheumatoid arthritis* and *Sjögren's syndrome.* In *amyloidosis,* there is deposition of amyloid protein in the skin and subcutaneous tissue, which leads to vascular fragility, especially about the orbits and upper torso. The "raccoon eyes" appearance of such patients is characteristic.

Mixed Defects

A number of conditions impair the hemostatic apparatus at multiple levels. Chronic renal failure, chronic liver disease, and consumption coagulopathies are the most important examples. *Uremia* interferes with platelet function and causes deficiencies in production of clotting factors. Dialysis helps correct the bleeding tendency, which ranges from purpura and mucous membrane bleeding to gastrointestinal hemorrhage. Uremic patients often experience prolonged oozing from arterial and venipuncture sites.

Patients with severe *chronic liver disease* no longer make adequate amounts of vitamin K-dependent clotting factors. The PT becomes prolonged and does not correct with parenteral administration of vitamin K. In addition, fibrinogen production suffers, and that which is made is defective. Patients with portal hypertension may become thrombocytopenic from platelet sequestration in the spleen, though, by itself, this rarely causes bleeding. The formation of varices further increases the risk of hemorrhage (see Chapter 71).

Disseminated intravascular coagulation occurs in the setting of illness that causes exposure of blood to tissue thromboplastin (*e.g.,* snake bite, extensive burn, serious infection, cancer). Activation of the extrinsic pathway in the microcirculation consumes clotting factors and platelets; it leads to bleeding that ranges from minor petechiae to hemorrhage. The condition is rarely encountered in the office setting.

DIFFERENTIAL DIAGNOSIS

The causes of a bleeding diathesis can be organized according to the subdivisions of the hemostatic apparatus: platelet function, platelet number, intrinsic pathway, extrinsic pathway, and vessels (Table 80-1). Differential diagnosis proceeds by identifying which segment of the clotting system is at fault (see following discussion).

WORKUP

When faced with a patient complaining of easy bruising or bleeding, the clinician needs to ascertain the likelihood of an underlying defect in hemostasis. Bleeding from multiple sites, easy bruising, spontaneous bleeding, ecchymoses greater than 3 cm in diameter, or prolonged bleeding after a surgical or dental procedure strongly suggest a bleeding diathesis. Before embarking on a detailed evaluation in the office, one should be sure there is no serious hemorrhage or major volume depletion. Inquiry is required into dyspnea, lightheadedness, marked postural fatigue, and observed quantity of blood loss. A quick check of skin color, skin temperature, and postural signs will provide added evidence of intravascular volume status and degree of anemia. Once the presence or risk of severe hemorrhage is ruled out, the outpatient evaluation can commence.

The first task is to try identifying which segments of the hemostatic system are at fault. This determination, along with an assessment of whether the condition is acquired or hereditary, can greatly help focus the evaluation (Table 80-2).

History. One needs a full history of the bleeding problem, including its onset, course, precipitants, manifestations, associated family history, and drug history. Bleeding that is petechial, purpuric, or limited to the mucous membranes suggests a platelet disorder, as does the occurrence of bleeding that is immediate and transient. Nosebleeds or menorrhagia may be presenting complaints. Vascular purpuras can have a similar presentation. In contrast, patients with major defects in the coagulation cascade (*e.g.,* those with hemophilia) report spontaneous bleeding, which may be into joints or soft tissue or present as hemorrhage from the gastrointestinal or genitourinary tracts. When bleeding in hemophiliacs follows trauma, it may initially be delayed, since primary hemostasis is provided adequately by blood vessels and platelets; brisk bleeding or persistent oozing may then ensue.

Onset of bleeding problems in childhood as well as a positive *family history* provide strong presumptive evidence of a hereditary etiology. However, as many as 30% of hemophiliacs give no family history of bleeding. Eighty-five percent of hereditary coagulation disorders are due to factor VIII deficiency; another 10% are due to low levels of factor IX. Since these are sex-linked conditions, their presence in a male patient raises the index of suspicion.

A thorough review of the patient's *medications,* both those

Table 80-1.   Differential Diagnosis of Bleeding

Qualitative Platelet Disorders	
Defective adhesion	Von Willebrand's disease; high doses of semisynthetic penicillins and cephalosporins
Defective aggregation	Glanzmann's thrombosthenia; high doses of semisynthetic penicillins and cephalosporins
Defective activation	Nonsteroidal anti-inflammatory drugs; dipyridamole; cardiopulmonary bypass
Defective acceleration	Factor V deficiency
Quantitative Platelet Disorders	
Thrombocytosis	Myeloproliferative disease
Thrombocytopenia	
Decreased production	Thiazides, alcohol, viral infection, marrow failure, megaloblastic anemia, myelophthisic process
Increased destruction	Quinidine, methyldopa, sulfa, phenytoin, barbiturates, lupus, infection, ITP, chronic lymphocytic leukemia
Increased sequestration	Hypersplenism
Intrinsic Pathway Defects	
Factor VIII defiency	Hemophilia A
Factor IX deficiency	Hemophilia B
Factor XI deficiency	Ashkenazi Jews
Extrinsic Pathway Defects	
Vitamin K–dependent factor deficiency	Poor diet, cholestasis, hepatocellular failure, coumarin, broad-spectrum antibiotics
Vascular Defects	
Connective tissue fragility	Age, Cushing's syndrome, scurvy, purpura simplex
Hereditary defect	Marfan's syndrome, Rendu-Weber-Osler disease
Drug-induced	Procaine penicillin, sulfa, thiazides, quinine, iodides, coumarin
Paraproteinemia	Myeloma, macroglobulinemia, cryoglobulinemia
Connective tissue disease	Lupus, rheumatoid arthritis, Sjogren's syndrome
Multiple Defects	
Uremia	
Chronic hepatocellular failure	
Disseminated intravascular coagulation	

prescribed and those available over-the-counter, is essential. Particular note should be taken of drugs that are capable of interfering with platelet function (nonsteroidal anti-inflammatory agents, semisynthetic penicillins, cephalosporins, dipyridamole), causing thrombocytopenia (*e.g.,* thiazides, alcohol, quinidine, methyldopa, sulfa, phenytoin, barbiturates), or inhibiting coagulation factor synthesis (coumarin).

Presence of a recent or *concurrent illness* that might affect hemostasis ought to be given particular attention, including chronic liver disease, uremia, viral infection, connective tissue disease, myeloproliferative states, and paraproteinemias.

Physical Examination. After taking the vital signs and checking for significant volume depletion, one can proceed with a systematic examination. General appearance is noted for cushingoid habitus and marfanoid appearance. On ex-amination of the skin, the size, number, and location of any *purpuric lesions* should be recorded, and note made of whether they are *petechial* (less than 3 mm) or *ecchymotic* (greater than 3 mm). Purpura represents bleeding into the skin, usually the result of vessel breakage or leakage. Petechial lesions occur with thrombocytopenia, qualitative platelet disorders, and vascular defects. Petechial rashes are also a hallmark of vasculitis, but the lesions in vasculitic cases are characteristically palpable, tender, pruritic, and surrounded by an erythematous flush (see Chapter 175). One can readily distinguish petechiae from nonpurpuric erythematous skin lesions by noting their failure to blanch when compressed with a glass slide.

Blanching lesions must not be dismissed too hastily, because they may be *telangiectasias,* which are an important clue to Rendu–Weber–Osler syndrome. Ecchymoses occur-

Table 80-2. Differentiating Platelet, Coagulation, and Vascular Disorders

CLINICAL FEATURES	PLATELET	COAGULATION	VASCULAR
Onset	Immediate	Delayed	Immediate
Duration	Short	Prolonged	Variable
Precipitant	Trauma	Often spontaneous	Variable
Site	Skin, mucous membranes, GI	Joints, muscle, viscera	Skin, GI tract
Family history	Absent	Usually present	Usually absent
Drug related	Often	Rarely	Sometimes
Sex predominance	Often female	Usually male	Usually female
Response to focal pressure	Usually effective	Ineffective	Effective
Platelet count	Normal, low, or excessive	Normal	Normal
Prothrombin time	Normal	Abnormal in cases of factor II, VII IX, and X deficiency	Normal
Partial thromboplastin time	Normal	Abnormal with factor VIII or IX deficiency	Normal

ring in areas subject to trauma are a common finding in normal people; however, ecchymotic lesions greater than 6 cm in the absence of major trauma are likely to represent an underlying bleeding problem. The skin is also noted for signs of chronic liver disease (spider angiomata, jaundice).

The mucous membranes are examined for bleeding, the lymph nodes for enlargement, the abdomen for hepatosplenomegaly, and the joints and muscles for hematomas and hemarthroses. Rectal and pelvic examinations are conducted for evidence of bleeding.

Laboratory Studies. Although the history and physical examination often provide important clues regarding etiology, laboratory investigation helps to classify the cause of the bleeding more definitively. Preliminary testing should include a PT, PTT, platelet count, and bleeding time. The *PT* best assays the extrinsic clotting system; the *PTT,* the intrinsic one. The PT and PTT may miss mild factor deficiencies (when levels are in excess of 25% of normal). The PTT will be prolonged in the absence of a bleeding diathesis when there is a deficiency of factor XII, kininogen, or prekallikrein.

The *platelet count* will formally document a quantitative problem. Finding platelets on a examination of a peripheral smear is good preliminary evidence of adequate quantity. The *bleeding time* is the best screening test of platelet function, and the *Ivy method* is the standard technique for its performance. A cut is made in a relatively avascular area of the forearm, utilizing a template to ensure an incision of 1 cm in length and 1 mm in depth, while venous return is obstructed with a blood-pressure cuff inflated to 40 mm Hg. Blotting paper is applied to the edge of the incision; a normal result is cessation of blotter-detected oozing by 9 minutes. Recent use of aspirin or another nonsteroidal anti-inflammatory agent will produce a modest prolongation in the bleeding time, although this usually does not represent a sig-

nificant risk of bleeding unless there is a pre-existing bleeding diathesis.

The need for further laboratory testing is determined by initial findings. A prolonged bleeding time in the setting of a normal platelet count, normal PT, and normal PTT is an indication to test for a qualitative defect in platelet aggregation, especially if there is no recent history of taking a nonsteroidal anti-inflammatory drug. *Aggregation study* is conducted by adding an aggregating substance such as ADP, epinephrine, collagen, or thrombin to a platelet-rich plasma sample. If the bleeding time and the PTT are prolonged, then *ristocetin-induced agglutination* of platelets can be obtained to check for von Willebrand's disease. Aggregation is normal in von Willebrand's disease, but the platelets fail to agglutinate. Aggregation and ristocetin studies are best ordered in consultation with a hematologist.

SYMPTOMATIC MANAGEMENT AND PATIENT EDUCATION

Patients with a clinically insignificant laboratory abnormality deserve detailed reassurance that they have adequate hemostasis. For example, the patient with a minor prolongation of bleeding time on preoperative testing yet no prior history of bleeding problems is unlikely to have anything more serious than recent salicylate exposure. Functional hemostasis will usually be preserved and no special precautions or further action (other than repeating the bleeding time) need be taken. However, the patient with a clinically important bleeding diathesis requires some basic advice, even as evaluation proceeds. The nature of the advice depends upon the type of bleeding problem at hand.

Vascular Defects. Reassurance can be given to patients with purpura simplex and senile purpura. Occasionally, these patients take large doses of vitamins C and K in hopes of lessening their easy bruisability; such self-treatment measures are without proven efficacy and only add unnecessary expense. Nonsteroidal anti-inflammatory agents may exacerbate their cosmetic problem and can be withheld if the easy bruising disturbs the patient, but they ought not be avoided if there is an important indication for their use. Patients with recurrent bleeding from more serious vascular disease (*e.g.,* hereditary hemorrhagic telangiectasia) should be advised to avoid any agent that might compromise hemostasis. Bleeding episodes respond to compression if the rest of the hemostatic system is kept intact. Patients with vascular defects often suffer iron deficiency from recurrent bleeding; the resulting anemia responds well to oral iron (see Chapter 84).

Platelet Disorders. Those with a known qualitative platelet disorder and a history of bleeding should be counselled to avoid salicylates and nonsteroidal agents. Patients who have no history of bleeding problems prior to nonsteroidal use can probably continue on the agent, provided the bleeding is clinically unimportant and the indication for drug use compelling. However, the drug should be stopped in anticipation of a major surgical procedure.

Patients with platelet counts less than 50,000 are at risk for posttraumatic bleeding and should be advised to put off surgery, dental extraction, and contact sports until the problem is corrected. Use of stool softeners and a soft toothbrush are recommended. Those with counts below 20,000 are at risk for serious spontaneous bleeding and require hospitalization. While work-up is in progress to identify an etiology, all but the most essential medications should be halted, with substance exposures (solvents, insecticides, alcohol) limited and nonsteroidal anti-inflammatory drugs prohibited.

Clotting Factor Problems. Most patients on coumarin who exhibit bleeding from excessive anticoagulation need only hold their dose for a few days to allow the PT to drift back into safe therapeutic range (see Chapter 85). Vitamin K should not be used to accomplish correction of the PT, unless anticoagulation is no longer desired; it is difficult to quickly re-anticoagulate a patient who has recently received large doses of vitamin K. Urgent need to correct the PT without impairing future anticoagulation efforts can be met by administering fresh frozen plasma.

Those with poor intake or *malabsorption of vitamin K* can be treated with oral vitamin K supplements (2.5 to 10 mg/day) or parenteral doses (10 to 25 mg IM) in addition to attending to the underlying cause of the malabsorption (see Chapter 58). Patients with severe hepatocellular failure will not respond to vitamin K because synthetic function has been compromised (see Chapter 71).

The patient and family with *hemophilia* face life-long problems. Detailed discussion of the management of such patients is beyond the scope of this chapter, but basic management includes specifying guidelines for permissible physical activity and teaching proper first aid. If the severity of bleeding has been only mild to moderate, then one can encourage participation in noncontact sports and other activities that have little risk of injury. The goal is to allow as much normal activity as possible. *First aid* treatment of an acute hemarthrosis should be learned by the family. One immobilizes the joint and applies ice packs to reduce pain and swelling. Splinting and elastic bandages can help ensure that a position of good joint function is maintained.

Pain control is important. Aspirin and related nonsteroidal agents must be avoided. Judicious use of acetaminophen and codeine work well when given in adequate doses for short periods of time. The primary physician should not try to aspirate a hemarthrosis; there is high risk of further bleeding and introducing infection.

Administration of *factor VIII* concentrates has been the mainstay of therapy, used for acute bleeding episodes and prior to surgery and dental work. Screening prospective blood donors for HTLV-III antibody greatly reduces the risk of transmitting the AIDS virus to hemophiliacs; however, many have already contracted the illness (see Chapter 142). *Desmopressin,* an analogue of vasopressin, is being used in place of factor VIII for treatment of patients with mild to moderate hemophilia or von Willebrand's disease and is proving effective for both acute bleeding episodes and prophylaxis. If future studies support these encouraging results, desmopressin should offer hemophilia patients an alternate means of treatment.

Genetic counselling is an important component of hemophiliac care. Definitive identification of women who are carriers of the hemophilia gene has been difficult, but DNA analysis techniques offer hope of improved identification to facilitate genetic counselling.

INDICATIONS FOR ADMISSION AND REFERRAL

Bleeding problems carry the potential for serious harm and bear very careful evaluation and monitoring. If there is any doubt as to the severity of the condition, prompt hospital admission should be considered. Patients who manifest volume depletion, gross bleeding, bleeding from multiple sites, or change in mental status require emergency admission. The otherwise well-appearing person with a dangerously low platelet count (less than 20,000), absence of platelets on smear or a markedly prolonged bleeding time is best evaluated and monitored in the hospital. Hemophiliacs with acute bleeding require emergency factor VIII transfusion.

Referral or consultation with a hematologist can be very helpful when a patient with clinical bleeding is suspected of having a qualitative platelet disorder. Proper test selection and interpretation will be facilitated. Referral is also indicated for patients with unexplained, clinically significant clotting factor deficiencies, severe thrombocytopenia, or suspected hemophilia or von Willebrand's disease.

A.H.G.

ANNOTATED BIBLIOGRAPHY

Antonarakis SE, Waber PG, Kittur SD et al: Hemophilia A: Detection of molecular defects and of carriers by DNA analysis. N Engl J Med 313:842, 1985 (*A report of DNA analysis of the factor VIII: C gene, providing an accurate method of carrier detection, which had previously been problematic.*)

Barber A, Green D, Galluzzo T et al: The bleeding time as a preoperative screening test. Am J Med 78:761, 1985 (*110 of 1941 preoperative bleeding times were prolonged, but in only 27 was the prolongation unexpected, and in only 2 was the bleeding time greater than 20 minutes. The authors conclude that routine screening of preoperative patients is not warranted; moreover, prolongation is not strongly predictive of excessive surgical blood loss.*)

Burns TR, Saleem A: Idiopathic thrombocytopenic purpura. Am J Med 75:1001, 1983 (*Good review that emphasizes new developments, such as significance of platelet-associated IgG.*)

de la Fuente B, Kasper C, Rickles FR et al: Response of patients with mild and moderate hemophilia A and von Willebrand's disease to treatment with desmopressin. Ann Intern Med 103:6, 1985 (*A report indicating that the vasopressin analogue is both effective and safe in treatment and prevention of bleeding episodes; a series of 68 cases.*)

Kitchens CS: The anatomic basis of purpura. Prog Hemostasis Thromb 5:21, 1980 (*An interesting discussion of purpura from the perspective of blood vessel structure and function.*)

Levine PH: The acquired immunodeficiency syndrome in persons with hemophilia. Ann Intern Med 103:723, 1985 (*Reviews prevalence, risk factors, and prevention.*)

Lind SE: Prolonged bleeding time. Am J Med 77:305, 1984 (*The bleeding time continues to be the best screening test of platelet function.*)

Ratnoff OD, Jones PK: Laboratory detection of the carrier state for classic hemophilia. Ann Intern Med 86:521, 1977 (*Details the standard method of carrier detection.*)

Suchman AL, Griner PF: Diagnostic uses of the activated partial thromboplastin time and prothrombin time. Ann Intern Med 104:810, 1986 (*Screening PTs and PTTs add little to screening in the absence of a history of bleeding. Normal PT and PTT rule out a clotting factor abnormality in the patient with a bleeding problem.*)

81
Evaluation of Lymphadenopathy
HARVEY B. SIMON, M.D.

Of the nearly 600 lymph nodes throughout the body, only a few are normally palpable, including small nodes in the submandibular, axillary, and inguinal regions. Nevertheless, lymphadenopathy is a very common presenting symptom. Most often, adenopathy indicates benign, self-limited disease; this is particularly true in children and young adults, who are more prone to reactive lymphatic hyperplasia. Despite this, patient concern is often substantial, due to worry about serious infectious processes (*e.g.,* AIDS) on one hand and neoplastic diseases on the other. A systematic evaluation of lymphadenopathy will provide reassurance as well as a correct diagnosis. A critical decision for the primary physician is when to refer the patient for lymph node biopsy.

PATHOPHYSIOLOGY AND CLINICAL PRESENTATION

Small lymph nodes in the neck, axilla, and groin may be palpable in normal individuals. Palpable nodes in other regions or any node exceeding 1 cm in size should be regarded as potentially abnormal. Inflammation and infiltration are responsible for pathologic enlargement. Although size alone is not itself diagnostic, nodes in excess of 3 cm suggest neoplastic disease. Localized lymphadenopathy may represent spread of disease from an area of drainage. Of particular importance are palpable supraclavicular nodes. The left one, which is sometimes referred to as the "sentinel" node, is in contact with the thoracic duct, which drains much of the abdominal cavity. The right supraclavicular node drains the mediastinum, lungs, and esophagus.

In addition to lymphadenopathy, abnormalities of the lymphatic system may present in other ways. Lymphangitis, appearing as red, warm streaks along the course of superficial lymphatic networks, suggests an acute inflammatory response to pyogenic infection in the drainage area; staphylococci and streptococci are frequently responsible. Lymphadenitis, presenting as a tender, warm, soft, rapidly enlarging node, has similar significance and often reflects acute pyogenic infection of the node itself. Lymphedema results from interruption of lymphatic drainage; surgical node dissection, radiotherapy, or fibrosis due to chronic infections such as filariasis or lymphogranuloma venereum are causes of lymphedema.

DIFFERENTIAL DIAGNOSIS

The causes of lymphadenopathy can be conveniently considered in terms of location of the enlarged nodes (Table 81-1). In children and young adults, most adenopathy is due to reactive hyperplasia and is less likely to represent serious pathology than is its occurrence in adults.

WORKUP

A number of fundamental questions should be raised in every case of lymph gland enlargement.

Table 81-1. Important Causes of Lymphadenopathy

GENERALIZED LYMPHADENOPATHY	LOCALIZED LYMPHADENOPATHY
Infections	*Anterior Auricular*
Mononucleosis	Viral conjunctivitis
AIDS	Trachoma, posterior auricular
AIDS-related complex (ARC)	Rubella
Toxoplasmosis	Scalp infection
Secondary syphilis	
	Submandibular or Cervical (Unilateral)
Hypersensitivity Reactions	Buccal cavity infection
Serum sickness	Pharyngitis (can be bilateral)
Phenytoin and other drugs	Nasopharyngeal tumor
Vasculitis (lupus, rheum. arthritis)	Thyroid malignancy
Metabolic Disease	*Cervical Bilateral*
Hyperthyroidism	Mononucleosis
Lipidoses	Sarcoidosis
	Toxoplasmosis
Neoplasia	Pharyngitis
Leukemia	
Hodgkin's disease (advanced stages)	*Supraclavicular, Right*
Non-Hodgkin's lymphoma	Pulmonary malignancy
	Mediastinal malignancy
	Esophageal malignancy
	Supraclavicular, Left
	Intra-abdominal malignancy
	Renal malignancy
	Testicular or ovarian malignancy
	Axillary
	Breast malignancy or infection
	Upper extremity infection
	Epitrochlear
	Syphilis (bilateral)
	Hand infection (unilateral)
	Inguinal
	Syphilis
	Genital herpes
	Lymphogranuloma venereum
	Chancroid
	Lower extremity or local infection
	Any Region
	Cat-scratch fever
	Hodgkin's disease
	Non-Hodgkin's lymphoma
	Leukemia
	Metastatic cancer
	Sarcoidosis
	Granulomatous infections

History and physical examination often provide critical information and the answers to many of these queries.

1. Is the palpable mass indeed a lymph node? A variety of other structures, including enlarged parotid glands, cervical hygromas, thyroglossal and branchial cysts, hemangiomas, abscesses, lipomas, and other tumors may on occasion be confused with lymphadenopathy.

2. Is the lymphadenopathy acute or chronic? Clearly, lymph node enlargement due to acute viral or pyogenic infections becomes less likely as the days and weeks pass, and granulomatous inflammation (sarcoid, tuberculosis, fungal infection) and neoplastic disease become greater worries. Even so, chronicity alone is not always a harbinger of serious disease, for on occasion reactive hyperplasia can persist for many months.

3. What is the character of the enlarged node itself? Tender, mobile nodes most often reflect lymphadenitis or lymphatic hyperplasia in response to acute inflammation. Firm, rubbery, nontender nodes may be found in lymphoma. Painless, stone-hard, fixed, matted nodes suggest metastatic carcinoma.

4. Is the adenopathy localized or generalized? Numerous systemic processes, including *infections* (*e.g.,* infectious mononucleosis and other viral infections, toxoplasmosis, secondary syphilis); *hypersensitivity reactions* (serum sickness, reactions to phenytoin [Dilantin] and other drugs, and vasculitis, including systemic lupus erythematosus and rheumatoid arthritis); *metabolic diseases* (hyperthyroidism and various lipidoses), and *neoplasia* (especially leukemia) can produce generalized lymphadenopathy. However, Hodgkin's disease is usually unicentric in origin and spreads to contiguous regional nodes, so that generalized adenopathy is rare except in very advanced disease. While certain non-Hodgkin's lymphomas may be multicentric, generalized adenopathy is also a late finding and is usually asymmetric, unlike the earlier and more symmetric adenopathy of some leukemias, such as chronic lymphocytic leukemia.

Generalized adenopathy, particularly if accompanied by weight loss, fever, or other constitutional symptoms, should raise the question of *AIDS* or *AIDS-related complex.* Male homosexuals, intravenous drug abusers, hemophiliacs and other multiply-transfused individuals, and Haitians are at particular risk (see Chapter 142).

Localized adenopathy should raise additional possibilities, depending on the area involved. For example, *submandibular* lymphadenopathy, which is perhaps the most common type of adenopathy, frequently results from pharyngitis (viral, streptococcal, gonococcal) or head and neck or intraoral infection. While these benign processes vastly predominate, it should be remembered that patients with Hodgkin's disease most often present with cervical lymphadenopathy. *Preauricular* adenopathy may be a component of "occuloglandular fevers" due to adenoviral conjunctivitis, sarcoidosis, tularemia, cat scratch disease, and other processes. *Posterior auricular* or *posterior cervical* adenopathy frequently reflects infections of the scalp, but may also be prominent in systemic processes, such as rubella or toxoplasmosis. While *anterior cervical* lymphadenopathy often results from head and neck infections, isolated supraclavicular node enlargement is more indicative of metastatic malignancy; the *right supraclavicular* nodes drain the mediastinum, esophagus, and thorax, while *left supraclavicular* adenopathy (Virchow's node) is suggestive of primary intra-abdominal neoplasia. *Axillary* nodes become enlarged in response to upper extremity infection, but breast cancer must be considered as well. Although enlarged *epitrochlear* nodes are traditionally associated with secondary syphilis, this finding reflects generalized lymphadenopathy in lues; epitrochlear lymphadenopathy can be seen in many other systemic processes, as well as in response to hand infections. *Inguinal* lymphadenopathy is much more common. Inguinal nodes are palpable in most normal individuals, but they can enlarge substantially in infections of the genitalia or perineum, as well as in lower extremity infections.

5. Are there associated systemic or localizing symptoms or signs? Fever, rash, weight loss, sore throat, dental pain, genital inflammation, and infections of the extremities are clues that may be particularly helpful. Of these symptoms, night sweats and weight loss are suggestive of granulomatous and neoplastic disease. Ear, nose, and throat symptoms suggest reactive lymphatic hyperplasia secondary to viral or localized bacterial infection.

A careful examination of the skin for a primary inoculation site may provide the clue to a diagnosis of processes such as cat scratch disease or tularemia. Careful examination for scalp infections, dermatophytes, and scabies may be rewarding. Similarly, the finding of hepatomegaly, splenomegaly, or both may be of great significance (*e.g.,* mononucleosis, sarcoidosis). Sternal tenderness can be present in leukemia.

6. Are there unusual epidemiologic clues? To cite a few examples, patients exposed to cats may develop cat scratch disease or toxoplasmosis, which may also result from eating poorly cooked meat. Travel to the southwest United States may suggest the possibility of plague. An appropriate travel history or exposure to bird droppings may suggest fungal infection, as may lacerations sustained while gardening, in the case of sporotrichosis. Contact with wild rodents may result in tularemia, as may tick bites. A history of exposure to tuberculosis may be an important clue to scrofula. More commonly, community outbreaks may provide clues to the diagnosis of streptococcal pharyngitis or rubella, while a history of sexual exposure may raise the question of gonorrhea, syphilis, genital herpes, or lymphogranuloma.

Laboratory studies need not be very elaborate. A *complete blood count* with *differential* is almost always indicated and may be a valuable clue to detection of infectious mononucleosis, other viral processes or toxoplasmosis (lymphocytosis, atypical lymphocytosis), pyogenic infection (granulocytosis), hypersensitivity states (eosinophilia), or malignancies (anemia, abnormal granulocytes). Leukopenia can be a clue to AIDS.

If pharyngitis or cervical or submandibular adenopathy is present, a *throat culture* is mandatory; it should be remembered that while these are routinely processed for streptococci, special Thayer–Martin medium must be used as well if gonococci are suspected. *Urethral* or *cervical cultures* and smears should also be obtained if gonorrhea is a potential cause of inguinal lymphadenopathy. Blood cultures are indicated in the rare cases of suspected plague, tularemia, or brucellosis, or if the clinical picture suggests staphylococcal or streptococcal lymphadenitis.

Serologic tests may be of great value; the *heterophil* and *serologic tests for syphilis* are obvious examples. *HTLV-III antibody testing* can facilitate diagnosis of patients with AIDS-related complex (see Chapter 142). In addition, a serum sample can be frozen during the acute phase of the illness to be submitted with a later convalescent phase serum specimen for *antibody titers* of various viruses, fungi, and *Toxoplasma*. Brucellosis may also be diagnosed serologically. Serological tests, including *antinuclear antibodies* and *rheumatoid factor,* may suggest a noninfectious process such as collagen-vascular disease. A different form of immunologic test, the delayed *hypersensitivity skin test,* can be useful in the evaluation of possible tuberculous lymphadenitis. Reliable skin tests are available for coccidioidomycosis and tularemia. On the other hand, cutaneous anergy may suggest sarcoidosis or lymphoma but is nonspecific. If available, a *Kveim skin test* may be helpful in the evaluation of sarcoidosis (see Chapter 48). Skin testing may be very helpful in the diagnosis of cat-scratch disease, but like the Kveim test, the necessary antigen is available only on a research basis in selected centers.

A variety of blood chemistries may help in selected cases. Elevations of *uric acid* may reflect lymphoma or other hematologic malignancies. Liver function tests are of particular value; while abnormalities may be present in a great variety of illnesses that produce lymphadenopathy (ranging from mononucleosis to sarcoidosis to malignancy), they do provide an additional parameter to follow, and may suggest liver involvement, which can be further evaluated by biopsy.

Among radiologic studies, the *chest x-ray* is particularly valuable, since hilar adenopathy may be present in patients with enlargement of peripheral nodes. Hilar adenopathy may also be detected on chest x-rays in the absence of peripheral lymphadenopathy. Sarcoidosis, lymphoma, fungal infection, tuberculosis, or metastatic carcinoma (particularly from a lung primary) should be among the diagnostic considerations. Mediastinoscopy may be required for diagnosis. On occasion, lymphomatous retroperitoneal or intra-abdominal nodes may enlarge enough to present as an abdominal mass. When lymphoma is a serious possibility, or when staging is necessary in known lymphoma or Hodgkin's disease, studies such as abdominal *computed tomography* can be used to detect enlargement of the retroperitoneal nodes; bone marrow biopsy may also be indicated (see Chapters 82 and 83).

In addition to the studies outlined above, careful *observation* over a period of time may be very useful diagnostically, since in many cases benign lymphadenopathy will regress spontaneously even if no etiologic diagnosis has been made. But if adenopathy persists over a period of weeks, if the nodes are enlarging, or if neoplastic disease seems likely, biopsy should be performed.

Lymph node biopsy should be considered as the most direct approach to the diagnosis of lymphadenopathy. Although the majority of such procedures are technically easy and can be accomplished under local anesthesia, this is an invasive test and should be employed only when simpler approaches have failed to provide a diagnosis and there is suspicion of a therapeutically important etiology, such as TB, lymphoma, cancer, sarcoid, or cat-scratch disease. In one retrospective study, weight loss, night sweats, nodes > 2cm, and abnormal chest x-ray were the strongest prebiopsy predictors of such important disease. In the case of fluctuant nodes, *needle aspiration* can be used to diagnose infectious processes in some cases.

The node to be biopsied should be selected with care; if generalized adenopathy is present, it is best to avoid inguinal or axillary nodes when possible, because reactive hyperplasia in these areas may make interpretation difficult. In general, enlarged supraclavicular nodes have the highest diagnostic yield. When possible, excisional biopsy is preferred. At the time of biopsy, tissue should be submitted for appropriate bacteriologic smears and cultures, as well as for histologic study. Touch preps may be useful. Special stains for bacteria, mycobacteria, and fungi may be helpful, as may specific stains for unusual processes such as PAS stains for Whipple's disease or lipidosis, and Congo red stains for amyloid. Interpretation of lymph node pathology can be quite difficult and requires careful study by experienced observers. With such study, benign processes such as toxoplasmosis or cat-scratch disease can be suspected histologically, and detailed analysis of serial sections may reveal lymphomas that are not diagnosed with less intensive pathologic study. Finally, if pathologic study reveals reactive hyperplasia or is nondiagnostic, patients should be followed carefully, since up to 25% may eventually exhibit an illness responsible for the lymphadenopathy, most often lymphoma.

ANNOTATED BIBLIOGRAPHY

Abrams DI, Lewis BJ, Blackstead JH et al: Persistent lymphadenopathy in homosexual men: Endpoint or prodrome? Ann Intern Med 100:801, 1984 (*Seventy homosexual men with adenopathy and constitutional symptoms, but without the opportunistic infections or neoplasia diagnostic of AIDS. It is not known how many of these patients with AIDS-related complex go on to develop the full syndrome.*)

Greenfield S, Jordan MC: The clinical investigation of lymphadenopathy in primary care practice. JAMA 240:1388, 1978 (*A systematic algorithmic approach to the work-up of peripheral lymphadenopathy in the ambulatory setting.*)

Lalle AM, Oski FA: Peripheral lymphadenopathy in childhood. Am J Dis Child 132:357, 1978 (*A retrospective study of 75 lymph node biopsies in patients younger than 18. Fifty-five percent were nondiagnostic, 28% showed granulomatous inflammation, and 17% showed lymphoproliferative disorders. Clinical findings correlated poorly with pathologic diagnosis.*)

Petricciani JC: Licensed test for antibody to human T-lymphocyte virus Type III: Sensitivity and specificity. Ann Intern Med 103:726, 1985 (*Reports sensitivity ranges from 0.93 to 0.99 and specificity 0.99.*)

Saltzstern SL: The fate of patients with nondiagnostic lymph node biopsies. Surgery 58:659, 1965 (*A retrospective study of lymph node biopsies in 177 adult males. In 68 patients, the indication for biopsy was lymphadenopathy; 52% of these were nondiagnostic, but 17% of patients with nondiagnostic biopsies subsequently developed lymphoma. Supraclavicular node biopsies had the highest diagnostic yield.*)

Schroer KR, Fransilla KO: Atypical hyperplasia of lymph nodes: A follow-up study. Cancer 44:115, 1979 (*Of patients with nondiagnostic lymph node biopsies, 25% to 60% were found within a few months to have lymphoma, cancer, connective tissue disease, or infection. Emphasizes importance of follow up.*)

Sinclair S, Beckman E, Ellman L: Biopsy of enlarged superficial lymph nodes. JAMA 228:602, 1974 (*A retrospective pathologic study of 135 lymph node biopsies performed because of undiagnosed lymphadenopathy. Sixty-three percent of the biopsies were diagnostic; 50 patients had lymphoma, 14 carcinoma, 6 tuberculosis, 1 histoplasmosis, 7 acute lymphadenitis, and 1 Dilantin sensitivity. Of the 50 patients with nondiagnostic biopsies, 25% developed a disease related to the indications for biopsy, which was most often lymphoma, and which usually occurred within 8 months of the initial biopsy.*)

Slap GB, Brooks JSJ, Schwartz JS: When to perform biopsies of enlarged peripheral lymph nodes in young patients. JAMA 252:1321, 1984 (*A retrospective study of 123 patients up to the age of 25 who underwent lymph node biopsy. A predictive model was developed to determine before biopsy which patients were likely to have "treatable" causes of adenopathy.*)

82

Approach to the Patient with Hodgkin's Disease

JACOB J. LOKICH, M.D.

Hodgkin's disease must be considered an uncommon malignancy in that the annual incidence is approximately three cases per 100,000 population, or a total of approximately 7,000 cases annually. However, the disease is essential to recognize and properly manage because it affects young people and is often curable. Peak incidence is between the ages of 20 and 40 (with a second peak over 60). The primary physician has an important role in staging the disease, coordinating plans for management, and delivering follow-up care on an outpatient basis.

PATHOLOGY, CLINICAL PRESENTATION, AND COURSE

The histology of Hodgkin's disease incorporates four categories: lymphocyte predominance, nodular sclerosis, mixed cellularity, and lymphocyte depletion. *Lymphocyte predominance* occurs in 10% to 15% of patients, *nodular sclerosis* in 20% to 50%, mixed cellularity in 20% to 40%, and *lymphocyte depletion* in 5% to 15%. In about 15% of cases, classification is difficult and requires expert interpretation of the histology. In all instances the *sine qua non* of diagnosis is the pathognomonic *Reed-Sternberg cell*.

The clinical presentation of the disease most commonly involves cervical or mediastinal adenopathy, which is asymmetrical and asymptomatic; however, any area containing lymph nodes may be the site of presentation, including the axilla and the inguinal region. The nodes are characteristically firm and nontender; they often are matted, but may be discrete and freely movable. Fever, weight loss, night sweats, or alcohol-induced pain may develop and almost always represents advanced stage disease.

Conceptually, Hodgkin's disease is *unicentric* in origin and progresses by contiguous extension along lymphatic pathways. This pattern of evolution is in contrast to non-Hodgkin's lymphomas, which are multicentric and associated with more advanced stages of disease at initial presentation.

The differential diagnosis of Hodgkin's disease includes infectious mononucleosis, AIDS, and other nonbacterial adenopathies in the young (see Chapter 81). In the elderly, other malignancies are a common diagnostic consideration; they are particularly suspect in the presence of a fever of unknown origin.

Staging at time of presentation is important for determination of prognosis and choice of therapy (Table 82-1).

Table 82-1. Hodgkin's Disease: Stages, Relative Incidences, and Prognosis

STAGE	DEFINITION	RELATIVE INCIDENCE (%)	THERAPY	5-YEAR SURVIVAL (%)*	5-YEAR RELAPSE-FREE (%)*
Stage I	Confined to single node-bearing area	30	Radiation	86.0	72.5
Stage II	Confined to two contiguous node-bearing areas; on one side of diaphragm	25	Radiation	93.6	69.0
Stage III	In nodal areas on both sides of the diaphragm	25	Radiation and chemotherapy	81.3	61.1
Stage IV	Visceral lesions (liver, lung) *not in* contiguity with nodes	20	Chemotherapy	39.0	26.9
Special Categories					
E	Visceral extranodal disease in continuity with nodes. For example, lung mass extending out from hilum		Radiation +/− chemotherapy		
B	Symptoms of fever, weight loss, or sweats		Chemotherapy +/− radiation		

* Survival and disease-free figures for each stage combine patients with A and B disease. (Kaplan HS, Rosenberg S: Management of Hodgkin's disease. Cancer, 36:796, 1975)

Stage I is defined as disease confined to a single node-bearing area; *stage II* involves two contiguous node-bearing areas on the same side of the diaphragm; *stage III* is nodal involvement on both sides of the diaphragm; and *stage IV* represents visceral (liver, lung parenchyma, bone) lesions. Additional subcategories have been developed for patients with intra-abdominal disease. *Stage III$_1$* represents disease confined to the upper abdomen; it is generally microscopic. *Stage III$_2$* designates disease extending into the pelvis with grossly involved nodes or bulky retroperitoneal disease.

The special category designated *E* (for extranodal) was created because of data indicating that involvement of an organ contiguous to a lymph node-bearing area has a distinctly better prognosis than does visceral involvement that is hematogenous. Nonetheless, the prognosis is not as good as it would be if there were no organ involvement.

Early (stages I and II) and advanced (stages III and IV) Hodgkin's disease are relatively equally distributed in terms of frequency. More sophisticated staging by pathologic as well as clinical procedures generally tends to advance the stage of disease. Approximately 20% of patients will have *fever, night sweats,* or a *significant loss of weight.* These systemic symptoms are incorporated into the staging system because they are important determinants of prognosis. When absent, the designation is *A;* when any of the three is present, the designation is *B.* Patients with pruritus only are no longer included in the B group.

The prognosis of Hodgkin's disease has improved dramatically with the advent of careful staging and improved radiation technology and chemotherapy programs. Overall 5-year survival is 80%; 60% experience 5-year relapse-free survival when all stages of disease are combined (see Table 82-1).

PRINCIPLES OF MANAGEMENT

Staging

Staging (Table 82-2) is critical to design of a therapeutic program and estimation of prognosis. *Clinical staging* involves assessment of history, physical examination, and radiologic findings. However, most treatment decisions require *pathologic staging,* which includes biopsy evidence of disease extent. History should ascertain presence of fever, night sweats, or weight loss. Careful palpation of all lymph nodes and assessment of liver and spleen size are important, though enlargement discovered by physical examination does not necessarily indicate involvement by the disease. One-half of patients with a palpable spleen do not have histologic splenic involvement, and one-quarter with normal-sized spleens do.

The principal staging procedures include chest x-ray, computed tomography (CT), lymphangiography, and bone marrow biopsy. All patients should have a *plain film* of the chest, because some of the most common forms of Hodgkin's disease involve the mediastinum. *CT of the chest* provides definition of any mediastinal, hilar, or paravertebral adenopathy.

Lymphangiography was developed to detect occult disease below the diaphragm by visualizing the retroperitoneal nodes. Unfortunately, the test has a low sensitivity, with a false-negative rate of 20%; this limits its utility for staging. When strict radiologic criteria for nodal involvement are used, specificity reaches 95%, with less than 5% false-positives noted. Thus, a positive study is helpful, but a negative lymphangiogram does not rule out disease below the diaphragm and requires use of a more definitive staging procedure. Moreover, even if the test is positive, it does not detect involvement of the liver or spleen, which is an important de-

Table 82-2.   Staging Procedures for Hodgkin's Disease

STUDY	INDICATION
Radiographic Studies	
Chest radiography	All patients; tomograms if mediastinal or hilar disease
Lymphangiogram	*Only if* (a) no clinical evidence of infradiaphragmatic disease, (b) no mass or lung disease, or (c) no advanced stage signs or symptoms (B)
Abdominal CT	Complements lymphangiogram; same indications
Surgical Studies	
Laparoscopy	Preferable to laparotomy in presence of B symptoms. To identify liver pathology
Laparotomy	Stage I or II disease and no symptoms
Hematologic Studies	
Bone marrow biopsy	Only if clinical stage IIB or more
Liver function tests Complete blood count ESR, serum copper, leukocyte alkaline phosphatase	Usefulness unclear

terminant of therapy. Lymphangiography carries a small risk of pulmonary insufficiency related to extravasation of dye in the lung parenchyma, and it should not be performed in those with severe lung disease. Lymphangiography should be performed in all patients with clinical stage I or II disease without B symptoms, particularly those patients in whom laparotomy is scheduled, in order to identify the lymph nodes to be removed. About 25% of patients classified clinically are reclassified on the basis of lymphangiogram results.

Abdominal CT complements lymphangiography by providing anatomic information about nodes in areas not well visualized by lymphangiography (mesentery, porta hepatis, celiac, and para-aortic regions). CT cannot detect microscopic disease and gives less information than the lymphangiogram about nodal architecture. Radionuclide scans of the liver and bone have not proved useful for routine use.

Bone marrow biopsy is a useful staging procedure in patients with systemic symptoms or disease beyond stage II, being positive in up to 20% of such patients. Since disease in the marrow is often focal, multiple biopsies are necessary to avoid sampling error. Marrow aspiration is never useful. A positive marrow classifies the disease as stage IV, and makes laparotomy unnecessary. Patients with clinical stage I or IIA disease have never been reported to have positive marrow biopsies, but stage IIB is associated with marrow involvement in 9% of patients.

Staging laparotomy is generally performed in patients who clinically have stage I or II disease. The procedure includes wedge biopsy of the liver, splenectomy, and examination of the lymph nodes in contiguous chains, exclusive of mesenteric nodes. The operation has a low mortality rate (0.5%) and negligible early morbidity. However, patients who receive radiation and chemotherapy after splenectomy are at some

risk (21% in one series) for fulminant sepsis, with its attendant 50% mortality; those who undergo splenectomy but do not receive combination therapy appear to be much less vulnerable to serious infection. Because of the risk of serious infection, only those who will have their treatment program altered by the results of laparotomy should undergo the operation. Patients who are candidates for laparotomy require tracheal tomography to be sure no mediastinal lesions are compressing the trachea and capable of causing airway obstruction during intubation for surgery.

The staging laparotomy has the advantage of allowing more precise definition of the extent of disease, thereby guiding more rational therapeutic approaches. Laparotomy frequently results in reclassification of patients into different disease stages and consequent alterations in therapeutic programs. In a series of 114 patients who underwent staging laparotomy, 18 received less irradiation, 10 received more, 2 were given radiation instead of chemotherapy, and 4 received chemotherapy instead of radiation. Two other advantages of laparotomy with splenectomy are that radiation to the left upper quadrant can be avoided and in women the ovaries can be moved out of the way of a radiation therapy portal. At the present time, laparotomy is indicated in all patients with stage I or II disease without symptoms. In clinical stage III disease, the issue of laparotomy is controversial. Chemotherapy is being employed more commonly in stage III, so that pathologic confirmation by laparotomy may not be necessary for determining choice of therapy.

Laparoscopy has been advocated as a less invasive means of identifying liver involvement in patients with a high probability of disease below the diaphragm, for example, those with B symptoms. Liver biopsy specimens are taken from suspicious areas under direct visualization. Laparoscopy is superior to percutaneous liver biopsy (20% yield vs. 5%), but its yield does not quite match that of open biopsy performed during staging laparotomy. Few patients with Hodgkin's disease that involves the liver are free of systemic complaints; on the other hand, neither hepatomegaly upon physical examination or scan nor elevated alkaline phosphatase levels identify patients likely to have positive biopsies.

Many other tests for staging of Hodgkin's disease lack sensitivity and/or specificity. Such is the case for liver and spleen scans, bone scans, and gallium scans, which are not indicated in routine staging. Complete blood count, alkaline phosphatase, and sedimentation rate are similarly nonspecific. The use of the erythrocyte sedimentation rate, serum copper, and leukocyte alkaline phosphatase as indices of disease activity and extent is promoted by various investigators, but all of these tests represent nonspecific approaches to evaluating the patient with Hodgkin's disease.

In sum, the history is reviewed for characteristic systemic symptoms; the physical examination focuses on lymph-node bearing areas. A chest x-ray is obtained, as is lymphangiography and abdominal CT in patients who are clinically in stage I or II. If the patient is clinically in stage I or II and would be treated by radiation, a staging laparotomy should be performed to identify occult disease below the diaphragm. Until it becomes possible to predict more accurately who is likely to have occult disease in the abdomen, one must rely on the laparotomy. In instances where systemic symptoms are present, a laparoscopy and bone marrow biopsy can be performed as preliminary studies; if either is positive, the need for laparotomy is obviated. Lymphangiography produces too many false negatives to be relied upon without intra-abdominal evaluation and, even if positive, fails to provide information about the liver and spleen, which is necessary for selecting radiation therapy, chemotherapy, or both.

Treatment

Although selection of treatment modality is the province of the oncologist, it is important for the primary physician to be cognizant of the most common treatment regimens and their outcomes. Therapy for Hodgkin's disease has resulted in a cure rate which is substantial in all stages. For patients with stage IA and IIA disease, *local radiotherapy* to contiguous node-bearing areas has resulted in an 85% to 90% cure rate. *Total nodal radiation therapy* has been used in stages IB and IIB, delivered at a dose of 3500 to 4500 rads over a 3- to 4-week period through a portal referred to as the "mantle" for chest radiation and the "inverted Y" for intra-abdominal lymph nodes. Stage IB and IIB patients have a 70% to 75% chance of cure with such radiation therapy. Sometimes chemotherapy is added when there is a large mediastinal mass, systemic symptoms, or contiguous extranodal disease; optimal therapy in such instances remains a subject of debate.

Radiotherapy as a single modality has been employed for patients with stage III disease, particularly in asymptomatic

stage III_1A disease, and the cure rate is in the range of 50% to 60%. More recently, Hodgkin's disease distributed on either side of the diaphragm (stage III) has been treated with a combined approach of radiation therapy and chemotherapy and with chemotherapy alone.

The *chemotherapy* of Hodgkin's disease is a milestone in the development of cancer therapy. The Mustargen, Oncovin, prednisone, procarbazine (*MOPP*) therapeutic program developed in 1965 at the National Cancer Institute has served as a prototype for the development of combination chemotherapy, as it is known today, for many malignant diseases. The program is based on the identification of four agents with individually distinctive mechanisms of antitumor activity. Their side effects are nonadditive, thus minimizing drug-related morbidity. Response rates for stage IIIB and IV disease are in the 80% range, and complete remission of disease is the rule.

By manipulation of dosages and schedules of drugs, sophisticated chemotherapy can be delivered conveniently to outpatients. Potentially curative therapy in patients with advanced disease in the stage IV category has become possible for approximately 50% of the patients who enter complete remission. MOPP therapy is administered for 6 months, at which time restaging is carried out; in the absence of residual disease, therapy is discontinued.

Over 50% of patients *relapse* after complete remission with MOPP therapy. Retreatment with MOPP may induce a second remission if the disease-free interval was over 12 months. An alternative chemotherapeutic approach was developed for the substantial numbers of patients who *relapse* after radiation and subsequent MOPP therapy. The combination referred to as ABVD incorporates Adriamycin, bleomycin, vinblastine and DTIC, or diaminotriazenoimidazole (Carboxamide). This noncross-resistant regimen is employed in patients who are MOPP-resistant, and, more recently, in combination with MOPP either as an alternative sequence or as a compact therapy following a course of MOPP therapy. The response rate is comparable to that achieved with MOPP therapy; the durability and potential for cure are not yet established, but long-term, disease-free survival appears to be uncommon.

Among the adverse effects of treatment are sterility, secondary malignancy, and increased susceptibility to infection. MOPP produces *sterility* in over 80% of males so treated. Sperm-banking is indicated prior to initiation of therapy. The incidence of sterility is lower with ABVD. Risk of *secondary malignancy* (e.g., acute non-lymphocytic leukemia) occurring within 5 to 10 years of treatment is increased and is greatest in patients over age 40 who receive combined modality therapy, especially when MOPP is used. Other chemotherapy-related side effects include severe emesis, bone marrow suppression, and neuropathy.

The risk of overwhelming *pneumococcal sepsis* associated with splenectomy can be lessened by use of polyvalent *pneumococcal vaccine*. The vaccine is often given prior to splenectomy but can be administered following surgery; antibody response is just as adequate after splenectomy. However, antibody production is blunted if chemotherapy is begun within 10 days of vaccination.

MONITORING THERAPY

Periodic examination of involved nodes is the simplest means of judging response to therapy. Many laboratory parameters have been developed but offer little advantage over physical examination and chest x-ray. The need for periodic restaging is a judgment to be made in consultation with the oncologist. Patients receiving MOPP require close surveillance (see Chapter 89). Patients being treated with radiation should be watched for bone marrow suppression, and, when lung fields are involved, radiation pneumonitis and thyroid dysfunction.

The likelihood of *late relapse* (36 months or more after completion of therapy) is small, but large enough to warrant continued monitoring. Recent figures from Stanford showed a risk of late recurrence of 12.9%; patients with stage I disease or nodular sclerosis histology showed the highest rates of late relapse. Unirradiated nodes were the most common site of relapse. Use of adjuvant chemotherapy did not appear to alter the risk of late relapse. Eighty-eight percent of relapses at Stanford were detected by history, physical examination, or chest x-ray; abdominal CT may also help detect late disease. Careful late follow-up is warranted, even after 3 years. Response to retreatment is good.

Another group at risk for recurrence are patients presenting with a large mediastinal tumor; local recurrence is typical. Monitoring is done by checking visceral sites near node-bearing areas.

PATIENT EDUCATION

Many patients will greet the diagnosis of Hodgkin's disease with dread, equating it with carcinoma and a fatal outcome. Without raising false hopes, the physician can point to the excellent 5-year survival rates and the high percentage of individuals who are disease-free after 10 years. Patients who have undergone splenectomy should be advised to have polyvalent pneumococcal vaccine before undergoing chemotherapy or radiation, which inhibits immune response. Since chemotherapy can cause permanent sterility, it is important to review this prospect with the patient and family before embarking on treatment. Pretherapy sperm storage has been advocated. An encouraging report of a retrospective study indicates that women successfully treated for Hodgkin's disease are capable of bearing phenotypically normal children.

INDICATIONS FOR CONSULTATION AND REFERRAL

Hodgkin's disease is an excellent example of a condition requiring the advice and coordination of many specialists.

The primary physician needs to consult the oncologist, surgeon, and radiation therapist to plan staging and selection of a therapeutic program; yet, with their help, he can provide the major portion of ongoing care.

ANNOTATED BIBLIOGRAPHY

Aisenberg A: The staging and treatment of Hodgkin's disease. N Engl J Med 299:1288, 1978 (*In a series of 75 patients with clinical stage I or II disease, one-third were reclassified to clinical stage III on the basis of a positive lymphangiogram, and another one-third on the basis of a staging laparotomy.*)

Bagley C, Roth J, Thomas L et al: Liver biopsy in Hodgkin's disease. Ann Intern Med 76:219, 1975 (*Yield of percutaneous biopsy was half that obtained by laparoscopy or laparotomy.*)

Canellos GP, Come SE, Skarin AT: Chemotherapy in the treatment of Hodgkin's disease. Semin Hematol 20:1, 1983 (*A comprehensive review of approaches to chemotherapy for all stages of the disease.*)

Coker DD, Morris DM, Coleman JJ et al: Infection among 210 patients with surgically staged Hodgkin's disease. Am J Med 75:97, 1983 (*The overwhelming pneumococcal sepsis syndrome is uncommon in splenectomized patients in the absence of a predisposing factor, such as extremes of age or increasing stage of disease.*)

Fisher RI, DeVita VT, Hubbard SP et al: Prolonged disease-free survival in Hodgkin's disease with MOPP reinduction after first relapse. Ann Intern Med 90:761, 1979 (*Patients who relapse after at least 12 months of remission induced by MOPP may respond with another remission to retreatment with MOPP.*)

Greenberg LH, Wong YS, Richardson AP Jr et al: Combination chemotherapy of Hodgkin's disease in private practice. JAMA 221:261, 1972 (*This unusual report of the application of sophisticated combination chemotherapy in the private practice of medicine attests to the safety and comparability of therapeutic results to the more complex large institution trials.*)

Herman TS, Hoppe RT, Donaldson SS et al: Late relapses among patients treated for Hodgkin's disease. Ann Intern Med 102:292, 1985 (*A report from the Stanford cohort indicating that prolonged surveillance for late relapse is necessary, because rate of relapse was substantial (12.9%). Survival after treatment for late disease was good and similar to that for early relapse.*)

Horning SJ, Hoppe RT, Kaplan HS et al: Female reproductive potential after treatment for Hodgkin's disease. N Engl J Med 304:1377, 1981 (*Reports retrospectively on 103 women, finding that even after intensive treatment programs, women successfully treated for Hodgkin's can become pregnant and deliver phenotypically normal children.*)

Kadin ME, Glatstein E, Dorfman RF: Clinicopathologic studies of 117 untreated patients subjected to laparotomy for the staging of Hodgkin's disease. Cancer 27:1277, 1971 (*A follow-up of the initial report of the use of laparotomy in staging patients with Hodgkin's disease, which has become a standard procedure. The use of laparotomy as a determinant of therapy is not specifically emphasized, but the low complication rate is indicated.*)

Pedersen-Bjergaard Larsen SO: Incidence of acute nonlymphocytic leukemia, preleukemia and acute myeloproliferative syndrome up to 10 years after treatment of Hodgkin's disease. N Engl J

Med 307:965, 1982 (*Seventeen cases of leukemic complication occurred among 312 patients. Despite the observed relatively high risk, especially among older patients, the rate of death from progressive Hodgkin's disease, nonleukemic complications, and unrelated causes still exceeds the rate of leukemia-related deaths.*)

Rosenberg SA, Kaplan HS: The evolution and summary results of the Stanford randomized clinical trials of the management of Hodgkin's disease: 1962–1984. Int J Radiat Oncol Biol Phys 11: 5, 1985 (*A summary report from one of the leading centers for treatment of Hodgkin's disease.*)

Siber GR, Gorham C, Martin P et al: Antibody response to pretreatment immunization and post-treatment boosting with bacterial polysaccharide vaccines in patients with Hodgkin's disease. Ann Intern Med 104:467, 1986 (*Antibody response was not affected by timing of immunization relative to splenectomy, but was blunted if chemotherapy was begun within 10 days of immunization. No spontaneous rebound was seen one year after therapy and no increase with booster vaccination.*)

Santoro A, Bonadonna G, Bonfante V et al: Alternating drug combinations in the treatment of advanced Hodgkin's disease. N Engl J Med 306:770, 1982 (*This prospective randomized trial, although yet to be independently confirmed, is a well-designed and probably definitive study addressing the optimal application of chemotherapy for Hodgkin's disease.*)

Santoro A, Bonfante V, Bonadonna G: Salvage chemotherapy with ABVD in MOPP-resistant Hodgkin's disease. Ann Intern Med 96:139, 1982 (*The use of ABVD achieved a 59% complete response rate in patients resistant to MOPP chemotherapy, 38% of whom are disease-free at 5 years. Long-term complications may be less profound with ABVD therapy.*)

Wagener DJT, Burgers MV, Dekker W et al, for the EORTC Radiotherapy-Chemotherapy Cooperative Group: Sequential non-cross-resistant chemotherapy regimens (MOPP and CAVmP) in Hodgkin's disease stage IIIB and IV. Cancer 52:1558, 1983 (*Alternating three or four drug regimens for treatment of malignancy may increase the curability potential in Hodgkin's disease [as well as other malignancies] based on preventing the development of tumor cell resistance.*)

83
Approach to the Patient with Non-Hodgkin's Lymphoma

JACOB J. LOKICH, M.D.

Non-Hodgkin's lymphoma is twice as common as Hodgkin's disease, with 15,000 new cases annually and an incidence of 6 per 100,000 population. There are multiple subtypes, each with specific immunologic and pathologic characteristics and a distinctive clinical presentation and therapeutic response. Non-Hodgkin's lymphoma strikes much later than Hodgkin's disease; peak incidence is in the fifth decade. Prognosis is considerably less favorable in terms of long-term cure, although survival and responsiveness to therapy are substantial.

The role of the primary care physician is to carry out staging and help design and implement a therapeutic program in conjunction with the oncologist.

PATHOLOGY, CLINICAL PRESENTATION, AND PROGNOSIS

In contrast to Hodgkin's disease, the pathologic characteristics of a non-Hodgkin's lymphoma are major determinants of prognosis and response to therapy, while stage at time of presentation is of somewhat less importance. The categories outlined in Table 83-1 represent a composite of classification schemes based on those of Rappaport and others. Classification schemes continue to evolve; an international one has defined 13 separate types of lymphoma, grouping them according to prognosis. General acceptance and application of the international classification are not uniform.

Nodal architecture, cell type and differentiation are key histologic features that influence prognosis and response to therapy. Distribution and stage are of lesser importance than in Hodgkin's disease; most patients present with widespread disease (stage III or IV). Immunologic characterization is of etiologic interest, but its clinical significance remains unclear at the present time.

Architecture refers to the arrangement of tumor cells within the lymph node at the time of pathologic analysis. Two patterns predominate: nodular and diffuse. The *nodular* pattern indicates a favorable prognosis (see Table 83-1) and a substantial likelihood of response to therapy, be it total body irradiation or single-drug chemotherapy. In contrast, *diffuse* histology is associated with shorter survival, even though the response rate to combination chemotherapy is significant; however, one subtype with diffuse histology, diffuse lymphocytic, well-differentiated lymphoma, has a good prognosis.

Cell type and differentiation also influence prognosis and therapeutic response. The clinical course of the *well-differentiated lymphocytic* type is indolent, with a median survival of 7 years. Of the cell types *lymphoblastic, histiocytic,* and *mixed lymphocytic-histiocytic,* only the histiocytic type is potentially curable, with a response rate to combination che-

Table 83-1. Pathologic Categories in Non-Hodgkin's Lymphoma

CATEGORY	RESPONSE TO CHEMOTHERAPY	SURVIVAL
Architectural Distribution		
Nodular	40%–50%	Long
Diffuse	60%–80%	Short
Cell Type (Differentiation)		
Lymphoblastic	60%–80%	Unestablished
Histiocytic	50%–60%	20% Long-term
Mixed	60%–80%	Unestablished
Variants		
Immunoblastic	Variable	Unknown
Hairy cell	Variable	Long

motherapy of 50% to 60% and cure achieved in 20% to 30%. *Immunoblastic* lymphomas are in a special category, having an unpredictable prognosis and demonstrating variable responsiveness to chemotherapy. A distinctive variant is the *hairy cell* lymphoma, characterized by splenomegaly, a leukemic phase, and an excellent prognosis.

Distribution and stage have some influence on prognosis, although, as noted earlier, the vast majority of patients present with *disseminated* disease (stages III and IV). *Localized* and *regional* lymphomas (stages I and II respectively) account for less than 10% of cases. Non-Hodgkin's lymphomas can occur in nodal sites, in viscera, or in both. *Extranodal disease* is often solitary and likely to be confined to the organ of origin. Waldeyer's ring, bone, and upper gastrointestinal tract are the most commonly involved extranodal sites, accounting for up to 15% of cases in some series. Extranodal disease can have a favorable prognosis, particularly in the absence of nodal involvement. Five-year survival rates are as high as 30% to 50% irrespective of pathologic type. A unique site of extranodal disease is the central nervous system, especially the epidural space, leptomeninges, and cerebral hemispheres. The propensity for developing CNS lymphoma is related to histologic type (lymphoblastic), distribution (marrow spread), and age (younger patients).

The staging system for lymphoma is identical to that used for Hodgkin's disease (see Chapter 82), with the exception that there are no categories for symptoms or designations for contiguous visceral involvement or splenic disease.

PRINCIPLES OF MANAGEMENT

Staging

Although pathologic typing is most important to clinical decision-making, staging helps to determine prognosis and affects the selection and intensity of treatment. Unlike Hodgkin's disease, non-Hodgkin's lymphomas are multicentric in origin and can appear in discontinuous lymph node chains.

Physical examination requires evaluation of all node-bearing areas, including such sites as the epitrochlear area, Waldeyer's ring, and preauricular nodes. Liver and spleen are commonly enlarged when involved. Routine staging is conducted with *chest radiographs* and *bone marrow biopsy* (especially in patients with follicular histology). Bilateral or multiple bone marrow biopsies can identify occult stage IV disease. In a series of 131 patients, 27% had positive biopsies when more than one marrow site was sampled. Aspiration is inadequate, since the false-negative rate is 30%; a solid bone marrow specimen is essential.

Patients with clinical stage I or II disease (confined to one regional area above the diaphram) should undergo a *lymphangiogram* or *computed tomography (CT) of the abdomen and pelvis.* For lymphangiography, the reported false-negative rate ranges from 8% to 33% and the false-positive rate from 11% to 17%. CT is proving superior to lymphangiography, particularly for detection of disease in the pelvis and retroperitoneum; it will probably replace the older procedure. *Lumbar puncture* should be considered in patients at risk for CNS spread (*i.e.,* those with marrow involvement, lymphoblastic histology, or young age).

Several staging procedures are unnecessary. *Laparotomy* is not indicated because the yields from lymphangiogram, CT, and bone marrow biopsy are so high that rarely do the findings from laparotomy influence clinical decision making. Gallium scanning is also not very helpful.

Therapy

Chemotherapy is the predominant mode of treatment for non-Hodgkin's lymphoma (Table 83-2) because most patients already have widespread disease at the time of initial clinical presentation. It may be administered as a single agent or as a complex multidrug regimen. Radiation plays a role in management of localized disease.

Focal Disease. Radiation therapy is reserved for patients with stage I disease manifested by localized nodal or extranodal involvement. Total body irradiation has been employed, but only on an investigational basis for patients with nodal histology and stage III distribution.

Indolent Disease. Management of patients with asymptomatic, indolent disease characterized by confinement to the lymph nodes, nodular histology, and well-differentiated cell type is a subject of ongoing debate. Many monitor these patients and withhold treatment until they become symptomatic. A single agent applied intermittently for symptoms or high-grade disease may achieve control for long periods of time; some patients survive for up to 10 years. Some employ single-agent chemotherapy at the time of initial presentation, and a few treat aggressively from the outset with combination chemotherapy. Results of long-term clinical trials will provide much needed data on the optimal approach.

Table 83-2.   Therapeutic Approaches to Non-Hodgkin's Lymphomas

INDICATION	TREATMENT
Localized disease (stage I or IE)	Radiation to the involved field
Well-differentiated lymphocytic disease, nodular or diffuse	Controversial, though most follow expectantly
Diffuse disease (with exception of that which is well differentiated)	Multi-agent chemotherapy
Histiocytic and mixed cell types	Multi-agent chemotherapy
Lymphoblastic disease	Multi-agent chemotherapy
Investigational:	
Nodular stage III	Total body irradiation
Nodular	Interferon
Indolent disease (well-differentiated, lymphocytic, focal, or diffuse)	Single or multidrug chemotherapy
B-cell lymphomas	Monoclonal antibody, alone or as a pretreatment for autologous bone marrow transplantation

Progressive Disease. Multidrug therapy is indicated for patients with symptomatic or rapidly progressive disease, particularly if they have a histiocytic cell type or diffuse nodal architecture. Response rates with multidrug therapy approach 95%, with median survival in excess of 2 years. For some subgroups, combination chemotherapy may result in cure for 20% to 40% of patients.

Drug Regimens. The original three-drug regimen COP (cyclophosphamide, Oncovin, and prednisone) continues to be used and is administered at 3- to 4-week intervals and utilizes either oral or intravenous cyclophosphamide. In patients who fail to respond to COP or who relapse after initial response, secondary therapy is employed, using non–cross-resistant drugs such as bleomycin and doxorubicin. Secondary responses in high-grade lymphomas are invariably shorter in duration. In recent years, more intensive first echelon combination chemotherapy regimens have been tried with the hope of maximizing chances for complete or at least prolonged remission. Typically five drugs are used (*e.g.,* BACOP); such regimens are designed to allow continuous therapy, and have been particularly effective in inducing response in patients with histiocytic lymphoma, even achieving cure in some, despite advanced disease.

Investigational therapies being explored include use of monoclonal antibodies, autologous bone marrow transplantation, and interferon. Since most lymphomas are of B-cell origin, identification of a specific antigen allows development of a *monoclonal antibody* against the tumor cell. Monoclonal antibodies have induced remissions but are associated with development of immune responses against the immunoglobin in some patients. Another approach is to perform *autologous bone marrow transplantation* after treating the marrow with monoclonal antibodies to purge tumor cells from the marrow. Clinical trials with interferon are underway; partial remissions have been achieved in patients with nodular lymphomas.

MONITORING THERAPY

Monitoring patients on chemotherapy requires close surveillance (see Chapter 87). Relapse or recurrence generally develops in the areas of previous disease (in contrast to Hodgkin's disease, in which relapse is in extranodal or visceral sites). Relapse typically occurs within 12 to 18 months of initiating treatment. Watching for development of neurologic symptoms is particularly important in those with a predisposition to CNS spread (see above).

PATIENT EDUCATION

The strong likelihood that chemotherapy-induced sterility will occur, at least temporarily, needs to be discussed with the patient. Fortunately, this disease occurs more frequently in older age groups (in contrast to Hodgkin's disease), for whom reproductive capacity is less likely to be an issue. Return of spermatogenesis is seen in some patients, beginning about 2 years after completion of chemotherapy. Potency and libido are unaffected.

The encouraging results of chemotherapy, even in patients with advanced disease, provide new hope. As with Hodgkin's disease, the patient can be given a fairly accurate assessment of his prognosis after careful histologic study and staging have been carried out. Often the prognosis is far better than the patient's fearful expectations and can be shared profitably.

INDICATIONS FOR REFERRAL

Management of the patient with lymphoma needs to be a cooperative venture from the start, with the primary physician working closely with the oncologist experienced in lymphoma. Selection of treatment modality requires the judgment of one who is familiar with available protocols, which are still undergoing revision. Although consultation and referral are essential, the primary physician can assume responsibility for long-term management as soon as a treatment plan is devised. Working closely with the oncologist, the patient's personal physician can administer and monitor the chemotherapy program on an outpatient basis, maintain continuity, and provide psychologic support.

ANNOTATED BIBLIOGRAPHY

Aisenberg AC: Cell lineage in lymphoproliferative disease. Am J Med 74:679, 1983 (*A detailed discussion of designating lymphomas on the basis of T- or B-cell origin.*)

Anderson T, Chabner BA, Young RC et al: Malignant lymphoma. Histology and staging of 473 patients at the National Cancer Institute. Cancer 50:2699, 1982 (*A review of histology and staging in a retrospective series, with emphasis on relationship to prognosis and response to therapy.*)

Brunning R, Bloomfield C, McKenna R et al: Bilateral trephine bone marrow biopsies in lymphoma and other neoplastic diseases. Ann Intern Med 82:365, 1975 (*Reports a 37% yield on bilateral samples; 11 of 50 samples were positive only on one side, demonstrating the need for bilateral procedure.*)

Castillino R, Billingham M, Dorfman R: Lymphographic accuracy in Hodgkin's disease and malignant lymphoma with a note on the "reactive" lymph node as a cause of most false-positive lymphograms. Invest Radio 9:155, 1974 (*A prospective study with 114 non-Hodgkin's lymphoma patients. The false-negative rate was 8% and false-positive rate 11%. Most false-positives resulted from misreading a reactive lymph node.*)

Chabner BA et al: Sequential nonsurgical and surgical staging of non-Hodgkin's lymphoma. Ann Intern Med 85:149, 1976 (*Helps define approach to staging, based on studies at the National Cancer Institute.*)

Coleman M: Chemotherapy for large-cell lymphoma: Optimism and caution. Ann Intern Med 103:140, 1985 (*A review of the excellent progress in treating this form of lymphoma.*)

Ezdinli E et al: Comparison of intensive versus moderate chemotherapy of lymphocytic lymphomas: A progress report. Cancer 38:1060, 1976 (*Emphasizes the importance of nodular vs. diffuse histologic pattern and, in a relatively large group of patients [273], demonstrates the potential need for conservative single-agent therapy in some patients.*)

Fisher RI, DeVita VT, Hubbard SM et al: Diffuse aggressive lymphomas: Increased survival after alternating flexible sequence of ProMACE and MOPP chemotherapy. Ann Intern Med 98:304, 1983 (*The use of alternating non–cross-resistant chemotherapy achieves a 74% complete remission rate, with 90% of this group [with this specific histologic subgroup] achieving the possibility of cure.*)

Foon KA, Maluish AE, Abrams PG et al: Recombinant leukocyte A interferon therapy for advanced hairy cell leukemia. Am J Med 80:351, 1986 (*An example of utilizing interferon for treatment of lymphoma.*)

Horwich A, Peckham M: "Bad risk" non-Hodgkin's lymphomas. Semin Hematol 20:35, 1983 (*A comprehensive review of prognosis and approach to treatment for patients with unfavorable histologic subtypes.*)

National Cancer Institute: Classification of non-Hodgkin's lymphomas: Summary and description of a working formulation for clinical usage. Cancer 49:2112, 1982 (*An international effort to construct a new working classification scheme.*)

Portlock CS: "Good risk" non-Hodgkin's lymphomas: Approaches to management. Semin Hematol 20:25, 1983 (*A review of approaches to treating indolent forms of lymphoma.*)

Proceedings of the National Conference on Lymphomas and Leukemias: Cancer (Suppl.) 421(2), 1978 (*A comprehensive review of the state of the art of diagnosis and therapy in the hematologic neoplasms, including Hodgkin's and non-Hodgkin's lymphomas, as viewed from the perspective of individuals who have been most influential in developing concepts in management.*)

Sherins R, DeVita V: Effect of drug treatment for lymphoma on male reproductive capacity. Ann Intern Med 79:216, 1973 (*Azoospermia is not uncommon [10 of 16 in this series] after chemotherapy. Potency and libido are maintained; spermatogenesis may return, but only after more than 2 years after drug therapy.*)

84

Management of Common Anemias

Anemias that result from deficiencies of iron, folate, and B_{12} are common in primary care practice. The relative ease with which one can replace the deficient substance sometimes leads to correction of the anemia without sufficient attention to the underlying cause. Complicating the issue is inappropriate self-treatment with large doses of iron and vitamins. The primary care physician needs to be knowledgeable about the evaluation of anemias (see Chapter 78) and the indications for and proper use of iron, B_{12}, and folate replacement therapies.

IRON DEFICIENCY ANEMIA

Iron deficiency anemia is extremely common, occurring in about 10% to 15% of premenopausal women. The condition is particularly likely to be a manifestation of underlying disease when it occurs in males and in the elderly (see Chapter 78). It helps to assess whether there is inadequate intake, poor absorption, increased loss, or a combination of factors responsible for the anemia. Knowing the most economical, effective, and best tolerated forms of supplemental iron facilitates design of an optimal replacement therapy program.

Clinical Presentation and Course

In menstruating women, the balance between dietary iron intake (1 mg per day) and loss (15 mg per month) is precarious. Low-grade anemia, especially when losses from pregnancy (approximately 500 mg) are not made up, is common. However, the many vague complaints in otherwise healthy menstruating women that are attributed to "low iron" have not been found to correlate with the severity of the anemia or to respond to its correction in controlled studies.

Iron deficiency anemia is usually slow in onset, allowing for compensatory changes such as increases in 2,3-DPG and cardiac output to minimize symptoms. When blood loss has been rapid or the anemia severe (hemoglobin below 7 g/100 ml), patients are likely to become symptomatic, especially if cardiopulmonary reserve is limited. Replacement therapy is required in such cases, regardless of etiology. Also, the occasional patient with severe iron deficiency who presents with glossitis, angular stomatitis, koilonychia or esophageal web improves upon correction of the deficiency. Whether or not the menorrhagia sometimes seen with iron deficiency is corrected by iron is a subject of debate. Patients who have undergone subtotal gastrectomy and gastrojejunostomy have up to a 60% chance of incurring iron deficit due to loss of acid-secreting capacity, rapid gastric emptying, and bypass of the duodenum. Pregnancy is almost certain to produce iron deficiency, since a net loss of over 500 mg of iron occurs. Iron deficiency from chronic GI blood loss has been documented in long-distance runners.

Unless the cause of the iron deficiency is removed, recurrence rates are high, even when treatment is prescribed. In a series of 100 cases, 29 relapses were noted; in 24 instances, inadequate iron was being taken; in 12, blood loss continued in excess of iron therapy, and in 4, malabsorption was documented.

Principles of Management

As noted above, the importance of identification and treatment of the underlying etiology cannot be over emphasized, especially when the anemia is found in a man or an elderly patient. The severity of the anemia does not indicate the seriousness of the cause. Indications for iron replacement are tempered by the fact that symptoms are often minimal and the morbidity from a mild anemia is low. Moreover, as noted previously, correction of the iron deficit is not certain to alleviate the host of vague complaints often attributed to it. Nevertheless, replacement therapy makes sense when (1) the patient is symptomatic and has a limited cardiopulmonary reserve, (2) the anemia has become moderately severe (hemoglobin 8–9 g per 100 ml), (3) the patient is pregnant, (4) the patient had a subtotal gastrectomy and gastrojejunostomy, (5) continued heavy blood loss is anticipated, or (6) the patient is recovering from megaloblastic anemia.

Oral iron is preferred; the ferrous form is better absorbed than the ferric one. Absorption occurs best under conditions of low *p*H in the proximal small bowel. Phytates and phosphates found in food bind iron and reduce absorption. When iron tablets are taken with meals, a 40% drop in absorption can be demonstrated. Absorption also varies according to the severity of the deficit. About 20% of an oral dose is taken up initially, but absorption falls to 5% after 1 month of therapy, even though the anemia remains incompletely corrected.

Most ferrous salts have equivalent rates of absorption and produce similar rates of hemoglobin replenishment. *Choice* is a matter of cost and side effects; the degree of gastrointestinal upset is a function more of the iron content of the tablet than of the form of ferrous salt used. Slow-release preparations have been touted as producing fewer side effects and requiring only once-daily administration. However, they dissolve slowly and can bypass the proximal small bowel before significant absorption has occurred. There is no evidence they are worth the extra cost, which is about ten times that of ferrous sulfate. Some preparations contain ascorbic acid with the claim that the acid facilitates absorption, especially in patients with achlorhydria; such patients respond quite adequately to ferrous sulfate alone, probably because of the excess amount of iron available.

The *recommended dose* for iron deficiency is 300 mg of ferrous sulfate, three times daily. Although taking iron with a meal reduces absorption, it also lessens disagreeable gastrointestinal symptoms such as nausea and epigastric discomfort. Constipation and diarrhea are frequently reported as well, but are less a function of the amount of iron available for absorption. About 25% of patients report side effects.

The *response* to iron is apparent within 10 days of initiating therapy; a reticulocytosis is first noted, followed by a rise in the hemoglobin concentration of 0.1 to 0.2 g per 100 ml per day. Several weeks of therapy are required to bring the hemoglobin level back up to normal, and replenishing iron stores may take months. However, speed is not an issue unless blood loss is rapid, in which case blood transfusion rather than iron therapy is the treatment of choice. The response to parenteral iron therapy is no more rapid than that seen with oral preparations.

Parenteral iron has a very limited role. It should be used only in patients who have had an adequate trial of oral iron and shown a genuine intolerance to all available preparations. Patients with inflammatory bowel disease may require parenteral iron due to the irritant effect of oral iron and the need to take large doses in order to keep up with blood loss. Parenteral iron has also been suggested for patients with malabsorption, but most are able to absorb a sufficient amount of oral iron. Intramuscular administration has been associated with development of sarcomas at injection sites and should be avoided. Fatal anaphylatic reactions and asthma have been produced by all parenteral forms of iron administration. If parenteral iron must be used, it should be administered by the intravenous route, beginning with a very small test dose and continuing with a slow drip; a syringe with epinephrine should be drawn up at the same time and kept on hand.

Patient Education and Prevention of Iron Deficiency

Patients need to be instructed on the best means of minimizing gastrointestinal side effects in order to maximize compliance. Starting with a small dose, for example, 300 mg per day, of ferrous sulfate and building to 900 mg per day avoids initial intolerance. Taking iron just after eating may also help. It needs to be made clear that therapy has to be continued on a regular basis for weeks and often months.

Prevention of iron deficiency is most important in those with increased needs, that is, pregnant women and young children. The average American diet contains 12 mg of iron per 2000 calories. Twenty percent is absorbed by markedly iron-deficient patients and 5% to 10% by others; thus, about 0.6 to 1.2 mg is taken up under normal circumstances each day. Daily requirement for men and postmenopausal women is 0.5 to 1.0 mg per day, indicating that dietary intake should suffice. However 1.5 mg per day is needed by menstruating women and 2.5 mg per day by pregnant women. Iron-rich foods can be used to avoid the need for iron supplements. Fish, meat (particularly liver), and iron-enriched cereals and bread are excellent sources. Eggs and green vegetables are also high in iron, but the iron is unavailable for absorption because it is bound to the phosphates and phytates present in these foods.

When diet alone seems inadequate and needs are very high, as in pregnancy, a once-daily dose of 150 to 300 mg of ferrous sulfate is recommended to avoid significant iron deficiency. It must be emphasized that most people who eat a balanced diet do not require iron supplements. Taking widely promoted supplements that contain iron, vitamins, and minerals is expensive and unnecessary in most instances.

VITAMIN B₁₂ DEFICIENCY

Vitamin B_{12} deficiency can result from inadequate intake, impaired absorption, increased requirements, or faulty utilization. Poor intake is distinctly rare, occurring mostly in ultra-strict vegetarians who refrain from eating eggs and dairy products as well as meat. Most cases of B_{12} deficiency are due to pernicious anemia; the lack of intrinsic factor compromises absorption. Absorption can also impaired by disease of the terminal ileum, by bacterial overgrowth from stasis, and by gastrectomy. Faulty utilization is uncommon, occurring with genetic defects in synthesis of transcobalamin, the plasma protein used for B_{12} transport.

Clinical Presentation and Course

Irrespective of etiology, B_{12} deficiency leads to a slowly evolving *megaloblastic anemia, glossitis,* and *neuropathy.* Although megaloblastic anemia and glossitis also occur with folic acid deficiency, the neuropathy is distinctive. Symptoms are unlikely to begin until the serum B_{12} level falls to less than 80 to 100 pg/ml. Due to body's large B_{12} storage capacity, onset of clinical manifestations may take months to years to develop. Macrocytosis is usually the first manifestation and can precede anemia by as much as 1 to 2 years. Neurologic symptoms are usually a late development but can occur in the absence of anemia. Classically, they include symmetrical paresthesias in the hands and feet, progressing to ataxia from loss of vibratory and position sense as the posterior columns of the spinal cord become involved. However, neurologic presentations may be confusing; cortical lesions can ensue, leading to perversions of taste and smell, irritability, and central visual scotomata. If left untreated, neurologic deficits may become permanent.

In *pernicious anemia,* there may be coincident thyroid disease, rheumatoid arthritis, vitiligo, or gastric cancer. *Achlorhydria* after histamine stimulation is characteristic. Diagnosis is usually made by the Schilling test, utilizing exogenous intrinsic factor to help document its absence (see Chapter 78).

Principles of Management

For the vast majority of cases, treatment consists of administering *parenteral vitamin B_{12}.* There are a host of therapeutic regimens, all of which are quite adequate. For example in a commonly utilized program for patients with pernicious anemia, patients are initially treated with 100 to 1000 µg of IM cyanocobalamin or hydroxocobalamin daily for up to 2 weeks, followed by the same dose twice weekly for another month, and then once a month for the remainder of the patient's life. If neurologic symptoms are present, a twice-monthly dose is recommended for six months. Some argue that 1000 µg doses are unnecessary, because only 100 µg can be effectively utilized at one time, with the remainder being excreted in the urine. However, because of its low cost and safety, doses in excess of 100 µg are often given. Hydroxocobalamin is better bound to serum proteins and less rapidly excreted; it need be given only half as frequently. In practice, either form of B_{12} suffices. Oral B_{12} preparations are of little value, except in patients with poor intake. Absorption of oral B_{12} in most patients is problematic and unpredictable.

There is a discrepancy between the recommendation for monthly injections and the body's known capacity to store several year's worth of B_{12}. Retrospective data suggests that after replenishment of body stores, such frequent injections are unnecessary; prospective studies are underway. In the meantime, it is probably best to continue with a monthly regimen, especially in patients with neurologic sequelae. Compliance with a monthly injection program is often poor; having the visiting nurse or family member give the injection is helpful and far less inconvenient than a monthly office visit.

The response to treatment can be dramatic, with marked reticulocytosis beginning within 72 hours and rapid improvement in neurologic deficits. However, neurologic deficits that have persisted for 12 to 18 months in spite of therapy are probably permanent. During recovery, patients who were severely B_{12} depleted can develop serious *hypokalemia* as potassium is taken up by new red cells. The serum potassium level should be monitored and supplements provided if it falls below normal.

There is no need for *folic acid* supplementation. In fact, the inappropriate use of a large pharmacologic dose of oral folate (*e.g.,* 5 mg) might partially correct and mask a B_{12} deficiency and put the patient at risk for an acute, marked deterioration of neurologic function if B_{12} is not given. There is no harm if the patient takes folate in addition to B_{12}, but this is rarely necessary unless diet is extremely poor.

Patients with B_{12} deficiency due to disease of the terminal ileum or bacterial overgrowth require treatment directed at the underlying bowel problem (see Chapter 65).

Many well-intentioned physicians have used parenteral vitamin B_{12} as a nonspecific therapy for patients bothered by fatigue and other vague symptoms. Although there is little risk in giving such therapy, there is no evidence it has any beneficial effect. The temporary symptomatic improvement reported by some patients represents the placebo effect of an intramuscular injection. Such therapy is misleading and should be abandoned in favor of a more comprehensive and etiologic approach to the patient's underlying problems, be they medical or psychologic (see Chapters 6, 222, 223, 226).

FOLIC ACID DEFICIENCY

Most folic acid deficiency results from inadequate intake, although occasionally increased need or impairment of absorption or utilization is encountered. *Dietary deficiency* is in part a consequence of limited capacity to store folate; within 3 months of assuming an inadequate diet, megaloblastic changes and anemia can develop. Foods rich in folate include green vegetables (asparagus, lettuce, spinach, broccoli), liver, yeast, and mushrooms. Excessive boiling of vegetables in water can remove a substantial amount of available folic acid. Alcoholism is responsible for many cases of inadequate intake.

Impaired absorption is seen in the context of ileal disease (*e.g.,* tropical and nontropical sprue, heavy giardial infestation), short bowel syndrome, and phenytoin use. *Increased demand* takes place in the setting of pregnancy, severe hyperthyroidism, hemolytic anemia, malignancy, and florid psoriasis. *Utilization* is *hindered* by use of methotrexate; triamterene and trimethoprim have similar though less marked effects on dihydrofolate reductase. Patients undergoing hemodialysis experience substantial folic acid *loss,* necessitating replacement therapy.

The *clinical presentation* of folic acid deficiency is one of megaloblastic anemia, sometimes accompanied by glossitis. Anemia occurs within 3 to 4 months of the onset of deficiency. Diagnostic features include a low serum folate level (less than 15 ng/ml) and a marked reticulocytosis in response to physiologic doses (200 μg) of folic acid. Response to treatment

with folic acid is prompt. There are no neurologic deficits associated with folic acid deficiency.

Management

Most forms of folic acid deficiency, even malabsorptive types, can be overcome by orally administering pharmacologic doses of folic acid (1 to 2 mg per day). Four to five weeks of treatment will usually reverse the anemia and replenish body stores. When the underlying cause persists (*e.g.,* malabsorption, malignancy, psoriasis, hemodialysis), chronic therapy is indicated. Patients taking methotrexate can be given folinic acid, which bypasses inhibition of dihydrofolate reductase. As noted above, nonspecific use of folic acid for treatment of a megaloblastic anemia is ill-advised, since it may mask an underlying B_{12} deficiency and precipitate neurologic symptoms.

A.H.G.

ANNOTATED BIBLIOGRAPHY

Adverse effects of parenteral iron. Medical Letter, 19:35, 1977 (*Recommends extreme caution in use of these agents due to risks of sarcomas with intramuscular injection and anaphylaxis reported with all parenteral forms of therapy.*)

Brise H, Hallberg L: Influence of meals on iron absorption in oral iron therapy. Acta Med Scand (Suppl.) 171:376, 1962 (*Absorption fell 40% when oral iron was taken with meals.*)

Cook JD: Clinical evaluation of iron deficiency. Semin Hematol 19: 6, 1982 (*An updated review of classic data on the problem.*)

Crosby W: Who needs iron? N Engl J Med 297:543, 1977 (*Terse review of iron requirements and need for supplements.*)

Elwood P, Williams G: A comparative trial of slow-release and conventional iron preparations. Practitioner 204:812, 1970 (*No therapeutic advantage found for the slow-release preparations.*)

Fry J: Clinical patterns and course of anemias in general practice. Br Med J 2:1732, 1961 (*Recurrence rate of iron deficiency was 30% after treatment.*)

Kerr D, Davidson S: Gastrointestinal intolerance to oral iron preparations. Lancet 2:489, 1958 (*An early description of GI side effects of oral preparations.*)

Linnell JC, Matthews DM: Cobalamin metabolism and its clinical aspects. Clin Sci 66:113, 1984 (*Draws correlations between elements of B_{12} metabolism and clinical conditions.*)

Oral iron. Medical Letter, 20:45, 1978 (*Menstruating and pregnant women may need iron supplements; ferrous sulfate is least expensive and no less effective or less well tolerated than other preparations.*)

Savage D, Lindenbaum J: Relapses after interruption of cyanocobalamin therapy in patients with pernicious anemia. Am J Med 74:765, 1983 (*Provides data pertinent to determining optimal frequency of therapy.*)

Wood M, Elwood P: Symptoms of iron deficiency anemia: A community survey. Br J Prev Soc Med 20:117, 1966 (*The correlation between hemoglobin concentration and symptoms was poor. Iron therapy produced no statistically significant improvement in complaints.*)

85

Outpatient Oral Anticoagulant Therapy
ROBERT A. HUGHES, M.D.

Oral anticoagulant therapy with coumarin derivatives has become a major therapeutic tool in the prevention of fibrin thrombus formation. Approximately 300,000 patients are stricken annually by thromboembolism—over 50,000 die. A great deal of morbidity and mortality could be avoided by timely anticoagulation. It is important to know (1) indications for therapy, (2) how to initiate and maintain patients on oral anticoagulants in the outpatient setting, (3) common complications, and (4) drugs and conditions that interfere with or potentiate the anticoagulant's effect.

MECHANISM OF ACTION

Warfarin and other coumarin derivatives act by inhibiting the action of vitamin K in the normal carboxylation of coagulation factors II, VII, IX, and X. Noncarboxylated coagulation factors, known as PIVKAs (proteins induced by vitamin K antagonism), fail to participate effectively in the coagulation reaction. The warfarin-induced decline in active, carboxylated coagulation factors is a function of the half-life of each factor, which varies from 5 hours for Factor VII to 72 hours for Factor II. The prothrombin time (PT) may be prolonged after only 2 to 3 days of therapy, but this represents primarily depression of Factor VII and the extrinsic clotting cascade. Full anticoagulant effect is only achieved after all factors, including the intrinsic clotting cascade, are comparably depleted after 5 to 7 days of therapy, and the partial thromboplastin time (PTT) is also prolonged.

INDICATIONS

Therapy is indicated in conditions having a high risk of thrombus formation and subsequent embolization. However, there are few well-controlled studies documenting conditions with a high incidence of thromboembolism that can be significantly reduced by oral anticoagulant therapy. Nevertheless, the consensus is that *mitral stenosis* complicated by *atrial fibrillation* (see Chapter 23), *deep vein thrombophlebitis* (see Chapter 30), *pulmonary embolization, systemic embolization,* and implant of an *artificial prosthetic heart valve* are indications for oral anticoagulant therapy. Other conditions felt by many to be indications for oral anticoagulant therapy, though less well established, include transient ischemic attacks (see Chapter 165), chronic and paroxysmal atrial fibrillation

in the elderly (see Chapter 23), congestive cardiomyopathy (see Chapter 27), and ventricular aneurysm. There is no evidence that atherosclerotic heart disease is prevented by use of coumarin anticoagulants.

CONTRAINDICATIONS

Contraindications to the use of oral anticoagulants need to be considered in the context of urgency of anticoagulation, risk and seriousness of potential complications, and duration of therapy. Patients with previous *central nervous system bleeding,* recent *neurosurgery,* or *frank bleeding* should not receive warfarin. Important relative contraindications include active peptic ulcer disease, chronic alcoholism, blindness (unless in supervised situations), bleeding diathesis, and severe hypertension. When taken early in pregnancy, coumarins may cause birth defects; when they are used at delivery, fetal hemorrhage can occur. Heparin should be used in place of warfarin during early pregnancy and childbirth. Embarking on oral anticoagulant therapy is unwise when follow-up cannot be readily maintained, when laboratory facilities for accurately measuring the prothrombin time are inadequate, or when the patient is unreliable.

METHODS OF INITIATING AND MONITORING THERAPY

Patients with acute pulmonary embolization, deep vein thrombophlebitis, or acute systemic embolization should be admitted for immediate parenteral administration of heparin, to be followed by oral warfarin therapy. Other patients are in less urgent need of immediate full anticoagulation and can be safely started on a warfarin program as outpatients. One method of *initiating outpatient therapy* is to prescribe 10 mg of warfarin daily for the first 3 days; the prothrombin time is measured on the third day. At 10 mg per day, it takes a mean of 5 days to reach therapeutic range. The dose is subsequently adjusted or maintained to achieve a prothrombin level of 1.5 to 2 times control. Recently, controlled trials have suggested that a lower therapeutic range of 1.4 to 1.6 times control may be just as effective for thrombophlebitis of the leg as the higher therapeutic range, yet cause fewer bleeding complications. The efficacy of low-range therapy has not been proved for other indications, but is occasionally used for patients felt to be at higher risk of bleeding.

Once the desired level of anticoagulation is achieved, *monitoring* is carried out by measuring the PT once every 3 to 4 weeks. In about 85% of patients, dosage adjustments over time are unnecessary; in 15% they are. Since it is impossible to predict who will and who will not need adjustments, the PT should be checked every 3 to 4 weeks, the schedule being rigorously enforced.

There are many possible *methods of dosage adjustment.* One that is designed to maximize safety and avoid wide swings in prothrombin time utilizes 10% changes in weekly dose, unless PT is grossly out of range. For example, if the patient is taking 7.5 mg per day, the weekly dose is 52.5 mg. If the prothrombin time is too low, the dose is increased so that on 2 of the 7 days, the patient takes 10 mg, and 7.5 mg the other 5 days. The prothrombin time is then measured weekly for the next 2 weeks.

Outpatient anticoagulation requires facilities for accurate prothrombin time measurement, reliable collection of samples, and the ability to contact patients promptly. Careful monitoring and follow-up are essential to the safety and success of any outpatient anticoagulation program. At the beginning of therapy, patients can benefit considerably from a session with a nurse who can instruct them in the use of warfarin, answer questions, test understanding, and provide informative booklets for them to take home. The importance of close monitoring and patient education cannot be over-emphasized. If the patient fails to keep his appointment for a prothrombin time test, he should be contacted immediately. A computer system can provide reminders so that no patient is lost to follow-up. To further simplify therapy and avoid confusion, scored 5-mg tablets of sodium warfarin can be used exclusively. Commercial laboratory services are sometimes employed to draw samples at home for patients who have difficulty coming to the office for frequent PT determinations.

COMPLICATIONS

Reports on the incidence of *bleeding complications* in patients on long-term anticoagulant therapy have been variable. Several series have demonstrated that the incidence of hemorrhage severe enough to require hospitalization or transfusion should occur in less than 5% of patients who are carefully monitored. Unfortunately, the risk of serious bleeding is not always linked to excessive prolongation of the prothrombin time and can occur even with the prothrombin time in therapeutic range. Older patients generally experience a higher incidence of complications.

Patients with prothrombin times in the therapeutic range (*i.e.,* 1.5 to 2 times control), who bleed from the urinary tract, rectum, or vagina while on anticoagulant therapy should be considered to have an *underlying pathologic process* until proven otherwise. In several series, a lesion responsible for the bleeding was detected in over 50% of patients. Often it was an occult malignancy in the bladder or colon.

In rare instances, *hemorrhagic necrosis of skin* has been reported in women and cyanotic toes in men—all with prothrombin times in therapeutic range. The mechanism of this complication remains unclear.

CONDITIONS AND MEDICATIONS THAT INCREASE OR DECREASE ANTICOAGULANT EFFECT OF WARFARIN

Drugs that potentiate the effect of warfarin may do so by preventing synthesis or absorption of vitamin K, displacing warfarin from binding sites, inhibiting microsomal degradative enzyme activity, increasing catabolism of clotting factors, or impairing platelet function (Table 85-1). Hepatocellular failure results in impaired synthesis of clotting factors and albumin; cholestasis makes for less efficient absorption of vitamin K. Both conditions are capable of prolonging the prothrombin time and potentiating the effects of warfarin.

Anticoagulant effects are decreased by agents that induce microsomal enzymes, decrease absorption of warfarin, or increase synthesis of clotting factors or binding proteins (see Table 85-1). Moreover, coumarins will cause a decrease in the metabolism of tolbutamide and phenytoin by competing for the same degradative enzymes. The prothrombin time should be measured when any change in drug program is made, and it should be followed closely thereafter.

Table 85-1. Common Drugs That Interact with Oral Anticoagulants

DRUG	MECHANISM
Agents Potentiating the Anticoagulant Effect of Warfarin	
Alcohol	Decreased metabolism during acute intoxication
Allopurinol	Inhibition of microsomal enzymes
Anabolic steroids	Unknown
Chloral hydrate	Displacement of binding sites
Chloramphenicol	Inhibition of microsomal enzymes
Clofibrate	Displacement from binding sites
Indomethacin	Impairment of platelet function
Phenylbutazone	Displacement from binding sites
Salicylates	Impairment of platelet function
Sulfonamides (including trimethoprim–sulfa combinations)	Unknown
Thyroxine	Increased catabolism of clotting factors
Agents Decreasing the Anticoagulant Effect of Warfarin	
Barbiturates	Induction of microsomal enzymes
Cholestyramine	Decreased absorption
Oral contraceptives	Increased synthesis or activity of some clotting factors
Glutethimide	Induction of microsomal enzymes
Rifampin	Induction of microsomal enzymes

INDICATIONS FOR CONTINUATION AND TERMINATION OF THERAPY

Therapy should be continued indefinitely in patients with valvular disease with atrial fibrillation, systemic embolization, or artificial heart valves. In other instances, there are few data on proper duration of therapy. In deep venous thrombosis, most experts recommend continuation of therapy for approximately 3 to 6 months; the same is true in pulmonary embolization. Deep vein thrombophlebitis or pulmonary emboli that recur after 6 months of treatment are usually followed by retreatment for a period of 12 months. If a serious bleeding problem develops in a patient on anticoagulant therapy, the prothrombin time can be corrected promptly by administration of *fresh frozen plasma*. This is the preferred mode of therapy. Parenteral administration of *vitamin K* is also effective, though it may take longer to have an effect (up to 5 hours) and can cause refractoriness to warfarin if prompt reinstitution of anticoagulant therapy is attempted. The decision to discontinue anticoagulant therapy in the context of bleeding needs to be individualized. The risk of hemorrhage has to be balanced against the risk of serious embolization.

PATIENT EDUCATION

Avoidance of unnecessary morbidity depends on thorough patient education. Prior to initiation of outpatient therapy, the patient and responsible family members need to learn the name of the medication, the dose, time of day to be taken, need for routine check of PT, necessity of avoiding alcohol and aspirin-containing compounds, and they must be able to recognize signs of bleeding such as melena and spontaneous ecchymoses. Teaching undertaken by the nurse, as well as distribution of helpful booklets detailing proper use of the drug, are essential components of the patient education effort. Any patient who is incapable of understanding the instructions or deemed unreliable should not be placed on therapy, since the risks of hemorrhage probably outweigh any possible benefits. The one exception is the patient who can be closely supervised by family members or health care professionals.

ANNOTATED BIBLIOGRAPHY

Breckinridge A: Oral anticoagulant drugs: Pharmacokinetic aspects. Semin Hematol 15:19, 1978 (*Excellent discussion of newly understood mechanisms of vitamin K antagonism.*)

Brozovic M: Oral anticoagulants in clinical practice. Semin Hematol 15:27, 1978 (*Recent review of all aspects of anticoagulant management.*)

Coon WW, William PW: Hemorrhagic complications of anticoagulant therapy. Arch Intern Med 133:386, 1974 (*A review of 3800 courses of anticoagulant treatment, detecting bleeding in 6.8%. Frequency of bleeding increased with intensity of treatment as reflected in prothrombin time. More than half of the patients with bleeding had an identifiable lesion responsible for the bleeding.*)

Davis FB, Estruch MT, Samsonn-Corvera EB et al: Management of anticoagulation in outpatients. Arch Intern Med 137:197, 1977 (*Details of operating a centralized anticoagulant clinic; less than 5% incidence of major complications.*)

Deykin D: Warfarin therapy. N Engl J Med 2833:691, 1970 (*Excellent discussion of warfarin's actions, metabolism, and interactions with other drugs.*)

Feder W, Auerback R: Purple toes: An uncommon sequela of oral coumarin drug therapy. Ann Intern Med 55:911, 1961 (*A complication seen in 1% of patients, all men with PT in range.*)

Forfar, JC: A 7-year analysis of haemorrhage in patients on long-term anticoagulant treatment. Br Heart J 42:128, 1979 (*Documents incidence of major hemorrhage as less than 5% and examines potential risk factors.*)

Hall JG, Paull RM, Wilson KM: Maternal and fetal sequelae of anticoagulation during pregnancy. Am J Med 68:122, 1980 (*Updates recommendations for therapy during pregnancy, namely heparin for first and third trimesters and warfarin during the second trimester.*)

Hull R, Hirsch J, Jay R et al: Different intensities of oral anticoagulant therapy in the treatment of proximal-vein thrombosis. N Engl J Med 307:1676, 1982 (*Elegant controlled trial demonstrating the efficacy of low-range therapy for deep vein thrombophlebitis.*)

Koch-Weser J, Sellers EM: Drug interaction with coumarin anticoagulants. N Engl J Med 285:487, 1971 (*Good summary of the many possible potentiating and inhibiting interactions.*)

Mackie M, Douglas A: Oral anticoagulants in arterial disease. Br Med Bull 23:177, 1978 (*Critical review of the evidence for coumarin use in coronary, cerebral, rheumatic, and peripheral vascular disease; 95 references.*)

O'Reilly RA, Aggeler PM: Studies on coumarin anticoagulation: Initiation of therapy without a loading dose. Circulation 38:169, 1968 (*At 10 mg per day, it took a mean of 5.2 days to achieve therapeutic range; using 15 mg per day, it took 2.7 days. No bleeding problems were encountered compared to frequent problems when larger (25 mg) initial doses are used.*)

O'Reilly RA, Motley CH: Racemic warfarin and trimethoprim–sulfamethoxazole interactions in humans. Ann Intern Med 91:34, 1979 (*A prospective study showing potentiation of warfarin effect.*)

Petitti DB, Strom BL, Melmon KL: Duration of warfarin anticoagulant therapy and the probabilities of recurrent thromboembolism in hemorrhage. Am J Med 81:255, 1986 (*A case review study of 370 patients with positive venography showed that anticoagulation beyond 6 weeks was associated with a linearly increasing risk of hemorrhage but no apparent protection against recurrent thromboembolism.*)

Verhagen H: Local hemorrhage and necrosis of skin and underlying tissues during anticoagulant therapy with dicumarol. Acta Med Scan 148:453, 1954 (*A very rare but important complication, occurring in women whose PTs were in range.*)

Wessler S: Drug prophylaxis for arterial thromboembolism, 1981. JAMA 246:2484, 1981 (*Excellent review of the respective roles of anticoagulant therapy versus antiplatelet therapy in light of most recent clinical trials. Argues that only established indications for anticoagulants are atrial fibrillation with mitral stenosis, prosthetic heart valves, deep vein thrombophlebitis, pulmonary embolization, and systemic embolization.*)

B
Oncology

86
Evaluation of the Unknown Primary Tumor
JACOB J. LOKICH, M.D.

In up to 15% of patients presenting with malignancy, the initial manifestation is metastatic disease in the absence of an evident primary tumor. The discovery often prompts an extensive search for the tumor of origin in the hope that a treatable form of cancer will be found. The advent of improved noninvasive diagnostic methods has made outpatient evaluation by the primary physician more practical than ever before. Evaluation must be undertaken with an understanding that the probability of finding the primary tumor is small (less than 15% in most series) and the prognosis poor even in cases where a primary tumor is discovered.

A tumor is designated as a tumor of unknown origin (TUO) after meeting two criteria: the tissue is histologically confirmed to be malignant and a primary tumor of the organ is ruled out. In addition, routine screening must fail to identify the primary source, and a very late metastasis (as occurs in breast cancer, melanoma, and renal cell carcinoma) ruled out. Common sites of presentation include the lung, liver, bone, and lymph nodes. When a primary is discovered, the most frequent sites of origin prove to be the pancreas, liver, bowel, and stomach.

The evaluation of a TUO can prove expensive and uncomfortable. Assessment is guided by the principle of looking for treatable disease. Careful and thorough histopathologic evaluation of the tissue obtained should be completed before undertaking a search for the primary tumor. Extensive staging is usually unwarranted, since the tumor is already metastatic.

CLINICAL PRESENTATION

A TUO may present in the lung as a solitary nodule or recurrent pleural effusion (see Chapters 39 and 40). Mediastinal TUOs, often present with catastrophic secondary complications, such as dysphagia, stridor or respiratory difficulty, or superior vena cava syndrome. In bone, TUO may appear as a lytic or blastic lesion of axial skeleton, long bones, or skull. An isolated hard lymph node is another common presentation (see Chapter 80), as is a hepatic nodule or focal defect on liver scan.

DIFFERENTIAL DIAGNOSIS*

In patients without a prior malignancy, the *new pulmonary nodule* indicative of tumor may represent a primary tumor of the lung or a synchronous metastasis from another site (see Chapter 40). The same is true for a nodule in patients with a prior malignancy (see Chapter 42). If breast cancer is the previous malignancy, there is a 70% to 80% chance that the pulmonary shadow on radiographic examination represents a synchronous metastasis; if colon cancer is the previous malignancy, 50% of such patients will have a new primary tumor in the lung; and finally, if Hodgkin's disease is the previous primary tumor, the pulmonary lesion will be Hodgkin's disease in almost all instances.

Recurrent *pleural effusions* are a common complication of mesothelioma and various metastatic pleural lesions (see Chapter 39). *Mediastinal tumors* are usually from lung or breast or spread of lymphoma. In bone, *osteoblastic lesions* are observed primarily with breast, prostate, and lung cancers and, less commonly, with thyroid cancer and lymphoma. These must be distinguished from osteogenic sarcoma, chondrosarcoma, and Ewing's sarcoma, which are the treatable primary bone tumors. *Focal defect on liver scan* may be due to granulomatous disease, benign hepatomas, and primary hepatic malignancies, as well as a metastatic lesion. *High cervical nodes* may be associated with submucosal nasopharyngeal tumor or may represent a site of metastasis from a tumor within the oral cavity. *Axillary adenopathy* suggests a metastasis from the ipsilateral breast, and *inguinal nodes* develop metastases from the genitalia or perineal structures (see Chapter 81).

WORKUP

The most important general principle in evaluating a patient with TUO is to search carefully for *treatable tumor*. In men, the most common treatable tumor is prostatic cancer;

---

* See individual chapters noted for full differential diagnoses of each of these entities.

in women the most amenable to therapy are breast and ovarian cancers. Cancers of the testicles, thyroid, and lung (small cell type) are less prevalent, but also responsive to therapy and important to look for. Patients with undifferentiated carcinoma must be evaluated for lymphoma, which has become a most treatable malignancy (see Chapters 82 and 83).

A number of other tumors are routinely sought, even though they are untreatable or respond less than optimally to chemotherapy or radiation. These include pancreatic cancer, gastric and colonic cancer, and renal-cell carcinoma. Recognition and treatment of the asymptomatic primary tumor does not improve longevity. The expense and discomfort incurred by the many diagnostic studies ordered in search of them can be avoided if the physician remembers to look primarily for the treatable malignancy (Table 86-1).

The second major principle in evaluation of a TUO, is that, after a metastatic lesion has been identified, it is *unnecessary to stage* the patient for other sites of metastases, since the incurable nature of the tumor has already been revealed. Thus, the patient who presents with a pulmonary nodule and is found to have breast cancer as a primary source does not require a liver scan to document the presence of liver disease. Treatment in patients with cancer is determined first and foremost by stage of disease, but once metastases have been identified, the tumor is sufficiently staged. The prime consideration for therapy becomes the presence of symptoms.

Before investigation for a treatable primary tumor is initiated, a thorough evaluation and a *histologic diagnosis* of tumor must be made on tissue obtained from the metastatic site. Most commonly, a specific tissue type is identified, although the histopathologic origin of the tumor may be undifferentiated carcinoma, or simply malignant tumor. It must be noted that biopsied tissue fixed in formalin and sectioned reveals architectural relationships as well as cytologic detail. Cytologic examination of an aspirated fluid or of an aspirated solid mass lesion yields malignant-appearing cells without any architectural relationships. Moreover, cytologic preparation may misrepresent nuclear and cytoplasmic abnormalities, which can be induced by inflammation or drugs. Therefore, in patients with serositis and pleural or peritoneal effusions, the cytologic diagnosis should be confirmed by tissue diagnosis.

The histologic designation of *adenocarcinoma* does not definitively establish the primary source of the tumor. Any organ may develop a glandular malignancy. The distinction on histologic grounds between an adenocarcinoma of the ovary, the stomach, the lung, or the breast is possible, but other methods may be needed. The estrogen receptor protein (ERP) assays are useful because ERP has been identified only in breast cancer and in a small number of nonmammary tumors, such as uterus and ovary.

The histologic designation *undifferentiated carcinoma* presumes a level of anaplasia, which cannot be used to reliably identify the origin of the malignancy. Subjecting additional tissue to electron microscopy, surface marker typing, and special histochemical staining for intracytoplasmic and intranuclear inclusions may provide additional clues. Immunohistologic staining detects such diagnostically important substances as prostatic acid phosphatase, alpha-fetoprotein, and chorionic gonadotropin (see Chapter 141).

Table 86-1.   Tumors and Responsiveness to Chemotherapy

TUMOR	RESPONSE RATE	TREATMENT
Responsive		
Breast	40%–60%	Hormone, CMF, A
Ovary	60%–70%	Platinum, alkylating agents
Prostate	60%–70%	Hormones
Head, neck	50%–70%	Bleomycin, platinum, 5-FU
Esophageal, anus	50%–70%	FU, Mitomycin C
Testicular	80%–100%	Platinum, vinblastine, bleomycin
Lymphoma	80%	COP, CHOP, VP-16, MOPP, ABVD
Sarcoma	30%	Doxorubicin
Neurosecretory	30%–50%	Streptozocin, DTIC, doxorubicin
Marginally Responsive		
Colon, other GI tumors	10%–15%	5-Fluorouracil
Melanoma	10%–15%	DTIC
Hepatoma	20%	Doxorubicin
Unresponsive		
Renal, lung, brain		

Further workup is determined, in part, by the site of presentation and histologic findings (see below). Nevertheless, all patients should undergo a careful *physical examination,* with special emphasis on the breasts, uterus, and ovaries in women and prostate and testicles in men. Every patient needs a rectal examination and stool test for occult blood. Routine use of radiologic contrast studies is wasteful unless there is clinical evidence of bowel or urinary tract disease. A *chest x-ray* and, perhaps, *abdominal CT* (to search for an occult retroperitoneal malignancy) are among the few radiologic studies of potential value. In women, *mammography* and *pelvic ultrasonography* are indicated. Most blood tests are not helpful, but a few serologic markers of treatable cancers deserve consideration, including the acid phosphatase (prostatic fraction), alpha-fetoprotein, and HCG-beta subunit.

The patient with a *solitary pulmonary nodule* is often evaluated for the presence of tumor outside the lung before it is determined that the nodule represents a tumor. The first task is to confirm the diagnosis of malignancy; this involves consideration of transpulmonary needle aspiration vs. bronchoscopic fiberoptic brushing vs. thoracotomy (see Chapters 40 and 42). Whether the tumor is associated with a prior malignancy or not, thoracotomy is generally indicated when it is necessary to maximize the histopathologic information, as well as to remove all known tumor, or to stage and establish the extent of disease by direct observation. A needle aspiration may yield cytologic information but does not identify the tumor's site of origin. Furthermore, the tissue obtained cannot be evaluated by electron microscopy, surface marker typing, or special staining.

Pleural effusions due to malignancy can be diagnosed cytologically, though there are pitfalls. Mesothelioma, a primary tumor of the pleura, may be mistaken for adenocarcinoma when cytologic specimens are used. Often a pleural biopsy in conjunction with aspiration is more informative, especially when granulomatous disease is also under consideration (see Chapters 39 and 47). A diagnosis of adenocarcinoma in cytologic fluids does not identify the primary source; for these patients, diagnosis should be approached by searching for treatable tumors.

Mediastinal malignancies that produce symptoms of dysphagia, respiratory difficulty, or superior vena cava syndrome are almost invariably due to primary lung cancer, metastatic breast cancer, or lymphoma. All can be rather well managed by local radiation therapy and do not warrant extensive evaluation and search for the primary tumor.

The identification of a *bony lesion* that is radiographically characteristic of neoplasia should be followed up with a biopsy of the area. If the lesion is inaccessible or is amenable to biopsy only with difficulty, an alternate first step is to obtain a routine bone marrow biopsy from the iliac crest. The vast majority of patients with bony metastases have multiple lesions that often invade the bone marrow. The second crucial step is to obtain a bone scan in order to identify other sites of tumor that may be more easily accessible to a fluoroscopically guided biopsy. Having established a histologic diagnosis of malignancy in the bone, the search for the primary should, as always, be confined to focusing on treatable tumor.

Bony metastases are generally not treated systemically; for the most part they are palliated locally by radiation therapy when symptoms arise. Therefore, in the absence of symptoms, the bone lesions may simply be monitored unless a definitively responsive tumor, such as prostate or breast cancer, can be identified.

Hepatic TUOs are usually diagnosed by liver biopsy. Most are adenocarcinomas. Once an adenocarcinoma in the liver has been identified, it is unnecessary for therapy to order an upper GI series, small bowel follow-through, barium enema, colonoscopy, pancreatic endoscopy, or gallbladder series. None of the tumors that arise in any of these sites, once metastatic to the liver, are sufficiently treatable with systemic therapy to warrant establishing the diagnosis. Furthermore, patients with hepatic metastases have a life expectancy of less than six months. Prophylactic surgery of the primary tumor is not indicated unless significant antitumor effect can be demonstrated in the metastatic disease. Assessment for antitumor effect should be scheduled to occur at 4 to 6 weeks, if cytotoxic chemotherapy is utilized. Only if marked response is documented is search for the primary tumor warranted.

Lymph nodes in the cervical, axillary, and inguinal sites occasionally harbor an unknown primary tumor. For the most part, lymph node lesions are drainage areas for a TUO in a contiguous organ (see Chapter 81).

Cervical lymph nodes are first biopsied to determine the histopathologic category of tumor. If an epidermoid carcinoma is found, then extensive otolaryngologic evaluation of the nasopharynx, retropharynx, and oral cavity must be performed, including blind biopsies of the base of the tongue and the nasopharynx. If no definite primary is identified, the carcinoma must be managed by either radiation or lymph node dissection on the ipsilateral site. The carcinoma is cured in 20% to 35% of patients. Other tumors that may be metastatic to cervical nodes include those of the sinuses and salivary glands; if the histopathology is adenocarcinoma, the sinuses or the salivary glands may be the primary source. If the histologic studies indicate lymphoma, then the diagnosis and staging approach are altogether different (see Chapters 82, 83).

Axillary nodes that histologically manifest adenocarcinoma are most commonly associated with mammary cancer. Even in the presence of a normal mammogram, mastectomy may sometimes be necessary because identification of the primary tumor can be difficult. The diagnosis may be assisted by performing ERP assays on any tissue obtained from the axilla that appears to be a carcinoma (see Chapter 121).

Inguinal adenopathy is approached diagnostically and therapeutically in much the same manner as cervical adenopathy. The presence of an epidermoid carcinoma or adenocarcinoma may be treated by local radiation therapy bilaterally if there is no evidence of an anal or prostatic lesion on blind biopsy. If inguinal node biopsy identifies a lymphoma, there is no need for lymphangiography, particularly in the presence of adenopathy at sites above the diaphragm. Lymphangiography alone is never a diagnostic procedure and only occasionally a staging procedure, since it generally cannot determine therapy. It invariably requires histologic confirmation, particularly in the presence of lymphangiographically positive lymph nodes (see Chapters 82, 83).

TREATMENT

When the primary remains unknown (as is the case in the vast majority of patients), the therapeutic approach to the patient may be based on a prudent estimate of the most likely treatable tumor (see Table 86-1). If the pathologic type is undifferentiated, treatment is directed toward the most responsive tumors in this class, namely, lymphoma and germ-cell neoplasms. Metastatic adenocarcinoma in men can be treated as metastatic prostate cancer, and in women as metastatic ovarian or breast cancer, since these are the most treatable tumors. Metastatic prostate cancer has a 40% to 60% response rate to hormonal therapy (see Chapter 141). Carcinoma of the breast has a similar response rate to therapy; modalities include hormonal treatment for some patients and chemotherapy for others (see Chapter 121).

Asymptomatic patients need not be treated when the primary remains unknown. Radiation may provide reasonable palliation for localized symptomatic disease, especially that which involves bone, mediastinum, or lymph nodes.

ANNOTATED BIBLIOGRAPHY

Copeland EM, McBride CM: Axillary metastases from unknown primary sites. Ann Surg 178:25, 1972 (*The breast is the most common primary source in woman with an undifferentiated axillary lesion, but alternatives include primary melanoma or adnexal tumors of the extremity.*)

Fitzpatrick PJ, Kotalik JF: Cervical metastases from an unknown primary tumor. Ther Radiol 110:659, 1974 (*Radiation therapy for cervical lymph nodes in an unknown primary tumor may result in a cure rate of more than 40%, in spite of inability to identify the primary tumor source. Emphasis on the site of cervical node involvement and the technique of radiation therapy produces optimal therapeutic effect.*)

Greco FA, Vaughn WK, Hainsworth JD: Advanced poorly differentiated carcinoma of unknown primary site: recognition of a treatable syndrome. Ann Intern Med 104:547, 1986 (*Patients with poorly differentiated histology and tumor in the mediastinum, retroperitoneum, and lymph nodes responded well to chemotherapy with cisplatin-based combination chemotherapy.*)

Legg MA: What role for the diagnostic pathologist. N Engl J Med 305:950, 1981 (*An editorial reviewing the contributions from pathologic examination of tissue specimens.*)

McMillan JH, Levine E, Stephens RH: Computed tomography in the evaluation of metastatic adenocarcinoma from an unknown primary site. Radiology 143:143, 1982 (*A retrospective series comparing CT to other radiologic modalities and finding CT superior.*)

Nystrom JS, Weiner JM et al: Metastatic and histologic presentations in unknown primary cancer. Semin Oncol 4:53, 1977 (*The most common primary tumor site above the diaphragm proved to be the lung; below the diaphragm it was the pancreas.*)

Nystrom JS, Weiner JM et al: Identifying the primary site in metastatic cancer of unknown origin: Inadequacy of roentgenographic procedures. JAMA 241:381, 1979 (*Standard x-ray studies proved too insensitive to detect the primary lesion.*)

Smith PE, Krementz ET, Chapman W: Metastatic cancer without a detectable primary site. Am J Surg 113:633, 1967 (*In more than 70% of the cases, a primary tumor site was not established, in spite of extensive diagnostic evaluation. The survival was longest in those patients with undifferentiated tumor.*)

Zaren HA, Copeland EM, III: Inguinal node metastases. Cancer 41:919, 1978 (*One percent of more than 2200 patients with inguinal node metastases had an unknown primary tumor; in them, survival and possible cure was obtained in 50% by surgical excision alone. In only one of the 22 patients with an unknown primary tumor was the primary tumor found.*)

87

Approach to Staging and Monitoring

JACOB J. LOKICH, M.D.

Staging and monitoring are essential components of cancer management. Staging is performed to assess the extent of disease, and it is used to help determine prognosis and therapy. Monitoring serves to detect the reappearance or progression of cancer and contributes importantly to updating prognosis and revising treatment plans. Staging and monitoring procedures are determined by tumor type, its natural history, response to therapy, and characteristic pattern of spread. The frequency and duration of monitoring depend on the rate of disease recurrence.

If the primary physician is to be responsible for the management of the cancer patient, he must be able to stage and monitor disease. This task requires knowledge of the indications for and limitations of the many available laboratory tests and radiologic procedures, so that important decisions about test and procedure selection can be made effectively, and unnecessary expense and discomfort avoided.

STAGING TERMINOLOGY

The general classification of staging is based on the anatomic distribution of disease. It is broadly categorized as *local* (confined to a visceral site); *regional* (extension within the local site, with or without involvement of contiguous lymph nodes); or *distant* (generally hematogenous metastases beyond the regional scope, which precludes treatment that uses local surgical removal). This staging system is translated into *T* for tumors, *N* for nodes, and *M* for metastases. Subcategories may be developed depending upon the size of the tumor (T-1 to 3); the number or fixation of the lymph nodes (N-1 to 2); and the presence or lack of metastases (M-0 or 1).

PRINCIPLES AND PROCEDURES OF STAGING

Staging procedures are selected predominantly on the basis of the malignancy's characteristic pattern of local and metastatic spread. The type of tumor and the natural history of its rate of growth are other determinants of the staging strategy. For example, sarcomas metastasize hematogenously, usually to lung, and rarely proceed to lymph nodes. Thus, lung tomography is an important staging tool for sarcomas, while lymphangiography is not.

Two other important factors in the selection of a staging procedure are the sensitivity and specificity of the test (see Chapter 2) for the particular tumor in question.

Radiographic Procedures. The most frequently used for determining the extent of disease include computed tomog-

raphy (CT), ultrasonography, radionuclide scanning, lymphangiography, and metastatic series bone films. Their principal limitation is inability to detect disease less than 1 cm in diameter (see Table 87-1).

Computed tomography represents an important advance; it provides not only improved detection of tumor, but also quantitation. By virtue of its enhanced resolution power, *chest CT* has proven superior to conventional full lung tomography for detection of pleural, mediastinal, and parenchymal lesions (see Chapter 86). The test is particularly useful for staging patients with sarcomas or testicular cancers, malignancies with high rates of lung metastasis. *CT of the abdomen* permits enhanced evaluation of the retroperitoneum, permitting identification of enlarged lymph nodes that were previously undetectable by other means (see Chapters 82 and 83). Moreover, CT has improved the search for and quantitation of tumor in the pancreas, liver, and pelvis as well as helping to guide needle biopsy. *CT of the brain* has eliminated the need to conduct invasive studies in search of CNS metastases. Although sensitivity for detection of lesions in the posterior fossa was low for first-generation CT scanners, later machines give better views of the area, as do *magnetic resonance* scanners. Magnetic resonance techniques have considerable promise and offer the advantage of no radiation exposure; the literature should be followed for developments in their application to staging and monitoring.

Ultrasonography is more useful for detection of intra-abdominal disease, than for quantitation. It is especially effective as a means of identifying pancreatic and retroperitoneal lesions that are more than 2 cm in diameter. Ultrasonography accurately distinguishes solid masses from cystic ones, a capability of importance in evaluation of pelvic, testicular, and thyroid nodules (see Chapters 114, 130, and 95). It can also help guide needle biopsy.

Radionuclide scanning, especially of the liver and brain, has been overutilized for staging cancer. In many areas of

Table 87-1. Radiographic Procedures in Cancer Staging

PROCEDURE	TUMOR TYPES	FALSE-POSITIVE	FALSE-NEGATIVE	COMMENT
Computed Tomography				
Chest	Sarcoma, testicular, lung cancer	20%	5%	False-positive related to identification of granulomas not representing tumors. Ideal for mediastinum assessment.
Abdomen	Lymphoma, testicular, ovarian cancer	<5%	10%–15%	May replace lymphangiography for testicular cancer but not for lymphomas or Hodgkins disease
Lymphangiography	Hodgkins disease, lymphomas, testicular cancer	20%	10%–20%	Standard only for Hodgkins disease

the body, the technique offers only low levels of sensitivity and specificity, greatly limiting its clinical usefulness. *Hepatic scanning* is frequently ordered to stage gastrointestinal cancers, but rarely detects disease that is not predicted on the basis of abnormal liver function tests (*e.g.,* an elevated alkaline phosphatase) or clinical hepatomegaly. Furthermore, a large percentage of abnormal hepatic scans represent secondary drug effects or incidental inflammatory disease. True-positive liver scans are found in less than 1% of patients with otherwise operable primary breast or colon cancer; routine liver scanning for metastases is unwarranted in these conditions. *Brain scanning* is of low sensitivity and has been replaced in most instances by CT.

One useful radionuclide technique is the *bone scan,* an exquisitely sensitive means of detecting abnormalities of bone physiology and far superior to skeletal x-rays. Nevertheless, diagnostic confirmation by standard radiographs, and occasionally by biopsy, is necessary. Bone scanning allows earlier detection than conventional x-ray metastatic series, though this does not necessarily translate into prolonged survival. The test should be used in the initial evaluation of primary tumor to determine therapeutic approach or later to evaluate bone pain or other symptoms. It can document spread in patients with clinical suspicion of advanced disease of the prostate, breast, and lung (oat cell carcinoma).

Standard radiographs, such as the *metastatic series,* have a high false-negative rate and are relatively insensitive, though false-positive rates are relatively low. *Contrast studies,* such as intravenous pyelography, venography, and angiography, are infrequently applied to staging, although they may aid in planning surgery. Conventional chest tomography has been supplanted by chest CT (see above), which has a lower false-negative rate.

Lymphangiography was developed primarily for the evaluation of retroperitoneal lymph nodes in the staging of Hodgkin's disease, but it has been similarly employed for lymphoma. The usefulness of the test for staging has declined because treatment no longer depends heavily on its findings (see Chapters 82 and 83). In lymphoma, the test has been replaced by abdominal CT, though it is still used for staging in Hodgkin's disease.

Gallium scanning grew out of an attempt to develop an agent that would localize within tumors. However, sensitivity and specificity proved poor because the nuclide also readily enters inflamed tissue. Nevertheless, the test is recommended by some for staging melanoma and lymphoma. The discomfort of the study, which requires frequent enemas, and its high false-negative rate relegate it to infrequent use.

Tumor Markers have been sought with the hope of obtaining a more sensitive means of tumor detection, enabling earlier identification of metastatic disease and recurrence. Radiologic techniques usually require a mass of at least 1 cm in size. Although tumor-specific monoclonal antibodies may soon revolutionize tumor marker technology, only a limited number of markers are presently of proven clinical utility: carcinoembryonic antigen, alpha-fetoprotein, human chorionic gonadotropin, CA125, and CA19-9.

Carcinoembryonic antigen (CEA) is present in both normal and malignant tissue; serum levels in excess of 2.5 ng/ml are suggestive of tumor, but the test is too nonspecific for screening. Its most useful application is in early detection of recurrence, especially for cancers of the colorectum, breast, and lung (see Chapters 73, 121, and 42). The consensus is that serial CEA determinations are the best currently available noninvasive means for identifying recurrent colorectal cancer after surgery.

Alpha-fetoprotein (AFP) has been found in high serum concentrations in association with hepatomas and embryonal testicular tumors (see Chapter 141). Although lacking sufficient specificity for diagnostic purposes, repeat AFP determinations can be used to monitor for disease recurrence and assess adequacy of treatment. *Human chorionic gonadotropin (hCG)* is another useful tumor marker for germ-cell tumors of the testes and ovaries. Monitoring of its beta-subunit provides information similar to that provided by the AFP. *Acid phosphatase* elevations occur in up to 80% of patients with prostate cancer that has spread to bone; elevations may occur in the absence of bone metastasis. Identification of a prostatic fraction has improved the test's specificity.

Tumor markers derived from monoclonal antibody techniques include *CA19-9,* which is elevated in cancers of the gastrointestinal tract, and *CA125,* produced by 80% of epithelial ovarian cancers. CA125 appears to correlate with the clinical course and is useful for monitoring. The specificity is high; it is being tested as a diagnostic tool.

Surgical Procedures. Surgical staging of cancer has evolved from *lymph node dissection* procedures. Lymphadenectomy was initially undertaken in patients with breast cancer and malignant melanoma to eliminate contiguous sites of disease. For both tumors, however, it has been demonstrated that lymphadenectomy at the time of surgery for the primary lesion does not extend survival, but does serve as a prognostic determinant (Table 87-2).

Lymph node evaluation of distant disease has become a recognized staging procedure. For example, scalene node biopsy is sometimes performed in patients with primary tumors of the cervix or testicle. In a small proportion of patients, metastases to distant lymph node sites are demonstrated; the identification of distant metastases is important to the management of the primary tumor (see Chapter 141).

Laparotomy and *laparoscopy* have been used in the evaluation of Hodgkin's disease and, more recently, in the evaluation of ovarian cancer to detect abdominal disease. Laparotomy and splenectomy are recommended for the staging

Table 87-2.   Surgical Procedures in Staging Evaluation of Cancer

PROCEDURE	TUMOR	COMMENTS
Scalene node biopsy	Lung, testicle, cervix	Diagnostic; 10% positive in stage II disease
Lymphadenectomy	Breast, melanoma, head, and neck	May be therapeutic but more specifically prognostic
Laparoscopy	Hodgkin's disease, esophagus, ovary	Allows limited access to abdominal contents; has high false-negative rate
Laparotomy	Hodgkin's disease, melanoma, ovary	Definitively evaluates the abdomen and allows for debulking and splenectomy

of Hodgkin's disease in patients with potential disease below the diaphragm, helping to delineate the radiation portals as well as to move the ovaries out of the port of radiation therapy. For patients who already have evidence of disease below the diaphragm (positive CT, lymphangiography, palpable inguinal nodes, or splenomegaly), the evaluation of the abdomen should be confined to laparoscopy and biopsy of the liver. Patients with clinical disease below the diaphragm and, particularly, patients with B symptoms have a high incidence of secondary complications following laparotomy and splenectomy (see Chapter 82).

PRINCIPLES AND PROCEDURES OF MONITORING DISEASE

Once the extent of disease is determined and treatment initiated, monitoring begins. As noted earlier, the frequency and duration of monitoring are dependent upon the rate of disease recurrence. The procedures selected are based in part on tumor type, response to therapy, stage of disease, and pattern of metastasis. Test sensitivity and specificity are also important.

Local or Regional Disease. Patients with local or regional disease may be monitored by routine physical examinations supplemented by careful examination of the disease site at 3-month intervals for the first year following operation, and at 4-month intervals for the second year. Thereafter, follow-up may be accomplished at 6-month intervals for a minimum of 5 years. By and large, most tumors will recur at a maximum rate during the first 2 years following the initial operation—if in fact they are destined to recur. Three malignancies are notorious for late recurrence: breast carcinoma, melanoma, and renal-cell carcinoma. In some patients with these tumors, the lag period before the development of detectable metastases may extend beyond 10 years from initial diagnosis.

Periodic evaluation of patients with regional disease who have undergone curative primary therapy should be directed less at detecting the presence of asymptomatic metastases, and more at finding new primary tumors in the involved organ (Table 8-3). Identification of asymptomatic metastases by radionuclide scanning is of little use, because the early detection and treatment of asymptomatic metastatic disease does not necessarily improve survival.

Metastatic Disease. Follow-up examinations for patients with metastatic disease who receive systemic therapy should be performed at intervals determined by the time expected for an objective clinical response. For hormonal therapy of breast cancer, clinical evidence of response may take as long

Table 87-3.   Periodicity of Follow-up Examination Following Local Surgery for Colon (Dukes B$_2$ and C) and Breast (Stage II) Cancers

TUMOR	INCIDENCE OF SUBSEQUENT METASTASES (%)	INCIDENCE OF NEW (SECOND) 1° (%)	EXAMINATION	FREQUENCY OF EXAMINATIONS
Colon	70	5	Barium enema	Every 2 years
			Sigmoidoscopy or colonoscopy	Every 3 years
			CEA	Every 6 months
			Liver scan	Not indicated
Breast	70	10	Mammogram	Every 1–2 years
			Bone scan	Not indicated
			Metastatic series	Not indicated

as 3 months to appear. The effects of cytotoxic chemotherapy may be seen rapidly, for example, within two courses of treatment or 4 to 6 weeks. This is particularly true for exquisitely responsive tumors such as breast, testicular, ovarian, and oat-cell carcinomas.

Patients with metastatic disease receiving palliative systemic therapy should be examined for evidence of new disease. Unnecessary chemotherapy-induced morbidity can be avoided if ineffective palliative systemic therapy is discontinued at the first signs of new disease. Response to therapy may be objectively demonstrated after a predictable interval, but new growth or spread may be noted on earlier examination.

An important corollary to the monitoring of patients with metastatic disease on systemic therapeutic regimens is to define the most objective site of disease to be followed and to avoid additional staging procedures if they do not alter the therapeutic plan. For example, a patient with hepatic metastases from primary breast cancer need not endure a bone scan unless there is bone pain or fracture. The tumor is already established as being incurable, and therapy is determined by the presence of liver metastases. Alternatively, the patient with bony metastases that are difficult to monitor may undergo selective staging in order to identify a more measurable marker of metastatic disease, such as plasma carcinoembryonic antigen.

ANNOTATED BIBLIOGRAPHY

Bast RC, Jr, Klug TL et al: Radioimmunoassay using a monoclonal antibody to monitor the course of epithelial ovarian cancer. N Engl J Med 309:883, 1983 (*An important application of this new technology to tumor monitoring.*)

Beard DB, Haskell CM: Carcinoembryonic antigen in breast cancer. Am J Med 80:241, 1986 (*A review of CEA's role in breast cancer; especially useful in patients with advanced disease.*)

Fletcher RH: Carcinoembryonic antigen. Ann Intern Med 104:66, 1986 (*A critical review, pointing out the limitations of its usefulness.*)

Friedman MA, Resser KJ, Marcus FS et al: How accurate are computed tomographic scans in assessment of changes in tumor size? Am J Med 75:193, 1983 (*Documents the sensitivity of CT for determining changes in size; authors argue the test is the best means available.*)

Galasko CSB: The value of scintigraphy in malignant disease. Cancer Treat Rev 2:225, 1975 (*A comprehensive assessment of the technical features of scintigraphy and its application to monitoring malignant disease. The identification of tumor-specific, tumor-searching agents is reviewed in relationship to other uses of radionuclide scanning in malignant disease.*)

Gerard G, Rossi DR: Nuclear magnetic resonance imaging of the brain. Hosp Pract 19:143, 1984 (*A broad review of MR that includes consideration of its use in detecting brain metastases.*)

Lokich JJ: Carcinoembryonic antigen (CEA): A monitor of therapy for breast and colon cancers. Am Fam Physician 17:173, 1978 (*The author promotes the application of CEA as a tumor associating antigen in specific clinical settings with specific tumor categories.*)

Lokich JJ: Tumor markers: Hormones, antigens, and enzymes in malignant disease. Oncology 35:54, 1978 (*The general considerations of tumor markers as specific monitors of malignancy are reviewed, and specific recommendations regarding the realistic application of tumor markers are presented.*)

McMillan JH, Levine E, Stephens RH: Computed tomography in the evaluation of metastatic adenocarcinoma from an unknown primary site. Radiology 143:143, 1982 (*A retrospective study comparing CT to other diagnostic modalities. CT was superior.*)

O'Connell MJ, Wahner HW, Ahmann, DL et al: Value of preoperative radionuclide bone scan in suspected primary breast carcinoma. Mayo Clin Proc 53:221, 1978 (*It is emphasized that localized disease uncommonly reveals a positive bone scan that would be a determinant of future therapy. Specific guidelines for the timing of bone scans in breast cancer are outlined.*)

Sears HF, Gerber FH, Sturtz DL et al: Liver scan and carcinoma of the breast. Surg Gynecol Obstet 140:409, 1975 (*The specific lack of usefulness of liver scans in 100 patients with carcinoma of the breast in this series may be extended to other tumors. It is, therefore, rarely useful to employ liver scans in patients who have other sites of documented extension of their disease or who lack hepatomegaly, liver pain, or abnormal liver function tests.*)

Smalley RV, Malmud LS, Ritchie WGM: Preoperative scanning: Evaluation for metastatic disease in carcinoma of the breast, lung, colon, bladder, and prostate. Semin Oncol 7:358, 1980 (*A critical analysis of radionuclide, ultrasound, and computed tomographic scanning that realistically assesses the precise usefulness of these tests in relation to the staging and natural history of these particular tumors.*)

Van Dyke JA, Stanley RJ, Berland LL: Pancreatic imaging. Ann Intern Med 102:212, 1985 (*A detailed review that discusses use of CT in documenting presence and extent of tumor.*)

Veronesi R et al: Inefficacy of immediate node dissection in melanoma of the limbs. N Engl J Med 297:627, 1977 (*This specific reference to the use of lymphadenectomy in malignant melanoma as a prognostic, rather than as a therapeutic procedure is an example that may be extended to other tumors in which lymph node dissection is employed routinely as a staging device.*)

Wittes RE, Yeh SDJ: Indications for liver and brain scans: Screening tests for patients with oat cell carcinoma of the lung. JAMA 238:506, 1977 (*The lack of usefulness of liver and brain scans in the staging of patients with oat-cell carcinoma is reviewed in a singular experience.*)

88

Comprehensive Care of the Cancer Patient

JACOB J. LOKICH, M.D.

The treatment of cancer has become multifaceted, involving the interdigitation of physician support with surgery, radiation, cytotoxic agents, and, most recently, biologic response modifiers. The role of the primary physician is pivotal; most cancer patients can remain at home with their families and receive optimal therapy on an outpatient basis when there is a primary physician working closely with a cancer center or local specialist in cancer management. Only when radiation therapy, blood product transfusions, or experimental protocols are used is it essential for the patient to go to a cancer treatment center.

Curative treatment that focuses on the primary tumor site has traditionally been the province of surgery, with radiation and chemotherapy relegated to palliative roles. More recently, radiation and chemotherapy have been employed as adjuvants for local disease, enhancing the capability of surgery to cure. Moreover, radiation therapy has proved to be curative in early Hodgkin's disease (see Chapter 82) and cervical cancer (see Chapter 122). The role of immune therapy is currently undergoing clinical trial.

In order to provide effective care to the cancer patient, the primary physician should have a thorough understanding of the natural history of the tumor in question and its potential responsiveness to surgery, radiation, and drug therapy. Skillful management requires proper staging and monitoring (see Chapter 87), knowledge of the indications, limitations, and adverse effects of each treatment modality (see Chapters 88 and 89), formation of a supportive alliance with patient and family, provision of symptomatic relief and pain control (see Chapter 91), and access to expert advice.

COMMUNICATING THE DIAGNOSIS

For most patients, the diagnosis of cancer evokes images of pain, suffering, mutilation, and certain death. These basic fears are so intertwined with the word "cancer" that confirmation of the diagnosis places extreme emotional stress on the patient and his family. It is in managing this anguish that the physician plays a most important role. The physician often represents the one person to whom the patient and family can turn and must be not only the source of scientific and medical expertise but also the provider of emotional support and understanding. It is important to recognize that cancer affects not only the patient but also his family, who must grieve and resolve their own fears and anxieties. The physician is frequently obliged to deal with many members of the family, often at differing levels of need for information and support. By virtue of his long-standing relationship with the patient and family, the primary physician is in an ideal position to provide effective support.

It is always difficult to give bad news. Physicians sometimes avoid telling the patient the diagnosis in accurate and specific terms at the outset, resorting to such euphemisms as "lump," "mass," and "lesion." Further inhibiting communication may be the ill-advised, though well-intentioned insistence of family members that the diagnosis be kept from the patient out of fear of precipitating a severe depression. Such concerns are usually ill-conceived. It is rare that ignorance of the diagnosis or prognosis is helpful for the patient or family. Quite the contrary. Well-informed patients deal better with their illness and treatment regimens. The candor facilitates development of trust between patient and medical staff and breaks down the barrier that often isolates the cancer patient from his family.

More important, the patient who is unaware of the diagnosis and prognosis may not resolve important issues in his life. He may continue to have unrealistic plans or persistently uncomfortable relationships with other members of his family, which might otherwise be resolved if all were to understand the prognosis. Similarly, the uninformed family is unable to express its grief gradually over time, and death may appear to be sudden. The resulting unresolved grief may profoundly affect the surviving family members (see Chapter 223).

Common misconceptions about cancer include the certainty of death, intractable pain, and erosive, disfiguring disease. In order to avoid needless worry, it is essential at the outset to address these common concerns directly, even if the patient does not express them.

The goal in communicating the diagnosis and prognosis is to be accurate without destroying all hope. First and foremost, the words "cancer" and "malignant tumor" should be used at the outset of the interview and not avoided, although constant repetition of the terms is usually unnecessary. The term "fatal" ought to be omitted in discussions of prognosis, for it implies little hope of control. When informed of an incurable malignancy, the patient and family want to know "How much time is left?" A rough estimate may be necessary if the patient must arrange his affairs, but, if possible, the physician should avoid indicating a specific period of time, because it is apt to be inaccurate. Preferably, the physician should direct the patient toward realistic therapeutic approaches and reinforce his role in living instead of dying.

The family certainly needs full and frequent reports of the patient's status and prognosis. Patients often pass through a sequence of emotions that have been characterized by Kubler-Ross. These include periods of denial, hostility, anger, hope, depression, and finally acceptance. The physician often has much impact in determining the length of any one phase before the patient accepts living with cancer. The physician's role in this aspect of treatment is as important to maintaining the patient's quality of life as is any other therapeutic modality.

PATIENT AND FAMILY REACTIONS

Patient reactions at the time of presentation of the diagnosis depend on preconceived ideas about cancer and what the specter of cancer suggests to them. Denial, hostility, rejection of loved ones, regression to immaturity, and withdrawal represent the most common reactions.

Hostility is occasionally an early reaction to the diagnosis. Anger may be directed against the medical team for the delayed diagnosis or for inadequate attention, as well as toward family members, who may be viewed as not particularly upset and happy to finally "get their way." This phase is generally transient, receding as the patient comes to recognize the reality of the situation and the need for family and physician. Hostility is difficult for both patient and doctor and may be intense enough to lead the physician and family to reject the patient emotionally. If recognized, this reaction should be allowed to run a natural course without withdrawing support.

Infantile regression is an accentuated response commonly occurring in the patient with a dependent personality. It also develops as a reaction-formation in patients who were overly independent before their illness. If it is more than transient, infantile regression must be mitigated by providing a parental figure who will be, on the one hand, supportive and, on the other hand, stern and demanding. Infantile regression places an inordinate burden on the family, who are called upon to provide extraordinary amounts of support.

Withdrawal is an extreme form of regression. Often tinged with elements of hostility. Direct confrontation is essential for the patient who withdraws; constant encouragement and the setting up of goals for achievement (such as ambulation, planning trips, or visiting friends) are critical.

Denial of the diagnosis is generally a transient reaction. When denial is mild, the physician may need only to reinforce his remarks with re-presentation of the facts or provision of objective and tangible evidence. However, in some patients, denial is extreme and functions as a crude psychologic defense mechanism, necessary for sustaining the psyche. A constant onslaught of evidence and reinforcement of the diagnosis or prognosis may be counterproductive and is not justified.

The *reactions of the family* are critical to the patient's well-being and to aiding the health care team in providing maximum support. Thus, the physician must be concerned with the family's responses to the patient and to the diagnosis. Not uncommonly, complete families—wives, husbands, and children—may be alienated by the patient, who disallows them the opportunity to resolve their confusion. Such alienation, which may approach pathologic proportions, can be understood with the help of the physician. A frequent family reaction is to provide smothering protection in compensation for guilt over previous misunderstandings with the patient and the need to resolve such differences. Again, the physician can help alleviate such pathologic reactions.

PSYCHOLOGIC REACTIONS TO CANCER TREATMENT

The patient who enters treatment for cancer is subjected to a reinforcement of the diagnosis and a rekindling of the fears regarding threats to self-esteem and self-image. The latter may be particularly demoralizing if the cancer treatment involves bodily disfigurement or a physical limitation that is either cosmetically mutilating or functionally disabling. Thus, the patient who requires a mastectomy, jaw resection, amputation, or colostomy faces a significant and frightening change in self-image. The distortions that are incorporated into the patient's unconscious perhaps as a result of real or imagined experiences with friends, are potentially devastating. Often these distortions are unrealistic and unsubstantiated, but, more importantly, they may be unexpressed. The physician must inquire into the patient's concerns and offer a realistic appraisal in order to minimize unnecessary anguish (see Chapter 1). Patient education is a most important component of the approach to dealing with the stress of therapy. It additionally serves to cushion the stress by allowing the patient to intellectualize about the disease and its treatment. In this "demythologizing process" patient fears are identified and dealt with openly. Often the result is a more acceptable view of one's illness and treatment. Educational materials may facilitate the task. For example, booklets are available from the National Cancer Institute (NCI) that address questions that the patient may have about various types of therapy (*e.g., Chemotherapy and You,* NCI-HEW Publication No. 76-1136). Detailed explanation of the therapy in terms of its effect on the tumor as well as its potential side effects allows the patient to approach treatment realistically. Support groups have also proven valuable.

LOCAL TUMOR THERAPY: SURGERY AND RADIATION

Surgery has traditionally assumed the dominant role in the management of cancer. Diagnosis is established and confirmed by surgical biopsy, and cure may be effected by operation. Nonetheless, there has recently been a shift in emphasis toward minimizing surgical procedures, particularly when the prognosis is determined by factors such as distant metastases, and when salvage by secondary local modalities can be accomplished. Four standard surgical operations have been scaled down in many cases to less radical procedures to lessen chances of morbidity:

1. Lymph node dissection for malignant melanoma (see Chapter 171)
2. Limb amputation for osteogenic sarcoma
3. Ostomy and AP resection for rectal cancer (see Chapter 73)
4. Radical mastectomy for breast cancer (see Chapter 121)

Although controversial, the surgical approach to these lesions may be modified by the addition of local therapy (*e.g.,* radiation) or systemic therapy (*e.g.,* cytotoxic agents).

Radiation therapy has become more effective due to development of high-energy linear accelerators and technical improvements in delivery, which have lowered rates of morbidity and increased rates of survival and local control. There are at least two tumors for which radiation therapy is now the local therapy of choice: early stages of Hodgkin's disease (see Chapter 82) and carcinoma of the cervix (see Chapter 122). Radiation in conjunction with surgery may be curative in some tumors when administered pre- or postoperatively. In other malignancies the combined application of radiation and either surgery or chemotherapy may promote palliation and chances for long-term survival, although rarely achieving cure (see Chapter 90).

ADJUVANT OR COMBINED THERAPY OF LOCAL OR REGIONAL CANCER

Adjuvant therapy involves the addition of chemotherapy or radiation to surgical procedures. The rationale for adding

radiation therapy is primarily to promote local control of presumed residual microscopic tumor. In theory, chemotherapy functions as an adjuvant modality because of the possibility that tumor cells are released into the circulation at the time of surgery. In addition, adjuvant chemotherapy may be effective because it affects existing micrometastases at a time when they are rapidly proliferating and likely to be quite drug sensitive.

Adjuvant therapy has been proposed or is part of ongoing trials for treatment of a number of cancers (Table 88-1); at present it is a proven and established therapy for carcinomas of the breast and rectum. In breast cancer, premenopausal women with positive lymph nodes and pathologic stage II disease have benefited from the addition of chemotherapy. It has reduced the incidence of recurrence and prolonged disease-free survival to 4 years (see Chapter 121). Patients with rectal cancer that extends beyond the bowel wall (so-called Duke's B_2 or C lesions) have shown reduced local recurrence rates and possibly increased survival time with the use of radiation therapy (see Chapter 73). The role of preoperative radiation therapy in comparison to postoperative radiation therapy has not been definitely established (see Table 88-1).

For the vast majority of tumors, local or regional disease is incurable in spite of adjuvant modalities. Only 15% of patients with stage II malignant melanoma survive 5 years; less than 5% of patients with lung, renal cell, and pancreatic cancers that are regionally advanced show long-term survival. Thus chemotherapy, immune therapy and radiation are not generally employed as adjuvant modalities for these tumors, unless used investigationally.

For some tumors, such as testicular cancer (see Chapter 141), osteogenic sarcoma, or Hodgkin's disease (see Chapter 82), the role of ancillary modalities is important in extending survival time and limiting morbidity of regional disease.

With the advent of more effective cytotoxic drugs and

Table 88-1.   Stage and Category of Tumors That Require
Adjuvant Chemotherapy or Radiotherapy

TUMOR	STAGE	ADJUVANT MODALITY	STATUS
Breast cancer	II	Chemotherapy (CMF)	Established for premenopausal women
Lung cancer	I	Immune therapy	Unestablished
Colon cancer	B_2/C	Chemotherapy (5-fluorouracil + nitrosourea) Immune therapy	Unestablished; clinical trials ongoing
Rectal cancer	B_2/C	Radiation	Established for postoperative radiotherapy; preoperative radiotherapy speculative
Ovarian cancer	I, II	Chemotherapy and radiation	Unestablished; ongoing trials
Testicular cancer	II	Chemotherapy (vinblastine, bleomycin, 1-CPDD)	Unestablished; ongoing trials

the use of radiation to sterilize local sites of tumor with minimal morbidity, the combined approach to local, regional, and even advanced cancers should become an increasing part of standard management. Currently, the application of forms of therapy ancillary to surgery must await the outcomes of ongoing clinical trials.

MANAGEMENT OF ADVANCED METASTATIC CANCER

The management of advanced disease is largely palliative, and involves systemic therapy provided by *cytotoxic drugs.* Chemotherapeutic regimens have become increasingly sophisticated and complex, but also more effective due to development of new agents and multiple-drug regimens (see Chapter 89). Decisions concerning use and timing of cytotoxic therapy in advanced disease are difficult, because of the potential morbidity associated with such therapy and the frequent lack of established benefit in promoting cure or even in prolonging survival. The decision to use chemotherapy in advanced disease is often a philosophical one, based on the feelings of patient, family, and physician.

Any decision to employ chemotherapy should involve an analysis of host tolerance as well as potential tumor responsiveness. Most important, the use of chemotherapy must be preceded by informed consent of the patient, who should be aware of the side effects as well as the potential for response. A common misconception is that the drugs invariably create morbidity and prolong life only at the cost of agonizing discomfort. In fact, when effective, chemotherapy can improve the quality of life as well as prolong it and, when it is ineffective, it will not necessarily induce more than transient morbidity.

In addition to these considerations, the primary indications for the use of chemotherapy in advanced disease include:

1. A probability of tumor responsiveness to chemotherapy greater than 30% for a partial response and greater than 5% for a complete response
2. Progressive tumor growth during a period of observation (*e.g.,* pulmonary nodules doubling in less than 30 days)
3. Symptomatic metastatic disease (*e.g.,* pleural effusion)

Within these guidelines, cytotoxic therapy can be administered with a reasonable risk-benefit balance.

The use of *experimental drug therapy* should be reserved for:

1. Patients who have failed with known effective drugs (*i.e.,* those drugs with a response rate > 30% and established ability to prolong survival)
2. Patients who wish to have or insist on a new form of treatment
3. Patients who have a measurable parameter to monitor for judging effectiveness of therapy

Biologic response modifiers utilizing agents such as interleukin-2 and interferon, are new forms of systemic treatment, designed to promote a generalized response that can affect tumors at any site. They are often included in the classification of chemotherapy, which is also systemic. Such therapy remains a highly experimental form of treatment, to be administered predominantly, if not exclusively, as a part of clinical trials at regional cancer centers. The use of intralesional BCG may be effective in small, superficial cutaneous lesions.

MANAGEMENT OF THE PRETERMINAL PHASE

"Terminal cancer" is an expression commonly employed by both patients and physicians, but with distinctly different definitions. Strictly defined, "terminal cancer" means that death will ensue within a 4-week period. The physician should avoid using the term "terminal" in talking with the patient or family. Not infrequently, patients may absorb the label and yet live for months or even years. The term imposes upon the family and the patient a tremendous stress, often resulting in withdrawal.

The physician's role in the terminal phase is a crucial one. It is essential to remain sensitive to all the patient's needs and specifically, to the patient's need to know that his physician is always available. If the patient is at home, frequent home visits may be enormously appreciated. It may be helpful to allow the patient to come to the office once or twice a week, even though there are no specific medications to be administered.

It is not incumbent upon the physician to reinforce the inevitability of death to patients who have entered a preterminal or terminal state and are sustaining hope for a reversal of the tumor. More important, however, during this period, the family must be apprised precisely in order to allow them to pass through the grieving process successfully.

The approach to preterminal care has begun to include more emphasis on comfort measures and care at home or in a hospice, where hospital routines and studies are omitted in favor of psychologic and symptomatic support. Relief of pain is an essential component of effective preterminal care (see Chapter 91).

PSYCHOTROPIC DRUG THERAPY

The use of psychotropic drugs for cancer patients has not been scientifically evaluated, but in many instances such drugs have a beneficial effect. For example, *tricyclic antidepressants* may be helpful in alleviating somatic symptoms of depression. If there is no contraindication, they should not be withheld on the basis of the common clinical misconception that "the patient is appropriately depressed, considering the diagnosis and prognosis" (see Chapter 223).

In recent years, hallucinogens and other consciousness-altering drugs have been used in terminal patients to promote euphoria and an acceptance of death. Such drugs are currently under investigation for use in terminal illness. The literature should be followed for developments in this very interesting area.

NUTRITION AND PAIN CONTROL

See Chapters 74 and 91 for discussions of nutrition and pain control.

ANNOTATED BIBLIOGRAPHY

Cullen JW, Fox BH, Isom RN (eds): Cancer: The Behavioral Dimensions. New York, Raven Press, 1976 (*Three papers focusing on coping with cancer and the difficulties of the physician and the patient in the presentation and the confrontation with the diagnosis of cancer represent an extensive personal experience by the three authors [JCB Holland, MJ Krant, and JN Vettese]. This is a useful introduction to the experience of patient issues in dealing with cancer.*)

Gates C: Psychodynamics of the Cancer Patient. In Lokich J (ed): Primer of Cancer Care. Boston, GK Hall, 1978 (*Based on the central concept that self-esteem is the singular aspect of the ego that must be supported and maintained. The impact of cancer on the ability of the patient to relate to his surroundings, to his closest friends and family members, and to his own goals and aspirations is assessed. The author specifically identifies a means of recognizing the anxiety states associated with cancer diagnosis and awareness.*)

Gates C, Hans P: Psychologic complications of cancer and its treatment. In Lokich J (ed): Clinical Cancer Medicine. Boston, GK Hall, 1979 (*Case histories detail patient reaction to the process of dying and living with cancer and the inherent difficulties in enduring treatment. The practical use of psychotropic drug therapy is described.*)

Gilbert HA et al: Evaluation of radiation therapy for bone metastases: Pain relief and quality of life. Am J Roentgenol 129:1095, 1977 (*A study of 158 patients, revealing considerable success in achieving palliation. Mean survival was 1 year after therapy, indicating that relief of pain was worthwhile, since patients lived for a considerable period of time.*)

Golden S, Horwich C, Lokich J: Chemotherapy and You. Department of Health and Welfare Publication (NIH) 76-1136 (*This pamphlet originally produced at the Sidney Farber Cancer Institute is available for patient use from the National Cancer Institute and serves as a layman's introduction to the concept of chemotherapy and its potential effects.*)

Goldie JH, Goldman AJ, Gudauskas GA: Rationale for the use of alternating non-cross-resistant chemotherapy. Cancer Treat Rep 66:439, 1982 (*The theoretical basis for modern multi-drug regimens.*)

Kaplan HS: Radiotherapeutic advances in the treatment of neoplastic disease. Isr J Med Sci 13:808, 1977 (*A comprehensive discussion and review of the applications of radiation therapy in treatment of cancer.*)

Krant MJ: The hospice movement. N Engl J Med 299:547, 1978 (*A thoughtful presentation of the methods and issues involved with this approach to terminal care.*)

Lokich J: Telling the diagnosis. In Lokich J (ed): Primer of Cancer Care. Boston, GK Hall, 1978 (*Through the use of multiple examples, the author describes a selected group of patient reactions to the diagnosis of cancer and clarifies the pros and cons of the informed patient, emphasizing the need to increase awareness in order to allow the patient and the family to resolve differences and to settle at some point of equilibrium.*)

Schabel FM, Jr: Rationale for adjuvant chemotherapy. Cancer 39: (Suppl) 2875, 1977 (*Discusses the biologic reasons for use of adjuvant therapy.*)

Spiegel D, Bloom JR, Yalom I: Group support for patients with metastatic cancer. Arch Gen Psychiatry 38:527, 1981 (*Documents benefits of support group interactions.*)

Staquet M: Cancer Therapy: Prognostic Factors and Criteria of Response. New York, Raven Press, 1975 (*A comprehensive interpretation of the natural history of solid tumors and hematologic malignancies and the impact of therapy on survival as well as objective tumor regression.*)

Weichselbaum R, Goebbels R, Lokich J: Complications of therapy. In Lokich J (ed): Clinical Cancer Management. Boston, GK Hall, 1979 (*A comprehensive review of the acute as well as chronic effects of chemotherapy and radiation therapy and a discussion of the reversibility of such effects as well as the mechanism of induction.*)

89

Principles of Cancer Chemotherapy

JACOB J. LOKICH, M.D.

The availability of chemotherapy for the cancer patient represents an important contribution to patient management. However, because the drugs are not selective, it is necessary to consider the adverse effects of therapy as well as their antitumor effects. The judicious use of chemotherapy involves a delicate balance of the two.

Chemotherapy has become a concern of the primary care physician as more cancer patients are managed on drug regimens outside of the hospital. Design of the chemotherapy program requires the expertise of the oncologist, for drug regimens are constantly being revised and new agents developed. However, it is often the primary physician who must follow the patient on a day-to-day basis and manage the entire range of medical and emotional problems encountered (see Chapters 74, 91) even though close cooperation with the oncologist is important. The role of the primary physician requires that he know the general indications for chemotherapy and the major toxic and adverse side effects of the commonly employed agents. He must evaluate response to therapy and alleviate side effects. In some instances, he may be called upon to administer chemotherapeutic agents, necessitating familiarity with proper dosage, route and technique.

PRINCIPLES OF THERAPY

Indications and Types of Regimens

There are three principal applications for chemotherapy: as a preoperative therapy, as adjuvant or postoperative therapy, and as palliative therapy for advanced disease. *Preoperative chemotherapy* is used to treat tumors that are moderately sensitive and responsive to drugs. The goal is to decrease the tumor bulk and make possible a more conservative surgical approach than would otherwise be possible. Determining the responsiveness of the individual tumor to drug therapy may also provide a more rational basis for long-term adjuvant treatment.

Postoperative adjuvant therapy has not yet been established as a standard form of treatment for most tumors; it is undergoing assessment for use in a number of tumors. The rationale behind giving chemotherapy to patients who have had what appears to be curative surgery is the frequency of distant micrometastases and local recurrences. Animal studies suggest that vigorous chemotherapy applied at this stage may be more successful than when delayed until clinically evident tumor has developed.

Chemotherapy of advanced disease has evolved from a strictly palliative role to a curative one in some instances, often in combination with radiation and surgery. This change has resulted from the discovery of increasingly effective chemotherapeutic agents and the development of *multi-drug regimens* that have increased not only the response rate, but also the duration of the response and the percentage of patients who enter a complete clinical remission. Single-agent regimens are still being employed, but mostly as adjuvant therapy or when a cancer is uniquely sensitive to a single drug, such as dactinomycin (Actinomycin D) for choriocarcinoma.

The treatment of advanced disease with chemotherapy has been variably successful; there are a number of effective tumor-specific regimens (see Table 89-1). In the absence of an established therapy (or research protocol), the asymptomatic patient should not be a candidate for chemotherapy, especially if the disease or the lesion cannot be measured by standard criteria. For the most part, the role of chemotherapy in advanced disease remains palliative. Patients who have an objective response, with at least partial tumor regression, usually live longer than those who achieve no response. Patients whose disease stabilizes according to objective criteria fare no better than patients who achieve no response. Therefore, when it can be objectively determined that a tumor has not regressed by 50% or more, therapy should be stopped or changed to an alternative drug regimen; the patient is unlikely to benefit from continued therapy.

The most active drugs in the management of cancer are the *alkylating drugs* and *doxorubicin* (see below). The combined use of these drugs, may be effective in a broad section of tumors, including lung, breast, and ovarian cancer, as well as in the hematologic malignancies. Consequently, for desperately ill patients with an *ill-defined tumor,* the combination may be employed as a first-line chemotherapy with a salutary effect.

The component drugs of combination regimens share important characteristics: they are each active against the specific tumor, have different modes or mechanisms of action on the tumor, have variant toxicities, and act at different sites in the cell cycle. This has permitted increased effectiveness without increased toxicity.

Sequential therapy has been found to be associated with a lower response rate than is maximal therapy that employs all active agents simultaneously at the outset of therapy. When chemotherapy is introduced sequentially or when second-line drugs are employed after failure of an initial program or a relapse, response is less likely. The tumor behaves in resistant fashion. Explanations advanced to explain this phenomenon include emergence of drug-resistant cell lines, slowed rate of growth, and membrane alterations.

Meaningful response to chemotherapy is usually observed within two courses of treatment. Only rarely does continued treatment in the absence of initial response result in an increased appreciation of response; usually, more therapy is unwarranted. To determine whether or not chemotherapy may be effective, one should schedule initial follow-up to take place within 2 months of the initiation of treatment.

Adverse Effects

The principal factor prohibiting the generalized application of chemotherapy is that the majority of cytotoxic drugs have a relative *lack of selectivity* for the tumor cell, resulting in a *narrow therapeutic index.* This factor, combined with the fact that there is a steep dose–response relationship for most cytotoxic effects, generally results in some form of host toxicity.

Cytotoxic drugs can adversely affect normal cell populations with rapid turnover, such as those of the bone marrow, hair follicles, and gastrointestinal mucosa. Bone marrow suppression, alopecia, and gastroenteritis are frequently encountered shortly after initiation of chemotherapy. For example, onset of acute marrow suppression is common 7 to 10 days after therapy and may last about 1 week.

Table 89-1. Combination Chemotherapy Regimens in Management of Cancer

PROGRAM	TUMOR	DOSE SCHEDULE	RESPONSE RATE (%)
CMF	Breast	See Chapter 121	
Cytoxan–Adriamycin	Ovary, breast	See Chapter 122	60–80, 40–60
		Every 28 days	
MOPP	Hodgkin's disease	M, 6 mg/m^2, day 1 and 8	80
		O, 1 mg/m^2, day 1 and 8	
		P, 100 mg/m^2 for 10 days	
		Pr, 50 mg for 10 days	
		Every 30 days	
COP; CVP	Non-Hodgkin's lymphoma	C, 100 mg/m^2 for 10 days	60
		O, 1 mg/m^2, day 1 and 8	
		P, 50 mg for 10 days	
		Every 28 days	
ABVD	Hodgkin's disease	A, 25 mg/m^2	80
		B, 10 mg/m^3, day 1 and 14	
		V, 6 mg/m^2	
		D, 200 mg/m^2	
		Every 28 days	
VBP	Testicular	V, 0.02 mg/kg, day 1 and 2	80–100
		B, 15 mg/m^2, day 1 and 8	
		Pt, 20 mg/m^2, day 1 to 5	

M = Mustargen, O = Oncovin, P = Prednisone, P = Procarbazine, C = Cyclophosphamide
A = Adriamycin, B = Bleomycin, V = Vinblastine, D = DTIC, Pt = Cisplatin

The most common chronic effect of cytotoxic therapy is cumulative *suppression of the bone marrow.* Among patients who are now living as a consequence of more effective therapy, marrow suppression represents a universal phenomenon that affects the stem-cell population and may lead to chronic thrombocytopenia, anemia, and leukopenia.

The most serious risks of chemotherapy are *leukopenia* leading to overwhelming sepsis and *thrombocytopenia* resulting in hemorrhage. Uniformly, leukopenia and thrombocytopenia are dose-related and may be prevented or lessened by dose adjustment in patients who have marginal marrow reserve due to marrow invasion, age, or prior therapy. Nonetheless, the goal of most chemotherapeutic regimens is to induce some degree of leukopenia, for it serves as a measure of cytotoxic effect and as a guideline to dosage.

Of concern is the increasing evidence that *secondary malignancies,* such as acute leukemia, may develop in patients treated with alkylating agents. Although the accumulating evidence grows increasingly compelling, the risk of treatment remains outweighed by its benefits.

Alopecia is a concomitant effect of only four drugs: nitrogen mustard, cyclophosphamide, vincristine, and doxo-rubicin. It is usually partial, but with doxorubicin the hair loss is generally total. Alopecia begins approximately 2 weeks after initiation of treatment and is complete by 4 to 6 weeks. It is always transient, and hair often grows during the course of treatment; however, total restitution does not take place until chemotherapy is stopped.

The *gastrointestinal toxicity* of chemotherapy can be debilitating; nausea and vomiting are common. However, with the judicious use of antiemetics, sedatives, behavioral conditioning, and compassionate support, the adverse gastrointestinal effects can be minimized. The chemotactic trigger zone of the brain stem is exquisitely sensitive to a variety of chemotherapeutic agents and activates the emesis center, resulting in the nausea and vomiting. The best approach to the vomiting, therefore, is to suppress the trigger zone and emesis center. Phenothiazines and other antiemetics are used for this purpose (see Chapter 74).

Cytotoxic Chemotherapeutic Agents

Cytotoxic drugs have been grouped into five categories based on their mechanism of action or the chemical derivation of the drug (Table 89-2).

Table 89-2. Cytotoxic Chemotherapeutic Drugs

CLASS	PROTOTYPE	ADMINISTRATION	ADVERSE EFFECTS
Alkylating drug	Cyclophosphamide	Intravenous, oral	Hemorrhagic cystitis
Antimetabolite	5-Fluorouracil	Intravenous	Gastrointestinal
Antibiotics	Doxorubicin (Adriamycin)	Intravenous	Cardiomyopathy
	Bleomycin	Intramuscular, intravenous	Interstitial pneumonitis
Plant alkaloid	Vincristine	Intravenous only	Neurotoxicity
Miscellaneous	Nitrosoureas	Intravenous, oral	Marrow failure
	Cisplatin	Intravenous	Renal failure

The Alkylating Agents are a large group that include cyclophosphamide, nitrogen mustard, chlorambucil (Leukeran), phenylalanine mustard (L-PAM, Alkeran), and mitomycin C. All of the alkylating drugs are commercially available. The most commonly used drug in this class is *cyclophosphamide,* which may be administered intermittently either by injection at 3-week intervals or as a 7- to 10-day course of oral medication. The alkylating agents in general have a broad spectrum of antitumor activity, and cyclophosphamide has been effective against many tumors. The alkylating agents with the fewest side-effects (except for myelosuppression) are L-PAM and chlorambucil. There is no known advantage of one schedule or route of drug administration over another.

The Antimetabolites include 5-fluorouracil, methotrexate, and the antileukemic drugs cytosine arabinoside, hydroxyurea, and 6-mercaptopurine. These drugs interfere with synthesis of DNA and, therefore, have greatest effect on rapidly growing cells. The antimetabolites are uniformly and rapidly metabolized or excreted in the urine; therefore, they must be administered frequently. They are most effective when administered as a 24-hour or continuous infusion. *5-Fluorouracil* is the prototype and has been extensively applied in gastrointestinal cancer. The drug is best administered intravenously for 5 to 7 days, and repeated at 5- to 6-week intervals. High-dose *methotrexate* therapy has been combined with leucovorio (a reduced form of folic acid) to overcome drug resistance and "rescue" normal cells that would otherwise by damaged by the methotrexate-induced inhibition of folate reductase.

The Antibiotics include dactinomycin, doxorubicin, and bleomycin. Doxorubicin (Adriamycin) is an anthracycline antibiotic with a spectrum of activity comparable to the alkylating drugs. In combination with the alkylating drugs, doxorubicin appears to be synergistic in antitumor effect. The drug has a cumulative toxic effect on the heart that results in a cardiomyopathy, limiting the maximum cumulative dose to 450 to 500 mg/m^2. Periodic radionuclide scanning of the heart is indicated once the cumulative dose exceeds 300 mg/m^2; the drug is halted if a 15% decrease is noted in the ejection fraction. *Bleomycin,* a polypeptide antibiotic mixture, causes pulmonary fibrosis, an effect that may be dose-related or, occasionally, idiosyncratic. As a result, the maximum cumulative dose for bleomycin is 200 mg/m^2. Measurement of the pulmonary diffusion capacity is the most sensitive means of early detection. A decrease to below 40% of predicted is a sign of lung injury.

The Plant Alkaloids are mitotic inhibitors. They are primarily the *vinblastine* and *vincristine* derivatives of the periwinkle plant. These drugs are always administered intravenously and most commonly on a weekly basis. Their chief adverse effects are cumulative neurotoxicity (seen with vincristine), which recedes slowly with drug withdrawal, and marrow suppression (vinblastine). A new plant derivative is *etoposide,* an agent with activity against lymphomas, small-cell carcinoma of the lung, and testicular cancer. Adverse effects include marrow suppression; it can cause hypotension if injected rapidly.

Miscellaneous or Mixed Mechanism agents include two important drugs: nitrosoureas and cisplatin. The *nitrosoureas* are alkylating drugs that cross the blood–brain barrier. They have a unique, delayed marrow-suppressive effect that necessitates a specific drug schedule with a long hiatus between administered courses (6 weeks). *Cisplatin* has primary activity in testicular and ovarian cancers and probably squamous tumors of the bladder. It is administered at 3- to 4-week intervals primarily in combination with other drugs. It can cause renal failure in patients inadequately hydrated and has been associated with ototoxicity and neurotoxicity.

MANAGEMENT RECOMMENDATIONS

Administration of cancer chemotherapeutic drugs by the primary care physician requires a specific understanding of preferred routes of administration. Particularly important is awareness of the potential hazard of *extravasation* associated with certain intravenously administered agents (Table 89-3). In each instance, extravasation results in tissue irritation and secondary inflammation leading to ulceration and necrosis,

Table 89-3. Drugs that Require Slow Intravenous Administration and the Careful Avoidance of Extravasation

Actinomycin D
Doxorubicin
Mitomycin C
Cisplatin
Nitrogen mustard
Vincristine

which not uncommonly require surgical grafting and débridement. In the event of extravasation, the local area may be injected with *cortisone* preparation, and *ice* applied. The actual inflammation and necrosis may not occur for 3 to 10 days following injection, although pain is generally present early on. Repeated intravenous use of such drugs, often results in sclerosis and endothelial deterioration, particularly when small-caliber veins are used for infusion. The agents used should go into large-bore veins in the antecubital fossa or higher.

Traditionally, chemotherapy is delivered according to a schedule of *intermittent boluses,* with the patient receiving an injection of the maximum tolerated dose at weekly or monthly intervals. However, it was suspected that agents with a short half-life or effects limited to one part of the cell cycle might prove more effective if administered as a *continuous infusion,* especially when used against solid tumors, which characteristically have only a small proportion of cells in cycle and metabolically active at any point in time. Major advances in infusion technology have made continuous drug administration possible, utilizing reliable portable infusion pumps. Continuous infusion has greatly reduced the frequency and severity of gastrointestinal side-effects. Therapeutic efficacy has been demonstrated; trials comparing continuous therapy with standard bolus administration are underway.

Multiple drug regimens are designed first and foremost for convenient outpatient administration. The dose and schedule of the component drugs are adjusted to minimize side effects (see Table 88-1).

Suppression of Chemotherapy-Induced Vomiting requires identifying the pattern of emesis. Some agents cause vomiting

Table 89-4. Schematic for Management of Chemotherapy-Induced Emesis

Day prior to therapy
Mild tranquilizer with or without tricyclic compound

Day of therapy
Phenothiazine spansule or suppository
Normal food intake (to minimize retching on an empty stomach, which produces muscle cramps and pain)
1 hour prior to anticipated emesis, 200 to 400 mg barbiturate plus phenothiazine to sedate
Phenothiazine at 3- to 4-hour intervals if vomiting exceeds four discharges per hour

that begins approximately 30 to 45 minutes following injection. In other regimens, particularly Cytoxan and Adriamycin, the vomiting begins 4 to 5 hours after injection. The approach to antiemetic use should be based on time of emesis. An important cause of vomiting is the conditioned vomiting response, which in time becomes more severe than that induced by drug therapy. This pattern of vomiting develops following the second or third course of emesis-inducing cancer treatment; it is characterized by anxiety and anorexia the day before therapy and a conditioned response that may be precipitated by little more than driving down the street on which the therapy center is located. This form of emesis is best treated by tranquilizers for 1 to 2 days prior to treatment. Other forms of antiemetic support include metoclopramide for cisplatin-induced emesis, haloperidol in the setting of combination chemotherapy, and lorazepam and desensitization for psychogenic emesis (see Chapter 74). In many instances, sedation and phenothiazines suffice for chemotherapy-induced emesis (Table 89-4).

Management of Bone Marrow Suppression requires adjustments in dose and timing of chemotherapy. Generalized marrow suppression is common. The pattern of suppression is a function of the type of drug, its dose and schedule (Table 89-5). Nitrosoureas, for example, induce thrombocytopenia more often than leukopenia and do so in delayed fashion at 21 days, with recovery sometimes not achieved until day 35. Dose adjustments for subsequent courses of therapy are based on the nadir day's levels.

In monitoring patients on chemotherapeutic regimens, the anticipated nadir days for blood counts are the most crucial times to obtain follow-up complete blood counts. In patients who develop leukopenia, the observation period ought to be intensified, depending upon the level of the count and the presence of associated fever or sepsis (Table 89-6). Dose adjustment for the subsequent course of therapy is therefore based on the nadir level. The goal of treatment should be to maintain intermittent white blood counts at between 2000 and 3000 cells/mm. Dose escalation or reduction is not necessary if a blood count is maintained at this level at nadir time. A small number of drugs have absolutely no effect on the bone marrow (see Table 89-5), but the majority have some impact with variation in the time of the nadir count and the duration of marrow suppression.

EVALUATION OF RESPONSE TO THERAPY

Monitoring patients on chemotherapeutic regimens for adverse effects is performed in concert with evaluation of the effectiveness of treatment (see also Chapter 87). Objective tumor measurements are often difficult to define, but generally the oncologist depends on them to gauge response to therapy (Table 89-7).

The criteria of response are often difficult to evaluate because partial responses may be influenced by nontumor fac-

Table 89-5. Chronologic Patterns of Marrow Suppression Secondary to Chemotherapy

AGENT	NADIR DAY	DURATION
Nonsuppressive Drugs		
Bleomycin		
Vincristine		
Streptozotocin		
Corticosteroids		
DTIC		
Marrow-Suppressive Drugs		
1. *Alkylating drugs*		
Cyclophosphamide		
Nitrogen mustard	5–8	Variable
Mitomycin C	Delayed	Cumulative
2. *Antibiotics*		
Doxorubicin	12–14	5 days
Dactinomycin		
3. *Antimetabolites*		
5-Fluorouracil	5–10	<5 days
Cytosine arabinoside		
Methotrexate		
4. *Natural products*		
Vinblastine	8–12	3 days
5. *Others*		
Nitrosoureas	14–28	Cumulative
Hydroxyurea	Variable	
Procarbazine	Variable	

Table 89-7. Criteria of Response to Therapy

Survival
Measured from time of diagnosis, metastasis, or initiation of treatment in days, weeks, or months, to be compared by median (as opposed to mean) to a randomized control or historical control not receiving treatment or receiving alternative treatment. Survival as a measurement of time may also be supplemented by a time measurement of diagnosis to point of recurrence and is translated as disease-free survival.

OBJECTIVE REDUCTION IN TUMOR

Partial response
Equals a 50% reduction in the product of the maximum perpendicular diameters of the most easily measurable lesion without increase in other lesions and with a minimum duration of 4 weeks.

Complete response
Equals a 100% reduction in all evidence of tumor for minimum of 4 weeks without appearance of new lesions.

Stable disease
Equals a less than 25% decrease in measurable disease without development of other lesions.

No response (progressive disease)
Equals a more than 25% increase in the size of the lesion or the development of new lesions.

Improvement
Equals a 25%–50% reduction in the product of maximum perpendicular diameters lasting at least 4 weeks.

tors. In addition, some forms of metastatic disease simply cannot be measured, such as osseous metastases and, particularly, osteoblastic lesions. There are established criteria for some metastatic patterns, such as hepatomegaly where the criterion for response is a 30% decrease in the sum of measurements made below the costal margin at the midclavicular and midxiphoid lines. Peritoneal masses, pleural effusions, and skin ulcerations are not considered amenable to evaluation. Ultrasonography and computed body tomography have helped quantify lesions in the retroperitoneum.

Tumor markers have facilitated objectively gauging response to therapy. Sequential monitoring of marker serum levels correlates well with tumor mass and often predicts recurrence before it becomes clinically evident. Human cho-

rionic gonadotropin, carcinoembryonic antigen, and some of the markers derived from monoclonal antibody techniques (*e.g.,* CA 19-9) are among the clinically useful markers (see Chapter 87). Other biochemical parameters, such as alkaline phosphatase and the various hepatic enzymes, have been uniformly inadequate to evaluate the effectiveness of treatment.

PATIENT EDUCATION

The ability to tolerate chemotherapy is enhanced by a strong and trusting patient–doctor relationship. Fully educating the patient and his family about diagnosis, prognosis, and the rationale and side-effects of planned treatment can greatly facilitate the development of trust and confidence (see Chapter 88). Concerns about alopecia, sterility, gastrointestinal upset, and other side-effects should be elicited and di-

Table 89-6. Management of Leukopenia and Chemotherapy

WHITE BLOOD COUNT (WBC) AT NADIR	MONITORING SCHEDULE	CHEMOTHERAPY DOSE
1000–2000	Repeat in 1 week	Allow recovery to >3000, treat with 100% dose
500–1000	Observe on outpatient basis daily until WBC is same on consecutive days	Allow recovery to >3000, treat with 50% dose
100–500	Hospitalize for observation	Allow recovery to >4000, treat with 25% dose

rectly addressed. The probability of response also deserves review. A comprehensive educational effort appropriate for the patient's level of understanding allows him to participate meaningfully in decision making and encourages a sense of partnership in the undertaking, an attitude that can help sustain one through this often difficult time.

INDICATIONS FOR REFERRAL

Chemotherapy programs are in a constant state of revision as new combinations are tried and new agents developed. Each patient's treatment program must be designed in conjunction with an oncologist. When such expertise is not locally available, patients may have to travel to a regional center for therapy. Computer-based chemotherapy protocol advisory systems are under development to help provide expert input where it may not be otherwise available.

ANNOTATED BIBLIOGRAPHY

Carlson RW, Sikic BI: Continuous infusion or bolus injection in cancer chemotherapy. Ann Intern Med 99:823, 1983 (*The rationale and clinical trials of a new schedule for delivery of cancer chemotherapeutic agents is reviewed for a number of agents demonstrating substantial amelioration of adverse effects.*)

Chabner, BA et al: The clinical pharmacology of antineoplastic agents. N Engl J Med 292:1107, 1159, 1975 (*Excellent review of pharmacokinetics, toxicities, and drug interactions.*)

Comis RL, Kuppinger MS, Ginsberg SJ et al: Role of single-breath carbon monoxide diffusing capacity in monitoring the pulmonary effects of bleomycin in germ-cell tumor patients. Cancer Res 39: 5076, 1979 (*A reduction to less than 40% of predicted suggests onset of pulmonary fibrosis.*)

Golden S, Horwich A, Lokich J: Chemotherapy and you. Department of Health and Welfare Publication (NIH) 76-1136 (*This pamphlet originally produced at the Sidney Farber Cancer Institute is available for patient use from the National Cancer Institute and serves as a layman's introduction to the concept of chemotherapy and its potential effects.*)

Goldie JH, Goldman AJ, Gudauskas GA: Rationale for the use of alternating noncrossresistant chemotherapy. Cancer Treat Rep 66:439, 1982 (*An interesting discussion of the theoretical basis for combination chemotherapy.*)

Gottdiener JS, Mathisen DJ, Borer JS et al: Doxorubicin cardiotoxicity: Assessment of late left ventricular dysfunction by radionuclide cineangiography. Ann Intern Med 94:430, 1981 (*A 15% reduction in ejection fraction strongly suggested onset of cardiomyopathy.*)

Hickam DH, Shortliffe EH, Bischoff MB et al: The treatment advice of a computer-based cancer chemotherapy protocol advisor. Ann Intern Med 103:928, 1985 (*Report of an experimental computer-based advisory system.*)

Jolivet J, Cowan KH, Curt GA et al: The pharmacology and clinical use of methotrexate. N Engl J Med 309:1094, 1983 (*A comprehensive and clinically helpful review.*)

Loehrer PJ, Einhorn LH: Drugs five years later: Cisplatin. Ann Intern Med 100:704, 1984 (*Excellent review for the generalist.*)

Lokich JJ, Bothe A, Fine N et al: The delivery of cancer chemotherapy by constant venous infusion. Cancer 50:2731, 1982 (*The crucial technologic issues of venous access and ambulatory infusion pumps are addressed in detail for protracted infusion cancer chemotherapy.*)

Penta JS, Poster DS, Bruno S et al: Clinical trials with antiemetic agents in cancer patients receiving chemotherapy. J Clin Pharmacol 21 (suppl):11s, 1981 (*A good review of available therapies.*)

Sallen SE et al: Antiemetics in patients receiving chemotherapy for cancer: A randomized comparison of tetrahydrocannabinol and prochlorperazine. N Engl J Med 302:135, 1980 (*Tetrahydrocannabinol proved to be effective and was often preferred to prochlorperazine for relief of drug-induced emesis in young patients.*)

Schein P: Long-term effects of cytotoxic and immune suppression therapy. Ann Intern Med 82:84, 1978 (*A detailed review of the mechanisms and duration of adverse effects of cytotoxic agents on various organ systems.*)

Weichselbaum R, Goebbels R, Lokich J: Complications of therapy. Lokich J (ed): Clinical Cancer Management. Boston, GK Hall, 1979 (*A comprehensive review of the acute as well as chronic effects of chemotherapy and radiation therapy and a discussion of the reversibility of such effects as well as the mechanisms of induction.*)

Young RC, Ozols RF, Myers CE: The anthracycline antineoplastic drugs. N Engl J Med 305:139, 1981 (*Detailed discussion of doxorubicin and related compounds.*)

90
Principles of Radiation Therapy

Modern radiation therapy represents an important means of achieving local and regional control of malignancy, as well as providing palliation. When given with the intent of controlling disease and attempting cure, it is termed "radical;" when given for symptomatic relief, it is designated as "palliative." Although the design and implementation of such therapy is the responsibility of the radiation oncologist, the primary physician has an important role in monitoring the patient, and providing support. As such, one needs to be familiar with basic aspects of radiation therapy and its side effects.

PRINCIPLES OF MANAGEMENT

Response to Irradiation

There is exponential killing of both tumor and normal cells after an initial sublethal accumulation of radiation. The *response curves* of cells in culture are remarkably similar, with most of the difference in "radiosensitivity" due to the greater number of actively dividing cells in malignant tissue.

Response to irradiation is also affected by the volume of the tumor. Except for uniquely radiosensitive tumors (lymphomas and seminomas), the greater the tumor's volume, the more radioresistant it will be. Part of the reason for this resistance is *tissue hypoxia*. Oxygen facilitates the cytotoxic effect of x-rays. Hypoxic cells are about three times more refractory to irradiation than are cells treated in the presence of oxygen. Interior areas of large tumors can become hypoxic and relatively refractory to radiation. However, as the tumor shrinks, its hypoxic cells gain better access to oxygen, making them more susceptible to radiation if doses are given in sequential fractionated fashion (see below).

Charged particle beams are less dependent on oxygen for their cytotoxic action than are x-rays and represent another means of treating large, poorly vascularized tumors. Compounds that will sensitize hypoxic tumor cells and improve their response to radiation therapy are under investigation.

The amount of radiation that can be safely directed at a malignancy is limited by the tolerance of the organs surrounding it. Radiation damage can be particularly injurious when it affects the heart, liver, brain, intestines, bone marrow, kidneys, or lung (see below). Usually, trade-offs must be made between therapeutic benefits and adverse effects.

The probability of radiation-induced complications depends on how narrow the difference is between the dose needed for control of the tumor and the dose that causes injury to normal tissue. (The ratio of the two doses is termed the *therapeutic ratio*.) Conversely, the greater the difference in doses, the better the likelihood of beneficial effect.

Dose fractionation, shielding, and use of computed tomography for precise definition of tumor volume have helped limit the adverse effects of radiation therapy. *Fractionating* the dose helps to widen the margin of safety and improve selective killing of tumor cells. Normal cells repair sublethal radiation damage more effectively than do tumor cells. Most fractionation programs provide about 200 rads per treatment, applied five times per week. *Shielding* helps protect vital organs adjacent to the portal from radiation exposure. Often, custom-fabricated lead shields are made when there is risk of irradiating normal tissue abutting the tumor. *CT scan* has improved delineation of the tumor volume and surrounding anatomic structures so that the target can be more precisely defined. *Simulation* reproduces the geometry of the actual radiation portal, helping to ensure that only the desired tissue is irradiated. Work is in progress to develop compounds that will preferentially protect normal cells.

Clinical Applications

Radiation is applied for cure and control as well as to achieve palliation. It may be the sole treatment, an alternative therapy, or combined with other modalities (Table 90-1).

As Sole or Alternative Therapy. In some instances, such as stage I Hodgkin's disease (see Chapter 82), x-ray therapy is the treatment of choice. In others, such as localized breast cancer (see Chapter 121) or early head and neck cancers, it represents an alternative to surgery. When surgery and radiation provide similar rates of cure and control, choice depends largely upon the impact of treatment on the patient.

As Combination Therapy. Radiation therapy has several qualities that make it a good complement to *surgery*. Its capacity to reduce tumor bulk and destroy microscopic disease facilitates surgical removal and local control. By allowing use of lower radiation doses and less radical surgery, combination therapy minimizes side-effects. Adjuvant radiotherapy directed at regions of potential spread, such as lymph nodes, makes radical exploration unnecessary.

Whether to give radiation before, during, or after surgery depends upon several practical and theoretical issues. Favoring preoperative treatment are the need to reduce tumor size for easier resection and desirability of sterilizing tumor cells that might be spread during surgery. Moreover, postoperative irradiation may be less effective if the vascular bed is surgically reduced and oxygen delivery impaired. Factors favoring postoperative treatment include promptness of surgery and destruction of any remaining microscopic disease. Intraoperative treatment allows one to displace normal abdominal organs (which are quite intolerant to irradiation) and better target diseased tissue.

Radiation in combination *with chemotherapy* to achieve cure is established for advanced stages of Hodgkin's disease (see Chapter 82) and is being explored in patients with small cell carcinoma of the lung (see Chapter 42). It helps to sterilize sites of initial involvement and treat areas not readily accessible to chemotherapy, such as the brain and testes. Although results appear promising, toxicities can be additive. Marrow suppression is the limiting problem. There are other instances of additive adverse effects: cytoxan and radiation produce hemorrhagic cystitis: methotrexate and x-ray cause mucositis of the oral cavity; and MOPP plus radiation lead to increased risk of leukemia. Some drugs enhance radiation reactions in normal tissues, even when given up to a year after radiotherapy. Adriamycin is the most prominent example of a drug producing this "recall phenomenon."

At present, the optimal strategies for application of combined modality therapy remain unsettled. The literature should be followed for results of studies now ongoing.

As Palliative Therapy. Radiation serves an important function in providing symptomatic relief to some patients with incurable disease. For those tumors that respond to chemotherapy or hormonal therapy, radiation should be held in reserve. However, if there is localized tumor not sensitive to other modalities, radiation may be worth consideration. Palliative treatment is reserved for symptomatic patients; "prophylactic" treatment of asymptomatic lesions yields little benefit. For example, painful *bony metastases* from such tu-

Table 90-1. Applications of Radiotherapy

TUMOR	COMMENTS
Radiation Therapy Alone is Curative	
Hodgkin's disease	Stages IA and IIA; 94% 10-year survival
Lymphoma	Stage I only; 90% 5-year disease-free survival
Cervical cancer	Curative for early disease; 65% 5-year disease-free survival for invasive disease
Testicular cancer	Seminomas
Head and neck cancer	Early stage disease (T1); results comparable to surgery with less functional and cosmetic loss
Radiation Combined with Another Modality is Potentially Curative	
Uterine cancer	With surgery; good results for stages I, II, and III; 70% to 90% 5-year survival
Head and neck cancer	With surgery in more advanced cases
Soft tissue sarcomas	In combination with surgery
Breast cancer	In combination with limited resection; excellent control of local recurrence
Rectal cancer	With surgery, marked improvement in survival
Radiation Therapy is Palliative	
Prostate cancer	5-year disease-free survival as high as 70% for stage B disease; drops to 36% for stage C disease
Lung cancer	For unresectable non–small-cell disease
Brain metastases	Especially as a prophylactic measure
Ovarian cancer	Exact role of radiation unsettled
Bony metastases	For painful lesions unresponsive to chemoRx
GI cancers	For unresectable gastric, pancreatic, and esophageal cancers, results are fair; better for colon cancer when combined with surgery

mors as breast and prostate respond well; within 2 to 3 weeks of a relatively short course of radiotherapy (2 weeks), many patients experience relief from bone pain.

Adverse Effects

As noted previously, normal cells tolerate radiation better than do malignant cells. However, the degree of tolerance varies greatly (see Table 90-2); tissues having high rates of turnover are among the most vulnerable. Tolerance to radiotherapy decreases as dose is increased. The *dose limit* for a tissue can be expressed as the cumulative dose that produces a 5% incidence of toxicity when radiation is delivered in 200 rad fractions, 5 days per week. Beyond the dose limit, the incidence of toxicity rises quickly.

The bone marrow is the most radiosensitive tissue, with *marrow suppression* developing when exposure exceeds 250 rads. At such low doses, suppression is usually transient. The lungs are also quite sensitive to irradiation. *Pneumonitis* starts to appear when the dose surpasses 2500 rads; the incidence reaches 100% at doses of 4000 rads. Onset is usually within 6 to 12 weeks, characterized by dyspnea, hypoxemia, and a "ground glass" appearance on chest x-ray. Restrictive defects and chronic hypoxemia follow if fibrosis sets in, which typically takes place over the ensuing 6 to 24 months. Treatment is mainly supportive. High-dose steroids and oxygen can al-

eviate symptoms during the acute phase; there is no treatment once fibrosis occurs. The best approach is prevention by carefully limiting the radiation portal.

Nephrosclerosis is the renal response to doses in excess of 2000 rads. *Hepatitis* is a consequence of doses to the liver

Table 90-2. Serious Adverse Effects of Radiotherapy

TISSUE	ADVERSE EFFECT	DOSE LIMIT (≤5%) (TOXICITY) IN RADS
Bone marrow	Marrow suppression	250
Kidneys	Nephrosclerosis	2000
Lungs	Pneumonitis	2500
Liver	Hepatitis	3000
Heart	Pericarditis	4500
Spinal cord	Infarction	4500
Intestines	Ulceration	4500
Skin	Dermatitis, sclerosis	5500
Brain	Infarction	6000

(Chabner BA: Principles of cancer therapy. In Wyngaarden JB, Smith LH (eds): Cecil's Textbook of Medicine, 16th ed, p. 1034. Philadelphia, WB Saunders, 1982)

above 3000 rads. Gastrointestinal *ulceration* followed by perforation or fibrosis are complications of bowel doses exceeding 4500 rads. *Pericarditis* and *spinal cord infarction* are risks of 4500-rad doses to the heart and spinal cord respectively. The skin can tolerate as much as 5500 rads; *dermatitis* becomes a problem at higher doses; the brain can withstand up to 6000 rads before the risk of *infarction* begins to rise.

The minor and temporary side-effects of radiation therapy can be quite disabling unless anticipated and dealt with. *Nausea* occurs with abdominal irradiation; onset can be as soon as 1 to 2 hours after treatment. Prior administration of prochlorperazine helps to lessen gastrointestinal upset. Small frequent feedings are better tolerated than large ones. If nausea and vomiting become problems, the daily dose can be scaled back or treatment temporarily halted. Head and neck irradiation may cause dryness in the mouth and *difficulty* with *mastication* and *swallowing.* Use of blenderized meals or liquid dietary supplements can help to maintain adequate caloric intake. *Diarrhea* resulting from bowel radiation responds to diphenoxylate (Lomotil) and loperamide. *Skin care* is commonly overlooked. Although use of megavoltage machines has cut skin exposure to 30% of the total dose delivered, avoidance of heat and excessive sun exposure helps preserve the integrity of irradiated skin.

PATIENT EDUCATION

Patients undergoing radiation therapy need plenty of emotional support. The fears associated with cancer are compounded by the awesome machinery and concerns about exposure to radiation. Patients who are well informed tolerate therapy better than those who are not. Answering questions and addressing concerns about the rationale for radiation therapy, the side-effects to be expected, and how they will be controlled are essential to the successful conduct of a radiation therapy program. Knowing that treatment can be adjusted to one's tolerance to therapy is reassuring, as is knowledge that one does not become radioactive from therapy (a common misconception).

COORDINATION OF CARE

Conducting a radiotherapy program is the province of the radiation therapist, carried out in the context of an overall treatment plan designed by the oncologist in consultation with the primary care physician. The primary physician can ensure that the therapeutic program is well suited to the patient's needs and carefully monitored. A multidisciplinary team approach works best for the patient when there is an individual on the team whom the patient feels he can always turn to for advice and help; in many instances this important role can be best carried out by the primary care doctor.

A.H.G.

ANNOTATED BIBLIOGRAPHY

Abe M, Takahashi M, Yabumoto E et al: Clinical experiences with intraoperative radiotherapy for locally advanced cancers. Cancer 45:40, 1980 (*Details results and limitations.*)

Fletcher GH: The evolution of the basic concepts underlying the practice of radiotherapy. Radiology 127:3, 1978 (*Discusses the development of combination therapy utilizing radiation as one component.*)

Klingerman MM: Preoperative radiation therapy in rectal cancer. Cancer 36:691, 1975 (*An example of preoperative radiotherapy.*)

Kohn HI, Fry RJ: Radiation carcinogenesis. N Engl J Med 310:504, 1984 (*A review that includes a terse, informative section on the risks associated with cancer radiotherapy.*)

Montague ED, Fletch GH: The curative value of irradiation in the treatment of nondisseminated breast cancer. Cancer 46:508, 1980 (*An example of curative radiotherapy.*)

Peschel RE, Fischer JJ: Optimization of the time-dose relationship. Semin Oncol 8:38, 1981 (*A discussion of fractionation.*)

Prosnitz LR, Kapp DS, Weissberg JB: Radiotherapy. N Engl J Med 309:771,834, 1983 (*A comprehensive two-part review that emphasizes recent treatment results and basic principles of radiation therapy; 157 references.*)

Weissberg JB: Role of radiation therapy in gastrointestinal cancer. Arch Surg 118:96, 1983 (*Good overview of this difficult area.*)

91

Management of Cancer-induced Pain

JACOB J. LOKICH, M.D.

Relief of pain is an essential objective in the treatment of the cancer patient. It is indeed a tragic situation when relentless pain is superimposed upon a fatal outcome. In most instances, effective amelioration of pain can be achieved with proper use of analgesics. Unfortunately, undertreatment of pain is common.

The primary physician is the person to whom the patient most often turns for pain relief. One must know not only the appropriate treatments and their limitations, but also how to support the cancer patient and minimize the emotional suffering that is invariably intertwined with the perception of pain (see Chapter 88).

PATHOPHYSIOLOGY AND CLINICAL PRESENTATIONS

The pain syndromes associated with cancer can be separated into acute and chronic clinical states, and the acute pain syndromes further subdivided (Table 91-1). The major pain syndromes are more often than not a prelude to the incurable stage of illness, but may precede the terminal phase by a substantial interval.

Peripheral Nerve Compression Syndromes. The relatively uncommon nerve compression syndromes result in pain in the shoulder or arm (brachial plexus), buttocks and perineum (sacral plexus), lumbar area (paraspinal nerves), and mouth or face (trigeminal nerve). All are secondary to nerve entrapment and, occasionally, nerve invasion by tumor growth.

Nerve Root Compression Syndromes. Pain originating in the back and radiating down an extremity is characteristic of root compression. When there is an associated neurologic deficit, it suggests the possibility of evolving cord compression. The tumor most commonly extends either from the retroperitoneal space or from a contiguously involved bony structure. Bone scans or radiographs often demonstrate lytic or blastic lesions. Compression syndromes may also occur as a consequence of vertebral body collapse secondary to tumor without direct tumor compression of the nerve.

Osseous Pain Syndromes. Metastases to the bony skeleton may cause pathologic fractures; the development of pain in a bony site is invariably secondary to interruption of the cortex, which may or may not be observed radiographically. Common sites are vertebra, long bones, pelvis, and skull.

Another form of osseous metastasis involves the bone marrow or medullary cavity. Intramedullary tumor is characteristic of leukemia, but may also be observed in some solid tumors, particularly malignant melanoma. These produce a pain syndrome characterized by diffuse bone sensitivity in the presence of normal bone x-rays.

Abdominal Pain Syndromes. Abdominal pain may develop as a consequence of intestinal obstruction; cramping pain is characteristic (see Chapter 53). Ascites can be uncomfortable as a consequence of abdominal distention. Hepatic metastases may cause pain by distending the liver capsule or irritating the peritoneal surface secondary to tumor necrosis. The latter is often associated with a friction rub.

Thoracic Pain Syndromes. Pain associated with thoracic disease is generally a consequence of local invasion of the intercostal nerves. Pleuritic pain may develop if the malignancy spreads to involve the pleura. Direct invasion of a contiguous bony structure may result in local or referred pain.

Special Pain Syndromes. The *phantom limb syndrome* characteristically develops following amputation in patients with osteogenic sarcoma, especially in those who have endured the tumor over a long period. Persistence of phantom limb pain may lead to narcotic dependence. It is only after

Table 91-1. Classification and Types of Cancer-related Pain

SYNDROME	CAUSES OR ANATOMIC SITE	COMMON CANCERS
Peripheral nerve compression or entrapment	Brachial plexus	Breast
	Sacral plexus	Rectum
	Paraspinal nerves	Pancreas
	Trigeminal nerve	Mouth
Nerve root compression	Paraspinal tumor or vertebral collapse	Breast
		Lung
		Myeloma
Osseous lesions	Pathologic fractures or intramedullary expansion	Breast
		Prostate
		Lung
Abdominal lesions	Obstruction	GI tumors
	Hepatic metastases	
	Ascites	
Thoracic lesions	Pleuritis or intercostal neuritis	Lung
Special pain forms		
Phantom limb	Reverberating neurocircuit	Sarcoma
Herpes zoster	Neuralgia	Hodgkin's disease
Hypertrophic pulmonary osteoarthropathy	Periarticular distal extremities	Lung Sarcoma

a protracted period of time that the reverberating neural circuit is eventually exhausted.

Herpes zoster (shingles) occurs in patients with hematologic malignancies, particularly Hodgkin's disease, the non-Hodgkin's lymphomas, and chronic lymphocytic leukemia. Postherpetic pain may persist in the absence of typical skin lesions; herpes zoster should be suspected in patients complaining of pain in a dermatomal distribution (see Chapter 192).

Hypertrophic pulmonary osteoarthropathy (HPO) produces a periarticular pain syndrome that develops in patients with primary or metastatic tumors of the lung and mesotheliomas. The mechanism of the periarticular pain is unclear (see Chapter 41).

PRINCIPLES OF MANAGEMENT

Optimal selection of pain relief measures requires identification of the pathophysiologic process responsible for the discomfort. Rational therapy can then be instituted. Often a multifaceted approach is necessary. Psychological support, control of tumor, analgesics, neurosurgical procedures, and behavioral methods are among the important modalities for treatment of cancer-induced pain (Table 91-2).

Support. The importance of psychological support from both physician and family cannot be overemphasized. The personal role of the primary physician is vital to successful control of pain. The understanding and concern given are as central to effective pain relief as are tumor control and proper analgesic use (see Chapter 88).

Control of Tumor. For pain directly related to the tumor, the most important therapeutic maneuver is the introduction of *tumor-specific therapy.* Surgery and radiation therapy are the principal modalities for the treatment of localized malignancy. Adjuvant therapy, employing chemotherapy or radiation, is also being utilized. Advanced metastatic cancer is treated with cytotoxic drugs for palliation of symptoms (see Chapter 89).

Even if disease is widespread, *local surgical excision* may be necessary for tumors that cause pain because of size, fixation of underlying muscle, distention of the subcutaneous tissue, or localized secondary infection. For example, patients with fungating tumors of the breast may benefit from removal of the breast ("toilet mastectomy"); this achieves a modicum of pain control and minimizes secondary infection.

Lesions of the extremities producing similar local complications (*i.e.,* pain, disfigurement, secondary infection, or poor function) may be considered for local surgical control; amputation is rarely justified or necessary. Local cryosurgery or electrocautery and more recently laser treatment will remove the lesion with a minimum of morbidity and permit maintenance of the limb.

Drug Therapy. Control of cancer pain often requires use of *narcotics.* Regularly scheduled *oral* administration of narcotics is the most effective means of controlling *chronic* pain. *Parenteral* narcotic use should be reserved for treatment of severe *acute* pain. The narcotic doses necessary to achieve control of chronic pain can be reduced when intake is on a scheduled basis; regular use prevents pain from reaching severe intensity. To withhold narcotics until the patient is very uncomfortable or to use them in subtherapeutic doses makes little sense in patients with limited life expectancy. When narcotics are deemed necessary, they should be used in full pharmacologic doses as often as needed to achieve freedom from pain, an attainable and important goal.

Analgesics can be classified on the basis of effectiveness (Tables 91-3 and 91-4). For moderate pain, *codeine* offers excellent analgesia at low cost. Expensive combination preparations containing *oxycodone* offer no advantage over codeine alone. *Morphine* is the prototype narcotic analgesic. It is effective orally as well as parenterally. Chronic oral use of morphine was pioneered by English hospice physicians who prepared a sweetened solution of morphine, cocaine, phenothiazine, and alcohol (the "Brompton solution") for oral use on a regular basis. Results were gratifying, with excellent relief and a minimum of unwanted sedation attained by most of their terminally ill patients. Later studies found that the cocaine was unnecessary to ensure alertness; regular intake permitted use of less sedating narcotic doses.

Some have argued that *heroin* is better than morphine and should be made available. It has a slightly shorter onset of action and is indeed more potent on a weight-for-weight basis (about 2.5 times more potent). However, it is less well suited for chronic oral use, because of its short half-life and the resultant need for frequent doses. Side-effects are identical. Its availability would probably do little to improve management of pain in terminally ill patients. In fact, there are considerably more potent orally active narcotic agents available to the physician (see Table 91-4).

Table 91-2. Approaches to Therapy of Cancer-related Pain

1. Psychological support
2. Tumor control
3. Drug therapy
   a. Nonaddictive analgesics (anti-inflammatory drugs)
   b. Narcotic analgesics
   c. Psychotropic drugs
4. Neurosurgical ablative procedures
   a. Dorsal rhizotomy
   b. Sympathectomy
   c. Percutaneous cordotomy
   d. Chemical hypophysectomy
5. Unproven methods of pain management
   a. Hypnosis
   b. Acupuncture
   c. Behavior modification

Table 91-3. Analgesic Drugs

LEVEL	DRUG	SCHEDULE (STARTING)	COMMENT
I	Aspirin	600 mg q4–6h	Can enhance narcotic benefit
	Other NSAIDs* *e.g.,* ibuprofen	400 mg q6h	Can enhance narcotic benefit
	Acetaminophen	600 mg q4h	Can enhance narcotic benefit
II	Codeine	30–60 mg q4–6h	Inexpensive; effective for moderate pain
	Oxycodone	5 mg q4–6h	Expensive; usually in combination preparations
III	Meperidine	100 mg q3h	Relatively ineffective orally
	Morphine	2–5 mg q3–4h	Effective; modest cost
	Methadone	5 mg q4–6h	Longer half-life than morphine
	Heroin		Not available; no advantages
	Hydromorphone	2 mg q4–6h	Potent orally; expensive

* Nonsteroidal anti-inflammatory drugs.

Hydromorphone is one such potent narcotic agent, being very effective orally and several times more potent than morphine (see Table 91-4). Although expensive, it is very useful in instances where morphine does not suffice. Being more potent than morphine, it also makes possible use of a smaller injected volume, an important advantage in the emaciated patient who requires parenteral analgesia. *Methadone* has also proven useful, having a longer duration of action than morphine and being very active orally. *Meperidine* is commonly prescribed for oral use, but it is relatively inactive when taken by mouth and also short-acting; thus not particularly good for chronic pain control. *Pentazocine* (Talwin) has narcotic antagonist qualities and should not be used for chronic pain.

Several agents can enhance the effect of narcotics and, when used in conjunction with them, may allow use of smaller narcotic doses or improve pain control. The *nonsteroidal anti-inflammatory agents* (see Chapter 153) have such an effect, perhaps through their inhibition of prostaglandin synthesis.

Table 91-4. Relative Potency of Narcotic Analgesics

DRUG	TRADE NAME	EQUIVALENT DOSAGES (mg)
Morphine sulfate		10
Heroin		3
Hydromorphone	Dilaudid	1–5
Oxycodone	In Percodan	15
Meperidine*	Demerol	100 (orally)
Methadone*	Dolophine	10
Codeine		60
Pentazocine*	Talwin	50

* Synthetic narcotic.

Aspirin is the prototype, but other agents in this class (*e.g.,* ibuprofen, naproxen) also have analgesic qualities that augment control of severe pain. By themselves, these agents rarely suffice.

The *tricyclic antidepressants* (see Chapter 223) not only help to counter the reactive depression associated with cancer pain, but also have an analgesic effect, perhaps through their effect on seratonin metabolism and endorphine production. As noted above, *stimulants* (*e.g.,* dextroamphetamine) can be used to counter the somnolence sometimes associated with high-dose narcotic use. When sleep is a problem, a nighttime dose of a *benzodiazepine* (see Chapter 228) can help. Adding such agents to a narcotic program should be done only when necessary; multidrug regimens increase the likelihood of side-effects.

Dosages and dose schedules need to be constantly reviewed to ensure adequate pain control and prevention of over- or underdosing. Tolerance may develop to narcotic agents, necessitating an escalation of dose or dose frequency. Concern about drug abuse in cancer patients is unwarranted; none has been documented among patients receiving regularly scheduled narcotics. PRN schedules appear to encourage psychologic dependence.

No patient should have to endure pain if effective analgesia is available. Patients may require 10 mg or more of morphine as often as every hour to control intractable pain. Again, the dose should be administered on a schedule (not PRN) and increased as tolerance develops. Patients endure their condition much better when they know that maximum pain relief is available to them. All members of the health care team and family need to be informed of the patient's analgesic needs in order to avoid reluctance on the part of pharmacist, nurse, or family to dispense the necessary type and amount of medication.

Neurosurgical Procedures. A proportion of patients with metastatic cancer will have a slowly growing tumor, which may be associated with chronic refractory pain in conjunction with prolonged survival. In these patients, determining the source of pain and controlling it with analgesics are often difficult. In such cases, neurosurgical procedures are resorted to. Before such extreme measures are utilized, it is important to characterize the pain as precisely as possible to avoid mistaking a psychogenic component for an organic one. Treating the latter while ignoring the former is bound to end in failure and unnecessary suffering. When there is confusion as to the nature of the pain, a *nerve blockade* can serve an important diagnostic function. There are three types of blocks: sensory, sympathetic, and motor. By employing control solutions of normal saline in addition to titered solutions of anesthetic, the physician can determine the source of pain and, if organic, classify it into sensory, sympathetic, or motor nerve involvement.

Neurosurgical procedures are indicated only when (1) pain is uncontrolled by narcotic analgesics, (2) tumor control allows prediction of substantial longevity, and (3) functional status is significantly compromised by pain.

Rhizotomy is successful in 50% of patients with malignancy; efficacy is not necessarily predicted by the success of a peripheral nerve block. *Chordotomy* is presently done percutaneously, avoiding general anesthesia and allowing for precise delineation of the pain tracts. Electrical chordotomy or radiofrequency chordotomy achieves long-term pain control in 40% to 70% of patients. However, chordotomy, particularly the open surgical approach, is associated with potential functional loss, necessitating a discussion with the patient of the risks involved. Lateralization or regionalization of the pain syndrome makes chordotomy an important therapeutic option.

Finally, *hypophysectomy* induced by a chemical injection procedure (so-called alcohol-induced adenolysis) has been employed in limited numbers of patients in this country. Pain control may be related to the opioid peptides or endorphins in the hypothalamic area and is not necessarily related to the responsiveness of the tumor to hormonal ablation.

Behavioral therapies for pain control are a new approach to treatment. The influence of operant conditioning on the threshold for perception and tolerance to pain is well-established. *Behavior modification* or deconditioning may, therefore, have a role in pain control. Other investigational methods are *hypnosis* and *acupuncture,* which have been demonstrated to have some effect, particularly in the relief of chronic pain syndromes.

Many considerations are important when behavioral methods are introduced. First, one needs to be certain that specific organic causes and the anatomic lesion are attended to. Behavioral therapy should never be the singular treatment, but it may help when applied in conjunction with more standard forms of treatment. Second, the effects of these therapies are usually transient and require reinforcement. The pain syndrome becomes refractory unless a concomitant deconditioning or unlearning process is occurring. Finally, the identification of appropriate patients is crucial. Those unlikely to respond tend to be older, more control-oriented, committed to religious or rigid ideals, cynical, or hostile. Younger patients and those involved in meditation or astrology are likely to be sympathetic to and benefit from a behavioral approach.

MANAGEMENT RECOMMENDATIONS FOR SPECIFIC PAIN SYNDROMES

Peripheral Nerve Compression. The specific therapeutic approach to all such syndromes is the application of local antitumor therapy (for the most part, radiation treatment) to induce regression of the tumor. The nerve compression syndromes are, however, generally associated with a resistant tumor that has invaded along the nerve sheaths, and palliation is often only temporary.

Nerve Root Compression. The distinction between direct tumor compression and osseous inpingement on the nerve is often difficult, but local radiation is the treatment of choice. The absence of improvement following radiation therapy suggests that bony compression is the major component. Structural support by orthopedic measures, including brace or corset splinting, may be salutary.

Bone Pain and Pathologic Fractures. Fractures of weight-bearing bones should be prophylactically immobilized by surgery in conjunction with radiation therapy that is instituted for therapy of bone pain. Pathologic fractures of nonweight-bearing sites with or without symptoms should be managed with radiation therapy. In either instance, rapid healing follows treatment of responsive tumors such as those of breast or prostate.

Abdominal Pain. In most instances of intra-abdominal pain, the effectiveness of the antitumor treatment is limited, making analgesic drug therapy essential. Obstruction is an indication for surgery.

Thoracic Pain. When there is invasion into a local bony structure, radiation therapy is indicated. Neurosurgical procedures may be needed later. Hypertrophic pulmonary osteoarthropathy can cause considerable discomfort, but rapid resolution of the pain is achieved with removal of the intrathoracic process either by surgery or radiation therapy. The narcotic requirement in patients with HPO is inordinate and generally necessitates thoracic surgical intervention, regardless of the presence of metastases.

ANNOTATED BIBLIOGRAPHY

Bonica J (ed.): International Symposium on Pain. In Advances in Neurology, Vol. 4. New York, Raven Press. 1974 (*An extensive review of the basic biology and pathophysiology of pain mechanisms, including the diagnosis and therapeutic approaches to pain. A review of the psychologic approaches, including hypnosis, operant conditioning, and behavioral modification adds to the comprehensive nature of the symposium.*)

Brechner VL, Ferrer-Brechner T, Allen GD: Anesthetic measures in management of pain associated with malignancy. Semin Oncol 4:99, 1977 (*A general and practical review of the neurosurgical approaches to pain as well as the local anesthetic approach. Specific emphasis on the pain due to perineal, Pancoast, and pancreatic tumors, presented in sequential management steps.*)

Catalano RB: The medical approach to management of pain caused by cancer. Semin Oncol 2:379, 1975 (*Thorough review of pathophysiology and detailed discussion of available narcotics.*)

Health and Public Policy Committee, American College of Physicians: Drug therapy for severe, chronic pain in terminal illness. Ann Intern Med 99:870, 1983 (*A clinically useful and wise statement on providing effective pain control; includes a terse review of medications.*)

Hourde RW: Rational use of narcotic analgesics for controlling cancer pain. Drug Ther 10:63, 1980 (*Useful review of narcotic therapy: includes details on use of specific agents.*)

Kaiko RF, Wallenstein SL, Rogers AG et al: Analgesic and mood effects of heroin and morphine in cancer patients with postoperative pain. N Engl J Med 304:1501, 1981 (*Heroin showed no unique advantages over morphine.*)

LaRossa JT, Strong MS, Melby JC: Endocrinologically incomplete transethmoidal trans-sphenoidal hypophysectomy with relief of bone pain in breast cancer. N Engl J Med 298:1332, 1978 (*A possible clinical translation of the data developing with regard to encephlan localization in the hypophysis. The lack of a hormonal mechanism for analgesia suggests an intrinsic mechanism in the hypophysis as the vehicle for analgesia, thus implicating a role for encephlans.*)

Marks RM, Sachar EJ: Undertreatment of medical inpatients with narcotic analgesics. Ann Intern Med 78:173, 1973 (*Provides evidence suggesting that "refractory" pain is often due to inadequate doses and PRN use.*)

Reuler JB, Girard DE, Nardone DA: The chronic pain syndrome; misconceptions and management. Ann Intern Med 93:588, 1980 (*Discusses the failure to provide adequate pain relief for terminally ill patients.*)

92

Complications of Cancer: Oncologic Emergencies, Malignant Effusions, and Paraneoplastic Syndromes

JACOB J. LOKICH, M.D.

The complications of cancer are great in number and variable in degree of urgency. They range from commonly experienced gastrointestinal difficulties (see Chapter 74) and pain syndromes (see Chapter 91) to true emergencies, stubborn malignant effusions, and the uncommon, but important paraneoplastic phenomena. Most oncologic emergencies and malignant effusions are consequences of anatomic spread. Paraneoplastic syndromes result from hormonal and immunologic disturbances. The primary care physician's important role in monitoring the cancer patient requires familiarity with the early presentations of these complications, many of which are amenable to intervention. In most instances, hospital admission for inpatient treatment will be necessary.

ONCOLOGIC EMERGENCIES

The anatomic spread of tumor is capable of causing serious complications, including superior vena cava syndrome, spinal cord compression, and constrictive pericarditis. Other adversities associated with malignancy ensue from a combination of tumor invasion and metabolic/immunologic effects (*e.g.,* hypercalemia, fever, and susceptibility to infection).

Superior Vena Cava Syndrome

The superior vena cava syndrome is usually caused by extrinsic compression of the superior vena cava. The majority of cases are due to bronchogenic carcinoma, lymphoma, and metastatic disease. The earliest manifestation is asymptomatic, unexplained *distention of the neck veins*. Late signs include swelling of the face, neck, and upper extremities, plethora, shortness of breath, and persistent headache. If untreated, thrombosis and neurologic deficits may develop. Diagnosis is confirmed by finding a mass on chest X-ray in the right superior mediastinum or hilar area. Venography and other flow studies are unnecessary in most instances.

At one time it was considered essential to treat the mass

immediately with emergency radiotherapy. Now, the view is one of urgency rather than emergency. A host of tumors with different degrees of radiosensitivity and, occasionally, benign processes may be responsible for the condition. The first task is to attempt a tissue diagnosis (see Chapter 40) before instituting radiotherapy. Invasive study may be appropriate, if the result will alter therapy. For example, chemotherapy may be preferred in some cases due to small-cell carcinoma or lymphoma (see Chapters 42 and 83).

Optimal therapy depends on the underlying diagnosis, prior treatment, and overall clinical status of the patient. Diuretics and corticosteroids can occasionally diminish local symptoms, but the effect is transient and no substitute for more definitive therapy. There is no benefit from the use of heparin. The occurrence of superior vena cava syndrome does not worsen the prognosis (if adjusted for stage of disease).

Spinal Cord Compression

Extradural or epidural cord compression occurs in approximately 5% of patients with cancer. It is a true emergency, with early diagnosis and treatment essential to preventing serious, permanent neurologic damage. The majority of epidural compressions result from bony metastases in the vertebral bodies extending into the epidural space. Less frequently, metastatic tumor reaches the epidural space by direct extension through the intravertebral foramina. Malignancies with a propensity to spread to bone (*e.g.,* lung, breast, prostate, myeloma, lymphoma, melanoma, and renal-cell carcinoma) are associated with the greatest risk of cord compression.

In over 90% of cases, the initial symptom is *back pain,* often radicular in nature. The course is progressive; weakness and sensory deficits follow. Sphincter incontinence is a late development, unless the cauda equina is the initial site of compression. *Plain films* of the spine should be obtained in all cancer patients with back pain. If films are normal in the area of pain and there are no neurologic deficits, no further work-up need be carried out, but the patient should be followed closely. If bone films are abnormal or if there are neurologic deficits, then a *myelogram* is indicated. The frequency of abnormal myelograms in cancer patients with back pain approaches 50%. Use of a nonresorbable dye, such as iophendylate (Pantopaque); allows for convenient follow-up films without repeated injection of dye. *Computed tomography with metrizamide* is an acceptable alternative.

Patients with suspected cord compression require prompt hospitalization and consultation with physicians skilled in managing this emergency condition. *Corticosteroids* and *irradiation* are mainstays of therapy, with surgical *decompression* indicated when there is rapid deterioration of neurologic function. Prognosis depends on the extent of neurologic damage at the time of presentation. Patients who are ambulatory have a 60% to 80% chance of leaving the hospital able to walk; those with paraplegia have less than a 20% chance of regaining their ability to walk.

Hypercalcemia

Malignancy is a common cause of hypercalcemia (see Chapter 96). Cancers of the breast, lung (epidermoid and squamous cell), cervix, esophagus, head and neck, myeloma, and hypernephroma are important etiologies. The mechanism is a function of tumor type. For example, in breast cancer, the complication results from bony metastasis, with lysis of bone and release of calcium. For epidermoid cancers, production of a PTH-like substance in the absence of bony lesions is responsible.

Monitoring the serum calcium provides the simplest means of early detection. Initially the patient is asymptomatic. Later such nonspecific symptoms as *weakness, fatigue, lethargy, nausea, and constipation* ensue. If the hypercalcemia progresses, it will lead to an osmotic diuresis manifested by *thirst and polyuria.* The electrocardiogram may undergo change, with *prolongation of the PR* interval, *shortening of the QT* interval, and *widening of the T wave.* Dysrhythmias become a risk at very high calcium levels. Calcium potentiates the effects of digitalis and can trigger digitalis toxicity.

Hospitalization is needed if one decides to treat the hypercalcemia. (When it occurs in the setting of terminal illness, therapy may not be indicated.) One begins with *intravenous saline,* followed by use of *furosemide* to accelerate saline diuresis. For hypercalcemia due to osteoclastic bone resorption, *mithramycin* provides good control by inhibiting the process; although effective, it must be given parenterally and refractoriness occurs. *Corticosteroids* provide some benefit in cases of myeloma, lymphoma, and metastatic breast cancer. Long-term control mandates treatment of the underlying tumor.

Fever in the Setting of Neutropenia

Infection ranks as the leading cause of death in patients with leukemia and the cause of death in half of those with lymphoma and solid tumors. Malnutrition, immune dysfunction, mechanical compromise, and lowered neutrophil count (mostly due to cytotoxic therapy) all contribute to the high risk of mortality from infection. Neutropenia is defined in cancer patients as granulocyte counts below 500 per ml, the minimum necessary to counter infection.

Patients who develop a fever during periods of neutropenia should be considered infected until proven otherwise. The majority of neutropenic cancer patients with fever will have a bacterial infection (often due to a gram-negative organism). The possibility of viral, fungal, or parasitic infection is increased in those with leukemia, chronic steroid therapy, or prolonged broad-spectrum antibiotic coverage.

Often, neutropenic patients lack the usual signs of inflammation, making it hard to determine the site of infection at the time of presentation. Bacteremia without an identifiable primary site and pneumonitis lead the list of presentations. Onset of fever in the neutropenic patient is an indication for *prompt hospitalization,* regardless of whether or not there are any additional signs of infection. The mortality in such patients ranges from 18% to 40% within the first 48 hours.

Once admitted, cultures of urine, sputum, and blood samples will be needed, as will samples of material from any suspicious site (*e.g.,* cerebrospinal fluid). In the absence of an identified pathogen, broad-spectrum antibiotic therapy (usually an aminoglycoside and a broad-spectrum semisynthetic penicillin) is instituted. Studies on the use of single-agent, broad-spectrum antibiotics, such as the new generation of cephalosporins, are ongoing.

Short-term prognosis for patients treated early and aggressively is good. Sixty to 90% of neutropenic, febrile cancer patients will recover from their infection with aggressive use of antibiotics.

Cardiac Tamponade

Life-threatening tamponade may arise as a complication of malignancy. The pace may be indolent or rapid, depending on the progression of the underlying tumor. Cardiac compression in the setting of malignancy may occur from tumorous encasement, malignant effusion, or scarring from radiation-induced pericarditis. Cancers associated with tamponade include breast, lung, lymphoma, leukemia, and melanoma. In some instances, signs of pericarditis (see Chapter 14) will precede symptoms. The presence of *pulsus paradoxus* strongly suggests significant tamponade. Unexplained neck vein elevation, narrowed pulse pressure, inspiratory distention of neck veins or a pericardial friction rub should raise suspicion. Unfortunately, a pericardial friction rub is often absent in cases of tamponade caused by a malignant pericardial effusion. The usual accompanying symptoms (dyspnea, weakness, chest discomfort, cough) are nonspecific. *Cardiac ultrasonography* is the most sensitive and specific noninvasive test for documenting the problem and its physiologic significance. Detection of tamponade necessitates urgent hospitalization for *pericardiocentesis.* When the degree of tamponade is unclear or there is still a question about the diagnosis, it is best to conduct further evaluation on an inpatient basis and proceed to right heart catheterization.

MALIGNANT EFFUSIONS

Some malignant effusions can be life threatening (*e.g.,* those in the pericardium—see above). Others are an important source of discomfort and disability. For example, malignant ascites can lead to marked abdominal distention and respiratory compromise; treatment is supportive (see Chapter 71). Malignant pleural effusions from pleural implants or lymphatic obstruction can impair respiration. Lung, breast, and ovarian cancers are important causes of pleural implants; lymphomas lead to lymphatic obstruction. Optimal therapy is systemic treatment of the malignancy. Repeat thoracenteses are ineffective and associated with considerable morbidity. Definitive local therapy demands placement of an indwelling chest tube for several days to allow thorough drainage and closure of the third space. Instillation of a sclerosing agent (*e.g.,* tetracycline) after drainage promotes the scarring process and helps to limit reaccumulation of exudate (see Chapter 42).

PARANEOPLASTIC SYNDROMES

Ectopic Hormone Syndromes

Small-cell (oat-cell) carcinoma of the lung is the archetypical tumor capable of ectopic hormone production. A variety of other tumors may behave in similar fashion. One or more polypeptides may issue forth from the tumor, leading to such complications as Cushing's syndrome and inappropriate ADH secretion.

Cushing's Syndrome develops in approximately 5% of patients with small-cell carcinoma of the lung, although some degree of ectopic ACTH production may take place in as many as 80% of patients with the tumor. The clinical syndrome can be subtle and is usually not manifested by the typical cushingoid appearance, but rather by metabolic and immunosuppressive effects, such as severe, recalcitrant *hypokalemia* and *impaired resistance* to infection. The hypokalemia requires extraordinary doses of supplemental potassium and use of spironolactone. Serum and urinary ketosteroids are especially abundant, with some patients demonstrating virilization. Metabolic inhibitors of adrenal hormone synthesis have been tried; success has been variable. Prognosis is very poor; medial survival is less than 2 months.

Hyponatremia (Syndrome of Inappropriate Antidiuretic Hormone [SIADH]) occurs in small-cell carcinoma patients with twice the frequency of Cushing's syndrome (about 10% of cases). The earliest manifestations are hyponatremia and renal sodium wasting; the urine osmolality is inappropriately elevated. If the serum sodium falls to very low levels, confusion and disorientation may ensue. Treatment includes use of *lithium carbonate* or *demeclocycline,* two agents that counter the action of antidiuretic hormone. *Restriction of free water* intake also helps to restore the serum sodium level. Hypertonic saline infusions are to be avoided, since these patients, although not edematous, tend to be volume overloaded. However, diuretics are contraindicated due to sodium depletion. SIADH is rapidly reversible with effective *treatment of the underlying tumor.*

Hypercalcemia usually is a consequence of bony metastases (see above), but may also arise from ectopic production of proteins that affect calcium metabolism, such as parathyroid hormone, prostaglandins, and cyclic AMP-stimulating factors. Lymphomas are unique in their ability to make osteoclastic activating factor. Because symptoms may not develop until the serum calcium becomes markedly elevated, routine monitoring of the serum calcium is the best means of early detection and is worthwhile in tumors having a high frequency of this complication. Control of the tumor is the primary means of countering the hypercalcemia, but hydration, diphosphonates, and mithramycin are among the measures helpful for acute management (see Chapter 96).

Hyperthyroidism and Acute Thyrotoxicosis have resulted from ectopic production of chorionic gonadotropin (which functions like thyroid-stimulating hormone). Choriocarcinomas are the main source of the overproduction. Patients can present with all the typical hypermetabolic manifestations of thyrotoxicosis. The use of beta-blocking agents is only modestly effective; primary treatment must be directed at the tumor.

Immunologically Mediated Paraneoplastic Syndromes

A series of syndromes, mostly neurologic in nature, have been linked to aberrations in immune function. The precise identification of the mediator or immune complex has not been possible in all instances; at times, the link to an immune mechanism is merely speculative.

Myasthenic (Eaton–Lambert) Syndrome occurs in patients with small-cell carcinoma of the lung and characteristically results in proximal muscle weakness of the limbs. Its electromyographic pattern is distinct from that of true myasthenia, being characterized by facilitation and an increasing evoked muscle potential. Clinical management includes use of *guanidine.*

Remote Neurologic Syndromes are believed to have an immunologic basis. The most common is a nonmyasthenic form of *proximal muscle weakness.* A more centrally occurring syndrome is *subacute cerebellar degeneration,* with injury to the Purkinje cells; it has been associated most commonly with small-cell carcinoma of the lung. A *motor neuron disease* similar to amyotrophic lateral sclerosis has been identified on rare occasions, as has a necrotizing myelopathy; bronchogenic carcinoma is often the underlying malignancy in such cases. Unlike the ectopic hormone syndromes, effective treatment of the tumor does not lead to a reversal of the remote neurologic syndromes.

Nephrotic Syndrome. Some patients with Hodgkin's disease develop massive edema with proteinuria and hypoalbuminemia. The renal lesion appears as an accumulation of immune complexes along the basement membrane. The nature of the antigen is unknown. The problem does not respond to steroid therapy, but does regress with control of the underlying malignancy.

Paraneoplastic Syndromes of Unknown Etiology

A host of other purportedly paraneoplastic syndromes have been described, linked to malignancy by their receding with effective treatment of the underlying tumor. Identification of a tumor secretory product or other mechanism has not yet occurred.

Hypertrophic Pulmonary Osteoarthropathy presents with the findings of digital clubbing and tenderness along the distal long bones. Most commonly, the syndrome occurs in the setting of primary or metastatic lung tumors. Radiographically, x-rays of the long bones show an elevation of the periosteum, and radionuclide scanning demonstrates a distinctive pattern of increased uptake along the cortical margins. The exquisite pain accompanying these changes is relieved by removal of the tumor. The mechanism of the syndrome remains unknown.

Cachexia. In some tumors (*e.g.,* those of the lung and pancreas) there is profound wasting, far out of proportion to the tumor burden. Some wasting is a consequence of increased catabolism and decreased anabolism. What triggers these events remains unknown, but disproportionate weight loss suggests a mechanism beyond simple metabolic demand of the tumor (see Chapter 74).

Hyperpyrexia and Tumor-Related Fever have been observed in patients with hepatic metastases, typically from colon cancer, and also as a manifestation of the "B" syndrome associated with Hodgkin's disease. The release of pyrogens from tumor has been proposed as the cause of fever, but other possibilities include the inability to detoxify endogenous endotoxin and an alteration in metabolism of fever-producing steroids. Control can be accomplished by use of *nonsteroidal anti-inflammatory agents.*

Cutaneous Paraneoplastic Syndromes

Cutaneous paraneoplastic syndromes are quite rare, but important to recognize as clues to the presence of internal malignancy. They may be a consequence of hormone secretion, such as the hyperpigmentation or *melanosis* that occurs with ACTH-producing tumors or the *necrotizing erythema* seen with glucagon-secreting malignancies of the pancreas. Proliferation of *seborrheic keratoses* can be a sign of internal malignancy; *acanthosis nigricans* or freckling and hyperpigmentation in the axillary folds suggest neurofibromatosis and intestinal cancer. *Acquired ichthyosis* is associated with lymphomas and several other tumors.

ANNOTATED BIBLIOGRAPHY

Ahmann FR: A reassessment of the clinical implications of the superior vena cava syndrome. J Clin Oncol 2:961, 1984 (*Argues that diagnostic workup is safe and useful for proper selection of treatment modality; based on a review of over 1800 cases.*)

Barron KD, Rodichok LD: Cancer and disorders of motor neurons. Adv Neurol 36:267, 1982 (*A good overview of the neurologic paraneoplastic syndromes affecting motor function.*)

Friedman MA, Slater E: Malignant pleural effusions. Cancer Treat Rev 5:49, 1978 (*Comprehensive review; covers pathophysiology and management.*)

Hainsworth JD, Workman R, Greco A: Management of the syndrome of inappropriate antidiuretic hormone secretion in small cell lung cancer. Cancer 51:161, 1983 (*Antitumor chemotherapy resulted in resolution of the SIADH in 16 or 17 patients.*)

Lokich JJ: The frequency and clinical biology of the ectopic hormone syndromes of small cell carcinoma. Cancer 50:2111, 1982 (*Small cell carcinoma represents the most common tumor associated with ectopic hormone production. This series emphasizes the relative infrequency of the syndromes and the clinical correlation of SIADH and CNS metastasis.*)

Minna JD, Bunn PA: Paraneoplastic syndromes. In DeVita VT, Hellman S, Rosenberg SA (eds): *Cancer: Principles and Practice of Oncology*, pp 1797–1842. Philadelphia, JB Lippincott, 1985 (*A detailed review with an extensive bibliography.*)

Rodichok LD, Harper GR, Ruckdeschel JC et al: Early diagnosis of spinal epidural metastases. Am J Med 70:1181, 1981 (*Early diagnosis achieved by performing myelography on patients with back pain and abnormal spinal films.*)

7

Endocrinologic Problems

93
Screening for Diabetes Mellitus

Diabetes is, after obesity and thyroid disease, the most common metabolic disorder seen by the primary care physician; eight to ten diabetic patients are seen in the office every week in the average primary care practice. Patients' concerns about the possible need for insulin injections and about such well-known complications as blindness, impotence, and premature vascular disease make diabetes one of the most feared diagnoses. Detection campaigns and advertising have further heightened public awareness. Diabetes screening is commonly requested by patients, even in the absence of symptoms. Although there is no question that treatment effectively reduces symptoms associated with the metabolic derangements induced by diabetes, benefits of treatment initiated in the asymptomatic phase have not been demonstrated. On the other hand, labeling a patient "diabetic" on the basis of a nonspecific screening test may be harmful. Uncertainty about the natural history of the disease and its complications does not allow definitive recommendations regarding screening for, or early treatment of, diabetes.

EPIDEMIOLOGY AND RISK FACTORS

Diabetes mellitus is heterogeneous. A number of pathophysiological mechanisms cause the destruction of beta cells in the islets of Langerhans that is responsible for the clinical syndrome of type I or insulin-dependent diabetes mellitus (IDDM). The etiology and pathogenesis of type II or non-insulin-dependent diabetes mellitus (NIDDM) may be even more heterogeneous, with multiple lesions including a blunted beta cell response to insulin, a defect at the insulin receptor, and a defect in hepatic uptake of glucose contributing to glucose intolerance. Depending on the diagnostic criteria used, the prevalence of all types of diabetes in the United States is between 3% and 7%; type II diabetes is five to ten times more common than type I diabetes.

Type I Diabetes (IDDM). Type I diabetes is generally manifest in childhood or early adulthood. It is not inherited; only 20% of patients with IDDM have a first degree relative with diabetes. However, a predisposition to IDDM, apparently mediated through the immune system, is inherited. This pathologic predisposition to autoimmune destruction of the beta cells has been linked to the presence of certain HLA antigens, some of which are also associated with other autoimmune diseases, including Hashimoto's thyroiditis and Addison's disease. Conversely, other HLA antigens seem to be associated with protection against diabetes. Overall, the risk of eventually developing diabetes in a sibling of a patient with IDDM is between 3% and 6%. However, the risk for siblings can be defined by comparing HLA antigens with those of the index case. Although siblings who are HLA identical to the diabetic patient face a risk of diabetes 25 times greater than the general population, relative risk for those who share no antigens or are haplo-identical is only two or three. The role of autoimmune destruction of beta cells in many patients with IDDM is attested to by the presence of islet cell antibodies on a large proportion of newly diagnosed cases. Islet cell antibodies can also be detected in nondiabetic relatives of patients with IDDM. The specificity of antigen assays is debated and the prognostic significance of the finding is uncertain.

At least in some cases, islet cell destruction is the result of viral infection, perhaps initiating the autoimmune response. Coxsackie viruses, particularly Coxsackie B4, have been most strongly implicated. Mumps, cytomegalovirus, Epstein–Barr virus (EBV), and hepatitis virus have also been associated with IDDM. The role of viral infection has been linked to a seasonal variation in incidence of IDDM and has raised questions about a relationship between socioeconomic status and risk of IDDM, but the evidence is equivocal.

Type II Diabetes (NIDDM). Type II diabetes has a much stronger genetic component than IDDM; concordance in identical twins is greater than 90%. The genetic link is not related to HLA antigens, and islet cell antigens are no more prevalent than in the general population.

The overwhelming risk factor for NIDDM is overnutrition and resulting obesity. Eighty percent of adult diabetics are obese or have a history of obesity. Among adults who are at least 25% over their ideal body weight, one out of every five has elevated fasting blood sugar levels, and three out of every five have abnormal glucose tolerance tests. Obesity increases insulin levels and decreases the concentration of insulin receptors in tissue, including skeletal muscle and fat. The relationship between concentration of insulin receptors and glucose tolerance is modified, however, by intracellular sequences following insulin binding that are poorly understood. Exercise increases the concentration of insulin receptors, and a sedentary lifestyle is associated with glucose intolerance. Steroids reduce receptor affinity for insulin, as does uremia and hepatic failure. Other drugs can impair glucose tolerance by further diminishing the sluggish response of beta cells to glucose. These include thiazide diuretics, beta-adrenergic blockers, alpha-adrenergic stimulants, and phenytoin. Prostaglandin inhibitors, including indomethacin and salicylate, may increase beta cell release of insulin.

Persons with impaired glucose tolerance (IGT) are also at greater risk of frank NIDDM (see below). Although long-term follow-up studies indicate that as many as one half of those with IGT will have normal glucose tolerance tests 5 to 10 years later, somewhere between 1% and 5% of these patients become diabetic each year.

Approximately 1% to 2% of previously euglycemic women develop glucose intolerance during pregnancy. The fetal hyperglycemia and hyperinsulinemia that accompany maternal diabetes results in increased neonatal morbidity and mortality and the increased birthweight common in infants of diabetic mothers. This *gestational diabetes* in the mother resolves postpartum for 90%, but more than half of these will eventually develop NIDDM.

NATURAL HISTORY OF DIABETES AND EFFECTIVENESS OF THERAPY

Diabetes mellitus is so heterogeneous that descriptions of its natural history are difficult. This problem has historically been confounded by studies that have defined diabetes using varying degrees of glucose intolerance. In 1979, the National Diabetes Data Group was convened to define criteria for the diagnosis of diabetes. In addition to defining diagnostic criteria, which have since been widely accepted, the group suggested new designations for persons with glucose intolerance who do not meet criteria for frank diabetes. The term *impaired glucose tolerance* is reserved for patients with glucose tolerance between normal and frank diabetes. As already noted, the natural history of impaired glucose intolerance is variable; between 1% and 5% develop frank diabetes in any year but as many as one half have exhibited *normal* glucose tolerance when retested 10 or 15 years later in follow-up studies. Patients with impaired glucose tolerance are at increased risk for developing the macrovascular complications resulting from accelerated atherogenesis. However, unless glucose intolerance progresses to frank diabetes, they do not develop characteristic diabetic microangiopathy.

Vascular and neurologic complications occur in an unpredictable pattern, reflecting again the heterogeneity of diabetes. The incidence of complications clearly tends to increase with the duration of clinical diabetes. This is reflected in mortality rates for diabetics. When compared with age-matched nondiabetics, rates for diabetics increase with duration of known disease. In one study of patients followed for up to 25 years, the increase in risk with duration was greater after age 40 and among women. However, long-term studies of patients followed for as long as 40 years have indicated that clinical evidence of microvascular disease, atherosclerosis, or neuropathy may occur in only 20% to 40% of insulin-dependent patients. In general, complications occur with similar frequency in patients with noninsulin-dependent disease if duration of known disease is considered.

Coronary artery disease is the most common cause of death among diabetics. Autopsy studies indicate that coronary disease is two to three times more common among diabetics than nondiabetics. Not surprisingly, coronary disease is more prevalent in patients who have had the disease longer. Peripheral vascular disease is also very common among diabetics; clinical studies have indicated a prevalence of about 60%. Diabetics in the Framingham Study were shown to be four to five times more likely to have intermittent claudication and two to three times more likely to suffer the morbid consequences of stroke than nondiabetics. Complications seem to be more clearly related to duration than to severity of diabetes.

Data regarding the incidence of retinopathy among diabetics are conflicting, presumably reflecting both differences in populations studied and definitions of retinal abnormalities. In general, the incidence of retinopathy increases with duration regardless of age at onset. Prevalence ranges of 40% to 80% have been reported among patients with known diabetes lasting 20 to 30 years. Neovascularization or malignant retinopathy is more common among long-term, younger insulin-dependent diabetics.

Renal disease has been reported in 15% to 80% of autopsies among diabetics. Renal failure is the cause of death in 6% to 12% of diabetic patients. Prevalence estimates vary widely from study to study, but it is clear that the risk of glomerulosclerosis with clinically evident functional impairment increases dramatically with the duration of the disease.

Although duration of glucose intolerance and associated metabolic abnormalities can be related to many of the complications of diabetes, the variability of the natural history must be kept in mind. It has been argued that all complications, including specific microangiopathic changes, have been identified in patients without evident glucose intolerance. Whether or not the morbidity and mortality associated with the complications can be influenced by therapy is a matter of long-standing debate (see Chapter 100, Approach to the Patient with Diabetes Mellitus). Some have argued that close control of glucose levels results in fewer and later complications. Others point out the heterogeneity of diabetes and the variable incidence of complications independent of glucose control. It has been argued that close control may involve selection of cases in which complications are less likely to develop because of the milder nature of the diabetes itself. Regarding screening, there is no evidence that therapy of asymptomatic patients with chemical diabetes offers any benefit.

By these criteria, at least one of the following conditions must be met to establish the diagnosis of diabetes in the non-pregnant adult:

1. Presence of classic symptoms of diabetes with unequivocal elevations of glycemia (random *plasma* glucose ≥200 mg/dl); or
2. Fasting plasma glucose ≥140 mg/dl or fasting venous (or capillary) whole blood glucose ≥120 mg/dl *on more than one occasion;* or
3. Abnormal oral glucose tolerance test (OGTT) performed under standardized conditions (75-g glucose load with blood measurements performed every 30 minutes for 2 hours). Both the 2-hour level and at least one other sample must exceed 200 mg/dl.

It should be remembered that any criteria for the diagnosis of diabetes based on glucose level are, by necessity, arbitrary. The sensitivity and specificity of the tests will depend on the arbitrary levels chosen. The principal effect of the NDDG criteria, which require higher levels than were commonly used in the past, has been to increase the specificity of the criteria at the expense of sensitivity. This trade-off reflects the judgment that little benefit can be expected from aggressive identification and treatment of early or mild degrees of glucose intolerance, *and* that the label *diabetes* can engender substantial anxiety and morbidity.

Despite widespread acceptance of these *diagnostic* tests, the indications for OGTT and for any blood glucose measurements to *screen* the asymptomatic person is controversial.

Some have advocated the use of hemoglobin A$_{1c}$ measurements for screening and diagnosis of diabetes. However, in population-based studies, fasting glucose levels have been found to be more sensitive and more specific.

CONCLUSIONS AND RECOMMENDATIONS

- Diabetes mellitus is a common but heterogeneous condition. The most important risk factor of IDDM is family history with diabetes in a twin, sibling, or parent. Family history is even more predictive for NIDDM, but the most important risk factor is obesity. Persons with a history of gestational diabetes or with impaired glucose tolerance are also at risk of developing frank diabetes.
- The natural history of diabetes and the incidence of complications is highly variable. The incidence of diabetic complications increase with duration of disease. Whether or not close control of glucose levels with available modes of insulin therapy influences the severity of diabetic complaints remains a matter of debate. Although the weight of opinion favors some beneficial effect of close control in patients with symptomatic diabetes, there is no evidence that therapy of asymptomatic, nonpregnant patients with diabetes or impaired glucose tolerance offers benefit. Therefore, the routine measurement of blood glucose levels to screen asymptomatic, nonpregnant adults for diabetes is not recommended.

A.G.M.

ANNOTATED BIBLIOGRAPHY

Ellenberg M: Diabetic complications without manifest diabetes. JAMA 183:926, 1963 (*Early review. Virtually any of the common "complications" can precede detectable abnormalities in carbohydrate metabolism.*)

Garcia MJ, McNamara PM, Gordan T et al: Morbidity and mortality in diabetics in the Framingham populations. Diabetes 23:105, 1974 (*Insulin-dependent diabetic women have the greatest relative mortality. Increased mortality among diabetics is not entirely explained by associated obesity, hypertension, and hyperlipidemia.*)

Hirohata T, MacMahon B, Root HF: The natural history of diabetes. I. Mortality. Diabetes 16:875, 1967 (*Excess mortality of diabetes increases with age of onset and is higher in females than in males.*)

Mulrow CD, Lichtenstein MJ: Blood glucose and diabetic retinopathy. J Gen Intern Med 1:73, 1986 (*A critical appraisal of evidence concluding that the case for tight control is weak.*)

National Diabetes Data Group: Classification and diagnosis of diabetes mellitus and other categories of glucose intolerance. Diabetes 28:1039, 1979 (*Report of consensus panel, including diagnostic criteria.*)

O'Sullivan JB: Age gradient in blood glucose levels: Magnitude and clinical implications. Diabetes 23:713, 1974 (*Mean fasting levels increase 2 mg per 100 ml per decade, postprandial at 4 mg per 100 ml per decade.*)

O'Sullivan JB, Mahan CM: Prospective study of 352 young patients with chemical diabetes. N Engl J Med 278:1038, 1968 (*Only 32% of those with chemical diabetes by Fajans and Conn criteria progressed to overt diabetes within 10 years.*)

Paz-Guevara AT, Hsu T-H, White P: Juvenile diabetes mellitus after 40 years. Diabetes 24:559, 1975 (*Insulin-induced hypoglycemia was the most common complication. The prevalence of compli-*

cations was significant visual impairment in 50%; nephropathy in 59%; neuropathy in 50%; peripheral vascular disease in 40%; and major cardiac complications in 20%.)

Wagener D, Sacks JM, LaPorte RE et al: The Pittsburgh study of insulin dependent diabetes mellitus: Risk for diabetes among relatives of IDDM. Diabetes 31:136, 1982 (*Risk of sibling eventually developing IDDM is generally low, but is much higher when HLA antigens are identical.*)

Warram JH, Krolewski AS, Gottlieb MS et al: Differences in risk of insulin dependent diabetes in offspring of diabetic mothers and diabetic fathers. N Engl J Med 311:149, 1984 (*By the age of 20, 6% of offspring of males with IDDM had diabetes whereas only 1% of offspring of women had the disease.*)

Winegrad AI, Greene DA: The complications of diabetes mellitus. N Engl J Med 298:1250, 1978 (*A brief review of variability of complications and implications for etiologic hypotheses*).

94
Screening for Thyroid Cancer

Cancer of the thyroid is a relatively rare disease with a low mortality rate. Approximately 10,000 cases are diagnosed each year in the United States; the number of deaths caused by the tumor is about 1000 annually—only 0.2% of cancer deaths. Nevertheless, this disease has major significance for the primary physician because of its iatrogenic relationship to childhood irradiation of the head and neck. A high prevalence of thyroid cancer, diagnosed after a long latent or asymptomatic period, has repeatedly been documented among patients exposed to such irradiation. The appropriate approach to the evaluation and management of radiation-exposed patients remains a subject of debate.

EPIDEMIOLOGY AND RISK FACTORS

Generally, the incidence of thyroid cancer increases with age. This is particularly true of tumors with anaplastic or follicular histopathologies and of the medullary carcinomas derived from the parafollicular cells. The most common tumors, with papillary histopathology, have a bimodal age-specific incidence with peaks in the 30s and late in life. Thyroid tumors occur more than twice as frequently in females. Whites seem to be at greater risk than blacks. Wide variations in thyroid cancer prevalence at autopsy have been reported internationally, with the highest rates reported from Japan. Approximately 20% of the rare medullary carcinomas are familial.

The major identifiable risk factor for the development of thyroid cancer is a history of external irradiation of the head and neck. External irradiation was used as early as 1907 to shrink an enlarged thymus in infancy. During the 1920s and subsequently until the 1950s, it was used extensively for treatment of enlarged tonsils and adenoids, cervical adenitis, mastoiditis, sinusitis, hemangiomas, tinea capitis, and acne. Concern about ill effects began to mount in 1950 when a history of neck irradiation was noted in 9 of 28 cases of childhood thyroid cancer with a latency period of 5 or more years. Further documentation followed, and radiation to the neck was discontinued. In 1973, attention focused on the issue again when 40% of a series of adults with thyroid cancer were found to have a history of irradiation. Clearly, the latent period between exposure and diagnosis of cancer could be measured in decades. It was also clear that the exposed population at risk was substantial—estimates ranged from one million to two million individuals—and largely unidentifiable.

Successive reports focused on the risk among exposed individuals. Large studies indicated that more than 25% had detectable thyroid abnormalities; the prevalence of cancer was estimated at 7% to 9%. These figures must, however, be considered in light of information available regarding the prevalence of thyroid abnormalities including carcinoma in the general population.

At least one investigation has questioned the value of thyroid screening in persons with a history of radiation exposure based on the legitimate questions that can be raised about the effects of sampling bias and observer bias on results of most studies. In a small retrospective cohort study comparing irradiated persons with siblings or patient-selected controls, the investigators found no difference in prevalence of malignant and nonmalignant thyroid abnormalities. This study has in turn been challenged, however, because of its own potential biases and limited power.

Preliminary evidence suggests that some radiation-exposed persons may be at greater risk than others. Radiation during infancy may be most carcinogenic, with cancer risk decreasing as age at the time of radiation increases. Although the threshold dose for cancer risk appears to be low, risk may be greatly increased for persons who received multiple treatments.

NATURAL HISTORY OF THYROID CANCER AND EFFECTIVENESS OF THERAPY

The prevalence of occult carcinoma of the thyroid is not well defined. Autopsy studies have indicated that prevalence ranges from 5% to 13%. An often quoted study showing an overall prevalence of 5.7% found highest age-specific rates in the fifth and sixth decades.

A high prevalence of asymptomatic thyroid cancer is not surprising in light of the benign clinical course of most thyroid tumors after diagnosis. Follow-up studies have determined that probability of survival depends on tissue type and age of the patient. For localized papillary carcinoma, survival approximates that of age-matched controls; in one large study, there were no deaths among patients under 40 during 10 to 15 years of follow-up. The course of follicular cancer is only slightly more aggressive. Anaplastic tumors, on the other hand, run a rapid clinical course to death.

The relatively high prevalence of occult thyroid cancer presumed to be present, in general, raises a number of questions about the significance of tumors found during the evaluation of patients with radiation exposure. It is worth noting that in the largest study, conducted at Michael Reese Hospital in Chicago, 47% of the tumors were incidental findings identified after surgery was recommended because of palpable or scan abnormalities. That is, 29 of 60 cancers were not found in or near the benign nodule that prompted surgery. There is no evidence indicating that tumors found in patients with past radiation exposure are more likely to result in morbidity or mortality than occult tumors found in the general population. However, they do have a high frequency of recurrence.

SCREENING AND DIAGNOSTIC TESTS

The sensitivity of history-taking in identifying persons at risk is not known. Many who were irradiated during early childhood may be unaware of their exposure. Physical examination of the thyroid gland is often difficult, and the palpable nodule is a nonspecific finding that can be found in 4% to 7% of the adult population. Thyroid scan is more sensitive in detecting thyroid abnormalities, but, since it fails to distinguish between benign and malignant disease, is even less specific. A number of studies indicate that physical examination itself becomes more sensitive after scanning is performed and the physician is aware of scan results.

Large studies utilizing both multiple examinations and ^{99m}Tc scanning indicate that 60% of thyroid abnormalities (identified by either or both modalities) will be identified by palpation alone. Scanning alone will be more than 95% sensitive. However, palpable abnormalities appear to be more specific for cancer. In one study of patients with palpable nodules who ultimately had thyroidectomy, the prevalence of cancer was 34%, compared with 19% among patients who went to surgery on the basis of scan abnormalities alone. Physical examination was nearly 80% sensitive in identifying thyroids containing cancers. Cancers found in glands with scan abnormalities alone were often incidental, unrelated to the scan abnormality.

The availability of high-resolution ultrasonography has increased our capacity to identify small thyroid nodules. However, no specific sonographic criteria distinguish between benign and malignant nodules.

Attempts to use measurements of serum thyroglobulin as a screening test for thyroid cancer have not been successful.

Despite poor specificity, thyroglobulin abnormalities are disappointingly insensitive.

When abnormalities are detected on examination or scan, additional diagnostic steps are indicated. The palpable nodule accompanied by a hypofunctioning area on scan is considered by some an indication for surgery. In some centers, needle biopsy of the nodule has become the preferred approach to patients with, as well as those without, a history of irradiation. While some physicians would operate on the basis of scan abnormalities alone, careful follow-up examination with reservation of surgery for palpable abnormalities has been recommended as a prudent alternative. An alternative explanation for scan abnormalities should be considered and thyroid function and the status of antithyroid antibodies determined. Needle biopsy is generally recommended in cases of diffuse thyroid enlargement when it is important to rule out thyroiditis or when the patient is a poor surgical risk (see Chapter 95).

When physical examination or scan findings are questionable, some physicians have used suppression of the thyroid for 3 to 6 months in an effort to shrink normal thyroid tissue, thereby increasing the sensitivity of the examination for autonomous nodules. Although this remains a reasonable approach when cancer risk is low, it must be kept in mind that regression following thyroid hormone suppression is neither perfectly sensitive nor highly specific for thyroid cancer. There are case reports of confirmed carcinomas that had apparently responded to suppression therapy; only a minority of nodules that do not respond prove to be malignant. On the basis of animal experiments, long-term thyroid suppression as prophylaxis for thyroid cancer has also been advocated for all patients with an exposure history or, more selectively, those with questionable scans.

CONCLUSIONS AND RECOMMENDATIONS

- Childhood irradiation is an important risk factor for thyroid carcinoma that may be diagnosed as long as 35 years after exposure.
- The prevalence of thyroid abnormalities among the estimated one to two million patients with an exposure history is about 25%. The prevalence of thyroid cancer has been estimated to be 7% to 9%.
- The significance of occult thyroid cancer in exposed patients is not known. There appears to be a high prevalence of occult tumors in the general population.
- Identification of patients at risk is an important part of history-taking.
- Patients at risk should be carefully examined yearly or at least every 2 years. Scanning is not necessary in the absence of palpable abnormalities. If scanning is performed, low radiation dose methods should be used (^{99m}Tc or ^{123}I).
- In general, surgery should be reserved for patients with palpable abnormalities of the gland. Needle biopsy may be

preferred in cases where a single nodule has been identified. Multiple examinations by experienced examiners may be necessary. Thyroid suppression may increase the sensitivity of thyroid palpation. Repeat examination of patients with normal examination but abnormal scan should be performed yearly.

A.G.M.

ANNOTATED BIBLIOGRAPHY

Arnold J, Pinsky S, Ryo UY et al: ^{99m}Tc-pertechnetate thyroid scintigraphy in patients predisposed to thyroid neoplasms by prior radiotherapy to the head and neck. Radiology 115:653, 1975 (*Documents higher sensitivity but very low specificity of technetium scanning.*)

Beahrs OH, Upton AC, Land CE et al: Irradiation to the head and neck area and thyroid cancer. JAMA 244:337, 1980 (*A commentary refuting the negative conclusions of Royce et al.*)

Crile G, Jr, Esselstyn CB, Jr, Hawk WA: Needle biopsy in the diagnosis of thyroid nodules appearing after irradiation. N Engl J Med 301:997, 1979 (*An important editorial citing data that support a conservative approach for those with nodules.*)

Favus MJ, Schneider AB, Stachura ME et al: Thyroid cancer occurring as a late consequence of head-and-neck irradiation. Evaluation of 1056 patients. N Engl J Med 294:1019, 1976 (*An important paper. Of 1056 patients, 16.5% had nodular disease on palpation, another 10.7% on technetium scanning. Estimated prevalence of carcinoma of 9%.*)

Gharib H, Goeller JR, Zinsmeister AR et al: Fine needle aspiration biopsy of the thyroid. Ann Intern Med 101:25, 1984 (*Of nearly 2000 patients with solitary nodules, 17% had suspicious cytologic findings; of these, 24% had malignant lesions.*)

Gonzalez-Villalpando C, Frohman LA, Bekerman C et al: Scintigraphic thyroid abnormalities after radiation. Ann Intern Med 97:55, 1982 (*Palpable and nonpalpable thyroid nodules were much more common among patients with prior radiation exposure than among controls.*)

Maxon HR, Saenger EL, Thomas SR et al: Clinically important radiation-associated thyroid disease: A controlled study. JAMA 244:1802, 1980 (*A retrospective cohort study with potentially serious bias problems. Most notable for finding that repeated doses of radiation dramatically increased risk.*)

McTiernan AM, Weiss NS, Daling JR: Incidence of thyroid cancer in women in relation to reproductive and hormonal factors. Am J Epidemiol 120:423, 1984 (*Despite the impact on the production of thyroid-stimulating hormone, pregnancy and use of exogenous estrogens had little or no effect on the risk of thyroid carcinoma in this case-control study.*)

National Cancer Institute: Information for physicians on irradiation-related thyroid cancer. CA 26:150, 1976 (*Good summary with recommendations.*)

Refetoff S, Lever EG: The value of serum thyroglobulin measurement in clinical practice. JAMA 250:2352, 1983 (*A review. No value in cancer screening.*)

Rojeski MT, Gharib H: Nodular thyroid disease. Evaluation and management. N Engl J Med 313:428, 1985 (*An extensive, critical review.*)

Royce PC, MacKay BR, DiSabella PM: Value of postirradiation screening for thyroid nodules. JAMA 242:2675, 1979 (*A controversial retrospective cohort study that found no difference in prevalence of benign or malignant thyroid disease in radiation-exposed persons and controls.*)

Sampson RJ, Woolner LB, Bahn RC et al: Occult thyroid carcinoma in Olmstead County, Minnesota: Prevalence of autopsy compared with that in Hiroshima and Nagasaki, Japan. Cancer 34:2072, 1974 (*Prevalence of 5.6% among 157 autopsies of clinically occult thyroid cancer. Highest age specific prevalence between 40 and 60.*)

Schneider AB, Favus MJ, Stachura ME: Plasma thyroglobulin in detecting thyroid carcinoma after childhood head and neck irradiation. Ann Intern Med 86:29, 1977 (*Thyroglobulin levels not found to be very useful.*)

Schneider AB, Favus MJ, Stachura ME et al: Incidence, prevalence and characteristics of radiation-induced thyroid tumors. Am J Med 64:243, 1978 (*Further follow-up from Michael Reese Hospital and Medical Center demonstrating a high [36%] incidence of new thyroid tumors after surgery. Thyroid suppressive therapy appeared to prevent recurrences.*)

Schneider AB, Recurrent W, Pinsky SM: Radiation-induced thyroid carcinoma. Ann Intern Med 105:405, 1986 (*Describes the clinical course of Michael Reese cohort at 10 years' mean follow up; a high frequency of recurrent disease noted. Small nodules managed conservatively.*)

VanHerle AJ, Rich P, Ljung BE et al: The thyroid nodule. Ann Intern Med 96:221, 1982 (*An extensive review of the diagnostic value of fine needle aspiration, thyroid scanning, and ultrasonography including an analysis of alternative sequencing strategies; fine needle aspiration followed by scan in patients with cytologically suspicious lesions is recommended.*)

Woolner LB, Beahrs OH, Black BM et al: Classification and prognosis of thyroid carcinoma: A study of 885 cases observed in a 30-year period. Am J Surg 102:354, 1961 (*Noninvasive disease without significant morbidity or mortality.*)

95
Evaluation of Thyroid Nodules

Thyroid nodules are an extremely common phenomenon, clinically, radiographically, and histologically. A palpable thyroid nodule can be detected in 4% to 7% of the adult population. The prevalence of nodules in autopsy series approaches 50%, a figure that is approximated by patients undergoing modern high-resolution, real-time ultrasonography of the thyroid. The incidence of thyroid nodules increases with age and neck irradiation; it is 6 to 9 times more common in women than in men.

The principal objective in evaluating thyroid nodules is to distinguish the patient with a malignant lesion from one with a benign mass. Among patients with thyroid nodules who come to surgery, thyroid cancer is found in about 10% to 20%; the fraction increases to 30% to 50% if there has been radiation exposure. One wants to identify for consideration of surgery patients with a high risk of malignant disease and avoid operations in those with little risk of cancer (see Chapter 94). To accomplish this task, the primary physician must be skilled in the detection of thyroid lesions by physical examination and capable of designing a cost-effective evaluation of the palpable thyroid nodule. Knowledge of the indications for and utilities of scanning, ultrasonography, and fine-needle aspiration are particularly important.

PATHOPHYSIOLOGY AND CLINICAL PRESENTATION

Thyroid nodules may be single or multiple, with and without underlying disturbances of hormonal homeostasis. A solitary nodule is usually the more worrisome one, because it may represent a malignancy; on occasion a malignancy can arise in a multinodular gland.

Benign and malignant thyroid nodules are usually asymptomatic and discovered by the patient or examining physician. Large nodules may cause a cosmetic problem or compress an adjacent structure. The nodules are usually painless unless rapid growth, inflammation, or hemorrhage occurs and produces significant discomfort.

Solitary Nodule. Solitary thyroid nodules represent benign adenomas, carcinomas, or multinodular etiologies in which only a single nodule is palpable. *Benign adenomas* account for most nonmalignant truly solitary nodules. The majority are *follicular*. Growth is typically slow, extending over many years. Follicular adenomas rarely become large enough to encroach on the trachea or esophagus. TSH receptors are present in most, making them hormonally responsive. The majority of adenomas do not produce much thyroid hormone; their radioiodine uptake on scan is also

limited, giving the appearance of a *"cold" nodule.* Most thyroid cysts are benign adenomas that have necrosed and degenerated; they also appear as cold nodules on scan.

A few follicular adenomas produce such substantial quantities of thyroid hormone that the patient presents with thyrotoxicosis (see Chapter 101). This is particularly true for adenomas that grow to over 3 cm in diameter. These function autonomously, suppress TSH (which renders the rest of the gland atrophic), and appear as a *"hot" nodule* on thyroid scan. A *"warm" nodule* represents an adenoma that produces sufficient thyroid hormone to suppress the rest of the gland, but not enough to cause hyperthyroidism.

Thyroid *carcinomas* are uncommon; the current incidence is 2.5 per 100,000 population per year. They are more frequent in women than in men. *Papillary carcinomas* are the most common and account for 60% to 70% of all thyroid malignancies. The lesions are slow growing, spread to local lymph nodes, and metastasize late; as a result, prognosis is good. *Follicular carcinomas* make up another 15% to 20% of thyroid cancers. Lymph node metastases may occur without invasion of the thyroid capsule; this occurrence does not alter prognosis. Hematogenous spread is early, and initial presentation is often from a metastasis to lung or bone. On radioiodine scan, most thyroid carcinomas present as "cold" nodules, failing to take up iodine, though on technetium scan a rare malignant nodule will take up the radionuclide. On ultrasonography, most cancers are solid, though occasionally a mixed cystic and solid appearance is encountered. *Anaplastic carcinomas* comprise another 10% to 12% of cases; these are very invasive, usually inoperable, and fatal within 1 year.

Medullary carcinomas, derived from the parafollicular cells of the thyroid, may occur as an autosomal dominant disease, as in familial medullary cancer and multiple endocrine neoplasia types II and III in conjunction with pheochromocytoma. The malignancy often presents as a thyroid nodule located in the upper half of the thyroid gland. It can be multicentric, especially in the familial forms. At least 50% of medullary carcinomas of the thyroid occur sporadically. Calcitonin, produced by the parafollicular of "C" cells, is a tumor marker for medullary carcinoma.

Multiple Nodules. *Hashimoto's thyroiditis,* an autoimmune condition, is the leading cause of goiter in the United States. Pathologically, there is lymphocytic infiltration, formation of germinal centers, fibrosis, and Hürthle cell change involving follicular epitheial cells. Antimicrosomal antibodies are found in 70% to 95% of patients. About one third experience a progressive loss of glandular function and eventually become hypothyroid, though this is not inevitable. Hyperthyroidism is noted in patients who have concurrent Graves' disease. The gland is characteristically firm and either lobulated or diffusely enlarged.

Multinodular goiter (sporadic goiter) is believed due to minor defects in hormone synthesis, though its precise pathophysiology remains poorly defined. After Hashimoto's disease, it is the most common cause of a multinodular gland in adults. Although the gland may first enlarge diffusely, it typically evolves into a multinodular goiter as areas of the thyroid undergo degenerative changes. Nodules may also develop when colloid accumulates in hyperplastic cells (*colloid cysts*). Uptake of radioiodine on scan is heterogenous; some areas may not take up iodine and appear "cold." The thyroid gland feels less firm than it does in Hashimoto's disease. Goiter due to *iodine deficiency* (endemic goiter) is rare in the United States, but may have a similar appearance, though iodine uptake on scan is generally elevated.

Subacute lymphocytic thyroiditis appears to be another autoimmune thyroid disease, producing a goiter resembling that of Hashimoto's thyroiditis. This self-limited condition has been noted with particularly high frequency among *postpartum women*, who experience onset within 3 to 6 months of delivery. There is transient hyperthyroidism followed by a period of hypothyroidism. Resolution occurs within 6 to 12 months. Many experience recurrences, especially with subsequent pregnancies. Sometimes there is little glandular enlargement; when it does occur, the gland's appearance and feel are identical to that of Hashimoto's thyroiditis. Antimicrosomal antibodies can be found in the serum. Radioiodine uptake on scan is low or absent.

Thyroid cancer or *lymphoma* may arise in a multinodular gland, though this is very uncommon. Cervical adenopathy, hoarseness (due to recurrent laryngeal nerve compression), and the continued enlargement of a "cold" nodule on thyroid scan are distinguishing features of the clinical presentation. A history of neck irradiation or family history of thyroid cancer (suggestive of the multiple endocrine neoplasia syndrome) are risk factors. The nodule may be tender if the tumor is rapidly growing (as with lymphoma), a finding atypical of other multinodular goiters.

DIFFERENTIAL DIAGNOSIS

The vast majority of solitary nodules are benign, even among those that fail to take up radionuclide on thyroid scan (see below). Hashimoto's thyroiditis accounts for most cases of multinodular goiter in the United States. (See Table 95-1.)

WORKUP

History can help determine the risk of malignancy. Although definitive assessment cannot be made by history and physical examination alone, these elements of the evaluation can provide important information regarding risk and need for biopsy or excision. *Age, sex,* and a *history of neck irradiation* are most helpful. The incidence of malignancy among patients with thyroid nodules is considerably higher in males than in females, although women make up a greater proportion of those with thyroid cancer. Moreover, the incidence of thyroid cancers in patients with nodules is greatest in those under age 40, especially if they have previously been subjected to head or neck irradiation.

Symptoms suggestive of local invasion, such as hoarseness, dysphagia, and obstruction, may be manifestations of malignancy but also occur with benign lesions. The same holds true for a new nodule or one that is growing rapidly in a multinodular gland that is otherwise unchanged. In fact, many thyroid cancers are slow growing and may have been present for years; duration is not particularly useful for distinguishing benign from malignant disease. However, a history of living in an iodine-deficient area, goiter, or intake of goitrogens such as lithium, turnips, or beets favors a benign lesion, as do age greater than 40, female sex, and family history of goiter. Symptoms of hypothyroidism or hyperthyroidism argue against malignancy, as does sudden growth or sudden onset of neck pain, which suggest subacute thyroiditis or hemorrhage into a benign adenoma.

Physical Findings are not particularly useful for distinguishing benign disease from malignancy, with a few exceptions. The presence of a firm, irregular large nodule (>2 cm in diameter) that is fixed and fails to move with swallowing does point towards cancer, as does associated cervical adenopathy. Multiple nodules suggest a benign condition, such as multinodular goiter; risk of malignancy is greater in a gland with a solitary nodule. The consistency of the tissue may not be diagnostic, because malignancy may be present in soft nodules (*e.g.,* papillary carcinomas that have undergone cystic degeneration).

Laboratory Studies. Since history and physical examination rarely provide a diagnosis, laboratory study takes on considerable importance. Scanning, ultrasound, and fine-needle biopsy have been the major diagnostic modalities employed. Thyroid radionuclide scanning has been quite popular. [123]I is preferred since it produces the least radiation exposure. An appreciation for its lack of specificity has emerged. While most malignant disease has the appearance of a "cold" nodule on scan and accounts for about 15% of all "cold" nodules, the occurrence of uptake in the nodule rule out malignancy. One can say only that there is an increased chance of malignancy if the nodule appears "cold" on scan.

Ultrasonography represents another heavily utilized noninvasive diagnostic approach, often used in combination with radionuclide scan. Patients with a "cold" nodule on scan are commonly referred for ultrasound to determine if the nodule

Table 95-1. Causes of Thyroid Nodules

CAUSE	APPEARANCE OF NODULE ON ^{123}I THYROID SCAN
Solitary Nodule	
Adenoma	
Nonfunctioning	Absent or low uptake
Functioning	Moderate uptake, remainder of gland normal
Toxic	"Hot" nodule with remainder of gland without uptake
Cyst	No uptake
Follicular carcinoma	No uptake
Papillary carcinoma	No uptake
Anaplastic carcinoma	No uptake
Medullary carcinoma	No uptake; may be multicentric; upper part of the gland
Lymphoma	No uptake
Congenital anomaly	No uptake
Multiple Nodules	
Hashimoto's thyroiditis	Heterogenous uptake
Multinodular goiter	Heterogenous uptake, including areas without uptake
Subacute lymphocytic thyroiditis	Low or absent uptake diffusely
Cancer in a multinodular goiter	Cold nodule that continues to enlarge

is cystic (and more likely to be benign) or solid and at significant risk for malignancy. Although the technique is quite good at distinguishing cystic from solid lesions, and new high-solution technology can detect ever smaller lesions, it too lacks specificity. Not all malignancies are confined to the solid group; moreover, there are no clearly defined architectural criteria for malignant lesions. Combined data show that 21% of solid lesions, 12% of mixed lesions, and 7% of purely cystic ones are malignant. Thus, like scanning, the technique lacks the specificity one would like to have optimally to select patients for surgery. Work is ongoing to better distinguish nodules on the basis of fine architectural detail.

With the failure of scanning and ultrasound to provide adequate specificity, *fine-needle biopsy* has emerged as the preferred study for selection of patients who require surgical excision. Specificity ranges from 70% when patients with "suspicious" readings are included in the group in need of surgery, to over 90% if they are not. Compared to use of ultrasound and scan, fine-needle biopsy has reduced by half the number of patients who undergo operations needlessly, doubled the incidence of malignancy in surgically excised nodules, and reduced costs by over 25%. The procedure is safe and inexpensive. Shortcomings include the need to have an experienced surgeon perform the procedure, an experienced pathologist interpret the aspirate, the possibility of a sampling error, and the difficulty of interpreting a "suspicious" result. Differentiating benign Hürthle cell and follicular neoplasms from their malignant counterparts is difficult because the biopsy provides only cytologic information, not

histologic. At present, it is recommended that all patients with suspicious lesions undergo surgical removal.

With a few exceptions, ancillary laboratory studies are usually of little help. When *thyroid indices* reveal hypofunctioning or hyperfunctioning of the gland, one has presumptive evidence against malignancy. *Antimicrosomal antibody titers* are useful in suspected Hashimoto's and subacute lymphocytic thyroiditis. Rarely, an incidental plain film of the neck may demonstrate punctate calcifications indicative of the psammoma bodies seen in papillary carcinoma or the shell-like calcification characteristic of a benign lesion. A very high *erythrocyte sedimentation rate* in the setting of an acutely tender gland is very suggestive of subacute granulomatous thyroiditis. With the exception of an elevated serum *calcitonin* in medullary thyroid cancer, there are no markers for thyroid cancer. Thyroglobulin elevations do occur with cancer, but also with benign nodular thyroid disease. A calcitonin determination is indicated when there is a strong family history of thyroid cancer. Response to *TSH suppression* (by administration of thyroid hormone) is not a reliable diagnostic test, because carcinomas as well as adenomas may shrink when TSH secretion is inhibited.

In sum, a fine-needle biopsy provides the best means of evaluating a thyroid nodule. In a patient with a solitary nodule, it is the diagnostic procedure of choice. If the necessary expertise for its performance and interpretation are unavailable, the combination of radionuclide scanning and ultrasound is a less specific but reasonable alternative. Scanning also plays a role in localization for biopsy and follow-up. If radionuclide scanning is performed, low dose methods should be used (^{99m}Tc or ^{123}I).

Patients with multinodular glands usually do not require biopsy unless there is increased concern for cancer due to neck irradiation, cervical adenopathy, rapid growth of a single nodule in an otherwise stable gland, or onset of recurrent laryngeal nerve palsy. Most cases are due to *Hashimoto's thyroiditis* and can be diagnosed by obtaining thyroid antibody determinations. High titers of *antimicrosomal antibodies* correlate best with biopsy-proven disease. Antithyroglobulin titers are less useful. There is an increased risk of *lymphoma* of the thyroid in patients with Hashimoto's disease, mandating *needle biopsy* of the gland if there is an enlarging tender goiter, a goiter enlarging on thyroid hormone, or enlargement of a cold area on thyroid scan.

Further Evaluation of the Benign Adenoma. When a lesion is found to be a benign adenoma, the question arises as to whether or not it functions autonomously and thus poses the risk of toxicity. Diagnosis of autonomous function is achieved by performing *serial radionuclide scans* and demonstrating little change in uptake when comparing scans taken before and after *stimulation by TRH* or *suppression by thyroid hormone.* Adenomas less than 2 cm in size rarely change much in size or function and can be followed. Those greater than 3 cm are at risk for progressing to toxicity within a few years. Observation rather than ablation is now preferred for the smaller, low-risk lesions. Annual determination of the nodule's size and hormonal output usually suffices. Every 5 years scanning can be repeated to see if there is increasing suppression of extranodular tissue function, a sign of impending toxicity. Other signs include size greater than 3 cm, rise in serum T3 to the upper limits of normal, and decreasing responsiveness to stimulation or suppression.

SYMPTOMATIC THERAPY

Patients with benign lesions who are otherwise healthy can be given a trial of exogenous thyroid hormone therapy in an attempt to decrease the size of the nodule. Reduction in size also can occur with some cancers and should not be interpreted as a sign of a benign etiology. Approximately 10% to 30% of patients with nontoxic nodular goiters will show a decrease in nodule size when treated with doses of L-thyroxine sufficient to suppress TSH. The rationale is that suppression of TSH should diminish nodule size in those lesions that are TSH responsive, *e.g.,* follicular adenomas and Hashimoto's thyroiditis. The required dose of L-thyroxine is often slightly supraphysiologic, that is, 0.2 to 0.3 mg daily, though one should begin with small doses (0.05 mg/day) and increase gradually (see Chapter 102). Thyroid hormone therapy is not indicated in the elderly or in those with underlying coronary disease. It is unknown whether therapy prevents increase in nodule size in patients who have not achieved a decrease.

Patients with *autonomously functioning solitary adeno-mas* that are at high risk for becoming toxic (greater than 3 cm in diameter, serum T3 at upper limit of normal, increasingly unresponsive to TRH stimulation and thyroxine suppression) should be considered for prophylatic *ablative therapy.* Ablation is mandatory for those with autonomous nodules that have already become toxic. One needs to choose between surgery and radioiodine. *Surgery* represents a definitive approach with low risk if done by a skilled thyroid surgeon. Young patients are the best candidates. *Radioiodine* is simpler and usually the treatment of choice in the elderly. The theoretical risk of inducing cancer in the remaining thyroid tissue makes radioiodine a less attractive option for young people, though no increase in incidence of malignancy has been reported. A palpable nodule often remains after irradiation; it is of no consequence other than cosmetic. The patient needs to be monitored for development of posttreatment hypothyroidism.

Multinodular goiters often do not shrink much because they are composed of a great deal of fibrous tissue. Bothersome *large cysts* may require surgical removal, but smaller ones can be aspirated as necessary. Hormone therapy has no effect on recurrence of thyroid cysts after aspiration.

PATIENT EDUCATION

The primary care physician should counsel and closely follow patients with previous head or neck radiation (see Chapter 94). Regular follow-up is important in any patient with a nodule, and the patient should be instructed to call if there should be a change in size, development of lymphadenopathy, pain, dysphagia, or hoarseness.

The patient with an autonomous nodule or a multinodular goiter should be advised to avoid substances containing high concentrations of iodine (medications, kelp, radiographic contrast media), because they may precipitate thyrotoxicosis. If a contrast study is necessary, the patient should be started on a betablocking agent 10 days before the study.

INDICATIONS FOR REFERRAL

Detection of a solitary thyroid nodule in a clinically euthyroid patient should prompt a referral to a consultant skilled in performing thin-needle biopsy of the thyroid. Encountering a worrisome nodule (see above) in a patient with a multinodular gland represents another indication for consideration of biopsy. Patients with a toxic or large (>3 cm) autonomously functioning adenoma require consultation for discussion of ablative therapy. Those with goiters unresponsive to thyroid hormone that are causing obstruction or cosmetic discomfort may be surgical candidates.

A.H.G.

ANNOTATED BIBLIOGRAPHY

Ashcraft MW, Van Herle AJ: Management of thyroid nodules. Head Neck Surg 3:216, 297, 1981 (*A two-part review of 22 series, pro-*

viding important data on yields of tests and correlating them with surgical findings.)

Baker BA, Gharib H: Correlation of thyroid antibodies and cytologic features in suspected autoimmune thyroid disease. Am J Med 74:941, 1983 (*Antimicrosomal antibodies correlated best with biopsy-proven disease.*)

Crile G, Jr, Esselstyn CB, Hawk WA: Needle biopsy in the diagnosis of thyroid nodules appearing after radiation. N Engl J Med 301: 997, 1979 (*An editorial summarizing the usefulness of this diagnostic method.*)

Gershengorn MC, McClung MR, Chu EW et al: Fine-needle aspiration cytology in the preoperative diagnosis of thyroid nodules. Ann Intern Med 87:265, 1977 (*Thirty-three patients who had aspiration biopsy and excisional biopsy were assessed. Satisfactory aspiration specimens were obtained in 97%. The diagnosis of malignancy was made in nine, seven were correct, and there was one false-positive and one occult carcinoma unrelated to the clinical nodule. Eighteen aspirations were interpreted as benign. There was one false-negative.*)

Gharib J, Goellner JR, Zinsmeister AR et al: Fine-needle biopsy aspiration biopsy of the thyroid. Ann Intern Med 101:25, 1984 (*Addresses the difficult issue of what to do with the "suspicious" finding.*)

Hamburger JI: The autonomously functioning thyroid adenoma. N Engl J Med 309:1512, 1983 (*An editorial summarizing diagnosis and treatment.*)

Hamburger JI: The various presentations of thyroiditis. Ann Intern Med 104:219, 1986 (*Authoritative review with detailed discussions of Hashimoto's and subacute thyroiditis; 51 references.*)

Hamburger JI: Lymphoma of the thyroid. Ann Intern Med 99:685, 1983 (*A clinical review drawing attention to the relation between the condition and Hashimoto's thyroiditis; provides indications for biopsy.*)

McCowen KD, Reed JW, Fariss BL: The role of thyroid therapy in patients with thyroid cysts. Am J Med 68:853, 1980 (*Treatment with hormone did not prevent recurrence of cysts after aspiration.*)

Rojeski MT, Gharib H: Nodular thyroid disease. N Engl J Med 313: 428, 1985 (*Useful review, especially of evaluation methods; 115 references.*)

Ross DS, Ridgeway EC, Daniels GH: Successful treatment of solitary toxic thyroid nodules with relatively low-dose iodine-131, with low prevalence of hypothyroidism. Ann Intern Med 101:488, 1984 (*Reports excellent results with no hypothyroidism being induced.*)

Van Herle AJ, Rich P, Ljung BB et al: The thyroid nodule. Ann Intern Med 96:221, 1982 (*Suggests that fine-needle biopsy supplemented by scan is the best means of evaluating thyroid nodules.*)

Warner SC: Modalities of medical therapy for nodular goiter. In Warner S, Ingbar S (eds.): The Thyroid, p 525. New York, Harper & Row, 1978 (*A critical discussion of thyroxine therapy.*)

96

Evaluation of Asymptomatic Hypercalcemia

SAMUEL R. NUSSBAUM, M.D.

The advent of automated laboratory screening has led to the increased recognition of asymptomatic individuals with hypercalcemia. In addition, patients with nonspecific complaints, such as fatigue, weakness, abdominal discomfort, and constipation, may have hypercalcemia discovered during biochemical testing. Mild hyperparathyroidism is usually the explanation for these often inadvertently recognized calcium elevations. Hypercalcemia may also herald other important underlying diseases, such as malignancy or sarcoidosis. Asymptomatic hyperparathyroidism is not necessarily a benign condition. Long-standing action of parathyroid hormone on its target tissues (bone and kidney) may lead to skeletal loss and impairment of renal function.

The primary physician must be able to interpret an abnormal calcium value, diagnose its cause, and, if hyperparathyroidism is present, decide whether surgery or medical therapy is warranted.

PATHOPHYSIOLOGY AND CLINICAL PRESENTATION

The serum calcium concentration is maintained within narrow limits by parathyroid hormone. The precision of calcium homeostasis is related to the vital function of calcium for neuromuscular function, membrane function, hormonal secretion, and hormone action. The free or ionized portion of serum calcium is responsible for its physiologic actions. Slightly less than 50% of serum calcium is in the form of free calcium ions. The remainder is bound to plasma proteins, mostly albumin. Globulins can also bind serum calcium. Calcium binding by serum proteins is pH-dependent; increased binding occurs at alkaline pH and explains the common symptom of paresthesias that occur in conjunction with hyperventilation. The normal range for serum calcium is 8.5–10.4 mg/dl or 4.7–5.2 mEq/L. True hypercalcemia requires an increase in the ionized fraction of serum calcium; a convenient correction factor to apply to total serum calcium is to subtract or add 1 mg/dl to the calcium concentration for every 1.0 g/100ml of serum albumin lower or higher than 4.0 g/100ml.

Hyperparathyroidism increases with age, peaking in the fourth through sixth decades of life, and is more common in women than men by approximately a 6:4 ratio. It is not certain whether the increased recognition of disease relates to biochemical screening of patients with no symptoms or non-specific symptoms such as weakness or fatigue or whether there is an increase in the disease, possibly as a result of head and neck irradiation in infancy.

The majority of patients with hyperparathyroidism do not have symptoms. The "classic" disease presentation of hyperparathyroidism with "stones, bones, abdominal groans, and psychic moans" representing an incidence of renal stones as high as 60%, skeletal fracture and bone pain of osteitis fibrosa cystica, a possible but somewhat controversial increase in peptic ulcer disease and pancreatitis, and a spectrum of psychiatric disease has been replaced by a more subtle and nonspecific presentation. Fatigue, weakness, mild gastrointestinal symptoms including constipation and abdominal pain, changes in intellectual performance, and depression may all be manifestations of hypercalcemia or excessive parathyroid hormone. Hypercalcemia can lead to a renal concentrating defect and increased urination, as well as to an increase in calcium oxalate stones, particularly in patients with increased 1,25 dihydroxyvitamin D levels and urinary calcium excretion in excess of 300–350 mg per 24 hours. Often nonspecific symptoms of hyperparathyroidism are recognized only after successful parathyroid surgery when the patient describes an improved sense of well-being.

The hypercalcemia of hyperparathyroidism is caused by increased osteoclastic bone resorption mediated though parathyroid hormone, as well as an increase in gut calcium absorption. Pathologically, approximately 80% of patients are found to have a single parathyroid adenoma, whereas 20% have four-gland hyperplasia. Parathyroid cancer accounts for approximately 1% of all hypercalcemia attributed to excess parathyroid hormone secretion.

Hyperparathyroidism may be observed in familial settings, such as the autosomal dominant multiple endocrine neoplasia (MEN) type I and type II syndromes. In MEN I, parathyroid hyperplasia occurs in conjunction with adenomas of the pituitary and pancreas; in MEN II, parathyroid hyperplasia may occur with medullary cancer of the thyroid and bilateral adrenal pheochromocytoma. *Familial hypocalcuric hypercalcemia,* which causes hypercalcemia as often as multiple endocrine neoplasia type I, is associated with varying parathyroid gland hyperplasia at surgery and, importantly, is not cured by surgery. Urinary calcium excretion is often less than 100 mg/24 hours.

Patients with "*normocalcemic hyperparathyroidism*" often have serum calcium levels at the upper limit of normal, which on repeated determinations will fluctuate into the frankly elevated range. Although many textbooks suggest *thiazide diuretics* may cause hypercalcemia, it is likely that these individuals have mild hyperparathyroidism. Their serum calcium rises as thiazide limits urinary calcium excretion.

Malignancy is the second most frequent cause of hypercalcemia and the most common among hospitalized patients;

cancers of the breast and lung lead the list of malignant etiologies, accounting for 50% to 80% of such cases. The incidence of hypercalcemia during the course of breast cancer ranges from 18% to 42%; in lung cancer from 6% to 16%. Other malignancies associated with hypercalcemia include multiple myeloma (incidence 30% to 100%), squamous cell carcinomas of the head and neck (2%), lymphoma, and leukemia (1%) and genitourinary cancer (1%).

The mechanisms of hypercalcemia in malignancy are under active investigation. Accelerated bone resorption is the usual cause. However, hypercalcemia can occur without bony metastases as a result of humoral factors that bind to parathyroid hormone receptors and activate adenyl cyclase, giving the biochemical profile of hyperparathyroidism.

Hypercalcemia in malignancy represents a diverse spectrum of diseases and mediators; in some patients with lymphoma and leukemia, increased 1,25 dihydroxyvitamin D with increased gut calcium absorption is implicated.

Hypercalcemia is rarely the sole presenting manifestation of an underlying malignancy. The presence of hypercalcemia in malignancy indicates a grim prognosis, as 60% of these patients will be dead in 3 months.

Higher levels of serum calcium (greater than 14 mg%) are more often associated with malignancy, although levels of calcium as high as 20 mg% may be seen in *parathyroid crisis* caused by large parathyroid adenomas, often in the clinical setting of intercurrent medical illness. Hypercalcemia in these situations is exacerbated by dehydration caused by the loss of renal concentrating ability in hypercalcemia and immobilization. Immediate medical attention must be directed to this life-threatening clinical situation.

In *sarcoidosis,* absorption of calcium from the gut increases due to enhanced production of 1,25 dihydroxyvitamin D, the biologically active form of vitamin D. The granulomatous tissue contains the hydroxylase enzyme capable of converting inactive vitamin D to its active form.

Vitamin D intoxication and *milk-alkali syndrome* are being seen increasingly with the popularization of calcium and vitamin D to avert osteoporosis. Hypercalcemia occurs when an excess of 100,000 units of vitamin D and an excess of 5 grams of calcium are consumed each day.

The *thiazide diuretics* cause a transient mild increase in serum calcium, generally within the normal range. As noted earlier, a sustained increase in serum calcium beyond 10 days implies underlying metabolic bone disease, usually hyperparathyroidism. Some investigators have used thiazides as a provocative test for hyperparathyroidism in patients with borderline hypercalcemia. *Theophylline excess* is another pharmacologic etiology.

Hyperthyroidism is associated with mild elevations in serum calcium in approximately 20% of individuals due to increased skeletal turnover. *Immobilization* in young individuals who have not completed skeletal growth, and in patients with Paget's disease may cause severe hypercalcemia.

Lithium therapy for manic-depressive illness can cause hypercalcemia. It is unclear whether these individuals taking lithium have altered calcium set-point for PTH secretion. Addison's disease may be associated with hypercalcemia because the dehydration and elevation in albumin leads to an erroneous assessment of the free serum calcium.

DIFFERENTIAL DIAGNOSIS

In the ambulatory primary care setting, hypercalcemia is most often noted as an incidental laboratory finding during multiphasic screening. With the advent of multiphasic biochemical screening at the Mayo Clinic in 1974, the number of newly recognized patients with hypercalcemia (the majority of whom were ultimately determined to have hyperparathyroidism) increased from an annual incidence of 7.8/100,000 to 51/100,000. Hyperparathyroidism is overwhelmingly the most likely etiology for hypercalcemia in the medically well, asymptomatic patient. In a Swedish population survey, 15,903 persons were screened for hypercalcemia. Ninety-five had hypercalcemia, with hyperparathyroidism being suspected in 88 patients and confirmed surgically in 57 of the 59 who underwent neck exploration for cure of hyperparathyroidism.

Malignancy, granulomatous diseases, hyperthyroidism, Addison's disease, and excess ingestion of vitamin D and calcium are the cause of most other cases. Primary hyperparathyroidism accounts for more than 60% of hypercalcemic patients and is extremely likely to be the explanation for hypercalcemia should it be found that an elevation of serum calcium was recognized in the preceding years. Occasionally there is an underlying multiple endocrine neoplasia syndrome or hypocalciuric hypercalcemia.

WORKUP

Prior to costly laboratory evaluation, a repeat calcium determination is indicated to confirm the elevation. Ordering serum albumin and globulin levels helps assure the elevation is not artifactual due to elevated protein binding of calcium. Hypercalcemia that appears ephemeral may be spurious, caused by prolonged application of the tourniquet at the time of blood drawing. Should hypercalcemia be confirmed, then evaluation can proceed.

History. In the "asymptomatic" patient, subtle manifestations of hyperparathyroidism, such as fatigue, weakness, lethargy, arthralgias, nonspecific gastrointestinal complaints, impairment of intellectual performance, and depression should be specifically sought. Associated conditions such as hypertension, gout, pseudogout, and nephrolithiasis ought to be noted. A history of increased urination may indicate calcium-related defects in urine-concentrating ability. Symptoms of underlying malignancy, particularly of breast (see Chapter

121), lung (see Chapter 42), and hematologic malignancies should be pursued. Review of antacids, food additives, and health food store preparations may uncover excessive ingestion of vitamin D or calcium. Symptoms of hyperthyroidism (see Chapter 101) also need checking.

Physical Examination in the totally asymptomatic patient is generally unrevealing; however, a careful search for signs of malignancy (breast mass, lymphadenopathy, bone tenderness) and sarcoidosis (lymph node enlargement, abnormalities on lung exam) should be undertaken. There are no readily apparent signs of hyperparathyroidism; band keratopathy is rarely visible without the slit lamp.

Laboratory Studies. When hyperparathyroidism is under consideration, serum electrolyte and phosphate concentrations can provide indirect evidence of the diagnosis. Fasting hypophosphatemia, hyperchloremia, and mild metabolic acidosis suggest the diagnosis. This is because parathyroid hormone induces renal phosphate and bicarbonate wasting. Although a chloride-to-phosphate ratio of 33 has been advocated, it may also be seen in patients with humoral hypercalcemia of malignancy. A normal serum phosphate does not exclude the diagnosis of hyperparathyroidism; and hypophosphatemia can be observed in malignancy. Furthermore, phosphate must be measured in the fasting state, as glucose causes an intracellular shift in phosphate. *Alkaline phosphatase* elevation implies increased osteoblastic activity and can be seen in malignancy, hyperparathyroidism with PTH bone disease, and Paget's disease. Rather than proceeding with laboratory determinations that exclude the myriad causes of hypercalcemia, the most direct approach to the diagnosis of hypercalcemia is the measurement of parathyroid hormone.

In principle, an elevated *parathyroid hormone (PTH)* concentration or an inappropriately "normal" level in the setting of hypercalcemia should indicate hyperparathyroidism. However, most PTH assays detect the biologically inactive carboxyl-terminal segment of the molecule, which derives from hepatic cleavage and clears through renal excretion. In the setting of renal insufficiency, this metabolic fate of parathyroid hormone can lead to a falsely elevated PTH determination.

Additionally, many radioimmunoassays recognize factors that have been implicated in humoral hypercalcemia of malignancy, although the elevation in PTH is minimal for the more marked degree of calcium elevation. Recently, radioimmunoassays for intact parathyroid hormone have been introduced. These assays overcome the inadequacies of previous carboxyl-PTH assays in the setting of renal insufficiency, and do not give false-positive results in hypercalcemia associated with malignancy. Some investigators measure urinary cyclic AMP as a bioassay for PTH effect; however, several malignancies also produce factors that stimulate c-AMP.

Although *anemia* and an *elevated sedimentation* rate can

be seen in severe hyperparathyroidism with osteitis fibrosa cystica, these laboratory findings are more suggestive of multiple myeloma, the diagnosis of which requires a serum *immunoelectrophoresis* (IEP), or occasionally, a urine IEP for light chain secretion by myeloma. A *chest x-ray* with the findings of hilar adenopathy or pulmonary parenchymal abnormalities, in conjunction with an elevated *angiotensin converting enzyme,* is indicative of sarcoidosis. The hypercalcemia of sarcoidosis may be made more severe following an interval of sun exposure and may require more sophisticated diagnostic studies, including diffusing capacity, a hydrocortisone suppression study in which hydrocortisone 40 mg TID for 10 days normalizes the hypercalcemia of sarcoidosis, and even bronchoscopy or mediastinoscopy with biopsy for histologic confirmation (see Chapter 48).

A *bone scan* will detect the skeletal metastases of breast and squamous cell cancer; however, hyperparathyroidism is often associated with a generalized increase in skeletal uptake of imaging radionuclides. *Skeletal x-rays* may show lytic lesions of metastases or myeloma, and although x-rays are frequently normal in hyperparathyroidism, the finding of *subperiosteal bone resorption* is specific for and diagnostic of hyperparathyroidism.

Familial hypocalciuric hypercalcemia should be considered and excluded by finding a 24-hour *urinary calcium excretion* over 80 to 100 mg. *Thyroid hormone* determinations (see Chapter 10), particularly total triiodothyronine by radioimmunoassay, and measurements of serum cortisol following Cortrosyn should be performed if there is a history suggestive of hyperthyroidism or Addison's disease. A *2,5-hydroxyvitamin D assay* will unequivocally allay concerns of excessive vitamin D intake.

PRINCIPLES OF MANAGEMENT

Hyperparathyroidism

The physician needs to decide with the patient if surgical cure is appropriate. The decision regarding surgical cure must take into account the natural history of hyperparathyroidism. Certainly, if a patient is symptomatic with recurrent kidney stones or parathyroid bone disease, or if the serum calcium is markedly elevated (in excess of 12.5–13.0 mg%), then surgical cure is generally necessary. However, often the patient is asymptomatic or minimally nonspecifically symptomatic with mild hypercalcemia.

Prospective studies have attempted to ascertain which patients with asymptomatic disease and minimal elevation of serum calcium will develop end-organ adverse effects, particularly deterioration in skeletal and renal function. Only in rare instances did recurrent nephrolithiasis, pancreatitis, or hypercalcemic crisis develop. The major consequence of untreated disease was a decline in skeletal mass, which may predispose to fracture. There is no way to predict who will

suffer these effects. Moreover, routine skeletal x-rays and alkaline phosphatase measurements are insufficient for long-term follow-up; more sophisticated measurement of bone loss must be performed utilizing *bone densitometry* (either by the photon absorption method or by CT scan of spinal bone density). Marked urinary calcium elevation can predict development of nephrolithiasis.

Surgical Treatment for cure of hyperparathyroidism should be a serious consideration in young and middle-aged patients because of the likelihood of progression of skeletal disease, particularly in women who must anticipate the synergistic effects of menopausal bone loss. The cost of medical surveillance, which includes yearly or biannual assessment of renal function and skeletal mass, may surpass the cost of surgical cure after 5 to 10 years of follow-up studies.

Prior to surgery, localization of the parathyroid adenoma is helpful even to the skilled surgeon. Ultrasonography and technesium-thallium scanning using computer programs that subtract thyroidal uptake of technesium have localized parathyroid adenomas in approximately 70% of patients preoperatively. Anatomic localization by selective angiography or less commonly by venous sampling is generally only reserved for patients in whom neck exploration by an experienced parathyroid surgeon fails to cure the disease.

In patients who do not undergo surgical cure for hyperparathyroidism, several *medical alternatives* exist. These alternatives may help limit nonspecific symptoms of hyperparathyroidism and, more importantly, may prevent the often-seen skeletal loss. *Oral phosphate* therapy, particularly when moderate hypophosphatemia exists, lessens fatigue and weakness, reduces urinary calcium excretion thereby reducing the likelihood of renal stones, and may lead to calcium-phosphate deposition in bone. Serum calcium is lowered by oral phosphate, given as 250 mg to 500 mg of neutral phosphate four times daily. The most common side effect of this therapy is dose-related frequent bowel movements, which are often preferred to the constipation of hyperparathyroidism. Phosphate should be very cautiously administered in renal insufficiency; the proven calcium-phosphate solubility product of 65 might be exceeded.

Estrogen therapy given to postmenopausal women may normalize serum calcium and improve bone histology and represents a reasonable therapeutic option in older women in whom contraindications for estrogen therapy do not exist (see Chapter 158).

Symptomatic Management. As previously discussed, truly symptomatic hyperparathyroid patients should undergo surgery. Patients who are on medical therapy for hypercalcemia with phosphate or estrogen and patients who are on no therapy but are being monitored for the development of skeletal or renal disease should be instructed to maintain a *fluid intake* of at least 2 liters daily and to report to their physician during an illness that might lead to dehydration and the worsening of hypercalcemia. *Furosemide* and a *high salt intake* may limit the elevation of serum calcium. More severe and often symptomatic hypercalcemia requires hospitalization with hydration, forced saline diuresis, and often mithramycin to limit osteoclastic resorption of bone.

Management of hypercalcemia associated with *malignancy* includes treatment of the underlying malignancy with chemotherapeutic drugs (see Chapter 92). Drugs, such as aspirin and indomethacin, initially thought to be useful in the setting of humoral hypercalcemia of malignancy, have generally proven ineffective. *Oral phosphate* therapy, outpatient use of *mithramycin* (25 μg/kg intravenously every several weeks), and *glucocorticoid therapy* have been of benefit in selected patients. *Sarcoidosis* associated with hypercalcemia responds to alternate day *prednisone* therapy.

INDICATIONS FOR REFERRAL

One cannot predict which patients with hyperparathyroidism will develop progressive complications of their disease. Therefore, recommendations for which patients should be referred for surgical cure cannot be rigidly applied. The decision for surgical cure is dependent on the patient's preferences, his access to skilled surgical care, his willingness to undergo yearly surveillance for end-organ consequences of excess parathyroid hormone, the cost of long-term surveillance, the patient's ability to undergo surgery and the hope that nonspecific manifestations of hyperparathyroidism (including control of hypertension) will improve.

Surgical cure is warranted for all persons under age 40, for individuals who have a cortical bone density of two standard deviations below normal, and for patients with urinary calcium excretion over 350–400 mg in 24 hours, implying, on a restricted calcium intake, that a negative calcium balance is occurring. Cure rates for the initial neck exploration, in experienced surgical centers that employ preoperative localization, are better than 90%. Patients in whom surgical cure is planned should be referred to surgeons experienced in the complexities of parathyroid surgery not only for cure of potential hyperplasia and discovery of the parathyroid adenoma in an unusual location, but also to avert complications of recurrent laryngeal nerve injury and hypoparathyroidism.

PATIENT EDUCATION

Several recommendations will prevent the likelihood of more severe hypercalcemia in patients with mild hyperparathyroidism. Adequacy of fluid intake and prevention of dehydration that might occur during an acute gastrointestinal illness should be encouraged. Although, thiazide diuretics and calcium administration have been discouraged, thiazides may limit hypercalciuria and renal stone disease, and dietary calcium actually decreases parathyroid hormone secretion

and limits negative calcium balance in many patients. Patients should be encouraged to remain active and avoid immobilization. The necessity of surveillance for parathyroid hormone-induced skeletal disease and the delineation of symptoms that might represent manifestations of hyperparathyroidism (such as symptoms of nephrolithiasis and pancreatitis) should be carefully reviewed.

The patient who prefers to postpone surgical therapy ought to be advised that current clinical evidence suggests a 50% likelihood for requiring surgery over the next 5 to 10 years, often at a time of increased risk due to the development of other medical illnesses.

ANNOTATED BIBLIOGRAPHY

Bilezikina JP: The medical management of primary hyperparathyroidism. Ann Intern Med 96:198, 1982 (*Reviews the variable natural history of the disorder in asymptomatic patients advising observation for those who remain without symptoms or signs.*)

Broadus AE, Horst RL, Lang R et al: The importance of circulating 1,25-dihydroxyvitamin D in the pathogenesis of hypercalciuria and renal-stone formation in primary hyperparathyroidism. N Engl J Med 302:421, 1980 (*A clinical study that defines a subgroup of patients with hyperparathyroidism who are most likely to form renal stones because of elevated 1,25 vitamin D levels, leading to increased gut absorption of calcium and more marked degrees of hypercalciuria.*)

Bone HG, Snyder WH, Pak CY: Diagnosis of hyperparathyroidism. Ann Rev Med 28:111, 1977 (*Emphasizes the changing clinical presentation of the disorder resulting from detection of the disease in the asymptomatic or early phases.*)

Boonstra CE, Jackson CE: Hyperparathyroidism detected by routine serum calcium analysis—Prevalence in a clinic population. Ann Intern Med 63:468, 1965 (*In a population of over 25,000, 67 patients with hypercalcemia were identified. Thirty-one had hyperparathyroidism, though only eight were symptomatic. In only four was hypercalcemia the presentation of an underlying malignancy.*)

Christensson T, Hellstrom K, Wengle B et al: Prevalence of hypercalcemia in a health screening in Stockholm. Acta Med Scand 200:131, 1976 (*In a population of over 15,000, 95 patients were confirmed to have hypercalcemia, with probable hyperparathyroidism in 88.*)

Heath III, H, Hodgson SF, Kennedy MA: Primary hyperparathyroidism incidence, morbidity and potential economic impact in a community. N Engl J Med 302:189, 1980 (*An examination of the incidence, and clinical and economic consequences of the finding of hypercalcemia in Rochester, Minnesota from 1965–1974, emphasizing increased case finding with the advent of multiphasic biochemical screening and the increasing recognition of the disease in older women.*)

Insogna KL, Mitnick ME, Stewart AF et al: Sensitivity of the parathyroid hormone–1,25 dihydroxyvitamin D axis to variations in calcium intake in patients with primary hyperparathyroidism. N Engl J Med 313:1126, 1985 (*Parathyroid function may be suppressed by dietary calcium in some patients with hyperparathy-*

roidism. Perhaps we should be encouraging increased calcium intake in nonhypercalciuric patients?)

Marcus R, Madvig P, Crim M et al: Conjugated estrogens in the treatment of post-menopausal women with hyperparathyroidism. Ann Intern Med 100:633, 1984 (*Estrogen therapy normalized serum calcium and decreased bone turnover in ten women with hyperparathyroidism for up to two years.*)

Marx SJ, Attie MF, Levine M et al: The hypocalciuric or benign variant of familial hypercalcemia: Clinical and biochemical features in fifteen kindreds. Medicine 60:397, 1981 (*A genetic, clinical, and physiologic review of familial hypocalciuric hypercalcemia.*)

McPherson ML, Prince SR, Atamer ER et al: Theophylline-induced hypercalcemia. Ann Intern Med 105:52, 1986 (*Documents elevations in the settings of both excess and therapeutic theophylline levels.*)

Mundy GR, Cove DH, Fisken R: Primary hyperparathyroidism: Changes in pattern of clinical presentation. Lancet I:1317, 1980 (*An acute hypercalcemic syndrome in elderly patients was the presentation for 14% of 207 hypercalcemic patients discovered in a population of 1 million in Birmingham, England during a 5-month period.*)

Mundy GR, Ibbotson KJ, D'souza SM: The hypercalcemia of cancer. Clinical implications and pathogenic mechanisms. N Engl J Med 310:1718, 1984 (*A current review of the pathogenesis of humoral hypercalcemia of malignancy, with emphasis on the authors' research on transforming growth factors.*)

Mundy GR, Wilkinson R, Heath DA: Comparative study of available medical therapy for hypercalcemia of malignancy. Am J Med 74: 421, 1983 (*Oral phosphate and mithramycin were found to be more effective than glucocorticoids, EHDP, or indomethacin for hypercalcemia of malignancy.*)

Scholz DA, Purnell DC: Asymptomatic primary hyperparathyroidism: 10 year prospective study. Mayo Clin Proc 56:473, 1981 (*With all its limitations of difficulty with patient follow-up and lack of noninvasive measure of bone density, this study represents the best information on the natural history of mild, asymptomatic hyperparathyroidism.*)

Simeone JF, Mueller PR, Ferucci JT et al: High-resolution real-time sonography of the parathyroid. Radiology 141:745, 1981 (*Ultrasonography may demonstrate the location of a parathyroid adenoma in 70–80% of patients.*)

Stewart AF, Horst R, Deftos LJ et al: Biochemical evaluation of patients with cancer-associated hypercalcemia. Evidence for humoral and non-humoral groups. N Engl J Med 303:1377, 1980 (*The "classic" study segregating patients with humoral hypercalcemia, often without bone metastases, from patients with metastatic disease, utilizing nephrogenous cyclic AMP as a useful marker for humoral hypercalcemia. This entity is biochemically indistinguishable from primary hyperparathyroidism.*)

97
Evaluation of Hypoglycemia

Hypoglycemia is defined statistically as a serum glucose concentration less than 45 mg per 100 ml, though glucose levels may fall to as low as 35 mg per 100 ml in normal asymptomatic women and in normal men during prolonged exercise. A low serum sugar leads to clinical manifestations only if symptoms of neuroglycopenia or an adrenergic response ensue, an occurrence that depends on factors other than just the serum glucose concentration. Unfortunately, most of the symptoms resulting from hypoglycemia are very nonspecific and resemble complaints expressed by anxious or depressed patients (*e.g.,* tiredness, lightheadedness, nervousness, irritability, palpitations, tremulousness). Stimulated by articles in the lay press, patients with a host of such functional complaints come to physicians wondering if they have "hypoglycemia." Many seek a medical explanation to account for their symptoms; the vast majority have underlying emotional problems unrelated to serum glucose levels.

The primary physician needs to identify the patient whose symptoms are indeed related to hypoglycemia and determine the underlying cause. Postprandial hypoglycemias represent annoying but harmless conditions; the fasting hypoglycemias are more worrisome. One should have an effective evaluation strategy that will detect and efficiently workup the occasional patient with true hypoglycemia, yet avoid unnecessary studies in the large number of patients who have no underlying hypoglycemic condition.

PATHOPHYSIOLOGY AND CLINICAL PRESENTATION

Hypoglycemia can result from increased insulin secretion, enhanced glucose utilization, or inadequate functioning of one or more compensatory glucoregulatory mechanisms. When hypoglycemia occurs, the liver responds with increased glycogenolysis and glyconeogenesis, stimulated by glucagon and epinephrine, which activate hepatic phosphorylase. In addition, the pituitary secretes growth hormone (which inhibits utilization of glucose by muscle and enhances lipolysis) and ACTH (which promotes adrenal glucocorticoid production). The increased cortisol acts to stimulate gluconeogenesis and diminish muscle uptake of glucose.

There is no threshhold glucose concentration that invariably triggers symptoms. Many people with blood sugars between 35 and 45 mg/dl are completely asymptomatic. In fact, over 20% of normal patients demonstrate serum sugars below 50 mg/dl during glucose tolerance testing. The clinical presentation of chemical hypoglycemia depends on the rapidity and magnitude of the fall in blood sugar, as well as the absolute nadir of the serum glucose concentration. However, the lower the serum sugar and the more rapid the fall, the more likely symptoms will ensue. Hypoglycemic symptoms are typically categorized as *neuroglycopenic* (confusion, lethargy, visual disturbances, behavioral changes, impaired performance of routine tasks) or *catecholamine-mediated* (anxiety, tremulousness, headache, palpitations, sweats). Adrenergic symptoms characteristically accompany acute, rapid falls in blood sugar, especially if levels drop to concentrations below 40 mg/dl. Neuroglycopenic symptoms can develop in the absence of premonitory adrenergic complaints.

The hypoglycemias can be classified pathophysiologically as postprandial or fasting. In the *postprandial* variety, the fall in glucose results from an abnormal response to the intake of food. In the *fasting* (*postabsorptive*) hypoglycemias, symptoms occur in the fasting state or after prolonged exercise.

Functional reactive hypoglycemia is a postprandial form of hypoglycemia, characterized by an onset of neuroglycopenic and adrenergic symptoms several hours after a meal in conjunction with a simultaneously low serum glucose. Its pathogenesis remains unclear, and debate continues as to even its existence. Some have suggested that it be called *idiopathic postprandial syndrome*. Hypotheses advanced to explain the condition range from increased insulin sensitivity to decreased release of counterregulatory hormones; insulin secretion is normal. The suspicion that intake of sweets may precipitate symptoms is supported by the finding in many patients with documented reactive hypoglycemia of falls in blood sugar after a glucose load, but not after consumption of a mixed meal.

The oral glucose tolerance test (OGTT) shows a normal pattern for the first two hours, followed by a fall in serum glucose to below-fasting levels at *3 to 5 hours* in conjunction with development of hypoglycemic symptoms. Since there is no precise definition of what constitutes a "low" serum glucose (levels used range from 35 to 45 mg/dl), diagnostic criteria remain a bit vague. Some authorities believe too many patients are labelled as having this condition. Consensus remains elusive. The diagnosis should be considered only when symptoms accompany a low blood sugar; an isolated low postprandial glucose concentration does not suffice.

Adult-onset diabetes may also result in postprandial hypoglycemia. A diabetic glucose tolerance curve is noted on OGTT during the first 2 to 3 hours, followed by transitory hypoglycemia between hours 3 and 5. Insulin release is found to be sluggish, with levels inappropriately high for the level of serum glucose at hand. Fortunately, the majority of adult-onset diabetics do not experience reactive hypoglycemia on glucose tolerance testing.

About 10% of *postgastrectomy* patients are bothered by postprandial hypoglycemia. Rapid entry of glucose into the small bowel excessively stimulates still unidentified gut factors that trigger release of too much insulin. Hypoglycemia and neuroglycopenic symptoms appear 2 to 3 hours postprandially—earlier than in reactive hypoglycemia. Symptoms should not be confused with those of the dumping syndrome (see Chapter 58), which consist of nausea, fullness, and weakness coming on within an hour of eating.

Fasting hypoglycemias that result from autonomous insulin secretion, overuse of exogenous insulin, or defects in glycogenolysis and gluconeogenesis generally worsen with fasting or exercise. *Insulinomas* represent a rare but important cause of uncontrolled insulin production and account for the large majority of patients with endogenous hyperinsulinemia. Over 85% of insulinomas are benign islet-cell tumors. The clinical presentation can be confusing, and levels of serum glucose are not always low after an overnight fast. In a series of 39 patients with proven islet-cell tumors, just about half had glucose levels above 60 mg per 100 ml after 10 hours of fasting; in 20%, this level persisted for a full week with the patient on a regular diet. Thus it should be no surprise that clinical presentations may be highly variable in timing and severity. For example, in a Mayo Clinic series of 60 patients with insulinomas, the timing of symptoms was equally divided between early morning, late afternoon, and several hours following a meal. The only valid generalization is that fasting and exercise may precipitate symptoms; profound degrees of hypoglycemia may result. In the Mayo clinic series, a combination of diplopia, blurred vision, sweating, palpitations, and weakness occurred in 85%. Confusion or abnormal behavior occurred in 80%, amnesia occurred in half, and 10% experienced seizures.

Other causes of fasting hypoglycemia include excess doses of *exogenous insulin, sulfonylurea* administration, and defects in glycogenolysis or gluconeogenesis (as in severe pituitary or adrenal insufficiency, end-stage liver disease, and severe alcoholism complicated by poor nutrition).

Two groups of nonhypoglycemics must be differentiated from patients manifesting genuine falls in glucose in conjunction with symptoms. One group is composed of anxious and depressed individuals who have multiple bodily complaints of a functional or psychophysiologic nature (see Chapter 226). The most common symptoms include fatigue, headache, spasms, palpitations, numbness, sweating, and mental dullness. They attribute their symptoms to "hypoglycemia" in order to explain their difficulties and avoid the psychosocial issues at hand. Requests for glucose tolerance testing are frequent. A second group is bothered by postprandial symptoms very similar to those experienced by patients with reactive hypoglycemia, yet in the context of normal serum sugar levels. The pathophysiology of this alimentary variant is unknown.

DIFFERENTIAL DIAGNOSIS

The differential diagnosis of true hypoglycemia can be organized around whether it is fasting or postprandial (Table 97-1). The hypoglycemias most commonly encountered in the outpatient setting are postprandial and include functional

Table 97-1. Important Causes of Hypoglycemia in Ambulatory Patients

CAUSE	CLINICAL MANIFESTATIONS/DIAGNOSIS
Postprandial (Reactive)	
Functional reactive	Normal OGTT for first 2 h, then fall in glucose between 3 and 5 h
Postgastrectomy	Hypoglycemia and symptoms 2–3 h after eating
Adult-onset diabetes	Diabetic pattern in first 2 hrs of OGTT, then fall in glucose at 3–5 hrs
Fasting (Postabsorptive)	
Surreptitious insulin use	Medical personnel; high concentration of plasma insulin, low C-peptide level
Surreptitious oral agent use	High insulin, high C-peptide; (+) for high serum drug level
Insulinoma	Symptoms provoked by fasting or exercise; inappropriately high plasma insulin and high C-peptide at the time of low serum glucose
Alcohol abuse	6–24 h after a bout of heavy alcohol consumption and no food intake

reactive hypoglycemia, postgastrectomy syndrome, and adult-onset diabetes. The most common forms of fasting hypoglycemia are due to excessive doses of insulin or sulfonylureas. End-stage liver disease, alcoholism complicated by poor nutrition, Addison's disease, and hypopituitarism are causes of impaired glycogenolysis or gluconeogenesis that may result in hypoglycemia. Rare etiologies include insulinomas and pelvic or retroperitoneal neoplasms. In rare cases of severe hypothyroidism or chronic renal failure, there may be hypoglycemia.

WORKUP

Since most patients who present with adrenergic or vague psychoneurologic symptoms suffer from something other than hypoglycemia (*e.g.,* anxiety, depression, or even undiagnosed hyperthyroidism), the first task is to document a clear relationship between the patient's complaints and a low serum glucose concentration. A blood sugar at the time of symptoms is essential. Criteria for diagnosis of hypoglycemia include (1) symptoms consistent with neuroglycopenia (blurred or double vision, confusion, odd behavior, lethargy) or adrenergic stimulation (anxiety, tremulousness, headache, palpitations, sweats); (2) low serum glucose concentration at the time of symptoms; and (3) relief of symptoms when glucose level is raised to normal. Once hypoglycemia has been established, the evaluation proceeds to determining whether the condition is postprandial (and thus relatively harmless) or fasting (potentially more ominous).

History. Even before hypoglycemia is confirmed by blood sugar, there are important historical clues that can help determine who needs to be evaluated. The *timing* of symptoms should be carefully explored. The report of neuroglycopenic or adrenergic symptoms occurring consistently before breakfast, after exertion, or 3 to 5 hours postprandially suggests a truly hypoglycemic etiology, especially if symptoms abate with eating. Neuroglycopenic symptoms may be vague and

can occur in the absence of adrenergic complaints (especially in patients with fasting hypoglycemia); one should be careful not to mistake them for those of a functional or psychologic condition.

Detailed inquiries into *associated symptoms* and psychosocial status are essential and may serve to detect an underlying depression, anxiety problem, or thyroid disorder. For example, a story of early morning awakening, chronic fatigue, appetite and libido disturbances in conjunction with a history of personally significant losses provide strong presumptive evidence for *depression* (see Chapter 223). Paroxysms of anxiousness, palpitations, difficulty getting air in, and chest tightness unrelated to meals suggest a *panic attack disorder* (see Chapter 222). The presence of heat intolerance, weight loss in spite of normal food intake, constant nervousness unrelated to meals, and skin and hair changes point to *hyperthyroidism* (see Chapter 101).

Once nonhypoglycemic etiologies have been eliminated, one should search for additional historical clues of potential diagnostic value. Knowing the relation of symptoms to meals, fasting, and exercise helps distinguish fasting from reactive hypoglycemia. If symptoms occur in the fasting state and/or after exercise, one needs to inquire into *use of insulin* and *oral hypoglycemic agents.* A person making surreptitious use of such drugs is likely to deny any intake, but a *vocational history* of medical or paramedical work should raise one's index of suspicion. A check into recent *binge drinking* in conjunction with absent food intake identifies alcohol-induced hypoglycemia.

Patients with insulinomas report few symptoms other than those related to their hypoglycemia, which worsens after prolonged fasting (*e.g.,* just before breakfast or late in the afternoon, especially after exercising). The occurrence of neuroglycopenic symptoms (blurred vision, diplopia, sweats, confusion, poor memory) during these periods should raise suspicion of the diagnosis. Cases in which the fasting hypoglycemia is due to end-stage liver disease, adrenal insufficiency, or marked hypopituitarism are usually self-evident, with symptoms of the underlying condition (see Chapters 71, 18, and 109) dominating the clinical presentation. If symptoms occur postprandially, it is essential to ask about *diabetes,* a history of *gastric surgery,* and heavy use of *sweets.*

Physical Examination. In most cases of hypoglycemia there are few physical findings. However, the patient ought to be checked for alcohol on the breath, needle marks at common insulin injection sites, jaundice, hyperpigmentation, visual field defects, signs of hyperthyroidism (see Chapter 101), goiter, upper abdominal surgical scar, ascites, and other signs of cirrhosis (see Chapter 71). A full neurologic examination is essential to rule out a focal neurologic injury.

Laboratory Studies. The objective is to document the correlation between symptoms and a low serum glucose concentration. Without such documentation, one cannot make a diagnosis of physiologically significant hypoglycemia. A *serum glucose* determination drawn at the time of symptoms is essential for the diagnosis.

For patients suspected of having postprandial hypoglycemia, the 5-hour *oral glucose tolerance test* (*OGTT*) might be obtained if more evidence seems necessary. Steps to prevent erroneous results include intake of at least 250 mg of carbohydrate per day for 3 days prior to testing, use of an indwelling venous catheter (*e.g.,* a butterfly needle with heparin lock), and sampling every 30 minutes. Most importantly, additional blood samples should be drawn at the moment symptoms begin, meaning that the patient should stay in the office for the full 5 hours of the test to allow for prompt sampling. As noted, use of a mixed meal rather than glucose for the carbohydrate load might lead to a different result.

Fasting hypoglycemias can be identified by withholding food and exercising the patient. An *overnight fast* of 10 hours will often cause a fall in the glucose levels to less than 60 mg per 100 ml in the majority of patients with fasting hypoglycemias, but not in those with the reactive types. Extending the fast 4 more hours causes a drop below 50 mg per 100 ml in a greater percentage of patients, and by 24 hours, glucose level is about 35 mg per 100 ml in most. Occasionally, *72 hours of fasting* are required for demonstration of hypoglycemia. Since exercise promotes a fall in serum glucose, it may be used in conjunction with fasting to bring out hypoglycemia and precipitate symptoms. Two-thirds of the patients with insulinomas will develop hypoglycemia within 24 hours; fewer than 5% will have to fast for 72 hours.

Concurrent determination of *plasma insulin levels* when the patient is symptomatic will help document that excess insulin is the etiologic factor. When there is a question of factitious hypoglycemia due to self-administration of excess insulin, a *"C"-peptide* assay can be helpful if available. In the synthesis of endogenous insulin, the C-peptide is formed as proinsulin is split. Low C-peptide levels in the presence of high serum insulin concentrations indicate exogenous insulin use. High C-peptide and plasma insulin levels suggest hy-

perinsulinism due to an endogenous source, but surreptitious use of oral agents can produce a similar picture; collection of urine and serum samples to test for sulfonylurea and its metabolites can settle the issue when the question arises.

Need for additional studies in the patient with fasting hypoglycemia depends on suspicion of other etiologies. Cortisol and ACTH determinations are indicated if hypopituitarism or adrenal insufficiency is suggested by clinical findings. Extensive liver function tests may be superfluous if the patient is floridly jaundiced, but the prothrombin time and serum albumin are good measures of hepatocellular function and are worth obtaining (see Chapter 71).

It is essential that the physician avoid mislabeling a patient as hypoglycemic, especially when an individual already misattributes his symptoms to "low sugar." The incidental discovery of a blood sugar level below 60 mg per 100 ml on a random determination certainly does not warrant the diagnosis. In all likelihood, the patient is normal. The diagnosis requires concurrent demonstration of symptoms and very low serum glucose levels.

SYMPTOMATIC MANAGEMENT

Treatment of most fasting hypoglycemias requires attending directly to the underlying etiology. Those with postprandial etiologies may respond to dietary interventions. Patients with *functional reactive hypoglycemia* have been advised to try frequent feedings (six per day), diets high in protein and low in carbohydrate, and reductions in consumption of concentrated sweets. Some report symptomatic improvement, although there are no controlled studies establishing the efficacy of any of these dietary manipulations. A patient who demonstrates hypoglycemia after a glucose load but not after intake of a more balanced meal might be the logical candidate for restriction of sweets.

Those suffering from postgastrectomy hypoglycemia have been treated with anticholinergic agents to delay gastric emptying and intestinal motility; results are fair at best. Other approaches with some reported success include reversal of a 10 cm segment of the jejunum, use of beta-blocking agents, and pectin administration.

PATIENT EDUCATION

Patients without clinical evidence of hypoglycemia or its causes should be told that glucose tolerance testing is not indicated. A few will insist that they undergo the GTT and probably should have the test to avoid their roaming from one doctor to another.

A number of patients will initially refuse to accept the fact that hypoglycemia is not responsible for their symptoms; the attribution had served to explain a variety of functional symptoms for the patient. One needs to explore with these people their concerns and discuss other causes that might be responsible, including anxiety and depression (see Chapters 222 and 223).

A.H.G.

ANNOTATED BIBLIOGRAPHY

American Diabetes Association: Statement on hypoglycemia. Diabetes Care 5:72, 1982 (*A consensus statement of criteria for diagnosis of functional reactive hypoglycemia.*)

Charles MA, Hofeldt F, Shackeldord A et al: Comparison of oral glucose tolerance tests and mixed meals in patients with apparent idiopathic postabsorptive hypoglycemia. Diabetes 30:465, 1981 (*Mixed meals did not result in hypoglycemia; a glucose load did.*)

Chaiyapon C, Freinkel N, Nagel TC et al: Plasma C-peptide and diagnosis of factitious hyperinsulinism. Ann Intern Med 82:201, 1975 (*The finding of low C-peptides is helpful in diagnosing factitious hyperinsulinism.*)

Fajans SS, Floyd JC: Fasting hypoglycemia in adults. N Engl J Med 294:766, 1976 (*A physiologically oriented review of fasting hypoglycemia with a table of causes organized around pathophysiologic mechanisms.*)

Freichs H, Creutzfeldt W: Hypoglycemia I. Insulin-secreting tumors. Clin Endocrinol Metabol 5:747, 1976 (*Well done review.*)

Gastineau CF: Is reactive hypoglycemia a clinical entity? Mayo Clin Proc 58:545, 1983 (*A example of the debate surrounding the issue.*)

Lev-Ran A, Anderson RW: The diagnosis of postprandial hypoglycemia. Diabetes 30:996, 1981 (*Data and discussion on diagnosis of reactive hypoglycemia, with a focus on what is a "low" glucose level.*)

Merimee TJ, Tyson JE: Stabilization of plasma glucose during fasting—Normal variations in two separate studies. N Engl J Med 291:1275, 1974 (*Established that women have lower blood sugars and may normally have blood sugars in the 40s. Glucose levels must fall below 35 mg per 100 ml to be significant.*)

Permutt MA, Kelly J, Bernstein R et al: Alimentary hypoglycemia in the absence of gastrointestinal surgery. N Engl J Med 288:1206, 1973 (*An early report.*)

Scarlett JA, Mako ME, Ruberstein AH et al: Factitious hypoglycemia: Diagnosis by measurement of serum C-peptide and insulin-binding antibodies. N Engl J Med 297:1029, 1977 (*Documents the usefulness of these measures in patients who administer insulin surreptitiously.*)

Yeager J, Young RT: Nonhypoglycemia as an epidemic condition. N Engl J Med 291:907, 1974 (*A succinct discussion of how to manage patients with self-diagnosed "hypoglycemia."*)

98
Evaluation of Hirsutism

SAMUEL R. NUSSBAUM, M.D.

Hirsutism in women is characterized by excessive growth of hormone-dependent pubic, axillary, abdominal, chest, and facial hair. A patient may present when her hair growth is regarded as excessive or more coarse, long, or pigmented than that of others in her societal, geographic, or racial environment. For example, Mediterranean women are among the more hirsute of Caucasians, yet, in their country of origin, the excess hair is rarely considered unattractive and few seek medical attention. However, women of the same Mediterranean background living in the United States occasionally present to physicians concerned about their body hair; for them hirsutism may connote a loss of femininity or sexuality in a society preoccupied with stereotyped perceptions of beauty.

Virilization is manifest by temporal hair recession, acne, deepening voice, increased muscle mass, and clitoromegaly. In contrast to hirsutism, it often represents important underlying endocrine pathology.

When confronted with women with excessive hair growth, the primary care physician must decide whom to evaluate for underlying endocrine disease, and whom to reassure or treat symptomatically to reduce hair growth. Women with signs of virilization, with progressive hair growth beginning after age 25, and with associated amenorrhea should undergo endocrine evaluation.

PATHOPHYSIOLOGY AND CLINICAL PRESENTATION

Hair follicles are located over the entire body except for the palms and soles. Hair growth is of two types: lanugo (neonatal) or vellus hair is soft, unpigmented, and rarely more than 2 cm long. Terminal hair is coarse, pigmented, and grows in excess of 2 cm. A survey of college women revealed that one quarter had easily noticeable facial hair, one third reported hair extending along the linea alba from the pubic area (male escutcheon) and 17% had periaureolar hair. Three-quarters of women over age 60 have a measurable growth of facial hair.

Hirsutism has familial, ethnic, and racial patterns. Eastern European women are more hirsute than Scandanavian women; white women are more hirsute than black women, who have more body hair than Asian women.

The hormonal stimulus for hair growth is 5-alpha dihydrotestosterone, a potent testosterone metabolite derived from the peripheral conversion at the hair follicle of testosterone by 5-alpha reductase. Delta-4 androstenedione (A), and dehydroepiandrosterone (DHEA), produced by the ovaries and adrenal glands, are the precursors for 50% to 70% of circulating testosterone in women; the remainder of testosterone is secreted directly by the ovaries or occasionally by the adrenals.

Hirsute women generally have increased production rates of the relatively weak androgens, DHEA and A, or of the more potent androgen, testosterone. Serum measurements of total concentrations of androgens reflect sex steroid hormone binding to sex hormone-binding globulin: however, only the free fraction, which for testosterone is 1% of total testosterone, is biologically active. The source of enhanced androgen production may be the ovary, the adrenal gland, or both.

The majority of women with isolated hirsutism have an *inherited condition* of increased ovarian androgen production of either testosterone or androstenedione. *Polycystic ovary disease* (PCO) may present with menstrual abnormalities and infertility accompanying the hirsutism (see Chapter 109). Women with PCO may have enlarged ovaries with multiple follicular cysts, but may also have normal-sized ovaries. They have abnormal gonadotropin dynamics with increased LH to FSH ratios, and elevated testosterone levels, often only appreciated when unbound serum testosterone is measured. The adult onset, attenuated or partial forms of *congenital adrenal hyperplasias* are being increasingly recognized as causes of hirsutism. These disorders, inherited as an autosomal recessive trait closely linked to the HLA gene, may be associated with menstrual abnormalities. Clinically, glucocorticoid insufficiency does not occur in this syndrome, which is most commonly due to partial deficiency of the 21 hydroxylase enzyme. Androgen excess may accompany *hyperprolactinemia* as prolactin stimulates androgen production, particularly DHEA (see Chapter 111).

The virilized patient will often have testosterone levels of greater than 200 ng%. Etiologies include *ovarian hyperthecosis,* which may be seen in association with the syndrome of acanthosis nigricans and insulin resistance, and *ovarian tumors,* including arrhenoblastoma and hilar-cell tumors. Virilization may be seen as a feature of *Cushing's syndrome,* especially if the underlying cause of Cushing's syndrome is an adrenocortical carcinoma. Other causes of Cushing's syndrome are more likely to cause excess hair growth and typical cushingoid features without true virilization.

Drugs are sometimes responsible for hirsutism: oral contraceptives containing androgenic progestogens (see Chapter 118), phenytoin, glucocorticoids, diazoxide, and minoxidil have most often been implicated in an increase in nonandrogenic hair. There is a generalized increase in body hair in *anorexia nervosa* (see Chapter 230). Manipulation of and *trauma* to the hair follicle such as that which occurs with tweezing may be responsible for local coarse growth of hair.

DIFFERENTIAL DIAGNOSIS

The causes of excessive hair growth in women can be divided into those causing isolated hirsutism and those capable of producing true virilization. Most etiologies are conditions in which there is overproduction of androgens or androgenic precursors by either the ovaries or adrenals (see Table 98-1).

WORKUP

A paramount objective in the evaluation of hirsutism is to identify the woman who is likely to have important underlying endocrine pathology and is in need of detailed investigation.

History must include inquiry into *symptoms of virilization* (voice change, temporal hair recession, increased muscle mass, and acne); progression, particularly with sudden increase in hair growth after age 25; amenorrhea or changes in menstruation; and development of hypertension. A detailed *drug history,* covering the use of oral contraceptives, phenytoin, and other neuroleptics, should be obtained. A *family history* of hirsutism in mother, grandmothers, aunts, and sisters is generally reassuring to both physician and patient.

Physical Examination is studied for evidence of virilization, including temporal and vertical scalp *hair loss,* deep *voice,* acne, increase in *muscle mass,* and *clitoromegaly.* Cushing's syndrome should be suspected when centripetal obesity, muscle wasting with myopathy, and violaceous striae are encountered. Patients with oligomenorrhea require careful pelvic examination for the presence of bilaterally enlarged cystic ovaries; however, a significant number of women with polycystic ovary physiology will not have palpable ovarian

Table 98-1.   Differential Diagnosis of Hirsutism and Virilization

Isolated Hirsutism
Inherited
Polycystic ovary disease
Adrenal hyperplasia
Hyperprolactinemia
Cushing's syndrome
Drugs (oral contraceptives, phenytoin, glucocorticosteroids minoxidil, diazoxide)
Anorexia nervosa
Trauma to the hair follicle (focal thickening of hair; not true hirsutism)

Virilization
Ovarian hyperthecosis
Ovarian tumors (arrhenoblastoma and hilar cell)
Cushing's syndrome (especially that due to adrenal carcinoma)

abnormalities. Women with virilization may have palpable adrenal carcinomas or ovarian tumors.

Laboratory Studies. An abundance of costly endocrinologic hormonal assays may be performed in the evaluation of hirsutism. To avoid the expense of unnecessary testing, it is important to clinically define the likely diagnostic considerations and the goals of therapy for hirsutism so that appropriate hormonal evaluation may be obtained rather than the indiscriminate measurement of all ovarian and androgen sex steroids and pituitary hormones.

Familial Hirsutism. A young woman of Southern European ancestry who complains of minimal increase in facial hair, yet has regular menses and a family history of similar degrees of hirsutism need not undergo extensive endocrinologic studies. Conversely, patients with virilization, amenorrhea, or progressively worsening hirsutism deserve more extensive assessment.

Suspected Polycystic Ovary Disease. When amenorrhea or oligomenorrhea, obesity, and hirsutism occur, especially in the context of infertility, polycystic ovary disease needs to be considered. Since pelvic examination may not reveal bilaterally enlarged cystic ovaries, laboratory testing is necessary to confirm the clinical suspicions for PCO. Testosterone, particularly *unbound testosterone,* and *LH:FSH ratios* are increased. Because increased androgens suppress sex hormone–binding globulin, measurement of unbound or free serum testosterone is more valuable than measurement of total testosterone. Free testosterone correlates best with testosterone production rates. Because testosterone secretion is episodic, *three serum samples* taken 15 minutes apart may be pooled for immunoassay.

The attenuated or partial congenital adrenal hyperplasias (most often 21-OH deficiency) can be determined by demonstration of a *hyperresponsiveness of plasma 17-hydroxyprogesterone* measured one hour following the administration of 25 µg of Cortrosyn (synthetic ACTH 1-24). Although these patients represent a minority of hirsute women, there are no distinguishing clinical features of this entity that sets it apart from the more common PCO syndromes. *Prolactin* should be measured in women with oligo-amenorrhea.

Cushingoid Appearance. Patients having clinical features of Cushing's syndrome should undergo screening studies with either a *24-hour determination of urinary free cortisol or overnight dexamethasone suppression.* Twenty-four hour urinary free cortisol, the more specific study, is greater than 100 µg in Cushing's syndrome. *Urinary 17-ketosteroids* will be elevated in adrenocortical carcinoma. For overnight dexamethasone suppression, the patient is given 1 mg of dexamethasone at midnight, and a plasma cortisol is obtained at approximately 8:00 A.M. the next day. Cortisol should be suppressed to less than 5 µg per 100 ml. If either the urinary free cortisol is elevated or suppression of elevated cortisol by dexamethasone fails to occur, more extensive dexamethasone

testing to determine the likelihood and etiology of Cushing's syndrome needs to be pursued.

Virilization. When virilization is present, *serum testosterone* and *urinary 17-ketosteroids* should be measured. Serum testosterone will be greater than 200 ng% in women with masculinizing ovarian or adrenal neoplasms. Measurement of 17-ketosteroids will detect elevated adrenal androgens, such as androstenedione and dehydroepiandrosterone in adrenal cortical carcinoma. Although both the adrenal and ovaries can biosynthesize all androgenic steroids, the best measurement of adrenal hormanal production is *DHEA-sulfate,* with greater than 90% arising from the adrenal gland. Androstenedione is biosynthesized equally by adrenal and ovary glands.

SYMPTOMATIC MANAGEMENT AND PATIENT EDUCATION

Alternative approaches to the management of hirsutism include (1) supportive reassurance that there is no important underlying endocrine disease; (2) cosmetic manipulations such as bleaching, waxing, use of depilatories, and electrolysis; (3) medical therapy with estrogens or glucocorticoids directed at suppressing ovarian and adrenal hormone overproduction; (4) medical therapy directed at antagonizing the action of androgens at the receptor level, and (5) definitive curative therapy of underlying diseases such as Cushing's syndrome or masculinizing ovarian neoplasms.

Some women can be most effectively cared for with the *reassurance* that their hirsutism has no serious underlying cause and that it will not impair sexuality or fertility. If a woman is concerned about her appearance, cosmetic manipulation or medical therapy is appropriate.

Hair may be bleached with 6% *hydrogen peroxide* solution or commercially available cream bleaches. Shaving removes unwanted hair; however, because hair grows at the rate of 1 mm per day, "stubble" appears within several days. *Epilation* with tweezers or hot wax may retard hair growth for several months, but has the risk of low-grade folliculitis. *Chemical depilatories* may require the use of low concentration hydrocortisone topically to prevent irritation. *Electrolysis,* the only permanent method of hair removal, involves electrocoagulation and destruction of the hair root. It is a costly and time-consuming process and should be performed only by a licensed electrologist.

Estrogen and progestin combination *oral contraceptives* suppress ovarian and adrenal androgen production by decreasing FSH and LH. Estrogens increase sex hormone-binding globulin, compete with the cytosolic receptor for dihydrotestosterone, limit (along with progestogens) endometrial hyperplasia in hyperandrogenic PCO patients, and are an ideal therapy in women who also want highly effective contraception. Oral contraceptives containing 35 µg of ethinyl estradiol or 50 µg of mestranol reduce androgen levels, whereas oral contraceptives that contain low amounts of estrogen are less effective. The least androgenic progestins such as norethindrone 1 mg or ethynodiol acetate in combination with mestranol and ethinyl estradiol are preferred. If androgen and clinical responses to these therapies, determined at 3 months, are inadequate, an oral contraceptive containing higher amounts of estrogen should be used. Side-effects of these drugs, including increased risks for thromboembolism, stroke, and myocardial infarction (see Chapter 118) must be reviewed with the patient. A decrease in hirsutism is usually not evident for 3 to 6 months; a decrease in the rate of hair growth is noted initially, followed by a transformation to lighter, finer hair.

If androgens are of adrenal origin, *glucocorticoids* may reduce hirsutism and may lead to induction of ovulation in a subset of hirsute women. Adrenal suppression with a concomitant decrease in androgens can be best accomplished by administration of 1 mg of dexamethasone given at bedtime. A potential concern for this therapy is suppression of the hypothalamic–pituitary–adrenal axis, with diminished glucocorticoid response to stress.

Newer approaches antagonize testosterone action at the target tissue. *Spironolactone,* an antihypertensive diuretic, decreases androgen levels by decreasing testosterone biosynthesis as well as antagonizing its action on the hair follicle. Doses as high as 100 mg twice daily have been shown to diminish hirsutism during a 3-month observation interval, but may cause menstrual disturbances. One might begin therapy with 50 mg twice daily, given from the 4th through 22nd day of each menstrual cycle. Cyproterone acetate, available in Europe, has peripheral antiandrogenic, antigonadotropic and strong progestational activity. Its side effects of loss of libido, fatigue, nausea, and irregular menstrual bleeding seem to be increased over those of spironolactone. *Cimetidine,* a histamine-2 receptor antagonist, competes with androgens for target tissue binding; it appears to be less effective than spironolactone.

Because androstenedione is converted to testosterone in fatty tissue, and because androgen production rates are increased in obesity, *weight reduction* is an adjunct to all therapies for hirsutism.

INDICATIONS FOR REFERRAL

Patients with virilization and elevated testosterone levels require evaluation by an endocrinologist and gynecologist, since a virilizing tumor may be present. If polycystic ovary syndrome is present and if infertility is an issue, referral for clomiphene therapy and evaluation for endometrial hyperplasia by endometrial biopsy is appropriate. Hyperprolactinemia necessitates coronal computer tomographic or magnetic resonance imaging scanning to recognize a prolactinoma or pathologic process interrupting dopaminergic inhibition of prolactin. Patients with Cushing's syndrome should be referred for endocrinologic ascertainment of its pituitary, adrenal, or ectopic ACTH origin.

ANNOTATED BIBLIOGRAPHY

Bardin CW, Lipsett MB: Testosterone and androstenedione blood production rates in normal women and women with idiopathic hirsutism or polycystic ovaries. J Clin Invest 46:891, 1967 (*A higher secretion of ovarian testosterone occurs in PCO and hirsute women when contrasted to nonhirsute women who have testosterone produced from conversion of androstenedione.*)

Biffigandi P, Massucchetti C, Molinatti GM: Female hirsutism: Pathophysiological considerations and therapeutic implications. Endocr Rev 5:498, 1984 (*The most current discussion of adrenal and ovarian androgen overproduction and therapeutic approaches to hirsutism.*)

Chetkowski R, DeFazio J, Shamunki I et al: The incidence of late onset CAH due to 21-hydroxylase deficiency among hirsute women. J Clin Endocrinol Metab 58:595, 1984 (*Of 83 unselected hirsute women undergoing ACTH stimulation testing, only one patient was identified as having late onset congenital adrenal hyperplasia. Clinical characteristics more often seen with late onset CAH are reviewed.*)

Chrousos GP, Loriaux DL, Mann DL et al: Late-onset 21-hydroxylase deficiency mimicking idiopathic hirsutism of polycystic ovary disease. Ann Intern Med 96:143, 1982 (*Late-onset congenital adrenal hyperplasia is an HLA-linked autosomal recessive disorder representing between 6% and 12% of hirsute women only recognizable with ACTH stimulation testing.*)

Cumming D, Yang JC, Rebar RW et al: Treatment of hirsutism with spironolactone. JAMA 247:1295, 1984 (*Clinical responses and side-effects of spironolactone therapy are studied in 39 hirsute patients. Responses to spironolactone were observed as early as 2 months; side-effects were limited to several days of diuresis.*)

Ettinger B, Goldfield ED, Burrill KC et al: Plasma testosterone stimulation-suppression dynamics in hirsute women; correlation with long-term therapy. Am J Med 54:195, 1973 (*An article showing the effectiveness of estrogen-progestagen combinations in the treatment of hirsutism.*)

Forbes AP: Endocrine function in hirsute women. N Engl J Med 294:665, 1976 (*Editorial that accompanies the paper by Kirschner, Zuker, and Jespersen [see later entry].*)

Givens JR: Hirsutism and hyperandrogenism. Adv Intern Med 21: 221, 1976 (*A comprehensive review of androgen excess in the production of hirsutism.*)

Kirschner MA, Bardin CW: Androgen production and metabolism in normal and virilized women. Metabolism 21:667, 1972 (*An excellent review of androgens, their metabolism, and the differential diagnosis and evaluation of the virilized woman.*)

Kirschner MA, Zuker IR, Jespersen D: Idiopathic hirsutism—An ovarian abnormality. N Engl J Med 294:637, 1976. (*Although 20 of 44 women had suppression of plasma testosterone and androstenedione with dexamethasone, the ovaries were the predominant source of androgen production.*)

McKnight E: The prevalence of "hirsutism" in young women. Lancet 1:410, 1964. (*An epidemiologic study showing prevalence of hirsutism among college students.*)

Vigersky RA, Hehlman I, Glass AR et al: Treatment of hirsute women with cimetidine. N Engl J Med 303:1042, 1980. (*Cimetidine produced a decrease in rate of hair growth in 4 of 5 women; none had a decrease in serum androgen levels. Cimetidine, therefore, blocks androgen action by inhibiting the binding of dihydrotestosterone androgen receptors.*)

99
Evaluation of Gynecomastia

Gynecomastia is defined as enlargement of the male breast due to increase in glandular tissue. It is unilateral in a third of cases and may cause pain. It must be distinguished from simple obesity. Some patients are concerned about loss of masculinity or the possibility of breast cancer. Others may not have recognized the change and come to the physician at the suggestion of friends or family. Gynecomastia is a normal transient physiologic event in 70% of pubertal boys; its prevalence in adults is less than 1%. The physician must thoroughly investigate the cause, for it may be a manifestation of serious illness, such as adrenal or testicular cancer, cirrhosis, or hyperthyroidism. In most instances the etiology is more benign, and the tasks are to allay fears and help the patient decide about treatment.

PATHOPHYSIOLOGY AND CLINICAL PRESENTATION

Gynecomastia represents an estrogen-mediated phenomenon, leading to breast tissue proliferation. It is countered by androgen, and it can result from increased testicular or adrenal secretion of estrogens, increased conversion of testosterone and androstenedione to estradiol and estrone, estrogen-producing tumors, gonadotropin-producing tumors, and estrogen ingestion. Klinefelter's syndrome is an example of increased estrogen secretion. In heart failure, there is increased shunting of testosterone and androstenedione to the periphery, where they are converted to estrogens. In cirrhosis and hyperthyroidism, there is also increased peripheral conversion. Much of the conversion takes place in fatty tissue. HCG-producing tumors stimulate testicular production of estradiol. Teratomas of the testes and carcinomas of the lung, pancreas, and colon are known sources of ectopic HCG. Spironolactone is one of the more commonly used drugs with estrogenic effects. The gynecomastia of puberty is believed to be linked to a high estradiol:progesterone ratio, though this is controversial. Numerous other drugs are associated with gynecomastia, operating directly through hormonal stimulation or indirectly by inhibiting androgen production or effect (*e.g.,* cimetidine).

The clinical presentation is usually a noticeable increase in breast tissue. Tenderness may be noted in a third of patients, but actual pain is less frequent. Enlargement is usually central and symmetrical, though it is occasionally eccentric. Idiopathic and drug-induced gynecomastias are usually unilateral, while pubertal and hormonal etiologies often cause bilateral change. It may be that asymmetry is a more accurate description than unilateral enlargement, judging from the

prevalence of bilaterally histologic but not clinically evident gynecomastia in autopsy series.

There are a few distinctive clinical presentations. In Klinefelter's syndrome, gynecomastia develops around puberty in a patient with long limbs, small, firm testes, infertility, and normal or deficient secondary sex features. In cirrhosis, patients present with loss of libido, loss of body hair, and testicular atrophy (see Chapter 71). Carcinoma of the male breast is distinct from gynecomastia; it is characterized by a unilateral, eccentrically located firm mass that may be fixed. Male breast cancer is rare; it is generally not more frequent in patients with gynecomastia, though there is a higher incidence in Klinefelter's syndrome.

DIFFERENTIAL DIAGNOSIS

Seventy percent of healthy pubertal males have transient gynecomastia, which regresses in 1 to 2 years (see Table 99-1). Testicular or adrenal tumors are rare in this age group. The gynecomastia of Klinefelter's syndrome also presents around puberty. In one series, 15% of all young patients with gynecomastia had primary hypogonadism.

The two most common causes of gynecomastia in adults are drugs and alcohol-related liver disease. Estrogens, androgens, spironolactone, digitoxin, phenothiazines, amphetamines, reserpine, methyldopa, isoniazid, imipramine, phenytoin, heroin, cimetidine, and marijuana have all been

Table 99-1.   Differential Diagnosis of Gynecomastia

Increased Estrogen Production
Klinefelter's syndrome (with decreased androgen production)
Primary testicular damage
Ectopic HCG secretion by tumor (lung, pancreas, colon, testes)
Adrenal carcinoma
Leydig's cell tumor

Increased Peripheral Conversion
Cirrhosis
Hyperthyroidism (also increased sex hormone–binding globulin)

Decreased Androgen Production
Anticancer drugs
Bilateral orchiectomy

Antiandrogenic Activity
Spironolactone
Cimetidine

Estrogenic Activity
Digitoxin
Exogenous estrogen

associated with gynecomastia, although the association is tenuous in some. In one series, 22% of patients had a history of taking a drug associated with gynecomastia, and 26% had alcoholic liver disease.

Recovery from malnutrition due to severe illness, as seen with hemodialysis or congestive heart failure, may be associated with breast changes. A number of hyperthyroid patients have gynecomastia. Tumor-related gynecomastia is feared, but rare; tumors capable of HCG production include those of lung, liver, pancreas, colon, and stomach. Feminizing adrenal, testicular, and pituitary tumors are very rare causes of gynecomastia. In just under 10% of cases, a probable cause is not identified. Gynecomastia must be distinguished from carcinoma of the male breast.

WORKUP

History. Onset, location, duration, and course deserve note. The most important aspect is a detailed inquiry into drug use, including alcohol consumption, use of cimetidine, spironolactone, or digitoxin. Any symptoms of hyperthyroidism (see Chapter 101) or hepatocellular failure (see Chapter 71) or changes in libido, skin, voice, testicles, or hair should be elicited. Weight loss, change in bowel habits, history of heart failure or dialysis, headaches, and visual field disturbances should be ascertained.

Physical Examination often provides helpful clues. Arm span greater than height suggests Klinefelter's syndrome. One needs to look at the skin for jaundice, spider angiomas, pallor, changes in texture, and decreases in pubic and axillary hair. The eyes are checked for exophthalmus, and the neck is palpated for goiter. The breast examination requires distinguishing the glandular texture of true gynecomastia from the fatty consistency of breast enlargement related to obesity; asymmetry or nodules deserve note. The question of malignancy in the breast tissue must always be considered in gynecomastia. If the enlargement is unilateral and eccentric, or if the breast feels particularly firm or nodular, biopsy should be performed. Any signs of heart failure (see Chapter 27) and hepatocellular disease (see Chapter 62) should be noted. The abdomen must be palpated for masses, and the stool tested for occult blood. The testicles are examined for atrophy and nodules.

Laboratory Studies. Gynecomastia is not due to puberty, drugs, hyperthyroidism, hepatocellular failure, or another obvious cause requires further evaluation. Laboratory testing ought to begin with measurement of serum gonadotropin levels. High concentrations are consistent with testicular failure, Klinefelter's syndrome, and HCG-secreting tumors. Ectopic HCG production can be identified by finding elevated serum HCG levels. To check for Klinefelter's syndrome, a buccal smear is obtained and examined for chromatin positivity (Barr bodies). If negative, the diagnosis is most likely primary testicular failure or a chromatin-negative variant of Klinefelter's syndrome. More worrisome are patients with low gonadotropin concentrations. If accompanied by elevations in serum estrogens, adrenal cancer, and Leydig cell tumor of the testes must be ruled out. Patients with normal gonadotropin and sex hormone levels of are unlikely to have a serious underlying condition and can be followed expectantly with periodic reevaluation.

SYMPTOMATIC MANAGEMENT AND PATIENT EDUCATION

Removal of the offending drug usually produces regression of breast enlargement within a month or two. Gynecomastia that accompanies puberty or refeeding after starvation is a transient phenomenon that can be managed by providing reassurance. Treatment of hyperthyroidism will usually improve gynecomastia. Gynecomastia attributable to alcoholic liver disease or Klinefelter's syndrome is not likely to respond to any treatment. When HCG-secreting tumors are discovered, resection of the tumor is indicated if possible.

The persistence of gynecomastia may produce cosmetic problems. Patients who are considerably bothered by breast enlargement may elect to undergo mastectomy, but this should be accomplished only after the etiology has been elucidated. There is no evidence that antiestrogen drugs such as clomiphene are useful in adults, though they may have a role in puberty.

When a benign etiology such as drug-induced gynecomastia is discovered, it is comforting to reassure the patient that the condition is not a reflection of loss of maleness or a carcinomatous process. It must be remembered that some conditions that produce gynecomastia may reduce potency; this situation must be confronted and discussed with the patient. There is no evidence of carcinomatous degeneration in gynecomastia except in Klinefelter's syndrome. Pain, irritation, or social problems that may arise should be dealt with symptomatically and sympathetically.

A.H.G.

ANNOTATED BIBLIOGRAPHY

Bannagan GA, Hajdu SI: Gynecomastia: Clinicopathologic study of 351 cases. Am J Clin Pathol 57:431, 1972. (*The histologic appearance of fibrous gynecomastia relates to duration, irrespective of etiology. Idiopathic and drug-induced gynecomastias are usually discrete and unilateral, while endocrine and pubertal gynecomastias are bilateral.*)

Braunstein GD, Vaitukaitis JL, Carbone PP et al: Ectopic production of human chorionic gonadotropin by neoplasms. Ann Intern Med 78:39, 1973. (*HCG was found in 60 of 828 patients with established neoplasms.*)

Carlson HE: Gynecomastia. N Engl J Med 303:795, 1980 (*Reviews the causes of gynecomastia and associated clinical conditions as well as carcinoma of the male breast.*)

Gordon GG et al: Effect of alcohol (ethanol) administration on sex-hormone metabolism in normal men. N Engl J Med 295:797, 1976 (*Alcohol caused a decrease in testosterone production as well as limiting the LH response.*)

Jensen RT, Collen MJ, Pandol HD: Cimetidine-induced impotence and breast changes in patients with gastric hypersecretory states. N Engl J Med 308:883, 1983 (*Fifty percent of 22 patients with Zollinger–Ellison syndrome developed impotence, breast tenderness, and/or gynecomastia during treatment with high doses of cimetidine; these side-effects disappeared when cimetidine was replaced by ranitidine.*)

Knott D, Bidlingmaier R: Gynecomastia in male adolescents. J Clin Endocrinol Metab 4:187, 1975 (*Discussion of mechanisms.*)

Rose LI, Underwood RH, Newmark SR et al: Pathophysiology of spironolactone-induced gynecomastia. Ann Intern Med 87:398, 1977 (*A review of mechanisms of spironolactone-induced gynecomastia.*)

Williams MW: Gynecomastia, its incidence, recognition and host characterizations in 447 autopsy cases. Am J Med 34:103, 1963 (*An interesting pathologic study, revealing a 40% incidence of histologic gynecomastia, though only four cases involved clinically obvious enlargement.*)

Wilson JD, Aiman J, MacDonald PC: The pathogenesis of gynecomastia. Adv Intern Med 25:1, 1980 (*A detailed review of mechanisms.*)

100

Approach to the Patient With Diabetes Mellitus

SAMUEL R. NUSSBAUM, M.D.

Diabetes mellitus is the most prevalent endocrinologic problem in primary care practice. The condition affects between 2 million and 10 million people in the United States, with an annual incidence reported in community-based studies of about 130 new cases per 100,000 population. The primary physician is in the unique position to provide comprehensive care to the diabetic. Goals include elimination of symptomatic hyperglycemia and ketosis and prevention (to the extent possible) of vascular complications. Management requires thoughtful, skillful, and meticulous care, especially of the patient with complications.

The challenge is to design a program that is safe, practical, and acceptable to the patient. Important decisions include determining when drug therapy is necessary, selecting between insulin and oral hypoglycemic agents, and deciding how aggressively to control the blood sugar. Practical tasks include creation of an effective means for diabetic surveillance and provision of education and encouragement that enables the patient to become a partner in management.

PATHOPHYSIOLOGY, CLINICAL PRESENTATION, AND COURSE

Definitions and Classification. Diabetes mellitus is a syndrome of diverse etiologies characterized by hyperglycemia, a relative or absolute deficiency of insulin or a resistance to the action of insulin, and a propensity to develop microvascular and macrovascular disease. The *diagnosis* of diabetes is made by finding a *fasting plasma glucose of greater than 140 mg%* on two or more occasions in the absence of metabolic stress. If fasting blood glucose is between 100 and 140 mg%, the diagnosis can be made on the basis of a 75-g oral glucose tolerance test showing a *2-hour postprandial glucose of greater than 200 mg%*. It is no longer appropriate to assign labels of "chemical," "latent," or "borderline" diabetes. These designations were based on clinically and prognostically insignificant abnormalities on glucose tolerance testing. However, in pregnancy, even minor degrees of glucose intolerance can be important (see below).

The common forms of diabetes may be classified into two broad categories, which differ in their genetic background, etiology, and clinical manifestations. *Type I diabetics* are severely *insulin deficient,* ketosis prone, and require insulin to live; their onset is typically in youth but may occur at any age. Persons with the more common *type II diabetes,* with obesity as a frequent concomitant, are *neither insulin dependent nor ketosis prone.* The incidence of type II diabetes increases with age but may occur in young individuals.

Pathogenesis. The pathogenesis of diabetes is incompletely understood; however, there is a genetic determinant in both type I and type II diabetes. Studies of monozygotic twins demonstrate a very strong *genetic influence* in type II diabetes with 90% of twins exhibiting diabetes within 5 years of each other; whereas in type I diabetes, almost half of the twin pairs failed to develop diabetes even after intervals of 10 to 20 years. Yet the concordance rate of 50% is greater then the approximately 6% concordance rate for siblings. The incidence of type I diabetes is strongly associated with a variety of markers known to be on chromosome 6, whereas type II diabetes shows no such linkage. *Beta cell autoimmunity* is present in type I but not in type II diabetics. In patients with type II diabetes, 60% to 80% of whom are obese, there is considerable heterogeneity in the insulin secretory response and the degree of *insulin resistance.* Glucose intolerance in these patients may be worsened by infection, stress, thiazides, glucocorticoids, and pregnancy. Excess secretion of growth hormone, cortisol, catecholamines, or glucagon may result in glucose intolerance, as can diseases that destroy a substantial portion of the pancreas (*e.g.,* chronic pancreatitis, hemochromatosis, and cystic fibrosis).

Clinical Manifestations. Diabetes is often discovered as an incidental finding on screening urinalysis or blood sugar. Occasionally, the diagnosis is made during the workup of cardiovascular, renal, neurologic, or infectious disease. A complication such as myocardial ischemia, stroke, intermittent claudication, impotence, peripheral neuropathy, proteinuria, or retinopathy may be the initial manifestation. Sometimes, fatigue is the predominant symptom. Only in a minority of cases is the textbook presentation of polyuria, polydypsia, and polyphagia with weight loss encountered.

The major complications of diabetes are vascular, neuropathic, infectious, and ocular. Diabetic vascular disease includes both microangiopathic and atherosclerotic varieties. Large and medium sized vessels may develop *premature atherosclerosis,* leading to coronary ischemia, stroke, and peripheral arterial insufficiency. The pathophysiology remains poorly understood, and it is unclear to what degree this predisposition is modifiable by normalization of blood sugar. Some patients seem to be more susceptible than others, regardless of degree of blood sugar control. Correction of other cardiovascular risk factors, such as smoking, hypertension, and hyperlipidemia, appears important to the prevention and limitation of this complication.

Diabetic *microvascular disease* leads to nephropathy, retinopathy, and mononeuritis. Diabetic *nephropathy* is a major cause of renal failure. Currently, 25% of new dialysis patients are diabetic. The pathologic renal changes are glomerular basement membrane thickening and mesangial proliferation; they appear to develop independent of each other and are believed to be causative of impaired renal function. Mesangial proliferation correlates strongly with the onset of proteinuria and hypertension. With persistent proteinuria, hypertension becomes established and glomerular filtration begins to decline at the rate of 1 ml/min/month. The risk of developing nephropathy correlates with duration of disease. Thirty to fifty percent of type I diabetics and 6% to 9% of type II patients will eventually develop renal failure. Tight control of the blood glucose can reduce mild proteinuria in insulin-dependent diabetics who do not yet have renal insufficiency, but in the presence of significant proteinuria (>500 mg/day), near normalization of the plasma glucose does not slow the rate of renal deterioration. Bladder dysfunction and resultant urinary tract infections also contribute to renal impairment.

Retinopathic changes (see Chapter 208) are microvascular in nature and pathologically similar to those that occur in the kidney. The risk of retinopathy is related to duration of diabetes; after 20 years of diabetes, all age groups show a 75% to 80% prevalence of retinopathy. The relation of retinopathy to degree of blood glucose control is unsettled; there are conflicting data. Other ophthalmologic complications of diabetes include reversible changes in lens configuration induced by wide fluctuations in plasma glucose; this may cause transiently blurred vision. In addition, cataracts and glaucoma occur with increased frequency (see Chapters 206 and 207).

Diabetic *neuropathy* may lead to a peripheral sensory deficit, autonomic dysfunction, or a mononeuritis. Mechanisms include myoinositol depletion in nerve cell membranes (which prolongs conduction time) and hyperglycemia-induced sorbitol accumulation in nerve tissues that have a polyol pathway for metabolism of glucose (*e.g.,* Schwann cells). Microangiopathic changes decreasing blood supply to the myelin sheaths are believed responsible for the mononeuropathy. The *peripheral neuropathy* is predominantly sensory, reducing sensation in the lower extremities and capable of progressing to cause pain and dysesthesias. *Autonomic neuropathy* most commonly presents as impotence. Gastrointestinal motility disturbances, orthostatic hypotension, and urinary retention are other potential manifestations. Autonomic neuropathy is almost always seen in association with distal polyneuropathy; its occurrence decreases life expectancy. Diabetic *mononeuropathy* involves discrete cranial or peripheral nerves, singly or as a mononeuritis multiplex. The most commonly affected cranial nerves are III and VI. In contrast to other diabetic neuropathies, there is near complete resolution of mononeuropathies within 1 year of onset.

There appears to be an *increased susceptibility to infection,* which may result from impaired leukocyte function. Cellulitis and candidiasis occur, with infections of ischemic foot lesions especially serious since they may lead to osteomyelitis and loss of limb. Urinary tract infections are common in patients with an autonomic bladder (see Chapters 132 and 133).

PRINCIPLES OF MANAGEMENT

Although the goals of therapy in diabetes are normalization of carbohydrate metabolism and prevention of multisystem complications that may result from hyperglycemia, the *optimal degree of control* of blood sugar remains a subject of controversy. The unresolved question is whether restoration of glucose to near normal will reduce the serious consequences of diabetes. The extent to which complications are related to the degree of hyperglycemia, a coexistant metabolic abnormality, or a hereditary propensity is a source of much debate.

Both laboratory and clinical studies have produced contradictory evidence. The hypothesis that normalization of hyperglycemia will prevent or delay the microvascular and macrovascular complications of diabetes finds support from animal studies. Other experimental studies have shown physiologic improvement in visual function, but some data suggest that clinical retinopathy may worsen with tight control. Tight control has been associated with improvement in nerve conduction, but not with clinical improvement in sensation or autonomic function. As noted earlier, mild degrees of proteinuria may be reversed, but renal failure is inevitable once significant proteinuria develops.

To scientifically and more definitively examine the "glucose hypothesis," a randomized, prospective, 10-year multicenter study of intensive therapy versus conventional therapy was begun in 1983. This Diabetes Control and Complication Trial will enable a comparison of endpoints such as retinopathy and neuropathy between two groups—one tightly controlled and one treated in a conventional manner. It should help resolve the issue of whether the maintenance of a normal metabolic state in diabetes prevents complications.

Although normalization of blood sugars to nondiabetic postprandial and fasting levels is an ideal objective, it is difficult to achieve with available means. The risk of tight control is an increase in hypoglycemic reactions. The goal of glucose normalization may be achieved within the next decade as the biotechnology to create small, implantable glucose sensors and insulin delivery systems is further refined.

Diet

The cornerstone of therapy for all overweight and type II diabetics is *weight reduction* through calorie restriction. Achieving ideal body weight is the single most important goal for the physician to encourage and advance to achieve metabolic control in the patient. Weight loss has been shown to enhance the sensitivity of peripheral insulin receptors to endogenous insulin and reduce requirements for administered insulin. It is not possible to predict the exact improvement in glucose control from each pound lost, but a reduction of only 7 to 10 pounds often improves glucose tolerance.

Most type II diabetics can have hyperglycemia controlled by the achievement of ideal body weight; however, such weight reduction is often a difficult goal to sustain, requiring a permanent restriction in caloric intake. An effective exercise program will enhance weight loss because of the increase in caloric use. Recent clinical research indicates that obese individuals may require fewer calories to maintain body weight. Rigidly developed and prescribed diets should be supplanted by diets that are adapted to the patient's lifestyle but encourage gradual, and hopefully sustained, weight reduction of approximately 1 to 2 pounds each week (see Chapter 229).

Diet *composition* for type II diabetics is less critical than achieving ideal body weight. In mild glucose intolerance, isocaloric increases in carbohydrate up to 80% actually improve

glucose tolerance, particularly when complex carbohydrate, high-fiber diets are consumed. Hypertriglyceridemia secondary to the increase in carbohydrates has not been a problem, and in several studies, triglycerides and cholesterol have fallen substantially. Recent studies support the concept that all carbohydrates are not similar; some sources of starch, such as potato, have a greater effect on hyperglycemia than do carbohydrates in beans or wheat. Even the inclusion of sucrose or ice cream in mixed meals does not adversely affect glucose control.

High-fiber diets, generally associated with a higher intake of complex carbohydrates and decreased intake of refined carbohydrates and animal fats, are associated with low prevalence of diabetes mellitus. *Increase in fiber content* of the diet with unprocessed natural foods that include cereals, grains, fruits, and vegetables results in improved glucose tolerance in type II diabetics and decreased insulin requirements in type I diabetics. The mechanism for this improvement in glycemic control is likely the delayed absorption caused by fibers such as guar and pectin.

Patients who are not taking insulin do not require elaborate exchange systems, careful timing of meals, or other special dietary accomodations.

Patients on Insulin. For type I *insulin-requiring diabetics* who are at ideal body weight, the essential aspect of dietary therapy is the *regularity of caloric intake* and the spacing of meals. Three meals, supplemented by snacks midmorning, midafternoon, and before bed are needed to provide a source of glucose during the sustained presence of exogenously administered insulin. The commonly utilized American Diabetic Association diets recommend $2/9$ of calories at breakfast, $2/9$ at lunch, $4/9$ at dinner, and $1/9$ as snacks. The timing of meals must match peak insulin effects and activity schedules; increased activity requires increased food intake or a decrease in insulin dosage to prevent hyperglycemia. *Simple sugars* are generally restricted because they worsen postprandial hyperglycemia; however, patients should carry a source of simple sugar, such as fruit juice or sugar candy, to limit an insulin reaction.

Exercise

Exercise has beneficial effects on glucose control in diabetes. In the well-controlled diabetic, it increases glucose consumption and improves glucose tolerance by increasing insulin receptor number and affinity. There are several precautions regarding exercise in diabetic patients. The increased absorption of insulin from an exercising limb may precipitate hypoglycemia in patients on insulin; therefore, the abdomen should be used as the site for insulin injection. Because of the possibility of underlying ischemic heart disease, an exercise EKG (see Chapter 10) should be obtained prior to the commencement of a rigorous exercise program in a sedentary diabetic.

Drug Therapy

When reduction to ideal body weight fails to achieve reasonable control of blood sugar or amelioration of symptoms, the patient is unable to lose weight, ketosis is present, or gestational diabetes occurs, then drug therapy is indicated.

Oral Agents. With the introduction of second generation sulfonylureas, oral hypoglycemic agents are being increasingly utilized in the management of diabetes. However, opinion remains divided on the effectiveness of these compounds in achieving glycemic control. There is no evidence that long-term use of oral hypoglycemic agents can reduce the premature morbidity and mortality of diabetes. The sulfonylureas acutely increase insulin release; whereas in the long term, the hypoglycemic actions of these drugs are based on actions at the receptor or post-receptor level.

Although oral agents lower blood sugar in approximately 60% to 70% of diabetics, their safety has been questioned. The findings of the *University Group Diabetes Project* (*UGDP*) *study* revealed an *increased* rate of *cardiovascular death* in patients on long-term tolbutamide therapy. This unanticipated result from a study that was designed to determine whether control of blood glucose prevents or delays vascular disease in type II diabetics has given rise to considerable ongoing controversy about the design of the 12-center UGDP study, and the application of the tolbutamide findings to other first and second generation sulfonylureas such as chlorpropamide, glyburide, and glipizide. The UGDP report states: "The findings of the study indicate that the combination of diet and tolbutamide therapy is no more effective than diet alone in prolonging life. Moreover, the findings suggest that tolbutamide and diet may be less effective than diet alone or diet and insulin, at least in so far as cardiovascular mortality is concerned." Independent biometric review of the UGDP study's design and data analysis—despite criticisms that include baseline inequalities among treatment groups after randomization, the use of standard dosages of tolbutamide that led to under- and overtreatment, and unmonitored variables, especially smoking—have confirmed the UGDP conclusions.

At the present time, available oral hypoglycemic agents have a limited role in the treatment of diabetes. Patients with symptomatic hyperglycemia who cannot take insulin because of infirmity, vision loss, or unwillingness to administer injections and symptomatic, overweight patients who are entering a program of weight reduction are candidates for therapy with sulfonylureas. If weight reduction should fail, then these drugs might best be abandoned in favor of insulin.

Two *second generation oral hypoglycemic sulfonylureas* are available for treatment of type II diabetics: *glyburide* (Micronase, Diabeta) and *glipizide* (Glucotrol). These sulfonylureas stimulate the release of insulin from pancreatic beta cells, increase the number of insulin receptors, and correct defects in postreceptor insulin action. Glyburide and glipizide are nonionically bound to plasma proteins and have less variation in their bioavailability than the earlier oral agents. Both are inactivated by the liver. Glyburide is excreted in bile and urine, offering a potential advantage over glipizide in patients with renal insufficiency. In contrast to chlorpropamide, neither glyburide nor glipizide causes the syndrome of inappropriate secretion of antidiuretic hormone, and only rarely causes disulfiram (Antabuse)-like effects. Like their predecessors, they may have their effects potentiated by sulfonamides, salicylates, and clofibrate or inhibited by coumadin. Generally, a patient can be started on 2.5 to 5.0 mg of glyburide or glipizide once daily, increasing the dose to as much as 20 mg daily, monitoring blood sugars and hemoglobin A_{1C} (see below). Occasionally, patients who have become refractory to earlier sulfonylureas may benefit by substitution with glyburide or glipizide.

Insulin is the drug therapy of choice for diabetics who develop ketosis, for symptomatic type II diabetics who cannot be controlled by diet alone, and for diabetics in whom near-normalization of blood sugar is a goal of therapy.

PREPARATIONS. Since 1971, *"single peak" insulin,* prepared by chromatographic systems that result in an insulin containing 300 to 3000 ppm of proinsulin, has been the most commonly utilized commercial preparation. This routinely used insulin, available in short-, intermediate-, and long-acting preparations, is a mixture of beef and pork insulins. In 1980, insulins *highly purified* by high-performance liquid chromatography and containing less than 1 ppm of proinsulin were introduced. In 1982 *human recombinant insulin* was approved by the FDA. As long as these two insulin preparations remain costly, the indications for their use are limited to individuals who develop local reactions at the site of injection, insulin allergy or resistance, or lipoatrophy, or who need insulin for only a limited time. With increasing purity of insulins, there has been a decline in the incidence of local reactions, insulin allergy, and immune resistance, but it is not yet certain that the greater purity of the newer insulins is clinically significant. In some patients, human insulin may be absorbed more rapidly and have a shorter duration of action than animal insulins. Although antibody formation against human insulin is less than that against insulin from animal species, there is a measurable increase in anti-insulin antibodies in a minority of patients treated with the recombinant preparation.

Insulin is available in short-, intermediate-, and long-acting preparations. Intermediate types of insulin, *NPH* and *lente,* with peak actions at 6 to 12 hours and 24-hour duration of insulin effect, are the most commonly used. Short-acting insulins, *CZI* and *semilente,* have an earlier onset and peak (2 to 4 hours) action. Long-acting insulins, *protamine-zinc insulin* and *ultralente* insulin, may have greatest utility in intensive insulin therapy programs to provide basal release of insulin in conjuction with multiple injections of short-acting insulin.

PROGRAMS (SEE TABLE 100-1). The majority of *type II diabetics* can be reasonably controlled with a *single dose of intermediate insulin* in the morning before breakfast. Approximately one third of patients have either a delayed or early response to intermediate insulins. About 15% are *early* or *type A responders;* they experience their peak insulin effect shortly after noon and become hypoglycemic in the early afternoon. Their insulin program consists of *splitting the dose* of intermediate insulin into two parts: two thirds given in the morning and one third administered prior to dinner. Occasionally, supplementation with a short-acting insulin is necessary in the morning and evening.

Another 15% of diabetics on insulin are *late* or *type C responders,* having a delayed response with the nadir of blood sugar occurring between 10 PM and 5 AM. These patients require a reduction in intermediate-acting insulin and the *addition of a short-acting insulin* to the morning dose. An additional small evening dose of short-acting insulin may be necessary if postprandial hyperglycemia is a major problem in the early evening.

For the two thirds of patients who respond adequately to intermediate-acting insulin, *greater glucose control* may be achieved by *dividing* the total daily insulin dose into injections before breakfast and before dinner. To further improve control and minimize excursions of glycemia, this schedule is sometimes supplemented by small amounts of *short-acting insulin,* which can be mixed in the same syringe.

There is increasing emphasis on *intensive insulin programs* to achieve near-normalization of blood sugar as a treatment objective in motivated, carefully selected patients, facilitated by the teaching and widespread use of home blood glucose monitoring (HBGM) (see below). In addition, open-loop *pump therapy,* represents an attempt to duplicate the normal physiologic pattern of insulin release. Insulin infusion devices and multiple daily injections are being widely applied in gestational diabetes and in difficult-to-control, type I diabetics. This therapeutic approach requires patient motivation and sophistication, close monitoring, and careful supervision to be safe and effective. Several studies emphasize that comparable control of glycemia can be achieved by insulin pump and conventional intensive therapy. The major advantage of insulin pumps revolves around ease of frequent insulin administration. Complications include catheter infection, inadvertent catheter displacement from the skin, and cost.

A typical *intensive insulin program* utilizing subcutaneous injections to emulate physiological insulin release, is to administer ultralente insulin at 6 PM and semi lente or CZI insulin before meals and prior to sleep. This therapy requires self-monitoring of glucose to adjust dosage schedules. Additionally, a 3 AM blood glucose would ensure that nocturnal hypoglycemia is not occurring.

These therapeutic programs enable the normalization of serum *hemoglobin A_{1C},* a useful indicator of long-term glucose control (see below). The major *complication* of intensive insulin therapy is frequent and more severe *hypoglycemia.* Since the ultimate benefit of normalization of blood glucose in preventing diabetic complications remains to be determined (except in pregnancy), the only firm indication for intensive

Table 100-1. Common Insulin Regimens

STANDARD REGIMENS Response to Insulin	Regimen
Early (type A)	⅔ dose intermediate insulin before breakfast
	⅓ dose intermediate insulin before dinner
Normal (type B)	Full dose of intermediate insulin before breakfast
Late (type C)	Reduced dose of intermediate insulin plus a short-acting insulin before breakfast
	Small dose of short-acting insulin before dinner, if postprandial evening hyperglycemia occurs
TIGHT CONTROL REGIMENS* Degree of Control	Regimen
Tight	Divide total daily intermediate insulin dose into injections before breakfast and before dinner
Very tight	Add to each of the intermediate insulin doses a small dose of short-acting insulin

* Intended for normal insulin reactors (type B) only.

therapy is pregnancy. Young, sophisticated, motivated patients without established complications may also be considered for this intensive therapy.

INITIATION OF INSULIN THERAPY can be carried out safely on an ambulatory basis as long as the patient is reliable, nonketotic, and not severely hyperglycemic with intercurrent illness. Treatment should be initiated with 10 to 15 units of an intermediate-acting insulin and increased by approximately 2 units each day depending on urine, or preferably, blood sugar monitoring performed by the patient. Double-voided urine glucose determinations, commonly used in the past, have limitations (see below).

TECHNIQUE. Insulin is injected subcutaneously where it is absorbed directly into the circulation. The abdomen and limbs serve as convenient *injection sites,* with rotation among sites used to minimize lipoatrophy and discomfort. Rotation among multiple abdominal injection sites is preferable to limb injections in athletically active diabetics because of the possibility of more rapid insulin absorption from an exercising limb. Insulin, best *stored* in the refrigerator, may be left at room temperature for up to 12 hours without loss of biopotency.

DEGREE OF CONTROL. Most endocrinologists agree that it is desirable to achieve the best glycemic control possible. However, in the absence of proven limitation of diabetic complications, the question remains whether tight control can be accomplished safely and whether the means of insulin administration currently available are compatible with an individual's lifestyle and personal choices for therapy. Whereas an intelligent, well-motivated, reliable individual can be taught to regulate daily insulin dosages, less adept patients risk hypoglycemic reactions when tight control is attempted. Reasonable glycemic control in these patients might be considered a fasting blood glucose of less than 150 mg%, and postprandial blood glucose of less than 200 mg%.

WORSENING HYPERGLYCEMIA (SEE TABLE 100-2). in a patient taking a previously adequate dose of insulin requires prompt attention. Although important changes in caloric intake or failure to take insulin properly may be the explanation for worsening hyperglycemia, occult infection (especially in the urinary tract), coronary ischemia, severe emotional stress, steroid use, and Somogyi phenomenon (rebound hyperglycemia) must be investigated. A recently recognized phenomenon, worsening hyperglycemia in the early morning hours, is caused by the growth hormone surges that occur during sleep. An intermediate-acting insulin given at bedtime can provide excellent coverage for this early morning hyperglycemia.

The *Somogyi phenomenon* may be mistaken for inadequate control, because of the rebound hyperglycemia and possible ketosis that occurs after insulin-induced hypoglycemia. The hypoglycemia usually goes unnoticed because it occurs at night or, because there is severe autonomic neuropathy. Hypoglycemia is followed by several days of poor control. Clues to recognizing nocturnal hypoglycemia include night sweats, poor sleep, nightmares, and morning headaches. Urinary monitoring reveals negative urinary glucose and ketones in the evening followed by trace urinary sugar and large ketones in the morning. The best way to recognize the Somogyi effect is to be cognizant of its potential existence and to obtain a blood glucose at a time of suspected hypoglycemia. Appropriate therapy, which involves slowly decreasing the dosage of insulin, may be commenced after documenting hypoglycemia. If detection is impractical, a diagnostic trial of treatment may be used to confirm the clinical suspicion. Doses of insulin should be decreased slowly each day rather than precipitously because a dramatic decrease in insulin dosage will lead to worsening hyperglycemia.

In uncommon instances, *insulin resistance* is the cause of poor control. It is arbitrarily defined as the requirement for greater than 200 units of insulin daily. Insulin resistance seen in obesity is caused by a decrease in the number of insulin receptors from acanthosis. Restoring normal weight represents the best treatment. Classic insulin resistance is immunologically mediated by antibodies directed at bovine or porcine insulin, or against protamine or protamine insulin complexes. For patients with immunological insulin resistance, switching therapy to a lente insulin preparation or to human recombinant insulin may be advantageous. At times, high-dose glucocorticoids (80–100 mg of prednisone daily) may be necessary to treat insulin resistance. Most patients respond to steroid therapy, which can often be rapidly tapered. Immunological insulin resistance is often seen in individuals who have been receiving insulin in intermittent treatment programs. In patients who will receive insulin for only limited intervals (such as during myocardial infarction or during weight reduction for obesity), human insulin represents the best choice of therapy to limit antibody development.

INSULIN REACTIONS occur when food intake is delayed or diminished, increased physical activity is undertaken, or insulin dose is excessive. The symptoms of *hypoglycemia* include those associated with increased sympathomimetic activity: sweating, palpitations, tremor, and weakness. *Neuroglycopenic symptoms* of fatigue and changes in mentation

Table 100-2. Important Causes of Worsening Hyperglycemia During Insulin Therapy

Inadequate dose
Increased caloric intake
Failure to take insulin properly
Occult infection (especially urinary tract)
Coronary ischemia
Severe emotional stress
Use of corticosteroids
Somogyi phenomenon
Insulin resistance
Growth hormone surge in early morning

may also be seen when there is a less precipitous decline in blood sugar. Profound hypoglycemia may lead to loss of consciousness. If autonomic neuropathy is present, or if a patient is taking a beta-adrenergic blocking drug, many hypoglycemic symptoms will be masked and mental confusion may be the paramount symptom.

Insulin allergy, represented by cutaneous reactions to insulin in approximately 5% of patients and only rarely manifest by urticaria, angioedema, or anaphylaxis, may also be treated by a change to human insulin administered with antihistamines. Desensitization may be necessary if systemic allergic manifestations have occurred.

INSULIN AND SURGERY. Insulin management of the diabetic patient during surgery is to allow modest hyperglycemia and assiduously avoid hypoglycemia and ketosis. The preoperative medical evaluation is critical because the majority of perioperative complications relate not to hyperglycemia or hypoglycemia, but rather to coexisting cardiac or renal disease. Many insulin programs for operative management have been advanced; in general, the dose of insulin should be reduced by approximately one third to one half on the morning of surgery with carbohydrate being supplied by intravenous 5% dextrose at 150 ml/hour. Surgery should, if possible, be performed early in the day, with postoperative monitoring of blood sugar and renal function. An EKG should be obtained because of the higher incidence of silent myocardial ischemia and infarction in diabetics. Until the patient is eating, insulin dosages may need to be decreased, unless increased secretion of counterregulatory hormones (such as growth hormone, cortisol, and catecholamines) worsens hyperglycemia and necessitates an increase in dose.

Management of Complications

It is currently unproven that controlling hyperglycemia will limit or prevent the microvascular, macrovascular, and renal complications of diabetes. Consequently, it is more important that all associated risk factors for the development of coronary artery disease and renal failure be meticulously controlled. Energies spent on the cessation of smoking, the control of hypertension, and the reduction of hypercholesterolemia are much more vital for the patient than attempting to control blood sugar more tightly.

Renal Failure. Although the progression to renal failure may be inexorable once heavy proteinuria of greater than 3 g/day occurs, the primary care physician may still be able to prevent the renal insufficiency that is associated with bladder dysfunction secondary to autonomic neuropathy, the deterioration in renal function that occurs with pyelonephritis and acute papillary necrosis, and the contrast-induced acute renal failure that occurs in diabetics with moderate to advanced renal insufficiency. Prompt and aggressive treatment of urinary tract infections (see Chapters 132 and 140), therapy

to limit urinary retention that increases the risk for infection (see Chapter 133), control of hypertension that is often accelerated as renal function declines (see Chapter 21), and avoidance of unnecessary contrast studies will help control avoidable renal insults. Necessary dye studies require maintaining hydration, using as small a dye load as possible, and administering mannitol following study. Nephrotoxic antibiotics and cyclooxygenase inhibitors (*e.g.,* the nonsteroidal anti-inflammatory agents) should be avoided.

Recent experimental evidence suggests that the increased glomerular filtration rate in early diabetic nephropathy can be normalized with *protein restriction* to 0.5 g/kg/day. Over the past decade, the outlook for the diabetic receiving hemodialysis or renal transplantation has improved, although the mortality rate for diabetics on these treatment modalities remains higher than that of nondiabetics. Combined renal and pancreatic transplantation offers promise. Chronic ambulatory *peritoneal dialysis* has been used for diabetic patients because of concerns that the heparin used for hemodialysis may lead to a worsening of diabetic retinopathy. However, early information suggests higher infection rates in diabetic patients on chronic peritoneal dialysis.

Peripheral Vascular Disease. See Chapter 29 for a discussion of peripheral vascular disease.

Foot Problems. Because of vascular insufficiency and neuropathy, diabetics have unique foot care problems. Meticulous foot care is essential for the prevention of cellulitis, osteomyelitis, and amputation (see Chapter 29). Feet must be kept clean, interdigital spaces dry, calluses pared down, and toenails carefully trimmed. Frequent inspection for skin breakdown and cellulitis by the patient needs to be stressed, as does the importance of wearing properly fitting shoes. Prior to bathing, the diabetic patient should use his hands to ascertain the water temperature to prevent scalding injuries that may occur because of loss of temperature sensation in the lower extremities. The diabetic patient who is incapable of foot care or who has had a foot infection must see a podiatrist regularly.

Neuropathy. Neuropathic *pain* has been treated with phenytoin, carbamazepine, and combinations of tricyclic antidepressants and phenothiazines, but no singularly effective treatment program has emerged. *Phenytoin* seems to have the least toxicity and should be tried first. The *postural hypotension,* impotence, and urinary retention associated with autonomic neuropathy are usually permanent. Postural hypotension may respond to the synthetic mineralocorticoid *Florinef* (see Chapter 18). If sexual performance is limited by *impotence,* and anxiety and depression (which are often superimposed on neurological dysfunction) are excluded, sexually incapacitated patients can be considered for implantation of a *prosthesis* (see Chapters 131 and 225).

Enteropathy. Gastrointestinal motility problems, which include *gastroparesis* and *diabetic* (often nocturnal) *diarrhea,* can be difficult to treat. Small, frequent feedings and cholinergic drugs such as *metoclopramide* may lessen symptoms caused by gastroparesis. Patients with diarrhea due to bacterial overgrowth of the bowel can be treated with a trial of a broad spectrum antibiotic (*e.g.,* ampicillin). Fortunately, nocturnal diarrhea, refractory to therapy, often resolves spontaneously.

Diabetics should have regular dental examinations because of their higher incidence of *pyorrhea* and abscesses, which may also worsen diabetic control.

Ophthalmopathy. Diabetic *retinopathy* is the most important systemic disease causing blindness. Proliferative retinopathy accounts for the majority of cases of blindness among type I diabetics, whereas *macular edema* from nonproliferative retinopathy accounts for the majority of cases of blindness in type II diabetics. Photocoagulation with laser therapy has resulted in retarding visual loss by 50% (see Chapter 208). Cataracts and glaucoma are also important complications (see Chapters 206 and 207 for management).

Glucose Intolerance and Pregnancy

Fetal hyperglycemia contributes to excessive fetal growth, which increases the risks of birth trauma, asphyxia, neonatal respiratory distress syndrome, and *in utero* deaths. In addition, there is an increased need for cesarean section. Maintenance of blood sugars in the physiologic range (60 to 120 mg%) takes on added importance during pregnancy, because the complications of fetal hyperglycemia can be prevented and perinatal mortality reduced to that of nondiabetics. Even nondiabetic pregnant women who develop an otherwise insignificant degree of hyperglycemia (2-hour postprandial blood sugars in the range of 140 to 160 mg%) show an increased risk of macrosomia and its complications. Women with postprandial readings in excess of 165 mg% have an increased incidence of diabetes in later life.

The importance of glucose intolerance during pregnancy has led to the recommendation by the American Diabetic Association that all pregnant women be screened for glucose intolerance by the 24th to 28th week of gestation using a 50-g oral glucose load, which can be given at any time of day. Patients with a 1-hour serum glucose in excess of 140 mg% should be given a 100-g glucose tolerance test and treated if the level is greater than 165 mg% at 2 hours. Some argue on the basis of studies showing increased fetal risk with previously "normal" levels of glucose intolerance (120 to 160 mg%) that even more modest elevations are grounds for therapy, at least with dietary measures.

All patients with glucose intolerance should be treated with diets that limit simple sugars and total calories (35 to 38 calories/kg of ideal weight before pregnancy). Repeat testing of the blood sugar every 1 to 2 weeks until delivery is indicated. Patients showing fasting sugars in excess of 105 mg% or postprandial levels greater than 120 mg% should be considered for insulin therapy; consultation with a diabetologist is indicated.

For diabetic patients already on insulin, adjustments in dose may be necessary. During the first trimester, the type I diabetic needs a reduction in insulin, because insulin requirements decrease and there is a heightened risk of hypoglycemia. In the second trimester, the type I diabetic requires more insulin as the diabetes becomes more labile and the chances of ketoacidosis (with its associated risk of fetal death) rise. Third trimester dose requirements usually do not change, but the increase in glomerular filtration rate can lower the tubular threshold for glucose and make urine testing unreliable. Within a few hours of delivery, insulin requirements fall considerably, returning fully to prepregnancy levels within 1 to 2 weeks. Optimal control is facilitated by use of home glucose monitoring (see below).

Monitoring

Monitoring can be divided into two categories: control of glycemia and observation for signs of systemic complications.

For Control of Glycemia. The traditional means of monitoring was the *double-voided urine* test for glucose and ketones, usually performed before breakfast and before the evening meal in patients taking insulin. The technique requires voiding fully, then voiding again ½ hour later and testing the urine sample by means of tape or tablets for a colorimetric response that indicates the urine glucose and ketone concentrations. The correlation between urine and serum glucose concentrations is approximate at best and varies from patient to patient and from time to time in the same patient because of differences and changes in renal tubular threshold for glucose, renal blood flow and urine volume. Moreover, the test is compromised in patients with bladder dysfunction who have a postvoid residual.

HOME GLUCOSE MONITORING represents a marked improvement in monitoring. The patient obtains a finger-stick sample of capillary blood, which is tested for glucose concentration by colorimetric reading of a reagent strip to which a drop of blood is applied. Both meters and color charts are available for making the glucose determination. Measurements are most useful for patients on insulin therapy. Frequent measurements, both fasting and at several intervals postprandially, are valuable at the time of starting or adjusting an insulin program and also during periods of illness or worsening control. Most patients can be taught the method; there are numerous devices that automatically perform the finger-stick. Once a stable insulin dose is achieved, a single measurement need be taken only once every several days; typically it is obtained before breakfast. Patients who are capable of adjusting their own insulin doses can use home monitoring to keep their sugars in the mid-100 range. Home monitoring does not obviate the need to carefully inform the patient about symptoms of hyperglycemia and hypoglycemia (see below).

HEMOGLOBIN A_{1C} is the glycosylated form of hemoglobin in the red cell. The degree of glycosylation parallels the glucose concentrations the red cell has been exposed to over its life-span. Thus, its measurement allows an assessment of overall glycemic control for the preceding 2 to 3 months; it correlates well with frequent blood glucose determinations. Levels of less than 8.0% indicate blood sugars of less than 200 mg%; values of 11% to 12% correlate with glucose levels in excess of 300 mg% and indicate poor carbohydrate control. This test has superceded the *random blood sugar* as the best means of assessing control over time. For the patient with mild non-insulin-dependent diabetes, a periodic hemoglobin A_{1C} will suffice for monitoring glycemic control. Patients on insulin require acute as well as chronic measurements of blood sugar.

Checking for Complications. Patients with diabetes should have a biannual office evaluation that includes a check of the blood pressure for elevation; the skin for infection; the eyes for background retinopathy (see Chapter 208); the cardiovascular system for evidence of carotid, coronary, and peripheral vascular disease; and the feet for ischemic lesions. The evaluation should conclude with a careful neurologic examination for signs of neuropathy. Of particular importance is the need to test for an vigorously treat other risk factors for vascular disease, such as hypertension (see Chapter 21), hypercholesterolemia (see Chapter 22), and smoking (see Chapter 49). Laboratory monitoring should include a urinalysis for proteinuria and sediment and a BUN and creatinine for estimation of renal function. A diabetic summary sheet placed in the patient's record helps to quickly note the extent, severity, and progression of the disease and its complications.

Teaching the patient to watch for skin, eye, neurologic, and cardiovascular changes is an important part of the monitoring effort (see below).

PATIENT EDUCATION

The success of a program for metabolic control depends on patient compliance. Because *weight reduction* to ideal body weight is the most important therapy we can offer type II diabetics, instruction in *diet* and healthy foods should take place in a setting that includes the patient and his family. Sample diets can be obtained from the American Diabetic Association. Self-imposed caloric restriction in diabetics is to be discouraged. The emphasis on diet therapy for the type II diabetic should focus more upon caloric restriction than actual percentages of carbohydrate or obsession with simple sugars.

The patient receiving insulin requires continuous education. Many hospital-based practices and several office practices have utilized a diabetes-teaching nurse to give patients careful instruction in drawing up insulin into the syringe (particularly if the patient is visually impaired), to teach insulin injection techniques and the complications of excess insulin administration, and to be readily available for telephone communication with patients. Some physicians consider deliberately giving their patients mild insulin reactions so that the patient may appreciate his or her unique warning symptoms of hypoglycemia. For severe, out-of-hospital hypoglycemia, a syringe with glucagon for intramuscular injection is given to the patient in the event that the patient becomes profoundly hypoglycemic. Oral administration of juices in the unconscious and obtunded patient may lead to pulmonary aspiration.

The importance of skin and foot care must be emphasized (see Chapter 29). Referral of elderly diabetics with vision loss to podiatrists for footcare is indicated.

INDICATIONS FOR ADMISSION AND REFERRAL

Patient care programs that encourage communication between patients and health care professionals reduce the need for hospitalizations for dehydration, marked hyperglycemia, ketoacidosis, and infection. Acute hospitalization for intravenous fluids is necessary for diabetic patients with protracted nausea and vomiting who are becoming dehydrated and hyperglycemic. Often cellulitis of the foot requires intravenous antibiotic therapy, as does acute pyelonephritis. In general, elderly diabetic patients with pneumonia or urinary tract infections benefit from brief hospitalizations. Referral to an endocrinologist is indicated for the diabetic with insulin resistance, and for the diabetic who has marked excursions in blood sugar with frequent hypoglycemia and hyperglycemia. When proteinuria is in the nephrotic syndrome range, and creatinine is beginning to rise above 2.5, referral to a nephrologist for consideration of dialysis or transplantation is necessary. Indications for coronary artery bypass grafting are not different for the diabetic. Because of the rapidity and severity of cholecystitis and ascending cholangitis, cholecystectomy for cholelithiasis may be a reasonable clinical course to follow. Ophthalmological referral is indicated when background diabetic retinopathy first becomes evident.

THERAPEUTIC RECOMMENDATIONS

- The diagnosis of diabetes mellitus should be suspected and confirmed by fasting blood sugar, or if necessary by glucose tolerance testing in individuals who (a) have polyuria, polydipsia, weight loss, and visual changes that may be due to the hyperosmolar effects of hyperglycemia; (b) are overweight and have a strong family history of diabetes; (c) have significant risk factors for the development of coronary artery disease such as hypertension, smoking, and hypercholesterolemia; and (d) have unexplained neuropathy, proteinuria, renal insufficiency, or peripheral vascular disease. Pregnant women should have fasting blood sugar determination early in pregnancy and blood sugar measured following 50 g of glucose by the 24th to 28th week of gestation, particularly if there is a family history of diabetes.

- Until the results from ongoing multicenter clinical studies on the effectiveness of tight control reducing complications of diabetes are known, it is more important to reduce all other risk factors for the development of atherosclerosis and to encourage exercise and healthful diet than it is to rigidly adhere to the goal of achieving a particular blood sugar concentration.
- The cornerstone of therapy in type II diabetes is weight reduction to ideal body weight. The composition of the diet, per se, is less important but should include a high polyunsaturated:saturated fat ratio, low cholesterol, and complex carbohydrate. Low-protein diets may be beneficial in averting diabetic nephropathy.
- In patients who continue to be symptomatic despite diet therapy of diabetes, or continue to have fasting blood sugars above 180 mg%, insulin therapy, with an intermediate acting insulin preparation (lente or NPH) should be commenced. Newly treated diabetics should receive human insulin, because of less insulin allergy, insulin resistance, and antibody development. This recommendation assumes a reduction in cost of human recombinant insulin.
- The newer oral hypoglycemic sulfonylureas with the advantage of once daily administration (glyburide and glypizide) should be considered in individuals who will not consider insulin self-injection, who cannot safely administer insulin because of visual loss, or who will only require therapy for a brief interval because of successful weight reduction.
- In young, medically sophisticated, motivated patients who have not developed diabetic complications, intensive insulin therapy should be considered.
- Daily monitoring of control is most effectively accomplished by home blood glucose determinations. Long-term glucose control is most accurately assessed by hemoglobin A_{1C} measurements three or four times yearly. Home blood glucose testing is an important component of the education of diabetic patients, aiding their modification of insulin schedule and dosage following exercise or change in dietary intake. Causes for worsening hyperglycemia (see Table 100-2) should be carefully investigated.
- A comprehensive physical exam and history should be obtained at least annually, searching for evidence of the development of coronary artery disease, cerebrovascular disease, peripheral vascular disease, diabetic neuropathy, renal insufficiency, proteinuria, and retinopathy.
- The development of proteinuria should lead to more careful monitoring of renal function. Consider use of low-protein

diets and tighter control of hyperglycemia. When the serum creatinine reaches 3 mg%, obtain nephrology consultation regarding candidacy for dialysis or transplantation.
- Exert caution in use of iodinated contrast agents.
- Diabetics who have findings of background retinopathy or who have been diabetic for 10 years should be referred to ophthalmologists for indirect ophthalmoscopy and, if necessary, fluorescein angiography.
- Foot care in diabetics with neuropathy and vascular insufficiency should be emphasized, with consideration of podiatric care in this group of patients.

ANNOTATED BIBLIOGRAPHY

Arky R: Current principles of dietary therapy of diabetes mellitus. Med Clin North Am 62:655, 1978 (*An overview of dietary methods of controlling diabetes.*)

Brenner BM: Hemodynamically mediated glomerular injury and the progressive nature of kidney disease. Kidney Int 23:647, 1983 (*The Zatz and Brenner investigations suggest increased renal blood flow and the mesangial capillary proliferative reaction to this increased blood flow, not glycemic control, is the pathogenesis of diabetic renal disease.*)

Bressler R, Galloway JA: Insulin treatment of diabetes mellitus. Med Clin North Am 62:663, 1978 (*An update of the authors' 1971 paper, which describes the various glycemic responses to intermediate insulins. A very helpful paper on beginning insulin therapy.*)

Brown MJ, Asbury AK: Diabetic neuropathy. Ann Neurol 15:2, 1984 (*A concise review of myriad clinical presentations of diabetic polyneuropathy.*)

Campbell PJ, Bolli G, Cryer P et al: Pathogenesis of the dawn phenomenon in patients with insulin dependent diabetes mellitus. N Engl J Med 312:1473, 1985 (*Physiological studies implicating growth hormone, not catecholamines, in the pre-awakening rise in glucose.*)

Gabbe SG: Gestational diabetes. N Engl J Med 315:1025, 1986 (*An editorial reviewing the condition and the new data suggesting complications even with modest degrees of hyperglycemia.*)

Gerich JE: Sulfonylureas in the treatment of diabetes mellitus—1985. Mayo Clin Proc 60:439, 1985 (*A general review of the pharmacology and a comparison of the sulfonylureas in the treatment of diabetes.*)

Jenkins DJA, Thomas DM, Wolever MS et al: Glycemic index of foods: A physiological basis for carbohydrate exchange. Am J Clin Nutr 34:362, 1981 (*An analysis of the glycemic effects of various carbohydrates; beans lead to less hyperglycemia than potatoes or corn.*)

Judzewitsch RG, Jaspan JB, Polonsky KS et al: Aldose reductase inhibition improves nerve conduction velocity in diabetic patients. N Engl J Med 308:119, 1983 (*Although aldose reductase inhibitors improve nerve conduction time, there is no evidence that this soon-to-be-introduced class of drugs reverses the painful neuropathies.*)

Kahn CR: Insulin resistance: A common feature of diabetes mellitus. N Engl J Med 315:252, 1986 (*An editorial examining the clinical significance of insulin resistance both for pathogenesis and for treatment.*)

Miller LV, Goldstein J: More efficient care of diabetic patients in a community hospital setting. N Engl J Med 286:1388, 1972 (*Demonstrates the importance of communication between patient and health care provider in reducing acute hospitalizations for diabetes.*)

Molnar GD et al: Methods of assessing diabetic control. Diabetologia 17:5, 1979 (*A discussion of traditional urinary glucose monitoring as newer approaches to self-monitoring are being introduced.*)

Mulrow CD, Lichtenstein MJ: Blood glucose and diabetic retinopathy. J Gen Intern Med 1:73, 1986 (*A meta-analysis of available studies on the association between control and its complications. No significant relation was found.*)

Nathan DM, Singer DE, Hurxthal K et al: The clinical information value of the glycosylated hemoglobin assay. N Engl J Med 310:341, 1984 (*Hemoglobin A_{1C} can be used to accurately determine average mean blood sugars in a clinical population in which physicians caring for the patients were, at times, misled by other monitoring information presented by the patient.*)

Raskin P, Rosenstock J: Blood glucose control and diabetic complications. Ann Intern Med 105:254, 1986 (*An extensive review of data supporting or refuting the two hypotheses of the microvascular complications of diabetes. (1) These complications are genetically determined and independent of glucose control. (2) Long-term hyperglycemia is responsible for the subsequent development of diabetic microangiopathy. The authors review preliminary data from the Steno, Kroc, Oxford, New Haven, and Dallas studies and conclude that once retinopathy has developed, its progression may not be altered by intensive insulin therapy.*)

Rizza R: New modes of insulin administration: Do they have a role in clinical diabetes? Ann Intern Med 105:126, 1986 (*An editorial that discusses risks and benefits of intensive insulin therapy. It includes an up-to-date bibliography.*)

Sherwin RS, Taborlane WV: Metabolic control and diabetic complications. In Olefsky JM, Sherwin RS (eds): Diabetes Mellitus: Management and Complications. New York, Churchill Livingstone, 1985 (*Excellent and readable discussion concerning control and complications. An extensive bibliography.*)

Symposium on Biosynthetic Human Insulin Diabetes Care 4:139, 1981 (*From molecular biology to clinical studies with human recombinant insulin.*)

Tallarigo L, Giampietro O, Penno G et al: Relation of glucose tolerance to complications of pregnancy in nondiabetic women. N Engl J Med 315:989, 1986 (*Even limited degrees of glucose intolerance during pregnancy were associated with increased risks of macrosomia and its attendant complications.*)

Tattersall RB: Patient self-monitoring of blood glucose and refinements of conventional insulin treatment. Am J Med 70:177 (*Changes in insulin administration programs can be accomplished by introducing self-monitoring of blood glucose.*)

Teutsch SM, Herman WH, Dwyer DM et al: Mortality among diabetic patients using continuous subcutaneous insulin-infusion pumps. N Engl J Med 310:361, 1984 (*With numerous studies showing equivalent glucose control with intensive conventional therapy and pump therapy, there is a small but real concern for death, perhaps caused by excessive insulin administration.*)

Wilson RM, Clark P, Barkes H et al: Starting insulin treatment as an outpatient. JAMA 256:877, 1986 (*Presents data indicating this is both safe and cost effective.*)

Zatz R et al: Predominance of hemodynamic rather than metabolic factors in the pathogenesis of diabetic glomerulopathy. Proc Natl Acad Sci USA 82:5963, 1985 (*Data supporting increased renal blood flow as the pathophysiological mechanism for mesangial proliferation.*)

101
Management of Hyperthyroidism

Hyperthyroidism is the clinical expression of a heterogeneous group of disorders that produce elevations of free thyroxine (FT_4) and/or triiodothyronine (T_3). Well-recognized forms of hyperthyroidism are diffuse toxic goiter (Graves' disease), toxic multinodular goiter, and toxic uninodular goiter. The prevalence of hyperthyroidism is not precisely known, but the condition occurs in women eight times more often than in men. Approximately 15% of recognized cases occur in persons over the age of 60; the clinical presentation of hyperthroidism in the elderly is often atypical. The primary physician should be able to recognize hyperthyroidism and design a therapeutic program appropriate to the patient's age, clinical condition, and personal preferences. The indications and limitations of surgery, radioiodine therapy, and antithyroid agents must be understood.

PATHOPHYSIOLOGY, CLINICAL PRESENTATION, AND COURSE

The primary physiologic alteration in hyperthyroidism is excess secretion of thyroid hormone, which stimulates calorigenesis, catabolism, and enhanced sensitivity to catecholamines. This produces the classic picture of heat intolerance, nervousness, tremor, increased appetite, weight loss, excessive sweating, lid lag, stare, and muscle weakness. Diarrhea may also occur.

In the *elderly* thyrotoxic patient, the characteristic manifestations of hyperthyroidism may be absent and the clinical picture dominated instead by apathy, weight loss, and otherwise unexplained atrial fibrillation. This apathetic hyperthyroidism of the elderly has been mistaken for depression and occult malignancy.

Elevations in alkaline phosphatase and angiotensin-converting enzyme may accompany thyrotoxicosis and persist even after treatment. The pathophysiologic significance of these elevations remains unclear, but the findings might suggest thyroid disease and save extensive workup when other explanations for their occurrence are lacking.

In *Graves' disease,* an autoimmune mechanism appears to be responsible for the overproduction of thyroid hormone. A deficiency of thyroid-specific suppressor T-cell lymphocytes allows production of a thyroid-stimulating antibody (TSAb) which binds to thyrotropin receptors and triggers excess thyroid hormone synthesis. Graves' disease accounts for close to 90% of hyperthyroidism seen in those under age 40.

Infiltrative *exophthalmos* and *pretibial myxedema* are characteristic physical manifestations. It used to be thought that the eye findings could occur independently of the hyperthyroidism, but careful observations have uncovered subclinical exophthalmos (increased intraocular pressure on upward gaze) in almost all Graves' disease patients tested. Eye involvement is probably an inevitable complication of the disease and may result from the same factor that triggers the glandular changes. Unfortunately, eye findings may worsen with treatment of the hyperthyroidism.

The thyroid gland in Graves' disease is diffusely enlarged and a bruit may be heard in severe cases. The classic symptoms and signs of thyrotoxicosis are common. The skin is velvety and the hair silky. Onycholysis, vitiligo, and gynecomastia are found in some cases and may suggest the diagnosis. Cardiac complications are infrequent, due to the relative youth of the patient population, but a reversible cardiomyopathy has been identified, manifested by a fall in ejection fraction with exercise. Heart failure is rare, but impaired exercise tolerance is often reported, perhaps caused by the decrease in ejection fraction.

The clinical course waxes and wanes, with exacerbations and remissions of unpredictable duration. After many years, mild hypothyroidism may ensue, especially in patients with small goiters and mild hyperthyroidism at the time of onset.

Toxic multinodular goiter (Plummer's disease) accounts for most cases of hyperthyroidism in middle-aged and elderly persons. The condition is often associated with a long-standing simple goiter. The gland is clinically and pathologically indistinguishable from that of nontoxic multinodular goiters. Cardiovascular symptoms may dominate the clinical presentation; new onset of heart failure, atrial fibrillation, or angina is not uncommon and reflects the high prevalence of coexisting organic heart disease in this older population. In a series of 85 hyperthyroid patients between ages 60 and 82, two-thirds experienced heart failure and 20% reported angina. Only a minority evidenced the more typical symptoms of hyperthyroidism; for example, less than 11% had polyphagia.

On the other hand, 33% suffered from anorexia, and constipation was as prevalent as diarrhea. Lid lag may be noted on occasion, but exophthalmos does not occur. Sometimes apathy and weight loss are the most prominent clinical features and can be so profound as to suggest occult malignancy or severe depression.

Elderly patients with large nodular goiters have demonstrated an increased risk of developing thyrotoxicosis upon exposure to *iodides.* The problem is most prevalent among patients who come from areas of low iodine intake (*e.g.,* Europe) and has a self-limited clinical course. Laboratory findings include a low radioactive iodine (RAI) uptake and no antithyroid antibodies.

The autonomously functioning *single toxic nodule* presents clinically much like the toxic multinodular goiter. The principal difference is the finding of a "hot" nodule surrounded by suppressed gland on radioiodine thyroid scan. The larger the nodule, the greater its propensity to cause thyrotoxicosis, with risk quite high once the nodule reaches 3 cm in diameter. Often, onset of toxicity is first manifested by an isolated increase in serum T_3; later T_4 levels rise. Sometimes hemorrhagic infarction terminates the overproduction of hormone and limits the progression to thyrotoxicosis.

T_3 toxicosis is an important entity to consider when patients with clinically apparent hyperthyroidism have normal T_4 levels. The condition has been reported in association with both diffuse and nodular goiters. Clinical presentation is no different from hyperthyroidism due to elevations in T_4. Isolated elevations in T_3 concentration may also occur in euthyroid patients who have no underlying thyroid disease (see below).

Transient hyperthyroidism may occur in association with subacute or chronic thyroiditis, due to uncontrolled release of hormone. The clinical manifestations of hyperthyroidism are usually mild. The course is self-limited, and hypothyroidism often ensues. *Subacute thyroiditis* typically follows a viral illness, producing a tender multinodular gland. The occasional case associated with hyperthyroidism is abrupt in onset in conjunction with thyrotoxic symptoms. The erythrocyte sedimentation rate is high, and thyroid scan characteristically shows little or no uptake of radioiodine. *Chronic thyroiditis (Hashimoto's)* is a common autoimmune cause of goiter (see Chapter 95), but hyperthyroidism is neither frequent nor permanent. It may be due to coexisting Graves' disease in some cases. There are high titers of antibodies to microsomes and thyroglobulin. Prevalence is highest in middle-aged women and among the elderly, where it may go unrecognized. The gland feels rubbery and is enlarged, sometimes asymmetrically. Hypothyroidism eventually develops in a substantial number of cases.

Postpartum (subacute lymphocytic) thyroiditis, a previously unappreciated but surprisingly frequent problem (incidence as high as 5% in one series) can precipitate transient mild hyperthyroidism. Onset is within 3 to 6 months of delivery and often is mistaken for anxiety due to the stress of caring for a new child. The gland is nontender and may resemble that of Hashimoto's thyroiditis (see Chapter 95). RAI uptake is low and antithyroid antibodies detectable, suggesting an immunologic mechanism. The condition may persist for months before eventually resolving. A period of hypothyroidism may occur before the condition ceases (see Chapter 102). It tends to recur with subsequent pregnancies.

Clinical hyperthyroidism in the context of a normal-size gland raises the possibility of an unusual cause such as pituitary neoplasm, HCG-producing tumor, struma ovarii, and excess intake of exogenous thyroxine or iodide.

DIAGNOSIS

Clinical recognition of hyperthyroidism can sometimes be difficult, especially when symptoms are mild or when the condition occurs in the elderly or pregnant patient. Reliable radioimmunoassays and equilibrium dialysis techniques for quantitation of serum thyroid hormone levels have greatly facilitated accurate diagnosis.

An elevation in the serum *free T_4* or *free T_4 index* (an excellent proxy for the free T_4, calculated by multiplying the serum T_4 by the T_3 resin uptake) is the cornerstone of diagnosis. Measurement of the serum *total T_3* is indicated when the patient is clinically thyrotoxic, yet the free T_4 is normal or only slightly elevated. Routinely ordering a serum T_3 in the evaluation of suspected hyperthyroidism is probably wasteful, because T_3 toxicosis is uncommon.

Overreliance on thyroid hormone levels can be misleading. *Euthyroid hyperthyroxemia* occurs when there is an increase in thyroid-binding globulin (*e.g.,* pregnancy, estrogen use, liver disease), which produces an increase in total T_4, while the free T_4 remains normal. More confusing are euthyroid states with increases in free T_4 as well as total T_4. Patients with autoantibodies against thyroid hormones may manifest surprisingly high free hormone levels due to interference by these immunoglobulins with the standard radioimmune assays for thyroid hormones. Acute medical, surgical, and psychiatric illnesses as well as intake of high-dose propranolol, amiodarone, and gallbladder dyes can impair peripheral conversion of T_4 to T_3, leading to rises in free T_4 concentration in conjunction with a reduction in T_3. An unexpectedly normal or low T_3 level in a patient who is clinically euthyroid yet has elevations in T_4 and free T_4 should raise the suspicion of euthyroid hyperthyroxemia. The T_3 concentration helps in the differentiation. TRH testing might also be useful.

TRH stimulation testing can aid interpretation of equivocal thyroxine levels. In patients with genuine hyperthyroidism, the TSH response to TRH is minimal or absent. This reflects suppression of the pituitary by elevated levels of thyroid hormone. However, cortisol hypersecretion can also suppress TSH response to TRH, simulating the pattern seen with hyperthyroidism. TRH stimulation testing is usually unnecessary, but remains among the most sensitive of tests for detection of hyperthyroidism and is useful in difficult or confusing situations.

New, very sensitive *immunoradiometric assays (IMRA)* for thyrotropin (TSH) hold much promise for improved diagnosis of hyperthyroidism. The absence of detectable TSH by IMRA has the same diagnostic significance as an absent TSH response to TRH. A normal TSH level by IMRA rules out hyperthyroidism and obviates the need for TRH-stimulation testing. In a few situations, the absence of TSH by IMRA is not diagnostic of hyperthyroidism (use of exogenous thyroid hormone and euthyroid patients with an autonomously functioning thyroid nodule). Overall, the advent of IMRA testing for TSH is an important advance and may prove to be the best screening test for hyperthyroidism. The literature should be followed for studies examining the utility of the assay.

The *thyroid scan* aids evaluation of the thyrotoxic patient with a nodular goiter. *Whole-body scanning* will identify the rare case of extrathyroidal hormone synthesis, such as a struma ovarii or a hyperfunctioning metastasis from a thyroid malignancy. *Serum thyroglobulin* determination serves as an elegant yet simple means of detecting the patient surreptitiously taking thyroid hormone. Exogenous hormone use results in suppression of thyroglobulin synthesis.

PRINCIPLES OF THERAPY

The goals of therapy are to correct the hypermetabolic state with a minimum of side effects and with smallest incidence of hypothyroidism. For definitive therapy, one must choose among antithyroid drugs, radioiodine, and thyroidectomy. Beta-blocking agents are useful for prompt, temporary control of hyperadrenergic symptoms. Hyperthyroidism should not go untreated, particularly in the elderly who are at risk for cardiovascular complications. Moreover, not only are symptoms uncomfortable, but thyrotoxic crisis may ensue if the untreated patient unexpectedly encounters a severe stress such as emergency surgery or acute sepsis.

Therapeutic Modalities

Beta-Blocking Agents provide excellent, prompt symptomatic relief from many of the catechol-mediated manifestations of hyperthyroidism (*e.g.,* tremor, palpitations, heat intolerance, nervousness). Control is often achieved within a few days. These drugs frequently serve as the first line of therapy and as preoperative treatment. They are also of value to treat cardiac complications, such as atrial fibrillation (see Chapter 23) and angina (see Chapter 25). Heart failure that is strictly rate-related will benefit from beta blockade, but that due to myocardial pathology will worsen with such therapy; consequently, it must be applied with care in the elderly and those with pre-existing heart disease (see Chapter 27).

Of the beta blockers, propranolol remains the most widely used for control of hyperthyroidism, but other agents in this class (*e.g.,* atenolol, metoprolol, nadolol) demonstrate comparable efficacy. Those with a long half-life (see Chapter 25) are particularly useful for patients who are to undergo surgery. They all work by blocking the adrenergic effects of thyroid hormone and have no clinically significant direct antithyroid effect, except (as noted previously) at high doses, where they are capable of slowing the peripheral conversion of T_4 to T_3. Since these drugs do not interfere with thyroid hormone secretion, they need to be prescribed in conjunction with other treatment modalities for more definitive therapy of hyperthyroidism. Adequacy of dose is determined by monitoring the resting and exercise heart rates, as well as the degree of symptomatic relief.

One important benefit from beta-blockade is the ability to proceed safely with thyroid surgery within 1 to 2 weeks. Antithyroid drugs (see below) require 6 to 8 weeks of preoperative treatment. The addition of *potassium iodide* to beta-blocker therapy produces more rapid and greater preoperative control of patients with Graves' disease who are to undergo thyroidectomy; it is especially useful in those who fail to achieve adequate control on beta-blockers alone, as defined by a resting pulse of less than 90 beats/min and a blunting of exercise-induced tachycardia.

Antithyroid Drugs. *Methimazole* and *propylthiouracil* (*PTU*) are the most important antithyroid agents. PTU acts by interfering with the synthesis of thyroxine and blocking peripheral conversion of T_4 to T_3, though at conventional doses, this latter effect is probably not clinically important. Methimazole does not have any peripheral effect, but is more potent; the doses used are one-tenth those for PTU. Biochemical response to the antithyroid drugs is detectable within 1 to 2 weeks; clinical response typically takes 4 to 8 weeks.

These antithyroid agents are useful for treatment of Graves' disease, preoperative control, therapy prior to and following radioiodine ablation, and long-term treatment of children, adolescents, and young adults. Initial PTU therapy averages 300 mg per day, given in divided doses every 8 hours; for methimazole, the starting dose is 15 mg/day, which can be given as a single dose since its half-life is much longer. Once clinical and biochemical control are attained, the dose is tapered to the lowest amount needed to maintain a euthyroid state. Usually, treatment is continued for 12 to 24 months, then halted to see if relapse occurs.

PTU induces remission in approximately 50% of patients with Graves' disease who are treated for 1 to 2 years, but one-third to one-half of those who respond will relapse. Reports of a remission rate of 40% after only 3 to 5 months of antithyroid therapy suggest that a shorter course of treatment

might be almost as effective. The risk of inducing hypothyroidism is low. Patients who relapse or fail to achieve remission need to be considered for radioiodine or surgical therapy.

Common adverse effects include skin rash, fever, and arthralgias; these are usually not of major clinical significance. However, the rare (0.3% to 0.6% of patients), but potentially fatal complication of *agranulocytosis* necessitates careful patient selection and close monitoring of therapy. The risk of agranulocytosis increases with age, (beginning around age 40) and is independent of dose for PTU, but dose-dependent for methimazole. Onset is usually within 2 months, rarely beyond 4 months. No patients taking less than 30 mg per day of methimazole have been reported to develop agranulocytosis, making this drug the safer of the two.

Close monitoring for agranulocytosis is important, but only during the first 4 months of therapy. Mild leukopenia is common, occurring in up to 10% of patients; its occurrence does not require halting treatment. If the leukocyte count falls below 1500 per cc, therapy should be withheld.

Properly monitored, antithyroid therapy is a reasonable treatment modality, especially for younger patients; it needs to be used with more caution in the elderly. Although PTU is more widely prescribed, methimazole appears preferable in terms of cost, hematologic side-effects, and ease of administration. PTU might be preferable during pregnancy and breast feeding (see below).

Potassium iodide (SSKI) was initially prescribed by Plummer to prepare patients for thyroid surgery. Iodides interfere with the synthesis and release of thyroxine from the thyroid gland. SSKI is less effective than the more modern antithyroid drugs, but, as noted earlier, is useful as an adjunct to beta-blocking or antithyroid therapy prior to thyroid surgery. Prolonged use of iodides has been associated with an occasional, paradoxical rise in thyroid hormone output. Thus, they are best utilized for preoperative control in patients who require a second drug to counter the hyperthyroidism and in those who have a contraindication to use of beta-blockers and other antithyroid medications.

Radioactive Iodine (131I) represents an important form of ablative therapy, first introduced in 1942 and widely used today. It is indicated in Graves' disease when antithyroid drugs do not suffice, in elderly or noncompliant patients, in those with solitary toxic nodules, and in those with contraindications or a reluctance to undergoing surgery. Advantages include established efficacy, relative safety, and ease of administration. Disadvantages are delay in controlling symptoms and high incidence of ensuing hypothyroidism.

Hypothyroidism is the most common complication. High-dose radioiodine provides predictable relief but a high incidence of early hypothyroidism (70% in the first year). Low-dose regimens have a lower early risk of hypothyroidism (15% in the first year) but provide less control of the disease (50% still hyperthyroid at one year). Long-term follow-up studies of patients given low-dose treatment indicate a steady increase in the cumulative incidence of hypothyroidism (75% at 11 years), suggesting that its early advantages fade with time. Regardless of dose used, the risk of eventual hypothyroidism requires that patients be regularly re-evaluated, typically at 6-month intervals.

The concern that radioiodine would lead to long-term *radiation injury* has not been borne out. The gonadal radiation dose from ^{131}I therapy is small, the equivalent of that from a barium enema or an IVP. There is no evidence of increased rates of birth defects or thyroid cancer. Available retrospective cohort studies have evaluated patients treated as long as 30 years ago.

Surgery represents the most direct ablative approach to hyperthyroidism. The objective is to reduce thyroid mass sufficiently to cure the hypermetabolic state without inducing a hypothyroid condition. Unfortunately, there is a substantial incidence of permanent hypothyroidism, and smaller but perceptible risks of hypoparathyroidism and laryngeal paralysis. Moreover, hyperthyroidism may recur despite subtotal thyroidectomy in Graves' disease. Prior preparation of the patient with antithyroid drugs is required to avoid precipitating thyroid storm. Surgery is particularly useful for relieving esophageal obstruction; cosmesis and pregnancy are other indications. It is also a choice when antithyroid drugs fail or produce complications, or when patients are noncompliant. Young patients with moderate to severe disease do particularly well. However, ^{131}I is increasingly replacing surgery, because it is a less expensive and less morbid therapy.

Choice of Therapy

Graves' Disease. For *elderly* patients, *radioactive iodine* is the treatment of choice. For *middle-aged adults* with mild disease and relatively small glands, *antithyroid drugs* represent an effective mode of therapy. A short-term course of beta-blocker and/or antithyroid drug therapy are indicated to establish a euthyroid state in patients who are to undergo surgical or isotopic ablation therapy.

Consensus is less evident in the case of optimal treatment for a *young adult.* A survey of 54 thyroidologists found that for a 19-year-old patient with moderate hyperthyroidism and a gland three to four times normal size, two-thirds favored an initial course of *antithyroid medication,* one-quarter preferred radioiodine, and the remainder surgery. For a 29-year-old patient, about half would treat initially with antithyroid medication and about half with *radioiodine;* surgery was a distant third. If hyperthyroidism recurred after an initial course of antithyroid drugs, about half would recommend *surgery* and half ^{131}I. Despite the absence of evidence for long-term genetic risk, concern persists over giving ^{131}I to patients in their reproductive years.

With a host of alternative therapies available, each with its own advantages and disadvantages, it is important to in-

dividualize treatment according to the patient's needs, capabilities, and clinical status. There is still no specific therapy for the underlying immunopathologic process of Graves' disease; until there is, one must settle for treating the resultant hyperthyroidism.

One consequence of the inability to etiologically treat Graves' disease is the lack of effective therapy for *exophthalmos.* Severe exophthalmos may respond to very high doses of corticosteroids (*e.g.,* 120 to 150 mg per day of prednisone) or require surgical decompression. Precipitation of hypothyroidism has been known to worsen the condition, making careful monitoring of control essential.

Solitary Toxic Nodule. Radioiodine is the treatment of choice for elderly patients with this condition. Since the rest of the gland is suppressed by the hyperfunctioning nodule, the incidence of posttreatment hypothyroidism is far less than that seen with treatment of Graves' disease. Optimal radioiodine dose remains a subject of debate. A relatively low dose of ^{131}I (5–15 mCi) has recently been reported to achieve excellent results with minimal adverse effects. Over 75% of patients became euthyroid by 2 months and over 90% within 6 months. Posttreatment hypothyroidism was very rare. Surgical removal may be preferable in young patients.

Hyperthyroidism in Pregnant and Nursing Patients. The choice is between antithyroid drugs and surgery, because radioiodine is contraindicated (it crosses the placenta and concentrates in the fetal thyroid). Antithyroid drug therapy is considered safer than surgery, with surgery reserved for refractory cases and patients who refuse to take their medication. Among the *antithyroid agents, PTU* is preferred; methimazole has been associated with aplasia cutis in the fetus. The risk of drug crossing into the placenta and inducing hypothyroidism in the fetus is small and not strictly dose-related, but precipitation of hypothyroidism in the mother can compromise the fetus and should be avoided. Pregnant women with Graves' disease may transfer large amounts of thyroid-stimulating antibody to the fetus and induce fetal thyrotoxicosis, even after thyroid ablation. Testing the newborn for thyrotoxicosis is essential in this setting. There is no evidence that treatment of pregnant thyrotoxic patients leads to impaired intellectual development in the offspring. The optimal antithyroid drug regimen for fetal thyroid status appears to be one that maintains maternal free T_4 levels near the upper limit of normal.

Breast-feeding mothers can transfer antithyroid medication in the milk, but the amount is small, especially with use of PTU, and not likely to induce significant hypothyroidism. However, discussions of potential risks and need for careful monitoring are important.

Short-term use of *beta-blocking agents* and/or *iodides* provide prompt, effective, and safe control of thyrotoxic symptoms. Symptoms improve within 2 to 7 days. Longer term use of these agents is more problematic. Beta-blocking drugs have been linked to intrauterine growth retardation, small placenta, postnatal bradycardia, and hypoglycemia. Nevertheless, the complication rate is low and use during pregnancy is generally safe. Extended use of iodides is riskier, with large, obstructing fetal goiters reported.

Surgery is usually reserved for the patient who has failed or is a bad candidate for medical treatment. Operative mortality, though low, still exceeds that associated with drug therapy. Prior to subtotal thyroidectomy, preoperative medical therapy is indicated to attain control and prevent thyroid storm.

Thyroiditis. Hyperthyroidism due to thyroiditis can be managed symptomatically with *beta-blocking agents,* because spontaneous resolution is the rule. Aspirin and occasionally corticosteroids are indicated in subacute thyroiditis to control inflammatory symptoms.

PATIENT EDUCATION

Patients with hyperthyroidism are often relieved to know that their "nervousness" is due to an underlying medical illness rather than an emotional problem and that it will improve with therapy. Patients who are taking antithyroid agents need to be instructed on prompt reporting of symptoms suggestive of agranulocytosis (*e.g.,* fever, chills), especially during the first 4 months of therapy. Those with prominent exophthalmos should be warned to come at the first sign of diplopia or visual impairment. Hyperthyroid mothers taking antithyroid drugs and eager to breast-feed their infants need not be prohibited from breast-feeding, as long as one takes the time to explain the potential risks and the importance of careful monitoring. Patients treated with radioiodine should be informed to watch for symptoms of hypothyroidism.

INDICATIONS FOR REFERRAL AND ADMISSION

Patients who are candidates for ^{131}I therapy should have a thyroid scan and be seen by the endocrinologist or radiation therapist for calculation of the dose of ^{131}I to be administered. Consultation with an endocrinologist is also indicated in the management of the pregnant or lactating hyperthyroid patient and the individual with severe exophthalmos. Referral for consideration of surgical therapy is indicated when the patient is pregnant, has obstruction to swallowing, desires cosmetic improvement, or fails antithyroid drug therapy. Hospital admission is needed if heart failure, rapid atrial fibrillation, or angina develops.

THERAPEUTIC RECOMMENDATIONS

- For initial symptomatic therapy, as well as to prepare for thyroid surgery, begin a beta-blocking agent (*e.g.,* propranolol 80 mg/day). Increase dose daily until symptoms are controlled. Use with extreme caution, if at all, in patients with underlying heart failure.
- Add potassium iodide (60 mg tid) in the preoperative patient if beta-blockade does not suffice to promptly control symptoms (*e.g.,* resting heart rate >90 and persistence of exercise-induced tachycardia). Do not use for prolonged period of time; in particular, no more than 10 days in the pregnant patient.
- For patients with Graves' disease, add an antithyroid agent (*e.g.,* methimazole 10 mg tid) to beta-blocker therapy. Continue both for 4 to 8 weeks and then taper the beta-blocker as the antithyroid agent takes hold. Adjust antithyroid drug dose according to clinical status and thyroid indices (see below). Use the lowest possible dose that maintains biochemical and biologic control. Take special care and monitor use closely if given to pregnant, nursing, or elderly patients (see below).
- Monitor therapy by clinical status (*e.g.,* degree of heat intolerance, tremor, appetite, weight, resting heart rate) and serum level of free T_4; obtain a TSH determination to monitor for overtreatment and development of hypothyroidism.
- Continue antithyroid therapy for 3 to 5 months and then taper to see if remission has been attained. If relapse occurs, consider a resumption of antithyroid therapy for 12 to 24 months or a switch to another treatment modality.
- Check the leukocyte count of patients on antithyroid agents every 2 to 4 weeks during the first 4 months of therapy, then every 4 to 6 months. Stop therapy if the count falls below 1500 neutrophils per ml. (Risk of agranulocytosis is greatest in the elderly and those taking PTU or more than 30 mg per day of methimazole.)
- Consider ^{131}I therapy for patients with solitary toxic nodules, elderly patients with Graves' disease and other patients with Graves' disease who cannot be maintained on antithyroid drugs. During the 2- to 3-month period that it takes for the radioiodine to exert its full effect on the gland, continue beta-blockade. Six months after onset of treatment and at 6-month intervals thereafter, check TSH for development of hypothyroidism.
- Treat pregnant thyrotoxic patients with an antithyroid agent; PTU is preferred (starting dose is 100 mg tid); the drug can be used with acceptable safety in the patient who is eager to breast-feed, but only after the risks are fully explained and understood. Careful monitoring of thyroid status in both mother and baby is essential. Maintain pregnant patient's free T_4 levels near the upper limit of normal.
- Refer for consideration of surgery patients with neck obstruction, poor compliance in taking medication, a contraindication to or failure of antithyroid drug therapy, or a cosmetic concern. Young patients do particularly well. If surgery is contemplated, continue antithyroid or beta-blocking therapy up to the moment of surgery. Monitor for postoperative hyperthyroidism.

- Treat patients with transient hyperthyroidism due to thyroiditis symptomatically with a beta-blocking agent until the condition resolves on its own.

A.H.G.

ANNOTATED BIBLIOGRAPHY

Borst GC, Eil C, Burman KD: Euthyroid hyperthyroxemia. Ann Intern Med 98:366, 1983 (*A detailed review of the mechanisms and syndromes causing elevations in thyroid hormone levels while the patient remains clinically euthyroid; 229 references.*)

Brown J et al: Autoimmune thyroid disease—Graves' and Hashimoto's. Ann Intern Med 88:279, 1978 (*Considers pathogenesis, diagnosis, and therapy.*)

Burrow GN: The management of thyrotoxicosis in pregnancy. N Engl J Med 313:562, 1984 (*A terse, but clinically useful review; 49 references.*)

Chopra IJ, Hershman JM, Pardridge WM et al: Thyroid function in nonthyroidal illnesses. Ann Intern Med 98:946, 1983 (*Discusses the changes in thyroid hormone levels and their consequences in nonthyroidal illness.*)

Cooper DS: Which antithyroid drug? Am J Med 80:1165, 1986 (*Favors methimazole over PTU for most cases.*)

Cooper DS, Goldminz D, Levin AA et al: Agranulocytosis associated with antithyroid drugs. Ann Intern Med 98:26, 1983 (*Increasing age and dose of methimazole were associated with increased risk; the risk with use of PTU was independent of dose.*)

Dunn JT: Choice of therapy in young adults with hyperthyroidism of Graves' disease. Ann Intern Med 100:891, 1984 (*Results of a survey of 54 thyroidologists; much diversity of recommendations, though antithyroid agents were the preferred approach.*)

Feek CM, Sawers JS, Irvine WJ et al: Combination of potassium iodide and propranolol in preparation of patients with Graves' disease for thyroid surgery. N Engl J Med 302:883, 1980 (*The combination provided superior control preoperatively.*)

Forar JC, Muir AL, Sawers SA et al: Abnormal left ventricular function in hyperthyroidism. N Engl J Med 307:1165, 1982 (*Provides evidence for a reversible cardiomyopathic state directly related to excess thyroid hormone.*)

Forar JC, Miller HC, Toft AD: Occult thyrotoxicosis: A correctable cause of "idiopathic" atrial fibrillation. Am J Cardiol 44:9, 1979 (*Many of the patients in this series with unexplained AF had normal serum thyroid hormone levels, but were diagnosed by their abnormal TSH response to TRH indicative of hyperthyroidism.*)

Gamblin GT, Harper DG, Galentine P et al: Prevalence of increased intraocular pressure in Graves' disease. N Engl J Med 308:420, 1983 (*Reports evidence of frequent subclinical eye involvement, suggesting it is an invariable part of the disease.*)

Greer MA, Kammer H, Bouma DJ: Short-term antithyroid drug therapy for the thyrotoxicosis of Graves' disease. N Engl J Med 297:173, 1977 (*A 3- to 5-month course of therapy was nearly as effective as the standard 1- to 2-year course of treatment.*)

Holm LE, Dahlqvist I, Israelsson A: Malignant thyroid tumors after iodine-131 therapy. N Engl J Med 303:188, 1980 (*No increase in frequency or risk were noted in this cohort study with a mean follow-up period of 13 years.*)

Irvine WJ et al: Spectrum of thyroid function in patients remaining in remission after antithyroid drug therapy for thyrotoxicosis. Lancet 2:179, 1977 (*In some patients, spontaneous euthyroidism or hypothyroidism followed discontinuation of therapy.*)

Kaplan KM, Utiger RD: Diagnosis of hyperthyroidism. Clin Endocrinol Metab 7:97, 1978 (*Critical review of available diagnostic tests.*)

Mariotti S, Martino E, Cupini C, et al: Low serum thyroglobulin as a clue to the diagnosis of thyrotoxicosis factitia. N Engl J Med 307:410, 1982 (*The test is a simple means of distinguishing such patients from others with hyperthyroidism; no glandular production leads to absent thyroglobulin levels in the serum.*)

Momotani N, Noh J, Oyanagi H et al: Antithyroid drug therapy for Graves' disease during pregnancy. N Engl J Med 315:24, 1986 (*A Japanese study suggesting that the optimal antithyroid regimen for the fetus is one that maintains maternal free T_4 in the mildly thyrotoxic range.*)

Ross DS: New sensitive immunoradiometric assays for thyrotropin. Ann Intern Med 104:718, 1986 (*An editorial suggesting the test is very sensitive for diagnosis of hyperthyroidism and may prove to be the best screening test for the condition.*)

Ross DS, Ridgway EC, Daniels GH: Successful treatment of solitary toxic thyroid nodules with relatively low dose iodine 131, with a low prevalence of hypothyroidism. Ann Intern Med 101:488, 1984 (*Reports excellent efficacy and safety; argues that high doses are unnecessary.*)

Sakata S, Nakamura S, Miura K: Autoantibodies against thyroid hormone or iodothyronine. Ann Intern Med 103:579, 1985 (*Autoantibodies distort the results of radioimmunoassays of serum hormone levels, but do not seriously interfere with gland function; a comprehensive review: 95 references.*)

Sridama V, McCormick M, Kaplan EL et al: Long-term follow-up of compensated low-dose ^{131}I therapy for Graves' disease. N Engl J Med 311:426, 1984 (*Low-dose ^{131}I treatment gave less control and yet no major reduction in long-term development of hypothyroidism.*)

Strakosch CR, Wenzel BE, Row VV et al: Immunology of autoimmune thyroid disease. N Engl J Med 307:1499, 1982 (*Good review: 79 references.*)

Utiger RD: Beta-adrenergic antagonist therapy for hyperthyroid Graves' disease. N Engl J Med 310:1597, 1984 (*An editorial summarizing the use of beta-blockade as well as other modalities for treatment of Graves' disease.*)

102
Management of Hypothyroidism

The development of accurate and relatively inexpensive techniques for diagnosis of hypothyroidism and the availability of levothyroxine have greatly facilitated management of hypothyroidism. The majority of hypothyroid patients have primary disease of the thyroid gland, with chronic (Hashimoto's) thyroiditis, idiopathic thyroid atrophy, previous ^{131}I therapy, and subtotal thyroidectomy being the leading causes. As much as 5% of the elderly population manifests evidence of hypothyroidism, most of it resulting from thyroiditis. Less common etiologies include neck irradiation, iodide administration, and use of lithium or para-aminosalicylic acid. Pituitary insufficiency can result in secondary hypothyroidism. Rarely, hypothalamic disease is the source of difficulty. The prevalence of hypothyroidism increases with age. Women are more frequently affected than are men. Sometimes, a patient comes for evaluation, having been prescribed a thyroid preparation for unclear reasons; a decision regarding continuation of the drug is necessary. The primary physician should be able to determine when replacement therapy is indicated and to provide it with safety and precision.

PATHOPHYSIOLOGY, CLINICAL PRESENTATION, AND COURSE

The clinical manifestations of hypothyroidism reflect the decreases in metabolic rate and sensitivity to catecholamines that result from insufficient circulating thyroid hormone. Early symptoms are gradual in onset and may occur before serum free thyroxine levels fall below normal limits (thyroid-stimulating hormone is elevated). The patient typically complains of fatigue, moderately dry skin, heavy menstrual periods, slight weight gain, or cold intolerance. These symptoms are followed over the next few months by reports of very dry skin, coarse hair, hoarseness, continued weight gain (though appetite is minimal), and slightly impaired mental activity. Later, depression may be evident.

In late stages, hydrophilic mucopolysaccharide accumulates subcutaneously, producing the myxedematous changes that characterize this severe form of the disease; the skin becomes doughy, the face puffy, the tongue large, expression dull, and mentation slow, even lethargic. Muscle weakness, joint complaints, diminution in hearing, and carpal tunnel syndrome are also found. Daytime sleepiness in severely myxedematous patients suggests that obstructive sleep apnea may be occurring.

On examination, the thyroid gland is not palpable unless there is a goiter, which may be due to thyroiditis, hereditary defects in thyroxine synthesis, or use of iodides, PAS, or lithium. The heart may show signs of dilatation or an effusion. Bowel sounds are diminished, and the relaxation phase of the deep tendon reflexes is slowed or "hung up." A mild anemia may be present (see Chapter 77) and hypercholesterolemia is often noted. In severe cases of myxedema, dilutional hyponatremia occurs as a result of inadequate renal blood flow. A warning of impending myxedema coma is a rise in arterial pCO_2, which takes place as the respiratory drive weakens.

In secondary hypothyroidism there may be signs of concurrent ovarian and adrenal insufficiency, such as loss of axillary and pubic hair, amenorrhea, and postural hypotension. Myxedematous changes tend to be less marked than with primary hypothyroidism.

The onset of hypothyroidism is, in most instances, gradual and its course progressive. At times, hyperthyroidism precedes hypothyroidism as in various forms of thyroiditis (see Chapter 101), but eventually the disease or its treatment decreases thyroid reserve. Studies of *pregnant women* have revealed a previously unappreciated form of *transient thyroiditis* that occurs 3 to 6 months after delivery. First, symptoms of mild hyperthyroidism, mistakenly attributed to "tension," occur, followed by fatigue and depression resulting from onset of hypothyroidism. The symptoms resolve spontaneously over 2 to 3 months, but tend to recur with subsequent pregnancies. An incidence of up to 5% has been reported. Drugs that have an antithyroid effect produce a rapid but reversible form of hypothyroidism.

Regardless of etiology, changes in laboratory parameters may precede clinical manifestations. The earliest development is an increase in thyroid-releasing hormone (TRH). The TRH induces secretion of thyroid-stimulating hormone (TSH) and an increase in basal TSH levels. At this stage, many patients have thyroid hormone levels that remain "within normal limits," yet may already be mildly symptomatic. Shortly thereafter, free thyroxine decreases, and the onset of more prominent symptoms follows.

PRINCIPLES OF MANAGEMENT

Diagnosis. When the diagnosis is in question, the first step should be to *stop all thyroid medications*. Patients who are taking a thyroid preparation but lack documentation of hypothyroidism can stop replacement therapy without serious risk. Abrupt cessation of exogenous thyroid hormone therapy is not dangerous, as long as there is no prior history of severe hypothyroidism; adequate and prompt (though submaximal) responses of the pituitary and thyroid gland occur when hormone intake is halted. It takes about 5 weeks for full function to return, at which time testing for hypothyroidism can be carried out.

The diagnosis of *primary hypothyroidism* is readily achieved by demonstrating a *low free T_4* (or low free T_4 index) and an *increased TSH*. The TSH is the more sensitive indicator of primary hypothyroidism and the test of choice. The range of normal for the free T_4 is wide. A single free T_4 determination may not detect the patient who has a modest yet physiologically important decline in hormone level, because the serum concentrations may remain within normal limits. Moreover, antithyroid antibodies can interfere with the commonly used immunoassays and produce falsely high or low readings, depending on the type of assay used. Nevertheless, the free thyroxine level is a better measure of thyroid function than *total T_4,* which is affected by changes in protein binding.

Often, measurement of total T_3 is routinely ordered as part of a battery of thyroid function tests. The assay is expensive to perform, and the results correlate poorly with thyroid status, affected by such events as a fall in peripheral conversion of T_4 to T_3, which is common in the elderly. The serum cholesterol and radioactive iodine uptake are also insensitive tests that contribute little to the diagnostic evaluation.

Secondary hypothyroidism should be suspected when the TSH level is inappropriately low in the setting of clinical hypothyroidism. To test pituitary reserve, one can give TRH and note the TSH response. In secondary hypothyroidism, there is little increase in TSH, whereas in primary hypothyroidism and in hypothalamic disease a surge in TSH secretion occurs.

Treatment of mild to moderate hypothyroidism is best done gradually, because hypothyroid patients are very sensitive to the effects of thyroxine. An excessive rate of replacement may cause palpitations, tremor, nervousness, or even angina. Full replacement doses of L-thyroxine average between 100 and 150 μg per day. These doses are lower than those previously listed because contemporary L-thyroxine preparations are more potent than previous ones. Schedules for treatment depend on age, the presence of cardiac disease, and the severity of symptoms. Young, otherwise healthy patients can be started on 50 μg per day of thyroxine. This dosage can be increased in 25- to 50-μg increments every 2 weeks until a euthyroid state is achieved.

In patients over age 50 who are at risk for coronary disease, more cautious replacement is indicated. Thyroid medication may produce angina, sinus tachycardia, or arrhythmias (particularly atrial fibrillation) in patients with underlying coronary artery disease. It may be necessary to initiate therapy in these patients with 25 μg per day. If angina or cardiac symptoms occur, the dosage of thyroid hormone should be reduced; when increments are resumed, the dosage should be increased more slowly. Some advocate the concurrent administration of propranolol to protect the heart from overstimulation by thyroid replacement. This may be particularly useful in patients with angina. However, adequate control of angina usually necessitates settling for incomplete correction of hypothyroidism.

Despite the potential risks, it has been standard practice to administer thyroid replacement therapy to coronary disease patients before surgery, out of concern for their response to anesthesia and the stress of an operative procedure. It is now clear that mildly to moderately hypothyroid patients with coronary disease can safely undergo urgent surgery (including bypass procedures) without prior replacement. The rate of complications is no greater than that for nonhypothyroid patients, and the cardiac risks are lessened. Careful preoperative anesthesia planning is essential.

L-thyroxine is the agent of choice for replacement therapy on the basis of uniform bioavailability, cost, safety, and ease of monitoring therapy (the serum T_4 level directly reflects the dosage utilized). The onset of effect is gradual; the agent's half-life is about 24 hours, making once-a-day therapy possible. Some of the drug is converted peripherally to T_3, making it unnecessary to use the more expensive preparations, which contain mixtures of T_4 and T_3. The use of exogenous T_3 is considered inadvisable for replacement purposes, especially in older patients, because it causes rapid increases in metabolic rate and oxygen demand and can precipitate angina. Moreover, its short half-life produces wide swings in T_3 levels and requires frequent administration. For these reasons, many physicians find it best to switch patients from older thyroid hormone preparations and T_3 to L-thyroxine.

L-thyroxine has its own shortcomings, such as occasional reports of variation in biologic activity and tablet content of some commercial preparations. Patients who have inadequate serum thyroid levels when taking what ought to be an adequate dosage should be switched to another brand of L-thyroxine.

Adequate replacement should result in resolution of fatigue, loss of excess weight, and reversal of autonomic symptoms. The first signs of response are modest loss of weight, increase in pulse rate, and resolution of constipation. Myxedematous skin changes, pleural and pericardial effusions, and elevated creatine phosphokinase levels also normalize, but require more time. Most patients feel better within 2 weeks, and clinical resolution is usually complete by 3 months.

Laboratory *monitoring* of replacement requires measurement of TSH, T_4, and free T_4. *TSH* is best for determining the adequacy of the replacement dosage to correct hypothyroidism, but it cannot distinguish excessive from physiologic thyroxine doses. A *free T_4* or T_4 level will detect excesses, except during the first 6 months of treatment, when reduced metabolic clearance of thyroid hormone causes elevated serum thyroxine concentrations in patients who are not thyrotoxic. Serum thyroxine levels obtained during the first 6 months of therapy are not reliable guides to proper replacement dosage and, if ordered at all, should be interpreted only in the context of the patient's clinical status.

Once a stable replacement dosage is achieved, twice-yearly assessments are probably sufficient. Any upward adjustments in dosage should be made in small increments.

The treatment and monitoring of *secondary hypothyroidism* must take into account the lack of TSH response and probable coexistence of adrenal and ovarian hypofunction. Because thyroid replacement and the resultant rise in metabolic rate can precipitate addisonian crisis, adrenal function should be assessed with an ACTH stimulation test before replacement therapy is prescribed in any patient suspected of having secondary hypothyroidism. Treatment with cortisone acetate should precede L–T_4 replacement.

Therapy for primary hypothyroidism is continued indefinitely.

THERAPEUTIC RECOMMENDATIONS

- Stop any exogenous thyroid or antithyroid medication if reason for use is unclear.
- Confirm the diagnosis of hypothyroidism with TSH and free T_4 determinations.
- If the TSH is not appropriately elevated, test for pituitary insufficiency.

Primary Hypothyroidism

- If possible, stop all drugs with potential antithyroid effect (*e.g.,* iodides, PAS, lithium).
- Begin replacement with L-thyroxine, initiating therapy with 50 μg per day in most patients, but using 25 μg in those with clinical coronary disease.
- Increase the dosage by 25 to 50 μg every few weeks, according to clinical response, tolerance of side-effects (*e.g.,* tremor, angina, or arrhythmias), and TSH and free T_4 levels. Elderly patients and those with coronary disease may require smaller, more gradual increments in dosage.
- Patients with mild to moderate hypothyroidism and underlying coronary disease need not receive replacement therapy before urgent surgery. However, careful anesthesia planning is necessary.
- Average replacement dosages are in the range of 100 μg to 150 μg per day of L-thyroxine. L-thyroxine is the drug of choice. Combination preparations containing T_3 are unnecessary, since T_4 is converted peripherally to T_3.
- Therapy can be monitored by measurement of TSH and free T_4. The TSH is needed to detect undertreatment, and the free T_4, overtreatment. However, hormone measurements during the first 6 months may be high because of reduced hormone metabolism.

- Patients with low serum levels who are taking what ought to be adequate replacement dosages should be switched to another brand of L-thyroxine.

Secondary Hypothyroidism

- Perform an ACTH stimulation test to assess adrenal reserve. If it is low, give cortisone acetate *before* providing thyroid replacement.
- Replace thyroid hormone as for primary hypothyroidism.
- Monitor therapy by following clinical signs and free T_4.

PATIENT EDUCATION

Euthyroid patients who are inappropriately placed on exogenous thyroid for treatment of fatigue or obesity are often reluctant to give up the medication. Documenting that their thyroid status is perfectly normal is an essential first step to taking them off the medication successfully. Often a request from the physician to temporarily halt thyroid hormone for 5 weeks to measure TSH and free T_4 is agreed to. Usually there is little change in how the patient feels, and this helps to convince the patient that exogenous hormone is unnecessary.

Hypothyroid patients need to be warned of the danger of increasing their medication too rapidly or of taking more than is prescribed. Unfortunately, some patients adjust their dosages on the basis of other symptoms they mistakenly attribute to hypothyroidism, for example, those of depression. All patients should be instructed to measure and record their weight regularly and report any unexplained change of 5 pounds or more.

It is imperative that the patient and family be instructed in the signs of worsening hypothyroidism. Hypothyroid patients have been known to stop taking their thyroid medication. The importance of continuing therapy indefinitely must be emphasized to the patient and persons close to him.

A.H.G.

ANNOTATED BIBLIOGRAPHY

Amino N, Mori H, Iwatani Y et al: High prevalence of transient post-partum thyrotoxicosis and hypothyroidism. N Engl J Med 306:849, 1982. (*The initial report of this phenomenon, from Japan; the incidence was 5% and it was attributed to an autoimmune thyroiditis.*)

Brown ME, Refetoff S: Transient elevation of serum thyroid hormone concentration after initiation of replacement therapy in myxedema. Ann Intern Med 92:491, 1980. (*Transient elevations were noted during the first 6 months, which limited the usefulness of the T_4 and free T_4 for determinating the optimal replacement dosage.*)

Cooper DS, Halpern R, Wood L et al: L-thyroxine therapy in subclinical hypothyroidism. Ann Intern Med 101:18, 1984. (*Docu-*

ments that symptoms are actually common in such patients and that replacement therapy is helpful in eliminating them.)

Hennessey JV, Evual JE, Tseng Y-C et al: L-thyroxine dosage: A re-evaluation of therapy with contemporary preparations. Ann Intern Med 105:11, 1986. (*Newer preparations are more potent, requiring lower replacement doses.*)

Hurley JR: Thyroid disease in the elderly. Med Clin North Am 67: 497, 1983. (*Comprehensive review; high prevalence of hypothyroidism is found in this age group.*)

Inada M et al: Estimation of thyroxine and triiodothyronine distribution and the conversion rate of thyroxine to triiodothyronine in man. J Clin Invest 55:1337, 1975. (*Most T_3 derives from peripheral conversion of T_4, both in normal individuals and in hypothyroid patients. These data suggest that replacement therapy using T_3–T_4 mixtures is unnecessary and that L-thyroxine should suffice.*)

Klein I, Levey GS: Universal manifestations of hypothyroidism. Arch Intern Med 144:123, 1983. (*Detailed review of clinical presentations.*)

Krugman L, Hershman J, Chopra I et al: Patterns of recovery of the hypothalamic–pituitary–thyroid axis in patients taken off chronic thyroid therapy. J Clin Endocrinol Metab 41:70, 1975. (*Full recovery of pituitary and thyroid responsiveness to TRH occurred in euthyroid patients 5 weeks after withdrawal of chronic thyroid hormone therapy.*)

Levine HD: Compromise therapy in the patient with angina pectoris and hypothyroidism. Am J Med 69:411, 1980. (*Details the difficulties in adequately controlling angina in the context of fully correcting the hypothyroidism.*)

Rootwelt K, Solberg HE: Optimum laboratory test combinations for thyroid function studies, selected by discriminant analysis. Scan J Clin Lab Invest 38:477, 1978. (*The free T_4 and TSH are the best studies for detection of hypothyroidism; serum cholesterol, RAI uptake, and other tests commonly ordered were of little use.*)

Rosenbaum RL, Barzel US: Levothyroxine replacement dose for primary hypothyroidism decreases with age. Ann Intern Med 96: 53, 1982. (*Levothyroxine dose needed for complete replacement appeared to be inversely correlated with age.*)

Sawin CT, Surks MI, London M et al: Oral thyroxine: Variation and biologic action in tablet content. Ann Intern Med 100:641, 1984. (*Serum thyroxine levels fell when patients were switched from Levothroid to Synthroid due to a 20% to 30% lower thyroxine content of Synthroid. This difference has been corrected, but is an example of what sometimes occurs.*)

Sakata S, Nakamura S, Miura K: Autoantibodies against thyroid hormones. Ann Intern Med 103:579, 1985. (*Unexpectedly low serum T_4 or free T_4 levels may be due to the presence of autoantibodies interfering with the assay; TSH will be normal.*)

Stock J, Sarks M, Oppenheimer J: Replacement dosage of L-thyroxine in hypothyroidism. N Engl J Med 290:529, 1974. (*Mean replacement dosage needed was 169 μg, as determined by return of TSH levels to normal. T_3 levels were close to normal after the use of T_4, demonstrating peripheral conversion of T_4 to T_3 and lack of need to supply T_3.*)

103

Glucocorticosteroid Therapy

The therapeutic potency of glucocorticosteroids has led to their widespread and, sometimes, indiscriminant use. A number of questions must be addressed before steroid therapy is initiated: (1) Is the underlying disorder of such severity that the benefits of therapy outweigh the substantial risk of serious side-effects? (2) Will prolonged treatment be required, or will a brief, limited course suffice? (3) Have alternative, less morbid therapies been maximally utilized? (4) Does the patient have any underlying condition that will worsen on steroid therapy or predispose him to drug-induced complications? (5) Can alternate-day therapy be utilized?

The primary physician must decide when and how to institute steroid therapy, whether to use daily or alternate-day treatment, and how to withdraw chronic glucocorticoid treatment safely.

ADVERSE EFFECTS

The adverse effects of glucocorticosteroid therapy are a function of dosage and duration of use. A few are irreversible; fortunately, most resolve within several months of terminating therapy.

Suppression of the hypothalamic–pituitary–adrenal (HPA) axis is among the most important consequences of chronic glucocorticoid use. An incompletely resolved issue is how long and at what dosage therapy must be given to suppress the HPA axis to a clinically significant degree. Most data suggest that clinically important HPA suppression does not occur until dosages in the range of 20 to 30 mg of prednisone are taken daily for at least 2 to 4 weeks, although reduced responsiveness to exogenous ACTH stimulation and metyrapone have been noted after as few as 5 days initiation of steroid treatment.

Daily physiologic dosages of glucocorticosteroids (*e.g.,* 5 to 7.5 mg of prednisone) given in the morning do not cause suppression of any consequence, but if the same dosages are given at night, normal diurnal cortisol secretion is inhibited. Dosages just above the physiologic range are suppressive after about a month of use. Alternate-day therapy utilizing short- or intermediate-acting preparations taken at 8 A.M. every other day does not induce clinically significant HPA suppression. Neither does a cyclic program of 5 days of daily therapy followed by 2½ weeks off therapy. However, cycles of 2 weeks on/2 weeks off do lead to HPA suppression. A single daily pharmacologic dosage of glucocorticoid produces less HPA suppression than does the same dosage divided over the course of the day.

After chronic use of pharmacologic dosages, it takes about 12 months for full recovery of the HPA axis to occur (as measured by response to exogenous ACTH, metyrapone, or insulin tolerance testing). Hypothalamic–pituitary function returns first, beginning 2 to 5 months after cessation of suppressive therapy, and is manifested by appropriate plasma ACTH levels that demonstrate a normal diurnal pattern. Signs of adrenal recovery become evident at 6 to 9 months, with return of the baseline serum cortisol to normal; maximal adrenal response to ACTH does not reappear until 9 to 12 months.

Laboratory data on suppression and recovery of HPA activity are relatively abundant, compared with the scant amount of clinical information available on how long a patient is at risk for serious adrenal insufficiency after cessation of steroid use. Most guidelines for replacement therapy in times of stress are based on the results of laboratory investigation, though clinical data are beginning to accumulate. There is no proven method for accelerating the restoration of normal HPA function once inhibition has occurred. The administration of ACTH does not appear to speed adrenal recovery.

A number of other important metabolic and endocrinologic problems result from chronic corticosteroid use. *Negative nitrogen balance* (due to inhibition of protein synthesis and enhancement of protein catabolism) is believed to be partially responsible for reduced muscle mass, weakness, thinning of the skin, and striae formation. *Glucose intolerance* is common. Mechanisms include increases in peripheral insulin resistance, gluconeogenesis, glucagon secretion, and substrate availability. Usually the glucose intolerance is mild, does not lead to ketosis, and resolves when therapy is stopped. In patients who develop carbohydrate intolerance, the effect appears to be dose-related. *Fat redistribution* accounts for the characteristic truncal obesity and cushingoid appearance. This change as well as negative nitrogen balance are minimized by using alternate-day therapy or administering daily physiologic doses each morning, but not by using ACTH or daily pharmacologic glucocorticoid dosages.

Enhanced susceptibility to infection results from the anti-inflammatory and immunosuppressive actions of corticosteroids. Bacterial infections are common. Candidiasis and aspergillosis sometimes result. Herpes zoster, varicella, vaccinia, and cytomegalovirus are the principal viral infections encountered in patients on steroids. Reactivation of tuberculosis is a well-recognized risk (see Chapter 47).

Osteoporosis develops when large steroid doses are used over prolonged periods. The incidence is unknown because measuring skeletal mass accurately is difficult and expensive. The precise relationship between dosage, duration of use, and risk of osteoporosis remains unclear, though, there is some suggestion that alternate-day therapy minimizes the chance of serious osteoporosis. Patients with a predisposition to osteoporosis, such as menopausal women and immobilized individuals, appear to be among the most susceptible. The axial skeleton is affected more than the limbs, and vertebral compression fractures may result. *Aseptic necrosis* of the femoral head and other bones is a well-recognized but rare skeletal complication; sometimes it may be due to the underlying illness for which corticosteroids are being given, as is the case in rheumatoid arthritis.

The relationship between *peptic ulceration* and glucocorticoid therapy remains unresolved. Multiple, randomized controlled trials have produced conflicting results, as have two major meta-analyses examining pooled data from such trials (see Chapter 64). Even if steroids do cause ulcers, the risk is small. Hotly debated is the degree to which risk is a function of dosage and duration of exposure. Prolonged use of high dosages appears to confer the greatest chance of ulceration, though only in the range of a 1% to 2% increase in incidence. Antacids and food do not interfere with absorption of oral steroid preparations.

Myopathy may be seen in patients on chronic therapy when large dosages are utilized. Proximal muscle wasting and weakness of the lower extremities are characteristic; patients complain of difficulty climbing stairs. Average time of onset is 5 months into treatment. Muscle enzymes are normal. The condition is reversible. Exercise may help minimize it.

Psychological and *behavioral changes* are of considerable importance, and are particularly common in the elderly. The reported incidence is as high as 25% to 40% of patients receiving steroid therapy. Increased appetite, mild euphoria, and changes in sleep patterns are rather common at the beginning of treatment. Psychoses, which are not predictably related to dosage or duration of therapy, can occur; they slowly respond to reduction or cessation of steroid use. Some clinicians argue that the patient's premorbid personality plays a role, while others deny this. Steroid therapy can exacerbate previous psychiatric disease.

Posterior subcapsular cataracts are reported in 10% to 35% of cases. They are usually dosage- and duration-dependent. A few require removal; most do not. *Hypertension* and *fluid retention* with peripheral edema are more common when agents with mineralocorticoid effects are used (see Table 103-1), and are not dependent on preexistence of elevated blood pressure. Again, dosage and duration of therapy are important factors. *Electrolyte derangements* are common, especially hypokalemia. *Acute pancreatitis* is noted with increased frequency in patients taking corticosteroids. *Acne* is seen more often with ACTH use than with glucocorticoids, because of stimulation of adrenal androgen production, but the problem does bother patients on corticosteroids. *Panniculitis* is unique to iatrogenic Cushing's syndrome.

PRINCIPLES OF THERAPY

The cardinal principle of steroid therapy is to obtain the maximal therapeutic benefit while minimizing the compli-

Table 103-1. Commonly Used Glucocorticoids

DURATION OF ACTION	GLUCOCORTICOID POTENCY*	EQUIVALENT GLUCOCORTICOID DOSE (MG)	MINERALOCORTICOID ACTIVITY
Short-acting			
Cortisol (hydrocortisone)	1	20	Yes†
Cortisone	0.8	25	Yes†
Prednisone	4	5	No
Prednisolone	4	5	No
Methylprednisolone	5	4	No
Intermediate-acting			
Triamcinolone	5	4	No
Long-acting			
Betamethasone	25	0.60	No
Dexamethasone	30	0.75	No

* The values given for glucocorticoid potency are relative. Cortisol is arbitrarily assigned a value of 1.

† Mineralocorticoid effects are dose related. At dosages close to or within the basal physiologic range for glucocorticoid activity, no such effect may be detectable.

Adapted from Axelrod L: Glucocorticoid therapy. Medicine 55:39, 1976)

cations and potential problems inherent to interfering with normal hypothalamic–pituitary–adrenal function. Steroids usually do not cure disease or alter its natural history; rather they suppress the inflammatory response or modify the immunologic abnormality. Steroid treatment is in some sense symptomatic, and therefore one must carefully weigh the perceived therapeutic benefit against the potential risks.

A short course of steroid therapy (7 to 14 days) can be very useful in selected situations (*e.g.,* acute asthma, contact dermatitis) and is relatively free of adverse effects (appetite stimulation and restlessness are the major ones). There are no long-term consequences. The decision to initiate more prolonged steroid therapy requires greater consideration of the risks, which are more substantial.

Selection of Agent. Once it has been determined that the potential benefits outweigh the probable risks of therapy, the physician faces the task of deciding which agent to use, for how long, at what dose, and in what schedule. Minimizing HPA suppression is a major consideration and best accomplished by using a short-acting agent, such as prednisone (see Table 103-1), on an alternate-day schedule, at the smallest possible dosage for the shortest period of time. It is also preferable, when anti-inflammatory or immunosuppressive effects are desired, to use a preparation that has the least mineralocorticoid activity (see Table 103-1), and it is certainly important to continue using maximal nonsteroidal therapy, so that the steroid dosage prescribed is the lowest one possible.

Prednisone and prednisolone are identical in action. Prednisone is rapidly metabolized to prednisolone by the liver. Oral prednisolone is preferred in patients with liver failure.

Although ACTH does not cause clinically significant HPA

suppression or adrenal atrophy, it must be given parenterally, and there is no way to know how much glucocorticoid effect is obtained from a given dosage. These disadvantages, as well as induction of mineralocorticoid and androgenic effects, limit its usefulness. ACTH has not been shown to be superior to prednisone, although it is used preferentially by many neurologists for exacerbations of multiple sclerosis.

Alternate-Day Therapy. Most conditions that require corticosteroid treatment can be adequately managed with *alternate-day therapy,* although it is often necessary to begin with a program of daily steroids when symptoms are severe and the disease is very active. Important advantages of alternate-day treatment are avoidance of significant HPA suppression and minimization of cushingoid side-effects, without a substantial loss of anti-inflammatory activity. It appears that the anti-inflammatory effects of glucocorticosteroids persist longer (up to 3 days) than the undesirable metabolic effects. Other adverse effects that are reduced or eliminated by an alternate-day schedule include inhibition of delayed hypersensitivity, susceptibility to infection, negative nitrogen balance, fluid retention, hypertension, and psychological and behavioral disturbances.

Alternate-day therapy by itself will not prevent HPA suppression if a long-acting steroid preparation is used (*e.g.,* dexamethasone). Moreover, therapy must be truly alternate-day, with the total dosage given first thing in the morning every other day; intermittent therapy or doses given throughout the day every other day do not preserve HPA responsiveness.

Although daily steroid therapy is often required to bring florid disease under control, alternate-day treatment is as effective, or nearly as effective, in maintaining control. Only temporal arteritis and case reports of fulminant ulcerative colitis and pemphigus vulgaris have been found to require daily steroid doses to maintain control of symptoms and disease activity. In fulminant ulcerative colitis, high-dosage, alternate-day therapy has not been tried in a systematic fashion. Among the conditions found to respond well to alternate-day corticosteroids are certain forms of the nephrotic syndrome (see Chapter 139), sarcoidosis (see Chapter 48), myasthenia gravis, and asthma (see Chapter 45).

Once daily steroid treatment has achieved control of disease activity, it is advisable to attempt switching the patient to alternate-day therapy. The objective is to maintain the same total steroid dosage while gradually increasing the dosage on the first day and decreasing it on the second day, so that a point is reached where a double dose is given every other day, with no drug given in between. How fast the changeover can be made varies, depending on the activity of the underlying disease, the duration of therapy, degree of HPA suppression, and the patient's cooperativeness. A rough guideline for switching to alternate-day therapy is to make changes in increments of 10 mg of prednisone (or its equivalent) when the daily prednisone dosage is greater than 40 mg, and in 5-mg increments when the daily dosage is between 20 and 40 mg. Below 20 mg per day, the change ought to be in amounts of 2.5 mg. The interval between changes ranges from 1 day to several weeks and is determined empirically, based on clinical response. It is important to keep in mind that most patients who have been on a daily steroid program for more than 2 weeks probably have some degree of HPA suppression.

Daily Therapy. When *daily therapy* is necessary, HPA suppression can be minimized by having the patient take the entire dosage first thing in the morning and by using a short-acting glucocorticoid at the lowest possible dosage. Daily single-dose regimens may be as effective or nearly as effective as divided-dose regimens in controlling underlying illness; however, in contrast with alternate-day therapy, manifestations of Cushing's syndrome are not prevented.

Withdrawing Therapy. The abrupt withdrawal of patients from daily steroid therapy after more than a month at dosages in excess of 20 to 30 mg of prednisone per day can precipitate adrenal insufficiency, a flare-up of the underlying illness, or a withdrawal syndrome. There is no way to speed HPA recovery, nor are there specific schedules for reducing the dosage. One must monitor disease activity and decrease the dosage empirically in small amounts, watching for flare-up of disease or signs of adrenal insufficiency such as hypotension and gastrointestinal distress.

One empirical approach to reducing the dosage toward physiologic levels is to make changes in decrements of 10 mg of prednisone or its equivalent every 1 to 3 weeks, as long as the dosage is above 40 mg. Below 40 mg, the decrement is 5

mg. Once a physiologic dose of prednisone is reached (5 to 7.5 mg per day), the patient can be switched to 1-mg prednisone tablets or the equivalent dosage of hydrocortisone, so that further reductions in dosage can be made in smaller steps than is possible using 5-mg prednisone tablets. Weekly or biweekly reductions can then be carried out in steps of 1 mg of prednisone at a time, as permitted by disease activity.

During the tapering process, some patients develop a *steroid withdrawal syndrome,* characterized by depression, myalgias, arthralgias, anorexia, headaches, nausea, and lethargy. Studies have failed to show a relationship between these symptoms and low cortisol or 17-hydroxycorticosteroid levels. In most instances, complaints are reported when levels are normal or even elevated, but falling rapidly. HPA responsiveness has also been found to be normal in many of these patients. The mechanisms responsible for this syndrome are unknown, but seem to be linked to the rapidity with which dosage is tapered.

At times of anticipated stress, such as preoperatively, when it is necessary to know what the status of the HPA axis is and whether or not supplementary steroid therapy is needed, an *ACTH stimulation test* can provide an indication of adrenal reserve. Because adrenal response is the last component of the HPA system to return, testing of suppression can be done with ACTH stimulation. A test injection of synthetic ACTH (*e.g.,* Cortrosyn) is given intravenously; if in 1 hour the serum cortisol is greater than 18 μg per 100 ml, there is no need to supplement for stress. The response of the serum cortisol to intravenous ACTH stimulation corresponds to the cortisol level that can be expected from such stresses as general anesthesia and surgery.

If the patient cannot mount an adequate cortisol response, or testing is impractical because of urgency or unavailability of agents or assays, corticosteroid supplementation should be given for acute stress. Even minor illnesses such as gastroenteritis, influenza, or pharyngitis are indications for an additional 100 mg of hydrocortisone per day in divided doses. This will also suffice for minor surgical procedures such as dental extraction. During major stress, such as trauma or surgery, the patient should be given 100 mg of hydrocortisone every 6 to 8 hours. The need to continue supplementation can be evaluated by repeat ACTH stimulation testing.

PATIENT EDUCATION

Steroids should be used with caution in patients whose reliability or intelligence is in question, because of the risk of HPA suppression and adrenocortical insufficiency. Individuals on alternate-day therapy need instruction on the importance of keeping to the every-other-day schedule and taking their medication around 8 A.M. so as to minimize the risk of suppression. Patients on suppressive dosage of steroid should be informed of the need for steroid supplementation when there is stress or illness and should wear an identification bracelet stating they take a corticosteroid. Patients must understand the need to contact the physician and to increase steroid dosage when subjected to physiologic stress. The family can be given a prepackaged syringe containing dexamethasone phosphate, 4 mg, to be injected intramuscularly if the patient should become unconscious or so ill he cannot take steroids by mouth.

Many patients are fearful or reluctant to be taken off chronic steroid therapy because of concern for recrudescence of the underlying illness or because malaise is experienced as the drug is tapered. A detailed review of the side-effects of prolonged therapy is necessary so that the rationale for reducing the dosage and the desirability of eventually discontinuing corticosteroids are understood and appreciated. Any change in dosage and schedule should be written out. When chronic, daily, high-dosage therapy is required, the psychological impact of adverse effects (*e.g.,* cushingoid features) can be lessened by forewarning the patient of their likelihood and at least partial reversibility.

THERAPEUTIC RECOMMENDATIONS

- Use glucocorticoids only when other forms of therapy have been used in maximal dosages and proven inadequate, and when the risks of steroid use are outweighed by the therapeutic benefit expected.
- Add the least possible dosage of corticosteroid to the ongoing treatment program, but *do not replace* previous therapy with steroid treatment when there is partial benefit from nonsteroidal agents.
- Add antacids to the program of patients who will be taking high dosages for prolonged periods of time. The antacid can be taken at the same time as the steroid.
- Steroids can be taken with food; absorption is not impaired.
- When anti-inflammatory or immunosuppressive effects are desired, use a preparation with the fewest possible mineralocorticoid effects (*e.g.,* prednisone). ACTH offers few advantages and a number of disadvantages; it must be given parenterally, and it stimulates mineralocorticoid and androgen production.
- Try initiating therapy on an alternate-day basis if symptoms are not severe; HPA suppression and cushingoid effects are thus avoided. Most conditions respond as well, or nearly as well, to alternate-day doses as to daily ones, though there are exceptions.
- If alternate-day therapy is not successful or symptoms are severe, daily therapy ought to be used. Try to give the entire dose in the morning to minimize HPA suppression.
- Since HPA suppression may occur after as little as 20 mg to 30 mg of prednisone given daily for 7 to 10 days and may not completely return to normal for 9 to 12 months, patients on daily pharmacologic doses should be advised

of the need to supplement their steroid intake when under stress or experiencing an acute illness; 100 mg per day of hydrocortisone or its equivalent should be prescribed in divided doses. It usually suffices for minor illnesses; 100 mg of hydrocortisone every 8 hours is needed for trauma or surgery. Give the patient's family a prepackaged syringe containing 4 mg of dexamethasone for intramuscular emergency use. ACTH stimulation testing can be performed to assess the adequacy of adrenal reserve.

- Initiate withdrawal of steroids by moving from a divided-dose schedule to a once-daily morning dose and from daily dose schedules into alternate-day therapy. Condensing divided doses into a single daily dose can usually be done rather quickly, but moving from daily to alternate-day therapy must be gradual and requires monitoring for flare-up of underlying disease and adrenal insufficiency.
- To switch from a daily to an alternate-day corticosteroid program, one increases the dosage on the first day and decreases the dosage on the second day by the equivalent of 10 mg of prednisone if the daily dosage is above 40 mg, and by 5 mg if the daily dosage is below 40 mg. Below 20 mg, the increment is 2.5 mg. The interval between changes in dosage is determined empirically, based on clinical status of the patient. The endpoint of switching occurs when the previous entire 2-day dosage is given once every other day.
- Tapering of alternate-day therapy can proceed in 10-mg decrements when the dosage is above 40 mg and 5-mg steps when it is below 40 mg. Rapidity of tapering is limited by recrudescence of disease activity and development of symptoms of withdrawal or adrenal insufficiency; it is determined empirically. Once the dosage is down to 5 mg of prednisone, switch to 20 mg of hydrocortisone or 1-mg prednisone tablets and reduce the dosage in decrements of 2.5 mg of hydrocortisone or 1 mg of prednisone.
- At a dosage level of 10 mg of hydrocortisone, check the 8:00 A.M. cortisol level. If it is greater than 18 μg per 100 ml, stop exogenous steroids; otherwise, continue therapy and do ACTH stimulation testing to determine if it is safe to taper the dosage.
- If withdrawal symptoms are a problem on alternate-day therapy, a small morning dose of hydrocortisone, 10 to 20 mg, given on the off day may help alleviate symptoms without prolonging HPA suppression.

A.H.G.

ANNOTATED BIBLIOGRAPHY

Anatruda TT Jr, Hurst MM, D'Esposo ND: Certain endocrine and metabolic facets of the steroid withdrawal syndrome. J Clin Endocrinol Metab 25:1207, 1965 (*The steroid withdrawal syndrome is not due to inadequate serum levels of steroid: a classic study.*)

Axelrod L: Glucocorticoid therapy. Medicine 55:39, 1976 (*A superb review concentrating on the duration of suppression of the pituitary-*

adrenal axis, the relative merits of single-dose therapy, alternate-day therapy, and the fact that ACTH has not been demonstrated superior to orally administered glucocorticoids; 188 references.)

Byyny RL: Withdrawal from glucocorticoid therapy. N Engl J Med 295:30, 1976 (*A protocol for withdrawal is suggested which is eminently reasonable and feasible.*)

Dale DC, Fauci AS, Wolff SM: Alternate day prednisone, leukocyte kinetics and susceptibility to infections. N Engl J Med 29:1154, 1974 (*An important study establishing that alternate-day steroid therapy leaves leukocyte counts, inflammatory responses and neutrophil half-life normal, compared with daily steroid therapy, which causes significant reductions.*)

Fujieda K, Reyes FI, Blankenstein J et al: Pituitary–adrenal function in women treated with low doses of prednisone. Am J Obstet Gynecol 137:962, 1980 (*As little as 5 mg per day can cause detectable but not clinically significant suppression of the adrenal-pituitary axis.*)

Graeber AL, Ney RL, Nicholson WE et al: Natural history of pituitary adrenal recovery following long-term suppression with corticosteroids. J Clin Endocrinol Metab 25:11, 1965 (*A classic paper, which showed that patients on glucocorticoids for 1 to 10 years had full restoration of function generally within 1 year, that hypothalamic–pituitary function was restored during the initial 2 to 5 months, that 17-hydroxycorticosteroids returned to normal during months 6 to 9 [probably a response to supranormal levels of ACTH], and that from 9 months on all responses to testing were essentially normal. The study provides no information about recovery following shorter courses of glucocorticoids.*)

Meikle AW, Tyler FH: Potency and duration of action of glucocorticoids. Effects of hydrocortisone, prednisone and dexamethasone on human pituitary–adrenal function. Am J Med 63:200, 1977 (*A paper that demonstrates the prolonged suppressive effect of dexamethasone on the pituitary–adrenal axis. The intrinsic potency and relative rate of disappearance from plasma are the two most important factors determining the relative potency of orally administered glucocorticoids.*)

Messer J, Reithman D, Sacks HS et al: Association of adrenocorticosteroid therapy and peptic ulcer disease. N Engl J Med 309:21, 1983 (*Meta-analysis of 71 controlled clinical trials of corticosteroid therapy. The conclusion drawn from the pooled data is that corticosteroids do increase the risk of peptic ulcer and gastrointestinal hemorrhage. However, while the relative risk for these complications was 2, the absolute risk was quite small. Approximately 1% in control patients and 2% in treated patients.*)

Morimoto Y, Oishi T, Hanasaki N et al: Relative potency in acute and chronic suppressive effects of prednisone and betamethasone on the hypothalamic–pituitary–adrenal axis in man. Endocrinol Jpn 27:659, 1980 (*Long-acting agents are far more suppressive than short-acting ones.*)

Rae SA, Williams IA, English J et al: Alteration of plasma prednisolone levels by indomethacin and naproxen. Br J Clin Pharrmacol 14:459, 1982 (*Nonsteroidal agents may displace prednisolone from binding sites and raise the free fraction, thus augmenting effect.*)

Streetend HP: Corticosteroid therapy complications and therapeutic implications. JAMA 232:1046, 1975 (*A short review of the likely complications associated with the therapeutic use of glucocorticoids.*)

Webb J, Clark TJ: Recovery of plasma corticotrophin and cortisol levels after three-week course of prednisolone. Thorax 36:22, 1981 (*HPA axis remained clinically intact after a 3-week, high-dosage program.*)

Zamkoff K, Kirshner J, Cass D et al: Adrenal response to serial cosyntropin stimulation after repeated high-dose prednisone administration in patients with lymphoma. Cancer Treat Rep 65: 563, 1981 (*A program of 5 days on, 2½ weeks off does not cause significant HPA suppression.*)

8

Gynecologic Problems

104
Screening for Breast Cancer

Breast cancer is among the most common malignancies afflicting women. Internationally, its incidence varies widely; rates in North America and northern Europe are five to six times higher than those in Asia and Africa. More than 120,000 women develop breast cancer each year in the United States, accounting for more than one in four cancer diagnoses among women. Of these, 40,000 eventually die of the disease, accounting for one in five female cancer deaths. The lifetime probability that an American woman will develop breast cancer is approximately 9%. As high as this rate is, many women overestimate it, probably because four out of five women have seen breast cancer in a relative or acquaintance.

Despite diagnostic and therapeutic advances, mortality rates for breast cancer have changed little in the past 30 years. The high incidence, morbidity, and mortality associated with the disease, coupled with the importance of the breasts to many women's self-image, make breast cancer one of the most feared tumors. It is also one of the rare conditions for which screening benefits have been documented, at least for some women. The primary care provider deals with breast tumor screening and diagnosis or associated fears on a daily basis.

EPIDEMIOLOGY AND RISK FACTORS

The epidemiology of breast cancer has been studied extensively. Risk factors for the disease include the following.

Age. Risk of breast cancer increases throughout life for American women. Nevertheless, it is not uncommon in women under 40 in whom approximately 20% of cases occur. The median age at the time of diagnosis is 54 years, and 45% of cases occur after age 65.

Reproductive History. Generally, there is an inverse relationship between breast cancer risk and parity, but maternal age at the time of first full-term pregnancy may be the most important variable. Independent of parity, an early age at first birth may reduce the risk compared with that for no pregnancy, whereas a late first birth may increase the risk. In a woman with high parity, whose first birth occurs before the age of 20, the risk of breast cancer is half that of a nulliparous woman and one third that of the woman with one or two births after the age of 30. An aborted pregnancy does not affect cancer risk. The effect of lactation on risk, if any, is minor.

Menstrual History. Both late menarche and early natural menopause reduce breast cancer risk. Women who experienced menarche after age 16 have half the risk of those who experienced it earlier. Women in whom menopause occurred before age 45 have half the risk of those in whom menopause occurred after age 55. Women in whom early menopause is surgically induced seem to be similarly protected.

Family History. A family history of breast cancer, whether among maternal or paternal relatives, increases the risk to two to three times that of the general population. Relatives of women with bilateral disease have an even higher risk.

History of Benign Breast Disease. The relative risk of breast cancer is twofold to threefold greater in women who have a history of benign breast disease. Some have estimated higher relative risks and others have questioned whether or not benign breast disease confers any additional risk. The question is complicated by many issues, most of which relate to definitions of benign breast disease. Recent evidence indicates that a substantial majority of women with benign breast disease worrisome enough to prompt biopsy have nonproliferative changes and are not at increased risk for eventual breast malignancy. In one study, women with proliferative disease without atypical hyperplasia accounted for 26% of breast biopsies and had a twofold increase in risk;

those with atypical hyperplasia had a fivefold increase in risk but accounted for only 4% of all biopsies.

Mammographic Findings. The appearance of breast tissue on mammographic examination has been related to risk of subsequent malignancy, but this association has been questioned. In 1975, Wolfe advanced a classification system that divided breasts into four categories based on mammographic appearance: *N1, P1, P2,* and *DY.* The lowest-risk class, *N1,* includes breasts that are essentially replaced by fat. The two *P* classes include breasts with increasingly prominent ducts, believed to be at intermediate risk. *DY* denotes severe involvement with dysplasia. In the early studies, Wolfe estimated 20-fold to 30-fold increased risk in cancer in DY breasts compared with *N* breasts. These findings have not been replicated. Although some investigators have found associations between the DY pattern and subsequent cancer, the estimates of relative risk have been much lower and substantially affected by patient age. Other investigators have found no relationship between mammographic pattern and cancer risk.

History of Previous Malignancy. Approximately 10% of women who survive for 10 years following the diagnosis of breast cancer will have a second primary malignancy, usually in the contralateral breast. Increasing popularity of breast-sparing surgery for minimal breast cancer may increase the incidence of second breast cancers among survivors with more breast tissue at risk. Women with a history of endometrial carcinoma have slightly increased risk of breast cancer.

Diet, Drugs, and Other Factors. A number of observations suggest that breast cancer risk is influenced by diet, particularly consumption of fats. Unsaturated fats promote breast tumors in animal models. Geographic differences and associations between dietary intake and cancer provide supporting evidence, but the hypothesis remains unproved. Low levels of vitamin A have also been tentatively linked to small increases in risk. Obesity has been consistently linked to minor increases in risk. The role of drugs is controversial. A link between reserpine and breast cancer has been discredited. An association between either oral contraceptive use or postmenopausal exogenous estrogens and breast cancer has not been demonstrated. Because smoking decreases urinary levels of endogenous estrogens, it has been postulated that smoking might reduce the incidence of breast cancer. This has not been borne out by epidemiologic investigations.

NATURAL HISTORY OF BREAST CANCER AND EFFECTIVENESS OF EARLY THERAPY

Little can be said with certainty about the natural history of breast cancer. The few observational studies of untreated breast cancer have shown widely variable tumor doubling times ranging from less than a week to more than 6 months.

The mean duration of the preclinical phase of the disease has been estimated to be 20 months. Estimates of lead time, from the Health Insurance Plan (HIP) of Greater New York screening trial, have been 7 months at the initial screening examination and approximately 1 year for subsequent screenings at yearly intervals.

It is particularly difficult to judge the benefit of early treatment of breast cancer because of the widely variable course of the disease after diagnosis at any stage. Biologic determinism as the major influence on outcome has been widely debated. Many studies have shown that there is no clear relationship between survival rates and the length of time the patient delayed seeking medical attention after becoming aware of the tumor, despite the drop in 5-year survival rates from 85% to about 50% when there is nodal involvement.

Data from the HIP randomized breast cancer screening trial, however, suggest substantial benefits of screening. After 10 to 14 years of follow-up, breast cancer mortality was 25% to 30% lower in the study group that received yearly screening by x-ray mammography and physical examination. This reduction was evident in women over 50 but not in those between 40 and 49.

SCREENING METHODS

Breast Self-Examination has been a mainstay of prevention programs. Through the years, 90% of tumors have been detected by patients. A recent survey conducted by the American Cancer Society found that two thirds of women performed breast self-examination in the past year. However, most were not performing the procedure monthly and were not spending sufficient time to do it correctly. Age, education, marital status, having been instructed by a health professional, regular professional breast examinations, and a family history of breast cancer have all been shown to influence breast self-examination behavior.

Some still question the effectiveness of self-examination in the early detection of disease. All agree that effectiveness depends on breast size and other characteristics. Small or poorly supported pendulous breasts are most suitable. Examination of large, well-supported breasts is difficult for both patients and physicians. All women should be taught systematic breast examination techniques and advised to use them on a monthly basis. Seven to 10 days after menses is the best time for premenopausal women; postmenopausal women can pick a regular calendar date, such as the first of each month. Breast self-examination should be particularly stressed for women who are at high risk and those with breasts that are anatomically suitable.

Physical Examination is extremely important and should never be neglected. It is often not appreciated that much of the benefit evident in the HIP study was derived from the physical examination rather than from mammography; only

44% of cancers in women aged 50 to 59, and 19% of those in women aged 40 to 49, were found on mammography alone. It is widely acknowledged that current mammographic techniques are much more sensitive than those used in the HIP study. Nevertheless, physical examination and mammography remain complementary procedures; a substantial proportion of cancers, particularly among younger women, will be missed by physicians who rely too heavily on mammography and thereby neglect careful, systematic inspection and palpation of the breasts. A number of studies have demonstrated that the proportion of lesions confined to stage I at the time of diagnosis is higher for tumors discovered during routine physical examination than for those presenting symptomatically or found during breast self-examination.

Mammography is a valuable aid in the diagnosis of breast masses (see Chapter 110) and as a screening test. Its precise role in general screening remains somewhat controversial. There are conflicting recommendations regarding which women should be screened and the frequency of mammography in different age groups.

The HIP study provided a rigorous test of the hypothesis that regular screening by means of physical examination and mammography can reduce breast cancer morbidity and mortality. After 14 years of follow-up, benefit has been conclusively demonstrated among women aged 50 to 59 who showed a 25% to 30% reduction in breast cancer mortality compared with women randomized to the nonscreened control group. The remaining questions are: Does the screening benefit extend to other age groups, particularly younger women in whom mammography has been shown to be less sensitive and specific and who may be more adversely affected by repeated radiation exposure? and How much of the benefit is attributable to mammography rather than physical examination of the breasts?

Data from the Breast Cancer Detection Demonstration Projects (BCDDP) derived from screening nearly 300,000 women in 29 centers in the United States are frequently cited to support both the contribution of mammography to screening and the extension of screening to younger women. Of more than 3500 cancers detected by BCDDP examinations, 42% were found by mammography alone; these cancers were more likely to be stage I lesions. Approximately 32% of cancers were found in women under age 50; of these, 35% were detected by mammography alone. BCDDP data also provide a clear indication of how much mammographic techniques have improved following the HIP study. Whereas mammography had a sensitivity of 60% in the HIP program for cancers in the age 50 to 59 cohort, sensitivity for the same group was 92% in the BCDDP.

Improvements in technology have also reduced risks of radiation. Although it was once asked if regular use of mammography might induce more cancers than it would detect for cure, best current estimates indicate that exposure of 1 million women to 1 rad would produce only six excess cancers

after a latent period of 10 to 15 years; the risk of naturally occurring breast cancer is more than 1000-fold greater. Mammography can be performed now with considerably lower radiation exposure. The two widely available techniques are xeromammography and screen-film mammography, which require 0.4-rad and 0.2-rad exposure, respectively.

The findings of the BCDDP and the improved safety of mammography have moved the American Cancer Society to modify recommendations that had previously urged annual mammography only for women older than 50 years. Current recommendations include a "baseline" study between ages 35 and 40, followed by mammograms at intervals of 1 to 2 years between ages 40 and 49 as well as annual mammography beginning at age 50. Although these recommendations are supported by strong evidence, it must be kept in mind that BCDDP participants were self-selected and there were no controls. The wisdom of these recommendations will be tested by the results of a Canadian randomized trial designed to determine the benefits of mammography in younger women and to distinguish between the effects of screening mammography and screening physical examination. Useful follow-up information from the Canadian National Breast Screening Study should be available in 1990.

Other Modalities may be useful in the diagnosis of symptomatic breast disease, particularly a breast mass (see Chapter 110), but mammography is the only imaging technique shown to be efficacious for screening asymptomatic women to detect clinically occult malignancy.

CONCLUSIONS AND RECOMMENDATIONS

- Breast cancer is common. Although risk factors allow identification of subgroups at particularly high risk, women without risk factors are nonetheless at substantial risk and should receive regular, periodic screening.
- Evidence indicates that early diagnosis leads to substantial reduction in mortality.
- Self-examination should be taught to all women by the primary care provider. The technique should be emphasized when the woman is at high risk and has breasts that are suitable for effective self-examination.
- Physical examination is an important element of screening. It should be performed in all women at yearly intervals, more frequently in high-risk populations.
- Mammography has been proven to be beneficial in women older than 50 years. When possible, it should be performed on an annual basis in this group. A baseline mammogram at age 35 to 40 followed by regular mammograms at 1- to 2-year intervals beginning at age 40 have also been recommended. Although this is a reasonable approach, the benefits have not been proven and the primary physician should be mindful of the potential harm produced by an imperfect test, including overdiagnosis and false reassurance, as well as risks associated with repeated radiation exposure.

A.G.M.

ANNOTATED BIBLIOGRAPHY

Adami HO, Malker B, Holmberg et al: The relation between survival and age at diagnosis in breast cancer. N Engl J Med 315:559, 1986 (*Women age 45 to 49 seem to have the best prognosis with relative survival declining markedly in women whose cancer is diagnosed in later years.*)

Bennett SE, Lawrence RS, Fleischmann KH et al.: Profile of women practicing breast self-examination. JAMA 249:488, 1983 (*Breast self-examination was more common among women to whom technique had been demonstrated, with a maternal history of breast disease; education and practice of other preventive health activities were not associated with breast self-examination.*)

Berg JW: Clinical implications of risk factors for breast cancer. Cancer 53:589, 1984 (*Makes the important point that "low-risk" women still face substantial risk of breast cancer, that is, approximately 6%.*)

Bland KI, Buchanan JB, Mills DL et al: Analysis of breast cancer screening in women younger than 50 years. JAMA 245:1037, 1981 (*Of 163 cancers detected among 10,128 asymptomatic women, 34% were in women younger than 50.*)

Breast Cancer Detection Demonstration Project: Five year summary report. CA, 32:4, 1982 (*A summary of screening results in more than 300,000 women.*)

Brinton LA, Hoover R, Fraumeni JF Jr: Epidemiology of minimal breast cancer. JAMA 249:483, 1983 (*In this case control study, epidemiologic associations for small and larger invasive tumors were similar: family history, age at first live birth, history, oophorectomy, and obesity. In situ cancer was associated with family history and age at first childbirth but not with oophorectomy or obesity.*)

Brisson J, Merletti F, Sadowsky NL et al: Mammographic features of the breast and breast cancer risk. Am J Epidemiol 115:428, 1982 (*Did find a five-fold risk of cancer in women with Wolfe's DY pattern compared with those with the N pattern. Risk was influenced by age.*)

Check WA: Can mammographic parenchymal patterns foretell breast cancer? JAMA 244:221, 1980 (*Reviews the basis for the controversy.*)

Council on Scientific Affairs, AMA: Early detection of breast cancer. JAMA 252:3008, 1984 (*Council recommendations on the use of mammography, identical to those of the American Cancer Society, as well as breast biopsy.*)

Dupont WD, Page DL: Risk factors for breast cancer in women with proliferative breast disease. N Engl J Med 312:146, 1985 (*Among 3303 women followed for a median of 17 years after benign breast biopsy, 134 developed breast cancer; 70% who had nonproliferative histologies were not at increased risk of cancer.*)

Evans JS, Wennberg JE, McNeil BJ: The influence of diagnostic radiography on the incidence of breast cancer and leukemia. N Engl J Med 315:810, 1986 (*Data from a closed population and a mathematical model lead to conclusion that incidence of radiation-induced breast cancer is low.*)

Foster RS, Costanza MC: Breast self-examination practices and breast cancer survival. Cancer 53:999, 1984 (*Women who had practiced self-examination had better survival rates following cancer diagnosis.*)

Helmrich SP, Shapiro S, Rosenberg L et al: Risk factors for breast cancer. Am J Epidemiol 117:35, 1983 (*A large case control study confirming increased risk associated with age at first birth as well as independent effects of parity, a history of benign breast disease, positive family history of breast cancer, Jewish religion, and 12 or more years of education.*)

MacMahon B, Cole P, Brown J: Etiology of human breast cancer: A review. J Natl Cancer Inst 50:21, 1973 (*Extensive review of risk factors [excluding drug history] as well as etiologic hypotheses with 178 references.*)

Mettlin C: Diet and the epidemiology of human breast cancer. Cancer 53:605, 1984 (*Reviews the evidence linking dietary fat intake to risk of breast cancer.*)

Miller AB: Routine mammography and the National Breast Screening Study. Can Med Assoc J 130:259, 1984 (*Reviews the objectives of this important study designed to answer the questions about screening women younger than 50 and the marginal value of mammography in women older than 50.*)

Miller AB, Bulbrook RD: The epidemiology and etiology of breast cancer. N Engl J Med 303:1246, 1980 (*A succinct review from the Multidisciplinary Project on Breast Cancer of the International Union Against Cancer.*)

Moskowitz M: Screening for breast cancer: How effective are our tests? CA 33:26, 1983 (*A valuable review of sensitivity, specificity, and predictive values of mammography when clinical circumstances indicate high, intermediate, or low probability of cancer.*)

Rosenberg L, Schwingl PJ, Kaufman DW: Breast cancer and cigarette smoking. N Engl J Med 310:92, 1984 (*A case control study that detected no association between cigarette smoking and breast cancer, thereby refuting the hypothesis that the lowered estrogen levels resulting from smoking could protect against this malignancy.*)

Shapiro S, Goldberg JD, Hutchinson GB: Lead time in breast cancer detection and implications for periodicity of screening. Am J Epidemiol 100:357, 1974 (*Average duration of preclinical disease previously estimated to be 20 months. Lead time estimated to be 1 year—7 months at the initial examination and 11 to 13 months at subsequent screenings.*)

Shapiro S, Venet W, Strax P et al.: Ten to fourteen year effect of screening on breast cancer mortality. J Natl Cancer Inst 69:349, 1982 (*Latest results from the randomized HIP trial.*)

The Cancer and Steroid Hormone Study of the Centers for Disease Control and the National Institute of Child Health and Human Development: Oral contraceptive use and the risk of breast cancer. N Engl J Med 315:405, 1986 (*A large case control study that found no association between birth control pill use and breast cancer.*)

Verbeek ALM, Hendricks JH, Peeters PH et al: The mammographic breast pattern and the risk of breast cancer. Lancet 1:591, 1984 (*No difference in relative risk using the Wolfe classification.*)

Willett WC, McMahon B: Diet and cancer—an overview. N Engl J Med 310:633, 1984 (*Reviews the relationship between vitamins and trace elements and various cancers as well as the association between fiber and dietary fat and colon cancer and between dietary fat and breast cancer.*)

105
Screening for Cervical Cancer

Cancer of the cervix is the second most common malignancy among women. In the United States, the annual incidence of invasive cervical cancer is 15,000, and annual mortality is 8000. The incidence of carcinoma in situ is three times that of invasive disease. There is a very long asymptomatic period during which cytologic detection is possible. Early therapy is often curative. Appropriately, the Pap smear is one of the most widely used cancer screening tests.

EPIDEMIOLOGY AND RISK FACTORS

Age and sexual activity are the principal risk factors for cervical cancer.

The age-specific prevalence rates for carcinoma *in situ* follow a bimodal distribution with the dominant, first peak of about 6 per 1000 women occurring in the 30 to 45 age group. A second peak of about 5 per 1000 occurs after age 60. The highest carcinoma *in situ* incidence rates are in the 25 to 29 age group. The prevalence of invasive carcinoma is highest in older age groups, rising precipitously after 50. A breakdown in host barriers at the time of menopause has been proposed as an explanation for the decreased *in situ* and increased invasive prevalence rates observed in these patients.

Many factors have been associated with cervical neoplasia. Most are related to sexual activity. First intercourse at a young age (*e.g.,* prior to age 18) and multiple sexual partners (four or more) are the factors most consistently associated with high risk. Increasing parity, poor personal hygiene, a history of venereal disease, an uncircumcised partner, and a high number of sexual partners of the husband or regular sexual partner have also been linked to cervical cancer. The extremely low risk of cervical neoplasia in women who have never had intercourse and the consistent association with variables that define sexual exposure has sparked several hypotheses about cervical cancer as a venereal disease. The strongest evidence points to herpes simplex type II virus and human papilloma virus, particularly types 16 and 18, as potential venereally transmitted oncogenic agents. It is now thought that the combination of exposure to such agents and the presence of susceptible cervical epithelium leads to cervical neoplasia. The recent appreciation that normal immature squamous epithelium in the transformation zone of the cervix is particularly sensitive to herpes simplex and papilloma virus infections may explain some of the long-observed epidemiologic correlates of cervical cancer. Immature squamous cells are present in the developing transformation zone

following menarche and during remodeling of the transformation zone following pregnancy. Women who are sexually active early in life and who have multiple pregnancies may be more likely to come in contact with oncogenic agents when their cervical epithelium is susceptible to infection. This theory would also explain the twofold to fourfold increase in risk of dysplasia and carcinoma *in situ* in women exposed *in utero* to diethylstilbestrol. Persistent susceptibility to oncogenic agents may stem from immature metaplastic squamous cells that arise in the areas of cervical and vaginal adenosis frequently found in women exposed to diethylstilbestrol (see Chapter 107).

Other factors have been associated with cervical neoplasia, but it is difficult to control for sexual exposure. The incidence of cervical cancer is decreased in Jewish women and increased in black women. In the latter case, socioeconomic status may be the most important predictor, inasmuch as the racial disparity is eliminated when socioeconomic factors are controlled. Smoking has been identified as a potentially important independent risk factor for cervical cancer in a number of studies that controlled for both sexual activity and socioeconomic status. Although the issue remains controversial, the weight of current evidence supports the association. One theory holds that smoking may make women more susceptible to the oncogenic effects of herpes viruses.

The most compelling risk information comes from the Pap smear itself, in that the risk of carcinoma is 100 times greater in women with dysplasia than in those with a normal cervix.

NATURAL HISTORY OF CERVICAL CANCER AND EFFECTIVENESS OF THERAPY

Cervical cancer classically presents with intermenstrual bleeding prompted by coitus or douching. Symptoms invariably occur late in the course of the disease. Epidemiologic evidence indicates that the natural history of cervical neoplasia should be viewed as a progression from mild dysplasia, through carcinoma *in situ,* to invasive carcinoma. Only a minority of mildly dysplastic lesions progress to carcinoma. It is not clear that carcinoma *in situ* invariably becomes invasive, but epidemiologic data suggest that progression occurs in the vast majority of cases. Both of these premalignant lesions, which are referred to together as cervical intraepithelial neoplasia, are reliably detected by cytologic techniques.

The mean duration of the detectable asymptomatic period, as estimated from incidence and prevalence rates, is very long. The mean duration of carcinoma *in situ* varies with age but averages about 10 years. The duration of asymptomatic invasive carcinoma is 5 years for all age groups. It should be emphasized that these are estimated means; the proportion of cervical cancers that become invasive early in their development is not known.

There is no doubt that the earlier the clinical stage of the tumor when detected and treated, the better the prognosis. Survival for carcinoma *in situ* treated with hysterectomy is essentially 100%. But the uncertainty about the natural course of carcinoma *in situ* must be kept in mind. Relative 5-year survival rates for localized and regional invasive carcinoma are about 80% and 40% respectively. The 5-year experience of one screening program demonstrated that 86% of cases detected by cytologic screening were limited to regional invasion, while only 44% of those presenting symptomatically were in this early stage.

SCREENING METHODS AND DIAGNOSTIC TESTS

There are three techniques of cell collection for Papanicolaou staining and cytologic screening of the cervix. The easiest is aspiration from the vaginal pool. More sensitive, but requiring visualization of the cervix with a vaginal speculum, are endocervical swabbing and cervical scraping. The sensitivity of the vaginal aspirate technique has been reported in a range from 62% to 92% in the presence of invasive carcinoma and from 31% to 70% in the presence of carcinoma in situ. The range of reported sensitivities for swabbing is 82% to 92% and that for scraping, 86% to 100%. There is no consistent difference in detection rates between invasive carcinoma and carcinoma *in situ* with the swabbing and scraping techniques.

Recent reports indicate that sensitivity in actual practice may be substantially lower because of poor cell collection technique or faulty interpretation. It is currently recommended that two cell smears be taken for each test: one taken from the endocervical canal, with either a pipette or cotton swab, and one scraped with a spatula from the os of the cervix, which contains the squamous–columnar junction or transformation zone. Smears should be interpreted by an experienced cytopathologist.

The specificity of cytologic diagnosis is very high. In a 2-year period, 151 of 25,000 cytologic examinations of the cervix performed at the Massachusetts General Hospital were read as positive. Eighty percent of these women had uterine cancer. Clearly, more than 99% without disease had negative smears. This high specificity limits the costs associated with false-positive results.

The frequency of cervical cancer screening is currently controversial. Because of the usual long duration of the asymptomatic detectable period of cervical intraepithelial neoplasia, which is easily controlled and cured when detected, the American Cancer Society has moved away from its previous recommendation of annual Pap smears. The ACS now recommends Pap smears every 3 years after two successive negative smears 1 year apart at age 20 and 21, or younger if the patient is sexually active. The purpose of the short first interval is to improve sensitivity of the first screening effort. Screening is recommended until age 65. Although the ACS acknowledges that women who are at high risk because of early age at first intercourse, multiple sexual partners, or other risk factors may need to be tested more frequently, it argues that the decision about test frequency depends on the duration of the asymptomatic detectable disease rather than a woman's individual risk.

The recommendations of the Canadian Task Force on Cervical Cancer Screening reflect more concern with anecdotal evidence that a greater proportion of carcinoma *in situ* among younger women may be rapidly progressive. The reconvened task force recently changed its recommendations and now argues that women who have had sexual intercourse should be screened annually between 18 and 35 years of age. Pap smears every 5 years are recommended for women age 35 to 60 years. Screening is not recommended for women who have never had intercourse.

Cytologic smears are not read as simply positive or negative. A widely adopted classification system for cytologic findings appears in Table 105-1. Women whose smears show moderate to severe dysplasia, carcinoma *in situ,* or invasive carcinoma should be referred to a gynecologist experienced in the use of the colposcope. Colposcopic examination will allow the gynecologist to select sites for biopsy and determine the limits of the lesion. This will allow informed choice between conservative measures such as electrocautery and cryotherapy, which are used increasingly frequently, and more traditional measures such as conization and hysterectomy. Such decisions will be based not only on the size, location, and histology of the lesion but also on the patient's age, parity, reliability for follow-up, and other considerations.

CONCLUSIONS AND RECOMMENDATIONS

- The high prevalence, long mean duration of asymptomatic detectable disease, and availability of a highly specific

Table 105-1.   Classification of Cytologic Findings

Findings inadequate for diagnosis
Findings essentially normal
Atypical cells present suggestive of (specify)
Cytologic findings consistent with:
Cervical intraepithelial neoplasia
Grade 1 (mild dysplasia)
Grade 2 (moderate dysplasia)
Grade 3 (severe dysplasia to carcinoma in situ)
Invasive squamous-cell carcinoma
Endometrial carcinoma
Other cancer (specify)

screening test make cervical cancer screening an important task for all primary care providers.

• Known risk factors, including early sexual activity and high number of sexual partners, allow selection of high-risk patients and populations.

• Because of the long duration of preinvasive, detectable disease in women of reproductive age, annual screening in the absence of specific risk factors may be unnecessary. Two screens with a short interval (6 months to 1 year) are indicated to reduce the number of false-negative prevalence cases. The interval between subsequent screens can be lengthened for low-risk individuals. The presence of a risk factor, particularly in the menopausal or postmenopausal patient, is an indication for more frequent (*i.e.*, yearly) screening.

• A cytologic smear positive for cancer or severe dysplasia is an indication for referral to a gynecologist for further evaluation, including appropriate biopsies.

• A doubtful smear—suggestive of mild dysplasia—can be further evaluated by the nongynecologist. If a concurrent infection is evident, the smear should be repeated following specific treatment of the infection. If no infection is present, the smear may be repeated after a 3- to 6-month interval. Persistently abnormal smears should be referred for colposcopy or biopsy.

A.G.M.

ANNOTATED BIBLIOGRAPHY

Canadian Task Force on Cervical Cancer Screening Programs: Cervical cancer screening programs: summary of the 1982 Canadian task force report. Can Med Assoc J 127:581, 1982 (*A carefully reasoned argument followed by specific recommendations accompanied by editorial.*)

Crum CP, Ikenberg H, Richart RM et al: Human papillomavirus Type 16 in early cervical neoplasia. N Engl J Med 310:880, 1984 (*HPV 16 virus was isolated from condylomata of the uterine cervix, which contained abnormal mitotic figures and appeared to be precursors of invasive cancer of the cervix.*)

Devesa SS: Descriptive epidemiology of cancer of the uterine cervix. Obstet Gynecol 63:605, 1984 (*Documents a decline in cervical cancer mortality in all age groups accompanied by a sharp rise in incidence of diagnosis of carcinoma in situ.*)

Kashgarian M, Dunn JE: The duration of intraepithelial and preclinical squamous cell carcinoma of the uterine cervix. Am J Epidemiol 92:211, 1970 (*Detailed analysis of incidence and prevalence data from Memphis study providing estimates of preclinical duration of disease.*)

Massachusetts Department of Public Health: Papanicolaou testing—Are we screening the wrong women? N Engl J Med 294:223, 1976 (*Points out high frequency of screening of young women with low risk.*)

Richart RM: The patient with an abnormal pap smear—Screening techniques and management. N Engl J Med 302:332, 1980 (*Reviews cytologic detection of cervical cancer precursors as well as newer diagnostic and therapeutic approaches utilizing colposcopy and cryotherapy.*)

Richart RM, Vaillant HW: Influence of cell collection techniques upon cytological diagnosis. Cancer 18:1474, 1965 (*Reviews sensitivities of endocervical swabbing, cervical scraping, and vaginal aspirate techniques.*)

Schachter J, Hill EC, King EB et al: Chlamydia trachomatis and cervical neoplasia. JAMA 248:2134, 1982 (*This case control study indicates the relative risk of antichlamydial antibody for cervical neoplasia was approximately 2. Association to herpes simplex virus type II was not detected.*)

Trevathan E, Layde P, Webster LA: Cigarette smoking and dysplasia and carcinoma in situ of the uterine cervix. JAMA 250:499, 1983 (*A case control study suggesting substantially increased risk of cervical cancer among young women who smoke cigarettes.*)

Winkelstein W, Shillitoe E, Brand R et al: Further comments on cancer of the uterine cervix, smoking and herpes virus infection. Am J Epidemiol 119:1, 1984 (*An analytic review of evidence linking cervical cancer risk to smoking and herpes virus infection concluding that the evidence is strong.*)

106
Screening for Endometrial Cancer

More than 95% of the cancers of the uterine corpus are adenocarcinomas arising from the endometrium. In the United States, endometrial cancer is a more common problem than invasive cervical cancer. Approximately 36,000 cases occur among American women each year. There is some evidence that increases in the incidence of endometrial cancer are parallel to the increased life span among American women, and until recently, to the increased use of exogenous estrogens among postmenopausal women. Most cases occur in women in whom risk factors are well defined. The tumors often present symptomatically at a time when cure is still possible. Diagnostic tests suitable for indiscriminate screening are not available. It is the responsibility of the primary care provider to be aware of the risk factors and limitations of diagnostic tests, to elicit the pertinent history, and to respond to worrisome symptoms.

EPIDEMIOLOGY AND RISK FACTORS

Advancing age is the single most important risk factor for endometrial cancer. Most tumors occur during the sixth and seventh decades; fewer than 5% occur before age 40. The risk is increased among first-degree relatives of patients with endometrial cancer. Epidemiologic studies have also shown an association with cancer of the breast and cancer of the colon. Case-control studies have also demonstrated a surprisingly high prevalence of obesity and glucose intolerance among patients with endometrial cancer. Between 20% and 80% of patients with tumors were obese, depending on the definition of obesity used in different studies. Up to 40% of patients were found to have diabetes mellitus; this relationship is less clear, partly because of varying definitions of diabetes and the likely correlation with obesity.

Epidemiologic, clinical, and experimental data indicating that estrogens, either endogenous or exogenous, play a principal role in the etiology of endometrial carcinoma have been mounting in recent years. The histologic precursor of endometrial cancer is atypical endometrial hyperplasia. Retrospective studies have indicated a progression from cystic hyperplasia through adenomatous hyperplasia to atypical hyperplasia, associated with unopposed estrogen effects. Prospective studies have demonstrated a cumulative incidence of carcinoma of 10% among patients with atypical endometrial hyperplasia.

A number of clinical syndromes that include ovarian estrogen excess have been associated with the increased risk of endometrial cancer. Postmenopausal women with estrogen-secreting tumors have been reported to have a 10% to 24% incidence of endometrial cancer. There is also a high incidence of cancer in patients with polycystic ovary disease; 19% to 25% of young women with endometrial carcinoma have underlying Stein Leventhal syndrome. It is likely that less well-defined abnormalities of estrogen control explain the association of endometrial cancer with menstrual abnormalities and infertility. Approximately half of all women with endometrial carcinoma and 20% to 30% of married women with endometrial carcinoma are nulliparous.

The principal estrogen in postmenopausal women is estrone, which is peripherally converted from androstenedione produced in the adrenal glands. Peripheral conversion of androstenedione to estrone has been shown to be increased in patients with endometrial cancer, and estrone to estradiol ratios are higher. Peripheral conversion by adipose cells may be the explanatory link between obesity and endometrial cancer.

A number of recent retrospective case-control studies indicate that the use of estrogens postmenopausally substantially increases the risk of endometrial cancer. Rates of endometrial cancer among estrogen users ranged from 4 to 14 times those among control patients in various studies. Several studies have demonstrated a dose-response relationship, in that use of estrogen for longer periods of time was associated with greater risk. It has been argued that the association between estrogens and endometrial cancer can be explained in part by a greater likelihood of detection of preexisting tumors in women for whom estrogens are prescribed. Implications of this link between exogenous estrogens and endometrial cancer

for treatment of menopausal symptoms are discussed in Chapter 117. Recent case-control data suggest a decreased risk among users of combination birth control pills but an increased risk among women exposed to Oracon, a sequential pill containing a relatively large amount of the potent estrogen ethinyl estradiol and a weak progestogen.

NATURAL HISTORY OF ENDOMETRIAL CANCER AND EFFECTIVENESS OF THERAPY

Postmenopausal bleeding, by far the most common symptom associated with endometrial cancer, must always be pursued aggressively. Clinical studies have indicated that, depending on patient selection, cancer is the explanation in from 10% to 70% of women who present with postmenopausal bleeding. In one review of more than 400 presentations of bleeding at least 2 years after menopause, 16% of patients had endometrial cancer. The likelihood of malignancy increased with the span of years since menopause.

In a series of more than 500 patients with endometrial cancer from the Mayo Clinic, nearly all presented with postmenopausal bleeding or similar symptoms; only 3% of the tumors were detected in asymptomatic women. In this series, there was little if any correlation between the duration of symptoms and the clinical stage of the tumor at the time of diagnosis. The prognosis for endometrial cancer is generally favorable. In the Mayo series, a 75% 5-year survival rate was reported.

DIAGNOSTIC TESTS

Available data suggest that endometrial cancer presents with symptoms early in its natural history. There is little evidence that cytopathologic screening can appreciably advance the time of diagnosis in most patients. The diagnosis of endometrial cancer can be made on the basis of a Pap smear of cells aspirated from the vaginal pool or scraped from the cervical os. However, a number of studies have indicated that the sensitivity of the Pap smear in the diagnosis of endometrial cancer is only 70% to 80%. A retrospective review of patients with endometrial cancer who had Pap smears during the year prior to diagnosis found that only 18% had smears that were suggestive of cancer.

Jet wash and other techniques have been advocated for more direct sampling of the uterine cavity. However, one study of patients without suspected cancer showed that cells extracted with this technique provided a diagnosis in only 3 of 7 cases of adenocarcinoma. None of the tumors that eventually proved to be early and focal were detected by the jet wash method.

In the largest reported effort to detect asymptomatic endometrial cancer, 2007 women, 80% of whom were postmenopausal, were screened using both vaginal pool Pap smear and an endometrial sampling technique. Satisfactory samples could be obtained in only 86% of women. Ten cancers occurred: eight were detected by endometrial samples, one was detected by vaginal pool smear, and one was missed. Endometrial sampling proved to be painful for most patients, and the authors noted difficulty in interpreting endometrial cytology. The authors were unable to conclude that such screening would be either acceptable or effective in lowering endometrial cancer morbidity and mortality.

SUMMARY AND CONCLUSIONS

Endometrial carcinoma is a source of substantial morbidity and mortality and has well-defined risk factors. Evidence indicates that endogenous and exogenous estrogen stimulation plays an etiologic role. Although Pap smears potentially advance the diagnosis of cervical cancer, there are no tests as suitable for endometrial cancer screening. A prompt diagnostic workup, including endometrial biopsy, must be initiated by the primary care provider in patients presenting with postmenopausal bleeding.

A.G.M.

ANNOTATED BIBLIOGRAPHY

Antunes CMF, Stolley PD, Rosenshein NB et al: Endometrial cancer and estrogen use. N Engl J Med 300:9, 1979 (*Overall sixfold risk in estrogen users. Increased risk with dosage and duration. Stage 0 and 1 tumors are more common in estrogen users.*)

Burke JR, Lehman HF, Wolf FS: Inadequacy of Papanicolaou smears in the detection of endometrial cancer. N Engl J Med 291:191, 1974 (*Only 18% of Pap smears taken within a year of presentation with endometrial cancer were suggestive of malignancy.*)

Centers for Disease Control Cancer and Steroid Hormone Study: Oral contraceptive use and the risk of endometrial cancer. JAMA 249:1600, 1983 (*Combination pill use for more than a year showed a protective effect in this case-control study, particularly among nulliparous women.*)

Horwitz RI, Feinstein AR: Alternative analytic methods for case-control studies of estrogen and endometrial cancer. N Engl J Med 299:1089, 1978 (*Points out the potential of bias in casefinding but does not refute increased risk.*)

Jick H, Walker AM, Rothman KJ: The epidemic of endometrial cancer: A commentary. Am J Public Health 70:264, 1980 (*Reviews the time series and cross-sectional data supporting the association between estrogen therapy and endometrial cancer and estimates 15,000 cases attributable to estrogens during the period 1971–1975.*)

Koss LG, Schreiber K, Moussouris H et al: Endometrial carcinoma and its precursors: Detection and screening. Clin Obstet Gynecol 25:49, 1982 (*Vaginal pool and endometrial sampling were used to screen 2007 women; results were inconclusive.*)

Lucas WE: Causal relationships between endocrine-metabolic variables in patients with endometrial carcinoma. Obstet Gynecol Surv 29:507, 1974 (*Exhaustive review with 255 references.*)

Mack TM, Pike MC, Henderson BE et al: Estrogens and endometrial cancer in a retirement community. N Engl J Med 294:1262, 1976 (*Retrospective study indicating risks of approximately eight times the control risks for estrogen users.*)

Malkasian GD, McDonald TW, Pratt JH: Carcinoma of the endometrium. Mayo Clin Proc 52:175, 1977 (*Detailed review of 523 cases with 74% 5-year survival rate.*)

Pachecho JC, Kempers RD: Etiology of postmenopausal bleeding. Obstet Gynecol 32:40, 1968 (*Sixteen percent of 401 women with postmenopausal bleeding had endometrial cancer.*)

Rodrigues MA et al: Evaluation of endometrial jet wash technique in 303 patients in a community hospital. Obstet Gynecol 43:392, 1974 (*Only three of seven cases detected; none of three focal tumors detected.*)

Smith DC, Prentice R, Thompson DJ, Hermann WL: Association of exogenous estrogen and endometrial carcinoma. N Engl J Med 293:1164, 1975 (*Case-control study showing 4.5 times greater risk among exposed women.*)

Weiss NS, Sayvetz TA: Incidence of endometrial cancer in relation to the use of oral contraceptives. N Engl J Med 302:551, 1980 (*Case-control study suggesting decreased endometrial cancer risk among users of combination birth control pills but increased risk among users of Oracon, a particular brand of sequential pills. Accompanying editorial is noteworthy.*)

Weiss NS, Szekely DR, Austin DF: Increasing incidence of endometrial cancer in the United States. N Engl J Med 294:1259, 1976 (*Cross-sectional data indicating sharp increases in incidence during the 1970s.*)

Wynder EL, Escher GC, Mantel N: An epidemiological investigation of cancer of the endometrium. Cancer 19:489, 1966 (*Extensive retrospective study indicating obesity is a major risk factor.*)

Ziel HK, Finkle WD: Increased risk of endometrial carcinoma among users of conjugated estrogens. N Engl J Med 293:1167, 1975 (*Case-control study showing risk increasing with duration of exposure.*)

107
Vaginal Cancer and Other Effects of Diethylstilbestrol Exposure

Vaginal cancer is a rare disease, accounting for approximately 1% of gynecologic malignancies. More than 90% of vaginal cancers are squamous cell tumors. Elderly women are at greatest risk, and because of the extensive lymphatic drainage of the vagina, the 5-year survival rate is only 20% to 25%.

Of greater concern to the primary care provider is adenocarcinoma, or clear-cell carcinoma of the vagina, which occurs in young women who were exposed to diethylstilbestrol or other synthetic estrogens *in utero.* Although these tumors are quite rare, the population at risk is large. Increasing public awareness and concern bring many patients to their doctors with questions regarding diethylstilbestrol exposure. The anxiety among exposed persons has been heightened by reports of other abnormalities of the genital tract, including some that may affect reproductive function. The primary physician must understand the risks that follow diethylstilbestrol exposure as well as the natural history of the associated conditions if he is to counsel and evaluate these patients appropriately.

DIETHYLSTILBESTROL AND ABNORMALITIES OF THE GENITAL TRACT

Diethylstilbestrol is a synthetic estrogen first produced in 1938. After early studies indicated it was helpful in preventing spontaneous abortion, it and other synthetic estrogens were used extensively from the 1940s until 1971 in pregnant women at risk for miscarriage. It has been estimated that between 100,000 and 160,000 women born between 1960 and 1970 were exposed to diethylstilbestrol or similar drugs *in utero.* Because these agents were used more extensively in the 1940s and 1950s, well over 1 million women are estimated to have been exposed.

In 1970, a cluster of cases of the then very rare adenocarcinoma of the vagina, occurring in daughters who had been exposed to DES *in utero,* was reported from Massachusetts General Hospital. Since that time, the association has been confirmed, and several hundred cases of clear-cell carcinoma have been recorded and investigated. A history of

DES exposure has been elicited in approximately two thirds of all cases of malignancy.

A subsequent prospective study of 110 exposed women detailed the abnormalities of the cervix and vagina that can be found in women at risk, in addition to clear-cell carcinoma. Vaginal adenosis, the presence of glandular epithelium in the vagina, was found in 35% of exposed women, but in only 1% of matched controls. Cervical erosion was present in 84% of exposed women and in only 38% of controls. Gross structural abnormalities of the cervix were found in 22% of exposed women, but were not found among controls. No cases of carcinoma were identified in this study. The cumulative incidence of carcinoma in exposed daughters is not known; estimates of from 1 per 1000 to 1 per 10,000 have been made. All abnormalities of the vagina and cervix identified to date occur more commonly in women who were exposed early *in utero.* The embryonic development of the female genital tract begins as early as the 4th week of gestation and is completed by the end of the 18th week. Patients exposed early during this period (*i.e.,* the 4th to 18th week) are most likely to have the epithelial changes and structural abnormalities.

While tumors have been identified in preteenage patients as young as 7, more than 90% of tumors have been found in daughters 14 or older. The peak incidence of tumors occur between the ages of 14 and 20, suggesting that the period of greatest risk occurs when the abnormal vaginal or cervical epithelium is stimulated by ovarian hormones with the onset of puberty. It is too early to say with certainty whether the decreased incidence after age 21 indicates a true decrease in risk with age or is a result of the current age distribution of the cohort at risk.

Recent findings from the National Collaborative Diethylstilbestrol Adenosis (DESAD) Project indicate that women exposed to the drug *in utero* have a twofold to fourfold increase in risk of cervical and vaginal dysplasia over nonexposed controls. The incidence of dysplasia and carcinoma *in situ* was correlated with the area of squamous metaplasia, an immature form of normal squamous epithelium that arises in areas of adenosis. When squamous metaplasia was confined to the os or inner half of the cervix there was no increased risk. The relative risk of dysplasia for exposed women was influenced by sexual activity; those who initiated sexual activity at an early age and those with multiple partners were at greater risk. It has been postulated that the increased risk among women exposed to diethylstilbestrol derives from the greater prevalence and extent of squamous metaplasia. It is presumed that these immature squamous cells, like the immature cells of the transformation zone (see Chapter 105), are particularly susceptible to oncogenic agents such as herpes viruses or human papilloma viruses.

Questions have also been raised about the ability of diethylstilbestrol-exposed offspring to conceive. A high prevalence of uterine and fallopian tube abnormalities has been described in case series of exposed women who have undergone hysterosalpingography. A controlled cohort study from the DESAD Project, however, found no difference in fertility between exposed and control subjects. Once pregnant, however, diethylstilbestrol-exposed women were 70% more likely to have an unfavorable outcome of pregnancy. Nevertheless, more than 80% of such women had at least one full-term live birth during the course of the study.

Genital abnormalities and infertility have also been described in male offspring of mothers who took diethylstilbestrol early in pregnancy. It is likely that these findings were influenced by selection and ascertainment biases; the only controlled study addressing this question found no differences in rates of genitourinary abnormalities, infertility, or testicular cancer in exposed and nonexposed men.

SYMPTOMS AND NATURAL HISTORY OF VAGINAL CANCER AND EFFECTIVENESS OF THERAPY

The natural history of clear-cell carcinoma is still unfolding. Most cases present with abnormal vaginal bleeding or discharge, but because of increasing public and professional awareness, an increasing percentage of cases are detected in the asymptomatic stage. Adenosis has been found in proximity to adenocarcinoma in more than 95% of cases, and is therefore considered a malignant precursor by some. Transitions from adenosis to carcinoma have not, however, been documented.

Limited follow-up information indicates that clear-cell carcinoma is an aggressive tumor. Metastases have been found at the time of surgery in 17% of cases of stage 1 disease and in the majority of cases of stage 2 disease. Short-term follow-up of registry cases of clear-cell carcinoma has indicated that recurrence, death, or both occur in approximately 25% of patients.

It is too early to know whether or not cervical dysplasia and carcinoma *in situ* in diethylstilbestrol-exposed young women has the same natural history as in nonexposed women (see Chapter 105). However, it seems prudent to follow such patients with vigilance and yearly Pap smears.

DIAGNOSTIC TESTS

Although the discovery of abnormal cytology has led to the detection of some cases of clear-cell carcinoma, the Pap smear has been shown to have a relatively low sensitivity (80%) for detecting this lesion. This may be explained by the relatively high degree of differentiation of the neoplastic cells, which may resemble endocervical cells. The cells may also be obscured by a heavy polymorphonuclear infiltration. The initial examination of a woman exposed *in utero* to diethylstilbestrol or similar drugs must therefore include, in addition to direct inspection of the vagina and cervix and cytologic sampling, careful Schiller's iodine staining and biopsies of areas that appear red or fail to stain with the iodine solution. Colposcopy is a complementary procedure. It is particularly useful in patients with abnormal iodine staining or cytology. Colposcopy should be performed by an experienced gynecologist.

Despite the poor sensitivity of the Pap smear for clear-cell cancer, Pap smears should be done yearly in all women with an exposure history. This is especially important in light of the increased risk of dysplasia and cervical cancer, particularly among women with risk factors related to sexual activity.

CONCLUSIONS AND RECOMMENDATIONS

- As many as 1 million women are at risk for abnormalities of the genital tract, including clear-cell adenocarcinoma, because of *in utero* exposure to diethylstilbestrol or other synthetic estrogens.
- Risk of malignancy among exposed women is low. Nevertheless, because of the significant morbidity and mortality associated with these tumors, careful case finding and evaluation are indicated. Because routine screening procedures such as the Pap smear are inadequate, patients at risk must be identified by careful history-taking if they are to receive proper evaluation and counseling.
- It is recommended that exposed daughters with symptoms such as vaginal discharge or bleeding be examined promptly regardless of age. Asymptomatic daughters with a history of exposure should have an initial evaluation at age 14 with subsequent yearly examinations.
- More frequent examinations are advised when extensive epithelial changes are present. When possible, such examinations should be performed by a gynecologist experienced in the use of the colposcope.

A.G.M.

ANNOTATED BIBLIOGRAPHY

Barnes AB, Colton T, Gunderson J et al: Fertility and outcome in pregnancy in women exposed in utero to diethylstilbesterol. N Engl J Med 302:609, 1980 (*Fertility was not affected by DES exposure; there was, however, an increased risk of unfavorable outcome of pregnancy associated with DES exposure—the relative risk was 1.69.*)

Heinonen OP: Diethylstilbestrol in pregnancy: Frequency of exposure and usage pattern. Cancer 31:573, 1973 (*Drug utilization data for 1960s indicated that 100,000 to 160,000 women born in the United States during that decade were exposed in utero.*)

Herbst AL, Kurman RJ, Scully RE, Poskanzer DC: Clear-cell adenocarcinoma of the genital tract in young females. N Engl J Med 287:1259, 1972 (*Registry report of 91 cases 2 years after the initial report of 7 clustered cases in Cancer in 1970.*)

Herbst AL, Poskanzer DC, Robboy SJ et al: Prenatal exposure to stilbestrol: A prospective comparison of exposed female offspring with unexposed controls. N Engl J Med 292:332, 1975 (*Prospective examination of 110 exposed and 82 unexposed females. No cancers were found, but adenosis and other abnormalities were common among exposed individuals.*)

Herbst AL, Scully RE, Robboy SJ: Effects of maternal DES ingestion on the female genital tract. Hosp Pract (October) 1975 (*General review with update of registry cases.*)

Johnston GA Jr: Health risks and effects of prenatal exposure to diethylstilbesterol. J Fam Pract 16:51, 1983 (*Succinct review of structural and neoplastic abnormalities of the genital tract that have been linked to diethylstilbestrol.*)

Leary FJ, Resseguie LJ, Kurland LT et al: Males exposed in utero to diethylstilbesterol. JAMA 252:2984, 1984 (*Careful urologic and fertility evaluation of exposed and unexposed controls showed no increase risk of abnormalities.*)

Robboy SJ, Noller KL, O'Brien P et al: Increased incidence of cervical and vaginal dysplasia in 3,980 diethylstilbestrol-exposed young women. JAMA 252:2979, 1984 (*The incidence of dysplasia and CIS was 15.7 versus 7.9 per 1000 person-years in exposed and nonexposed women, respectively.*)

108

Evaluation of Abnormal Vaginal Bleeding

Vaginal bleeding that occurs at an inappropriate time or in an excessive amount may be a sign of important pathology or simply a manifestation of a functional disorder. In postmenopausal women, cancer is the principal concern, accounting for about 25% of cases in this age group. A number of confusing terms have been used to describe the timing, duration, and amount of abnormal bleeding, including polymenorrhea (frequent but regular episodes of uterine bleeding), menorrhagia (bleeding normal in timing but excessive in amount and duration), metrorrhagia (excessive, prolonged bleeding occurring at irregular intervals), and epimenorrhea or intermenstrual bleeding (occurring between otherwise normal menstrual periods).

The primary physician needs to distinguish the patient with dysfunctional bleeding from one likely to have pelvic pathology and to decide when referral for a dilatation and curettage (D&C) or other diagnostic procedure is indicated. The task is particularly important and often difficult in the perimenopausal woman, because the alteration in menstrual activity coincides with the time that the incidence of malignancy increases.

PATHOPHYSIOLOGY AND CLINICAL PRESENTATION

Dysfunctional bleeding is defined as abnormal bleeding in the absence of tumor, inflammation, or pregnancy. The pathophysiology varies with the age of the patient. In teenagers, immaturity of the hypothalamic–pituitary–gonadal axis is often responsible. In women of reproductive age, emotional or physical stress may alter hypothalamic–pituitary function and disturb the menstrual cycle. Abnormal bleeding results from ovarian dysfunction with inadequate progesterone production due to alterations in luteinizing hormone–follicle-stimulating hormone (LH–FSH) secretion. In the perimenopausal woman, bleeding accompanies anovulation due to onset of "senile" ovarian failure.

Unruptured ovarian follicles persist, and functioning corpora lutea are absent. The endometrium shows hyperplasia resulting from unopposed estrogen effect; there is little if any secretory pattern because of the lack of progesterone. Ovulation does not occur, and anovulatory bleeding results when progesterone production returns or excessive proliferation results in sloughing of the overstimulated endometrium. This condition results in irregularity of the menstrual interval, periods of amenorrhea, and episodes of very heavy and prolonged bleeding when the heavily built-up endometrium finally sheds.

Anatomic lesions of the uterus, tubes, and ovaries can result in abnormal vaginal bleeding. In general, ovulation continues in such cases, and the normal menstrual intervals are preserved, but there is intermenstrual bleeding or excessive menstrual blood loss. *Uterine fibroids* are the most common cause and are estimated to occur in 30% of women over the age of 35; they account for about one third of cases. Only those fibroids that are submucosal in location and involve the uterine cavity lead to bleeding. Since they are so common, they may coexist with another cause of abnormal vaginal bleeding. Periods are often very heavy. *Carcinoma of the cervix* is among the most important sources of abnormal bleeding, though it accounts for only about 3% of cases. Bleeding is often postcoital, typically intermenstrual, and described as slight spotting. It results from surface ulceration, which may occur in early stages of the disease (see Chapter 112). *Cervical polyps* and *cervical erosions* resulting from cervicitis present similarly, with slight spotting noted intermenstrually, especially after coitus. *Adenocarcinoma of the endometrium* is an important cause of bleeding in the postmenopausal woman, but almost 20% of cases are detected in menstruating women, though very rarely before 40. Heavier than normal periods, as well as intermenstrual blood loss, are noted. Initially, the intermenstrual problem is reported as a watery discharge containing small amounts of blood. *Ovarian tumors,* whether benign or malignant, rarely result in abnormal bleeding, unless they are endocrinologically active.

Retained products of gestation represent a very common cause of abnormal uterine bleeding after abortion; blood loss is often heavy. *Ectopic pregnancy* is characterized by delay of the regular period, followed by spotting, often in conjunction with unilateral pelvic pain. Intraperitoneal hemorrhage results if tubal rupture occurs, but this happens in fewer than 5% of cases. A careful menstrual and contraceptive history is most useful.

Pelvic inflammatory disease may alter the normal pattern of menstrual bleeding by disturbing ovarian function, as well as affecting the endometrial surface (see Chapter 115). *Intrauterine devices* also alter the endometrial surface and can be similarly responsible for heavy menstrual bleeding or intermenstrual bleeding (see Chapter 118). Even *tampon* use may lead to minor vaginal bleeding.

Bleeding may be associated with *hypothyroidism* or *hyperthyroidism;* these can produce abnormally heavy periods. *Oral contraceptives* can cause intermenstrual spotting, so-called breakthrough bleeding (see Chapter 118). *Bleeding diatheses* or *iron deficiency* may present as abnormally heavy periods (see Chapter 80).

DIFFERENTIAL DIAGNOSIS

Abnormal vaginal bleeding can be broadly divided into anatomic, dysfunctional, inflammatory, endocrinologic, and hematologic etiologies with vaginal, uterine, tubal, and ovarian sources (see Table 108-1).

WORKUP

History. One should first attempt to establish whether or not any vestige of menstrual regularity remains, since hematologic and anatomic lesions (with the exception of pregnancy) usually do not interfere with ovulation. Dysfunctional bleeding of the anovulatory type is suggested by complete irregularity of menstrual periods and months of amenorrhea. It is useful to assess the severity of bleeding (for example, by inquiring into the number of pads used); but such information is more helpful for management than for diagnosis. More

Table 108-1.   Important Causes of Abnormal Vaginal Bleeding

Anatomic Lesions
1. Uterine fibroids
2. Cervical erosions
3. Cervical polyps
4. Retained products of gestation
5. Ectopic pregnancy
6. Carcinoma of the endometrium
7. Carcinoma of the cervix
8. Ovarian neoplasms
Dysfunctional Bleeding
1. Immaturity or senescence of the hypothalamic–pituitary–ovarian axis
2. Inadequate luteal phase
3. Ovarian senescence
4. Endometriosis
Inflammation/Irritation
1. Pelvic inflammatory disease
2. Intrauterine devices
3. Tampon use
Endocrine Disturbances
1. Hyperthyroidism
2. Hypothyroidism
3. Oral contraceptive use
Hematologic Disturbances
1. Bleeding diatheses
2. Iron deficiency
3. Anticoagulation therapy

important is obtaining information on the patient's normal menstrual cycle, its duration, frequency, and intensity, and how the current bleeding pattern compares with it. The presence of postcoital bleeding, trauma, an IUD, hormone or drug use, recent abortion, unprotected intercourse, breast engorgement, morning sickness, emotional stress, weight loss, iron-deficiency anemia, symptoms of hypothyroidism, easy bruising, abdominal pain, or dyspareunia can be useful for determining etiology. Shoulder pain representing diaphragmatic irritation from abdominal bleeding may be reported.

Physical Examination. Assessment of vital signs should include a check for postural drop in pressure, suggesting significant loss of intravascular volume. Pallor, skin changes indicative of hypothyroidism, petechiae, or purpura need to be noted. A thorough speculum and bimanual pelvic examination is essential, with particular care taken to note any cervical erosions, uterine or adnexal masses, or focal tenderness.

Laboratory Studies. A Pap smear of the cervix is mandatory for proper assessment of cervical lesions. Vaginal cytologic sampling is especially important in older women, because endometrial cancer is a concern. Acetic acid may need to be added to cytology preservative if the smear sample is bloody.

In patients of reproductive age, pregnancy is always a possibility. Serum should be tested for presence of beta-subunit of human chorionic gonadotropin (HCG); beta-subunit determination is the most sensitive test for pregnancy (see Chapter 109). A complete blood count will help assess the severity of blood loss, and a peripheral smear may show signs of iron deficiency. Evaluation for a bleeding diathesis is indicated in the presence of petechiae or purpura and should include a platelet count, bleeding time, prothrombin time, and partial thromboplastin time (see Chapter 80). A TSH and free T_4 will detect hypothyroidism (see Chapter 102). A cervical culture for gonorrhea as well as for other pathogenic organisms is needed in the patient with pain on motion of the cervix and adnexal tenderness (see Chapter 115); an elevated sedimentation rate supports a suspicion of pelvic inflammatory disease. When a mass is detected on pelvic examination, an ultrasound examination can help with localization and in determining whether the lesion is solid or cystic (see Chapter 114).

INDICATIONS FOR REFERRAL

Any patient with abnormal vaginal bleeding who has a mass lesion, an abnormal Pap test, or a high risk for carcinoma of the cervix or endometrium (see Chapters 105 to 107) should be referred to a gynecologist. The consultation is especially important for any postmenopausal woman who experiences the new onset of staining or bleeding. Perimenopausal and postmenopausal patients will usually require a D&C to ensure the absence of malignancy. In one retrospective series, 23% of women with postmenopausal bleeding were found to have endometrial carcinoma. Immediate hospital admission and gynecologic consultation are essential if ectopic pregnancy is a possibility, because life-threatening hemorrhage is a real, albeit slight, risk. The same applies in cases of recent abortion, because placental tissue may be retained. Bleeding in pregnancy is a definite indication for an emergency obstetric consultation. Nonpregnant women who are not bleeding heavily can be referred on an ambulatory basis.

SYMPTOMATIC MANAGEMENT AND PATIENT EDUCATION

Symptomatic management of dysfunctional bleeding can be accomplished by the primary care physician. Dysfunctional bleeding can be stopped in most patients by administration of progestational agents. *Ethinyl estradiol* (Estinyl), 0.05 mg once to three times daily, can be administered to control bleeding, followed by *medroxyprogesterone* (Provera), 10 mg daily for 7 days, then discontinued for 1 week to await bleeding. A period of observation for the return of normal cycles should follow. If bleeding recurs and precipitating factors such as drugs or emotional stress have been ruled out, maintenance hormonal therapy may be employed. In patients who do not desire pregnancy, estrogen–progestin combination pills may

be used (see Chapter 118). Patients who would like to conceive should be referred. In young patients with anovulatory dysfunctional bleeding, oral contraceptives may regularize periods and control blood loss, but will not alter the underlying cause.

Correction of any iron deficiency (see Chapter 84) or hypothyroidism (see Chapter 102) should be carried out, and any pelvic infection treated (see Chapter 115).

When anovulatory bleeding is diagnosed, it is important for the patient to know that reproductive capacity is not lost, that the condition is usually self-limited, and that the possibility of malignancy is low under the age of 40. Directing attention to any contributing situational stresses may prove beneficial. Patients experiencing breakthrough bleeding on low-dosage estrogen oral contraceptives need to be queried to be sure they are strictly adhering to their regimen (see Chapter 118). If they are taking the medication on schedule, switching to another preparation with a slightly greater estrogen dosage is indicated.

The perimenopausal patient who is being referred to the gynecologist usually ought to be told that further assessment for the possibility of malignancy is necessary. When discussed openly, the concerns that most patients already harbor can be addressed and often lessened, since the majority of cases are not likely to be cancerous.

A.H.G.

ANNOTATED BIBLIOGRAPHY

Aksel S, Jones GS: Etiology and treatment of dysfunctional uterine bleeding. Obstet Gynecol 44:1, 1974 (*A study to determine specific FSH and LH patterns associated with dysfunctional uterine bleeding.*)

Goldfarb JM, Little AB: Abnormal vaginal bleeding. N Engl J Med 302:666, 1980 (*Reviews pathophysiology, diagnosis, and treatment of anovulatory bleeding.*)

Isaacs JH, Ross FH: Cytologic evaluation of the endometrium in women with postmenopausal bleeding. Am J Obstet Gynecol 131: 410, 1978 (*A retrospective series of 143 women with postmenopausal bleeding found endometrial carcinoma in 23%. A prospective study in 69 showed good correlation of endometrial cytology with curettage results, but 1 out of 9 carcinomas was missed.*)

Quick AM: Menstruation in hereditary bleeding disorders. Obstet Gynecol 28:37, 1966 (*An excellent discussion of the role of hematologic pathology in abnormal menstrual bleeding.*)

Reyniak JV: Dysfunctional uterine bleeding. Reprod Med 17:293, 1976 (*A thorough review of the problem.*)

Scommegna A, Dmowski WP: Dysfunctional uterine bleeding. Clin Obstet Gynecol 16:221, 1973 (*Another comprehensive review.*)

Shane JM, Naftolin F, Newmark SR: Gynecologic endocrine emergencies. JAMA 231:393, 1975 (*A succinct review of gynecologic endocrine emergencies that cause uterine bleeding.*)

Weissberg SM, Dodson MG: Recurrent vaginal and cervical ulcers associated with tampon use. JAMA 250:1430, 1983 (*Case reports plus review of the literature of what may be a frequent cause of minor abnormal vaginal bleeding.*)

109
Evaluation of Secondary Amenorrhea

Amenorrhea is defined as the absence of menstruation in a woman of reproductive age. In the United States, the mean age for menarche is 13.3 years (range, 11 to 17); the mean age for menopause is 49 (range, 35 to 55). Primary amenorrhea is defined as failure of menstruation to occur by age 17. Secondary amenorrhea is defined as cessation of established menses for 6 months or more. In an epidemiologic study of an unselected population, the incidence of secondary amenorrhea was 3.3%.

The primary physician is frequently consulted by the otherwise asymptomatic woman who has missed a period or two. Recent discontinuation of oral contraceptives and fear of pregnancy are commonly encountered. One needs to be able to recognize the common causes of secondary amenorrhea, realize when simple counseling is sufficient, and know when to initiate a more extensive workup, such as gonadotropin assays and radiologic evaluation of the sella.

PATHOPHYSIOLOGY AND CLINICAL PRESENTATION

Amenorrhea reflects an interruption in the regulation of menstruation. In a normal menstrual cycle, FSH stimulates development of follicles and production of estradiol, which causes the endometrial lining to increase in width and the glands to elongate. At midcycle, there is an FSH–LH surge triggered by high estrogen levels and a small increase in serum progesterone. Ovulation occurs, and estradiol and progesterone are produced by the corpus luteum. Under the influence of progesterone, the endometrial glands become secretory. In the late luteal phase, estradiol and progesterone decline, the stroma becomes edematous, and the blood vessels necrose, resulting in menstrual bleeding.

In secondary amenorrhea, inadequate gonadotropic activity may result from hypothalamic or pituitary disease, ovarian failure, local disease of the uterus with normal endocrine function, obstruction of the cervix, or androgen excess.

Hypogonadotropic or Eugonadotropic Conditions

Functional Amenorrhea. In the majority of women with secondary amenorrhea, FSH and estrogen stimulation are normal, but cyclic LH secretion is lost. Alterations in the hypothalamic–pituitary axis are believed to be responsible, triggered by emotional stress, concurrent illness, sudden weight loss, use of drugs, or any other significant physical stress. This so-called functional amenorrhea occurs in such situations as starting school or a new job, severe illness, anxiety over pregnancy, crash dieting, strenuous athletic training, or with the use of birth control pills, phenothiazines, or a host of other drugs. The problem is particularly prevalent among young professional women who work long hours, eat lightly, and engage in vigorous daily aerobic exercise. Patients suffering from anorexia nervosa experience a similar problem. Loss of cyclic LH production may also cause mild hirsutism and acne because of simulation of ovarian androstenedione, testosterone, and estrogen. Prolonged stress may eventually lead to loss of LH release. The amenorrhea noted after oral contraceptive use rarely last more than 6 months, unless there is a history of a previous menstrual disorder. The incidence of postpill amenorrhea lasting beyond 6 months is less than 1%.

Pituitary Tumors, mostly in the form of *prolactin-secreting microadenomas,* are another hypogonadotropic form of secondary amenorrhea, responsible for as much as 20% of cases. Prolactinomas cause amenorrhea by interfering with the normal cyclic discharge of gonadotropin-releasing hormone from the hypothalamus. Rhythmic release of FSH and LH ceases and amenorrhea ensues. Prolactinomas occur either as macroadenomas (>10 mm in diameter) or as microadenomas (<10 mm). The natural history of these lesions is not well understood, but 10-year follow-up studies show only a small fraction (5% to 15%) of microadenomas enlarge in size. In most, the tendency is toward a decrease in prolactin production and return of ovulation. About 10% of microadenomas enlarge symptomatically during pregnancy, a development that can be well controlled by medical therapy (see below). Patients with microadenomas have otherwise normal pituitary function; those with macroadenomas exhibit loss of other pituitary functions.

Idiopathic Hyperprolactinemia is clinically and endocrinologically indistinguishable from microadenomatous disease, with the exception that there is no discernable tumor on computed tomographic (CT) scan of the sella, and prolactin levels tend to be lower (<150 ng/ml). As with microadenomas, the condition exhibits little tendency to progress to tumor formation or to increasing elevations of prolactin. Regardless of the cause, hyperprolactinemia leads to secondary amenorrhea, infertility, and, in some cases, galactorrhea (see Chapter 111); the accompanying hypoestrogenemia can result in bone demineralization.

Chromophobe Adenomas are a less common cause of amenorrhea. Failure to menstruate can be the presenting complaint before the tumor has enlarged sufficiently to cause hypothyroidism and other manifestations of hypopituitarism. Headache and visual field loss are late signs of the expanding mass lesion. Some chromophobes are associated with excess prolactin producton. An important cause of severe hypopituitarism is postpartum necrosis (Sheehan's syndrome), which develops in the setting of an obstetrical accident. Onset of hypopituitarism may be insidious, with failure to lactate or resume periods being initial manifestations. Symptoms of panhypopituitiarism usually follow.

Polycystic Ovarian Disease (Stein–Leventhal syndrome) is characterized by amenorrhea, infertility, hirsutism, and obesity in conjunction with bilaterally enlarged, polycystic ovaries. Persistent LH secretion is believed to be a major factor. Infertility (found in about 75% of cases), is a common symptom, followed by hirsutism (70%) and amenorrhea (50%).

Bilateral Ovarian Tumors rarely destroy enough ovarian tissue to cause amenorrhea, but granulosa-cell tumors, which produce excess estrogen, and arrhenoblastomas, which synthesize excess androgen, may be repsonsible for amenorrhea.

Endometrial Scarring from radiation therapy, septic abortion, or overly vigorous curettage can produce adhesions that obliterate the uterine cavity (Asherman's syndrome). Similarly, cervical trauma can result in scarring.

Endocrinopathies are important causes, for example, *uncontrolled diabetes mellitus,* especially in the setting of insulin resistance. When control is adequate, periods are normal, but flagrantly poor control manifested by polyuria, polydipsia, and polyphagia can be complicated by amenorrhea. Marked *hypo-* and *hyperthyroidism* are accompanied by amenorrhea in many instances; other thyroid symptoms are usually evident and often dominate the clinical presentation. Mild hypothyroidism may lead to hyperprolactinemia and amenorrhea. *Cushing's syndrome* is another endocrinologic cause of suppressed periods; symptoms of cortisol excess are usually obvious by the time amenorrhea is present.

Hypergonadotropic Conditions

Menopause represents the most common form of hypergonadotropic amenorrhea. In the United States the average age for menopause is 50 years (range, 40 to 60). Manifestations include hot flashes, night sweats, and decreased vaginal secretions. LH and FSH levels are elevated. Such findings in a woman under the age of 40 without evidence of other endocrine dysfunction are indicative of *premature menopause* due to ovarian failure. Early menopause also presents in the setting of *polyendocrine deficiency,* a presumed autoimmune disease characterized by adrenal, pancreatic, and thyroid hy-

pofunction. The condition is hereditary, transmitted in autosomally recessive fashion. *Radiation* injury and cancer *chemotherapy* are iatrogenic sources of ovarian failure.

DIFFERENTIAL DIAGNOSIS

The causes of secondary amenorrhea can be divided pathophysiologically into conditions association with pituitary–hypothalamic dysfunction (hypogonadotropic amenorrhea) and those representing ovarian dysfunction (hypergonadotropic amenorrhea) (see Table 109-1). The most common etiology, excluding pregnancy and menopause, is functional amenorrhea. Hyperprolactinemia may account for as many as 20% of cases.

WORKUP

Evaluation (see Fig. 109-1) ought to begin by first ascertaining if the patient is pregnant. A simple *HCG precipitation slide test* performed on a first morning voided urine is more than 90% sensitive when performed 6 weeks after the last menstrual period. If the test is negative and suspicion persists, it can be repeated in a week, when the HCG concentration will have risen, or serum can be drawn immediately for the more sensitive β-subunit determination.

Once the pregnancy issue is settled, evaluation for other etiologies can proceed. Among the less common causes of amenorrhea, but of greatest consequence to long-term survival, are occult neoplasms of the sellar region. Unlike ovarian or adrenal tumors, these may present with few symptoms other than amenorrhea, making diagnosis difficult unless a high index of suspicion is maintained. However, embarking on an elaborate workup in every patient with amenorrhea is bound to be wasteful, because the incidence of pituitary tumors is so low. High-risk patients who deserve detailed endocrinologic and radiologic study need to be identified.

Table 109-1. Differential Diagnosis of Secondary Amenorrhea

Hypogonadotropic Conditions (may also be eugonadotropic)
Functional (stress, concurrent illness, anorexia)
Prolactinoma
Idiopathic hyperprolactinemia
Pituitary tumor other than prolactinoma (*e.g.,* chromophobe)
Pituitary or hypothalamic destruction (*e.g.,* postpartum necrosis)
Polycystic ovary disease
Ovarian tumor
Endometrial scarring
Uncontrolled diabetes
Thyroid disease
Cushing's syndrome

Hypergonadotropic Conditions
Menopause
Premature menopause
Polyendocrine deficiency
Chemotherapy
Ovarian irradiation

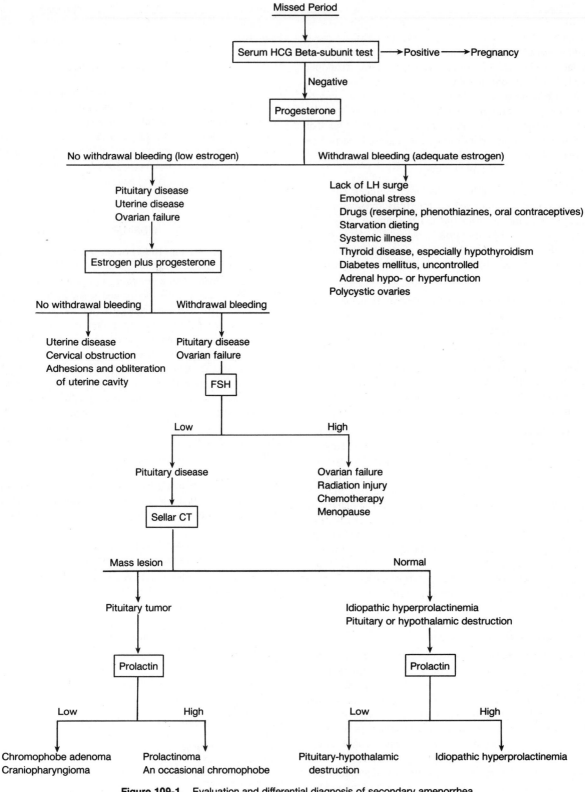

Figure 109-1. Evaluation and differential diagnosis of secondary amenorrhea.

History. A menstrual history that includes age of onset, character of normal cycles, timing of missed periods, and any prior pregnancies or abortions should be obtained. Detailed inquiry into any emotional problems, changes in eating and exercise habits, dieting, and drug use is required. The patient should be asked about concurrent stress factors, including recent changes in school, job, family, or social relationships. History of sexual activity, contraceptive use, and symptoms of pregnancy should be pursued. The patient also needs to be asked about headaches, breast discharge, change in body hair pattern, and symptoms of thyroid or adrenal disease.

Physical Examination should include assessment of weight, secondary sex characteristics, and skin; any signs of thyroid or adrenal disease ought to be noted as should any signs of virilization or hirsutism. The breasts are checked for evidence of galactorrhea, masses, or darkening of areola (as seen in pregnancy). On pelvic examination, it is important to check for any clitoromegaly, evidence of estrogenization of vaginal mucosa, appearance of the cervix, patency of the canal, and size of the uterus and ovaries. Rectopelvic examination will help differentiate cul-de-sac masses from feces or a retroflexed uterus.

When history and physical examination are unremarkable and pregnancy has been ruled out, one needs to decide whether or not further evaluation is indicated at that time. The nonpregnant woman who has missed one or two periods, has a normal physical examination and is involved in a stressful situation such as the first year of college or boarding school, a new job, or a new city can be observed for 6 months before further workup is planned. If periods have not returned by 6 months and there is no obvious emotional stress to account for the problem, further assessment is indicated.

Laboratory Studies. The first step in a more detailed assessment (see Fig. 109-1) is to determine if there is sufficient estrogen effect. If there is, it indicates that amenorrhea is due to a disturbance of cyclic LH secretion and progesterone production. Estrogen effect can be assayed by the administration of *exogenous progesterone,* which will result in withdrawal bleeding if estrogen secretion has been adequate. To test the response to progesterone, medroxyprogesterone (Provera) can be administered orally, 10 mg per day for 5 days, and withdrawal bleeding awaited. Another way to assess estrogen effect is to note the pattern made by *cervical mucus* on a glass slide; the mucus from a patient with normal estrogen levels has a fernlike pattern.

Patients in whom withdrawal bleeding occurs have adequate estrogen, suggesting that the problem involves a lack of LH surge or is due to polycystic disease (if in conjunction with hirsutism, obesity, and infertility). The vast majority will have a "functional" type of amenorrhea resulting from temporarily disturbed LH secretion of hypothalamic origin.

Assessment for polycystic ovary disease can be done noninvasively by ultrasonography, though persistently elevated *LH levels* are very suggestive of the diagnosis, if the patient is obese, hirsute, or infertile. Laparoscopy can be reserved for difficult cases. Patients with normal estrogen effect do not require testing for Cushing's syndrome unless there is clinical evidence of excess cortisol. The same is true for diabetes and thyroid disease, although occult hypothyroidism may trigger an increase in prolactin, which interrupts menses. Thus a TSH is probably worth ordering, though hyperprolactinemia is usually accompanied by low estrogen levels.

Failure of the progesterone to induce bleeding implies inadequate endogenous estrogen production or target organ failure. These patients require a more extensive evaluation for the possibility of pituitary disease, uterine pathology, or inadequate ovarian function.

If bleeding follows administration of estrogen plus progesterone, either the problem is at the hypothalamic–pituitary level, and an evaluation for tumor is required, or the difficulty resides with the ovaries. Measurement of *FSH level* will distinguish between these; a four- to fivefold elevation in FSH points to an ovarian etiology, low FSH to pituitary disease.

Amenorrheic women with a low FSH and suspected pituitary disease require both neuroanatomic and endocrine studies. *CT scan* of the sella turcica has emerged as the anatomic study of choice, replacing all previous diagnostic modalities. Advanced scanners have the resolution power to detect lesions a few millimeters in diameter (at the expense of a slight decrease in specificity). Endocrinologic study of patients with suspected pituitary disease begins with a *serum prolactin* determination. To avoid making a false-positive diagnosis of a hyperprolactinemic condition, the prolactin determination should be done with the patient off all medications known to stimulate prolactin secretion, including estrogens, phenothiazines, and reserpine. L-dopa, nicotine, and ergotamine reduce prolactin output and may mask or blunt an elevation.

Patients with a mass lesion and a high prolactin level have a prolactinoma (an occasional patient will have a chromophobe adenoma); those with a pituitary mass and no prolactin elevation have a nonprolactin-secreting pituitary tumor. Patients with no mass lesion visible by CT and a high prolactin level are designated as having idiopathic hyperprolactinemia. Those with low prolactin are likely to have suffered postpartum necrosis or another form of pituitary or hypothalamic damage. Further evaluation of pituitary function is readily achieved by measurement of trophic hormone levels, especially *TSH,* which tends to fall after LH and FSH decline.

SYMPTOMATIC THERAPY

Patients with functional amenorrhea need only advice and reassurance (see below), for their periods are likely to return shortly. There is no medical need to reestablish menstrual cycles unless the patient is uncomfortable living with the uncertainty of waiting for menstrual flow to resume.

Hyperprolactinemic patients with microadenomas or idiopathic disease can achieve restoration of normal ovulation and menstruation with *bromocriptine* in 95% of instances. Bromocriptine is a dopamine agonist that halts prolactin secretion. It can restore fertility and has been found safe for use in patients who desire to become pregnant. Surgery is no longer deemed necessary for patients with a microadenoma, unless there is documentation by CT of an enlarging tumor mass. Monitoring during pregnancy is especially important, because a small percentage of prolactinomas will grow during that time. Patients found on initial or subsequent workup to have a large mass or clinical/biochemical evidence of pituitary compromise require referral for consideration of surgery.

Patients with hypergonadotropic hypogonadal types of secondary amenorrhea are candidates for *estrogen* and *progesterone* replacement therapy. Such measures will prevent osteoporosis, hot flashes, and atrophic vaginitis from setting in prematurely. Estrogen (ethinyl estradiol, 20 μg/day or conjugated estrogens 0.625 mg/day) is given, with progesterone added for 10 days of each month in women with an intact uterus, to induce adequate shedding of endometrial tissue.

PATIENT EDUCATION

The first priority is to inform the patient who presents with one or two missed periods as to whether or not she is pregnant. Sometimes this essential communication is forgotten. In addition, the primary physician can reassure the patient with functional amenorrhea that menstrual bleeding is not essential for health and that periods usually return within a few months, often soon after resolution of a stressful situation. Patients whose amenorrhea followed use of oral contraceptives can be reassured that they have not been rendered infertile and that normal ovulatory periods resume in more than 99% of patients by 6 months. If conception is not desired, the need for mechanical contraception should be stressed, because the incidence of spontaneous ovulation is high in functional amenorrhea.

INDICATIONS FOR REFERRAL

Patients found to have ovarian failure, suspicion of Stein–Leventhal syndrome, or uterine scarring should be sent to the gynecologist for further evaluation. Virilization deserves consultation with the gynecologist and endocrinologist, though serum testosterone, androstenedione, and urinary 17-ketosteroid levels can be obtained prior to referral. Further evaluation of a large pituitary neoplasm should be done in conjunction with the endocrinologist and neurosurgeon. Patients with idiopathic hyperprolactinemia or a microadenoma (especially those desiring to become pregnant) should have an endocrinologic consultation for confirmation of the diagnosis, counselling, and consideration of need for bromocriptine therapy. In any patient in whom amenorrhea of unclear etiology has persisted for 12 months, the opinion of a subspecialist may be reassuring to both patient and primary physician.

A.H.G.

ANNOTATED BIBLIOGRAPHY

Boyar R, Kapen S, Weitzman E et al: Pituitary microadenoma and hyperprolactinemia. N Engl J Med 294:263, 1976 (*Secondary amenorrhea with hyperprolactinemia and no galactorrhea. Microadenomas found on polytomograms.*)

Friedman CI, Barrows H, Kim MH: Hypergonadotropic hypogonadism. Am J Obstet Gynecol 145:360, 1983 (*Differential diagnosis and evaluation; based on a series of 29 cases.*)

Fries H et al: Epidemiology of secondary amenorrhea. II. A retrospective evaluation of etiology with special regard to psychogenic factors and weight loss. Am J Obstet Gynecol 118:473, 1974 (*A comprehensive discussion of the epidemiology of secondary amenorrhea related to weight loss and stressful life events.*)

Frisch RE, Gotz-Welbergen AV, McArthur JW et al: Delayed menarche and amenorrhea of college athletes in relation to age of onset of training. JAMA 246:1559, 1981 (*Documents associations between training, weight loss, and amenorrhea.*)

Jacobs JS: Prolactin and amenorrhea. N Engl J Med 295:954, 1976 (*Discusses significance of prolactin evaluation in assessment of amenorrhea.*)

Koppelman MC, Jaffe MJ, Rieth KG et al: Hyperprolactinemia, amenorrhea and galactorrhea. Ann Intern Med 100:115, 1984 (*Provides important data on the natural history of these conditions.*)

McDonough PG: Amenorrhea—Etiologic approach to diagnosis. Fertil Steril 30:1, 1978 (*A comprehensive review using hypergonadotropic, hypogonadotropic, and androgen excess as the physiologic organization of the differential diagnosis.*)

Melmed S, Braunstein GD, Chang RJ et al: Pituitary tumors secreting growth hormone and prolactin. Ann Intern Med 105:238, 1986 (*A comprehensive review of pathophysiology, diagnosis, and treatment; 167 references.*)

Molitch ME: Pregnancy and the hyperprolactinemic patient. N Engl J Med 312:1364, 1985 (*Excellent review, especially for those who counsel hyperprolactinemic women.*)

Nakano R, Hashiba N, Kotsuji F: A schematic approach to the workup of amenorrhea. Fertil Steril 28:229, 1977 (*A good description of sophisticated endocrine tests used in the precise determination of amenorrhea.*)

Neufield M, KacLaren N, Blizzard R: Autoimmune polyglandular syndromes. Pediatr Ann 9:154, 1980 (*A good description of these syndromes and their autoimmune pathophysiology.*)

Pettersson F, Fries H, Nillius SJ: Epidemiology of secondary amenorrhea. I. Incidence and prevalence rates. Am J Obstet Gynecol

117:80, 1973 (*A sample of 2000 Swedish women with a 1-year incidence of 3.3% and a prevalence of 4.4%. A relationship to oral contraceptives was found in 16% of the women with amenorrhea.*)

Robinson AG, Nelson PB: Prolactinomas in women: Current therapies. Ann Intern Med 49:115, 1983 (*An editorial providing guidelines for therapy.*)

Shearman R, Fraser I: Impact of new diagnostic methods on the differential diagnosis and treatment of secondary amenorrhea. Lancet 1:1195, 1977 (*A prospective series of 90 women who had at least 12 months of secondary amenorrhea; 39% had hyperprolactinemia; 11% had pituitary tumors, and most had galactorrhea or hyperprolactinemia.*)

Shearman RP: Prolonged secondary amenorrhea after oral contraceptive therapy. Lancet 2:64, 1971 (*A review of the syndrome of postpill amenorrhea.*)

Vance ML, Evans WS, Thorner MB: Bromocriptine. Ann Intern Med 100:78, 1984 (*Comprehensive review of the drug; includes 134 references.*)

110
Evaluation of Breast Mass or Discharge

A solitary or dominant breast mass or an abnormal breast discharge may be a harbinger of breast cancer, the most common malignancy among women. Because such a finding, whether discovered by the patient or by her physician, will raise legitimate fears, the primary physician must be able to proceed with deliberate speed in reaching a diagnosis that excludes carcinoma.

PATHOPHYSIOLOGY AND CLINICAL PRESENTATION

The breast is a complex organ composed of epithelium that forms acini and ducts, fibrous tissue that provides support, and fat. It is exquisitely sensitive to its hormonal milieu. Estradiol stimulates proliferation of epithelial cells and accompanying increases in periductal vascularity. Progesterone induces the development of acini and opposes the mesenchymal actions of estrogens. With each menstrual cycle, the breast exhibits its own cycle of proliferation and desquamation of duct lining. But the response of epithelium, fibrous tissue, and fat to the same hormonal stimulation is variable. Certain areas of the breast may overshoot in the monthly preparation for pregnancy, causing thickening of the breasts and lumpiness. The overgrowth may involve proliferation of fibrous tissue alone or also involve epithelial cells of the ducts and glands, leading to fibroadenomas or ductal dysplasia. Lumps can also be caused by the collection of fluids, essentially colostrum or dissolved cellular debris, which form microcysts or macrocysts.

Although the variable response of tissue to physiologic proliferative and involutional hormonal stimuli is responsible for most benign masses, there are other causes. Infection, usually associated with duct obstruction, can result in an inflammatory mass. Blunt trauma can lead to hematoma formation.

Approximately 20% of solitary or dominant breast masses are cancers.

Nonmilky unilateral breast discharges may reflect local inflammatory or neoplastic lesions, most of which are benign.

Approximately 5% of women with a breast discharge have cancer; one in four of those who have a bloody discharge have cancer. Bloody discharge due to carcinoma may present in the absence of a breast mass.

DIFFERENTIAL DIAGNOSIS

The differential diagnosis of a breast mass, with or without associated discharge, is confusing because of lack of agreement or standardization in clinical and pathologic terminology, particularly regarding the cystic and proliferative changes generally referred to as fibrocystic disease. These changes can be found clinically in approximately 50% of women during their reproductive years and histologically in 90%. Most investigators currently believe that benign breast disease, including neoplasms such as fibroadenomas and intraductal papillomas as well as fibrocystic disease, represents a spectrum of responses to normal hormonal stimulation rather than distinct diseases.

Masses may represent proliferative changes in epithelial or mesenchymal tissue or fluid-filled cysts. The most common discretely palpable mass is the fibroadenoma; multiple fibroadenomas may be present in 10% to 15% of cases. Approximately 20% of solitary or dominant breast masses are breast cancers.

A serous or bloody discharge may occur with fibrocystic disease. Intraductal papillomas are often too small to be palpable and, therefore, often present with nipple discharge. Duct ectasia in fibrocystic disease can produce discharge with or without a palpable mass. If a mass is present, it should be biopsied.

WORKUP

Much is made of the clinical characteristics of breast masses in estimating the probability of malignant disease. Easy mobility within the breast, regular borders, and a soft or cystic feel on palpation all suggest a benign process. However, these signs are not reliable; 60% of cancers are freely movable, 40% have regular borders, and 40% feel soft or cystic. Using these data and estimating that 90% of benign lesions have "benign" physical findings, Mushlin has estimated the change in probability of cancer based on these findings. Assuming that 20% of all masses are malignant, a fixed mass has about a 50% chance of being malignant. The most important point derived from this analysis is that a benign finding reduces the probability of cancer no further than to approximately 10%. In the presence of multiple nodules and diffuse thickening consistent with fibrocystic changes in a young woman, reexamination after a short interval or ultrasonography to document a cystic lesion is a reasonable approach, but a persistent solitary or dominant nodule requires biopsy.

Mammography is a valuable diagnostic test in the woman over 30 with breast symptoms, but it must be emphasized that a negative mammogram does not obviate the need for biopsy of a clinically suspicious breast mass. Studies in which the most advanced techniques were used by the most experienced clinicians have repeatedly indicated that mammography has a false-negative rate of 8% to 10%. Mammograms should be obtained prior to biopsy or preoperatively for any woman undergoing breast surgery. The preoperative study may help to delineate the lesion and identify any occult lesions in the ipsilateral or contralateral breast.

Ultrasonography can be used to distinguish between a cystic and a solid palpable mass, especially in women under 30. An alternative is *needle aspiration,* guided by simple palpation. Needle aspiration of solid as well as cystic lesions, with cytologic examination of the material obtained, is sometimes a means to avoid open biopsy. In one large study, the procedure was accomplished successfully and satisfactory specimens were obtained from only 64% of patients. Among these, however, sensitivity was 87% and specificity was 99%.

Other imaging techniques have, as yet, limited roles. Thermography has proved to be insufficiently sensitive and specific. Computed tomography may localize clinically occult lesions noted but not readily localized on mammography. The potential roles of transillumination, digital radiography, and magnetic resonance imaging are currently being investigated.

SYMPTOMATIC MANAGEMENT

Women with a breast mass or discharge generally have no symptoms that need therapy. The woman with painful breasts associated with fibrocystic disease can be assured that symptoms will improve with the cyclical decrease in hormonal stimulation. Because a number of studies have linked consumption of caffeine and methylxanthines to severe fibrocystic disease, women can be advised to abstain from coffee and other caffeine-containing beverages. A number of aggressive regimens have been used to treat severe fibrocystic disease, including the antiestrogen tamoxifen, the antigonadotropin danazol, and vitamin E. These approaches have been insufficiently evaluated and cannot be recommended at this time. Women with a breast mass or discharge are more concerned with the possibility of breast cancer than they are with symptoms. A prompt, efficient diagnostic evaluation is the best medicine.

PATIENT EDUCATION

Women who present with a breast mass or discharge should be advised that the great majority of such lesions are benign. The nature of fibrocystic breast disease, its extremely high prevalence, and its natural history should be explained. Focusing on this common benign condition, while still insisting on more definitive diagnostic measures when indicated, will provide needed reassurance for most patients.

A.G.M.

ANNOTATED BIBLIOGRAPHY

Atkins H, Wolff B: Discharges from the nipple. Br J Surg 51:602, 1964 (*A review of 203 cases from the Breast Clinic at Guys Hospital; 171 cases without a lump had histologic examination with 71 cases of fibroadenosis, 43 of direct papilloma, 21 of papillary cyst adenomas, and only 14 carcinomas. A treatment plan is proposed.*)

Berkowitz GS, Kelsey JL, Livolsi VA et al: Oral contraceptive use in fibrocystic breast disease among pre- and postmenopausal women. Am J Epidemiol 120:87, 1984 (*A case-control study that did not detect a protective effect of oral contraceptive use.*)

Ernster VL: The epidemiology of benign breast disease. Epidemiol Rev 3:184, 1981 (*A thoughtful review emphasizing the problem of case definition and reviewing evidence that has linked benign breast disease with age, race, socioeconomic status, menstrual and reproductive characteristics, family history of breast cancer, obesity, endogenous hormone levels, and exogenous hormone use.*)

Hislop TG, Threlfall WJ: Oral contraceptives and benign breast disease. Am J Epidemiol 120:273, 1984 (*This retrospective cohort study on oral contraceptive use had a protective effect against benign breast disease.*)

Kopans DB, Meyer JE, Sadowsky N: Breast imaging. N Engl J Med 310:960, 1984 (*Reviews imaging techniques including mammography, ultrasonography, thermography, and NMR. Discusses reasons for limited sensitivity and specificity for each technique.*)

Love SM, Gelman RS, Silen W: Fibrocystic "disease" of the breast A nondisease? N Engl J Med 307:1010, 1982 (*A critical review of clinical and histologic definitions of fibrocystic disease in a careful exploration of its role as a risk factor for breast cancer.*)

Mushlin AI: Diagnostic tests in breast cancer. Ann Intern Med 103:

79, 1985 (*A superb review, logical and carefully reasoned, of test characteristics with recommendations based on diagnostic probabilities. Accompanies a position statement of the American College of Physicians in the same issue.*)

Odenheimer DJ, ZunZunegui MV, King MC et al: Risk factors for benign breast disease: A case control study of discordant twins. Am J Epidemiol 120:565, 1984 (*Positive association was found between benign breast disease and coffee consumption; oral contraceptive use and greater body mass were inversely associated.*)

Parazzini F, Vecchia CL, Franceschi S et al: Risk factors for pathologically confirmed benign breast disease. Am J Epidemiol 120: 115, 1984 (*This case-control study found identical risk factors for benign and malignant breast disease and did not detect a protective effect for oral contraceptives or body mass.*)

111
Evaluation of Galactorrhea

Discharge of milk or colostrum from the breast is an abnormal finding except in late pregnancy and the postpartum period. When a woman presents with galactorrhea, the possibility of an occult pituitary neoplasm must be evaluated.

PATHOPHYSIOLOGY AND CLINICAL PRESENTATION

The pathophysiology of *galactorrhea* is not well understood; it has only a limited relationship to hyperprolactinemia. In the common, idiopathic form of galactorrhea, menses are normal and 85% of such patients have normal prolactin levels. The cause of galactorrhea is believed related to local breast factors after the capacity for lactation has been induced previously by childbirth or another stimulus. Galactorrhea in conjunction with *amenorrhea* is often associated with high prolactin levels, but only 20% of patients with hyperprolactinemia have galactorrhea. Galactorrhea occurs when high levels of prolactin act on a breast primed by estrogen and progesterone, accounting for its occurrence just after pregnancy or use of oral contraceptives. Prolactin secretion may increase as a result of an autonomously functioning prolactinoma, or because of agents acting on the hypothalamus; for example, thyroid-releasing hormone (TRH) may stimulate prolactin, accounting for the association of galactorrhea with hypothyroidism.

The importance of galactorrhea is its relationship to *hyperprolactinemia* and the association of hyperprolactinemia with pituitary adenomas. In one study of 235 patients with galactorrhea, all those with prolactin values above 300 ng/ml had pituitary neoplasms; 57% of those with values above 100 ng/ml had tumors. In the same series, 6 women with prolactin levels in the normal range of 1 to 20 ng/ml were found to have adenomas, but 4 had acromegaly and 1 had had prior radiotherapy, so only 1 patient without acromegaly and with a normal serum prolactin had an untreated tumor.

Galactorrhea may be first noted as an isolated finding by the patient or discovered during the physical examination. Amenorrhea may or may not be concurrent. Occasionally, the patient is discovered to have galactorrhea during an infertility workup. Less frequently, patients present with other symptoms, such as headache or visual symptoms associated with pituitary adenomas.

DIFFERENTIAL DIAGNOSIS

The differential diagnosis of galactorrhea includes idiopathic cases, pituitary tumors, drug use, and hypothyroidism. The largest single group of patients (32% in one series) have the idiopathic variety, with normal periods and normal prolactin levels. The hypothalamic pituitary causes of galactorrhea include prolactin-producing pituitary adenomas, the empty sella syndrome, and, less commonly, craniopharyngiomas or pinealomas. About one third of patients with galactorrhea and amenorrhea are found to have neoplasms. Persistent galactorrhea after childbirth accounts for less than 10% of cases. Drugs associated with galactorrhea include oral contraceptives, tranquilizers (phenothiazines, benzodiazepines, haloperidol), and, less commonly, reserpine, methyldopa, isoniazid, and imipramine. Primary hypothyroidism is a definite cause. Galactorrhea has also been associated with heroin addiction.

Various local factors (*e.g.,* chest trauma or breast manipulation) as well as central lesions (*e.g.,* head trauma, sarcoidosis) have been noted in association with galactorrhea.

WORKUP

The workup for galactorrhea should include questioning about recent pregnancy, abortion, current presence or absence of normal menstrual periods, symptoms of hypothyroidism, and presence of headache or visual complaints. A careful review of drug use, particularly oral contraceptives and major tranquilizers, needs to be pursued. Physical examination ought to include a careful examination of the breast, although no increased risk of breast cancer has been found in patients with galactorrhea. Confrontation testing of the visual fields and fundoscopic examination are important, though usually normal. Any signs of hypothyroidism (see Chapter 102) should be noted, and confirmed by ordering a TSH and free T_4.

The development of prolactin assays and the occasional association of galactorrhea with high prolactin levels and pituitary tumors have made prolactin testing a very important adjunct to assessment; however, prolactin levels may be affected by stress, time of day, sleep, or breast stimulation. Accuracy is enhanced by placing a catheter in the patient's vein and having the patient rest in a recumbent position for an hour before a morning sample is drawn. The patient with galactorrhea and amenorrhea is at increased risk for a pituitary neoplasm and should be prolactin tested.

Computed tomography (CT) of the sella turcica should be obtained in any patient with a markedly elevated prolactin level or symptoms and signs suggestive of pituitary adenoma. Formal visual field evaluation by an ophthalmologist or optometrist should be performed in patients with abnormal sella turcica films.

From a practical standpoint, regular menses and a normal prolactin level in a patient with galactorrhea make the likelihood of a clinically important pituitary tumor remote. Patients in whom the likelihood of tumor is low can be followed carefully with periodic determinations of prolactin, usually at 1-year intervals; if prolactin levels become elevated, CT of the sella can be ordered.

SYMPTOMATIC MANAGEMENT

Symptomatic management of galactorrhea depends on the degree of concern shown by the patient. In patients who are not bothered by the discharge, no treatment is indicated except for explanation, follow-up, and discontinuation of drugs associated with the production of galactorrhea. In patients with idiopathic galactorrhea who are bothered by the discharge, the most effective treatment is the use of ergot derivatives; their dopaminergic effects lower prolactin secretion, may lessen galactorrhea, and often restore regular menses.

PATIENT EDUCATION

Patients with galactorrhea may be worried about cancer. Fear that may be engendered by the possibility of a pituitary adenoma can be lessened by explaining the slow growth and good prognosis associated with the majority of prolactinomas.

The patient with galactorrhea and amenorrhea should be informed that numerous options for induction of fertility are available and that these may be pursued according to the patient's wishes. By providing accurate information, moral support, and close follow-up, the primary physician can prevent a great deal of unnecessary suffering.

A.H.G. and A.G.M.

ANNOTATED BIBLIOGRAPHY

Adler RA: The evaluation of galactorrhea. Am J Obstet Gynecol 127: 569, 1977 (*A useful diagnostic classification.*)

Boyd AE, Reichlin S, Turksoy RN: Galactorrhea-amenorrhea syndrome: Diagnosis and therapy. Ann Intern Med 87:165, 1977 (*High basal prolactin levels [150 mg/ml] that increase by 100 mg/ml after TRH or chlorpromazine are suggestive of tumor.*)

Frantz AG: Prolactin. N Engl J Med 298:201, 1978 (*A well-synthesized review; 17 references.*)

Gomez F, Reyes FI, Faiman C: Nonpuerperal galactorrhea and hyperprolactinemia. Clinical findings, endocrine features and therapeutic responses in 56 cases. Am J Med 62:648, 1977 (*A superb review emphasizing that many cases are without precise diagnosis; prolactin suppression tests were of no value and prolonged observation remains essential. Pituitary adenomas were found in 17, myxedema in 2, and phenothiazine in 6; 27 were considered dysfunctional.*)

Hooper JH, Welsh VC, Shackleford RT: Abnormal lactation associated with tranquilizing drug therapy. JAMA 178:506, 1961 (*An incidence of abnormal lactation of 26% was found in 100 women receiving tranquilizers; the effect was dose dependent.*)

Kleinberg DL, Noel GL, Frantz AA: Galactorrhea: A study of 235 cases, including 48 pituitary tumors. N Engl J Med 296:589, 1977 (*A comprehensive review finding a 2% incidence of pituitary tumors overall and 34% in connection with amenorrhea. The largest group, 32%, had idiopathic galactorrhea without amenorrhea. Ergot derivatives are an effective treatment.*)

Koppelman MC, Jaffe MJ, Rieth KG et al: Hyperprolactinemia, amenorrhea and galactorrhea. Ann Intern Med 100:115, 1984 (*Excellent review of the problem.*)

Reichlin S: The prolactinoma problem (editorial): N Engl J Med 300: 313, 1979 (*A succinct statement on the implication of discovering approaches to treating small prolactin-secreting pituitary adenomas.*)

112
Evaluation of Vulvar Pruritus

Vulvar itching in young women is annoying, but rarely a sign of serious illness; in older women it may be a manifestation of malignancy. A specific cause can usually be identified, making etiologic treatment possible. The primary physician needs to be aware of the common vulvar irritants, inflammatory conditions, and infestations as well as the appearance of early malignancy so that use of nonspecific therapies and delay in detection of carcinoma are avoided.

PATHOPHYSIOLOGY AND CLINICAL PRESENTATIONS

In the genital area only the vulvar and perineal skin have sensory receptors that trigger the sensation of itching when irritated. The mucosa of the vagina and cervix are not innervated in such a manner. Of the many etiologies of vulvar pruritus, squamous *carcinoma of the vulva* is the most ominous. The typical patient is elderly; 70% of cases appear in women over 60 years of age; however, the condition may appear at any age, and recent data suggest an increasing incidence of carcinoma *in situ* among younger women. Squamous-cell carcinoma of the vulva may present with single or multiple papules or macules, which can be confluent or discrete, usually on the labia majora or minora. The lesions can be red, white, or pigmented and may be in multiple locations on the labia. They typically arise on the vulvar skin in areas already long-involved with premalignant change (see below). Spread is to inguinal and deep pelvic nodes. Occasionally, a patient with carcinoma complains of a lump or an ulcerated lesion. Itching may be intense, sometimes in conjunction with a slightly bloody discharge. Delay in presentation is common; often the patient gives a history of unsuccessful trials of topical agents for symptomatic relief from itching. Epidemiologically, there is an association with early menopause, obesity, diabetes, and nulliparity.

Premalignant skin changes, referred to as *vulvar dystrophies,* present as thickened white-gray lesions; formerly, such lesions were labelled *leukoplakia.* They are often edematous, fissured, or excoriated and accompanied by a secondary inflammatory reaction. The red areas are more likely than the white ones to contain dysplastic cells. When there is no atypia on histologic examination, the risk of cancer is nil. Sometimes there is scaling, erythema, or a thin, pale, wrinkled appearance, as in *lichen sclerosus,* which may contain atypical cells. *Paget's disease* of the vulva is a diffuse scaling process involving the anal region as well; in 5% of cases, there is an underlying adenocarcinoma. Vulvar dystrophies progress over a period of years mimicking vulvitis or even urinary tract infection because of the superficial burning from contact with urine.

Atrophic vaginitis may produce considerable itching. The mucosa is red and thin; sometimes a mild discharge is present. It occurs postmenopausally from lack of estrogen and is seen in women who have undergone oophorectomy as well as in normal menopause (see Chapter 117).

Infectious forms of vaginitis are often very itchy, such as those due to *Candida* and *Trichomonas.* In candidal vulvovaginitis the vulva is erythematous, with a sharp scalloped border demarcating the area of involvement. "Satellite" lesions are characteristic, as is the cheesy discharge of the associated vaginitis (see Chapter 115). Intense vulvar inflammation also occurs with trichomonal infection, but there are no satellite lesions and the discharge tends to be thin, yellow-brown, and malodorous.

Infestations with mites or lice are very uncomfortable. *Scabies* produces papular lesions and itching, which may occur anywhere on the body; involvement of the skin between the fingers is very characteristic but not always present. *Pediculosis* is confined to areas covered by hair, since eggs are deposited on the hair shafts (see Chapter 194).

Irritations caused by scratching, maceration, and chemical agents are common. Deodorants, soaps, douching agents, bubble baths, and contraceptive foams may incite allergic reactions or chemical irritations, leading to itching. Some patients habitually scratch themselves, but often the precipitant is inadequate hygiene; the warm moist environment and chafing fosters maceration of skin in conjunction with the itching and scratching. Cutaneous candidiasis may arise in such an environment, especially when the patient is pregnant or diabetic. Pantyhose exacerbate the problem, as does urinary incontinence. Women who shave their pubic hair are often bothered by pruritus.

DIFFERENTIAL DIAGNOSIS

In young women, vaginitis, pediculosis, scabies, chemical irritants, poor hygiene, use of pantyhose, and allergic reactions are the major etiologies of vaginal itching. The same etiologies apply to older women, but atrophic vaginitis and vulvar carcinoma also become major considerations. Premalignant conditions include lichen sclerosus and Paget's disease. Any condition capable of causing pruritus may present with vulvar itching. Primary cutaneous candidiasis is common among obese diabetic women.

WORKUP

It is important to inquire about vaginal discharge, maceration, skin rash, urinary incontinence, vulvar lesions, and other sites of itching. Possible irritants and allergens need to be identified, such as creams, soaps, bubble baths, vaginal deodorants, douches, and contraceptive foams. The sexual history or presence of genital itching in partners or roommate may suggest infection or infestation. Information related to the duration of the problem and responses to prior treatments can be useful. Presence of an ulceration or nodule that has persisted or grown should be ascertained.

The vulva and perineal skin is inspected for macules, papules, scaling, erythema, ulcerations, pigmented lesions, hypopigmentation, excoriation, rash, lice, and mites. A close look at the hair shaft may reveal lice eggs (nits), which are pathognomonic of the infestation (see Chapter 194). A speculum examination helps to identify any vaginitis or discharge (see Chapter 115). Inguinal nodes should be palpated. A smear of the discharge for identification of an organism and a urinalysis for glycosuria are the major laboratory studies needed. Any suspicious lesions should be referred for biopsy; lesions can be stained with toluidine blue to direct selection of biopsy sites.

SYMPTOMATIC MANAGEMENT, PATIENT EDUCATION, AND INDICATIONS FOR REFERRAL

The management of vulvar pruritus is most likely to be successful when a specific etiology can be identified. Self-treatments and use of potentially irritating soaps or creams ought to be stopped. Incontinent patients will benefit from washing and using protective pastes such as zinc oxide. Biopsy-proven lichen sclerosus without atypia may respond to 2% testosterone propionate cream applied two or three times a day for a period of 6 months. Hyperplastic dystrophy without atypia often responds to topical corticosteroid therapy within 6 weeks. Treatments of vaginitis and mite or lice infestations are detailed in Chapters 115 and 194. Atrophic vaginitis may require a topical estrogen cream (see Chapter 117).

When poor hygiene or excessive moisture are suspected to be contributing to the problem, the patient should be instructed to avoid tight garments such as pantyhose and to use absorbent white cotton underwear.

Occasionally, an antihistamine sedative may be used at night to relieve itching and break the itch-scratch cycle. In the absence of infection or other specific etiology, hydrocortisone cream or lotion might be tried. While vaginitis is treated with a specific agent, application of topical hydrocortisone may facilitate symptomatic relief. Persistence of any suspicious lesion requires referral for consideration of biopsy.

A.H.G.

ANNOTATED BIBLIOGRAPHY

Friedrich EG Jr: Lichen sclerosus. J Reprod Med 17:147, 1976 (*Topical testosterone may be an effective treatment.*)

Friedrich EG Jr: Vulvar pruritus—A symptom, not a disease. Postgrad Med 61:164, 1977 (*An excellent review.*)

International Society for Study of Vulvar Disease. Committee on Terminology: New nomenclature for vulvar disease. Obstet Gynecol 47:122, 1976 (*The introduction of "dystrophy" to substitute for a confusing collection of terms.*)

Kaufman RH: Hyperplastic dystrophy. J Reprod Med 17:137, 1976 (*The risk of malignancy is low and is present only in cases that show atypia.*)

Sobel JD: Vulvovaginal candidiasis: What we do and do not know. Ann Intern Med 101:390, 1984 (*Discusses the perplexing and sometimes intractable problem of recurrent incapacitating vulvovaginal candidiasis.*)

Woodruff JD, Julian C, Puray T et al: The contemporary challenge of carcinoma in situ of the vulva. Am J Obstet Gynecol 115:677, 1972 (*Emphasizes need for early diagnosis.*)

113
Medical Evaluation of Dyspareunia and Other Female Sexual Dysfunctions
ANN B. BARNES, M.D.

DYSPAREUNIA

Dyspareunia, or painful intercourse, is probably more common than physicians realize because patients may not volunteer the complaint. It often requires an aware and sympathetic clinician to uncover the problem. Pain on intercourse may be the presentation of pelvic disease or a symptom that disrupts a marriage. The primary physician is often in the best position to evaluate the causes and manage the problem.

Pathophysiology and Clinical Presentation

Several pathogenic mechanisms may be responsible for painful intercourse. They include inflammatory lesions, failure of lubrication, anatomic problems, and psychological conflicts. Pain can arise from friction against inflamed tissue or by jarring of deeper inflamed parametrial structures. Failure of normal vaginal lubrication may produce pain or spasm. Physical impediments to penile penetration of the vagina may be due to surgery, inflammation, or anatomic variants. The psychological mechanisms of dyspareunia reflect a variety of conflicts, fears, and hostility (see Chapter 225).

In premenopausal women, inadequate lubrication because of too little foreplay is among the most frequent causes of dyspareunia. In postmenopausal patients, atrophic vaginitis is an important factor. Scant production of vaginal secretions may also reflect fears, misunderstandings, marital conflicts, and hostilities. Concern about venereal disease and cancer are other common underlying issues that can inhibit normal lubrication.

Dyspareunia may be due to anatomic difference between partners, especially when the woman's vagina is functionally or anatomically small. A tight or thick hymenal ring, marked vaginal constriction, or partial fusion of the labia can cause pain on intercourse.

Irritation of the vulva caused by tight-fitting clothes, lack of hygiene, or infection is found in patients complaining of *pain on intromission.* Fungal vulvovaginitis and bacterial infection of the vagina, cervix, and Bartholin's gland duct are common (see Chapter 115). A cyst of the Bartholin's gland duct occurs when mechanical irritation and the attendant inflammatory reaction obstruct the ductal lumen. Viral vulvitis from herpes vaginalis is usually so painful that intercourse is not attempted. Condylomata can be painful and may bleed, but usually do not inhibit intercourse.

Deep dyspareunia may occur with endometriosis, ovarian cysts, adhesions, and pelvic inflammatory disease. These sources of pain on intercourse cause difficulty when penetration is deep. Penile thrusting moves the entire uterus, with resultant pulling on the peritoneum. Acute or defervescing pelvic inflammatory disease or endometritis will produce pain even on gentle motion.

A thin vulvar surface and vaginal mucosa are less resilient and less resistant to trauma. These vaginal changes take place in women who are anorexic, breast-feeding, or menopausal, or who have had pelvic irradiation.

Vaginismus, defined as involuntary spasm of the perineal muscles induced by any attempt at physical penetration, is an important, though uncommon, cause of dyspareunia.

Differential Diagnosis

The causes of dyspareunia can be listed according to whether there is pain on intromission or on deep penetration (Table 113-1).

Workup

One needs to determine whether dyspareunia occurred with the first effort at intercourse or has developed recently secondary to organic change or a situational problem. The patient should be asked whether pain occurs before penetration, on penetration, or only after deep penetration. It is important to establish whether the patient can insert a tampon without pain; if she can, mechanical obstruction is unlikely. A history of previous surgery, pelvic inflammatory disease, or radiation may suggest the etiology. Failure to localize the site of coital pain suggests psychogenic dyspareunia. A history of sexual fears, time spent on foreplay, and feelings toward the partner should be sensitively obtained (see Chapter 225). Interviewing the husband or sexual partner is essential to an adequate evaluation. The duration of dyspareunia should be determined, because symptoms that have existed for years

Table 113-1. Important Causes of Dyspareunia

PAIN GREATEST ON INTROMISSION	PAIN GREATEST ON DEEP PENETRATION
Inadequate lubrication	Pelvic inflammatory disease
Size discrepancy in partners	Ovarian cyst
Incompletely ruptured hymen	Endometriosis
Bartholin's gland cyst	Pelvic adhesions
Stricture	Relaxation of pelvic support
Inadequate episiotomy	
Vaginitis	
Atrophy of vaginal and vulvar tissue	
Vaginismus	

may not resolve even after a medical condition is identified and corrected.

The most important part of the workup is pelvic examination. The physician should inspect for signs of vulvovaginitis, atrophic vaginitis, narrowed introitus, cervicitis, and congenital abnormalities. Observation of involuntary spasm on attempted examination suggests vaginismus. Palpation may identify a uterine mass, a retroverted uterus, or tenderness. The cervix should be manipulated to see if pain is produced. Examination for loss of pelvic support, rectocele, or cystocele is needed. A smear should be obtained for cervical cytology to detect underlying malignancy.

A complete blood count, sedimentation rate, and cervical culture are indicated when there is evidence on physical examination suggesting pelvic inflammatory disease (see Chapter 115). Pelvic ultrasonography may be indicated to help define a suspected pelvic mass. Referral to a gynecologist for laparoscopy is indicated when endometriosis, adhesions, or an adnexal mass is under consideration.

Symptomatic Management, Patient Education, and Indications for Referral

The patient without organic pathology who is troubled by inadequate lubrication should be sympathetically reassured that she is healthy and provided advice, which may include insisting on more prolonged foreplay and use of a water-soluble lubricant jelly (*e.g.,* Lubafax). Contraceptive creams should not be used for lubrication because they often cause dehydration and may worsen soreness. Oral-genital foreplay, trying different positions for coitus, and guiding the man's penis for insertion are other suggestions that can be made. The *postmenopausal* woman with an atrophic vaginal mucosa can be given estrogen cream to use topically on an intermittent basis (see Chapter 117).

If there is an underlying vaginal or pelvic infection, it should be treated and the patient advised to refrain temporarily from intercourse (see Chapters 115 and 116). A cyst of the Bartholin's gland duct may spontaneously drain following frequent warm soaks in the bathtub, which sometimes relieves the obstruction; marsupialization by a gynecologist may be required to provide adequate drainage if the cyst is badly inflamed and infected. Patients troubled by pain from herpes simplex infection can obtain relief with use of acyclovir (see Chapter 138).

Patients bothered by pain on deep penetration may be more comfortable lying on one side during coitus so that deep penetration is limited.

Retained suture material in episiotomy scars, vulvar islands of adenosis (ectopic columnar epithelium), or nerve endings previously damaged by herpetic infection may require local excision for relief of pain.

The patient with a narrow introitus should be referred to a gynecologist for a trial of vaginal dilators. Vaginismus may be managed by education, relaxation, and Kegel exercises, all of which are usually best accomplished by an experienced therapist or sex therapy clinic.

Failure to succeed in identifying or relieving dyspareunia should prompt referral to the gynecologist. This ought to be done only after a thorough evaluation has been performed, the sexual history has been elicited, any infection treated, advice on sexual technique has been provided, and lubricants have been tried. Referral to a psychiatrist or sex therapist, involving both partners, might also be considered. Nevertheless, constant education and reassurance as to the lack of physical danger associated with the symptom are important when there is no evidence of underlying disease. The patient's fears and concerns must be sensitively explored and specifically addressed, as must any marital discord (see Chapter 225).

EXCITEMENT AND ORGASMIC PHASE DYSFUNCTIONS

Medical causes of female sexual dysfunction beyond those resulting in dyspareunia have only recently been explored in systematic fashion. Data are still sketchy but are beginning to accumulate. Psychogenic etiologies still predominate (see Chapter 225).

Excitement phase problems beyond inadequate lubrication are manifested by poor libido. Drug-induced decrease in sexual desire has been identified and is similar to that seen in men. Antihypertensive agents that cross the blood–brain barrier (*e.g.,* reserpine propranolol, and methyldopa) sometimes diminish libido. Oral contraceptives, particularly the sequential variety (which are no longer marketed), have depressive and libido-reducing side-effects in about 5% to 10% of women who use them. Antidepressants, minor tranquilizers, alcohol, phenothiazines, hypnotics, and opiates have been linked to reduction in libido, though it is unclear if it is the underlying emotional problem rather than the drug that is more at fault. Libido is a very sensitive indicator of general physical health, and any intercurrent illness will blunt it. The third trimester of pregnancy often produces a diminution in desire. There is no evidence that estrogen deficiency has an impact on libido, but androgen deficiency does. Loss of androgen synthesizing capacity (*e.g.,* by hypophysectomy or adrenalectomy) can lead to losses of desire and capacity for orgasm.

Orgasmic dysfunction from medical causes is seen in patients who previously functioned normally. In one study, loss of orgasmic capacity among diabetic women was found to have a 35% prevalence. Excitement phase functions were normal, and the severity of the problem correlated with du-

ration of the diabetes. As with excitement phase problems, any illness can interfere with this phase of sexual activity. Usually the problem is global when illness is present, and all sexual functioning is reduced. Correlations between individual disease states and isolated orgasmic dysfunction remain to be further elucidated.

An increasingly common problem is the use of *cytotoxic chemotherapy* in young women with malignancies. A marked loss of libido, lack of lubrication, hypoestrogenism from ovarian failure and inhibition, as well as hot flashes may occur. The depression that accompanies confronting a chronic, malignant disease, combined with the fatigue that follows surgery and chemotherapy, further distresses patients and impairs sexual functioning. Marital problems may ensue. Patient and partner need to be informed of these side-effects of therapy prior to its use and be supported through therapy. For some women, these side-effects are sufficient reason to decline or discontinue such medication. Other women may experience few such side-effects and need to be encouraged to sustain contraceptive practices to avoid harm to a developing fetus.

A.H.G.

ANNOTATED BIBLIOGRAPHY

Chapman RM, Sutcliffe SB, Malpas JS: Cytotoxic-induced ovarian failure in women with Hodgkin's disease I and II. JAMA 242: 1877, 1979 (*Study of sexual function in 41 women.*)

Fordney DS: Dyspareunia and vaginismus. Clin Obstet Gynecol 21: 205, 1978 (*A comprehensive review emphasizing behavioral therapy and the role of sex clinics; includes 36 references.*)

Huffman JW: Office gynecology: Relieving dyspareunia. Postgrad Med 59:223, 1976 (*A useful overview.*)

Kolodny R: Sexual dysfunction in diabetic females. Diabetes 20:557, 1971 (*Isolated orgasmic phase dysfunction identified in 35%.*)

Lamont JA: Vaginismus. Am J Obstet Gynecol 131:632, 1978 (*A review of the presentation and treatment of 80 patients with vaginismus.*)

Levine SB, Rosenthal M: Marital sexual dysfunction: Female dysfunctions. Ann Intern Med 86:588, 1977 (*Good review for the generalist, with emphasis on definition of dysfunctions.*)

Solberg D, Butler J, Wagner N: Sexual behavior in pregnancy. N Engl J Med 288:1098, 1973 (*Third-trimester is associated with reduced libido.*)

Story N: Sexual dysfunction resulting from drug side effects. J Sex Res 10:132, 1974 (*Antihypertensive agents that cross the blood–brain barrier are an important cause of reduced libido.*)

Sutcliffe SB: Cytotoxic chemotherapy and gonadal function in patients with Hodgkin's disease. Facts and thoughts. JAMA 242:1898, 1979 (*Comments on treatment of side-effects of chemotherapy.*)

114
Approach to the Patient with Menstrual or Pelvic Pain

Pelvic pain is a major source of concern and morbidity in women. Dysmenorrhea or painful periods affect approximately half of menstruating women at some time, and an estimated 10% are incapacitated by the problem, with much time lost from work and school. Acute episodes of pelvic pain are also common and may represent potentially serious pathology. The primary physician should be able to distinguish pain of a functional nature from that due to infection or an anatomic lesion, and know when referral to the gynecologist or urgent hospital admission is indicated. Moreover, one should be able to provide the young woman bothered by dysmenorrhea and premenstrual complaints with rational and effective therapy.

PATHOPHYSIOLOGY AND CLINICAL PRESENTATION

Acute Pain. Pelvic pain of acute onset may result from pelvic inflammatory disease, ectopic pregnancy, torsion of the tube or ovary, rupture of an ovarian cyst, or extrapelvic pathology such as acute appendicitis or ureteral stone. *Pelvic inflammatory disease* (PID) usually causes little pain until infection has spread from the cervix through the lymphatics into the parametria and fallopian tubes. The process may not occur until weeks or even months after initial contact with an infected partner. The consequent acute salpingitis is characteristically bilateral, though one side may be more involved than the other, and peritoneal signs may follow if pus escapes from the tube and soils the overlying peritoneum. The gonococcus was once considered the predominant offending organism, but more careful bacteriologic investigation based on culdocentesis or laparoscopic sampling of fallopian tubes has revealed other organisms that can produce the infection, often in conjunction with the gonococcus. It is estimated that gonorrhea accounts for a third to a half of pelvic inflammatory disease; other agents commonly implicated include alpha strep, *E. coli, Chlamydia trachomatis, Mycoplasma,* and anaerobic organisms such as *Bacteroides* (see Chapter 115). Mixed infection is common. The PID associated with *Chlamydia* tends to be less acute in onset than that due to gonorrhea, but is more likely to result in ectopic pregnancy and infertility. Infection with both *Chlamydia* and *N. gonorrhoeae* has been documented in a substantial fraction of patients with both salpingitis and endometritis.

There is a striking association between menstrual periods and onset of gonococcal PID, suggesting that spread from the cervix may occur during menstruation. Prior gonorrhea appears to increase the likelihood of nongonococcal PID, possibly by causing tubal damage. The recurrent nature of PID may be due to fallopian tube damage that impairs bacterial clearance. Pelvic inflammatory disease can be provoked by abortion, endometrial biopsy, hysterosalpinograms, D & C, and hysterectomy. The use of an intrauterine device (IUD) increases the risk of PID, particularly in nulliparous women.

Ectopic pregnancy is a much feared cause of acute pelvic pain, since catastrophic hemorrhage may ensue from tubal rupture. In most cases, the period is delayed by 1 to 2 weeks, followed by recurrent spotting. Severe hemorrhage occurs in fewer than 5% of cases, causing sudden severe pain and hypotension. There may be mild, unilateral tenderness in those cases without bleeding. Patients with previous PID are at greater risk for ectopic pregnancy.

Torsion of the tube with or without ovarian involvement is seen mostly in young women, many of whom have otherwise normal adnexa. Severe, acute unilateral pain and distention are found without an elevation of white count, fever, or increased sedimentation rate, unless complicated by ischemic necrosis.

Ovarian cysts may spontaneously rupture or twist on their pedicles. Rupture can be associated with marked blood loss, thereby presenting in a fashion similar to that of a ruptured ectopic pregnancy. More commonly, only small amounts of fluid or blood are released, causing milder, often recurrent, discomfort. Torsion of the pedicle can lead to ischemic gangrene of a cyst and present as acute unilateral pelvic pain with local peritoneal signs, fever, and leukocytosis. Sometimes the twisting reverses itself spontaneously and only mild intermittent symptoms result.

Periodic or Chronic Pain. Conditions predisposing to recurrent or chronic pelvic pain are generally less ominous than those responsible for acute pain. Common etiologies include primary dysmenorrhea, endometriosis, adenomyosis, chronic pelvic inflammatory disease, intrauterine devices, ovarian cysts, and fibroadenomas.

Dysmenorrhea represents the major source of periodic pelvic pain. It is labeled "primary" when unaccompanied by recognizable pelvic pathology and "secondary" when it occurs in the setting of an underlying gynecologic problem, such as endometriosis, PID, or IUD use. Primary dysmenorrhea typically begins at the time of onset of ovulatory periods and tends to diminish after the first pregnancy. Secondary dysmenorrhea has a later onset and parallels the disease process responsible for it. The prevalence of primary disease is difficult to establish because of the absence of precise diagnostic criteria, the almost universal experience of menstrual cramping, and the wide variability of responses to similar degrees of pelvic discomfort.

It was thought that psychological factors played an etiologic role in primary dysmenorrhea. Now it is recognized that the pain results from high-intensity uterine contractions triggered by prostaglandins. Patients experience cramping pain in the pelvis, lower abdomen, and/or back, coinciding with the start of menstrual bleeding. The cramps can last from minutes to hours; they cease as menstrual flow ends. At times, headache, nausea, vomiting, and/or diarrhea accompany the cramps. All such symptoms have been reproduced by administration of prostaglandin F_2 and blocked by nonsteroidal anti-inflammatory drugs that inhibit prostaglandin synthesis. Episodes of secondary dysmenorrhea may begin a few days before menstruation and worsen or even diminish with onset of bleeding, depending on the underlying etiology.

Premenstrual syndrome. Other symptoms seemingly unrelated to prostaglandin activity are often noted in the late luteal phase of the menstrual cycle and frequently attributed to the dysmenorrhea syndrome. Complaints include irritability, fatigue, bloating, food cravings, constipation, inability to concentrate, mood swings, and depression. Such symptoms have been labelled the premenstrual syndrome (PMS), since they tend to come on 7 to 10 days before the onset of menstruation and, for the most part, cease with onset of flow. Most authorities believe premenstrual syndrome to be pathophysiologically distinct from dysmenorrhea, unrelated to prostaglandin metabolism, and unresponsive to nonsteroidals. Like dysmenorrhea, this syndrome has been attributed to psychological factors and treated unsuccessfully with psychotherapy. Personality testing done during symptomatic periods does reveal abnormalities, but retesting at other stages of the menstrual cycle shows resolution of changes, suggesting that psychological factors may be a manifestation rather than a cause of the problem. Etiology remains unknown. Current investigations center on neuroendocrine factors. Hypotheses that have failed to be substantiated in clinical trials include progesterone deficiency, dietary factors, and vitamin deficiencies. PMS continues to be a major source of temporary disability for a substantial portion of otherwise healthy menstruating women.

Endometriosis, one of the known causes of secondary dysmenorrhea, is seen mostly in women aged 25 to 45, many of whom are nulliparous; the mean age at time of diagnosis is 37. The condition is due to the presence of functioning ectopic endometrial tissue, located in such places as the ovaries, uterosacral ligaments, cul de sac, and peritoneum. The origin of the ectopic tissue is unclear. Pain can begin days or even a week before menstruation, tends to subside with bleeding, and is usually bilateral, deep-seated, or aching, with radiation to the rectum or perineal region. There is often a history of infertility, dyspareunia, or menorrhagia.

A retroverted and fixed uterus or nodular uterosacral ligaments are sometimes detectable on physical examination. Symptoms of endometriosis depend on actively functioning endometrial tissue, but bear no relationship to the amount of endometrial tissue present. The condition resolves with menopause, but often hysterectomy is resorted to.

Adenomyosis is related to endometriosis in that there is ectopic endometrial tissue, but it is localized to the myometrium and occurs mostly in older women. Incidence is greatest in women 41 to 50. The condition can cause menorrhagia, dysmenorrhea, and an enlarged, sometimes tender, uterus. Pain is referred to the back and rectum as the uterus enlarges. Endometrial carcinoma is found with slightly increased frequency in patients with adenomysosis.

Chronic pelvic inflammatory disease is another source of secondary dysmenorrhea with exacerbation of pain occurring around the time of menstruation. A history of previous venereal disease, dyspareunia, menstrual irregularity, backache, rectal pressure, or pelvic pain with fever is often obtained. The physical examination typically reveals tender, thickened adnexal organs; bilateral involvement is characteristic, though one side may predominate.

Intrauterine devices are an important source of secondary dysmenorrhea and heavy bleeding. The rate of removal because of bleeding and pain ranges from 4% to 15%. The crampy menstrual pain can occur in previously normal patients who never experienced dysmenorrhea; parity has little impact, but bleeding seems to be worse in women whose periods were scanty before IUD insertion.

Benign neoplasms, predominantly dermoid cysts, cystadenomas, and uterine fibroids may produce a chronic aching localized to one side of the pelvis. The pain may be intermittent, secondary to periodic leakage of irritant contents, or, occasionally, chronic. Chronic intermittent discomfort that is worse at the time of ovulation or in the latter half of the cycle is sometimes a feature of benign ovarian lesions. The majority of benign cystic or solid ovarian tumors are painless unless complicated by torsion or rupture, which can produce severe acute abdominal pain. Pain is a rather late feature of cervical, uterine, ovarian, or tubal malignancy.

Strictly speaking, *mittelschmerz* or intermenstrual pain is not a form of dysmenorrhea because it occurs in midcycle at the time of ovulation. It is more common on the right side than the left and may be accompanied by bleeding. There is some evidence that the ovary is the source of the blood loss. The pain, believed due to distention of the ovarian capsule, is harmless but annoying and a source of concern.

In the large number of patients who have significant pelvic complaints but in whom no disease is found on repeated examinations, including laparoscopy, a diagnostic classification of *enigmatic pelvic pain* has often been utilized. This syndrome has been characterized as occurring in premenopausal women who have usually borne children. The pain is described as dull; it is localized to the suprapubic area or one or both of the iliac fossae, with frequent referral to the medial aspect of the thighs. Discomfort is usually worse before menstruation, and deep dyspareunia is often reported. Discharge and menorrhagia are sometimes noted; gastrointestinal symptoms are rare.

DIFFERENTIAL DIAGNOSIS

The causes of pelvic pain can be organized into acute, chronic, and recurrent categories, with these in the latter group subdivided according to their relationship to the menstrual period (see Table 114-1). Uterine hypoplasia and retroverted uterus are no longer considered causes of dysmenorrhea.

WORKUP

For the patient with acute pain, the first task is to assess the need for immediate hospitalization, because some etiologies are potential medical emergencies. A rectal temperature and a check for postural changes in blood pressure or pulse indicative of significant volume depletion are essential. The abdomen is examined for evidence of peritonitis. Speculum examination is performed for detection of vaginal discharge, bleeding, and any cervical pathology. Bimanual palpation should establish that the pain is pelvic in origin, help to further localize the problem, and identify any masses or distorted anatomy. Exquisite pain on motion of the cervix is a classic finding in acute PID, but the sign is indicative only of generalized pelvic irritation and not pathognomonic for PID. Rectovaginal examination should not be overlooked, because gastrointestinal pathology or a cul de sac mass may be discovered.

Table 114-1.   Important Causes of Pelvic Pain

Acute Pain
1. Pelvic inflammatory disease
2. Ectopic pregnancy with rupture
3. Twisted fallopian tube, ovary, or ovarian cyst
4. Ruptured ovarian cyst
5. Extrapelvic disease (*e.g.,* appendicitis)

Recurrent Pain with Menstruation
1. Primary dysmenorrhea
2. Endometriosis
3. Adenomyosis
4. Chronic pelvic inflammatory disease
5. Intrauterine devices

Recurrent Pain Unrelated to Menstruation
1. Mittelschmerz
2. Leaking ovarian cysts

Chronic Pain
1. Psychogenic pain
2. Malignancy
3. Benign neoplasms
4. Enigmatic pelvic pain

The necessary laboratory studies for acute pelvic pain are few, but should be obtained promptly. A complete blood count (CBC), differential, sedimentation rate, urinalysis, and serum HCG beta-subunit pregnancy test in any woman of reproductive age are of greatest utility. Urine HCG testing is less sensitive; a negative urine HCG test within the first 6 weeks after the last menstrual period does not rule out the diagnosis of ectopic pregnancy.

Any patient with high fever, postural signs, or peritoneal signs should be sent directly to the hospital, even before laboratory results are available or a detailed history elicited. However, even if the situation is urgent, a few historical facts can help establish the diagnosis. Inquiry is needed into any delay in menstrual period, dyspareunia, IUD use, shaking chills, abnormal vaginal discharge or bleeding, recent abortion, and location and spread of pain. Development of generalized severe pain is a worrisome symptom indicating possible peritoneal involvement, especially in conjunction with a rigid abdomen and absent bowel sounds. Unilateral pain suggests a local tubal or ovarian problem, whereas bilateral involvement is more indicative of PID or another cause of diffuse pelvic irritation. Gastrointestinal and urinary symptoms such as constipation, nausea, vomiting, diarrhea, flank pain, and dysuria need to be asked about to avoid mistaking appendicitis, acute pyelonephritis, or ureteral stone for a pelvic etiology.

If the pain is chronic or recurrent, a more detailed history should be obtained during the office visit. The relationship of the pain to the menstrual cycle is of central importance. Radiation of the pain may give a clue to its origin. Pain due to cervical, uterine, or vaginal pathology is often referred to the low back or buttock, while that which is tubal or ovarian in origin is generally localized to one side and referred to the medial aspect of the thigh. Menstrual and obstetrical history should be elicited in detail. Any emotionally stressful situations should be elucidated. It is essential to find out what the patient understands about menstruation and identify any gaps in her knowledge. A detailed pelvic examination needs to be carried out, looking in particular for adnexal thickening, cervical discharge, uterine masses, fixation of any structures, ovarian masses, and focal tenderness.

Laboratory studies beyond a CBC, SED rate, examination of any vaginal discharge, and urinalysis contribute little to the evaluation unless a mass is felt, in which case ultrasonography is indicated to confirm the finding, better localize it, and distinguish a solid from a cystic lesion. Laparoscopy or D&C may become necessary to establish a diagnosis.

SYMPTOMATIC MANAGEMENT AND PATIENT EDUCATION

Patients with *dysmenorrhea* can achieve good symptomatic control of pelvic pain with PRN use of a *nonsteroidal anti-inflammatory drug* (NSAID). These drugs are believed to provide benefit by a combination of prostaglandin synthesis inhibition and nonspecific analgesia. Over-the-counter formulations of the NSAID ibuprofen are available in 200-mg strength; 200 to 400 mg every 4 to 6 hours provides good relief from pelvic pain. Most other NSAIDs are similarly effective, and many will be available in over-the-counter formulation for nonprescription use. NSAIDs are well tolerated. The most common side-effect is GI upset (see Chapter 153). Adverse gynecologic effects include occasional reports of menstrual delays and dysfunctional uterine bleeding in patients taking 400 mg tid of ibuprofen regularly for 3 days before onset of menstrual flow. Fluid retention also occurs. A mild analgesic such as acetaminophen can be added if additional analgesia is desired.

The woman with primary dysmenorrhea should be told that her examination is normal and that there is no evidence of any worrisome gynecologic pathology. An explanation of the mechanism of cramping may be helpful and provides a rational basis for therapy. Taking time to clear up misconceptions and answer questions about menstruation can be very productive, especially in younger patients. It is sometimes comforting to explain that many women experience relief as they grow older, but it should be pointed out that there is no controlled evidence to support the notion that childbirth will predictably resolve the problem.

Since primary dysmenorrhea occurs with ovulation, it can also be treated with oral contraceptives (see Chapter 118), which will suppress ovulation and relieve cramps in 80% to 90% of patients. Progestins may also inhibit ovulation but are not as effective clinically in alleviating symptoms, perhaps because of their prostaglandin-stimulating effect. Occasionally, a teenager will complain of menstrual pain as an excuse to obtain oral contraceptives.

NSAIDs are not effective for the symptoms of *premenstrual syndrome*. Other therapies that have been tried include vitamins, progesterone, tranquilizers, antidepressants (in the absence of true underlying depression), diuretics, diet programs, exercise, lithium, bromocriptine, danazol, and lithium. None of these has ever been proven in controlled study to be of value. Improvement has been achieved experimentally with use of a gonadotropic-releasing hormone agonist; the implications for therapy are unclear at the present time, but the literature should be followed closely for developments. In the meantime, patients should be counselled to avoid unscrupulous clinics, programs, and products that claim to treat PMS; there is no treatment. Psychiatric evaluation need not be advised, unless the patient also exhibits symptoms of emotional distress unrelated to the menstrual cycle. Reassurance that PMS is not a sign of serious underlying psychopathology or reproductive endocrine disease can be comforting and help the patient to cope. Use of tranquilizers and other psychotropic drugs is to be avoided.

Pain due to IUD use may be sufficient grounds for removal. Therapy for most causes of secondary dysmenorrhea require gynecologic referral, but PID ought to be treated promptly by the primary physician (see Chapter 115).

INDICATIONS FOR REFERRAL

Patients with a mass lesion detected on physical examination should be referred, though a pelvic ultrasound study may be worth obtaining prior to the visit to the gynecologist. Suspicion of chronic pelvic inflammatory disease, endometriosis, adenomyosis, ovarian cyst, or any other condition that might be better assessed by laparoscopy should lead to consultation with the gynecologist, who may be able to provide reassurance to both patient and primary physician as well as to determine if further assessment is necessary. Surgical therapy for primary dysmenorrhea (involving dilatation of the fibromuscular tissue at the level of the internal os, presacral neurectomy, or uterosacral ligament resection) is worth considering only in severe cases if all other forms of treatment have failed and the patient is severely incapacitated by her symptoms. Hysterectomy is a last resort for patients with secondary amenorrhea who have already fulfilled their reproductive potential.

A.H.G.

ANNOTATED BIBLIOGRAPHY

Budoff PW: Zomepirac soldium in the treatment of primary dysmenorrhea syndrome. N Engl J Med 307:714, 1982 (*A placebo-controlled double-blind study demonstrating efficacy of a NSAID in treatment of dysmenorrhea.*)

Beard RW, Belsey EM, Lierberman BA et al: Pelvic pain in women. Am J Obstet Gynecol 128:566, 1977 (*A study comparing 18 patients with pain and normal laparoscopy and a group with documented pathology; a higher incidence of necrotic qualities was found in patients with pain and no evident pathology.*)

Dingfelder JR: Prostaglandin inhibitors: New treatment for an old nemesis. N Engl J Med 307:746, 1982 (*An editorial examining the pathophysiology and treatment of primary dysmenorrhea, with emphasis on prostaglandins.*)

Enigmatic pelvic pain (editorial). Br Med J 2:1041, 1978 (*A review of the difficult problems of managing pelvic pain in the absence of detectable pathology.*)

Muse KN, Cetel NS, Futterman LA et al: The premenstrual syndrome: Effects of "medical ovariectomy." N Engl J Med 311: 1345, 1984 (*An intriguing double-blind placebo-controlled study showing that use of an experimental GnRH agonist is effective in providing symptomatic relief.*)

Progesterone for premenstrual syndrome. Med Lett 26:101, 1984 (*Concludes there is no evidence that progesterone or any other available remedy is of proven value for treatment of premenstrual syndrome.*)

Trobough GE: Pelvic pain and the IUD. J Reprod Med 20:167, 1977 (*A thorough review of the role of IUDs in producing pelvic pain; includes 36 references.*)

Vaitukaitis JL: Premenstrual syndrome. N Engl J Med 311:1371, 1984 (*An editorial summarizing the status of current knowledge and lack thereof concerning this perplexing condition.*)

Wasserheit JN, Bell TA, Kiviat NB et al: Microbial causes of proven pelvic inflammatory disease and efficacy of clindamycin and to-

bramycin. Ann Intern Med 104:187, 1986 (Chlamydia and N. gonorrhea *often occurred together.*)

Ylikorkala O, Dawood MY: New concepts in dysmenorrhea. Am J Obstet Gynecol 130:833, 1978 (*A solid and comprehensive review on which rational therapy can be designed; includes 119 references.*)

115

Approach to the Patient with a Vaginal Discharge

Vaginal discharge is among the most common gynecologic complaints the primary physician is asked to evaluate. Some degree of discharge is normal, but complaints of dysuria, offensive odor, staining, itching, or accompanying rash point to a pathologic etiology. Uncomplicated vaginal discharge rarely presages serious illness, but can be an irritating and recurrent problem for the patient. The primary physician should be able to identify the cause of the discharge by its appearance and simple laboratory tests as well as detect venereal transmission and underlying disease. Management of vaginitis requires proper choice of antimicrobial agents. Patient education is necessary to reduce recurrences.

PATHOPHYSIOLOGY AND CLINICAL PRESENTATION

The normal vaginal discharge consists of desquamated vaginal epithelial cells, lactic acid, and secretions from cervical glands. An abnormal discharge may result from infection with bacteria, yeasts, or parasites. Atrophy secondary to estrogen deficiency produces a mucosa more vulnerable to injury. Inflammation produces desquamation of cells and stimulates glandular secretion from the cervical area. Other pathogenic factors, such as foreign bodies, trauma, recent surgery, alteration of the normal vaginal flora by antibiotic use, and chemical irritants, may disrupt or inflame the vaginal mucosa, increasing the amount of discharge. Rarely, neoplastic change produces an increase in discharge.

The clinical presentation of vaginitis involves a discharge that is notable because of its amount, color, or odor. Clinical presentation depends in part on the underlying etiologic agent.

Trichomoniasis is reported in 3% to 15% of asymptomatic women seen in private practice and in up to 50% to 75% of prostitutes. The prevalence among women attending gynecology clinics is approximately 15% to 20%. Sexual transmission of trichomoniasis is well established; peak incidence occurs in woman between the ages of 16 and 35. The most prominent symptom is pruritus; it is the sole complaint in 25% of patients; another 50% may seek treatment for pruritus and discharge while 25% are symptom-free. Vulvar edema may result and give rise to dyspareunia. Dysuria accompanies

infection in approximately one fifth of cases. Physical examination generally reveals erythema, edema, and occasionally characteristic petechial hemorrhages or frank excoriations of the external genitalia. Vaginal discharge may be copious and is usually frothy and foul-smelling.

Vulvovaginal candidiasis is very common. Yeast is often recovered as a commensal organism. In one private practice study, the incidence of candidiasis was 8.5% and of these individuals, 25% were asymptomatic. A common complaint is vulvar pruritus. Symptoms are usually rather rapid in onset, occurring shortly before menstruation when the pH of the vagina falls. On physical examination, erythema, edema, and excoriation are often prominent; sometimes there are pustules apparent on the skin. The discharge is typically thick, white, somewhat adherent, and often described as resembling cottage cheese or milk curd.

Gardnerella vaginitis used to be referred to a "nonspecific vaginitis" before the predominant causative organism, *Gardnerella vaginalis* (also known as *Hemophilus vaginalis*) was isolated and found to be the etiologic agent in more than 90% of cases. Anaerobes may also contribute to the problem. The clinical picture tends to be one of mild discomfort, though in 10% to 20% of cases the vaginal burning and itching are more pronounced. Sometimes patients note a disagreeable odor, though not the fishy one typical of *Trichomonas* infection. The discharge ranges from grayish to occasionally a creamy yellow or yellow-green color. Wet-mount of the discharge shows short, motile rods and characteristic "*clue cells*" (vaginal epithelial cells with a stippled or granulated appearance due to the adherence and uniform spacing of bacilli on their surfaces).

Gonorrhea presents with acute infection of the urethra, vagina, cervix, and occasionally Bartholin's glands (see Chapter 116). Onset of symptoms occurs after about a week of incubation, though much longer delays are not uncommon. Dysuria, frequency, vaginal discharge, pelvic discomfort, and dyspareunia are among the focal complaints. The condition produces a thick, purulent, profuse, creamy, irritating discharge involving the cervix, vagina, and urethra. Wet prep of the discharge is nonspecific, revealing many leukocytes and bacteria. A finding of gram-negative intracellular diplococci on Gram stain of the discharge is diagnostic and present in about 50% of cases.

Mycoplasma infection of the female urogenital tract produces a rather nonspecific clinical picture of discharge and mild discomfort. The organism is found in about 10% of patients with "nonspecific vaginitis." Often, mycoplasma infection coexists with one of the more common causes of vaginitis and results in persistence of symptoms and discharge despite seemingly appropriate treatment, one of the few clues to its presence. Special culturing techniques are needed for isolation of the organism. Debate continues as to its importance as a pelvic pathogen.

Atrophic vaginitis accounts for much of the vaginal discharge and discomfort experienced by postmenopausal women. Lack of estrogen leads to loss of all but the basal cell layer of the vaginal epithelium, which leaves it a thinned-out, ineffective mucosal barrier against infection and inflammation of the submucosal tissue. Symptoms include vaginal and vulvar burning, soreness, and occasional bleeding or itching. External burning on urination is sometimes noted; it results from localized irritation of raw and inflamed mucosa, rather than from infection of the urinary tract. Examination of the vaginal mucosa reveals a thin, erythematous surface and scant watery discharge.

Condyloma acuminata (venereal warts) are due to viral infection resulting in multiple papillary proliferations on the vulva, vagina, and less frequently, the cervix. A profuse, irritating vaginal discharge and secondary vulvitis are common in severe cases. Florid cases involving the vagina or cervix are associated with an increased risk of cancer (see Chapter 105).

Mucopurulent cervicitis due to *Chlamydia trachomatis* is becoming an epidemiologically important condition, in some studies exceeding the combined prevalences of gonococcal and nongonococcal urethritis in men. The condition is characterized by yellow-white mucopurulent discharge emanating from the cervical os, in conjunction with 10 or more WBC/microscopic field (high-power oil-immersion) on Gram-stain examination. Erythema, friability, and ectocervical ulceration are common. The risk is proportionate to the number of sexual partners.

Type 2 herpesvirus causes bullous lesions on the vulva, vagina, and cervix (see Chapter 191). It is transmitted venereally, and findings begin to appear within 3 to 7 days. Cervical involvment occurs in 75% of cases, producing ulceration, friability, and a grayish exudate in conjunction with a profuse watery discharge. Patients with mild infection may be entirely asymptomatic. Previous type 1 herpesvirus infection elsewhere in the body blunts the clinical manifestations of type 2 infection. Many cases are accompanied by trichomonal, candidal, or gonococcal infection.

Chronic cervicitis ensues from extensive chronic infection in a badly lacerated cervix, torn during childbirth. Mixed vaginal flora multiply in the area, giving rise to a mucopurulent, alkaline, irritating, and often malodorous discharge. The irregular cervix appears edematous, grossly inflamed, and eroded. The irritating discharge may lead to a secondary vulvovaginitis.

Cervical eversion from childbirth permanently exposes the endocervical epithelium, which can cause a slight nonirritating mucoid secretion. *Cervical erosions* and ulcerations may be the consequence of local trauma (*e.g.,* pessary) or chemical irritation from douches or topical contraceptives. The constant chafing from uterine prolapse can have a similar effect on the cervix. A nonspecific inflammatory discharge may develop.

Cervical polyps and cancer may be heralded by vaginal discharge or bleeding. However, most cause no symptoms until late in the course of the disease (see Chapters 105 and 122).

DIFFERENTIAL DIAGNOSIS

The most common cause of an abnormal vaginal discharge is infection by *Candida, Trichomonas, Gardnerella, N. gonorrhea,* or *Chlamydia.* Occasionally, the etiology is herpesvirus cervicitis, condyloma acuminata, or *Mycoplasma* infection.

If an infectious etiology is not identified, irritants and foreign bodies must be considered. The most common irritants are IUDs, condoms, spermicidal foams, creams, deodorants, sprays, soaps, and excessive douching. Foreign bodies include tampons, sexual implements, and laminaria. Discharge may be increased postoperatively after an episiotomy, hysterectomy, conization, or cauterization. Cervicitis may be produced by infection, erosion, or eversion. Postmenopausal women with estrogen deficiency may have atrophic vaginitis causing abnormal discharge and increased susceptibility to infection. Neoplasms of the vulva, vagina, or upper genital tract as well as cervical polyps and uterine fibroids may produce excessive discharge.

A number of cases are misattributed to infection, when a number of women who complain of excess discharge merely have physiologic midcycle cervical mucus production or an increased perception of the normal mucosal discharge.

WORKUP

History should ascertain the onset of the discharge, its appearance, amount, odor (if any) and associated symptoms. Need for a pad or tampon is a sign of excessive discharge. A sexual history is important, with emphasis on the number of partners (pertinent to risk of chlamydial infection) and any known exposure to venereal disease or a partner with a penile discharge or lesion. The relationship of the discharge to phase of the menstrual cycle, coitus, vaginal delivery, pessary, or medication use should be noted. Inquiry into associated symptoms such as dysuria, pruritus, pain, dyspareunia, and skin rash provides additional information. Known allergies need to be reviewed in conjunction with use of douches, bubble baths, soaps, or genital deodorants. Symptoms suggestive of diabetes and the recent or current use of antibiotics or corticosteroids need to be considered in a search for alterations in vaginal flora or host defenses. Any self-treatment should be carefully inquired about.

Physical examination begins with careful inspection of the vulva, vagina, and cervix for erythema, erosion, edema, excoriation, bulli, condyloma, maceration, atrophy, prolapse, and foreign bodies. A careful look at the cervix during speculum examination is most important, with any discharge, erosion, ulceration, polyp, mass, or laceration being noted. The finding of cervical mucopus raises the question of chlamydial infection, especially if it appears yellow against the background of a white cotton swab. The discharge is noted for color, consistency, and odor, which can often provide useful clues to etiology (see Table 115-1). On bimanual examination, one checks for tenderness on cervical motion and adnexal and uterine masses.

Laboratory Studies. A *wet-mount* examination of the discharge is simple and potentially diagnostic. A fresh sample is placed on a microscope slide to which a drop or two of normal saline is added, and a cover slip is placed over the suspension. The slide is examined before the sample dries to search for diagnostically useful findings such as the motile flagellated trichomonads, "clue cells," and yeast forms. Although the sensitivity of the wet mount for detection of *Trichomonas* is low (25%), the finding is very specific and permits immediate diagnosis. Clue cells have been found in 44% of patients with *Gardnerella* infection and in 18% of those who do not; their presence is suggestive, but not diagnostic; their absence does not rule out the diagnosis. Adding a drop of *10% KOH* to a sample of the discharge aids in the recognition of *Candida.* The KOH dissolves most cellular material except for the filamentous hyphae and budding forms of *Candida;* the sensitivity of the test ranges from 40% to 80%. Gram stain even has an even higher sensitivity for detection of *Candida.*

When gonorrhea is suspected, *Gram stain* of the discharge is worth considering; its sensitivity is about 50%. The finding of intracellular gram-negative diplococci is potentially diagnostic (see Chapter 116). Gram stain is also useful in identifying mucopurulent cervicitis due to chlamydial infection. The presence of more than 10 WBC/oil-immersion field suggests the diagnosis and distinguishes chlamydial cervicitis from that due to gonorrhea and herpetic disease.

Further suspicion of *Chlamydia* infection can be tested for quickly by *direct immunofluorescent staining;* if this is unavailable, a culture may be necessary (see Chapter 136). *Culture* is also essential in the setting of suspected gonorrhea, both for antibiotic sensitivity testing and for diagnosis. The

discharge must be plated immediately onto a Thayer-Martin plate to ensure recovery of the organism. A swab of the discharge is sent to the laboratory for further culturing when *Gardnerella* or other bacterial pathogens are a diagnostic consideration.

Determination of the discharge's *pH* has some value in diagnosis of a vaginal discharge, but there is considerable overlap among etiologies (see Table 115-1). Nevertheless, some clinicians keep a roll of litmus paper handy for quick pH testing and use the information adjunctively.

A few general laboratory studies are often helpful. A *CBC* and *sedimentation rate* are indicated if pain is present and pelvic inflammatory disease possible. *Urinalysis* should be obtained to check for pyuria and bactiuria, especially if there is concurrent dysuria. A 2-hour postprandial *blood sugar* is indicated if *Candida* recurs. However, occult diabetes is rarely the cause. A *Pap smear* should be done, recognizing that it may be abnormal in the presence of inflammation. In patients who are certain to return for follow-up, it may be reasonable to defer the Pap test until the vaginitis or cervicitis has been treated.

SYMPTOMATIC MANAGEMENT

Trichomonal Vaginitis. Asymptomatic vaginal or urethral colonization with this parasite is common, and probably does not require therapy (see Table 115-1). An occasional mild case responds to douching with 1 tablespoon vinegar per pint of water. If vaginal discharge, itching, and irritation are marked, *metronidazole* (Flagyl) is the treatment of choice, though some controversy surrounds prolonged or repeated use because of the carcinogenicity noted in animal studies. This drug is probably most effective if administered orally in a dosage of 250 mg tid for 10 days, but a one-time dose with 2.0 g by mouth has been shown to suffice when the male partner is also treated. Some authorities advocate simultaneous treatment of male sexual partners; others treat the male only if the female relapses. Treatment of the male partner is most effective when there is a single sexual partner. It may be optimal to culture the male and restrict treatment to those in whom a *Trichomonas* infection has been documented by culture. Because of the disulfiramlike effects of metronidazole, patients should be instructed to avoid alcohol intake while taking the drug.

Metranidazole is contraindicated in the first trimester of pregnancy because of the risk of fetal malformation. Intravaginal clotrimazole given for 1 week can relieve symptoms and cures some patients, though it is less effective than metronidazole. Douches should be avoided.

Candidal Vaginitis. Precipitants such as use of broad-spectrum antibiotics, oral contraceptives, or corticosteroids or the presence of diabetes or pregnancy need to be treated, as does the organism itself. Use of *nystatin* vaginal supposi-

Table 115-1. Common Causes of Vaginal Discharge

AGENT	PREDISPOSING FACTORS	SYMPTOMS	SIGNS (INCLUDING DISCHARGE)
Trichomonas	Sexually active Frequent douching	Malodorous discharge, itching, dysuria and dyspareunia	Vulvar irritation, gray to green malodorous (fishy) discharge, vaginal inflammation with petechiae pH 4.5–6.0
Candida	Pregnancy, recent use of broad-spectrum antibiotics, diabetes mellitus, oral contraceptives and corticosteroids	Musty odor, white discharge, dyspareunia, postcoital burning, pain with washing or sitting	Vulvar erythema, possibly pustules or excoriation, white cheesy, curdlike discharge pH 4.0–4.7
Gardnerella	Sexually active Estrogen use	Malodorous thin discharge, occasionally itchy but may be asymptomatic	Turbid thin pasty discharge adheres to vaginal walls, rarely pools in posterior fornix pH 5.0–5.5
Gonococcus	Sexually active History of VD Multiple partners	Discharge—profuse often foul-smelling; fever, pain, dyspareunia, frequently dysuria, itching	Purulent heavy cervical discharge; fever, cervical and pelvic tenderness, adnexal mass
Herpes vaginalis	Sexually active Prior infection Multiple partners	Pain, dysuria, urinary retention dyspareunia, itch, fever	Mild discharge, blisters on vulva, vesicular lesions on vagina and cervix, fever, inguinal adenopathy, sometimes secondary bacterial infection with profuse discharge
Atrophic vaginitis	Postmenopause Surgical castrate	Itching, burning, dysuria, dyspareunia secondary to dryness, bleeding	Vulvar, urethral inflammation, pale, thin vaginal mucosa
Chlamydia trachomatis	Multiple partners	Vaginal discharge, occasionally asymptomatic	Cervical erosion, mucopus (yellow and thick) from cervical os >10 WBC/field

tories once a day for 14 days has been the mainstay of treatment for *Candida*. Generic nystatin is the least expensive of available therapies, but it must be taken for longer than newer agents, and the suppository tablets can be messy. Topical nystatin is available in combination with other antibacterial agents or corticosteroids. These preparations offer little added efficacy and should rarely be used; they are expensive and associated with an increased incidence of adverse reactions. The introduction of synthetic imidazoles *clotrimazole* (Lotrimin), *miconazole* (Monistat), and *butoconazole* (Femstat) has provided alternative agents for topical treatment of candidiasis. One advantage is a shorter course of treatment necessary for cure (3 to 7 days). The imidazoles are safe for use during the second and third trimesters of pregnancy, but most authorities advise avoidance during the first trimester.

Symptomatic relief from the discomfort of the infection can sometimes be obtained by using witch hazel compresses or cool water and hastened by application of nystatin or a synthetic imidazole cream to the vulva. The patient should avoid irritant soaps, pantyhose, and hot baths, and should

TRANSMISSION	DIAGNOSIS	TREATMENT
1. Venereal with reservoir in male urethra 2. Families 3. Autogenous reinfection	1. Wet-mount with motile flagellated parasite and many polys 2. Occasionally appears in Pap smears 3. Culture	Metronidazole 2 g dose
1. Usually endogenous with predisposing factors 2. Possible venereal 3. Infection from GI tract	1. KOH stain shows hyphae and buds 2. Culture on Nickerson medium	Nystatin for 14 days or a synthetic imidazole (*e.g.,* clotrimazole, butoconazole) 3–7 days
1. Local factors 2. Venereal from asymptomatic males 3. Families	1. Wet-mount—clue cells (bacilli within epithelial cells) 2. Vaginal culture	Metronidazole 500 mg bid for 7 days
1. Venereal	1. Gram-negative intracellular diplococci 2. Culture on Thayer-Martin medium	Amoxicillin 3 g plus probenecid 1 g
1. Venereal 2. Close contact with infected person	1. Multinuclear giant cells on scraping 2. Rise in convalescent serum antibody titers	Acyclovir 200 mg 5–7/day for 5–7 days
1. Endogenous involutional process	1. Minimal estrogen effect on mucosa measured by maturation index 2. Low serum estradiol and high FSH	Estrogen cream topically
1. Venereal	1. (+) swab test (presence of mucopus) 2. >10 WBC/field 3. Direct immunofluorescence test 4. Culture	Tetracycline 500 mg qid for 7 days

substitute cotton for nylon underwear. Sometimes prolonged therapy, treatment of consorts, eradication of intestinal sources, and prophylactic measures do not totally eradicate infection. Chronic maintenance therapy may be necessary. The etiology of recurrent disease is poorly understood.

Gardnerella Vaginitis. It used to be common practice to treat "nonspecific" vaginitis with sulfonamide vaginal creams. Results were frequently disappointing, which is not surprising given that *Gardnerella* (*Hemophilus vaginalis*) is usually the causative organism. *Metronidazole,* 500 mg bid for 7 days, is the treatment of choice. *Amoxicillin,* 500 mg tid for 7 days, is an alternative. Single-dose metronidazole regimens are less effective. Treatment of the partner is needed only if there are recurrences.

Mucopurulent Cervicitis resulting from *Chlamydia* responds well to *tetracycline,* 500 mg qid for 7 days. Sulfisoxazole, 500 mg qid for 10 days, is the alternative. Partners should be treated to stem the growing spread of this infection.

Atrophic Vaginitis. The approach is to treat any superimposed infection and then to restore the integrity and resilience of the vaginal mucosa. The latter goals are best achieved by topical use of estrogen cream (see Chapter 117).

Gonorrhea. Treatment of choice is *amoxicillin,* 3 g once, preceded by 1 g of probenecid, or *ceftriaxone,* 125 to 250 mg IM once (see Chapter 116). Consorts need to be treated.

Herpes Genitalis responds to *oral acyclovir,* 200 mg five to seven times per day for 5 to 7 days, followed by a prophylactic program in patients with recurrent disease (see Chapter 138).

PATIENT EDUCATION AND INDICATIONS FOR REFERRAL

Advice regarding sexual activity and need for the partner to be checked or treated is commonly sought. Abstention from sex, or at least use of a condom, should be advised for patients with trichomonal, chlamydial, or *Gardnerella* infection. In such cases, the male partner needs to come in for consideration of treatment. It is especially important that patients with chlamydial infection be treated in order to stem the quasi-epidemic that exists for this condition; the same pertains for patients with gonorrhea. There is no evidence that treating male partners of patients with recurrent or persistent vulvovaginal candidiasis is effective.

Patients with physiologic vaginal discharges appreciate knowing that the condition is harmless and self-limited. They should be advised to avoid douches, irritant soaps, bubble baths, genital deodorants, nylon panties, wet bathing suits, and prolonged wearing of pantyhose. Patients who complain of unpleasant odors in the absence of proven pathology usually improve with the reestablishment of good personal hygiene.

Referral is needed for patients with suspicious cervical or vaginal lesions, especially erosions and ulcerations that fail to clear with treatment of a known pathogen. Colposcopy and biopsy are indicated (see Chapter 122).

A.H.G.

ANNOTATED BIBLIOGRAPHY

Brunham RC, Cho-Chou K, Stevens CE et al: Therapy for cervical chlamydial infection. Ann Intern Med 97:216, 1982 (*Tetracycline is effective.*)

Brunham RC, Paavonen J, Stevens CE et al: Mucopurulent cervicitis. N Engl J Med 311:1, 1984 (*An important paper on the clinical manifestations and diagnosis of this common condition.*)

Butoconazole for vulvovaginal candidiasis. Med Lett 28:68, 1986 (*Finds the agent as effective as, and similar in price to, other synthetic imidazole agents; good summary of available topical agents.*)

Corey L, Holmes KK: Genital herpes simplex virus infection. Ann Intern Med 98:973, 1983 (*A good review, best for its sections on clinical manifestations and course; section on therapy is dated.*)

Davis BA: Vaginal moniliasis in private practice. Obstet Gynecol 34: 40, 1969 (*A review of 1001 consecutive patients, revealing an 8.5% incidence of* Candida *that was asymptomatic in 25%. Pregnancy, oral contraceptives, antibiotics, and steroids increase the incidence.*)

Kaufman RH: The origin and diagnosis of "nonspecific vaginitis." N Engl J Med 303:637, 1980 (*Argues that evidence now supports* Hemophilus *vaginalis as the organism responsible for "nonspecific" vaginitis.*)

Pheifer TA, Forsyth PS, Durfee MA et al: Nonspecific vaginitis: Role of *Hemophilus vaginalis* and treatment with metronidazole. N Engl J Med 298:1429, 1978 (*Corynebacterium vaginale* [Hemophilis vaginalis] *was isolated from 94% (17 out of 18) of symptomatic patients compared with 1 out of 18 normal controls. Sulfonamide was found ineffective, while metronidazole was effective in 80 of 81 patients with nonspecific vaginitis.*)

Rein MF, Chapel TA: Trichomoniasis, candidiasis and the minor venereal diseases. Clin Obstet Gynecol 18:73, 1975 (*A thorough review of the clinical characteristics and sensitivity of diagnostic approaches to the major causes of vaginitis; 54 references.*)

Sobel JD: Vulvovaginal candidiasis. Ann Intern Med 101:390, 1984 (*An editorial summarizing the state of current knowledge and addressing the difficult issue of the patient with persistent or recurrent disease.*)

Spiegel CA et al: Anaerobic bacteria in nonspecific vaginitis. N Engl J Med 303:601, 1980 (*Reports that certain anaerobes act with H. vaginalis as causes of nonspecific vaginitis.*)

Treatment of sexually transmitted diseases. Med Lett 28:23, 1986 (*Excellent and authoritative summary; includes latest CDC recommendations.*)

Zuspan FE: Management of patient with vaginal infections. J Reprod Med 9:1, 1972 (*An invitational symposium, the opinions of a number of experts are offered in this article.*)

116
Approach to the Patient with Gonorrhea
HARVEY B. SIMON, M.D.

The incidence of gonorrhea has declined slightly since 1975, yet it still remains an all-too-common problem. More than 900,000 cases were reported in the United States in 1983, but, because of underreporting, it can be safely estimated that at least 3 million cases occur annually. Gonorrhea is most prevalent among teenagers and young adults, especially those in the inner city; but the infection crosses all age and socioeconomic barriers.

The great majority of patients with venereal disease present to an ambulatory care facility, and should be diagnosed and treated in this setting. At the same time, the physician must be alert to serious systemic complications requiring hospitalization. In addition, patient education is critical to prevent inadequate treatment and recurrent infections. Finally, the responsibility of the physician must extend beyond the diagnosis and treatment of an individual patient to the identification and treatment of sexual contacts who may otherwise harbor and further disseminate these infections.

PATHOPHYSIOLOGY AND CLINICAL PRESENTATION

The clinical features of gonorrhea differ greatly in the male and female.

In the male, clinical symptoms usually follow within 2 to 10 days of sexual exposure. The risk that a male will acquire gonorrhea following a single exposure to an infected partner is approximately 35%. Absence of symptoms does not indicate absence of infection. Indeed, up to 10% of infected males are asymptomatic carriers of the gonococcus and are fully capable of transmitting the disease. In the male, gonorrhea is principally an infection of the anterior urethra, and hence the major symptom is purulent *urethral discharge,* often accompanied by urinary frequency and dysuria. Although spread of infection to the *prostate* or *epididymis* is uncommon in the antibiotic era, gonococci occasionally gain entry into the *bloodstream* to produce disseminated infection.

In the female, the *cervix* is the favored site of gonococcal infection. However, up to 25% of women with gonococcal infection are asymptomatic and must be identified through epidemiologic casefinding. When symptoms do occur, cervical discharge is most common. While the vagina itself is usually spared, the gonococcal infection may spread downward from the cervix to produce *urethritis,* presenting as dysuria and frequency. Infection of *Bartholin's glands* presents as labial swelling and pain, and rectal infection presents as anorectal discomfort. If, on the other hand, gonococcal infection spreads upward from the cervix, more serious processes may develop. Such upward spread is particularly likely at the time of menstruation and can produce a variety of syndromes. Gonococcal *endometritis* can cause pelvic pain and abnormal vaginal bleeding, while *salpingitis* characteristically leads to fever, chills, leukocytosis, and a tender adnexal mass. Both systemic and pelvic signs and symptoms are even more pronounced in frank *pelvic peritonitis,* and further intraperitoneal spread may produce gonococcal *perihepatitis* with right upper quadrant pain and tenderness.

Primary extragenital infections are being encountered more frequently as a result of changing sexual practices. Gonococcal infection of the pharynx is usually asymptomatic, but can present as an acute *exudative pharyngitis,* with fever and cervical lymphadenopathy. Gonococcal *proctitis* is also most often asymptomatic, but can present as proctitis with anorectal discomfort, tenesmus, or rectal bleeding and discharge.

Gonococcal infection invariably begins with the direct infection of a mucosal surface during sexual activity. Organisms may then gain access to the bloodstream to produce *bacteremia* and systemic spread of infection. This is most common in women, especially at the time of menstruation, but it occurs in males as well. Symptoms of the primary gonococcal infection may be absent, making the diagnosis more difficult.

A common manifestation of bacteremic gonococcal infection is the "*dermatitis–arthritis syndrome.*" Patients have fever, chills, and other constitutional symptoms. Skin lesions are an important clue to diagnosis; these are typically pustular, hemorrhagic, or papular, are few in number, and tend to be most common on the distal extremities. *Tenosynovitis,* especially involving the extensor surfaces of hands and feet, and *migratory polyarthritis* are typically seen. During the early stage of systemic infection, blood cultures are often positive, but joint cultures are characteristically negative. Later in the course of untreated patients, however, gonococci can produce frank *septic arthritis;* these patients have less fever, no skin lesions, and negative blood cultures, but more impressive joint swelling and pain, often with purulent synovial fluid in which gonococci can be demonstrated by Gram stain or culture. In rare instances, gonococci can produce *osteomyelitis* or even life-threatening bacterial *meningitis* or *endocarditis.*

DIFFERENTIAL DIAGNOSIS

The organisms besides *N. gonorrhoeae* capable of producing female genital infections include *Chlamydia, Gardnerella, Trichomonas,* and *Candida* (see Chapter 115). The differential diagnosis of gonococcal salpingitis and peritonitis mainly encompasses the causes of nongonococcal pelvic inflammatory disease (PID) (see Chapter 114), but other conditions, such as appendicitis, ectopic pregnancy, hemorrhagic ovarian cysts, and endometriosis can produce similar clinical findings and often require urgent therapy very different from that of PID. In the male, the causes of nongonococcal urethritis enter the differential diagnosis (see Chapter 129). Gonococcal infection also needs to be considered among the causes of pharyngitis (see Chapter 218) and proctitis (see Chapter 61).

WORKUP

The diagnosis of gonorrhea requires a high index of suspicion and a careful sexual history. Physical examination in men with urethritis is usually normal except for purulent urethral discharge. In asymptomatic women, the physical examination is normal, but cervicitis may produce cervical inflammation, discharge, and marked cervical tenderness. Adnexal tenderness and fullness are signs of salpingitis, and may be unilateral or bilateral in women with gonorrhea. Tubal abscesses may be suspected because of a palpable mass, and rebound tenderness is a sign of pelvic peritonitis.

Pelvic inflammatory disease resulting from organisms other than the gonococcus may present similarly. Clinical features favoring the gonococcus include purulent cervical discharge, onset early in the menstrual cycle, no previous history of PID, and exposure to a male with urethritis.

A properly made *Gram stain* of the urethral discharge can be a highly reliable diagnostic tool. A Gram stain is considered "positive" when biscuit-shaped gram-negative diplococci are seen within polymorphonuclear leukocytes; "equivocal" if diplococci are only extracellular or if intracellular organisms are morphologically atypical; and "negative" if no diplococci are found. Sensitivity of the Gram stain is >95% in symptomatic men but declines to 50% to 60% in those with asymptomatic urethral infection. Gram stains are much less reliable in cervical, rectal, and pharyngeal infections.

In both sexes, *cultures* confirming the diagnosis of gonorrhea are mandatory. *Neisseria gonorrhoeae* is a very fragile and fastidious organism that requires special handling in the laboratory. The gonococcus is readily killed by drying, so all cultures must be plated promptly. Ideally, this should be done by the physician at the time of examination by streaking the swab across the surface of the culture medium in a Z-shaped pattern. Special culture media must be used. Although chocolate agar has been the traditional medium used, a modified *Thayer-Martin medium* is preferred for specimens obtained from genital, anal, or pharyngeal sites because the addition of antibiotics to this medium suppresses the growth of nonpathogenic *Neisseria* species and other bacteria. The culture medium should be at room temperature at the time of inoculation. Because the gonococcus requires a high CO_2 concentration to grow, cultures should be promptly incubated in a candle jar or CO_2 incubator. When this is not possible, the cultures should be planted on modified Thayer-Martin medium in bottles with a 10% CO_2 atmosphere. These bottles should be kept capped until the moment of inoculation and should be held in an upright position when open to prevent the loss of CO_2, which is heavier than air.

In the male, cultures of the anterior urethra suffice unless homosexual contacts are suspected, in which case cultures of the anal canal and pharynx are also indicated. In the female, the endocervix should be cultured by inserting a swab into the cervical os through a speculum that has been lubricated only with water. In all women, rectal cultures are indicated because rectal infection can result simply from direct spread of infection from the genital tract. When pharyngitis is suspected, throat culture is mandatory. When acute arthritis is present, joint fluid should be obtained by arthrocentesis and should be evaluated with cell counts, sugar and protein determinations, Gram stain, and culture. Blood cultures are indicated in patients with fever, skin lesions, and tenosynovitis or arthritis.

PRINCIPLES OF MANAGEMENT

The therapy of gonorrhea has undergone dramatic changes over the past 40 years. During this time, there has been a steady increase in the *penicillin resistance* of the gonococcus, so that the currently recommended dosages of penicillin are 30 times greater than the initial regimen used with success in 1943. Until recently, this penicillin resistance was just a matter of degree, since it was based on chromosomal mutations decreasing the permeability of the cell wall to penicillin and other antibiotics. Simply increasing the dosage of penicillin sufficed.

A new form of penicillin resistance was recognized in 1975, when gonococcal strains were isolated that resisted the effects of even massive doses of penicillin by producing *penicillinase*. These strains were found to contain beta-lactamase-producing plasmids. In the United States, infection with a plasmid-containing strains was initially sporadic and limited to prostitutes and persons who had traveled to Southeast Asia. However, since 1979 the number of such infections has increased 500% and is no longer limited to a few groups of patients. Many strains are also resistant to tetracycline. Even more recently, very high-level, chromosomally mediated penicillin resistance has emerged in several states, with sustained outbreaks noted in Oregon, Tennessee, and New Mexico.

Because of the emergence and spread of highly resistant strains, no single regimen any longer suffices for all situations. The Centers for Disease Control (CDC) and the World Health Organization (WHO) have issued new recommendations for the treatment of gonorrhea to account for these changes in antibiotic sensitivity and for regional differences in the organisms encountered. A set of "Group A" regimens has been devised for use in areas where gonococci remain chromosomally sensitive to antibiotics and the penicillinase-producing strains account for fewer than 1% of the isolates. "Group B" regimens are for use in areas where antibiotic resistance results in a greater than 5% failure rate with "Group A" regimens or penicillinase-producing strains account for 5% or an increasing percentage of isolates. These recommendations are superimposed on differences in treatment program necessitated by the clinical type of gonorrhea encountered (see Table 116-1).

Uncomplicated Gonorrhea (Including Urethritis, Cervicitis, and Rectal Infection). The Group A regimen is a single dose of *amoxicillin* (or ampicillin) plus *probenecid* (given to delay renal drug clearance and prolong therapeutic serum levels). *Intramuscular procaine penicillin G* plus probenecid is necessary for pharyngeal gonorrhea or gonorrhea in ho-

mosexual men, because of reduced efficacy of amoxicillin in these settings. The procaine penicillin regimen is also effective against incubating syphilis, for which homosexual men are at particular risk. Because many heterosexual patients with gonorrhea have coinfection with *Chlamydia trachomatis* (figures range from 20%–40%, many authorities recommend following therapy for gonorrhea with a program of *doxycycline* (or *tetracycline*) for heterosexual patients. Young men with epidydimitis may have either gonorrhea or chlamydial infection and should receive this treatment regimen as well. Doxycycline is more expensive than tetracycline, but patient compliance is better with doxycycline because the drug need be taken only twice daily. Tetracycline used to be an effective alternative to amoxicillin, but is no longer considered a first-line treatment because of increasing drug resistance. Moreover, the drug is substantially less effective than penicillin G in women and in those with rectal gonorrhea. For penicillin-allergic patients and those who fail penicillin therapy, a single intramuscular dose of *spectinomycin* is recommended. It is ineffective in pharyngeal infection.

In areas experiencing penicillin resistance, the Group B regimen consists of spectinomycin or the "third-generation" cephalosporin *ceftriaxone,* given as a single-dose intramuscular injection. Ceftriaxone has a long half-life and proven

Table 116-1.   Outpatient Treatment of Gonorrhea

TYPE OF GONORRHEA	LOW PROBABILITY OF ANTIBIOTIC RESISTANCE	HIGH PROBABILITY OF ANTIBIOTIC RESISTANCE
Uncomplicated gonorrhea	Amoxicillin, 3 g PO (or ampicillin, 3.5 g, plus probenecid, 1 g both orally once; or	Ceftriaxone, 250 mg IM or
		Spectinomycin, 2 g IM; plus
	Procaine Pen G, 4.8 mU IM plus probenecid, 1 g orally;* or	Doxycycline, 100 mg bid po for 7 days (or tetracycline, 500 mg qid po for 7 days)‡
	Spectinomycin, 2 g IM;† plus	
	Doxycycline, 100 mg bid po for 7 days (or tetracycline, 500 mg qid po for 7 days)‡	
Disseminated infection	Same as for uncomplicated disease in patients with mild disease, a definite diagnosis, good compliance, and ensured careful follow-up; otherwise, inpatient admission for parenteral therapy is indicated	
Pelvic inflammatory disease	Program listed below is only for nonpregnant patients with mild disease, a definite diagnosis, and ensured follow-up; all others require hospitalization:	Same as for no drug resistance
	Cefoxitin, 2 g IM plus probenecid, 1 mg po; plus	
	Doxycycline (as above)‡	

* Regimen of choice for homosexual men and patients with pharyngeal infection.

† For patients allergic to penicillin or in those who have failed penicillin therapy.

‡ To treat likely simultaneous *Chlamydia trachomatis* infection; this is not for treatment of the gonorrhea *per se.*

(Adapted from Hook EW, Holmes KK: Gonococcal infections. Ann Intern Med 102:229, 1985)

effectiveness *in vitro* against penicillinase-producing strains of *N. gonorrhoeae.* Neither chlamydial infection nor incubating syphilis is adequately treated by cephalosporin therapy.

Disseminated Gonococcal Infection. Patients with evidence of disseminated infection require more intensive therapy. For those with the arthritis-dermatitis syndrome, initial therapy consists of at least 3 days of *intravenous penicillin G* followed by 7 days of orally administered *ampicillin.* If hospitalization for intravenous therapy is logistically difficult or impractical, the patient is very reliable, the diagnosis is clear-cut, and the case is mild, outpatient treatment with ampicillin alone is acceptable, as long as close follow-up is provided. Intravenous cefoxitin, cefotaxime, or ceftriaxone is indicated for disseminated infection caused by penicillinase-producing strains. Gonococcal osteomyelitis, meningitis, and endocarditis are much more serious infections, necessitating high-dose, prolonged parenteral antibiotic therapy.

Pelvic Inflammatory Disease (PID). Mild cases of PID can be treated with the same program used for uncomplicated gonorrhea. However, many cases of PID are caused by multiple organisms, including *Chlamydia, Mycoplasma,* anaerobes, and/or bowel flora, and it may be preferable to administer a single dose of *cefoxitin* followed by a course of *doxycycline* or tetracycline. Patients treated on an outpatient basis must be closely monitored to ensure compliance and efficacy. Hospitalization should be seriously considered if the diagnosis is not completely certain and the possibility of a surgical illness has not been ruled out. In addition, patients who are pregnant, toxic, suspected of having a pelvic abscess, or frank peritonitis, or who are unresponsive to oral therapy should be hospitalized. Patients who are both *pregnant* and *penicillin-allergic* present a difficult problem. Cephalosporins are usually effective but may cause allergic reactions. *Erythromycin* is safe, but less effective. Spectinomycin is effective, but its safety for the fetus has not been established.

Monitoring. In all patients with gonorrhea, it is mandatory to test for cure by follow-up urethral, cervical, and anal cultures 1 to 2 weeks after therapy is completed. Organisms isolated from patients who are treatment failures should be submitted for testing to determine whether or not they are producing penicillinase.

All patients with gonorrhea should have serologic testing for syphilis. Seronegative patients treated with procaine penicillin do not require follow-up serologies because this regimen is effective for incubating syphilis; however, patients receiving amoxicillin, ampicillin, tetracycline, or spectinomycin do require repeat serologic testing in 3 months. All cases of gonorrhea should be reported to the appropriate local health department. Because many patients are asymptomatic, vigorous case finding represents the only present means of controlling this epidemic.

THERAPEUTIC RECOMMENDATIONS

Therapeutic recommendations are summarized in Table 116-1.

PATIENT EDUCATION AND PREVENTION

The importance of completing a full course of therapy must be emphasized. Single-dose regimens have greatly simplified treatment of gonorrhea, but proper therapy should also include a 7-day antibiotic course directed against chlamydial infection, which is reaching epidemic proportions. Just as important is a return visit within 1 week for reculturing of all possible sites to evaluate response to therapy.

Preventive measures include attention to *case finding* and health education. When the patient is a symptomatic male, all sexual contacts within the previous 2 weeks ought to be notified and treated. This will result in reaching more than 90% of partners likely to be infected. However, if the patient is an asymptomatic male or a female, then all contacts within the previous 60 days should be notified to reach 90% of the people at risk. *Health education* vis-à-vis high-risk sex (multiple partners, intercourse with a patient having a purulent discharge, or recent history of untreated gonorrhea) seems not to be have been very effective over the years, but the fear of AIDS (see Chapter 142) has done much to encourage safer sexual activity.

Properly used barrier methods of contraception are effective means of preventing gonorrhea. *Condoms* do not permit transmission of the gonococcus or *Chlamydia.* The diaphram may also offer some protection, especially when used with a *vaginal spermicide* containing nonoxynol-9, the active ingredient in many preparations.

INDICATIONS FOR ADMISSION

Patients with disseminated disease who are febrile, unreliable, or have evidence of osteomyelitis, endocarditis, or meningitis must be hospitalized. The same is true of the woman with pelvic inflammatory disease who appears toxic, pregnant, unlikely to comply, or suffering from pelvic pain of unclear etiology in association with peritoneal signs.

ANNOTATED BIBLIOGRAPHY

Barnes RC, Holmes KK: Epidemiology of gonorrhea: Current perspectives. Epidemiol Rev 6:1, 1984 (*A detailed review discussing trends in the incidence of gonorrhea and patterns of antibiotic susceptibility as well as priorities for case finding and control.*)

Cunningham FG, Hauth JC, Strong JD et al: Evaluation of tetracycline or penicillin and ampicillin for treatment of acute pelvic inflammatory disease. N Engl J Med 296:1380, 1977 (*A study of 197 women showed that both regimens were effective. Notably, pelvic abscess developed ten times more often in nongonococcal PID.*)

Eschenbach DA, Buchanan TM, Pollock HM et al: Polymicrobial etiology of acute pelvic inflammatory disease. N Engl J Med 293: 166, 1975 (*An excellent study of the microbiology of acute pelvic inflammatory disease.*)

Eschenbach DA, Harnisch JP, Holmes KK: Pathogenesis of acute pelvic inflammatory disease: Role of contraception and other risk factors, Am J Obstet Gynecol 128:838, 1977 (*An excellent review of the increased risk of PID in patients with IUDs, particularly in nulliparous women.*)

Handsfield HH, Lipman TO, Harnisch JP et al: Asymptomatic gonorrhea in men. N Engl J Med 290:117, 1974 (*An important study showing that asymptomatic males can be prolonged urethral carriers of N. gonorrhoeae and may be an important reservoir of infection. All sexual contacts of patients with gonorrhea should be cultured, whether male or female and whether symptomatic or not.*)

Hook EW, Holmes KK: Gonococcal infections. Ann Intern Med 102:229, 1985 (*Authoritative review: recommended reading for all primary physicians: includes 157 references.*)

Hutt DM, Judson FN: Epidemiology and treatment of oropharyngeal gonorrhea. Ann Intern Med 104:655, 1986 (*Procaine Pen G was effective, as was a two-dose ampicillin program, but not a single-dose therapy.*)

Jick H, Hannan MT, Stergachis A et al: Vaginal spermicides and gonorrhea. JAMA 248:1619, 1982 (*This descriptive study suggests a protective effect against gonorrhea of vaginal spermicides.*)

Kelaghan J, Rubin GL, Ory HW et al: Barrier-method contraceptives and pelvic inflammatory disease. JAMA 248:184, 1982 (*A case-control study detecting a relative risk of 0.6 for women using barium methods compared with others for pelvic inflammatory disease.*)

Klein EJ, Fisher LS, Chow AW et al: Anorectal gonococcal infection. Ann Intern Med 86:340, 1977 (*A clinical review of rectal infections in women and homosexual males.*)

McCormack WM: Treatment of gonorrhea—Is penicillin passé? N Engl J Med 296:934, 1977 (*A lucid summary of the basic mechanisms, epidemiologic patterns, and therapeutic complications of antibiotic-resistant gonococci.*)

O'Brien JP, Goldenberg DL, Rice PA: Disseminated gonococcal infection: A prospective analysis of 49 patients and a review of pathophysiology and immune mechanisms. Medicine 62:395, 1983 (*A comprehensive study of 49 patients and review of the literature.*)

Platt R, Rice PA, McCormack WM: Risk of acquiring gonorrhea and prevalence of abnormal adnexal findings among women recently exposed to gonorrhea. JAMA 250:3205, 1983 (*The incidence of gonorrhea infection among women with one definite exposure, two definite exposures, and more than two exposures was 50%, 86%, and 100%. Upper genital tract involvement appeared to be a common early complication.*)

Rinaldi RZ, Harrison WO, Fan PT: Penicillin-resistant gonococcal arthritis. A report of 4 cases. Ann Intern Med 97:43, 1982 (*A sobering report, since most gonococci that disseminate are penicillin-sensitive. These four patients responded to spectinomycin or cefoxitin.*)

Treatment of sexually transmitted diseases. Med Lett 28:23, 1986 (*Authoritative recommendations for the management of gonorrhea and other sexually transmitted diseases.*)

Wasserheit JN, Bell TA, Kiviat NB: Microbial causes of proven pelvic inflammatory disease. Ann Intern Med 104:187, 1986 (*Chlamydia and N. gonorrhoeae were often present, as were anaerobes, mycoplasmas, and facultative organisms.*)

117

Approach to the Menopausal Woman

Menopause is a difficult stage for women in our society because of the emphasis on youth. Although many of the emotional and physical changes blamed on menopause are actually more general manifestations of aging and not tied to decreased estrogen levels, the cessation of menstruation has major symbolic significance and, as a result, many symptoms and complaints are attributed to it. The naive hope that taking exogenous estrogen would protect the user from normal aging, coronary disease, and other conditions has for the most part proven ill-founded. Moreover, a disturbing association between estrogen therapy and increased risk of endometrial cancer has appeared, in addition to previous concern about cardiovascular complications.

If one uses the generally accepted definition of menopause as a full year without menstrual flow in a previously menstruating woman, then the incidence of menopause is 10% by age 38, 20% by age 43, 50% by 48, 90% by 54, and 100% by age 58. In addition, the prevalence of surgically induced menopause is estimated to be 25% to 30% of women in their mid-50s.

The primary physician can do a great deal to help women pass through this potentially trying stage with confidence and dignity. It is important to provide relief from disabling symptoms, such as severe hot flashes, while avoiding unnecessary exposure to estrogen therapy and its attendant risks.

PHYSIOLOGY AND CLINICAL PRESENTATION

The essential cause of menopause is decreased estrogen production by the aging ovaries, resulting in cessation of menses and rise in gonadotropins. Some estrogen production continues, but its source is primarily peripheral conversion of delta-4-androstenedione. The diagnosis of menopause is confirmed by a marked increase in the gonadotropins; maximum levels of FSH and LH occur within 1 to 2 years of onset and remain high for 10 to 15 years. The physiologic events are identical in surgically induced menopause, but the time course is shorter, with FSH and LH rising to high levels within 20 to 30 days. Approximately 25% of women do not experience any symptoms, perhaps because of nonovarian sources of estrogen production.

Hot flashes, believed to be related to rate of estrogen withdrawal and resultant vasomotor instability, are among the most specific of menopausal symptoms. An uncomfortably warm sensation radiates upward from the chest to neck and face and lasts seconds to a few minutes before subsiding. Eating, exertion, emotional upset, and alcohol are known precipitants. As many as 20 episodes per day occur; in most patients, the condition lasts for 2 to 3 years but may continue for 6 years or more. Prevalence of severe, disabling hot flashes ranges from 10% to 35% of menopausal women. No link between emotional makeup and symptoms has been demonstrated, though it is clear that the flashes can be very distracting and cause considerable misery and upset.

Other clinical manifestations of estrogen decline include *atrophy* of the *vaginal mucosa* and vulvar epithelium. The vagina becomes smaller and less compliant; lubrication decreases. Women may present with complaints of itching, discharge, bleeding, or painful intercourse. The uterus becomes smaller, but this causes no symptoms. The urethra becomes atrophic, and perineal bacteria colonize the area, increasing the risk of urethritis and dysuria. Of interest is the finding that sexually active women show less vaginal atrophy. Whether this is a cause or effect is unclear.

There is no evidence that estrogen decline is responsible for the increased incidence of *cardiovascular disease* that parallels the menopause. Studies on the effects of estrogen replacement therapy on cardiovascular morbidity and mortality are conflicting (see below).

Osteoporosis represents an important consequence of estrogen decline; decreased activity, inadequate nutrition, and the aging process also contribute, to varying degrees. Although irreversible, osteoporosis can be prevented by prophylactic administration of estrogen (see Chapter 158).

Various functional and psychological symptoms such as headache, nervousness, and depression, which frequently occur during the climacteric, are more a reflection of the emotional stress attending this difficult stage of life than a result of a change in hormonal milieu. Some women report feeling better emotionally on estrogen therapy, but this probably represents a placebo effect. No specific psychiatric problems have been found to be linked specifically to menopause.

The cosmetic changes associated with aging have been attributed by some to a decrease in estrogens, but clinical evidence is to the contrary. Breast atrophy, loss of skin turgor, and redistribution of fat to the abdomen and thighs have not

been shown to be influenced by estrogen therapy and most likely are part of the more general process of aging.

PRINCIPLES OF MANAGEMENT

The objectives are to alleviate any disabling symptoms that result from estrogen deficiency and to provide support for the host of emotional and functional problems that may accompany this phase of life.

Estrogen Replacement Therapy. Because much of the medical morbidity of menopause (*e.g.,* osteoporosis) relates to estrogen deficiency, the clinician and patient are faced with the difficult decision of when to use replacement therapy. This necessitates consideration of risks and benefits.

RISKS. The major risk associated with use of systemic estrogen is malignancy. Epidemiologic data show an increased incidence of *endometrial carcinoma* in menopausal patients taking estrogen regularly (see Chapter 106). Risk appears independent of other known factors or the type of estrogen preparation used ("natural" versus synthetic), but correlates with dosage and duration of estrogen treatment and declines with cessation of therapy. For example, dosages of 0.625 to 1.25 mg of conjugated estrogens cause a seven-fold rise in the incidence of endometrial cancer when taken daily for 2 to 4 years. Case-control studies reveal an incidence of 4.5 to 13.9 times that of nonusers.

Estrogens cause cystic hyperplasia of the endometrium, a premalignant condition. Prolonged, continuous use makes for excessive stimulation, leading to malignant change. Fortunately, the tumors induced by estrogen therapy in postmenopausal women tend to be of low grade and in early stages when detected.

One way suggested to overcome excessive endometrial stimulation is to periodically add a *progestegin* to the estrogen program. Progestegins cause sloughing of the endometrium, leaving very few glands to uninterruptedly proliferate and undergo hyperplasia. Available clinical studies suggest that adding a progestin to a program of long-term estrogen therapy does help reduce the risk of endometrial cancer.

Disadvantages of progestin use include the return of light to moderate menstrual periods and an undesirable alteration in serum lipoproteins (low-density lipoprotein elevation, high-density lipoprotein reduction; see Chapter 22) that might be responsible for the increased risk of cardiovascular disease reported with use of high doses. Controlled, prospective, large-scale, long-term studies are needed to better determine safety and efficacy.

Whether or not postmenopausal estrogen therapy alters the risk of *breast cancer* remains a subject of debate. Some data suggest that it raises the risk, but other studies show no such risk. The reader is urged to watch the literature for further studies bearing on this important question. Women with breast cancers that have estrogen receptors do experience stimulated tumor growth with estrogen exposure; those without receptors improve with estrogen (see Chapter 121).

There are also conflicting data regarding the effects of estrogens on *cardiovascular morbidity* and *mortality.* The two major prospective studies currently available have produced opposite results—one shows an increase in risk of heart disease, the other shows a decrease. Further examination of these studies and new data will be required to clarify this most important issue. The answer will have a major impact on the overall safety of estrogen use in menopausal women. A worsening of cardiovascular prognosis will greatly overshadow any benefit from prevention of osteoporosis. A salutory effect will greatly enhance the value of the medication. For the present, caution is urged. There does not appear to be an increased risk of *thromboembolism* among menopausal women on estrogen replacement, but patients with known peripheral vascular disease who are given estrogens should be monitored closely.

Other adverse effects of exogenous estrogen include fluid retention, blood pressure elevation, gallstones (due to a change in bile cholesterol content), glucose intolerance, and headaches. Often there is recurrent uterine bleeding.

Given such a list of potentially serious adverse effects and some important risks still poorly defined, the primary physician must exert care and judgment in selecting patients for estrogen therapy. Treatment should be reserved for patients incapacitated by estrogen deficiency symptoms or at very high risk for one of its serious complications. Currently, most recommendations regarding use are based on an analysis that is neutral regarding cardiovascular risk. As noted previously, recommendations could change markedly when this risk is better defined. Whenever estrogen therapy is used, it should be prescribed at the lowest possible dosage for the shortest period of time. The decision to use estrogens needs to be made with full consideration of the patient's willingness to undertake the risks in exchange for specified benefits. One woman may be willing to accept the risk of endometrial cancer in return for prevention of disabling osteoporosis; another might not.

DISABLING HOT FLASHES severe enough to functionally incapacitate the patient are a reasonable indication for estrogen treatment. In most instances, the problem is self-limited, but symptomatic relief during the year or two that symptoms are most severe can mean much. A program of conjugated estrogen taken daily for 3 weeks, with 1 week off, will prevent hot flashes. The daily dose ranges from 0.3 to 1.25 mg; often a low dosage is quite adequate. Every 3 to 6 months, one should attempt to taper and discontinue therapy. In places where the winters are cold, year-round therapy may be avoidable. If treatment is going to be for less than 1 year, addition of a progestin is probably not necessary but ought to be considered in those requiring more prolonged estrogen therapy.

POSTMENOPAUSAL OSTEOPOROSIS can be prevented by long-term prophylactic estrogen therapy (see Chapter 158). Controlled studies have shown decreased rates of vertebral, wrist, and hip fractures. Exercise and good nutrition, ensuring adequate calcium and vitamin D intake, also slow osteoporotic changes, but not as effectively as estrogen. Nevertheless, the addition of 1.0 to 1.5 g of dietary calcium carbonate per day will compensate for the intestinal malabsorption of calcium that results from estrogen deficiency and will retard bone loss, especially when combined with regular exercise. Vitamin D treatment is not beneficial unless serum levels of 25-OH vitamin D are low. Small doses (400 units/day) are helpful in preventing vitamin D deficiency in elderly women; large doses are unnecessary. Risk factors for postmenopausal osteoporotic fractures include thin body build, premature surgical menopause, cigarette smoking, and heavy alcohol use. Prolonged bed rest is a potent stimulus of osteoporosis.

Since the condition is largely irreversible and resumes once therapy is stopped, treatment must be initiated prophylactically in the perimenopausal period and continued indefinitely. Ten to 15 years of therapy are not uncommon, and even more prolonged therapy is likely in the future as the average life span increases. For women willing to accept the increased risk of endometrial cancer and tolerate the uncertain cardiovascular risk in return for the best possible means of preventing osteoporosis, estrogen therapy in conjunction with exercise and modest dietary calcium supplementation offers the best option. A program of cyclical therapy is prescribed. Efficacy of therapy can be measured by bone densitometry. Addition of a progestin to the long-term estrogen program is advocated as a means of limiting the risk of endometrial cancer (see above). Progestin is added on days 15 to 25 of a 25-day estrogen program each month. Women who are reluctant to take estrogen should be encouraged to engage in an exercise program and maintain an adequate calcium intake.

Patient selection for prophylactic estrogen therapy against osteoporosis remains problematic (see Chapter 158). It would be optimal to select only those at greatest risk, but aside from a positive family history and the other epidemiologic risk factors mentioned earlier, there are no clinical means of reliably and inexpensively making this determination. *Bone densitometry* studies are expensive; results correlate well with risk of vertebral fracture, but not with that of hip fracture, a more devastating consequence of osteoporosis. Moreover, a single study at the onset of menopause that shows little osteoporosis does not guarantee against rapid matrix thinning in the future. Repeat studies are more informative, but further raise the cost of evaluation, which is prohibitive when multiplied by the size of the population at risk. The development of very inexpensive yet reliable measures of bone density that correlate with risk will greatly aid in selection of patients for treatment. The hand and heel studies being promoted commercially are worthless.

Experimental approaches to treatment of osteoporosis include use of sodium fluoride, calcitonin, and 1,25-dihydroxy vitamin D.

ATROPHIC VAGINITIS responds well to topical estrogen cream, which restores turgor to the vaginal mucosa. Some systemic estrogen absorption does take place, although its consequences are uncertain. The risk of adverse estrogen effects (see above) must still be considered a possibility, though probably to a lesser degree than with the use of systemic therapy. To maximize safety, topical treatment should be prescribed for the shortest time possible and only for women who suffer from severe symptoms clearly attributable to atrophic vaginitis (*e.g.,* inability to engage in intercourse, painful vaginal burning, or discharge). Milder symptoms (*e.g.,* mild dryness with intercourse) may respond well to use of a water-soluble vaginal lubricant and obviate the need for estrogen. A typical estrogen program is daily topical application for 3 weeks, followed by 1 week off, using from one half to a full applicator of estrogen cream (*e.g.,* 2 g–4 g of conjugated estrogens). Careful monitoring for signs of endometrial cancer (see below) is important. Once symptoms have resolved, therapy should be discontinued; usually 1 to 3 months of treatment suffices.

MONITORING. Patients who undergo estrogen therapy require careful monitoring. Endometrial cancer is unlikely to cause discomfort in its early stages, but unexplained vaginal staining or bleeding is an important clue that necessitates a workup (see Chapter 108). Actually, one of the unquantified risks of estrogen therapy is the increase in frequency of endometrial biopsies and D&C procedures.

Other Measures. Many problems of menopausal women can be handled safely without resorting to replacement therapy. For example, painful coitus due to vaginal atrophy can be prevented by use of a water-soluble lubricant. Muscle tone, appearance, and sense of well-being can be improved by a carefully tailored program of gentle exercises, including walking and swimming. Multiple bodily complaints such as fatigue, headache, and arthralgias should be investigated systematically. If an underlying depression is discovered, specific treatment should be undertaken (see Chapter 223). Patients troubled by preexisting emotional and/or physical problems are probably going to have more difficulty as they grow older, necessitating continuation and enhancement of treatment as they pass such important milestones of aging as menopause.

PATIENT EDUCATION

Since the emphasis in our society is on youth and vitality, the physician has an important supportive role to play in helping the menopausal woman to adjust psychologically and maintain her sense of self-worth and well-being. Discussion of the physiologic consequences of menopause and their clinical manifestations can give the patient a rational basis for understanding her own symptoms and properly attributing them. This might save many anxious phone calls and office visits. One can take advantage of this milestone to interest the patient in a program of regular exercise, attainment of ideal weight, and cessation of such self-destructive habits as smoking. The woman needs to know that any incapacitating symptoms due to lack of estrogen can be controlled and that many are self-limited. During the perimenopausal period, women should be reminded to use contraception because ovulation and unwanted pregnancy may occur. Reassurance that capacity for normal sexual activity will continue after menopause is often tremendously comforting. Lack of need for special vitamin supplements should be pointed out, since the lay press heavily encourages their use and this unnecessary expense can be considerable.

If estrogen therapy is being considered, the patient must share in the decision with full awareness of the potential risks and benefits. Patients on estrogen therapy must be reminded to stop the estrogen for 5 to 7 days each month and not to increase the dose on their own. The need for regular follow-up and prompt reporting of any abnormal vaginal bleeding, breast masses, leg swelling, and so on must be emphasized.

THERAPEUTIC RECOMMENDATIONS

- Estrogen therapy should be reserved for incapacitating hot flashes, increased risk of osteoporosis, and symptomatic atrophic vaginitis. The decision to treat with estrogens should be made jointly by the physician and patient.
- If prescribed, systemic estrogen should be used in the minimal effective dose (usually the equivalent of 0.625 mg of conjugated estrogens daily for osteoporosis prophylaxis and 0.3 mg/day for hot flashes), for as short a time as possible (rarely more than 1 or 2 years for hot flashes, but more than 10 years for prophylaxis of osteoporosis). The need for continued treatment should be constantly reevaluated. When estrogens are used for hot flashes, it is suggested that discontinuation be attempted during winter months.
- Therapy should be cyclical (21 days on, 7 days off if not using concomitant progestin therapy; 25 days on, 5 days off if using progestin) to prevent uninterrupted stimulation of the endometrium.
- Some authorities suggest adding a progestin (*e.g.,* medroxyprogesterone acetate [Provera], 2.5–10 mg/day) during the last 10–12 days of the estrogen cycle to reduce endometrial buildup. The cardiovascular safety of long-term intermittent progestin use is unknown (progestins cause unfavorable elevations in LDL cholesterol and decreases in HDL cholesterol).
- Estrogen therapy cannot replace lost bone, so it is not a therapy for reversing established osteoporosis. Patient selection for prophylactic treatment of osteoporosis needs to be individualized and carefully considered (see Chapter 158).

- Severe atrophic vaginitis with dysuria or dyspareunia will respond to topical estrogen, which should be given for no more than 3 weeks at a time; topical therapy applied as little as once or twice a week may be effective. Systemic absorption occurs, but its effect is uncertain. Milder cases, with painful coitus only, can be treated with a water-soluble lubricant (*e.g.,* Lubafax).
- Medical surveillance of patients on estrogen is mandatory. Blood pressure measurement, breast and pelvic examination, and Pap smear should be done every 6 months. When a woman requires estrogen for more than a year, a referral to a gynecologist should be made for consideration of endometrial biopsy, which is advocated by some clinicians.
- Uterine fibroids, hypertension, diabetes, and hypertriglyceridemia are relative contraindications to estrogen use and demand careful monitoring. A history of myocardial infarction, pulmonary embolism, thrombophlebitis or malignancy of breasts or uterus generally precludes treatment with exogenous estrogens.

A.H.G.

ANNOTATED BIBLIOGRAPHY

Ballinger CG: Psychiatric morbidity and the menopause: Clinical features. Br Med J 1:1183, 1976 (*A description of psychiatric symptoms during the menopause.*)

Boston Collaborative Drug Surveillance Program: Surgically confirmed gallbladder disease, venous thromboembolism and breast tumors in relation to postmenopausal estrogen therapy. N Engl J Med 290:15, 1974 (*Postmenopausal estrogen therapy increases risk of gallstones, but not of thromboembolism or breast tumor.*)

Bush TL, Cowan LD, Barrett-Conner E et al: Estrogen use and all-cause mortality. Preliminary results from the Lipid Research Clinics program follow-up study. JAMA 249:903, 1983 (*A decrease in risk of cardiac mortality is found, contradicting the findings of Gordon et al below.*)

Cummings SR, Black D: Should menopausal women be screened for osteoporosis? Ann Intern Med 104:817, 1986 (*A good consideration of the major issues, including excellent review of the literature; 89 references.*)

Gordon T, Kannel WB, Hjortland ML et al: Menopause and coronary heart disease. The Framingham Study. Ann Intern Med 89:157, 1978 (*A doubled risk in postmenopausal women on hormones is found.*)

Hillner BE, Hollenberg JP, Pauker SG: Postmenopausal estrogens in prevention of osteoporosis. Am J Med 80:1115, 1986 (*A decision-analysis study that argues in favor.*)

Horsman A, Jones M, Francis R et al: The effect of estrogen dose on menopausal bone loss. N Engl J Med 309:1405, 1985 (*Documents a dose-related inhibition of cortical bone resorption.*)

Jick H, Watkins RN, Hunter JR et al: Replacement estrogens and endometrial cancer. N Engl J Med 300:218, 1979 (*Long-term estrogen users in a large Seattle group practice showed an annual risk of 1% to 3% for users and a risk less than one tenth as great for nonusers. A reduced incidence of endometrial cancer paralleled the downward trend in the use of replacement estrogens.*)

Judd HL, Meldrum DR, Deftos LJ et al: Estrogen replacement therapy: Indications and complications. Ann Intern Med 98:195, 1983 (*A symposium presenting a balanced view of the indications and side-effects associated with estrogen replacement therapy.*)

Kaufman DW, Miller DR, Rosenberg L et al: Noncontraceptive estrogen and the risk of breast cancer. JAMA 252:63, 1984 (*Case-control study suggesting that noncontraceptive estrogens do not increase the risk of breast cancer.*)

Leiblum S, Bachmann G, Kemmann E et al: Vaginal atrophy in the postmenopausal women. JAMA 249:2195, 1983 (*Less vaginal atrophy was apparent in sexually active women compared with sexually inactive women; women with less vaginal atrophy had higher levels of estrogens and gonadotrophins.*)

MacDonald PC: Estrogen plus progestin in postmenopausal women. N Engl J Med 305:1644, 1981 (*An editorial on the issue that is favorable on the endometrial carcinoma issue, but raises the question of unknown cardiovascular risk.*)

MacDonald PC: Estrogen plus progestin in postmenopausal women: Act II. N Engl J Med 315:959, 1986 (*An editorial critical of adding progestin to estrogen therapy for postmenopausal women.*)

Padwick ML, Pryse-Davies J, Whitehead MI: A simple method for determining the optimal dosage of progestin in postmenopausal women receiving estrogens. N Engl J Med 315:930, 1986 (*Adjustment of dose to induce withdrawal bleeding on or after day 11 of a 12-day progestin program was associated with a secretory endometrium.*)

Rosenbert L, Armstrong B, Jick H: Myocardial infarction and estrogen therapy in postmenopausal women. N Engl J Med 294:1256, 1976 (*No increase in risk of myocardial infarction.*)

Smith DC, Prentice R, Thompson D et al: Association of exogenous estrogen and endometrial carcinoma. N Engl J Med 293:1164, 1975 (*Among the first reports of the association of endometrial cancer with estrogen use.*)

Wenz AC: Psychiatric morbidity and menopause (editorial). Ann Intern Med 84:331, 1976 (*Psychiatric symptoms are not a function of estrogen deficiency.*)

Whitehead MI, Townsend PT, Pryse-Davies J et al: Effects of estrogens and progestins on the biochemistry and morphology of the postmenopausal endometrium. N Engl J Med 305:1599, 1981 (*The original report on progestins counteracting the effects of estrogen.*)

118
Approach to Fertility Control

The ideal contraceptive is perfectly safe, effective, inexpensive, acceptable, and available. None exists. The efficacy of individual contraceptive agents is expressed in several ways. *Theoretical effectiveness* refers to the ability of the medication, device, or procedure to prevent pregnancy if applied under ideal conditions. *Use effectiveness* combines theoretical effectiveness with inherent patient-related lapses in application. *Extended use effectiveness* adds the dimension of time. All are important aspects of evaluation of approaches to fertility control.

The primary physician should be knowledgeable about the effectiveness, difficulties, and adverse effects of available contraceptive methods to help the patient or couple intelligently select the one that suits them best.

NATURAL METHODS

Natural methods of birth control do not meet the demands of most sexually active individuals in industrialized societies. Faithfully practiced *rhythm,* with daily basal body temperature recording, usually results in one pregnancy every 2 years or at least one more child than planned by the couple by their late thirties. Rhythm practiced by abstinence according to menstrual dates is less effective. Rhythm controlled by following the cervical mucus cycle is confounded by infections, dietary changes, douching habits, oral medications, patient understanding of her anatomy, and availability of testing materials. One needs to understand reproductive anatomy and physiology and to have privacy to conduct such tests. These ingredients are unavailable to many Americans. The *amenorrhea of lactation* is useful, but the duration of ovarian inactivity in an individual is hard to predict or follow. *Withdrawal* is probably the most commonly used natural contraceptive technique. Unfortunately, sperm migration from the female perineum occasionally occurs, as does some discharging of semen prior to ejaculation.

BARRIER CONTRACEPTIVES

Condoms have extended use effectiveness. Pregnancies may occur in 3 per 100 couples per year using condoms, which means that properly used, this method is 97% effective. For a few cents more than the cheapest devices, high-quality thin condoms are available, use of which is accompanied by very little loss of sensation. The condom is inexpensive and widely available. It requires no medical intervention or prescription. Failure by means of rupture is rare, but easily rec-

ognized. An often overlooked benefit is the condom's imperviousness to such infectious agents as gonococci, HTLV III virus, *Chlamydia,* and herpes simplex virus.

Diaphragms are synthetic rubber barriers mounted on covered rims that deny access of sperm and penis to the anterior vaginal wall and cervical os. There are three widely used rims: all flex, coil spring, and flat spring. These have minor differences in characteristics and provide alternatives for fitting a variety of women. The largest diaphragm that will cover the cervix and anterior vagina from the pubis symphysis to the posterior fornix, without uncomfortably stretching the rest of the vagina, should be selected. The diaphragm should not be so big that the penis could get between the pubic symphysis and its rim, nor so small that it is beyond the reach of the exploring finger. The vagina has no bony limitations and will continue to stretch with sexual activity, so that size checks are warranted in the first year and at 2- to 3-year intervals thereafter. Parturition will also alter the size of the vagina. Only massive weight changes of 25% of body weight or more require refitting of diaphragms, despite popular belief.

Diaphragms with a small amount of spermicidal cream or jelly, properly used, are 97% effective; that is, similarly to condoms, three pregnancies per 100 fertile women per year would be expected. The cream facilitates insertion but need not be used in the large amounts recommended by the manufacturers, as it is unpleasantly messy. The diaphragm is worn for 6 hours after the last coital event, since this is the length of time during which sperm motility persists. It may be worn for longer periods of time, but like all vaginal contraceptives, will then become associated with an unpleasant odor. It may also be worn while the patient is swimming or during menstruation.

The diaphragm must be fitted to the individual woman by a physician, nurse, or trained technician. The cost of the diaphragm is reasonable, but manufacturers advocate massive use of creams, which adds to the expense. The patient must have some understanding of her anatomy and not be concerned about exploring her reproductive organs. Some adolescents reject the diaphragm as representing premeditated sexual intercourse, which they find less acceptable than spontaneous events. Women in their twenties seldom voice such a complaint. Some women cannot be adequately fitted with a diaphragm for anatomical reasons. The cervix may not protrude into the vagina adequately (absent pars vaginalis). The cervix may be displaced posteriorly by retroversion or extreme anteversion.

Spermicidal Creams and Jellies may have a high theoretical effectiveness, but lesser use effectiveness. Most contain nonoxyl-9 as the spermicidal agent. The physical nature of the creams and jellies and difficulty in their application often result in inadequately smearing the cervical os, so that sperm invasion is not prevented. Both men and women complain of the dehydrating effect of spermicidal agents and may report burning sensations. Nonoxyl-9 has the added advantage of being toxic *in vitro* to gonococci, *Chlamydia,* and other genital pathogens; some clinical evidence suggests an *in vivo* effect as well. *Foams* have better physical properties allowing more adequate smearing of the cervical os; however, foams are effective for short periods of time only, and reapplications are necessary. This increases their cost. They also contain nonoxyl-9 and will cause irritation. Although failure rates as high as 50% have been reported in some studies, others claim a 97% success rate, with only three pregnancies per 100 fertile women per year. *Encapsulated foams* compared to foams applied through applicators are far less successful because the capsule may not be inserted deeply enough into the vagina or may not disintegrate at the appropriate interval to smear the cervical os adequately. Foams have the advantage of being readily accessible in both supermarkets and drugstores and do not require medical instruction or prescription.

Cervical caps are individually molded to a particular cervix and are difficult to apply repeatedly. Their use requires an extensive amount of physician and nurse teaching, and they are more costly than diaphragms. For these reasons, they have found little general application.

Vaginal Contraceptive Sponges represent a more convenient, though slightly less effective, barrier method of contraception than the diaphragm. The sponge is smaller and thicker than the diaphragm, being made of hydrophilic polyurethane foam with 1 g of the spermicide nonoxynol-9 incorporated within it. Mechanisms of contraceptive action include release of spermicide, blocking of the cervical os, and absorption of semen. The sponge has an indentation on one surface to fit over the cervix. It is moistened with a few teaspoons of tap water and inserted high into the vagina. Once inserted, it is protective for 24 hours, regardless of how many episodes of intercourse occur. For maximum protection, the sponge needs to be left in at least 6 hours after intercourse. The product has a woven polyester strap attached to one side to aid in removal.

Twelve-month pregnancy rates with use of the sponge average 16% in the United States (range: 10%–27%); this compares with 12% for use of the diaphragm. The spermicide nonoxynol-9 has been used for years as the active ingredient of most spermicidal foams, jellies, and creams. There is one report of a possible increase in congenital anomalies and spontaneous abortions in women using spermicidal agents, but other studies have failed to confirm it. No evidence exists of a significant increase in birth defects in the children of women using spermicides. Nonoxynol-9 may contain trace amounts of residues that are known carcinogens; moreover, the carcinogen 2,4-toluenediamine can form as a contaminant during the polymerization of polyurethane. Precautions have been taken to prevent formation of contaminants, and careful analyses have failed to detect any carcinogens in the sponge. If any carcinogens were present, they would be in such small concentrations as to make them unlikely to increase the risk of cancer.

Mild side-effects include vaginal dryness during intercourse resulting from absorption of secretions by the sponge, mild local irritation in those sensitive to the spermicide, and odor from leaving the sponge in too long. If the sponge is placed incorrectly, the strap may be hard to reach and the sponge difficult to remove. However, no episodes of toxic shock have been reported to date (only polyacrylate rayon products have been associated with the pathogenesis of toxic shock).

The sponge is available without prescription and popular with many women because of its convenience and simplicity of use. The safety of long-term use and risks from misuse remain to be determined; no serious complications have emerged so far.

INTRAUTERINE DEVICES (IUDs)

The idea of inserting materials into the uterine cavity to prevent nidation is ancient. Nevertheless the precise mechanism of IUD action remains unknown. What appears to be important is the area of surface contact. Copper enhances effectiveness. The 1% to 5% first-year pregnancy rates with IUD use are among the lowest attainable from a birth control method and comparable to those of oral contraceptives. The lack of need for constant compliance greatly enhances efficacy. Another advantage is the lack of systemic effects, a major problem with oral contraceptives (see below). A major limitation to efficacy is expulsion, which is particularly frequent in nulliparous women. The overall expulsion rate is 19 per 100 women per year, lower with copper devices. Occasionally it is necessary to remove an IUD because of bleeding or pain, which occurs at a rate of about 11% per year; copper devices are better tolerated by nulliparous women.

The confirmation of a markedly increased risk of tubal infertility associated with IUD use has greatly discouraged IUD placement as a means of safe birth control, especially among nulliparous women. Not all IUDs demonstrate equally high risk of infertility. In one large study, risk was greatest in users of the Dalkon shield; it decreased somewhat in users of the Lippes loop and Saf-T-Coil; risk with use of copper-containing IUDs was normal except in nulliparous women with more than one sexual partner.

Clinical or subclinical pelvic inflammatory disease is believed to account for the tubal infertility. Insertion of the IUD results in transient introduction of bacteria into the uterine cavity; normal host defenses usually clear them within a few days, except in the case of the Dalkon shield. The string used for insertion and retrieval of the IUD is made of slippery monofilament, which may act as a conduit between the never-sterile vagina and the usually sterile endometrial cavity. Risk of pelvic inflammatory disease in nulliparous sexually active women with an IUD has been found to be seven times that for similar women not using an IUD; for parous women the risk is three times greater.

In view of the infertility risk, IUD use is best confined to multiparous women and nulliparous women with a single sexual partner. The nulliparous woman considering an IUD as a means of birth control should be fully informed of the risk of tubal infertility before any decision is made regarding its use. Only copper-containing IUDs should be used.

ORAL CONTRACEPTIVES

Combinations of synthetic estrogens and progesterones have been found to have use effectiveness rates that exceed most estimates of effectiveness of condoms, diaphragms, and IUDs. Although some note failure rates may be as high as 5% to 10%, most report only one to three pregnancies per 100 users per year. The combination pill appears to prevent cyclic FSH and LH release, which are required for ovulation. At the present time, combination pills consist of ethinyl estradiol and norethindrone, mestranol, and norethynodrel, ethinyl estradiol and norgestrel, or mestranol and ethynodiol diacetate. Packets are made up for taking the pills from the fifth day of the menstrual cycle for the subsequent 21 days; some packets have placebos, so that one pill is taken daily.

Preparations. More than two dozen combination preparations are available in the United States. In general, it is most useful to renew any prescription with which a patient is satisfied, as long as the patient has no new symptoms or habits that warrant discontinuation of any oral contraceptive.

Because the risk of cardiovascular problems appears to increase with estrogen dosage and progestin potency, emphasis in recent years has been on use of preparations that have the lowest effective estrogen dose (20 μg–35 μg ethinyl estradiol) and the least progestin potency. Epidemiologic studies show cardiovascular risk increases with use of estrogen dosages over 50 μg; under 50 μg, adverse cardiovascular effects are rare (see below). Fortunately, efficacy of 30 μg to 35 μg of estrogen for prevention of pregnancy is about the same as that of 50 μg of estrogen.

It is best to begin with a pill containing 35 μg of either mestranol or ethinyl estradiol. The lowest possible progestin dosage will not only reduce cardiovascular risk, but also help minimize bothersome side-effects such as increased appetite, steady weight gain, acne, and depression. Patients who have a history of symptoms suggesting hyperresponsiveness to en-

dogenous estrogens (premenstrual breast engorgement and soreness, cyclic weight gain, heavy periods) may benefit from a preparation containing a progestin with minimal estrogenic effect, and perhaps some antiestrogenic or androgenic qualities. Similarly, a patient bothered by acne or hirsutism should not be given a preparation with an androgenic progestin (see Table 118-1). Other side-effects such as nausea seem related to estrogen content.

The disadvantages to using lower-dose agents are higher rates of spotting, breakthrough bleeding, and amenorrhea. Moreover, women who use oral contraceptives containing less than 30 μg of estrogen may experience a greater chance of pregnancy. In an attempt to improve on rates of breakthrough bleeding and pregnancy associated with low-estrogen/weak-progestin formulations, manufacturers have developed *biphasic* (e.g., Ortho-Novum10/11) and *triphasic formulations* (e.g., OrthoNovum7/7/7, Triyorinyl, Triphasil). The rationale is to more closely mimic normal ovarian patterns. Efficacy is similar to other low-estrogen/weak-progestin preparations; no controlled evidence to date suggests that they are superior in terms of breakthrough bleeding. All low-dose preparations need to be taken religiously to be maximally effective and to minimize the chances of breakthrough bleeding.

It is helpful to become familiar with four or five pills and their minor differences, rather than use the most recently marketed combinations. Providing the patient with full, understandable information at the initiation of therapy will ward off many anxious phone calls. In particular, if one pill is missed, it can be made up by doubling the dose for the next 1 or 2 days, but barrier contraception is recommended for the remainder of the cycle. If three or more consecutive pills are missed, the pills should be stopped altogether, allowing withdrawal bleeding to occur, and then started 1 week after the last pill is taken. However, failure to take oral contraceptives regularly is an indication for trying another form of birth control.

Patients require follow-up care yearly, checking for headaches, hypertension, breast masses, cervical abnormalities, phlebitis, and signs of cardiovascular or cerebrovascular disease.

Physicians are generally unaware of the high discontinuation rate among oral contraceptive users. Factors involved include the patient's perceptions of need and attitudes about

Table 118-1. Effects of Synthetic Progestins*

ESTROGENIC	ANDROGENIC
Norethynodrel	Norgestrel
Ethynodiol	Norethindrone
All others have none	Norethindrone acetate
	Ethynodiol
	Norethynodrel (has none)

* In order of decreasing potency.

taking medications that affect the sex organs. Oral contraceptives may cost several dollars a month and require a medical prescription, important barriers for adolescents. Despite these factors and known side-effects, birth control pills continue to be the most used, safest birth control method for most women under 30. The pill's relative safety is most apparent in countries where the risk of dying in childbirth is high.

Adverse Effects. The major hazards of oral contraceptives are cardiovascular. The relative risks of cardiovascular events in users compared with nonusers are reported to be 4 to 11 times greater for thromboembolism, 4 to 9.5 times greater for thrombotic stroke, 2 times greater for hemorrhagic stroke, and 2 to 12 times greater for myocardial infarction. Mortality from myocardial infarction rises sixfold in women over 40 who are smokers. The overall excess death rate annually has been estimated to be 20 per 100,000, with risk concentrated in women over 35, especially if they smoke cigarettes and have used oral contraceptives for 5 years or more. Division of data at 35 years of age is arbitrary, and it would be prudent to assume that risk gradually increases with age. Increased rate of infarction persists even after discontinuation of long-term use. Progestin potency is also associated with increased cardiovascular risk, probably because of its ability to raise LDL cholesterol and lower HDL cholesterol (see Chapter 9).

Any population of women provided with oral contraception will show a rise in mean blood pressure in about 3 months. Prospective studies have found that the incidence of *hypertension* increases two- to sixfold in users compared with nonusers. Patients with hypertension are at increased risk and should not use oral contraceptives. It is wise to check blood pressure before renewing a patient's prescription. The progesterone in the birth control pill, like the progesterone in the secretory phase of the menstrual cycle, increases aldosterone secretion, and estrogen increases renin substrate.

There is a twofold increase in the risk of *gallbladder disease* in users compared with nonusers, because of increased cholesterol saturation of bile. The frequency of gallstones appears to rise after 2 years' usage and to reach a plateau after 4 to 5 years' usage. This risk must be balanced against the increased risk of gallbladder disease associated with multiparity. Another hepatobiliary problem is development of highly vascular *hepatic adenomas,* which can rupture spontaneously, resulting in serious hemorrhage, isolated cases have appeared in the literature. In cases, most patients were using the pill more than 5 years. The actual risk is unknown. Finally, estrogen use has been associated with *cholestatic jaundice,* but oral contraceptive use does not worsen cases of mild viral hepatitis and need not be discontinued unless cholestasis or hepatocellular injury is severe.

At present, there is no evidence of increased risk of *cancer* from use of oral contraceptives by premenopausal women. A large multicenter case-control study has demonstrated that long-term oral contraceptive use in women of reproductive age confers no increased risk of breast cancer compared with that of other methods of delaying first pregnancy. However, the growth of certain cancers may be stimulated by estrogens; these include carcinoma of the breast (see Chapter 121), cervix, and endometrium (see Chapter 122). Most studies have shown diminished incidences of fibroadenomas, ovarian and endometrial cancers, and benign fibrocystic disease of the breast in pill users.

There appears to be an increased risk of *congenital malformations* with inadvertent exposure of the fetus to birth control pills in early pregnancy, but this is a subject of continued dispute. Masculinization of the fetus was reported with earlier pill preparations.

Metabolic and *endocrinologic effects* are numerous. Thyroid-binding globin levels increase, which in turn raises the serum thyroxine level. Glucose tolerance falls as circulating growth hormone rises and peripheral resistance to insulin occurs. Triglyceride levels increase, sometimes dramatically, with the concurrent boost in lipoprotein production.

A few miscellaneous effects are worth noting. Birth control pills increase the frequency of *migraine headache* in patients with prior migraine attacks. Anecdotal reports of *exacerbation of lupus erythematosus* appear in the obstetric literature. Sensitivity to sunlight and chloasma (mask of pregnancy) are seen in some users and fade with discontinuation.

A number of gynecologic conditions are affected by use of these agents; effects may be beneficial or detrimental. Patients with menstrual irregularities prior to oral contraceptive use will have regular pill-induced periods while taking the medication. Upon discontinuation of the pills, some will revert to their previous irregularity. Rarely, *amenorrhea* due to ovarian suppression will persist for several months, even a year (see Chapter 109). Usually, menses return promptly, and fertility rates in the first 3 months of discontinuation are increased. Occasionally, a patient will notice nipple discharge (nonpuerperal lactation) with use of oral contraceptives. The mechanism is not clear. No increased incidence of pituitary prolactinomas has been observed.

Many patients with *dysmenorrhea* find marked relief with oral contraceptives (see Chapter 114). If the dysmenorrhea is associated with endometriosis, the response is variable, with many patients complaining of exacerbation of symptoms rather than relief.

With these side-effects in mind, absolute and relative contraindications can be listed (Table 118-2). Patients exposed to diethylstilbestrol have used birth control pills with no evidence to date of either beneficial or deleterious effects.

"Morning-After Pill." Large doses of estrogen (50 mg of diethylstilbestrol daily for 5 days or ethinyl estradiol, 0.5 mg twice a day for 5 days) will result in withdrawal bleeding, denying the conceptus an environment for nidation. Such doses usually cause nausea, and antiemetic medication is

Table 118-2.   Contraindications of Oral Contraceptives

Absolute Contraindications
1. Thromboembolic disorders, cardiovascular disease, thrombophlebitis, or a past history of these conditions or other conditions that predispose to them
2. Markedly impaired liver function from severe hepatitis, alcoholism, etc.
3. Known or suspected estrogen-dependent neoplasm (cancers of the breast, endometrium, etc.)
4. Undiagnosed genital bleeding
5. Known or suspected pregnancy

Relative contraindications
1. Migraine headache
2. Hypertension
3. Familial hyperlipidemia
4. Epilepsy
5. Uterine leiomyoma
6. History of idiopathic obstructive jaundice of pregnancy
7. Smoking one-half pack or more per day
8. Diabetes mellitus
9. Severe heart disease
10. Patient unreliability
11. Age > 35 years

needed. Provided that nidation has not already occurred, this therapy may work. However, failures are reported.

ABORTION

Studies by Planned Parenthood have not found that a substantial number of American women rely on abortion as the sole method of birth control, nor has any trend to such a reliance been noted. Rather, abortion is used as a backup when other methods fail. Frequently, the necessity for an abortion initiates effective contraceptive use, particularly in those under 20 years of age. No adverse effect of first-trimester-induced abortion on future childbearing has been demonstrated. The effect of second-trimester abortions in rupturing cervical tissue is controversial. Rarely, an anomalous cervix may become incompetent, requiring cerclage if the patient wishes to carry future pregnancies to term. Morbidity and mortality in teenagers from induced abortion is lower than in older women.

OVERALL RISKS

Used alone by women 30 and under, condoms, diaphragms, IUDs, birth control pills, and first-trimester abortion have a mortality risk of 1 to 2 per 100,000, significantly lower than the 12 per 100,000 delivery-related risk rate. After age 30, the risk of birth control pills rises, especially in smokers, but is still less than the morbidity and complications of childbearing without fertility control. The lowest level of mortality is achieved by a combination of contraception with access to early abortion.

STERILIZATION

In 1965, one third of the married couples in the United States used oral contraception, sterilization, or IUDs. By 1975, almost three quarters used one of these methods. Sterilization is now the most frequently used method of contraception among couples married for a decade or more, as well as among couples who have had all the children they want.

Vasectomy is the simplest and safest means of sterilization. Only a few surgical instruments and local anesthesia are required. The procedure may be done in a clinic, doctor's office, ambulatory surgical day care unit, or hospital. The procedure does not lead to impotence; rather, men with problems associated with impotence may blame vasectomy. It takes about 90 days of average ejaculatory activity to completely empty the spermatic cord and accessory glands of residual sperm. Thus, the vasectomy subject should have a postoperative semen analysis before he is considered sterile. Alternative methods of birth control should be used in the interim. Circulating antibodies to sperm may be induced by foreign proteins as well as by sperm. The effect of elevated sperm antibodies on a man's health is not clear, but has been the subject of much concern. Retrospective cohort study of more than 10,000 vasectomized men fails to support such concerns; no serious immunopathologic consequences of vasectomy were noted. Further evidence of safety emerges from use-control and cohort studies showing no relationship between vasectomy and cardiovascular disease. The only adverse effects are an increased risk of epidydimitis–orchitis and testicular changes leading to infertility (see below). Vasectomy still appears safe and effective, and is the least expensive form of permanent sterilization. Recanalization when ends of the vas are tied too closely together may account for failures. Reanastomosis may be carried out with microsurgical techniques; however, only about one third of patients undergoing reanastomosis father live-born children. The causes of diminished fertility are multifactorial and include damage to nerves adjacent to the vas, the development of interstitial fibrosis within the testicle, and age.

Procedures on the Fallopian Tubes. In 1975, 2% of women 25 to 34 years of age underwent tubal sterilization. In the ensuing decade, the rate has increased markedly. Surgical division of the fallopian tubes after delivery is easily accomplished, either with normal vaginal delivery or with cesarean section. The procedure adds 1 to 2 days to the patient's hospitalization. Procedures that leave the two ends of the fallopian tubes in close proximity (Pomeroy technique, in which a suture ties a knuckle of tube and the apex of the knuckle is excised) may have a failure rate of 2%. Other methods that leave the two severed ends well separated have less than 1% failure rates. When there is concern for the survival of the newborn, postpartum sterilization is contraindicated.

Vaginal tubal ligation is usually not done postpartum through the vagina because of the increased vascularity and the risk of sepsis. A skilled obstetrician-gynecologist can do interval sterilizations under local anesthesia, usually in a day care or hospital facility. However, leiomyoma, endometriosis, or previous infection may obstruct the approach to the tube.

The *minilaparotomy* involves a small abdominal incision of 1 to 2 inches done under local anesthesia through the peritoneum. Each fallopian tube is identified, ligated, and divided. The incision is closed with resorbable sutures, and a bandage is applied. The patient is able to go home within a few hours.

These methods have the advantage of simplicity and require commonly used instruments. They have been taught to surgical technicians in Third World countries. Such procedures may be unsuitable in an obese or anxious patient. In fact, other methods are more commonly used in the United States.

Laparoscopy requires expensive special instrumentation and an experienced gynecologist or surgeon. Although it can be done under local anesthesia, general endotracheal anesthesia is more commonly used. A preparatory D&C is usually done (as many patients consider themselves sterile at the time the appointment is made) in anticipation of, rather than after, laparoscopy. A fiberoptic endoscope is inserted through a subumbilical incision, and a second instrument accompanies the endoscope or is inserted through the pelvic incision. The tubes are cauterized or both cauterized and divided. Alternatively, plastic rings or clips are used to occlude them. Cauterization has the lowest failure rate; however, clips are advocated as being less likely to cause damage to bowel. In fact, complications and failures with clips are often remedied by cauterization. Furthermore, the half-life of the plastic materials used for occlusion has not been clearly defined, and very little 5-year data are available.

In experienced hands, laparoscopy is highly effective with minimal risk in a healthy woman. Most insurance carriers will pay for such procedures, though some require a euphemistic indication such as "recurrent situational anxiety." Laparoscopy may be accomplished on a 1-day basis, although most hospitals do not offer day care facilities. The patient may be expected to continue her normal menstrual life and menopause. Anastomosis of severed fallopian tubes is accomplished by careful surgical procedures with or without optical magnification. However, as with vasectomy, the rate of achieving patency is higher than that of live births. Motivating factors, patient age, concurrent disease, or attitudes of the partner as well as surgical technical details account for the low fertility rate.

In general, tubal sterilization should be considered irreversible. The procedure is indicated when the patient requests it. Many requests for anastomosis of divided tubes come when the procedure is initially advocated by a physician or partner. A woman of 23 with three children may be firm in her desire for sterilization, whereas a woman of 34 with five children may be unwilling to consider it. On the average, women are 28 to 30 years old at the time of tubal sterilization; 88% are married, 6% have never been married.

The federal government will not reimburse for sterilization done at the time of abortion, because the combined procedure has been found to be more hazardous than either done separately. The rare instance in which this does not hold true is the patient in whom the risk of anesthesia is unduly high, such as a woman with myasthenia gravis. There is no federal reimbursement for sterilization of minors or mentally incompetent patients. Though awkward in individual cases, on the whole, such regulations have been necessary to prevent widespread abuse of easily accomplished, low-risk surgical procedures done without due respect for the patient's understanding or desires. In addition the government will not pay for hysterectomies done solely for the purpose of sterilization. The public acceptability of sterilization is suggested by government reports of women interviewed in 1970 and reinterviewed in 1975; one half had changed their method of birth control, and most of these changed to sterilization.

CHOICE OF METHOD

The choice of birth control is best viewed in terms of the patient's age and family expectations. *Unmarried adolescents and women in their early twenties* may use oral contraceptives with a high degree of safety and acceptability. Contraindications are infrequent in this age group, and the cost, in general, is not beyond their reach. Diaphragms may be as effective, but often are less acceptable. Though less effective, the sponge is convenient and, as such, more likely to be used. Condoms and foam are adequate as long as they are always available. Their use depends on motivation, which can be lacking at times. IUDs are effective, but the risk of pelvic sepsis that may affect future childbearing is a concern.

For sexually active *26- to 35-year-olds,* birth control pills, diaphragms, and condoms may be equally effective, and choice is simply a matter of preference. Sponges have the advantages of convenience and safety, but with some compromise of efficacy. IUDs may be a reasonable choice for parous women aware of the small risk of pelvic inflammatory disease and willing to seek help promptly at the first sign of infection. The smoker should be asked to stop tobacco use if she wants to use oral contraceptives. Many patients in this age group have completed their families and request sterilization. Nulliparous women in this age group who desire sterilization present a problem to many health care providers. If the patient is not well known to the clinic or physician, one can suggest she practice contraception for a year, then undergo sterilization if she still wants to. When such advice is given, perhaps half the patients return for the procedure. The others go elsewhere or change their minds.

For *women over 35,* the risk of birth control pills makes them a less desirable choice than the other methods discussed. *The woman over 40* is not a candidate for oral contraception.

Moreover, she may have a leiomyoma, making IUD insertion difficult. Though she is near the menopause, sterilization often relieves recurrent anxiety associated with risk of pregnancy. An ECG and chest x-ray are important preoperative procedures in such women undergoing general endotracheal anesthesia.

PATIENT EDUCATION

There are few areas in primary care in which patient education is so important to decision making. Diagrammatic and written material is available from most commercial distributors of contraceptive products, Planned Parenthood, many women's advocate organizations, the American College of Obstetrics and Gynecology, and the American Medical Association. It is most important that information be clearly written in the patient's native language, and that the patient be given an opportunity to ask questions and demonstrate her understanding.

The need to offer sympathetic and nonjudgmental counseling cannot be overemphasized. Regardless of the physician's personal views on abortion and birth control, the patient should be able to obtain factual information from her primary care physician or be referred to someone who is willing to provide the information and care desired.

INDICATIONS FOR REFERRAL

Patients may need or request referral for counseling on emotional responses to sexual activity and contraceptive techniques. Referral to a social worker, sex therapist, or psychiatrist with an interest in the area may be useful, but thorough discussion between the primary physician and patient usually suffices.

When a surgical procedure is being considered, the patient should meet with the gynecologist to discuss the issue in more detail. Referrals of medically uncomplicated patients may be made by phone. For patients with known medical problems, a careful history and physical examination and written referral to the specialist are helpful, so that the risks of the various procedures may be carefully discussed and therapy individualized. Patients who seem unable to use any form of birth control offered may also be referred to any of the above-named specialists, in the hope that an alternative approach will enhance motivation.

A.H.G.

ANNOTATED BIBLIOGRAPHY

Barnes AB, Cohen E, Stoeckle JD et al: Therapeutic abortion: Medical and social sequels. Ann Intern Med 75:881, 1971 (*Summarizes impact on the patient from medical and social perspectives.*)

Cates W, Schultz KF, Grimes DA: Risks associated with teenage abortion. N Engl J Med 309:621, 1983 (*Teenagers had lower rates of morbidity or mortality from induced abortion than older women.*)

The Centers for Disease Control Cancer and Steroid Hormone Study: Long-term oral contraceptive use and the risk of breast cancer. JAMA 249:1591, 1983 (*Large multicenter case control study detecting no increased risk associated with oral contraceptive use compared with other methods of delaying first pregnancy.*)

The Centers for Disease Control Cancer and Steroid Hormone Study: Oral contraceptive use and the risk of endometrial cancer. JAMA 249:1600, 1983 (*A large multicenter case-control study detecting a significant protective effect for oral contraceptive use with a relative risk of developing endometrial cancer of 0.5; protective effect was most notable for nulliparous women.*)

The Centers for Disease Control Cancer and Steroid Hormone Study: Oral contraceptive use and the risk of ovarian cancer. JAMA 249:1596, 1983 (*This multicenter case-control study demonstrated a significant protective effect with a relative risk of 0.6 for oral contraceptive uses against ovarian cancer.*)

Collaborative Group for the Study of Stroke in Young Women: Oral contraception and increased risk of cerebral ischemia or thrombosis. N Engl J Med 288:871, 1973 (*The incidence of thrombotic stroke showed a ninefold increase among women using oral contraceptives; hemorrhagic stroke showed less dramatic, but still significant, increase.*)

Cramer DW, Hutchinson JB, Welch WR et al: Factors affecting the association of oral contraceptives and ovarian cancer. N Engl J Med 307:1047, 1982 (*Prior use of birth control pills appeared to provide long-lasting protection against ovarian cancer among subjects aged 40 through 59 years.*)

Cramer DW, Schiff I, Schoenbaum SC et al: Tubal infertility and the intrauterine device. N Engl J Med 312:941, 1985 (*Risk of infertility was high in users of the Dalkon shield and other non-copper-containing IUDs.*)

Edmondson HA, Henderson B, Benton B: Liver cell adenomas associated with use of oral contraceptives. N Engl J Med 294:470, 1976 (*A study of 42 women with matched controls showed a dramatic rise in incidence of liver adenomas, correlated with prolonged use of pills that are more likely to contain mestranol as the synthetic estrogen.*)

Flickinger CJ: The effects of vasectomy on the testis. N Engl J Med 313:1283, 1985 (*An editorial summarizing current state of knowledge; no serious adverse consequences other than infertility.*)

Goldacre MJ, Holford TR, Vessey MP: Cardiovascular disease and vasectomy. N Engl J Med 308:805, 1983 (*A report of both a case-control study and a cohort study that did not demonstrate a relationship between vasectomy and cardiovascular disease.*)

Jarow JJ, Budin RE, Dym M et al: Quantitative pathologic changes in the human testis after vasectomy. N Engl J Med 313:1252, 1985 (*The development of interstitial fibrosis occurred with increased frequency and correlated with development of infertility.*)

Jick H, Hannan MT, Stergachis A et al: Vaginal spermicides and gonorrhea. JAMA 248:1619, 1982 (*This descriptive study suggests a protective effect against gonorrhea of vaginal spermicides.*)

Kaufman TW, Watson J, Rosenberg L et al: The effect of different types of intrauterine devices on the risk of pelvic inflammatory disease. JAMA 250:759, 1983 (*A case-control study demonstrating an overall relative risk of pelvic inflammatory disease of 8.6 among current users of IUDs and 1.6 for past users. Risk was highest for users of the Dalkon shield and lowest for users of copper-containing devices; editorial.*)

Kelaghan J, Rubin GL, Ory HW et al: Barrier-method contraceptives and pelvic inflammatory disease. JAMA 248:184, 1982 (*A case-control study detecting a relative risk of 0.6 for women using barrier methods compared with others for pelvic inflammatory disease.*)

Kopit S, Barnes AB: Patients' response to tubal division. JAMA 236:2761, 1976 (*Of 197 patients who underwent tubal division, 93.5% said they would make the same choice again. Those who were regretful could not be readily identified by any preoperative characteristic such as age, parity, or marital status.*)

LeBolt SA, Grimes DA, Cates W: Mortality from abortion and childbirth. JAMA 248:188, 1982 (*A pair of studies indicating that women are about seven times more likely to die from childbirth than from legal abortion and that available data are likely to be biased in the direction that overestimates abortion risks relative to the risks of childbearing.*)

Massey FJ, Bernstein GS, Ofallon WM et al: Vasectomy and health. JAMA 252:1023, 1984 (*Retrospective cohort study of over 10,000 vasectomized men that does not support concerns about serious immunopathologic consequences of vasectomy.*)

Mills JT, Parsonnet J, Tsai Y-C et al: Control of production of toxic-shock-syndrome toxin by magnesium ion. J Infect Dis 151:1158, 1985 (*Relates toxin production to magnesium chelation by polyacrylate rayon.*)

Mishell DR: Current status of intrauterine devices. N Engl J Med 312:1984, 1985 (*Recommends limiting use to copper-containing types in parous women and nulliparous women willing to risk infertility.*)

Sartwell PE, Stolley PD: Oral contraceptives and vascular disease. Epidemiol Rev 4:95, 1982 (*A succinct review of the literature including a discussion of benefits as well as risks of oral contraceptive use.*)

Shy KK, McTiernan AM, Daling JR et al: Oral contraceptive use and the occurrence of pituitary prolactinoma. JAMA 249:2204, 1983 (*Case-control study detecting no increased risk of prolactinoma among prior users of oral contraceptives.*)

Slone D, Shapiro S, Kaufman DW et al: Risk of myocardial infarction relation to current and discontinued use of oral contraceptives. N Engl J Med 305:420, 1981 (*A case-control study suggesting that increased risk of myocardial infarction persists after discontinuation of long-term use of oral contraceptives.*)

Stadel BV: Oral contraceptives and cardiovascular disease. N Engl J Med 305:612, 1981 (*An extensive review assessing the risk attributable to oral contraceptive use.*)

Svensson L, Westrom L, Mardh P: Contraceptives and acute salpingitis. JAMA 251:2553, 1984 (*Among women with the first episode of salpingitis observed through the laparoscope, women taking oral contraceptives had milder degrees of inflammation than women using IUDs or using no birth control.*)

Vaginal contraceptive sponge. Med Lett 25:78, 1983 (*Concludes it is a safe, convenient, but less effective barrier method than the diaphragm.*)

Wahl P, Walden C, Knopp R et al: Effective estrogen/progestin potency on lipid/lipoprotein cholesterol. N Engl J Med 308:862, 1983 (*Low-estrogen/high-progestin birth control pills increase low-density lipoprotein cholesterol while high-estrogens/low-progestin preparations, as well as estrogen use in postmenopausal women, were associated with elevated high-density lipoprotein cholesterol.*)

119
Approach to the Infertile Couple

PATHOPHYSIOLOGY AND CLINICAL PRESENTATION

Any disorder involving the male or female reproductive system may interfere with function to a degree sufficient to cause infertility.

Fertility rates are affected by socioeconomic circumstances, disease patterns, war, and use of contraceptive techniques; they vary from place to place. Fertility may be measured by the census of live-born children in a population, but the variations do not inversely reflect infertility. Epidemiologic data on involuntary infertility are inadequate. Social scientists' data on samples of populations lack medical documentation. Data from infertility clinics lack documentation of the patient selection process and the population from which the patients are drawn. Estimates of infertility in populations of industrialized nations vary from 5% to a high of 22%.

The primary physician is often the first to be consulted by the couple unable to conceive. Although the usual request is to find or rule out a medical cause for the problem, there is also a need to identify any psychological or socioeconomic barriers to conception. Treatment is frequently carried out by individuals specializing in infertility, but the primary care physician should become proficient in performing the initial assessment and knowing when referral is indicated. Principal tasks include providing accurate advice and uncovering treatable etiologies.

Men

Infertility in the male can be classified in terms of gonadal, gonadotropic, anatomic, and functional etiologies and considered according to whether they present with azoospermia, oligospermia, or normal sperm counts.

Azoospermic Etiologies. Patients with *primary hypogonadism (e.g.,* Klinefelter's syndrome) have azoospermia, a low testosterone, and elevations of LH and FSH. Those with *isolated germinal compartment failure* (as from adult mumps or irradiation) are also azoospermic, but manifest normal testosterone, normal LH, and elevated FSH. *Hypogonadotropic hypogonadism* also causes azoospermia. It may be congenital or acquired. Patients present with azoospermia and low levels of FSH, LH, and serum testosterone. Congenital disease is often associated with anosmia. *Pituitary tumors* account for much of the acquired disease; often the other manifestations of panhypopituitarism dominate the clinical picture. *Drugs* (including alcohol and marijuana) can interfere with hypothalamic–pituitary function. Azoospermia in association with normal levels of LH, FSH, and testosterone characterize *retrograde ejaculation* (due to diabetes or drugs) and *obstruction* of the ejaculatory system. Absence of seminal fructose, produced by the seminal vesicles, is a sign of *congenital obstruction* of the seminal vesicles and vas deferens; the vas deferens may be absent. Most other types of obstruction are more proximal, giving normal testicular size and normal semen fructose.

Oligospermic Etiologies. Patients with a large *varicocele* may present with the typical "bag of worms" appearance to the testicle, but at times the only manifestation is a faint pulsation along the spermatic vein upon Valsalva or coughing. The varicocele may be unilateral (usually on the left) or bilateral. There is no correlation between size of the varicocele and degree of infertility. Testicular size may be reduced, even though the scrotal contents appear enlarged. The mechanism by which varicocele results in infertility remains undetermined; some even question the association, but repair of the varicocele by spermatic vein ligation often restores normal sperm quantity and function and, more important, corrects the infertility. Another large group of oligospermic patients with normal FSH, LH, and testosterone have no detectable pathology and are labeled "idiopathic." Patients with *primary gonadal insufficiency* have low testosterone and elevations of LH and FSH along with oligospermia. *Selective damage* to the *germinal elements* of the testicles (as in chemotherapy or irradiation) produces oligospermia in conjunction with normal testosterone, normal LH, but an elevated FSH. In *acquired hypothalamic–pituitary disease* with some function preserved, FSH and LH are low to low normal and testosterone is low; prolactin may be elevated because of a pituitary tumor. In *partial androgen resistance,* testosterone and LH are elevated while FSH remains normal. Gynecomastia develops as a result of excess estradiol production by the testicle and peripheral conversion of testosterone.

Etiologies with Normal Sperm Counts. Most patients demonstrate abnormal sperm morphology or motility and suffer from many of the same conditions as those with oligospermia (*e.g.,* varicocele). In addition, *genitourinary tract infection* may cause such qualitative sperm changes; leukocytes sometimes appear in the semen. *Antisperm antibodies* are noted in some patients, but the relationship between antibodies and infertility has not been established. *Impotence* ranks as a leading, though frequently overlooked, etiology. Hormone concentrations and sperm parameters are usually normal in "functional" types (though depression and situational stress can transiently reduce sperm counts); in organic etiologies of impotence, these parameters reflect the under-

lying pathology (see Chapters 131 and 225). Anatomic anomalies, such as proximal location of the urinary meatus, may lead to infertility because of deposition of sperm and semen too far from the cervical os.

Women

Ovulatory Disorders are among the most frequent causes of failure to conceive. Any of the many causes of amenorrhea (see Chapter 109) may be responsible. A few deserve elaboration. *Polycystic ovaries* accompanied by low estrogen production with or without hirsutism, virilism, or obesity will produce severe difficulties, including infertility; when this condition is associated with moderate to high estrogen levels, infertility may be less of a problem. *Inadequate follicular development* with consequently inadequate corpus luteum formation is estimated to occur with 4% of all ovulations and is claimed to occur in as many as 20% of infertile women. *Endometriosis* is found in 8% to 15% of infertility clinic populations. The person with *testicular feminization* (testosterone insensitivity) is typically attractive in appearance and has well developed breasts, but lacks pubic and axillary hair, ovaries, and a competent uterus.

Tubal Disorders closely follow ovulatory difficulties as sources of infertility. *Pelvic inflammatory disease,* particularly nongonococcal in origin, is the most serious problem. A prospective study of 415 patients with pelvic inflammatory disease confirmed by laparoscopy and followed with repeat laparoscopy revealed that of those with a single episode of salpingitis, 12.1% had tubal occlusion; of those with two infections, 35% had occlusion; and of those with three or more, 75% had occluded tubes. Other pelvic infections and abdominal infections (such as a ruptured appendix in childhood) may lead to *tubal adhesions.* Infections associated with IUDs are a problem. Postpartum infection has an unusually frequent association with tubal occlusion. Infections following induced abortion, particularly if inadequately treated (*e.g.,* with inappropriately low doses of antibiotics), unrecognized, or not brought to medical attention, may lead to infertility. Unfortunately, oil-based radiopaque dyes used for uterotubograms (hysterosalpingograms) in some countries have also been associated with adhesions. Uncommon causes in the United States are pelvic trauma from vehicular accidents, ulcerative colitis, regional ileitis, tuberculosis, and schistosomiasis. In general, processes that cause adhesions rather than tubal epithelial damage seem to have a better prognosis.

Uterine Problems play a role in infertility less frequently. *Congenital anomalies,* such as absence or duplication of the uterine fundus, often present as repeated pregnancy wastage. Complete duplication of cervix and uterus tends to diminish fertility, but less so than anomalies causing distortion of a single uterine cavity. Septate and deeply arcuate uteri may be more useful after hysteroscopic or operative repair. Urinary tract anomalies are estimated to occur with 25% of congenitally abnormal uteri. They are found more frequently in the completely duplicated situation or when one side of the mullerian duct is missing. *Leiomyoma uteri* may distort or obstruct the uterine cavity. Resection and re-resection have been surprisingly successful. The *forgotten IUD* is occasionally a cause of infertility. The role of uterine glycosaminoglycan in stimulating conversion of sperm proacrosin to acrosin, a step necessary for sperm penetration of the zona pellucida, is an area of current investigation.

Cervical Factors are attributed to as many as 20% of the female infertile population. *Cervical incompetence* may account for repeated abortion or later trimester pregnancy losses. The incompetence can result from inadequate innervation, disturbances in synthesis or breakdown of prostaglandin, or defects in muscle and collagen fibers. Incompetence of the cervix may also compromise its role in resisting the entry of infectious agents into the sterile uterine cavity. The role of *cervical mucus* is little understood. Its physical characteristics in cystic fibrosis seem an obvious factor. The importance of cervical mucus antibodies and proteins as a cause of infertility is under investigation, and it is the focus of much speculation.

Vaginal Factors are occasionally implicated as the cause of infertility. An intact or nearly *intact hymen,* a septum, or a constricting ring in the upper vagina can limit access to the cervix. Total absence of the vagina is only rarely associated with sufficient development of the cervix and uterus to allow fertility at all. As a site of *infection,* the vagina may prove to be an important cause of pregnancy wastage. *Trichomonas, Candida albicans, Chlamydia, Mycoplasma, Gardnerella,* streptococci, and gonococci are all associated with cervical and vaginal discharge (see Chapter 115); their role in vaginally related obstructions to conception is not clear, though their role in pregnancy wastage is established. When these organisms lead to pelvic inflammatory disease, they become more clearly accountable for infertility.

Viral *infections* of the *vulva* and *labia,* particularly herpes vaginalis and condyloma accuminata (see Chapters 191 and 193) are usually only temporary impediments to fertility. Vulvar surgery *per se* need not cause infertility. Similarly, paralysis or hemipelvectomy may or may not be blamed for infertility; much of the impediment derives from the social and emotional impact of these conditions.

Both Partners

Interpersonal problems (see Chapter 225) are an important etiologic factor. The desire for children may not be shared equally by both partners. This may be overt, with one partner seeking medical assistance to persuade the other. More often, it is covert. There may be anxiety over how family respon-

sibilities will interfere with career development, or one partner may not want to lose the economic and social freedom of a childless couple. Sometimes one partner may be concerned about sharing the other's affection with a child. Some may feel inadequate or unwilling to assume parental duties. Such concerns can lead to sexual inactivity or frigidity. Transient situational problems arise. The young professional person may be under considerable job pressure; travel may interfere with optimal moments for insemination. Acknowledged or unrecognized homosexual preference may also interfere with fertility.

Controversy surrounds the role of *genital Mycoplasma infection* in the genesis of infertility. In one study, if the husband was culture positive, treatment of the infertile couple for *Mycoplasma* led to a 60% pregnancy rate if the infection was eradicated versus a 5% rate when it was not. Other studies fail to show any association between the *Mycoplasma* infection and infertility. The reader is urged to watch for further studies on this issue.

DIFFERENTIAL DIAGNOSIS

Male factors account for 30% to 40% of cases. Reports from infertility clinics list 40% due to a varicocele; 40% as idiopathic; 10% from primary testicular failure; 9% with genital tract obstruction; 1% due to coital disorders; and 0.5% due to hypothalamic pituitary disease. Among female factors, ovulatory disturbances account for 40%, tubal disorders for 10% to 30%, cervical factors for 20%, and uterine factors for 8%. Tables 119-1 and 119-2 list some of the most important etiologies.

WORKUP

Initial Evaluation

Since the prognosis even for untreated couples is favorable (see below), an extensive "infertility workup" need not be undertaken on first visit, unless the couple is in their mid- to late 30s, has been unable to conceive in spite of trying steadily for over a year, or has a similar good reason to hasten the pace of evaluation. Otherwise, a reasonable approach to the first visit is to limit the assessment to a careful general history and physical examination, checking for such important causes as endocrinopathy, tumor, genitourinary tract infection, anatomic disorder, and interpersonal problems.

In the Male. History should include inquiry into drug and medication use (marijuana, alcohol, antihypertensive agents), urethral discharge, headache and other symptoms of panhypopituitarism (see Chapter 109), history of radiation exposure, mumps, toxin exposure, and systemic illnesses (especially diabetes with associated retrograde ejaculation). A sexual history that reviews the marital relationship, sexual techniques, potency, and frequency of intercourse is also important.

Table 119-1. Differential Diagnosis of Male Infertility

Azoospermic Etiologies
Primary hypogonadism
Hypogonadotropic hypogonadism
  Idiopathic
  Pituitary tumor
  Drugs
Nonendocrine problem
  Obstruction
  Retrograde ejaculation
  Germinal compartment failure (*e.g.*, irradiation)

Oligospermic Etiologies
Primary gonadal insufficiency
  Chemotherapy
  Irradiation
  Infection (adult mumps)
Acquired pituitary or hypothalamic insufficiency
  Early tumor (*e.g.*, prolactinoma)
  Drugs (alcohol, marijuana, antihypertensive agents)
Varicocele
Partial androgen resistance
Idiopathic

Normospermic Etiologies
Genitourinary tract infection
Abnormal sperm motility
Abnormal cervical mucus interaction
Idiopathic (includes patients with antisperm antibodies)
Impotence

Physical examination begins with noting general appearance and any signs of underandrogenization (decreased body hair, gynecomastia, eunuchoid proportions). The scrotum is examined for testicular size, presence of a varicocele, hypospadias, and absent vas deferens. Small testes (less than 4.0 cm in longest diameter) are consistent with primary testicular failure and pituitary–hypothalamic insufficiency. A Valsalva maneuver performed while the patient is standing will help

---

Table 119-2. Differential Diagnosis of Female Infertility

Ovulatory
Genetic disorders
Hypothalamic dysfunction
Pituitary insufficiency
Inactive or polycystic ovaries
Endometriosis

Tubal
Infection, PID
Adhesions
Postsurgery

Uterine
Congenital malformations
Fibroids (repeated abortion)

Cervical and Vaginal
Poor mucus quality from infection, trauma, or estrogen deficiencies
Anatomic abnormalities

Vulvar
Infections

---

reveal a small varicocele. The urethra is observed for discharge and the prostate and seminal vesicles for tenderness and other signs of infection. If a pituitary condition is suspected, visual field testing by confrontation might reveal an important field defect; a normal study does not rule out a mass lesion. Testing deep tendon reflexes may uncover delay in relaxation suggestive of hypothyroidism (see Chapter 102).

In the Female. *History* focuses on the menstrual history, age at menarche, and pregnancy history. Inquiry into any surgery or deliveries should be made; if any biopsies were done, pathology reports need to be obtained. The history and *physical examination* should include a search for evidence of a concomitant medical problem, such as thyroid disease (rarely a cause when it is not clinically obvious), diabetes mellitus, long-standing renal disease, or use of antihypertensive medications. A careful pelvic examination is essential, taking special note of any palpable adnexal, ovarian, or tubal mass or thickening of the uterosacral ligaments. During the pelvic examination, the patient's response to the procedure may provide an opportunity to inquire into her feelings about sexual intercourse as well as to observe anatomic impediments.

Both Partners. An empathetic, supportive, nonjudgmental exploration of the marital relationship is essential; it is often best done by interviewing the couple together (to observe their interactions) as well as each partner separately.

Further Evaluation

Couples with no evidence of serious pathology on initial evaluation can be reassured and informed that more than half of such couples go on to conceive without the aid of treatment. Those who have been trying to conceive for less than 1 year can be advised to delay further evaluation until 12 months have passed, provided they are willing to do so and have no compelling reason for proceeding directly to more extensive testing. Couples who have failed to conceive after continuously trying for 12 months, or who insist on further workup at the time of immediate visit, can undergo a set of basic laboratory studies to more fully define the problem and guide further evaluation and treatment.

In the Male. The first test to perform is a *sperm count.* Counts are expressed as number per milliliter of semen (the lower limit of the "normal" range is 20×10^6). *Semen volume* is also a useful measure; less than 1.5 ml may be inadequate to buffer vaginal acidity. Patients with normal counts might have qualitative studies of the sperm performed (*motility, morphology, cervical mucus interaction*), although these studies are often more useful for identifying the infertile individual than for defining a specific course of therapy (see below).

Patients with azoospermia and oligospermia are candidates for serum gonadotropin (*LH* and *FSH*) and *testosterone* levels, because of the possibility of an underlying endocrinopathy. Proper sampling technique is important to avoid misleading results. One draws three serum samples 20 minutes apart and pools them for LH, FSH, and testosterone determinations. As noted above, the pattern of the results helps characterize the problem. A primary gonadal problem produces high gonadotropins and low or low-normal testosterone; a pituitary–hypothalamic etiology is suggested by low gonadotropins and low testosterone.

The patient with suspected pituitary disease needs a *prolactin level* and *CT scan* of the sella turcica to search for a tumor. An elevated prolactin in the setting of a normal CT may be due to a drug-induced problem, but CT should be repeated in 6 months to be sure an early tumor has not been missed. Patients with normal concentrations of LH, FSH, and testosterone and oligospermia have either a varicocele or an idiopathic disease. Similar hormone levels and azoospermia raise the question of obstruction. A *semen fructose* may be informative in this setting. Although *antisperm agglutination antibodies* are commonly measured, the utility of such a determination is unclear at the present time.

In the Female a *postcoital examination* is a useful way to initiate the next phase of the infertility evaluation. The woman is asked to come for her appointment within 6 hours of coitus in the midcycle or second half of the menstrual cycle. If her partner is unable to respond on demand, the appointment is simply rescheduled. Repeated failure may provide a clue to the presence of difficulties involving the marital relationship, social circumstances, or a partner's physical well-being.

A specimen should be obtained from the cervical os, placed on a glass slide, and observed under high power. Five or more motile sperm found in the specimen confirms her partner's competence. Most physicians also look at a sample from the vaginal vaults, particularly if the cervix is directed away from the dependent parts of the vagina, as is seen in uterine retroversion. A negative postcoital test means very little and can occur even though the man is fertile. However, a repeated failure does justify a request for an examination of the partner (see above), and sometimes an analysis of the semen is revealing.

If the patient complains of amenorrhea or oligomenorrhea, a *maturation index* may be obtained. In this procedure, the vaginal wall is scraped, the scrapings are applied to two separate microscopic slides, and the slides are submitted in preservative for cytologic examination. A low maturation index shows few mature superficial squamous cells and suggests a lack of estrogen stimulation. A high maturation index shows that 20% to 50% of the superficial squamous cells are mature, and represents evidence that estrogen is present in amounts sufficient to mature the vagina, although the amounts may still be inadequate for production of withdrawal bleeding from the endometrium.

To establish ovulatory capacity, *serum progesterone* can be drawn on days 21 to 23 of the cycle, when the level should be two to four times its baseline. Endometrial biopsy may also be useful, but is more expensive, more painful, and may remove the long-awaited pregnancy. *Temperature charts* can also be used to identify ovulatory cycles; each morning the patient records oral temperature, using a special thermometer graduated in tenths (not two-tenths) of degrees Fahrenheit. Since this procedure is a constant daily reminder of one's infertility, it may be more depressing than helpful.

If the serum progesterone is low or the menstrual periods are so infrequent that it is impractical to obtain a progesterone level, one should assess pituitary function by ordering *serum prolactin, FSH,* and *LH* determinations. The findings of an elevated serum prolactin is an indication for CT scan of the skull to define the sella turcica in search of a pituitary tumor or empty sella syndrome (see Chapter 109). Elevations of luteinizing hormone and follicle-stimulating hormone suggest ovarian failure. Ovarian failure, whether caused by genetic factors, disease, or treatment such as cancer chemotherapy or radiation, is presently untreatable.

If the FSH alone is elevated beyond the normal range for the ovulatory woman, the problem lies in ovarian response; the patient should be referred to an endocrinologist or gynecologist interested in endocrinology for further investigation; there may still be some chance of pregnancy.

If there is an isolated LH elevation, the test should be repeated with careful attention to the day of the menstrual cycle to exclude the ovulatory peak. With the repeat LH, the serum free and total testosterones and androstenedione should be ordered; increased levels of these in the context of persistently high LH suggest polycystic ovary syndrome.

A *pelvic ultrasound* study can be a useful preliminary step in identifying a pelvic mass, particularly in distinguishing a cystic lesion from a solid one. If after the initial history, physical examination, postcoital test, and serum progesterone, it is evident that tubal or uterine factors are most likely to be causing infertility, a *uterotubogram* (hysterosalpingogram) may be helpful if a uterine anomaly seems likely. However, in the presence of recent or even long-past pelvic inflammatory disease, it may cause a recrudescence, adding to the infertility problem.

Intravenous pyelogram is sometimes used in selecting patients for uterotubograms, but the identification of an absent kidney or duplicated urinary structure does not automatically mean that there must be mullerian duct anomalies in an infertile woman and need for a uterotubogram. There should be positive evidence on physical examination or a history of pregnancy wastage.

Laparoscopy is presently one of the more useful procedures in the investigation of infertile women. Adhesions are most commonly found. Endometriosis, an unpalpable fibroid, or polycystic ovaries may also be discovered. Often tubal patency and position may be confirmed more accurately than by radiologic investigation. Not to be forgotten is the importance of negative findings.

PRINCIPLES OF MANAGEMENT AND INDICATIONS FOR REFERRAL

Studies from infertility clinics have shown that many couples go on to conceive without treatment (*e.g.,* 44% of those with ovulation deficiency, 61% of those with endometriosis, tubal defects, or seminal deficiencies, and 96% of those with cervical factors or idiopathic infertility). A conservative approach of watchful waiting is reasonable in such cases, provided there is no evidence of tumor, infection, anatomic defect, or serious endocrinopathy. Counseling can be a very important adjunct (see below).

When the workup suggests causative organic pathology, an appropriate referral for confirmatory testing and design of a treatment program is indicated. The continued participation of the primary physician in the care of the couple ought to remain, but the subtleties of specialized care that some types of infertility treatment require argue for referral rather than for treatment by the primary physician. Successful referral depends to a large extent on proper patient selection.

Men. Urologic referral is indicated for the male partner with a varicocele, a neurologic or anatomic cause of impotence that might benefit from a *prosthesis* (see Chapter 131), or a suspected acquired obstructive defect. Treatment of obstruction requires a urologist skilled in *microsurgical techniques,* as does *vasectomy reversal.* Neurosurgical and endocrinologic consultations become essential when prolactin levels are elevated or CT scan reveals signs of a pituitary tumor. Sometimes *bromocriptine* will control a prolactinoma and obviate the need for surgery. Men with idiopathic hypogonadotropic hypogonadism might benefit from consultation with a reproductive endocrinologist for consideration of *gonadotropin-releasing-factor therapy.* Patients with idiopathic oligospermia (no evidence of a varicocele; normal LH, FSH, and testosterone) are often treated with *clomiphene* or another type of antiestrogen therapy. The advice of a reproductive endocrinologist is essential in this situation, because there are no well-controlled, long-term studies to guide therapy. Expertise in *artificial insemination* may be of help to patients with otherwise refractory qualitative sperm defects. Patients with retrograde ejaculation might also effect pregnancy with artificial insemination, using semen recovered in the urine.

Men who have quantitatively and qualitatively normal sperm and normal LH, FHS, and testosterone levels pose a challenge. Either the wife is the infertile one, or an inapparent etiology remains. Some investigators have postulated that antisperm antibodies are responsible for the infertility and suggest repeated short courses of high-dose corticosteroid therapy in patients with detectable antibody titers. There is no controlled evidence that such treatment is effective. Sub-

clinical infection, especially with mycoplasmas, has been suggested as a cause. Culturing both partners and treating the couple if one partner is culture positive has produced impressive results in only one study; others find no link between *Mycoplasma* and infertility. There is no evidence that vitamins (A, E, and C), zinc, thyroid hormone, or a host of other drugs and home remedies are at all useful in men with normospermia or oligospermia. Artificial insemination has been proposed as a therapy, though data on increased rates of pregnancy are lacking. There are no known treatments for patients with gonadal failure or androgen insensitivity.

Women. As noted earlier, the woman with "functional" anovulatory periods is quite likely to resume ovulating without therapy and needs only counseling at the time of initial evaluation. There is no available treatment for the woman with ovarian failure, but when an isolated FSH elevation is noted, help might be afforded by the reproductive endocrinologist. The patient suspected of having polycystic ovary disease (isolated LH elevation, high testosterone, cystic ovarian mass on ultrasoography) needs gynecologic referral; *surgical reduction* of the cystic mass may permit ovulation. When there is suspicion of endometriosis, a gynecologic referral is helpful for confirmation of the diagnosis, as is consultation with a gynecologic endocrinologist to see if the patient warrants *danazol* therapy to achieve fertility. Patients with a history of pelvic inflammatory disease and suspected tubal scarring ought to be further evaluated by a gynecologist experienced in *tubal reconstruction.* Those with signs of a pituitary tumor (elevated prolactin and/or mass on CT) require endocrinologic consultation; bromocriptine may suffice if the mass is small (see Chapter 109); if the tumor appears large, the neurosurgeon should join the effort. The anovulatory patient who continues to be frustrated in her attempts to conceive may be a candidate for *clomiphene;* again, expert opinion on its use is necessary to ensure safe administration.

Both Partners. When referral is indicated, patients should be encouraged to ask questions and voice their concerns to the specialist. If a working relationship is not developed, the primary physician may be helpful in finding an alternative. Patients with prolonged infertility (3 to 4 years) become discouraged and will seek alternative opinions. Here, the primary physician can help by inquiring into the expertise of the subsequent specialists. It is particularly important in the referral for tubal repair to select a gynecologist skilled in the procedure, since success rates vary considerably and results are often discouraging. Yet, it is unusual for women with tubal occlusion to refuse surgery; even with the slimmest chance of success, most women still will choose surgical repair.

PATIENT EDUCATION

Patients are eager for information about their chances of conceiving. In providing reassurance to the couple who has no evidence for an irreversible or serious etiology, one can share with them the published findings from infertility clinics, which show that 25% to 35% of couples achieve conception within 1 to 2 years of registration; the percentages continue to rise over the next 4 to 5 years. There is a slight decrease in fecundity after 30 and a marked decrease after age 35. There appears to be no difference in prognosis between infertile couples who have conceived in the past and those who have never conceived. The prognosis for women who experience recurrent spontaneous abortions is better than the approximately 20% live birth rate previously estimated. Patients with ovulatory problems do reasonably well; those with tubal problems have more difficulty. In some series, pregnancy following tubal surgery occurred in 10% of patients, whereas following minimal procedures, 79% of couples achieved a live birth. Anastomosis of surgically divided vas deferens or fallopian tubes by a specialist is highly successful in achieving patency, but overall, only about one third of such procedures are followed by a live birth. Couples whose infertility involves multiple factors do less well than those in whom only one factor is present.

Whenever an evaluation comes out normal, it is important to reassure patients about their normality, particularly if one harbors guilt or fear about an episode of infidelity, a previous abortion, an out-of-wedlock pregnancy, or some other factor.

The investigation of infertility provides an opportunity to educate patients about normal human reproduction. This area is still omitted from many school curricula, and is inadequately covered in others. Education for both partners about the menstrual cycles, frequency of coitus, and male and female sexual attitudes and responses may provide the cure.

Infertility studies may be the necessary impetus for encouraging the couple to take better care of themselves and follow any medical regimens attentively. Infertility may also lead to reconsideration and redesign of treatment regimens for other problems (*e.g.,* antihypertensive agents and cancer therapy may interfere with conception; see Chapters 21, 89, and 90, respectively).

The couple that is still unsuccessful after a year of trying can be given some reassurance as they begin to undergo evaluation. Nearly one quarter of such couples achieve pregnancy within 3 months, and half do so within the year.

Infertility resulting from lack of privacy because of the presence of a child or in-laws needs to be approached with careful and understanding explanation, perhaps in conjunction with a family member, clergy, or mental health professional. A home visit may sometimes be helpful in delineating the problem and suggesting solutions. Despite the patient's frequent efforts to medicalize social problems, there may be no medical solution; instead, attention may need to be directed to the home environment and marital relation.

A.H.G.

ANNOTATED BIBLIOGRAPHY

Aral SO, Cates, W: The increasing concern with fertility. JAMA 250: 2327, 1983 (*An analysis of the demographics of infertility and explanations for increased demand for infertility services.*)

Collins JA, Wrixon W, Janes LB et al: Treatment-independent pregnancy among infertile couples. N Engl J Med 309:1201, 1983 (*A retrospective review of more than a thousand couples, which indicates that the potential for a spontaneous cure of infertility is high.*)

Cook ID: The natural history and major causes of infertility. In Diczfalusy A (ed): The WHO Symposium on Advances in Fertility Regulation. Copenhagen, Scriptor, 1977 (*A hard to obtain but most useful overview of the problem.*)

Diugnan NM, Jordan JA, Couglan BM et al: One thousand consecutive cases of diagnostic laparoscopy. J Obstet Gynecol Br Cwlth 79:1016, 1972 (*There are many series on laparoscopy, but this is one of the most useful. The role of ovarian biopsy, however, is not supported by most other authors.*)

Gorry GA, Pauker SG, Swartz WB: Diagnostic importance of the normal finding. N Engl J Med 298:486, 1978 (*Emphasizes the value to the patient of a normal finding.*)

Gump DW, Gibson M, Ashikaga T: Lack of association between genital mycoplasmas and infertility. N Engl J Med 310:937, 1984 (*A study limited to women with involuntary infertility that did not find an association between prior pelvic inflammatory disease and the presence of* Mycoplasmas; *the presence of* Myoplasma *was infrequent, leading the authors to question the role of genital* Mycoplasma *as a cause of infertility.*)

Hurley DM, Brian R, Outch K et al: Induction of ovulation and fertility in amenorrheic women by pulsatile low dose gonadotropin-releasing hormone. N Engl J Med 310:1069, 1984 (*Thirteen of 14 women resistant to clomiphene therapy achieved pregnancy with subcutaneous pulses of GnRH.*)

Masters WH, Johnson VE: Human Sexual Response. Boston, Little, Brown, 1966. (*The classic modern work on the physiology and pathophysiology of sexual activity.*)

Mueller BA, Daling JR, Moore DE et al: Appendectomy and the risk of tubal infertility. N Engl J Med 315:1506, 1986 (*Risk increased only in cases of ruptured appendix.*)

Schwartz D, Mayaux MJ: Female fecundity as a function of age. N Engl J Med 306:404, 1982 (*Data from more than 2000 attempts at artificial insemination suggest a slight but significant decrease in fecundity after 30 years of age and a marked decrease after 35 years.*)

Swerdloff RS, Overstreet JW, Sokol RZ et al: Infertility in the male. Ann Intern Med 103:906, 1985 (*A comprehensive yet practical review of the pathogenesis, evaluation, and treatment; 132 references.*)

Toth A, Lesser ML, Brooks C et al: Subsequent pregnancies among 161 couples treated for T-mycoplasma genital tract infection. N Engl J Med 308:505, 1983 (*A prospective study convincingly demonstrating the importance of eradicating T-mycoplasma infection in the treatment of infertility.*)

120

Approach to the Woman with an Unwanted Pregnancy

ANN B. BARNES, M.D.

The woman who suspects an unwanted pregnancy often calls on her primary physician soon after a period is missed to have the diagnosis confirmed. To provide assistance, the physician needs to know the resources available in the community for abortions, prenatal care, placement, and the indications and risks of various abortion methods, as well as the woman's emotional makeup and social situation. An unwanted pregnancy, especially in the younger patient, is a reflection of the need for patient education in reproductive matters, which should be carried out at the time of the medical encounter to prevent recurrences.

CLINICAL PRESENTATIONS

The presentations of women with unwanted pregnancies are as varied as all human experience. However, certain patterns occur that reflect stress points as well as socioeconomic pressures that touch each individual similarly. A pregnancy may reassure a woman of her unique ability and her potential continuity. The decision to abort is usually a practical one. Few women "want" an abortion. Few perceive a risk; the risk of dying in childbirth is not a deterrent to sexual relations or pregnancy. Indeed, it is hard to tell the sick cardiac patient that she is not capable of carrying a pregnancy to term and that for her safety the pregnancy should be aborted. No woman, no matter how ill, likes to be told she "can't be a woman."

A number of presentations are particularly important because of their psychosocial circumstances and ramifications for prevention of future pregnancy.

In both rural and urban areas, *incest* persists to a greater extent than most professional people assume. It may occur between father and daughter, but frequently involves a mother's boyfriend or second husband and a child. Brother and sister pregnancies also occur. Often the mother is so offended by the implications of the incest that she will never appear with the pregnant youngster. The pregnant youngster is confused, scared, and may be unaware of what is going on. Usually it is beyond a physician's capability to change the social situation from which such a pregnancy arose, but encouraging the patient to have an IUD inserted at or after the procedure or prescribing birth control pills may prevent a future pregnancy even if the social setting cannot be improved.

Adolescent women are no different from young men in their perception of risks—"Oh it will never happen to me," or "I can do it once and it will be OK." Other teenagers feel unwanted or unloved and see a pregnancy as providing a companion who will want them and love them. The impracticality of this dream may be stressed, and usually parental permission for abortion is promptly forthcoming. Such young women are likely to become pregnant repeatedly, as medical intervention can seldom affect the surrounding circumstances.

Other young women are angry at their parents and see a pregnancy as a way of getting even or "really hurting" them. They may not be eager for any abortion that is arranged by their parents, and often are not enthusiastic participants in prenatal care either. That the fate of the unborn might be similar to their own sometimes sways their decisions as to whether or not to continue the pregnancy.

The 15-year-old unmarried couple who come together are charming in their innocent trust, but may be masking substantial personal problems.

Most second-trimester abortions are done on teenagers. The number decreases each year, but because the complications of the procedure increase with the passing weeks of gestation, this remains an important problem. At first, there may be a problem of denial, but denial is usually hard to sustain after two missed periods. Then there is the problem of how to get help. Many teenagers are uninformed on such matters and often turn to their uninformed peers. Perhaps an older sister, a friend, or an older brother will be able to provide information. Alternatively, a suspicious mother will drag her daughter to the doctor. Such patients provide monosyllabic histories and may even mumble or not answer inquiries at all.

The *older teenager* or 20-year-old often presents early with an unwanted pregnancy, and simply wants to "get it over with." Such patients are often able to accept office curettage (menstrual extraction) with little difficulty and minimal or no anesthesia. Contraception is usually accepted with alacrity.

The 20-year-old who presents in the second trimester often signals marked ambivalence. Counseling, including an opportunity for her to express her mixed feelings, is especially necessary.

The *rape victim* may be repulsed at the thought of a baby inside her from such a horrible experience. She may present near or after 12 weeks, and may not be able to cooperate in either the pelvic examination or other care.

Women in their *30s* and *40s* seek abortion with the same air of practicality as younger women, but are often touched with a tinge of remorse that there may not be many more opportunities for motherhood ahead. This attitude is as common in unmarried as in married women. Others come for abortion forced by the economic reality of childbearing. Often the husband has made the economic decision and the pregnant woman accepts it as the best course, but is far from eager. At this time, such women are not receptive to the suggestion of permanent sterilization.

Patients undergoing amniocentesis for genetic counseling do so on the assumption that they would accept induced abortion, which usually would occur between 20 and 24 weeks gestation, often after they have experienced fetal movement (quickening). The feeling of being a failure and unable to have a normal child will add to the normal hormonally induced depression that follows any pregnancy termination and requires supportive care. Sometimes there is a touch of anger with the sadness, and the primary physician will be asked to arbitrate the advice of the genetic counselor and the obstetrician.

One of the saddest situations involves the *previously infertile woman* when she comes to have taken away that which she wanted most for as many as 5 or 10 years, because of such issues as economic problems, or change of attitude of an aging spouse.

Patients who present for *repeat abortions* tend to generate feelings of frustration in health care personnel. They may return because they made the same mistake again, or because they tried a different form of birth control that was not properly explained or has failed. Other women need to reassure themselves of their fertility; in such cases, no form of birth control will work. A few lack motivation for any self-help. Others may be prostitutes, earning cash for a drug or alcohol habit. Others are severely ill mental patients. There is little evidence that the pregnancy affects the course of the mental illness or that the mental illness will affect the outcome of the pregnancy, except insofar as their illness affects their socioeconomic status and ability physically to care for themselves.

PRINCIPLES OF MANAGEMENT AND PATIENT EDUCATION, AND INDICATIONS FOR REFERRAL

Diagnosis. One must first confirm the diagnosis of pregnancy. A *first morning voided urine* is collected about 40 days from the last menstrual cycle (LMP) or 10 days after the first missed period and saved in a clean container. Usually the specimen will contain sufficient human chorionic gonadotropin (HCG) for a positive slide test. It is important to practice the test several times before utilizing it, to ensure that the test is done correctly. A positive or negative pregnancy test of this nature does not by itself prove or disprove a pregnancy, but rather must be interpreted in conjunction with the patient's signs and symptoms. The patient may complain of some nausea; often breast tenderness is the first clue the patient can recount. It is particularly important to repeat the test or obtain the more expensive determination of the *serum beta-subunit of HCG* if the patient thinks she is pregnant and urinary pregnancy tests are repeatedly negative. In general, if a woman thinks she is pregnant, she should be considered so until proven otherwise.

Counseling. Once the diagnosis is confirmed, the physician needs to explore with the patient her feelings about the pregnancy. A nonjudgmental, unbiased, supportive approach to the woman coming for help is essential to an effective outcome. For the woman who is certain that she does not want the child, a thorough review of available options is indicated. Although the issue of what to do about an unwanted pregnancy remains one of the most controversial and emotional questions of our time, the primary care physician should be knowledgeable about and capable of objectively discussing all available alternatives, ranging from continuing with the pregnancy, to abortion. If the physician has moral reservations about the patient's preferences, then the patient needs a referral to a competent physician who is willing to respect her preferences and provide care to her. The worst possible situation is for the woman (often, an adolescent) to be made to feel ashamed, abandoned, and cut off from help. Such feelings often lead her to turn away from medical care and resort to such desperate measures as criminal abortion, abandonment of a newborn, or the abuse of an unwanted child. Knowing what community resources are available to the patient and helping her to choose among psychologically and medically sound options represents a tremendously important primary care responsibility.

Therapeutic Abortion. Since abortion is an important option, the primary physician needs to be knowledgeable about its indications, safety, and consequences. It remains one of the leading means of dealing with an unwanted pregnancy. When performed under proper conditions, it is safe and does not alter one's chances of normal childbearing (at least for up to two therapeutic abortions). There may be an individual situation in which a weakened cervix results, but this is rare. Risk is lower for teenagers undergoing abortion than it is for older women.

The earlier an abortion is performed, the less the risk of complications. However, the risk increases each week of pregnancy, and approaches the risk of term delivery after the

13th week; nevertheless, there may be some time to resolve conflicts, make practical economic arrangements, or find the most appropriate resource within the community. Though most abortions are done in the state in which the patient resides, availability of services is inconsistent, and some patients may have to travel long distances to unfamiliar surroundings. Planned Parenthood and the National Organization for Women usually have a list of referral centers and local resources. Local medical societies are less often helpful, although the district offices of the American College of Obstetrics and Gynecology are usually well informed.

It takes about 1000 operative procedures, many under local anesthesia, to provide enough experience for an individual physician to develop skill commensurate with the national average complication rate. Thus, referring the patient to an experienced facility may be wiser than asking an associate who only occasionally does abortions to help out. However, Planned Parenthood or a direct call may clarify whether a new physician has just started or a waiting list is too long for a particular patient's needs.

Local and general anesthesia have the same rate of complications. Local anesthesia is associated with febrile and convulsive morbidity; general anesthesia with hemorrhage, cervical injury, and uterine perforation. General anesthesia usually costs more, but can still be used on a 1-day ambulatory basis. Patients with venereal disease are particularly at risk for febrile complications. Patients should be tested for blood type, and immune globulin (RhoGAM or mini-RhoGAM) should be given to Rh-negative women (15% of the population). The postabortion period is also a good time for rubella immunization. The cervix may not prevent introduction of bacterial infection into the sterile uterine cavity for about 2 weeks following abortion; consequently, abstinence from coitus should be advised for this period. Longer periods of abstinence are usually unacceptable to the patient. All abortion facilities encounter patients who have coitus with a partner eager to console immediately following an abortion.

If products of conception are retained, bleeding and fever usually do not occur for about 3 days; then cramping pain, a tender uterus, and temperature elevation, possibly with an elevated white count and sedimentation rate, will be found. Repeat curettage with oral, or possibly intravenous, antibiotics, is indicated. Passage of fetal parts may spontaneously resolve the problem; however, this is not dependable.

Uterine perforation is usually recognized at operation. If it is not, it may lead to peritonitis, hemorrhage, or even prolapse of bowel through the uterus and cervix with obstructive symptoms. If a perforation is recognized at operation, bed rest, careful monitoring, and intravenous or liquid diet will often resolve the hazard, averting the need for exploratory surgery.

First-trimester abortions are done with cervical dilatation over 8 to 12 hours with *laminaria* insertion or with dilators after anesthesia is administered. Following dilatation, *suction*

curettage is carried out. Evidence is accumulating that suggests the slower laminaria dilatation may diminish the frequency of cervical malfunction in future pregnancies.

After 12 weeks, the fetal parts no longer can be removed with ease through a cervix dilated with standard dilators. Loss of blood may be excessive and the procedure incomplete. Second-trimester abortion usually requires dilatation by insertion of several *dilateria* (laminaria japanica [Japanese seaweed] gas-sterilized). These are hydrophilic, swell on absorption of water, and gently dilate the cervix to 14 mm to 18 mm in diameter. However, dilateria connect the never-sterile vagina with the sterile endometrial cavity and its contents. Furthermore, the uterine contents are removed from the normal maternal defenses to infection. Usually the abortion relieves this risk of sepsis, but some women get infections and, thus, some abortions are covered by prophylactic intravenous or oral antibiotics. Coverage should be directed against bowel flora. The abortion is carried out within 12 to 14 hours after laminaria insertion, usually with large *suction* instruments. At present, data from the Centers for Disease Control indicate that this is the safest method of abortion up to 20 weeks. It is unusual for abortions to be done between 20 and 24 weeks. Legal intervention is required after 24 weeks.

Hysterotomy has the highest complication rate and appears unjustified at the present time. Furthermore, because the uterus is small, the uterine incision traverses the fundus, putting the patient at risk for rupture in subsequent pregnancy.

Laparoscopic sterilization at the time of induced abortion has been shown to be more hazardous than either procedure performed separately.

Despite these hazards, legal abortions are safer than normal deliveries. Abortions in the hands of the inexperienced physician or outside the legal channels of care are a serious risk. With financial discrimination against certain segments of the population, and threats against clinics providing legal abortions, it is not surprising to hear of *criminal abortions,* again. The major risks associated with criminal abortion are very high incidences of sepsis and hemorrhage. The signs of complications usually appear within 3 days, but often the patient does not present for treatment until 7 to 10 days after abortion. The history is usually not forthcoming, or the patient says she fell down the stairs and started to bleed. A complete physical examination is required. The punched-out, clean, clear ulcers of potassium permanganate tablets on opposing vaginal mucosal surfaces are a familiar indication of illicit attempts at self-abortion. Complete blood count, differential, and blood cultures are essential; intravenous colloid or blood products are often needed. An upright KUB x-ray may indicate free air in cases of uterine perforation or suggest gas gangrene if coathangers or unsterile metal probes were used.

It is unusual for women undergoing pregnancy termination, even teenagers and incest and rape victims, to require formal psychiatric referral. The primary physician, in association with a psychiatric social worker, often can provide appropriate supportive counseling and discussion of the psychosocial ramifications. The positive impact that understanding and support by the primary physician can have during this trying period should not be ignored or underestimated.

Adoption represents a very important alternative for patients who cannot see themselves undergoing an abortion, but who feel it is impossible for them to care for a child. This option is supported by a number of religious groups and actually is an underutilized option, especially in teenage pregnancies. The psychological difficulty of carrying a child to term and then having to give it up stands as the major emotional barrier, but may be a relatively easy one to overcome when the mother is a young teenager with many future opportunities for child rearing. The demand for an adopted newborn child remains very high. The patient interested in putting a child up for adoption will benefit from referral to the appropriate community adoption agency. The father of the baby should also be involved in the referral.

Keeping the Child represents a change in the patient's initial view; it may emerge as a realistic option if the main reason for not wanting the child is a social situation that is amenable to change (*e.g.,* the father of the baby decides to marry the patient and support the new family). For this to be a viable option, the social situation needs to be conducive and the patient (especially the teenager) needs to understand and accept the enormous demands an infant will make on her. Having a baby will profoundly alter her life and her economic circumstances; she needs to be prepared for these changes. Teenage pregnancy promises to be one of the most serious social problems of this decade, as a source of poverty and child neglect.

Birth Control. Individualized instruction on reproductive processes and contraception (see Chapter 118) can be effective when given at the time the patient presents for abortion, at the abortion, and following the procedure. About one half of patients who undergo therapeutic abortion return for follow-up. However, unwed women who have a delivery and place the child for adoption frequently do not return for their postpartum checkups, and they have an 80% risk of returning with another unwanted pregnancy within 2 years. On the other hand, 80% of abortion patients are found to be using contraception appropriately after the procedure. The number of abortions arising out of lack of awareness of contraceptive needs or methods emphasizes the need for public education as well as informing the individual.

ANNOTATED BIBLIOGRAPHY

Alan Guttmacher Institute: Family Planning Perspectives (*An ultimate source of research and opinion.*)

American College of Obstetricians and Gynecologists, Chicago, Pertinent *Technical Bulletins* (*Current practice guidelines recommended in the United States by a specialty organization.*)

Boston Women's Health Book Collective: Our Bodies, Ourselves. New York, Simon & Schuster, 1984 (*Consumer writers; useful alternate resource to professional publications.*)

Cates W, Schulz KF, Grimes DA: Risks associated with teenage abortion. N Engl J Med 309:621, 1983 (*When data are adjusted according to gestational age, teenagers have lower rates of morbidity and mortality from induced abortion than older women.*)

Centers for Disease Control: Abortion Surveillance (*A source that is continually updated to provide current information.*)

121
Management of Breast Cancer
JACOB J. LOKICH, M.D.

Breast cancer is one of the most common malignancies in the United States; it is estimated that 1 in 11 women will contract the disease. This solid tumor is also among the most responsive to therapy. Unfortunately, in spite of the expanded therapeutic armamentarium for breast cancer, survival and potential for cure of these lesions remain relatively unchanged. However, the advent and implementation of effective screening measures (see Chapter 104) and the application of adjuvant chemotherapy in the early stages of disease has resulted in modestly improved rates of survival.

The treatment of local disease is in the process of evolution, with greater emphasis being placed on treatments that preserve the breast. Still there is much debate over the best means of treating curable primary breast cancer. The primary physician has several important roles to play in the management of breast cancer, including initial evaluation, explaining treatment options, and participation in the monitoring and treatment of the patient with advanced disease.

CLINICAL PRESENTATION AND COURSE

As many as 90% of breast cancers are discovered by the patient. *Stage I* disease is defined as a primary tumor of less than 2 cm in diameter and no axillary lymph node involvement (see Table 121-1). Approximately 55% of patients with primary breast cancer now present with stage I disease, in

Table 121-1. Curability of Breast Cancer by Stage

STAGE	TUMOR EXTENT	10-YEAR DISEASE-FREE SURVIVAL (%)
I	Confined to breast	70–80
II	Involves the axillary nodes	20–40
III	Tumor > 5 cm; nodes > 2 cm; with or without fixation	<5
	Inflammatory	0

part because of improved screening methods. *Stage II* disease is still considered a localized disease, but now there is involvement of axillary lymph nodes. About 25% of patients with *clinical* stage I disease turn out to have pathologic stage II disease on sampling of the axillary nodes. Interestingly, a similar percentage of patients with clinical stage II disease (palpable axillary lymph nodes) turn out to have no tumor in the nodes on pathologic examination. In stage III disease, there is extensive tumor (>5 cm) at the primary site and lymph nodes are >2 cm with or without fixation. In stage IV there are distant metastases.

Another important category is the so-called *minimal breast cancer.* Included in this designation are small lesions often discovered by mammography. They tend to be intraductal carcinomas pathologically and are considered forms of carcinoma *in situ* or lobular carcinomas without invasion.

Prognosis. The course of breast cancer is largely a function of the pathologic stage of tumor at the time of presentation. Of patients with a tumor less than 5 cm in size and confined to the breast, 70% can expect to live 10 years. With axillary node involvement, the rate of survival decreases according to the number of nodes involved. Among patients with stage II cancer, those with four or more nodes have a 10-year survival of 10% to 20%; those with three or fewer have a 10-year survival of close to 50%. For stage III disease, the cure rate is less than 5%. Within stage III, there is a subcategory of inflammatory breast cancer, a very virulent form unresponsive to therapy and uniformly fatal. Patients with minimal breast disease have very limited risk for involvement of the axillary nodes and strong likelihood of cure without need for radical surgery or extensive radiation therapy (see below). Nonetheless, a proportion do develop metastases if left untreated.

In addition to the stage of tumor and tumor size, *estrogen receptor* and *progesterone receptor* status affect the prognosis. Patients with stage I or stage II disease whose tumors have estrogen or progesterone receptors, or both, have a better prognosis than those with the same stage of disease whose tumors are receptor negative.

Breast cancer may metastasize to almost any site in the body, but five general categories have been distinguished by Smalley and coworkers, which are correlated with predictable response to therapy and prognosis (Table 121-2). It is evident that even in patients with metastatic disease, median survival may exceed 3 years, and there does not have to be significant change in quality of life when palliative radiation and chemohormone therapy are used throughout that period (see below). Today more than 50% of patients with metastatic breast cancer may respond to therapy, but only a small portion (perhaps fewer than 10%) show complete regression. The median duration of response is not more than 12 to 18 months.

The clinical course of breast cancer is unique in that metastatic lesions may develop after a long period of freedom from disease, even after as long as 20 years. Thus, 5 years without evidence of metastatic spread does not indicate cure.

PRINCIPLES OF MANAGEMENT

The therapeutic options for women diagnosed by an incisional or excisional biopsy have expanded in recent years, accompanied by greater patient participation in choice of therapy. It is no longer justified to perform a biopsy and immediate mastectomy under the same anesthesia. Patients should be fully informed of the diagnosis, promptly staged, and advised of the therapeutic options.

Staging. Staging procedures at the time of diagnostic surgery should include a *chest x-ray* and *alkaline phosphatase.* Pathologic examination of axillary nodes is necessary, because, as noted previously, palpation of nodes for evidence of involvement is fraught with the danger of false-positive and false-negative determinations; 25% of palpable nodes are histologically negative, while nonpalpable nodes are positive in 25% to 40% of patients. Thus, *regional node dissection* or sampling is important. Patients with pathologic stage II and those with primary tumors greater than 3 cm in diameter are at increased risk of metastases. Their staging should include a *radionuclide bone scan. Liver scan* should be obtained only in patients with hepatomegaly or an elevated serum alkaline phosphatase.

Table 121-2. Patterns of Recurrence and Survival in Breast Cancer

PATTERN	INCIDENCE (%)	MEDIAN TIME (MONTHS) Relapse	MEDIAN TIME (MONTHS) Survival
Multiple metastases	19	9	4
Pulmonary	12	36	18
Bone	26	15	29+
Effusions*	16	39	44
Skin and subcutaneous†	26	15	27+

* + Minor skin nodules.

† + Minor bone metastases.

Treatment of Localized Disease. In recent years, treatment of operable breast cancer has evolved toward procedures that conserve breast tissue. At present there are two major therapeutic options backed by extensive evidence of efficacy: (1) total mastectomy and (2) partial mastectomy (lumpectomy or quadrantectomy) followed by irradiation. The effectiveness and morbidity of each procedure must be discussed with the patient so that an informed decision can be reached.

Complete mastectomy (total or modified radical) involves removal of all breast tissue and axillary lymph nodes. Ten-year follow-up studies have demonstrated that the procedure provides "cure" of localized disease in 80% of stage I cases and 25% to 35% of stage II cases. Removal of the entire breast also precludes the risk of a second primary tumor in the same breast and helps to establish whether or not there are any other foci of tumor at the time of initial treatment. In addition, the extent of tumor in the lymph nodes can be readily determined.

Partial mastectomy with radiation therapy involves removal of a section of breast; and axillary dissection is performed on all patients. Local recurrence rates appear to be comparable to, if not better than, those achieved by surgery alone. The 10-year survival rate has not been determined. Thus, direct comparison of long-term results with those of complete mastectomy is not yet possible. However, 5-year survival rates in prospective randomized controlled studies closely match, if not exceed, those for total mastectomy.

Thus, women with breast cancer have two nearly equivalent treatment options. Complete mastectomy offers established 10-year effectiveness and a high rate of cure. Partial mastectomy plus irradiation provides a cosmetic advantage, by preserving much of the breast tissue, and at the same time offering a seemingly equal, though not yet proven, chance at long-term cure. In essence, the woman has to choose between known efficacy and greater preservation of breast tissue. This is a personal decision that the primary care physician can help the patient reach by exploring how important cosmetic preservation is to her and by avoiding such inadequate terms as "radical," "simple," and "lumpectomy." Not all patients with localized disease are candidates for partial mastectomy plus radiation. Radiotherapy can be difficult in patients who are older, have pendulous breasts, or have a primary lesion of greater than 4 cm. Proper resection that ensures tumor-free margins with good preservation of breast tissue is very difficult in patients found to have two widely separated primary lesions or diffuse microcalcifications on mammogram.

Adjuvant chemotherapy is undergoing extensive clinical trials for patients with stage II disease, because it is believed that such patients have a high risk of micrometastases at the time of mastectomy. Preliminary data indicate that the greatest benefit is in premenopausal women. The adjuvant programs used in clinical trials are cyclophosphamide, methotrexate, and 5-FU (CMF) and other regimens that include adriamycin. Patients with negative nodes and those with positive nodes who are over the age of 60 have not experienced improved survival with such regimens. However, postmenopausal patients appear to achieve some benefit from adjuvant therapy consisting of the anti-estrogen tamoxifen. Ongoing clinical trials will help clarify efficacy. At this time, patients with localized breast cancer should not routinely receive adjuvant chemotherapy unless under the aegis of a research protocol.

Monitoring. Patients undergoing definitive local therapy should be monitored with an extensive examination at 3-month intervals for the first 2 years, at 4-month intervals for the second 2 years, and every 6 months thereafter. Monitoring should include a complete history and physical, with very careful examination of the other breast, which is at increased risk of developing a second primary tumor. A mammogram should be obtained annually. Follow-up examination of the bones should be undertaken only in patients who develop symptoms of bone pain. The crucial concern in monitoring patients with breast cancer is the increased risk of a second primary tumor, which may also be curable. The identification of early metastatic disease is inconsequential, because systemic therapy should be used only in patients with either rapidly growing tumor or symptomatic disease.

Treatment of Advanced Disease. Advanced disease includes not only distant metastases in bone, lung, or liver but also extensive regional tumor, the so-called neglected primary tumors of the breast. Patients with extensive regional tumor have a surprisingly favorable prognosis; the prolonged time of survival already achieved indicates that the malignancy is relatively low grade. Many of these tumors are responsive to hormonal management as well as local radiation therapy. The concomitant use of these two therapies may be associated with a long or protracted life expectancy.

Stage III breast cancer (inoperable local disease confined to the skin, breast, or lymph nodes) may be treated in the following sequence: (1) biopsy for histologic confirmation and receptor assays; (2) systemic therapy, either hormone or chemotherapy, to determine the effectiveness of the systemic treatment and to reduce the bulk of tumor; and (3) local therapy, which may be either mastectomy followed by radiation therapy or radiation therapy alone. The median length of survival after effective treatment is 18 to 24 months.

The management of advanced metastatic breast carcinoma is determined in part by sites of metastases, age (menopausal status), and receptor status. The decision to treat and the timing of therapy depend on the presence or absence of symptoms and the growth rate of the tumor. There are three categories of therapy for advanced breast cancer: hormone therapy, chemotherapy, and combination therapy.

Hormone therapy. The decision to use hormone therapy and prediction of response depend to a large extent on hormone receptor status. A tumor is deemed hormone dependent if it contains a sufficiently high concentration of estrogen receptor protein (ERP) in the cytoplasm and if there is no defect in the cascade for effecting steroid hormone action. Simply the presence of receptors does not guarantee response. The same holds true for progesterone receptors; tumors having such receptors are more hormonally responsive. The presence of receptors does not indicate which hormone treatment will be effective; either estrogen withdrawal or supplementation may work.

The sites of disease most often associated with hormone response are pulmonary nodules, pleural effusions, osseous lesions, and cutaneous disease. There is a very remote likelihood of response to hormonal manipulation in patients with hepatic metastases, lymphangitic pulmonary involvement, brain metastases, or skin lesions en cuirasse.

Hormone management also depends on menopausal status (see Table 121-3). The least responsive group is perimenopausal. From the time of *menopause* to 5 years afterward, the response to ablation or estrogen supplements is meager. These patients have been treated with *androgens,* with a response rate of 20% or less. Androgen therapy is associated with significant side-effects of masculinization and is therefore used rather sparingly. *In premenopausal* patients, tumor develops in a setting of estrogen abundance; consequently, ablative procedures are almost invariably used; *oophorectomy* is associated with a response in 40% to 50% of patients. The response may last for 6 to 12 months, and upon relapse, *adrenalectomy* is usually performed.

In *postmenopausal patients,* the tumor develops in an estrogen-depleted environment; therefore, *estrogen* has been the first hormonal manipulation to be employed. A response may be achieved in 40% to 50% of patients, but in 20% of patients, tumor growth may be exacerbated. *Tamoxifen* is replacing estrogen as the usual first line hormonal therapy

because of lesser side-effects; progestational agents are often the second line before the introduction of estrogens.

Following an initial response to hormonal therapy, a relapse usually occurs, but a subsequent secondary response is not uncommon. Patients initially treated with estrogen may, upon relapse, be managed with estrogen withdrawal and sustain a second response. Later they may be reinduced with maximal doses of estrogen or with an alternative hormone preparation, such as progesterone or androgens. For the most part, such secondary responses are short-lived and are not of the quality of the initial response. It is important to recognize that the effect of hormonal therapy on tumor bulk may not be observed for 1 or 2 months, even though the agent may begin working immediately. Relief of bone pain is much more rapidly achieved.

Hormonal therapy occasionally results in exacerbation of bone pain or tumor growth. The mechanism is not known. In a small percentage of these patients, the opposite hormonal maneuver (*i.e.,* ablation or supplementation) may induce an antitumor effect. In some institutions, patients are monitored in the hospital for a 10-day period to determine whether or not tumor stimulation and serious hypercalcemia occurs.

The development of drugs for use in place of adrenalectomy has eased the burden of treatment for patients with advanced disease. *Tamoxifen,* a competitive inhibitor of endogenous estrogen, binds to estrogen receptors and achieves an antitumor effect by an unknown mechanism. The drug has a low rate of toxicity and a response rate comparable to that of other forms of hormone therapy. *Aminoglutethimide* inhibits synthesis of steroids in the adrenal glands and conversion of peripheral androgens to estrogens. For patients with advanced breast cancer it has been used as a "medical adrenalectomy." Patients on aminoglutethimide need concomitant hydrocortisone supplementation.

Chemotherapy should be considered in patients with advanced disease after hormonal manipulations have failed or when they are deemed inappropriate (receptor-negative patients). However, the likelihood of response is reduced when the tumor has proven resistant to other forms of treatment. The chemotherapeutic regimens most commonly used to manage advanced disease include CMF and combination regimens with doxorubicin (see Table 121-4). Alopecia and gastrointestinal upset are common side-effects (see Chapter 89). Response rates range from 30% to 80% with a median duration of response of almost 8 months. When a patient becomes resistant to one regimen, a second one is instituted that does not utilize any of the previously used drugs. Patients who fail conventional chemotherapy are candidates for experimental agents.

Combination therapy, which makes use of hormonal manipulations and multidrug programs, has been advocated on the basis of a possible synergistic interaction. Recent results in receptor-positive postmenopausal women are encouraging.

Monitoring. Any readily measurable manifestation of

Table 121-3.   Hormonal Management
of Advanced Breast Cancer

HORMONE/ABLATION	INDICATION	RESPONSE RATE (%)
Estrogen*	Postmenopausal	40–50
Progesterone	Postmenopausal	30–40
Androgen	Perimenopausal	15–30
Antiestrogen†	Pre- and postmenopausal	30–40
Aromatase inhibitor‡	Pre- and postmenopausal	30–40
Oophorectomy	Premenopausal	30–40
Adrenalectomy	Pre- and postmenopausal	30–40
Hypophysectomy	Pre- and postmenopausal	30–40

* Diethylstilbesterol or estinyl.

† Tamoxifen (Nolvadex).

‡ Aminoglutethimide (Cytadren).

Table 121-4.   Chemotherapeutic Regimens in Management of Advanced Breast Cancer

REGIMEN	DOSE	ROUTE	SCHEDULE	RESPONSE RATE (%)
CMF*				30–60
Cyclophosphamide	100 mg	Oral	For 10 days, every 28 days	
Methotrexate	30 mg/m^2	Intravenous	Days 1 and 8	
Fluorouracil	300 mg/m^2	Intravenous	Days 1 and 8	
C-A†				40–80
Cyclophosphamide	500 mg/m^2 or 100 mg	Intravenous Oral	Every 3 weeks Days 3–6	
Doxorubicin (Adriamycin)	50 mg/m^2	Intravenous	Every 3 weeks	
A-V				40
Doxorubicin	60 mg/m^2	Intravenous	Every 3 weeks	
Vincristine	1.5 mg/m^2	Intravenous	Every 3 weeks	
CAF				40–60
Cyclophosphamide	100 mg	Oral	For 10 days	
Adriamycin	50 mg/m^2	Intravenous	Days 1 and 8	
Fluorouracil	500 mg/m^2	Intravenous	Days 1 and 8	
CMFVP				40–80
(Cooper regimen)	Variable	Variable	Variable	

* Low-dose regimen.

† In all doxorubicin regimens, the doxorubicin is discontinued beyond a 450 mg/m^2 cumulative dosage.

metastatic disease can be followed to gauge response to therapy. When there is none, carcinoembryonic antigen (CEA) or the breast tumor-associated antigen (CA-153) can serve as a useful marker for response in those patients who have elevated levels.

Radiation therapy. Breast cancer is exquisitely responsive to irradiation. Common patterns of recurrence that require palliation include metastatic *bony* lesions and local *cutaneous* implants. The latter may develop as small subcutaneous implants and then coalesce to form a tumor en cuirasse with secondary obstruction to dermal lymphatics and enormous lymphedema. The pain and incapacity from this complication of breast cancer are significant and may be avoided by local radiation therapy at a time when tumor on the chest wall is minimal.

Metastatic bony lesions are present in more than 60% of patients with breast cancer; the lytic lesions in particular, are associated with pain. Local radiation therapy at relatively low doses of 2000 to 3500 rads may abort the pain, although persistent structural defects as a consequence of cortical bony erosion may necessitate orthopedic support and even internal fixation for weight-bearing bone structures.

Another important role for radiation therapy is in palliation of patients who develop metastatic brain lesions; these occur in more than 10% of patients. The radiation sensitivity and responsiveness of the tumor make this form of therapy an excellent treatment modality for brain metastases. An extended period of survival can be achieved.

PATIENT EDUCATION

Most patients with breast cancer fear disfigurement and loss of their physical attractiveness almost as much as they are concerned about survival. Informing the patient of the impressive advances in both the type of treatment needed for localized disease (see above) and reconstructive efforts (including reconstruction of the nipple) should help to ease the very substantial dread that accompanies the diagnosis of breast cancer, especially in younger, sexually active women. Eliciting and addressing concerns of disfigurement can be very comforting and an important part of the overall supportive effort of the primary physician (see Chapter 88).

ANNOTATED BIBLIOGRAPHY

Fisher B, Bauer M, Margolese R et al: Five-year results of a randomized clinical trial comparing total mastectomy and segmental mastectomy with or without radiation in the treatment of breast cancer. N Engl J Med 312:665, 1985 (*A prospective, randomized study demonstrating the efficacy of segmental mastectomy plus radiation and its comparability to [if not superiority over] total mastectomy.*)

Harris JR, Hellman S, Kinne DW: Limited surgery and radiotherapy for early breast cancer. N Engl J Med 313:1365, 1985 (*A report of a concensus workshop on the technical details of the surgery and radiotherapy to be used in this approach to treatment.*)

Haskell CM, Sparks FC, Graze PR et al: Systemic therapy for metastatic breast cancer. Ann Intern Med 86:68, 1977 (*The UCLA conference reviews adjuvant therapy as well as hormone therapy for advanced disease and emphasizes the role of estrogen receptor protein and other clinical factors in predicting response.*)

Kiang DT, Gay J, Goldman A et al: A randomized trial of chemotherapy and hormonal therapy in advanced breast cancer. N Engl J Med 313:1241, 1985 (*Evidence that combination therapy may be useful in postmenopausal patients with receptor-rich tumors.*)

McGuire WL, Horwitz, KB, Zara, DT et al: Hormones in breast cancer. Metabolism 27:487, 1978 (*A detailed review of hormone receptor proteins and their implications for therapy.*)

Mueller CB: Surgery for breast cancer: Less may be as good as more. N Engl J Med 312:712, 1985 (*An editorial summarizing the issue of optimal treatment for localized disease.*)

Smith IE, Harris AL, Morgan M et al: Tamoxifen versus aminoglutethimide in advanced breast carcinoma. A randomized crossover trial. Br Med J 283:1432, 1981 (*The roles of the antiestrogen and the adrenal blocker are evaluated in a prospective trial, which demonstrates that they are equally effective [30% response rate] and that secondary responses to the alternative drug are achieved with both agents.*)

122
Management of the Woman with Genital Tract Cancer

JACOB J. LOKICH, M.D.

Cancers of the genital tract account for about 20% of cancers in women and 12% of cancer deaths. They range from the very readily detectable and curable carcinoma of the cervix to the very problematic ovarian carcinoma, with its tendency to remain inconspicuous until very late. Endometrial carcinoma has come to be one of the most common genital cancers of the postmenopausal years; much interest has developed in the relationship between the use of estrogens and the risk of this malignancy (see Chapter 106). Treatment of women with genital tract cancer is usually the province of the oncologist and gynecologist, but the primary physician remains an important part of the collaborative effort. Patient counseling, monitoring, and management of ongoing medical problems are among the important responsibilities.

CARCINOMA OF THE CERVIX

The incidence of invasive cervical carcinoma peaks in the fifth and sixth decades; however, most patients with the disease now present in their 20s and 30s with the precursor lesion, carcinoma *in situ,* thanks to early detection from use of the Pap smear (see Chapter 105). Among the risk factors are early sexual exposure, multiple sexual partners, and multiple genital tract infections.

Principles of Management

Diagnosis. Postcoital bleeding should raise suspicion for the diagnosis. In most cases of early disease, the patient is asymptomatic and, as noted above, detection is by screening Pap test. Diagnosis requires biopsy confirmation of a sufficiently abnormal Pap test or grossly suspicious-looking lesion. Patients with only mild dysplasia seen on the Pap smear can be followed without biopsy, but require periodic reevaluation to be sure there is no progression to more serious dysplasia.

If there is ongoing infection, it should be treated and the Pap smear repeated. Patients with moderate dysplasia seen on Pap smear are at greater risk and should be referred for further evaluation by the gynecologist. Cervical biopsy guided by colposcopy or Schiller testing (application of iodine to the cervical epithelium to identify abnormal areas by their failure to stain) helps to determine the significance of the abnormal Pap smear. The Pap smear is adequate for screening, but not for grading pathologic change. Colposcopic examination in skilled hands may obviate the need for biopsy.

Staging. Although staging will be carried out by the gynecologist, a reasonable estimation of disease extent can be made by pelvic examination; it should include careful palpation to see if there is lateral extension to the vagina or pelvic wall. Bimanual and rectopelvic examinations are helpful in this regard. Palpating lymph nodes helps in detecting distant metastasis.

Treatment. Moderate dysplasia is usually treated with cautery or laser therapy directed at the suspicious site(s). Severe dysplasia is usually treated with conization, as is carcinoma *in situ,* though some recommend hysterectomy when preservation of the uterus for childbearing is unimportant to the patient. Cryosurgery with repeat colposcopic examination and other conservative measures have been utilized; studies on their long-term effectiveness are ongoing. Microinvasive disease (less than 3 mm below the basement membrane) is treated with total hysterectomy. Stage IB cancer responds well to radium application and external radiation, or to radical hysterectomy and pelvic node dissection; results are comparable, although surgery allows preservation of ovarian function and vaginal flexibility. Both techniques are curative. Patients with disease extending beyond the cervix are treated with radium implantation and external beam irradiation. Stage IV treatment is individualized.

Patient Education

The fact that carcinoma of the cervix is potentially curable and early disease well treated without compromising child-bearing makes education of the young woman with carcinoma *in situ* or severe dysplasia particularly important to ensure that she is not lost to follow-up because of fear. Older patients presenting with more invasive disease can still obtain some comfort from knowing the prognosis remains very favorable for most stages of this disease.

CARCINOMA OF ENDOMETRIUM

Uninterrupted administration of exogenous estrogens in the postmenopausal period, particularly in the absence of progestin (see Chapter 117), risks induction of cystic and adenomatous hyperplasia, which are considered premalignant changes. Other risk factors include nulliparity and obesity (perhaps resulting from the ability of adipose tissue to convert circulating androstenedione into estrogen). The sixth and seventh decades represent periods of peak incidence. Post-menopausal bleeding (defined as uterine bleeding occurring 6 months after the onset of menopause) may be the only early clue to the development of this tumor. Occasionally, a mass is felt on routine pelvic examination.

Principles of Management

Diagnosis. Suspicion of the diagnosis mandates gyne-cologic referral for curettage and pathologic evaluation. When there is confusion as to whether a pelvic mass is ovarian or uterine, ordering a pelvic ultrasound examination can help make the distinction noninvasively (see Chapter 114).

Staging. Prognosis is a function of the extent of disease as well as of histologic type. The gynecologist will attempt to determine if the problem is confined to the uterine corpus or extends into the cervix and beyond.

Treatment. Patients with the premalignant change of ad-enomatous hyperplasia are usually advised to undergo hys-terectomy because of the risk of developing cancer; however, a second option is progestin therapy followed by repeat cu-rettage. Patients with stage I or stage II disease (confined to the uterus) have curable disease, treated by the combination of hysterectomy and irradiation. The precise type of radiation therapy depends on histologic type and degree of spread; in-tracavitary as well as external beam treatments are considered. The treatment of stage III disease (spread beyond the uterus but within the pelvis) is individualized, determined by findings on laparotomy. Patients with more advanced disease are in-operable and treated with radiation, progestins, or chemo-therapy for palliation. The use of progesterone for endometrial cancer has been advocated, although the data in the literature are predominantly anecdotal. Responses are achieved for the most part in patients with pulmonary nodules, and not in patients who have pelvic extension of the tumor or who have received prior radiation therapy. More than 50% of patients have responded to chemotherapy using cyclophosphamide (Cytoxan) and doxorubicin (Adriamycin). This combination regimen should be considered the standard form of treatment for patients who do not have a comorbid problem, such as heart disease, that precludes the use of either the alkylating drugs or doxorubicin.

Patient Education

Patients who are considering estrogen therapy for treat-ment of postmenopausal osteoporosis need to consider the risk of developing endometrial cancer. Although patients who do develop cancer from estrogen therapy are often detected early at a curable phase of illness, the disease still represents a serious consequence of an elective form of therapy. Adding a progestin to the estrogen program helps prevent unopposed endometrial proliferation and development of cystic hyper-plasia; but progestins unfavorably alter serum lipoproteins and are associated with an increased risk of cardiovascular disease. Only women willing to undertake such risks should be considered candidates for postmenopausal replacement therapy (see Chapters 117 and 158).

OVARIAN CARCINOMA

Ovarian cancer is the fifth leading cause of cancer death among women and a difficult disease to deal with. Initial manifestations may be very vague, typically nonspecific gas-trointestinal complaints that seem to persist in the absence of objective evidence for bowel disease. There is no adequate screening test, although the tumor-associated antigen CA 125 has been elevated in more than 80% of patients with ovarian cancer. Its potential as a diagnostic test is under investigation. At the time of presentation (which might be heralded by an abdominal or pelvic mass or development of ascites), almost 70% of patients have already reached stage III (spread to the upper abdomen). Disease limited to the ovaries is considered stage I and, if confined to the pelvis, stage II. Ascites and bulky peritoneal tumor are frequent manifestations. Precise staging necessitates a meticulous laparotomy to assess the diaphragmatic surface as well as the omentum and other intra-abdominal sites. Of the 18,000 new cases discovered annually, more than two thirds will die. Therapy is effective in reducing tumor bulk, but cure is still limited. The disease most com-monly recurs within the abdominal cavity; monitoring can be accomplished by ultrasonography and other imaging techniques, although miliary implants on the serosal surface may go undetected.

Principles of Management

Although the tumor is quite responsive, its bulk and spread limit the results of treatment. *Surgery* for ovarian cancer often necessitates "debulking" or tumor removal. Omentectomy as well as total abdominal hysterectomy and bilateral salpingo-oophorectomy are performed, in addition to the reduction of tumor masses throughout the abdominal cavity. This is believed to lessen the host–tumor burden and increase the effectiveness of ancillary or adjunctive therapeutic modalities, such as radiation or chemotherapy.

Radiation therapy to the pelvis or to the abdomen (for patients with disease that extends beyond the pelvis) has been advocated as a routine adjunct to surgery. The impact on survival has not been established. The rationale for abdominal and pelvic irradiation is based on the fact that ovarian tumors not infrequently cause recurrent ascites and bowel obstruction, leading to progressive inanition as a consequence of malabsorption and protein sequestration in the abdominal space.

The alkylating drugs have been the mainstay of systemic therapy for ovarian cancer. The simplest regimen uses one drug, such as melphalan or phenylalanine mustard. When alkylating drugs are employed in intermittent courses— monthly or over 6 weeks—30% of patients with extensive abdominal tumor respond, and a substantial proportion of patients achieve a complete response for an extended period of time. Recently, the combination of an alkylating drug with doxorubicin (Adriamycin) or cis-platinum has achieved response in up to 80% of patients. The effect on survival of combination chemotherapy regimens, compared with that of single-agent regimens, has yet to be established, but complete clinical remission rates of 30% to 40% are reported. The regression of disease, confirmed by "second-look" operations, suggests that multimodality and multidrug therapies should be the standard approach to ovarian cancer.

A unique type of chemotherapy, peritoneal infusion, has been employed in ovarian cancer, because of the unusual pattern of intra-abdominal dissemination. The "belly bath," or peritoneal infusion of chemotherapy, allows bathing of the superficial tumor cell implants in a drug solution over an interval of 3 to 4 hours, much like a dialysis procedure. The effectiveness of this approach remains to be determined.

Because tumors can be widespread and difficult to monitor, a better means of determining response to therapy has been sought. Monoclonal antibody CA 125 has shown promise as a means of monitoring in patients with ovarian cancer.

Patient Education

Patients with ovarian cancer have a long and difficult clinical course. Mortality rates are high and tumor bulk leads to considerable morbidity. Women with this disease and their families need all the support, interest, and comprehensive care that one can muster (see Chapter 88).

ANNOTATED BIBLIOGRAPHY

Barber HRK: Ovarian cancer. CA 36:149, 1986 (*An excellent and detailed review for the clinician, with considerable attention to the difficult care issues associated with this disease.*)

Bast RC, Klug TL, St John E et al: A radio-immunoassay using a monoclonal antibody to monitor the course of epithelial ovarian cancer. N Engl J Med 309:883, 1983 (*The use of tumor markers to detect as well as monitor patients with malignancy has been difficult even with the tumor-associated antigen CEA. This ovarian antigen has both specificity and sensitivity and may be developed successfully.*)

Crum CP, Ikenberg H, Richart RM et al: Human papillomavirus type 16 and early cervical neoplasia. N Engl J Med 310:880, 1984 (*Identifies one of the precursors to cervical cancer.*)

Decker DG, Fleming TR, Malkasian GD et al: Cyclophosphamide plus cis-platinum in combination: Treatment program for Stage III or IV ovarian carcinoma. Obstet Gynecol 60:481, 1982 (*The two most effective agents for ovarian cancer; reinforces the essential role of multiple agents in cancer treatment.*)

Gusberg SB: The changing nature of endometrial cancer. N Engl J Med 302:729, 1980 (*Examines the increased incidence of the disease with estrogen use and describes its clinical course and treatment.*)

Howell SB, Pfeifle CE, Olshen RA: Intraperitoneal chemotherapy with melphalan. Ann Intern Med 101:14, 1984 (*A description of the "bath" approach to chemotherapy for advanced ovarian cancer.*)

Richardson GS, Scully RE, Nikrui N et al: Common epithelial cancer of the ovary. N Engl J Med 312:415, 1985 (*Authoritative state-of-the-art review.*)

Richart RM: The patient with an abnormal Pap smear. N Engl J Med 302:332, 1980 (*A discussion of evaluation and the new options made possible by colposcopy and cryotherapy.*)

9

Genitourinary Problems

123
Screening for Syphilis
HARVEY B. SIMON, M.D.

Syphilis, like tuberculosis, has become dramatically less prevalent since the introduction of effective antibiotic therapy in the 1940s. As a result, manifestations of the disease have become less familiar to practitioners. If a patient is not identified and treated during the primary or secondary stages of the disease, the infection becomes latent and is identifiable only by means of laboratory tests until late, often irreversible, clinical manifestations appear. The prevention of destructive cardiovascular and neurologic lesions by means of appropriate screening for latent syphilis is an important task for the primary physician. Because false-positive results are common and are potentially traumatic for the patient, it is critical that the sensitivities and specificities of the various serologic tests be understood.

EPIDEMIOLOGY AND RISK FACTORS

With the exception of infection *in utero* or, very rarely, by means of blood transfusion, syphilis is transmitted exclusively by direct sexual contact with infectious lesions. It follows that risk increases with sexual activity. Since syphilis is readily treated with antibiotics, it is less common in populations with access to medical care. The reported incidence of syphilis among nonwhites in the United States is 20 times that among whites. Rates are highest in urban areas. It must be remembered, however, when comparing incidence rates in different populations, that case reporting has been shown to be more complete in public clinics than among private practitioners. The age-specific incidence rates parallel those of gonorrhea, with the peak incidence for both diseases occurring between ages 20 and 25. A diagnosis of gonorrhea, nongonorrheal urethritis, or another sexually transmitted disease should be considered a risk factor for syphilis. Presumably because they tend to have multiple sexual contacts,

homosexuals are at particularly high risk. In the United States, nearly 40% of all males with primary, secondary, or early latent syphilis reported being either homosexual or bisexual.

The importance of an accurate sexual history in determining risk of syphilis is obvious. Patients with early syphilis report an average of three recent sexual contacts. The probability that a known contact will develop syphilis has been shown to be approximately 50%.

NATURAL HISTORY OF SYPHILIS AND EFFECTIVENESS OF THERAPY

Treponema pallidum enters the bloodstream within a few hours after innoculation through intact mucous membranes or abraded skin. A primary lesion occurs at the site of the innoculation between 10 and 90 days after contact. This incubation period depends on the size of the innoculum, but is usually less than 3 weeks. The painless chancre usually resolves within 4 to 6 weeks, ending the *primary stage*. The *secondary stage* is usually heralded by a maculopapular rash that appears approximately 6 weeks after the primary lesion has healed. When the rash subsides, after 2 to 6 weeks, the untreated patient enters the *latent stage* (arbitrarily divided into *early latent* for the first 2 years and *late latent* thereafter).

Because anorectal or vaginal chancres are not likely to be brought to medical attention, primary syphilis is usually not diagnosed among homosexual men or among women. While more than 40% of syphilis cases are detected in the primary stage among heterosexual males, only 23% and 11% respectively, are detected in the primary stage among homosexual males and among females.

Natural history studies from Oslo and Tuskegee indicate that approximately one third of untreated syphilitics will develop clinically manifest tertiary disease and that autopsy evidence of cardiovascular syphilis can be found in more than half. In the retrospective Oslo study, 10% of patients had clinically evident cardiovascular syphilis, 7% neurosyphilis, and 16% gummatous disease. The incidence of cardiovascular syphilis was higher and that of neurosyphilis was lower in the prospective Tuskegee study.

Factors that influence the progression to clinical tertiary disease are incompletely understood. Congenital syphilis or disease contracted before age 15 does not predispose to cardiovascular tertiary disease. In general, late complications seem more likely to occur among untreated men than women.

The antibiotic regimens recommended in Chapter 138 are highly effective in eradicating early syphilis. If response to therapy is appropriately monitored by following the quantitative VDRL titer, the risk of late complications is virtually eliminated. Antibiotic treatment of late syphilis has less predictable results. Improvement among patients with general paresis has been reported in 40% to 80% of cases. Not surprisingly, structural cardiovascular changes caused by syphilis are not reversed by antibiotic treatment.

SCREENING AND DIAGNOSTIC TESTS

Serologic tests for syphilis depend on reactions to either a nonspecific reaginic antibody or to a specific antitreponemal antibody. The former tests include the sensitive and easily automated rapid plasma reagin test (RPR) and the quantitative VDRL flocculation test. Although these tests are virtually 100% sensitive during the secondary stage of syphilis, their sensitivity is only 70% during primary, latent, or late disease. Their specificity is approximately 70% during all stages. Acute false-positive reactions, which revert to negative within 6 months, may follow acute infections or vaccinations. Chronic false-positive reactions can be expected among patients with autoimmune disease, as well as among drug addicts and the elderly. Approximately 15% of patients with systemic lupus erythematosus (SLE), 25% of drug addicts, and 10% of people over 70 have false-positive reactions. The more expensive antitreponemal tests are both more sensitive and specific. The most commonly used is the fluorescent treponemal antibody absorption test (FTA-ABS). It has a sensitivity of 85% in primary disease, 100% in secondary disease, and 98% in latent or late disease. Although it is highly specific, false positives do occur, but the results are generally interpreted as borderline. Such equivocal results are more likely during pregnancy or in patients with SLE. The *Treponema pallidum* immobilization test (TPI) is less sensitive than the FTA-ABS but essentially 100% specific for past or present treponemal infection.

CONCLUSIONS AND RECOMMENDATIONS

- Syphilis is now a relatively uncommon disease. Nevertheless, screening for latent disease is simple, and the late man-

ifestations of syphilis are entirely preventable if treatment is instituted early.

- Many patients have been screened routinely at the time of marriage, during prenatal care, prior to giving blood, or on hospital admission. Frequent screening is unnecessary, but the nonreactivity of sexually active individuals, particularly those with multiple sex partners, should be documented at approximately 5-year intervals. Special indications for screening include contact or infection with other sexually transmitted diseases and pregnancy.

- Nontreponemal tests such as the RPR or VDRL are appropriate for screening because of their sensitivity and simplicity. FTA-ABS and other treponemal tests should be reserved for confirming a diagnosis suspected on the basis of clinical presentation or positive nontreponemal tests.

ANNOTATED BIBLIOGRAPHY

Clark EG, Danbold N: The Oslo study of the natural course of untreated syphilis. Med Clin North Am 48:613, 1964 (*A restudy of case material of untreated syphilis collected from 1891 to 1910.*)

Drusin LM, Topf-Olstein B, Levy-Zombek E: Epidemiology of infectious syphilis at a tertiary hospital. Arch Intern Med 139:901, 1979 (*Although only 37% of patients admitted to New York Hospital had routine admission serologic screening for syphilis, 245 new cases of syphilis were discovered over a 2-year period. The authors recommend routine testing for all hospital admission, but the cost-effectiveness of screening all patients versus testing high-risk groups is not discussed.*)

Hart G: Syphilis tests in diagnostic and therapeutic decision making. Ann Intern Med 104:368, 1986 (*An evaluation of available tests, with consideration of their sensitivity and specificity.*)

Jaffe HW: The laboratory diagnosis of syphilis. Ann Intern Med 83: 846, 1975 (*A review of diagnostic tests including discussion of the RPR.*)

Mascola L, Pelosi R, Blount JH: Congenital syphilis. Why is it still occurring? JAMA 252:1719, 1984 (*Of the 159 cases of congenital syphilis reported in the United States in 1982, 50 occurred in Texas. This study of the 50 Texas cases points out that persistence of this preventable disease reflects a failure of health-care delivery and prenatal screening.*)

Rockwell DH, Yobs AR, Moore MB Jr: The Tuskegee study of untreated syphilis. Arch Intern Med 114:792, 1964 (*Report of a prospective study of untreated syphilis in 412 black males in its 30th year. Notable for the ethical questions raised as well as the natural history of syphilis.*)

Sparling PF: Diagnosis and treatment of syphilis. N Engl J Med 284: 642, 1971 (*An extensive review of both diagnostic tests and treatment schedules.*)

Waring GW: False-positive tests for syphilis revisited. The intersection of Bayes' theorem and Wassermann's test. JAMA 243:2321, 1980 (*A reminder that as the incidence of a disease declines, so does the specificity of its screening test. The overall sensitivity of a positive STS was calculated at 85%.*)

124
Screening for Asymptomatic Bacteriuria and Urinary Tract Infection

When urinary tract infection is associated with symptoms, the early resolution of these symptoms and the resulting reassurance of the patient is justification enough for treatment that involves little risk. However, efforts to detect and treat asymptomatic bacteriuria are based on the assumption that treatment reduces the likelihood of subsequent morbidity due to symptomatic infection, sepsis, or chronic renal disease. The risk of such complications depends on the clinical situation, including the age and sex of the patient. For some, risk is well defined, and treatment is indicated; for others, the most significant morbidity may be related to the side-effects of inappropriate treatment. It is therefore critical that the physician appreciate the different implications of bacteriuria in different settings.

EPIDEMIOLOGY AND RISK FACTORS

The prevalence of bacteriuria depends on age and sex. Among neonates, positive cultures are found in about 1% of both males and females. During school-age years, the prevalence among boys is as low as 0.03%, compared with 1% to 2% among girls. Prevalance among females increases by 1% of the population per decade; throughout the childbearing age, the prevalence is 2% to 4% and by age 50, it has reached 5% to 10%. Geriatric males are almost as likely to have bacteriuria as females because of the high incidence of prostate and other urologic disease and subsequent instrumentation in this group. Prevalence in these older age groups reaches 15%.

The greater susceptibility of younger women and girls can be explained anatomically, in that a short urethra allows easier access to the bladder, facilitating colonization by perineal organisms. Risk increases with local trauma associated with sexual activity and the relaxation of pelvic supporting structures with age. Anatomic changes may also explain the slightly higher prevalence of bacteriuria (2% to 4%) among pregnant women. Alternatively, since users of birth control pills have a similarly increased risk, this prevalence may reflect estrogen-mediated dilatation of the urethra.

It must be kept in mind that prevalence figures indicate the extent of bacteriuria at a single point in time. Since risk factors are shared by many and bacteriuria frequently resolves spontaneously as well as after therapy, the cumulative prevalence of bacteriuria is higher. By age 30, approximately 25% of women have experienced symptoms consistent with urinary tract infection.

Structural abnormalities, including obstruction of the urethra or ureters, significant vesicourethral reflux, neurologic lesions, and foreign bodies are important additional risk factors for bacteriuria.

NATURAL HISTORY OF ASYMPTOMATIC BACTERIURIA AND EFFECTIVENESS OF THERAPY

Asymptomatic and symptomatic urinary tract infections have the same epidemiologic correlates. Asymptomatic infections can become symptomatic; bacteriuria can persist after symptoms have resolved. Ninety percent of women with bacteriuria have had symptoms some time in the past, nearly 70% within the preceding year. While both asymptomatic and symptomatic infections can resolve spontaneously, the urine is more likely to become sterile after treatment. Approximately 80% of women with bacteriuria have sterile urine after appropriate antibiotic treatment. However, follow-up studies indicate that only 55% of those treated will have sterile urine at the end of 1 year. Sterile urine developed spontaneously in fully 36% of untreated bacteriuric women during the same period. Significantly, women who had recurrences of infection after treatment were more likely to have associated symptoms than those who had persistent or relapsing bacteriuria. Symptomatic infection recurs within 3 years in 40% of women.

The importance of chronic or recurrent bacteriuria in the etiology of chronic renal failure has been deemphasized as diverse noninfectious etiologies for the pathologic findings of interstitial nephritis have been recognized. Patients with bacteriuria are more likely to be hypertensive. They are also more likely to have identifiable abnormalities on IVP, including small kidneys, delayed excretion, caliceal dilation and blunting, ureteral reflux, stones, and other obstructive lesions. However, chronic renal failure rarely occurs as a complication of urinary tract infection in the absence of structural abnormalities. Evidence indicates that such abnormalities predispose patients to both chronic renal failure and recurrent infection. Definitive studies that address this important question have not yet been performed.

In addition to symptomatic urinary tract infection and chronic renal disease, the clinician must also be concerned with the possibility that chronic asymptomatic infection is a potential source of disseminated infection, such as endocarditis. This danger is particularly likely in the male patient with prostate disease and infection who requires instrumentation. Bacteremia has been documented in as many as 50% of males whose urine is infected at the time of the procedure; it is relatively rare when the urine is sterile.

In elderly populations, asymptomatic bacteriuria has been associated with increased mortality rates. Obviously, such increased rates may be due either to bacteriuria or to other factors that increase the risk of both bacteriuria and death. Recent evidence suggests the latter; at least one study found no difference among elderly women and men with and without bacteriuria when comorbidity such as cancer was controlled.

Special risks are associated with bacteriuria during pregnancy. Asymptomatic bacteriuria, defined by either repeated recovery of greater than 10^5 CFU/ml in voided urine or positive suprapubic aspirates, occurs in approximately 5% of pregnancies. Among women with bacteriuria identified early in pregnancy, there is a 40% incidence of acute pyelonephritis without prophylactic treatment. Women with bacteriuria are nearly twice as likely to deliver a low birth weight infant. Their relative risk of perinatal infant mortality has been estimated at 1.6. Randomized trials of treatment of asymptomatic bacteriuria of pregnancy have demonstrated efficacy in reducing the incidence of pyelonephritis and low birth weight delivery.

SCREENING AND DIAGNOSTIC TESTS

Asymptomatic bacteriuria is a laboratory diagnosis that requires careful definition. Because voided urine is easily contaminated by urethral and (in women) perineal flora during micturition, cultures of clean voided urine must be cultured quantitatively. The probability of infection in a patient whose specimen contains 10^5 CFU/ml is nearly 100% for males but only 80% for females. Two such positive cultures in a female increase the probability of infection to 95%. False-negative findings are more likely if the patient is undergoing vigorous diuresis, if the urine is unusually acidic (pH 5.5), or if the specimen was inadvertently contaminated with antibacterial detergents. Spurious positive cultures are more common, because of unclean collection technique, contaminated collection equipment, or failure to promptly culture the urine.

A single culture of urine collected on urethral catheterization with $\geq 10^5$ CFU/ml has a predictive value of infection of 95%. Catheterization should be limited to patients requiring relief of obstruction or those who absolutely cannot cooperate with collection techniques. The risk of introducing infection during catheterization may be as high as 5%. The risk of inducing bacteremia in men with an infected urinary tract approaches 50%. When suprapubic percutaneous bladder aspiration is used in young children or to resolve confusing problems in the adult, infection can be presumed if any bacterial growth other than that of skin contaminants occurs.

Nonquantitative approaches to diagnosis include microscopic examination for bacteria and clinical tests of bacterial activity such as the reduction of nitrate to nitrite. These and the less specific signs of urinary tract inflammation such as pyuria, hematuria, and proteinuria may be helpful in making a presumptive diagnosis in the symptomatic patient. They may also indicate the need for urine culture when incidental abnormalities are detected in the asymptomatic patient. Confirmation of infection with quantitative culture technology should always precede a therapeutic decision in the absence of symptoms.

CONCLUSIONS AND RECOMMENDATIONS

- Bacteriuria, both symptomatic and asymptomatic, is a common phenomenon with well-defined risk factors.
- Treatment is moderately effective in the short run, but because of high rates of spontaneous recurrence and resolution, the likelihood that bacteriuria will be noted with longer follow-up is not significantly influenced by short-term therapy.
- Symptomatic infections are generally not prevented by treatment of asymptomatic bacteriuria in nonpregnant women.
- Although an association exists between bacteriuria and renal abnormalities, there is no evidence that this is an etiologic relationship. Furthermore, there is no evidence that treatment of infection in the absence of urinary tract abnormalities will prevent progressive renal disease.
- Screening for asymptomatic bacteriuria is recommended only in selected high-risk populations including (1) pregnant women; (2) elderly males with clinical prostatism or other urologic abnormalities, particularly before and after required instrumentation; (3) all patients recently catheterized; (4) patients with known renal calculi or other structural abnormalities of the urinary tract.

A.G.M.

ANNOTATED BIBLIOGRAPHY

Asscher AW, Sossman M, Waters WE et al.: The clinical significance of asymptomatic bacteriuria in the nonpregnant woman. J Infect Dis 120:17, 1969 (*Controlled trial of treatment of asymptomatic bacteriuria. Concludes that screening for bacteriuria in nonpregnant women is unlikely to be of value.*)

Freedman LR, Seki M, Phair JP: The natural history and outcome of antibiotic treatment of urinary tract infections in women. Yale J Biol Med 37:245, 1965 (*Short-term follow-up cultures overestimate benefits of treatment.*)

Gower PE, Haswell B, Sidaway ME, deWardener HE: Follow-up of 164 patients with bacteriuria of pregnancy. Lancet 1:990, 1968 (*Fewer than 20% of those not treated in this study incurred pyelonephritis.*)

Kass EH, Zinner SH: Bacteriuria and renal disease. J Infect Dis 120: 27, 1969 (*Exhaustive review of the links between bacteriuria and renal disease. Authors conclude that a causal relationship has been demonstrated in cases of pyelonephritis in pregnancy and bacteremia postcatheterization but not in progressive renal disease among adults.*)

Kunin CM, Polyak F, Postel E: Periurethral bacterial flora in women. JAMA 243:134, 1980 (*Intensively monitored small cohort of women with and without history of UTI. The most notable finding is a high frequency of asymptomatic bacteriuria with spontaneous resolution in both groups.*)

Nordenstam GR, Brandberg CA, Oden AS et al.: Bacteriuria and mortality in an elderly population. N Engl J Med 314:1152, 1986 (*A 9-year cohort study finding no difference in mortality among women with and without bacteriuria; also, no difference among men when those with cancer were excluded.*)

Platt R: Quantitive definition of bacteriuria. Am J Med 75:44, 1983 (*Discusses trade-offs between sensitivity and specificity and recommends different colony count cutoffs for different clinical situations.*)

Pollock HM: Laboratory techniques for detection of urinary tract infection and assessment of value. Am J Med 75:79, 1983 (*Reviews techniques both for determining the presence of bacteriuria and for localizing urinary tract infection.*)

Stamm WE: Prevention of urinary tract infections. Am J Med, 76: 148, 1984 (*Thoughtful review of risk factors and preventive approaches; recommends screening only for pregnant women.*)

Takahashi M, Loveland DB: Bacteriuria and oral contraceptives. JAMA 227:762, 1974 (*Fifty percent higher prevalence among oral contraceptive users.*)

125
Screening for Prostatic Cancer
JOHN D. GOODSON, M.D.

Prostatic carcinoma is perhaps the most common malignancy among men in the United States. The lifetime probability that a man will incur clinical prostatic cancer is between 5% and 6%, but the probability of death due to prostatic cancer is approximately 2%. Even the patient with clinically evident disease is more likely to die of something else. Pathologic studies indicate that occult prostatic cancer is even more prevalent than these figures suggest.

The physician faces a great deal of uncertainty in making clinical decisions about prostatic cancer. The tumors are exceedingly common and have the potential to cause significant morbidity and mortality. They also have a variable, often indolent course and a higher prevalence in those whose health is often more limited by coincident diseases. The clinician should be aware of the unpredictable natural history of the disease and the limitations of therapy when considering the use of screening tests for prostatic cancer. Fortunately, the only accepted screening procedure is part of the routine physical examination.

EPIDEMIOLOGY AND RISK FACTORS

The incidence of prostatic carcinoma increases with age. Reports of age-specific prevalence range from 5% to 15% during the sixth decade, 10% to 30% during the seventh decade, and 20% to 50% or higher after age 70. Such prevalence estimates have increased over the years as detailed histologic study of glands removed at surgery has become more common. Clinical detection of prostatic cancer is highest in whites of northern European origin and American blacks. A history of prostatitis does not seem to be a risk factor, but benign prostatic hypertrophy may predispose the patient to malignant disease. There is no clear etiologic relationship to environmental factors, socioeconomic status, fertility, or endogenous androgen level. Regional variations in the prevalence of prostatic cancer reflect either differences in unidentified environmental factors or variation in case detection methods.

NATURAL HISTORY OF PROSTATIC CANCER AND EFFECTIVENESS OF THERAPY

Unfortunately, the biologic behavior of prostatic carcinoma varies widely, making individual cases unpredictable. In most of the reported cases of prostatic cancer, the patient presents with symptoms of urinary tract outflow obstruction such as hesitancy, frequency, nocturia, and loss of stream volume and force. In up to 20% of cases, presentation includes signs or symptoms of early metastasis such as bone pain.

Approximately 50% of isolated prostatic nodules found on routine rectal examination in the asymptomatic patient are subsequently proven to be malignant. Such presentations account for 10% of all prostatic cancers. Another 10% of cases are discovered incidentally during microscopic examination of glandular tissue after removal for reasons other than suspected malignancy.

The clinical course after diagnosis is remarkably variable and depends on the degree of histologic differentiation of the tumor more than on the extent of disease. Most incidentally discovered tumors have well-differentiated isolated malignant foci. Even without treatment, survival in these patients is the same as that in age-matched controls. A minority of latent tumors have diffuse poorly differentiated histology. Prognosis in these cases is nearly as poor as in those with metastases at presentation. The mean duration of the asymptomatic stage of prostatic cancer has been estimated to be between 10 and 30 years, but it is apparent that a substantial number of cases with poorly differentiated tumors are on the short end of the distribution. It is also clear that tumors can run a very aggressive course after they become clinically manifest. In some older series, the median survival from diagnosis to death in untreated patients was less than 2 years.

This variability in natural history makes assessment of the efficacy of therapeutic interventions difficult. Some have argued that early and aggressive intervention with surgical extirpation of involved tissue and radiation therapy to involved areas may prolong survival in patients in whom the tumor is isolated to the gland or is locally metastatic. However, no form of intervention applied to asymptomatic patients, either with latent carcinoma or carcinoma found on biopsy of a suspected malignant nodule, has been shown to improve survival. In older patients, most oncologists withhold treatment until symptoms of obstruction or metastasis develop. More aggressive therapy is reserved for patients without serious comorbid conditions.

SCREENING AND DIAGNOSTIC TESTS

Careful digital examination of the rectum is the only practical screening technique for prostatic carcinoma. The finding of a hard (similar in consistency to the tip of the nose), stony, and asymmetric prostate is highly suggestive of malignancy. Fixation to adjacent tissue and a loss of the lateral prostatic sulcus suggests local metastasis. The isolated prostatic nodule, though possibly an indication of localized disease, is a nonspecific finding. It occurs in up to 5% of men over 50 years of age and 10% of men over 70. Approximately 50% of such nodules are prostatic cancers.

Although acid phosphatase is found in normal hyperthrophied or malignant prostatic tissue, measurement of serum levels is not a sensitive test for early disease. Elevated levels are found in 80% of individuals with bony metastasis, but in only 5% to 15% of those with localized disease. Measurement of acid phosphatase levels has a reported specificity of greater than 90%. The physician should be aware, however, that transient elevations of less than 24 hours' duration can occur following prostatic massage of the hypertrophied nonmalignant gland. Although radioimmunoassay for prostatic acid phosphatase has an increased sensitivity for early disease, its poor specificity limits its usefulness as a screening test.

CONCLUSIONS AND RECOMMENDATIONS

- Routine yearly rectal examination is recommended for the detection of asymptomatic prostatic nodules. Stool obtained should be tested for the presence of occult blood as a screen for early colorectal cancer.

- Prostatic nodules in younger patients should be referred for biopsy. Nodules in elderly patients or those with comorbid conditions should be followed at 6-month intervals and biopsied only if the size increases or symptoms of outflow obstruction or bone pain appear.

- Although radioimmunoassay or counterimmunoelectrophoretic techniques for determining acid phosphatase levels may allow more sensitive detection of early disease, routine screening is not recommended on the basis of currently available data regarding benefits of early detection. Routine chemical determination of acid phosphatase is not sensitive enough to detect early disease.

ANNOTATED BIBLIOGRAPHY

Armenian HK, Lilienfield AM, Diamond EL, Bross ID: Relation between benign prostatic hyperplasia and cancer of the prostate. Lancet 2:115, 1974 (*Retrospective analysis of patients with BPH showed a 5.1 relative risk for prostatic cancer compared with age-matched controls.*)

Blackard CE, Millinger GT, Gleason DF: Treatment of Stage I carcinoma of the prostate: A preliminary report. J Urol 016:729, 1971 (*No difference in survival of patients with localized carcinoma treated surgically or hormonally, or with no therapy at all.*)

Chodak GW, Schoenberg HW: Early detection of prostate cancer by routine screening. JAMA 252:3261, 1984 (*Results of a screening program: 5% of 811 men were advised to have biopsies; 25% had cancers.*)

Fleischmann J, Catalona WJ, Fair WR et al.: Lack of value of radioimmunoassay for prostatic acid phosphotase as a screening test for prostatic cancer in patients with obstructive prostatic hyperplasia. J Urol 129:312, 1983 (*None of the patients with an abnormal screening test actually had cancer.*)

Gittes RF: Serum acid phosphatase and screening for carcinoma of the prostate. N Engl J Med 309:852, 1983 (*An editorial retrospective pointing out the lack of screening utility of serum acid phosphatase measurements primarily because of poor sensitivity in early disease and nonspecificity including frequent elevation in patients with benign prostatic hypertrophy.*)

Guinan P, Bush I, Ray V et al.: The accuracy of the rectal examination in the diagnosis of prostate carcinoma. N Engl J Med 303:499, 1980 (*Finds the rectal examination to be the most efficient test with a sensitivity of 69% and specificity of 89%. Accompanying article cautions about limits of RIA acid phosphatase screening.*)

Heaney JA, Chang HC, Daley JJ et al.: Prognosis of clinically undiagnosed prostatic carcinoma and the influence of hormonal therapy. J Urol 118:283, 1977 (*Survival among patients with incidentally found moderate or poorly differentiated carcinoma was significantly reduced. Survival in patients with well-differentiated carcinoma was unchanged.*)

Hudson PB, Stout AP: Prostatic cancer. NY State J Med 351, 1966 (*Fifty-two percent of prostatic nodules were malignant.*)

Hutchison GB: Epidemiology of prostatic carcinoma. Semin Oncol 3:151, 1976 (*Excellent review of epidemiologic data.*)

Klein LA: Prostatic carcinoma. N Engl J Med 300:824, 1979 (*An excellent review. A detailed approach to each stage of prostatic malignancy is outlined.*)

Rullis I, Shaeffer JA, Lilien OM: Incidence of prostatic carcinoma in the elderly. Urology 6:295, 1975 (*Two thirds of males over 80 had prostatic cancer.*)

Snowdon DA, Phillips RL, Choi W: Diet, obesity, and the risk of fatal prostate cancer. Am J Epidemiol 120:244, 1984. (*Obesity and animal product consumption may increase the risk of fatal prostate cancer three- to fourfold.*)

Watson RA, Tang DB: The predictive value of prostatic acid phosphatase as a screening test for prostatic cancer. N Engl J Med 303:497, 1980 (*Points out the necessarily low predictive value of RIA-PAP screening due to a not-insignificant false-positive rate and the low prevalence of disease in an asymptomatic population.*)

126
Screening for Cancers of the Lower Urinary Tract

Lower urinary tract cancers include tumors of the renal pelves, ureters, bladder, and urethra. These lesions can logically be considered together because of similar cell types—more than 95% consist of transitional cells, squamous cells, or a combination of the two—and because of common epidemiologic correlates.

Cancer of the lower urinary tract is viewed by many primary physicians as a relatively benign tumor that principally affects the elderly. Nevertheless, approximately 40,000 new cases occur each year in the United States; 10,000 deaths per year can be attributed to bladder cancer. The lifetime probability of incurring cancer of the bladder is approximately 2% for white males and 1% for white females.

Risk factors, including a strong association with occupational exposure, have been well defined. A weaker association with tobacco use has more recently been demonstrated. Screening tests are available. Although there is still insufficient understanding of the natural history of bladder cancer to allow specific screening recommendations, the physician must understand the epidemiology of these tumors as well as the potential costs and benefits of various screening practices.

EPIDEMIOLOGY AND RISK FACTORS

Cancer of the lower urinary tract is a tumor of older age groups; in the United States, the mean age at the time of diagnosis is 68 years. The incidence increases at a constant rate during adult life, varying from 1 per 100,000 per year at age 20 to 200 per 100,000 per year at age 80 for white males. Females have approximately one third the risk of males. In the United States, whites are twice as likely to have bladder tumors as nonwhites. Urban dwellers, too, have consistently been shown to have a higher incidence of lower urinary tract tumors compared with people who live in rural or suburban areas.

The most notable risk factor for development of lower urinary tract cancers is occupational exposure to aromatic amines, first noted in England in 1895. Subsequently, dyestuff workers were shown to have a 10-fold to 50-fold increased risk of bladder carcinoma. Compounds most closely associated with bladder carcinogenesis include 2-naphthylamine and benzidine. Recent case-control studies indicate excess risk among men who worked with dyestuffs, rubber, leather, or painting or other organic chemicals. It has been estimated that these occupational exposures are responsible for 18% of bladder cancer cases. As little as 2 years' exposure may be sufficient to increase the risk, but the time between exposure and subsequent cancer may be as long as 45 years.

Smoking has been implicated as a risk factor for bladder cancer in many studies, most of which indicate that smokers have a twofold increase in risk over nonsmokers. Other suggested risk factors include pelvic irradiation, which was used in the past for dysfunctional bleeding, heavy coffee consumption, and abuse of phenacetin-containing analgesics.

NATURAL HISTORY OF LOWER URINARY TRACT CANCERS AND EFFECTIVENESS OF THERAPY

The natural history of lower urinary tract tumors is not well defined. Prognosis at the time of diagnosis depends on both clinical stage, defined by depth of penetration and extent of metastases, and histologic grade of the tumor. There is often close correlation between depth of penetration and histologic grade. Urothelial tumors are grossly subdivided into papilloma, papillary carcinoma, and transitional cell carcinoma. These gross morphologic distinctions have histologic counterparts that are highly predictive of 5-year survival. Grade 1 papillary carcinoma (papilloma) has a 5-year cure or clinical control rate of approximately 95%. Grade 2 papillary carcinoma (papillary carcinoma) has a 5-year survival rate of only 25%. The outlook for Grade 3 papillary and infiltrating carcinoma (transitional cell carcinoma) is worse. Prognosis for patients with squamous carcinoma is also very poor, unless the tumor is well differentiated. Clinical staging systems that distinguish between levels of tumor penetration of the bladder have also been shown to have good prognostic value. Overall, about 50% of patients with treated bladder cancer survive for 5 years. However, multiple synchronous and asynchronous tumors are the rule in lower urinary tract cancer, contributing to morbidity and eventual mortality.

Hematuria is the most common presentation of lower urinary tract cancer. Other symptoms suggestive of cystitis may also occur. Although it has been claimed that 75% of tumors promptly diagnosed after a first episode of hematuria are localized, little data on this subject are available. The likelihood that screening tests, including urinalysis and urinary cytology, would significantly advance the time of diagnosis is likewise unproven. A progression from urothelial atypia to sessile carcinoma *in situ* or papilloma to higher grade malignancy has been postulated. Studies of the natural history of urothelial carcinoma *in situ* indicate that the majority of lesions progress to more malignant forms. Although early lesions are much less likely to be detected cytologically, 3.7% of detected tumors were *in situ* in one study. The usual synchronous and asynchronous multiplicity of such tumors makes it difficult to assess the benefits of early detection.

SCREENING TESTS

Urinary cytology is the most specific screening test for lower urinary tract cancers. Reports of the sensitivity of cytology in detecting bladder carcinoma vary from 50% to 90%. Studies have consistently demonstrated that sensitivity increases with the grade of malignancy. Although invasive transitional-cell carcinoma can regularly be detected with 90% or greater sensitivity, sensitivity rates for papillomas and papillary carcinomas range from 0% to 50%.

Studies of cytologic screening of high-risk populations have been conducted. In one such study, screening of 285 exposed workers produced positive results in 31, 10 of whom had the diagnosis of cancer confirmed at cystoscopy. Within 4 years, 11 additional tumors developed among the 21 cytology-positive, cystoscopy-negative patients. Cystoscopy was also performed in the 254 workers with negative cytologic findings; only 1 case of bladder cancer was diagnosed on that examination. In general, the specificity of urinary cytology depends on the skill of the cytologist. False-positive rates as low as 1% and as high as 20% have been reported.

The value of other urinary sediment abnormalities, particularly hematuria, has not been well defined. In one study of cytologic detection, hematuria was absent in 50% of true-positive cytologic diagnoses.

Cystoscopy and radiographic procedures cannot be considered screening tools. They should be reserved for patients who present with symptoms suggestive of urinary cancer or who have positive cytologies. Frequent follow-up cystoscopies are also a part of the postoperative care of the patient with bladder cancer.

CONCLUSIONS AND RECOMMENDATIONS

- Lower urinary tract cancer is associated with significant morbidity and mortality.
- Risks of occupational exposure to dyestuffs, rubber, leather and leather products, and paint and organic chemicals have been well defined. Smoking is associated with a smaller, but significant, increase in risk.
- Urinary cytology is an imperfect but useful screening test for high-risk groups.
- There is no evidence that screening significantly advances the time of diagnosis in an individual case or that early treatment influences the outcome. Nevertheless, because of the relatively high specificity and lack of morbidity associated with cytologic screening, identification of patients at high risk because of occupational exposure, with subsequent yearly cytologic screening, is indicated. Screening of asymptomatic smokers without risk of occupational exposure is not recommended.

A.G.M.

ANNOTATED BIBLIOGRAPHY

Cole P: Coffee-drinking and cancer of the lower urinary tract. Lancet 1:1335, 1971 (*Further case-control data identifying the association between coffee-drinking and cancer of the lower urinary tract, particularly among women.*)

Cole P, Hoover R, Friedell GH: Occupation and cancer of the lower urinary tract. Cancer 29:1250, 1972 (*Case-control study identifying excess risk among five occupation categories: dyestuffs, rubber, leather and leather products, paint, and organic chemicals. There was no identifiable risk in those who worked with nonorganic chemicals, petroleum, or printing.*)

Cole P, Monson RR, Haning H et al.: Smoking and cancer of the lower urinary tract. N Engl J Med 284:129, 1971 (*Case-control data indicating that smokers have a two-fold greater risk of developing bladder cancer.*)

Foot NC, Papanicolaou GN, Holmquist ND, Seybolt JF: Exfoliative cytology of urinary sediments (a review of 2,829 cases). Cancer 11:127, 1958 (*Sensitivity of 62% in detecting tumors of renal pelves, bladder, or ureters, 8% in renal tumors, and 15% in prostatic tumors; high specificity.*)

Jewett HJ: Cancer of the bladder. Diagnosing and staging. Cancer 32:1072, 1973 (*Good, brief review of presenting symptoms and staging.*)

Kantor AF, Hartge P, Hoover RN et al: Urinary tract infection risk of bladder cancer. Am J Epidemiol 119:510, 1984 (*A case-control study detecting a relative risk for bladder cancer of two among those with a history of three or more UTIs.*)

Matanoski GM, Elliott EA: Bladder cancer epidemiology. Epidemiol Rev 3:203, 1981 (*Extensive review of descriptive epidemiology as well as risk factors including smoking, coffee-drinking, use of sugar substitutes, as well as occupational exposures.*)

Melamed MR, Koss LG, Ricci A et al: Cytohistological observations on developing carcinomas of the urinary bladder in men. Cancer 13:67, 1960 (*Documents cytologic identification of latent bladder cancer in patients with occupational exposure.*)

Morrison AS, Buring JE: Artificial sweeteners and cancer of the lower urinary tract. N Engl J Med 302:537, 1980 (*A case-control study that did not detect a significant association between use of artificial sweetners and excess risk of lower urinary tract cancer.*)

Tweeddale DN: Urinary Cytology. Boston, Little, Brown, 1977 (*Detailed text with chapters on pathology of urinary tract tumors and clinical value of cytology that are useful for the generalist.*)

127

Evaluation of the Patient with Hematuria

LESLIE S.-T. FANG, M.D.

Virtually every disease of the genitourinary tract can produce hematuria. The primary physician may encounter a patient complaining of gross hematuria or may find microscopic hematuria on routine examination of the urine. Sometimes the etiology is a harmless condition, especially when there is asymptomatic microscopic hematuria in an otherwise healthy, young patient. At other times, hematuria may be the only symptom of genitourinary neoplasia. Its presence demands careful consideration and often a thorough investigation to ascertain the underlying etiologic factors. One needs to be able to initiate an effective workup, and decide how comprehensive and invasive it ought to be; this includes deciding when referral for urologic evaluation or renal biopsy is necessary.

PATHOPHYSIOLOGY AND CLINICAL PRESENTATION

Normally, fewer than 1000 red blood cells are excreted in the urine each minute. Microscopic hematuria ensues if the rate of excretion rises to 3000 to 4000 red blood cells per minute; 2 to 3 red blood cells per high-power field will appear on microscopic examination of the urine. If the excretion rate exceeds 1 million red blood cells per minute, macroscopic or gross hematuria will result. Definitions of clinically significant hematuria are somewhat arbitrary; however, greater than 10 red blood cells per high-power field is considered by many a reasonable cutoff point for separating benign etiologies from potentially serious pathology.

Any intrinsic lesion within the genitourinary tract involving the kidneys, ureters, bladder, prostate, or urethra can produce hematuria. Hematuria may also result from periurethral problems in the pelvis or colon, systemic diseases, bleeding diatheses, and use of certain drugs (*e.g.,* cyclophosphamide).

Symptoms associated with hematuria may provide important clues to etiology. The flank pain of renal colic is usually secondary to renal calculi, but may occasionally be associated with the passage of clots. Frequency, dysuria, urgency, and suprapubic pain occur with inflammatory lesions of the lower urinary tract. Dull flank pain with fever and chills may accompany pyelonephritis (see Chapter 132). Occasionally, complaints such as fever, rash, or joint pains may indicate an underlying systemic disease. Uncommonly, hematuria occurs without any associated symptoms, though the majority of cases have a definable cause. When a thorough

workup fails to reveal an etiology, the patient is said to have "essential hematuria." Renal biopsy of such patients often shows minimal glomerular or interstitial disease. Long-term prognosis of these patients is excellent.

In view of the high incidence of structural lesions associated with hematuria, a thorough workup to establish the etiology is necessary regardless of the mode of presentation.

DIFFERENTIAL DIAGNOSIS

Intrinsic genitourinary lesions involving the kidneys, ureters, bladder, prostate, and urethra can all produce hematuria. The diagnoses from a series of 1000 referred cases of gross hematuria and from a study of 500 referred cases of microscopic hematuria are tabulated in Tables 127-1 and 127-2. Gross hematuria is most commonly associated with inflammatory lesions and neoplasms; in this series, infection accounted for 34% and neoplasms accounted for 31%. Benign prostatic hypertrophy accounted for another 12.5% of the diagnoses. Microscopic hematuria was most commonly associated with infection and benign prostatic hypertrophy, the former being the final diagnosis in 28% of the patients.

Rarely, periureteral inflammatory lesions in the appendix, colon, or pelvic structures produces microscopic hematuria. On occasion, a systemic illness such as lupus erythematosus, bacterial endocarditis, or rheumatic fever is the source of hematuria. Blood dyscrasias (*e.g.,* hemophilia, sickle cell disease, polycythemia vera, and leukemia), and hemorrhagic disorders (*e.g.,* thrombocytopenic purpura and various coagulation defects) can be responsible for red cells in the urine.

Drugs such as anticoagulants, salicylates, methanamine preparations, and sulfonamides have been known to cause hematuria. Cyclophosphamide can induce hemorrhagic cystitis or microscopic hematuria (see Chapter 89). Hematuria in a patient on anticoagulants requires thorough evaluation because an underlying urologic lesion is often found (see Chapter 85).

Fever, strenuous exercise, and long-distance running are among the harmless etiologies of microscopic hematuria in otherwise healthy patients. If a thorough workup fails to reveal an etiology, the patient is said to have "essential" hematuria.

Conditions occasionally mistaken for hematuria include menstrual bleeding and the intake of substances that can darken the urine, such as beets, rhubarb, and the drugs pyridium and rifampin.

Table 127-1. Diagnosis in 1000 Referred Cases of Gross Hematuria

DIAGNOSIS	PATIENT (%)
Kidneys	15.0
Tumor	3.5
Infection	3.0
Calculus	2.7
Trauma	2.0
Obstruction	1.5
Others	2.3
Ureters	6.5
Calculus	5.3
Tumor	0.7
Others	0.5
Bladder	39.5
Infection	22.0
Tumor	14.9
Others	2.6
Prostate	23.6
Benign hyperplasia	12.5
Infection	9.0
Tumor	2.1
Urethra	4.3
Stricture	1.7
Calculus	1.3
Others	1.3
Essential Hematuria	8.5

(Source: Lee LW, Davis E et al: Gross urinary hemorrhage: A symptom, not a disease. JAMA 153:782, 1953)

Table 127-2. Diagnosis in 500 Referred Cases of Asymptomatic Microscopic Hematuria

DIAGNOSIS	PATIENT (%)
Kidneys	6.2
Calculus	3.4
Cyst	1.2
Hydronephrosis	0.6
Tumor	0.4
Others	0.6
Ureters	0.8
Calculus	0.4
Ureterocoele	0.4
Bladder	8.6
Infection	6.6
Tumor	1.8
Others	0.2
Prostate	23.6
Benign hyperplasia	23.6
Urethra	23.4
Infection	21.2
Calculus	1.8
Others	0.4
Essential Hematuria	44.0

(Source: Greene LF, O'Shaughnessy EJ Jr, Hendricks ED: Study of 500 patients with asymptomatic microhematuria. JAMA 161:610, 1956)

WORKUP

A repeat urinalysis is worthwhile in patients suspected of having a self-limited or trivial cause for their hematuria, such as low-grade infection, menstrual period, or vigorous exercise. However, in the absence of a good explanation, the finding of an abnormal number of red blood cells on a urinalysis should be taken seriously, even if a repeat urine is clear. A urinary tract malignancy may present in just this manner.

History is of paramount importance in narrowing the scope of the workup. History of trauma ought to direct attention to possible renal, ureteral, or urethral injury. Massive hematuria is usually associated with bladder neoplasm, benign prostatic hypertrophy, or trauma. Passage of large bulky clots implicates the bladder as the source, while long shoestring-shaped clots suggest a ureteral origin. Past history of analgesic excess makes analgesic nephropathy a possibility. A prior history of nephritis requires consideration of chronic nephritis as the etiology of the hematuria. Family history of renal diseases may suggest polycystic kidney disease or hereditary ne-

phritis. Harmless, self-limited forms of microscopic hematuria are suggested by a recent history of strenuous exercise, long-distance running, or a minor febrile illness.

Physical Examination should include observation of any fever, hypertension, rash, purpura, petechiae, friction rub, heart murmur, or joint swelling. Presence of hypertension suggests renal parenchymal disease. The abdomen has to be examined carefully for enlargement of one or both kidneys, liver, or spleen. Thorough examination of the prostate in the male and the pelvis in the female is essential.

Laboratory Testing begins with a careful examination of the *urinary sediment.* Presence of white cells and bacteria favors a diagnosis of cystitis; white cell casts imply the presence of pyelonephritis or interstitial nephritis. Red cell casts strongly suggest glomerulonephritis. A urine specimen should be sent for routine *culture* when there is pyuria (see Chapter 132). Culture for urine acid-fast bacillus needs to be obtained if sterile pyuria and hematuria persist.

The need for further workup is determined by the probability of important underlying pathology. For example, a patient over age 50 is at increased risk for urinary tract cancer; it must be ruled out. On the other hand, an otherwise healthy young patient with an unremarkable history, a normal physical examination, and a benign urinary sediment need not undergo invasive testing, since the likelihood of malignancy or other serious pathology is low. In a major population study, the frequency of clinically significant urologic disease in patients with asymptomatic microscopic hematuria was 2.3% with only 0.5% having bladder or renal cell carcinoma; malignant lesions were found almost exclusively in patients over the age of 50.

A *three-glass test* (see Chapter 137) can be done to attempt to identify the site of the bleeding. Initial hematuria is usually associated with anterior urethral lesions such as stenosis and urethritis. Terminal hematuria usually arises from a lesion in the posterior urethra, bladder neck, or trigone. Total hematuria is associated with lesions at the level of the bladder or above.

Renal function is checked when there is suspicion of renal parenchymal disease. In those with proteinuria, a *24-hour urine collection* for *creatinine* and *protein* determinations should be done to assess renal function and quantitatively assess the degree of proteinuria. Heavy proteinuria (greater than 3 g per 24 hours) is usually associated with glomerular lesions (see Chapter 128). In the presence of renal colic, the urine should routinely be strained to detect the presence of calculi or papillae. Three, first-void morning urine specimens are sent for *cytology* in patients over age 40 with hematuria, because such people are at increased risk for a neoplasm. Normal cytologies do not rule out a malignancy (see Chapter 126); cystoscopy is indicated if suspicion remains. *Flat plate* and *upright films* of the abdomen are obtained and carefully examined to ascertain renal size and detect the presence of calcifications.

If these tests fail to define the origin of the hematuria, an *intravenous pyelogram* with *nephrotomograms* should be done. Renal and ureteral abnormalities can be defined accurately. A *postvoid film* should be obtained to assess the amount of postvoid residual urine in order to estimate the degree of bladder neck obstruction. *Ultrasonography* or *computerized body tomography* are useful to differentiate a solid mass from a cystic lesion if the differentiation cannot be made on nephrotomograms. *Renal angiography* is reserved for evaluation of possible renal trauma, suspicious renal masses, and possible arteriovenous malformations.

If there is clinical evidence of glomerular disease (red cell casts, heavy proteinuria), *immunologic studies* should be performed and a renal biopsy considered. The immunologic tests of diagnostic use include ANA, anti-DNA antibodies, and complement levels (C_3, C_4) for the diagnosis of systemic lupus erythematosus (see Chapter 128); ASLO titer, antistreptokinase, antihyaluronidase, and complement levels for the diagnosis of poststreptococcal glomerulonephritis; serum and urine immunoelectrophoresis for the diagnosis of multiple myeloma; serum IgA level for patients suspected of having Berger's disease (IgA nephropathy) or Henoch-Schonlein purpura; and serum antiglomerular basement membrane antibodies for patients suspected of having Goodpasture's syndrome.

INDICATIONS FOR REFERRAL

In a patient over age 50, if a distinct lesion is still not defined or there is suspicion of a bladder lesion, it is necessary to proceed to *cystoscopy* (see Chapter 126). The procedure is particularly useful during periods of active bleeding. Careful examination of the ureteral orifices for bleeding and biopsy of suspicious lesions are essential.

Referral to the nephrologist for consideration of *renal biopsy* should be carried out in patients with evidence of glomerulonephritis. Renal biopsy is indicated only for the establishment of a diagnosis that will affect the selection of therapy (see Chapter 128) and should be reserved for patients with clinical evidence of glomerular disease. Rarely, renal biopsies may be indicated if the preceding studies have not led to a diagnosis.

PATIENT EDUCATION

It is essential to impress on the patient the necessity of a complete evaluation of hematuria. The high incidence of potentially curable neoplasms in patients over the age of 50 (see Chapter 141) makes thorough investigation in this group mandatory.

ANNOTATED BIBLIOGRAPHY

Chen BT, Ooi BS, Tan KK et al: Causes of recurrent hematuria. Q J Med 41:141, 1972 (*Series of 82 patients.*)

Froom P, Ribak J, Benbasset J: Significance of microhematuria in young adults. Br Med J 288:20, 1984 (*One thousand members of the Israeli Air Force were studied for 15 years, showing 387 incidences of microhematuria; 161 individuals had microhematuria on two more occasions, 58 of whom had persistent changes and were studied, including an IVP, which found 6 cases of urolithiasis. Only one case of malignancy was found during this 15-year follow up.*)

Greene LF, O'Shaughnessy EJ Jr, Hendricks ED: Study of 500 patients with asymptomatic microhematuria. JAMA 161:610, 1956 (*Diagnoses in 500 cases of microscopic hematuria.*)

Kincaide-Smith P: Exercise-related hematuria. Br Med J 285:1595, 1982 (*A succinct review of this relatively common phenomenon.*)

Koehler PR, Kyaw MM: Hematuria. Symp Radiol Intern Med 59: 201, 1975 (*Radiologic evaluation of patients with hematuria.*)

Kudish HG: Determining the cause of hematuria. Postgrad Med 58: 118, 1975 (*Good overview of etiologies and diagnostic considerations.*)

Lee LW, Davis E et al: Gross urinary hemorrhage: A symptom, not a disease. JAMA 153:782, 1953 (*Diagnosis in 1000 cases of gross hematuria.*)

Mohr DN, Offord KP, Owen RA et al: Asymptomatic microhematuria and urologic disease: A population-base study. JAMA 256: 224, 1986 (*Asymptomatic microhematuria was found in 13% of adult men and postmenopausal women in Rochester, Minnesota. The frequency of serious urologic disease was only 2.3% with fewer than 1% with a malignancy. Serious disease tended to be associated with a high grade of hematuria.*)

128

Evaluation of the Patient with Proteinuria

LESLIE S.-T. FANG, M.D.

Normal individuals excrete less than 150 mg of urinary protein each day; the mean is 40 mg to 50 mg. Excretion in excess of 150 mg per 24 hours is classified as clinically significant proteinuria. Causes range from benign conditions, such as exercise and orthostatic proteinurias, to glomerulonephritis with rapidly deteriorating renal function. Office evaluation is frequently prompted by an incidental finding of proteinuria on routine urinalysis. The objective of the outpatient workup is to establish the presence of significant proteinuria, search noninvasively for treatable underlying conditions, and select patients who need referral for renal biopsy.

PATHOPHYSIOLOGY AND CLINICAL PRESENTATION

Small amounts of protein (2 mg–8 mg per 100 ml) are normally found in the urine of healthy individuals, but at a concentration below that detectable by routine methods. Two thirds of this protein is low-molecular-weight globulin of serum origin; the remainder is albumin and nonserum protein.

Significant proteinuria can occur through a number of mechanisms:

1. Increased glomerular permeability;
2. Increased production of abnormal proteins small enough to pass freely through the glomerulus (*e.g.,* Bence Jones protein);
3. Decreased tubular reabsorbtion (*e.g.,* due to interstitial nephritis);
4. Lower urinary tract disease, including infection;
5. Fever, heavy exertion, congestive failure, postural changes, and surgical trauma—all believed to be related to changes in renal blood flow.

Proteinuria can present as an isolated asymptomatic finding on urinalysis, as edema of unknown etiology, or as part of the clinical picture in a patient with known renal or systematic disease. Patients excreting less than 2 g of protein daily are more likely to be *asymptomatic.* Asymptomatic proteinuria in young, healthy individuals (especially men) may be related to *posture.* In such cases, a substantially greater fraction of protein is excreted in the upright position than when recumbent. The finding may be evanescent or persistent. Even when persistent and accompanied by minor glomerular changes, the condition has an excellent prognosis as long as there are no associated abnormalities of the urine sediment. In many individuals with fixed or persistent postural proteinuria, the condition resolves after a few years; in others it remains. Long-term (20-year) follow-up studies of patients with fixed orthostatic proteinuria show no development of progressive renal impairment.

Heavy proteinuria can lead to progressive declines in the serum albumin level and plasma oncotic pressure and formation of *edema.* When more than 3.5 g of protein are excreted per day and the serum albumin falls to less than 3.0 g per 100 ml, *nephrotic syndrome* is said to be present. Serum cholesterol is often increased in these patients, and lipiduria is common. Clinically, the edema that forms usually begins in the medial aspect of the ankles, but on occasion there may only be *periorbital puffiness.*

Other presenting symptoms reflect associated renal dysfunction or underlying systemic diseases.

DIFFERENTIAL DIAGNOSIS

Asymptomatic Proteinuria. Proteinuria without other abnormalities in an asymptomatic patient can be transient or persistent (see Table 128-1). *Transient* proteinuria can occur in association with exercise, orthostatic changes, lower urinary tract diseases, and occasionally fever or congestive failure. *Persistent* proteinuria occurs in patients with mild glomerular or tubular pathology.

Symptomatic Proteinuria. Heavy proteinuria resulting in nephrotic syndrome is usually the result of glomerular disease

Table 128-1. Differential Diagnosis of Proteinuria

Asymptomatic-Transient
Exercise
Upright posture
Lower urinary tract disease (*e.g.,* infection)
Fever (occasionally)
Congestive heart failure (occasionally)

Asymptomatic-Persistent
Idiopathic
Fixed postural type
Mild glomerular injury
Mild tubular injury

Symptomatic
Glomerular disease (see Tables 128-2 and 128-3)
Severe tubular disease (see Table 128-4)

(Table 128-2), but can occassionally occur with severe tubular injury.

Intrinsic glomerular diseases account for 75% of the conditions causing nephrotic syndrome. In adults, *membranous glomerulonephritis* is the most common histologic abnormality seen on the biopsies of patients with nephrotic syndrome. In the remaining 25%, nephrotic syndrome is associated with systemic illnesses that can produce glomular pathology (Table 128-3). Among these illnesses, diabetes mellitus, systemic lupus erythematosus, and amyloidosis are the most commonly encountered. Rarely, marked proteinuria may be seen in tubular disorders (Table 128-4).

WORKUP

Most workups begin with a *dipstick* check of a *random urine* sample. The test is specific for albumin and can detect concentrations in excess of 30 mg per 100 ml. A negative test does not rule out significant proteinuria, since excretion may be intermittent or composed of protein other than albumin. Also, false negatives can occur if dilute specimens are used. Therefore, note of the specific gravity should be made along with the test results. False-positive dipstick reactions can be seen in patients with dehydration, gross hematuria, and those receiving large doses of nafcillin or cephalosporins. A positive test should be repeated on a separate urine sample before proceeding with further evaluation.

A *24-hour urine collection* is the only satisfactory quantitative method for determining significant proteinuria. The adequacy of collection can be judged by simultaneous determination of total urinary creatinine. Depending on muscle mass, the total 24-hour urine creatinine should be 15 mg to 24 mg kg. Recent reports indicate some progress in developing quantitative estimates of heavy proteinuria using a spot urine sample. For now, 24-hour collection remains necessary.

Once significant proteinuria is established, the evaluation is tailored to whether the patient is asymptomatic or symptomatic. In *asymptomatic proteinuria,* several urinalyses should be performed to determine if the proteinuria is transient or persistent. *Transient orthostatic,* or *exercise-induced proteinuria,* is benign and may occur in the absence of underlying disease, usually in young adults. In such cases, invasive procedures and extensive workups should be avoided. *Persistent asymptomatic proteinuria,* on the other hand, is associated with a high incidence of renal pathology and warrants the same investigation as in patients with symptomatic proteinuria.

Table 128-2.   Glomerular Diseases Causing Nephrotic Syndrome

Membranous glomerulonephritis
Minimal change disease
Focal and proliferative glomerulonephritis
Membranoproliferative glomerulonephritis

Table 128-3.   Systemic Diseases Causing Nephrotic Syndrome

Common Causes of Nephrotic Syndrome
Diabetes mellitus
Systemic lupus erythematosus
Amyloidosis
Less Common Causes of Nephrotic Syndrome
Infection (subacute bacterial endocarditis, shunt infection, malaria, syphilis, hepatitis, schistosomiasis)
Toxins (heroin, mercury, bismuth, gold, penicillamine)
Uncommon Causes of Nephrotic Syndrome
Allergens (bee stings, serum sickness)
Mechanical causes (constrictive pericarditis, renal vein thrombosis, obstruction of inferior vena cava)
Malignancy (Hodgkin's disease, lymphoma, and other tumors)
Pregnancy
Congenital (Fabry's disease, nail-patella syndrome, Alport's disease)

History. In symptomatic proteinuria, the history should be reviewed for known renal disease, streptococcal infection, drug allergies, toxin exposure, diabetes, hypertension, analgesic intake (especially phenacetin-containing compounds), urinary tract infections, and family history of renal disease.

Physical Examination. Erect and supine blood pressure should be measured, and the patient checked for skin rash, retinopathy, adenopathy, tricuspid valve disease, congestive heart failure, constrictive pericarditis, abdominal masses or organomegaly, periorbital, sacral, and ankle edema, prostatic enlargement, and signs of joint inflammation.

Laboratory Studies. Once the presence of significant proteinuria has been established, the history taken, and physical examination performed, certain laboratory studies can be very helpful and should be obtained in most patients:

- *Urinalysis* with *examination* of the *sediment* is the single most important test and should be done on a freshly collected specimen. Red cell casts indicate glomerulonephritis (though the absence of erythrocytes on one sample does not rule out glomerulonephritis). White cell casts are found in pyelonephritis and interstitial nephritis. Oval fat bodies are due to lipiduria in patients with nephrotic syndrome. A negative or weakly positive dipstick test combined with a positive sulfosalicylic test for protein suggests the presence of myeloma protein in the urine, since the dipstick is specific for albumin only. Collecting a urine sample upon arising

Table 128-4.   Tubular Disorders Associated with Proteinuria

Analgesic abuse
Pyelonephritis
Fanconi's syndrome
Cadmium and mercury poisoning
Balkan's nephropathy
Lowe's syndrome
Hepatolenticular degeneration

and another after being continuously upright for 2 hours helps distinguish the patient with orthostatic proteinuria from one with a more ominous etiology.

- *Creatinine clearance* is best for determination of renal function; it approximates the glomerular filtration rate. A serum creatinine and a 24-hour urine collection for urinary creatinine levels are simultaneously obtained. Random *BUN* or *creatinine* serum levels are less accurate than a clearance determination, but are useful for following the patient once the creatinine clearance is known.
- *KUB* can be used to judge kidney size, which may help to elucidate etiology (*e.g.,* small, shrunken kidneys suggest significant chronic, bilateral disease). *Intravenous pyelogram* is essential for the diagnosis of chronic pyelonephritis and is an excellent means of determining kidney size. It also gives an estimate of individual kidney function, based on how well each concentrates and excretes the contrast material. When creatinine clearance is reduced by more than 75%, the kidneys may not concentrate the contrast medium sufficiently for visualization. Contrast-induced acute renal failure is a risk in patients with underlying renal disease, especially in those with diabetes, multiple myeloma, and renal insufficiency. *Renal ultrasound* studies may be more appropriate in these patients.
- *Complete blood count* will identify any anemia resulting from severe subacute or chronic renal insufficiency. Anemia is also present at some point in all cases of myeloma.
- *The serum albumin level* is worth monitoring, since it correlates inversely with the severity of proteinuria.
- *The protein selectivity index* is useful for diagnosis and therapy in patients with nephrotic syndrome. Proteinuria is considered selective when urine contains large amounts of proteins of low molecular weight. A high degree of selectivity in patients with nephrotic syndrome suggests minimal change disease, which is responsive to corticosteroids.

More specific investigations for individual conditions are indicated only when clinical or laboratory data suggest a particular underlying condition. For example, if there is evidence of glomerular disease (*e.g.,* red cell casts, heavy proteinuria), then immunologic studies are needed (see Chapter 126). A wasteful "pan scan" should not be ordered initially.

INDICATIONS FOR REFERRAL

At times, the diagnosis may remain unclear, even after extensive laboratory testing. In such instances, a referral for *renal biopsy* is indicated if the result will have important therapeutic or prognostic implications. Most causes of glomerulonephritis do not respond to therapy; thus, biopsy is of academic interest only. However, at times it will be impossible to rule out the treatable forms of glomerulonephritis, such as minimal change disease and, perhaps, idiopathic membranous nephropathy. When faced with this situation, the primary physician should consult with a nephrologist to help decide the usefulness of a biopsy.

PRINCIPLES OF MANAGEMENT AND PATIENT EDUCATION

Asymptomatic Proteinuria. *Transient proteinuria* is, by and large, benign. Patients should be reassured; therapy is not warranted. On the other hand, *persistent proteinuria* is more often associated with renal pathology. However, idiopathic and fixed orthostatic forms of proteinuria that occur as isolated findings without other associated abnormalities have been found to have excellent prognoses in prospective studies with 5 to 20 years of follow-up. These patients should be carefully followed with checks of blood pressure and urine annually, and referred to a nephrologist for consideration of renal biopsy if the urine sediment becomes abnormal or the blood pressure begins to rise.

Symptomatic Proteinuria. In proteinuria associated with systemic diseases such as multiple myeloma, diabetes, or systemic lupus erythematosus, treatment should be directed toward the underlying disease (see Chapters 100 and 144). In proteinuria secondary to renal disease, therapy depends on the renal pathology defined by biopsy.

In patients with *nephrotic syndrome,* general measures that can provide symptomatic relief include *sodium restriction* and the judicious use of *diuretics.* Specific therapeutic interventions that have been of benefit include the use of *corticosteroids* and *immunosuppressive agents* in children and adults with *minimal change disease.* Recent studies have shown *alternate-day steroids* to be of some benefit in nephrotic syndrome secondary to *membranous glomerulonephritis.* A randomized prospective study indicated that patients receiving alternate-day steroid therapy for a 3-month period had a lower incidence of progression of renal disease than patients receiving placebo. Because alternate-day steroid therapy for 3 months carries a fairly low morbidity, it should be considered in patients with biopsy-proven membranous glomerulonephritis.

Recent data have also suggested that *dietary protein restriction* may be of benefit in preventing progression of renal disease. Patients with renal diseases that are known to progress (*e.g.,* focal sclerosis) may benefit from restriction of protein intake to 40 g to 60 g per day. These patients should be closely followed to ensure reasonable nitrogen balance.

ANNOTATED BIBLIOGRAPHY

Abuelo JG: Proteinuria: Diagnostic principles and procedures. Ann Intern Med 98:186, 1983 (*A terse review with detailed discussion of patients with isolated proteinuria.*)

Ginsberg JM, Chang BS, Matarese RA, Garella S: Use of single voided samples to estimate quantitative proteinuria. N Engl J Med 309:

1543, 1983 (*An attempt to identify significant proteinuria from a spot urine sample; those with a protein/creatinine ratio of greater than 3.5 were likely to have significant proteinuria.*)

Glassock RJ: Postural (orthostatic) proteinuria: No cause for concern. N Engl J Med 305:639, 1981 (*An editorial summarizing the condition and arguing that reassurance and monitoring are all that are necessary.*)

Heinemann HO, Maack TM, Sherman RL: Proteinuria. Am J Med 56:71, 1974 (*A good discussion of the pathogenesis of proteinuria.*)

Madaio MP, Harrington JT: The diagnosis of acute glomerulonephritis. N Engl J Med 309:299, 1983 (*A useful guide to further evaluation, once glomerulonephritis is suspected; emphasis is on complement levels.*)

Robinson RR: Idiopathic proteinuria. Ann Intern Med 71:1019, 1969 (*Short review of idiopathic benign proteinuria.*)

Robinson RR: Orthostatic proteinuria: Definition and prognosis. Kidney 4:1, 1971 (*Review of pathogenesis and prognosis of orthostatic proteinuria.*)

Smith FG, Stanley TM, McIntosh RM: The nephrotic syndrome: Current concepts. Ann Intern Med 76:463, 1972 (*Detailed definition of nephrotic syndrome and the renal pathologic conditions that can result in nephrotic syndrome.*)

Springberg PD, Garrett LE, Thompson AL Jr et al.: Fixed and reproducible orthostatic proteinuria: Results of a 20-year follow-up study. Ann Intern Med 97:516, 1982 (*Prognosis was excellent, with no renal impairment developing in the vast majority.*)

129

Evaluation of Penile Discharge

JOHN D. GOODSON, M.D.

Urethral discharge in the male can range from a relatively trivial moistening of the penile meatus to copious purulent fluid associated with severe dysuria and secondary urinary retention. The number of known causes is limited, and the most important responsibility of the primary physician is to distinguish gonococcal from nongonococcal etiologies so that appropriate therapy can be initiated and complications avoided. In the older patient, malignancy must be excluded, especially if the discharge is bloody.

PATHOPHYSIOLOGY AND CLINICAL PRESENTATION

Numerous bacterial and nonbacterial organisms can invade the mucosal lining of the male urethra. Slightly less than half the urethritis seen in urban venereal disease clinics is due to gonococcal infection. The patient with *gonococcal urethritis* usually presents with a 2- to 4-day history of dysuria and penile discharge. The discharge is thick and purulent; on Gram stain, polymorphonuclear leukocytes and gram-negative intracellular diplococci are the characteristic findings. Systemic gonococcemia develops in approximately 3% of patients.

In contrast, patients with *nongonococcal urethritis* (NGU) present with symptoms of longer duration, occasionally 3 to 4 weeks. The discharge is mucoid and frequently scant. On Gram stain, polymorphonuclear leukocytes and pleomorphic extracellular gram-negative and gram-positive organisms may be seen. Only 20% of ambiguous Gram stains (rare extracellular gram-negative diplococci) will be shown by subsequent culture to represent gonococcal infection.

Nongonococcal urethritis also develops from infection by organisms with low levels of tissue invasiveness. *Chlamydia trachomatis* accounts for about 40% of such cases; often female partners are found to have mucopurulent cer-

vicitis. Prevalence of chlamydial infection is greatest among heterosexuals under age 25. Most present with discharge and/or dysuria, but about 25% manifest neither symptoms nor leukocytes on urethral swab.

Infection with *Ureaplasma urealyticum* (formerly referred to as T-strain mycoplasma) is probably another important cause of nongonococcal urethritis. Although debate about its etiologic role has persisted for decades, the data linking it to nongonococcal urethritis are becoming more and more convincing. *Trichomonas vaginalis* and *Candida albicans* occasionally cause nongonococcal urethritis.

Reiter's syndrome is a relatively common connective tissue disorder of unknown etiology characterized by conjunctivitis or iritis, acute symmetrical polyarthritis, circinate balanitis, keratodermia blennorrhagica, mucosal ulcerations, and urethritis. One or a combination of symptoms may be present at any one time (see Chapter 144). Many of these patients present with a mucoid or purulent penile discharge and mild dysuria; eye, joint, or skin complaints occasionally accompany the urethritis. The histocompatibility antigen HLA-B27 is found in up to 96% of these patients versus in 10% of controls. Whether this histocompatibility antigen correlates with a predisposition to viral, bacterial, or other infections that subsequently lead to the symptom complex is still unknown.

Trauma and *acute prostatitis* can also produce discharges. A bloody discharge suggests lower genitourinary tract *neoplasm,* though prostatitis may be responsible for the problem (see Chapter 137).

DIFFERENTIAL DIAGNOSIS

The differential diagnosis of urethral discharge can be divided into infectious and noninfectious causes (Table 129-

Table 129-1. Causes of Urethral Discharge in Males

Infectious Causes
Neisseria gonorrhoeae
Chlamydia trachomatis
Candida albicans
Trichomonas vaginalis
Ureaplasma urealyticum
Noninfectious Causes
Reiter's syndrome
Trauma
Cancer of lower genitourinary tract

1). The known infectious causes are *Neisseria gonorrhoeae, Chlamydia trachomatis, Candida albicans,* and *Trichomonas vaginalis.* The noninfectious causes are *Reiter's syndrome,* trauma, and malignancy of the lower urinary tract.

WORKUP

History. The duration and character of the discharge can be informative. A spontaneous purulent discharge usually indicates gonococcal infection; a scant mucoid discharge points toward a nongonococcal etiology. Inquiry should be made concerning symptoms of localized gonorrheal infection (pharyngitis, proctitis), of systemic gonococcemia (arthritis, punctate skin lesions, sepsis), or Reiter's syndrome (polyarthritis, dermatitis, conjunctivitis).

A careful search for sexual contacts who have gonorrhea or mucopurulent cervicitis is important in the historical evaluation of all patients with a penile discharge; however, both female and homosexual male consorts can be asymptomatic.

Physical Examination should be checked for systemic signs of gonococcemia and Reiter's syndrome. Fever, punctate, centrally hemorrhagic, necrotic skin lesions, tenosynovitis, and polyarthritis suggest gonococcemia. Reiter's syndrome can be manifest by any combination of conjunctivitis, iritis, mucosal ulcerations (oral or meatal), circinate balanitis (ulceration and erythema on the penile glans), keratoderma blennorrhagica (pustular or hyperkeratotic lesions on the soles of the feet), and acute symmetrical polyarthritis (knees, ankles, heels, and sacroiliac joints), in addition to urethritis.

Laboratory Studies. Since the clinical presentations of patients with gonococcal and nongonococcal urethritis often overlaps, all patients with penile discharge must be carefully evaluated to exclude gonococcal infection. The *Gram stain* and routine *culture* of the *urethral discharge* for gonorrhea are essential to accurate diagnosis. The finding of gram-negative intracellular diplococci is highly predictive of gonococcal urethritis with greater than 95% sensitivity, while mixed gram-negative and gram-positive pleomorphic extracellular organisms or simply leukocytes and no visible organism are

suggestive of a nongonococcal etiology. A "*wet*" *saline preparation* and a *KOH preparation* should be done in ambiguous cases to screen for the presence of *Trichomonas* and *Candida,* respectively. All patients should have a *gonorrhea culture* and *serology for syphilis* regardless of Gram stain results. There is no role for routine *culture* for *U. urealyticium* and *C. trachomatis,* because such cultures are expensive and not widely available. Recent studies using *direct immunofluorescence staining* for rapid diagnosis of *Chlamydia* are encouraging. Treatment is usually begun on clinical grounds. When routine cultures and Gram stains are not diagnostic and an empiric trial of treatment for nongonococcal urethritis is unsuccessful, a culture for *Chlamydia* or *Ureaplasma* may be useful. When there is reasonable suspicion of Reiter's syndrome, the patient can be checked for the presence of *HLA-B27* histocompatibility antigen.

Undiagnosed or bloody discharge warrants *cytologic examination* of the discharge and urine for neoplastic cells and referral to a urologist for possible cystoscopy.

PATIENT EDUCATION

Patients with gonococcal urethritis and NGU must be told that the successful treatment of the disease depends on the eradication of the infecting organism in all sexual contacts. All partners must be screened regardless of complaints and treated in the same fashion as the symptomatic patient. The asymptomatic sexual partner appears to be a reservoir for reinfection for both heterosexuals and male homosexuals. The female homosexual partner does not seem to play a role in reinfection.

Treated patients should be strongly encouraged to return for follow-up culture and to seek medical attention immediately if symptoms return.

There are no firm data concerning abstinence from intercourse during the treatment period, but it seems reasonable to suggest 2 to 5 days of treatment before sexual activity is resumed.

SYMPTOMATIC MANAGEMENT

Treatment must be etiologic to be effective (see Chapter 136).

ANNOTATED BIBLIOGRAPHY

Arnett FC, McClusky OE, Schacter BZ et al: Incomplete Reiter's syndrome: Discriminating features and HLA-B27 in diagnosis. Ann Intern Med 84:8, 1976 (*Description of 13 patients who presented primarily with oligoarticular asymmetric arthritis. The diagnosis of Reiter's syndrome was suspected because of the presence of HLA-B27 in 12.*)

Bowie WR, Alexander ER, Stimson JB et al: Therapy for nongonococcal urethritis. Ann Intern Med 95:306, 1981 (*Detailed culture of NGU patients yielded* U. urealyticum *and/or* C. trachomatis *in nearly 80% of cases. Relapse rates were no different for short [7 days] or long [21 days] treatment courses.*)

Jacobs NJ, Kraus SJ: Gonococcal and nongonococcal urethritis in men. Ann Intern Med 82:7, 1975 (*Ninety-eight percent of the specimens that were definitely positive for gonococcus on Gram stain were culture positive. Ninety-seven percent that were definitely negative were culture negative. Twenty-one percent of stains that were equivocal were gonococcal culture positive.*)

Morris R, Metzger AL, Bluestone R et al: HLA-B27-A clue to the diagnosis and pathogenesis of Reiter's syndrome. N Engl J Med 290:554, 1974 (*Ninety-six percent of patients with Reiter's syndrome were HLA-B27 positive.*)

Nettleman MD, Jones RB, Roberts SD et al: Cost effectiveness of culturing for *Chlamydia trachomatis.* Ann Intern Med 105:189, 1986 (*A decision-analysis study favoring empiric treatment over culturing first.*)

Schacter J: Chlamydial infections. N Engl J Med 298:428, 1978 (*Excellent review of the role of chlamydial organisms in genitourinary infection.*)

Stamm WE, Koutsky LA, Benedetti JK et al: *Chlamydia trachomatis* urethral infections in men. Ann Intern Med 100:47, 1984 (*A study of the prevalence, risk factors, and clinical manifestations; 25% had no signs or symptoms.*)

Tam MR, Stamm WE, Handsfield JJ et al: Culture-independent diagnosis of *Chlamydia trachomatis* using monoclonal antibodies. N Engl J Med 310:1146, 1984 (*Describes the direct fluorescent antibody test for rapid diagnosis.*)

Taylor-Robinson T, McCormack WM: The genital mycoplasmas. N Engl J Med 302:1003, 1980 (*Excellent review.*)

130
Evaluation of Scrotal Pain, Masses, and Swelling

A mass, generalized enlargement, or acute pain involving the scrotum may be noted by the patient or discovered incidentally on physical examination. Patients with scrotal complaints are often concerned about loss of sexual function and the possibility of cancer. The primary physician needs to be able to promptly recognize torsion and epididymitis and to differentiate benign masses from those suggestive of malignancy, which require referral for urologic evaluation.

PATHOPHYSIOLOGY AND CLINICAL PRESENTATION

Almost all *testicular neoplasms* are malignant and of germ cell origin. The metastatic lesion may be histologically different from the primary lesion; on occasion, extensive metastasis occurs with little evidence of the primary tumor. Fortunately, these tumors are not common, accounting for fewer than 1% of all deaths from neoplasms in men; however, they are the third most frequently found tumor in men between ages 20 to 34, having an estimated incidence of 2 to 3 per 100,000 men. Incidence is increased in those with an undescended testicle and remains high even if orchiopexy is performed or the testicle is removed; the risk seems to be genetically determined.

Typically the tumor presents as a hard, heavy, firm, nontender testicular mass that does not transilluminate, but sometimes the lesion is smooth or even resilient in nature, leading to confusion with benign etiologies even though it blocks transmission of light. Although these lesions are usually painless, about 20% cause some discomfort in the scrotum, especially if there is hemorrhage into the tumor. Metastasis may result in a palpable left supraclavicular node or epigastric mass. A few of these malignancies produce chorionic gonadotropin or estrogen, leading to gynecomastia (see Chapter 99).

Nontesticular, intrascrotal malignancies are usually firm and do not transilluminate.

Testicular torsion presents with acute pain and a firm tender mass in a young patient. The intense pain may be associated with nausea and vomiting and may be confused with an abdominal process. The condition is most prevalent among adolescent boys and becomes much less common in adulthood. There may be no history of antecedent trauma.

Trauma produces acute testicular pain and swelling similar to torsion or infection. It does not predispose to cancer.

Mumps orchitis is usually seen 7 to 10 days after parotitis and is most often unilateral in association with fever, swelling, pain, and tenderness. On occasion parotitis is absent.

Cystic masses containing fluid or sperm often develop spontaneously. They are slow-growing, usually painless, and may be large and fluctuant. *Hydroceles* are cystic accumulations of clear or straw-colored fluid within the tunica vaginalis or processus vaginalis. *Spermatoceles* are intrascrotal cysts containing sperm that derive from the small tubules of the epididymis. The space between the testicle and tunica vaginalis may also fill with fluid secondary to impaired drainage or inflammation.

In *epididymitis,* which often occurs secondary to prostatic infection and sometimes in association with carcinoma of the testes, the epididymis is cordlike, tender, swollen, and palpably distinct from the testicle.

Varicoceles arise from incompetent venous valves. They occur on the left in 97% of cases, because the left spermatic vein empties directly into the renal vein, resulting in transmission of considerable hydrostatic pressure into the scrotum when the valves are incompetent and the patient stands. Varicoceles have a "bag of worms" appearance and are usually nontender; they decrease in size when the patient is recumbent.

Inguinal hernias can lead to scrotal enlargement as bowel tracks through the inguinal canal and pushes down into the scrotum.

DIFFERENTIAL DIAGNOSIS

The differential diagnosis of a soft painlessly enlarged scrotal mass includes hydrocele, spermatocele, nonincarcerated bowel herniating into the sac, and nonincarcerated generalized edema. Painful scrotal swelling is caused by epididymitis, orchitis, torsion of the cord, trauma, or, less commonly, hemorrhage into tumor. A firm, hard, nontender testicular nodule or a smooth one that cannot be transilluminated represents carcinoma till proven otherwise.

WORKUP

History. It is important to determine whether or not the lesion is painful, how long it has been present, and whether there has been any change, recent trauma, inguinal hernia, prostatitis, or mumps. A history of an undescended testicle raises the possibility of testicular cancer. Age may be helpful in diagnosis; for example, epididymitis is much more common in older patients than is torsion, which occurs in the 15-to-40 age group. A complaint of heaviness usually means tumor, hydrocele, or epididymitis. It is important for therapeutic purposes to establish whether or not infertility has been a problem, as may occur with some varicoceles (see Chapter 119).

Physical Examination. The principal task is to determine if the problem is testicular or extratesticular. The scrotum must be carefully inspected and palpated. Inspection should include note of any erythema, masses, hernias, or varices. To palpate the scrotal contents properly, one should stand to one side and use both hands, one to support the testicle and the other to feel and identify each structure. The head of the epididymis is usually situated above the testis; the body and tail run posteriorly and are separately palpable.

One should try to assess whether a lesion is cystic or solid, testicular or nontesticular. Transillumination with a penlight in a darkened room is needed to help determine whether the lesion is cystic or solid. Cystic lesions allow transmission of light in most instances, although a bloody exudate may not. A mass that appears extratesticular and cystic is most likely benign and either a spermatocele, a cyst of the epididymis, or hydrocele. If it is hard, does not transilluminate, or is reported to be steadily growing, tumor must be considered and urologic evaluation is necessary even if the mass appears

to be extratesticular. In patients suspected of having testicular tumors, a careful physical is needed because more than 50% present with metastatic disease. The breasts should be checked for gynecomastia, the abdomen for masses, and the supraclavicular lymph nodes for enlargement. Inguinal adenopathy does not suggest testicular tumor because the testicular lymphatics drain into the para-aortic nodes. Scrotal nontesticular lymphatics drain into the inguinal nodes.

Laboratory Studies. When a mass is noted, an *ultrasound* examination can help determine whether the lesion is testicular or extratesticular, solid or cystic; in uncertain cases, it is worth obtaining. Measurement of tumor markers, such as *HCG* and *alpha fetoprotein,* have been more useful for monitoring recurrence (see Chapter 141) than for diagnosis; a positive result is very suggestive, but a negative one does not rule out cancer.

A *urinalysis* is helpful in all cases for detection of pyuria or bacteriuria suggestive of an infectious process. Semen analysis should be performed only when infertility is a concurrent complaint. A right-sided varicocele or suddenly appearing left-sided varicocele requires further evaluation because of the possibility of venous obstruction or renal carcinoma; in such cases an *intravenous pyelogram* is indicated.

Summary. An acutely painful, swollen scrotum requires urgent assessment because if torsion of the testes is present, permanent damage may occur within hours. Acute epididymitis and torsion are the two main causes. Epididymitis is suggested by its occurrence most often in men over age 40, a more gradual onset in the context of urinary tract symptoms, a tender boggy prostate gland, a tender cordlike epididymal mass, or a urinalysis revealing pyuria and bacteriuria. The finding of a firm tender mass of acute onset in a young patient must be considered torsion till proven otherwise. Urgent urologic consultation is necessary to determine whether or not the scrotum should be explored. Sometimes it can be very difficult to distinguish torsion from epididymitis on clinical grounds, and surgical exploration is mandatory.

PATIENT EDUCATION AND SYMPTOMATIC MANAGEMENT

The patient with a nontender cystic, clearly extratesticular mass can be reassured that the lesion is not a cancer. Concern about fertility sometimes arises. Fertility is compromised only occasionally in a patient with a varicocele. The reassurance can be most comforting.

Most hydroceles and cystic lesions do not require therapy, but the patient should be instructed to return if the enlargement becomes uncomfortable or interferes with intercourse. The patient should understand that surgery is an option that will not threaten virility or fertility. Patients may want a hydrocele removed for cosmetic reasons or relief of discomfort. Aspiration of a hydrocele is to be avoided. Patients with inguinal hernias that are at risk of causing bowel strangulation should be advised to have them repaired (see Chapter 63).

INDICATIONS FOR REFERRAL

Referral to a urologist should be swift in cases of torsion, because surgical exploration must not be delayed if a viable testicle is to be preserved. Patients in whom tumor is suspected also need prompt surgical evaluation, because early disease is almost 100% curable. Any mass that cannot be confidently defined as cystic and as separate from the testicle should be subjected to a urologist's examination. Whenever a testicular malignancy is suspected, exploration should be conducted through an inguinal incision. Trans-scrotal biopsy may cause spillage of tumor into the scrotum and areas of lymphatic drainage. A patient with varicocele should be referred if it does not deflate when he lies down, is painful, or is associated with infertility. Referral to a general surgeon is needed for the patient with a poorly reducible hernia.

A.H.G.

ANNOTATED BIBLIOGRAPHY

Anderson T, Waldmann TA, Javadpour N et al: Testicular germ-cell neoplasms. Ann Intern Med 90:373, 1979 (*A review of advances in diagnosis and therapy, with detailed discussion of tumor markers.*)

Beccia DJ, Krane RJ, Olsson CA: Clinical management of nontesticular intrascrotal tumors. J Urol 116:476, 1976 (*Even extratesticular masses may be malignant.*)

Essenhigh DM: Scrotal swelling. Practitioner 212:216, 1974 (*A succinct review of scrotal lesions organized around the anatomy.*)

Gott LJ: Common scrotal pathology. Am Fam Physician 15:165, 1977 (*A good discussion of the diagnosis and management of common scrotal lesions.*)

Hainsworth JD, Greco FA: Testicular germ cell neoplasms. Am J Med 75:817, 1983 (*A comprehensive review with a good discussion of evaluation as well as therapy; includes 121 references.*)

Haynes BE, Bessen HA, Haynes VE: The diagnosis of testicular torsion. JAMA 249:2522, 1983 (*An important review emphasizing the importance of early diagnosis, the clinical differential diagnosis, and the value of nuclear scans and Doppler studies.*)

131
Medical Evaluation and Management of Male Sexual Dysfunction

Approximately 10% of medical outpatients are experiencing sexual dysfunction at any one time. In recent years, the primary physician has taken a more active role in evaluation and management of sexual problems as a result of advances in understanding of sexual pathophysiology and increases in the number of patients openly complaining of sexual difficulties. One is frequently called on to distinguish organic from psychogenic etiologies and to initiate corrective measures. The workup of any sexual problem requires thorough investigation from both physical and psychological perspectives (see also Chapter 225). It is estimated that up to 50% of impotence is organic in origin, a number that is bound to increase as the mean age of the population rises.

NORMAL AND PATHOLOGIC PHYSIOLOGY AND CLINICAL PRESENTATIONS

Normal responses to erotic stimuli may be organized into three categories: (1) a general response mediated by the autonomic nervous system resulting in increases in pulse rate and blood pressure and a diminution of auditory and visual senses; (2) an erectile response; and (3) ejaculation.

The erectile response may occur from one of two erectile centers in the body: the psychic (or cortical) erectile center and the reflex (or spinal) erectile center. Visual, auditory or olfactory sensations will produce erection by stimulating the psychic erectile center located in the cerebral cortex. Tactile stimulation of the penis produces afferent impulses carried by the internal pudendal nerve, which synapses in the reflex erectile center (sacral cord segments, 2, 3, and 4), and from there efferent impulses pass over the pelvic nerves (nervi erigentes) to the parasympathetic plexuses. These impulses produce dilation of the arterioles of the corpora and closure of the arteriovenous shunts, leading to development of an erection. The shunts permit arterial bypass of the corpora in the flaccid state. Adequate testosterone levels are essential to attainment of an erection as well as to maintenance of libido.

Continued stimulation of the glans results in a summation of stimuli, triggering ejaculation. First there is elevation and closure of the internal vesical sphincter, followed by expulsion of secretions from the prostate, vas deferens, and seminal vesicles. The presence of ejaculatory fluid in the posterior urethra promotes still another reflex through the pudendal nerve, which causes rhythmic contraction of the striated perineal musculature and expulsion of the semen through the urethra.

Orgasm consists of all the coordinated sensations resulting from the sequence of events described previously. The ejaculatory response appears to be a function of the sympathetic nervous system and is entirely separate from the mechanism of erection, which is dependent on the parasympathetic nervous system. Erection may occur in the quadriplegic with a cervical fracture or dislocation of the spinal cord, because the reflex center below the lesion is still intact, though the psychic center above has been isolated. This explains why neurologic lesions of the lower spinal cord involving the reflex erectile center, especially those of the sacral cord, can result in organic impotence.

It is not clinically useful to label all problems related to male sexual function as "impotence." Rather, each dysfunction should be classified according to the specific impairment of sexual physiology involved. Male sexual dysfunctions can be divided into disorders of erection and ejaculation. *Impotence* denotes the inability to obtain or maintain an erection. *Premature, retarded,* or *retrograde ejaculation* describes difficulties with the orgasmic phase of sexual activity. When there is a prior history of normal sexual functioning, the disorder is termed "secondary"; if satisfactory erection and ejaculation have never been achieved, it is labeled "primary."

It is important to recognize that most normal men have occasional episodes of erectile failure, especially at times of stress, fatigue, or distraction. Only when the rate of failure to achieve successful coital connection approaches 25% of opportunities is it proper to invoke the clinical diagnosis of impotence.

Lesions in any part of the sexual apparatus, its blood supply, or innervation may produce a problem in sexual function. Among the most tragic of lesions are traumatic *spinal cord injuries* resulting in paraplegia. Fortunately, capacities for erection and even ejaculation are often preserved; however, erections are totally abolished when there is complete local destruction of spinal segments S_2 to S_4 or their roots. Some degree of reflex erection can usually occur in all other cord injuries above this level. The higher the location of the lesion, the better the chances of a good erection. About 60% of paraplegics regain penile erections 1 to 24 months after injury. The percentage of erections is higher if the injury is above T_{11}, lower if below. Ejaculation is rare when the lower thoracic and upper lumbar segments (approximately to L_3) of the cord are so extensively damaged that the nearby sympathetic components are destroyed. Sexual sensation is abolished with transection anywhere above the sacral level. Following tactile stimulation, a paraplegic must look to confirm that reflex erection has occurred. Ejaculation can be documented only by feeling wetness with the fingers. Orgasm must be identified by feeling for perineal muscle contractions. Herniated intervertebral disks and metastatic cancer of the vertebral column, especially between T_{10} and L_5, which cause local swelling and destruction of spinal cord tissue, may produce a similar clinical picture.

A second group of common lesions involves the autonomic fibers of peripheral nerves, with diabetes and surgical procedures most often responsible. One out of four young men with *diabetes* is believed to develop impotence, and another 10% have some impairment in potency. The forerunner of erectile impotence in the diabetic is most often retrograde ejaculation. The presence of dry orgasm or milky postcoital urine augurs that potency may be extinguished within a year. There are substantial indications that diabetic impotence is due to peripheral neuropathy affecting the parasympathetic pelvic plexuses, nervi erigentes, and so on. Some observers implicate premature *arteriosclerosis* or *secondary hypogonadism.*

Surgical procedures often leave the patient with sexual dysfunction following transection of autonomic fibers. In *simple prostatectomy,* whether transurethral, suprapubic, or retropubic, erectile impotence is only occasional and is a function of age, prior potency, extent of surgical dissection, and psychological expectations. However, more than 80% of patients undergoing simple prostatectomy, regardless of the type of procedure performed, will develop some degree of retrograde ejaculation as a result of surgical destruction of the internal sphincter mechanism at the bladder neck. The surgically destroyed or the neurologically incompetent internal sphincter allows retrograde flow of seminal fluid into the bladder, producing a dry emission. Normal ejaculation will not occur under these circumstances, because the external sphincter tightens to retain urine. Simple perineal prostatectomy has a much higher incidence of impotence because of unavoidable direct dissection of parasympathetic fibers along the posterior capsule. Open *perineal biopsy* and posterior urethral reconstruction can result in impotence; transperineal or transrectal needle biopsy of the prostate does not. *Radical prostate, bladder,* or *colorectal surgery* can produce impotence as a result of surgical damage to the pelvic autonomic nerves, notably the nervi erigentes as they course through the perirectal, retroperitoneal tissues. Following radical *retroperitoneal lymph node dissection* for testicular tumors, young men may develop ejaculatory failure as a result of bilateral resection of the para-aortic sympathetic ganglia, but rarely erectile impotence. *Bilateral sympathectomy* of lumbar ganglia at L_1 will inhibit ejaculatory capacity, but not orgasmic sensation, in more than half of cases.

Prostatic disease plays a variable role as a source of sexual difficulty. *Prostatitis* may cause painful ejaculations and even hematospermia. Premature ejaculation and postcoital fatigue occur, but impotence is not characteristic. *Benign prostatic hypertrophy* does not interfere with sexual functioning. Impotence may be the first sign bringing the patient with cancer of the prostate to the physician. Advancing centrifugal growth of neoplastic tissue in the posterior lobe of the prostate may induce local swelling and destruction of the parasympathetic fibers that run along the posterolateral aspect of the prostate. *Compulsive vesiculoprostatitis* represents a chronic congestive syndrome of gradual onset, which may appear to result in progressive weakening of the quality of erection, although complete erectile impotence is not a primary part of the syndrome. The condition often occurs with habitual self-inhibited masturbation in an adult, lifelong limitation of sexual activities to heavy petting, chronic coitus interruptus with a sexually inert partner, or habitually hastened acts fraught with anxiety related to threatened interruptions. Other symptoms of this psychosomatic syndrome may include sacroiliac ache, irritating sensations in the glans penis, urinary urgency and frequency, minor weakness of the urinary stream, overflow prostatorrhea (especially after straining), and sometimes hematospermia.

Very obvious performance problems ensue from *penile* or *urethral damage.* Pelvic fractures, resulting from crash injuries in which the posterior urethra is ruptured, cause impotence in 25% to 30% of cases. Nonperformance may result from painful intromission associated with *Peyronie's disease, balanitis,* acute *gonorrhea, herpes genitalis,* or *phimosis.* Hypospadias with a downward chordee of the shaft can preclude intercourse. With *priapism,* erection may be only partial and insufficient for intercourse because irreversible fibrosis of the corpus cavernosum has occurred. A large hernia or hydrocele may mechanically interfere with coitus, although potency should be intact.

Many *drugs* can interfere with sexual function by affecting autonomic transmission or libido. Drug effects are often unpredictable and may vary from patient to patient and with dosage and duration; they are usually reversible by reducing or discontinuing the medication. *Antihypertensives* are frequently to blame (see Chapter 21), with diuretics, methyldopa, clonidine, beta blockers (*e.g.,* propranolol), and reserpine leading the list. Although most antihypertensives have been implicated, the calcium-channel blocker nifedipine, beta-blockers, which do not readily cross the blood–brain barrier (*e.g.,* atenolol), and angiotensin-converting enzyme inhibitors (*e.g.,* captopril and enalapril) appear to interfere the least with sexual function. *Ganglionic blocking agents* may inhibit parasympathetic activity from the sacral segments of the cord or sympathetic activity from the sympathetic chain. Parasympathetic inhibitors produce impotence, while sympathetic inhibitors result in faulty ejaculation. *Psychotropic agents* may also be responsible for unpredictable forms of sexual dysfunction. The *phenothiazines* suppress central sympathetic activity; they are capable of producing such side-effects as decreased libido, impaired ejaculation, erectile impotence, and retrograde ejaculation. The *anticholinergic effects of tricyclic antidepressants* may interfere with erection. Large doses of *alcohol* can acutely depress the sexual reflexes to the point of abolishing them. The chronic alcoholic is usually impotent because of either the direct toxic effect of the alcohol or the high blood level of circulating estrogens seen in alcoholic liver disease. *Exogenous estrogen* therapy may have a similar effect of diminishing the libido.

Drug abuse involving barbiturates, heroin, morphine, or methadone can result in major disturbances of sexual po-tency; most are reversible. Marijuana, amyl nitrite, hashish, and lysergic acid diethylamide may heighten the perception of the sexual experience, but do not specifically increase or decrease potency. Amphetamines, in moderate users, may increase libido and delay orgasm, thus prolonging the sexual act; however, impotence often occurs with chronic, heavy use. Cocaine increases sexual excitability in males and females, but side-reactions including a flight of ideas may interfere with sustained sexual performance. Episodes of painful priapism may develop in chronic users.

Impaired potency and reduced libido are often features of *endocrinopathies. Addison's disease* tends to lead to loss of libido and to impotence. *Cushing's syndrome,* except when due to adrenal carcinoma, impairs libido and potency after an initial period (weeks or months) of marked increase. Untreated *hypothyroidism* may diminish libido; in severe cases, a degree of impotence exists. *Acromegaly* leads to early potency impairment and premature extinction of function; decline in function is frequently preceded by a hyperlibidinal period. *Hypogonadism,* whether a result of chromosomal, pituitary, or testicular disorders, involves nondevelopment or regression of the secondary male sex characteristics along with feeble libido and waning potency. Conditions associated with *elevations* in serum *prolactin* concentration have been shown to produce impotence, even in the setting of normal testosterone levels. Reduction in prolactin restores erectile function.

Vascular insufficiency is becoming a more widely recognized source of impotence in older men. Unexplained, progressive weakening of erection can be the first symptom of aortoiliac vascular disease (see Chapter 17). Impairment of blood flow by atheromatous narrowing occurs at or near the bifurcation of the abdominal aorta and the iliac arteries immediately distal. Almost 40% of men with stenosis and nearly 75% of those with occlusion develop impotence. Some of the younger men can initiate erection, but are unable to maintain it. Symptoms of claudication in association with impotence, aortic or femoral bruits, and diminished peripheral pulses describe the Leriche syndrome.

Zinc deficiency is touted in the lay literature as a possible cause of impotence, with health food stores promoting zinc preparations. Although zinc replacement has benefited impotent dialysis patients, the frequency of such severe hypozincemia in most other patients is probably very low. More study of the issue is needed, especially in patients taking diuretics, which may lower zinc concentrations.

DIFFERENTIAL DIAGNOSIS

In a review of 165 men with sexual dysfunction seen at the Cleveland Clinic, 51% were found to have functional disorders, 47% had organic disorders, and 2% had incomplete evaluations (see Table 131-1). Peak incidence of sexual dysfunction occurred between the ages of 50 and 59. Of those

Table 131-1. Major Organic Causes
of Sexual Dysfunction

CAUSE	PERCENTAGE OF PATIENTS (N = 77)
Diabetes mellitus	41.5
Vascular insufficiency	16.8
Peyronie's disease	15.5
Hypogonadism	12.9
Postsurgical impotence	10.3
Neurologic disease	9.0
Trauma	7.7
Medications	3.8
Priapism	2.5
Excessive alcohol abuse	1.2

(Source: Montague DK, James RE Jr, DeWolfe VG, Martin LM: Diagnostic evaluation, classification, and treatment of men with sexual dysfunction. Urology 14(6):545, 1979. A report from a referral practice.)

suffering from organic sexual dysfunction, diabetes mellitus accounted for 41.5%. In 16.8%, sexual dysfunction was due to vascular insufficiency. Those with Peyronie's disease (15.5%) could not penetrate because of marked chordee or inability to achieve sufficient erection. In 12.9%, hypogonadism, resulting from low levels of serum testosterone, was a factor. In 10.3%, impotence followed a variety of surgical procedures. Sexual dysfunction secondary to various neurologic diseases occurred in 9%.

The Cleveland Clinic data represent the experience of a referral practice. Reports from primary care practice reveal higher frequencies for medications and alcohol as etiologies of sexual dysfunction, but not a substantially greater prevalence of psychological disease.

The widespread use of drugs affecting the autonomic nervous system makes pharmacologic agents an epidemiologically important source of impotence and ejaculatory disturbances. Table 131-2 provides a listing of some of the more important etiologies of secondary impotence and ejaculatory disturbances.

Many patients, especially the elderly, suffer from multifactorial sexual dysfunction. Both psychological and organic factors are often present and, in many instances, more than one medical etiology is involved.

WORKUP

History can be instrumental in evaluating sexual dysfunction, particularly in identifying psychogenic and organic causes. Since an intact nervous system, blood supply, and sexual apparatus are necessary to achieve an erection, any occurrence of erection and ejaculation, even if rare, suggests that the problem may be more emotional rather than organic. However, it is important to recognize that in the early phases of organically determined impotence, many patients retain some erectile function and are more likely to report a decrease in number of erections, rapid detumescence after penetration or inability to obtain a sufficiently hard erection for intercourse. Further confusing the issue, early organic disease almost always triggers performance anxiety. Finally, the absence of an erection does not rule out a psychogenic cause, but usually one is able to elicit from patients with a psychogenic etiology a story of an occasional erection (particularly on awakening from sleep). Thus, even if an emotional etiology is suspected, every patient needs to be questioned thoroughly in a search for evidence of an underlying medical problem contributing to or causing the sexual dysfunction. Of primary importance are a history or symptoms of diabetes, antihypertensive or tranquilizer use, prostate surgery, alcohol abuse, claudication, urethral discharge, and concurrent neurologic deficits. Detailed description of the specific difficulty with sexual performance is needed to determine whether erection, ejaculation, or both are affected.

Physical Examination can provide helpful clues to etiology. For example, postural fall in blood pressure may be a sign of autonomic insufficiency, and characteristic skin changes may alert one to the presence of thyroid disease, Addison's disease, or Cushing's syndrome. The flaccid penis ought to be inspected for tumor, inflammation, or phimosis of the foreskin and the hard plaques of Peyronie's disease along the dorsolateral aspect of the shaft. If possible, assessment of the erect penis should be attempted, especially if disease of the shaft is suspected, so that precise information on degree of chordee or erectile weakness can be obtained. Testicles and prostate are checked for size, masses, nodules, and tenderness. Small soft testes suggest hypogonadism. Intrascrotal pathology such as varicocele, hydrocele, or inguinal hernia may mechanically interfere with performance and can be readily detected by a careful examination (see Chapter 130).

The aorta and femoral arteries need to be palpated and auscultated for signs of bruits and other occlusive disease when there is a history of claudication (see Chapter 17). Neurologic assessment includes testing for pain sensation in the genital and perianal areas and a check of the bulbocavernosus reflex. This reflex is achieved when the anal sphincter contracts around the examining finger upon squeezing the glans. A positive response indicates that $S_{2,3,4}$ are intact. Other aspects of neurologic function also deserve thorough testing, looking for cortical, brain stem, cord, or peripheral deficits.

Laboratory Studies. Ordering a routine battery of tests is rarely cost-effective. Moreover, there is no single test or set of tests that "rules out" organic disease.

Monitoring for *nocturnal penile tumescence* serves to confirm loss of erectile function in the patient who reports

Table 131-2.   Important Organic Causes of Secondary Sexual Dysfunction

CAUSE	EFFECT		
	Decreased Libido	*Impotence*	*Ejaculatory Failure*
Drugs			
Alcohol	+	+	+
Amphetamines		+	
Antidepressants		+	
Antihypertensive agents (methyldopa, clonidine, beta blockers, diuretics, reserpine)		+	
Barbiturates		+	
Cocaine		Priapism with chronic abuse	
Guanethidine	+		+ (Retrograde)
Methadone		+	
Phenothiazines	+	+	+
Cord Lesions			
Well above T_{11}	Sensation abolished		+/−
Below T_{11}	Sensation abolished	+	+
Peripheral Autonomic Neuropathy			
Diabetes		+	+ (Retrograde)
Surgical Procedure			
Simple prostatectomy (all approaches)		Occasional	+ (Retrograde)
Perineal prostatectomy		+	
Open perineal biopsy		+	
Radical prostatectomy, bladder or rectal surgery		+	
Radical retroperitoneal node dissection			+
Bilateral sympathectomy			+
Prostatic Disease			
Benign prostatic hypertrophy		No effect on function	
Cancer of the prostate		+	
Vesiculoprostatitis		+/−	
Prostatitis			Painful
Penile and Urethral Lesions			
Pelvic fractures		+	+
Hypospadias			+
Priapism			+
Phimosis, herpes, balanitis		Painful intromission	
Peyronie's disease		Painful intromission	
Hernia or hydrocele		Interferes with coitus	
Endocrine–Metabolic Disease			
Addison's disease	+	+	
Cushing's syndrome	+	+	
Hypothyroidism	+	+/−	
Acromegaly		+	
Hypogonadism	+	+	
Hyperprolactinemia		+	
Zinc deficiency (severe, in dialysis patients)		+	
Vascular Disease			
Aortoiliac insufficiency		+	

total absence of erections, even on awakening from sleep. The physiologic basis for testing at night is the observation that 80% to 95% of young men experience erections during REM sleep; although the percentage falls with age, nocturnal monitoring represents the most sensitive available means of testing for intactness of the erectile apparatus.

A simple, inexpensive, yet remarkably reliable method of detecting nocturnal tumescence is the *"postage stamp test."* The patient is instructed to snugly wrap a ring of postage stamps around the flaccid penis at night before going to bed, and to moisten the overlapping stamps to seal the ring. A positive test is finding breakage along the perforations on awakening in the morning. More expensive gauges are available, consisting of plastic wires that break at different tensile strengths, which helps to determine the degree of tumescence and the strength of erection.

The absence of nocturnal tumescence indicates advanced organic disease and remains the "gold standard" for organic impotence; however, in early organic disease some erectile function may persist. Thus, demonstration of tumescence does not negate the need for further medical evaluation.

Patients with a family history of diabetes, polyuria, or urinary incontinence should have a *2-hour postprandial serum glucose* or a hemoglobin A1C determination (see Chapter 93). Many argue that every impotent patient should be tested. Because neurogenic bladder dysfunction is associated with diabetic impotence, a *postvoid residual* or cystometrogram (see Chapter 131) may be of help if glucose intolerance shows up on testing; yet doubt remains as to its role in the development of impotence.

An alternative test for neurologic impairment is measurement of *sacral nerve reflex latency time.* One applies an electrical stimulus to the penile shaft and measures the time it takes for contraction of the bulbocavernosal muscles to occur. A time in excess of 35 milliseconds is strongly suggestive of pathology in the nerves comprising the sacral reflex arc.

Many diabetic and elderly patients are likely to have underlying vascular disease. Those who report claudication or other symptoms of arterial insufficiency (see Chapter 17) are candidates for noninvasive measurement of aortoiliac and penile blood flow. *Doppler ultrasonography* is an excellent means of quanitifying aortoiliac flow (see Chapters 17 and 29). *Plethysmography* and Doppler have been used to judge penile perfusion, with the former considered superior because of its ability to assess flow in all vessels in a cross-section of the penis rather than in a single vessel. Angiography is hard to justify in the absence of reconstructive surgical approaches to the problem.

Hypogonadism accounts for a substantial fraction of patients with organic impotence. Testing for *LH* and *testosterone* is important in patients with small, soft testicles or other evidence of an endocrinopathy. Pooled samples of each (obtained 30 to 60 minutes apart) are necessary to avoid a sampling error from the large oscillations in serum concentration that can occur every few hours. A low or low-normal serum testosterone in the setting of a high LH level indicates primary hypogonadism; if concentrations of both are low, pituitary–hypothalamic disease becomes a major consideration.

High testosterone levels occur with hyperthyroidism. Patients with this finding or other manifestations of either hyper- or hypothyroidism require measurement of *thyroid indices* (see Chapter 101). Many patients with low testosterone levels are treated with testosterone replacement therapy. Failure to respond to replacement therapy may be due to high *prolactin* concentrations, which then need to be measured. Many patients with high prolactin levels harbor anterior pituitary or hypothalamic pathology.

The usefulness of a serum zinc determination is yet to be proven, except perhaps in dialysis patients. The literature should be followed to see if more widespread measurement has physiologic meaning and therapeutic implications.

Patients who report absence of normal ejaculations can be tested for retrograde ejaculation by examining a *postintercourse urine sample* for the presence of sperm.

SYMPTOMATIC MANAGEMENT AND PATIENT EDUCATION

When a specific and treatable etiology is uncovered (*e.g.,* endocrinopathy, genitourinary tract infection, medication, alcoholism, prostate disease), treatment efforts should focus on the condition rather than on the impotence *per se.* Fortunately, a number of organic etiologies are reversible and even the castrated patient can look forward to recovery of sexual function with use of replacement therapy. Most patients with *hypogonadism* will respond to *testosterone* therapy, at least during the initial 6 months of treatment. Limiting factors include such side-effects as sodium retention, prostatic enlargement, gynecomastia (from peripheral conversion to estrogens), and polycythemia. Patients on *antihypertensive medications* implicated in impotence might benefit from a trial of dose reduction, or switching to an angiotensin-converting enzyme inhibitor (*e.g.,* captopril), a calcium-channel blocker (*e.g.,* nifedipine), or a relatively selective beta-blocking agent (*e.g.,* atenolol) (see Chapter 21). A period of trial and error will necessitate patience on the part of both physician and patient.

A number of urologic conditions are quite amenable to therapy. At least temporary relief from the acute discomfort of *prostatosis* ensues from repeated prostatic *massage* (see Chapter 135). Selected patients with *Peyronie's disease* are candidates for *plaque resection* and replacement with a dermal skin graft. Ability to perform sexually may return following removal of a large hydrocele or repair of an inguinal hernia. Even *cord lesions* due to tumor can be sufficiently reduced by *irradiation* or *decompression surgery* to help the patient regain some sexual function, at least temporarily. Patients recovering from routine *simple prostatectomy* (either transurethral or suprapubic) can be reassured that potency and ability to engage in coitus are likely to return within 4 to 6 weeks after surgery.

Those with *vascular insufficiency* have yet to achieve consistently successful results from reconstructive surgery, unless the obstruction lies within the aortoiliac vessels, a condition that responds well to *bypass-graft* surgery (see Chapter 29). Experimental symptomatic therapies for vascular impotence, such as self-injection of vasoactive substances into the corpus cavernosum or use of the alpha-antagonist yohimbine remain to be proven safe and effective.

Although many causes of organic impotence are amenable to etiologic therapy, a number of leading etiologies are not. For example, *diabetic impotence* caused by autonomic neuropathy is usually not reversible, even with reestablishment of tight glucose control (see Chapter 100). The same is true for *penile vascular insufficiency.* When the patient expresses a serious need to regain his capacity to engage in coitus, the patient and physician need to discuss the option of a *penile prosthesis.* Of the three types of prostheses currently available, the simpler ones (the semirigid and adjustable malleable types) have proven the most satisfactory. They are least likely to fail and have the fewest complications associated with their implantation and use. Although it might seem the most "natural," the inflatable prosthesis has somewhat higher breakdown and complication rates (the reservoir tends to leak, infection is a risk, and repeat surgical revisions are sometimes necessary). Overall, patient and sexual partner satisfaction with prostheses are in the range of 80%, with little difference reported among users of the various types.

Most patients with organic etiologies develop *performance anxieties* when their ability to engage in sexual intercourse becomes impaired. The onset of anxiety can result in full loss of function in a patient who is only partially compromised physiologically. In such instances, patient and partner should come in for supportive counseling, both to remove blame and inappropriately exclusive psychological attributions and to educate as to prognosis and available therapy.

INDICATIONS FOR REFERRAL

Patients with urologic disease should have a urologic consultation to see if they are candidates for surgical correction. Those who are psychologically prepared and eager to have prosthetic surgery will benefit from consultation regarding the benefits and risks of implantation. Referral is best made to a urologist experienced in performing the implantation and counseling prospective patients. Patients found to have symptomatic, critical aortoiliac disease by Doppler study require evaluation by a vascular surgeon (see Chapter 29). Endocrinologic advise is indicated in patients with elevated prolactin levels, primary hypogonadism (low testos-

terone, high LH), or evidence of pituitary–hypothalamic disease (low LH concentrations). Patients suspected of harboring a cord lesion need urgent neurologic consultation. Psychiatric referral is useful when the patient with organic disease decompensates psychologically and fails to respond to supportive psychotherapy given by the primary physician (see Chapter 225). Premature referral to a psychiatrist before an appropriate medical evaluation is complete should be avoided, for it runs the risk of inappropriately labeling the condition as purely psychological and alienating the patient.

A.H.G.

ANNOTATED BIBLIOGRAPHY

Abelson D: Diagnostic value of the penile pulse and blood pressure. A Doppler study of impotence in diabetics. J Urol 113:636, 1975 (*This paper provides early research data on penile circulation in diabetics who report sexual impotence.*)

Barry JM, Blank B, Boileau M: Nocturnal penile tumescence with stamps. Urology 15:171, 1980 (*An early report of this clever technique.*)

Beaser RS, VanderHoek C, Jacobsen AM et al: Experience with penile prostheses in the treatment of impotence in diabetic men. JAMA 248:943, 1982 (*Eighty percent reported satisfaction.*)

Carter JN, Tyson JE, Tolis G et al: Prolactin-secreting tumors and hypogonadism in 22 men. N Engl J Med 299:847, 1978 (*An important report on the association of hyperprolactinemia and impotence.*)

Cass AS, Godec CJ: Urethral injury due to external trauma. Urology 11:607, 1978 (*This short paper provides statistical reference to the degree of impotence following urethral injury from external major trauma.*)

Collins WE, McKendry JBR, Silverman M et al: Multidisciplinary survey of erectile impotence. Can Med Assoc J 128:1393, 1983 (*A report on causes of impotence as seen in primary care practice.*)

Deutsch S, Sherman L: Previously unrecognized diabetes mellitus in sexually impotent men. JAMA 244:2430, 1980 (*Twelve percent of impotent men with no prior evidence of diabetes had abnormal glucose tolerance tests.*)

Fischer C, Gross J, Zuch J: Cycle of penile erection synchronous with dreaming (REM) sleep. Arch Gen Psychiatry 12:29, 1965 (*The original report of the association of REM sleep with nocturnal erections.*)

Frosch WA: Psychogenic causes of impotence. Med Asp Human Sexual 12:57, 1978 (*This article differentiates between psychogenic and organic causes of impotence and provides an easy method for obtaining information from the history.*)

Karacan I: Advances in the diagnosis of erectile impotence. Med Asp Human Sexual 12:85, 1978 (*This excellent article summarizes the use of nocturnal penile tumescence studies.*)

Karafin L, Kendall RA: Psychosomatic problems in urology. In Urology, Chapter 29. Hagerstown, MD, Harper & Row, 1977 (*This chapter provides a broad review of the sexual problems seen in a typical urologic practice.*)

Lange PH, Duffy M, Braatz GA et al: A comparison of functional and cosmetic results among penile prostheses. J Urol 131:307A,

1984 (*All three types were equally acceptable; a good paper to review for counseling patients.*)

Levine SB: Marital sexual dysfunction: Introductory concepts. Ann Intern Med 84:448, 1976 (*This paper, written by a psychiatrist, clearly outlines the emotional forces contributing to marital sexual dysfunction.*)

Machleder HI: Sexual dysfunction in aorto-iliac occlusive disease. Med Asp Human Sexual 17:125, (May) 1978 (*This paper outlines the various vascular diseases and their relationship to sexual dysfunction.*)

Mahajan SK, Abbasi AA, Prasil AS et al: Effect of oral zinc therapy on gonadal function in hemodialysis patients. Ann Intern Med 63:357, 1982 (*A well-documented instance of zinc therapy proving effective.*)

Masters WH, Johnson VE: Human Sexual Inadequacy. Boston, Little, Brown, 1970 (*This excellent complete textbook provides a thorough description of cases in all categories of sexual inadequacy. It is less technical than their first book, Human Sexual Response.*)

Montague DK, James RE Jr, DeWolfe VG et al: Diagnostic evalu-

ation, classification, and treatment of men with sexual dysfunction. Urology 14:545, 1979 (*A review.*)

Morley JE: Impotence. Am J Med 80:897, 1986 (*A comprehensive review of medical aspects; includes some editorializing, but is useful clinically; 72 references are included.*)

Oliven JF: Clinical Sexuality: A Manual for the Physician and the Professions ed 3. Philadelphia, J B Lippincott, 1974 (*This textbook is a superb manual that covers all phases of sexuality. It is well organized and provides a wealth of clinical, psychiatric, and therapeutic information.*)

Prout GR, Jr: Succinct description of the pathophysiology of retrograde ejaculation. Med Asp Human Sexual 12:131, 1978 (*This brief discussion clearly describes a common condition following simple prostatectomy.*)

Slag MF, Morley JE, Elson JK et al: Impotence in medical clinic outpatients. JAMA 249:1736, 1983 (*Of more than 1000 clinic outpatient males, 34% admitted to having erectile dysfunction; nearly half agreed to evaluation. A diagnosis was possible in more than 90%; the most common etiology was drug effect.*)

132

Approach to Dysuria and Urinary Tract Infections in Women

LESLIE S.-T. FANG, M.D.

Among adult women, urinary tract infection is the most common of all bacterial infections. Between 20% and 30% of women will have a urinary tract infection in their lifetime, and 40% of women with one infection will have a recurrence. Thus, urinary tract infections represent a significant source of morbidity among women. For the primary physician, evaluation should be directed at the detection of any anatomic abnormalities that may predispose the patient to recurrent infections; therapy should be aimed at the eradiction of infection to minimize morbidity.

PATHOPHYSIOLOGY AND CLINICAL PRESENTATION

Current evidence suggests that most episodes of urinary tract infection in adult women are secondary to *ascending infection*. Bacteria reach the bladder through the urethra and may then ascend to the kidneys through the ureters. Hematogenous spread has rarely been implicated in the pathogenesis of urinary tract infections.

Bacteria that commonly cause urinary tract infection are found in the periurethal area in up to 20% of adult women. This *colonization* of the *vaginal introitus* has been shown to be the essential first step in the production of bacteriuria and plays an important role in recurrent urinary tract infections. Entry of bacteria into the bladder through the relatively short female urethra can occur spontaneously, but urethral trauma

such as that associated with *sexual intercourse* has also been incriminated. Serial determinations of urine bacterial counts before and after sexual intercourse demonstrated significant increases following 30% of the intercourse episodes. Transient bacteriuria therefore occurs frequently in the sexually active female.

The establishment of a bladder infection depends on the virulence of the bacteria introduced, the number of organisms introduced, and, most important, a lapse in the normal host defense mechanisms. A number of *host defense mechanisms* normally act together to decrease the likelihood of infection. Normal voiding eliminates some organisms. Certain chemical properties of the urine are antibacterial; urine with a high urea concentration, low pH, and high osmolarity supports bacterial growth poorly. The most important host defense mechanism resides in the ability of the bladder mucosal surface to phagocytose bacteria coming into contact with it. Vaginal epithelial cell characteristics also contribute. Susceptibility to urinary tract infection correlates with increases in cellular bacterial adhesiveness. Abnormalities in these host defense mechanisms will result in recurrent and complicated urinary tract infections.

In approximately 30% of cases of sustained bladder infection, further extension of the infection through the ureters into the kidneys can occur. The presence of *reflux* will increase the chance of the infection ascending. Once infected urine gains access to the renal pelvis, it can enter the renal parenchyma through the ducts of Bellini at the papillary tips, and then spread outward along the collecting ducts, leading to parenchymal infection.

Clinical Syndromes

Urinary tract infections are associated with a number of clinical syndromes, ranging from acute urethral syndrome to pyelonephritis. Most are accompanied by dysuria, frequency, urgency, and suprapubic or flank discomfort. Other features distinguish one from the other.

Acute urethral syndrome (symptomatic abacteriuria) occurs in about 10% to 15% of women who present with symptoms suggestive of urinary tract infection. Patients in this catagory have fewer than 10^5 organisms per cubic centimeter on urine culture; in addition, urinalysis is usually unimpressive, with few white cells and no bacteria. These patients divide into two groups: approximately 70% have some degree of pyuria (>2–5 WBC per high-power field in a centrifuged sample) and true infection, either with bacterial counts <10^5 organisms or with *Chlamydia trachomatis;* the remaining 30%, without pyuria, do not have such infection, and the etiology of their dysuria is unknown. Only those without pyuria have proven to be truly abacteriuric.

Asymptomatic bacteriuria. See Chapter 124 for a discussion of this syndrome.

Symptomatic bacteriuria, in the form of cystitis or pyelonephritis, is the most common of the clinical syndromes. *Cystitis* has traditionally been thought to present primarily as frequency, urgency, dysuria, and bacteriuria. *Pyelonephritis,* on the other hand, is generally believed to be associated with fever, flank pain, and systemic symptoms such as nausea and vomiting. Unfortunately, numerous investigations have shown that the ability to differentiate between bladder and kidney infection on clinical grounds alone is quite limited. Studies using bilateral ureteral catheterization to directly localize the site of infection have demonstrated that many patients with upper tract infection present with symptoms supposedly characteristic of lower tract infection. Moreover, patients whose infection is limited to the bladder may occasionally have fever, flank pain, and systemic symptoms usually associated with pyelonephritis. Thus, the traditional clinical clues are, at best, imprecise for identifying the site of infection.

Recurrent infections may occur in some patients. Two basic patterns of recurrences are recognized: *relapse,* in which the original organism is suppressed by antimicrobial therapy and then reappears when the antibiotic is stopped; and *reinfection,* in which the original organism is eradicated by antimicrobial therapy, and the recurrence is due to the introduction of a new bacterial strain. Approximately 80% of recurrences are due to reinfection. Ureteral catheterization studies have demonstrated that the majority of reinfections

occur in patients in whom infection is restricted to the bladder, whereas the majority of relapses occur in patients with renal parenchymal infection.

Groups frequently bothered by recurrent infections include (1) sexually active women, who report a temporal relationship of urinary symptoms to intercourse, (2) patients with compromised host defenses because of underlying systemic illness or residual urine in the bladder, (3) patients with upper tract infections, and (4) pregnant females.

The consequences of recurrent uncomplicated infections are, for the most part, minimal and rarely result in progressive renal impairment. However, patients with infections in the setting of vesicoureteral reflux, pregnancy, or diabetes are at greater risk. *Vesicoureteral reflux* is associated with residual urine in the bladder, ascending infection, chronic pyelonephritis, and high risk of renal scarring leading to focal glomerulosclerosis, proteinuria, and progressive renal failure. Patients most likely to have vesiculoureteral reflux are those who report a long history of urinary tract infections, beginning in childhood. Urinary tract infection during pregnancy has been linked by some to increased rates of fetal complications and prematurity, especially when the infection occurs within 2 weeks of delivery. The mother has an enhanced risk of pyelonephritis. Patients with diabetes show increased susceptibility to upper tract infection.

DIFFERENTIAL DIAGNOSIS

Dysuria. The differential diagnosis of dysuria is limited to *urinary tract infections,* vaginitis, and urethritis. Patients with *vaginitis* may occasionally be mistaken as having urinary tract infection. Vaginal discharge, "external" discomfort (from urinary irritation of inflamed labial tissue), absence of frequency or urgency, and negative urine cultures distinguish vaginitis from urinary tract infection. Women with dysuria and absence of bacterial growth on routine urine culture may have *urethritis* due to *Neiserria gonorrhea, Trichomonas vaginalis, Candida albicans,* or *Herpes simplex,* although, as previously noted, most cases will be due to *Chlamydia trachomatis.* Presence of pelvic pain, vaginal discharge, cervicitis, or vesicular eruptions suggest such an etiology (see Chapter 115).

Pyuria typically accompanies gonococcal and trichomonal etiologies, as well as chlamydial infection. Patients with acute urethral syndrome and no pyuria may have dysuria on the basis of *local trauma* or *irritation* rather than infection, as may occur in postmenopausal women secondary to dessication of vaginal and urethral tissue.

Flank Pain. Patients with *renal calculi* or *embolic infarction* may present with flank pain and hematuria, mimicking *pyelonephritis.* Unlike in urinary tract infection, urine cultures are sterile and no bacteria are seen on Gram stain.

WORKUP

The pace, extensiveness, and order of the evaluation are largely dictated by the patient's clinical presentation. Candidates for outpatient evaluation include dysuric patients with no evidence of systemic toxicity or obstruction.

Acutely Ill Patients

Those presenting with fever, flank pain, and systemic symptoms require prompt evaluation for the possibility of urinary tract obstruction with superimposed infection. Such patients should be questioned about a history of diabetes, sickle cell anemia, and excessive analgesic abuse; patients with these problems are at higher risk of renal papillary necrosis and subsequent obstruction by sloughed papillae. Likewise, a history of renal calculi is cause for concern in this setting. The patient with any of these risk factors who appears toxic on examination (high temperature, prostration), restless, and markedly tender in the costovertebral angle requires immediate hospitalization and early urologic evaluation to rule out obstruction. Infection behind an obstruction constitutes a medical and urologic emergency necessitating urgent therapeutic intervention.

Dysuric Patients

History. The acutely dysuric woman ought to be questioned about vaginal discharge, external irritation on urination, or pain on intercourse, to sort out the vaginal etiologies of dysuria from those referrable to the urinary tract. Also helpful is a sexual history for risk factors of chlamydial urethritis, including new sexual partners, one with a penile discharge or recent urethritis, mucoid vaginal discharge, or gradual onset of symptoms. A recent history of gonorrhea or exposure to it should also be checked.

Physical Examination involves a temperature determination, percussion of the costovertebral angles to test for tenderness, palpation of the suprapubic region for discomfort and distention, and a careful pelvic examination, noting any urethral discharge, vaginal erythema, discharge or atrophy, cervical erosions, or vesicles.

Laboratory Studies begin with a careful *urinalysis* and Gram stain of the unspun urine. Proper collection of the urine specimen is essential; the *clean-voided technique* has withstood the test of time and minimizes contamination from vaginal and labia sources.

The *female patient* is told to straddle or squat over the toilet and to spread the labia with the nondominant hand. This position is maintained throughout collection. With the other hand the vulva is swabbed front to back with three sterile gauze pads soaked in sterile water or with a sponge soaked in a mild nonhexachlorophene soap. A small amount of urine is then passed. This is a urethral specimen and can

be saved if bacterial or protozoan urethritis is suspected. More urine is voided and collected in a sterile cup. Alternatively, the patient can be told to slide the cup into a freely flowing stream to collect a true midstream specimen. The adequacy of collection can be confirmed by examining for epithelial cells; their presence indicates vulvar or urethral contamination.

With an elderly patient, the assistance of a family member or a nurse may be needed. When repeated contamination is suspected, straight catherization of the bladder can be done with relatively little risk.

Examining the urine promptly minimizes artifactual findings. The finding of *pyuria* (>2–5 WBC per high-power-field on examination of a spun sediment) is indicative of urinary tract infection and predictive of a response to antibiotic therapy. The absence of pyuria suggests a vaginal cause for the dysuria or a noninfectious variant of the acute urethral syndrome. The presence of one organism on high-power-field examination of an Gram-stained unspun urine sample represents clinically significant bacteriuria ($>10^5$ organisms/cc).

Urine is sent for *culture*. The traditional criterion for infection has been a colony count of $>10^5$ organisms per cubic centimeter. Studies using suprapubic aspirates and catheter specimens found that half of dysuric women with "negative" urine cultures by the traditional criterion, were truly infected, although the colony counts were in the range of 10^2 to 10^5. Subsequent studies have demonstrated that colony counts of more than 10^2 obtained on clean-voided specimens from acutely dysuric women are diagnostic of true coliform infection. Many such women who previously were labeled as having symtomatic abacteriuria fall into this catagory. As noted earlier, the presence of pyuria identifies those who are infected and will respond to antibiotics.

The need to obtain a urine culture on every acutely dysuric woman with mild to moderate symptoms has been challenged. The vast majority of organisms that cause infection in this group are sensitive to the antibiotic regimens commonly prescribed (see below). Even when disk-sensitivity testing designates an organism as "resistant" to an antibiotic, the resistance is only relative and the organism is usually susceptible to the much higher antibiotic concentrations found in the urine. With encouraging results from small-scale prospective studies, some authorities suggest basing the decision to treat with antibiotics and selection of agent on the results of urine sediment examination and Gram stain, reserving urine culture for patients with a recurrence or report several urinary tract infections within the past year.

When urine culture is obtained, familiarity with important urinary pathogens facilitates interpretation of culture results. The most common urinary pathogen is community-acquired urinary tract infection is *E. coli*. Occasionally, the other gram-negative rods are responsible. Of the gram-positive organisms involved in urinary tract infection, enterococci, *Staphylo-*

coccus aureus, and Group B streptococci are common isolates. Less appreciated as a urinary pathogen is *S. saprophyticus,* a coagulase-negative staphylococcus frequently found to cause urinary tract infections in female outpatients. Diphtheroids, lactobacilli, and alpha-hemolytic strep represent contaminants.

Recurrent infection raises the specter of a structural lesion. However, as already noted, the vast majority of recurrences are due to reinfection in the absence of upper tract disease or other pathology. Studies examining the role of *intravenous pyelography* in patients with recurrent infection have demonstrated low-yield for influencing therapy. Radiographic and urologic evaluations should be reserved for patients in whom anatomic abnormalities are suspected. Currently recommended for intravenous pyelography are those who *fail to respond* to appropriate antimicrobial therapy and those with *relapsing infections.* If evidence of reflux is suggested by intravenous pyelography, a voiding cystourethrogram should be done to document the degree of reflux. Urologic evaluation is indicated when urethral meatal stenosis is strongly suspected (see Chapter 133).

PRINCIPLES OF THERAPY

Acutely Ill Patients presenting with fever, chills, flank pain, nausea, and vomiting should be hospitalized and started on *parenteral antibiotics,* with selection based on the type of organism identified on urine Gram stain. If the organism is a *gram-negative rod,* an antibiotic with adequate coverage of Enterobacteriaceae (such as *ampicillin* or *trimethoprim-sulfamethoxazole*) should be used initially until the sensitivity of the causitive organism is ascertained. *Gram-positive cocci* seen on urine Gram stain often prove to be enterococci, which are also sensitive to ampicillin, as is *S. saprophyticus.* Failure to respond to an appropriate antibiotic suggests an anatomic abnormality and the need for radiologic evaluation.

Uncomplicated Urinary Tract Infection (Mild to Moderate Symptoms). Most patients with mild to moderate symptoms and *gram-negative rods* on urine Gram stain respond to *single-dose* antimicrobial therapy, using either a sulfonamide or a penicillin derivative, which will cover more than 90% of Enterobacteriaceae found in the community. Single-dose treatment with *amoxicillin* (3 g orally), *trimethoprim-sulfa* (two double-strength tablets), *kanamycin* (500 mg IM), and *sulfisoxazole* (2 g orally) appears to be equally effective. In contrast, results with three different cephalosporins—cephaloridine, cefadroxil, and cefaclor—have been less impressive.

With single-dose therapy, the incidence of side-effects that require medical intervention is less than 2%, significantly less than that observed with 10- to 14-day therapy. Problems associated with a conventional course of antibiotic therapy (*e.g.,* vaginal candidiasis, rash, diarrhea, poor compliance, emergence of resistant organisms, and high cost) are greatly reduced.

Patients with mild to moderate symptoms who are less likely to succeed with single-dose therapy are those with diabetes, a history of relapses, an episode of pyelonephritis, more than three urinary tract infections in the past year, or immunocompromise. In the setting of mild to moderate symptoms, such patients might best be given a conventional course of antibiotics, with a follow-up culture obtained within 2 to 4 days of completing therapy. The same pertains to patients with mild symptoms and white cell casts on examination of the urine sediment.

Relapse. Patients who experience a recurrence of symptoms shortly after a single-dose regimen, or do not respond in the first place, are likely to have subclinical upper tract infection (pyelonephritis) and often fail with a conventional *10- to 14-day course* of an effective antimicrobial agent. In fact, failure to respond to single-dose therapy has proven to be a reliable clinical criterion for upper tract disease, correlating well with results from such localization techniques as antibody coating. More prolonged treatment (4 to 8 weeks) is usually necessary in these patients.

Acute Urethral Syndrome. Patients *with pyuria,* no bacteria on Gram stain and no clinical evidence for chlamydial, gonococcal, or other venereal forms of urethritis can be treated with *single-dose antibiotic therapy* in the same manner as any patient with lower tract infection. Alternatively, they can be treated with *trimethoprim-sulfa* (one single-strength tablet bid for 10 days) or *doxycycline* (100 mg bid for 10 days); the latter is effective against *Chlamydia* and gonococci as well as most common urinary pathogens. Recurrences are common in patients with acute urethral syndrome.

Patients *without pyuria* do not respond to antibiotics; *symptomatic therapy* with fluids and urinary analgesics such as phenazopyridine (pyridium) is usually prescribed.

Recurrent Infections. Patients bothered by frequent recurrences are potential candidates for prophylactic measures. The clinical setting is again important in selecting the appropriate form of therapy. Recurrences in *sexually active women* are, as noted earlier, most likely to represent reinfection with a new organism. *Prophylaxis* with a *single-tablet nocturnal dose* of ampicillin, nitrofurantoin, or trimethoprim-sulfa has proven effective in minimizing the frequency and severity of recurrences. In *older patients* with bladder distention, postvoid residual urine and recurrent reinfection, prophylactic therapy with *nightly trimethoprim-sulfa* (one-half single-strength tablet qhs) usually suffices and works better than regimens using sulfisoxazole or mandelamine and ascorbic acid. In patients with defined anatomic abnormalities, such as significant reflux or nephrolithiasis, surgical correction to decrease the severity and frequency of recurrences requires consideration.

Table 132-1.   Antibiotic Regimens for Urinary Tract Infections in Women

CLINICAL SITUATION	REGIMEN
Acutely ill and toxic patient	Hospitalization; parenteral antibiotics; TMS or ampicillin if Gram stain shows GNR; ampicillin if it shows GPC
Uncomplicated UTI	Single-dose TMS (2 double-strength tablets) or amoxicillin (3 g) if Gram stain shows GNR; amoxicillin if it shows GPC
Relapse	Same drug as for uncomplicated UTI, but continued for 4 to 8 weeks
Acute urethral syndrome with pyuria	TMS as for uncomplicated UTI or 10-day course with 1 single-strength tablet bid, or doxycycline 100 mg bid for 10 days
Acute urethral syndrome without pyuria	No antibiotics
Recurrent infection Sexually active	Prophylaxis with nocturnal single-tablet dose of ampicillin or TMS
Elderly patient with large postvoid residual	Prophylaxis with nightly dose of TMS (half of a single-strength tablet)
Pregnancy	Ampicillin, amoxicillin, and oral cephalosporins have proved safe; nitrofurantoin safe for the fetus, but potentially toxic for the mother

TMS = trimethoprim sulfamethoxazole
GNR = gram-negative rod
GPC = gram-positive cocci
UTI = urinary tract infection

Treatment of the Pregnant Patient. Treatment of symptomatic urinary tract infection in pregnancy is recommended because of an increased risk of upper tract infection in the mother and potential injury to the fetus (low birth weight, prematurity). Antibiotics proven safe for use in pregnancy include ampicillin, amoxicillin, and oral cephalosporins. The combination preparation amoxicillin–clavulanic acid (Augmentin) is recommended for use against organisms demonstrating resistance to multiple drugs. Nitrofurantoin has also been used without evidence of fetal toxicity; however, its associated risk of inducing peripheral neuropathy, pulmonary fibrosis, and hepatic injury in adults makes it a less preferrable choice.

THERAPEUTIC RECOMMENDATIONS

Table 132-1 summarizes therapeutic recommendations for urinary tract infections.

INDICATIONS FOR REFERRAL OR ADMISSION

Hospitalization is indicated in patients with severe symptoms such as rigors, high fever, flank pain, nausea, and vomiting. Patients with suspected obstruction and those unable to maintain oral intake also require hospitalization. Referral to a urologist is indicated if a surgically correctable anatomic abnormality is detected or suspected.

PATIENT EDUCATION

Certain general measures are important in minimizing the possibility of recurrent infection. The patients should be instructed about increasing fluid intake during symptomatic periods and maintaining urine flow around the clock. Patients with urinary tract infections temporally related to sexual intercourse would probably benefit from voiding after intercourse. Those with relapses and reinfections should be convinced of the importance of the follow-up visits for repeat urinalysis and culture after each course of therapy.

ANNOTATED BIBLIOGRAPHY

Fowler JE, Pulaski ET: Excretory urography, cystography and cystoscopy in the evaluation of women with urinary tract infection. N Engl J Med 304:462, 1986 (*A prospective study showing a very low yield for such studies in the evaluation of women with two or more recent infections.*)

Komaroff AL: Acute dysuria in women. N Engl J Med 310:368, 1984 (*A useful review that emphasizes the importance of pyuria as a sign of infection and a predictor of response to therapy; good discussion of the acute urethral syndrome; 106 references are included.*)

Komaroff AL: Diagnostic decision: Urinalysis and urine culture in women with dysuria. Ann Intern Med 104:212, 1986 (*Argues that the urinalysis is the most reliable indicator of treatable infection, with urine culture of limited value except in cases of suspected upper tract infection.*)

Kunin CM: Duration of treatment of urinary tract infection. Am J Med 71:849, 1981 (*A thoughtful discussion that emphasizes matching duration of treatment with the natural history and consequences of the infection.*)

Latham RH, Running K, Stamm WE: Urinary tract infections in young adult women caused by staphylococcus saprophyticus. JAMA 250:3063, 1983 (S. saprophyticus *was the second most common cause of UTIs, accounting for 11% among 72 college women.*)

Schaeffer AJ, Jones JM, Dunn JK: Association of in vitro escherichia coli adherence to vaginal and buccal epithelial cells with susceptibility of women to recurrent urinary tract infection. N Engl J Med 304:1062, 1981 (*Data suggesting that susceptibility may be related to factors other than the structural abnormalities that clinicians often look for.*)

Stamm WE, Counts GW, Running KR et al: Diagnosis of coliform infection in acutely dysuric women. N Engl J Med 307:463, 1982 (*Argues that 10^5 organisms/cc is too insensitive a criterion for infection in this setting.*)

Stamm WE, Running K, McKevitt et al: Treatment of acute urethral syndrome in women. N Engl J Med 304:956, 1981 (*A placebo-controlled study documenting the efficacy of doxycycline.*)

Stamm WE, Wagner KF, Cimsel R et al: Causes of the acute urethral syndrome in women. N Engl J Med 303:409, 1980 (*Patients with pyuria had infection with coliforms,* S. saprophyticus, *or C. trachomatis:* those without pyuria had no organism isolated.)

Stamm WE, Counts GW, Wagner KF et al: Antimicrobial prophylaxis of recurrent urinary tract infections. Ann Intern Med 92:770, 1980 (*Prophylaxis with trimethoprim-sulfa, trimethoprim, and nitrofurantoin were compared with placebo in a double-blind trial. All agents proved effective and well-tolerated, and did not produce the emergence of resistant strains of* E. coli.; *however, once prophylaxis was stopped, there was no residual prophylactic benefit.*)

Stamm WE, McKevitt M, Counts GW: Is antimicrobial prophylaxis of urinary tract infections cost effective? Ann Intern Med 94:251, 1981 (*Prophylaxis became cost-effective when women had three infections per year and the cost per office visit was $42.*)

133
Approach to Incontinence and Other Forms of Lower Urinary Tract Dysfunction

JOHN D. GOODSON, M.D.

Patients with lower urinary tract dysfunction may present with incontinence, hesitancy, dribbling, loss of stream volume or force, frequency, or urgency. Such complaints are particularly prevalent among the elderly and a common problem in primary care practice. An efficient and parsimonious evaluation strategy is essential, given the large number of possible etiologies and available studies.

Incontinence can have a major impact on one's life and family. At the least, it is an embarrassment and inconvenience. Constant incontinence can predispose to local skin breakdown, serious infection, and social isolation. The primary physician must be attuned to the nature of the problem and the needs of the patient and family, to design and implement an effective treatment program. Substantial progress has been made in the management of incontinence, and one should be familiar with available treatment strategies and their indications.

PATHOPHYSIOLOGY AND CLINICAL PRESENTATION

The detrusor muscle of the bladder is normally under simultaneous sympathetic and parasympathetic control. During the *filling* phase, *sympathetic* tone predominates while parasympathetic tone is inhibited. The internal bladder sphincter tightens under alpha-adrenergic influence, and the detrusor relaxes under beta-adrenergic influence. During voluntary *emptying, parasympathetic* stimulation produces detrusor contraction; at the same time sympathetic tone decreases, the external sphincter of the pelvic floor relaxes, and abdominal muscles tighten. Normally the urethra is oriented to the bladder so as to facilitate continence. With the initiation of voluntary voiding, the urethrovesicular angle changes so as to permit full drainage. Complete bladder emptying depends on unimpeded flow.

The process of voiding usually begins with a sensation of bladder fullness mediated by proprioceptive fibers in the detrusor. A reflex arc between the detrusor and the brain stem initiates and amplifies bladder contraction by parasympathetic stimulation. This arc is under cortical inhibition. Voiding occurs with the release of inhibition and voluntary relaxation of the pelvic external sphincter.

Incontinence. The pathophysiology and clinical presentations of incontinence can be divided on clinical and mechanistic grounds into catagories of detrusor instability, sphincter or pelvic incompetence (stress incontinence), reflex incontinence, overflow incontinence, and functional incontinence. Clinically, two or more processes frequently coexist to varying degrees in the same patient.

Detrusor instability is characterized by reduced bladder capacity resulting from excessive and inappropriate detrusor contraction. For many, the condition appears to arise as a concomitant of *aging,* although the mechanism is unclear. In some, it seems to be the result of *decreased cortical inhibition* of detrusor contraction. Loss of cortical input can ensue from such conditions as cerebral infarction, Alzheimer's disease, brain tumor, and Parkinson's disease. For others, the detrusor overactivity is linked to *bladder irritation* from such causes as trigonitis (a common accompaniment of cystitis), chronic interstitial cystitis, postradiation fibrosis, and detrusor hypertrophy from outflow tract obstruction. Patients note a few moments of warning, frequent episodes of urgency, moderate to large volumes, and nocturnal wetting. Postvoid residual is small; perineal sensation and sacral reflexes are intact.

Sphincter or pelvic incompetence (stress incontinence) is usually a consequence of *pelvic floor laxity* and the most common cause of urinary incontinence in women. Less frequently, it develops from *partial denervation* that reduces sphincter tone. Pelvic laxity is seen as a concomitant of normal aging and after difficult or multiple vaginal deliveries or direct perineal injury. In some cases, a cystocele forms and further impedes control. Estrogen deficiency in females reduces the competency of the internal sphincter and can also cause urethral symptoms (dysuria and frequency). In men, pelvic incompetence may result from prostatic surgery, although in most the abnormality resolves within 6 months if innervation remains largely intact. Patients complain of incontinence, which occurs predominantly at times of straining (coughing, laughing, sneezing, lifting bundles). There is loss of small to moderate volumes of urine, very infrequent nighttime leakage, and little postvoid residual.

Reflex incontinence derives mostly from *spinal cord damage* above the sacral level. Interference with sensation and coordination of detrusor and sphincter activity due to inhibited or absent central control leads to detrusor spasticity and functional outlet obstruction. The patient is unable to sense the need to void. Spinal cord injury is the most common cause. Diabetes, multiple sclerosis, tabes dorsalis, and intrinsic or extrinsic cord compression from tumor or disk herniation are also important etiologies. Reflex incontinence takes place day and night with equal frequency and without warning or precipitating stress. Volumes are moderate, and voiding is frequent. Voluntary sphincter control and perineal sensation are reduced; sacral reflexes remain intact.

Detrusor hypotonia (overflow incontinence) results from either long-standing *outlet obstruction, detrusor insufficiency,* or *impaired sensation.* The bladder becomes hypotonic, flaccid, and distended. Voiding consists primarily of overflow spillage. In outflow tract obstruction (most often from long-standing prostatic hypertrophy), the detrusor is constantly overstretched and gradually becomes incapable of generating sufficient pressure to ensure bladder emptying. Retrograde flow of urine and increased ureteral pressures can compromise renal function if the condition is left uncorrected. Often, detrusor insufficiency is a consequence of lower motor neuron damage, as occurs with injury to the sacral cord or development of peripheral neuropathy. Importantly, numerous medications (*e.g.,* anticholinergics, antidepressants) can reduce detrusor tone. Distinguishing clinical characteristics include a palpably distended bladder and a large postvoid residual. Patients void frequently, especially after fluid loads and diuretics. A history of incomplete emptying, slow or interrupted flow, hesitancy, and need to strain are reported. Injury to either peripheral nerve (as in diabetes or vitamin B_{12} deficiency) or sacral cord may be accompanied by losses of perineal sensation and sacral reflexes.

Functional incontinence refers to situations in which physical or mental disability makes it impossible to void independently, even though the urinary tract may be intact. Patients with disabling illness or simply an acute change to a bedridden state may be unable to maintain sufficient control over lower urinary function to avoid incontinence. Sedating drugs in such situations may only exacerbate the problem. Patients who are aware of their condition will describe their unsuccessful attempts to maintain continence. Patients with frontal lobe dysfunction due to cortical degenerative disease or normopressure hydrocephalus may be unaware of their own voiding and, therefore, functionally incontinent. Rarely, a severely disturbed patient is deliberately incontinent.

Urinary Frequency in Conjunction with Dysuria. Frequency accompanied by dysuria is a common presentation of lower *urinary tract infection.* Inflammation of the bladder trigone and urethra are responsible for most acute symptoms. Chronic interstitial cystitis, acute urethral syndrome, and prostatosis have been implicated as causes in cases without identifiable infection, although some of these may be due to inapparent infection with *Chlamydia* (see Chapters 129 and 140). *Carcinoma* of the bladder trigone or urethra is a rare but important cause of dysuria, frequency, and symptoms of outflow tract obstruction.

Urinary Frequency in Conjunction with Difficulty Voiding. When associated with slow stream, hesitancy, and a sense of incomplete emptying, frequency is likely to be a manifestation of *outflow tract obstruction* (extrinsic or intrinsic). At first, the patient may notice only minor slowness of stream. If the obstruction persists, bladder instability may ensue causing frequent voiding of small volumes, followed later by chronic distention and overflow incontinence (see above). Strictures, tumor (especially prostatic enlargement), and occasionally stones are responsible for most cases of obstruction. In the setting of severe constipation, the rectal vault can become sufficiently impacted that it actually blocks the urethra and prevents bladder emptying. *Alpha-adrenergic agents* and *beta-blockers* can increase sphincter tone and impair voiding acutely, especially when used in patients with preexisting lower urinary tract dysfunction. *Drugs with anticholinergic effects* may interfere with bladder contraction.

Urinary Frequency and Polydipsia. When frequency presents in association with increased thirst, it suggests a diabetic condition leading to increased urine volume and the resultant polyuria. *Diabetes mellitus* is distinguished by significant glycosuria (see Chapter 100). *Neurogenic (idiopathic central) diabetes insipidus* is manifested by sudden onset, craving for huge volumes of cold water, and prodigious urine outputs (5 to 10 liters/day). Inability to concentrate the urine after overnight fluid deprivation and response to parenteral antidiuretic hormone (ADH), with formation of a concentrated urine, characterize the condition. Patients with *nephrogenic diabetes insipidus* differ from those with the neurogenic variety in that their kidneys do not respond to intrinsic or parenteral ADH. Hypercalcemia, lithium therapy, and pregnancy are precipitants of the acquired variety. Patients with *psychogenic polydipsia* may be hard to distinguish from those with nephrogenic diabetes insipidus because they have washed out their renal concentrating system and also do not adequately respond to parenteral ADH. They do respond normally to fluid deprivation, a diagnostically useful finding, although some patients with neurogenic disease respond in a similar fashion.

Isolated Urinary Frequency may be a manifestation of reduced bladder capacity, as well as a presentation of mild diabetes mellitus, mild diabetes insipidus, a minor urinary tract infection, or bladder irritation. A large *extrinsic* or *intrinsic mass* impinging on the bladder can reduce its capacity and produce more frequent urination, usually of small volumes, distinguishing it from other forms of polyuria. Pelvic surgery, chronic interstitial cystitis, or irradiation can have a similar effect by reducing bladder capacity. Patients who surreptitiously abuse *diuretics* rarely complain of frequency, but those who take them for therapeutic purposes are often bothered by the side-effect.

DIFFERENTIAL DIAGNOSIS

The differential diagnosis of incontinence can be classified according to clinical presentation and mechanism (see Table 133-1). The differential diagnosis of dysuria and frequency is that of urinary tract infection and its related syndromes (see Chapters 132 and 140). Most of those with difficulty voiding are men with prostatic enlargement (see Chapter 135). Among other causes of difficulty voiding are drugs (anticholinergics, beta-blockers, sedatives), urethral stricture, congenital valves, stone, tumor, pelvic abscess, and fecal impaction. Causes of urinary frequency in the absence of other urinary tract symptoms include diabetes mellitus, diabetes

insipidus, psychogenic polydipsia, diuretics, and bladder compression.

WORKUP

The evaluation of incontinence and other lower urinary tract symptoms requires assessment of the major neuromuscular and anatomic elements involved in maintaining urinary continence and flow. Much can be gleaned from the history and physical examination, which provide important clues to the underlying pathophysiology and precipitants.

History. For the assessment of incontinence, one cannot overemphasize the importance of a detailed history, with emphasis on the circumstances, precipitants, timing, frequency, and volume of urine loss, the presence of warning symptoms, and intactness of perineal and bladder sensation. When the history is sketchy, asking the patient or family to keep a *diary* of events and contributing factors can be of considerable help.

Several clinical pictures are indicative of mechanism. Incontinence triggered only by straining indicates stress incompetence, though an occasional patient with overflow incontinence will report leakage under similar circumstances. Patients with overflow differ in that they also experience frequent loss of small volumes without warning or straining and are bothered by nocturnal episodes. A history of long-standing obstructive symptoms suggests an etiology for the overflow physiology.

In contrast to those with overflow disease, patients who suffer from frequent episodes of urgency, lose small amounts of urine, yet retain perineal sensation are likely to be suffering from detrusor instability. Although they may have a few moments of warning, they too report nocturnal incontinence. When this is accompanied by dysuria, a search for urinary tract infection is indicated (see Chapters 132 and 140). Frequent small voidings and urgency are also consistent with a small bladder from extrinsic compression.

Reflex incontinence is suggested by a strong history of spinal cord injury, diabetes, multiple sclerosis, or dementia and marked neurologic deficits. Severe loss of cortical function is also a precipitant of detrusor instability. The patient who reports marked distress at wetting himself in bed because of an inability to get to the toilet is likely to have a functional etiology, especially if there is a history of recent physical disability and confinement to bed.

Regardless of history and type of underlying pathology, the patient and family should be carefully quizzed about medications, especially those with anticholinergic, alpha-adrenergic, beta-blocking, or tranquilizing effects (*e.g.,* tricyclic antidepressants, major and minor tranquilizers, decongestants, and antihypertensives).

Patients with isolated urinary frequency need to be asked about increased thirst, a feature consistent with diabetes mellitus and diabetes insipidus. Compulsive water drinkers with

Table 133-1. Important Causes of Incontinence

TYPE	MECHANISM	CHARACTERISTICS
Detrusor Instability Bladder infection Irradiation Chronic cystitis Detrusor hypertrophy CNS disease (dementia, stroke)	Unstable detrusor due to bladder irritation or loss of cortical inhibition	Warning; frequent episodes; nocturnal wetting; small postvoid residual; intact reflexes; normal sensation
Stress Incontinence Pelvic laxity Perineal injury Aging Estrogen deficiency Autonomic neuropathy Urologic surgery	Inadequate sphincter	Upon straining; small to moderate volumes; rarely at night; small postvoid volume

Reflex Incontinence
Spinal cord disease
 	
Multiple sclerosis
 	
Disk herniation
 	
Tumor
	Upper neurologic tract disease
	  Spinal cord injury
	  Severe cortical disease
		No warning or precipitants; severe neurologic disease; episodes can occur day and night; frequent; moderate volumes; loss of control and sensation; reflexes intact

Overflow Incontinence Outflow obstruction Diabetes B$_{12}$ deficiency Sacral cord lesions Peripheral neuropathy Tabes dorsalis Medications	Bladder outlet obstruction, lower motor neuron injury, or impaired sensation; toxic impairment of detrusor contraction	Distended bladder; hx of obstructive sx; frequent loss of small volumes; loss of reflexes and sensation if due to neurologic injury; large postvoid residual
Functional Incontinence Acute illness Psychiatric disease Medications	Inability to reach toilet in time	Functionally impaired patient

psychogenic polydipsia may deny their intake of water but do not report nocturia, a feature of both diabetes mellitus and diabetes insipidus. Sudden onset of intense thirst for ice-cold water is very suggestive of diabetes insipidus. Also important is inquiry into use of diuretics. Any excessive use of coffee, tea, or alcohol should be noted.

Those with symptoms of slow stream and hesitancy are likely to have outflow obstruction and should be checked for prostatism, stricture, stone, tumor, and fecal impaction.

Physical Examination. For the patient with incontinence, the examination begins by noting general appearance and any lack of attention to personal hygeine. A careful urogenital examination is essential and includes palpating and percussing the bladder suprapubically after voiding for distention and

masses; one also checks the *rectum* for impaction and *prostatic enlargement.* Absence of palpable prostatic enlargement does not rule out obstruction, especially in a patient with obstructive symptoms; median lobe encroachment on the urethra is often not palpable. Moreover, the degree of prostatic enlargement does not correlate with severity of obstruction.

The woman with stress incontinence should be placed in the lithotomy position and her *pelvic motion* and continence noted during cough or Valsalva maneuver. Testing for stress incontinence is best done with the bladder full, unless the problem is severe and requires little provocation. The *vaginal mucosa* is noted for presence of atrophic changes (red, thin mucosa with a watery discharge) indicative of inadequate estrogenization. A *bimanual examination* completes the evaluation, with note taken of any uterine or adnexal masses.

Neurologic control of voiding needs to be assessed to determine if there are any deficits above, within, or distal to the autonomic reflex arc. Checking the *bulbocavernosus reflex* tests the integrity of the arc. Normally squeezing the clitoris or glans penis will cause anal sphincter contraction. Lack of response suggests interruption. Another means of testing the arc is to note *anal sphincter tone.* Since control of the anal sphincter is similar to that of the bladder, the examiner can indirectly estimate its competence by checking the anal tone on rectal examination and by noting the patient's ability to contract the sphincter voluntarily. Loss of sphincter tone in a patient who retains sensation suggests a motor neuron lesion within the arc.

Perineal sensation is also tested; if it is lacking, yet sacral reflexes are preserved, reflex incontinence from a lesion above the arc is suggested, such as one due to diabetes, multiple sclerosis, or spinal cord injury. Patients with loss of both sensation and reflexes are likely to have overflow incontinence because of neurologic injury to the reflex arc. Incontinent patients who retain their reflexes and sensation suffer from detrusor instability, stress incontinence, overflow incontinence, or a functional problem.

A mental status examination is usually not necessary to detect underlying dementia in the patient with incontinence; in most cases the condition is quite apparent by the time incontinence occurs.

Laboratory Studies. Often a careful history and examination are sufficient to arrive at a working diagnosis of the patient with lower urinary tract symptomatology. A *urinalysis* and a few simple chemistry studies (*BUN, creatinine, and glucose*) are appropriate for most patients. Patients with overflow incontinence require a *serologic test for syphilis.* If dysuria or frequency is a problem, a clean-voided urine specimen ought to be sent for *culture.* Patients with evidence suggestive of outflow tract obstruction should have an *intravenous pyelogram* to identify the site of blockade. The test allows an estimate of postvoid residual and identifies any detrusor hypertrophy, bladder diverticula, or intravesicular prostate enlargement, useful signs of significant bladder outflow tract obstruction. *Pelvic ultrasonography* offers a noninvasive method of assessing postvoid residual and prostate size. *Straight catheterization* after voiding is a simple office technique for determining residual volume, a useful measure when overflow incontinence is in question. A volume over 50 ml is abnormal. The *voiding cystourethrogram* is indicated when urethral obstruction is suspected; it can document and localize the site and nature of the blockade.

The *cystometrogram* (CMG) is helpful in determining the functional characteristics of suspected neurogenic abnormalities. Normal individuals sense bladder filling between 100 cc and 200 cc, have a nonurgent desire to void at 250 cc to 350 cc, and experience detrusor contraction at 400 cc to 550 cc. A spastic bladder will demonstrate a small capacity and recurrent uninhibited contraction (see Fig. 133-1, line *B*). An atonic bladder will show a large volume and little contractile force (see line *C*).

Measurement of *urine flow rates* provides information on outflow obstruction and aids in monitoring for progression. The normal curve (see Fig. 133-2, line *A*) shows an early peak flow rate while the curve of the obstructed bladder manifests a delayed and reduced flow rate (see line *B*).

Patients with polyuria should be checked for glycosuria, hypercalcemia, and hypokalemia. Those with normal levels need a test of urine concentrating ability by measuring *urine osmolality* after 8 hours of *fluid restriction* (usually overnight). Normal persons and those with psychogenic polydipsia should be able to concentrate their urines to over 700 milliosmoles/liter after 8 hours of fluid restriction. Inability to concentrate requires further testing that includes measurement of serum osmolality before and after water restriction and parenteral administration of ADH. Direct measurement of ADH may be helpful.

More sophisticated urodynamic testing is useful in the unusual case when the exact mechanism of detrusor, reflex, or sphincter dysfunction needs to be clarified.

MANAGEMENT OF INCONTINENCE

Management is best guided by the mechanism(s) responsible for the patient's incontinence, the patient's overall medical and mental status, and the capabilities of the family or caretakers. However, some general measures apply to all incontinent patients:

- Restrict fluid loads, coffee, tea, and alcohol.
- Limit the use of diuretics, and if necessary, give them in the morning.

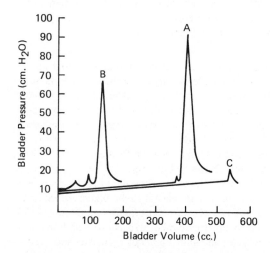

Figure 133-1. Cystometrogram findings. (*A*) Normal pressure-volume relationship; (*B*) the uninhibited neurogenic bladder; (*C*) the atonic bladder.

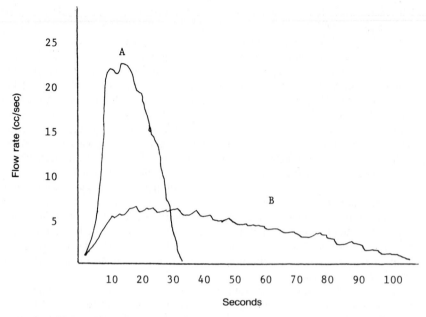

Figure 133-2. Urinary flow studies. (*A*) Normal voiding (*B*) obstructed voiding. The area under each curve represents the volume voided.

- Use of anticholinergic drugs for nonurologic purposes should be done with care and in the lowest possible dosages.
- Avoid use of indwelling catheters because of the risk of infection, exacerbation of detrusor instability, and leakage around its periphery.
- Avoid use of condom catheter, except for short, well-supervised periods.
- Advise use of an adsorbent pad for patients with refractory symptoms and recommend that it be changed frequently to prevent skin maceration.
- Prescribe drug therapy always in divided doses.

Detrusor Instability. Before initiating symptomatic therapy, one should attend to treatable etiologic factors, such as outflow obstruction or chronic bladder irritation. In most instances, the cause cannot be identified or it is not amenable to definitive treatment, making symptomatic relief the major objective. Much can be done.

- Teach the patient to void at regular, frequent intervals. Over time, the intervals can be increased.
- Provide a bedside commode or urinal for the elderly patient who may not be able to make it to the bathroom in time.
- Initiate a trial of a tricyclic agent such as imipramine (10–100 mg/day in divided doses) or an agent with both smooth-muscle relaxant and anticholinergic properties such as oxybutynin (2.5–5 mg tid). Lower doses can be effective in the elderly without inducing untoward central nervous system side-effects.

- A calcium-channel blocker such as nifedipine (10 mg tid) may also help and is better tolerated in the patient with coexistent coronary artery disease or hypertension. The choice of agent is determined in part by the patient's other medical problems (see Table 133-2).
- Agents may be combined in some situations.

Stress Incontinence responds well to a number of simple measures, beginning with exercises to strengthen the perineal muscles that terminate the urinary stream; estrogen cream can also help. Surgical approaches are reserved for patients with persistently incapacitating difficulty.

- Instruct the male patient to exercise by voluntarily contracting the anal sphincter slowly 15 times once or twice a day.
- Instruct the female patient in the Kegel exercises (see Table 133-3).
- Advise a trial of vaginal tampon use in female patients; be sure the tampon is changed at least daily.
- If there is evidence of atrophic vaginitis, prescribe a topical estrogen cream (see Table 133-2). Apply it daily for the first 3 weeks and then once or twice weekly thereafter to maintain sufficient estrogenization to restore internal sphincter tone in postmenopausal women. Continuous use is discouraged in women with intact uteri due to increased risk of uterine cancer. Oral estrogens with or without a progestin are an alternative (see Chapter 117).
- Prescribe the alpha-adrenergic agonist phenylpropanolam-

Table 133-2.   Some Drugs Used to Treat Incontinence

DRUGS	DOSAGE RANGE	ACTION	SIDE-EFFECTS	POSSIBLE CONTRAINDICATIONS
Detrusor Instability				
Imipramine hydrochloride (Tofranil)	10–25 mg qd to qid	Decreases detrusor and increases internal sphincter tone	Dry mouth, blurred vision, constipation, postural hypotension, palpitations	Anatomic obstruction, cardiac arrhythmias, hyperthyroidism, glaucoma, hepatic or renal disease, pregnancy
Oxybutynin chloride (Ditropan)	2.5–5 mg qd to qid	Decrease detrusor tone	Same	Same
Detrusor Atony				
Bethanechol chloride (Urecholine)	5–25 mg bid to qid	Increases detrusor tone	Salivation, flushing, abdominal cramps, diarrhea, sweating	Anatomic obstruction, asthma, ganglionic blocker therapy (guanethadine), peptic ulcer, hyperthyroidism, age
Prazosin	1–5 mg bid to qid	Decreases internal sphincter tone	Lightheadedness	Postural hypotension
Spincter Incompetency				
Imipramine hydrochloride (Tofranil)	10–25 mg qd to qid	Decreases detrusor and increases internal spincter tone	See above	See above
Estrogen cream (in women) (Premarin)	qd initially then biw, tiw	Increases internal spincter tone	Uterine cancer, possibly breast cancer, hypertension, cholelithiasis, glucose intolerance, thromboembolic disease	Uterine or breast malignancy, uterine fibroid tumors
Phenylpropanolamine	25 mg qd to qid	Increases internal spincter tone	Abdominal distress, insomnia, palpitations, nervousness	Hypertension, hyperthyroidism, glaucoma
Reflex Incontinence				
Prazosin	1–5 mg bid to qid	Decreases internal sphincter tone	See above	See above

ine (50–100 mg/day in divided doses) for patients who need more than exercises. The agent is especially useful in the presence of weakened pelvic muscles and following surgical instrumentation of the urethra. It can be found in most over-the-counter cold remedies.

- Try a course of imipramine (10–100 mg/day in divided

Table 133-3.   Kegel Exercise Program for Women

1. During pelvic examination, request patient to tighten around the examining finger in order to estimate the strength of the pubococcygeus muscle. Ask the patient to "stop a bowel movement" or "stop the flow of urine."
2. Request that patient repeat this maneuver and observe for effectiveness. Repeat instruction if necessary.
3. Instruct patient to interrupt the flow of urine at each voiding for 5 to 10 seconds and then to resume voiding.
4. Instruct patient to repeat pelvic muscle contraction slowly and fully 10 to 15 times a day.
5. Reexamine the patient monthly for 3 months to evaluate the effectiveness of the exercises and to assess the strength of the external sphincter. Reinstruct if necessary.

doses) for those with symptoms of both bladder irritability and stress incontinence.

- A penile clamp may be necessary in men who do not respond to other measures.

Reflex Incontinence.   One of the main problems in many of these patients is a dyssynergy between bladder contraction and sphincter relaxation resulting in ureteral reflux and the potential for hydronephrosis; the bladder needs to be decompressed, and an alpha-adrenergic blocking agent or mechanical maneuvers may help. For frequent urination, the mechanical measures and behavioral techniques are similar to those for detrusor instability.

- If there is bladder–sphincter dyssynergy, try pharmacologically decompressing the bladder by giving prazosin (2–20 mg per day in divided doses) or a muscle relaxant such as diazepam (5–10 mg/day in divided doses).
- Check for postvoid residual; if it is present, consider a prophylactic antibiotic program to prevent recurrent urinary tract infection.

- Agents used for detrusor instability (see above) may be helpful. A sphincterotomy may be required to assure bladder emptying.

Overflow Incontinence. The first priority is to definitively treat any mechanical obstruction or reversible neurologic deficit (*e.g.,* herniated disk, B_{12} deficiency), followed by efforts to reduce the postvoid residual and prevent infection. If there is a fixed obstruction, it must be removed before other therapy can proceed.

- Once the obstruction has been relieved, place an indwelling catheter or repeatedly catheterize the patient for 10 to 14 days to decompress the bladder.
- If this does not restore bladder function, then teach the patient to void while performing a Credé maneuver (suprapubic external compression) or Valsalva maneuver.
- Add the alpha-blocker prazosin (2–20 mg/day in divided doses) to reduce sphincter resistance.
- Add bethanechol (25–125 mg/day in divided doses) to augment bladder contraction.
- Monitor the effects of these agents by checking postvoid residuals; patients with a residual in excess of 300 cc require repeat catheterizations on an intermittent basis.
- Treat obstructed patients who cannot undergo surgery with a trial of prazosin as above.
- Initiate antibiotic prophylaxis (see Chapters 124 and 132) in patients with a significant (>100 cc) and persistent postvoid residual.

Functional Incontinence. The prime effort is to ease the patient's access to a urinal, bed pan, or commode. Bedside placement is the obvious solution. For more disabled patients, an indwelling catheter must be considered, especially in women.

PATIENT EDUCATION

Incontinence is a problem that can be hard for both the patient and the family. The primary care physician must explain the nature of the problem so that everyone has an understanding of its cause and no one blames the patient for being incontinent. The need to provide the patient and family with palliative relief early in the course of the evaluation makes it important to teach symptomatic measures even before the workup is completed. Use of adult diapers, pads, and scheduled voiding times, plus elimination of xanthine-containing beverages and alcohol, and rescheduling of medication intake can do much to lessen symptoms and the stress on patient, family, and caretakers. If a penile clamp is used, teaching of proper skin care is essential to prevent breakdown. If chronic or intermittent Foley or condom catheterization is needed, a strict protocol for usage must be developed.

INDICATIONS FOR REFERRAL

The incontinent patient with a suspected cord lesion or other form of neurologic injury should be promptly referred for neurologic consultation. Urologic referral is needed in cases of outflow tract obstruction, especially those severe enough to cause a hypotonic bladder and a large postvoid residual (over 100 ml). The risk of ureteral reflux and development of hydronephrosis makes definitive therapy essential. Women with refractory stress incontinence are candidates for reconstructive surgical efforts; referral should be made to a surgeon experienced with correcting pelvic incompetence. Those with stubborn detrusor instability or hypotonia are potential candidates for some of the newer biofeedback therapies. Patients with severe sphincter dyssynergy and reflex incontinence may need a sphincterotomy if all else fails.

ANNOTATED BIBLIOGRAPHY

Badenoch AW: Chronic interstitial cystitis. Br J Urol 43:718, 1971 (*Short clinical review of an unusual syndrome. The primary symptoms are frequency and suprapubic pain relieved by voiding.*)

Burgio KL, Whitehead WE, Engel BT: Urinary incontinence in the elderly. Bladder-sphincter biofeedback and toilet training skills. Ann Intern Med 104:507, 1985 (*A report of encouraging results using behavioral methods.*)

Castro JE, Griffith HLJ: The assessment of benign prostatic hypertrophy. J R Coll Surg Edinb 17:194, 1972 (*Technique for calculation of urethral caliber based on flow rates and bladder pressure.*)

Haber PA: Urinary incontinence. Ann Intern Med 104:429, 1986 (*An editorial emphasizing the importance of incontinence in general internal medicine practice.*)

Khanna OP: Disorders of micturition. Urology 8:316, 1976 (*Excellent review of bladder neuropharmacology and various treatment modalities.*)

Meares EM: Bacterial prostatitis vs "prostatosis." JAMA 224:1372, 1973 (*"Prostatosis" produces symptoms of outflow obstruction without evidence of infection. Treatment is palliative.*)

Messing EM, Stamey TA: Interstitial cystitis. Urology 12:381, 1978 (*The diagnosis of interstitial cystitis should be considered in women with persistent lower urinary tract symptoms and negative cultures and urine cytologies. Diagnosis and treatment are discussed.*)

Resnick NM, Yalla SV: Management of urinary incontinence in the elderly. N Engl J Med 313:800, 1985 (*Terse clinically useful review with considerable discussion of clinical presentation and evaluation, as well as management; 71 references are included.*)

Stern P, Valtin H: Verney was right, but . . . N Engl J Med 305: 1581, 1981 (*An editorial on the approach to workup of diabetes insipidus; underscores the pitfalls and problems.*)

Turner-Warwick R, Whiteside CG: Clinical urodynamics. Urol Clin North Am 6:1, 1979 (*The entire issue is devoted to the subject of urodynamics.*)

Wein AJ, Raezor DM, Benson GS: Management of neurogenic bladder dysfunction in the adult. Urology 8:432, 1976 (*Review of the surgical and nonsurgical options in the treatment of the neurogenic bladder.*)

Williams ME, Pannill FC: Urinary incontinence in the elderly. Ann Intern Med 97:895, 1982 (*The most clinically relevant review.*)

134
Approach to the Patient with Nephrolithiasis
LESLIE S.-T. FANG, M.D.

Nephrolithiasis is a significant medical problem incurring substantial morbidity and cost. One autopsy series estimated the prevalence as 1.12%. In most industrialized countries, 1% to 3% of the population may be expected to have a calculus at some time. The annual frequency of hospitalization for nephrolithiasis is estimated at 1 per 1000 population. In the outpatient setting, the primary physician may encounter patients with a history of renal calculi, asymptomatic nephrolithiasis, or acute colic. Others may present with hematuria or urinary tract infection. One needs to identify the nature of the stone and any precipitating factors, prevent further stone formation, and know when referral for surgical intervention or lithotripsy is needed.

PATHOPHYSIOLOGY AND CLINICAL PRESENTATION

Two major groups of factors are important in the pathogenesis of stones: (1) changes that increase the urinary concentration of stone constituents and (2) physiochemical changes.

Increase in Concentration can occur with reductions in urinary volume or increases in excretion of calcium, oxalate, uric acid, cystine, or xanthine.

CALCIUM-CONTAINING STONES. The majority of calcium-containing stones contain calcium oxalate; hypercalciuric and hyperoxaluric states promote their formation.

Hypercalciuric states can be categorized into three groups: increased gut absorption of dietary calcium, increased resorption of calcium from bone, and presence of a renal calcium leak. Combinations of these factors can be at play in certain clinical settings. *Hyperoxaluria* is less common than is hypercalciuria. It may result from increased absorption of dietary oxalate, as occurs in small bowel disease; from increased endogenous production of oxalate resulting from a genetic deficiency in enzymes in the glyoxalate pathway or of pyridoxine (an important cofactor in glyoxalate metabolism); or rarely, from markedly increased ingestion of oxalate or one of its precursors.

MAGNESIUM AMMONIUM PHOSPHATE STONES (STRUVITE). Struvite formation occurs in an *alkaline* environment and is almost invariably associated with *urinary tract infection* produced by a urea-splitting organism.

URIC ACID STONES. Hyperuricosuric states are seen in patients with primary and secondary *gout*. Occasionally, persistently *acid urine* promotes uric acid stone formation even in the absence of increased urinary uric acid concentration. In myeloproliferative disorders and during chemotherapy, significant hyperuricosuria can occur, and uric acid stones can form if adequate urine flow and alkalinization are not maintained.

CYSTINE STONES. Cystine stones are found exclusively in patients with cystinuria. These people have an inherited disorder in which renal and gastrointestinal transport of cystine, ornithine, lysine, and arginine is abnormal.

XANTHINE STONES. These occur in the setting of xanthinuria, an extremely rare genetic disorder of purine metabolism associated with a deficiency of xanthine oxidase. Rarely, xanthine stones may be seen in patients taking xanthine oxidase inhibitors for treatment of uric acid disorders.

Physicochemical Factors that have been identified as important in stone formation include changes in *urinary pH* and urinary concentrations of potential *inhibitors* of stone formation, such as magnesium, citrate, organic matrix, and pyrophosphate. As noted earlier, alkaline pH favors struvite formation, and acidic pH facilitates formation of uric acid and xanthine stones.

High urinary concentrations of magnesium, citrate, pyrophosphate, and certain anions are potent inhibitors of stone formation. Deficiencies in one or more of these inhibitors have been identified in some patients with recurrent stones.

Three *major theories* have been advanced to explain stone formation and growth. The *matrix-nucleation* theory suggests that some matrix substances (*e.g.,* urate) form an initial nucleus for subsequent stone growth by precipitation. The *precipitation-crystallization* theory suggests that when the urinary crystalloids are present in a supersaturated state, precipitation and subsequent growth occur. The *inhibitor-absence* theory postulates that the deficiency of one or more of numerous agents known to retard stone formation leads to nephrolithiasis. Evidence for and against each of these theories has been collected; multiple factors may be involved in any given patient.

Clinical Presentation is one of pain, bleeding, or silent obstruction. *Renal "colic"* is typically a constant unilateral pain, abrupt in onset, localized to the flank when a stone sits in the upper tract, and radiating into the groin when one lodges in the lower portion of the ureter. The presentation may be mistaken for pyelonephritis and occasionally for abdominal and pelvic processes, but the initial workup should rapidly lead to the correct diagnosis.

Any *obstruction* that occurs is usually transient and of no lasting significance; however, in some instances it persists and may be silent and progressive. Occasionally, asymptomatic calcareous calculi are detected on abdominal x-rays taken for other reasons. Calculi extending from one renal calyx to another (staghorn calculi) can result in renal failure.

Hematuria, especially the microscopic type, often accompanies urolithiasis. Occasionally an episode of gross hematuria ensues.

The Natural History of stone formation is still not clearly delineated. The likelihood of *recurrence* of calcium stones with time was examined prospectively in one study of patients who formed single stones. An exceedingly high incidence of recurrence was found, with a mean time to recurrence of 6.78 years. With time, the incidence of cumulative recurrence approached 100%. Recurrence took place early in half of the patients, but could take up to 20 years in others.

Other studies have found a more benign course. In one, a group of 101 patients was followed for an extended period (mean 7 years); additional stone formation was observed in only a third of the patients. These differences in recurrence rates undoubtedly reflect heterogeneity among patients in the respective referral groups. In any case, the incidence of recurrence is high enough to justify evaluation and consideration of preventive treatment.

Most kidney stones pass spontaneously; however, 10% to 30% do not, and may cause continuing pain, infection, or obstruction.

DIFFERENTIAL DIAGNOSIS

In the United States, about two thirds of all renal calculi are composed of either calcium oxalate or calcium oxalate mixed with calcium phosphate (Table 134-1). Struvite or magnesium ammonium phosphate stones occur almost exclusively in patients with urinary tract infections resulting from urea-splitting *Proteus* species, and contitute about 15% of stones analyzed. Stones of pure uric acid account for another 8%. Other stones occur infrequently and are composed of cystine, xanthine, and salicates.

The disease states associated with nephrolithiasis are best categorized according to the type of stones formed. In many instances, stone formation is a manifestation of a systemic disease (see Table 134-2).

WORKUP

In the evaluation of the patient with recurrent nephrolithiasis, knowledge of the stone composition is essential to rational management. Obtaining the stone for analysis is the single most important study; therefore, urine should be strained for stones when renal colic is present. Ideally, studies of the stone should include the use of quantitative chemical analyses in addition to crystallographic examination.

History. When there is no stone available for analysis, certain aspects of the clinical history can be helpful in the evaluation. The *age* of the patient at onset of nephrolithiasis should be obtained because metabolic disorders such as hyperoxaluria, cystinuria, xanthinuria, and renal tubular acidosis are often associated with stones at an early age; idiopathic calcareous nephrolithiasis and primary hyperparathyroidism commonly occur after age 30. The *sex* of the patient can also be helpful; idiopathic nephrolithiasis is common in males, whereas primary hyperparathyroidism is more common in females. A *past history* of stones is invaluable if their composition has been previously determined. Any prior history of systemic illnesses (*e.g.,* sarcoidosis or cancer) and any prior urinary tract infections should be noted. *Family history* of nephrolithiasis may suggest a hereditary metabolic disorder. Careful *dietary history* should also be taken to rule out excessive oxalate or calcium intake (*e.g.,* leafy green vegetables, tea, calcium-containing antacids). It is important to check

Table 134-1.   Types of Renal Calculi

CRYSTAL NAME	CHEMICAL NAME	FREQUENCY (%)
Whewellite	Calcium oxalate monohydrate	
Weddelite	Calcium oxalate dihydrate	33
Apatite, pure	Calcium phosphate	4
Mixed	Calcium oxalate and phosphate	34
Brushite	Calcium phosphate	2
Struvite	Magnesium ammonium phosphate	15
Uric acid	Uric acid	8
Cystine	Cystine	3

(Source: Prien EL: Urol Clin North Am 1:229, 1974)

Table 134-2. Important Conditions Associated
With Nephrolithiasis

Calcium Stones
Increased gastrointestinal calcium absorption
  Primary hyperparathyroidism
  Sarcoidosis
  Vitamin D excess
  Milk-alkali syndrome
  Idiopathic nephrolithiasis

Increased bone calcium resorption
  Primary hyperparathyroidism
  Neoplastic disorders
  Immobilization
  Distal renal tubular acidosis

Renal calcium leak
  Idiopathic hypercalciuria

Hyperoxaluria
  Small bowel disease
  Enzymatic deficiency
  Pyridoxine deficiency
  Increased ingestion

Magnesium Ammonium Phosphate Stones
Alkaline environment
  Urinary tract infection due to urea-splitting organism

Uric Acid Stones
Increased uric acid production
  Primary gout
  Secondary gout (myeloproliferative disorder, chemotherapy)

Cystine Stones
Inherited disorder of amino acid transport

Xanthine Stones
Xanthine oxidase deficiency

Use of xanthine oxidase inhibitor

for use of *drugs* that would promote calcium or uric acid excretion (*e.g.,* furosemide, probenecid).

Physical Examination is not particularly revealing in most cases, but should be checked for evidence of a systemic disease, such as sarcoidosis (lymphadenopathy, organomegaly) or cancer (adenopathy, breast mass, etc.).

Laboratory Evaluation should include a *urinalysis* for determination of pH and an examination of urinary sediment for crystals. An alkaline pH suggests infection with ureasplitting organisms and struvite formation. Inability to acidify the urine pH below 5.3 despite systemic acidosis suggests renal tubular acidosis. Serum ought to be obtained for determinations of calcium, uric acid, BUN, and creatinine and a *24-hour urine* collected for creatinine, calcium, uric acid, and oxalate.

Repeated determinations of *fasting serum calcium and phosphorus* are necessary if primary hyperparathyroidism is suspected. *Serum albumin* should be determined at the same time, since 40% to 45% of the serum calcium is protein-bound. If the serum calcium is elevated and hyperparathyroidism is suspected clinically, confirmation of the diagnosis

can be made by obtaining a *simultaneous PTH* determination, which should reveal an inappropriately elevated level. (see Chapter 96). If the clinical presentation suggests a rare cause of nephrolithiasis, such as cystinuria or xanthinuria, special 24-hour collections of urine should be sent for study.

Roentgenographic evaluation includes a *KUB* and an *intravenous pyelogram*. The flat-plate radiograph of the abdomen can provide an estimate of renal size and is important in detecting the presence of small radiopaque stones. Staghorn calculi usually denote magnesium ammonium phosphate or cystine stones. The latter usually have a more laminated appearance. *Intravenous pyelogram* (IVP) provides better details of any renal abnormalities that may be present, as well as the level of the obstruction caused by the renal calculus. *Renal ultrasound* examination is useful for detecting hydronephrosis, but it is not a substitute for the IVP in the initial workup of urolithiasis.

The laboratory evaluation permits identification of stones and hyperexcretory states and therefore allows rational therapy.

PRINCIPLES OF MANAGEMENT

Because of the high incidence of stone formation and its attendant morbidity, preventive therapy is indicated in all patients with nephrolithiasis.

In general, maintenance of dilute urine by means of vigorous fluid therapy around the clock is beneficial in all forms of nephrolithiasis. Between 2 liters and 3 liters of fluid need to be taken daily. Specific therapy should be tailored to the type of stones involved.

Calcium-Containing Stones. Any underlying primary hyperparathyroidism should be treated surgically when feasible (see Chapter 00). Vitamin D excess and milk-alkali syndrome are readily correctable by cessation of intake. Steroids have been found to be effective in patients with sarcoidosis (see Chapter 48).

Patients with *hypercalciuria* require *limitation* of *dietary calcium,* including careful avoidance of dairy products. *Thiazides* decrease urinary calcium excretion; and hydrochlorothiazide, 50 mg given twice a day, has been found to be effective. Primary hyperparathyroidism has to be ruled out prior to the use of thiazides to avoid hypercalcemia. *Phosphates,* in the form of neutral sodium phosphate (500 mg qid) or cellulose phosphate, have been used to decrease absorption of calcium and found to be effective in decreasing stone formation. Diarrhea and extraskeletal calcifications are the major side-effects of phosphate therapy.

Patients with *hyperoxaluria* need to have their intake of *dietary oxalate limited.* Tea, rhubarb, and many green leafy vegetables should be avoided. Dietary calcium, on the other hand, should not be restricted, since calcium has been shown to cause increases in urinary excretion of oxalate. In the rare patient with pyridoxine deficiency, replacement would improve the hyperoxaluric state.

Studies in those patients with *no identifiable metabolic disorder* have demonstrated drastic reduction in new stone formation when given *allopurinol* and a *thiazide.* In one study, *30* such patients formed 6 stones, compared with a predicted 31.8 stones, during a 1- to 7-year follow-up period. The use of allopurinol is based on the supposition that sodium hydrogen urate crystals are reasonable heterogeneous nuclei for calcium oxalate crystal growth.

Magnesium Ammonium Phosphate Stones. These are often very large and may have to be removed surgically. Acidification of the urine with ascorbic acid, along with a prolonged course (often, at least 2 months) of appropriate *antibiotic treatment* to eradicate any *Proteus* urinary tract infection, is essential for the prevention of recurrences of struvite. Controlled study of the urease inhibitor *acetohydroxamic acid* has demonstrated an ability to forestall stone growth and facilitate sterilizing the urine. However, the drug causes many adverse side-effects (*e.g.,* hemolysis, leukopenia, and thrombophlebitis) and should not be used without consultation.

Uric Acid Stones. *Hydration* to maintain copious urine flow, *allopurinol* therapy, and *alkalinization* of the urine are the mainstays of therapy. The solubility of uric acid is a hundred times higher at pH 7 than at pH 4.5, and every attempt should be made to maintain an alkaline urine by giving 100 mEq to 150 mEq of *bicarbonate* every 24 hours in divided doses. In patients with myeloproliferative disorders undergoing chemotherapy, prophylactic uses of allopurinol, saline diuresis, and alkalinization should eliminate the incidence of uric acid stone formation.

Cystine Stones. Copious urine flow and maintenance of urinary pH above 7.5 are important in preventing and dissolving cystine stones. *D-penicillamine* has also been shown to be effective, but significant side-effects may be encountered.

Xanthine Stones. Limitation of dietary purines, maintenance of urine flow, and maintenance of very high urine pH (greater than 7.6) minimize difficulties. Prophylactic alkalinization and forced diuresis should be employed in patients with myeloproliferative disorders on xanthine oxidase inhibitors.

In addition to the therapeutic interventions outlined, several other less well-evaluated modes of therapy have been advocated. Administration of *magnesium oxide* may improve the solubility of urinary oxalate. It has been suggested that *methylene blue* is an effective inhibitor of calcium oxalate stone formation. In an uncontrolled study, administration of *potassium citrate,* an inhibitor of calcium-stone formation, was associated with a very low incidence of new stone formation. The drug comes in a wax matrix formulation; other

potassium salts in such formulations have caused ulceration and bleeding in the upper GI tract.

INDICATIONS FOR ADMISSION AND REFERRAL

In a patient with renal colic, the needs for hospitalization and other intervention are dictated by the clinical presentation. Patients with mild to moderate pain can be managed as outpatients with oral analgesics, and instructed to maintain a high fluid intake and urine output around-the-clock. These patients should be told to strain the urine to retrieve calculi for stone analysis.

Patients with severe pain, nausea, and vomiting need hospitalization for intravenous hydration and pain control. In these patients, KUB and IVP are indicated to localize and determine the extent of the obstruction. In the majority of cases, stones will pass spontaneously. Patients with severe symptoms and persistent obstruction beyond 3 to 4 days should be referred for urologic evaluation.

Patients presenting with fever, chills, and symptoms of renal colic require hospitalization and prompt intervention. If the presence of an infection behind an obstructed ureter is indeed confirmed, antibiotic coverage (see Chapter 132) and surgical decompression are mandatory.

In recent years, surgical intervention for nephrolithiasis has changed with the introduction of *lithotripsy* (stone fragmentation) techniques. The stone is shattered by subjecting it to focused ultrasonic shock waves, delivered either percutaneously through a nephrostomy or extracorporeally. These techniques are less invasive than conventional surgical lithotomy and have important roles in selected patients.

Extracorporeal shock-wave lithotripsy is quickly becoming the treatment of choice for fragmentation and removal of simple stones in the kidney and upper ureters. Its very low complication rate and high degree of efficacy are rapidly eliminating the need for surgical lithotomy in the few centers where the lithotriptor is currently available. Because the equipment to perform the procedure is expensive and not yet widely available, *percutaneous* ultrasonic lithotripsy represents an acceptable alternative, and may be the preferred initial therapy for upper tract stones lodged in the ureter for more than 4 to 6 weeks. However, extracorporeal lithotripsy has a lower complication rate than the percutaneous method and, when available, is the treatment of choice for simple stones. Percutaneous methods are often reserved for large (>2.5 cm) stones.

The expense and operator skill required for these technologies will limit their availability to regional centers. Patients with documented stones, especially those located in the upper tracts and kidney, causing continuous pain, infection, or obstruction should be referred to such centers for consideration of lithotripsy.

PATIENT EDUCATION

Meticulous care must be taken in giving dietary instructions. Lists of foods high in calcium or oxalate should be provided to help guide the patient's choices. Instructions should also be given to help patients divide their fluid intake evenly to maintain a dilute urine at all times. As noted previously, a fluid intake of 2 liters to 3 liters/day is needed to help minimize stone formations. Patients who need to alkalinize their urine ought to be instructed in how to measure urinary pH with litmus test tapes. Long periods of immobilization should be avoided, and appropriate fluid intake should be prescribed if such situations are anticipated.

ANNOTATED BIBLIOGRAPHY

Coe FL, Keck J, Norton ER: The natural history of calcium urolithiasis. JAMA 238:1519, 1973 (*Retrospective study indicating that calcium urolithiasis is a recurrent disease incurring significant morbidity.*)

Ettinger B, Tang N, Citron JT et al: Randomized trial of allopurinol in the prevention of calcium oxalate calculi. N Engl J Med 315: 1386, 1986 (*A double-blind controlled study demonstrating that allopurinol is effective in prevention of recurrent calcium stones.*)

Health and Public Policy Committee, American College of Physicians: Lithotripsy. Ann Intern Med 103:626, 1985 (*A terse summary of the evidence on the method's safety and efficacy. Endorses extracorporeal lithotripsy as the treatment of choice for upper tract simple stones of less than 2.5 cm that cause persistent pain, infection, or obstruction; percutaneous lithotripsy is viewed as a reasonable alternative when the extracorporeal method is unavailable.*)

Pak CYC, Britton F, Peterson R et al: Ambulatory evaluation of nephrolithiasis. Am J Med 69:19, 1980 (*An attempt to classify stone patients according to their underlying pathophysiology, using readily available ambulatory serum and urine determinations.*)

Pak YCY, Fuller C: Idiopathic calcium-oxalate nephrolithiasis successfully treated with potassium citrate. Ann Intern Med 104:33, 1986 (*An uncontrolled study that is cited here as an example of work being done with inhibitors of stone formation; requires controlled studies to draw conclusions on safety and efficacy.*)

Pak CYC, Sakhaee K, Crowther C et al: Evidence justifying a high fluid intake in treatment of nephrolithiasis. Ann Intern Med 93: 36, 1980 (*A fluid intake of 2 liters to 3 liters/day was associated with a reduced propensity for crystallization of calcium salts.*)

Smith LH: Medical evaluation of urolithiasis: Etiologic aspects and diagnostic evaluation. Urol Clin North Am 1:241, 1974 (*Discussion of the importance of adequate medical history, laboratory data, and stone analysis in the evaluation of stone disease.*)

Strauss AL, Deutch L, Parks JH: Factors that predict relapse of calcium nephrolithiasis during treatment. Am J Med 72:17, 1982 (*A prospective study demonstrating the importance of urinary volume and degree of calciuria in determining risk of relapse.*)

Thomas WC Jr: Medical aspects of renal calculus disease. Treatment and prophylaxis. Urol Clin North Am 1:261, 1974 (*Discussion of therapeutic programs directed to alter urine in such a way that it becomes undersaturated with respect to the offending crystalloid.*)

Williams HE: Nephrolithiasis. N Engl J Med 290:33, 1974 (*Excellent review of pathogenesis and treatment of renal calculi.*)

Williams JJ, Rodman JS, Peterson CM: Randomized double-blind study of acetohydroxamic acid in struvite nephrolithiasis. N Engl J Med 311:760, 1984 (*An example of a trial using a urease inhibitor: it proved efficacious, but the incidence of adverse effects was high.*)

135

Management of Benign Prostatic Hypertrophy

JOHN D. GOODSON, M.D.

Benign prostatic hypertrophy (BPH) is a nearly ubiquitous condition in aging American males and is a frequent cause of urinary tract outflow obstruction. The primary physician must distinguish BPH from the other causes of outflow obstruction (see Chapter 133), determine its severity, and design a therapeutic approach that will provide symptomatic relief, preserve renal function, and prevent infection.

PATHOPHYSIOLOGY

Benign prostatic hypertrophy arises from nodular hyperplasia of prostatic stromal, epithelial, and muscular elements. Growth is primarily centered in the periurethral glandular tissue, but frequently the lateral lobes show significant enlargement. The etiology of age-related prostatic hyperplasia is still unknown, though it is reasonably well established that androgenic changes at the cellular level have a major influence. Unfortunately, it is not known which specific hormonal manipulations are efficacious in reversing or slowing the process. In white males, symptoms from BPH are unlikely to emerge before the age of 55 whereas in black males, the disease may become manifest 10 years earlier.

Regardless of the lobe(s) involved, BPH is manifest clinically by urinary tract outflow obstruction or infection. As the gland enlarges, urine flow through the urethra diminishes and muscular hypertrophy of the bladder ensues. Bladder emptying is usually incomplete. The resulting residual urine predisposes to infection. Numerous saccules or bladder herniations form between the thickened overlapping muscular bands that compose the detrusor. These diverticula are incompletely emptied with voiding, further predisposing to infection. Ureteral dilatation is common in advanced cases of chronic retention because of increased bladder pressure. Hydronephrosis and renal deterioration may follow shortly thereafter.

When the detrusor is no longer able to generate sufficient pressure to overcome urethral obstruction, bladder failure occurs, and urinary retention develops. If there is a large fluid load or the contratile function of the bladder is otherwise impaired by anticholinergic or sympathomimetic drugs, the patient may be unable to void (see Chapter 133).

The hypertrophied prostate is highly vascularized and predisposed to bleeding; painless hematuria is not uncommon.

The complications of chronic retention caused by BPH include hydronephrosis, loss of renal concentrating ability, diminished hydrogen ion excretion (with systemic acidosis), and renal failure.

CLINICAL PRESENTATION AND COURSE

Patients with clinically significant urethral *obstruction* due to BPH generally present with hesitancy, loss of stream force, frequency, nocturia, double voiding, and dribbling. It is most common for patients to have a waxing and waning symptomatic course with very gradual deterioration over several years. Sometimes, urinary tract *infection* is the first indication of outlet obstruction. *Hematuria* may be an early symptom of BPH, but neoplasm must always be excluded. Malignancy is also a concern when a new nodule occurs. Unfortunately, the acid phosphatase is inadequate for detection of early cancer; palpation remains the most effective means (see Chapter 125).

The rectal examination of the prostate is, unfortunately, of little help in assessing the degree of obstruction resulting from gland enlargement, though it does provide a reasonable estimate of overall gland volume. Normally, one can readily feel over the top of the gland; this becomes more difficult as the gland enlarges. The inability to palpate the distal margins of the gland generally indicates massive enlargement (more than three times normal size).

BPH in the elderly can have protean manifestations. It may cause so-called *silent prostatism,* which can produce a lower abdominal mass because of bladder enlargement; confusion, anorexia, a palpable kidney, anemia, and a bleeding diathesis secondary to hydronephrosis and uremia; altered medication requirements, as a consequence of diminished renal clearance; and incontinence related to overflow.

PRINCIPLES OF MANAGEMENT

Assessment. In cases of urinary outflow obstruction from BPH, the clinician must determine the extent to which the patient is bothered by his symptoms. For some, frequency and nocturia significantly interfere with a restful night of sleep, while for others they are a minor inconvenience. It is generally best to see the patient repeatedly over a 3- to 6-month period to get a general sense of how his symptoms are progressing before making any major therapeutic decisions. The elderly require special attention because their symptoms may be poorly expressed or confusing.

A *BUN, creatinine,* complete *blood count,* and *urinalysis* should be obtained on all patients to assess renal function. Observation of the patient while he is voiding may be helpful. *Straight catheterization* after voiding is a simple office procedure that can give a direct assessment of bladder emptying; more than 50 cc to 100 cc of residual urine is abnormal.

In most patients, an *intravenous pyelogram* (IVP) should also be obtained to assess upper and lower tract function. With obstructing prostatic enlargement, excretory films frequently demonstrate bladder wall trabeculations and a significant intravesicular prostatic component. The postvoiding film shows any residual urine volume. A *voiding cystourethrogram* (VCUG) gives a better portrayal of bladder wall diverticula, trabeculations, and residual urine volume.

A *cystometrogram* (CMG) can be added to the evaluation when there is a need to screen for a coincident abnormality of bladder function. Urinary flow studies have recently become more widely available. The tests are useful in assessing true flow rates in patients whose symptoms are variable and difficult to interpret (*e.g.,* the elderly or mentally impaired) and as a means of objectively following patients with moderate obstruction who do not clearly need surgery (see Chapter 133).

Treatment. Many patients with symptomatic BPH can be managed conservatively. Repeated *prostatic massage* (three to four times over a 2-week period) and frequent intercourse are felt to reduce obstruction. Any prostatic infection should be treated (see Chapter 137).

The patient should be told to *void frequently* and to avoid beverages that are likely to produce a diuresis (coffee, tea, alcohol), particularly before bed. Diuretics should be taken early in the day to avoid nocturnal bladder distention. Drugs, such as anticholinergics, mild tranquilizers, and antidepressants, that can exacerbate the symptoms of bladder outflow obstruction should be used only with great care.

Patients with any acute change in symptomatology, such as a dramatic increase in frequency or the development of incontinence, must be evaluated immediately. In such cases, the bladder may be acutely distended. The risk of infection and renal deterioration is very high, and prompt attention with hospitalization is indicated. It is generally agreed that the acutely distended bladder should be decompressed slowly (in amounts of 200 cc–300 cc over several hours) to reduce the risk of hemorrhagic cystitis.

Surgical therapy is indicated in patients with deterioration of bladder or renal function, as evidenced by large postvoid residuals, hydronephrosis on IVP, repeated urinary tract infections, or increasing BUN and creatinine. It is more difficult to assess the subjective inconvenience BPH causes the individual patient. Clearly, some men are greatly troubled by outflow obstruction but have little demonstrable deterioration in bladder or renal function. The identification of patients in whom surgery would be helpful depends on the careful clinical assessment by the primary physician and an experienced consulting surgeon.

Transurethral resection of the prostate (TURP) is a procedure that is associated with low morbidity and that is useful in patients with mildly to moderately enlarged glands and in older, debilitated patients. A retropubic or a *suprapubic prostatectomy* may be required if the gland is substantially enlarged. All of these operations have a low mortality rate (less than 1% for TURPs). Most patients are able to maintain sexual potency regardless of the surgical approach used, although temporary dysfunction may occur (see Chapter 131). Incontinence is unusual, except following radical surgical procedures, but up to 6 months may be required for patients to regain full spincter control. Retrograde ejaculation and infertility are universal complications of prostatic surgery and should be discussed with the patient prior to operation.

If, for reasons of age or concomitant disease, a patient is considered inoperable, chronic Foley or suprapubic *catheter drainage* may be necessary. *Antiandrogrens* and antiestrogens may come to play a role in the medical therapy of BPH, but such therapies must still be considered experimental.

Most prostatic operations leave a substantial amount of prostatic tissue in place; postoperative patients must still be screened for the development of malignancy (see Chapter 125). Furthermore, since residual prostatic tissue will continue to hypertrophy, renal function and patient symptomatology must be monitored in all patients, so that any return of obstructive symptoms will be detected.

MANAGEMENT RECOMMENDATIONS

- All patients should have a baseline BUN, creatinine, complete blood count, and urinalysis.

- An IVP is necessary to assess upper tract function and the clinical severity of obstruction. A CMG can be done to assess bladder muscle function.

- Urine flow rates are useful when symptomatology is confusing or ambiguous.

- Most patients can be followed expectantly, unless there is evidence of obstruction, sepsis, or deterioration in renal function. Fluid loads and drugs that affect bladder function must be avoided. Infection should be treated promptly (see Chapter 140).

- Surgical consultation should be obtained early. The decision to operate is contingent on symptomatology, bladder and renal function, the risk of infection, and objective evidence of obstruction.

ANNOTATED BIBLIOGRAPHY

Castro JE, Griffiths HLJ: The assessment of patients with benign prostatic hypertrophy. JR Coll Surg Edinb 17:190, 1972 (*No correlation was found between gland size or symptoms and calculated urethal area.*)

Castro JE, Griffiths HLJ, Edwards DE: A double-blind, controlled, clinical trial of spironolactone for benign prostatic hypertrophy. Br J Surg 58:485, 1971 (*Seventy-six percent of patients treated with placebo had symptomatic improvement at 6 months, illustrating the subjectivity of symptoms.*)

Finestone AJ, Rosenthal RS: Silent prostatism. Geriatrics 26:89, 1971 (*Seven cases illustrating the protean presentations of BPH in the elderly.*)

Finkle AL, Prian DV: Sexual potency in elderly men before and after prostatectomy. JAMA 196:125, 1966 (*Eighty-four percent of patients who were potent preoperatively maintained potency after prostatectomy [TURP, perineal, suprapubic]. The highest level of impotency occurred with the perineal approach.*)

Gittes RF: Serum acid phosphatase and screening for carcinoma of the prostate. N Engl J Med 309:851, 1983 (*An editorial arguing that the test is inadequate for detection of stages A and B disease.*)

Schoenberg HW, Gutrich JM, Cote R: Urodynamic studies in benign prostatic hypertrophy. Urology 14:634, 1979 (*Urodynamic studies are most useful in following patients, either prior to or after surgery.*)

Wilson JD: The pathogenesis of benign prostatic hypertrophy. Am J Med 68:745, 1980 (*Excellent review of the hormonal basis of BPH.*)

136

Management of Nongonococcal Urethritis

JOHN D. GOODSON, M.D.

Nongonococcal urethritis (NGU) has surpassed gonorrhea as the prime form of urethritis in the male. It can occur as an isolated infection or in conjunction with gonorrhea. In about half of all instances, infection with *Chlamydia trachomatis* is responsible for the condition; *Ureaplasma* (formerly T-strain mycoplasma) and Reiter's syndrome account for much of the remainder. Evaluation of urethritis primarily requires distinguishing gonococcal disease from NGU (see Chapter 129); further assessment is usually unnecessary to initiate therapy, although new diagnostic methods facilitate rapid identification of the important pathogen *C. trachomatis.*

Because chlamydial infection is becoming the most common sexually transmitted disease among heterosexuals in the United States and a potential source of female infertility and infant morbidity, the primary physician needs to be cognizant of its clinical manifestations (*e.g.,* NGU), epidemiologic importance, and antibiotic treatment.

CLINICAL PRESENTATION AND COURSE

Regardless of etiology, the clinical presentation of NGU is rather stereotypical. Compared with gonococcal urethritis, NGU tends to be an indolent illness; dysuria is not as severe, and the discharge is less purulent, sometimes scanty, or even absent. The urethral Gram stain shows some neutrophils and, at most, a few mixed organisms, helping to distinguish NGU from gonococcal infection (see Chapter 129).

Chlamydial infection is most common among young heterosexual males with multiple consorts; prevalence appears to be higher among blacks than whites. As many as one half to one third of men with chlamydial urethritis are asymptomatic; some even lack abnormal numbers of leukocytes on Gram stain. In up to 20% of patients presenting with gonococcal urethritis, there is mixed infection, involving both gonococci and *Chlamydia.* Mixed infection is suggested when individuals experience persistence of symptoms if treated only for the gonorrhea, despite clearing of gonococci from repeat Gram stains and cultures.

As much as 40% of NGU has been attributed to infection with *Ureaplasma urealyticum.* Persistence of symptomatic urethritis after appropriate antibiotic treatment of NGU has been linked to tetracycline-resistant strains of *Ureaplasma.* However, most recurrent NGU is due to reinfection from an untreated sexual partner rather than from infection with a resistant organism.

Reiter's syndrome is characterized by various combinations of conjunctivitis, iritis, acute asymmetrical polyarthritis (see Chapter 143), circinate balanitis, keratodermia blennorrhagica, mucosal ulcerations, and urethritis. Many patients present first with the urethritis, though involvement of other organ systems is frequently present in subclinical form or soon materializes within a few weeks. There is some evidence that *C. trachomatis* infection is capable of triggering Reiter's syndrome in susceptible men and that an exaggerated immune response may play a role in the condition's pathogenesis.

NGU used to be considered a condition limited to males. In recent years, female counterparts of NGU have been identified, including mucopurulent cervicitis (see Chapter 115) and acute urethral syndrome (see Chapter 132), both of which are closely linked to chlamydial infection. *C. trachomatis* is also an important cause of pelvic inflammatory disease, leading to infertility and ectopic pregnancy. There is a very high prevalence (almost 70%) of chlamydial infection among female partners of men with chlamydial NGU.

NGU may wax and wane over several weeks; spontaneous resolution can occur. Complications of NGU are uncommon. Prostatitis and epididymitis have been reported in untreated or poorly treated cases. On occasion, epididymitis is a concomitant finding. (About half of epididymitis cases in the United States are due to gonococcal infection and the remainder to *Chlamydia.*) Most patients with Reiter's syndrome experience a self-limited illness, although a minority progress to chronic or recurrent symptoms in conjunction with bouts of arthritis.

DIAGNOSIS

Every male patient with a urethral discharge or complaint of dysuria should have a *Gram stain* of a urethral specimen, and the specimen should be *cultured for gonococci.* If there is spontaneous discharge, this material can be used; otherwise, a sterile swab should be inserted into the penile meatus to obtain a specimen for stain and culture. Alternatively, the urethral fraction of a voided bladder urine specimen, the VB_1 fraction (see Chapter 137), can be collected and centrifuged; the resulting pellet is then Gram-stained and cultured.

If no definite gram-negative intracellular diplococci are seen on Gram stain, then a tentative diagnosis of NGU is appropriate. The diagnosis is confirmed by a negative gonococcal culture. It is not practical to *culture* for *Chlamydia* or *Ureaplasma,* because of the expense, technical difficulty, and 2- to 3-day delay in obtaining results. However, more rapid, less expensive detection of *Chlamydia* is possible using a *direct fluorescent antibody* method to stain smears of urethral discharge. An *enzyme immunoassay* of secretions is also available. The former is more sensitive and specific, the latter cheaper and better suited for laboratories that process large numbers of specimens.

PRINCIPLES OF MANAGEMENT AND THERAPEUTIC RECOMMENDATIONS

Because chlamydial infection accounts for 50% of NGU, ranks as the most common sexually transmitted disease among heterosexuals in the United States, and represents a potential source of morbidity to female partners and their infants, all patients with NGU should be treated, regardless of whether or not definite identification of the organism has been achieved. Female partners of NGU patients should be tested; if testing is not available, they too should be treated for presumptive chlamydial infection. Male homosexual partners should be tested. Treatment of asymptomatic male homosexual partners of the patient with NGU is not deemed necessary because of the reduced incidence of *Chlamydia* infection in this population.

The Centers for Disease Control recommendation for treatment is *tetracycline,* 500 mg qid for 7 days, or *doxycycline,* 100 mg bid for 7 days. Patients who cannot take tetracycline (*e.g.,* pregnant women) can be treated with *erythromycin,* 500 mg qid for 7 days or 250 mg qid for 14 days. These regimens are effective not only against *Chlamydia,* but also against *Ureaplasma. Sulfamethoxazole,* 1 g bid for 10 days, has a lower response rate, but can be used in patients unable to tolerate other agents.

Persistent symptoms of NGU after a course of tetracycline therapy can prompt a repeat course of therapy, especially if there has been a partial response. An alternative is to use erythromycin for the second course of therapy. Recurrent disease is most often due to reinfection.

Prevention of infection can be accomplished by using barrier methods of contraception. Heterosexual men with multiple partners should be encouraged to use prophylactics.

ANNOTATED BIBLIOGRAPHY

Bell TA, Grayston JT: Centers for Disease Control guidelines for prevention and control of *Chlamydia trachomatis* infections. Ann Intern Med 104:524, 1986 (*A terse, but excellent summary of a more detailed CDC document: this 3-page paper is essential reading for every primary care physician.*)

Martin DH, Pollack S, Kuo CC: *Chlamydia trachomatis* infections in men with Reiter's syndrome. Ann Intern Med 100:207, 1984 (*Documents infection and an exaggerated immune response in some patients who go on to develop Reiter's syndrome: not definitive, but nevertheless intriguing data.*)

Stamm WE, Koutsky LA, Benedetti JK et al: *Chlamydia trachomatis* urethral infections in men. Ann Intern Med 100:47, 1984 (*Details prevalence, risk factors, and clinical manifestations: from a sexually transmitted disease clinic.*)

Stimson JB, Hale J, Bowie WR et al: Tetracycline-resistant *Ureaplasma urealyticum:* A cause of persistent nongonococcal urethritis. (*An important cause of persistent illness, though not responsible for most recurrences.*)

Tam MR, Stamm WE, Handsfield JJ et al: Culture-independent diagnosis of *Chlamydia trachomatis* using monoclonal antibodies. N Engl J Med 310:1146, 1984 (*Describes the direct fluorescent antibody test for rapid diagnosis of chlamydial infection.*)

Taylor-Robinson D, McCormack WM: The genital mycoplasmas. N Engl J Med 302:1003, 1980 (*A comprehensive two-part review detailing the role of* Ureaplasma *infection in NGU and other genital infections.*)

137

Management of Acute and Chronic Prostatitis

JOHN D. GOODSON, M.D.

Prostatitis is the most important cause of urinary tract infection in men. Chronic prostatitis is a common infection that can cause persistent and annoying symptoms, while acute prostatitis is less common but potentially much more serious. Both conditions require accurate recognition and treatment by the primary physician; prompt initiation of therapy is especially important for acute prostatitis.

CLINICAL PRESENTATION, PATHOPHYSIOLOGY, AND COURSE

Bacterial prostatitis may ensue from ascending urethral infection, reflux of infected urine, extension of rectal infection, or hematogenous spread. Gram-negative bacilli (predominantly *E. coli*) and enterococci account for most of the single isolates obtained from culture. Occasionally, *Chlamydia, Ureaplasma,* a virus, or *trichomonas* is the etiologic agent. *Ureaplasma* has been isolated from 13.7% of patients with chronic prostatitis, suggesting the organism may be more important than previously suspected and might account for some cases previously labeled as "nonbacterial." Accurate data is difficult to obtain from cultures; contaminants are common.

Acute Prostatitis. The condition is readily identified by the onset of diminished urine flow, perineal pain, dysuria, and fever. On gentle rectal examination, the gland is enlarged, exquisitely tender and boggy. Abdominal examination occasionally reveals striking bladder distention. Some patients may appear toxic at the time of presentation.

Chronic Prostatitis. In older men, the symptoms are generally those of bladder outflow obstruction. Patients complain of frequency, dribbling, loss of stream volume and force, double voiding, hesitancy, and urgency. Younger men more often complain of dysuria, dribbling and intermittent discomfort in the perineum, low back, or testicles. Some patients present initially with hematuria, hematospermia, or painful ejaculations. Rectal examination usually reveals an enlarged prostate with a variable amount of asymmetry, bogginess, and tenderness. Untreated or incompletely treated chronic prostatitis is characterized by recurrent symptomatic exacerbations, though these may be separated by long asymptomatic intervals.

Both acute and chronic prostatitis can cause urinary tract and systemic complications. The acutely infected gland may lead to renal parenchymal infection or bacteremia. Rarely, acute infection will progress to a well-defined abscess of the gland. Chronic infection can produce small prostatic stones, which may serve as a nidus for further inflammation and recurrent symptomatic bouts of infection.

Prostatosis mimics the presentation of chronic prostatitis, but cultures are negative and microscopic examination of expressed prostatic secretions shows no white cells. Etiology is unknown. The term *prostatodynia* has been suggested for this condition.

DIFFERENTIAL DIAGNOSIS AND WORKUP

Acute prostatitis is readily evident by the clinical presentation and exquisitely tender prostate found on rectal examination. However, chronic prostatitis presents a more difficult diagnostic problem, often resembling, in clinical presentation, other common forms of urinary outflow tract obstruction, such as benign prostatic hypertrophy (see Chapter 135), prostatic carcinoma (see Chapter 141), and urethral stricture (see Chapter 133). The lower urinary tract irritative symptoms associated with chronic prostatitis may be seen with bladder carcinoma (see Chapter 141), sphincter dyssynergy, and neurogenic bladder (see Chapter 133).

Since history and physical examination are often inadequate for making a diagnosis of prostatitis, one needs to examine *expressed prostatic secretions (EPS)* and obtain *quantitative bacterial localization cultures* to garner more definitive evidence. Urines representing urethral, bladder, and postprostatic massage specimens (labeled VB_1, VB_2, and VB_3) are collected (see the appendix), in addition to any expressed prostatic secretions (EPS) that can be obtained as a result of massage. Vigorous massage should be avoided in patients with severe acute prostatitis, because of the risk of inducing bacteremia. Gram stain of the EPS or the spun VB_3 specimen will often demonstrate organisms or white blood cells (>20 WBC per high-power field is abnormal). Cultures of the EPS and VB_3 should show significant growth (greater than 5,000 colonies/ml), while the VB_1 and VB_2 should be sterile or have a colony count that is one order of magnitude less. Direct culture of the prostate through the rectum or the urethra has not proved reliable. Culture for *Chlamydia* and *Mycoplasma* requires special techniques and should be reserved for difficult or protracted infection.

Older men without evidence of infection, yet bothered by lower urinary tract irritative symptoms, should have urine cytologies performed to help exclude a bladder malignancy. A bladder carcinoma located in the trigonal region may present in such a fashion. Cystoscopy is indicated when the diagnosis is not confirmed by urine culture data.

PRINCIPLES OF MANAGEMENT

Acute Prostatitis accompanied by severe pain, high fever, rigors, and marked leukocytosis requires hospitalization for intravenous antibiotic therapy. Achievement of high tissue drug levels is essential. Such patients should be examined gently for the presence of a fluctuant prostatic mass suggestive of an abscess, which may necessitate surgical drainage. Less toxic patients can be treated as outpatients with an oral antibiotic program. Trimethoprim–sulfa, doxycycline, and carbenicillin indanyl sodium work well. Three weeks of therapy are recommended to prevent acute infection from becoming established. Most other antibiotics effective against gramnegative rods (*e.g.,* ampicillin and amoxicillin) penetrate the acutely inflamed prostate well and work satisfactorily in the acute phase of illness, but less so in subacute and chronic states.

Chronic Prostatitis is more difficult to eradicate, partly because of the poor penetration by oral antibiotics into the prostate (see below). Even 4 to 12 weeks of therapy with trimethoprim–sulfa (which penetrates reasonably well and is effective against most of the offending organisms) may not suffice in curing the infection; success rates are in the range of 30% to 70%. Although erythromycin diffuses well into the gland, it is not particularly effective against many of the pathogenic organisms.

Curative antibiotic therapy is indicated by the elimination of bacteria from prostatic fluid. Since the gland's secretions are normally acidic (pH 6.5–7.4), the most efficacious drugs are those that readily penetrate membranes (lipid-soluble) and are ionically trapped (basic). Trimethoprim and erythromycin have these characteristics. Animal studies have demonstrated good prostatic fluid levels for both. With chronic infection, the prostatic fluid becomes alkaline, a situation that tends to reduce trimethoprim concentrations. As a result, some men are not cured even by prolonged courses of antibiotic therapy. Trimethoprim is more effective than erythromycin against gram-negative bacteria and consequently is preferred. The combination of trimethoprim and sulfamethoxazole, a sulfa drug with a similar half-life, acts synergistically on a wide range of gram-negative and gram-positive infections, with the notable exception of enterococci. As noted earlier, ampicillin and most other antibiotics enter the acutely inflamed prostate, but penetration of the chronically infected gland is uncertain. Carbenicillin indanyl sodium and doxycycline penetrate the prostate reasonably well.

The EPS and VB_3 should be inspected and cultured following the treatment period to determine the efficacy of therapy. A BUN and creatinine should be obtained at the initial visit and periodically thereafter depending on the chronicity and severity of symptoms. An intravenous pyelogram is indicated when there is evidence of renal deterioration or symptoms of persistent outflow obstruction.

Patients who achieve a partial response may be given a second extended course of treatment with the same antibiotic. Those failing to respond may benefit from switching to another antibiotic, such as a tetracycline preparation or erythromycin (both of which are active against *Ureaplasma* and other hard-to-identify organisms that sometimes play an etiologic role).

The relatively low cure rate achieved with antibiotics in chronic prostatitis requires that therapeutic goals be adjusted to the patient's age.

When a cure is not achieved in younger patients, antibiotic therapy is directed toward *suppression* of prostatic inflammation and prevention of upper tract infection or obstruction. One single-strength *trimethoprim-sulfa* tablet daily appears to be the most effective suppressive regimen. For older men, transurethral prostatic resection or total prostatectomy provides a surgical alternative when repeated courses of antibiotics fail. Both operations are associated with significant morbidity, including possible impotence or sterility and should be reserved for select patients. Recurrent infection associated with prostatic stones is an indication for removal of the gland.

Local Measures reduce symptoms in both acute and chronic infections. *Sitz baths* two to three times a day for 20 minutes can relieve perineal pain. The patient with a partial obstruction should be told to void while in a warm water bath with pelvic muscles relaxed.

The value of *prostatic massage* is a subject of debate. Many claim that prostatic massage will relieve gland congestion in chronic cases and should be repeated every 1 to 2 weeks. Massage of the acutely infected gland is contraindicated because it can produce bacteremia.

Stool softeners, antipyretics, analgesics, and bed rest are all helpful. The patient should avoid alcohol, coffee, tea, or other beverages that might produce rapid bladder expansion. The physician should discontinue or reduce the dosage, if possible, of anticholinergics, sedatives, and antidepressants, all of which can impair bladder function (see Chapter 133).

PATIENT EDUCATION

Patients should be advised of the chronic and relapsing nature of the disease and alerted to the early signs of infection in the upper urinary tract. They can also be reassured that isolated prostatitis does not cause infertility or impotence. Local symptomatic measures that can be suggested for symptomatic relief include sitz baths and voiding into a warm water bath. The importance of compliance with the prolonged antibiotic course needs to be stressed.

THERAPEUTIC RECOMMENDATIONS

- *Acute prostatitis* requires appropriate Gram stains, cultures of EPS and VB_3, and immediate treatment.
- For the nontoxic patient, the combination of 160 mg of trimethoprim and 800 mg of sulfamethoxazole twice a day orally is preferred. Ampicillin, 500 mg four times a day, tetracycline at the same dosage, doxycycline 100 mg twice a day, or carbenicillin indanyl sodium (1 g qid) would be reasonable alternatives in sulfa-allergic individuals. Treatment should be continued for 21 days.
- *Chronic prostatitis* requires a prolonged antibiotic course; 160 mg of trimethoprim and 800 mg of sulfamethoxazole orally twice daily for 6 weeks is recommended. After treatment, the patient should be followed closely for return of infections. A second antibiotic course of up to 12 weeks' duration may be necessary in partially responsive infectioins. Patients who fail to respond can be given a trial of a tetracycline (*e.g.,* doxycycline 100 mg bid for 6 weeks) or erythromycin (500 mg qid for 6 weeks), or carbenicillin indanyl sodium (1 g qid for 6 weeks).

INDICATIONS FOR ADMISSION AND REFERRAL

Patients with high fever, leukocytosis, and severe perineal pain need intravenous antibiotics, antipyretics, and analgesics; hospitalization is indicated. In the presence of marked outflow obstruction, suprapubic bladder decompression may be necessary. A fluctuant prostatic mass suggestive of an abscess may require surgical drainage. Until culture and sensitivity data are available, treatment of the toxic patient is directed toward gram-negative bacteria, utilizing parenteral ampicillin or gentamicin.

Patients with outflow tract obstruction or refractory chronic infection should have a urologic consultation.

ANNOTATED BIBLIOGRAPHY

Brunner H, Weidner W, Schiefer HG: Studies on the role of *Ureaplasma urealyticum* and *Mycoplasma hominis* in prostatitis. J Infect Dis 147:807, 1983 (*Thirteen percent of patients had rigorously documented* Ureaplasma *infection; more than 80% responded to tetracycline.*)

Drach GW: Problems in diagnosis of bacterial prostatitis: Gram-negative, Gram-positive and mixed infections. J Urol 111:630, 1974 (*Careful culture documentation of infection in 105 patients with prostatitis. Gram-positive organisms were found most frequently* [Staphylococcus aureus *and* Streptococcus] *but were felt to represent a more benign disease for which antibiotic suppression was not recommended. Gram-negative isolates were felt to increase the risk of urinary tract infection and suppression was recommended.*)

Drach GW, Fair WR, Meares EM et al: Classification of benign diseases associated with prostatic pain. Prostatitis or prostatodynia? J Urol 120:266, 1978 (*A letter to the editor discussing this confusing issue.*)

Drach GW, Nolan PE: Chronic bacterial prostatitis: Problems in diagnosis and therapy. Urol (suppl)27:26, 1986 (*Using strict criteria, only 20% of patients referred for evaluation of prostatitis had definitely positive cultures.*)

Fair WR, Crane DB, Schiller N et al: J Urol 121:437, 1979 (*Prostatic fluid from men with chronic infection was found to have a mean pH of 8.32 [basic]. This may explain why some men are not cured by trimethoprim and sulfamethoxazole since the trimethoprim would be ionically excluded.*)

Hensle TW, Prout GR Jr, Griffin P: Minocycline diffusion into benign prostatic hypertrophy. J Urol 118:609, 1977 (*Minocycline penetrates well into noninfected prostate.*)

Meares EM Jr: Infected stones of the prostate gland. Urology 4:560, 1974 (*Prostatic stones are found in 13.8% of men. Most are asymptomatic, but where recurrent infection is demonstrated, the gland and stones must be removed.*)

Meares EM Jr: Prostatitis syndromes. New perspectives about old woes. J Urol 123:141, 1980 (*An authoritative review of clinical prostatitis syndromes and their management.*)

Meares EM Jr: Long-term therapy of chronic bacterial prostatitis with trimethoprim-sulfamethoxazole. Can Med Assoc J 112:225, 1975 (*Twelve weeks of combination treatment produced an initially good response in 74%. Only 31% remained cured for a 30-month follow-up period.*)

O'Dea MJ, Moore SB, Greene LF: Tuberculous prostatitis. Urology 11:483, 1978 (*Tuberculosis may present in the prostate. Multiple biopsies are necessary to make the diagnosis.*)

Ristuccia AM, Cunha BA: Current therapy in antimicrobial therapy of prostatitis. Urology 20:338, 1982 (*Doxycycline and trimetho-*

prim alone are the preferred drugs. Though in vitro *spectrum is limited, the* in vivo *effectiveness of erythromycin may be good.*)

Smart CJ, Jenkins JD: The role of transurethral prostatectomy in chronic prostatitis. Br J Urol 45:654, 1973 (*Good results in treating chronic infection, but up to three operations may be required to remove all infected tissue. Recommended TURP for patients in whom sterility is not an issue.*)

Sporer A, Auerback O: Tuberculosis of the prostate. Urology 11:362, 1978 (*Tuberculosis of the prostate results from hematogenous dissemination of disease and is a frequent site of genitourinary involvement.*)

Stamey TA: Urinary Infections. Baltimore, Williams & Wilkins, 1972 (*Excellent chapter on male urinary tract infections.*)

Stamey TA, Meares EM Jr, Winningham DG: Chronic bacterial prostatitis and the diffusion of drugs into the prostatic fluid. J Urol 103:187, 1970 (*Discussion of the ideal drug for prostatic infection and the concept of ion trapping.*)

Thin RN, Simmons PD: Chronic bacterial and nonbacterial prostatitis. Br J Urol 55:513, 1983 (*The EPS leukocyte count for bacterial and nonbacterial prostatitis were no different. The test was highly specific but poorly sensitive.*)

Appendix: Urine and Prostatic Fluid Collections in Men

The appropriate diagnosis and management of infections involving the urinary tract depend on the correct identification of the responsible pathogen. The clinician must ensure the collection of urine specimens with a minimal amount of contamination. Careful patient instruction, adequate hydration, and assistance where necessary are essential to obtaining accurate, useful results.

Standard Clean-Voided Specimen

Specimen collection in the *male* varies with the clinical situation. When cystitis is suspected, the patient is traditionally instructed to retract the foreskin and clean the glans penis with three gauze pads or soap sponges. A small amount of urine is voided into the toilet and then a midstream specimen is collected. Recent data suggest that cleansing and retraction of foreskin make no difference if a midstream specimen is obtained. However, omitting these steps does lead to contamination of initial specimens. When urethritis or prostatitis is suspected, voided bladder specimens are indicated.

Voided Bladder Specimens

The patient retracts the foreskin and cleans the glans penis. The first 10 cc is collected and labeled VB_1 (voided bladder; see Fig. 137-1) and represents a urethral specimen, useful in cases of suspected urethritis (see Chapters 126 and 136). A midstream specimen is collected in the standard fashion. This specimen is labeled VB_2. The bladder must not be completely emptied. While the patient maintains foreskin retraction with

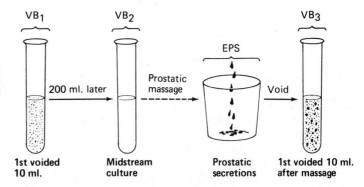

Figure 137-1. Segmented cultured of the lower urinary tract in the male. (Adapted from Meares EM, Stamey T: Bacteriologic localization patterns in bacterial prostatitis and urethritis. Invest Urol 5:492, 1968)

one hand, the physician massages the prostate with continuous strokes. The resulting prostatic fluid is collected in a sterile container labeled EPS (expressed prostatic secretion) and can be used for culture and Gram or acid-fast stain. If no fluid is obtained, the patient is instructed to milk the penis, starting from the base and moving toward the tip. Finally, if there is still no fluid, the patient is told to void another 10 cc into a sterile container. This specimen is labeled VB_3 and represents roughly a 100:1 dilution of prostatic fluid; it can be cultured or spun and stained. Vigorous prostatic massage can produce a transient bacteremia and should be avoided if acute prostatitis is suspected; if the patient has chronic prostatitis and known valvular heart disease, endocarditis prophylaxis may be necessary (see Chapter 11).

The EPS and VB_3 can be inspected under the microscope for the presence of fat globules, leukocytes, and organisms. If fewer than five leukocytes are seen per high-power field, bacterial prostatic infection is unlikely. A Gram stain should be prepared and examined, since it may aid in identifying the responsible organism. With bacterial prostatitis, growth will occur in VB_3 and EPS, but not in VB_1 and VB_2. When there is bacterial growth in both VB_2 and VB_3 samples, a prostatic infection may be masked by a bladder infection. In this situation antibiotics that sterilize the bladder contents but do not penetrate the prostate (*e.g.,* penicillin G, 500 mg four times a day orally, or Macrodantin, 100 mg three times a day orally) may be given for 2 to 3 days before specimen collection. With bacterial prostatic infection, the EPS will still grow organisms.

Urethral catheterization of the male is rarely required for culture and should be reserved for the symptomatic relief of marked outflow obstruction.

ANNOTATED BIBLIOGRAPHY

Lipsky BA, Inui TS, Plorde JJ et al: Is the clean-catch midstream void procedure necessary for obtaining routine urine culture specimens from men? Am J Med 76:257, 1984 (*The authors present data suggesting the answer is "no."*)

Meares EM, Stamey T: Bacteriologic localization patterns in bacterial prostatitis and urethritis. Invest Urol 5:492, 1968 (*Detailed description of methodology and rationale for voided bladder specimens.*)

138
Management of Syphilis and Other Venereal Diseases
HARVEY B. SIMON, M.D.

Syphilis

In 1943, the dramatic efficacy of penicillin treatment was established, and for the next 15 years the incidence of new cases of syphilis declined steadily to a low of about 6000 in 1957. Although *Treponema pallidum,* the spirochete that causes syphilis, has not developed resistance to penicillin, the incidence of syphilis has increased progressively in the last 20 years, largely because of a change in sexual mores, with many new cases occurring in adolescents, young adults, and homosexuals.

PATHOPHYSIOLOGY AND CLINICAL PRESENTATION

Man is the only natural reservoir of *T. pallidum.* Except for transplacental transmission, virtually all cases are acquired by sexual contact with persons having active infectious lesions. *T. pallidum* readily penetrates abraded skin and intact mucous membranes to multiply locally and disseminate through the lymphatics and bloodstream.

The course of syphilis can be divided into primary, secondary, latent, and tertiary phases. The lesion of *primary syphilis* is the chancre, which occurs at the site of inoculation about 3 weeks after exposure. The chancre is usually located on the genitalia, but depending on sexual practices, it can occur in the anal canal, on oral mucosa, hands, or even more unusual locations. The lesion begins as a small papule that enlarges and undergoes superficial necrosis to produce an ulcer with a clean base and sharp margins. The chancre is typically painless, and patients are free of constitutional symptoms, though regional nodes may be enlarged. The chancre is teeming with spirochetes and is highly infectious.

Even without therapy, the chancre will heal completely in 2 to 6 weeks. However, about 2 months after the primary infection, the features of secondary syphilis may appear. *Secondary syphilis* is a systemic disease. A flulike syndrome is common, as is generalized lymphadenopathy. The most characteristic feature of secondary syphilis is a generalized skin eruption. Lesions may be macular, papular, or papulosquamous, but tend to be symmetric and uniform in size; typically, the palms and soles are involved. Mucous patches and split papules often occur on the mucous membranes. Secondary syphilis can involve many other organs; clinical manifestations may include aseptic meningitis, hepatitis, nephritis, or uveitis. Patients with secondary syphilis are contagious.

As in primary syphilis, the manifestations of secondary syphilis resolve spontaneously even without therapy, although up to 25% of patients exhibit a brief relapse of secondary lesions. Untreated patients without active lesions are considered to have *latent syphilis.* About two thirds of these individuals remain entirely asymptomatic, but in the remaining one third, the lesions of tertiary syphilis develop, usually 10 to 40 years after primary infection. The major forms of *tertiary syphilis* include (1) cardiovascular, with aneurysmal dilatation of the ascending aorta and aortic insufficiency; (2) neurosyphilis, which may be asymptomatic or present as general paresis with disorders of intellect and personality, or as tabes dorsalis, with ataxic gait, impaired pain and temperature sensation, autonomic dysfunction, and hypoactive reflexes; (3) gummas, which are isolated, slowly progressive destructive granulomatous lesions of skin, bone, liver, or other organs.

Congenital syphilis occurs as a result of transplacental transmission of spirochetes during the second or third trimester of pregnancy. Fetal loss is about 60% and up to half of surviving infants have stigmata, which can result in serious permanent handicaps. Congenital syphilis can be prevented by prompt treatment of maternal infection.

DIAGNOSIS

Treponema pallidum cannot be cultured in the laboratory, but the diagnosis of syphilis can be made by direct visualization of treponemas from the chancre; however, this is a specialized technique that requires darkfield or fluorescent microscopy and very experienced observers. As a result, the diagnosis usually depends on clinical features and serologic testing. The most widely used serologic tests for syphilis use a lipoidal extract of mammalian tissues for the antigen. Examples include the VDRL, Hinton, and RPR tests. These are excellent screening tests, but the false-positive rate is as high as 20%, often as the result of unrelated infections or inflammatory diseases that produce hyperglobulinemia. More specific serologic tests use treponemal antigens and can be used to distinguish true-positive from false-positive results. The best of these treponemal tests is the FTA-ABS (fluorescent treponemal antibody absorption test).

Some patients with primary syphilis manifest falsely negative VDRL and FTA-ABS tests. False negatives are most likely to occur for patients with infections of less than 30 days' duration. Individuals with a suspicious primary lesion should have darkfield examination performed and serologic studies repeated in 10 to 14 days.

PRINCIPLES OF MANAGEMENT AND THERAPEUTIC RECOMMENDATIONS

The results of treatment of early syphilis are excellent. *Treponema pallidum* is very sensitive to *penicillin.* Because the organism multiplies slowly, the goal is to attain relatively low, but long-lasting, antibiotic levels. Present Public Health Service recommendations include the following:

- Early syphilis (incubating, primary, secondary, early latent stages): 2.4 million units of benzathine penicillin intramuscularly at a single session. Alternatively, one may give 600,000 units of procaine penicillin intramuscularly daily for 8 days. Penicillin-allergic patients may receive tetracycline or erythromycin, 500 mg by mouth four times a day for 15 days. Tetracycline is contraindicated in pregnancy.
- Syphilis of greater than 1 year's duration (latent or tertiary stages): benzathine penicillin, 2.4 million units intramuscularly for 3 consecutive weeks. Alternatively, patients may receive 600,000 units of procaine penicillin intramuscularly daily for 15 days. Substantially higher doses of penicillin should be used for neurosyphilis, which some feel necessitates intravenous penicillin at so-called meningeal doses. Penicillin-allergic patients should receive tetracycline or erythromycin, 500 mg by mouth four times a day for 30 days.

Immunity to syphilis is incomplete and reinfection may occur, especially in patients treated with penicillin within a year of infection. Follow-up of patients is essential. Quantitative VDRL assessments at 3, 6, and 12 months after treatment help determine adequacy of therapy for early syphilis. Antibody titer may decline more slowly in late syphilis and should also be checked at 24 months. Equally important is the reporting of cases to appropriate public health authorities, so that investigation of contacts can be carried out.

Gonorrhea

See Chapter 116 for a discussion of gonorrhea.

Herpes Genitalis

In addition to syphilis, gonorrhea (see Chapter 116), and nongonococcal urethritis (see Chapter 116), many other infections can be transmitted by sexual contact. The most common of these are viral infections. *Herpes genitalis* (see also Chapter 191) is caused by sexual transmission of *herpes simplex* virus, Type II. After a short incubation period averaging 2 to 10 days, vesicular lesions develop on the genitalia; these are penile lesions in the male; in the female they may affect the external genitalia or the vagina and cervix. The lesions ulcerate early, and although they may sometimes be asymptomatic, pain is often severe; regional lymphadenopathy and fever may be prominent. In most patients, herpes genitalis is self-limited, but the disease often pursues a relapsing course. Recurrent episodes tend to be progressively briefer and less severe. However, herpetic infection during pregnancy is particularly worrisome, since neonatal herpes can be a devastating disease, transmitted during birth by contact with infectious active cervical and vaginal lesions.

Acyclovir, an antiviral agent with selective activity against members of the herpes virus group, represents an advance in the treatment of genital herpes. A purine analog, acyclovir serves as a substrate for viral thymidine kinase, thereby interrupting viral DNA synthesis. Acyclovir is available in a 5% ointment for topical use as well as in both oral and intravenous preparations. Topical acyclovir decreases pain and other symptoms and reduces viral shedding in primary episodes of genital herpes, but treatment does not affect the recurrence rate, and ointment is ineffective in recurrent herpes. Patients with primary genital herpes may benefit from topical application of acyclovir ointment five times daily for 7 days. Oral acyclovir (200 mg) given five times daily for 7 to 10 days has a similar effect. Intravenous acyclovir produces symptomatic benefit, accelerates healing, and decreases viral shedding but does not prevent recurrences. However, hospitalization and intravenous treatment is rarely appropriate for patients with genital herpes.

Orally administered acyclovir is the treatment of choice for primary and recurrent genital herpes infections. Taking 200 mg five times daily for 7 to 10 days shortens clinical symptoms and reduces the period of viral shedding. However, the risk of recurrence is not diminished unless acyclovir therapy is continued indefinitely at a dosage of 200 mg two to five times daily. Seventy-five percent decreases in recurrence rates have been reported with continuous use. When acyclovir is discontinued, the pretreatment risk of recurrent attacks returns.

Suppressive therapy with acyclovir should be considered only for patients with frequent or disabling recurrences. Although acyclovir is a safe drug, the consequences of long-term use have not been fully evaluated. Resistant strains of *Herpes simplex* have been recovered from patients, but they are uncommon in clinical practice.

Condylomata Acuminata

Another viral disease that appears to be sexually transmitted is condylomata acuminata, or venereal warts. These typically present as painless papillomatous lesions of the moist mucocutaneous regions of the genitalia. Venereal warts can be treated with careful topical application of 20% podophyllum solution. However, the drug's disadvantages include toxicity to normal skin and a cure rate as low as 20%. Application of liquid nitrogen may be a more effective alternative. Cervical warts are associated with an increased risk of cervical cancer; those that persist require biopsy. All vaginal and cervical warts should be evaluated by Pap smear and/or colposcopy. Large lesions and those occurring intra-anally or vaginally may require cryotherapy, electrocoagulation, or excision (see Chapter 193).

Other Viral Infections

Although other viral infections, including cytomegalovirus and hepatitis, can be transmitted sexually (see Chapters 52 and 81), their major impact is not on the genital tract, and the great majority of cases are transmitted nonsexually.

Scabies and Pubic Lice

Cutaneous infestations with mites or pubic lice commonly result from intimate contact. Patients present with pruritus of the pubic region. The diagnosis of pubic lice or "crabs" is made by seeing the organism either with the naked eye or with a magnifying lens. Scabies, which is caused by mites, produces papules and burrows that may be scraped and examined microscopically in wet mounts to visualize the organism. Topical lotions, such as pyrethrins with piperonyl butoxide (Rid; and others) or 1% lindane (Kwell) are effective treatments. Bedding and clothing should be laundered.

Vaginitis

Although not strictly speaking a venereal disease, vaginitis (also see Chapter 115) may be perpetuated by sexual contact and may therefore require simultaneous treatment of male sexual partners. This is particularly true of trichomonal vaginitis, caused by the protozoan *Trichomonas vaginalis*. The diagnosis is made by direct microscopic examination of a wet mount of the vaginal discharge. *Metronidazole* is the treatment of choice. A single 2-g dose is effective when both sexual partners are treated simultaneously. The drug is contraindicated in the first trimester of pregnancy; clotrimazole (100 mg intravaginally qhs for 7 days) is an alternative.

"Nonspecific" vaginitis (bacterial vaginosis) results from an overgrowth of *Gardnerella* and anaerobic bacteria. Patients complain of an unpleasant discharge with a fishy odor, particularly noticeable when KOH is applied to a sample of the discharge on a slide. The vaginal pH is elevated (>4.5) and clue cells can be seen in wet mount (see Chapter 115). *Metronidazole* is the drug of choice (250 mg tid for 7 days); single-dose regimens are less effective than a 7-day course.

Vaginal candidiasis is only occasionally due to sexual transmission. The characteristic appearance of the organism is best seen on KOH smear of the discharge. Topical miconazole or clotrimazole (200 mg intravaginally of either agent at bedtime for 3 days) work well though recurrences are frequent. Cessation of systemic antibiotics or birth control pills may be necessary to prevent recurrences. Diabetic women have a slightly increased incidence of the condition.

Nongonococcal Urethritis and Cervicitis

Chlamydia trachomatis and *Ureaplasma urealyticum* are responsible for most cases of nongonococcal urethritis (see also Chapters 115 and 136). They cannot be differentiated on clinical grounds. An empiric course of tetracycline or erythromycin (500 mg qid of either drug for 7 days) usually suffices. Patients who do not respond to tetracycline therapy may have a tetracyline-resistant ureaplasmal infection and need a course of erythromycin. Relapse can be prevented by treating the patient's sexual partner.

Mucopurulent cervicitis represents another presentation of chlamydial infection, considered by some to be the female equivalent of nongonococcal urethritis. The "swab test" (demonstration of a thick yellow cervical discharge on a cotton swab) is considered highly suggestive of the diagnosis. Treatment is with a standard course of tetracycline for both the patient and her partner. *Acute urethral syndrome,* dysuria with "sterile" pyuria, is yet another manifestation of infection with *Chlamydia;* it responds to tetracycline (see Chapter 132).

Epidydimitis

Most epidydimitis (see Chapter 130) in young men results from sexually transmitted infection with *Chlamydia trachomatis or N. gonorrhoeae.* The condition is best treated with a course of single-dose amoxicillin (3 g) followed by a 10-day course of tetracycline (500 mg qid). Epidydimitis in older men and those who have undergone urinary tract instrumentation is usually a result of gram-negative rod infection of a nonsexual origin.

Chancroid and Granuloma Inguinale

The gram-negative bacillus *Hemophilus ducreyi* causes chancroid, which presents as dirty, shaggy, painful genital ulcers often accompanied by regional adenopathy. Single-dose therapy using four double-strength trimethoprim-sulfa tablets has proven to be highly effective. Ceftriaxone (250 mg IM once) and erythromycin (500 mg qid for 7 days) are also excellent modes of therapy.

Painless, slowly progressive genital ulcers are characteristic of *granuloma inguinale,* caused by the gram-negative bacterium *Donovania granulomatis. Tetracycline* or *erythromycin* is the treatment of choice. Both chancroid and granuloma inguinale are rare in temperate climates.

Lymphogranuloma Venereum

A microorganism belonging to the *Chlamydia* group of obligate intracellular parasites is the cause of lymphogranuloma venereum. In this disease, the primary genital lesion is a small, painless papule that heals spontaneously and often escapes notice. The major impact of the disease is on the regional lymphatics. Inguinal nodes enlarge and may suppurate to produce chronic draining sinuses. Scarring and lymphatic obstruction may result. Rectal fibrosis and strictures are late residua. Tetracycline (500 mg qid for 21 days) is the drug of choice; erythromycin and sulfonamides are alternatives.

ANNOTATED BIBLIOGRAPHY

Amsel R, Totten PA, Spiegel CA et al: Non-specific vaginitis. Diagnostic criteria and microbial and epidemiologic associations. Am J Med 74:14, 1983 (*A new look at this old problem, offering insights into its etiology and recognition.*)

Brunhan RC, Paavonen J, Stevens CE et al: Mucopurulent cervicitis—The ignored counterpart in women of urethritis in men. N Engl J Med 311:1, 1984 (*A study of "female NGU," often caused by* Chlamydia *and responding to tetracycline.*)

Corey L, Adams HG, Brown ZA, Holmes KK: Genital herpes simplex virus infections: Clinical manifestations, course, and complications. Ann Intern Med 98:958, 1983 (*A comprehensive overview of genital herpes.*)

Guinan ME, MacCalman J, Kern ER et al: The course of untreated recurrent genital herpes simplex infection in 27 women. N Engl J Med 304:759, 1981 (*A natural history study of the clinical course of the disease; done before acyclovir was available.*)

Hart G: Syphilis tests in diagnostic and therapeutic decision making. Ann Intern Med 104:368, 1986 (*A critical look at available diagnostic tests.*)

Laskin OL: Acyclovir. Pharmacology and clinical experience. Arch Intern Med 144:1241, 1984 (*A scholarly review of this important drug.*)

Lehrman SN, Douglas JM, Corey L et al: Recurrent genital herpes and suppressive oral acyclovir therapy. Ann Intern Med 104:786, 1986 (*There was neither a high frequency of acyclovir-resistant strains isolated nor a high incidence of recurrences due to resistant strains in patients on 4 months of suppressive acyclovir therapy.*)

McCutchan JA: Epidemiology of venereal urethritis: Comparison of gonorrhea and nongonoccal urethritis. Rev Infect Dis 6:669, 1984 (*A useful comparison of the two predominant varieties of urethritis.*)

Orkin M, Maibach HI: This scabies pandemic. N Engl J Med 298: 496, 1978 (*A detailed review of the clinical features of scabies.*)

Pheifer TA, Forsyth PS, Durfee MA et al: Nonspecific vaginitis: Role of *Haemophilus vaginalis* and treatment with metronidazole. N Engl J Med 298:1429, 1978 (*A provocative reappraisal of the common problem of nonspecific vaginitis.* Haemophilis vaginalis *was the etiologic agent in most patients. Traditional therapy with sulfonamide vaginal cream and orally administered doxycycline and ampicillin was ineffective. Oral metronidazole therapy was effective, but its efficacy must be weighed against its possible toxicity.*)

Plummer FA, Nsanze H, D'Costa LJ et al: Single-dose therapy of chancroid with trimethoprim-sulfametrole. N Engl J Med 309: 67, 1983 (*Four double-strength tablets taken as a one-time dose proved highly effective; a very practical therapy in low-compliance populations.*)

Rein MF, Chapel TA: Trichomoniasis, candidiasis, and the minor venereal diseases. Clin Obstet Gynecol 18:73, 1975 (*An overview of miscellaneous sexually transmitted diseases.*)

Rein MF: Treatment of neurosyphilis. JAMA 246:2513, 1981 (*An editorial review of the data supporting the use of high-dosage intravenous penicillin in neurosyphilis.*)

Sparling PF: Diagnosis and treatment of syphilis. N Engl J Med 284: 642, 1971 (*An excellent review of the serologic diagnosis and antibiotic management of syphilis.*)

Straus SE, Takiff HE, Seidlin M et al: Suppression of frequently recurring genital herpes. N Engl J Med 310:1545, 1984 (*A double-blind, placebo-controlled trial of oral acyclovir demonstrating suppression of recurrences in patients with a history of frequent recurrences.*)

139

Management of the Patient with Chronic Renal Failure

LESLIE S.-T. FANG, M.D.

Although diverse diseases can lead to chronic renal failure, the clinical manifestations and functional derangements are remarkably constant. Hemodialysis and transplantation have increased the capacity to prolong survival and function, but even with such advances in technology, the primary physician continues to have a very important role, being responsible for initial conservative management of the patient with decreasing renal function. The objectives are to prevent or minimize the complications of uremia in order to forestall the need for dialysis, monitor the disease, and judge when referral to the nephrologist is indicated for consideration of dialysis or transplantation.

PATHOPHYSIOLOGY, CLINICAL PRESENTATION, AND COURSE

Pathophysiology

Chronic renal failure can result from glomerular, vascular, or tubular disease. Congenital anomalies, infection, metabolic diseases, obstructive uropathy, and collagen vascular disease can all lead to renal insufficiency. Irrespective of underlying disease, the major clinical manifestations of chronic renal failure result from disturbances in such areas as electrolyte and fluid balance, elimination of metabolic wastes and other toxins, erythropoietin production, and blood pressure control. Considerable controversy exists about the contribution of urea and other toxins to the production of symptoms associated with chronic renal failure.

Fluid and Electrolyte Problems. These include hyperkalemia, volume overload, hypocalcemia, hyperphosphatemia, and metabolic acidosis. With moderate renal insufficiency, *urinary concentrating ability* is impaired, so that to handle the same solute load patients have to drink and excrete more water than normal. This results in polydipsia, polyuria, and nocturia. The ability to dilute urine is compromised with further renal impairment, producing isosthenuria and obligate fluid intake. As renal function continues to decline, oliguria supervenes. The situation is similar with sodium; moderate renal failure produces mild *salt wasting*. In the later stages, sodium excretion becomes limited, *salt retention* develops, and edema supervenes.

Potassium excretion is usually preserved until late in the course, when *potassium retention* occurs as oliguria develops and the ability of the distal tubule to secrete potassium is compromised.

Decreased renal function produces *phosphate retention, secondary hypocalcemia* and, consequently, *secondary hyperparathyroidism*. Decreased intestinal calcium absorption secondary to impaired hydroxylation of vitamin D also contributes to hypocalcemia.

Acidosis results from the compromised kidneys' inability to excrete urinary ammonium and, with further impairment, titratable acid. Acidosis also results from loss of bicarbonate.

Endocrine Problems. Impairment of renal endocrine function contributes to anemia, hypertension, and congestive failure, which may further compromise renal function. *Decreased erythropoietin* results in a mild to moderate normochromic normocytic anemia. Anemia also comes as a consequence of increased hemolysis and bleeding, aggravated by impaired platelet adhesiveness. *Increased renin* levels sometimes occur, causing modest hypertension and fluid retention. In addition to renal osteodystrophy, *secondary hyperparathyroidism* may lead to alterations in CNS calcium, which have been implicated in some of the neurologic manifestations of renal failure.

Clinical Presentation and Course

Early in renal failure, anorexia, lassitude, fatigability, and weakness are prominent symptoms. As renal failure worsens, the patient may complain of pruritus, nausea, vomiting, constipation, or diarrhea. Shortness of breath may occur secondary to cardiomyopathy and fluid overload. Edema, hypertension, and pericarditis are common late in the course. Neurologic manifestations include drowsiness, lethargy, peripheral myopathy, seizures and, terminally, coma.

The course of renal failure is punctuated by periods of rapid deterioration, often precipitated by dehydration or infection. The rate of progression depends on the underlying renal disease and the efficacy of conservative therapy. The rate of progression from moderate renal insufficiency appears to be more rapid for patients with diabetic nephropathy or severe hypertension and to be slower for patients with polycystic kidneys. However, progress to death or dialysis in patients with advanced renal failure (creatinine greater than 10) appears to be reasonably predictable, with a mean survival of 100 to 150 days.

PRINCIPLES OF MANAGEMENT

Conservative management of renal failure can prolong survival and preserve function outside the hospital. Principles of management involve compensating for the excretory, regulatory, and endocrine functions of the kidney. The goals of therapy are to reduce symptoms, slow progression of the underlying disease, and avoid preventable complications.

Protein Intake. The excretory function of the kidneys involves the removal of nitrogenous waste. The cornerstone of therapy is to reduce protein intake to prevent worsening of azotemia. Restricting proteins to 0.5 g/kg/day usually allows sufficient amounts for daily requirements while lessening progression of renal failure. By utilizing a diet high in *essential amino acids,* some investigators have been able to restrict proteins to 0.3 g/kg/day. Essential amino acids appear to be the most effectively utilized source of nitrogen.

Fluids and Electrolytes. Judicious fluid and electrolyte management is exceedingly important because patients with chronic renal failure have difficulty adjusting to variations of either excessive intake or rigid restriction of salt and fluids.

SODIUM. Prior to the late stages of renal failure, salt and fluid intake must be adequate to *match* the excess *losses* that occur as tubular functions begin to deteriorate. Restriction of intake can actually accelerate renal damage by causing decreased extracellular volume and reduced renal perfusion. Concentrating ability can be measured by determining the specific gravity of a first morning urine specimen, and sodium requirements can be estimated by testing a 24-hour urine collection for sodium excretion. In later stages, as excretion of sodium and water becomes limited, cautious sodium and fluid *restrictions* become necessary.

POTASSIUM. Since potassium excretion is preserved until late in the course of renal failure, there is usually no need to restrict its intake until oliguria sets in. However, it is prudent to *avoid* or at least use with caution *drugs* that predispose to potassium retention, such as potassium-sparing diuretics, potassium supplements, beta-adrenergic blockers, and nonsteroidal anti-inflammatory agents. Since acidosis worsens hyperkalemia, it should be corrected promptly. On the other hand, severe protracted hypokalemia can itself cause tubular damages; therefore, serum potassium should be monitored regularly and low levels corrected.

CALCIUM. Hypocalcemia and secondary hyperparathyroidism are best countered by reducing the elevations in serum phosphate that result from decreased renal excretion of the anion. The principle of therapy is to lower serum phosphate by reducing dietary sources, inhibiting absorption through administration of *aluminum hydroxide* antacids, and maintaining adequate calcium levels by pharmacologic doses of *vitamin D* and exogenous *calcium.* In advanced disease, renal hydroxylation of 25-vitamin D is impaired, necessitating use of 1,25-vitamin D. This will reduce the prevalence of secondary hyperparathyroidism and the consequent metabolic bone disease. However, there is some concern that excessive ingestion of aluminum-containing antacids may predispose to osteomalacia and neuropathy. In patients with severe hyperparathyroidism, partial parathyroidectomy should be considered. Hyperuricemia that precipitates symptomatic gouty attacks can be controlled by allopurinol (see Chapter 155).

ACIDOSIS. Correction of acidosis becomes desirable when the serum bicarbonate falls below 15 mEq/L. Any external acid loads, such as aspirin, vitamin C, or excess protein intake, should be removed. *Sodium bicarbonate* is given as long as the sodium load can be tolerated. The goal is to titrate the serum bicarbonate level to the 16 to 20 mEq/L range.

Hematologic Problems. Anemia in the patient with chronic renal failure may be severe enough to cause symptoms. *Androgens* have been shown to stimulate red cell production and can be used successfully in some patients. Others may require repeated transfusions. Repeated *transfusions* carry the risks of hepatitis (see Chapter 52) and sensitization to leukocyte HLA antigens, which may complicate finding a compatible cadaver donor for renal transplantation. On the other hand, transfusion prior to transplantation enhances subsequent graft survival. In many centers, prospective transplant candidates are being purposefully transfused prior to transplantation.

Patients with chronic renal failure should be cautioned to avoid antiplatelet drugs. Abnormalities in platelet function can be aggravated by drugs such as aspirin and other nonsteroidal anti-inflammatory agents (see Chapter 80). The abnormalities can be corrected by dialysis, administration of cryoprecipitates, or DDAVP. Uremia-induced megaloblastic changes are unresponsive to folate or B_{12}.

Cardiovascular Complications. As renal failure advances, these become frequent. The goal of treatment for *hypertension* is to decrease the blood pressure without reducing renal perfusion. The preferred anti-hypertensive agents are alphamethyl-dopa, hydralazine, prazosin, clonidine, and beta blockers. Diuretics, angiotensin-converting enzyme inhibitors, and ganglionic blockers may compromise the glomerular filtration rate.

The onset of congestive heart failure poses a very difficult problem, especially late in the course of the disease when the ability to excrete sodium may be very limited. *Salt restriction* and a trial of a *loop diuretic (e.g.,* furosemide) may be tried but are often insufficient. Digitalization must be done with care, since renal excretion of digoxin is compromised (see Chapter 27). *Dialysis* may be the only recourse in patients with refractory fluid overload.

Neuromuscular Difficulties. Lethargy, inability to concentrate, and asterixis improve with *protein restriction.* However, peripheral neuropathies often progress in spite of comprehensive conservation therapy. Muscle cramping and tetany respond to correction of hypocalcemia.

Itching, Hiccups, and Nausea. These symptoms are not life-threatening, but certainly contribute to the patient's misery and require attention. Pruritus can be quite stubborn, but topical agents for symptomatic relief help. *Prochlorperazine* is effective in lessening hiccups and nausea.

Adjustment of Medications and Avoidance of Nephrotoxic Agents. Doses of drugs and other substances that are excreted renally or are potentially nephrotoxic must be adjusted. This is one of the most crucial aspects of chronic renal failure management. *Digoxin* (see Chapter 27), *aminoglycoside* antibiotics, radiographic *contrast media, angiotensin-converting enzyme inhibitors,* and *nonsteroidal anti-inflammatory agents* are important examples of agents to be used with extreme care in uremic patients. Elderly azotemic patients, who are likely to have some degree of renovascular impairment, are particularly susceptible to agents that affect the renin-angiotensin system (*e.g.,* angiotensin converting-enzyme inhibitors) or inhibit renal prostaglandin production (*e.g.,* nonsteroidal anti-inflammatory drugs). Diabetics with underlying renal disease may experience acute deterioration in renal function from a dye load, such as may be administered for angiography or even pyelography.

Not all drugs that cause an elevation in serum creatinine are necessarily nephrotoxic. Cimetidine and trimethoprim compete with creatinine for tubular excretion; elevations in serum creatinine may ensue, especially in patients who are azotemic. Methyl dopa and cefoxitin interfere with some autoanalyzer measurements of creatinine and can give falsely elevated readings.

Aggravating Conditions. Of chief importance is early detection and correction of any condition that may further compromise renal function. Urinary tract infection, dehydration, gastrointestinal bleeding, and congestive heart failure are among the most common problems that can cause acute decompensation.

PATIENT EDUCATION AND SUPPORT

Successful therapy and good morale are strongly dependent upon a well-developed doctor-patient relationship. The patient must be educated about chronic renal failure and the rationale behind therapy, because compliance is central to successful conservative management, especially if the treatment requires dietary restrictions. Renal failure is a serious chronic disease, often precipitating depression, denial, anger, and noncompliance. The physician's patience, understanding, support, and interest are powerful but sometimes underutilized elements of the treatment program.

It is important to adapt the treatment program to the patient's psychologic style. In general, the patient should have a sense of control over his life by knowing the logic and purpose behind each therapy. Treatment alternatives must be presented honestly, completely, and optimistically. It is necessary to include the family in discussions about diet, medications, prognosis, and therapeutic options. Psychosocial management should aim at minimizing dependence and social isolation.

INDICATIONS FOR REFERRAL AND ADMISSION

Patients can generally be managed as outpatients, but referral to a nephrologist should be made when there is continued clinical deterioration in spite of maximal supportive therapy. As the serum creatinine approaches 10 mg/dl, mean survival drops to between 100 and 150 days, warranting consideration of dialysis or transplantation. Moreover, vascular access for hemodialysis needs to be constructed with 2 to 3 months of lead time to permit maturation of the fistula and revisions. Decisions regarding dialysis and transplantation require a comprehensive evaluation of the patient's medical, psychologic and social situation, necessitating a close working relationship among the patient, family, primary physician, and nephrologist.

The development of *continuous ambulatory peritoneal dialysis* (CAPD) offers an outpatient option with a high degree of independence for the patient and the physiologic advantage of a slow continuous dialysis process. Dialysate administrations are conducted through an indwelling abdominal catheter three to five times per day. Results are comparable to and sometimes better than those for hemodialysis. The main disadvantage is a substantial risk of peritonitis; fortunately, most cases are mild and can be managed on an outpatient basis through self-administration of antibiotics via the catheter.

Hospitalization may be required for control of fluid overload, hypertension, hyperkalemia, or infection. In general, the multiplicity of possible metabolic disturbances in the patient with chronic renal insufficiency demands careful follow-up and constant adjustments of the treatment program.

MANAGEMENT RECOMMENDATIONS

Protein and Calories

- 0.5 gm/kg/day of high-quality protein when the patient is symptomatic or acidotic, 0.5–0.75 gm/kg/day when the BUN is greater than 75, but the patient is asymptomatic.
- Maintain calorie intake at 40 to 50 cal/kg/day

Fluids

- With mild to moderate renal insufficiency, fluid restriction is not necessary unless there is concomitant hypertension or congestive heart failure.
- Restrict fluids only in the presence of oliguria. Intake should equal urine output and insensible losses.

Sodium

- With mild to moderate renal insufficiency, salt restriction is not necessary.
- In patients with hypertension or congestive heart failure, salt restriction to 4 g of sodium daily may be necessary.
- Restrict sodium in the presence of oliguria or congestive heart failure.

Potassium

- In hypokalemia, administer potassium supplements in low doses and check levels frequently. Do not maintain indefinite potassium supplementation.
- Avoid potassium-sparing diuretics in patients with moderate renal insufficiency.
- Monitor potassium frequently in oliguric patients. Treat levels greater than 6 mEq/liter and admit if ECG changes accompany levels greater than 6.5 mEq/liter. Mild chronic hyperkalemia is best treated with the use of exchange resins such as sodium polystyrene sulfonate (Kayexalate), given by mouth or instilled as an enema in sorbitol. Kayexalate exchanges sodium ion for potassium ion; therefore, be alert to possible sodium and volume overload.

Calcium and Phosphate

- Correct hyperphosphatemia with phosphate-binding antacids, usually 30–60 ml of aluminum hydroxide gel three times a day before meals.
- Symptomatic or severe hypocalcemia despite normalization of serum phosphate requires calcium supplements (*e.g.,* calcium carbonate 600 mg bid) and/or vitamin D in pharmacologic doses (*e.g.,* calcitriol 0.25 mg qd).

Acidosis

- Treat when serum bicarbonate concentration is less than 15 mEg/L.
- Remove external acid load.
- Treat acidosis with sodium bicarbonate, 600 mg twice daily initially, and titrate bicarbonate to the 16–20 mEg/L range. Follow serum potassium and calcium levels during treatment of acidosis, since both may fall.

Anemia

- Transfuse for high output failure or angina. Avoid unnecessary blood work and injections.
- Avoid antiplatelet drugs.
- Oral ferrous sulfate, 325 mg per day should be given to patients with iron deficiency.
- Weekly injections of nandrolone decanoate, 100 mg, can be administered to male patients.

Congestive Heart Failure

- Treat with restriction of salt.
- Add furosemide if congestive failure persists.
- Digoxin can be used, but frequent monitoring of digoxin levels is needed.

Itching, Hiccups, and Nausea

- Treat uremic complications by controlling the dietary protein intake.
- Prochlorperazine 5–10 mg orally four times daily may be effective for nausea.
- Itching may respond to menthol and phenol lotions or cholestyramine: recently, ultraviolet light has been used successfully.

Dialysis and Transplantation

- The conservative management outlined is directed toward the prolongation of the symptom-free period. When dietary therapy becomes intolerable or is no longer effective, dialysis or transplantation must be considered. Referral to a nephrologist is necessary at this point. The primary physician should continue to participate in the important decisions about dialysis and transplantation.

A.H.G.

ANNOTATED BIBLIOGRAPHY

Alfrey AC: The toxicity of the aluminum burden. Semin Nephrol 3: 329, 1983 (*Describes the neuropathic and bony effects attributed to the aluminum salts found in dialysate fluids and phosphate-binding antacids.*)

Baehler RW, Galla HJ: Conservative management of chronic renal failure. Geriatrics, September 1976, p. 46 (*A good review.*)

Bennett WM, Aronoff GR, Morrison G et al: Drug prescribing in renal failure. Am J Kidney Dis 3:155, 1983 (*Extensive tables and discussion of dosing guidelines for adults with renal failure, including those on dialysis.*)

Ciabattoni G, Cinotti GA, Pierucci A et al: Effects of sulindac and ibuprofen in patients with chronic glomerular disease. N Engl J Med 310:279, 1984 (*Provides evidence for impairment GFR by prostacyclin inhibitors such as the nonsteroidal anti-inflammatory drugs.*)

Feldman HA, Singer I: Endocrinology and metabolism in uremia and dialysis: A clinical review. Medicine 54:345, 1975 (*Excellent discussion of metabolic complications of uremia.*)

Fine RN, Terasaki PI, Ettenger RB et al: Renal transplantation update. Ann Intern Med 100:246, 1984 (*A comprehensive and recent review useful for the general internist.*)

Giordano C: Role of diet in renal disease. Hosp Pract November 1977, p. 113 (*A review of nitrogen metabolism, emphasizing reutilization of endogenous nitrogen with advice on dietary management of uremia.*)

Hendler ED, Goffinet JA et al: A controlled study of androgen therapy in anemia of patients on maintenance hemodialysis. N Engl J Med 291: 1046, 1974 (*A controlled crossover study demonstrating benefits of androgen therapy.*)

McCrary RF, Pitts TO, Puschett JB et al: Diabetic nephropathy. Am J Nephrol 1:206, 1981 (*A review of its natural history, prognosis, and treatment, with good discussion on the roles of dialysis and transplantation.*)

Mooradian AD, Morley JE: Endocrine dysfunction in chronic renal failure. Arch Intern Med 144:351, 1984 (*A short, but useful summary of the effects of chronic renal failure on endocrine function, including workup of these changes and therapy.*)

Quevedo SG, Young JH, Carrie BJ et al: Continuous peritoneal dialysis: Bridging the gap between evaluation and practice in chronic illness. Ann Intern Med 104:430, 1986 (*An editorial taking a critical look at the procedure and reports of its efficacy: makes a plea for incorporating the perspective of the patient's illness experience into decision-making.*)

Schwartz WB, Kassirer JP: Medical management of chronic renal failure. Am J Med 44:786, 1968 (*A symposium that remains a classic reference on the subject.*)

Volmer WM, Wahl PW, Blagg CR: Survival with dialysis and transplantation in patients with end-stage renal disease. N Engl J Med 308:1553, 1983 (*An examination of the survival experience of over 1000 patients: little difference found between groups treated with dialysis or transplantation: authors argue choice should be made on basis of factors other than survival.*)

140
Management of Urinary Tract Infection in Men

Urinary tract infection is rare in men under the age of 50, but occurs in almost 5% by age 70. In elderly debilitated patients confined to nursing homes, the prevalence may reach as high as 20% to 50%. Symptomatic urinary tract infection in young men suggests urethritis (see Chapter 129), prostatitis (see Chapter 137) or an anatomic defect in the urinary tract; identification of the underlying cause is relatively straightforward. By comparison, asymptomatic bacteriuria in the elderly patient is both more common and more perplexing.

The primary physician needs to know the clinical significance of bacteriuria in men, what type of workup is indicated, and what modes of therapy are most effective.

PATHOPHYSIOLOGY, CLINICAL PRESENTATION, AND COURSE

In young men, urinary tract infection ensues from a structural abnormality of the urinary tract (often congenital in nature) or represents infection of the prostate or urethra. Dysuria, frequency, and urgency accompany most forms, with urethral discharge characteristic of urethritis. Most cases of urethritis are venereal in origin and respond well to treatment (see Chapter 136). Prostatitis tends to be a more stubborn infection, often requiring prolonged antibiotic therapy (see Chapter 137). Those with an anatomic defect do not improve unless the structural problem is alleviated.

In elderly men, the development of a postvoid residual urine volume plays a major role in establishment of bacteriuria. Factors contributing to the residual volume include bladder dysfunction (see Chapter 133), outflow tract obstruction, concomitant illness, and the aging process. Condom catheters are widely used for incontinent elderly men and may contribute to the risk of infection, although the increased risk may simply reflect the high frequency of postvoid residual volumes in incontinent patients.

The *coliforms* account for the vast majority of the organisms isolated; enterococci are the cause in about 10% to 20%. In patients with infection due to a single organism, *E. coli* is the organism most often recovered. Multiple organisms are found in as many as a third of infected nursing home patients; *Proteus, Pseudomonas,* and *Providencia* are among the species found in mixed infections.

Elderly patients with bacteriuria may become quite ill, although the vast majority are asymptomatic. The usual manifestations of serious, symptomatic urinary tract infection may be absent, replaced by such vague findings as "failure to thrive" or worsening mental status. Gram-negative sepsis from a urinary tract source can be life threatening. On the other hand, asymptomatic bacteriuria can be a chronic, seemingly well-tolerated state. There is debate as to whether bacteriuria per se increases mortality; studies controlling for comorbid conditions show no increase.

One reason for the unresolved debate on the significance of bacteriuria in elderly men is the difficulty in definitively eradicating bacteria from their urinary tracts, especially in those who are debilitated and require nursing-home care. Both single-dose, conventional (10 day), and prolonged treatment programs (as long as 3 months) are associated with high rates of treatment failure and recurrent infection. The reasons for the refractoriness to treatment are not well understood, but may involve prostatic sequestration (chronic prostatitis has been found in over half of men with recurrent urinary tract infection) or the presence of a postvoid residual volume. Most recurrences represent relapses, with subsequent recovery of the same organism within 4 weeks of cessation of antibiotic therapy.

DIAGNOSIS AND WORKUP

In men, a diagnosis of urinary tract infection is justified upon isolation of a pure culture of 10^4 organisms per ml of urine. A midstream sample suffices for most clinical situa-

tions, but the expressed prostatic secretions (EPS) may need to be sampled when prostatitis is a consideration. Isolation of less than 10^3 organisms or mixed flora are generally felt to represent contamination. There is some debate regarding the significance of a urine sample containing a pure culture of 10^3 organisms per ml.

In the young man with urinary tract symptoms, searches for urethritis (see Chapter 129), prostatitis (see Chapter 137), and structural abnormalities are in order. Appropriate workup includes a thorough sexual history, checking for and gram-staining any urethral discharge, rectal examination of the prostate, Gram stain of the EPS, and intravenous pyelography (especially when there is a history of urinary tract infections in childhood or when the remainder of the workup is unrevealing).

In the elderly patient, assessment is best directed at elucidation of an underlying risk factor, such as a bladder dysfunction (see Chapter 133), prostatitis (see Chapter 137), or a form of outflow tract obstruction, such as prostatic hypertrophy (see Chapter 135).

PRINCIPLES OF MANAGEMENT

Symptomatic urinary tract infection in men should be treated. Standard 10-day regimens of *trimethoprim-sulfamethoxazole* (one double-strength tablet bid) or *amoxicillin* (500 mg tid) often produce symptomatic improvement; however, treatment is unlikely to be successful unless the *underlying precipitant* is corrected. If there is a large postvoid residual volume in the bladder, relapse is likely, even after a prolonged course of therapy; the same holds for patients with chronic prostatitis (see Chapter 137). In a large study of recurrent urinary tract infections in men, over half had a prostatic source.

Debate continues on whether to treat the *elderly* institutionalized male who has *asymptomatic bacteriuria.* The issue will remain moot so long as it continues to be virtually impossible to irradicate infection in such patients and the impact of infection on survival remains unknown. Again, attention to underlying risk factors (obstruction, bladder dysfunction, prostatitis) may be the most productive approach, rather than resorting to repeated courses of ever more potent antibiotics, which do little more than lead to the selection of drug-resistant strains. As noted above, whether or not condom catheter use precipitates infections remains unclear; however, an attempt at eliminating condom use for a period of time, if at all possible, is worth a try if there are no other precipitants evident.

A.H.G.

ANNOTATED BIBLIOGRAPHY

Dontas AS, Kasviki-Charvati P, Papanayiotou PC et al: Bacteriuria and survival in old age. N Engl J Med 304:939, 1981 (*A study of asymptomatic bacteriuria in elderly nursing home residents, showing a reduction in survival among those with infection compared to a group of uninfected residents.*)

Freedman LR: Urinary tract infections in the elderly. N Engl J Med 309:1451, 1983 (*An editorial discussing the unresolved issue of need to treat elderly men with asymptomatic bacteriuria.*)

Nicolle LE, Bjornson J, Harding GKM et al: Bacteriuria in elderly institutionalized men. N Engl J Med 309:1420, 1983 (*The data from this study suggest that treatment of asymptomatic bacteriuria is neither necessary nor effective; an example of a negative study on the subject.*)

Nordenstam GR, Brandberg CA, Oden AS et al: Bacteriuria and mortality in an elderly population. N Engl J Med 314:1152, 1986 (*A 9-year cohort study finding no difference in mortality among women with and without bacteriuria; also, no difference among men when those with cancer were excluded.*)

Smith JW, Jones SR, Reed WP et al: Recurrent urinary tract infections in men. Ann Intern Med 91:544, 1979 (*A study aimed at determining clinical characteristics and response to therapy. Found that half had underlying prostate infection, over 70% had E. coli as the organism, and most failed to respond to a standard 10-day course of therapy, whether symptomatic or not.*)

141
Management of Urinary Tract and Male Genital Cancers

JACOB J. LOKICH, M.D.

Cancers of the genitourinary tract in men are often localized, and if so, managed singularly by surgery or radiation. Unfortunately, advanced disease is common, requiring a team approach involving the surgeon, oncologist, radiotherapist, and primary physician. The responsibilities of the primary physician include prevention (particularly important in bladder cancer), screening for early disease (see Chapters 125 and 126), and counselling, supporting, and monitoring patients with advanced disease.

CARCINOMA OF THE PROSTATE

Epidemiology

Although by age 80 more than 50% of men have at least microscopic evidence of prostate carcinoma at autopsy, the condition should not be approached as an incidental finding because the morbidity and mortality rates are substantial. Carcinoma of the prostate is the third leading cause of death in men. There are an estimated 76,000 new cases annually. Incidence appears to be rising, particularly among older black men. No association with benign prostatic hypertrophy has been found. The relation of the disease to androgenic stimulation is suggested by the absence of the cancer in castrated men.

Clinical Presentation and Course

In 85% of cases, the tumor arises in the posterior lobe or lamella of the prostate, making detection by digital examination possible in many instances. However, only 30% of new cases are discovered by this means. Most present with symptoms of urethral obstruction; renal insufficiency from prolonged urinary tract obstruction ensues in a small, but not inconsequential, fraction. About 15% of patients have bone pain or other manifestations of metastatic disease as the presenting complaint. Osteoblastic metastases predominate; they can be painful and are the major cause of morbidity. Metastasis to regional lymph nodes is both common and usually asymptomatic; it may occur even when disease appears clinically to be confined to the gland (see later discussion) and before spread to bone.

Prognosis is a function of disease stage at the time of diagnosis. The majority of patients with prostate cancer will develop or demonstrate metastases at the time of initial presentation. However, only a third of the 76,000 new cases each year will die of the disease. Due to the advanced age of this patient population, many die of other conditions.

Staging

The staging of prostate cancer is done by clinical means and remains suboptimal due to the lack of methods that are sufficiently sensitive and noninvasive to effectively detect metastatic disease. At present, staging is conducted by careful *palpation* of the prostate to establish the extent of local tumor and by a *bone scan* to search for bony metastases. *Acid phosphatase* as well as lymphangiography, pelvic node dissection, and bone marrow biopsy have proven to be too morbid or too insensitive to justify routine use. For example, as many as 25% of patients with a normal acid phosphatase will have bony metastases.

Clinical staging frequently underestimates extent of disease. For example, digital examination has been found to under-stage about one third of patients thought to have disease limited to the prostate. Metastases to regional lymph nodes often go undetected and often occur before spread to bone.

Noninvasive assessment of lymph nodes by *lymphangiography* has proven inadequate due to poor visualization of obturator-hypogastric nodes, which are the only site of nodal disease in up to one-third of patients. *Pelvic lymphadenectomy* is the definitive means of establishing nodal disease, but its morbidity is substantial. The inadequacy of staging, in part, accounts for the oft-noted poor correlation between clinical stage and response to therapy. It is also the reason for the conflicting reports of treatment results that pervade the prostate cancer literature.

Attempts to compensate for the shortcomings of clinical staging and to better estimate the likelihood of metastatic disease include designation of subcategories within each stage and consideration of histologic pattern (patients with higher grade histology are more likely to harbor lymph node metastases).

A typical A, B, C, and D staging system is used. In *stage A,* there are no nodules or masses on palpation of the gland. Disease at this stage consists of malignancy found incidentally during prostatectomy for treatment of benign prostatic hypertrophy. *Stage A₁* represents microscopic foci of well-differentiated malignant cells; survival is the same as that of the population at large. *Stage A₂* denotes diffuse or poorly differentiated disease; this an aggressive tumor with a high risk of mortality if left untreated (as many as 25% of these patients have lymph node metastases).

In *stage B,* there is a palpable prostatic nodule noted on rectal examination. If the lesion is less than 1.5 cm in diameter and confined to one lobe, it is designated *stage B₁*. B₁ disease is usually confined to the gland and has a very good prognosis with treatment. If the palpable lesion is greater than 1.5 cm or extends beyond one lobe, it is considered *stage B₂*. Clinical stage B₂ has a 15% to 45% chance of having occult metastases to lymph nodes at the time of presentation; consequently, its prognosis is less favorable. Cure is still possible; failure to treat is potentially fatal.

In *stage C,* rectal examination reveals local extension beyond the prostate to the pelvic wall, seminal vessicles, or bladder neck. Bone scan is normal, suggesting localized disease, but 40% to 80% of patients at this clinical stage will have lymph node metastases. Thus many people who are clinically stage C already have metastatic disease and a poor prognosis. At present, there are no clinical means of distinguishing "true" stage C disease from more advanced cases.

In *stage D,* there are distant metastases, most often to bone; palliation is the most that can be expected. Some feel that the designation stage *D₁* is needed to identify patients with a small volume of metastatic disease limited to pelvic nodes who might be candidates for an attempt at curative therapy.

Principles of Management

Selection of treatment modality is determined by stage at the time of presentation:

Stage A₁. Patients with stage A₁ disease *need not be treated,* since survival is unaffected by the disease. Such patients require only periodic follow-up for symptoms or development of a prostatic nodule.

Stages A₂ and B. These patients are candidates for either surgery or irradiation. The 10-year survival rates are similar for both modalities (approximately 50%). For most patients, *irradiation* has emerged as the preferred treatment modality due to the lower risk of impotence and the absence of risk for urinary incontinence. *Radical prostatectomy* means almost certain impotence and a 5% to 10% chance of incontinence. Neither impotence nor incontinence is a problem with interstitial radiation conducted by surgical implantation. Factors favorable to radical prostatectomy are a small stage B lesion (less than 1.5 cm), well-differentiated histology, and the patient's willingness to put up with the adverse consequences of such surgery.

Stage C. Both irradiation and surgery provide excellent control of local disease. However, as already noted, many of these patients do not have localized disease; consequently, results are disappointing and hardly worth the morbidity of radical surgery unless disease is truly localized, which can be difficult to determine. Thus, *surgery* for stage C disease is becoming less common. *Irradiation* gives equally good control, with less risk of impotence and virtually no risk of incontinence. The 10-year survival rates for external beam irradiation and surgery are similar (approximately 30%); 5-year survival rates are slightly better for surgery than for radiation (60% vs. 40%). In the setting of systemic symptoms, hormonal manipulations (see below) may be of help.

Stage D. At the present time, the goal for this stage is palliation. Relief of localized bone pain can be achieved promptly with a short course of x-ray therapy, but the mainstay of treatment for symptomatic metastatic disease is hormonal manipulation.

Modalities range from orchiectomy to use of estrogens and antiandrogens. Therapy need not be instituted until the patient becomes symptomatic from metastatic disease, because survival is unaffected by when treatment is initiated.

Orchiectomy is the least morbid of the hormonal approaches; it results in significant tumor regression, manifested by reduction in size of the primary tumor and relief of bone pain. The procedure greatly reduces androgenic stimulation of the tumor, though it does not affect the adrenal source of androgens. Adrenalectomy and hypophysectomy have been used as tertiary hormonal measures. Before such ablative surgery is resorted to, exogenous hormone treatment deserves consideration.

Estrogens (diethylstilbestrol or ethinyl estradiol) are believed to work by decreasing gonadotropin levels, as well as by competitively inhibiting or blocking circulating androgens. Their effect is comparable to orchiectomy in inducing tumor regression. The combination of orchiectomy plus estrogen fares no better than when each is used alone. Moreover, patients failing to respond to orchiectomy are unlikely to benefit from estrogen.

A primary complication of estrogen therapy is *vascular thrombosis,* both arterial and venous. The risk becomes significant when high doses are used (>3 mg per day of diethylstilbestrol), especially in the elderly. For this reason, high-dose estrogen therapy is not advised; moreover, it is no more effective than moderate doses (*e.g.,* <3 mg per day of diethylstilbestrol). The high rates of arterial and venous thrombosis associated with estrogen use are perhaps a function of the hypercoaguable state of malignancy and advanced age. Concomitant use of aspirin or coumarin is sometimes prescribed to prevent such complications. *Gynecomastia* represents another estrogen side effect; it may be prevented by prophylactic low-dose breast irradiation.

An alternative hormonal approach involves use of *antiandrogens,* which act peripherally to inhibit androgenic effects. Though they do not induce a hypercoaguable state or gynecomastia, they can cause *impotence.* Undergoing clinical trials are *gonadotropin-releasing factor agonists (e.g.,* leuprolide). After causing a brief period of initial stimulation, they have the paradoxical effect of inhibiting LH and FSH release by the pituitary, which in turn reduces production of testosterone and adrenal androgens. There are a minimum of adverse effects, and clinical remissions have been documented in initial trials. Results are encouraging.

Much can be done to make the patient with advanced disease comfortable. In addition to the above palliative measures, use of adequate analgesia (see Chapter 91) should not be overlooked.

Monitoring. The serum *acid phosphatase* remains a convenient means of monitoring the effectiveness of treatment. It is elevated in up to 80% of patients with advanced disease. Although inadequate as a screening test for early disease (see Chapter 125) or as a staging technique (see above), it can be useful to monitor response to therapy if elevated at onset of treatment. An acid phosphatase fraction relatively specific for prostate cancer has been identified, but it shows elevations in only about 50% of patients with metastatic disease. Moreover, its quantitative level does not directly correlate with tumor burden. A radio-immunoassay for *prostate-specific* acid phosphatase is available, offering greater sensitivity with only minimal compromise of specificity. Although not appropriate as a screening test for early stages of disease (see Chapter 125), it may have a place in monitoring therapy; this remains to be established. Any specific correlation between marker and antitumor effect should incorporate additional objective and subjective parameters of tumor response.

For the asymptomatic patient under no current therapy, regular inquiry into development of *symptoms* has proven an economical yet effective means of monitoring; routine use of repeat blood tests and radiographic studies can become very expensive and should be considered only when the result will substantively alter clinical decision making.

Patient Education

Working in conjunction with the urologist, radiotherapist, and oncologist, the primary physician can play an important role in helping the patient to understand the various treatment options and their consquences. Patients who are deemed candidates for radical prostatectomy surgery need to clearly recognize the likelihood of impotence and the risk of incontinence.

Counselling is also important in patients who are being considered for orchiectomy. Patients are surprised and comforted to realize they will not undergo feminization upon removal of the testes.

TESTICULAR CANCER

Testicular cancer is the most common malignancy in men between the ages of 20 and 30 years and a major cause of death in this age group. Its seriousness and curability, both in early stages and, more recently, in advanced stages make it an important disease for the primary physician. One needs to encourage self-examination, screen young men during routine checkups (see Chapter 126), and help guide the patient with advanced disease through his illness.

Pathophysiology, Clinical Presentation and Course

Known predisposing factors are testicular atrophy (secondary to an undescended testicle) and Klinefelter's syndrome. Suspected risk factors include natural exposure to intrapartum estrogens, exposure to insecticides, and prior history of a testicular tumor. Trauma is not a known precipitant.

Almost all testicular cancers are germ-cell tumors. *Seminomas* account for 40% to 50%; most are confined to the testicle at the time of presentation. The remainder are termed *nonseminomatous germ-cell tumors* (NSGCT). These include *teratomas, choriocarcinomas, embryonal-cell carcinomas,* and *endodermal sinus tumors.* Many are of mixed cell type; their metastases may be less differentiated than the primary. Both groups commonly present as solid, painless, nontransilluminating testicular masses in young men (see Chapter 130). Some patients complain of "heaviness" in the scrotum; pain is less common. These tumors are rapidly growing and spread by the lymphatics and blood. Occasionally, the tumor is occult at the primary site with metastases already established. If chorionic gonadotropin is secreted (as may occur with several of the NSGCT), gynecomastia may be an initial complaint. Disease already established in the lung may present with cough or hemoptysis.

Diagnosis and Staging

A solid, nontransilluminating, painless testicular mass in a young man should be presumed to represent a primary testicular cancer. It needs to be assessed and treated by surgical removal of the testicle through an inguinal canal approach to minimize risk of seeding the scrotum, as might occur with a transscrotal operative procedure.

Staging procedures include a search for metastatic disease in the lung by *chest x-ray* and *computed tomography,* and in the lymph nodes, abdomen, and retroperitoneum by computed tomography of the retroperitoneum and abdomen. Previously, if there was no evidence of metastatic disease by these studies, an ipsilateral complete *lymphadenectomy* and contralateral partial lymphadenectomy to the level of the aortic bifurcation was considered mandatory for NSGCT, due to the high incidence of microscopic nodal involvement. However, lymphadenectomy is now being used less. Noninvasive staging may be followed by chemotherapy, with secondary surgical exploration to evaluate the retroperitoneum. Retroperitoneal lymph node dissection is unnecessary if the primary is a seminoma, since it so radiosensitive and highly curable.

Circulating *tumor markers* provide ability to detect occult disease. The *beta subunit of HCG* is always elevated in choriocarcinoma and in about half of the other NSGCT (its elevation is rare in pure seminoma, but a number of seminomatous cases have mixed disease and elevations in HCG). *Alpha-fetoprotein* is produced by about 80% of patients with embryonal-cell cancer. These markers are also an excellent means of monitoring response to therapy (see below).

Stage I involves disease localized to the testis. In stage II, there is spread beyond the testis to regional retroperitoneal lymph nodes; the subclass A has small- to moderate-sized metastases; subclass B designates massive adenopathy. In stage III, there are mediastinal or supraclavicular nodal metastases; in stage IV, extralymphatic spread.

Management

Treatment decisions are based on stage, histology, and tumor-marker levels. *Stage I seminomatous disease* is treated with *inguinal orchiectomy* followed by *retroperitoneal node irradiation.* The cure rate is close to 100%. Patients who relapse are candidates for combination chemotherapy, which is extremely effective (see below). Patients with *stage IIA* disease at time of initial presentation have their treatment fields extended to include irradiation of the *mediastinum* and *left supraclavicular nodes.* Cure rates are still close to 100% at this stage. Patients with IIB disease are more of a problem, requiring combination therapy with surgery, radiation, and, if necessary, chemotherapy for persistent disease.

Stages I and IIA NSGCT disease are treated with *surgery only.* Cure rates are in excess of 80%. Patients with stage IIB have a high probability of relapse and thus are candidates for chemotherapy, as are patients with more advanced stages of disease.

Multiple-agent chemotherapy represents an important breakthrough in treatment of testicular cancer. Even patients with metastatic disease have a chance for cure as a consequence of using *cisplatin* in conjunction with *vinblastine* and *bleomycin.* The ability to induce prolonged remission or even cure in patients with advanced disease is in excess of 80%. Adjuvant programs after surgery are unnecessary, because it is possible to cure most patients by use of chemotherapy if treated early in the course of relapse. Maintenance therapy after a course of treatment for disseminated disease is also not needed, due to the excellent and lasting response obtained by most patients.

Combined modality treatment with *"adjuvant" surgery* following chemotherapy is applied to patients with residual intraperitoneal or intrathoracic disease. If tumor markers are still elevated, another course of chemotherapy may be necessary to prevent relapse. Those with bulky tumors or very high marker levels may require salvage regimens utilizing high-dose cisplatin and other drugs such as *etoposide.*

Monitoring. Closely monitoring response to therapy is critical to achieving a successful result. As noted above, chemotherapy applied in the early phase of relapse is likely to be very successful, but much less so if treatment is delayed. *HCG* and *alpha-fetoprotein* serve as excellent means of detecting subclinical relapse and failure to respond to treatment. Resistance to therapy is suggested by an elevated serum marker level not falling to normal with therapy; its rise during follow-up indicates relapse. Patients having isolated elevations in tumor markers as the sole manifestation of relapse have nearly a 100% chance of cure when treated promptly with combination chemotherapy. In patients with advanced disease, a decline in HCG after initial chemotherapy is an excellent predictor of response to treatment.

Periodic physical examination for development of palpable adenopathy or an abdominal mass and *chest film* for thoracic metastases are important parts of the monitoring effort.

Patient Education

Treatment for testicular cancer is not without its adverse effects, which need to be reviewed with the patient prior to therapy. Retrograde ejaculation and subsequent infertility are consequences of lymph node dissection; erection is only rarely compromised. Radiation therapy is associated with a risk of decreased spermatogenesis in the remaining normal testicle, though shielding methods have reduced the radiation exposure and, consequently the period of infertility due to low sperm counts. Alopecia, sepsis, anemia, myalgias, and severe, though transient, nausea and vomiting are the important adverse effects of combination chemotherapy (see Chapter 89).

Cisplatin–induced renal toxicity is preventable with good hydration. There is a small (1% to 2%) risk of fatal pulmonary toxicity from bleomycin; another 2% to 3% experience irreversible pulmonary fibrosis; these effects are rare when cumulative dose is kept under 450 units.

CARCINOMA OF THE BLADDER

Bladder cancer strikes about 30,000 patients annually in the United States, causing about 10,000 deaths per year. Patients at increased risk include heavy smokers, those exposed industrially to naphthalene or aromatic amine antioxidants, and users of the drug cyclophosphamide. There are no long-term epidemiologic data on the relation between saccharin intake and bladder cancer, although animal studies suggest an association. The issue remains controversial (see Chapter 126).

Clinical Presentation and Course

Tumors of the bladder are usually detected when gross or microscopic hematuria is noted. In most instances the hematuria is painless and unassociated with dysuria, urgency, frequency, or voiding of small volumes of uninfected urine; however, older patients, especially men, with carcinoma-in-situ experience such symptoms in conjunction with hematuria.

Ninety percent of bladder cancers are transitional-cell carcinomas; squamous-cell tumors account for most of the others. A few are undifferentiated. Multiple tumors may arise simultaneously. Depth of invasion is the most important predictor of survival, though histologic grade is also a factor. Five-year survival with appropriate treatment is 95% for patients with carcinoma in situ, 60% for disease that invades the subepithelial connective tissue, 35% for superficial muscle invasion, 15% for deep muscle invasion, and nil for extension to the pelvis. Spread to the lymph nodes is common in patients with deep muscle invasion.

Diagnosis and Staging

Diagnosis begins with a urine specimen for cytology; midmorning sample is recommended by some because of degeneration of cellular material in urine that has been sitting in the bladder overnight. Suspicious cytology that is nondiagnostic warrants follow-up with *bladder washings,* which may be the only means of revealing an otherwise occult carcinoma in situ. *Intravenous pyelography* is obtained for evidence of an infiltrated bladder wall, a filling defect, or a bladder diverticulum. *Cystoscopy* completes the evaluation and includes biopsy samples from multiple sites.

Staging is performed by *cystoscopy* with *biopsy* and *bimanual rectal-abdominal examination* under anesthesia to determine depth of tumor penetration and infiltration into the bladder wall. Although almost half of patients with infiltration into deep muscle have spread to lymph nodes (which carries a poor prognosis), such spread is hard to detect without resorting to pelvic lymphadenectomy. Early spread involves the hypogastric and obturator nodes, which are not adequately visualized by pedal lymphangiography; moreover, inflamed nodes give false-positive results. A chest x-ray, alkaline phosphatase, and bone scan are commonly ordered to check for distant metastases.

Treatment

Noninvasive stages of disease are often curable with local measures. *Excision* at the time of cystoscopy in conjunction with fulguration represents a most effective form of therapy for early disease. In the setting of multiple tumors, the cytotoxic agent *thio-TEPA* can be instilled. Irradiation of the bladder can effect tumor regression, but the recurrence rate is high. Rapid recurrence of multiple lesions is an indication for combined *cystectomy* and *prostatectomy.* Diffuse carcinoma-in-situ with persistently positive washings despite treatment has a poor prognosis and may necessitate early cystectomy.

Infiltrative disease carries a poor prognosis due to the substantial likelihood of lymph node metastases (see above). Options include *partial bladder resection, cystectomy* with urinary diversion via an *ileal loop,* radical radiation and combination therapy. Although partial cystectomy has the attraction of preserving some of the bladder, only a few patients are suitable candidates. *Combination therapy* consisting of *preoperative irradiation* plus *cystectomy* is often utilized. Complications include a surgical mortality rate of 5%, postoperative problems necessitating a prolonged hospitalization in about one quarter and the possibility of need for revision of the ileal loop. Hyperchloremic metabolic acidosis sometimes occurs in these patients.

Those with *deeply invasive disease* are not candidates for surgery; external beam *megavoltage irradiation* provides a reasonable chance (50%) for local control and a small chance (no more than 25%) for cure. The rate of bowel and bladder complications is 10% to 15%. About half of these patients maintain sexual potency. In patients with *distant metastases, cisplatin* in conjunction with *cyclophosphamide* and *doxorubicin* have achieved substantial, but not lasting, regression.

Since many patients with bladder cancer present with advanced disease, the focus of treatment is often palliative. If not previously utilized, radiation can provide relief from pelvic and bone pain. The onset of ureteral obstruction and subsequent uremia presents a relatively comfortable means of dying to patients with advanced disease; relief of the obstruction is rarely indicated.

Monitoring of patients treated for early stage disease is essential. Surveillance cystoscopy and washings are conducted every 3 months during the first year and then at less frequent intervals.

Patient Education

The best treatment for bladder cancer is prevention. Risk factors such as smoking and occupational exposure should be addressed (see Chapter 126). Patients who are to undergo cystectomy need prior counselling about management of the ileal loop. Most adjust reasonably well to managing the stoma and bag. Stoma groups and teaching by a stoma nurse can be quite helpful.

RENAL CELL CARCINOMA (HYPERNEPHROMA)

Renal cancer is not particularly common, accounting for about 2% of all malignancies. However, it is a potentially curable disease, with about 15,000 new cases annually in the United States. The disease is notorious for its protean presentations, though painless hematuria is the most common, found in 50% to 75% of cases. Aching flank pain and a palpable mass are other classic, though far less frequent manifestations; they represent advanced disease. Unexplained weight loss, nausea and vomiting, fever of unknown origin, and a markedly elevated erythrocyte sedimentation rate are sometimes systemic clues of early disease, occurring in up to a third of patients. Paraneoplastic syndromes are associated with this disease, including polycythemia and hypercalcemia secondary to production of a PTH-like substance. The natural history of the tumor is unique, with spontaneous regression as well as long intervals before the appearance of metastases. Nevertheless, a major proportion of patients with hypernephroma present with or develop metastases.

A high index of suspicion is needed to make an early diagnosis of this disease. Patients suspected of harbouring a hypernephroma need a complete blood count, erythrocyte sedimentation rate (ESR), and urinalysis. Suggestive, though nondiagnostic findings include hematuria, normochromic, normocytic anemia, and markedly elevated ESR. The triad of fever, elevated ESR, and increased alpha-1 globulin is characteristic.

If suspicion remains high, radiologic evaluation should follow with *intravenous pyelography.* Finding a mass on IVP requires determining whether it is cystic (and therefore most likely benign) or solid; renal *ultrasound* offers an excellent means of making the distinction. In the 10% of instances where the lesion appears cystic by ultrasound but does not fullfil all ultrasonographic criteria for a cyst, radiologically guided *aspiration* of a suspected cyst can be utilized for confirmation. *Computed tomography* of a solid renal mass provides information on perinephric involvement, renal vein obstruction, and spread to the retroperitoneal nodes.

Tumor confined to the kidney is curable; when it extends beyond Gerota's capsule, prognosis is poor. Some authorities suggest that removal of the primary tumor may trigger regression of metastases, though the only evidence derives from case reports. Large series have failed to demonstrate

such an effect or an improvement in survival. Most argue that the primary tumor in patients with metastatic disease should be removed only for control of local pain or bleeding. Metastases to lung, bone, and brain are treated with chemotherapy or irradiation.

Effective chemotherapeutic regimens are lacking for this disease. Hormonal therapies (progesterone and androgens) have attained responses in about 20% of patients, but without prolonging survival. The use of interferon, a biologic response modifier (see Chapter 88), is undergoing evaluation.

ANNOTATED BIBLIOGRAPHY

Prostate Cancer

Bagshaw MA, Ray GR, Pistenma DA et al: External beam radiation therapy of primary carcinoma of the prostate. Cancer 36:723, 1975 (*A summary of the use of radiation therapy for carcinoma of the prostate employing high-dose extended field therapy in the Stanford University tradition. In the total population of more than 400 patients, the efficacy of radiation therapy appears comparable to surgery.*)

Barzell W, Bean MA, Hilaris BS et al: Prostatic adenocarcinoma: Relationship of grade and local extent to the pattern of metastases. J Urol 118:278, 1977 (*Suggests that local extent of disease can provide useful estimates of likelihood and pattern of metastases; clinical stage often underestimates extent of metastatic disease.*)

Blackard C: The Veterans Administration cooperative urological research group studies of carcinoma of the prostate: A review. Cancer Chemo Rep 59:225, 1975 (*A summary of the impact of estrogen therapy on prostate cancer in more than 3000 patients and an analysis of the effect of estrogen in inducing cardiovascular deaths. The controversial original publication by the VA study group is clarified.*)

Gittes RF: Serum acid phosphatase and screening for carcinoma of the prostate. N Engl J Med 309:852, 1983 (*The test has a relatively low sensitivity for detection of metastatic disease; even the newer assays have given disappointing results.*)

Guinan P, Bush I, Ray V, et al: The accuracy of the rectal examination in the diagnosis of prostatic carcinoma. N Engl J Med 303:499, 1980 (*It's imperfect and often underestimates the extent of disease, but it remains the most important means of early detection.*)

Huggins C, Hodges CV: The effect of castration, of estrogen and of androgen injection on serum phosphatases in metastatic carcinoma of the prostate. Cancer Res, March 22, 1941 (*This classic article presents the first awareness of the influence of hormones on prostate cancer and served as a basis for awarding the Nobel Prize to Charles Huggins.*)

Klein LA: Prostatic carcinoma. N Engl J Med 300:824, 1979 (*A comprehensive, thoughtful, and very useful review for the general reader.*)

Leuprolide Study Group: Leuprolide versus diethylstilbestrol for metastatic prostate cancer. N Engl J Med 311:1281, 1984 (*A trial of one of the new gonadotropin-releasing factor agonists; efficacy was similar to DES; produced fewer side effects.*)

Wilson CS, Dahl DS, Middleton RG: Pelvic lymphadenectomy for staging apparently localized prostatic cancer. J Urol 117:197, 1977 (*Makes the important point that there is often occult metastatic disease.*)

Testicular Cancer

Bosl GJ, Yagoda A, Golbey RB et al: Role of etoposide-based chemotherapy in treatment of patients with refractory or relapsing germ-cell tumors. Am J Med 78:423, 1985 (*This agent in combination with cisplatin was useful only in patients who had shown an initial response to cisplatin. An example of a therapeutic option in difficult cases.*)

Einhorn LH, Williams SD, Troner M et al: The role of maintenance therapy in disseminated testicular cancer. New Engl J Med 305:727, 1981 (*Effective chemotherapy has resulted in a reversal of the routine use of "adjuvant" chemotherapy at least for testicular cancer, in which virtually 100% of patients respond to treatment.*)

Einhorn LH, Donohue J: Cis-diamminedichloroplatinum, vinblastine and bleomycin combination chemotherapy in disseminated testicular cancer. Ann Intern Med 87:293, 1977 (*The original report on this most important advance in treatment of testicular cancer.*)

Fraley EL, Lange PH, Kennedy BJ: Germ-cell testicular cancer in adults. N Engl J Med 301:1370, 1420, 1979 (*Comprehensive review and good introduction for the general reader.*)

Lange PH, McIntire R, Waldmann TA et al: Serum alpha fetoprotein and human chorionic gonadotropin in the diagnosis and management of nonseminomatous germ-cell testicular cancer. N Engl J Med 295:1237, 1976 (*The original report of the utility of these tumor markers in staging and monitoring.*)

Picozzi VJ, Freiha FS, Hannigan JF et al: Prognostic significance of a decline in serum human chorionic gonadotropin levels after initial chemotherapy for advanced germ-cell carcinoma. Ann Intern Med 100:183, 1984 (*A fall in level was very predictive of an excellent long-term response to therapy.*)

Bladder Cancer

Heney NM, Ahmed SM, Flanagan MJ et al: Superficial bladder cancer: Progression and recurrence. J Urol 130:1083, 1983 (*Important data on clinical course.*)

Koontz WW: Intravesical chemotherapy for superficial bladder cancer. Urology 23(suppl):79, 1983 (*Useful in superficial disease.*)

Prout GR, Jr: Surgical management of bladder cancer. Urol Clin North Am 3:149, 1976 (*Comprehensive review.*)

Prout GR, Jr: Bladder carcinoma. N Engl J Med 287:86, 1972 (*An excellent review, though the treatment section is dated.*)

Radwin HM: Radiotherapy and bladder cancer: A critical review. J Urol 124:43, 1980 (*Thoughtful discussion.*)

Renal Cell Carcinoma

Clayman RV, Surya V, Miller RP et al: Pursuit of the renal mass: Is ultrasound enough? Am J Med 77:218, 1984 (*Ultrasound diagnosis of "cyst" obviates the need for further study.*)

Lokich JJ, Harrison JH: Renal cell carcinoma: Natural history and chemotherapeutic experience. J Urol 114:371, 1975 (*The association of paraneoplastic syndromes, splenomegaly, bilaterality of tumors, and delayed appearance of metastases is indicated. The lack of response to systemic forms of treatment is emphasized.*)

Richie JP, Garnick MB, Seltzer S et al: Computed tomography for diagnosis and staging of renal cell carcinoma. J Urol 129:1114, 1983 (*Details CT's role in workup.*)

142

Approach to the Patient with Acquired Immunodeficiency Syndrome (AIDS)

ROBERT T. SCHOOLEY, M.D.

AIDS represents one of the most difficult challenges in clinical medicine today. Often the primary physician is the first to encounter the patient, who may present with malaise, adenopathy, or fear of contracting the illness because of recent exposure. Although no definitive treatment is yet available, the primary physician must be knowledgeable about risk factors, clinical presentation, diagnostic methods, and the current status of therapy in order to provide the best advice, assessment, counselling, and support to patients with or at risk for the disease.

EPIDEMIOLOGY

At the time of this writing, approximately 20,000 U.S. cases of AIDS had been reported to the Centers for Disease Control. Ninety-three percent of these cases have occurred among members of three risk groups (homosexual men, intravenous drug abusers, and hemophiliacs receiving factor VIII concentrate) (Table 142-1). Many of the remaining cases involve either sexual partners of high-risk individuals, infants born of high-risk mothers, or recipients of blood products.

Table 142-1. AIDS Patients by Risk Group
(United States)

RISK GROUP	PERCENT OF CASES
Homosexual or bisexual men	74
Intravenous drug abuser	17
Hemophiliacs	1
Heterosexual contacts of high-risk individuals	1
Transfusion recipients	1
No apparent risk group	4

This distribution has not changed appreciably in the past three years.

AIDS was first recognized in U.S. cities in which large homosexual communities reside (New York, Los Angeles, San Francisco). The concentration of cases in these cities has become less pronounced with the gradual spread of the etiologic agent to other areas of the United States. AIDS has been identified in other parts of the world, including Haiti, Central Africa, and Western Europe. The epidemiology of the disease in Haiti and Central Africa differs somewhat from that observed in the United States in that there is much more evidence of heterosexual transmission in the third world than in the United States.

PATHOPHYSIOLOGY AND CLINICAL PRESENTATION

The newly described retrovirus human immunodeficiency virus (HIV), also known as human T-lymphotropic virus-III (HTLV-III) or lymphadenopathy associated virus (LAV), is the etiologic agent for AIDS. The agent can be isolated from blood, semen, saliva, or from several other sites. Despite the multiple sites from which it has been isolated, it is not a highly contagious agent; it is transmitted by intimate sexual contact, blood transfusion, or perinatal exposure.

The virus is tropic for lymphocytes of the T4 (helper/inducer) surface phenotype. Infection with the agent results in lysis of the infected lymphocyte. Depletion of lymphocytes of the T4 surface phenotype appears to be one of the central defects in the subsequent cascade, which results in profound cellular immunodeficiency in some infected individuals. It is also capable of infecting cells of the monocyte/macrophage lineage. Monocytes may serve as a reservoir for HIV after depletion of T4 lymphocytes. Monocytes may also serve as the vehicle by which the virus reaches the central nervous system.

It has become clear that infection with the agent is widespread among high-risk groups. This includes up to 70% of healthy homosexual men in San Francisco and up to 85% of hemophiliacs who have received factor VIII concentrate on a chronic basis. The majority of infected individuals appear to remain healthy for extended periods of time with or without measurable cellular immune defects. This large group of healthy carriers serves as the reservoir responsible for transmission of the virus to uninfected individuals. Carriers can be identified serologically (see below); once infected, the retrovirus remains with the host for life. It is not yet clear what factors account for the broad spectrum of clinical and immunologic outcomes for infected individuals, for example, why some individuals remain healthy carriers while others develop AIDS. At the present time, it is not possible to accurately predict the long-term outcome of the infection for a given individual.

Clinical manifestations of HIV infection are dependent on the degree of immunosuppression induced by the virus. *Primary infection* may be accompanied by a syndrome characterized by malaise, fever, a maculopapular eruption, and/or aseptic meningitis. This syndrome is usually self-limited, lasting 1 to 3 weeks, and follows exposure by 2 to 12 weeks. Many infected individuals, however, have no discernable clinical manifestations for long periods of time. Although these individuals remain carriers, they may or may not experience measurable cellular immune defects.

A subgroup of individuals develops *AIDS Related Complex (ARC)*. This clinically defined syndrome is a constellation of symptoms that are often identified in retrospect in patients who ultimately develop AIDS. The previous nomenclature for this syndrome (pre-AIDS) was changed to reflect the fact that only a minority of ARC patients develop AIDS. Most patients with ARC present with malaise, low-grade fever, and moderate diffuse lymphadenopathy. This may or may not be accompanied by other manifestations such as unexplained fever, diarrhea, and night sweats. A small minority of these patients recover; between 1% and 20% develop AIDS over a two-year period of time. The remainder retain ARC symptomatology for extended periods of time. It is not yet known what fraction of these individuals will develop AIDS, although currently emerging studies suggest the fraction will be appreciable. Clinical manifestations that may place ARC patients in a more worrisome prognostic group include oral thrush, hairy leukoplakia (a condition clinically resembling oral thrush but which appears to be due to an interaction between papilloma virus and Epstein-Barr virus), and disseminated herpes zoster. A number of immunologic studies have been proposed as being of predicitve value for the prognosis of ARC patients. At this writing, none of these is of sufficient precision for clinical application.

It is also clear that HIV is a neurotropic agent. As mentioned earlier, it appears that the virus reaches the brain very early in the course of primary infection. As in the case of the immunologic manifestations, the clinical impact of HIV upon the central nervous system is highly variable. Dementia, cognitive dysfunction, emotional lability, aseptic meningitis, peripheral neuropathy, and personality changes are among the clinical findings that are the result of the neurotropism of HIV. These findings may accompany, or even precede, all other manifestations of HIV infection. In addition to the difficulties these manifestations impose upon the patient and the primary care provider, the neurotropism further complicates the task of the development of effective antiviral agents.

Patients with Kaposi's sarcoma and early cases of pneumonia or central nervous system involvement may present in the outpatient setting. Although *Kaposi's sarcoma* may be cutaneous, lymphadenopathic, or visceral in distribution, most patients present initially with cutaneous lesions. The typical lesion is generally a nontender, nonpruritic, slightly raised, violaceous nodule or papule; definitive diagnosis is based on biopsy. The most frequent infectious complication of AIDS is *pneumocystis carinii* pneumonia. Most patients present with several days to several weeks of gradually increasing dyspnea or nonproductive cough, and fever. The chest x-ray may be interpreted as normal initially, but usually reveals an interstitial or nodular pattern. Any one of a number of other infectious agents (such as cytomegalovirus, *Mycobacterium avium-intracellulare,* mycoplasma pneumonia) may cause a similar clinical and radiographic picture. Definitive diagnosis is dependent upon the demonstration of *Pneumocystis carinii* organisms in bronchial washings, in tissue, or in touch preparations of bronchoscopically or surgically obtained tissue.

Involvement of the *central nervous system* is common among patients with AIDS. Patients may present with either focal or diffuse abnormalities. In addition to discrete neoplastic or infectious central nervous system complications in AIDS, a *progressive encephalopathy* has been observed in a significant percentage of AIDS patients. As noted earlier, these patients may present with intellectual impairment, emotional lability, or focal neurologic findings. Histopathologic findings include microglial nodules, but these are not specific for AIDS encephalopathy.

DIAGNOSIS

AIDS is also a clinically defined syndrome (see Table 142-2). The specific list of opportunistic infections and neoplasms that constitute the basis for the diagnosis of AIDS has undergone gradual evolution as understanding of the syndrome has developed. A great majority of AIDS patients present with *Pneumocystis carinii* pneumonia, Kaposi's sarcoma, *Toxoplasma gondii* encephalitis, or *Mycobacterium avium-intracellulare* infection. The diagnosis of an infection or neoplasm highly predictive of a defect in cellular immunity, in the absence of a known underlying immunodeficiency state, establishes the diagnosis of AIDS. HIV serology is needed in only in situations in which the particular tumor or infection is occasionally seen in the general population without known previously existing immunodeficiency. This circumstance is rare, however, and only includes such situations as Kaposi's sarcoma in individuals over the age of 65 or disseminated histoplasmosis. Many, but not all, AIDS patients will have had a period of malaise, night sweats, and low-grade fever (*e.g.,* ARC) for the two weeks to six months preceding the development of AIDS. The specific clinical presentation of an individual AIDS patient depends upon the infection or tumor that forms the basis of the diagnosis. It should be emphasized, both in terms of diagnosis and therapy that the *disease* is the cellular immunodeficiency; the infection or neoplasm serves simply as a clinical marker for the immunodeficiency state.

The diagnosis of AIDS is rather straightforward, once one of the infectious or neoplastic complications of the syndrome has developed. However, prior to the outbreak of opportunistic infection or malignancy, diagnosis may be difficult because primary infection and ARC resemble other conditions that are common in this population.

The rather nonspecific constellation of findings that form the basis for the diagnosis of ARC generates a broad group of differential diagnostic possibilities in patients suspected of having this diagnosis. *Epstein-Barr virus* (EBV) and *cytomegalovirus* (CMV) infections can each cause fever, lymphadenopathy, malaise, and several of the immunologic abnormalities noted in ARC and AIDS. Serologic diagnosis of a primary EBV infection may be made either by the demonstration of heterophile antibodies, or by the appropriate use of EBV-specific serologic studies. Primary CMV infection can be best diagnosed by the demonstration of a combination of a fourfold or greater rise in antibody to CMV and isolation of the virus from urine and buffy coat. Since both EBV and CMV are ubiquitous among patients at risk for AIDS, virus isolation studies should be interpreted with caution. Other causes of lymphadenopathy in this patient population include lymphoma, Kaposi's sarcoma, typical or atypical mycobacterial infection, or rarely, toxoplasmosis. The diagnosis of ARC rests on elimination of other causes of similar symptomatology in patients epidemiologically at risk for AIDS.

Table 142-2. Acquired Immunodeficiency Syndrome: Centers for Disease Control Surveillance Definition

1. Presence of reliably diagnosed disease at least moderately indicative of cellular immune deficiency (*e.g.,* Kaposi's sarcoma in a patient less than 60 years of age; pneumocystis pneumonia)
2. Absence of known causes of underlying immune deficiency and of any other reduced resistance reported to be associated with the disease (*e.g.,* immunosuppressive therapy, lymphoreticular malignancy)

WORKUP

History. Knowledge that a patient is in a group risk for AIDS radically changes the nature of the evaluation for a given clinical problem. Negative social attitudes about several of the groups of patients at risk for AIDS frequently raise impediments to communication between patients and health care providers. The profound impact of AIDS on the homosexual population has decreased somewhat the reluctance of gay men to communicate freely about sexual orientation with health care providers. Information about sexual orientation should be sought, but the ubiquity of HIV among the homosexual male population in the United States makes a detailed history about such factors as promiscuity and sexual techniques irrelevant. Such detailed questioning adds little useful information to the data base and frequently results in greatly increased anxiety about the physician-patient relationship.

Since many patients at risk for AIDS have read extensively about the disease or have known friends with the syndrome, history taking may be very straightforward once good rapport is established between patient and physician. A prior history of several to many sexually transmitted diseases may be elicited from many homosexual men with AIDS or ARC. These are relevant only in that several of the infections involve agents that become latent following primary infection, and that may result in major morbidity with waning cellular immunity (*e.g.,* cytomegalovirus and herpes simplex virus). As noted earlier, many, but not all, patients with AIDS will have experienced a period of malaise, weight loss, fever, or lymphadenopathy for weeks to months prior to the development of one of the specific manifestations of AIDS. Historical features differ from patient to patient, depending on the infectious or neoplastic process that brings the patient to the attention of the physician.

Physical Examination. With the exception of the rather stereotyped appearance of cutaneous Kaposi's sarcoma, there are no physical findings which are pathognomonic for AIDS. Many patients will show stigmata of weight loss, lymphadenopathy, or thrush associated with ARC. *Pneumocystis carinii* pneumonia, in particular, is often associated with a paucity of pulmonary physical findings. In all patients with, or suspected of having, HIV infection, a careful neurologic examination is in order in view of the frequent concurrent or subsequent development of intracranial infection or neoplasia and in view of the frequent involvement of the CNS by HIV.

Laboratory Studies. Routine laboratory studies are generally not particularly useful in making the diagnosis of AIDS. Many patients with AIDS, particularly those with opportunistic infections are lymphopenic. As noted above, HIV is tropic and lytic for lymphocytes of the T4 (helper/inducer) surface phenotype. Most AIDS patients are depleted of cells of the T4 surface phenotype and have both a relative and absolute decrease in the number of circulating lymphocytes bearing the T4 antigen. This finding is not specific for AIDS and may be found both in patients with ARC and in healthy HIV-infected individuals. Thus determination of the T4/T8 ratio is of little value in making the diagnosis of AIDS in an individual patient. Although T4/T8 ratios tend to be lower in HIV seropositive then HIV seronegative homosexual males, there is sufficient overlap between these groups that lymphocyte surface antigen studies should not be used as surrogate studies for HIV serology.

Several techniques for detection of *HIV antibodies* are available. The *ELISA technique* is the one which has achieved the most widespread use. There are several pitfalls in use of the ELISA about which health care providers need to be aware. Antibody titers to several HIV antigens may fall with progression from the healthy carrier state to AIDS. Thus, a negative test in a patient suspected of having AIDS does not rule out the diagnosis. It is also important that one be aware of the time required for seroconversion following infection. Although absolute limits are not currently available, it is believed that seroconversion may take up to 12 weeks. Furthermore, a small minority of HIV-infected individuals may not develop detectable antibodies to the virus. Thus, although negative serologic study for HIV antibodies decreases the likelihood significantly that an individual is infected with the virus, it does not totally rule out the possibility. High-risk individuals should still be counselled to avoid blood or organ donation, and to avoid sex that involves shared secretions with other individuals.

The ELISA may appear to be positive in individuals who are not virus infected. In the low-risk U.S. population, the false positivity rate for current ELISA techniques is less than 0.2%. False positivity is a particular problem when large populations at low risk are screened. Thus, until more specific techniques for HTLV-III serology become available, great care should be applied to utilize this laboratory study with forethought and planning.

The major diagnostic decision which faces physicians caring for patients with ARC relates to when to biopsy an enlarged lymph node. Although there are no formal guidelines that are universally applicable, early biopsy is not indicated for most patients. Lymph node biopsy is more productive in patients with painful or rapidly enlarging nodes or in patients with major constitutional symptoms. It is usually prudent to observe a patient on at least two occasions several weeks apart before proceeding to lymph node biopsy, unless significant systemic symptoms are present.

Management. Management of patients with, or at risk for, AIDS is both challenging and frustrating. The major task in management of worried individuals at risk for AIDS and of ARC patients is providing the patient with *emotional support and reassurance.* Given the current imprecision in predicting the subsequent course of healthy seropositive individuals and of ARC patients, reassurance often takes the form of availability and willingness to listen. Psychologic support of AIDS patients is even more difficult, in that virtually all patients are aware that the disease is ultimately fatal. The profound cellular immunodeficiency state makes precise prognostic statements extremely hazardous. As in the case with worried healthy and ARC patients, physician availability and longitudinal involvement is crucial for AIDS patients. Psychologic support structures are particularly difficult for AIDS patients who have not yet made risk factors known to loved ones. Even when risk factors are known, the profound implications of the diagnosis frequently result in the withdrawal of many friends and family members from further involvement with the patient. Successful management, thus, also requires that the physician communicate with family and loved ones about both the low level of contagiousness of the disease, and the prognosis of the illness.

Drug Therapy. Although specific therapy is available for most infectious agents causing morbidity for AIDS patients, it should be remembered that such therapy is directed at the symptom, not the disease. Although a patient may recover from a given infection, the immunodeficiency state persists and multiple simultaneous infectious complications usually ensue. Successful management of the disease will ultimately require the development of techniques for reconstitution of the immune response. This may be accomplished with antiviral drugs or immunomodulating agents, or it may require combined approach with both modalities. Promising therapies are under study.

PATIENT EDUCATION

Many individuals at risk for AIDS are better educated about the disease than the health care provider. The two areas about which the patients most frequently inquire are those of prognosis and contagiousness. As already noted, it is extremely difficult to offer an accurate prognosis for an individual patient. Although the median survival for patients presenting with opportunistic infections is 6 to 10 months, and that for patients with only Kaposi's sarcoma is 16 months, the extreme unpredictability requires caution on the part of the physician in providing a firm timetable for an individual patient. Prognostic information is even more difficult to provide for patients with ARC. Most ARC patients do not develop AIDS over a two-year period, but one cannot be certain who these individuals will be. Currently ongoing prospective studies may provide better criteria for predicting progression from ARC to AIDS than are currently available.

HIV should be regarded as an infectious but not highly contagious disease. Current recommendations to prevent nosocomial transmission, which are based on hepatitis B precautions, appear to be adequate. The agent is, however, quite transmissable by intimate sexual contact. Given the ubiquity of the agent among healthy gay men in the United States, it is likely that the bulk of the transmission of the agent to the uninfected individuals is accomplished by healthy HIV seropositive individuals who are unaware that they are shedding the virus in semen, saliva, or urine. Thus, it is prudent to recommend that gay men avoid sex that involves the sharing of bodily secretions. Social contact has not been shown to transmit the virus; therefore, overly restrictive isolation procedures provide no additional impediment spread of HIV and are extremely likely to deepen the feelings of isolation and abandonment that accompany this disease.

THERAPEUTIC RECOMMENDATIONS

There is currently no proven therapy that has any impact on the cellular immunodeficiency state exhibited by patients with ARC or AIDS. Therapy of infectious or neoplastic complications of AIDS treats symptoms, not the underlying disease.

ANNOTATED BIBLIOGRAPHY

Centers for Disease Control: Classification system for human T-lymphotropic virus type III/lymphadenopathy-associated virus infections. Ann Intern Med 105:234, 1986 (*A scheme for disease reporting and surveillance.*)

Conte JE: Infection with human immunodeficiency virus in the hospital. Ann Intern Med 105:730, 1986 (*Includes a discussion of biosafety considerations, many of which also apply in the outpatient setting.*)

Curran JW et al: Acquired immune deficiency syndrome associated with transfusions. N Engl J Med 310:69, 1984 (*Important risk.*)

Friedland GH, Saltzman BR, Rogers MF et al: Lack of transmission of HTLV-III/LAV infection to household contacts of patients with AIDS or AIDS-related complex. N Engl J Med 314:344, 1986 (*Household contacts are at minimal or no risk of infection.*)

Goedert JJ: Testing for human immunodeficiency virus. Ann Intern Med 105:609, 1986 (*Concise summary of diagnostic methods.*)

Ho DD, Rota TR, Schooley RT et al: Isolation of HTLV-III from cerebrospinal fluid and neural tissues of patients with neurologic syndromes related to the acquired immune deficiency syndrome. N Engl J Med 313:1493, 1985 (*Documents CNS disease.*)

Lederman MM: Transmission of acquired immunodeficiency syndrome through heterosexual activity. Ann Intern Med 104:115, 1986 (*An editorial on heterosexual risk.*)

Melbye M, Biggar RJ, Ebbesen P et al: Long-term seropositivity for human T-lymphocytotropic virus type III in homosexual men without the acquired immunodeficiency syndrome. Ann Intern Med 104:497, 1986 (*A high proportion become ill.*)

10

Musculoskeletal Problems

143
Evaluation of Acute Monoarticular Arthritis
DANIEL E. SINGER, M.D.

Acute monoarticular arthritis calls for a rapid diagnostic evaluation to rule out bacterial infection. The threat in such cases is joint destruction and disastrous septic sequelae. Certain noninfectious causes, notably crystal-induced arthritis, may also be quickly diagnosed and treated.

PATHOPHYSIOLOGY AND CLINICAL PRESENTATION

Many different diseases having different pathogenetic mechanisms may produce acute monoarthritis. These mechanisms can be broadly categorized as primarily inflammatory or noninflammatory. Noninflammatory etiologies include acute traumatic causes such as juxta-articular ligament or meniscus injury, frank bone fracture extending through to the joint space, or minor trauma in patients with impaired coagulation producing hemarthroses. A variety of mechanical disorders collectively referred to as "internal derangements" may produce chronic recurrent pain and noninflammatory effusion of the knee. Osteoarthritis, characterized by articular cartilage degeneration and adjacent bony sclerosis and proliferation, often produces chronic, gradually increasing joint symptoms but may present with an acutely painful joint with a noninflammatory effusion.

The inflammatory causes of acute monoarthritis include the more systemically dangerous entities.

1. *Septic arthritis* derives predominantly from hematogenous seeding of the synovium. Occasionally it results from direct extension from a site of trauma or from osteomyelitis. Among previously healthy, sexually active patients, *disseminated gonorrhea* is the most frequent etiology of joint infection. Women account for two-thirds of cases; pregnancy and menstruation appear to increase risk of dissemination. Dissemination occurs in about 1% to 3% of individuals with gonorrhea (see Chapter 116). Initially, there is a bacteremic stage with fever, polyarthralgias, transient scattered tendinitis, minimal joint effusion, necrotic skin lesions, positive blood cultures, and sterile joint fluid. This phase of the illness may be followed in several days by a septic joint stage, with monoarticular or occasionally polyarticular pain, marked joint swelling, and effusion. During the septic joint stage, gonococci can be recovered from the joint in about 50% of patients.

In *nongonococcal septic arthritis,* gram-positive organisms, especially *Staphylococcus aureus,* predominate. Enteric gram-negative bacteria also cause septic arthritis, particularly in chronically ill or hospitalized patients. Joint sepsis is more likely in patients with altered host defenses (diabetes, cirrhosis, immunodeficient states), previously damaged (*e.g.,* from rheumatoid arthritis), or prosthetic joints. Fever, chills and joint complaints are prominent. If the patient is very debilitated or immunosuppressed, fever may be indolent. The larger joints, particularly the knees, are most likely to be involved.

Articular destruction can be rapid. Within 10 days of nongonococcal infection, radiographic evidence of cartilage and bone damage may appear. Joint injury from gonococcal arthritis is less precipitous.

2. *Acute gout* is a common cause of acute monoarticular arthritis. Sodium urate crystals in the synovium incite a brisk inflammatory response after their ingestion by poly-

morphonuclear leukocytes. The condition is found most commonly among middleaged and older men. Onset is rapid, peaking within 12 to 24 hours. The metatarsophalangeal joint of the great toe is the classic site, but ankles, knees, wrists, and olecranon bursae are other important locations. Sodium urate crystals are found in the joint fluid; they are needlelike and negatively birefringent under the polarizing microscope.

Although the likelihood of a gouty attack increases with serum uric acid, the uric acid level is a poor way to diagnose gout except at the extremes. Alcoholic binges or new use of thiazide diuretics may precipitate gouty attacks. Rapid response to colchicine favors the diagnosis of gout or pseudogout.

3. *Pseudogout* resembles gout pathophysiologically, though clinical features differ. The condition results from crystals of calcium pyrophosphate inducing joint inflammation.

Under the polarizing microscope, synovial fluid will reveal the weakly positively birefringent rhomboid forms of calcium pyrophosphate. Chondrocalcinosis on x-ray is usually present. Pseudogout tends to occur in older patients and seems to be associated with hyperparathyroidism and hemochromatosis.

Other inflammatory processes that typically produce polyarthritis may present initially as monoarthritis. These include:

4. Rheumatoid arthritis (see Chapter 144)
5. Reiter's syndrome (see Chapters 129 and 144)
6. Ankylosing spondylitis (see Chapter 144)
7. Psoriatic arthritis (see Chapter 144)
8. The arthritis of inflammatory bowel disease (see Chapter 65)
9. The arthritis of sarcoidosis (see Chapter 144)

DIFFERENTIAL DIAGNOSIS

The most immediately important entities in the differential diagnosis of acute monoarthritis are infections, crystal-induced arthropathy and trauma. The gonococcus is the leading infectious agent, followed in frequency by gram-positive organisms (staphylococci, streptococci) and in compromised hosts by gram-negative coliforms. Gout and pseudogout are the important crystal-induced etiologies.

Several polyarticular diseases may initially present with one acutely inflamed joint or with symptoms that are greatest in a single joint. These monoarticular presentations of polyarticular disease are seen in rheumatoid arthritis, Reiter's syndrome, ankylosing spondylitis, psoriatic arthritis, the arthritis of inflammatory bowel disease, and sarcoidosis.

Despite the wide range of diagnostic possibilities, it should be appreciated that recent series of monoarthritis have revealed that the most prevalent diagnoses are osteoarthritis, septic arthritis, gout, and pseudogout.

WORKUP

History. The first objective is to establish whether or not the joint is infected. Although examination of the joint fluid is the single most important diagnostic test, history may provide useful information regarding the likelihood of infection as well as its source. Abrupt onset in conjunction with fever and chills points to a septic etiology, as does a history of skin lesions, vaginal or urethral discharge, gonorrhea exposure, diabetes, concurrent rheumatoid arthritis, joint prosthesis, immunosuppression, or previous trauma. Occurrence of acute trauma is suggestive of periarticular injury or hemarthrosis. A history of previous attacks suggests gout or pseudogout. Location is of some help diagnostically. Inflammation in the first MTP joint points to gout, especially in an elderly male; but in diabetics, extension of osteomyelitis into the joint must be ruled out. Associated back pain and stiffness raise the possibility of one of the spondyloarthropathies. The patient's age can be a helpful clue. Pseudogout is most common in older patients. Disseminated gonococcal infection is more common among young people. Reiter's syndrome and ankylosing spondylitis are also diseases of young people. Drug abuse suggests infection. Alcohol abuse predisposes to gout, trauma, and infection.

Physical examination should include a recording of the rectal temperature. Almost all patients with septic arthritis will be febrile. Low-grade fever may also be noted in gout and rheumatoid arthritis, but a high fever suggests infection. Inspection of the skin over the joint should focus on local trauma or infection. Examination of the rest of the skin should include a search for necrotic skin lesions on the extremities (indicative of disseminated gonorrhea), needletracks, tophi, rheumatoid nodules, pitting of the nails and other psoriatic manifestations, erythema nodosum, the hyperkeratotic blisters of keratoderma blennorrhagicum, and circinate balanitis. The eyes are examined for conjunctivitis and iritis, the fundi for signs of endocarditis, the mouth for mucosal ulceration, and the heart for murmurs.

All joints must be carefully examined to be certain that the problem is limited to one joint; inspection may reveal more than one inflamed area. It is important to be sure that the joint and not a periarticular structure is the site of the problem. Sometimes this distinction is impossible to make, but preservation of range of motion despite pain in the area reduces the likelihood of true joint involvement. The probability of a periarticular process is increased by finding localized tenderness not encompassing the entire joint space. The spine should be examined carefully for restriction of motion and tenderness, indicative of spondylitis. The genitalia need to be checked for purulent discharge.

Laboratory Studies. Aspirating and examining *joint fluid* is the single most important diagnostic procedure in the evaluation of acute monoarticular arthritis. A turbid appearance to the fluid points to an inflammatory etiology, blood suggests trauma or neoplasm, and a clear, straw-colored fluid is seen with degenerative disease and minor trauma. The fluid should be Gram-stained. It is most important to immediately culture the joint fluid onto proper media (including Thayer-Martin plates for detection of gonococci). Smears of the joint fluid may show organisms in the absence of a positive culture if antibiotics have already been taken. A repeat tap of the joint will improve the diagnostic yield of Gram stain and culture if the first arthrocentesis is negative.

Besides Gram stain and culture, synovial fluid should be examined for differential cell count and crystals. As described in Chapter 144, synovial fluid cell count can help distinguish inflammatory from noninflammatory conditions. WBC counts less than 1000/mm³ are noninflammatory. Higher WBC counts with predominantly neutrophils make inflammatory causes likely. From this perspective, gout and sepsis are the most inflammatory, with WBC counts often in the 50,000 plus/mm³ range. With sepsis, of course, one may aspirate frank pus. Crystal examination provides the most rapid and sure method of diagnosing gout and pseudogout. Other assessments of synovial fluid are less rewarding.

Cultures of the blood as well as of possible septic foci (*e.g.*, skin lesions, cervix) should be obtained if infection is a possibility. CBC may further suggest infection. The erythrocyte sedimentation rate can help separate inflammatory from noninflammatory causes. The serum uric acid level is useful only if extreme. X-rays of the involved and the contralateral joints should be obtained. They may reveal fractures, neoplasms, osteomyelitis, chondrocalcinosis, and so on. The presence of osteoarthritic changes does not make the diagnosis of osteoarthritis, but their absence makes osteoarthritis very unlikely. In most inflammatory monoarthritis, the early x-rays are not diagnostic, but they may serve as baseline studies for later comparison.

Despite optimal efforts, many cases of acute monoarthritis elude diagnosis. In one study, one-third were never satisfactorily diagnosed. Reassuringly, the majority of these patients improved or, at least, did not get worse. If infection, trauma, and, less importantly, crystal-induced arthritis are ruled out, the evaluation can be approached less hurriedly.

SYMPTOMATIC MANAGEMENT

Until a diagnosis is established, the patient may feel better with rest, immobility of the joint, and warm packs. If infection seems likely, parenteral antibiotic therapy aimed at the most probable bacteria should be begun while awaiting culture results. Use of anti-inflammatory agents should be postponed for at least 12 hours to allow for repeat arthrocentesis if the first one is nondiagnostic. If pain is unbearable and a diagnosis is not yet established, an analgesic without anti-inflammatory

effects (*e.g.*, codeine) may be used. After a second negative arthrocentesis, with infection not likely, it is reasonable to institute anti-inflammatory therapy even in the absence of a specific diagnosis.

In the proper circumstances, a therapeutic trial of IV colchicine may provide some diagnostic information. It should be appreciated that aspirin may prolong gout attacks. More definitive therapy will be based on the etiologic diagnosis (See Chapters 116, 153, 155).

INDICATIONS FOR REFERRAL AND ADMISSION

Septic arthritis requires hospital admission, treatment with intravenous antibiotics, and consultation with an infectious disease specialist. Cases of monoarticular arthritis that remain undiagnosed should be reviewed with a rheumatologist. Closed synovial biopsy or arthroscopy may be needed.

ANNOTATED BIBLIOGRAPHY

Bilka PJ: Physical examination of the arthritic patient. Bull Rheum Dis 20:596, 1970 (*An excellent discussion of the usefulness of physical examination.*)

Edeiken J: Arthritis: The roles of the primary care physician and the radiologist. JAMA 232:1364, 1975 (*Differentiates those conditions that have mainly clinical findings from those with specific roentgenographic manifestations.*)

Freed JF, Nies KM, Boyer RS et al: Acute monoarticular arthritis: A diagnostic approach. JAMA 243:2314, 1980 (*Discusses the prevalence of various diagnoses and which tests were useful. More than one-third of cases were never diagnosed.*)

Fries JF, Mitchell DM: Joint pain or arthritis. JAMA 235:199, 1976 (*An excellent flow chart–based article emphasizing judicious use of the laboratory.*)

Gelman MI, Ward JR: Septic Arthritis: A complication of rheumatoid arthritis. Radiology 122:17, 1977 (*Points out the problem of detecting superimposed infection and suggests radiologic criteria to help in identification.*)

Goldenberg DL, Reed JI: Bacterial arthritis. N Engl J Med 312:764, 1985 (*Reviews pathophysiology, risk factors, diagnosis, and therapy; emphasizes importance of early recognition and treatment.*)

Hansfield HH, Wiesner PJ, Holmes KK: Treatment of gonococcal arthritis-dermatitis syndrome. Ann Intern Med 84:661, 1976 (*High-dose IV penicillin G or oral ampicillin alone was effective.*)

Holmes K, Counts G, Beaty H: Disseminated gonococcal infection. Ann Intern Med 74:979, 1971. (*Arthritis occurred in 38 of 42 patients with disseminated disease. Classic paper describing the syndrome, with 141 references.*)

Mitchell WS, Brooke PM, Stevenson RD et al: Septic arthritis in patients with rheumatoid disease. J Rheumatol 3:124, 1976 (*Thorough discussion of pathophysiology and diagnosis.*)

Newman JH: Review of septic arthritis throughout the antibiotic era. Ann Rheum Dis 35:198, 1976 (*Little change in incidence or distribution of organisms. Poor prognosis is due to delay.*)

144

Evaluation of Polyarticular Arthritis

DANIEL E. SINGER, M.D.

The differential diagnosis of polyarticular complaints comprises a bewildering array of diseases. Nonetheless, the primary care physician can chart a simple, logical course that will minimize diagnostic error and maximize patient benefit. The initial evaluation should focus on answering the following basic questions:

1. Are the patient's complaints truly articular?
2. Is the arthritis inflammatory or degenerative?
3. Is the problem local or systemic?
4. How sick is the patient?

PATHOPHYSIOLOGY AND CLINICAL PRESENTATION

Polyarthritis can result from a degenerative, relatively noninflammatory process or from an inflammatory process. Noninflammatory forms of arthritis are, in most cases, the result of breakdown in joint cartilage and secondary mechanical disruption of the joint, as in degenerative arthritis. This may be a primary process or may be associated with an underlying disease, such as hemochromatosis. Uncommon mechanisms of nondegenerative noninflammatory joint injury include hemarthrosis, joint infarction, leukemic infiltration, and myxedematous changes.

Inflammatory arthritis results from the aggregation of inflammatory cells and their products in the joint space and synovium. Infection, gout, pseudogout, and the immunologically mediated diseases—rheumatoid arthritis, lupus, the spondyloarthropathies—all produce an inflammatory type of arthritis.

The typical features of the more common inflammatory arthropathies are given in Table 144-1.

DIFFERENTIAL DIAGNOSIS

Polyarticular disease may be inflammatory (see Table 144-1) or noninflammatory in origin. Osteoarthritis (OA) accounts for almost all noninflammatory cases, but hemophilia, sickle cell disease, leukemia, and myxedema may be responsible in rare instances.

WORKUP

Use of "Official" Criteria in Diagnosing Rheumatic Disease. Diagnosis in the rheumatic diseases often depends on a pattern of clinical findings rather than on some specific pathologic abnormality. As a result, criteria have been proposed to help objectify the diagnosis of rheumatoid arthritis (RA), systemic lupus erythematosus (SLE), and other related conditions. These criteria capture the essential features of the diseases and are necessary for epidemiologic and therapeutic studies. However, they should be applied cautiously to any given patient.

The American Rheumatism Association (ARA) criteria for RA stress chronicity (greater than 6 weeks), presence of symmetrical polyarthritis, positive rheumatoid factor, skin nodules, and consistent x-ray changes. Clearly, the patient who has RA at week 7 has had RA during weeks 1 through 6. Similarly, asymmetrical disease or even monoarticular arthritis can be due to RA. Thus, the diagnostic criteria are not perfectly sensitive, especially in the early phases of the disease. Nor are they highly specific; numerous other diseases can meet ARA criteria for RA. To increase specificity, the ARA has listed 20 conditions (including gout, SLE, scleroderma, and infections) whose presence invalidates the use of the criteria to diagnose RA.

The basic message for the clinician is that chronic inflammatory polyarthritis is often RA, but if there are atypical features (*e.g.*, lack of symmetry or lack of rheumatoid factor positivity) one needs to consider other causes.

The diagnosis of SLE poses similar problems. The so-called preliminary criteria for SLE are a list of 14 clinical features, of which 4 must be present for diagnosis. These include nondeforming polyarthritis or arthralgias, characteristic skin changes, evidence of serositis, hemolytic anemia, thrombocytopenia, and proteinuria. A study comparing these criteria against the diagnoses of experienced rheumatologists in cases of arthritis indicated that the hematologic manifestations, pleuritis, pericarditis, photosensitivity, and Raynaud's phenomenon correlated highly with the clinicians' diagnoses. In addition, the presence of a high titer ANA (a test which came into common use after the criteria were published) in conjunction with arthritis or any of the other clinical findings was highly predictive of SLE. The study emphasizes that for the individual patient, the diagnosis of SLE must be entertained when *any* of the clinical characteristics of the disease is associated with a positive ANA.

Table 144-1.   Common Inflammatory Polyarthritides

1. **Rheumatoid arthritis.** Female predominant subacute symmetrical polyarthritis often involving PIPs, MCPs, wrists. A.M. stiffness is characteristic. Rheumatoid factor positivity is found in approximately 75% of cases and is associated with nodules and more aggressive articular and extra-articular disease.

2. **Systemic lupus erythematosus.** Usually occurs in young women, with high prevalence in blacks. Characterized by symmetrical polyarthralgias or nondeforming arthritis, with malar rash, pleuritis, leukopenia, immune thrombocytopenia, hemolytic anemia, and glomerulonephritis. ANA is positive in nearly all cases. Renal disease and cerebritis are most life-threatening.

3. **Scleroderma.** Sclerodactyly and more general skin tightening, Raynaud's phenomenon, impaired esophageal motility, lung, heart, and renal involvement with malignant hypertension predominate. Articular symptoms are mild. ANA is frequently positive with a speckled pattern. The sensitivity of the ANA for scleroderma can be increased by using the newly available HEp-2 cell line as substrate.

4. **Psoriatic arthritis.** Peripheral form is characteristically asymmetrical, oligoarticular involving DIP joints, and may be very erosive. Spondylitic form can mimic ankylosing spondylitis but the extent of disease is less; HLA-B27 positivity is associated with the spondylitic form.

5. **Reiter's syndrome.** Primarily a disease of young men, defined by arthritis, nongonococcal urethritis, and ocular inflammation (conjunctivitis, iritis), although the latter two features may be fleeting and not simultaneous. It may follow bowel infections, for example, *Salmonella, Shigella*. Joints involved are often asymmetrical, lower extremity. Heel pain with plantar fasciitis and calcaneal periostitis is distinctive. Mild spondylitis and HLA-B27 positivity are common.

6. **Ankylosing spondylitis.** Recent studies question the previously observed male predominance. The disease is more severe and clear-cut in males. Inflammation of the joints and fibrous tissue of the spine with subsequent calcification and ossification produces the typical sacroiliitis and fused spine. Back pain that is worse with bed rest and improves with exercise, abnormal Schober's test and reduced chest expansion result. Uveitis, HLA-B27 are highly associated.

7. **Polyarticular gout.** Often, there is a past history of transient mono- or oligoarthritis; serum uric acid is usually but not necessarily elevated. Diagnosed by identifying urate crystals in synovial fluid (see Chapter 155).

8. **Pseudogout.** Calcium pyrophosphate crystal deposition disease: rarely polyarticular, patient often elderly, knee characteristically involved, cartilage calcification seen on x-ray; diagnosis made by identifying calcium pyrophosphate crystals in synovial fluid.

9. **Gonococcal arthritis.** Migratory polyarthritis and tendinitis that may lead to a frank infected joint and vesicular-pustular skin lesions. Diagnosis is made by culture of organism from cervix, urethra, or rectum as well as blood, skin, or synovial fluid (see Chapter 116).

10. **Acute hepatitis B arthritis.** Acute polyarthritis with urticarial skin lesions; occurs in preicteric phase and wanes as icteric phase develops. Diagnosed by laboratory evidence of hepatitis and hepatitis B antigen positivity (see Chapter 70).

11. **Lyme arthritis.** Recurrent or migratory arthritis that may become chronic. Typically follows the annular skin lesion erythema chronicum migrans, which develops at the site of a tick bite. The causative organism is a *Borrelia* species that is antibiotic-sensitive. Neurologic and cardiac manifestations occur. Diagnosis can now be made serologically.

Workup Strategy

The initial assessment of the patient who presents with polyarticular joint complaints should determine whether the complaints are truly articular, whether the underlying disease is inflammatory or not, whether it is systemic or focal, and whether vital organ function or joint integrity is endangered.

The answers to these questions can be provided by a careful history and physical examination supplemented by a complete blood count and erythrocyte sedimentation rate (see Table 144-2). Synovial fluid analysis is very helpful if an accessible effusion is present. The rest of the laboratory tests that are available for rheumatologic diagnosis are best used to modify one's initial impression, and are rarely helpful when used as a general rheumatologic screening procedure.

History. Patients complain of pain, stiffness, and loss of function. The physician should attempt to identify the anatomic basis of the symptoms by asking the patient to specify exactly where the pain is located, what aggravates it, and what functional loss has occurred. For the most part, joint symptoms are well localized and bear a logical relationship to the use of the joint. Hand involvement will reduce grip strength. Shoulder involvement prevents hair combing. Hip disease is characterized by difficulty in rising from a seated position, and in putting on shoes and stockings. Cervical spine involvment makes looking behind difficult. Neuropathic pain (see Chapter 161), bone pain, and myalgias are often confused with arthritis by the patient. These difficulties rarely have a specifically articular location and do not produce typical articular loss of function. For example, a common neuropathic

Table 144-2. Distinguishing Inflammatory From
Noninflammatory Articular Disease

	NONINFLAMMATORY	INFLAMMATORY
History	MCP and carpal joints rarely involved	MCPs and carpals often involved
	Little AM stiffness and much relief of pain with rest	AM stiffness is the hallmark; symptoms persist even without mechanical stress
	Few systemic effects	Patient often systemically ill, fatigued
	Little relief with antiinflammatory medications	Clear-cut benefit from aspirin
Physical Examination	MCP and carpal joints rarely involved	MCPs and carpals often involved
	Joints rarely warm, red, or swollen. Often merely bony enlargement	Synovitis is the central feature
	Extra-articular findings rare*	Extra-articular disease is common
Laboratory Tests	CBC is normal	Anemia and/or other abnormalities often present
	ESR < 30	ESR > 40
	RF and ANA usually negative	RF and/or ANA may be positive

* Throughout this chapter, noninflammatory arthritis has implied primary OA. This is usually the case. However, there are other diseases producing OA-like arthritis or a mildly inflammatory arthritis. These illnesses may have severe extra-articular manifestations. An example is the degenerative arthritis associated with hemochromatosis.

mimic of arthritis of the hands is the carpal tunnel syndrome. Here, poorly described pains in the hand may be associated with loss of grip strength. However, paresthesias, a sense of the hands being "ballooned" in size, aggravation of symptoms by sleep or driving, together with physical findings characteristic of median nerve entrapment will reveal the diagnosis.

After obtaining a specific description of the patient's complaints, one should ask in detail about other joints not mentioned. Complaints that initially appear to be monarticular may turn out to be polyarticular on further questioning. The *distribution* of involved joints can be relatively specific for certain diagnoses. Thus, symmetrical enlargement with pain and limitation of motion of the proximal interphalangeal joints (PIPs) and distal phalangeal joints (DIPs), without metacarpophalangeal (MCP) or wrist involvement and without an AM stiffness pattern, suggests osteoarthritis. As a general rule, involvement of MCPs, wrists, or elbows implies inflammatory disease and should strongly discourage a diagnosis of osteoarthritis, unless some clear predisposing antecedent trauma has occurred, for example, old fractures or a history

of working a jack-hammer. The distribution of joint involvement in rheumatoid arthritis is characteristically symmetrical and often includes the interphalangeal (IP), MCP, carpal, or metatarsophalangeal (MTP) joints. Temperomandibular (TM) joint arthritis is relatively specific for RA. Asymmetrical DIP disease characterizes the peripheral form of psoriatic arthritis. Bilateral heel pain suggests Reiter's syndrome and the other spondyloarthropathies. Overall, the pattern of joints involved best helps to distinguish OA from the inflammatory arthritides. Within the set of inflammatory arthritides, joint distribution suggests initial diagnostic possibilities.

Concurrent with establishing the distribution of involved joints, one should determine the *temporal pattern* of the disease. A chronic, subacute, additive process occurs in many cases of RA. Sudden, explosive, symmetrical polyarthritis, while found with RA, strongly suggests "serum sickness" diseases, for example, early hepatitis B infection or delayed penicillin allergy. Desultory arthralgias, arthritis, or tenosynovitis involving first one joint and then a second after the first's symptoms are receding typify gonococcal disease (see Chapter

116). A similar migratory pattern is noted in rheumatic fever. In establishing the temporal pattern, the physician should probe into the distant past as well. Has the patient ever had any other episodes of arthritis in the past? Gout may present as polyarthritis, but more often one uncovers a prior episode of podagra or other lower extremity monoarthritis (see Chapter 155). Young men with ankylosing spondylitis often give a history of unexplained mono- or oligoarthritis occurring in their teens.

A few questions are particularly helpful in deciphering the patient's articular complaints. First, are the involved joints stiff as well as painful, and if so, are they stiffer after rest or after activity? Inflammatory arthritis, in particular RA, is characterized by maximal stiffness after inactivity, so-called "AM stiffness." This stiffness persists for one or more hours. In contrast, osteoarthritis is characterized by maximal symptoms with use. If there is some stiffness with rest in OA, it passes quickly with activity. Second, have anti-inflammatory agents helped? RA patients reach for their aspirin as soon as they awaken, and they clearly feel worse if they miss a dose. The response in OA patients is much less dramatic. Third, has the patient noted joint redness, warmth, or swelling? The value of this question depends on the detail and credibility of the patient's response. A well-described "hot joint," as opposed to diffuse hand or foot swelling, probably indicates true inflammation, whether or not the current examination suggests arthritis. A negative response coupled with a negative examination suggests a noninflammatory and perhaps nonarticular etiology.

After determining the temporal and spatial pattern of the patient's illness, the physician should assess its *severity*. First, are there symptoms at night? Joint pain awakening the patient at night indicates a severe problem. Bone and neurologic pain may also occur at night. Second, what desired activities has the patient discontinued because of arthritis? The answer to this question depends on several factors, including the patient's premorbid level of activity, his attitudes toward work and pain, as well as the biologic severity of the disease. However, the answer reveals the overall impact of the illness and the urgency of the patient's complaint. Third, how systemically ill is the patient? Marked daily fatigue, the need for afternoon naps, weight loss, fever—all suggest active systemic illness.

Inflammatory arthritides are often associated with disease in other organ systems. Thus, a detailed review of systems is mandatory. In particular, one should ask about the new onset of Raynaud's phenomenon (a marker of scleroderma, SLE, and RA), the presence of nasopharyngeal ulcers, rashes, hair loss, fever or illness with sun exposure, or a history of pleuritis or pericarditis (all indicators of SLE). Chronically scratchy eyes or dry mouth suggests Sjögren's syndrome. A history of chronic or bloody diarrhea suggests inflammatory bowel disease (see Chapter 65). Dysuria, conjunctivitis, and balanitis are found in Reiter's syndrome (see Chapter 129). Details

about past or present psoriasis or unusual skin lesions (*e.g.,* erythema nodosum or the annular skin lesion of Lyme disease) will also aid diagnosis. Questions about family history are pertinent to the spondyloarthropathies, gout, and Heberden's nodes. In addition, it is critical to know what other medical problems the patient has had, what his medications are, and whether he uses alcohol or other drugs heavily.

The physician should appreciate the influence of *age, sex,* and *race.* The probabilities of different forms of arthritis vary with these determinants. SLE and RA for example, are female predominant, while Reiter's syndrome is male predominant. Onset of rheumatic fever or ankylosing spondylitis is nearly always before age 40. Peak incidence for SLE occurs in the premenopausal period, although later onset is not rare. The incidence of RA is less dependent on age, with new onset occurring in the elderly as well as in the young. Gout in women is mainly a postmenopausal disease; in men, it occurs at all adult ages. One point regarding race is worth noting. Despite the archetypal picture of a red butterfly rash on a Caucasian face, SLE is particularly common among black women, one study citing a prevalence of 1 in 250.

Physical Examination. The physical examination is basically a continuation of the same approach, documenting the pattern and type of joint involvement and the nature of any extra-articular disease. The myriad of extra-articular manifestations of arthritic diseases makes a detailed general physical examination mandatory. Certain aspects deserve emphasis. First of all, one should carefully palpate around the elbows, the Achilles tendons, and the pinnae searching for nodules and tophi. When pathologically confirmed, nodules and tophi are specific indicators of RA and gout, respectively. The nails should be examined for clubbing, which is associated with pulmonary osteoarthropathy and inflammatory bowel disease (see Chapter 41), and pitting, characteristic of psoriasis. In fact, nail pitting adjacent to erosive DIP arthritis can justify the diagnosis of psoriatic arthritis in the absence of any skin psoriasis. Fingertip atrophy with healed or active ulcers suggests severe Raynaud's syndrome, and should prompt a search for the calcinosis, subungual telangiectasias, and skin tightening of scleroderma. Other skin findings of value include the malar eruption of SLE, urticarial lesions of hepatitis B infection, the vesicular/pustular eruption of gonococcal infection (see Chapter 116), the nodules and palpable purpura of the vasculitides (see Chapter 175) and erythema nodosum. This last skin finding is often associated with painful periarticular inflammation about the ankles as well as with true arthritis and should prompt a chest x-ray looking for evidence of sarcoidosis. Erythema nodosum is also a finding in inflammatory bowel disease, and may be part of Behçet's syndrome. There are many other skin findings with the rheumatic diseases, attesting to the common parallel involvement of skin and synovium.

The eyes should be examined for conjunctivitis and iritis

(see Chapter 199), suggestive of Reiter's syndrome and spondylitis, and fundoscopic changes such as hemorrhages, exudates, and ischemic lesions consistent with systemic lupus and vasculitis. "Cotton-wool" exudates are the most common eye lesion in SLE. The oral and nasal mucosa should be examined for ulcers, which when painful suggest SLE or Behçet's syndrome, and when painless suggest Reiter's syndrome. Thyroid evaluation may reveal hypothyroidism, which can produce numerous musculoskeletal problems. Pleural or pericardial rubs are found in RA and SLE. Heart murmurs characterize rheumatic fever and SLE; mitral valve murmurs sometimes occur in SLE, and aortic regurgitant murmurs in the spondyloarthropathies. Splenomegaly is found in a variety of rheumatic diseases, including RA and SLE.

A detailed examination of the joints is very valuable in distinguishing periarticular from true articular disease, inflammatory from noninflammatory arthritis, and in objectively documenting which joints are abnormal. In general, the joint examination should assess the presence of tenderness, erythema, warmth, effusion, bony enlargement and mechanical abnormalities—such as limitation of motion, instability, subluxation, and tendon injury. An informative examination of the joints need take only a few minutes.

The primary physician is often faced with the problem of stiffness or pain in the hand. A valuable screening test for the presence of a joint or tendon abnormality is that of "curling." The patient is asked to extend the MCP joints and then maximally flex the PIP and DIP joints. This is quite different from making a fist, in which the MCPs are flexed as well. Curling is normal when a patient can bring his fingertips into apossition with his palm. Any limitation of motion in the PIP or DIP joints will interfere with curling. In addition, any inflammation along the entire length of the dorsal extensor tendons will also produce abnormal curling. As a sensitive but nonspecific test, curling is most useful in ruling *out* hand joint disease.

Another test that is useful but rarely performed by the general physician is Schober's test. Any patient with back pain or an arthritis pattern that suggests spondyloarthropathy should have this assessment of lumbar mobility. A mark is made on the patient's skin between the posterior iliac spines (the "dimples of venus") and another mark 10 cm above the first while the patient is standing upright. The patient is then asked to bend forward maximally. With normal lumbar flexion, the two marks should now be at least 15 cm apart. Schober's test is a nonspecific screening procedure. Any form of lumbar spine disease and even simple lumbar paraspinous muscle spasm may reduce lumbar flexion. However, when coupled with evidence of spine disease elsewhere—for example, abnormal chest expansion—an abnormal Schober's test can suggest ankylosing spondylitis. Similarly, an abnormal test in a patient complaining of hip or knee arthritis raises the probability of spondyloarthropathy.

Some forms of periarticular disease require particular attention. Bursitis and tendinitis commonly mimic arthritis. Subacromial bursitis and bicipital tendinitis can be confused with shoulder joint disease (see Chapter 147); lateral epicondylitis (tennis elbow) and olecranon bursitis for elbow joint disease (see Chapter 150); trochanteric bursitis (see Chapter 148) and anserine bursitis (see Chapter 149) for hip and knee disease respectively. Familiarity with these entities is essential to proper diagnosis and therapy.

Another important type of periarticular disease is that manifested by "frozen" joints and flexion contractures. Severe limitation of motion of a joint may occur with an intrinsically normal joint. Disuse due to neurologic disease or periarticular pain may lead to tightening of periarticular fibrous tissue and secondary contractures. The clinical presentation may be mistaken for arthritis, but normal joint x-rays and lack of indicators of inflammatory arthritis, plus an awareness of a predisposing illness, will lead to the correct diagnosis.

Laboratory Studies. A large number of laboratory tests, both simple and esoteric, are used in the evaluation of arthritic complaints. However, diagnostic hypotheses should be developed primarily from a detailed and directed history and physical examination. Diagnostic confusion that persists at the end of the physical examination is rarely resolved by laboratory results. The primary physician needs to know the indications and limitations of available studies.

SYNOVIAL FLUID ANALYSIS. If a synovial effusion is present in a patient whose diagnosis is still undetermined, it should be tapped. A white blood cell (WBC) count of greater than 3000 per mm^3 should be considered inflammatory; less than 1000 suggests OA or a mechanical derangement. A count between 1000 and 3000 is ambiguous. The presence of urate or calcium pyrophosphate crystals is diagnostic of gout and pseudogout respectively (see Chapter 143). Similarly, the diagnosis of joint infection is made by Gram's stain and positive cultures of joint fluid (see Chapter 143). Often, one obtains a synovial fluid WBC count of 5–20,000, without crystals, bacteria, or other distinctive attributes. All that one can conclude at that point is that the patient has inflammatory arthritis, type unspecified.

ERYTHROCYTE SEDIMENTATION RATE. The erythrocyte sedimentation rate (ESR) is useful as a screen for inflammatory disease and for monitoring therapy. In one study of patients with OA and RA, more than 90% of those diagnosed as having RA had an ESR greater than 30 (Westergren) while only 10% of those with OA had such a rapid ESR. These are crude figures and will vary with age and type of clinical presentation, as will the relative prevalence of OA and RA. The point of clinical usefulness is that a high ESR (*e.g.,* >40 mm/hr) suggests inflammatory disease. An ESR should be obtained on all arthritis patients.

RHEUMATOID FACTOR. Nearly all patients with polyarthritis are tested for rheumatoid factor (RF). RF is an immunoglobulin directed at the Fc fragment of the host's own immunoglobulin G. The exact relationship of RF and RA is a matter of great speculation. It is clear that one can have RA and be RF-negative, or conversely, one can be RF-positive and not have arthritis. In general, 70% to 80% of all patients meeting ARA criteria for RA are RF-positive. This, of course, means that almost 30% of RA patients are seronegative. Moreover, 5% to 15% (increasing with age) of so-called normals are RF-positive. The higher the titer of RF, the more likely the diagnosis of RA. RF negativity does not rule out RA nor does RF positivity rule it in. RF can also be positive in other connective tissue diseases and in chronic infections, for example, SBE. The RF test is most helpful in confirming the diagnosis of RA when one's probability of RA was high prior to the test.

ANTINUCLEAR ANTIBODY (ANA). The usual initial ANA is the *fluoresceinated ANA (FANA)*. Generally, rat or mouse liver cells are used as the test substrate over which the sample serum is run. A fluoresceinated antiserum against human immunoglobulin is then run over the sample to reveal any binding of the sample serum to substrate nuclei. The ANA is very sensitive but not very specific. More than 95% of patients diagnosed as having SLE are FANA-positive. Consequently, one is fairly safe in concluding that a patient who is FANA-negative does not have SLE. However, the FANA may be positive in drug-induced lupus, RA, scleroderma, and chronic hepatitis among other illnesses, and may be positive in normal individuals. Recent research has focused on the presence of antibodies to more homogeneous nuclear components. It seems that the presence of antibodies to native double-stranded DNA is a more specific indication of SLE than a positive FANA. As such, it would be a reasonable second test if the FANA were positive.

HLA TYPING. Over the past decade, much research has been devoted to the association between rheumatologic disease and HLA types. The most dramatic example of this is the relationship between HLA-B27 and ankylosing spondylitis. While 5% of the general population is B27 positive, 95% of patients with ankylosing spondylitis are B27 positive. Since the prevalence of ankylosing spondylitis is less than 1% of males, most B27 positive males will *not* have spondylitis (see Chapter 2). Therefore, HLA typing for B27 positivity is a sensitive but nonspecific test for spondylitis. A high percentage of patients with inflammatory spondylitis associated with Reiter's syndrome, inflammatory bowel disease, and psoriasis are also B27 positive. While the association of HLA-B27 with the spondyloarthropathies may say much about the mechanism of these diseases, the test itself has limited clinical value. The test neither rules in nor rules out inflammatory spondylitis. The diagnosis remains a clinical one, strongly based on x-ray evidence of spondylitis. The HLA-B27 antigen test is probably most useful in atypical cases, for example, those dominated by extraspinal findings.

URIC ACID LEVEL. Serum uric acid levels are obtained in most arthritis patients and too often serve as the primary basis for a diagnosis of gout. Definitive diagnosis requires observing urate crystals in the synovial fluid (see Chapter 143). A normal serum uric acid does not rule out the diagnosis of gout, nor does an elevated level rule it in.

X-RAYS. The question of appropriate x-rays is often raised. In osteoarthritis, joint x-rays are abnormal by the time the patient becomes symptomatic. However, the converse is not true. Degenerative changes are commonly found in asymptomatic joints. In new onset inflammatory arthritis, the x-ray may show only soft tissue swelling. As such, it serves more as a baseline examination than as a diagnostic test. In oligoarticular disease, the few involved joints should be x-rayed. In polyarticular disease, if no one joint is outstandingly worrisome, films of both hands and wrists assess the most joints for the least radiation. In cases of suspected spondyloarthropathy, films of the sacroiliac joints may provide definite evidence of sacroiliitis.

INDICATIONS FOR ADMISSION AND REFERRAL

The diagnosis of polyarticular arthritis may remain uncertain for a long period of time. For the most part, arthritis is not life threatening. Short-term risk to the patient is posed primarily by extra-articular disease. *The physician must assure himself that no active infection or vasculitis is present and that the patient's eyes, lungs, heart, kidneys, and other vital organs are not endangered.* Thus assured, he may approach the problems of diagnosis and therapy at a more relaxed pace on an outpatient basis; otherwise, hospitalization is needed.

Any patient with inflammatory polyarthritis who is systemically ill or who has vital organ involvement should be seen by a rheumatologist as soon as possible. When a patient with less serious illness remains undiagnosed after completion of the initial workup, referral to a rheumatologist may be appropriate. Patients with clear-cut osteoarthritis require referral only when severity warrants consideration of surgical therapy (see Chapter 154). In cases of RA, early consultation with a rheumatologist may be helpful in the design of a total therapeutic program (see Chapter 153).

SYMPTOMATIC THERAPY

Provided that acute gout and infection have been ruled out and pending results of the remainder of the initial evaluation, the patient bothered by symptoms of joint inflammation may be given aspirin at a dose of about twelve 325-mg tablets per day, or one of the newer nonsteroidal anti-inflammatory agents (see Chapter 147). Aspirin may aggravate gout, though other nonsteroidal anti-inflammatory agents are effective. Specific antimicrobials are needed to treat joint infection.

ANNOTATED BIBLIOGRAPHY

Anderson RJ: The diagnosis and management of rheumatoid synovitis. Ortho Clin North Am 6:629, 1975 (*An excellent, logical article outlining the main points of diagnostic and therapeutic concern in RA.*)

Beary JF, Christian CL, Sculco TP (eds): Manual of Rheumatology and Outpatient Orthopedic Disorders. Boston, Little, Brown & Co, 1981 (*This is an excellent, short source of information for office practice.*)

Brewerton DA et al: Ankylosing spondylitis and HL-A 27. Lancet, 1:904, 1973 (*One of the earliest reports of the association of ankylosing spondylitis and what is now known as HLA-B27.*)

Calin A: HLA-B27: To type or not to type? Ann Intern Med 92:208, 1980 (*A critical assessment of the use of B27 typing in clinical practice.*)

Fessel WJ: SLE in the community. Arch Intern Med 134:1027, 1974 (*This is the report in which the claim of a prevalence of 1/250 black women is made.*)

Harler NM, Franck WA, Bress NM et al: Acute polyarticular gout. Am J Med 56:715, 1974 (*A study of this uncommon presentation of a very common disease.*)

Kahn MA, Kahn MK: Diagnostic value of HLA-B27 testing in ankylosing spondylitis and Reiter's syndrome. Ann Intern Med 96: 70, 1982 (*Reviews the operating characteristics of this test as well as a Bayesian approach to its use.*)

Katz WA (ed): Rheumatic Diseases. Philadelphia: J. B. Lippincott, 1977 (*This text emphasizes the clinical problem rather than the disease. The first quarter of the text deals with the approach to given articular complaints, e.g., elbow problems, shoulder problems. Subsequently, individual disease entities are considered.*)

Keat A: Reiter's syndrome and reactive arthritis in perspective. N Engl J Med 309:1606, 1983 (*An extensive review of Reiter's syndrome including discussion of potential initiating infections, genetic predisposition, and clinical manifestations.*)

Kelley WN, Harris ED, Ruddy S et al (eds): Textbook of Rheumatology. Philadelphia, W. B. Saunders Co. 1981 (*This is the current dominant encyclopedic text.*)

Polley HF, Hunder GG: Rheumatologic Interviewing and Physical Examination of the Joints. Philadelphia: W.B. Saunders, 1978 (*A wonderfully useful short text on the physical examination of the joints. Excellent photographs and drawings.*)

Rodnan GP, Schumacher HR, Zvaifler NJ (eds): Primer on the Rheumatic Diseases. 8th ed. 1983 Arthritis Foundation, Atlanta, (*This is a useful "official" brief source.*)

Steere AC, Hutchinson GJ, Rhan DW et al: Treatment of the early manifestations of Lyme disease. Ann Intern Med 99:122, 1983 (*A concluding part of the triumphant tale of Lyme disease.*)

145

Evaluation of Back Pain
ROBERT J. BOYD, M.D.

Back pain is one of the leading causes of disability. Moreover, when a patient presents with back pain, serious underlying problems must be considered, because early recognition of tumor, infection, disc herniation, and vertebral compression fracture is essential to effective management and avoidance of permanent injury. After the description of lumbar disc herniation by Mixter and Barr in 1933, it became increasingly apparent that disc disease is frequently responsible for recurring mild low back discomfort and episodes of severe back pain with sciatica. Most back pain is due to musculoligamentous strain, degenerative disc disease, or facette arthritis, and will respond to symptomatic treatment. Occasionally, back pain may be due to problems originating outside the spinal axis. The frequency of back pain requires that the primary physician be skilled in its assessment and conservative management and knowledgeable about the indications for myelography and surgery.

PATHOPHYSIOLOGY AND CLINICAL PRESENTATION

The patient with *low back musculoligamentous strain* presents after a specific episode of bending, twisting, or lifting. The strain is usually severe and is associated with a feeling of something giving way in the lower back; the onset of pain in the lower lumbar area is immediate. There may be tearing of muscle fibers or distal ligamentous attachments of the paraspinal muscles, usually at the iliac crest or lower lumbar/upper sacral region. Resultant bleeding and spasm cause local swelling and marked tenderness at the site of injury. Pain radiates across the low back, often to the buttock and upper thigh posteriorly; radiation of pain into the lower leg is rare.

In *lumbar disc herniation,* there is often a several-year history of recurring mild mid-low back pain related to minor back strain, with symptoms clearing spontaneously within a few days. Attacks occur with increasing frequency and severity at intervals of several months to several years. Eventually, pain may radiate in the distribution of a lower lumbar nerve root, and bed rest may be needed in increasing amounts before symptoms resolve. Numbness, paresthesias, and weakness often develop in the areas supplied by the irritated nerve root.

The pathophysiology of disc disease is not completely understood. It is felt that lower lumbar disc degeneration and attritional changes are due to the concentration of stress at the lumbosacral level. Stresses result from the enormous longitudinal and sheer forces that are a consequence of upright posture and are aggravated by bending strain. The disc annulus may become injured, inflamed, and weakened, leading to localized back pain. Pain receptors in the longitudinal ligaments probably mediate the recurring attacks of local back pain. Eventually, the disc may become so weakened that it bulges posteriorly during relatively minor stress; compression and irritation of a lumbar nerve root result, and radicular symptoms develop. The clinical syndrome of back and leg pain in the distribution of a specific lumbar root is due to compression of an inflamed and sensitive root.

Disc herniation at the L_{4-5} or L_5 -S_1 level accounts for 95% of disc ruptures, with the L_5 and S_1 nerve roots affected, respectively. With S_1 root irritation, pain, numbness and paresthesias involve the buttock, posterior thigh, calf, lateral aspect of the ankle and foot, and lateral toes. Calf atrophy and a diminished or absent ankle jerk can occur as well as plantar flexion weakness. With L_5 root compression, pain radiates to the dorsum of the foot and great toe, and the only neurologic deficits may be extensor weakness of the great toe and numbness of the L_5 area on the dorsum of the foot at the base of the great toe (Fig. 145-1). In the rarer instance of high lumbar disc herniation, pain radiates to the anterior thigh, and the knee jerk may be diminished or absent. Quadriceps atrophy and weakness may be found, and reverse straight leg raising often reproduces the back and anterior thigh pain.

With lower lumbar disc herniations, there is often lumbar paraspinal muscle spasm that limits lumbar motions. There may be a list away from the side of the disc herniation, so-called sciatic scoliosis, and frequently there is tenderness of the lower lumbar spine and sciatic notch. Straight leg raising on the affected side is limited by back and leg pain that increases on ankle dorsiflexion at the extreme of straight leg raising.

Vertebral compression fracture in normal bone requires severe flexion-compression force and is acutely painful. Spontaneous vertebral body collapse, or pathologic fracture, is most commonly seen in elderly patients with severe osteoporosis (see Chapter 158), in patients on long-term steroids (see Chapter 103), and in cancer patients with lytic bony metastases. Usually there is a history of sudden back pain brought on by a minor stress. The discomfort is noted at the level of fracture, with local radiation across the back and around the trunk, but rarely into the lower extremities. The fracture is more likely to be in the middle or lower levels of the dorsal spine, which helps differentiate the problem from lumbar disc herniations, 95% of which occur at the L_4 or L_5 disc level.

The most common spinal tumor is *metastatic carcinoma,* which often presents with waist level or midback pain of insidious onset, gradually increasing in severity and aggra-

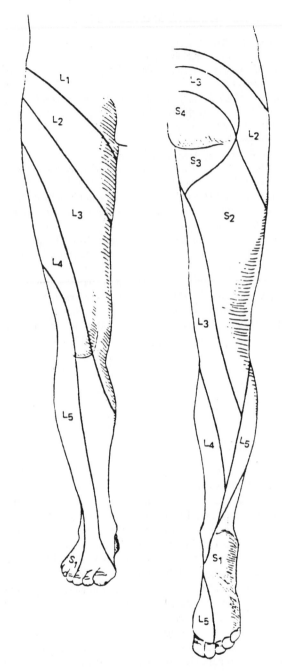

Figure 145-1.   Lower extremity dermatomes. (Finneson BE: Low Back Pain. Philadelphia, JB Lippincott, 1973)

vated by activity. Typically, the pain is not relieved by lying down, and night pain is frequent. The disc spaces are spared; disc space height is usually maintained, although collapse of the vertebral body due to destruction and weakening of bone is common. A history of previous malignancy and insidious increase in midback pain that is not relieved by lying down is highly indicative of metastatic tumor. Breast, lung, prostate, gastrointestinal, and genitourinary neoplasms frequently metastasize to the spine. Purely lytic lesions, which are often due to renal or thyroid carcinoma, are seen occasionally. *Myeloma* is the most common primary bone tumor involving the spine. Early in its course, the tumor may be difficult to differentiate from compression fracture due to osteoporosis.

Vertebral osteomyelitis is rare and involves the disc space as well as the vertebral bodies. It is usually hematogenous in origin but may occasionally follow a spinal procedure, such as lumbar puncture, myelography, discography, or disc surgery. Dull continuous back pain is the usual presentation, often in conjunction with low-grade fever and spasm over the paraspinous muscles. Tenderness to percussion over the involved vertebrae is common. A compression fracture or an *epidural abscess* may develop and result in root pain, weakness, and even paraplegia. The progression from spinal ache to paraplegia may be rapid, occurring over the course of a few days.

Ankylosing spondylitis usually occurs in young men; morning back stiffness is a prominent feature. Diminished chest expansion is the earliest physical finding. Occasionally there is a previous history of inflammatory bowel disease. The mechanism of the disease is unknown; spinal x-rays may be normal in its early phases. Initial radiologic changes occur in the sacroiliac joints and include narrowing of the joint space and reactive sclerosis; eventually obliteration of the space and fusion of the joint may occur. Over 90% of patients are HLA-B27 positive (see Chapter 144).

Spondylolisthesis denotes forward subluxation of a vertebral body. In adults, the condition results from degenerative changes and arthritis of the facet joints, usually at L_{4-5} or L_5-S_1, with forward slippage of 10% to 20% of the vertebral body diameter. About 70% of patients with spondylolisthesis have chronic low back pain; sciatica is infrequent. The pain is due to strain imposed on the ligaments and intervertebral joints.

Spinal stenosis has become better appreciated as an important cause of chronic low back and lower extremity complaints. It occurs in young people who have a congenitally narrowed lumbar spinal canal, and also in elderly individuals with osteoarthritic spurring, chronic disc degeneration, and facet joint arthritis. These changes narrow the canal and the neuroforamina, leading to root impingement and pain. The characteristic complaint is pain worsened by standing or walking and relieved by rest, especially by sitting or lying down and flexing the spine and hips. Patients report pain in the low back, gluteal region, or lower extremities; often it is bilateral. Numbness or weakness may accompany the pain in the legs. Because symptoms are worsened by walking and relieved by sitting down and resting, they can mimic vascular insufficiency and, in fact, are referred to as *"pseudoclaudi-*

cation." On exam, the spine actually demonstrates good range of motion and little focal tenderness; straight leg raising is normal. Minor neurologic deficits (*e.g.,* a diminished ankle jerk) may be present, but no pattern is characteristic.

Intraspinal tumors may present like herniated discs. However, marked progression of neurologic deficits despite adequate conservative therapy may be a clue to the existence of a tumor inside the spinal canal.

Extraspinal tumors may eventually cause root impingement and simulate sciatica due to disc disease. Tumors of the retroperitoneum, pelvis, and large bowel may extend to the roots. This is a very late development; metastases may occur earlier.

Depression may present with chronic low back pain. Often there is a history of previous back problems or onset at the time of a minor injury. Mild muscle spasm might be noted on physical examination; characteristically, the intensity of complaints and the degree of disability are much greater than the minor limitations found on examination. Multiple somatic symptoms are common (see Chapter 223). Many of these patients appear refractory to therapy, often unwilling to take an active role in their own treatment. Some even seem to derive a sense of legitimacy and self-worth from their suffering (see Chapter 226).

Malingering implies conscious deception for the sake of obtaining gain from being ill. Inconsistencies in symptoms and physical findings typify the malingerer. These often can be brought out by distracting the patient.

DIFFERENTIAL DIAGNOSIS

The differential diagnosis of back pain can be considered in terms of whether or not there is root pain. Conditions that produce root injury include lumbar disc herniation, spinal stenosis, late osteomyelitis, epidural abscess, compression fracture, intraspinal tumor, extraspinal neoplasms, and, occasionally, spondylolisthesis. Musculoligamentous strain, ankylosing spondylitis, most cases of spondylolisthesis, depression, and the very early phases of spinal osteomyelitis and epidural abscess usually cause back pain without root involvement. Occasionally a retroperitoneal neoplasm may be the source of difficulty.

WORKUP

History. In addition to elucidating mode of onset, location, radiation, aggravating and alleviating factors, and course of illness, one needs to inquire about fever, numbness, weakness, root pain, and recent injury. Previous therapy for back problems, recent lumbar puncture, concurrent illness, and chronic corticosteroid use also should be looked into. A discussion of emotional and social stresses is indicated when symptoms persist in the absence of obvious structural pathology. It is important to check for somatic symptoms of depression (see Chapter 223).

Physical Examination. The back should be examined with the patient unclothed, observing the back while the patient is standing for symmetry, muscle bulk, posture, and spinal curves. Spinal motions are assessed; flexibility is of greatest importance. One needs to look for muscle spasm and spinal segments that do not move freely. Description of what limits back motion is more important than estimating degrees of motion, which is imprecise at best. The spine is palpated for focal tenderness suggestive of tumor, infection, fracture, and disc herniation. Tip-toe and heel walking tests gross motor function of ankle plantar flexors (L_5-S_1 disc, S_1 root) and dorsiflexors (L_{4-5} disc, L_5 root) respectively. With the patient sitting, the knee jerks (L_{3-4}) and ankle jerks (S_1) are tested. With the patient supine, strength of the long toe extensor (L_5 root), cutaneous sensation, and straight leg raising are evaluated. The L_5 autonomous area of sensation is on the dorsum of the foot at the base of the great toe, S_1 autonomous sensory area is along the lateral border of the foot and the fifth toe (see Fig. 145-1). Thigh and calf circumferences are measured looking for evidence of atrophy, and lower extremity joint motions are tested. Abdomen, rectum, groin, pelvic visceral, and genitalia are examined, and peripheral pulses palpated. Femoral nerve sensitivity is usually present with higher lumbar ($L_{2,3,4}$) root irritation. The prone position allows palpation of the back and buttocks. Lower lumbar spine and sciatic notch sensitivity usually are found with lower lumbar disc problems.

Straight leg raising (*SLR*) is an important component of the assessment for disc disease. The maneuver is a sensitive test of disc herniation. SLR stretches the lower nerve roots; in the presence of disc herniation the additional root stretching causes impingement and pain. SLR is positive when leg or root pain is reported upon passively lifting the straightened leg with the patient supine. This should not be confused with hamstring muscle tightness, which can also cause discomfort on straight leg raising. Maximal L_5 and S_1 root movement occurs at 60–80° of SLR, whereas there is much less L_4 and minimal L_2 or L_3 movement. Thus a positive SLR is of maximal use in locating an L_5-S_1 or L_{4-5} disc, but its absence does not rule out herniation higher up.

Performing SLR on the opposite side also causes root movement. In the presence of a severely herniated disc, root pain may occur, especially with an L_5-S_1 disc. It is felt that a positive contralateral SLR test is specific for large disc herniation, suggesting an extruded disc fragment, though there may be a large percentage of false-negative results.

If severe pain is reported on elevation and resistance occurs, yet the leg can be raised another 20° or 30° when the patient is distracted, the test is "negative" and other causes of the pain should be sought, such as hamstring muscle tightness. Dorsiflexion of the ankle at the extreme of SLR may exacerbate the pain of disc herniation on SLR testing and is particularly useful when the SLR test is equivocal.

Laboratory Studies. For the majority of patients with low back pain, a careful history and physical examination usually suffice for diagnosis at the time of the initial office visit. Routinely obtaining *lumbosacral spine films* on every patient is low in yield and not cost-effective. The results are not very useful for clinical decision making. For example, the finding of normal disc spaces does not rule out the diagnosis of disc herniation. Moreover, a narrowed disc space does not distinguish between disc rupture and asymptomatic degeneration. The presence of osteophytes extending from the vertebral bodies indicates only long-existing disc degeneration and attempts at repair. Often lumbosacral films are more useful for reassuring the patient than for making a diagnosis. X-rays are also of little use in *early* osteomyelitis, because there are few radiographic abnormalities in the first week to 10 days, except for slight disc space narrowing; vertebral end-plate destruction and reactive bone formation develop later.

However, there are a number of situations in which back films are indicated at the time of the initial office evaluation, including suspicion of malignancy (age greater than 50, focal bone pain, history of malignancy), compression fracture (prolonged corticosteroid therapy, postmenopausal, or severe trauma), ankylosing spondylitis (limited spinal motion, sacroiliac pain), chronic osteomyelitis (low-grade fever, high sedimentation rate), significant trauma, and neuromotor deficits. When back pain is localized to the high lumbar or thoracic region, spinal films should be ordered, because compression fracture and metastic tumor are common in those areas and strain less so. Films may also be needed for patients seeking compensation for back pain.

If symptoms persist for several weeks despite conservative therapy, and disc herniation is suspected clinically, a *CT scan* may be of use to confirm the diagnosis and provide anatomic detail of some surgical value. CT is also needed when spinal stenosis is a diagnostic consideration.

Myelography is indicated when there are progressive neurologic deficits, such as loss of sphincter control or severe numbness and weakness of the lower extremities. The temptation to perform myelography in the patient with chronic refractory pain is strong, but the test should be reserved for patients with objective findings that are amenable to surgery or radiation therapy. *Electromyography* may be needed to document peripheral nerve deficits and help select patients who require myelography.

Bone scan is indicated for suspected metastatic disease of the spine and early osteomyelitis. An elevated sedimentation rate and increased uptake on technetium bone scan further suggest the diagnosis of osteomyelitis. Gallium scan and computerized axial tomography of the spine may be helpful in defining soft tissue involvement or abscess formation.

Immunoelectrophoresis (*IEP*) of serum and urine will diagnose most cases of myeloma. Crudely screening for myeloma with a CBC, erythrocyte sedimentation rate (ESR), and serum globulin level is probably sufficient when clinical suspicion is not high. The diagnosis must be suspected when back pain is accompanied by unexplained anemia and very high ESR. Nevertheless, such findings are quite nonspecific and may also be due to a chronic inflammatory process.

SYMPTOMATIC MANAGEMENT AND PATIENT EDUCATION

Acute Back Pain. Acute musculoligamentous strain, degenerative disc disease, and herniated lumbar disc with or without sciatica can usually be managed by bed rest; approximately 98% of patients respond favorably. The patient may be severely incapacitated by pain at rest as well as with movement. The acute discomfort usually persists for at least several days. Symptomatic measures consist of local heat or warm baths and use of mild analgesics. An oral narcotic analgesic such as codeine, 30 to 60 mg, is sometimes required every 4 hours for several days to achieve relief of severe acute pain. Most so-called muscle relaxants are actually minor tranquilizers; they have little direct effect on muscles but can be of help to the patient who cannot sleep. The patient should be advised to find the most comfortable position in bed; lying supine with pillows behind the knees and a low pillow for the head usually suffices. Lying on one's side with the hips and knees flexed is sometimes quite comfortable; lying prone is usually not.

The patient should be allowed up only to go to the bathroom, and rest should be continued until there is no discomfort in bed. Then, activity can be resumed gradually, beginning with getting up for meals and progressing to walking and sitting as tolerated. The patient should be prepared to return to bed promptly if significant pain recurs. Bed rest may be needed for as little as 2 days in patients with minor strain to as long as 2 to 3 weeks in those with evidence of disc herniations.

If pain remains severe and intractable after 3 weeks of strict bed rest, or if an important neurologic deficit develops, such as foot drop, gastroc-soleus or quadriceps weakness, or incontinence, hospitalization is indicated for enforced bed rest, myelography, and consideration of surgery.

A reasonable program of back care should be discussed when recovery from acute symptoms allows gradual mobilization and resumption of normal activities. The patient must understand that pain is a normal protective response to injury or inflammation; discomfort should be used as a guideline to determine the pace of increasing activity. However, minor discomfort, stiffness, soreness, or mild aching should not interfere with progressive mobilization.

If symptoms recur or marked pain develops in relation to a specific activity or level of activity, the patient should temporarily limit himself for several days. If pain increases within 24 hours of performing a new or greater level of activity, the activity should be halved each day until a tolerable level is reached, and then gradually increased. The patient can be encouraged to progress as rapidly as symptoms permit.

There are no studies documenting efficacy for chiropractic manipulation, diathermy treatments, or other quasimedical therapies. However, the benefit afforded the patient by a caring individual should not be underestimated.

Although acute symptoms will subside with rest, proper back care should become a way of life for the patient. The patient ought to be advised to avoid activities that cause pain as well as such potentially injurious actions as repetitive bending, heavy lifting (over 10 to 20 pounds), or shoveling snow. The patient must understand the limited goals of exercise, which are to restore and maintain the flexibility and strength of the back so that good posture can be attained and chances of recurrent injury minimized. Instruction sheets are often useful (see Figs. 145-2 and 145-3) to supplement instruction in the office. Mild daily exercise and more vigorous exercise two to three times a week are also encouraged. Walking briskly for 20 minutes once or twice a day, supplemented by swimming twice weekly for up to 30 minutes, fulfills such an exercise requirement; stationary bicycling or jogging can be substituted for swimming.

Chronic Back Pain. Patients with chronic refractory back pain and no clear anatomic deficits pose one of the most difficult long-term management problems encountered in primary care practice. Many of these patients do not take an active role in their own treatment and frustrate the efforts of physicians while continuing to complain of discomfort. Although there are no simple solutions to the management of such individuals, some important objectives can be achieved: identification and treatment of underlying psychopathology; avoidance of inappropriate tests, addictive medications, ineffective therapies, and unnecessary surgery; and preservation of the individual's capacity to function independently.

When a careful and thorough assessment fails to identify significant musculoskeletal pathology or neurologic deficits, diagnostic and therapeutic attention must be directed to the possibility of an occult depression or character disorder. Discovery of an underlying depression should be followed by consideration of tricyclic therapy (see Chapter 223). Recognition of a character disorder can lessen the frustration associated with trying to "cure" the patient. Therapeutic efforts are best directed at helping the patient to find ways other than suffering to achieve a sense of self-worth. Attempting to remove a person's one source of personal value (albeit maladaptive) is bound to be sabotaged by the patient, unless there is something to replace it (see Chapter 226).

Patients with chronic refractory back pain are at considerable risk for invasive testing (*e.g.*, myelography) and surgery, even though they may lack symptoms and signs that are considered proper indications for such procedures. The primary

How to get along
with your back

Sitting: Use a hard chair and put your spine up against it; try and keep one or both knees higher than your hips. A small stool is helpful here. For short rest periods, a contour chair offers excellent support.

Standing: Try to stand with your lower back flat. When you work standing up, use a footrest to help relieve swayback. Never lean forward without bending your knees. Ladies take note: shoes with moderate heels strain the back less than those with high heels. Avoid platform shoes.

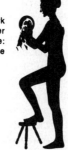

Sleeping: Sleep on a firm mattress; put a bedboard (¾" plywood) under a soft mattress. Do not sleep on your stomach. If you sleep on your back, put a pillow under your knees. If you sleep on your side keep your legs bent at the knees and at the hips.

Driving: Get a hard seat for your automobile and sit close enough to the wheel while driving so that your legs are not fully extended when you work the pedals.

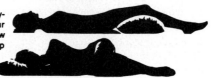

Lifting: Make sure you lift properly. Bend your knees and use your leg muscles to lift. Avoid sudden movements. Keep the load close to your body, and try not to lift anything heavy higher than your waist.

Working: Don't overwork yourself. If you can, change from one job to another before you feel fatigued. If you work at a desk all day, get up and move around whenever you get the chance.

Exercise: Get regular exercise (walking, swimming, etc.) once your backache is gone. But start slowly to give your muscles a chance to warm up and loosen before attempting anything strenuous.

See your doctor: If your back acts up, see your doctor; don't wait until your condition gets severe.

Figure 145-2. Sample instruction sheet describing care of the back. (McNeil Laboratories, Fort Washington, PA)

physician needs to protect these patients from unnecessary and potentially harmful interventions. One way to accomplish this objective is to arrange a consultation for the patient with an orthopedic surgeon or a neurosurgeon experienced in back problems, so that the patient does not feel the need to go "shopping around" for a surgeon.

Some patients will try chiropractors, acupuncturists, and other quasimedical practitioners. In double-blind controlled study, acupuncture has proved no better than placebo for treatment of chronic back pain. As noted above, there are no controlled studies on chiropractic manipulation for chronic back pain.

Exercises for low back pain

General Information:

Don't overdo exercising, especially in the beginning. Start by trying the movements slowly and carefully. Don't be alarmed if the exercises cause some mild discomfort which lasts a few minutes. But if pain is more than mild and lasts more than 15 or 20 minutes, *stop* and do no further exercises until you see your doctor.

Do the exercises on a hard surface covered with a thin mat or heavy blanket. Put a pillow under your neck if it makes you more comfortable. Always start your exercises slowly— and in the order marked—to allow muscles to loosen up gradually. Heat treatments just before you start can help relax tight muscles. Follow the instructions carefully; it will be well worth the effort.

Do exercises marked (X)

in numerical order

for _____ minutes

_____ times a day.

Take the medication

prescribed for you

_____ times daily

for_____ .

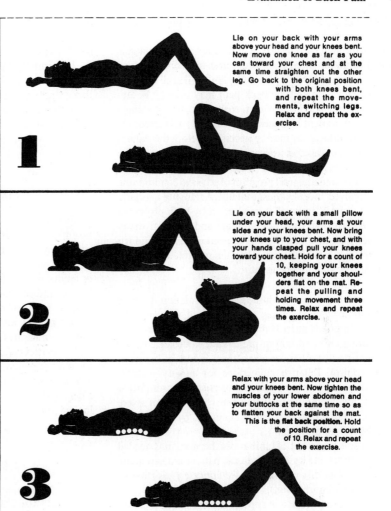

1 Lie on your back with your arms above your head and your knees bent. Now move one knee as far as you can toward your chest and at the same time straighten out the other leg. Go back to the original position with both knees bent, and repeat the movements, switching legs. Relax and repeat the exercise.

2 Lie on your back with a small pillow under your head, your arms at your sides and your knees bent. Now bring your knees up to your chest, and with your hands clasped pull your knees toward your chest. Hold for a count of 10, keeping your knees together and your shoulders flat on the mat. Repeat the pulling and holding movement three times. Relax and repeat the exercise.

3 Relax with your arms above your head and your knees bent. Now tighten the muscles of your lower abdomen and your buttocks at the same time so as to flatten your back against the mat. This is the **flat back position.** Hold the position for a count of 10. Relax and repeat the exercise.

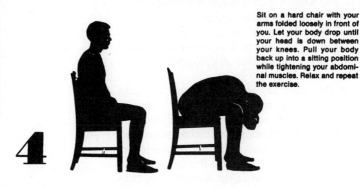

4 Sit on a hard chair with your arms folded loosely in front of you. Let your body drop until your head is down between your knees. Pull your body back up into a sitting position while tightening your abdominal muscles. Relax and repeat the exercise.

Figure 145-3. Sample instruction sheet describing exercises for low back pain (McNeil Laboratories, Fort Washington, PA)

Avoiding repeated use of narcotics for pain control is another important and difficult aspect of managing these patients. There may be repeated demands for strong analgesic agents, but unless there is an acute and reversible etiology for pain, the use of narcotics should be limited if at all possible. Many patients with chronic back pain may initially be unwilling to participate in their own treatment. Establishing a strong doctor–patient alliance (see Chapter 1) and attending to emotional difficulties may be necessary before the patient can be actively engaged in a program of self-help. Then advice that emphasizes good posture, proper body mechanics, postural exercises, and a general program of physical conditioning may be received more enthusiastically. Arranging regularly scheduled visits at intervals agreed upon by both physician and patient can help provide support and forestall many phone calls and unscheduled office appearances. Even though symptoms may not disappear, it is often possible to keep the patient functioning independently.

Surgical Treatment for lumbar disc herniation deserves consideration when disabling pain does not respond adequately to extended strict bedrest (of at least 2 to 3 weeks), when there is an important or progressive neurologic deficit in the lower extremities, or when there is loss of bowel or bladder control. Relative indications for surgery include: chronic disabling low back pain that persists after resolution of more acute symptoms; frequent acute recurrences of severe back pain that the patient cannot prevent by following a careful back care program.

If invasive treatment of lumbar disc herniation is needed to relieve intractable leg pain, then the patient is a candidate for either lumbar disc excision or *chemonucleolysis* (that is, chymopapain disc injection).

Lumbar disc injection is appropriate for surgical candidates who do not have mandatory requirements for open operation, such as massive disc herniation with cauda equina syndrome, major progressive neurologic deficit, calcified disc, extruded disc fragments that are not in continuity with the disc space, or pain due primarily to bony abnormalities rather than disc herniation. Chymopapain disc injection is not indicated for backache alone.

Chymopapain, a naturally occurring enzyme in papaya latex, acts to solubilize the nucleus pulposus of lumbar intervertebral discs by breaking down long-chain chondromucoprotein molecules. The enzyme has no important effect on collagen or connective tissue. The exact mechanism of pain relief is not understood, but it is felt that intradisc pressure is diminished by alteration of the water-binding characteristics of the nucleus, decreasing nerve root pressure with an effect very much like surgical disc excision. Hazards attendant to the use of this material include possible nerve damage from the technique of lateral needle placement, discitis, infection, and allergic reactions with anaphylaxis. The incidence of these complications is very low, and the drug is felt overall to be quite safe. Anaphylaxis has occurred in 1% to 2% of patients in large series, with very low mortality.

The initial enthusiasm for chymopapain use has waned, because many patients still experience back spasm and pain for several weeks postinjection, thus prolonging the recovery period to about the same duration as that for surgery. Nevertheless, in experienced hands the procedure represents a less invasive means of treating disablingly painful disc herniation.

INDICATIONS FOR REFERRAL

Patients with progressive neurologic deficits require prompt neurologic and surgical consultations. The same is true for individuals with acute vertebral collapse, particularly to assess stability of the fracture. Suspicion of osteomyelitis or epidural abscess is an indication for immediate hospitalization and infectious disease consultation; treatment must be early to be effective.

If a patient with refractory pain does not respond to conservative measures, referral to an orthopedist or neurosurgeon with a particular interest in back problems can be helpful. Even if the patient has no neurologic deficits and is thus not a surgical candidate, the referral can serve to reassure such a person that a surgically correctable lesion is not being overlooked, and that the efforts of the primary physician are appropriate.

ANNOTATED BIBLIOGRAPHY

Baker AS, Ojemann RG, Swartz MN, et al: Spinal epidural abscess. N Engl J Med 293:463, 1975 (*In a series of 39 patients, the typical progression was from spinal ache to root pain, followed by weakness and paralysis. Osteomyelitis was the cause in 38% and bacteremia in 26%.*)

Bickerstaff ER: Neurological Examination and Clinical Practice, 3rd. ed. Oxford: Blackwell Scientific Publications, 1975 (*A good text for additional information regarding details of the neurologic examination, including straight leg raising.*)

Deyo RA: Conservative therapy for low back pain. JAMA 250:1057, 1983 (*A review of 59 therapeutic trials and criticism of the methodologic standards used.*)

Deyo RA, Diehl AK: Lumbar spine films in primary care. J Gen Intern Med 1:20, 1986 (*A study on the use of selective ordering criteria to limit unnecessary x-rays.*)

Deyo RA, Diehl AK, Rosenthal M: How many days of bed rest for acute low back pain? N Engl J Med 315:1064, 1986 (*A randomized clinical trial showing that for patients without neuromotor deficits, 2 days of bed rest was as effective as 7.*)

Hadler NM: Regional back pain. N Engl J Med 315:1090, 1986 (*An editorial that provides an overview of the problem and suggests that patients may be the best judge of how long to rest in bed.*)

Hall S, Bartleson JD, Onofrio BM et al: Lumbar spinal stenosis. Ann Intern Med 103:271, 1985 (*Excellent review of this often overlooked etiology.*)

Hall H: Examination of the patient with low back pain Bull Rheum Dis 33:1, 1983 (*An organized approach.*)

Javid MJ, Nordby EJ, Ford LT et al: Safety and efficacy of chymopapain (chymodiactin) in herniated nucleus pulposus with sciatica. JAMA 249:2489, 1983 (*An important report on efficacy.*)

Larrienere RPT: Procedures for treatment by physical therapy. In The Low Back Patient. New York, Mason Publishers, 1979 (*A brief text outlining current concepts of physical therapy procedures and back care advice; well illustrated.*)

Liang M, Komaroff AL: Roentgenograms in primary-care patients with acute low back pain: A cost-effectiveness study. Arch Intern Med 142:1108, 1982 (*Cost is high, yield low when films ordered on a first visit.*)

Mendelson G, Selwood T, Kranz H et al: Acupuncture treatment of chronic back pain. Am J Med 74:49, 1983 (*A double-blind, placebo-controlled study showing no difference in results.*)

Meyer GA, Haughton VM, Williams AL: Diagnosis of herniated lumbar disc with computed tomography. N Engl J Med 299:1166, 1979 (*Visualization of disc herniation achieved by CT; one of the original reports.*)

Ruge D, Wiltse LL (eds): Spinal Disorders: Diagnosis and Treatment. Philadelphia, Lea & Febiger, 1977 (*This text includes a good discussion of spondylolisthesis and mechanical back problems.*)

146
Evaluation of Neck Pain
ROBERT J. BOYD, M.D.

The primary physician is often faced with the patient who complains of a stiff neck; most of the time the problem is musculoskeletal in origin. Although the majority of musculoskeletal etiologies are not serious, they can result in considerable discomfort. One should be able to provide symptomatic relief to the person with a minor neck problem and to identify the patient with a serious complication of cervical spine disease, such as root compression or cord injury, that requires surgical attention.

PATHOPHYSIOLOGY AND CLINICAL PRESENTATION

Severe *neck strain* is one of the most frequent causes of neck pain and usually results from a specific injury. Tearing of muscle fibers can cause bleeding, swelling, severe muscle spasm, and pain. Symptoms increase gradually over several hours, often becoming most severe the day following the acute event. The anterior or posterior ligaments of the cervical spine may be disrupted. When the injury is not complicated by root or spinal cord compression, there are no neurologic deficits.

Neck pain from *cervical paraspinal muscle spasm* is usually secondary to neck strain or prolonged, unconscious muscle contraction associated with emotional stress. The problem is usually self-limited, though it may recur. Muscles spasm also occurs with cervical arthritis and cervical disc disease.

Trauma or degenerative changes in the intervertebral discs or joint facettes can be a source of neck pain and result in ankylosis or subluxation of the cervical spine, termed *cervical spondylosis*. Immobility and consolidation of the joint may ensue. Usually the process is localized to the lower cervical levels, such as C_{4-5}, C_{5-6}, or C_{6-7}. Degenerative changes and spurring at the cervical disc spaces are prominent. The condition presents as recurring neck stiffness and mild aching discomfort, with progressive limitation of neck motion over months to years. Lateral rotation and lateral flexion of the neck toward the painful side are limited; pain is precipitated or increased by such motions.

Cervical disc degeneration can lead to narrowing of the neural foramina, causing *root impingement* and pain. Pain radiates in the distribution of the affected nerve root, and there may be associated paresthesias, numbness, and weakness. The C_5, C_6, and C_7 nerve roots are most often affected. C_5 root compression results in the development of pain, paresthesias, and numbness in the anterosuperior shoulder and anterolateral aspect of the upper arm and forearm; decreased biceps jerk and weakness of elbow flexion are found on examination. Compression of the C_6 nerve root produces symptoms in the dorsoradial aspect of the forearm and thumb, while C_7 impingement is denoted by altered sensation in the middle of the hand. The brachioradialis tendon reflex is affected by conditions altering C_5 and C_6, and the triceps jerk by injury to the C_7 and C_8 roots.

Whiplash is a lay term used to denote neck injury from an automobile accident. Typically, there is sudden hyperextension of the neck followed by flexion, resulting in musculoligamentous strain. Neurologic deficits are rare unless there is an accompanying cervical spine fracture leading to root or cord compression. The problem of neck pain is often complicated by concurrent legal proceedings.

DIFFERENTIAL DIAGNOSIS

The musculoskeletal causes of neck pain include muscle strain, muscle spasm, cervical spondylosis, and cervical root compression. Lymphadenopathy, thyroiditis (see Chapter 101), angina pectoris (see Chapter 14), and meningitis are important etiologies of cervical pain that may be mistaken for a musculoskeletal one.

WORKUP

History. Inquiry should focus on elucidating precipitating events, aggravating and alleviating factors (particularly specific neck movements), area of maximal tenderness, radiation of pain, presence of numbness or weakness in the extremities, course, past history of similar problems, and previous therapeutic efforts. One also needs to consider symptoms suggestive of coronary artery disease (see Chapter 14) or meningeal irritation.

Physical Examination must include full visualization of the neck, thorax, and upper extremities. Neck motions are assessed, including flexion-extension, left and right lateral flexion, and left and right rotation. Palpation must be carefully done to identify the point of local tenderness, which gives the best indication of the structure involved. The upper extremities should also be carefully examined, including evaluation of tendon reflexes, strength, sensation, range of motion, and pulses. Every patient with fever and neck pain needs to be tested for meningeal signs.

Laboratory Studies. Cervical spine x-rays are mandatory when there is root pain or a neurologic deficit, and should include AP, lateral, oblique, and flexion-extension views in

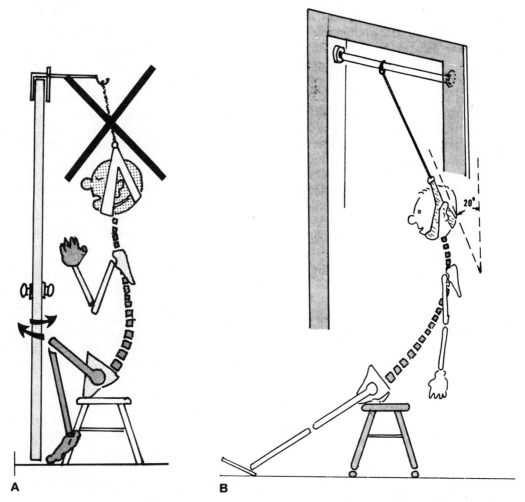

A   **B**

Figure 146-1. (*A*) Ineffective home door cervical traction. The patient is too close to the door to get the correct neck flexion angle. The door freely opens and closes, not permitting constant traction. The patient cannot extend the legs or assume a comfortable position. This type of home traction is not recommended. (*B*) Recommended home traction from chinning bar in the sitting position. (Cailliet R: Soft Tissue Pain and Disability, pp 129, 130. Philadelphia, FA Davis, 1977)

all cases to check for fracture, subluxation, narrowing of foramina, and soft tissue abnormalities. An electrocardiogram is needed when chest pain radiates into the neck and jaw, or the patient with isolated neck pain has risk factors for coronary disease.

SYMPTOMATIC MANAGEMENT

Neck pain due to minor muscle ligament strain is usually self-limited when aggravating activities are avoided. Heat and gentle massage may ease muscle spasm. There is no good evidence that injecting anesthetic into the tender body of a muscle in spasm speeds resolution of the problem. Injection may actually injure the muscle. Occasionally, a soft cervical collar is needed if symptoms persist. The collar should be worn for several days to a few weeks, and used at all times until pain clears. Once pain lessens, the collar can be worn at times when added support may be helpful, such as at night or when riding in a motor vehicle. So-called muscle relaxants are of limited value; they act predominantly by sedating the patient. Cervical traction is indicated for severe, chronic, or recurrent neck pain due to cervical spondylosis or disc herniation associated with radiculitis. Sitting cervical traction is employed at home for 20 to 30 minutes, 2 to 4 times a day, using 6 to 10 pounds of weight. The cervical traction apparatus needs to be carefully aligned, pulling slightly forward at an angle of about 20° to follow the natural line in the neck (see Figs. 146-1). Mild analgesics such as aspirin or acetaminophen, plus a mild tranquilizer such as chlordiazepoxide, may be helpful as well. If aspirin does not suffice, a trial with a more potent nonsteroidal agent (*e.g.,* naproxen or ibuprofen) might give better relief.

INDICATIONS FOR ADMISSION AND REFERRAL

If pain is intractable to conservative measures, if there is significant weakness in the upper extremity, or if there is evidence of cord pressure or long tract signs, neurosurgical or orthopedic referral is indicated. Surgery may be necessary when signs of cord injury are present, unless further cervical traction in hospital results in rapid improvement. Presence of meningeal signs is an obvious indication for urgent hospitalization.

ANNOTATED BIBLIOGRAPHY

American Medical Association: Skeletal muscle relaxants. *In* AMA Drug Evaluations, 3rd. ed. Littleton, MA, PSG Publishing Company, 1977, p. 1023 (*There is no evidence at the present time that sedative agents used as muscle relaxants have a direct muscle-relaxant effect; rather, the reduction in muscle tone may be dependent on their centrally acting sedative effects.*)

Bailey RW (ed.): The Cervical Spine. Philadelphia, Lee & Febiger, 1974 (*A good discussion of cervical spine problems emphasizing degenerative processes and trauma.*)

Cailliet R: Soft Tissue Pain and Disability. Philadelphia, FA Davis, 1977 (*Chapter 4 provides detailed discussion of soft tissue cervical problems.*)

Miller M, Gehweiler J, Martinez S et al: Significant new observations on cervical spine. Am J Roentgenol 130:659, 1978 (*An excellent recent article on x-ray abnormalities and cervical spine trauma.*)

Penning L: Normal movements of the cervical spine. Am J Roentgenol 130:317, 1978 (*An in-depth discussion of cervical spine biomechanics.*)

White A, Panjabi J: Basic kinematics of the human spine—Review of past and current knowledge. Spine 3:12, 1978 (*Review of kinetics, authoritative and current.*)

147

Approach to the Patient with Shoulder Pain

JESSE B. JUPITER, M.D.

The shoulder is a complex joint integrating 3 bones, 4 joints, and over 15 muscles. The shoulder's mobility exceeds that of all other joints, subjecting it to a wide range of stresses in both normal activity as well as in occupational and recreational pursuits. Shoulder pain and dysfunction are among the more common musculoskeletal complaints encountered in office practice. Successful treatment necessitates an accurate diagnosis; common nonspecific diagnoses such as "bursitis" and "tendinitis" can be misleading and delay appropriate therapeutic measures. Besides being capable of identifying an etiology, the primary physician needs to know how and when to utilize exercises, anti-inflammatory agents, and joint injection in order to provide safe and effective symptomatic relief.

PATHOPHYSIOLOGY AND CLINICAL PRESENTATION

Injury or degenerative change in the rotator cuff, bicipital tendon, or acromioclavicular joint can produce pain localized to the shoulder joint. Characteristically, there is focal tenderness and aggravation of pain on shoulder movement. Patients report difficulty dressing, combing their hair, or reaching up. Degenerative disease of the glenohumeral joint is uncommon; symptoms include mild stiffness, crepitus, and low-grade aching discomfort related to vigorous or sustained use. Pain originating in or about the shoulder may be referred to the upper arm or radiate to the neck, elbow, or forearm; it does not follow a specific cervical root distribution. Although pain originating in the neck may radiate to the shoulder, it is brought on by neck motion rather than by shoulder movement and is usually not affected by shoulder position. However, there may be poorly localized sensitivity to touch extending into the shoulder, vaguely simulating shoulder pathology (see Chapter 146).

Rotator Cuff Problems. The tendons of the cuff are subjected to considerable mechanical stress. Degenerative and attritional changes take place over time in the tendons and lead to structural weakening. Tendinitis and tears may ensue. Calcific deposits develop as degenerating tendon fibers become pulverized and collections of calcium salts form. These deposits may contribute to local mechanical irritation by causing a bulge in the tendon and decreasing the clearances under the acromion and coraco-acromial ligament. Fibrous scarring with limitation of motion often occurs as part of the repair mechanism.

Calcific tendinitis is frequent and commonly affects the supraspinatus tendon. Usually there is no major precipitating event. It can cause acute or chronic pain; initially the pain is localized to the vicinity of the greater tuberosity and acromion process. Pain is worsened by abduction and elevation of the shoulder joint. X-rays may demonstrate calcium deposits in the tendon.

Bursitis is rarely a primary condition; usually it is secondary to calcific tendinitis. The subdeltoid bursa lies just above the supraspinatus tendon. The acutely inflamed and bulging tendon may irritate the overlying bursa. In addition, calcium deposits in the tendon may evacuate into the subbursal space or rupture into the bursa; when such material ruptures into the bursa, pain and tenderness may be felt in the upper third of the humerus.

Tear. A weakened rotator cuff may tear spontaneously as a result of minimal trauma. Most patients with tears are over 40 and may present with surprisingly little pain. Pain over the deltoid, especially with overhead activities, plus weakness of shoulder elevation and external rotation, are diagnostic features. Muscle atrophy is commonly present. Local sensitivity is maximal over the greater tuberosity and rotator cuff (see Fig. 147-1). Passive range of motion is full. X-rays are normal or show a diminished subacromial space.

In *adhesive capsulitis,* or *frozen shoulder syndrome,* there is a characteristic symptom complex of pain and tenderness located diffusely about the anterior and posterior regions of the shoulder joint capsule. Active as well as passive motions of the glenohumeral joint are limited to a small pain-free arc. Glenohumeral motion slowly decreases over several weeks. The condition is often refractory to most forms of treatment, yet generally motion will improve with time.

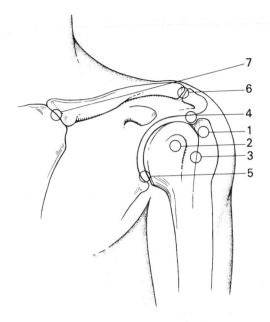

Figure 147-1. Trigger points. Palpable "trigger points" during the examination reveal the site of the pathology, corroborate the history, and indicate the type of therapy. (*1*) The greater tuberosity and the site of supraspinatus tendon insertion. (*2*) Lesser tuberosity, site of subscapularis muscle insertion. (*3*) Bicipital groove in which glides the bicipital tendon. (*4*) Site of the subdeltoid bursa. (*5*) Glenohumeral joint space. (*6*) Acromioclavicular joint. (*7*) Sternoclavicular joint. (Redrawn from Cailliet R: Shoulder Pain. Philadelphia, FA Davis, 1966)

Biceps tendinitis of the shoulder is less common than rotator cuff tendinitis, and often follows from overuse activities above the head that lead to subacromial impingement. Elbow flexion against resistance will usually reproduce the pain, which is over the anterior aspect of the shoulder and upper arm. Characteristically, there is tenderness localized to the area about the long head of the biceps, in the bicipital groove over the proximal anterior margin of the humerus (see Fig. 147-1).

Glenohumeral Joint Problems. The joint is subject to considerable stress and may develop arthritis or instability. *Instability* ensues from a posttraumatic capsular tear or stretch. The patient notes the shoulder "gives out" in conjunction with discomfort and weakness. *Dislocation* usually results from trauma to the shoulder while it is hyperextended. Dislocations are most often anterior and characterized by loss of the shoulder's rounded appearance. There is prominence of the acromion, limitation of movement by pain, and displacement of the humerus away from the trunk.

Arthritis of the joint causes symptoms at rest, exacerbated by shoulder use. The patient may note a "grinding" sound with motion. Muscle atrophy, "bone on bone" crepitation, and diminished motion are noted on examination. Rheumatoid disease will give a picture of symmetrical bilateral inflammatory changes.

Acromioclavicular Degenerative Lesions. Degenerative changes are seen in patients who do heavy labor or engage in contact sports. Pain arises with activities above and in front of the body and localizes to the acromioclavicular joint; tenderness is maximal over the joint and does not radiate.

Infection. The shoulder joint may become contaminated by an improperly performed injection and present with marked swelling, redness and fever.

Referred Pain. *Shoulder-hand syndrome* (also referred to as reflex sympathetic dystrophy) follows myocardial infarction, stroke, trauma, and a host of other events. The characteristic features are persistent burning, "causalgic" pain, diffuse tenderness, immobilization of the shoulder, and vasomotor changes in the hands. *Gallbladder disease* is suggested by pain at the tip of the scapula in conjunction with concurrent upper abdominal pain and tenderness. With *diaphragmatic irritation,* pain may be referred to the trapezius area running from the shoulder to the lateral aspect of the neck.

DIFFERENTIAL DIAGNOSIS

The causes of shoulder pain can be considered in terms of the structures that comprise the shoulder (see Table 147-1). The vast majority of nontraumatic shoulder complaints are related to tendinitis.

WORKUP

History. One should inquire about previous trauma or an inciting event, location and radiation of pain, specific lim-

Table 147-1. Important Causes of Shoulder Pain

Rotator Cuff
Calcific tendinitis
Subacromial impingement
Biceps tendinitis
Tear
Adhesive capsulitis

Glenohumeral Joint
Instability
Dislocation
Arthritis
Infection

Acromioclavicular Joint
Arthritis

Referred
Cervical spondylosis
Myocardial ischemia
Shoulder-hand syndrome (reflex sympathetic dystrophy)
Diaphragmatic irritation
Thoracic outlet syndrome
Gallbladder disease

itations of movement, associated neurologic deficits, aggravating and alleviating factors, previous history of shoulder problems, and therapies utilized. It is important to be sure there are no symptoms suggestive of angina, gallbladder disease, or diaphragmatic irritation. An occupational history is occasionally revealing, especially if the patient has engaged in heavy labor or sports.

Complaints suggestive of shoulder disease are a combination of pain, loss of mobility, and/or weakness. Pain associated with activities above the horizontal suggests subacromial impingement or acromioclavicular joint arthritis. Overuse syndromes are commonly associated with sporting activities involving throwing or racquet use. An occupational history such as wallpapering, painting, or carpentry would suggest rotator cuff pathology. The history of recent trauma may have resulted in a traumatic subdeltoid bursitis, whereas a past history of shoulder dislocations might suggest glenohumeral instability.

Physical Examination. The patient is comfortably seated and sufficiently disrobed to permit evaluation and comparison of both shoulders. Close *inspection* from both front and back may demonstrate asymmetry or deformity. For example, supraspinatus muscle atrophy would suggest either rotator cuff tear or suprascapular nerve pathology. The patient is instructed to place the involved shoulder *actively* through a *full range of motion* along with the contralateral limb for comparison. This includes forward flexion, extension, abduction, and internal and external rotation. Internal rotation is best recorded as the level at which the patient can reach posteriorly, such as buttock, thoracolumbar junction, and so on. The scapula is observed as the patient forward flexes the shoulder against resistance. Winging of the scapula is the result of serratus anterior muscle palsy.

The patient is instructed to point out specific *sites of tenderness.* Palpation by the examiner routinely should include the anterior aspect of the acromion, the acromioclavicular joint, the bicipital groove (which is best palpated with the humerus in about 10° of internal rotation), the greater tuberosity, and the cervical spine (Fig. 147-2). With the examiner's hand on the joint, the shoulder is *passively* put through a *range of motion* (Fig. 147-2). Limitations are noted as well as any palpable crepitation.

A manual *muscle test* is helpful, in particular, for comparison to the uninvolved shoulder. Inability to "shrug" the shoulder suggests trapezial muscle weakness, while weakness of forward flexion is associated with derangement of the rotator cuff (the supraspinatus, infraspinatus, and teres minor muscles). A *sensory* and *deep tendon reflex* examination of the upper extremity should be included in the routine shoulder evaluation. *Wright's maneuver* (evaluating the radial pulse at the wrist with the shoulder in external rotation and abduction) may uncover an underlying thoracic outlet syndrome. This test is considered positive if it reproduces shoul-

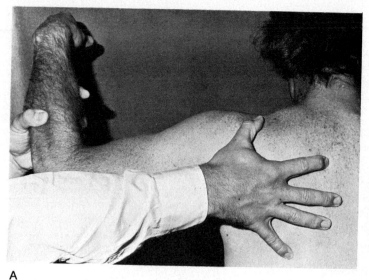

A

Figure 147-2. (A) Stabilization of the scapula while testing glenohumeral joint motion. (B) Normal range of adduction-abduction of the shoulder with and without scapular rotation. (C) Normal range of external-internal rotation with upper arm at 90 degrees and elbow held at right angle. (D) Normal range of flexion-extension of the shoulder with and without scapular rotation. (Katz WA: Rheumatic Diseases. Philadelphia, JB Lippincott, 1977)

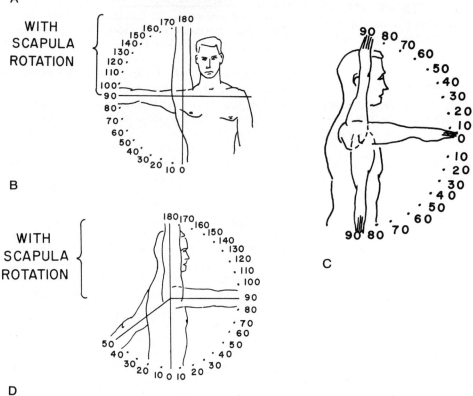

WITH SCAPULA ROTATION

B

WITH SCAPULA ROTATION

D

C

der and arm symptoms and the radial pulse is obliterated in this shoulder position.

DIAGNOSTIC MANEUVERS. Several other specific diagnostic maneuvers are helpful in the shoulder examination. The *impingement test* is performed by the examiner standing behind the patient and bringing the involved arm to the max-

imum degree of forward flexion with one hand while the other functions to depress the patient's shoulder girdle. If pain is elicited in the deltoid area or beneath the acromion, impingement of the greater tuberosity of the humerus against the undersurface of the acromium is likely. This can be further confirmed if an injection of 5 ml of xylocaine into the subacromial space relieves the symptoms. The same maneuver performed with the patient's elbow extended and the forearm supinated will accentuate the discomfort of bicipital tendinitis (Speed's sign).

A specific test for acromioclavicular joint pathology reproduces the patient's symptoms by bringing the involved arm across the body so that the *elbow touches* the *contralateral shoulder*. This can be further confirmed by repeating the maneuver after injecting the acromioclavicular joint with 1 ml of xylocaine using a 25-gauge needle to enter the joint.

Glenohumeral joint stability is best assessed with the patient supine. The involved arm is gently abducted, externally rotated, and held for one minute in this position. Laxity of the joint capsule will cause the patient to describe a feeling of joint instability and insecurity.

NECK, CHEST, HEART, AND ABDOMINAL EXAMINATIONS. Neck, chest, heart, and abdominal examinations are necessary in searching for sources of referred pain. Cervical disease is often mistaken for a shoulder problem. Cervical root compression is readily distinguished from intrinsic shoulder disease by the elicitation and reproduction of pain on neck motion to the side of complaint. Brachial plexus injury causing shoulder pain is associated with tenderness on deep pressure over the neurovascular bundle and scalene muscles of the supraclavicular fossa. Pain due to myocardial ischemia usually originates in the precordial region, but may present as shoulder or neck pain radiating into the arm. Relief with rest or nitroglycerin supports the diagnosis.

Laboratory Studies. Radiographs of the shoulder are mandatory in the initial evaluation. A *standard anteroposterior view* is helpful in ruling out underlying bone tumor, infection, or arthritis of either the glenohumeral or acromioclavicular joints. The anteroposterior view with the shoulder in *internal* and *external rotation* can best identify calcification. An *axillary view* is mandatory if dislocation is suspected; it will most clearly define the relationship of the humeral head to the glenoid fossa and is also helpful in assessing glenohumeral arthritis. Cervical spine films are needed when neck motion reproduces the shoulder pain or root compression symptoms are noted (see Chapter 146).

Shoulder arthrography is most helpful in identifying a suspected rotator cuff tear. Dye is injected directly into the glenohumeral joint and the joint is then mobilized. The presence of dye extravasated from the joint is highly suggestive of disruption of the rotator cuff.

When infection is suspected in the joint or joint capsule, *aspiration, Gram's stain* and *culture* are urgent so that definitive therapy can be initiated without delay (see Chapter 143). When a peripheral nerve deficit is discovered on neurologic examination, *electromyography* may help to better characterize the lesion. The need for an electrocardiogram, gallbladder study, chest fluoroscopy, or radionuclide scan is dictated by the presence and nature of referred pain and associated physical findings.

SYMPTOMATIC THERAPY

Acute Subacromial Impingement and Calcific Tendinitis. Acute subacromial impingement and calcific tendinitis will frequently respond to a 2- to 3-day trial of *rest,* avoidance of overhead activities, and *nonsteroidal anti-inflammatory agent* (*e.g.,* naproxen 375 mg bid or ibuprofen 600 mg tid). *Ice packs* applied for 15- to 20-minute periods during the first few days helps reduce the pain and swelling. If necessary, a *sling* is prescribed, but should not be worn for more than 3 to 4 days to offset the potential of adhesive capsulitis and restricted mobility.

Once the acute inflammatory phase has subsided, a supervised exercise program is begun. *Pendulum exercises* aid in maintaining joint mobility. With the patient bending forward at the waist, the arm is allowed to dangle and swing in forward-to-back, side-to-side, and circular pattern (see Fig. 147-3). Additional exercises such as "wall-climbing" (see Figure 147-4) are included as the pain subsides. The patient must be counselled to expect some mild discomfort with these exercises, as they are designed specifically to stretch the joint capsule. These exercises are performed for periods of 5 to 10 minutes 3 to 4 times each day.

In the case of severe acute calcific tendinitis, in which symptoms remain refractory, after 10 to 14 days, to the measures just described, a local *injection* of *corticosteroid* is often helpful. The point of maximum tenderness is carefully marked and the shoulder area prepared and draped under sterile conditions. One to 2 ml of xylocaine is injected to determine a clinical response. If the pain is diminished, a mixture of 3 to 5 ml of xylocaine and 40 mg of methylprednisolone (Depo-medrol) or an equivalent steroid is injected into the same area (see Fig. 147-5). Steroid injection may acutely worsen symptoms when the anesthetic wears off, but improvement is likely to follow within 48 hours. To avoid precipitating capsular atrophy, injections need to be limited to no more than once every 6 to 12 months. Care must be taken not to inject into the tendon; the goal is to deliver medication into the area around it.

Once joint mobility has been achieved, a program designed to strengthen the shoulder rotator muscles can be started under the supervision of a physical therapist. Orthopedic referral is appropriate if symptoms of subacromial impingement or calcific tendinitis persist beyond two months while following this therapeutic approach.

Adhesive capsulitis is difficult and often frustrating to treat; the course prolonged, and chances for full recovery unpredictable. The hallmark of treatment is an *active exercise program.* The patient is instructed to precede each session with the application of local heat, either by a heating pad or a warm shower for 15 to 20 minutes. Initially, one begins by lying supine and, using the contralateral hand, brings the involved shoulder into forward flexion. External rotation exercises are also begun; one holds a broom handle in both hands and moves from internal to external rotation. The pa-

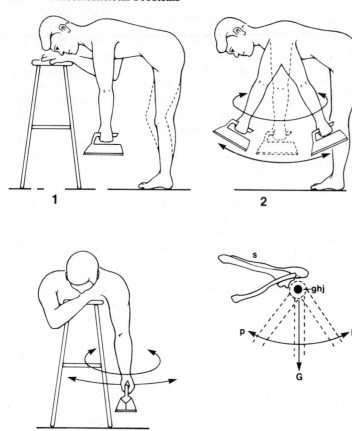

Figure 147-3. Active pendular glenohumeral exercise (so-called Codman exercises). (*1*) The posture to be assumed to permit the arm to "dangle" freely, with or without a weight. (*2*) The arm moves in forward-and-back sagittal plane, in forward and backward flexion. Circular motion in the clockwise and counterclockwise direction is also done in ever-increasing large circles. (*3*) The front view of the exercise showing lateral pendular movement actually in the coronal plane. The lower right diagram shows the effect of gravity, *G*, upon the glenohumeral joint, *ghj*, with an immobile scapula, *s*. The *p*-to-*p* arc is the pendular movement. (Redrawn from Cailliet, R: Shoulder Pain. Philadelphia, FA Davis, 1966)

tient should be encouraged to use the shoulder as much as possible for the normal activities of daily living. It is worthwhile for a physical therapist to keep a weekly or monthly log regarding the shoulder motion, as improvement is slow and usually in small increments; these objective signs of improvement help to lessen patient frustration. *Forceful manipulation* of the shoulder is rarely indicated and, in fact, *operative caspsulotomy* may be safer: the latter is infrequently needed; most patients will achieve a functional range of motion through a concerted but patient exercise program.

Torn Rotator Cuff. There is little chance for spontaneous healing of a torn rotator cuff. Despite this, many patients will respond to an exercise program designed to strengthen their shoulder rotator muscles. Repetitive steroid injections have no place in this disorder, as the cortisone, if anything, retards healing and will lead to an increase in the deterioration of the tendons.

Glenohumeral Arthritis. Conservative treatment of glenohumeral arthritis, whether secondary to osteoarthritis or inflammatory arthritis, utilizes nonsteroidal anti-inflamma-

tory medication and exercises to maintain a functional range of motion. The same exercises as those for adhesive capsulitis can be given to the patient to do on a daily or twice daily basis at home. Exercises directed at maximizing existing muscle strength are also prescribed, preferably with the supervision of a physical therapist. Improvements in total joint arthroplasty have offered a functional alternative to many patients refractory to medical management.

Acromioclavicular Arthritis. Anti-inflammatory medications and activity modification are often helpful in reducing the inflammatory component of acromoclavicular joint arthritis. At times, an injection of corticosteroid and xylocaine, done preferably under fluoroscopic control, may be of help. Rarely, surgery is required, and it consists of distal clavicular excision.

INDICATIONS FOR REFERRAL

Shoulder dislocation or instability, advanced acromioclavicular or glenohumeral joint arthritis, rotator cuff pa-

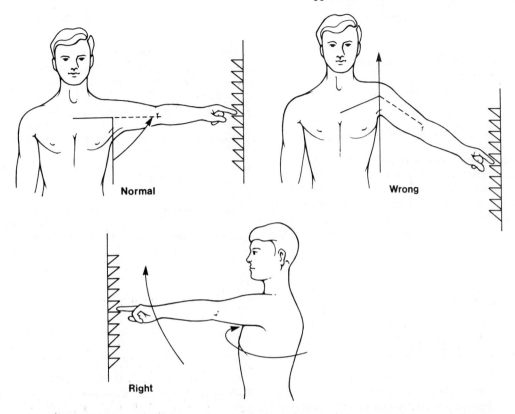

Figure 147-4. Correct and incorrect use of "wall-climbing" exercise. The wall climbing exercise frequently is done improperly. The normal arm climbs with normal scapulohumeral rhythm. When there is a pericapsulitis, the wall climb in abduction is done with "shrugging" of the scapula and accomplishes nothing. The wall climb should be started facing the wall and gradually turning the body until the patient is at a right angle to the wall. (Redrawn from Cailliet R: Shoulder Pain. Philadelphia, FA Davis, 1966)

Figure 147-5. Site of injection in acute calcific tendinitis. (*Left*) Region of supraspinatus insertion in the suprahumeral space. The region is palpable immediately below the overhanging acromion and by palpating the greater tuberosity just lateral to the bicipital groove of the humerus. (*Right*) Insertion of needle viewed from above. Two directions of entrance are shown, with the arrow depicting that shown in the anterior view. (Cailliet R: Soft Tissue Pain and Disability, p 161. Philadelphia, FA Davis, 1977)

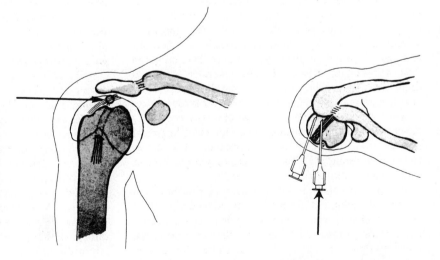

thology, and infection are best referred early to the orthopedic surgeon. Refractory subacromial impingement and associated tendinitis are indications for referral if resolution is not obtained with appropriate conservative treatment. Most of the other etiologies of shoulder pain can be managed, for the most part, by the primary physician.

PATIENT EDUCATION

The patient must be made to realize that thorough recovery from tendinitis requires active participation in the treatment program. Many individuals seek only relief from pain and expect oral or injectable medication to suffice. They must be told that repeated pain and limitation of function are bound to ensue if the exercise program is not taken seriously.

ANNOTATED BIBLIOGRAPHY

Bateman JE: The Shoulder and Neck. Philadelphia, W.B. Saunders, 1972 (*A good standard textbook for further reference.*)

Cailliet R: Shoulder Pain. Philadelphia, FA Davis, 1973 (*A clearly written and well-illustrated monograph that provides in-depth discussion of tendinitis.*)

Cave E, Burke J, Boyd R: Trauma Management. Chicago, Year Book Medical Publishers, 1974 (*In particular, Chapter 17 provides an excellent discussion of shoulder girdle injuries, including shoulder dislocations, for further reference.*)

Cogen L, Anderson RG, Phelps P: Medical management of the painful shoulder Bull Rheum Dis 32:54, 1982 (*Good review of therapy for the generalist.*)

Matsen FA: Biomechanics of the shoulder. *In* Frankel VH, Nordin M: Basic Biomechanics of the Musculoskeletal System. Philadelphia, Lea & Febiger, 1980, p. 221 (*Excellent review of mechanical aspects of the shoulder.*)

148
Evaluation of Hip Pain
ROBERT J. BOYD, M.D.

Hip pain can be a major source of misery for the patient and family. The joint is essential to locomotion and weight-bearing and is frequently subject to trauma and chronic mechanical stress. Assessment of hip pain requires determinations of severity and disability as well as etiology, because surgery is now a practical therapeutic option for disabled patients refractory to conservative measures.

PATHOPHYSIOLOGY AND CLINICAL PRESENTATION

The hip is supplied by the obturator, sciatic, and femoral nerves. Pain originating in or around the hip can be felt in the groin or buttock, with radiation to the distal thigh and anteromedial aspect of the knee. Occasionally, pain from the hip may be felt only in the thigh and knee. Pain occurs in the distribution of the L_2 and L_3 roots, and rarely is referred to the lower leg or foot. Conversely, pain due to a problem outside the hip may be referred to the hip if the lesion irritates the femoral, sciatic, or obturator nerve, or nerve roots. Extra-hip problems include herniation of high lumbar discs, spinal stenosis (see Chapter 145), retroperitoneal or pelvic tumor, and femoral hernia; aortoiliac insufficiency may also present with hip and buttock pain (see Chapter 17).

Hip pain may be focal or diffuse, depending on the extent to which the joint and surrounding structures are involved in the pathologic process. For example, bursitis is characterized by focal pain and tenderness over the site of the bursa; synovitis is more diffuse, involving the entire joint capsule. Stiffness, limitation of motion, limp, and crepitus are frequent

accompaniments of pain. Swelling is usually not evident and is difficult to detect, since the joint is buried deeply in soft tissues.

The major mechanisms of hip disease include cartilaginous degeneration, synovial inflammation, tendinitis and consequent bursitis, fracture, and ischemia.

Osteoarthritis. The hip is a major site of degenerative joint disease (see Chapter 154); the elderly are most affected. Onset is often insidious, beginning with minor aching or stiffness that may be unilateral or bilateral. Symptoms are characteristically exacerbated by prolonged standing, walking, or stair-climbing. Stiffness is present on getting up after long periods of sitting. The hip begins to loosen up on first moving about, but worsens with continued activity. As osteoarthritis gradually progresses, it results in decreasing hip motion, increasing stiffness, and increasing pain. A limp may develop as joint architecture is disrupted and weight-bearing becomes painful. The course of the disease is usually marked by spontaneous exacerbations and remissions.

On physical examination, the patient with substantial disease characteristically holds the leg in flexion, external rotation, and adduction. There may be an antalgic gait, positive Trendelenburg's sign (buttock falls when standing on opposite foot) indicative of abductor weakness, and limitation of hip motion, with or without crepitus. Pain, muscle spasm, and guarding occur when the examiner attempts to take the hip through the full range of motion. There may be buttock atrophy involving the gluteus maximus posteriorly and the gluteus medius more laterally. With severe degenerative arthritis of the hip, there may be a marked flexion deformity and pain in the hip joint even at rest.

Rheumatoid Arthritis. The hips are rarely affected in rheumatoid disease until other joints have become involved. Pain is characteristically bilateral and associated with morning stiffness, which lessens with activity. During flares of the disease, the hip joint is tender to palpation, and capsular fullness and thickening may be felt if effusion or chronic synovitis are present. Flexion contractures occur in advanced cases.

Ankylosing Spondylitis. The disease is unique among the spondyloarthropathies in that the hip is sometimes affected. Concurrent sacroiliac and spinal involvement is usually present and in itself may cause pain radiating into the hip or buttock (see Chapters 143 and 144).

Hip Fracture. This is most prevalent in the elderly, who are subject to frequent falls and osteoporosis. The femoral neck and intertrochanteric region are common fracture sites. There may be loss of normal surface architecture, acute joint deformity, severe pain, guarding and restriction of flexion and external rotation. Active straight-leg raising is impaired. X-rays are diagnostic.

Septic Arthritis. Joint infection in the hip most often follows hematogenous seeding (see Chapter 143). Since the joint is deep-seated, the ordinary signs of infection may not be readily evident. Fever, hip or knee pain (due to pain referral), and inability to bear weight are early symptoms. The thigh is often held in flexion, and a bulging, tender joint capsule may be palpable.

Idiopathic Avascular Necrosis. Aseptic necrosis of the femoral head is believed due to ischemia. The condition is most often seen in patients on chronic corticosteroid therapy. Alcoholics, patients with hemoglobinopathies, and those who work under conditions of increased atmosphere pressure are also at risk. Patients report gradual onset of focal pain and limitation of movement. X-rays are diagnostic; they show wedge-shaped areas of increased density and segmental collapse of the femoral head.

Bursitis. Inflammation of the bursa occurs as a consequence of trauma or spread of an inflammatory process. There is focal pain with tenderness over the bursa. *Trochanteric bursitis* is felt on the lateral aspect of the hip, posterior to the trochanter. Symptoms are increased by direct pressure or hip flexion and internal rotation. Pain may worsen at night and radiate down the leg to the knee. *Iliopectineal bursitis* causes pain on flexion and tenderness localized to the lateral border of Scarpa's triangle. *Ischiogluteal bursitis* presents with buttock pain that is worse on prolonged sitting, occurs at night, and occasionally radiates down the leg posteriorly, simulating sciatica.

Polymyalgia Rheumatica. This is a disease of the elderly, characterized by bilateral aching of the hips, thighs, and shoulders in conjunction with a very high sedimentation rate (see Chapter 156). Passive range of joint motion is usually preserved.

Pigmented Villonodular Synovitis. This uncommon granulomatous disease of the synovium presents with slowly progressive pain and limitation of movement. X-rays show large cystic areas about the hip joint, distinguishing the condition from degenerative joint disease.

Referred Pain. Any pelvic, abdominal, or retroperitoneal process irritating the obturator muscle can cause pain referred to the hip and worsened by internal rotation of the hip joint.

DIFFERENTIAL DIAGNOSIS

Hip pain is usually due to degenerative joint disease. Other causes include joint infection, avascular necrosis of the femoral head, bursitis, polymyalgia rheumatica, rheumatoid arthritis, and, rarely, ankylosing spondylitis, and villonodular synovitis. Pain may be referred to the hip from a lumbar or pelvic problem such as high lumbar disc herniation, retroperitoneal tumor or abscess, or obturator or femoral hernia. Aortoiliac insufficiency may present with hip and buttock pain.

WORKUP

History. One should ascertain the onset, location, and radiation of the pain as well as inciting and alleviating factors, and the presence of numbness or weakness. It is particularly important to inquire directly about trauma, involvement of other joints, morning stiffness, relationship of pain to activity, response to rest, steroid or alcohol use, and current infection or fever. There are a few pitfalls regarding history; for example, stiffness by itself is a nonspecific finding, because it may occur with degenerative disease as well as with rheumatoid involvement of the hip. The response to continued activity may be of more help; stiffness usually worsens in degenerative disease and lessens in rheumatoid arthritis. Bilateral cramping hip and buttock pain that comes on with walking and is relieved by rest may actually be a sign of vascular insufficiency rather than of joint disease.

Physical Examination. The hip should be looked at for deformities such as flexion or adduction contractures that are seen with rheumatoid disease, and for fixed external rotation, suggesting a fracture of the femoral neck. Gait is also important to check. The hip is then put through the full range of passive motion to detect crepitus, limitation of movement, flexion contracture, muscle spasm, or guarding. Normal range of hip flexion-extension is $-20°$ to $90°$ with the knee straight and $0°$ to $120°$ with the knee flexed. Normal adduction-abduction is $-20°$ to $90°$; normal internal-external rotation is

$-50°$ to $+50°$. Among the earliest limitations of movement in hip disease is internal rotation with the hip hyperextended. Palpation of the joint and individual bursae for focal tenderness and swelling is important for detecting a localized inflammatory process.

Circumference measurements should be made of the thigh at a fixed distance from a bony reference point such as the tibial tubercle of the knee, the anterior superior iliac spine, or the midpatella. Atrophy is suggestive of intrinsic hip disease. Femoral pulses need to be palpated for diminution and auscultated for bruits. Pelvic and rectal examinations are helpful in searching for tumors, which may cause referred pain. The back should be examined for evidence of L_{1-2} or L_{2-3} disc herniation (see Chapter 145). Neurologic assessment of the lower extremities is needed to test for weakness, sensory loss, and reflexes.

Laboratory Studies. *Hip x-rays* are essential to the assessment of hip pain. They may be diagnostic of degenerative joint disease, rheumatoid arthritis, avascular necrosis, or fracture. Weight-bearing films help one judge the severity of degenerative hip disease by disclosing the extent of joint space narrowing. Sacroiliac and spine films are needed if ankylosing spondylitis is under consideration (see Chapter 144). Other laboratory studies worth ordering are few in number. A CBC, sedimentation rate, and rheumatoid factor are useful if an inflammatory process is being considered (see Chapter 144). If a septic joint is suspected, aspiration for Gram's stain and culture is urgent (see Chapter 143).

SYMPTOMATIC THERAPY AND INDICATIONS FOR REFERRAL

Degenerative Disease. Simple treatment measures for relief of an acute exacerbation include bed rest, a nonsteroidal anti-inflammatory agent, limitation of sitting, and crutch or cane support. Once acute symptoms lessen, the patient can begin a program that includes avoidance of activities that specifically aggravate pain, rest periods of one hour twice daily with local heat to the hip, daily mild exercise of walking

short distances as tolerated, aspirin or acetaminophen regularly, cane support, weight reduction in the obese, and specific daily range of motion and strengthening exercises, preferably outlined by a physical therapist. Acute exacerbations of hip pain can often be managed effectively by a few weeks of bed rest and several weeks' use of a partial weight-bearing crutch. If conservative measures fail to control symptoms and the patient is active, surgery may be needed. Since results of hip reconstructive procedures are now quite good and the procedure has relatively low risk, referral for consideration of surgery need not be delayed indefinitely if symptoms are disabling and not well controlled by conservative measures. The need for reconstructive surgery must be a joint decision of patient, primary physician, and orthopedic surgeon.

Bursitis. Anti-inflammatory medication should be tried, (*e.g.,* naproxen 500 mg bid) for 1 to 2 weeks. If pain does not respond and if tenderness is well localized to a bursa, a local steroid injection can be given, using 2 ml of 2% lidocaine (Xylocaine) followed by 40 mg methylprednisolone (Depo-Medrol) in 1 ml injected into the tender area. Primary physicians who are unfamiliar with the technique of injecting a hip bursa should refer the patient to an orthopedist or rheumatologist. *Polymyalgia rheumatica* responds to low-dose steroids (see Chapter 156), and *rheumatoid arthritis* to nonsteroidal anti-inflammatory agents (see Chapter 153).

Hip fracture and *septic arthritis* are indications for immediate hospitalization.

ANNOTATED BIBLIOGRAPHY

Beckenbaugh R, Ilstrup D: Total hip arthroplasty—Review of 333 cases with long follow-up. J Bone Joint Surg 60(A):306, 1978 (*A carefully studied series of total hip replacement patients.*)

Burton KE, Wright V, Richards J: Patient's expectations in relation to outcome of total hip replacement surgery. Ann Rheum Dis 38:471, 1979 (*Often expectations are in excess of reality; preoperative counselling important.*)

Solomon L: Patterns of osteoarthritis of the hip. J Bone Joint Surg 58B, 1976 (*An excellent review with attention to precursor conditions as well.*)

149
Evaluation of Knee Pain
ROBERT J. BOYD, M.D.

The knee joint is frequently the site of trauma, degenerative disease, and rheumatologic conditions. Disability can be considerable because of inability to bear weight. The primary physician is called upon most often for minor acute injuries or chronic knee pain that limits mobility. Occasionally, an acute monoarticular arthritis is encountered. The popularity of jogging and especially long-distance running

has markedly increased the prevalence of acute and recurrent knee complaints.

PATHOPHYSIOLOGY AND CLINICAL PRESENTATION

Degenerative disease, trauma-induced soft tissue derangements, and inflammatory processes are the predominant mechanisms of knee pain in the adult. The pain is characteristically worsened by weight-bearing and may radiate into the anterior thigh, posterior calf, or pretibial region. An inflamed joint capsule produces diffuse pain; bursitis causes more focal discomfort; a tear in the meniscus may result in pain along the joint line (Fig. 149-1). Locking of the joint suggests a loose body or torn meniscus. Hip disease occasionally presents as knee pain (see Chapter 148).

Degenerative Disease. Changes often originate in the medial joint compartment and patellofemoral joint, related in part to mechanical stresses. The entire joint may be painful, but often the discomfort is localized to the anterior and medial portions of the knee. Prolonged standing or walking may precipitate or worsen symptoms. Mild stiffness is common on first arising in the morning and on getting up after a long period of sitting; it initially improves on moving about, but worsens with continued activity. Symptoms gradually progress, but may take many years to become disabling. Considerable degenerative change and joint destruction can occur before serious knee pain develops. Small effusions may appear after prolonged weight bearing, but few other signs or symptoms of inflammation occur.

Rheumatoid Disease. Rheumatoid arthritis commonly affects the knees. Pain, swelling, and morning stiffness are characteristic. Symmetrical polyarticular involvement is the rule, with joints in the hands, feet, ankles, and wrists often

affected. Symptoms wax and wane; the course is chronic (see Chapter 153). Other rheumatoid diseases can produce a similar picture (see Chapter 144).

Acute Monoarticular Arthritis. The knee is a frequent site of septic arthritis, gout, pseudogout, early rheumatoid arthritis, rheumatic fever, palindromic rheumatism, and disseminated gonorrhea. Usually there is the acute onset of unilateral swelling, pain, and generalized tenderness (see Chapter 143). Motion is limited and muscle spasm prominent.

Knee Sprain. Ligamentous injury caused by excessive joint strain is extremely frequent. Sprain injuries range from minor tears of a few fibers to complete tears of entire ligaments resulting in loss of joint stability. Mild sprains produce tenderness and local swelling without joint effusion or loss of joint stability. In moderate sprains, there is pain on stressing the joint, voluntary restriction of movement, some joint instability, and swelling due to an effusion. Severe sprains involve total loss of integrity and immediate swelling, marked joint instability, severe pain, and a large effusion. The collateral and cruciate ligaments are frequently injured in contact sports; ligamentous injuries are uncommon in joggers.

Degeneration or Tear of a Meniscus. An acute tear occurs as a result of excessive weight-bearing, twisting, or valgus or varus stress, and may be associated with partial or complete disruption of collateral or cruciate ligaments. There is usually a history of acute trauma and immediate swelling due to tissue disruption and bleeding. Joint locking may occur. If swelling does not develop until the next day, damage is likely to be confined to the meniscus and not involve the ligament; such swelling is due to a reactive joint effusion. Chronic internal derangements caused by degeneration or tear of the meniscus produce recurrent pain and swelling, and a knee that gives way, catches, or locks.

Chondromalacia Patellae. Degeneration of the posterior patellar cartilage is the cause of this condition. Dessication, thinning, fissure formation, and ultimately erosion of the cartilage occur. Mechanical factors are suspected, though unproven. Chondromalacia is the most common cause of knee pain in joggers. The patient presents with retropatellar aching that is worsened by standing up, climbing stairs, or any other form of bent-knee strain. There may be stiffness after inactivity, but there is usually no locking or giving way to the knee. Pain can be elicited by applying pressure against the patella with the knee actively extended. X-rays are normal until late stages, when the posterior surface of the patella becomes irregular and marginal osteophytes develop.

Baker's Cyst. Rupture of one of these popliteal fossa cysts can cause acute inflammation with pain, swelling, and limitation of knee flexion. The inflammation may extend down into the calf and simulate thrombophlebitis. Baker's cysts usually communicate with the knee joint space and most

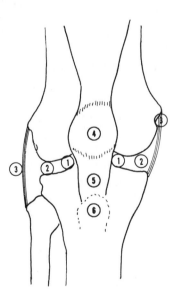

Figure 149-1. Tender sites of anterior aspect of the knee. (*1*) The site of painful fat pads; (*2*) Meniscus sites of tenderness; (*3*) Collateral ligament pain (medial and lateral); (*4*) Patellar pain and tenderness; (*5*) Infrapatellar bursal pain; (*6*) Tibial tubercle (Osgood–Schlatter's disease). (Cailliet R: Soft Tissue Pain and Disability, p 235. Philadelphia, FA Davis, 1977)

commonly occur in patients with osteoarthritis or rheumatoid disease. An unruptured cyst causes only mild aching and stiffness. Trauma may initiate a rupture.

Prepatellar Bursitis results from repeated trauma—hence, the name "housemaid's knee." Swelling, tenderness, and occasionally erythema over the prepatellar bursae are present. Bursitis of the suprapatellar and infrapatellar bursae have similar presentations, with findings localized to the bursal site.

Villonodular Synovitis is a granulomatous inflammatory condition of the synovium that lines the joints, bursae, and tendon sheaths. Etiology is unknown. It affects young adults, predominantly men, and presents with unilateral pain, persistent swelling, intermittent knee locking, and, occasionally, a palpable mass. Diagnosis requires arthroscopy or surgical exploration.

DIFFERENTIAL DIAGNOSIS

The list of conditions that can cause knee pain is extensive and includes those that cause polyarticular disease as well as those that are confined to the knee. A clinically useful classification system is to group etiologies according to whether they are acute or chronic, symmetrical or asymmetrical, and monoarticular or polyarticular (see Table 149-1).

WORKUP

History. Besides ascertaining the pain's quality, location, alleviating and aggravating factors, and associated symptoms such as swelling, redness, and warmth, it is necessary to determine if the problem is acute or chronic, symmetrical or asymmetrical, and mono- or polyarticular. By combining a careful description of the problem with a characterization of its pattern and chronicity, one can quickly focus the evaluation onto a relatively limited set of conditions having similar clinical presentations (see Table 149-1).

Acute Unilateral Knee Pain. One should inquire about trauma, jogging, locking, swelling, pain on climbing stairs, concurrent fever, purulent vaginal or urethral discharge, rash, recent strep infection or sore throat, heart murmur, morning stiffness, and urethritis or conjunctivitis (see Chapter 143). Any prior history of gout, sickle cell disease, or hemophilia should be checked for. When swelling is localized, it is important to determine the exact site, since it may be a clue to bursitis or a Baker's cyst.

Table 149-1.   Differential Diagnosis of Knee Pain

KNEE INVOLVEMENT							
ASYMMETRICAL				SYMMETRICAL			
ONE KNEE ONLY		ONE KNEE PLUS OTHER JOINTS		KNEES ONLY		SYMMETRICAL POLYARTHRITIS	
Acute	*Chronic*	*Acute*	*Chronic*	*Acute*	*Chronic*	*Acute*	*Chronic*
Sprain	Osteoarthritis	See Chap. 143		Rheumatoid arthritis	Osteoarthritis	See Chap. 144	
Strain	Baker's cyst			Juvenile RA	Chondromalacia patellae		
Acute gout	Chronic gout			Early phase of other rheumatoid diseases	Bursitis		
Meniscus tear	Chondromalacia patellae				Rheumatoid arthritis		
Early rheumatoid disease	Bursitis			Trauma			
Gonococcal arthritis	Meniscal injuries				Juvenile RA		
Septic arthritis					Chronic gout		
Reiter's syndrome					Neuropathic joints		
Bursitis					Hemophilia		
Pseudogout							
Pallindromic rheumatism							
Ruptured Baker's cyst							
Hemophilia							
Sickle cell disease							
Rheumatic fever							

(Adapted from Katz WA: Rheumatic Diseases. Philadelphia, JB Lippincott, 1977)

Chronic Unilateral Knee Pain. Questioning ought to cover previous or recurrent trauma, pain in association with prolonged walking, standing or climbing stairs, knee locking, crepitus, focal swelling and recurrent acute episodes or exacerbations.

Acute or Chronic Unilateral Knee Pain with Concurrent Asymmetrical Involvement of Other Joints. See Chapter 144.

Acute Bilateral Knee Pain. The focus of inquiry should be on the symptoms of rheumatoid disease (see Chapter 144) and recent trauma.

Chronic Bilateral Knee Pain. The questioning can be similar to that for chronic unilateral disease, but there should also be consideration of rheumatoid symptoms (see Chapter 144).

Acute or Chronic Bilateral Knee Pain with Concurrent Symmetrical Involvement of Other Joints. (See Chapter 144.)

Physical Examination. A complete physical examination must be performed because many systemic illnesses can present with knee pain. Skin and integument are examined for rash, clubbing, psoriatic changes, rheumatoid nodules, pallor, alopecia, and tophi; conjunctivae for erythema and petechiae; oral cavity for aphthous ulcers; lymph nodes for enlargement; chest for signs of consolidation and effusion, heart for murmurs and rubs; abdomen for organomegaly and tenderness; pelvis for vaginal discharge and adnexal tenderness; urethral for discharge and penis for balanitis. This is in addition to a thorough check of all joints and complete neurologic testing.

Examination of the knee should begin with a careful inspection for distortion of normal contours and irregular bony prominences at the joint margin. It is important to check for muscle atrophy. Measurements of knee, calf, and thigh circumferences can help quantitate the loss of muscle mass. Presence of an effusion needs to be determined; this is done by noting an increased knee circumference at midpatella and feeling for a distended fluctuant capsule with a fluid wave and ballotable patella. The joint line should be palpated for localized joint line tenderness suggestive of a meniscal tear. The McMurray and Apley tests are performed for suspected meniscal injury (see Fig. 149-2). The bursal regions should be assessed for focal tenderness and swelling indicative of bursitis.

Range of motion needs to be determined. The knees normally extend symmetrically 180°, and may hyperextend an additional 5° or 10°. Knee flexion is also symmetrical and limited to 135° to 170° by posterior soft tissue contact or by the heel striking the buttock. Collateral and cruciate ligaments

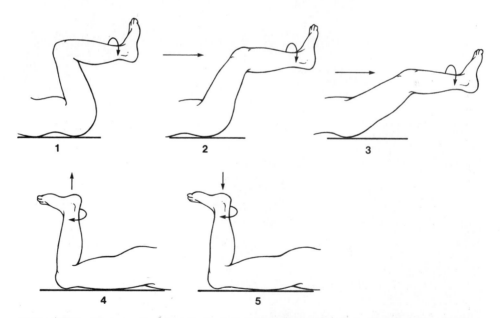

Figure 149-2. Meniscus signs (examination). (*1, 2, 3*) *McMurray test.* The patient is supine with knee flexed, heel touching the buttocks at the start. The leg is internally rotated for lateral meniscus testing or externally rotated for medial meniscus testing. Then the knee is fully extended. A painful click occurs if there is a meniscus lesion. The test is more meaningful in the first phase of knee extension. Full extension limitation does not indicate an anterior meniscus lesion. (*4, 5*) *Apley test.* The patient is prone. Leg is internally or externally rotated with simultaneous traction. Pain indicates a capsular or ligamentous lesion. Rotation with downward pressure that causes pain indicates meniscus lesion. (Redrawn from Cailliet R: Knee Pain and Disability. Philadelphia, FA Davis, 1973)

should be examined for stability. Collateral ligaments are tested by applying mediolateral valgus-varus strain with the knee in full extension and in 15° to 20° of flexion. Cruciate stability is determined by anterior-posterior displacement of the upper tibia on the fixed lower femur with the knee in extension and in 90° of flexion (Fig. 149-3).

Laboratory Studies. There is no set of "routine" laboratory studies for assessment of knee pain. When there is trauma, x-rays are needed to rule out fracture, and stress films are indicated to determine joint stability. Knee films are also indicated for suspected degenerative or rheumatoid disease. Weight-bearing films best demonstrate degree of joint obliteration. Acute monoarticular effusions require prompt arthrocentesis for Gram's stain and cultures to rule out a septic process (see Chapter 143). Joint fluid is sent for determinations of the white cell count, differential, and glucose, and is examined for crystals. Rheumatoid factor, sedimentation rate, antinuclear antibodies, uric acid, ASLO titer, and

HLA-B27 may be useful in evaluation of selected mono- and polyarticular problems (see Chapters 143 and 144).

SYMPTOMATIC THERAPY AND INDICATIONS FOR REFERRAL

Acute pain responds best to restriction of weight-bearing activities; only absolutely necessary walking is allowed, and kneeling, squatting, and stair-climbing are forbidden. Isometric quadriceps and hamstring exercises help prevent thigh weakness and atrophy. Aspirin may be quite helpful symptomatically when used in pharmacologic doses of 2 to 4 gm per day. Otherwise, any one of the other nonsteroidal antiinflammatory agents is a reasonable alternative (*e.g.,* naproxen 375 mg bid or ibuprofen 400 mg tid). If the problem is one of acute severe injury and pain, especially if the knee gives way or locks and there is a question of joint instability or internal derangement, prompt orthopedic referral is essential. Arthroscopy may be needed.

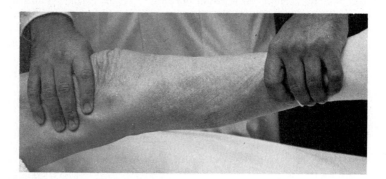

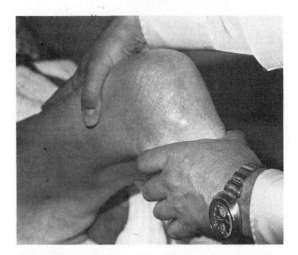

Figure 149-3.   (*Top*) Testing for lateral instability of the knee by fixating the lower femur with one hand and forcibly abducting and adducting the joint while grasping the leg. (*Bottom*) "Drawer sign" performed by drawing the upper tibia back and forth upon the fixated femur. (Katz WA: Rheumatic Diseases. Philadelphia, JB Lippincott, 1977)

ANNOTATED BIBLIOGRAPHY

Helfet AJ: Disorders of the Knee. Philadelphia, JB Lippincott, 1974 (*A good standard orthopedic text, including detailed discussion of the orthopedic aspects of knee problems.*)

Jackson RW, Dandy DJ: Arthroscopy of the Knee. New York, Grune & Stratton, 1976 (*Detailed description of arthroscopic technique as a guide to assessing knee problems.*)

Jones RE, Smith EC, Reisch JS: Effects of medial meniscectomy in patients older than 40 years. J Bone Joint Surg 60(A):783, 1978 (*Following meniscectomy for degenerative tears, there is a high incidence of osteoarthritis, and current feeling is that retention of as much of the meniscus as possible is important to protect the* compartment *from further articular cartilage stress and degeneration.*)

Laskin RS (ed): Symposium on disorders of the knee joint. Orthop Clin North Am 10(1):1, 1979 (*A discussion of problems affecting the knee joint.*)

Royer HR (ed): Sports injuries. Orthop Clin North Am 1(3):1, 1978 (*Further reference on management and assessment of athletic injuries.*)

Smillie IS: Injuries of the Knee Joint, 4th ed. New York, Churchill Livingstone, 1975 (*A classic text discussing traumatic knee problems in depth.*)

Watanabe M: Present state of arthroscopy. Int Orthop 2:101, 1978. (*Further information regarding use of arthroscopy in evaluating and managing knee problems.*)

150

Approach to Minor Orthopedic Problems of the Elbow, Wrist, and Hand

JESSE B. JUPITER, M.D.

As the physician of first contact, the primary care doctor encounters a host of minor upper extremity complaints that may be causing the patient considerable discomfort. Their quick recognition and proper treatment can save the patient an unnecessary referral and allow for prompt symptomatic relief.

ELBOW PAIN

The evaluation of elbow pain requires a careful correlation of the patient's presenting symptoms and the specific anatomic site. The elbow is particularly subject to overuse syndromes, inflammatory conditions, and localized nerve entrapments. A careful history and physical examination is often all that is required to reach an accurate diagnosis and formulate a treatment plan.

Lateral Epicondylitis ("Tennis Elbow"). This condition is the result of inflammation at the common tendinous origin of the extensor muscles of the forearm, in particular the extensor carpi radialis brevis, on the humeral lateral epicondyle. It is the result of repetitive overuse, such as with tennis players making backhand strokes or housewives knitting. The common denominator is a strong grasp during wrist extension. The patient complains of pain on the lateral aspect of the elbow. The physical examination reveals tenderness over the lateral epicondyle (see Fig. 150-1), pain with resisted wrist extension with the elbow extended, and symptoms reproduced by resisted extension of the elbow with the forearm pronated and the wrist palmarflexed. Radiographs are normal.

The management of epicondylitis consists of reduction of the inflammatory component, strengthening of the involved muscle, and awareness and avoidance of precipitating factors. It may take several weeks for pain to clear. Any painful activity is best avoided, including racquet sports, shaking hands, forceful use of the arm in hammering or unscrewing jars, or using a screwdriver. There is no certain way to prevent recurrences of epicondylitis related to playing tennis, but proper stroking of shots with a firm wrist and proper elbow positioning may be helpful. Elbow bands are often tried but usually are of limited value; however, sometimes they allow play when mild pain is present.

If symptoms do not clear with avoidance, systemic anti-inflammatory medication (*e.g.,* naproxen 375 mg bid or ibuprofen 600 mg tid for 1 week) should be tried. Local steroid injection may eventually be needed, though results may not be very dramatic. Injection is best reserved for refractory cases. The area of well-localized tenderness is carefully identified and injected with 1 ml of 2% lidocaine (Xylocaine), followed by injection of 20 mg of dexamethasone.

In most cases, a program of rest, ice applications, nonsteroidal anti-inflammatory medications, and a physical therapy program of friction massage, ultrasound, and exercises will be successful in reducing symptoms and permitting a return to function.

Medial Epicondylitis ("Golfer's Elbow"). This is similar to "tennis elbow" but involves the common forearm flexor origin at the humeral medial epicondyle. Occasionally seen in golfers, it more commonly is associated with certain man-

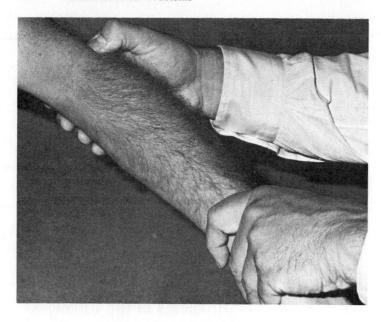

Figure 150-1. Technique of palpating the lateral epicondyle to elicit "point" tenderness typical of "tennis elbow." (Katz WA: Rheumatic Diseases. Philadelphia, JB Lippincott, 1977)

ual activities or household activities. The pain localizes to the region of the medial epicondyle and is reproduced by forcefully extending the elbow against resistance with the forearm supinated and the wrist dorsiflexed. Radiographs are normal. Treatment is the same as for lateral epicondylitis.

Calcific Periarthritis. This condition is the result of an inflammatory response to a deposition of hydroxyapatite crystals adjacent to the joint. It occurs mostly in patients with degenerative joint disease. Generally not associated with trauma, the patient presents with severe pain, localized tenderness, warmth, and swelling. Radiographs will demonstrate a dense, radio-opaque deposit adjacent to the joint. Nonsteroidal anti-inflammatory agents give prompt relief if taken early.

Olecranon Bursitis. The clinical presentation is a painful swelling over the posterior aspect of the elbow. The swollen bursa is usually fluctuant and will transilluminate light. Localized trauma or repetitive local pressure associated with certain occupations are the most common etiologies, but it can also be a manifestation of such inflammatory conditions as rheumatoid arthritis, gout, or sepsis.

Unless sepsis is suspected, one should avoid aspiration or corticosteroid injection, as they increase the possibility of introducing sepsis. Anti-inflammatory medication, a sling as needed, and local protection to avoid pressure are the basic treatment approaches.

Nerve Entrapment Syndromes. Pain in the elbow or forearm may be secondary to compression of the ulnar nerve in the cubital tunnel, the posterior interosseous nerve in the proximal forearm, or even median nerve compression in the

forearm or wrist (see later discussion). With ulnar nerve compression, pain may be found beneath the medial epicondyle, and the patient may experience numbness in the little and ring fingers. Intrinsic muscle weakness is also commonly found on examination. Posterior interosseous nerve compression presents in a similar fashion as tennis elbow, but symptoms are reproduced by extension of the middle finger against resistance. Treatment of ulnar nerve compression can be as simple as avoidance of leaning on the elbow. Use of a protective pad may help. Entrapment accompanied by atrophy requires referral.

Arthritis. The elbow is not a common site for osteoarthritis, but arthritis may be found in association with prior fracture or dislocation. In contrast, elbow involvement is common in rheumatoid arthritis. On examination, limitation of motion, swelling, and pain are common findings. Radiographs will demonstrate the extent of joint space involvement. Anti-inflammatory agents provide good relief (see Chapter 153).

Septic Arthritis. This is characterized by the sudden onset of pain, diffuse joint swelling, and erythema. Systemic symptoms are common. It is important to rule out underlying conditions such as diabetes mellitus, steroid treatments, or rheumatoid arthritis. Suspicion of sepsis requires hospital admission.

HAND AND WRIST PAIN

Carpal Tunnel Syndrome. Most commonly affecting middle-aged women, the condition typically causes nocturnal symptoms, including hand and wrist pain and paresthesias often relieved by shaking the hand. Numbness is common, affecting the middle or 3 radial fingers and occasionally the thumb. A number of systemic conditions are associated with carpal tunnel syndrome and include diabetes mellitus, hypothyroidism, inflammatory arthritis, and pregnancy.

Physical examination may reveal altered sensibility in the thumb, index, long, and radial side of the ring finger, although one may see changes only in one or two digits. Thenar (base of the thumb) muscle atrophy is present in prolonged or profound median nerve compression. A *Tinel's sign,* elicited by tapping over the median nerve at the wrist crease, consists of "electric shocks" or paresthesias in the median nerve distribution. *Phelan's test* is performed by having the patient palmar flex his wrist for one minute. It is considered positive and consistent with carpal tunnel syndrome if the patient's symptoms are reproduced by this test. A negative Phelan's or Tinel's sign does not necessarily rule out the presence of carpal tunnel syndrome. Definitive diagnosis can be made by *nerve conduction study* and *electromyography.* Testing is indicated if the diagnosis is unclear or if the condition persists and some numbness and/or weakness appears. In a patient with the condition, the electromyogram and nerve conduction study will demonstrate an increased motor or sensory latency, which is helpful in documenting the location and degree of nerve compression.

Conservative therapy for carpal tunnel syndrome consists of wrist splintage, control of any underlying systemic metabolic disorder, and occasional local injection of corticosteroids. A canvas cock-up or plaster wrist splint worn during sleep prevents wrist positions of extreme dorsiflexion or palmarflexion, which tend to increase the local compression within the carpal tunnel. In those patients with a significant flexor tenosynovitis, an injection of Xylocaine (1–2 ml) and dexamethasone (0.5–1 ml) directly into the carpal tunnel may be of value. The injection is placed just proximal to the transverse retinacular ligament in the wrist. If a paresthesia is elicited, a more superficial needle placement is made to avoid injecting into the nerve. Surgical intervention is considered if symptoms persist longer than 3 months, if there is associated thenar muscle atrophy, or if the motor or sensory latencies on the EMG and nerve conduction studies are extremely prolonged.

de Quervain's Tenosynovitis. On the dorsal aspect of the wrist, the extensor tendons to the hand and wrist course through six well-defined compartments. The first dorsal compartment contains the abductor pollicis longus and the extensor pollicis brevis and is located just proximal and radial to the anatomic "snuff box." A relatively common disorder is a nonspecific subacute or chronic inflammation of these tendons within the first dorsal compartment. Pain is exacerbated by use of the thumb and is reproduced by the patient grasping the thumb with the adjacent digits and ulnarly de-

viating and palmar flexing the wrist (Finkelstein's Test). This test distinguishes tendonitis from any underlying arthritis. The usual aggravating factor is excessive repetitive handwork, such as needlepoint, knitting, or peeling vegetables.

The majority of patients will respond to nonoperative treatment consisting of splintage and steroid injection. An injection preparation such as described for carpal tunnel syndrome is carefully placed within the first dorsal extensor compartment, which is somewhat more radial and volar than one might think. Care is exercised to inject just above the abductor pollicis longus. A removable plaster or orthoplast splint holding the wrist and thumb in slight dorsiflexion and radial deviation is worn for 10 to 14 days except for bathing. Nonsteroidal oral anti-inflammatory agents may also be of use. Failure to respond should be considered an indication for surgical referral.

Trigger Finger. Tenosynovitis is also commonly found involving the flexor tendons to the digits or thumb at the level of the metacarpophalangeal joints just proximal to the first annular pulley of the flexor tendon sheath. Snapping of the digit (triggering), which occurs with use, and inability to extend the proximal interphalangeal joint (locking) are the characteristic presenting complaints. Often the patient perceives the triggering to be at the level of the proximal interphalangeal joint. A palpable thickening of the flexor tendon may be felt at the level of the metacarpophalangeal joint in the palm.

Again, treatment consists of splintage, corticosteroid injection, and nonsteroidal anti-inflammatory agents. The steroid-Xylocaine combination is injected just proximal to the distal palmar crease where the first annular pulley of the flexor sheath is located. The involved digit or thumb is splinted in extension for 7 to 10 days except for bathing.

Calcific Tendinitis. Acute inflammation involving tendons or joints within the hand or wrist may be found in association with localized deposits of calcium hydroxyapatite crystals. The clinical presentation may be so striking as to raise the specter of an acute infection. The flexor carpi ulnaris tendon on the volar, ulnar aspect of the wrist is frequently involved. Radiographs may demonstrate amorphous, calcific deposits which may be seen to fragment and disappear on serial radiographs. Metabolic studies are normal.

Splintage and oral anti-inflammatory medications form the first-line treatments. Aspiration is advisable if concern exists regarding underlying infection or to obtain fluid for appropriate crystal analysis including uriate, calcium pyrophosphate dihydrate (CPPD), or calcium hydroxyapatite. If symptoms fail to improve within two weeks, steroid injection is advisable, with particular care taken not to inject directly into the tendon.

Ganglion Cysts. Ganglionic cysts are the most common mass occurring in the hand or wrist and may be found in a number of sites, including the dorsum of the wrist with its origin being the scapholunate ligament. Another common location is on the volar, radial surface of the wrist directly adjacent to and not to be confused with the radial artery. Ganglia are thought to be the result of an outpouching of the wrist capsule and contain fluid very similar to joint fluid. Their origin (stalk) is from the wrist joint, which explains the high incidence of recurrence with treatment methods such as aspiration or the traditional home remedy of striking the cyst with a heavy object, such as a Bible!

Most ganglia require no treatment. Aspiration with a large bore (16 or 19 gauge) needle is helpful when the diagnosis in doubt; however, even with steroid injection, the recurrence rate is high. Surgical treatment is indicated if the cyst is painful, the appearance is unsatisfactory, or concern is present regarding the exact nature of the mass.

Mucous Cysts. Associated with degenerative arthritis of the interphalangeal joints of the digits or thumb, mucous cysts are outpouchings of joint fluid similar to the wrist ganglion. Radiographs will show joint space narrowing and often marginal spurs or osteophytes. Osteophytes alone will be the etiology of the so-called Heberden's node at the distal interphalangeal joint and Bouchard's node at the proximal interphalangeal joint.

Arthritis. Degenerative joint disease commonly affects the carpometacarpal joint at the base of the thumb (see Chapter 154). Most often affecting women, the condition causes localized pain, decreased dexterity, and diminished grip strength. Pain and crepitation can be elicited by the examiner grasping the thumb metacarpal and compressing it onto the trapezium (grind test). Radiographic changes may vary from mild joint space narrowing to complete joint space loss, osteophytes, and loose bodies.

Once recognized, mild to moderate arthritis of the trapeziometacarpal joint of the thumb can be effectively managed with nonsteroidal anti-inflammatory medication and a molded splint worn 4 to 6 hours per day. The splint extends beyond the metacarpophalangeal joint but leaves the wrist free (a short opponens splint), it should be custom made by a trained occupational therapist.

The hand involvement in *rheumatoid arthritis* can vary from minimal pain and swelling to extensive deformity and joint destruction. Treatment includes pharmacologic and physical therapy measures (see Chapter 153). Tendon rupture is not uncommon; its occurrence should prompt early referral.

Hand Infections are potentially serious conditions, especially if they occur in a closed compartment. There are a variety of presentations. Infections around the fingernail are termed *panonychiae* and are usually caused by gram-positive organisms. Antibiotics and warm soaks suffice in mild, well-localized cases, but any spread requires referral for incisional drainage. A *felon* represents a more worrisome problem, since it is an infection in a closed compartment, the pulp space of the tip of the digit. The pulp will be swollen, exquisitely tender, and erythematous. If uncorrected, the edema can compromise arterial supply and lead to necrosis of the tip. Treatment includes incision, drainage, and antibiotics. Early referral to a hand surgeon is essential for definitive treatment. A less troublesome infection seen mostly in hospital personnel is *herpetic infection* of the finger tip, which is characterized by small vesicles along the pulp. It clears spontanously, though the patient is infectious until the vesicles clear.

Infectious flexor tenosynovitis presents with the digit symmetrically swollen, painful along the entire flexor sheath, held in a flexed posture, and tender with passive extension of the distal joint. Prompt recognition and surgical intervention are critical to preserve ultimate tendon function.

Puncture wounds, in particular human bites, may result in extremely virulent infection. Prompt and agressive wound care leaving the puncture site open, and antibiotic treatment may abort a more serious and destructive process. Animal bites, especially from dogs and cats, may transmit *Pasteurella multocida,* which in most instances is extremely sensitive to penicillin (see Chapter 195).

Summary

The localization of symptoms provides the keystone for evaluation. The examination should attempt to carefully localize the precise area of tenderness. A thorough functional exam, including active and passive motions of the wrist, digits, and thumb, sensory testing to light touch and pinprick, and specific flexor and extensor tendon function, should be part of every hand assessment. Standard AP and lateral radiographs are generally advisable in most cases. An EMG and a nerve conduction study are part of the workup for peripheral nerve compressions.

Nonspecific tenosynovitis and mild to moderate degenerative arthritis will generally respond to anti-inflammatory medication and simple splintage (see above). The patient with a hand infection, fracture, nerve compression, or mass should be referred to a hand specialist.

ANNOTATED BIBLIOGRAPHY

American Society for Surgery of the Hand: The Hand. Examination and Diagnosis, 2nd ed. New York, Churchill Livingstone, 1985 (*Concise, well-written, and well-illustrated; should be on the shelf of any physician who sees hand problems.*)

American Society for Surgery of the Hand: The Hand. Primary Care of Common Problems. (*A sequel to the above text; an excellent manual for anyone treating minor hand injuries.*)

Bernhang AM: The many causes of tennis elbow. NY State J Med 79(9):1363, 1979 (*An excellent overview of the subject.*)

Flatt AE: Care of the Arthritic Hand, 4th ed. St Louis, CV Mosby, 1983 (*Presents a comprehensive overview of arthritic problems in a well-written, interesting text.*)

151

Approach to Minor Orthopedic Problems of the Ankle and Foot

JESSE B. JUPITER, M.D.

Patients frequently consult primary physicians for advice and help regarding foot or ankle problems. Although some patients will require orthopedic referral for more detailed investigation and treatment, many can be substantially helped by the nonorthopedic physician who is knowledgeable about the diagnosis and treatment of common foot and ankle complaints. Such disorders are extremely prevalent and can incapacitate a patient. The primary care physician needs to be familiar with the basic types of foot and ankle complaints in order to effectively treat the minor etiologies and appropriately refer those problems that require the skills of the orthopedic surgeon.

FOOT PROBLEMS

Foot disorders are a major cause of disability in the work force. While often the result of normal activity, foot pain can also be precipitated by structural deformity or systemic disease. Environmental factors, such as shoe type and weight-bearing surface, add to the development and progression of symptoms.

Pathophysiology, Clinical Presentation, and Management

Anatomically, there are 26 bones in the human foot, equal to one quarter of those in the entire human skeleton, along with 100 or more ligaments, 12 extrinsic muscle insertions, and 19 intrinsic muscles. During gait, over two times the force of body weight is generated upon the foot. In normal gait, the foot assumes several roles, including that of a shock absorber, a mobile adaptor to accommodate uneven surfaces, and a rigid lever to propel the limb. Limitation or excess of these primary functions places the foot at risk for acquired mechanical trauma, with the prime candidates being the flat (pes planus) and high-arched (pes cavus) feet. Foot disorders are conveniently considered by anatomic zones: the digits, forefoot, and hindfoot. Office assessment is facilitated by familiarity with the location and manifestations of common foot problems (see Fig. 151-1).

Digital Problems. Complaints referrable to the toes usually are related to deformities. Most digital problems present as sagittal plane deformities; there are three types: *hammer-*

toes, mallet toes, and *claw toe.* Pain with or without a "corn" (clavus) is usually the primary complaint. Toe contractures develop secondary to muscle imbalances or are shoe-induced; they can be flexible or rigid. Shoes (prescription or commercial) that allow adequate room in the toe box area are the first line of treatment. If the contractures are flexible, digital splints may be helpful. In persistent or progressive disease, surgery may be necessary if foot pain compromises daily activity.

Forefoot Problems. (See Table 151-1 for a list of forefoot problems.) FIRST METATARSOPHALANGEAL JOINT. The most common deformity of this joint is the *hallux valgus* (*bunion*). It presents as a painful swelling on the dorsomedial aspect of the first metatarsal head associated with lateral drift of the toe. The deformity or a foot–shoe incompatibility may be the presenting complaint but, just as frequently, the patient presents with secondary problems adjacent in the forefoot, such as hammer toes or metatarsalgia. Hyperpronation (flat feet) as well as inappropriate shoes (high heels, pointed toe box) contribute to the development of the painful bunion, particularly in women.

On examination, a tender bursa is often present over the inner side of the head of the first metatarsal. The great toe itself may be deviated laterally and at times is not even passively reducible. Radiographs may show the underlying cause to be an increased angle between the first and second metatarsals (normal: 10° to 12°). This deformity is commonly seen in patients with rheumatoid arthritis.

Properly fitted shoes (commercial or custom made), bunion shields, and orthotic devices can affort symptomatic relief to many patients. Surgical intervention may be required to correct the structural deformity.

Hallux Limitus/Rigidus is characterized by limited or total loss of dorsiflexion of the first metatarsophalangeal joint and a dorsal "bunion." The patient usually complains of pain upon walking or problems with shoe fitting.

Physical examination reveals markedly limited mobility of the first metatarsophalangeal joint, especially on dorsiflexion (normal: 50° to 80° passively). Pain and crepitation are usually present. Radiographs reveal changes associated with degenerative joint disease, such as joint space narrowing, osteophytes, and sclerosis. Chronic gouty arthritis may resemble this condition.

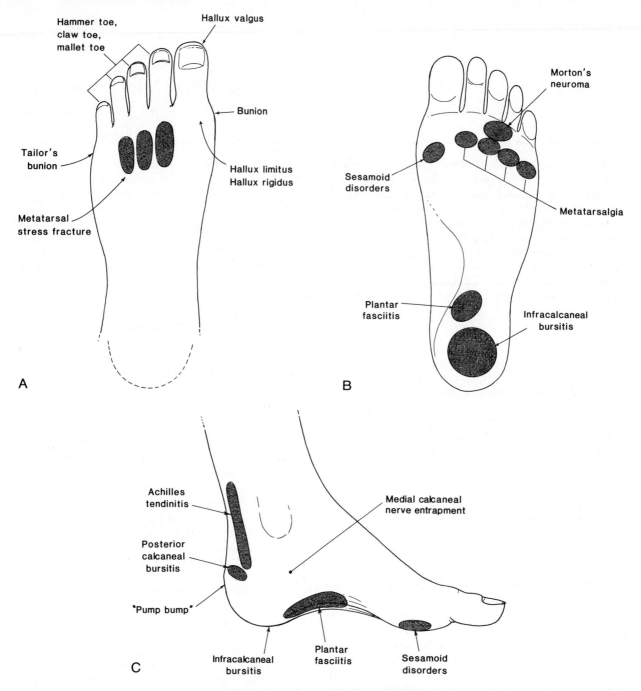

Figure 151-1. Sites of common foot problems.

The initial treatment should be directed at limiting the stresses on the joint. An orthotic with an extension under the great toe (Morton's extension), as well as a shoe with extra depth, should be prescribed. Limiting joint motion by stiffening the outer sole of the shoe (full-length steel shank)

may also help. Surgery involving either joint resection, replacement, or fusion is indicated when conservative treatment is unsuccessful.

SESAMOID DISORDERS. The first metatarsophalangeal joint contains two sesamoid bones (medial and lateral) that

Table 151-1. Common Causes of Foot Pain

Digital Deformities
Hammer toe
Claw toe
Mallet toes

Forefoot Pain—Great Toe
Hallux valgus (bunion)
Hallux limitus/rigidus
Sesamoid disorders

Forefoot Pain—Other Structures
Tailor's bunion (bunionette)
Metatarsalgia
Morton's interdigital neuroma
Metatarsal stress fracture

Rearfoot (Heel) Pain—Plantar
Plantar fasciitis
Infracalcaneal bursitis
Medial calcaneal nerve entrapment
Tarsal tunnel syndrome
Referred pain from subtalar arthritis or lumbosacral disc
   radiculopathy

Rearfoot Pain—Posterior
Posterior calcaneal bursitis
Exostosis ("pump bump")
Achilles tendinitis
Inflammatory arthritis

articulate plantarly with the first metatarsal and serve, to some degree, as a fulcrum in normal joint mobility. Excessive or abnormal stress about this area can lead to pain and inflammation (sesamoiditis), cartilage injury, or sesamoid fracture. There may be no obvious history of trauma, but sesamoid injuries are not uncommon among ballet dancers, joggers, aerobic dancers, and the like.

Localized pain and swelling are present on careful examination (plantar palpation). Radiographs should include, in addition to standard anteroposterior and lateral views, a sesamoid axial view, which is crucial for an accurate diagnosis. If a fracture is suspected, one must remember that bi- (or multi-) partate sesamoids are normal variants; a bone scan may be helpful in the diagnosis of fracture.

Treatment is directed towards providing rest and reducing the weight-bearing stresses in this area. A stiff sole, low heel shoe with a full-length shank and soft innersole may be all that is required to reduce stress on the sesamoids in mild cases. Orthotic devices may be of additional help. Infrequently, excision of the involved bone is required.

LESSER METATARSOPHALANGEAL JOINTS. The fifth metatarsal corollary to the bunion is the *bunionette,* which will also present as a painful deformity and foot–shoe incompatability. The lateral aspect of the fifth metatarsal head is tender with a local bursal swelling. Radiographs may show the primary defect to be an excessive angle between the fourth and fifth metatarsals or an enlarged fifth metatarsal head.

Alteration of shoe gear (*i.e.,* wider or stretched) usually helps, although surgical correction may be necessary.

Metatarsalgia. True metatarsalgia reflects pain with weight bearing in the vicinity of the lesser metatarsal heads. While this term is commonly used for any pain pattern in this area, it more accurately reflects an absence of other underlying conditions, such as interdigital neuroma, metatarsal stress fracture, metatarsophalangeal joint arthritis, or osteochondritis.

The metatarsals are tender to pressure and the plantar aspect of the foot (with the patient lying in the prone position) may reveal a protrusion in an otherwise flat forefoot surface. Hypermobility may also be found in the neighboring metatarsals. Often, a callus may develop directly beneath the involved metatarsal, creating additional discomfort.

A variety of conservative methods are employed to disperse weight away from the involved metatarsal, including soft innersoles, molded shoes with innersoles, metatarsal bars, and orthotic devices. On some occasions, as in deforming rheumatoid arthritis with dorsal dislocation of the metatarsophalangeal joints, surgical intervention (metatarsal head resection) is necessary and most rewarding.

Interdigital (Morton's) neuroma. Burning pain and cramping, most frequently involving the third and fourth toes, are characteristic symptoms of this lesion. Classically, the patient is a woman who reports that symptoms are aggravated by wearing closed shoes and relieved by removal of the shoe and forefoot massage.

The third intermetatarsal space is supplied by a common nerve trunk, receiving branches from both the medial and lateral plantar nerves. Compression and irritation of this trunk in a fibro-osseous ring formed by the metatarsal heads, the deep transverse intermetatarsal ligament, and the plantar weight-bearing surface are implicated in its etiology.

By compressing the forefoot and pushing up in the distal third intermetatarsal space, a "click" may be felt (Mulder's sign), with reproduction of the patient's symptoms.

Relief is sometimes achieved through wider shoes, a metatarsal bar, soft insoles, orthotic devices, nonsteroidal anti-inflammatory agents, and local anesthetic/steroid injections. Quite often, surgical excision is required.

Metatarsal stress fractures. Functional overload in a lesser metatarsal (usually the second or third metatarsal) may result in a march or fatigue (stress) fracture. The onset of symptoms is sudden and often without a history of trauma.

Palpation of the metatarsal shaft elicits pain over the site of injury. Four to 6 weeks post-injury, swelling can be palpated, reflecting the presence of a healing callus. Initially, radiographs are negative, but a bone scan may confirm the diagnosis early on.

Healing is uneventful if one avoids rigorous activities and wears a stiff-sole, low-heel shoe. Occasionally, a standard wooden postoperative shoe and an Unna boot compressive wrap are helpful in providing a more comfortable gait.

Rear Foot Problems. See Table 151-1 for a summary of rear foot problems.

PLANTAR HEEL PAIN. Plantar heel pain is seen in both young and old patients and can be disabling. It is often mistakenly attributed to "heel spurs," most of which are asymptomatic and unrelated to the pain.

Plantar fasciitis classically causes pain with the initial step taken upon getting out of bed in the morning. Often pain diminishes as the foot "stretches out," only to recur after periods of inactivity. Overuse syndromes, such as conditions caused by jogging, can contribute to small tears near the origin of the plantar fascia, with subsequent focal pain and localized inflammation.

Characteristically, tenderness can be elicited along the medial plantar aspect of the foot approximately three finger breaths distal to the posterior heel. Pain is increased with forced dorsiflexion of the digits during the examination. While radiographs often demonstrate a plantar spur at the anterior, inferior aspect of the calcaneus, this is usually not the etiology of the symptoms.

Orthotic devices tend to be the most effective form of management, although rest, ice, tendo-achilles stretching exercises, ultrasound, nonsteroidal anti-inflammatory agents, and local steroidal injections all have selective roles in the overall treatment. Rarely, surgical release of the plantar fascia is needed, but the operative results are not consistently good.

Infracalcaneal bursitis: In contrast to plantar fasciitis, this entity presents with an aching sensation in the direct *midplantar* aspect of the calcaneus, generally increasing with the duration of weight bearing. Symptoms are more pronounced as the day progresses.

Examination will reveal *point tenderness* directly under the midportion of the calcaneus. Localized warmth and swelling may be present. This localized lesion is most likely an inflamed bursa directly beneath the calcaneus.

Therapy includes local modalities such as ice, massage, nonsteroidal anti-inflammatory agents, and local steroidal injections. A soft heel pad, heel cup, or appropriately fabricated orthotic device to relieve direct impact on this region should be added.

Neurologic heel pain. Local or more *proximal nerve entrapment* is an important etiology of heel pain. For example, an entrapment of the medial calcaneal branch of the posterior tibial nerve in the region of the inferior calcaneus can mimic symptoms of inferior calcaneal bursitis. In this situation, however, one can elicit a proximal radiation *of pain* upwards toward the region of the tarsal tunnel beneath the medial malleolus. A positive Tinel's sign should be sought on examination. If local steroidal injection is not effective, resection of the medial calcaneal nerve branch may be required.

As the posterior tibial nerve courses behind the medial malleolus entering the fibroosseous tarsal tunnel, local compression of the nerve due to local trauma (sprain, fracture), a space-occupying lesion (varicosity, lipoma), or repetitive hyperpronation can result. Symptoms include paresthesias, dysesthesias, and nocturnal pain along the plantar aspect of the foot or anywhere along the distribution of the medial or lateral plantar nerves. Nerve conduction studies are not consistently abnormal in this "*tarsal tunnel syndrome.*" A foot surgeon should be consulted, although conservative treatment with orthotics and local steroidal injections may preclude the need for surgical release.

Lastly, neurologically related heel pain can be the result of a *radiculopathy* secondary to a herniated lumbosacral disc. Careful examination of the low back and neurologic testing including sensory and reflex function should be performed, especially when the cause of the pain is not readily apparent.

POSTERIOR HEEL PAIN. Two bursa are present at the posterior heel: a superficial bursa lying between the Achilles tendon and skin, and a deep bursa located between the tendon and the calcaneus. *Posterior calcaneal bursitis* results from structural and functional abnormalities of the rear foot or inappropriate shoe gear with a firm, unyielding heel counter. Pain can be elicited by compression of the heel cord and just anterior to its attachment and with passive dorsal and plantar flexion of the ankle. Several systemic inflammatory conditions (rheumatoid arthritis, ankylosing spondylitis, and Reiter's syndrome) can produce a similar clinical picture, as can a tear of the Achilles tendon and posterior calcaneal exostosis (see below).

The recommended treatment of acute posterior calcaneal bursitis begins with local measures such as application of ice in the first 24 hours, followed by moist heat, nonsteroidal anti-inflammatory medication, and rest. With a more chronic condition, a heel lift or orthotic device to control heel motion and heel counter adjustments of the shoe should be considered.

Exostosis. Posterior calcaneal exostosis ("pump bump") is most commonly seen in young women, presenting as a tender enlargement about the lateral dorsal aspect of the posterior calcaneus. Pain is aggravated by a firm heel counter. A thickened bursa may overlie a true exostosis of the calcaneus, which can be seen on a lateral radiograph.

The treatment of the acute, bursal inflammation parallels that of other types of heel bursitis already described. Resection of a posterior bony exostosis is reserved only for those cases where symptoms cannot be effectively controlled conservatively.

Achilles tendinitis. A common affliction of the athletic population, this problem reflects inflammation or small tears near the insertion of the Achilles tendon (or paratendon). Discomfort worsens during athletic activity, with subsequent swelling and stiffness.

On examination, there is tenderness to palpation of the tendon (often extending proximally), in association with a palpable fusiform swelling.

When acute, the first line of therapy is rest, even to the point of plaster immobilization. A heel raise, ultrasound, anti-inflammatory agents, heel cord stretching, and orthotics are helpful in the chronic phase.

Systemically Related Foot Disorders. The foot can mirror systemic disease. Vascular disorders with macro- or microvascular disorders can be the underlying etiology for a variety of foot problems, including ulcers and necrosis. Neurologic disorders can compromise both foot form and function. Systemic or metabolic disorders, including diabetes mellitus, gout, and rheumatoid arthritis, may all have profound effects on the foot requiring medical as well as orthopedic or podiatric treatment (see Chapters 29, 100, 153, and 155).

The Runner's Foot. The stress of repeated impact involved with athletic endeavors, such as jogging, predisposes the foot to significant mechanical trauma. All the specific entities discussed previously occur among runners. Just as important is the foot's biomechanical influence on the rest of the lower extremity. For example, the hyperpronated "flat" foot can cause excessive strain on the posterior tibial muscle and also increase the torque on the entire lower extremity, resulting in medial knee pain following prolonged jogging. If one does observe significant hypermobility or hyperpronation, it is best to mechanically support the foot with a molded orthotic. On the other hand, a rigid cavus-type foot deformity prevents normal pronation with stance. When engaged in running, the foot may lose its capacity to act as a shock absorber; increased shock will be transmitted up the entire lower extremity, even to the lower back region. Patients with this type of foot deformity may complain of leg, knee, and hip discomfort.

ANKLE

Ankle Sprain. A sprain is the most common ankle injury. Lesions range from minor ligamentous damage to complete tear or avulsion of the bony attachment, fracture and dislocation. A *strain* does not involve loss of joint stability or tearing of ligaments, whereas a sprain does. Sprain occurs when stress is applied while the ankle is in an unstable position, causing the ligaments to overstretch. During plantar flexion the joint is least stable and most susceptible to eversion or inversion forces. Such stresses are encountered during running or walking over uneven surfaces. Evaluation is facilitated by early presentation, because the event producing injury is likely to be remembered and swelling is confined to the site of injury.

Although all too often ankle *sprains* are considered minor injuries requiring little medical attention, experience has proven this concept to be misleading. While many sprains will heal with no residual disability, some do not. All reflect some degree of injury to one or several ligaments and may be classified as *first degree,* involving stretching of ligamentous fibers; *second degree,* involving a tear of some portion of the ligament with associated pain and swelling; and *third degree* implying complete ligamentous separation.

An *inversion injury* is the most common type of sprain, causing damage to the lateral ligaments. There is often a his-

tory of inversion during plantar flexion; a snap or tear may have been heard or felt. However, the history of injury is often inaccurate and may not be helpful in evaluating the extent of ligamentous damage. The careful physical examination is needed to identify the site and degree of injury, using one's fingertips to check the anterior capsule and medial and lateral ligaments (see Fig. 151-2). While significant edema commonly accompanies ligamentous injury, complete ligamentous and capsular disruption may produce remarkably little edema, due to extravasation into the surrounding soft tissue planes.

A useful sign of significant injury is the *anterior draw sign.* The sign maybe elicited by grasping the distal tibia in one hand and the calcaneous and heel in the other and sliding the entire foot forward. This is done with the ankle in both neutral as well as 30° of plantar flexion. Up to 2 mm of shift is normal. With disruption of the anterior or lateral ligaments, one sees upwards of 4 mm of anterior shift as the fibers of the anterolateral ligaments lie in anteroposterior direction. Passive inversion of the ankle produces pain. Swelling invariably occurs, usually anterior to the lateral malleolus at the onset; ecchymoses are common. Simple strain does not result in joint instability, whereas with a sprain, the joint loses stability and the talus tilts when the calcaneus is adducted (see Fig. 2). This produces a talomalleolar gap on the lateral aspect of the ankle. If swelling or pain interferes with evaluation, an x-ray assessment after nerve block may be needed to determine joint instability.

X-rays are useful in most cases of moderate to severe injury, helping to identify any associated skeletal injury in addition to assessing degree of ligamentous damage. Three standard views are obtained: AP, lateral, and mortice (an AP view with the ankle in 20° to 30° on internal rotation). In addition, a stress view is obtained (with the help of local anesthesia if necessary) to check for talar tilt. A tilt of greater than 15° is suggestive of lateral ligament injury; greater than 25° is diagnostic. One must always compare the tilt of one foot to the other to rule out underlying ligamentous laxity.

Control of swelling is the first and immediate priority of management, because effusion and hemorrhage further stretch and distend the joint and predispose to adhesions. An elastic bandage, ice water, and elevation are often helpful in controlling edema. The ankle should be placed in ice water for 15 to 20 minutes and then elevated. An ice pack may substitute for immersion. Cold application is repeated every few hours. X-rays can be done after taping, ice water, and elevation. A bulky, conforming, nonconstricting soft dressing may be applied.

Strains and mildly to moderately severe sprains are managed by repeated ice packs, followed within 48 hours by hot soaks. The soft dressing or elastic bandage is used for 1 to 2 weeks to control swelling and provide stability. In splinting the ankle, it should be kept in neutral or slightly everted position to avoid tightening the heel cord and other posterior

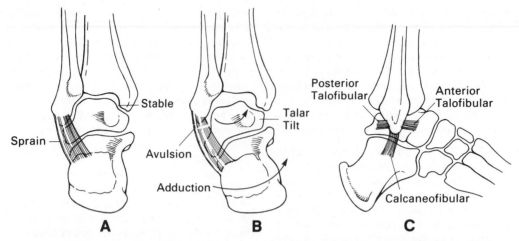

Figure 151-2. Lateral ligamentous sprain and avulsion. (*A*) Simple sprain in which the ligaments remain intact and the talus remains stable within the mortice. (*B*) Avulsion of the lateral ligaments; the talus becomes unstable and tilts within the mortice when the calcaneus is adducted. (*C*) Lateral ligaments of the ankle. The anterior talofibular and the calcaneofibular ligaments are the ligaments most frequently involved in inversion injuries. (Redrawn from Cailliet R: Foot and Ankle Pain. Philadelphia, FA Davis, 1968)

structures. Partial weight bearing is accomplished by utilizing a crutch until pain subsides. Nonweight-bearing exercises are started within 2 to 3 days of injury; these include active plantar flexion, dorsiflexion, toe flexion, inversion, and eversion.

Once pain subsides and swelling resolves, full weight-bearing can be resumed, often with use of a functional plastic "sprain brace." A number of commercially available designs can be obtained for these braces, and all function to support the ankle against the inversion and eversion stresses while, at the same time, allowing the ankle to dorsiflex and plantarflex. Running should be postponed another 1 to 3 weeks depending on severity of injury. With mild ligamentous laxity of the ankle and repeated minor sprains, proper taping to

support the lateral structures is indicated for athletic activity that involves contact, running, or jumping, particularly on uneven ground. Tape strips are applied from the medial aspect to the lateral aspect of the ankle (Fig. 151-3) to hold the heel and ankle in eversion and provide support. Exercises to strengthen the ankle evertors and high-laced leather supportive shoes may also be helpful.

Ankle sprain is a serious injury; if ligaments are torn and result in marked ankle instability (determined by examination under anesthesia or stress x-rays) surgical repair or at least cast immobilization for 4 to 8 weeks will be needed. Serious sprain requires prompt orthopedic referral to maximize chances of healing and restoration of joint stability.

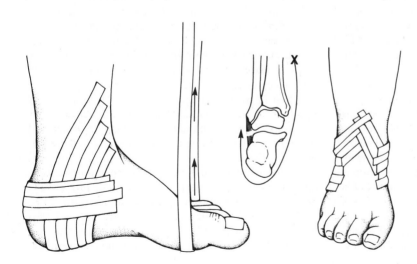

Figure 151-3. Taping a sprained ankle. The purpose of taping the ankle is to prevent further stretching of the injured ligaments until healing has occurred. The ankle must be inverted or everted to place the strained ligament at rest. The center figure depicts an avulsed lateral ligament. The tape here begins from inside and then runs under the foot to finish on the outer leg holding the heel *everted*. The horizontal strips minimize rotation of the forefoot. (Redrawn from Cailliet R: Foot and Ankle Pain. Philadelphia, FA Davis, 1968)

ANNOTATED BIBLIOGRAPHY

Cailliet R: Foot and Ankle Pain. Philadelphia, FA Davis, 1974 (*A concise, illustrated overview of foot and ankle disorders. Easy to read; has functional index for ready reference.*)

Ellison AE: Skiing injuries. In Ciba Clinical Symposia, Vol 29, 1977

(*Excellent discussion on examination and assessment of ankle injuries. Well illustrated.*)

Jahss MH (ed): Disorders of the Foot. Philadelphia, WB Saunders, 1982 (*The current definitive text on foot disorders. Although comprehensive, each chapter is well illustrated and well referenced.*)

152

Approach to the Patient with Asymptomatic Hyperuricemia

The detection of asymptomatic patients with hyperuricemia has increased markedly with the proliferation of multiphasic screening techniques. Hyperuricemia is defined as a serum uric acid concentration that exceeds the mean by at least two standard deviations. The mean, as determined by colorimetric assay (the most commonly used method) is 7.5 mg per 100 ml for men and 6.6 mg per 100 ml for women. By definition, 2.5% of the population is hyperuricemic; the consequences of being hyperuricemic and the need for lowering the uric acid are subjects of debate. Some have advocated prophylactic therapy in hopes of preventing acute gout, chronic tophaceous gout, stone formation, and renal failure. Others question the cost-effectiveness of such an approach and even the relationship of hyperuricemia to some of the adverse consequences attributed to it. The primary physician must decide when to treat the asymptomatic patient with an elevated uric acid.

PATHOPHYSIOLOGY AND CLINICAL PRESENTATION

Uric acid is the end product of purine metabolism. In man there is no pathway for further breakdown or uric acid; it must be excreted by the kidneys or the serum level will rise. The pathogenesis of hyperuricemia involves overproduction and/or underexcretion of urate. It is estimated that one-third of hyperuricemic patients are overproducers, that another third are underexcreters, and that the remainder have a combined deficit.

Overproduction of uric acid is especially marked in patients undergoing treatment for myeloproliferative and lymphoproliferative malignancies and in those with severe psoriasis. Rapid cellular turnover results in production of massive amounts of nucleic acid metabolites that are converted to uric acid. Overproduction may also develop from an increase in *de novo* purine synthesis, as occurs in patients with inborn errors of metabolism. Excessive dietary intake of purine-rich foods is rarely responsible for hyperuricemia, because dietary sources of purine make up only 10% of the uric acid pool.

Underexcretion of uric acid occurs if there is an overall decrease in glomerular filtration or a defect in tubular secretion of urate, or if another substance competes with urate

for tubular secretion. Thiazides are an important cause of decreased uric acid excretion; low doses of aspirin may also interfere with excretion. Fasting that results in ketosis also seems capable of transiently reducing urate excretion and raising the serum uric acid. Excessive intake of alcohol (greater than 100 gm per day of ethanol) has been found to produce hyperuricemia by increasing urate synthesis. The effect of alcohol was found in one study to be particularly prominent if the patient was fasting at the time of alcohol intake.

Well over 90% of hyperuricemic patients present asymptomatically; many are individuals subjected to multiphasic screening. Half of newly discovered patients in the Framingham study were taking thiazides. Just under 3% of hyperuricemic patients had elevations in uric acid secondary to a concurrent illness, such as a myeloproliferative disorder.

NEED FOR PROPHYLACTIC THERAPY

The need to treat patients with asymptomatic hyperuricemia continues to be controversial. The justifications cited for *prophylactic therapy* are founded on the belief that lowering the uric acid will prevent the development of acute gout, chronic gouty arthritis, gouty nephropathy, and urolithiasis. Such assumptions have been challenged by newer data that also help guide decision making.

Acute Gout. Two of the three existing population studies on the risk of acute gout in patients with hyperuricemia show that the higher the serum uric acid level, the greater the chance of an attack of acute gout. The incidence of acute gout in the Framingham study was 14% for men with a uric acid between 7.0 and 7.9 mg per 100 ml, 19% for those with a level between 8.0 and 8.9; and 80% when the level went above 9.0. However, only ten patients in the entire study population had a serum uric acid above 9.0 mg per 100 ml. Similar results were obtained in a large community study in Sudbury, Massachusetts. On the other hand, a study of 124 asymptomatic hyperuricemic patients followed in the Kaiser-Permanente system found no relationship between uric acid concentration and development of acute gout.

The costs of preventing attacks of acute gout include the

expense of medication and the risk of adverse drug effects. The cost of lifelong prophylactic therapy can reach several thousand dollars, because the mean age at time of detection is 35, and a year's worth of medication can cost well over $100. The prevalence of adverse drug reactions has been reported to be as high as 10% for probenecid and 25% for allopurinol. These costs appear excessive when compared to the safety, efficacy, and minimal expense of treating an acute attack of gout with an anti-inflammatory agent. It seems reasonable to wait until an acute attack occurs, rather than to subject the patient to lifelong prophylaxis, especially if the intervals between recurrences of acute gout are measured in years.

For Chronic Gouty Arthritis. The issue of prophylaxis for prevention of chronic gouty arthritis is of only minor importance, because almost all patients with this condition go through a stage of acute gouty attacks before developing chronic joint changes. Thus, asymptomatic patients are at little if any risk for silently falling victim to chronic gouty arthritis.

For Impairment of Renal Function. It is a common assumption that chronic hyperuricemia is potentially harmful to the kidneys and may result in progressive renal damage leading to azotemia. However, recent evidence does not fully support this belief. In a prospective Kaiser-Permanente study comparing 113 patients with asymptomatic hyperuricemia and 193 controls followed for 8 years, there was no significant difference in the incidence of azotemia for the two groups (1.8% versus 2.1%, respectively). The degree of azotemia that developed was always mild (serum creatinines were in the range of 1.3 to 1.7 mg per 100 ml).

In the same study, 168 patients with clinical gout were followed for 10 years; similarly, the incidence of azotemia was low and its severity mild. The development of azotemia was unrelated to the degree of control of hyperuricemia. In addition, the investigators studied the records of 1356 men aged 60 to 69 who were followed for 10 years; there were no deaths from renal failure that were attributable to hyperuricemia. The association between azotemia and hyperuricemia was further assessed by analysis of hyperuricemic patients and matched controls. Excluding those with hypertension, diabetes, and atherosclerosis, there were only three cases of azotemia in the hyperuricemia group and none in the matched controls; the difference was not statistically significant. In only two cases did hyperuricemia precede azotemia.

The investigators projected from their data that the long-term risk of clinically significant azotemia was minuscule until the uric acid level reached 13.0 mg per 100 ml in men and 10.0 mg per 100 ml in women. They estimated that only if such levels were sustained for 40 years would the risk of clinically important azotemia become substantial.

The Kaiser study is not the only one to show little evidence for hyperuricemia-induced renal impairment. A 12-year study

of 524 gouty patients found no relationship between hyperuricemia and renal function. A 3-year prospective study of hyperuricemic patients with and without renal failure showed no change in renal function when allopurinol was used to normalize the serum urate concentration. A study of hyperuricemic relatives of patients with clinical gout found normal insulin, creatinine, and hippurate clearances.

A frequently quoted study purporting to show a beneficial effect of lowering the serum uric acid level was uncontrolled and involved only ten patients, of whom all had chronic gout and many had high uric acid excretions. There was no change in serum creatinine during the 23-month mean treatment period of the study. The authors claim that deterioration of renal function was prevented by therapy, but if azotemia is as infrequent and mild as suggested by the Kaiser study, then it is no surprise that there was little change and one can hardly conclude that the effect was due to allopurinol therapy. Further investigations have helped elucidate the apparent relationship between gout and nephropathy. One study found a strong correlation between excessive lead stores and renal insufficiency in gouty patients. Another noted that coexisting hypertension, pre-existing renal disease, and ischemic heart disease accounted for all cases with renal impairment.

One group of hyperuricemic patients *is* at risk for renal failure. These are persons with myeloproliferative or lymphoproliferative disease. They may have a sudden increase in uric acid load after a course of treatment. The resultant hyperuricemia and extreme amount of uric acid excretion may lead to precipitation of uric acid crystals in the renal tubules and cause acute oliguric renal failure. Such patients require prophylaxis with allopurinol before receiving therapy for their proliferative disorder.

In sum, the preponderance of available data argues against the notion that asymptomatic hyperuricemia is associated with a substantial risk of clinically significant renal impairment or that attempts to lower the serum uric acid reduce the risk of azotemia. Moreover, patients with hyperuricemia *due to* renal failure are not at increased risk of renal damage from elevated serum urate.

For Nephrolithiasis. The risk of nephrolithiasis in patients with asymptomatic hyperuricemia was also addressed in the Kaiser study; it was found to be very small. Renal calculi occurred in 3 (2.6%) of 113 hyperuricemic patients and in 2 (1.1%) of 193 controls. In two of the hyperuricemic patients with stones, the stone was composed of calcium. The risk of developing a stone attributable to hyperuricemia was calculated to be less than 1% per year. Among gouty patients, the control of serum uric acid was the same in those who developed stones as in those who did not.

Factors other than hyperuricemia are believed to be important for stone formation. Family history of stone formation is contributory. Two of the three hyperuricemia patients with stones in the Kaiser study had a family history of nephrolithiasis. Urine acidity is a critical factor because the solubility of uric acid falls precipitously as the pH falls from 8.0 to 5.0. The amount of uric acid excreted in the urine per 24 hours has also been suggested as a cause; but careful studies have shown that the level of urinary uric acid is only a weak determinant of stone formation. However, dehydration can precipitate nephrolithiasis (see Chapter 134).

It is interesting to note that urolithiasis is rarely life threatening. In a study of 1700 patients with gout, only one patient experienced serious obstructive uropathy.

CONCLUSIONS AND RECOMMENDATIONS

- Asymptomatic hyperuricemia is associated with an increased risk of acute gouty arthritis, but the cost of prophylactic therapy in patients who have never had a single attack of gout greatly exceeds the cost of symptomatically treating an acute attack, should it occur.
- Treatment to prevent chronic tophaceous gout need not be started until clinical evidence of gout develops.
- There is insufficient evidence to justify prophylaxis for prevention of renal impairment unless the patient has a myeloproliferative or lymphoproliferative disorder and is about to be treated for it. The degree of azotemia that can be attributed to hyperuricemia is mild and clinically insignificant in most other instances.
- The risk of urolithiasis is sufficiently low to justify waiting for the development of a stone before initiating prophylactic therapy, unless the patient has a strong family history of nephrolithiasis.

A.H.G.

ANNOTATED BIBLIOGRAPHY

Batuman V, Maesaka JK, Haddad B et al: The role of lead in gout nephropathy. N Engl J Med 304:520, 1981 (*Detected a strong relationship between lead and nephropathy in patients with gout.*)

Burger LU, Yu TF: Renal function in gout—An analysis of 524 gouty subjects including long-term follow-up studies. Am J Med 59:604, 1975 (*Follow-up for 12 years showed that hyperuricemia alone had no deleterious effect on renal function in ambulatory patients with gout.*)

Coe FL: Hyperuricosuric calcium oxalate nephrolithiasis. Kidney Int 13:418, 1978 (*An interesting observation that 25% of patients with calcium oxalate stones hyperexcrete uric acid. The mechanism is not known, and allopurinol does not seem to reduce new stone formation.*)

Faller J, Fox I: Ethanol-induced hyperuricemia. N Engl J Med 307:1598, 1982 (*Ethanol increases urate synthesis.*)

Fessel JW: Renal outcomes of gout and hyperuricemia. Am J Med 67:74, 1979 (*A carefully done prospective study showing that the risks of renal failure and stone formation are very small and hardly justify prophylactic therapy.*)

Hall AP, Berry PE, Dawber TR et al: Epidemiology of gout and hyperuricemia—A long-term population study. Am J Med 42:27, 1967 (*The Framingham study; 14% of patients with uric acids of 7 to 7.9 mg, 19% with uric serum urates between 8 and 8.9, and 5 out of 6 patients with uric acids over 9 developed gouty attacks.*)

Klinenberg J: Hyperuricemia and gout. Med Clin North Am 61:299, 1977 (*A good review of the significance and treatment of both of these conditions.*)

Liang MH, Fries JF: Asymptomatic hyperuricemia: The case for conservative management. Ann Intern Med 88:666, 1978 (*A well-developed approach to asymptomatic hyperuricemia.*)

Maclaughlan MJ, Rodnan GP: Effects of food, fast, and alcohol on serum uric acid and acute attacks of gout. Am J Med 42:38, 1967 (*Fasting and consumption of over 100 g of alcohol raised urate levels. Acute changes in levels precipitated gouty attacks.*)

Paulus HE, Coutts A, Calabro JJ et al: Clinical significance of hyperuricemia in routinely screened hospitalized men. JAMA 211:277, 1970 (*An early but prophetic paper that argued that an abnormal laboratory finding does not confirm diagnosis or justify therapy.*)

Rastegar A, Their SO: The physiologic approach to hyperuricemia. N Engl J Med 286:470, 1972 (*An excellent review of the enzymatic defects that lead to increased uric acid.*)

Reif MC, Constantiner A, Levitt MF: Chronic gouty nephropathy: A vanishing syndrome. N Engl J Med 304:535, 1981 (*An editorial summarizing the data on the lack of a relation between renal injury and most forms of hyperuricemia.*)

Rosenfeld JB: Effect of long-term allopurinol administration on serial GFR in normotensive and hypertensive hyperuricemic subjects. Adv Exp Med Biol 41:581, 1974 (*Normalizing uric acid and following patients for 3 to 4 years produced no beneficial effect on renal function.*)

Yu TF, Berger LU: Impaired renal function in gout. Am J Med 75:95, 1982 (*Hyperuricemia alone did not affect renal function; renal insufficiency correlated best with coexisting hypertension, preexisting renal disease, and ischemic heart disease.*)

Yu TF, Gutman A: Uric acid nephrolithiasis in gout: Predisposing factors. Ann Intern Med 67:1133, 1967 (*A classic study of 305 gout patients correlating risk of stone formation with uric acid excretion, urine pH, serum urate level, and etiology.*)

153
Management of Rheumatoid Arthritis

Management of rheumatoid arthritis (RA) is a challenge because the disease is chronic, relapsing, potentially disabling, and without completely satisfactory methods of treatment. The problem is common. Population surveys indicate that 3% of females and 1% of males have definite or probable RA, based on the diagnostic criteria established by the American Rheumatism Association. Prevalence increases with age, and incidence peaks in the fourth decade. The estimated annual incidence ranges from 0.5 to 3 new cases per thousand per year. The objectives of therapy are to minimize pain and stiffness and preserve range of motion and muscle strength. The primary physician needs to be able to make optimal use of anti-inflammatory agents, know how to design and implement a program of supportive measures, and decide when referral is needed.

PATHOPHYSIOLOGY AND CLINICAL PRESENTATION

Rheumatoid arthritis is an immunologically mediated, chronic inflammatory disease of unknown etiology, manifested by a destructive arthritis of the diarthrodial joints. A genetically controlled, delayed hypersensitivity reaction to an as yet unidentified stimulus (perhaps an infectious agent, or a constituent of synovium or cartilage) appears to be the initial event. Important components of immunologic joint injury include T-cell lymphocytes, activated macrophages, and neutrophils releasing such mediators as interleukin-1, prostaglandins, collagenase, lysosomal enzymes, and oxygen-derived free radicals. In addition, rheumatoid factor is expressed by B-lymphocytes migrating into the inflamed joint. The clinical course is one of exacerbations and remissions.

Pathologically, the earliest change is synovial edema and dilatation of the small vessels, followed by new capillary formation, synovial proliferation, and infiltration by mononuclear cells. Neutrophils migrate into the joint space. As the inflammatory process progresses, the synovium becomes more hypertrophic, edematous, hypervascular, and further infiltrated by mononuclear cells. If exuberant granulation tissue (pannus) forms within the inflamed synovium, joint damage may ensue. Pannus is capable of eroding cartilage and bone, typically beginning at the joint margin, then spreading over the entire cartilaginous surface. Lysosomal enzymes released from within the pannus and latent colla-genases are believed to contribute to the direct erosive capacity. Often osteopenia is seen in subchondral bone adjacent to the involved joint even before the pannus has denuded the cartilage.

Initially, an effusion develops, distending the joint capsule. This is followed by damage to the articular surface and weakening of the capsule and periarticular ligaments. Secondary muscle atrophy results and leads to imbalance of opposing muscle groups. The net effect is an unstable, weak, swollen, subluxated joint. The synovium of tendon sheaths and bursae may also be affected by the inflammatory process, which leads to accompanying tenosynovitis and bursitis.

Clinical onset of RA is usually insidious, often beginning with vague *arthralgias, morning stiffness,* and *fatigue.* Frank signs of *articular inflammation* (swelling, pain, and warmth) soon follow. The small joints of the hands and feet—the proximal interphalangeals (PIP), metacarpophalangeals (MCP), and metatarsophalangeals (MTP)—are typically among the first to be involved, but knees, ankles, wrists, or elbows may also be affected early on. *Tenosynovitis* is common. Initially, the arthritis may be asymmetrical or may even present as a monoarticular arthritis, but symmetrical distribution supervenes in most instances and is characteristic of the disease.

In an occasional patient, RA is preceded by *palindromic rheumatism,* a condition characterized by repeated episodes of transient joint pain, swelling, and redness extending beyond the joint. The condition lasts a few hours to a few days, followed by complete resolution and no permanent joint injury. Fingers, wrists, shoulders and knees are most commonly affected. About 50% of these patients eventually develop typical RA.

Rheumatoid nodules appear in about 25% of patients with rheumatoid arthritis, usually as the disease progresses. These subcutaneous nodules are firm, nontender, and located principally along the extensor surface of the forearm and in the olecranon bursa. The appearance of rheumatoid nodules is an unfavorable prognostic sign, as is persistence of acute disease for more than 1 year, high serum titers of rheumatoid factor, and age under 20 at time of presentation.

Sustained joint inflammation lasting over a year leads to permanent erosion and loss of joint function. At first, the changes are partially reversible, but as cartilage and bone erode, the injury becomes permanent.

Clinical Manifestations

Hands and wrists. Characteristic hand deformities include ulnar deviation of the MCP joints, boutonniere deformities of the PIP joints, and swan-neck contractures of the fingers. In the wrists, there is often permanent loss of extension. A boggy, tender, dorsal wrist mass may result from tenosynovitis, and compression of the median nerve can occur. The subsequent *carpal tunnel syndrome* is usually reversible, but nerve damage is permanent by the time wasting of the thenar eminence is obvious.

Feet. Erosion of the metatarsal heads can lead to ventral subluxation. Increased weight-bearing on the inflamed heads and painful callus formation result. Erosive disease may be silent in the MTP joints.

Hips and knees. Involvement of these joints can be a source of much disability, because severe pain on weight bearing may result. Loss of internal rotation is the first change noted in the hip, followed by flexion contracture. One hip may predominate, even though the process is bilateral. In the knee, distention of the suprapatellar pouch by synovial effusion is common. If pressure rises rapidly, there can be herniation of the synovium with formation of a popliteal *Baker's cyst,* which can cause severe pain if it ruptures into the calf. Loss of full knee extension is followed by flexion contractures and gait difficulties.

Other joints. In the *elbow,* extension may be compromised, and olecranon bursitis is often present. *Shoulder* involvement presents as a subacromial or subdeltoid bursitis or as limitation of motion. Erosion of the rotator cuff leads to painful upward subluxation of the humeral head against the acromion. In the *cervical spine,* atlantoaxial subluxation is common, but usually asymptomatic. This development is potentially serious because it can lead to direct compression of the spinal cord or of the blood supply to the brain stem; fortunately, it is a rare event. When the *temporomandibular joint* is affected, there is pain on chewing or biting and difficulty in opening the mouth. *Avascular necrosis of the femoral head* and *vertebral osteoporosis* and collapse are usually a consequence of corticosteroid therapy.

Radiographic manifestations of early disease are soft tissue swelling around the joint and periarticular osteopenia. Relatively uniform narrowing of the joint space occurs as cartilage is destroyed. Periarticular subchondral erosion of bone is noted at the joint margin where pannus has developed. Finally, joint architecture is lost as the joint space is obliterated and erosion of subchondral bone progresses.

Extra-articular manifestations of rheumatoid arthritis develop mostly in patients with high titers of rheumatoid factor and persistent disease, so-called *sero-positive RA.* Pleural effusions with very low glucose concentrations and reduced complement can occur; there may or may not be accompanying pleuritic pain. Interstitial pulmonary changes, pulmonary nodules, and asymptomatic pericardial effusions are detected in some. Keratoconjunctivitis sicca (*Sjögren's syndrome*) has a strong association with RA, being found in up to 15% of patients. Splenomegaly is present in 5% to 10% of those with RA, and lymphadenopathy is not unusual. The combination of RA, splenomegaly, and neutropenia (*Felty's syndrome*) is noted in an occasional patient. Neutropenia may be severe, but the arthritis is often quiescent. Vasculitis is believed responsible for a number of systemic manifestations, including fever, mononeuritis multiplex, Raynaud's phenomenon, chronic leg ulcers, mucosal erosions of the gastrointestinal tract, focal ischemia of the digits, and necrotizing mesarteritis. The anemia of chronic disease is seen in a large percent of RA patients.

PROGNOSIS AND COURSE

It is difficult at the outset to predict the course of an individual case, although a high serum titer of rheumatoid factor, extra-articular manifestations, a large number of involved joints, age less than 30, and systemic symptoms all correlate with an unfavorable prognosis. Disease that remains persistently active for over a year is likely to lead to joint deformities and disability. Cases in which there are periods of activity lasting only weeks or a few months followed by spontaneous remission have a better prognosis. In one study, female sex and white race in patients under age 45 were associated with a somewhat less optimistic prognosis. Mortality for patients with RA is reported to be 2.5 times that of the general population. Infections and gastrointestinal problems are common, but mortality from cancer is unchanged.

Most published series on clinical course and prognosis are based on patients who were hospitalized or treated in arthritis centers, thus tending to overrepresent people with severe disease. A study of 200 such people followed for 9 years after discharge found 20.5% without significant disability, 41% moderately disabled, 27% severely crippled, and 11% dependent on others. This does not reflect the prognosis for the majority of rheumatoid arthritics treated exclusively as outpatients, many of whom carry a diagnosis of "probable" RA. Reviews suggest that over 50% of these patients remain fully employed after having disease for 10 to 15 years, with one-third having only intermittent low-grade disease, and another third experiencing spontaneous remission.

PRINCIPLES OF MANAGEMENT

The goals are to relieve stiffness and pain, preserve muscle strength and range of motion, and minimize progressive disability and deformity. There is no cure. A number of factors require consideration in design of a management program, including the patient's age, social and occupational responsibilities, emotional makeup, the activity and duration of disease, and results of prior therapies. A balanced, multifaceted approach to therapy is most likely to provide best results, because no single drug or treatment is by itself effective. The basic components of a program must include thorough patient education, adequate rest, proper exercise, and appropriate use of anti-inflammatory agents. Diet plays no role.

Nonpharmacologic Measures

Rest can be helpful, but in the patient with mild to moderate disease, complete bed rest is not only unnecessary but potentially harmful. Prolonged rest may lead to flexion contractures, osteoporosis, and muscle atrophy. Only the patient whose acute disease is severe enough to warrant hospitalization should be put to bed, in which case there is some benefit. However, a period of rest during the day can be of considerable benefit to less ill patients with persistently active disease, most of whom are usually bothered by fatigue.

Splinting. Selectively resting individual joints by splinting can help relieve pain and prevent contracture of severely inflamed joints. The principle is to maintain the joint in its physiologic position, especially during periods when the joint is stressed. Splinting of the wrist at night is the best example of this form of therapy. The patient with painful tenosynovitis of the wrist can be afforded a decrease in pain and prevention of flexion deformity with its attendant loss of grip. A wrist splint applied at night places the joint in 10° to 15° of extension. A cervical collar worn at night can provide similar relief when the cervical spine is involved. Deformed feet require specially constructed shoes.

Exercise helps to maintain range of motion and muscle strength. Again the goal is to minimize the chances of postinflammatory contractures. Exercises safely put involved joints through a full range of motion need to be taught to the patient. When pain is too severe for active exercises, isometrics can be performed, and passive exercises can be prescribed and carried out by a physical therapist. Prior application of *heat* or *cold* (either may work) will facilitate the exercise program. Hot baths, paraffin soaks, or ice packs are efficacious in loosening stiff joints for many patients. Moist heat is also useful in relieving pain and reducing the length of morning stiffness.

Exercises that utilize important muscle groups are prescribed in order to counteract the development of atrophy, strengthen periarticular tissues, and preserve joint stability. A judicious program of walking can play a similar role. Design and execution of an exercise program can be facilitated by the participation of a physical therapist. To protect the joint from damaging stress, the patient can be instructed in the use of implements that provide a mechanical advantage. Such "joint savers" are available commercially and are most helpful for tasks requiring use of the hands.

Pharmacologic Therapy

Anti-inflammatory Drugs. Agents in this category include aspirin and the other nonsteroidal anti-inflammatory drugs (NSAIDs). They provide pain relief by a nonspecific analgesic effect as well as by countering joint inflammation, but do not alter the course of RA.

ASPIRIN remains the cornerstone of pharmacologic therapy despite the much-promoted use of newer nonsteroidal anti-inflammatory drugs (NSAIDs). The drug remains the best proven and least expensive agent for treatment of RA. It decreases pain and lessens inflammation, although it has no effect on the course of the illness. The mechanism of action is believed related in part to the inhibition of prostaglandin synthesis. Serum levels of 15 to 20 mg per 100 ml are needed in adults under age 60 to effectively suppress the inflammation of rheumatoid arthritis. No standard dose predictably achieves this level, but usually at least 3.6 to 4.8 g per day are necessary.

The *dose* of aspirin can be increased to the point of tinnitus, which is a dependable sign of salicylate toxicity in adults. Temporary mild hearing loss also occurs, especially in the elderly, even at subtoxic doses. The most frequent adverse effects of aspirin are gastrointestinal. In an endoscopic study of 82 patients with RA receiving chronic aspirin therapy, 17% had gastric ulcers, 40% had erosions, and 76% had erythema of the gastric mucosa. One-third of patients with gastric ulcers had no symptoms. Frank bleeding occasionally occurs from gastritis or ulceration. Aspirin also inhibits platelet aggregation.

Many *preparations* of aspirin have been introduced with the hope of equaling regular aspirin's efficacy without causing its gastrointestinal side effects. Buffered aspirin does not appear to contain sufficient bicarbonate to prevent aspirin-induced gastric damage. In the endoscopic study just cited, the incidence of gastric ulceration among buffered aspirin users was 31%, compared to 23% for patients taking regular aspirin. Those who took enteric-coated aspirin had only a 6% incidence of ulceration (p < 0.005). Fasting salicylate levels were equal among all patients in the endoscopic study. However, the bioavailability of enteric-coated aspirin is delayed, resulting in slightly slower onset of pain relief when taken acutely.

OTHER SALICYLATES have been promoted. Choline salicylate (Arthropan) is less irritating to the stomach than regular aspirin, but also less effective and much more expensive. Several new salicylate tablets are being marketed, including magnesium salicylate, choline magnesium salicylate, and salsalate. There are insufficient data to determine whether these represent any improvement over aspirin.

NONSTEROIDAL ANTI-INFLAMMATORY DRUGS (NSAIDs) include ibuprofen, naproxen, fenoprofen, tolmetin, piroxicam, sulindac, and others. Many are derivatives of priopionic acid, and they act like aspirin to inhibit cyclo-oxygenase and impair prostaglandin synthesis; they also have analgesic properties. On a mg-per-mg basis, they are more potent than aspirin, permitting use of fewer tablets per day to achieve the same effect; however, efficacy does not significantly exceed that achieved by use of full aspirin doses (4.8 g per day). Although there is no available evidence that NSAIDs alter the course of disease, they do share with disease-modifying agents the ability to suppress production of IgM rheumatoid factor; this suggests the possibility of an immunoinhibitory effect.

Efficacy is a function of dose. In double-blinded, randomized cross-over study, there was no significant difference in efficacy among the six leading NSAIDs tested. Interestingly, patients had strong preferences for particular agents. This may be due to individual variation in the serum level attained by taking a given dose. In other comparison studies, differences in efficacy are usually a function of compliance with the drug regimen; patients using qd or bid agents often fare better than when using drugs requiring tid or qid dosing.

Side effects include gastrointestinal (GI) disturbances, prolongation of the bleeding time, mental confusion, and renal impairment. GI upset is the most frequently encountered of these, ranging from nausea or indigestion to frank bleeding from gastritis or peptic ulceration. Although the incidence of bleeding is less than that associated with plain aspirin, incidences of fatal gastrointestinal hemorrhage has been reported. Serious bleeding can occur with any one of these agents, as can peptic ulceration; risk of GI toxicity is particularly high with use of indomethacin. For most other NSAIDs, risk does not appear to correlate closely with dose, allowing increased dosage recommendations in recent years.

Hepatotoxicity is another important adverse effect; it resulted in the withdrawal of one agent (benoxaprofen). Cholestatic hepatitis has been reported with use of several other NSAIDs. Transaminase levels should be monitored, and the drug halted if levels rise above the upper limits of normal. Unlike aspirin, prolongation of the bleeding time is short-lived, because platelet cyclo-oxygenase inhibition quickly ceases with cessation of drug use.

Renal toxicity is believed related to impairment of renal prostaglandin synthesis (prostaglandins serve as important regulators of renal blood flow). Fluid retention and diminished sodium excretion are common with NSAID use. Prerenal azotemia, oliguria, and renal shutdown have been reported in patients with preexisting renal disease. Occasionally, control of hypertension will diminish with NSAID use. Risk of renal toxicity is greatest in the elderly, those with underlying cardiovascular or renal disease, and users of diuretics. Renal damage can ensue after only a few days of therapy, but is reversible with prompt cessation of use. Although there are reports that one agent (sulindac) may be slightly less nephrotoxic than others, most authorities feel all NSAIDs pose this risk, by virtue of their ability to inhibit prostaglandin

synthesis. Monitoring serum creatinine is advisable, especially in high-risk patients. No nephrotoxicity has been reported with prolonged, high-dose aspirin use.

The elderly are particularly susceptible to *alterations* in *cognitive function,* mood, and personality that sometimes accompany use of NSAIDs. Such neuropsychologic side effects are especially common with indomethacin. Confusion, poor memory, irritability, depression, lassitude, difficulty sleeping, and even paranoid behavior are among the reactions noted. Minor CNS effects, such as headache, dizziness, and lightheadedness are seen in patients of all ages.

Selection of an NSAID for use in RA requires some trial and error testing. Patients tend to respond best to one or two agents in particular; a 2-week trial at maximum dosage is the only way of determining the optimal agent for the individual patient. As noted earlier, response may be related to serum level attained, though at present serum level determinations are not available. Since frequency of side effects and efficacy are relatively similar, one can use cost and frequency of administration as bases for selection (see Table 153-1). *Aspirin* remains the least expensive but requires the greatest frequency of administration and most pills per day. Generic indomethacin is inexpensive, but frequency and severity of GI and CNS side effects limit its utility, especially in the elderly. *Generic ibuprofen* is the least expensive of the modern NSAIDs, but requires tid dosage. *Naproxen* is the least expensive of the bid formulations. Piroxicam offers once daily use, but is almost twice as expensive as naproxen and over 20 times the cost of aspirin.

Table 153-1. Nonsteroidal Anti-inflammatory Drugs

AGENT	STARTING DOSE FOR RA	RELATIVE COST
aspirin plain	900 mg qid	1.0
enteric coated		1.5
fenoprofen (Nalfon)	300 mg tid	11.5
ibuprofen (generic average)	400 mg tid	4.2
(Motrin)		7.4
indomethacin (generic aver.)	25 mg bid	5.2
(Indocin)		9.4
(Indocin SR)	75 mg qd	11.3
ketoprofen (Orudis)	50 mg tid	14.2
meclofenamate (Meclomen)	50 mg tid	17.5
naproxen (Naprosyn)	250 mg bid	13.4
piroxicam (Feldene)	10 mg bid or 20 mg qd	21.4
sulindac (Clinoril)	150 mg bid	16.0
tolmetin (Tolectin)	200 mg tid	11.8

(Adapted from Med Lett Drugs Ther 28:62, 1986)

Use of these agents is best reserved for patients unable to tolerate aspirin; sometimes they may be cautiously added to a program of aspirin therapy. Because their cost is high and they are not free of gastrointestinal side effects, they should not be used before a full trial of aspirin has been carried out, and salicylate levels in therapeutic range have been documented.

Disease-modifying Agents. For patients with active florid disease, NSAID therapy (which is mainly symptomatic) may not suffice. Symptoms persist and joint destruction may ensue. In an effort to slow progression and limit joint injury, disease-modifying agents (gold, d-penicillamine, hydroxychloroquine, and cytotoxic drugs) have been utilized. They appear to act by suppressing the immunologic response. These agents have no intrinsic anti-inflammatory or analgesic properties; as such they supplement rather than replace NSAID therapy. Although many of the studies on efficacy are marred by methodologic shortcomings, there is sufficient evidence that documents induction of partial clinical remission (complete remission is rare). Gold is among the most effective, demonstrating the ability to halt radiographically evident joint damage. These drugs are slow acting; clinical effect may not become evident until 3 to 6 months into therapy. Response rates of 50% are achieved within 3 to 6 months of initiating therapy, though many patients have to terminate treatment due to adverse drug effects. Serious toxicities include marrow suppression, nephropathy, and liver damage. Disease-modifying drugs can be used in conjunction with anti-inflammatory agents to provide a more comprehensive pharmacologic program to patients with severe active disease.

GOLD SALTS are used in patients with progressive erosive disease in an attempt to stop joint destruction. Gold is unique among drugs used to treat RA in that it has been shown to halt or even partially reverse articular erosion in up to 60% of cases, although the precise mechanism of action remains unknown. Decrease in inflammatory symptoms is noted in two-thirds of patients by the time the cumulative dose reaches 400 to 600 mg. Those who are going to respond do so by the time 1000 mg have been given. *Skin rashes* and buccal cavity mucosal ulcers represent minor adverse effects. Serious idiosyncratic reactions include *marrow suppression, glomerulonephritis, interstitial pneumonitis,* and *exfoliative dermatitis.* Consequently, treatment is begun slowly; each dose is preceded by urinalysis and complete blood and platelet counts. Gold is given intramuscularly by weekly injection using gold sodium thiomalate (Myochrysine) or aurothioglucose (Solganal). The former is sometimes associated with an immediate postinjection vasomotor reaction of warmth, erythema, and light-headedness.

Toxic reactions are not infrequent; the effects of gold are cumulative. If a skin rash occurs, the agent can be resumed at reduced doses following cessation for a few weeks to be sure a more generalized skin reaction does not set in. The first evidence of marrow suppression or nephropathy requires immediate cessation of therapy. Thrombocytopenia is reversible in early stages. Most patients who respond to gold are treated weekly until the cumulative dose reaches 1 gm; then administration is cut back to every other week until 1.5 gm is reached, at which point injections are given once a month. There are no clear indications as to when to stop therapy or how long to continue it.

AURANOFIN (RIDAURA), an oral gold formulation, has been developed. Its pharmacologic and immunologic actions are sufficiently different from those of parenteral gold to suggest that the drug is more than just another form of gold. Like parenteral gold, it retards disease progression. However, auranofin causes less renal and mucocutaneous toxicity than parenteral gold salts, but more diarrhea (which is dose-related) and other gastrointestinal reactions (*e.g.,* colitis). Often the GI side-effects cease with continued therapy, though a lowering of the dose may be necessary. Efficacy is less than that of injectable gold, but still significant in placebo-controlled studies. Auranofin's safety makes possible the consideration of gold therapy for severe early disease, even before erosive changes are noted. The combination of auranofin plus an NSAID may prove especially effective. Many studies on the use of auranofin are in progress. The literature should be followed for further data on safety and efficacy.

Auranofin is usually taken twice daily. It is safest to begin with a low-dose regimen for 6 months; if there is no response, a 3-month trial at higher dose is indicated before terminating therapy. The same hematologic, renal, and hepatic parameters as in parenteral therapy need to be monitored; testing is usually done on a monthly basis, more frequently if an abnormality arises.

PENICILLAMINE is another slow-acting drug used in RA patients with erosive disease; the agent may inhibit progression of joint destruction. In one study it retarded bony erosion. However, adverse effects are numerous and potentially serious; in one study, less than 30% of patients given the drug were able to continue with it for prolonged treatment. Fatal aplastic anemia, leukopenia, agranulocytosis, and thrombocytopenia can occur. Proteinuria is seen in 10% to 15% of patients, and may progress to the nephrotic syndrome. Rashes and autoimmune syndromes such as myasthenia gravis are reported. The drug should be reserved for those who fail to respond to aspirin and gold, and used only after consultation with a rheumatologist. It appears to be as effective as gold.

HYDROXYCHLOROQUINE can sometimes induce remissions; it is not as potent as gold or penicillamine. At least 4 to 6 weeks are needed before results are detectable. Use of hydroxychloroquine is reserved for chronic cases that lack active joint erosion but are uncontrolled by aspirin. Some rheumatologists recommend using the agent before resorting to gold because of its lower risk of adverse reactions. The major toxic effect is visual impairment (even blindness) due to drug accumulation in the retina. Although this complication is rare, its possibility limits dosage to 200 to 400 mg per day and makes regular ophthalmologic examinations advisable.

Immunosuppressive and Cytotoxic Drugs have been tried for treatment of refractory cases. Most controlled trials show only modest benefit, with no agents proving superior to gold, hydroxychloroquine, or penicillamine. Prolonged therapy with some agents in this class (*e.g., cyclophosphamide, azathioprine*) is associated with an increased risk of malignancy. However, a program of intermittent, low-dose, oral *methotrexate* seems promising and well tolerated; adverse effects include risk of irreversible hepatic injury and idiosyncratic pulmonary toxicity. Use of immunosuppressive/cytotoxic drug therapy should be reserved for patients with aggressive disease that fails to respond to other agents. Consultation with a rheumatologist familiar with its implementation is essential.

CORTICOSTEROIDS administered as a single *intra-articular injection* of a long-acting preparation may mean the difference between maintenance of daily activity and confinement, especially when a single large weight-bearing joint is inflamed. However, repeated steroid injections into the same joint may hasten its degeneration and increase the risk of infection. *Systemic* corticosteroids have a limited role in treatment because they cause osteoporosis, weaken joints by softening their ligamentous supports, and can produce aseptic necrosis of the femoral head. Moreover, their chronic use results in adrenal suppression and other important complications (see Chapter 103). The only clear-cut indication for systemic steroids is life-threatening extra-articular disease such as vasculitis, pericarditis, or alveolitis. Controversy surrounds systemic steroid use in patients with articular disease only. In extremely difficult situations, such as a flare-up of joint disease that threatens to totally disable the head of a household, some clinicians advocate a small nightly dose of 5 to 7.5 mg of prednisone to tide the patient over a difficult period.

Analgesics without anti-inflammatory effect have little role in RA. Occasionally a narcotic analgesic is resorted to for short-term pain control. Their regular use is to be avoided because of the risk of addiction in this chronic disease.

Total Lymphoid Irradiation and Apheresis

Total lymphoid irradiation and *apheresis* represent further attempts to inhibit the immunologic reaction. Uncontrolled studies of irradiation suggest some short-term benefit; long-term benefits and risks are unknown. The rationale behind plasmapheresis is to remove immune complexes and other mediators of the inflammatory process from the plasma. Placebo-controlled studies have failed to show significant benefit. Selective removal of lymphocytes from peripheral blood (*leukopheresis*) has yielded transient mild clinical improvement in refractory cases; there are no studies on long-term

effects. Irradiation and apheresis are unproven treatment modalities at the present time.

Surgery

Arthroplasty is an important component of therapy in patients with destroyed joints and marked disability. Hip and knee procedures are most successful; hand, wrist, elbow, and ankle reconstructions are less certain in outcome. There is a significant risk (25%) of a loosening of the hip prosthesis, even in the absence of active disease. Conventional surgical *synovectomy* is generally ineffective and results in loss of joint motion; however, arthroscopic synovectomy may permit control of particularly severe monoarticular disease involving the knee.

Unproven Modalities

A popular *diet* free of additives, preservatives, fruit, red meat, herbs and dairy products has been advocated as a treatment for RA. The only controlled, double-blind randomized study of this therapy failed to show any benefit in patients with long-standing, progressive active RA. *Biofeedback* is also without proven benefit, although it is helpful in patients with Raynaud's phenomenon. As noted earlier, exercise, rest, warm applications, and massage help maintain function, flexibility, and muscle strength.

Monitoring

Disease activity and response to therapy are monitored by reproducible measures such as duration of morning stiffness, sedimentation rate, number of tender swollen joints, strength of grip (measured with a blood pressure cuff), time needed to walk 15 meters, and ring size. The titer of rheumatoid factor does not correlate with disease activity, but does decrease with gold and penicillamine therapy if the patient responds.

The effective management of rheumatoid arthritis requires design and implementation of a comprehensive treatment program that is consistent with the patient's personality and fits well into his life-style and home environment.

PATIENT EDUCATION AND COUNSELLING

Telling the Diagnosis. For the patient with a potentially disabling disease such as RA, the act of telling the diagnosis takes on major importance. The goal is to satisfy the patient's informational needs regarding diagnosis, prognosis, and treatment without overwhelming him with an excessive amount of detail. This requires careful questioning and empathic listening to understand the patient's perspective, requests, and fears. Telling him more than he is intellectually or psychologically prepared to deal with (a common practice) risks making the experience so intense as to trigger withdrawal. On the other hand, failing to address issues of importance to the patient compromises the development of trust. The patient needs to know that the primary physician understands his situation and will be available for support, advice, and therapy as the situation arises. Encouraging the patient to ask questions helps to communicate interest and caring.

Discussing Prognosis and Treatment. Patients and family do best when they know what to expect and can view the illness realistically; uncertainty contributes heavily to the "disease" of RA. Many fear crippling consequences and dependency. The most common disease manifestations should be described; however, without building false hopes, the physician can point out that spontaneous remissions are frequent and that over two-thirds of patients live independently without major disability. In addition, it should be emphasized that much can be done to minimize discomfort and preserve function. A review of available therapies and their efficacy helps to overcome feelings of depression stemming from an erroneous expectation of inevitable disability. Guarded optimism is appropriate at the outset in all but the most actively aggressive situations. Even the patient with a poor prognosis (florid disease at the time of presentation, multijoint involvement) can derive comfort from knowing that he will be followed closely by his primary physician and any necessary consultants, all of whom are committed to maximizing his comfort and independence. A major fear is that of abandonment.

Dealing with Misconceptions. Several common misconceptions deserve attention. A substantial proportion of patients and their families feel guilty that they have done something to cause the illness. Explaining that there are no known controllable precipitants helps to eliminate much unnecessary guilt and self-recrimination. Another frequent misconception is the view that aspirin is too weak to work in a disease as severe as RA; when prescribed, patients may scoff at its use. Sometimes, physicians select a far more expensive, though no less effective NSAID instead of aspirin because they feel it is better for patient morale. Reviewing the difference between taking sporadic low doses of aspirin and near-toxic amounts often suffices to convince doubters and frees the physician to prescribe the most cost-effective therapy. The active participation of the patient and his family in the design and implementation of the therapeutic program helps to boost morale and ensure compliance, as does explaining the rationale for the therapies utilized.

Preserving a Sense of Self-worth. A major goal is to preserve the patient's sense of worth and independence. However, when fatigue, morning stiffness, or specific joint pathology interferes with the patient's capacity to perform usual work or home responsibilities, counselling will be necessary to recommend modification of work responsibilities and perhaps retraining. By utilizing occupational therapy, the treatment effort is geared to helping the patient maintain a meaningful work role within the limitations of his illness. The family plays an important part in striking the proper balance between dependence and independence. Its members need to be reminded to avoid overprotecting the patient (*e.g.,* a spouse might refrain from intercourse out of fear of hurting the patient) and to permit him to retain his sense of pride and ability to contribute to the family. Allowing the RA patient to struggle with a task is sometimes quite constructive.

Supporting the Patient with Debilitating Disease. Emphasis is on comfort measures (*e.g.,* an occasional hospitalization for rest and physical therapy) and supportive psychotherapy. Such individuals need help grieving for their disfigurement and loss of function. An accepting, unhurried, empathetic manner allows the patient to express his feelings. The seemingly insignificant act of touching does much to restore a sense of self-acceptance. Attending to pain with increased social support, medication, and a refocusing of attention onto function are useful. A trusting and strong patient–doctor relationship can do much to sustain a patient through times of discomfort and disability.

INDICATIONS FOR REFERRAL AND ADMISSION

The primary physician can usually provide for the continuous care of most patients with RA, even to the point of administering hydroxychloroquine or gold therapy. However, the occasional case that does not respond to maximal doses of aspirin or the newer nonsteroidal anti-inflammatory agents should be discussed with a rheumatologist before resorting to gold or hydroxychloroquine. Patients refractory to conventional therapy require referral to a rheumatologist for consideration of immunosuppressive therapy or penicillamine, as well as a general review of a patient's overall program.

Referral to a physical or an occupational therapist is basic to design of a good exercise program and should be made for every patient with active disease. Surgical referral is indicated for carpal tunnel syndrome that persists in spite of gold therapy and corticosteroid injection. Trigger finger deformity, tendon rupture with loss of manual dexterity, and refractory dorsal wrist effusions unresponsive after 6 months of therapy are also indications for surgery. Disabling hip or knee destruction with severe impairment of weight-bearing capacity deserves a surgical assessment regarding possible prosthetic joint replacement. Arthroscopic synovectomy may be needed for a single, very refractory joint that cannot be replaced.

When fever, floridly inflamed joints, severe pain, or marked extra-articular disease is present, hospital admission is an obvious requirement.

THERAPEUTIC RECOMMENDATIONS

- Aspirin is still the drug of first choice. It should be initiated in doses of at least 3 to 6 g per day, titrating the therapeutic response against the development of toxicity. Periodically check blood levels and adjust dose to maintain a therapeutic level of 15 to 20 mg per 100 ml in patients less than 60 years old.
- Use of a long-acting NSAID (*e.g.,* naproxen 375 mg) before bed can supplement aspirin therapy in patients bothered by severe morning stiffness.
- A lack of response, poor compliance, or intolerance to aspirin is a reasonable indication for trying one of the other nonsteroidal anti-inflammatory agents (see Table 153–1). When cost is an issue, ibuprofen is a reasonable agent to begin with. For convenience, naproxen is the least expensive of NSAIDs that allow bid administration.
- Since individual responses to the various NSAIDs are different, each should be tried separately for 2 weeks at maximum dose until a satisfactory drug is identified. Occasionally, aspirin and one of NSAIDS can be used together to permit a reduction in dose of aspirin if salicylate toxicity is a problem.
- Active erosive disease is an indication for initiating gold therapy. Such disease-modifying treatment is added to the ongoing program of anti-inflammatory therapy. Gold sodium thiomalate (Myochrysine) or aurothioglucose (Solganal) is started with a 10-mg intramuscular dose, followed by 25 mg the next week, and 50 mg weekly until definite improvement is observed or a cumulative dose of 1 gm of the salt is reached. Urinalysis and blood counts are monitored weekly. If no effect is observed after 20 weeks of therapy, gold therapy should be halted. Otherwise, injections every other week can be continued until 1.5 g is reached; then 50 mg per month is the maximal maintenance dosage.
- For less severe active disease, and perhaps for early severe disease before onset of erosion, the oral formulation auranofin is a reasonable consideration, since incidence of mucocutaneous and nephrotoxic reactions is lower than with parenteral gold. Starting dose is 3 mg bid or 6 mg once daily. GI upset is common; but if tolerated, the drug is continued for 6 months. If no response, then dose is increased to 3 mg tid for 3 more months of treatment. Biweekly monitoring of CBC, urinalysis, liver function tests, and platelet counts is needed in the first 3 months; later, monthly checks suffice.
- Patients with stubborn, nonerosive disease can be given hydroxychloroquine (maximum, 400 mg per day) for at least 8 weeks. Regular retinal examinations are required every 6 months if therapy is continued.
- Drug therapy should be initiated in conjunction with a program of daily range of motion and muscle-strengthening exercises and rest.
- Splinting may be applied, especially at night for the wrists, to support weakened joints and prevent flexion contractures.
- Heat can reduce pain and stiffness and is particularly helpful in the morning before the patient engages in activity.
- Penicillamine may be considered in refractory cases. Immunosuppressive therapy is investigational. For either, consultation with a rheumatologist is required.
- Intra-articular injection of a long-acting corticosteroid is indicated when a single refractory, inflamed joint prevents activity. An injectable suspension, such as triamcinolone acetonide 2.5 mg to 10 mg (depending on joint size) and a local anesthetic (*e.g.,* 1 ml lidocaine) is made up and injected into the joint space.
- Oral prednisone is reserved for only the most desperate situations. Short-term low-dose courses may suffice, such as 5.0 to 7.5 mg given in the evening.
- Psychologic support of the patient is essential, as is thorough instruction regarding the treatment program.

A.H.G.

ANNOTATED BIBLIOGRAPHY

Abruzzo JL: Auranofin: A new drug for rheumatoid arthritis. Ann Intern Med 105:275, 1986 (*An editorial summarizing indications and side effects; suggests an important role for the agent.*)

Altman RD, Gray R: Diagnostic and therapeutic uses of the arthroscope in rheumatoid arthritis and osteoarthritis. Am J Med 75:50, 1983 (*A useful review for the generalist on this important methodology.*)

Bardwick PA, Swezey RL: Physical therapies in arthritis. Postgrad Med 72:223, 1982 (*A discussion of the standard modalities of physical therapy and when to use them; notes ineffectiveness of biofeedback and electrical therapy.*)

Bombardier C, Vare J, Russell IJ et al: Auranofin therapy and quality of life in patients with rheumatoid arthritis. Am J Med 81:565, 1986 (*A multicenter trial documenting improvements in both synovitis and quality of life.*)

Clive DM, Stoff JS: Renal syndromes associated with nonsteroidal antiinflammatory drugs. N Engl J Med 310:563, 1984 (*Renal impairment emerges as one of the important adverse effects of NSAID use, especially in patients with underlying renal disease; a detailed review.*)

Coles LS, Fries JF, Kranines RG et al: From experiment to experience: Side effects of nonsteroidal anti-inflammatory drugs. Am J Med 74:820, 1983 (*An important paper for the clinician detailing the difference between reporting of side effects in clinical trials vs community use; their incidence is greater in community use than in clinical trials.*)

Decker JL, Malone DG, Haraoui B et al: Rheumatoid arthritis: Evolving concepts of pathogenesis and treatment. Ann Intern Med 101:810, 1984 (*An excellent review of disease mechanisms, with emphasis on immunologic issues.*)

Decker L: Apheresis and rheumatoid arthritis. Ann Intern Med 98:666, 1983 (*An editorial emphasizing the experimental nature of these therapies and the rather modest results obtained.*)

Dwosh IL, Giles AR, Ford PM et al: Plasmapheresis therapy in rheumatoid arthritis. N Engl J Med 308:1124, 1983 (*A double-blind, controlled, crossover trial showing no clinical benefit.*)

Epstein AM, Read JL, Winickoff R: Physician beliefs, attitudes and prescribing behavior for anti-inflammatory drugs. Am J Med 77: 313, 1984 (*Beliefs had little effect on prescribing behavior; attitudes did and helped to explain the very high frequency of prescribing proprietary non-steroidal agents in comparison to ASA.*)

Feigenbaum SL, Masi AT, Kaplan SB: Prognosis in rheumatoid arthritis. Am J Med 66:377, 1979 (*Identifies factors in 50 newly diagnosed patients under age 45 that seem to help predict outcome.*)

Fye KH: Conservative management of rheumatoid arthritis. West J Med 129:121, 1978 (*A good review emphasizing physical therapy and other nonsurgical aspects of care.*)

Iannuzzi L, Dawson N, Zein N et al: Does drug therapy slow radiographic deterioration in rheumatoid arthritis. N Engl J Med 309: 1023, 1983 (*A critical look at available studies on the efficacy of disease-modifying agents; finds that few studies are technically adequate to answer the question, though data supporting the efficacy of gold are among the best available.*)

Is all aspirin alike? *Med Lett, Drugs Ther,* 15:57, 1974 (*A succinct report on aspirin and its various forms.*)

Kaye RL, Hammand, AH: Understanding of rheumatoid arthritis—Evaluation of a patient education program. JAMA 239:2466, 1978 (*Evaluation of patient education, demonstrating behavioral changes; patients did not abuse joints as much, got more rest, and used medication more appropriately.*)

Lee P, Kennedy AC et al: Benefits of hospitalization in rheumatoid arthritis. Q J Med 170:265, 1974 (*A study of 30 indomethacin-treated patients showed moderate benefit from hospitalization.*)

Lipsky PE: Remission-inducing therapy in rheumatoid arthritis. Am J Med (supplement Oct 31):40, 1983 (*A useful review of this form of therapy; 129 references are included.*)

Masi AT: Articular patterns in the early course of rheumatoid arthritis. Am J Med 75:16, 1983 (*Patients with multijoint involvement at onset have a poorer prognosis than those with more limited disease.*)

Mills JA, Pinals RA, Ropes MW et al: Value of bed rest in patients with rheumatoid arthritis. N Engl J Med 284:453, 1971 (*Minimal benefit was obtained from enforced rest.*)

Pearson CM et al: Diagnosis and treatment of erosive rheumatoid arthritis and other forms of joint destruction. Ann Intern Med 82:241, 1975 (*A UCLA clinical case conference that emphasizes both medical and surgical therapy of destructive joint disease. It presents an excellent review of surgical procedures available for the rheumatoid patient.*)

Rogers MP, Liang MH, Partridge AJ: Psychological care of adults with rheumatoid arthritis. Ann Intern Med 96:344, 1982 (*An often overlooked area; many practical suggestions for effective personal care of both patient and family.*)

Silvoso GR, Ivey KJ, Butt JH et al: Incidence of gastric lesions in patients with rheumatic disease on chronic aspirin therapy. Ann Intern Med 91:517, 1979. (*An endoscopic study showing a high incidence of pathology; one-third of patients were asymptomatic. Provides uncontrolled data comparing various aspirin preparations.*)

Simon LS, Mills JA: Nonsteroidal anti-inflammatory drugs. N Engl J Med 302:1179, 1237, 1980 (*Reviews the pharmacology and role in therapy of nonsteroidal agents in comparison with aspirin.*)

Ward JR, Williams J, Egger MJ et al: Comparison of auranofin, gold sodium thiomalate, and placebo in the treatment of rheumatoid arthritis. Arthritis Rheum 26:1303, 1982 (*A placebo-controlled study showing both parenteral and oral therapy to be effective, with parenteral gold being the most effective, though also more likely to cause renal and mucocutaneous toxicity.*)

154
Management of Degenerative Joint Disease (Osteoarthritis)

Degenerative joint disease (DJD), the most prevalent arthropathy, is principally a consequence of aging. Prevalence is difficult to estimate; although 50% of adults show degenerative changes on x-ray, no more than 20% are symptomatic. However, DJD remains the most common cause of disability in the elderly. Because the condition is essentially irreversible, the goals of management are to provide relief from pain, minimize further damage to the involved joints, and keep the patient functioning independently.

PATHOPHYSIOLOGY AND CLINICAL PRESENTATION

Degenerative joint disease is characterized by degeneration of articular cartilage and reactive formation of new bone.

Unlike rheumatoid arthritis, the synovium plays only a secondary role. What causes the demise of the articular cartilage is incompletely understood. Available evidence suggests a combination of mechanical injury and age-related biochemical change such as an alteration in the glycosaminoglycan class of mucopolysaccharides. This change leads to a decrease in water content of cartilage. Fibrils become less resilient and more readily damaged by trauma; this change may allow penetration of synovial collagenases. It also appears that bone elasticity, which cushions normal trauma, is lost, allowing increased stress to be transmitted directly to the cartilage. Conditions that alter the mechanical relationships of joints—such as trauma, hypermobility, neuropathy, Paget's disease, and acromegaly—increase the likelihood that degenerative joint disease will develop.

Fissured hyaline cartilage is incapable of restoration. Eventually, the cartilage frays, shreds, and cracks. Underlying bone begins to be remodeled, with thickening of trabeculae; cyst formation is also seen. At the margins of the joint, hypertrophic spurs (osteophytes) eventually develop, followed by buttressing of adjacent cortical bone (osteosclerosis). The joint space narrows in an irregular fashion. There is little synovial reaction unless the degenerative process is very rapid, a piece of cartilage dislodges, or calcium pyrophosphate crystals form and incite an acute inflammatory response (pseudogout).

The patient with DJD typically complains of deep, aching joint pain that is aggravated by motion and weight bearing. In addition, there may be stiffness worsened by periods of inactivity. The involved joint can be enlarged due to osteophyte formation, but swelling is usually inconsequential, since soft tissue involvement and effusions are, in most instances, minimal. In later stages, pain occurs on motion and at rest in conjunction with stiffness. Nocturnal pain after vigorous activity is common. Patients with advanced disease suffer from pain on weight bearing and joint instability. Examination often reveals crepitus and discomfort on movement of the joint. Occasionally, slight warmth is noted in severely affected weight-bearing joints, but erythema and marked warmth are absent. Limitation of motion, malalignment, and bony protuberances from spurs are frequent findings.

The joints most commonly affected include the distal interphalangeal (DIP) joints of the hands, the carpometacarpal joint at the base of the thumb, the hips, the knees, and the cervical and lumbosacral spine.

DIP Joints. Disease in these joints is most common in middle-aged and elderly women, and sometimes proves to be quite painful and tender. A low-grade inflammatory response may accompany early rapid mucinous degenerative changes, giving the joint a tender, cystic inflammatory appearance. Later, osteophytes form, giving rise to the characteristic bony protuberances known as *Heberden's nodes.* All inflammatory activity resolves, leaving the joint nontender and with some limitation of motion. Occasionally, a similar process may affect the proximal interphalangeal joints, resulting in *Bouchard's nodes,* which may be mistaken for changes due to rheumatoid arthritis.

Thumbs. The base of the thumb, a site of much physical stress, is quite vulnerable to DJD. There is pain in the region of the thenar eminence and particularly over the carpometacarpal joint. Because the thumb is so important to manual dexterity, the development of arthritis at this site may be quite disabling. Grip becomes impaired and fine movements of apposition are restricted. Osteophytes are palpable and, in rare instances, may encroach upon the flexor tendon sheath, causing tenosynovitis.

Hips. Degenerative hip disease arises in young patients with congenital dislocations or slipped femoral capital epiphyses, and much later from wear and tear in the elderly. Unilateral or asymmetrical distribution is typical. Pain is reported deep in the hip, radiating into the anterior medial thigh, groin, or buttock. The site of radiation may be the only area of discomfort. At first, pain occurs only on weight bearing, but as DJD progresses, discomfort may become continuous and especially unbearable at night. Sexual intercourse is sometimes compromised. Loss of internal rotation during flexion is the earliest change and is as reliable as x-ray for diagnosis. The Trendelenburg test (see Chapter 148) is positive.

Knees. DJD of the knee produces pain that is localized to the joint and worsened by weight bearing. Crepitus is often marked, and range of motion reduced. A very small effusion may be noted. The joint appears enlarged and feels bony. On occasion there maybe very few physical findings, even though pain and x-ray changes are prominent.

Cervical Spine. DJD commonly involves the lower cervical spine (see Chapter 146). Although x-ray changes are frequent, most individuals are asymptomatic. Moreover, the correlation between symptoms and x-ray findings is often poor. The patient may complain of pain and stiffness in the neck, but sometimes only pain in the occiput, shoulder, arm, or hand is reported. In a few instances, scapular or upper anterior chest pain is produced. Osteophytes can protrude into the spinal foramina and impinge upon nerve roots, causing pain that radiates into the shoulder, upper arms, hands, and fingers (brachial neuralgia). At night, the patient may awaken with paresthesias and numbness is the arms that improve upon getting up and shaking them.

On examination, neck motion is restricted to some extent in all directions, and movement reproduces or aggravates symptoms. Reactive muscle spasm and tenderness are often present, and decreased sensation, weakness, and diminished reflexes occur when root compression is marked. However, even when symptoms of root compression are reported, neurologic findings may be scant and their absence does not rule out the complication.

Lumbosacral Spine. Degenerative changes in the lumbosacral spine involve the intervertebral discs and the apophyseal joints. With aging, the disc nucleus becomes brittle and less elastic. Herniation posteriorly or laterally through a defect in the disc annulus may occur and cause nerve root compression (see Chapter 145). Intervertebral spaces narrow and marginal osteophytes form. The apophyseal joints show typical secondary degenerative changes. The patient reports pain across the lower back with radiation into the buttock and posterior thigh, or down into the lower leg if root compression has occurred (see Chapter 145). Foreward flexion and extension are reduced, but lateral flexion is painless. Focal areas of tenderness are common and often due to spasm of the paraspinous musculature.

Other Sites. DJD may involve the great toe at the metatarsophalangeal joint, causing bony enlargement and a valgus deformity. Crepitus and pain in the temporomandibular joint are sometimes seen secondary to bruxism (grinding of the teeth because of anxiety or anger). Pain is reproduced by opening the mouth widely. Since DJD is not a systemic disease, there are no extra-articular manifestations nor any serum abnormalities; the sedimentation rate is normal, as is the synovial fluid in early disease. Radiographic findings are limited to the joints and include irregular narrowing of the joint space, sclerosis of subchondral bone, bony cysts, marginal osteophytes, and buttressing of adjacent bone.

COURSE

Degenerative joint disease is often progressive over months to years; significant disability may ensue, related to pain and restriction of motion. However, clinical remissions do occur, especially in the hands, neck, and back. It is important to note that progression is typically limited to a few affected joints and does not become widespread. A study of the natural history of untreated DJD of the knee in 71 patients found it to be especially progressive; the majority of patients ended up with pain at rest. Early onset of symptoms and varus deformity correlated with poor prognosis. Pain at rest and inability to use public transportation occurred over a period of 10 to 18 years. DJD of the hip also follows a relentless course. In most cases of DJD, symptoms in weight-bearing joints are exacerbated by obesity.

PRINCIPLES OF MANAGEMENT

There is no cure for osteoarthritis, but it helps to reduce stress imposed on the joint, maintain normal alignment, and treat pain and muscle spasm. Surgical intervention should be restricted to patients who do not respond to conservative management and are so disabled that they cannot function satisfactorily.

Rest. Some relief can be attained by partially resting the involved joint; this helps to reduce the stress imposed on it. Joint rest should be alternated with exercise; prolonged immobility greatly disturbs cartilage metabolism. A *cervical collar* can ease neck pain by supporting the spine and resting the paraspinous musculature. It may be necessary to continue use intermittently for many weeks before significant benefit is achieved. Cervical traction may also help (see Chapter 146). A *corset* or *brace* for the back may be similarly helpful.

Limiting the amount of walking a patient does will lessen stress on a weight-bearing joint, but can be counterproductive

because stiffness, muscle atrophy, and osteoporosis are accelerated, and the patient becomes demoralized from loss of independence and function. However, some relief can be provided without immobilization if the patient uses a walking cane, walker, or even forearm crutches. The cane is held on the side opposite the painful joint. Unnecessary strain such as stair climbing should be reduced. Bed rest is essential for relief of back pain (see Chapter 145) due to disc disease and facet joint arthritis.

Exercises. Strengthening the supporting muscles may help maintain proper joint alignment. Quadriceps exercises are among the simplest; they can be performed while sitting in a chair by extending the knee and holding the straightened leg horizontal. Isometric and active exercises for the neck improve muscle tone and may sometimes help in cases of painful cervical spine disease. Exercises for the abdominal and paraspinous musculature are useful for preventing back problems (see Chapter 145). Gentle walking, cycling, and swimming will improve the muscle groups of the hips and knees and provide considerable psychologic benefit. There is no evidence that manipulation is of any use. Excessive exercise may only exacerbate pain and cause further disruption of the joint.

Heat. Moist heat can give symptomatic relief from muscle spasm, though it has no effect on the disease itself. Diathermy and ultrasound units are expensive ways to delivering heat to deep-lying tissues. More than five or six treatments are unnecessary, though some patients derive considerable psychologic benefit and a sense of well-being from them.

Drugs. The progression of disease cannot be halted by available drugs, but they can offer symptomatic relief. Anti-inflammatory agents are used. Their effect is probably due as much to their analgesic properties as to their impact on inflammation, because the inflammatory component of DJD is usually a low-grade one. Since DJD is a chronic disease, any drug selected for use should be inexpensive and safe for long-term consumption. Narcotic analgesics should be used sparingly, and only for acute disabling pain. An individual's response to drugs is unpredictable, and it may be necessary to try several different agents. Intermittent use of drugs will sometimes suffice.

Because of its low cost, relatively low toxicity, and documented efficacy, *aspirin* remains an excellent first choice. It need not be given in the large doses needed in rheumatoid arthritis to suppress inflammation, but patients usually require 1.8 to 3.6 g per day. Sustained therapy is superior to intermittent use. Acetaminophen is an acceptable alternative for patients who do not tolerate aspirin; some patients find that they achieve quite acceptable pain relief with use of the drug.

The nonsteroidal, anti-inflammatory drugs (NSAIDs) such as *ibuprofen* (Motrin), *naproxen,* and a host of others (see Chapter 153) are quite helpful in patients who need more than aspirin or acetaminophen. Their disadvantages include high cost (as much as 30 times that of aspirin) and the risks of GI upset, nephrotoxicity, and CNS effects; the latter two are particularly common in the elderly (see Chapter 153). Like aspirin, the NSAIDs have both analgesic and anti-inflammatory effects; the degree of analgesia provided approximates that of equivalent doses of aspirin. NSAID doses for use in DJD are generally lower than those needed for inflammatory joint disease. However, their anti-inflammatory action may, in part, be responsible for some of their beneficial effect. The newer NSAIDs have obviated the need to rely on long-term use of *indomethacin,* which, although quite effective (especially for hip pain), has greater toxicity. *Phenylbutazone* and *oxyphenbutazone* are no longer recommended for use because of their high risk of marrow suppression and the availability of equally effective, safer drugs.

Antispasmodics are without effect, except for their tranquilizing action. Strong, potentially addicting *analgesics* such as *codeine* have a limited role, providing temporary relief for severe disabling disease when circumstances make it essential that the patient remain active. Obviously, prolonged use is contraindicated. *Propoxyphene* (Darvon) is taken by many patients with DJD, but its potential for dependence is considerable—similar to that of codeine—and its analgesic properties are no greater than low doses of aspirin.

The use of *intra-articular steroids* is controversial. Although widely utilized, there are no controlled studies documenting their efficacy. Moreover, repeated injections may accelerate degeneration of the joint. Thus the only time steroid injection should be considered is when there is a single disabling joint, refractory to other forms of therapy, and sufficiently inflamed to justify a trial of intra-articular steroids. *Acupuncture* has produced inconsistent results in double-blind studies, sometimes working, sometimes not. Results have not been sufficiently beneficial to warrant its inclusion in a treatment program.

INDICATIONS FOR REFERRAL

Physical and occupational therapists can be very helpful to patients with DJD in terms of teaching exercises, giving suggestions on performing the tasks of daily living, and providing psychologic support. A referral is indicated for most patients whose DJD interferes with their lives.

Surgical therapy, such as osteotomy, arthroplasty, removal of loose bodies, or joint replacement, deserves consideration in significantly disabled patients. Replacement of hip and knee joints has been particularly successful. Performing tibial or femoral osteotomy can produce long-term benefit by realigning weight-bearing stresses. The decision to refer for surgery must be made with an understanding of the risks involved and the need to undertake a vigorous postoperative exercise program. Surgery should be considered only in pa-

tients whose limitation of motion or pain has become so severe that it prevents them from living productively, and whose medical and emotional state make them reasonable candidates for the rehabilitative effort. They must be healthy enough to tolerate surgery and sufficiently motivated to carry out the exercise program needed to ensure full rehabilitation.

PATIENT EDUCATION

Patients need to know that DJD is not reversible; however, they should also be aware that pain can often be lessened and overall functioning preserved. Degenerative disease is not a generalized, systemic illness that produces crippling involvement of most joints. Moreover, those with cervical or lumbosacral disease can be given some hope for a spontaneous remission of severe pain. The need to reduce weight and strengthen supporting muscles should be stressed, as well as the importance of avoiding unnecessarily strenuous activity and addicting analgesics. Surgical options should be discussed with patients who have disabling disease of the hips or knees.

The physician's concern and support are essential to the successful management of any chronic disease, and especially one like DJD, in which the patient's response to the illness has much to do with its effect on his life. Return visits should be scheduled as frequently as needed to provide psychologic support. A strong doctor-patient relationship helps many patients to tolerate the disease and remain active.

THERAPEUTIC RECOMMENDATIONS

- Patients with disease of the hips or knees should be instructed to reduce excess weight, exercise regularly to strengthen quadriceps and hip muscles, and avoid excessive stress on these joints (*e.g.,* stair climbing). Gentle walking, swimming, or stationary cycling can be prescribed. Isometric exercises and use of a cane or crutches for reduction of weight bearing are preferred when severe pain limits joint motion. Absolute rest is inadvisable.
- Those with back pain should be instructed to obtain bed rest followed by exercises to strengthen supporting musculature (see Chapter 145). A corset or brace may help.
- Those with cervical pain can be given a soft cervical collar for support. It should be worn at all times, including during the night. Four weeks or more of use may be necessary. Cervical traction is also helpful (see Chapter 146).
- Drug therapy for reduction of pain should be instituted with aspirin, 1.8 to 3.6 g per day, given on a continuous basis at first. Acetaminophen may be tried in patients who are intolerant to aspirin, but a nonsteroidal anti-inflammatory drug (*e.g.,* ibuprofen 400 mg tid to qid or naproxen 250 to 375 mg bid) may be more effective.
- In general, use of narcotics should be avoided, because most pain is chronic. However, for an acute disabling exacerbation unrelieved by maximal doses of NSAID therapy, a

short course of an agent such as codeine sulfate (30 to 60 mg every 6 to 8 hours) may reduce pain sufficiently to allow the patient to function or sleep. Acupuncture has not proven sufficiently beneficial to recommend its use. Intra-articular injection of a corticosteroid is controversial, but may be considered if there is an inflammatory component to the arthritis and only a single joint is involved. Repeat injections exacerbate joint degeneration and are to be avoided.

- Referral for a surgical opinion should be restricted to the well-motivated patient who can tolerate major surgery and has refractory disease of a major weight-bearing joint that significantly interferes with lifestyle and ability to function satisfactorily.

A.H.G.

ANNOTATED BIBLIOGRAPHY

Dieppe PA, Sathapatayavong S, Jones HE et al: Intraarticular steroids in osteoarthritis. Rheum Rehab 19:212, 1980 (*A discussion of this controversial therapy.*)

Feinstein PA, Haberman ET: Selecting and preparing patients for total hip replacement. Geriatrics 32:91, July, 1977 (*A straightforward guide for the primary physician about total hip replacement.*)

Gaw AC, Chang LW, Shaw LC: Efficacy of acupuncture on osteoarthritic pain. N Engl J Med 293:375, 1975 (*A double-blind controlled study showing inconsistent results.*)

Greenfield S, Solomon NE, Brook RH et al: Development of outcome criterion and standards to assess the quality of care for patients with osteoarthrosis. J Chron Dis 31:375, 1978 (*An article that reviews the epidemiology of osteoarthritis, emphasizing the difficulty of assessing the efficacy of medical care for people with this disease.*)

Gresham GE, Rathey UK: Osteoarthritis in knees of aged persons: Relationship between roentgenographic and clinical manifestations. JAMA 233:168, 1975 (*A study showing that crepitus, decreased range of motion, pain, bone enlargement, and instability are more common in abnormal knees.*)

Hernborg JS, Nilsson BE: The natural course of untreated osteoarthritis of the knee. Clin Orthop 123:130, 1977 (*A study of 94 joints in 71 patients showing a generally unfavorable prognosis, with pain developing at rest in the majority of patients.*)

Huskinsson EC: The drug treatment of osteoarthritis. Scand J Rheumatol 43(suppl):57, 1982 (*A good review for the generalist.*)

Lawrence JS, Bremner JM, Bier F: Osteoarthrosis prevalence in the population and relationship between symptoms and x-ray changes. Ann Rheum Dis 25:1, 1966 (*A prevalence of minimal disease in 50% and more significant disease in 20%. Radiographic changes were associated with symptoms in all joints but the lumbar spine.*)

Leach RE, Baumgard S, Broom J: Obesity: Its relationship to osteoarthritis. Clin Orthop 93:271, 1973 (*Documents the increased risk of DJD involving weight-bearing joints in obese patients.*)

Mankin HJ: The reaction of articular cartilage to injury and osteoarthritis. N Engl J Med 291:1285, 1974 (*A good review of the biochemistry of cartilaginous change.*)

Solomon L: Patterns of osteoarthritis of the hip. J Bone Joint Surg 58:176, 1975 (*A detailed clinical and pathologic study of 327 cases of osteoarthritis that revealed normal cartilage failing under normal conditions as well as break-up of articular cartilage due to defective subchondral bone.*)

155
Management of Gout

Gout is among the most common causes of acute monoarticular arthritis (see Chapter 143). Estimates of prevalence in the United States range from 0.3% to 2.8% of the population; the condition is predominantly a disease of adult men. Inborn errors in purine metabolism and abnormalities in uric acid excretion (see Chapter 152) account for most cases of primary gout. The expanded use of agents that decrease uric acid excretion (*e.g.,* thiazide diuretics) has markedly increased the incidence of secondary gout. In the Framingham study, almost half of new cases were associated with thiazide use.

The primary physician should be able to promptly diagnose and treat acute gout, prevent recurrences, and minimize the chances of complications such as chronic gouty arthritis and nephrolithiasis.

PATHOPHYSIOLOGY AND CLINICAL PRESENTATION

Acute gout usually occurs after many years of sustained asymptomatic hyperuricemia. The greater the uric acid concentration, the greater the risk of an acute attack. The mean duration of the asymptomatic period is about 30 years. During this time there may be deposition of urate in synovial lining cells and possibly in cartilage as well. Acute gout develops when uric acid crystals collect in the synovial fluid as a result of precipitation from a supersaturated state or release from the synovium. Trauma, decline in temperature, fall in pH, dehydration, starvation, alcoholic binge, emotional or physical stress, and rapid change in serum uric acid concentration have all been implicated in the process. The pathogenesis of the inflammatory response appears to involve phagocytosis of crystals by leukocytes in the synovial fluid, disruption of lysosomes, release of enzymatic products, activation of the complement and kallikrein systems, and release of leukocyte chemotactic factor.

The typical attack of *acute gouty arthritis* is monoarticular and abrupt in onset, often occurring at night. Symptoms and signs of inflammation become maximal within a few hours of onset and last for a few days to a few weeks. Recovery is complete. The initial attack usually involves a joint of the lower extremity; in about half of patients the first metatarsophalangeal joint is the site of inflammation (podagra). The tarsal joint (located at the instep), ankle, and knee are other common sites of initial attacks. Later episodes may involve a joint of the upper extremity, such as the wrist, elbow, or finger; shoulder or hip involvement is rare. Over 80% of attacks occur in the lower extremity; 85% of patients have at least one episode of podagra. About 5% of acute gouty episodes are polyarticular. Some patients are normouricemic at the time of an acute attack.

The joint appears swollen and erythematous; periarticular involvement is also common. There may be a low-grade fever. During resolution, the skin overlying the affected joint often desquamates. The clinical presentation may simulate joint infection (see Chapter 143) or even cellulitis (see Chapter 188).

Interval gout follows the initial attack. There is an asymptomatic period that generally lasts for several years before a second episode of acute gout takes place. The original joint or another joint may be involved in subsequent attacks. Over time, the asymptomatic intervals between acute episodes shorten. In more advanced disease, polyarticular attacks are not uncommon, and resolution may be slower and less complete.

Chronic gouty arthritis (tophaceous gout) takes years to develop. Tophi are noted an average of 10 years after the initial attack of acute gout. The risk of chronic gout is a function of duration and severity of hyperuricemia. Tophi represent sodium urate collections surrounded by foreign body giant cell inflammatory reactions. They can occur in a variety of sites, including the synovium, subchondral bone, olecranon bursa, Achilles tendon, and subcutaneous tissue of the extensor surfaces of the arm. Eventually cartilage erodes, joints become deformed, and chronic arthritis ensues. The joints of the lower extremities and hands are most commonly affected. The process is insidious; the patient notes progressive aching and stiffness. Tumescences may develop over joints of the foot and cause difficulty with wearing shoes. Fortunately, the incidence of tophaceous gout has declined markedly with the introduction of effective antihyperuricemic agents. At present, less than 15% of patients with acute gout develop chronic gouty arthritis.

The incidence of *nephrolithiasis* among patients with clinical gout is small. In a prospective study from the Kaiser-Permanente system, the risk of new stone formation in a patient with new onset of gout was less than 1% per year. The probability of stone formation was unrelated to initial serum urate concentration or degree of uric acid control. The mean interval between onset of gout and passage of a stone was 5.5 years. Factors other than serum urate concentration are important to stone formation, and include family history of stone formation, urine pH, hydration status, and possibly the amount of renal uric acid excretion. Stone formation is rarely life-threatening, as demonstrated by one large 7-year study, in which only 1 of 1700 patients with gout developed obstructive uropathy due to urate lithiasis.

Chronic renal failure used to be viewed as a potential complication of long-standing hyperuricemia; however, recent data do not support this view. Data from controlled, long-term, prospective study of the question showed that azotemia was infrequent and, when it did occur, was clinically insignificant during the 10-year follow-up period. Projections based on this data indicate that there is no significant risk of clinically important azotemia until the serum uric acid reaches 13 mg per 100 ml in men and 10 mg per 100 ml in women *and* is sustained for 40 years. Most of the renal disease in gouty patients is fully attributable to concurrent hypertension, diabetes, cardiovascular disease, or underlying primary renal pathology. One study suggests lead toxicity may be a precipitant (see Chapter 152).

Acute renal failure can occur from the sudden extreme uric acid load that is produced in the early stages of treatment for lymphoproliferative and myeloproliferative diseases. Uric acid may precipitate in renal tubules and elsewhere in the urinary tract, leading to acute oliguria.

PRINCIPLES OF THERAPY

Acute Gouty Arthritis. Acute symptoms can be relieved by any one of a number of *anti-inflammatory drugs,* including colchicine, indomethacin, or one of the newer nonsteroidal agents such as ibuprofen or naproxen. Of these drugs, the newer nonsteroidals are better tolerated than colchicine or indomethacin.

Without treatment, an acute attack of gout usually resolves within 7 to 10 days, though severe episodes can last for weeks. Initiation of treatment with an anti-inflammatory agent at the very first sign of an acute attack produces a prompt and excellent therapeutic response. Delay of therapy is associated with less dramatic results. Symptomatic treatment is usually continued until symptoms have resolved.

Interval Gout. Although prophylactic therapy to prevent acute gouty arthritis is not necessary or cost-effective for patients with asymptomatic hyperuricemia (see Chapter 152), it may be worthwhile in patients who have had several attacks of acute gout, because the intervals between future recurrences are likely to shorten.

Colchicine is highly effective for prophylaxis and is commonly given for 3 to 6 months in conjunction with an agent that lowers the serum uric acid. Initiation of antihyperuricemic therapy without colchicine prophylaxis can precipitate an attack of acute gout. There are no definitive data on the ideal duration of colchicine therapy, but most authorities recommend that it be given for up to 6 months. Cost is minimal; a once-a-day dose suffices. Serious side effects associated with long-term colchicine use are rare, but include agranulocytosis, aplastic anemia, and myopathy. Consequently, prolonged colchicine use is to be avoided.

Antihyperuricemic agents are indicated in patients with repeated episodes of acute gout, because the risk of an attack is in part related to the degree of hyperuricemia. *Allopurinol* is currently the agent most widely used to lower the uric acid. It inhibits the enzyme xanthine oxidase and thus blocks the formation of uric acid. The half-life of allopurinol is about 3 hours, but its metabolites are biologically active for up to 30 hours. As a result, the drug can be given once daily. Serum urate levels fall within a week of initiating therapy. Toxic reactions are rare; rash is the most common side effect, and hepatocellular injury occasionally occurs in patients with renal failure. Reduction of dose is essential in the setting of renal insufficiency because of the risk of a fulminant toxicity syndrome (rash, fever, hepatitis, eosinophilia, and worsening renal failure). The drug is expensive. Colchicine is required during the initial phases of therapy. Allopurinol has no effect on acute gouty arthritis. Starting allopurinol within several weeks of an acute attack can precipitate a flare; initiation of therapy should be delayed under such circumstance.

A *uricosuric agent* is a reasonable alternative to allopurinol therapy as long as the patient does not demonstrate nephrolithiasis or hyperexcretion of uric acid (greater than 500 mg per 24 hours). *Probenecid* and *sulfinpyrazone* are the most commonly used uricosuric drugs. They work by blocking tubular reabsorption of uric acid. These agents are being used with less frequency because of the efficacy and safety of allopurinol, and their risk of precipitating nephrolithiasis. Moreover, at the onset of therapy, the uric acid excretion may reach extraordinary levels; consequently, it is essential that fluid intake be generous (2 to 3 liters per day) to minimize the chances of uric acid precipitation. Alkalinization of the urine to a pH of 6.6 is desirable but difficult to achieve. Colchicine is needed concurrently with uricosuric treatment to prevent an acute attack of gout.

The uricosuric action of probenecid and sulfinpyrazone is blocked by thiazides and low doses of salicylates; moreover, patients with renal failure do not respond to these drugs.

Dietary factors have received much attention, though only 10% of circulating purine is derived from dietary sources. Consequently, there is no need to restrict purine intake. However, reduction of excess weight (without fasting) and abstinence from excessive alcohol intake and binge drinking can help prevent future attacks.

Chronic Gouty Arthritis. Prevention or lessening of chronic tophaceous gout can be achieved by lowering the serum urate level to normal. Allopurinol is the drug of choice for patients with tophaceous gout. Tophi may begin to resolve after several weeks of therapy. Again, colchicine must be given concurrently because mobilization of urate deposits may trigger an acute attack. A uricosuric agent is a reasonable

alternative as long as there are no contraindications to its use, such as nephrolithiasis or excess uric acid excretion.

Nephrolithiasis. The patient with an established uric acid stone should be given allopurinol and instructed to keep well hydrated (see Chapter 134). Antihyperuricemic therapy for prevention of stone formation is indicated in gouty patients with a history of nephrolithiasis, a family history of kidney stones and, perhaps, extraordinary degrees of uric acid excretion (*i.e.,* greater than 1100 mg per 24 hours on a routine diet) (see Chapter 152). All patients should be instructed to avoid even temporary dehydration, especially if they live in warm dry climates.

Renal Failure. Gouty patients who drink moonshine or have an occupational exposure to lead should have their lead intake cut back drastically, since lead may lead to kidney damage. Lead has been implicated as one link between gout and chronic renal impairment. There is no proven renal benefit to lowering the serum or urinary uric acid, except in patients at risk for acute gouty nephropathy (see Chapter 83).

PATIENT EDUCATION

The importance of weight control (see Chapter 229), avoidance of excessive ethanol intake (see Chapter 224), and maintenance of good hydration need to be stressed. On the other hand, patients will often find it comforting to know that severe dietary restrictions are unnecessary. Fasting should be prohibited, since it might precipitate an acute episode of gout. Patients must be instructed to take their anti-inflammatory agent at the earliest sign of an attack.

THERAPEUTIC RECOMMENDATIONS

- At the first sign of an attack of acute gouty arthritis, a non-steroidal anti-inflammatory agent (*e.g.,* naproxen 500 mg bid) should be started; therapy is continued until symptoms resolve, and then tapered over 72 hours. Relief is usually prompt and effective. Delay in initiating therapy is associated with less dramatic results.

- Refractory cases of definite acute gout can be treated with intra-articular or systemic corticosteroids.

- For interval gout, when recurrences of acute attacks are becoming increasingly frequent, begin antihyperuricemic therapy using allopurinol (300 mg once daily) or a uricosuric agent (*e.g.,* probenecid 500 mg 1 or 2 times daily). Colchicine (0.6 mg/day) should be started at the time of antihyperuricemic therapy and continued for 3 to 6 months to prevent acute gout due to mobilization of urate deposits. Antihyperuricemic therapy helps prevent chronic gout and reduces the number of acute gouty attacks.

- Patients with renal insufficiency who take allopurinol are at risk for a serious toxicity syndrome and should have their allopurinol dose adjusted in proportion to the decrease in creatinine clearance.

- If a uricosuric agent is used, therapy should be initiated utilizing small doses (*e.g.,* 500 mg per day of probenecid) in conjunction with large volumes of fluid (2 to 3 liters per day) to prevent precipitation of uric acid in the urinary tract. Alkalinization of the urine to a pH of 6.6 is desirable during the first week of therapy, but is difficult to achieve; gram doses of sodium bicarbonate are required, supplemented by acetazolamide (250 mg) before bed.
- For chronic gout, allopurinol is the treatment of choice; again, colchicine is required during the first 6 months of therapy.
- Patients need to be instructed to take their anti-inflammatory agent at the first sign of an acute attack. An extra supply should be given for future episodes.
- Gradual reduction to ideal weight, decrease in alcohol intake, and avoidance of dehydration, binge drinking, and low-dose aspirin also need to be reviewed with the patient. Fasting should be discouraged, since it might precipitate an attack.
- Patients with clinical gout who require thiazide therapy should probably receive allopurinol. Asymptomatic patients with mild hyperuricemia on thiazide therapy do not need allopurinol (see Chapter 152).
- Gouty patients with exposure to lead ("moonshine" use, industrial contact) should be advised to greatly reduce their intake or exposure; there is risk of renal impairment.
- Hyperuricemia *per se* is not a risk for renal failure. No treatment is required.
- For gouty patients with urate nephrolithiasis, a strong family history of kidney stones, or marked uric acid excretion (greater than 1100 mg per 24 hours), allopurinol (300 mg once daily) and hydration are indicated. Long-term efforts to alkalinize the urine are impractical and need not be attempted.

A.H.G.

ANNOTATED BIBLIOGRAPHY

Bautman V, Maesaka JK, Haddad B et al: The role of lead in gouty nephropathy. N Engl J Med 304:520, 1981 (*A strong relationship was found between lead excretion during EDTA testing and serum creatinine.*)

Burger LU, Yu TF: Renal function in gout—An analysis of 524 gouty subjects including long-term follow-up studies. Am J Med 59:604, 1975 (*Follow-up for 12 years showed that hyperuricemia alone had no deleterious effect on renal function in ambulatory patients with gout.*)

Fessel JW: Renal outcomes of gout and hyperuricemia. Am J Med 67:74, 1979 (*A carefully done prospective study showing that the risks of renal failure and stone formation are very small and hardly justify prophylactic therapy.*)

Graham R, Scott JT: Clinical survey of 354 patients with gout. Ann Rheum Dis 29:461, 1976 (*An extensive epidemiologic review.*)

Hall AP, Berry PE, Dawber TR et al: Epidemiology of gout and hyperuricemia—A long-term population study. Am J Med 42:27, 1967 (*The Framingham study; 14% of patients with uric acids of 7 to 7.9 mg, 19% with uric serum urates between 8 and 8.9, and 5 out of 6 patients with uric acids over 9 developed gouty attacks.*)

Hande KR, Noone RM, Stone WJ: Severe allopurinol toxicity. Am J Med 76:47, 1984 (*A review of 78 cases; occurs in patients with renal insufficiency; requires dose reduction.*)

Maclaughlan MJ, Rodnan GP: Effects of food, fast, and alcohol on serum uric acid and acute attacks of gout. Am J Med 42:38, 1967 (*Fasting and consumption of over 100 gm of alcohol raised urate levels. Acute changes in levels precipitated gouty attacks.*)

Paulus HE, Coutts A, Calabro JJ et al: Clinical significance of hyperuricemia in routinely screened hospitalized men. JAMA 211:277, 1970 (*An early but prophetic paper that argued that an abnormal laboratory finding does not confirm diagnosis or justify therapy.*)

Rastegar A, Thier SO: The physiologic approach to hyperuricemia. N Engl J Med 286:470, 1972 (*Reviews what is known about enzymatic defects that lead to increased uric acid.*)

Rodnan GP, Robin JA et al: Allopurinol and gouty hyperuricemia: Efficacy of a single daily dose. JAMA 231:1143, 1975 (*A study that compared single 300-mg dose to divided doses, demonstrating that the once-daily dose of allopurinol is adequate.*)

Simkin PA: The pathogenesis of podagra. Ann Intern Med 86:230, 1977 (*Reviews the current state of understanding of the pathogenesis of gout.*)

Yu T, Gutman A: Uric acid nephrolithiasis in gout: Predisposing factors. Ann Intern Med 67:1133, 1967 (*A classic study of 305 gouty patients correlating risk of stone formation with uric acid excretion, urine pH, serum urate level, and etiology.*)

Yu TF, Berger LU: Impaired renal function in gout. Am J Med 75:95, 1982 (*Hyperuricemia alone did not affect renal function; renal insufficiency correlated best with coexisting hypertension, pre-existing renal disease, and ischemic heart disease.*)

156

Management of Temporal Arteritis and Polymyalgia Rheumatica

Temporal or giant cell arteritis is a vasculitic disorder of unknown origin that primarily affects people over the age of 60 and rarely occurs before 50. The incidence of temporal arteritis in one population study was 11.7 per 100,000, and its prevalence was 133 per 100,000. In an autopsy study of 389 unselected people, temporal arteritis was found in 1.7%. The importance of temporal arteritis derives from its potential to produce sudden irreversible blindness in approximately one-third of untreated patients.

Temporal arteritis has been reported in 40% of patients with polymyalgia rheumatica (PMR). The exact relationship between the two conditions has yet to be completely elucidated. PMR is characterized by proximal musculoskeletal discomfort and elevated sedimentation rate, often accompanied by fever, malaise, and weight loss. It affects patients over 50 and has a 2:1 predominance in females.

The primary physician needs to be alert to the possibility that these diseases may be present, because they can be subtle in presentation and easily dismissed as vague functional complaints. The associated risk of blindness makes recognition and treatment of prime importance. Because polymyalgia rheumatica may be accompanied by temporal arteritis, one needs to decide which patients with PMR require biopsy in search of arteritis.

PATHOPHYSIOLOGY AND CLINICAL PRESENTATION

Temporal arteritis is defined pathologically by histiocytic, lymphocytic, and giant cell infiltration of the walls of medium or large arteries. The internal elastic lamina is fragmented in conjunction with proliferation. The inflammatory process tends to be segmental and occurs predominantly, though not exclusively, in cranial arteries. The condition has many of the characteristics of an autoimmune process, but the precise pathophysiology remains to be elucidated.

The clinical presentations of *temporal arteritis* reflect direct inflammation of the arterial wall and ischemia secondary to vasculitic narrowing. Headache is reported in 44% to 98% of cases and is an initial symptom in 30% to 45%. The pain can be piercing or throbbing, often localized to the arteries of the scalp. A tender artery may be noted on combing the hair. Ischemic symptoms such as masseter claudication (jaw pain with chewing) occur in one-third to one-half of patients. Visual manifestations are due to vasculitis that may involve

the ophthalmic or posterior ciliary arteries. Blindness is usually a late symptom, occurring abruptly but frequently preceded by transient visual symptoms, such as amaurosis fugax. In early studies that included many untreated patients, visual loss occurred in 42% to 50%. Better recognition and prompt treatment has resulted in a drop in frequency of permanent visual loss to 5% to 10%. Constitutional symptoms of fatigue, malaise, anorexia, and weight loss occur in the majority of patients. Palpable, tender temporal or occipital arteries are sometimes encountered. A markedly increased erythrocyte sedimentation rate is highly characteristic of the disease; a normal sedimentation rate virtually rules out the diagnosis, though there are rare exceptions. A low-grade anemia of chronic disease is often present as well.

Polymyalgia rheumatica develops gradually over weeks or months. Pain and stiffness of periarticular structures of neck and shoulders is the presentation in two-thirds of cases, with hip and thigh involvement accounting for the other third. Many complain of shoulder and thigh involvement. Morning stiffness and pain with movement are highly characteristic; muscle strength is unimpaired. Synovitis has been documented histologically; muscle biopsies are usually normal or show minor inflammatory infiltrates. Low-grade fever, weight loss, and fatigue are commonly present for months before the diagnosis is made.

A PMR patient with headache, tender cranial artery or visual complaints is likely to have temporal arteritis. One study found temporal arteritis in 15 of 33 PMR patients who had such symptoms. However, most patients with symptoms solely of polymyalgia for 6 months do not later incur risk of blindness.

PRINCIPLES OF MANAGEMENT

Given the frequent association of temporal arteritis with PMR and the potential seriousness of temporal arteritis, one needs to decide on the need for temporal artery biopsy and steroid therapy. Headache and other arteritis symptoms help to identify those who will have positive biopsies. In the defined population studied by the Mayo Clinic, all patients with PMR found to have temporal arteritis had symptoms of arteritis. Though some rheumatologists advocate biopsy of all PMR patients, the data in support of such an approach are inconclusive. Some find it difficult to justify the costs and morbidity associated with biopsying all PMR patients, especially when the need for steroids in asymptomatic patients with positive biopsies is unclear. At the present time, it seems reasonable to defer temporal artery biopsy in those patients with PMR who have no symptoms of temporal arteritis and who can be depended on to report any. Should such symptoms arise, biopsy can be promptly performed. The risk to the patient in delaying biopsy until symptoms arise is probably very small, because symptoms almost always precede onset of visual loss.

Temporal artery biopsy has a considerable false-negative rate because the arteritis is often patchy in distribution. When clinical evidence is strong, yet biopsy is negative, treatment can proceed without obtaining pathologic confirmation. The false-negative rate can be minimized by obtaining a generous portion of the temporal artery at biopsy. Arteriography is sensitive but nonspecific and unreliable diagnostically, but may be helpful in choosing an area to biopsy, especially if the first attempt was unsuccessful.

Some authorities argue that biopsy can be omitted altogether when clinical evidence for temporal arteritis is compelling (*e.g.,* very high sedimentation rate, tender cranial artery, PMR). They proceed directly to steroid therapy.

The natural history of temporal arteritis is a self-limited one; most cases resolve within 2 years, though there is much individual variation. The disease should be treated initially with substantial daily doses of *prednisone* (40 to 60 mg per day). Daily therapy is needed; an alternate day schedule does not control the arteritis. The resolution of symptoms is characteristically prompt, and the sedimentation rate falls back to normal levels. The prednisone dose can be titrated against recurrence of symptoms and elevation of the sedimentation rate and should be reduced slowly toward a maintenance dose of 10 to 15 mg per day. The patient must be carefully watched for recurrence of symptoms and elevation of the sedimentation rate. It is sometimes possible to have the patient completely off steroids within a year. Data suggest that spontaneous remission may occur within 6 months, but in many cases activity persists for 2 to 3 years. Relapses have occurred in up to 20% when treatment was discontinued before 2 years had elapsed. In the Mayo Clinic series, blindness did not occur during relapses. Tapering should begin as soon as improvement is evident to minimize the adverse effects of prolonged high-dose steroid therapy (see Chapter 103).

Polymyalgia rheumatica without symptoms of arteritis can be treated with low-dose prednisone, beginning with 10 to 15 mg per day and tapering as the sedimentation rate falls and symptoms resolve. If improvement does not occur in 1 week, the diagnosis is probably incorrect. Characteristically, the condition responds dramatically to very small steroid doses. These dosages do not protect the patient from the complications of arteritis and require adjustment should vasculitic symptoms occur. However, it is very rare for blindness to occur if the sedimentation rate is normal. Treatment is

needed for an average of 12 months. In patients with mild PMR, switching within a month to a nonsteroidal anti-inflammatory agent (see Chapter 153) may suffice and minimize risks of chronic steroid therapy.

PATIENT EDUCATION

Patients with PMR must be told of the symptoms of arteritis and instructed to report their occurrence immediately. The rationale for daily prednisone therapy needs to be shared with the patient and family to ensure compliance. The usual precautions applicable to anyone on daily prednisone therapy should be reviewed (see Chapter 103).

INDICATIONS FOR REFERRAL

Before steroid therapy is undertaken, consultation with a rheumatologist is indicated if the temporal artery biopsy is negative but the clinical picture strongly suggests the diagnosis of temporal arteritis. Consultation is also indicated in cases of polymyalgia and temporal arteritis that do not respond to steroid therapy.

THERAPEUTIC RECOMMENDATIONS

- Diagnosis of suspected temporal arteritis should be established by confirmatory biopsy when there is clinical uncertainty, recognizing that a negative biopsy does not rule out the diagnosis.
- Patients with PMR and very strong clinical evidence of temporal arteritis (tender cranial artery, visual symptoms, headache, jaw claudication, high sedimentation rate) can be started immediately on prednisone therapy (see below); they do not require biopsy for confirmation of diagnosis.
- At present, there appears to be no justification for performing temporal artery biopsy in patients with PMR who do not have headache or other cranial symptoms suggestive of vasculitis, such as tender artery; onset of such symptoms (jaw claudication, visual disturbances, etc.) requires prompt biopsy and high-dose steroid therapy.
- Therapy for temporal arteritis is initiated with 60 mg of prednisone per day; tapering is started once the sedimentation rate has been substantially reduced and symptomatic control achieved. Daily prednisone therapy is required, usually for 18 to 24 months. Alternate day therapy does not suffice.
- Tapering can continue over a period of months, arriving at a minimal dose sufficient to keep the sedimentation rate normal and the patient free of symptoms.
- After 18 to 24 months, a cautious attempt at phasing out prednisone therapy can be undertaken; the patient is watched for recurrence of symptoms and rise in sedimentation rate.
- Polymyalgia rheumatica in the absence of temporal arteritis can be treated initially with low-dose prednisone (10 to 15

mg per day), which can be tapered once symptoms and elevated sedimentation rate have resolved. Therapy is commonly needed for 12 months; switching early (within 4 to 6 weeks) to a nonsteroidal anti-inflammatory agent (*e.g.,* ibuprofen 400 mg tid or naproxen 375 mg bid) may suffice to control symptoms and minimize risks of steroid therapy.
* The PMR patient needs to be instructed to report at once the onset of any symptoms suggestive of temporal arteritis (*e.g.,* visual disturbances, tender cranial artery, headache).

A.H.G.

ANNOTATED BIBLIOGRAPHY

Calamia KT, Hunder GG: Clinical manifestations of giant cell arteritis. Clin Rheum Dis 6:389, 1980 (*A useful paper on presentations and findings.*)

Chuang T-Y, Hunder GG, Ilstrup DM et al: Polymyalgia rheumatica; A 10-year epidemiologic study. Ann Intern Med 97:672, 1982 (*PMR is a relatively common disease in middle-aged and older persons; it runs a self-limited course.*)

Ettlinger RE, Hunder GG, Ward LE: Polymyalgia rheumatica and giant cell arteritis. Ann Rev Med 29:15, 1978 (*A review that tends to favor biopsy in PMR patients.*)

Fauchald P, Rygvold O, Osytese B: Temporal arteritis and polymyalgia rheumatica. Ann Intern Med 77:845, 1972 (*Documents the strong association between the two conditions.*)

Hall S, Persellin S, Lie JT et al: The therapeutic impact of temporal artery biopsy. Lancet 2:1217, 1983 (*Jaw claudication and a palpably tender temporal artery were strongly associated with a positive biopsy; fewer than 10% with a negative biopsy developed signs of arteritis.*)

Hamilton CR, Jr, Shelly WM, Tumulty PA: Giant-cell arteritis: Including temporal arteritis and polymyalgia rheumatica. Medicine (Baltimore) 50:1, 1971 (*Comprehensive review.*)

Healty LA: Giant cell arteritis (editorial). Ann Intern Med 88:710, 1978 (*A succinct statement encouraging a conservative approach to treating people with polymyalgia.*)

Horton BT, Magath TB, Brown GE: An undescribed form of arteritis of the temporal vessels. Proc. Staff Meetings Mayo Clin, 7:700, 1932 (*A classic description.*)

Hunder GG, Sheps SG, Allen GL, Joyce JW: Daily and alternate-day corticosteroid regimens in the treatment of giant cell arteritis. Ann Intern Med 82:613, 1975 (*Alternate-day steroids are not effective.*)

Huston KA, Hunder GG, Lie JT et al: Temporal arteritis, a 24-year epidemiologic, clinical and pathologic study. Ann Intern Med 88: 162, 1978 (*An epidemiologic survey detailing symptoms in an unselected population.*)

Klein RG, Hunder GG, Stanson AW et al: Large artery involvement in giant cell (temporal) arteritis. Ann Intern Med 83:806, 1975 (*Temporal arteritis can be a more generalized condition.*)

Layfer LF, Banner BF, Huckman MS et al: Temporal arteriography. Arthritis Rheum 21:780, 1978 (*Arteriography is a highly sensitive but nonspecific test for arteritis.*)

Sox HC, Liang MW: The erythrocyte sedimentation rate. Ann Intern Med 104:515, 1986 (*A review of the test's clinical utility, which is greatest for diagnosis of temporal arteritis and for monitoring response to therapy.*)

157
Management of Paget's Disease
SAMUEL R. NUSSBAUM, M.D.

Paget's disease of bone, or osteitis deformans, is a focal disorder of unknown etiology characterized by deformity of the bone's external contour and internal structure that results from excessive resorption and rapid new bone formation. The incidence of Paget's disease was reported to be 3.3% in an autopsy series and 0.1% to 4.0% in radiologic studies. The clinical presentation is variable. In the majority of cases, the diagnosis is made when the patient is asymptomatic. An elevated alkaline phosphatase is discovered on multiphasic screening, or x-rays of the pelvis, vertebrae, or skull show the hallmark radiolucent (osteolytic) areas with compensatory new bone formation. Symptomatic patients report pain in the back or lower extremities, disturbances of gait, increasing head size, hearing loss, and occasionally symptoms related to high output cardiac failure. The primary physician needs to be able to provide symptomatic relief and to know when to utilize agents that suppress osteoclastic activity.

PATHOPHYSIOLOGY AND CLINICAL PRESENTATION

The pathophysiologic mechanism of Paget's disease is excessive osteoclastic destruction and resorption of bone, followed by unregulated osteoblastic new bone formation. The process culminates in an abnormal pattern of lamellar bone with excessive local vascularity and an increase in fibrous tissue. The resultant bone, which is mechanically defective, distorted, and enlarged, leads to the cardinal manifestation of Paget's disease: bone pain and pathologic fractures. The initial stimulus for bone resorption remains unknown. Virus particles have been isolated from Pagetic bone, leading to speculation about an infectious etiology.

The exact mechanism of bone pain in Paget's disease is not understood, and its severity does not always parallel the extent of radiographic involvement. Pain is often exacerbated by weight bearing, muscular activity, or cold weather, and is often located over lytic areas of bone where active osteoclastic resorption is taking place. Bone pain is most common in the spine, pelvis, skull, femur, and tibia.

When the long bones of the lower limbs are affected by Paget's disease, deformity and bowing occur. Often the entire length of the tibia is involved, while the fibula is unaffected. Fractures of the long bones, common below the lesser trochanter of the femur and in the upper third of the tibia, result from the mechanical bowing and abnormal bone architecture. The skull is enlarged due to thickening of the calvarium, manifest in the frontal and occipital regions. Hearing loss occurs due to involvement of the ossicles in the middle ear, which impinge on the eighth cranial nerve in the temporal bone. Basilar invagination of the skull from its downward pressure on the atlas may cause compression of posterior fossa structures. Vertebral encroachment on the spinal cord or nerve roots may cause compression syndromes, including paraplegia.

High output congestive heart failure may occur in patients with extensive Paget's disease as a result of increased cutaneous blood flow to areas overlying pagetic limb involvement. Calcific periarthritis may mimic the symptoms of ankylosing spondylitis.

Hyperuricemia and gouty arthritis, hypercalciuria and renal calculi, and hypercalcemia precipitated by immobilization can occur. Osteogenic sarcoma is seen in 1% to 5% of patients with Paget's disease, rarely before age 50. Extensive and severe skeletal involvement increases the risk of osteogenic sarcoma, which is heralded by localized pain and bony enlargement and occurs more frequently in the upper extremities and skull.

Laboratory and radiographic evidence reflects the increased osteoblastic and osteoclastic activity of pagetic bone. Serum alkaline phosphatase, produced by osteoblasts, is elevated, as is the urinary hydroxyproline excretion, an index of osteoclastic resorption of bone matrix. A bone scan may show areas of increased technetium uptake before diagnostic changes are visible on standard x-rays.

PRINCIPLES OF THERAPY

Most patients with Paget's disease are asymptomatic and require no specific therapy. Localized mild bone pain can be controlled with analgesics; joint involvement usually responds to anti-inflammatory agents such as salicylates, or any of the newer nonsteroidal anti-inflammatory drugs (see Chapter 153). Treatment of more disabling Paget's disease is carried out utilizing agents which inhibit bone resorption. Calcitonin, diphosphonate, or mithramycin decrease osteoclastic resorption and lead to radiographic and clinical improvement.

Although there are no universal criteria for initiation of specific therapy, *indications for therapy* in Paget's disease include: (1) severe pain in pagetic areas, (2) compression of medulla, cauda equina, or auditory nerve with neurologic deficit, (3) high output cardiac failure, (4) hypercalcemia due to immobilization, (5) marked radiographic lytic lesions in long bones and skull representing risk of fracture or brain trauma, (6) multiple fractures, (7) prevention of disfigurement when the skull is extensively involved, (8) recurrent renal calculi due to hypercalciuria, (9) severe hyperuricemia and gout, (10) prophylaxis accompanying extensive orthopedic surgery to reduce vascularity of bone, and (11) prophylaxis when disease is of early onset in an area in which disabling deformity is likely to occur.

Calcitonin, diphosphonate, and mithramycin are the principal agents available for specific therapy. They decrease osteoclastic resorption of bone and have been shown to lead to dramatic relief of pain, relief of nerve entrapment syndromes (although auditory acuity does not improve if the ossicles of the middle ear are affected), decrease in cardiac output by a reduction in vascularity of bone and overlying skin, and healing of lytic radiographic lesions.

Salmon calcitonin (Calcimar) has been used successfully to treat Paget's disease. Its major disadvantages include intolerable nausea in some patients and the need to be given parenterally. It is started at 50 to 100 MRC units subcutaneously daily, depending on the severity of disease. Therapy is not only expensive but requires patient education and ability to learn self-injection techniques. With therapy, alkaline phosphatase and urinary hydroxyproline levels return to normal in one-third of patients and are decreased in another third; in the balance of cases, decreases are minimal or unsustained, as is symptomatic improvement. Antibodies against salmon calcitonin develop in approximately 50% of patients; occasionally there is neutralization of biologic activity and limitation of therapeutic effects. Patients who have developed antibodies against salmon calcitonin have had remissions when treated with human calcitonin. Calcitonin dosage may be reduced to 50 MRCU three times weekly when the disease is in remission. Current data suggest that a low dose needs to be continued indefinitely; otherwise relapse will occur.

Disodium etidronate (EHDP). Diphosphonate treatment also effectively inhibits bone resorption and has the advantage of being an oral therapy. It is given until a biochemical and clinical remission occurs, then discontinued, with recommencement of therapy at a time of relapse. Remissions achieved by use of the drug can last as long as 2 years. Though a useful drug, it has several drawbacks. It is costly; moreover, it may worsen symptoms. EHDP should not be used for more than 6 consecutive months, nor at a dose greater than 5 mg/kg/day, because prolonged therapy or higher doses (10 to 20 mg/kg/day) induces a mineralization defect that may lead to increased fracture rates in areas of lytic bone, as well as worsened bone pain. *Combined therapy with calcitonin* reduces bone turnover to normal in 80% of patients and is not accompanied by mineralization defects or increases in bone pain. It appears that calcitonin promotes mineralization and overcomes the adverse effect of etidronate. Combined therapy may prove to be an effective mode of treatment.

Mithramycin is a potent therapy for Paget's disease. Because of its acute though reversible renal, hepatic, and hematologic toxicities, the drug is reserved for patients with serious complications of Paget's disease, such as severe high output heart failure or hypercalcemic crisis. Thrombocytopenia can be particularly severe. The drug must be administered intravenously in doses of 15 to 25 μg/kg for 10 days, while monitoring urinary hydroxyproline for evidence of suppression of bone resorption.

Neurosurgical intervention is necessary in patients with spinal cord or nerve root compression syndromes. Orthopedic procedures such as total hip replacement and tibial or femoral osteotomy may help to restore mobility.

PATIENT EDUCATION AND INDICATIONS FOR REFERRAL

Patients should be instructed to drink at least 2 liters of liquid daily, especially if they are unable to keep active, because immobilization and dehydration can precipitate renal stone formation and hypercalcemia. Prompt neurosurgical consultation is warranted in patients who have evidence of nerve or cord compression. Orthopedic assessment is needed if the patient is severely immobilized by hip pain. Referral to an endocrinologist is needed if conventional medical therapy fails.

THERAPEUTIC RECOMMENDATIONS

- The majority of patients with Paget's disease are asymptomatic; they require no specific therapy but should be seen at yearly intervals for clinical assessment and alkaline phosphatase measurement.
- For relief of mild localized bone or articular pain, analgesics or anti-inflammatory agents can be used.
- Patients with severe bone pain, high output cardiac failure, hypercalcemia, multiple fractures, or risk of fracture, deformity or compression should be given calcitonin, 100 MRC units subcutaneously daily, *or* EHDP, 5 mg/kg per day orally. Choice of agent depends in part on capability of the patient to self-administer parenteral therapy.
- Two baseline measurements of alkaline phosphatase as well as skeletal x-ray survey or bone scan ought to be obtained at the outset of treatment to help later in gauging therapeutic

response. Serum alkaline phosphatase correlates well with disease activity; it can be followed at monthly intervals during therapy. Frequent bone scanning is unwarranted.

- When biochemical or clinical remission occurs, EHDP should be discontinued; however, intermittent therapy is worth consideration if symptoms recur. If calcitonin is being used, it should be reduced to 50 MRC units three times a week when remission is achieved.
- Avoidance of dehydration and immobilization is important for prevention of hypercalcemia and kidney stones. At least 2 liters of liquid should be taken daily, especially if the patient is inactive.
- If bone pain develops in a patient taking EHDP, skeletal x-rays should be obtained and consideration given to therapy with calcitonin.

ANNOTATED BIBLIOGRAPHY

Bijvoet OLM, Hosking DJ, Frijlink WB et al: Treatment of Paget's disease with combined calcitonin and diphosphonate (EHDP). Meta Bone Dis Relat Res 1:25, 1978 (*Twenty-five of 30 patients treated with a combination of calcitonin and EHDP obtained complete biochemical remission. Mineralization defects were not seen when EHDP was given with calcitonin.*)

Deuxchaisnes CN, Krane SM: Paget's disease of bone: Clinical and metabolic observations. Medicine 43:233, 1964 (*An extensive review of clinical manifestations of Paget's disease with a discussion of calcium balance and metabolic responses to fracture and immobilization.*)

Frank WA, Bries NM, Singer FR et al: Rheumatic manifestations of Paget's disease of bone. Am J Med 56:592, 1974 (*A discussion of the rheumatologic symptoms associated with Paget's disease.*)

Khairi MRA, Atman RD, DeRosa GP et al: Sodium etidronate in the treatment of Paget's disease of bone. A study of long-term results. Ann Intern Med 87:656, 1977 (*Demonstrates therapeutic efficacy of 5 mg/kg EDHP and complications of higher doses of EHDP.*)

Krane SM: Etidronate disodium in the treatment of Paget's disease of bone. Ann Intern Med 96:619, 1982 (*Definitive review of 5 years experience with the drug. Details the clinical efficacy of the drug and its risk of adverse effects.*)

Ryan WG: Paget's disease of bone. Ann Rev Med 28:143, 1977 (*A succinct review of Paget's disease, emphasizing treatment. There is a comprehensive bibliography.*)

Woodhouse NJ, Crosbie WA, Mohamedally SM: Cardiac output in Paget's disease: Response to long-term salmon calcitonin therapy. Br Med J 4(5998):686, 1975 (*A brief report documenting a fall in cardiac output in three patients with Paget's disease treated with salmon calcitonin.*)

158
Management of Osteoporosis
SAMUEL R. NUSSBAUM, M.D.

Osteoporotic fractures, particularly in aging women, represent a major health problem in industrialized nations. In the United States approximately 150,000 hip fractures occur annually in women over age 65 with 15% to 25% of these women experiencing excess mortality or needing long-term nursing home care. Current expenditures for hip fractures are in excess of 7 billion dollars yearly. Osteoporotic vertebral crush fractures, manifested by back pain, loss of height, and decreased ambulation are present in 5% to 10% of women by age 60 and 40% by age 80. The pathophysiological mechanisms for postmenopausal osteoporosis are imperfectly understood, but the means to ensure maximal skeletal growth and strength, prevent loss of bone mass, and noninvasively evaluate bone mass are now available. The primary care physician should educate women about prevention of osteoporosis and identify those who are at greatest risk of bone loss for consideration of therapy.

PATHOPHYSIOLOGY AND CLINICAL PRESENTATION

Osteoporosis is a reduction in the mass of bone per unit volume. Because a bone's strength is proportional to its density, the mechanical support of the skeleton is affected as bone mass declines. In contrast to osteoporosis, *osteomalacia* is characterized by a defect in the mineralization of the organic phase of bone.

The resorption and formation of bone is a continuous process throughout life; under physiologic circumstances, the rates of these processes are equal and coupled. Skeletal mass is usually maximal by age 35 and declines in women after age 40 and in men after age 50 when the rate of new bone formation does not equal the rate of bone resorption. The rate of decline in skeletal mass is most rapid in women within two years of menopause; the greatest loss of trabecular bone occurs in the femoral neck and lumbar vertebrae, sites of future fracture.

The explanations for the uncoupling of bone resorption and formation and development of osteoporosis remain speculative. Bone does not contain estrogen receptors; however, estrogens enhance calcium absorption by increasing 1,25 dihydroxyvitamin D and parathyroid hormone, while decreasing urinary hydroxyproline excretion. Fractional intestinal absorption of calcium in elderly persons is decreased. This decline in intestinal calcium absorption appears to be caused by a decrease in the formation of 1,25 dihydroxyvitamin D.

Epidemiologic studies have not demonstrated significant differences in calcium intake between normal and osteoporotic women. Factors that have been associated with an increased likelihood of developing osteoporosis include a family history of osteoporosis, fair skin, excess alcohol consumption, smoking, and lack of physical activity. Women in whom osteoporosis does not develop may have larger skeletal masses, which may be increased through physical activity.

Conditions other than aging that can lead to osteoporosis include Cushing's syndrome, exogenous glucocorticoid administration, chronic heparin therapy, thyrotoxicosis, hypogonadism, hyperprolactinemia, anorexia nervosa, and hyperparathyroidism. However, these diseases represent a small percentage of osteoporotic patients.

The progressive decline in skeletal mass (which may approach 50%) becomes clinically manifest when *fractures* are sustained spontaneously or after minimal trauma. A loss of height and developing kyphosis generally indicates vertebral compression fracture. Fractures most commonly occur in the sacral and lumbar vertebrae, the hip, the humerus, and the wrist. Back pain heralds new fractures. Although the incidence of new fractures tends to decrease with time, the clinical course and the frequency of fractures in individual patients cannot be predicted.

Osteopenia is a radiologic term that indicates a reduced amount of bone and encompasses both osteomalacia and osteoporosis. The characteristic radiographic finding in osteoporosis is the loss of horizontal vertebral trabeculae, accentuating the end-plates and resulting in biconcave "codfish" vertebrae. Pseudofractures, generally occurring in weight-bearing long bones, are pathognomonic for osteomalacia. The laboratory features of postmenopausal osteoporosis include normal serum levels of calcium, phosphate, vitamin D, parathyroid hormone, and alkaline phosphatase, though alkaline phosphatase may be elevated in the context of a healing fracture.

EVALUATION

Noninvasive Assessments of Bone Density. Increasing awareness of the consequences of osteoporosis, coupled with the development of noninvasive techniques for determining bone mass, has led to the screening of asymptomatic women for osteoporosis. Single photon absorptiometry of the forearm assesses cortical bone; dual photon absorptiometry of the spine measures both cortical and trabecular bone; and computed tomography (CT) of the spine assesses trabecular bone. Single photon absorption correlates well with bone ash weight, but not with spinal compression fractures. CT and dual photon bone density are better predictors.

Vertebral fractures are uncommon when vertebral bone density is greater than 1 g/cm^2 by dual photon absorptiometry or 100–110 mg/cm^3 by quantitative CT scanning. Unfortunately, the risk of hip fractures (the most morbid of pathologic fractures) does not correlate well with CT and dual photon bone densitometric measurements.

These tests are safe, acceptable to patients, and have predictive value for the development of spinal compression fractures; but, because they do not accurately predict the risk of hip fracture, they should not be routinely used in perimenopausal women. Moreover, a woman being treated with estrogen therapy in the perimenopausal period does not require routine measurements of bone mass. However, the woman at above average risk for the development of osteoporosis can be monitored for osteoporosis if rapidly declining bone density would lead to initiation of estrogen therapy. Additionally, patients being treated for osteoporosis may require bone density measurements to determine therapeutic efficacy.

PRINCIPLES OF THERAPY

The major goal in the management of osteoporosis is to minimize the loss of bone mass and the risk of fracture. Available therapies include estrogens and calcium supplements. If a fracture has occurred, symptomatic relief and attempts at halting further bone loss are indicated. An important issue is the need for prophylactic estrogen therapy.

Estrogen. The vast majority of patients with osteoporosis are postmenopausal women. Estrogen therapy may stop bone loss and even lead to skeletal accretion. Observational studies have consistently noted a 50% reduction in hip, wrist, and vertebral fractures in women who have used estrogen for at least 5 years after the menopause. Although estrogen therapy for osteoporosis has been advocated for three decades, only recently have controlled noninvasive studies of bone mass confirmed previous clinical observations. For example, patients treated with mestranol showed no further loss of bone mass and even slight bone accretion, contrasted with continued bone loss in patients given placebo. Unfortunately, if mestranol was discontinued, bone loss rapidly ensued. In a study utilizing quantitative CT bone density in surgically induced menopause, it was determined that 0.625 mg of conjugated estrogen is the necessary dose to prevent bone loss. A two-year study comparing calcium carbonate, conjugated estrogens, and placebo therapy in 60 postmenopausal women revealed that conjugated estrogens were superior to calcium carbonate in decreasing bone loss as determined by photon absorptiometry.

Adverse effects (see Chapter 117). There is an increased *risk of endometrial cancer* and an uncertain effect on the prevalence of breast cancer. The periodic administration of progestins may limit the increased rate of endometrial cancer. Women who dislike the withdrawal bleeding that occurs following estrogen and progestin therapy can use a progestin such as medroxyprogesterone (Provera) 10 mg for 7 days administered every 50 or 60 days. However, there is the possibility of increased cardiovascular risk incurred with progestin use (see Chapter 117).

Timing. Fracture rates and bone loss can be decreased by use of estrogen in postmenopausal women. However, once established, it is difficult to reverse the significant bone loss that occurs in the first few years of menopause. Consequently, if one is going to use estrogen to prevent osteoporosis, therapy should be initiated at the onset of menopause. Estrogen therapy needs to be continued indefinitely because skeletal loss will resume if treatment is halted.

Patient selection. There is no universal agreement as to which patients should be considered for prophylactic therapy with estrogen at the time of menopause. However, those with major risk factors (*e.g.,* family history of osteoporosis, a small frame, lack of exercise, low calcium intake, fair-skinned complexion, and smoking) are candidates for prophylactic therapy. Women who have a rate of decline in bone mass that is greater than age-matched controls also should receive estrogen therapy. When osteoporosis is clinically manifest by fractures or when osteopenia appears radiographically, at least 30% to 40% loss of bone mass has occurred and therapy with estrogen and supplemental calcium (see below) should be commenced.

Calcium and Vitamin D. Calcium carbonate in doses of 1.5–2.0 g/day helps preserve cortical bone mass; however, calcium therapy does not prevent bone loss to the degree that estrogen therapy does. Because dietary surveys indicate that the majority of young women are not consuming the RDA recommended 800–1000 mg of calcium each day, and because the fractional absorption of calcium decreases with aging, it is most reasonable to encourage supplementation of dietary calcium to 1.5 g/day in adolescent and young women and 2 g/day in older women. However, increasing calcium intake during early childhood and in young adult life has not conclusively been shown to lead to increased skeletal mass. Nevertheless, no complications from intake of 1–2 g of elemental calcium, such as renal stones or hypercalcemia, have been observed. Dietary calcium may be supplemented by drinking milk (250 mg of calcium per glass), eating dairy products, or taking calcium carbonate (250–500 mg qid; see Table 158-1). Larger doses of calcium carbonate, particularly in conjunction with vitamin D, may predispose the patient to hypercalcemia and hypercalciuric renal stone disease.

Vitamin D treatment is not useful for osteoporosis unless

there is concomitant vitamin D deficiency and osteomalacia, which actually are quite common in elderly patients (see below). Vitamin D is essential for bone accretion before menopause (see below).

Experimental Therapies. *Sodium fluoride.* Fluoride therapy leads to a striking increase in trabecular bone density if given in doses ranging from 40 to 60 mg/day. Cortical bone density continues to decline, and total body calcium and calcium balance do not change. Calcium supplementation is necessary to prevent fluoride-induced osteomalacia. Bursitis and GI side effects are common when 40 to 60 mg of NaF are used; these complications necessitate discontinuation of the drug in approximately one-third of patients. Although a study at the Mayo Clinic demonstrated a reduction in fractures in individuals receiving fluoride, a Scandanavian study demonstrated an increase in hip fractures in patients during high-dose fluoride treatment. Sodium fluoride therapy is still considered experimental by the FDA, because the dense fluorotic bone is abnormal both chemically and crystallographically and has undesirable mechanical properties *in vitro*. Currently trials of NaF in osteoporosis are underway to determine the role for fluoride in the treatment of osteoporosis.

Calcitonin. Daily subcutaneous injections of 100 units of salmon calcitonin in combination with oral calcium of 1000 mg daily will increase total body calcium in postmenopausal women by several percent, presumably reflecting an increase in skeletal mass. Changes in specific bones have been too small to measure. After a year there is no further increase in total body calcium, and it declines in parallel to untreated control patients. Calcitonin, therefore, is an expensive ($2500 per year) therapy to minimally increase the bone mass of postmenopausal women who are willing to administer daily injections.

Parathyroid hormone in combination with 1,25 dihydroxyvitamin D stimulates new bone formation, increases trabecular bone, and improves calcium balance while producing chemically and histologically normal bone without hypercalcemia. This approach is under active investigation.

Exercise. An important component of the preventive therapy of osteoporosis is ensuring maximal development of skeletal mass. The amount of bone accumulated premenopausally may be critical to the appearance of osteoporosis later in life, as evidenced by the low incidence of osteoporosis in black women (and in men), who have a greater skeletal mass than white women. Exercise and physical activity have been shown to increase skeletal mass and increase total body calcium. Physical activity, in conjunction with a 1500-mg calcium-supplemented diet and 400 units of vitamin D daily, offers the best hope for increasing skeletal mass during skeletal growth. However, exercise programs so intensive as to induce amenorrhea and estrogen deficiency (*e.g.,* competitive marathon running) may lead to osteoporosis.

Anabolic Steroids. Stanozolol 2 mg tid, a synthetic anabolic steroid, has been shown to preserve total body calcium and, by inference, bone mass. Side-effects are mild, but a reversible elevation of SGOT commonly occurs, even when treatment is given for only 3 weeks per month.

Fractures

In patients who have sustained vertebral fractures, bed rest and adequate analgesics should be prescribed until the acute pain of the fracture subsides, often within several weeks. Thereafter, ambulation and daily exercise, such as swimming and walking, should be encouraged as tolerated. Lifting and vigorous physical activity are best avoided. Attention to proper footwear, use of canes for support, and maintenance of an uncluttered home environment diminish the risk of further accidental trauma. Corsets and back braces, if comfortable, may facilitate ambulation in formerly bedridden patients. Individuals who have sustained fractures should then be treated for osteoporosis.

As noted earlier, the natural history of osteoporosis and compression fractures is not predictable in an individual patient. Symptomatic improvement cannot be used to measure the response to therapy because of the long fracture-free intervals. Noninvasive measurements of bone mass are needed to determine if bone loss has slowed or reversed with therapy.

Osteomalacia

Osteomalacia is defined as the inadequate deposition of calcium and phosphorus in bone tissue matrix. In recently conducted studies of hip fractures, at least 10% to 15% of patients were found to have osteomalacia on bone biopsy. The most frequent causes of osteomalacia (which should be suspected in all osteopenic patients), include *vitamin D deficiency* in elderly homebound patients who do not eat dairy products or go out in the sun, disorders of vitamin D metabolism, and gastrointestinal and hepatobiliary disease with *malabsorption.* Other causes include systemic acidosis and phosphate depletion resulting from impaired renal tubular phosphate reabsorption or excess aluminum hydroxide ingestion. Osteomalacia should be suspected in patients with hypocalcemia or hypophosphatemia, urinary calcium excretion of less than 100 mg/24 hours (unless the patient is taking thiazide diuretics), low 25-OH vitamin D levels, elevated parathyroid hormone, elevated alkaline phosphatase (unless this elevation can be explained by a recent fracture), premature osteopenia, and in osteopenic patients taking anticonvulsant therapy.

A 72-hour fecal fat determination revealing intestinal malabsorption, urine pH, 25-OH vitamin D, phosphate, calcium, and bicarbonate determinations often indicate the cause of the mineralization defect. In patients taking phenytoin or phenobarbital, hepatic conversion of vitamin D to

Table 158-1. Oral Calcium Preparations

PREPARATION	CALCIUM CONTENT	FORM	DOSE NEEDED TO ACHIEVE 1 g CALCIUM/DAY
Calcium lactate	300 mg/tab	Often in multivitamin; 300 mg tab	3⅓ tabs
Calcium carbonate	Approximately 200 mg/tab	Titralac	5 tabs
	Approximately 200 mg/tab	Tums	5 tabs
	250 mg/tab	Oscal	4 tabs
	500 mg/tab	Oscal	2 tabs
Calcium glubionate	115 mg/5cc	Neocalglucon, 480 ml	9 tsps
Milk	250 mg/8 oz	Whole milk	1 quart

25-OH vitamin D is impaired; resistance to the action of vitamin D on bone and gut also occurs. These patients, as well as the elderly patient with inadequate consumption of dairy products and sunlight exposure, have low levels of 25-OH vitamin D and secondary hyperparathyroidism.

In the absence of pseudofractures on x-ray, it is not possible to radiographically distinguish osteoporosis from osteomalacia. A bone biopsy (preceded by double tetracycline labeling) to observe for widened osteoid seams is necessary for the definitive diagnosis of osteomalacia. However, it is not feasible to perform bone biopsies on all osteopenic patients; moreover, osteomalacia responds dramatically to treatment with *dietary vitamin D, calcium,* and *phosphate* supplements. Consequently, bone biopsy should be reserved for patients in whom the diagnosis of osteomalacia remains uncertain. In such patients who are undergoing orthopedic procedures, biopsy, preceded by tetracycline labeling, should be performed at the time of surgery. If a 24-hour urinary calcium is greater than 100 mg/24 hours, osteomalacia is very unlikely.

THERAPEUTIC RECOMMENDATIONS

- Young people, especially pregnant women, should have a dietary intake of at least 1.0–1.5 g of calcium and 400 IU of vitamin D daily. A program of regular physical activity to stimulate accretion of skeletal mass should be encouraged.
- Postmenopausal women should receive 400 IU vitamin D daily and 2 g of calcium in their diet. A convenient form of dietary supplement is use of 250–500 mg calcium carbonate tablets (see Table 158-1).
- Women who have a family history of osteoporosis, or a history of physical inactivity, early menopause, or inadequate calcium intake should be considered for estrogen therapy beginning in the perimenopausal period.
- Estrogen therapy should be conducted using 0.625 mg of conjugated estrogens. The addition of progestins appears to lessen the risk of estrogen-associated endometrial cancer (see Chapter 117).

- Asymptomatic postmenopausal patients who are found to have radiographic osteopenia and no contraindications for estrogen therapy should have dual photon absorptiometry or CT quantitative bone density performed to quantify the reduction in skeletal mass, followed by treatment with estrogen, calcium, and vitamin D.
- Patients who have sustained fractures as a consequence of osteoporosis can be treated with bed rest and analgesics. When the pain subsides, ambulation can begin, followed by mild exercise such as walking or swimming. Avoidance of lifting and other weight-bearing stresses is advisable. These patients should receive treatment for osteoporosis with either estrogen or calcitonin.
- Estrogen therapy for postmenopausal osteoporosis is continued indefinitely, because bone loss resumes with cessation of treatment.
- Patients who are receiving therapy for symptomatic osteoporosis and postmenopausal women who are not receiving estrogen but are at increased risk for the development of osteoporosis should have a CT or dual photon bone mass measurement every 1 or 2 years.
- Individuals receiving phenytoin or phenobarbital should have vitamin D supplementation of 50,000 IU each 1 to 2 weeks.

ANNOTATED BIBLIOGRAPHY

Cummings SR, Black D: Should perimenopausal women be screened for osteoporosis. Ann Intern Med 104:817, 1986 (*A scholarly discussion and review of methods of assessing bone mass and their relationship to the incidence of clinical fractures.*)

Gambrell RD, Jr, Massey FM, Castaneda TA et al: Use of the progesterone challenge test to reduce the risk of endometrial cancer. Obstet Gynecol 55:732, 1980 (*Evidence that progestogen-induced withdrawal bleeding may prevent the development of endometrial cancer in postmenopausal women on estrogen therapy.*)

Genant, HK, Cann, CE, Ettinger B et al: Quantitative computed tomography of vertebral spungiosa: A sensitive method for detecting early bone loss after oophorectomy. Ann Intern Med 97:

699, 1982 (*Following surgical menopause, quantitative spinal CT detected bone loss within 6 months.*)

Horsman A, Gallagher JC, Simpson M et al: Prospective trial of estrogen and calcium in postmenopausal women. Br Med J 2: 789, 1977 (*Estrogen treatment prevents and calcium treatment retards postmenopausal bone loss when studied densitometrically and morphometrically, even when instituted an average of 6 years following menopause.*)

Horsman A, Jones M, Francis R et al: The effect of estrogen dose on postmenopausal bone loss. N Engl J Med 309:1405, 1983 (*Demonstrates a dose–response relationship between reduction in bone loss and dose of estrogen among postmenopausal women.*)

Jowsey J et al: Effect of continued therapy with sodium fluoride, vitamin D and calcium in osteoporosis. Am J Med 53:43, 1972 (*Fluoride, in conjunction with vitamin D and calcium, resulted in an increase in new bone formation without microscopic evidence of fluorosis.*)

Lindsay R et al: Long-term prevention of postmenopausal osteoporosis by estrogen. Lancet 1:1038, May 15, 1976 (*Evidence of increased bone mass even after delayed onset of estrogen therapy— 3 to 6 years postmenopause—is presented. This increase in bone mineral content occurs during the first 3 years of estrogen therapy.*)

Mazess RB: Non-invasive methods for quantitating trabecular bone. *In:* Avioli LV (ed.): The Osteoporotic Syndrome: Detection, Prevention and Treatment. New York: Grune and Stratton 1983, 85 (*A discussion of computed tomography and photon absorptoometry as methods of quantitating trabecular bone.*)

Nachtigall LE, Nachtigall RH, Nachtigall RD et al: Estrogen replacement therapy: I. A 10-year prospective study of the relationship to osteoporosis. Obstet Gynecol 53:277, 1979 (*Weiss [see later entry] and Nachtigall, in addition to several others, confirm the efficacy of perimenopausal estrogen administration by documenting a reduced incidence of fracture.*)

Notelovitz M, Ware M: Stand Tall! The Informed Woman's Guide to Preventing Osteoporosis. Gainesville, FL, Triad Publishing Co., 1982 (*A well-referenced, scholarly, but very readable account of the epidemiology and health aspects of osteoporosis. The discussions on exercise and diet may encourage women to build stronger skeletons; the discussion on estrogen will help many women select this prophylactic therapy.*)

Office of Medical Applications of Research, National Institutes of Health: Osteoporosis: Consensus conference. JAMA 252:799, 1984 (*A statement of the impact of osteoporosis on health care and recommendations for therapy by a panel of leaders in clinical bone and mineral research.*)

Quigley MM, Hammond LB: Estrogen-replacement therapy—Help or hazard. N Engl J Med 301:646, 1979 (*A brief review of current indications for estrogen replacement therapy in the menopause.*)

Richelson LS, Wahner HW, Melton LJ et al: Relative contributions of aging and estrogen deficiency to postmenopausal bone loss. N Engl J Med 311:1273, 1984 (*Bone loss in oophorectomized women was almost as great as that in postmenopausal women, indicating that estrogen deficiency rather than aging is the prominent cause.*)

Riggs, BL: Treatment of Osteoporosis with Sodium Fluoride: An appraisal. *In* Peck WA (ed.): Bone and Mineral Research Annual II. New York, Elsevier, 1984, 366 (*A review of the Mayo Clinic experience with NaF for reducing clinical fractures.*)

Recker RR, Saville RD, Heaney RP: Effect of estrogens and calcium carbonate on bone loss in postmenopausal women. Ann Intern Med 87:649, 1977 (*Estrogen and calcium treatment both led to a decrease in bone resorption. Estrogen was more effective than calcium by the technique of photon absorptiometry. Authors recommend calcium carbonate supplementation as a preventive measure.*)

Thomson DL, Frame B: Involutional osteopenia: Current concepts. Ann Intern Med 85:789, 1976 (*A comprehensive review of theories of pathogenesis and a critical evaluation of the limited success of therapeutic regimens. There is an extensive bibliography.*)

Weinstein MC: Estrogen use in postmenopausal women: Costs, risks and benefits. N Engl J Med 303:306, 1980 (*A structured analysis that includes a critical review of the literature regarding risks and benefits of postmenopausal estrogen therapy.*)

Weiss NS, Ure CL, Ballard JH et al: Decreased risk of fractures of the hip and lower forearm with postmenopausal use of estrogen. N Engl J Med 303:1195, 1980 (*A case control study indicating a reduction in fracture risk of 50%–60% among women treated for 6 or more years with estrogens.*)

Whedon GD: Osteoporosis. N Engl J Med 305:397, 1981 (*Editorial accompanying an article suggesting an impaired responsiveness of 1,25-dihydroxyvitamin D in older patients with osteoporosis. Discusses the clinical significance of this finding as well as our current knowledge base for the treatment of osteoporosis.*)

11

Neurologic Problems

159
Evaluation of Headache

It has been estimated that headaches generate almost 16 million patient visits in the United States annually and that 6% or 7% of the population suffer headaches that cause loss of time from work or school. Physicians and patients worry about headaches that are persistent, severe, or sudden in onset; tumor is a common concern when the headache persists. However, only the rare patient has a worrisome cause for headache; as a result, it is wasteful to subject all patients to extensive laboratory investigation. The primary physician's most immediate task is to identify on clinical grounds the occasional patient who requires aggressive workup.

PATHOPHYSIOLOGY AND CLINICAL PRESENTATION

Brain parenchyma is not sensitive to pain, but many intracranial and extracranial structures are. Intracranial sources of pain referable to the head include fibers of the fifth, ninth, and tenth cranial nerves, the dural arteries, the arteries of the circle of Willis, the major venous sinuses, and the dura at the base of the skull. Extracranial sites of headache include the skin, fascia, muscles, and blood vessels of the scalp, the upper cervical nerve roots, and the muscles of the neck. In general, pain that arises from an intracranial process above the tentorium is perceived in the frontal, temporal, or parietal region; pain originating from the posterior fossa and below the occiput is referred to the occiput. However, pain deriving from the posterior half of the sagittal sinus or upper aspect of the transverse sinus in the posterior fossa may be referred to the eye and forehead by way of the first division of the trigeminal nerve. In addition, the spinal tract and nucleus of the fifth cranial nerve plunge down into the area of the upper cervical roots; as a result, head pain may occur when upper cervical injury takes place.

The major mechanisms of headache are traction on pain-sensitive structures, inflammation of vessels and meninges, vascular dilatation, and excessive muscle contraction. A number of mechanisms may be operating simultaneously in a given case; patients frequently report being bothered by more than one type of headache.

Traction Headaches. Mass lesions that displace a pain-sensitive structure can produce head pain that is initially intermittent, unilateral, dull, and aching. The discomfort is often relieved by lying down and worsened by straining at stool, coughing, or bending over. Characteristically, the headache remains in the same location, but becomes progressive, with increases in duration and severity of pain over several months, in conjunction with subtle changes in mental status or development of focal neurologic deficits. A more generalized headache may develop if increased intracranial pressure ensues. Projectile vomiting is a late complication. Nocturnal awakening is common but not diagnostic.

About one-third of patients with *brain tumor* have headache as an early symptom. Initially, the headache may be the sole complaint unaccompanied by focal deficits. However, chronic headache due to a brain tumor is usually associated with an abnormality on neurologic examination. In a study of 165 patients with chronic headache followed for one year or more and subjected to computerized tomography (CT), there was no headache patient with a totally normal neurologic examination who had an abnormality on CT indicative of tumor.

Brain abscess can also cause a traction headache, especially in its later stages. Parenteral drug abuse, lung abscess, or parameningeal infection may serve as the source of infection. Fever and focal neurologic deficits are often absent. *Chronic subdural hematoma,* another important etiology, typically presents in subtle fashion, with head trauma followed by a symptom-free interval. The injury may be forgotten, but the patient begins to show mental status changes and, eventually, focal neurologic deficits. *Post-concussion headache* (see below) occurs in cases where the wrenching and displacement of pain-sensitive CNS structures from head trauma was severe enough to cause concussion.

Pseudotumor cerebri can mimic the clinical presentation of tumor. Characteristic features include onset in an obese, young woman, papilledema on exam, and compressed ventricles on CT.

Inflammatory Headaches. Meninges, sinuses, or cranial vessels may be involved. Tenderness of the involved structure is characteristic but is not invariable. *Meningitis* from infection or hemorrhage produces pain that is acute in onset, severe, generalized, and constant. Symptoms may be particularly intense at the base of the skull and aggravated by forward flexion of the neck. The headache of *giant cell arteritis* (temporal arteritis) is dull, aching, or throbbing. Initially it is localized to an involved vessel but can become diffuse; moreover, the inflamed artery may not always be tender or palpable. Jaw (masticatory muscle) claudication is often part of the clinical picture. Patients are elderly; some concurrently suffer from polymyalgia rheumatica. Sudden blindness is the most serious complication; it results from infarction caused by arterial occlusion (see Chapter 156).

Vascular Headaches. Abnormal vasodilatation produces headaches that are characteristically acute in onset and throbbing. *Migraine* is the most common form of vascular headache and is believed to involve vasoconstriction followed by vasodilatation of extracranial vessels. In addition, there are associated changes in circulating vasoactive agents such as serotonin, norepinephrine, prostaglandins, bradykinin, and histamine. Whether these changes are causal or reactive remains to be fully elucidated. Migraine presents in two forms: common and classical; the former can be unilateral or bilateral and is unaccompanied by prodromal symptoms; the latter is unilateral and preceded by transient disturbances in neurologic function (see Chapter 166). Prodromal symptoms have been ascribed to vasospasm and resultant transient ischemia. Patients may report scotomata, hemianopia, vertigo, diplopia, aphasia, even hemiplegia preceding onset of the headache. In rare instances these prodromal symptoms persist for 1 to 2 days, simulating a stroke. Both types of migraine are accompanied by nausea and photophobia. The headache is usually throbbing, though it may begin as a dull sensation and take a while to reach maximum intensity. It usually ends within 24 hours, but occasionally persists for 1 to 2 days. A family history of "sick headaches" is elicited in about 50%. Precipitants of migraine include emotional upset, menstruation, and, in some people, ingestion of tyramine- or tryptophan-rich foods (*e.g.,* ripe cheeses, red wine, or chocolate). Headache may occur shortly after or just prior to a period of psychologic stress. Some patients experience a paradoxical flare-up of migraine on weekends and vacations; the phenomenon is hypothesized to result from a fall in stress-induced endorphins (CNS substances with opiate qualities).

Cluster headaches are a poorly understood form of vascular headache occurring mostly in middle-aged men. They are characterized by nocturnal episodes of intense, unilateral searing, stabbing, or burning pain localized to the orbit and accompanied by lacrimation, nasal stuffiness, and facial flushing on the same side as the headache. In 20% to 40% there is also ipsilateral ptosis and miosis. Headache typically begins a few hours after going to bed, lasts about 1 to 2 hours, and repeats nightly for weeks to months. Then the headaches disappear, only to return again several years later. In about 10% attacks persist daily for 1 to 2 years. Stress and alcohol are believed to be precipitants, although alcohol is well tolerated between attacks. The exact mechanism of cluster headaches is unknown, but vasoactive substances are believed to have an important role. Abnormal cranial vasodilatation without prior vasoconstriction has been observed. Although the headache is classified as vascular, it is most often steady rather than throbbing.

Systemic infection and *fever* are common causes of cranial vasodilatation and diffuse, throbbing headaches. The headache that frequently accompanies a viral syndrome is typical of this type. Numerous *metabolic disturbances* and *drugs* may lead to vasodilatation and headache. A pounding headache is a prominent symptom of early carbon monoxide poisoning and a common complaint of patients who take nitrates for angina or vasodilators for other conditions.

Moderate to severe *hypertension* (diastolic pressures >110 mmHg) sometimes results in occipital headaches. The mechanism of the headache is unknown. The discomfort is worse in the morning and recedes as the day progresses. This headache resolves with correction of the hypertension and is not to be confused with the muscle contraction and psychogenic headaches that are responsible for most headaches that occur in hypertensive patients.

Arteriovenous malformation is a much feared cause of vascular headache. Acute rupture produces sudden severe meningeal irritation (see above). In the absence of any rupture, 10% to 15% of patients experience a chronic headache characterized by unilateral (always the same side) throbbing pain. Unlike migraine, there are no prodromal or associated symptoms. *Berry aneurysms* are silent until rupture, unless greater than 2 cm in which case they may cause a traction headache.

Muscle Contraction Headaches. Prolonged and excessive muscle contraction ranks among the leading causes of chronic and recurrent headache. Over 90% of these headaches are bilateral and are often described as a pressure or bandlike sensation about the head. The pain is dull and steady in most instances, worsening as the day progresses and sometimes accompanied by occipital and nuchal soreness. The headache may last days, weeks, or even months. Recording of myographic potentials from head and neck muscles reveals vigorous contractions in some but not all patients with this type of headache; vasoconstriction can also be detected. The mechanisms responsible for excessive muscle contraction have not been fully delineated, but anxiety, depression, and emotional conflicts are common precipitants. These factors may produce migraine headaches in the same patient. Muscle contraction headaches may also occur secondary to muscle strain from cervical spondylosis or temporomandibular joint disease (see below).

Psychogenic Headaches. Many psychogenic headaches are of the muscle contraction variety. However, others are unaccompanied by detectable changes in muscle contraction or blood flow. Depression, conversion reactions, and anxiety are among the causes. Some authorities postulate that such headaches represent somatic expressions of deep-seated conflict, and since the headache serves a psychologic function, it may become a way of life for the patient.

Psychogenic headaches are often described in flamboyant terms, without any clear or consistent pattern of timing, location, quality, or aggravating or precipitating factors. The pain may last for months or even years. Characteristically the patient uses vivid terms ("feels like an ax," or "lightning," or "something exploding") to depict the pain, yet does so without demonstrating any apparent discomfort. So psychologically engaging is the headache that many of these patients are unaware of their underlying emotional problems.

Postconcussion Syndrome (posttraumatic nervous instability) is a complicated state characterized by headache, neck pain, nervousness, emotional lability, crying spells, and inability to concentrate. The symptoms are suggestive of an agitated depression following trauma; the syndrome probably represents a variant of psychogenic headache. The correlation between severity of symptoms and seriousness of the injury is minimal. Often legal proceedings and litigation are pending. Because the headache is sometimes throbbing and reproduced by histamine, some authorities believe it has a vascular component.

Focal Pathology. Problems involving the eyes, sinuses, cervical spine, temporomandibular joints, or cranial nerves can be important sources of headache. *Eyestrain* is often blamed for headaches, though in most instances the attribution is incorrect. However, in an occasional patient, astigmatism can cause difficulty when there is prolonged use of the eyes for close work. It produces ocular muscle imbalance and sustained contraction of extraocular, frontal, and temporal muscles; aching discomfort about the orbit and the frontotemporal region results. Refraction corrects the problem. *Acute glaucoma* may produce sudden onset of an orbital headache accompanied by cloudy vision (see Chapters 200 and 206).

Sinusitis can lead to pain about the involved sinus and sensitivity of the overlying skin (see Chapter 217). The pain of sinusitis is sometimes described as throbbing in quality and may be worsened by bending over, thus superficially resembling a vascular or traction type of headache. Characteristic features include the headache's tendency to begin on awakening and to subside on standing up, only to worsen as the day progresses. Many patients with frontal muscle-contraction headaches attribute their problem to "sinus congestion" and self-treat with decongestants to no avail.

Headache is the most common presenting symptom of *cervical radiculopathy*. The pain arises from mechanical irritation of an upper cervical root. Findings on C-spine films are variable, ranging from normal to spondylosis. The pain is often localized to one side of the occiput or base of the skull, with tenderness to palpation. It may start in the neck and at times even radiate to the forehead or eye. The discomfort is described as nagging or aching and aggravated by neck movement. The headache tends to be worse upon awakening, perhaps related to unconscious neck motion during sleep. The mechanism of pain is believed to involve entrapment of upper cervical nerve roots as they course through toward the occiput among irritated nuchal ligaments and muscles.

Temporomandibular joint dysfunction has received much attention in the lay press as a common, yet often overlooked cause of chronic refractory headache. Organic joint changes occasionally do occur, but in most cases the problem is a psychophysiologic disturbance (without malocclusion). Chronic anxiety is very common among these patients, as is nocturnal grinding (bruxism) and jaw clenching. Such chronic involuntary oral habits are viewed as the source of masticatory muscle fatigue and spasm, leading to pain. Chronic, dull, aching unilateral discomfort may be described about the jaw, behind the eyes, in the ears, and even down the neck and into the shoulders. Jaw pain, clicking sounds, and difficulty opening the mouth in the morning are characteristic. Chewing may aggravate symptoms; locking of the jaw is common. On physical examination, masticatory muscle tenderness, mandibular hypomotility, and joint clicking and deviation on opening are noted. Molar prominences may be flattened from chronic teeth grinding.

Tic douloureux (trigeminal neuralgia) is one of the most severe pain syndromes known to man. Paroxysms of lancinating facial or cranial pain occur in middle-aged or elderly patients; these may last only a few seconds but can be excruciating and recurrent. The jaw, gums, lips, or maxillary region may be involved, and a trigger zone is characteristically located in the region (see Chapter 170).

DIFFERENTIAL DIAGNOSIS

The causes of headache can be considered in pathophysiologic terms (Table 159-1). Most serious acute headaches are of the inflammatory type, due to meningeal irritation from infection or hemorrhage, giant cell arteritis, or acute purulent sinusitis. Hypertensive encephalopathy and acute glaucoma are important noninflammatory causes of acute

Table 159-1.   Important Causes of Headache

Traction on Pain-Sensitive Structures
1. Brain tumor or pseudotumor cerebri
2. Brain abscess
3. Subdural hematoma
4. Cerebral edema (hypertensive encephalopathy)
5. Post concussion

Inflammation
1. Meningeal inflammation from infection or hemorrhage
2. Giant cell arteritis
3. Sinusitis

Vascular Dilatation
1. Migraine, common and classic varieties
2. Cluster headache
3. Drugs (e.g., vasodilators)
4. Metabolic disturbances (carbon monoxide poisoning, hypoglycemia)
5. Fever
6. Ateriovenous malformation

Muscle Contraction—Psychogenic Mechanisms
1. Depression
2. Anxiety
3. Conversion reaction
4. Post-traumatic instability
5. Cervical root irritation
6. Temporomandibular joint dysfunction

Miscellaneous
1. Cranial nerve disease (Trigeminal neuralgia)
2. Eyestrain
3. Acute glaucoma
4. Hypertension (moderate to severe)

headache; however, their associated symptoms usually overshadow the headache and dominate the clinical picture. Less worrisome acute headaches are of the nonmigrainous, vascular variety and include those due to high fever, nitrates, and other vasodilators, carbon monoxide poisoning, hypoglycemia, and drug withdrawal.

Most chronic or recurrent headaches result from vasodilatation, excess muscle contraction, or psychologic conflict. The more worrisome chronic headaches are caused by displacement and traction on pain-sensitive intracranial structures; causes include brain tumor, abscess, and chronic subdural hematoma. Diseases of the eye, sinus, cervical spine, temporomandibular joint, and cranial nerves must be considered when the etiology of a chronic or recurring headache remains elusive.

More than one type of headache may be present at a given time.

WORKUP

Acute Headache

History. This should include inquiry into onset, severity, location, and associated symptoms, especially neurologic deficits and fever. A previous history of headaches and head trauma should also be noted. The patient unaccustomed to having headaches who presents with the sudden onset of the worst headache ever experienced deserves prompt attention, particularly if fever, neck stiffness, ataxia, alteration in mental status, focal neurologic deficit, or visual impairment is reported. Diffuse headache in conjunction with a stiff neck and fever suggest acute meningitis. When acute headache and stiff neck occur in conjunction with ataxia of gait and profuse nausea and vomiting, a midline cerebellar hemorrhage needs to be considered. Cerebellar hemorrhage is uncommon, but early recognition is important because prompt treatment can be life saving. Hypertensive encephalopathy may be heralded by diffuse headache, nausea, vomiting, and altered mental status. Acute fever with fronto-orbital headache is suggestive of acute sinusitis. Eye pain and blurred vision raise the possibility of acute glaucoma (see Chapter 201). New onset of headache in an elderly patient requires consideration of temporal arteritis (see Chapter 156).

Acute throbbing headaches are mostly vascular in etiology; the patient needs to be asked about fever, vasodilator use, carbon monoxide exposure, drug withdrawal, and symptoms of hypoglycemia (see Chapter 97).

Physical Examination. The blood pressure and temperature should be checked for any elevations, the scalp for cranial artery tenderness; the sinuses for tenderness to percussion. Pupils are noted for loss of reactivity and the corneas for clouding (indicative of acute glaucoma); the disc margins for blunting, the neck for rigidity on anterior flexion, and the neurologic examination for ataxia, alteration of mental status, and focal deficits.

Laboratory Studies. Patients with meningeal signs require prompt hospitalization, especially if there is evidence of increased intracranial pressure. A lumbar puncture and examination of the cerebrospinal fluid are indicated to rule out an infectious etiology. If there is concern about raised intracranial pressure, an emergency computed tomographic (CT) study is the test of choice (if available), especially if a treatable lesion such as midline cerebellar hemorrhage is a consideration. Sinus films will identify an opacified area due to sinusitis, and an erythrocyte sedimentation rate should be markedly elevated if temporal arteritis is present. Few laboratory studies are necessary for assessment of a vascular headache, but a serum glucose is needed if hypoglycemia is a genuine concern, and a carboxyhemoglobin level is helpful if carbon monoxide poisoning is suspected.

Chronic and Recurrent Headaches

History. It is important to keep in mind that more than one kind of headache may be present; a full description of each type of head pain must be elicited. The quality of the headache, its location, and course over time are the historic features most helpful for identifying a headache of serious etiology. A dull, steady, recurrent, unilateral headache that occurs in the same area each time and progressively worsens in frequency and severity is suggestive of an intracranial mass lesion. In later stages, the headache may become bilateral and more generalized if intracranial pressure increases. Suspicion of a mass lesion necessitates inquiry into causes of brain abscess and subdural hematoma as well as concern about tumor. It is important to ask about chronic ear or sinus infection that has recently flared, parenteral drug use, and lung infection with abscess formation. Patients with brain abscess need not present with fever or focal neurologic deficits. Recent head trauma and a symptom-free interval between injury and onset of headache are characteristic of subdural hematoma; patients may show only subtle personality changes and be mistakenly thought to have a psychogenic problem.

Most throbbing, recurrent headaches are of vascular origin; migraine accounts for the vast majority. Transient neurologic symptoms preceding the headache, family history of "sick headaches," photophobia, nausea, vomiting, and hemicranial location are indicative of classic migraine. Sometimes the focal neurologic complaints that characterize certain auras may be confused with other causes of transient neurologic disturbances. Diagnosis and differentiation are aided by the subsequent occurrence of headache and complete resolution of symptoms within 24 to 48 hours. When headache is absent, diagnosis can be very difficult, but usually headache does occur and aural symptoms resolve with its onset.

Failure of prodromal symptoms to resolve at onset of headache does not rule out migraine, but one needs to consider other causes of transient neurologic deficit. The occurrence of a strictly unilateral vascular headache without such migrainous accompaniments as aura, nausea, or photophobia may be a clue for an A-V malformation, but only if the headache is *always* on the same side.

The presentation of common migraine can sometimes cause confusion, because there is no aura, family history is often negative (over 35% of patients report no family history of "sick headaches"), and the headache may be bilateral or shift sides. Nevertheless, the association of a recurrent throbbing headache with nausea and photophobia is quite suggestive; response to ergot further supports the diagnosis.

Headaches that are variable in quality and location, or constant over weeks to months but not relentlessly progressive in severity are likely to have a muscle contraction or psychogenic etiology. Often there is an underlying depression or anxiety state. It is important to ask about early morning awakening, inability to concentrate, fatigue, low self-esteem, loss of libido, and other somatic symptoms of depression (see Chapter 223), as well as acute and chronic psychosocial problems (see Chapter 222). The patient with a muscle contraction headache may complain of neck soreness, occipital

pain, or tightness about the head, typically worsening as the day progresses. When the description of the headache is dramatic, yet given without evidence of much physical distress, suspicion of a psychogenic etiology should be high. It is helpful to check into any recent minor trauma to the head or neck, which may precipitate a posttraumatic syndrome in the patient with an underlying depression. The diagnosis ought to be considered when an agitated patient reports varying types of discomfort that persist in the area of trauma long after evidence of injury. A nonvascular type of headache that lasts for years is also strongly suggestive of a psychogenic or muscle contraction mechanism.

Sometimes a story of headache awakening the patient from sleep is encountered. Although interruption of sleep by headache occurs in many patients with intracranial mass lesions, it is by no means pathognomonic of a traction headache; psychogenic, muscle contraction, and cluster headaches can do the same. If the interruption of sleep takes place on a daily basis at the same time each night for several weeks, the most likely diagnosis is a cluster headache. The presence of ipsilateral tearing and nasal congestion in conjunction with a piercing periorbital headache that lasts 2 to 3 hours is further evidence for cluster headache.

A chronic or recurrent frontal or periorbital headache of unclear etiology requires inquiry into symptoms of sinusitis (see Chapter 217), cervical spine disease (see Chapter 146), jaw difficulties, and astigmatism. Patients who get headaches after sustained periods of close-up reading should have their eyes checked for refractive errors. However, it is a mistake to blame recurring headaches on eyestrain unless the patient does prolonged close-up work and has a substantial refractive error, which upon correction, terminates the headache.

An occipital headache that is maximal on awakening in the morning and improves as the day progresses may have a hypertensive etiology, especially if it is not worsening as time goes on. However, an occipital headache that does progress in frequency and severity may be a symptom of a posterior fossa mass; an occipital lobe tumor may be mistaken for migraine because scotomata are sometimes produced that may simulate a migrainous aura.

Physical Examination. The temperature and blood pressure should be checked for elevation, the cranial arteries and sinuses for focal tenderness, the discs for blurring of the margins, and the visual fields for defects that are suggestive of a mass lesion along the visual pathways. The nasal cavity is examined for a source of discharge and the ears for signs of chronic otitis media (see Chapter 216); both are potential foci for parameningeal infection that could lead to brain abscess. The mouth is tested for a trigger zone indicative of trigeminal neuralgia, the teeth for signs of bruxism, and the temporomandibular joint for limitation of motion and crepitus.

The neck should be put through a full range of motion, taking note of any limitation of motion and palpating for focal tenderness or zones that reproduce head pain. Patients with muscle contraction headaches often have excessively taut muscles about the shoulders, neck, and occiput. A careful and complete neurologic examination is essential, because the finding of a fixed focal deficit is important evidence of intracranial pathology, especially in a patient with a headache that is progressively worsening.

Laboratory Studies. The patient who reports a chronic or recurrent headache that is getting worse with time deserves consideration for computed tomography (CT), especially if the headache has qualities suggestive of a traction mechanism or if there is an abnormality on neurologic examination. CT is the most sensitive neuroradiologic test for detection of a mass lesion; the false-negative rate is less than 10% and can be further reduced by prior injection of contrast. In a study of 168 ambulatory patients with chronic headache referred for CT, only those with an abnormality on neurologic examination proved to have a clinically important abnormality on CT. All patients with a normal neurologic assessment had normal CT as well as normal skull films, angiogram, or nuclide brain scan. In this study, neuroradiologic investigation was of very low yield in the upper middle-class population that composed the study group, and only served to increase the cost of care, unless one considers the value of a normal test result for the patient.

An occasional headache patient with an intracranial mass lesion may have a normal neurologic examination and little more than a masquerading symptom, such as persistent occipital-nuchal pain in a patient with a posterior fossa tumor. Consequently, the patient with a story that is very suggestive of a mass lesion is a reasonable candidate for CT. This is particularly true for the patient with a subdural hematoma, who may not demonstrate a focal deficit until late in the clinical course. The only manifestation in addition to headache may be a subtle personality change. Nevertheless, it is essential that there be careful selection of patients for CT in order to avoid overutilization of this expensive resource and unnecessary production of false-positive results (see Chapter 2).

Patients suspected of cervical root irritation will usually have normal C-spine films, which need not be ordered unless there are neurologic deficits or symptoms persist for weeks. A tender cranial artery in an older patient is an indication for obtaining a sedimentation rate and considering temporal arteritis (see Chapter 156).

In sum, the efforts taken to perform a careful history and physical examination are well worth the time, for these methods remain the best means available for the accurate diagnosis of headache.

SYMPTOMATIC MANAGEMENT AND PATIENT EDUCATION

Much of the anguish associated with chronic or recurrent headaches is due to concern about etiology. Tumor is a common fear. Although relief of symptoms may be a slow process, it should at least be possible to reduce unnecessary worry. A detailed history that includes eliciting the patient's concerns, combined with a thorough and careful physical examination and discussion of findings, is essential to providing meaningful reassurance. Occasionally, a very anxious patient will insist on a neuroradiologic procedure (*e.g.,* CT), but medically unnecessary testing can often be avoided if time is taken for careful assessment and explanation.

Muscle Contraction Headache. Heat and massage may help to ease muscle spasm due to prolonged, sustained muscle contraction. A mild analgesic such as aspirin or acetaminophen contributes to relief of pain and is superior in double-blind study to placebo, but many patients who come to physicians with muscle contraction headaches complain that such agents are of little help, and request stronger analgesics. It is important to avoid narcotic use in these patients, because symptoms are likely to be chronic. Most muscle relaxants that are employed for muscle contraction headaches (*e.g.,* chlordiazepoxide, methocarbamol [Robaxin]) have little or no direct action on skeletal muscle; they probably exert a beneficial effect by causing sedation and a lessening of anxiety.

Since many of these headaches are a response to environmental or intrapsychic stress, attention should be directed to these important precipitants (see Chapter 222). Many patients find that they tolerate stress better if they carry out a program of regular physical exercise (see Chapter 10). Relaxation techniques (see Chapter 222) help counter stress-induced symptoms. There is insufficient evidence to conclude that biofeedback provides any additional benefit for control of muscle tension headache. Temporomandibular problems respond to similar efforts. Patients should be advised against extensive surgical or dental therapies until simpler means have been given a thorough trial.

When cervical root irritation is the source of discomfort, a soft collar worn at night will often bring improvement (see Chapter 146).

Psychogenic Headache. There is no simple treatment for relief of psychogenic headache. Tricyclic antidepressants may help if there is an underlying depression (see Chapter 223), and settlement of pending litigation sometimes leads to a lessening of posttraumatic headache. For the patient in whom headache is a manifestation of a deep-seated conflict, psychotherapy is often necessary. Because the headache may last for months or years, it is important that narcotics and related agents (*e.g.,* propoxyphene), and agents that can be harmful if used in large cumulative doses (*e.g.,* phenacetin) be avoided. A number of popular headache remedies are combination agents that used to or even still do contain phenacetin; cumulative doses of 2 kg or more have been associated with renal papillary necrosis and interstitial nephritis.

Migraine. See Chapter 166.

INDICATIONS FOR ADMISSION AND REFERRAL

Any patient with evidence suggesting meningeal irritation, increased intracranial pressure, an A-V malformation, or malignant hypertension obviously requires prompt hospital admission. Less urgent situations in which an office consultation with a neurologist may be beneficial include episodes of transient neurologic dysfunction suspected of being migrainous, presence of symptoms suggestive of an intracranial mass lesion, and need for further reassurance in a patient with a muscle contraction or psychogenic headache. Dental consultation is indicated if temporomandibular joint problems appear refractory to conservative therapy. Detection of a tender cranial artery in an elderly patient with a high sedimentation rate should be followed by steroid therapy; if the clinical picture is ambiguous, surgical referral is indicated for biopsy to definitively diagnose temporal arteritis (see Chapter 156).

The ophthalmologist needs to be consulted at once if acute glaucoma is felt to be the cause of an acute orbital headache. If prolonged close-up work is resulting in headaches, a referral is in order for a vision check and assessment of the need for refraction.

Patients with psychogenic headache are sometimes reluctant to consider psychologic basis for their symptoms, but a psychiatric consultation for evaluation can often provide better definition of the conflicts that are troubling the patient than is possible in an office visit to a busy primary physician. The diagnostic consultation may also serve as an important learning experience for the patient vis à vis the importance of psychologic issues and the role of the psychiatrist in the therapeutic effort. However, it is important that a full medical evaluation be conducted before referral is made; otherwise the patient who believes there is a medical basis for the problem may view the referral as an inappropriate dismissal of his symptoms.

A.H.G.

ANNOTATED BIBLIOGRAPHY

Brenner C, Friedman AP, Merritt HH et al: Post-traumatic headache. J Neurosurg 1:379, 1944 (*A classic paper describing the syndrome.*)

Caviness VS, O'Brien P: Headache. N Engl J Med 302:446, 1980 (*An update on mechanisms of vascular headaches.*)

Committee on Classification of Headache: Classification of headache. JAMA 179:717, 1962 (*A helpful scheme based on disease mechanisms.*)

Friedman AP: Nature of headache. Headache 19:163, 1979 (*A useful summary of the important clinical features of common headaches.*)

Guralnick W, Kaban LB, Merrill RG: Temporomandibular-joint afflictions. N Engl J Med 299:123, 1978 (*The definitive paper on the subject: argues strongly against surgical therapy for patients with function disorders.*)

Health and Public Policy Committee, American College of Physicians. Biofeedback for headache. Ann Intern Med 102:128, 1985 (*Current evidence is insufficient to recommend its use in muscle tension and vascular headaches.*)

Larson EB, Omenn GS, Lewis H: Diagnostic evaluation of headache: Impact of computerized tomography. JAMA 243:359, 1980 (*Neuroradiologic evaluation of headache patients with normal neurologic examinations was expensive and clinically unrewarding.*)

Lieberman AN, Jonas S, Hass WK et al: Bilateral cervical carotid and intracranial vasospasm causing cerebral ischemia in a migrainous patient. Headache 24:245, 1984 (*Direct evidence for this suspected mechanism of prodromal symptoms.*)

Peters BH, Fraim CJ, Masel BE: Comparison of 650 mg aspirin and 1,000 mg acetaminophen with each other and with placebo in moderately severe headache. Am J Med 74:36A, 1983 (*Both gave equivalent relief and were clearly superior to placebo for headache pain.*)

Saper JR: Migraine: I. Classification and pathogenesis. JAMA 239:2380, 1978 (*Good review of mechanisms and presentations.*)

White KL: Testimony before the Senate Committee on Labor and Public Welfare, Subcommittee on Health. U.S. Senate, 94th Congress, second session, June 17, 1976. (*Provides statistics on epidemiology of headache and the disability it causes.*)

Wolff HG: Headache and Other Head Pain. New York: Oxford University Press, 1963 (*The classic work on headache; still very useful.*)

160
Evaluation of Dizziness

Dizziness can be one of the more frustrating complaints to assess, a task often made difficult by a vague history and a large number of possible etiologies, ranging from psychiatric disease and cardiovascular disorders to peripheral and central defects within the nervous system. However, with a bit of patience and careful attention to the history and physical examination, the primary physician can conduct a remarkably sophisticated clinical evaluation, one that will help direct further workup and treatment. In the setting of true vertigo, the goals are to distinguish central from peripheral disease, worrisome from benign etiologies.

PATHOPHYSIOLOGY AND CLINICAL PRESENTATION

The patient complaining of "dizziness" may be suffering from vestibular dysfunction, cardiovascular insufficiency, psychiatric illness, metabolic derangement, multiple sensory deficits, cerebellar disease, or a combination of problems.

Vestibular Disease

Patients with vestibular disease experience *true vertigo,* which is defined as a head sensation of abnormal movement, be it internal or in reference to one's surroundings. Descriptive terms include not only "spinning," but also "weaving," "seasickness," "ground rising and falling," "rocking," "things moving," and "merry-go-round" sensation. Nausea, vomiting, and diaphoresis accompany severe cases. Tinnitus and hearing loss indicate associated injury to the auditory component of the VIIIth nerve. Nystagmus is frequently found on examination (see below) or can be induced.

The vestibular problem may be central or peripheral; peripheral lesions include those which are cochlear or retrocochlear. Central lesions differ from peripheral ones in that they typically present with vertigo in association with other brainstem deficits; in peripheral disease, vertigo occurs in isolation except for accompanying tinnitus or hearing loss.

Peripheral Lesions. Benign positional vertigo is a common problem in the elderly, consisting of vertigo experienced only in specific positions. Onset is sudden, usually within a few seconds of assuming the triggering position. Symptoms cease after several minutes if the patient does not move, but will resume with further change in position. In most patients, the condition resolves within 6 months; recovery is usually complete. Head trauma sometimes results in this type of temporary vertigo. One suspected mechanism is development of a small fistula into the middle ear that allows changes of pressure in the middle ear to be transmitted to the inner ear, precipitating vertigo. Another possible explanation is cupulolithiasis: a piece of calcium from the internal apparatus breaks free into the endolymph and pressures the end organ. A more permanent form of positional vertigo results from vascular compression of the vestibular nerve. Patients with this condition suffer from constant positional vertigo and severe nausea; it has been labeled "*disabling positional vertigo*" to distinguish it from the more common forms of positional vertigenous disease.

Ménière's disease ensues from idiopathic endolymphatic hydrops, with damage to the hair cells from swelling of the semicircular ducts. Patients report tinnitus, pressure in the ear, and hearing loss in conjunction with vertigo. Episodes are paroxysmal, last minutes to hours, and then decrease in frequency after multiple attacks, only to recur in several months or years. Hearing loss and tinnitus usually accompany the episodes of vertigo and can be quite disabling.

Acute labyrinthitis develops as a consequence of viral infection involving the cochlea and labyrinth. The patient reports a viral upper respiratory syndrome followed by onset of vertigo, tinnitus, and hearing loss. Symptoms resolve entirely by 3 to 6 weeks, with no residual deficits. *Vestibular neuronitis* is believed to be the same illness, without any cochlear involvement; there is isolated vertigo, no hearing loss, and full clearing.

Ototoxins can injure the peripheral vestibular apparatus, although hearing impairment usually predominates. Streptomycin and gentamycin are among the VIIIth nerve toxins that are most injurious to the vestibular portion of the VIIIth nerve.

Acoustic neuroma (benign schwannoma of the VIIIth nerve) represents the most worrisome of the peripheral lesions, retrocochlear in location and distinguished from the others by its retrocochlear type of hearing loss (see below) and capacity to produce serious brainstem compression if untreated. Initially, symptoms may be indistinguishable from those due to other types of peripheral vestibular disease, starting out as mild hearing loss, tinnitus, and vague dizziness. However, the clinical course is progressive, which should raise suspicion. Nevertheless, only in late stages, as the expanding tumor compresses adjacent structures in the cerebellar-pontine angle, do other cranial nerve and brainstem deficits develop (*e.g.,* facial numbness and weakness). A decreased corneal reflex is one of the earliest signs of damage outside the internal auditory meatus.

Central Lesions. As already noted, these are accompanied in most instances by other brainstem symptoms. In addition, the vertigo and any accompanying nystagmus can be bidirectional or vertical, which does not occur in peripheral vestibular disease.

Multiple sclerosis (MS) causing focal demyelination in the vestibular pathways of the brainstem is an important central etiology of vertigo. The often transient nature of attacks (days to weeks) and subtlety of accompanying symptoms (slight facial numbness or huskiness of voice) may at first cause one to mistaken MS for one of the self-limited peripheral etiologies. Only with repeat episodes might the etiology become more evident. In the later phases of an acute attack, a central type of positional nystagmus may persist after the vertigo resolves. There are no characteristic features of the vertigo; attacks can be sudden, transient, recurrent, or persistent. Diagnosis depends on evidence of discrete CNS lesions and a course of recurrent dysfunction interspersed with remissions.

Vertebrobasilar insufficiency usually produces vertigo in conjunction with diplopia, sensory loss, dysarthria, dysphagia, hemiparesis, and other brainstem deficits. Self-limited episodes are manifestations of transient ischemic attacks. In about one quarter of cases, transient vertigo may be the initial and sole complaint; however, later episodes almost always include other brainstem symptoms.

Drugs that suppress the reticular activating system of the brainstem (*e.g.,* sedatives, anticonvulsants) can cause vertigo of a central nature, especially when taken in excess. Therapeutic doses of some drugs (*e.g.,* phenytoin) produce nystagmus.

Cardiovascular Disease

Cardiac and vascular insufficiency leading to inadequate cerebral perfusion can result in dizziness which patients tend to describe as "*lightheadedness*" or a sense of faintness (see Chapter 18). This form of dizziness is seen in patients with fixed or limited cardiac output, serious cardiac dysrhythmias, diminished vascular tone, or severe intravascular volume depletion. Symptoms characteristically worsen on standing and improve on lying down; postural change in blood pressure and pulse may be noted.

Multiple Sensory Deficits and Cerebellar Disease

These neurologic problems produce sensations of *impaired balance.* Patients report little difficulty when sitting, but become symptomatic upon walking or turning. Those with multiple sensory deficits are usually elderly and suffer from diabetes and other conditions that impair eyesight, position sense, and motor function. Symptoms are typically worse at night and improved by use of a cane or holding onto a railing. The patient with cerebellar disease also feels as if he *might fall;* physical examination is notable for ataxia and other cerebellar signs.

Psychiatric Illness

Patients with psychiatric difficulties complain of ill-defined dizziness ("I just feel dizzy"), constant "lightheadedness," or a "foggy" feeling. Depression, anxiety states, and psychosis, as well as the medications used to treat such conditions, are common precipitants. The precise mechanism of the lightheadedness is unknown, but is thought related to a confusional state induced by these illnesses or by the medications used to treat them. In the case of a panic attack leading to hyperventilation (see Chapter 222), the ensuing metabolic alkalosis may lead to paresthesias and lightheadedness.

Metabolic Disturbances

Alteration of CNS metabolic homeostasis can cause dizziness which resembles that due to inadequate cerebral perfusion. The patient complains of lightheadedness or feeling faint. Precipitants of acute symptoms include hypoglycemia, hypoxia, hypocarbia, hypercarbia, and drugs.

DIFFERENTIAL DIAGNOSIS

Conditions that cause dizziness can be grouped according to pathophysiologic mechanism (Table 160-1). Vestibular disease is divided into central and peripheral types. Central lesions are mostly due to basilar artery disease and multiple sclerosis. Peripheral causes include acoustic neuroma, benign positional vertigo, vestibular neuronitis, Meniere's disease, and ototoxic drugs.

Cardiac and vascular diseases are a second important group. Faintness on standing may be due to critical aortic stenosis, severe volume depletion, the use of antihypertensive drugs, autonomic insufficiency, or prolonged confinement to bed. Carotid sinus hypersensitivity results in inappropriate reduction of vascular tone.

Multiple sensory deficits are most common in diabetics and others with poor vision and peripheral neuropathies. Cervical spondylosis disturbs cervical sensory input and contributes to dizziness. The thick lenses used by patients following cataract surgery distort peripheral vision and can confuse their sense of position. Cerebellar dysfunction leads to a similar clinical presentation of gait unsteadiness.

Psychiatric problems are often associated with lightheadedness. Patients with anxiety, depression, and psychosis report feeling light-headed. At times, tranquilizers and antidepressants are responsible. Metabolic disturbances affecting the CNS have a similar presentation. Hypoxia, hypoglycemia, hypocarbia, and hypercarbia are among the most important.

In a study of 104 consecutive cases referred for evaluation of dizziness, 38% of patients had peripheral vestibular disease,

Table 160-1.   Differential Diagnosis of Dizziness

Vestibular Disease
1. Benign positional vertigo
2. Vestibular neuronitis and ototoxic drugs
3. Meniere's disease
4. Acoustic neuroma and other tumors of the cerebellopontine angle
5. Basilar insufficiency
6. Multiple sclerosis

Cardiac and Vascular Disease
1. Critical aortic stenosis
2. Carotid sinus hypersensitivity
3. Volume depletion and severe anemia
4. Autonomic insufficiency (drugs, diabetes)
5. Diminished vascular reflexes of the elderly

Multiple Sensory Deficits
1. Diabetes mellitus
2. Cataract surgery
3. Some cases of multiple sclerosis
4. Cervical spondylosis
5. Cerebellar disease

Psychiatric Illness
1. Anxiety
2. Depression
3. Psychosis

Metabolic Disturbances
1. Hypoxia
2. Severe hypoglycemia
3. Hypo- and hypercapnia

23% hyperventilation, 13% multiple sensory deficits, 9% psychiatric problems, and 5% cardiovascular or central neurologic illness.

WORKUP

History. The most important initial step in the evaluation of dizziness is to obtain the best possible description of the patient's experience and what he means by "dizziness." A history taken without leading questions or suggested descriptions is most likely to provide meaningful clues. *True vertigo* suggests *vestibular disease; faintness* that is *postural* or paroxysmal implies a *cardiovascular* disorder; constant *ill-defined dizziness* or lightheadedness unrelated to posture points towards a *psychogenic* etiology; a feeling of *poor balance* or disequilibrium typifies *multiple sensory deficits* and *cerebellar* causes.

If the patient complains of *vertigo,* the first task is to determine whether the lesion is *central* or *peripheral.* The most direct way of making the central vs. peripheral distinction is to inquire about brainstem symptoms (*e.g.,* diplopia, facial numbness, weakness, hemiplegia, dysphasia). Evidence of brainstem involvement rules out a peripheral lesion (with the exception of a very advanced acoustic neuroma compressing the cerebellar-pontine angle). The absence of brainstem symptoms does not rule out a central lesion, but makes its

probability very low. Even the very confusing picture of apparently isolated vertigo due to vertebrobasilar insufficiency or multiple sclerosis eventually becomes clearer as accompanying brainstem symptoms become more evident. The pattern of discrete CNS lesions and a course of recurrent episodes followed by remissions further suggest the diagnosis of MS (see Chapter 161).

In the patient with a suspected *peripheral lesion,* the focus turns to distinguishing *cochlear* from *retrocochlear* disease, that is, relatively benign etiologies from acoustic neuroma. The latter has a variable presentation and can initially mimic other peripheral types of vertigo. Episodes of vertigo, tinnitus, pressure in the ear, and hearing loss may take place, simulating Meniere's disease. However, the hearing loss is slowly and steadily progressive, rather than fluctuating or episodic. The development of brainstem symptoms (facial weakness or numbness) is a late occurrence and not very helpful for early diagnosis. When doubt still persists, physical examination and audiologic testing can be used to help make the cochlear/retrocochlear differentiation (see below).

With most other peripheral causes of vertigo, *timing* and *precipitating factors* help elucidate etiology. If symptoms occur only on change of *position* and last but a few moments, the diagnosis is benign positional vertigo, a condition mostly affecting people over 60. It may be a recurrent problem. A single bout of severe spontaneous vertigo, sudden in onset, sometimes after a *viral illness,* is usually vestibular neuronitis. When seen in the context of inner ear infection, it is properly called acute labyrinthitis. Some degree of positional vertigo may remain after the acute illness resolves. Meniere's disease is suggested by acute, recurrent paroxysms of vertigo that are accompanied by *tinnitus* and temporary *hearing loss.* Tinnitus, *pressure* in the ear, and hearing loss are episodic and may precede the other symptoms. Attacks can last for hours to days; residual positional vertigo occurs in 25% of cases.

Obtaining a thorough *drug history* is important. The ototoxic effects of the aminoglycoside antibiotics have been well documented; the diuretic ethacrynic acid also can cause eighth nerve injury, especially in patients with compromised renal function. Potent diuretics may be responsible for severe volume depletion. Vasodilators, phenothiazines, and antihypertensive agents can produce postural light-headedness. Antidepressants and minor tranquilizers cause some patients to feel dizzy.

When the complaint is light-headedness, it is worth asking if standing or turning brings on symptoms. If standing does, antihypertensive, tranquilizer, or antidepressant use should be investigated. During the examination, postural signs, carotid upstroke, and cardiac function should be evaluated, especially for signs of hemodynamically significant aortic stenosis. If turning worsens the situation, it is important to evaluate vision, search for other sensory deficits, and check for cerebellar signs (see below). If light-headedness is a constant sensation, an underlying psychiatric or metabolic disorder is likely. Anxiety and depression are frequent causes and warrant investigation (see chapters 222 and 223).

Physical Examination. General appearance can be quite informative. The overly anxious person will appear nervous and may sigh frequently during the interview. *Blood pressure* and pulse should be taken and noted for changes between readings taken in the *supine* and *standing* positions. The skin is examined for pallor, the eyes for *nystagmus* (remembering that a few beats of nystagmus on extreme lateral gaze are normal) and the ears for tympanic membrane lesions and *hearing acuity* (see below). The carotid arteries in the neck are checked for bruits (suggestive of cerebrovascular disease) and delay in upstroke (characteristic of severe aortic stenosis). A forceful, sustained left ventricular impulse, single second heart sound, and loud ejection quality murmur on cardiac examination also support a diagnosis of significant aortic stenosis (see Chapters 15 and 28).

A thorough and careful *neurologic examination* is essential, particularly when the possibility of central vestibular disease is being considered. Most important is examination for a brainstem lesion, which suggests central pathology or extrinsic compression by an acoustic neuroma. Cranial nerves V, VII, and X can be affected by a large acoustic neuroma pressing at the cerebellopontine angle of the brain stem. Testing of sensory function, peripheral vision, and gait often reveals multiple defects in elderly patients troubled by dizziness. The *Romberg test* (standing with feet together, eyes closed) will also be abnormal in such patients as well as in some with vestibular disease. The side to which the vertiginous patient sways has value in helping to localize the lesion. Cerebellar testing helps detect any ataxia.

Provocative maneuvers designed to trigger symptoms and reproduce the patient's complaint can be extremely useful. *Hyperventilating* for 2 minutes will reproduce the light-headedness that many call "dizziness." *Standing quickly* from a supine position will cause the susceptible patient to feel faint; turning quickly while walking can cause symptoms in the patient with multiple sensory deficits or cerebellar disease. The Barany maneuver and other forms of vestibular stimulation (see below) are indicated for those with vertigo.

Maneuvers which alleviate symptoms are also of diagnostic use. Getting up slowly lessens the faint feeling associated with cardiovascular causes; *paper bag rebreathing* reduces the light, giddy feeling that follows hyperventilation; *lying still* in one position may halt positional vertigo; touching the examiner's hand or using a *cane* to walk helps the patient with sensory deficits or cerebellar dysfunction. Withholding suspected drugs may be informative.

Simple office tests of hearing and stimulation of the vestibular apparatus can be very helpful in distinguishing central from peripheral disease, and cochlear from retrocochlear peripheral pathology. The *Rinne test* (see Chapter 210) identifies which VIIIth nerve is involved and helps differentiate between conductive and sensorineural hearing loss. Patients with a sensorineural hearing deficit may have a cochlear lesion or a retrocochlear one. The distinction can be made by testing *speech discrimination,* which is easily performed in the office by whispering a series of ten, two single-syllable, closely linked words (*e.g.,* baseball, ice cream) into the patient's ear while making a sound in the other ear to limit its participation. The patient is asked to repeat each whispered word. Correctly identifying fewer than 20% of the words is very suggestive of a retrocochlear lesion (which causes a disproportionate loss of speech discrimination); a score of 70% or better indicates the problem is cochlear. Scores in between these are indeterminate and necessitate formal audiologic testing (see Chapter 210).

Vestibular stimulation testing serves both as a good provocative test for reproducing symptoms (useful when the description of dizziness remains unclear) and as a means of distinguishing peripheral from central vestibular disease. The *Barany maneuver* (see Figure 160-1) is the least noxious of the standard forms vestibular stimulation. The patient starts in a sitting position on the examination table and lies down with his head extending over the edge of the table, tilted back and turned 45° to one side. The assumption of this position need not be overly abrupt, but it should be held for at least 30 seconds. The maneuver is repeated, this time turning the head 45° to the opposite side. A final time the test is repeated without turning the head.

The Barany maneuver provides simultaneous stimulation of all three semicircular canals. It is a useful provocative maneuver and potentially helpful in separating peripheral from central vestibular disease. One asks the patient to look straight ahead and watches for onset of nystagmus and reproduction of symptoms. If symptoms occur, one asks to which side do things seem to be spinning; if nystagmus ensues, one notes to which side the slow phase moves. Combining these results with findings from Romberg and Rinne testing, one can make a diagnosis of a peripheral lesion if (1) the slow phase of nystagmus moves toward the same side as the hearing loss; (2) the patient reports the spinning is away from the side of the hearing loss; (3) the Romberg test is positive and the patient sways toward the side of the hearing deficit. Absence of any one of these findings suggests a central lesion.

Laboratory Studies. *Electronystagmography* and audiologic testing are indicated when clinical and provocative data are insufficient to differentiate between central and peripheral causes of vertigo (see Chapter 210). If acoustic neuroma is suspected, then one should consider *brainstem auditory evoked response* testing. It represents the best audiologic means of differentiating cochlear from retrocochlear disease. In addition, *computed tomography* of the internal auditory canal and C-P angle should follow if evidence of a retrocochlear lesion emerges from audiologic testing. If basilar transient ischemic attacks are a concern because of transient, isolated vertiginous spells, it is felt by most authorities much safer to wait for confirmation by the appearance of accompanying brainstem symptoms than to hastily order angiography or anticoagulation.

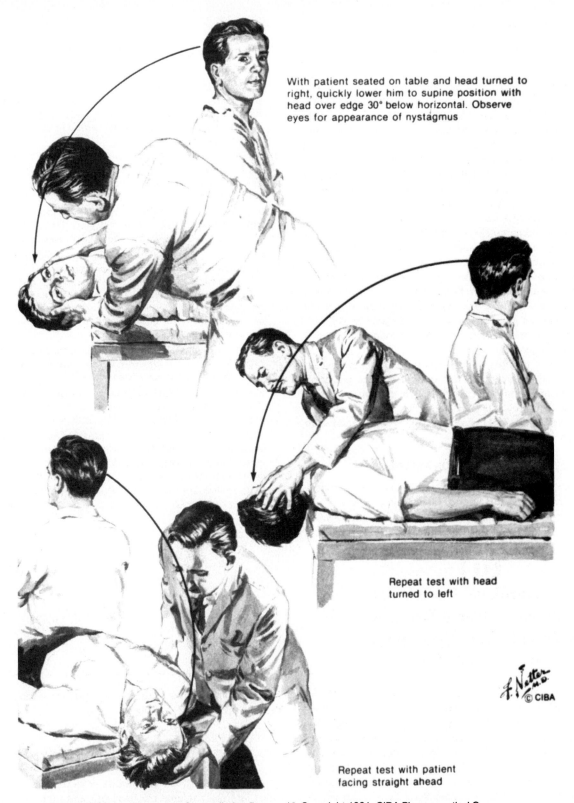

With patient seated on table and head turned to right, quickly lower him to supine position with head over edge 30° below horizontal. Observe eyes for appearance of nystagmus

Repeat test with head turned to left

Repeat test with patient facing straight ahead

Figure 160-1. Barany test for vestibular disease. (© Copyright 1981. CIBA Pharmaceutical Company, Division of CIBA-GEIGY Corporation. Reproduced with permission from Clinical Symposia by Frank H. Netter, M.D. All rights reserved.)

725

SYMPTOMATIC THERAPY AND PATIENT EDUCATION

Dizziness can be controlled in most instances. Therapy is aimed at the underlying pathophysiology. True vertigo responds to avoidance of precipitating positions and movements, use of meclizine 25 to 50 mg q6h PRN, and, if nausea and vomiting are not controlled by meclizine alone, promethazine 25 mg q6h PRN. These drugs are sedating and can cause drowsiness (which may be welcome in a patient having an acute attack, but is an adverse effect in treatment of chronic disease). Low-dose meclizine (12.5 mg tid) is quite effective in elderly patients and causes less sedation.

Cardiovascular faintness requires assuring adequate hydration, standing up slowly, and discontinuing or reducing offending drugs. The patient with critical aortic stenosis should undergo evaluation for surgery (see Chapter 28).

Psychogenic light-headedness may be refractory to symptomatic therapy. For acute hyperventilation, rebreathing into a paper bag is effective. Treatment with an antianxiety agent might help, but it can also cause symptoms (see Chapter 222). Patients with multiple sensory deficits are aided by use of a walker and good lighting.

The vast majority of people with dizziness have benign disorders. Symptomatic therapy combined with explanation and reassurance is always comforting. In particular, patients tolerate their problems better when they know that in most instances the symptom can be controlled or will resolve on its own.

INDICATIONS FOR REFERRAL

Neurologic consultation is indicated when there is concern about central vestibular disease or acoustic neuroma.

A.H.G.

ANNOTATED BIBLIOGRAPHY

Drachman DA, Hart CW: An approach to the dizzy patient. Neurology 22:323, 1972 (*In a series of 104 patients seen in a dizziness clinic, secure diagnoses were reached in 91%, with peripheral vestibular disease, hyperventilation, and multiple sensory deficits making up over two-thirds of cases. Article provides details of diagnostic measures.*)

Fisher CM: Vertigo in cerebrovascular disease. Arch Otolaryngol 85: 85, 1967 (*Argues that unaccompanied dizziness is unlikely to be vascular in origin and that it is safe to wait and watch for developments rather than risk anticoagulation or arteriography.*)

Hart GH, Gardner DP, Howieson J: Acoustic tumors: Atypical features and recent diagnostic tests. Neurology (NY) 33:211, 1983 (*Excellent discussion of making this difficult diagnosis.*)

Hitselberger WE: Tumors of the cerebellopontine angle in relation to vertigo. Arch Otolaryngol 85:95, 1967 (*In a series of 136 patients with surgically confirmed c-p angle tumors, only 25% had vertigo, only 12% had spontaneous nystagmus, but 92% had decreased response to caloric stimulation. The hearing loss associated with vertigo was progressive, distinguishing this condition from Meniere's disease.*)

Jannetta PJ, Moller MB, Moller AR: Disabling positional vertigo. N Engl J Med 310:1700, 1984 (*Report of a newly discovered form of vertigo linked to vascular compression of the vestibular nerve.*)

Schuknecht HF: Cupulolithiasis. Arch Otolaryngol 90:765, 1969 (*Calcium flecks were found, raising the question of an etiologic role in positional vertigo.*)

Schumacher GA: Demyelinating disease as a cause for vertigo. Arch Otolaryngol 85:93, 1967 (*Makes the important point that nothing in the character of vertigo due to multiple sclerosis is pathognomonic or even characteristic of central origin of vertigo.*)

Snow JB, Jr: Positional vertigo. N Engl J Med 310:1740, 1984 (*An editorial summarizing current methods in the evaluation of vertigo.*)

161
Focal Neurologic Complaints: Evaluation of Nerve Root and Peripheral Nerve Syndromes

AMY A. PRUITT, M.D.

Primary physicians are frequently asked to evaluate complaints of focal numbness, tingling, weakness, pain, or some combination of these. In general, major acute neurologic disease is not at issue during an office visit. Nevertheless, the broad range of outpatient complaints encountered encompasses lesions throughout the nervous system. Disorders of nerve roots and peripheral nerves in the upper and lower extremities are especially common. Several syndromes should be analyzable by the primary physician. Identification and localization of these problems can facilitate thorough neurologic evaluation and accurately segregate those cases that must be referred to a neurologist.

PATHOPHYSIOLOGY AND CLINICAL PRESENTATION

Many peripheral nerves, because of their superficial location, are easily injured mechanically, and others are vulnerable because of specific anatomic variants or because of alterations in anatomy caused by degenerative disease.

Upper Extremity Syndromes

Cervical Radiculopathy and Myelopathy. Age-related loss of water and elasticity in cervical discs leads to increased stress on vertebral bodies. Osteophytic spurs develop and may encroach on nerve roots (see Fig. 161-1). More serious but less common is encroachment on the spinal cord itself by progressive cervical spondylotic changes. Usually a combination of radiculopathy involving the C5, C6, or C7 roots (see Fig. 161-2) and myelopathy is present. The presence of cord compression due to spondylosis is indicated by radicular pain, variable weakness, diminished reflexes, and atrophy in the arms, with spastic weakness and hyperreflexia in the lower extremities.

It may be difficult to distinguish cervical spondylotic myelopathy from other progressive myelopathies, which include multiple sclerosis, subacute combined degeneration due to vitamin B_{12} deficiency, spinal tumor, syringomyelia, and amyotrophic lateral sclerosis. Suspicion of myelopathy should prompt referral to a neurologist.

Radiologic assessment usually includes cervical spine films. Unfortunately, nearly 50% of patients over age 50 show degenerative cervical spine changes on x-ray, and these do not correlate well with the degree of abnormality found clinically in either radiculopathy or myelopathy. Nevertheless, plain cervical spine films with oblique views to visualize the neural foramina are often informative. If the patient has only radiculopathy, a conservative trial of cervical traction is sometimes helpful (see Chapter 146). If myelopathy is suspected, myelography may be necessary to define the extent of compression, to rule out neoplastic lesions, and to assist the surgeon in a decision about decompressive laminectomy.

Brachial Plexus Neuritis. A painfully disabling condition, this syndrome develops in some patients after an immunization and presents with severe shoulder and upper arm pain followed by weakness which usually involves the upper roots of the plexus more than the lower ones. Prognosis is ultimately good, but recovery may be prolonged. Clinical examination reveals variable weakness and sensory loss in C5–T1 root distributions (see Fig. 161-2) with diminished deep tendon reflexes. Because of the involvement of many nerve roots, confusion with a cervical disc does not usually arise. Electromyography and nerve conduction studies help to localize the abnormality. Apical lordotic views of the chest should be obtained to rule out the possibility of neoplastic invasion of the plexus from an intrathoracic tumor.

Thoracic Outlet Syndrome. A cervical rib or bony abnormality of the first rib may lead to pressure on the subclavian artery or brachial plexus as it passes through the thoracic outlet (see Fig. 161-1). Diagnosis is primarily clinical and includes the presence of pain in the arm in certain positions, color changes in the hand, and a pattern of sensory loss and weakness most pronounced in the fourth and fifth fingers. Deep tendon reflexes are usually normal. The differential diagnosis includes Raynaud's phenomenon, ulnar nerve entrapment at the elbow, and compression of the brachial plexus from neoplasm or from fibrosis due to radiation.

Cervical spine films are extremely important to demonstrate cervical ribs or elongated transverse processes of C7. Electromyography may be entirely normal, but will help to exclude a defect at the elbow or a carpal tunnel syndrome. Ultrasonography of the subclavian artery with the arm held in different positions may help define the extent of compression.

Most surgeons advocate removal of the potentially constricting structures (cervical rib, fascial band to first rib, or first rib). Shoulder exercises to improve posture are often advised first, and orthopedic advice should be sought in each case.

Long Thoracic Nerve Entrapment. This nerve arises from the brachial plexus and innervates the serratus anterior. It is vulnerable to injury in workers who lift or push heavy loads, occurs after direct trauma from heavy backpacks, and may evolve over several months after the injury. The patient notes a change in the appearance of the shoulder, and examination reveals winging of the scapula. Most cases have a good prognosis.

Carpal Tunnel Syndrome. In this disorder, the median nerve is entrapped at the carpal tunnel (see Fig. 161-1) because of pressure from ligamentous thickening. Most cases are idiopathic, but the disorder may be seen with rheumatoid arthritis, pregnancy, acromegaly, hypothyroidism, fractures of the carpal bones, amyloidosis, and myeloma. A combination of pain, paresthesias, and numbness in the median nerve distribution is the earliest complaint, often worse at night (see Fig. 161-2). Later, muscle weakness (particularly of thumb abduction and opposition) occurs, and thenar atrophy may be seen. Importantly, aching pain can be felt as far up as the shoulder and should not distract the examiner's attention from the wrist. Tapping on the wrist may reproduce the pain (Tinel's sign).

Differential diagnosis includes radiculopathy from cervical spine disease, but the exact location of the pain should conform to the median nerve rather than to just one nerve root distribution. Electromyography and nerve conduction studies with motor and sensory conduction latencies of the median nerve provide the most useful data. While some cases respond to conservative therapy (wrist splints, anti-inflammatory medications), surgical relief is relatively easy and effective. Failure to respond to surgical therapy should prompt rechecking of the nerve conduction studies, careful re-examination, and consideration of the possibility of coexistent cervical spine disease or of median nerve compression higher in the forearm.

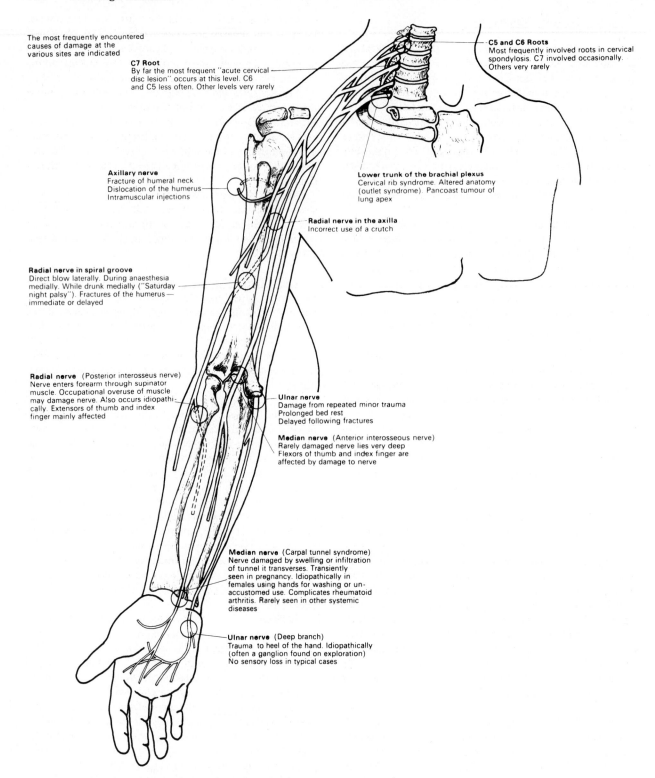

The most frequently encountered causes of damage at the various sites are indicated

C5 and C6 Roots
Most frequently involved roots in cervical spondylosis. C7 involved occasionally. Others very rarely

C7 Root
By far the most frequent "acute cervical disc lesion" occurs at this level. C6 and C5 less often. Other levels very rarely

Axillary nerve
Fracture of humeral neck
Dislocation of the humerus
Intramuscular injections

Lower trunk of the brachial plexus
Cervical rib syndrome. Altered anatomy (outlet syndrome). Pancoast tumour of lung apex

Radial nerve in the axilla
Incorrect use of a crutch

Radial nerve in spiral groove
Direct blow laterally. During anaesthesia medially. While drunk medially ("Saturday night palsy"). Fractures of the humerus — immediate or delayed

Radial nerve (Posterior interosseus nerve)
Nerve enters forearm through supinator muscle. Occupational overuse of muscle may damage nerve. Also occurs idiopathically. Extensors of thumb and index finger mainly affected

Ulnar nerve
Damage from repeated minor trauma
Prolonged bed rest
Delayed following fractures

Median nerve (Anterior interosseous nerve)
Rarely damaged nerve lies very deep
Flexors of thumb and index finger are affected by damage to nerve

Median nerve (Carpal tunnel syndrome)
Nerve damaged by swelling or infiltration of tunnel it transverses. Transiently seen in pregnancy. Idiopathically in females using hands for washing or unaccustomed use. Complicates rheumatoid arthritis. Rarely seen in other systemic diseases

Ulnar nerve (Deep branch)
Trauma to heel of the hand. Idiopathically (often a ganglion found on exploration) No sensory loss in typical cases

Figure 161-1. Peripheral nerve distribution to the upper limb. (Patten J: Neurological Differential Diagnosis. New York, Springer-Verlag, 1977)

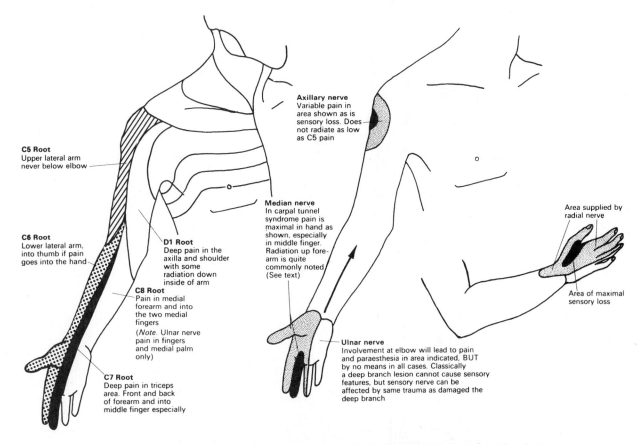

Figure 161-2. (*Left*) Distribution of root pain and paresthesia. (*Right*) Distribution of peripheral nerve pain and paresthesia. (Patten J: Neurological Differential Diagnosis. New York, Springer-Verlag, 1977)

Ulnar Nerve Entrapment. The most common location of ulnar entrapment is at the elbow (see Fig. 161-1). Causes include fracture deformities, arthritis, faulty positioning of the arm during surgery, or repetitive occupational or recreational trauma (*e.g.,* tennis). Sensation is usually spared in the forearm, but there is sensory loss in the fifth finger and half of the fourth (see Fig. 161-2). Wasting of the intrinsic muscles of the hand with weakness of grip occurs later. Nerve conduction studies can accurately localize the site of compression. If there is focal entrapment, repositioning of the nerve or elbow synovectomy may be necessary, but patients with trauma, diabetes, or the so-called "tardy" ulnar palsies (dysfunction developing late after injury) may not improve.

Radial Nerve Injuries. Compression of the radial nerve most often occurs in the axilla or the upper arm. It may be seen with improperly used crutches, with prolonged pressure during sleep (the Saturday night palsy), or as a result of direct injury. Wrist drop is the prominent feature. Vasomotor or atrophic changes are rarely present, and prognosis is good (recovery within 6 to 8 weeks).

Lower Extremity Syndromes

Lateral Femoral Cutaneous Nerve Compression. Also known as meralgia paresthetica, this syndrome involves a nerve formed by branches arising from the second and third lumbar roots. The nerve enters the thigh in close relation to the inguinal ligament, the anterior superior iliac spine, and the sartorius muscle insertion (Fig. 161-3). It is purely sensory and supplies the anterolateral and lateral aspects of the thigh almost as far as the knee (Fig. 161-4). Compression causes an extremely unpleasant, characteristic burning pain with increased cutaneous sensitivity. Sitting or lying usually provides relief, but standing or walking exacerbates the pain. The syndrome often occurs in obesity, in pregnancy, or when tight corsets are worn. It is more common in diabetics. Differential diagnosis includes a lesion of the second or third lumbar roots, usually associated with low back pain radiating

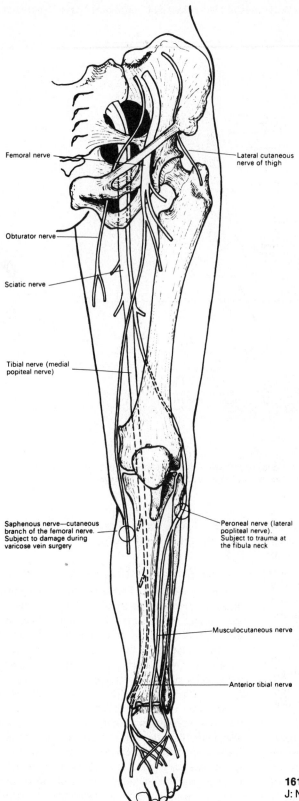

Femoral nerve

Lateral cutaneous
nerve of thigh

Obturator nerve

Sciatic nerve

Tibial nerve (medial
popliteal nerve)

Saphenous nerve—cutaneous
branch of the femoral nerve.
Subject to damage during
varicose vein surgery

Peroneal nerve (lateral
popliteal nerve).
Subject to trauma at
the fibula neck

Musculocutaneous nerve

Anterior tibial nerve

161-3. Peripheral nerve distribution to the lower limb. (Patten J: Neurological Differential Diagnosis. New York, Springer-Verlag, 1977)

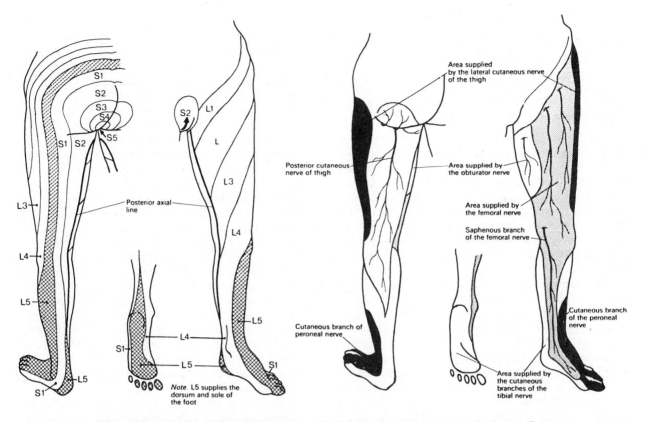

Figure 161-4. (*Left*) Lumbosacral dermatomes. (*Right*) Lower limb peripheral nerve distribution. (Patten J: Neurological Differential Diagnosis. New York, Springer-Verlag, 1977)

into the lower leg. Sensory changes in this case will extend further down the leg and more medially, and there is iliopsoas or quadriceps weakness. Weakness and reflex changes do not occur in meralgia paresthetica. The neuropathy tends to regress spontaneously, but weight loss should be encouraged.

Femoral Neuropathy. The femoral nerve derives from the second, third, and fourth lumbar roots. Its posterior division is the major innervation to the quadriceps and terminates as the saphenous nerve, which supplies sensation to the medial aspect of the leg as far as the medial malleolus (see Fig. 161-3). Onset of femoral neuropathy is frequently sudden, painful, and followed quickly by wasting and weakness in the quadriceps, loss of knee jerk, and sensory impairment over the anteromedial thigh (see Fig. 161-4). If there is also marked hip flexion weakness, the site of the lesion is usually in the lumbar plexus. Sensory symptoms in the saphenous distribution are uncommon in lesions of the main trunk of the femoral nerve.

Entrapment may occur in the inguinal region and from direct retroperitoneal compression by tumor or hematoma. However, the most common cause is presumed to be nerve infarction, seen usually in diabetics. A combination of thigh pain, weakness, and sensory deficit can be a manifestation of an isolated diabetic femoral neuropathy, although electromyographically, the involvement in such cases is frequently more widespread. While some improvement may occur, the patient is often left quite weak.

Sciatic Nerve Syndromes. The sciatic nerve arises from the lumbosacral plexus (L4 to S3) and terminates in the common peroneal and tibial nerves (see Fig. 161-3). The tibial nerve supplies gastrocnemius, plantaris, soleus, and popliteus muscles, while its extension into the calf, the posterior tibial nerve, supplies muscles of the calf. All these muscles are involved in plantar flexion. The common peroneal nerve divides into the superficial and deep peroneal nerves. The latter supplies the muscles that dorsiflex the foot and toes. The superficial peroneal nerve innervates the muscles that evert the foot.

Sciatic nerve compression may result from tumors within the pelvis or from prolonged sitting or lying on the buttocks. Gluteal abscesses and misplaced buttock injections have caused sciatic injury. Weakness of the gluteal muscles and pain in the sciatic notch area imply compression within the pelvis. Lesions just beyond the sciatic notch cause weakness in the hamstrings and in all the muscles of the lower leg.

Common peroneal compression usually occurs at the level

of the fibular head (see Fig. 161-3) and is seen in cachectic patients following prolonged bed rest, in alcoholics, in diabetics, and in patients placed in tight casts. Injury leads to faulty dorsiflexion and eversion of the foot, producing a characteristic footdrop with a slapping gait. Complete or partial recovery can be expected when paralysis results from transient pressure. Treatment consists of a foot brace and careful avoidance of compressive positions.

Lumbar Disc Syndromes. Compressive neuropathies of the lower limbs must be distinguished from the very common lumbar disc syndromes. In the lumbar region, the fourth and fifth discs are most frequently affected (*i.e.,* the discs between L4 and L5 vertebral bodies and between L5 and S1 vertebrae). The most common complaint is sudden onset of severe low back pain (see Chapter 145). The inciting event is often trivial, though heavy lifting or an acute twisting motion is sometimes reported. The pain is worsened by bending forward, sneezing, or straining.

The herniated disc can compress one or more nerve roots, but a disc herniation at a particular level generally causes a distinctive picture (see Chapter 145). *L4-5 disc herniation* usually affects the L5 root with pain over sciatic notch, lateral thigh, and leg, numbness of web of great toe and lateral leg, weakness of dorsiflexion of the great toe and foot, and no reflex changes (see Fig. 161-4). *L5-S1 disc herniation* catches the S1 root, producing pain down the back of the leg to the heel; numbness in the lateral heel, foot, and toe; weakness of plantar flexion; and loss of ankle jerk (see Fig. 161-4). Once the root level is defined, the usual course is a trial of bed rest and analgesia (see Chapter 145) unless there is pronounced weakness, uncontrollable pain, or bladder and bowel dysfunction. In these cases, acute myelography may be necessary to define the extent of disc protrusion and to rule out more unusual causes of lumbar radiculopathy such as neurofibroma.

WORKUP

Identification of the nerve root or peripheral nerve syndrome and precise localization of the neurologic lesion is possible in the office setting and, in most instances, does not require elaborate knowledge of neuroanatomy or extensive dependence on laboratory studies. Assessment is facilitated by determining (1) whether the problem is peripheral (in a nerve root or peripheral nerve) or central (in the cord or above); (2) whether the problem, if peripheral, is due to a lesion in the peripheral nerve or to nerve root injury; (3) whether there is evidence of cord compression (manifested by signs of myelopathy), particularly with upper extremity syndromes; (4) whether there is evidence (in other extremities) of more widespread peripheral neuropathy (*e.g.,* the diabetic patient with a femoral neuropathy who also has a diffuse peripheral neuropathy); and (5) whether the presence of weakness is due to a muscle or nerve lesion.

The neurologic examination should be organized to address these issues and answer the following questions:

1. Is the lesion upper motor neuron (UMN) or lower motor neuron (LMN)? Fasciculations, flaccidity, and the lack of reflexes indicate a LMN lesion and suggest that the disorder originates at the anterior horn cell or peripheral nerve level. Spasticity and increased reflexes are evidence for a lesion above the anterior horn cell that supplies the involved musculature. Thus, a cervical disc at the C6 level might decrease the biceps reflex and result in biceps weakness and atrophy, while causing increased reflexes and spasticity below that level.

2. Is the nerve dysfunction confined to one root or dermatome or to one peripheral nerve? A positive answer to this question suggests a compression neuropathy such as a radial, ulnar, or median nerve palsy. Findings of more generalized dysfunction such as diffusely decreased deep tendon reflexes, absent vibration sense at the ankles, and a stocking-glove pattern of sensory loss suggest a more diffuse peripheral neuropathy. Commonly seen forms of peripheral neuropathy include those associated with diabetes mellitus, excess alcohol consumption, toxin and drug exposure, and genetic diseases such as Charcot-Marie-Tooth atrophy. An electromyogram can localize the individual nerve abnormality and can confirm the presence of a generalized neuropathy.

3. Is the weakness due to nerve or to muscle disease? Weakness in conjunction with altered tendon reflexes and sensory loss suggests nerve disease. Primary muscle pathology results in preserved reflexes and normal sensation. Characteristic patterns of muscle weakness occur in the genetically determined muscular dystrophies. The toxic and metabolic myopathies produce largely proximal muscle weakness, in contrast to almost all primary nerve diseases, which affect distal musculature early and preferentially. Serum muscle enzyme elevations are seen in muscle disease, and some muscular disorders are associated with myotonia. The electromyogram coupled with nerve conduction studies can distinguish primary muscle disease from neuropathic processes.

Clinical identification of nerve root and peripheral nerve syndromes is often facilitated by selective use of radiologic, nerve conduction, electromyographic, and serologic studies (as detailed in discussions of each of the important syndromes). However, dependence on laboratory studies for initial assessment is usually not necessary.

INDICATIONS FOR REFERRAL AND ADMISSION

Evidence of acute spinal cord compression is an indication for immediate neurosurgical consultation and hospitalization. The patient with symptoms and signs of a slowly progressive myelopathy requires neurologic consultation, especially if myelography is being considered. A root or peripheral nerve compression syndrome usually needs surgical repair, and the patient with such a problem will need to see the neurosurgeon or orthopedist skilled in its treatment. Nevertheless, before referral, the primary physician should have localized the problem and instituted appropriate initial therapy.

ANNOTATED BIBLIOGRAPHY

Aguayo AJ: Neuropathy due to compression and entrapment. In Dyck PJ *et al* (eds): Peripheral Neuropathy. Philadelphia, W.B. Saunders, 1975, p. 688 (*Detailed discussion of the compression neuropathies.*)

Aids to the Diagnosis of Peripheral Nerve Injuries. 3rd ed. London, Her Majesty's Stationery Office, 1976 (*A classic; each muscle test is carefully illustrated and nerve innervation is beautifully diagrammed.*)

Chusid J: Correlative Neuroanatomy and Functional Neurology, 18 ed. Los Altos, Lange Medical Publications, 1977 (*Complete with numerous charts and diagrams, this is a succinct discussion of physiologic principles for the purpose of clinical diagnosis.*)

Dyck PJ: The causes, classification and treatment of peripheral neuropathy. N Engl J Med 307:283, 1982 (*A very short, but interesting review; good overview of a complex subject.*)

Keim HA: Low back pain. CIBA Clinical Symposia, 25(3): 1973 (*Well-diagrammed discussion of degenerative disc disease with excellent illustration of lumbar disc syndromes.*)

Warmolts JR: Electrodiagnosis in neuromuscular disorders. Ann Intern Med 95:599, 1981 (*A good review for the generalist of nerve conduction studies and electromyography.*)

162

Evaluation of Tremor

AMY A. PRUITT, M.D.

Tremor is best defined as a regular oscillation of a body part and must be distinguished from other rapid, involuntary movements. Many patients assume that the development of "shakiness" is a natural concomitant of aging. The physician must determine the significance of a variety of clinically similar tremors that may have widely dissimilar diagnostic, therapeutic, and prognostic implications. Workup involves differentiating the resting tremor of early parkinsonism from essential tremor and differentiating essential tremor from an exaggerated physiologic tremor. As new specific treatments are developed, accurate clinical distinction becomes increasingly valuable. Unfortunately, it may be difficult to differentiate tremors by clinical observation alone, and evaluation requires a working knowledge of simple electrophysiologic and pharmacologic characteristics.

PATHOPHYSIOLOGY AND CLINICAL PRESENTATION

The precise neural mechanisms of tremor remain unknown despite some clinicopathologic correlations, such as abolition of the parkinsonian and essential tremors by lesions in the ventrolateral nucleus of the thalamus. Drugs such as L-dopa, which are known to act centrally to increase catecholamines, may worsen essential tremor; this observation has led to the suggestion that beta-adrenergic blockers such as propranolol might exert their therapeutic action by central antagonism of beta-adrenergic receptors.

The patient most frequently reports the insidious onset of "shaking" of a limb. Very likely, he will have ignored the symptom's presence initially, assuming it was due to nervousness or fatigue. However, its steady progression brings him to see the physician. Tremors can be present during maintenance of a posture, at rest, or during an action (intention tremor).

Postural tremors are fine tremors with a frequency of 8 to 12 Hz; they occur normally in everyone during movement and while holding a fixed position. A true "physiologic" tremor is defined as one that does not produce symptoms and is within the given frequency range. It is unaffected by administration of propranolol or alcohol. The movement is usually invisible to the naked eye, but may become exaggerated by anxiety, coffee ingestion, or hyperthyroidism. Drugs, notably lithium and tricyclic antidepressants, may also accentuate this tremor. Amplitude and frequency vary among different people and in the same person at different times.

Intention tremors include those labeled essential (familial) and senile. *Essential tremor* may appear to be a variant or more extreme form of physiologic tremor. However, symptomatic essential tremors are of larger amplitude (hence, visible to the naked eye) and relatively slower frequency than genuine physiologic tremors. Their electromyogram (EMG) characteristically shows synchronous bursts of activity in antagonistic muscle groups. There often is a positive family history and the report of gradual progression; tremor is absent at rest and clearly present in the outstretched arms. It is accentuated by tasks that require precision (*e.g.,* writing, carrying full cups of liquid) and by phenothiazines and haloperidol. It is suppressed by alcohol and propranolol. *Senile tremor* has the same physiologic and pharmacologic qualities as essential tremor. It is usually first seen in the hands, often remaining there, but sometimes involving the head and legs as well. Essential tremor may begin at any time; senile tremor usually becomes apparent by the sixth or seventh decade.

A more dramatic action tremor is displayed by patients

with *cerebellar diseases* and is characterized by progressively increasing amplitude of the tremor as the patient brings the limb toward a target. In younger patients, this is most frequently caused by multiple sclerosis, but similar clinical states may be produced by cerebellar infarction, by degenerative disorders of the spinocerebellar pathways, and by chronic relapsing steroid-sensitive polyneuropathy. This tremor is multiplanar with large, irregular, and relatively slow (2–4 Hz) oscillations. The tremor often is worsened by alcohol. Propranolol has no effect, and no satisfactory therapy is available.

Rest tremors. The most common rest tremor in a relaxed, supported limb is that due to *Parkinson's disease.* It characteristically begins in the fingers and may later involve the arm and the leg. Flexion and extension of the fingers, abduction and adduction of the thumbs, and pronation and supination of the wrist produce the well-known "pill-rolling" movement. Frequently, this is the symptom that brings parkinsonian patients to the physician and may occur well in advance of bradykinesia or postural difficulties characteristic of the full-blown syndrome. It is important, of course, to distinguish this tremor from essential tremor, which demands a different treatment and portends a different prognosis. The parkinsonian tremor is slow (3–8 Hz), and its EMG, quite unlike that of essential tremor, shows alternating discharge in antagonistic muscle groups. This EMG activity is suppressed with voluntary movement.

A few parkinsonian patients may also have a typical action (essential) tremor, and L-dopa therapy may worsen it. Phenothiazines and haloperidol worsen the tremor-at-rest (see Chapter 167).

Other abnormal movements. The definition of tremor as a regular oscillation of a body part serves to distinguish it from other rapid, intermittent movements that bespeak a different neurologic state. For diagnostic, therapeutic, and prognostic purposes, several categories of abnormal involuntary movements should be distinguished from tremor. All of the following involuntary movements (and most true tremors) are greatly reduced or disappear altogether with sleep.

Tics are repetitive, coordinated, usually stereotyped movements that are seen widely in the population and increase in frequency in a given patient in response to stress. They usually involve face or hand muscles, may initially be a conscious mannerism, and usually can be suppressed by voluntary effort. *Hemifacial spasm* is a kind of oscillating movement usually beginning in a middle-aged or elderly person, localized to the facial muscles. It is thought to be due to degenerative lesions of the facial nucleus or peripheral nerve, but the exact mechanism is unknown, and treatment is unsatisfactory.

Asterixis is an irregular, skeletal muscle contraction that results in flapping of the hands, electromyographically coincident with brief pauses at irregular intervals. *Chorea* is an irregular, jerking movement usually involving the fingers and often accompanied by *athetosis,* in which writhing movements of limbs or trunk may be added. *Epilepsy partialis continuens* refers to a focal seizure in which continuous seizure activity may result in a somewhat rhythmic jerking of one body part. Sudden onset of the illness is the most useful distinguishing feature here.

Dyskinesias are rhythmic involuntary movements of the orofacial musculature resulting in tongue protrusion and chewing movements. These are important to recognize because of the frequency with which they occur as early manifestations of the tardive dyskinesia syndrome due to use of phenothiazines and other major tranquilizers.

DIFFERENTIAL DIAGNOSIS

Tremors can be divided clinically into postural, intention, and resting types. Most postural tremors are physiologic. Among the intention tremors are the essential, senile, and cerebellar varieties. Most resting tremors are due to Parkinson's disease. Tremors must be distinguished from other voluntary movements such as dyskinesias, tics, myoclonus, and athetosis.

WORKUP

History. Clinical assessment of tremor is greatly aided by first ascertaining the circumstances under which the tremor occurs. Some tremors are present during maintenance of a posture, some during rest, and others only during an action (the intention tremors). Careful questioning will often identify the type of tremor. Common diagnostic problems include distinguishing the resting tremor of early Parkinson's disease from an essential tremor and an essential tremor from an exaggerated physiologic one. All of these are common and some may, in fact, be present simultaneously in a given patient.

Physical Examination is directed primarily at determining whether the tremor is better or worse with activity. The patient should be asked to hold out his hands, to write, to perform rapid alternating movements, and to touch finger to nose repeatedly; the objective is to detect evidence of cerebellar or extrapyramidal disease. The patient should be observed discretely during the history and during other parts of the physical examination, because calling attention to the tremor may worsen it.

Laboratory Studies. If there is some question at the end of the examination as to whether the tremor is primarily resting or primarily action, a tremor recording (EMG) may be requested. Many parkinsonian patients will have no other extrapyramidal signs at the time they present with tremor. The EMG can separate the two types, sometimes confirming that both tremors are present simultaneously.

Diagnostic Trials. If the diagnosis of essential tremor is entertained, a family history should be sought. This tremor responds to small doses (80 to 120 mg per day) of propranolol, and the drug may be used in a diagnostic and therapeutic trial, provided there are no medical contraindications. Exaggerated physiologic tremor due to anxiety does not respond substantially to propranolol, although it has been observed that adding diazepam may further reduce essential tremor and, by its antianxiety effect, eliminate exaggerated physiologic tremor as well.

PATIENT EDUCATION AND INDICATIONS FOR REFERRAL

The etiology of the tremor and the fact that it can be controlled should be discussed with the patient. Avoidance of agents that worsen symptoms must be stressed. Patients with intention tremors and cerebellar signs must be referred to a neurologist since demyelinating or hereditary degenerative diseases may be responsible. Disabling tremors refractory to simple therapy may benefit from neurologic consultation.

SYMPTOMATIC MANAGEMENT

1. Essential or familial tremors respond to low, nonbeta-blocking doses of propranolol (80 to 120 mg per day).
2. Parkinson's tremor should be treated with anticholinergics or L-dopa-containing agents (see Chapter 167).
3. Physiologic tremors are unaffected by propranolol or alcohol but worsened by anxiety, coffee, hyperthyroidism, tricyclics, and lithium. A combination of diazepam and propranolol may lessen severe tremor due to anxiety.

ANNOTATED BIBLIOGRAPHY

Mawdsley C: Diseases of the central nervous system: Involuntary movements. Br Med J 4:572, 1975 (*Overview of abnormal movements with a brief differential.*)

Shahani BT, Young RR: Physiological and pharmacological aids in the differential diagnosis of tremor. J Neurol Neurosurg Psychiatry 39:772, 1976 (*Excellent detailed discussion of the EMG in diagnosis of tremor; very readable even without EMG training.*)

Winkler GF, Young RR: Efficacy of chronic propranolol therapy in action tremors of the familiar, senile, or essential varieties. N Engl J Med 290:984, 1974 (*The initial clinical trial.*)

163
Evaluation of Dementia
AMY A. PRUITT, M.D.

Dementia is a progressive loss of intellectual ability in which speech, memory, praxis, judgment, and mood may all be altered in varying proportions. There are an estimated 600,000 cases of advanced dementia in the United States, and milder degrees of altered mental status are very common in the elderly (15% of persons over 65 exhibit a degree of intellectual deterioration, according to some estimates). Each patient with dementia deserves careful workup, since as many as 15% may have conditions amenable to therapy. The primary physician should know how to distinguish dementia from other, more specific cortical deficits (aphasia, agnosia, etc.) and should be able to perform an adequate screening examination for potentially reversible disease.

PATHOPHYSIOLOGY AND CLINICAL PRESENTATION

Normal intellectual functioning requires appropriate reception of sensory perceptions, adequate association-making ability, and effective efferent mechanisms to express decisions and responses. Dementia is marked by progressive degrees of inability to adapt to the environment. The patient initially may be noted to have slight impairments in memory, atten-tion, and concentration (often excused or ignored by the family and, at least early in the course, concealed by the patient). Later, he may display impaired judgment on increasingly simple matters, inability to abstract or generalize, and personality change. This last symptom sometimes takes the form of a certain rigidity with perseveration, irritability, or confusion as a result of minor changes in environment. Still later, perception becomes distorted, and the patient is no longer aware of his deficits. Affective disturbances become more prominent, and depression frequently prevails over euphoria or agitation. Finally, the patient may lose interest in personal hygiene and nutrition, and is left helpless and disoriented.

The clinical presentation may be marked by specific signs of neurologic or medical disease (Table 163-1). However, all dementing processes can be distinguished by certain hallmarks. The *pace* of the illness is slowly progressive over a period of months to years; in rare instances the process is more rapid. The *pattern* of the disease is relentless, without stepwise decline or remission. Static, nonprogressive impairment of intellect is more accurately described as "mental retardation."

Table 163-1. Neurologic Diseases Associated
with Intellectual Dysfunction

DISEASE	PHYSICAL SIGNS	CLINICAL FEATURES
Alzheimer's disease (senile dementia)	Frontal lobe signs	Enlarged ventricles, cortical atrophy by CT scan
Normal pressure hydrocephalus	Gait disorder,* incontinence	Little cortical atrophy by CT scan
Atherosclerotic cerebrovascular disease (multiple strokes)	Focal deficits*	Episodic dysfunction consistent with multiple strokes
Parkinson's disease	Extrapyramidal signs*	Long-standing disease, extended duration of L-dopa therapy
*Intracranial tumor	Focal signs, papilledema	Subacute evolution, seizures possible
Neurosyphilis	Frontal lobe signs, optic atrophy, Argyll-Robertson pupils	Positive VDRL serum/CSF
Huntington's disease	Choreiform movements*	Family history
Creutzfeldt–Jakob disease	Myoclonus,* cerebellar signs, eye movement abnormalities	Subacute course; EEG specific, brain biopsy diagnostic
Multiple sclerosis	Brainstem signs, optic atrophy, spinal cord signs	Usually long-standing disease, episodic illness with remissions
Wilson's disease	Extrapyramidal signs,* hepatic dysfunction, Kayser-Fleischer rings*	Onset in adolescence or young adulthood, psychiatric disorders
Progressive supranuclear palsy	Failure of vertical gaze,* extrapyramidal signs*	Eye movement abnormalities; differentiate from other extrapyramidal disorders

* Invariable; all other physical signs are neither invariably present nor pathognomonic.

DIFFERENTIAL DIAGNOSIS

A useful way of organizing the differential diagnosis of dementia is to divide etiologies into those accompanied by signs and symptoms of medical or neurologic disease. The former includes hypothyroidism, vitamin B_{12} deficiency, thiamine deficiency, progressive multifocal leukoencephalopathy, the dementias associated with neoplastic disease, dementias associated with hemodialysis, and, perhaps inaccurately, "atherosclerotic dementia." This last entity is not a genuine dementia in the sense of progressive loss of all types of intellectual abilities. Instead, it is the end result of recurrent small strokes leading to multiple infarcts and focal neurologic deficits, which should be evident from the history and physical examination. In hypertensive patients, dementia may present in the form of pseudobulbar palsy following repeated lacunar strokes. Hallmarks of this disease are poor emotional control (inappropriate, excessive outbursts of laughing or crying), difficulty with gait, dysarthria, and bilateral signs of corticospinal tract (upper motor neuron) disease.

Neurologic diseases associated with dementia are listed in Table 163-1 and include Alzheimer's disease, normal pressure hydrocephalus, neurosyphilis, Creutzfeldt-Jakob disease (spongiform encephalopathy), Huntington's disease, intracranial tumor, late Parkinson's disease, Wilson's disease, progressive supranuclear palsy, and severe multiple sclerosis.

Most of these disorders present with specific, associated neurologic findings. However, *Alzheimer's disease* and *senile dementia,* the most common degenerative disorders, do not. They are pathologically and clinically identical except for age of onset (Alzheimer's disease being somewhat arbitrarily reserved for patients with onset at age less than 65.) It has been reported that 4.4% of people over 65 exhibit moderate to severe senile dementia and that about 66% of these fall into the category of idiopathic senile dementia. An additional 10% have a milder form of the disease. The brain is atrophied, the ventricles are enlarged, and evidence of severe vascular disease or infarction is minimal or absent. Neuropathologic study reveals neuronal loss, neurofibrillary tangles, and senile plaques whose extent does not correlate quantitatively with the degree of dementia. Similar changes are found in the brains of elderly people who are not demented. Etiology remains unknown.

Normal pressure hydrocephalus (NPH) deserves special mention both because of its reversibility and because of a tendency to overdiagnose the entity. The term refers to slow ventricular enlargement without cortical atrophy due to poor cerebrospinal fluid resorption. The brain literally becomes plastered against the skull. Most often, there is no known precipitant, but the condition can occur when there is blockage of CSF resorption due to meningitis or subarachnoid hemorrhage. Dementia, gait disturbance, and incontinence are the classic triad, presumably reflecting disease in areas most affected by ventricular enlargement, namely the frontal lobes and fibers that mediate sphincter and lower extremity function.

Conditions that resemble dementia and are often mistaken for it are schizophrenia, depression, and hysteria. The term delirium should be used to describe an acutely altered mental status often resulting from drug ingestion or withdrawal, fever, hypoxia, hypercapnia, encephalitis, hyperthyroidism, or metabolic abnormality.

Among patients presenting with dementia, Alzheimer's disease (including senile dementia) accounts for 50% to 60% of cases; vascular disease with multiple infarcts for 10% to 20%; brain tumors for 5%; 5%, unknown and 10%, all other causes.

WORKUP

The goal of the workup is to distinguish dementia from other causes of intellectual impairment, such as metabolic disorders and psychologic illness, and to identify the etiology of the dementia.

History. Detailed questioning should define the temporal course of the illness, ascertaining whether the process is indeed chronic and progressive and determining occurrence of past, focal neurologic insults. Specific inquiry is needed into previous gastric surgery (B_{12} deficiency), neck surgery (thyroid disease), meningitis, and subarachnoid hemorrhage (normal pressure hydrocephalus). A history of trauma, seizure disorder, and use of medications (particularly hypnotics, diuretics, anticonvulsants, or psychotropic medications) should be elicited. It is very important to probe the use of alcohol (see Chapter 224). A family history is crucial in identifying those patients with Huntington's disease. Additionally, the physician can form a general impression of the patient's psychologic state from the initial interview.

Physical Examination. Assessment begins with a mental status examination to confirm the presence of dementia. The complex faculties that constitute intellect are usually divided into testable, although not necessarily anatomically or pathologically exclusive, functions. Specific states which are not dementias (such as amnesias, aphasias, and agnosias) should be identified as well with these tests.

Immediate and remote memory are tested, as are reading, writing, calculating ability, and constructional capacity. Patients should be asked to recall a short story, to remember three items, to reproduce simple drawings, and to recite a list of digits. Ability to interpret proverbs or to discern similarities among objects offers insight into higher cortical functions. Judgment can be ascertained by presenting the patient with decision-requiring situations ("finding a stamped letter" or "seeing a fire in a theater").

Next, the physician should undertake specific neurologic and medical evaluation. Stigmata of alcoholism (see Chapter 224), renal disease (see Chapter 139), or other systemic processes should be sought. Frontal lobe signs such as grasp and suck should be elicited. Cranial nerve examination should be directed toward discovery of papilledema, visual field cut, optic atrophy, or abnormal pupillary reaction. Extraocular movements can be limited in supranuclear palsy. Nystagmus may indicate recent drug ingestion or the presence of brainstem disease (see Table 163-1). The motor examination should record the presence of abnormal movements and focal deficits. Parkinsonian facies, gait, and tremor, (see Chapter 167) may be encountered. Involuntary movements should be noted, such as tardive dyskinesias, tremors, asterixis, chorea, and myoclonus (see Chapter 162). Sensory examination may reveal parietal lobe disease with inattention to stimuli presented bilaterally, or evidence of peripheral neuropathy or combined system disease (B_{12} deficiency). Gait should be observed carefully; the small, rigid steps of frontal lobe gait apraxia can be distinguished from a wide-based cerebellar gait (alcohol being a major offender) or the "marche à petits pas" of Parkinson's disease.

Laboratory Studies. In most cases, the need for further studies is reasonably limited and involves few invasive procedures. The history and physical examination should limit the differential possibilities. The following guidelines outline evaluation, starting with the least invasive, least specific tests and progressing to the most invasive and specific ones. Baseline evaluation should include blood tests for electrolytes, urea nitrogen, thyroid function (see Chapter 101), syphilis (see Chapter 123), and complete blood count. The need for additional blood tests is dictated by history and physical examination findings and may include B_{12}, calcium, liver function studies, and toxic screen. A routine chest radiograph should be obtained if none has been performed recently.

At this point, the physician should select specific tests based on a knowledge of their yield in different situations. *Skull radiographs* may demonstrate an old (or new) skull fracture, which may be responsible for a seizure disorder or strengthen suspicion of alcohol ingestion. Calcium present in a subdural hematoma or tumor may be demonstrated (though these lesions are better seen with computerized tomography). *Electroencephalogram* (EEG) may be normal, even in advanced cases of dementia; nonspecific slowing of the baseline rhythm is common. Occasionally, the EEG may raise suspicions of a particular etiology: focal, delta slowing is seen with tumor; unilateral attenuation of voltage suggests subdural hematoma; excessive beta activity is consistent with drug ingestion; a seizure disorder may be demonstrated. Finally, Creutzfeldt-Jakob disease has a highly specific EEG pattern.

Lumbar puncture is frequently inconclusive, but is indicated when there is clinical suspicion of NPH, tertiary syphilis, or neoplastic invasion of the leptomeninges. Sugar, protein, cell count, gamma globulin, and serology for syphilis should be obtained. Serial lumbar punctures may be done to remove large volumes (30 ml) of CSF in the diagnostic assessment of strongly suspected NPH. Gait improvement may occur after repeated taps.

Computed tomography (CT scan) can answer many questions posed by the presence of dementia. Subdural hematomas and intracranial tumors can be readily identified. Huntington's disease is suggested by caudate nucleus atrophy. The CT scan can also distinguish between NPH and Alzheimer's disease or senile dementia. In the former, enlarged ventricles and little or no cortical atrophy are seen, while in the latter pronounced cortical atrophy is present as well as ventricular enlargement. The degree of cortical atrophy in NPH is not clearly correlated with response to shunting, and a neurologic opinion should be sought. Prospective studies of clinical course, CT scan, and response to shunt procedures are in progress.

Arteriography is not indicated in the primary evaluation of a dementia; it is best reserved for confirming intracranial tumor or a vascular lesion. Similarly, *brain biopsy* is a method of last resort indicated to confirm the diagnosis of herpes simplex encephalitis and occasionally to explain a subacute dementing process in a patient with atypical features of Alzheimer's or Creutzfeldt-Jakob disease.

For most patients, the workup can be accomplished by the internist. It consists of some screening blood work, a chest film, and, depending on precise circumstances, an EEG, an LP, and a CT scan. This requires about 3 days in the hospital, although the entire evaluation can be accomplished on an outpatient basis. Consultation with a neurologist should be sought for advice on interpretation of CT scans for normal pressure hydrocephalus or if focal neurologic signs are present.

No patient with progressive decline in mental faculties, particularly if he is under age 65, should be presumed to be the victim of an incurable process without evaluation. Careful history, physical examination, and a simple laboratory workup disclose the not infrequent patient whose course can be altered significantly.

Standardized mental-status tests can serve to further confirm a clinical impression of Alzheimer's disease. The currently utilized studies include the Information–Orientation–Concentration test, the Mini-Mental State test, and the Dementia Rating Scale. They have been validated and proven efficient and sensitive. The diagnostic criteria for the diagnosis of Alzheimer's disease established by the U.S. Department of Health and Human services requires the presence of dementia "established by clinical examination and documented by the Mini-Mental Test, the Dementia Scale or similar examination, with evidence of deficits in two or more areas of cognition; progressive worsening of memory and other cognitive function; no disturbance of consciousness; and absence of systemic disorders or other brain disease that in and of themselves could account for the deficits." The patient who meets such criteria has a better than 90% chance of having Alzheimer's disease.

SYMPTOMATIC MANAGEMENT AND COUNSELLING (See Also Chapter 168)

At the present time, there is no treatment for Alzheimer's disease or for patients with multi-infarct dementia. Although recent studies of patients with Alzheimer's disease suggest that CNS levels of acetylcholine may be diminished, attempts at dietary repletion with choline (usually in the form of lecithin supplements) have not proven effective. There is no evidence to support the widely promoted use of vasodilators in patients with dementia.

The use of sedative and psychoactive agents in the confused patient should be avoided unless extreme agitation hampers care. If such therapy is contemplated, only the lowest possible doses should be used. Patients who have emotional outbursts may respond to a small dose of *thioridazine* (10 to 25 mg qhs); those with depression to a tricyclic antidepressant (*e.g.*, desipramine 25 to 50 mg qhs). *Haloperidol* is often a first choice in the setting of delusions and hallucinations; doses in the range of 0.5 to 5 mg per day usually suffice, but the extrapyramidal side-effects of the drug (see Chapter 168) can limit its usefulness. If the only problem is occasional difficulty falling asleep, a short-acting benzodiazepine (*e.g.*, *lorazepam* or *triazolam*) can be given before bed on an as-needed basis. Beta-blocking agents and anticholinergics should be used with caution; they can lead to a deterioration in mental status.

An important task is helping the family maintain and care for the patient at home. The goal is to sustain the highest level of function possible, which is facilitated by promotion of an orderly home situation and a regular routine. Use of calendars, television, newspapers, and other means of orientation are important. Access to potentially dangerous appliances has to be limited; toilet facilities should be made especially convenient.

Families that are eager to care for the demented patient at home can often find help in local support groups and social service agencies, some of which may also provide day care and group therapy services. In addition, excellent handbooks are available (see Bibliography). When care at home begins to exhaust and strain the family, sensitive counselling can do much to help the family cope with the difficult decision regarding institutionalization.

ANNOTATED BIBLIOGRAPHY

Freemon FR: Evaluation of patients with progressive intellectual deterioration. Arch Neurol 33:658, 1976 (*A more general hospital series but comparable to that in Marsden and Harrison reference.*)

Hachinski VC, Lassen NA, Marshall J: Multi-infarct dementia. A cause of mental deterioration in the elderly. Lancet 2:207, 1974 (*Describes this syndrome, clearly differentiating it from Alzheimer's disease.*)

Katzman R, Karasu TB: Differential diagnosis of dementia, p 1030. In Fields W (ed): Neurological and Sensory Disorders in the Elderly. New York, Stratton Intercontinental Medical Book Corporation, 1975 (*Clinically oriented discussion.*)

Katzman R: Alzheimer's disease. N Engl J Med 314:964, 1986 (*Excellent review of all aspects; essential reading; 132 references.*)

Mace NL, Rabins RV: The 36-hour day: A family guide to caring for persons with Alzheimer's disease. Baltimore, Johns Hopkins' Press, 1981 (*Best book for families of patients; excellent instructional manual.*)

Marsden CD, Harrison MJG: Outcome of investigation of patients with presenile dementia. Br Med J 2:249, 1972 (*Specialized hospital with referral population; demonstrates relatively high incidence treatable causes of dementia. However, fails to define "cerebrovascular dementia."*)

Meier DE, Cassel CK: Nursing home placement and the demented patient. Ann Intern Med 104:98, 1986 (*Thoughtful discussion of the many difficulties and dilemmas posed in arranging care for demented patients.*)

Ojemann RG et al: Further experience with the syndrome of 'normal' pressure hydrocephalus. J Neurosurg 31:270, 1969 (*Classic report.*)

Stein SC et al: Normal pressure hydrocephalus: Predicting the results of cerebrospinal fluid shunting. J Neurosurg 41:463, 1974 (*Although the CT scan is being used more frequently for this purpose, the RISA scan is still essential, and norms for "allowable" cortical atrophy are not yet firm.*)

Strub RL, Black FW: The Mental Status Examination in Neurology. Philadelphia, F.A. Davis, 1977 (*Detailed description of the components of the examination.*)

Weiss J: The clinical use of psychological tests, p 41. In Nicoli AN (ed): Harvard Guide to Modern Psychiatry. Cambridge, Harvard University Press, 1978 (*Concise discussion of the use of these tests in distinguishing depression from dementia.*)

Wells CE (ed): Dementia. Contemporary Neurology Series, 2nd ed. Philadelphia, FA Davis, 1977 (*Best, thorough, overall reference.*)

164
Approach to the Patient With Seizures
AMY A. PRUITT, M.D.

The occurrence of a convulsion is a dramatic and frightening event; the experience is likely to trigger an immediate visit to the physician by an anxious family and a bewildered patient. The physician will need to plan for prevention of future episodes while orchestrating the diagnostic evaluation. Allaying fears and correcting misconceptions are also important tasks. Although an etiology for the majority of seizures is never found, a convulsion may represent a symptom of treatable underlying disease and deserves full evaluation. In addition, the event needs to be distinguished from other causes of loss of consciousness (see Chapter 18).

PATHOPHYSIOLOGY AND CLINICAL PRESENTATION

A seizure is the result of a sudden abnormal discharge from an area of the brain that, for reasons not entirely understood at present, appears to elude the control of normal inhibitory mechanisms that synchronize cerebral electrical activity. The activity of the initial focus may spread to other parts of the brain. Grand mal seizures and petit mal seizures presumably originate in subcortical structures. Any cerebral irritative lesion, whether vascular (such as previous stroke, arteriovenous malformation, or cortical vein thrombosis), neoplastic, or congenital (cyst or hamartoma), may produce clinical convulsive activity. In the majority of patients with epilepsy, no specific cause is ever determined, and pathologic examination after death reveals no diagnostic changes.

Generalized seizures are designated "major motor" or "absence" (petit mal). The term "major motor" includes both the true grand mal seizure, a convulsion without focal onset, and the other kinds of bilateral tonic-clonic convulsions that begin either as focal sensorimotor symptoms or as temporal lobe convulsions. When the onset is focal, the spread of symptoms may follow the cortical representation of body parts, with symptoms beginning, for example, in toes or fingers and spreading either up the leg or down the arm. Symptoms of temporal lobe epilepsy are legion and include motor automatisms, such as lip smacking or chewing, olfactory or gustatory hallucinations, and behavioral automatisms. Two-thirds of these patients experience generalized major motor convulsions at some time, and many have a distinctive personality, sometimes with psychotic manifestations. (See Table 164-1 for phenotypic classification of seizures.)

A number of misconceptions about clinical presentation require clarification. First, adults rarely seize with high fever; the presence of a temperature greater than 102°F does not suffice to explain the occurrence of a seizure. Second, seizures are rare during the initial presentation of an embolic stroke. However, 20% to 25% of patients who have had an embolic stroke may have seizures at some time after the event. Vascular lesions that are likely to have epilepsy as a sequela are emboli and cortical vein thrombosis, whereas subarachnoid hemorrhages and lacunar and thrombotic strokes rarely are succeeded by seizure activity. Third, alcohol withdrawal seizures occur between 7 and 48 hours after cessation of drinking, with a peak at 13 to 24 hours. They are preceded by a tremulous state in all patients and followed by delirium tremens in about 30%. Usually, only one or two convulsions occur, and status epilepticus is very rare. Alcohol exacerbates pre-existing epileptic foci. Alcohol withdrawal is more likely to produce seizures in an epileptic patient than in a normal person, and less drinking is needed to precipitate a seizure—an evening or weekend of binge drinking may suffice. Other drugs are associated with seizures, either when they are taken in overdose or when withdrawal occurs. These are summarized in Table 164-2.

Trauma is frequently invoked as a cause for seizures. However, a large Mayo Clinic study revealed that unless the trauma was quite severe (with loss of consciousness for more than one half hour, with a lobar hematoma, or with a depressed skull fracture) the incidence of posttraumatic seizures was not greater than that of the population as a whole. When there is a history of closed head trauma, epilepsy usually develops within 2 years if it is to do so, whereas with open head trauma (penetration of the dura), seizures may develop at any time after the original injury.

Table 164-1. Classification of Seizures

PHENOTYPE	EEG	ETIOLOGY*	PROGNOSIS	DRUG OF CHOICE IN ORDER OF PREFERENCE
Generalized				
Major Motor				
Grand mal	Normal, initially, in 20%; nonspecifically abnormal in 40%	Unknown in 85%	Age-related; overall, 25% seizure-free and off medications at 5 years	Phenytoin or carbamazepine, phenobarbital, sodium valproate
Focal onset (sensory or motor)	Focally abnormal in about 65%	Cause found in 33%	Related to etiology	Phenytoin or carbamazepine, phenobarbital
Temporal lobe onset	See below under partial seizures	Cause found in 50%	May be late result of multiple grand mal seizures; difficult to control	Phenytoin or carbamazepine *and* phenobarbital
Absence				
(petit mal)	80% have pathognomonic 3/second spike and wave pattern	Unknown autosomal dominant; normal EEGs in both parents in only 50%	Excellent; absences cease by age 20 in 50% but many continue to have grand mal seizures	Ethosuximide, sodium valproate, phenobarbital, trimethadione
Partial				
Simple (no loss of consciousness) motor or sensory	Focally abnormal in about 66%	Cause found in 33%	Related to etiology	Phenytoin or carbamazepine, phenobarbital,
Complex (TLE with or without loss of consciousness)	Awake; 50% abnormal; asleep; 85% abnormal	Cause found in 50%; trauma, neoplasm	15% seizure-free on medication; psychoses develop in 33% of idiopathic temporal lobe seizures	Phenytoin or carbamazepine *and* phenobarbital,

* These figures antedate widespread use of CT scanning in evaluation.

Table 164-2. Drugs Commonly Associated with Seizures

DRUGS	OVERDOSE SEIZURES	WITHDRAWAL SEIZURES	DOSE REQUIRED TO INDUCE SEIZURE
Alcohol	−	+	Depends on previous drinking or underlying epilepsy
Meperidine (Demerol)	+	+	2–3 g/day*·†
Propoxyphene (Darvon)	+	+	Variable
Pentazocine (Talwin)	−	−	May precipitate withdrawal from other opiates with as little as 100 mg
Barbiturates	−	+	>600 mg/day (short-acting)†
Meprobamate (Miltown)	−	+	>1.2 g/day†
Chlordiazepoxide, diazepam	−	+	Unknown—may have 7–8 day latency period
Phenothiazines, haloperidol	− But myoclonus may occur; may cause seizures in patients with old cortical focus	−	Variable

* Overdose seizure

† Withdrawal seizure

+ = occurs

− = does not occur

DIFFERENTIAL DIAGNOSIS

Several conditions can mimic seizures, by either causing acute focal motor deficits or by producing episodic loss of consciousness. Under the former should be considered transient ischemic attacks (either in the carotid or in the vertebrobasilar territory), migraine, and local pathology such as nerve compression. Under the latter are syncopal attacks of any etiology, including transient diminished cerebral perfusion from cardiac arrhythmias, transient ischemic attacks, and severe hypoglycemia, as with an insulin reaction.

The differential diagnosis of conditions responsible for a seizure is based largely on the age of the patient at the time of the first seizure. Idiopathic epilepsy is the most common etiology in children, but becomes increasingly rare in the late teenage and young adult population. Thereafter, an underlying lesion becomes increasingly likely; nevertheless, the infrequency of discovering a definite etiology may surprise some physicians. In a large retrospective study of patients with more than one documented seizure of any type, only 23% had a cause that became obvious after thorough investigation and a 10-year follow-up. Only 15% of seizures generalized from the outset had a demonstrable etiology, whereas underlying disorders could be found in almost 30% of seizures with a focal component. In the young adult population (18 to 45), the demonstrated causes were drugs (largely alcohol withdrawal), neoplasm, and trauma. In the older adult population, underlying pathology was divided roughly equally among neoplasm, trauma, and cerebrovascular accident.

WORKUP

The first objective in the workup is to distinguish seizure from other types of acute, transient, or focal neurologic deficits and loss of consciousness (see Chapters 18, 161, 165). In practice, distinguishing syncope from seizure may be difficult, and there are no definitive criteria. However, presence of aura, anatomic spread of symptoms, incontinence, overt tonic-clonic activity, postictal confusion, and report of a sudden loss of consciousness suggest seizure.

History requires an exact description of events from witnesses as well as from the patient. Questioning should include inquiry into presence of an aura, focal onset, loss of consciousness, and observed injury incurred during the convulsion. The physician should also ask about ingestion of drugs, alcohol consumption, cardiac arrhythmias, mitral or aortic valve disease, and previous malignancy, stroke, or trauma. A family history of convulsions is important to elicit, although idiopathic epilepsy becomes less common with increasing age.

Physical Examination. The physician may have the opportunity to perform the neurologic examination shortly after the seizure. A focal residual abnormality, such as paralysis of one arm (Todd's postictal paralysis), may suggest the initial focus even when the witnessed event was generalized. The examination should also include checking for head trauma, papilledema, carotid disease, cardiac dysrhythmias or valvular problems, and manifestations of alcohol abuse (see Chapter 224).

Laboratory Studies. Before embarking on a complex and expensive laboratory workup, one should be aware of the likely diagnostic yield of various procedures. The *skull series* rarely shows anything diagnostic, but films can be inspected for calcification (which sometimes occurs in several intracranial neoplasms, vessels, or congenital anomalies) and for evidence of skull fracture.

Familiarity with the *electroencephalogram* (EEG) is essential for proper evaluation of seizures; the major findings are summarized in Table 164-1. The EEG is always unequivocally normal in fully 20% of patients with purely grand mal seizures. It is nonspecifically abnormal (without localizing value) in another 40%. Either slow waves (described as "theta" or "delta" in EEG terminology) or spikes may be seen between seizures. Slow waves are somewhat more common with tumor, but the exact appearance of the EEG abnormalities provides no definitive clues. The EEG is somewhat more useful when there is a focal component to the convulsion; appropriate localization of spike activity occurs in about two-thirds of cases. The EEG may be of considerable use in detection of temporal lobe epilepsy. The likelihood of detecting the condition is increased by obtaining a *sleep study;* 85% to 90% of patients with temporal lobe epilepsy demonstrate appropriately localized abnormalities on the sleep EEG. The EEG picks up cortical disturbances; abnormalities of deep temporal lobe or diencephalic structures may not be evident on the usual EEG study.

After obtaining the EEG, the physician must decide whether to perform a *lumbar puncture.* Obvious contraindications include evidence of raised intracranial pressure, known tumor with high suspicion of CNS metastases, history compatible with intracranial neoplasm, and bleeding diathesis. If there are no major contraindications, most neurologists recommend performing a lumbar puncture. However, the diagnostic yield is quite low. The cell count is normal in 95% of patients with a first seizure, and sugar and protein concentrations are normal in 90% of CSF fluid samples obtained in these circumstances.

A *technetium brain scan* used to be included in every workup. It is a noninvasive procedure that is easily performed and may reveal serious intracranial pathology, particularly subdural hematomas. It has been supplanted by *computed cranial tomography* (CCT). Compared to radionuclide scanning, computed cranial tomography provides enhanced capability to visualize structural anomalies, but its utility in evaluations of patients with the new onset of seizure depends on the likelihood of an underlying anatomic lesion. At the present time, the following guidelines for evaluation seem reasonable:

1. For patients aged 16 to 30 years with a normal examination and a generalized convulsion, CCT is not essential.

2. In patients aged 31 years or older with normal examination and normal EEG, CCT may show an abnormality but in the vast majority, the test is unlikely to provide information essential to patient care. However, if there is no history of alcohol or drug abuse, CT deserves consideration.
3. Irrespective of age or seizure type, if neurologic examination is abnormal, CCT is useful and essential.
4. Electroencephalography remains an essential tool.

INDICATIONS FOR ADMISSION AND REFERRAL

It may be comforting for the physician confronted with the new onset of seizures to realize that patients with brain tumors usually have some evidence of tumor by history, physical examination, or EEG. In a prospective study of epilepsy in patients older than 50, 100% of patients who were subsequently shown to have a brain tumor had one or more of the following on initial evaluation: history of focal onset, abnormalities on neurologic examination, or abnormal EEG. Not every seizure patient must be referred to a neurologic specialist, but an abnormality in any of these initial studies should prompt consultation. Further diagnostic or therapeutic studies are indicated for these patients because they are at increased risk for serious underlying pathology.

The patient seen in the office with a first seizure can be sent home if there is a clear history of the use of alcohol or other drugs or withdrawal, provided the patient is medically stable. In these instances, further seizures are unlikely and hospitalization unnecessary. Otherwise, the evaluation of a first seizure is best performed in the hospital where the patient can be stabilized and observed; the frequency and severity of seizures, as well as the severity of the underlying cause, can never be known at first glance.

LONG-TERM OUTPATIENT MANAGEMENT

Long-term management of seizures is directed at the underlying disease, the resulting epilepsy, the side-effects of the medications, and the psychiatric and social effects of this chronic illness. In practice, the compromise between freedom from seizures and side-effects from medication is not always satisfactory. Because a correctable underlying etiology is not frequently found in epilepsy, most management involves symptomatic intervention by the physician.

NATURAL HISTORY

The prognosis of idiopathic epilepsy is dependent on both age at onset and type of convulsion (see Table 164-1). In general, patients with petit mal seizures have the best prognosis. These childhood-onset seizures cease by age 20 in over 50% of cases, but many patients then suffer from grand mal convulsions. Although statistics vary according to age at onset and type of seizure, on the average, 10 years after diagnosis,

61% of patients are seizure-free for 5 years (with or without medicine). The probability of remaining seizure-free is highest for patients who had idiopathic seizures that were generalized and for those who were diagnosed before 10 years of age. Eighty percent of recurrences will be within 5 years after stopping medication.

The prognosis for recurrence of seizures after a single convulsion has been studied by Hauser and others. Contrary to some other studies, they found that age, sex, type of seizure, and examination after the seizure did not affect the incidence of recurrence. Twenty-six percent of the patients had had a recurrent spell by 36 months, and there were no new cases of recurrent seizures after this date. The risk of developing recurrent convulsions increased with a family history of seizures or with an EEG that showed generalized spike and wave activity.

PRINCIPLES OF MANAGEMENT

The simplest management strategy is to become familiar with the use of one anticonvulsant as a first-line drug and to administer that drug by whichever route the patient can tolerate best. Although *diazepam* is often used for emergency management, it should never be the first drug for long-term seizure control. For most adults, the drug of choice is *phenytoin* (Dilantin). Intravenous or oral administration of this drug is acceptable, but intramuscular delivery results in unpredictable serum levels. Phenytoin is well-absorbed orally and has a serum half-life of 22 to 30 hours. An initial loading dose must be administered. Table 164-3 gives several loading schedules that result in therapeutic phenytoin levels, and demonstrates that failure to "load" the patient with medication results in a delay of as long as 2 weeks before therapeutic levels are reached.

The usual maintenance dose of phenytoin is 300 mg per day; blood level determinations are readily available in most laboratories. Therapeutic levels usually range from 8 to 20 mg per 100 ml. In most patients with epilepsy, phenytoin remains the drug of choice for long-term control. However, the medication has numerous side effects and interactions with other common medications (Table 164-4).

Table 164-3. Methods of Phenytoin Administration

TIME THERAPEUTIC RANGE REACHED (after initial dose)	ROUTE AND RATE OF ADMINISTRATION
20 minutes	1000 mg IV at 50 mg/min
4–6 hours	1000 mg PO, then 300 mg/day
23–30 hours	300 mg PO q8h × 3 doses; then 300 mg/day
5–15 days (no loading dose)	300 mg/day PO

Table 164-4. Phenytoin: Side Effects and Drug Interactions

Major Side-Effects

Dose-related: nystagmus, ataxia, dysarthria, blurred vision, decrease in measured total T_4

Duration-related: osteomalacia, peripheral neuropathy, anemia, cerebellar degeneration

Idiosyncratic: gingival hypertrophy, acne, hypertrichosis, encephalopathy

Rare, toxic: high, spiking fevers, exfoliative dermatitis, bone marrow depression, pseudo- and actual lymphoma lupus-like syndrome, teratogenesis during first trimester, neonatal coagulation defects

Interactions with Commonly Prescribed Drugs

Increased phenytoin levels with:
  Antimicrobials: chloramphenicol, INH
  Anticoagulants: coumadin
  Amphetamines (but seizure threshold decreased)
  Disulfiram (Antabuse)
  Alcohol: acute ingestion raises phenytoin levels, but see below
  Anti-inflammatory agent: phenylbutazone
  Anticonvulsants: ethosuximide; no consistent effect with simultaneous barbiturate administration
  Sedatives: chlordiazepoxide (librium), diazepam (valium, oxazepam (serax), clorazepam (clonopin)

Decreased phenytoin levels with:
  Alcohol: chronic ingestion

Phenytoin effects on levels of other drugs
  Insulin: may interfere with endogenous insulin release
  Quinidine: decreases quinidine effect at given dose
  Falsely low total T_4

If phenytoin fails to control the seizures, a second drug must be employed. *Phenobarbital* is the usual choice, and its administration should begin with 60 mg at bedtime or 30 mg two or three times a day. Patients may report increased sleepiness with larger doses, but with time they will be able to tolerate necessary dosage increases with acceptable side effects. There has been recent interest in higher dose monotherapy for seizure control. Thus, a patient who experiences convulsions with phenytoin level of 8–10 μg/ml may do better to have the phenytoin increased to give a level of 18–20 μg before a second medication is considered.

Carbamazepine (Tegretol) is also an excellent first-line drug for adult onset major motor seizures or for complex partial seizures. Many patients report less fatigue and better performance on this medication than on either phenytoin or phenobarbital. The usual adult dose is 200 mg two to four times per day. Major disadvantages of this medication include the necessity of multiple daily dosing because of the short half-life and the frequently required blood tests (weekly CBC and monthly liver function tests) because of the rare reports of aplastic anemia with this medication.

The patient who has *recurrent seizures* but says that he is taking his medication poses an important problem. Initial evaluation should include obtaining serum for anticonvulsant levels and persistent questioning to determine patient compliance with the regimen. Recent alcohol ingestion or addition of new medication may affect phenytoin levels (see Table 164-4). It is reasonable to administer 200 to 300 mg of phenytoin orally or intravenously if the history of compliance is unreliable and there is no nystagmus. Alternatively, the physician may elect to administer a second (or third) drug until laboratory results are known. Consultation with a neurologist is indicated in this situation.

Perhaps the most difficult aspect of epilepsy management is the long-term follow-up of a chronic seizure patient. The first obligation is the insurance of adequate anticonvulsant protection. Often this amounts only to yearly monitoring of anticonvulsant levels. Phenytoin has effects on the hematopoietic system related to duration of its use (Table 164-4), so that another useful yearly screen is a complete blood count to detect the development of megaloblastic anemia. No other routine tests are practical.

The physician will surely be asked when the medication can be stopped. As noted, the majority of patients with epilepsy, either idiopathic or with known etiology, do not achieve complete freedom from seizures when anticonvulsant medication is discontinued. Indeed, only about one-half are totally seizure-free with continuing therapy. This knowledge should temper the physician's willingness to attempt *discontinuation of medication*. Obvious contraindications to attempted withdrawal of medicine are recurrent seizures. Most neurologists would require a seizure-free interval of at least 1 year or, more likely, 2 years. The electroencephalogram is of little help in predicting which patients may successfully be weaned from their medicines. Clearly, a persistently abnormal electroencephalogram would make discontinuation of medication inadvisable.

PATIENT EDUCATION

Perhaps the most important obligation of the physician is his role as counselor, educator, and, sometimes, legal advocate. His is a long-standing relationship with a patient whose chronic disease is surrounded by an enormous amount of superstition, prejudice, and misunderstanding.

In addition to reviewing the prognosis with the patient, it is important to emphasize that even if seizures are not entirely controlled, most epileptics are able to lead productive lives. Fifteen to 25 percent of the nation's 4 million epileptics are unemployed, a figure three to four times higher than the national average. However, the few professions from which people known to suffer seizures are barred are those that require a chauffeur's or pilot's license.

The diagnosis of epilepsy imposes definite restrictions on the patient's life, which makes the certainty of diagnosis in a young, healthy person all the more imperative. *Driving laws* vary from state to state, but, in general, states require a seizure-free interval of at least 1 year before re-application for a driver's license may be made. Continued supervision by a physician is mandatory.

Apart from the impersonal considerations of driving permits and employment, the patient may feel that the diagnosis of epilepsy also bestows a social stigma. He may develop unnecessary fears and needlessly limit his life, because he does not understand his disease. The physician can help by recognizing and responding to his apprehensions and by educating him.

A patient may learn that he can tell when a seizure is about to occur; a headache, feeling of malaise, or another vague symptom may be present. Although such symptoms need not necessitate admission to a hospital, the patient can learn to avoid driving or other potentially dangerous activities at such times. Certain stimulants such as alcohol, coffee, and tobacco precipitate seizures, and the physician can legitimately recommend abstinence, at least from alcohol. Surgical procedures pose no special threat to the epileptic patient as long as his medications are not discontinued at any time.

There is considerable worry about *inheritance* of seizures. Epilepsy is hereditary, although the precise genetics are not known. One-quarter to one-third of patients with idiopathic epilepsy have a family history of seizures. Three percent of children of patients with idiopathic epilepsy develop seizures. Febrile convulsions also appear to be more common in children who have afflicted relatives. Although approximately one-half of these children will have a subsequent febrile convulsion, only one-quarter have a seizure without a high temperature. Six percent of the population will at some time have at least a single convulsion, so that the additional risk in children with febrile convulsions is about four times that of the general population.

Families of patients with epilepsy should know the fundamentals of emergency management of seizures. They should be instructed in the positioning that protects the airway and cautioned against insertion of the time-honored tongue blade. It should be emphasized that few seizures last long enough to impair cardiopulmonary function seriously, yet the families should understand the essentials of cardiopulmonary resuscitation.

Familiarity with the primary anticonvulsants and their side effects and sound understanding of the facts of epilepsy will enable the physician to control the physical disabilities of his patient's illness and to dispel the equally disabling fears that arise from this disturbing symptom.

THERAPEUTIC RECOMMENDATIONS

- Establish an etiologic diagnosis and treat the underlying cause, if possible. Symptomatic therapy can start while workup is in progress.
- To prevent further convulsions, begin with phenytoin in a loading dose of approximately 1000 mg over the first day

(see Table 164-3). This is usually done while the patient is hospitalized, but can be done on an outpatient basis. Maintenance dosage of 300 mg per day can then be started. Adjust the dose to achieve a therapeutic level, in the range of 8 to 20 mg per 100 ml in most laboratories.

- If phenytoin is ineffective or if adverse reactions to this drug develop, add phenobarbital at 60 mg before bed.
- If seizures persist, check the serum levels of the anticonvulsants and inquire into alcohol and other drug use; administer additional phenytoin if there is a low level of anticonvulsant or add a second or third agent. This is an indication for referral to a neurologist.
- Once seizures are controlled, continue the medication for at least 1 year; if the patient remains seizure-free, a cautious attempt at tapering the medication can be made.
- Teach the patient how to recognize the warning signals of a seizure and what to do to minimize injury; instruct him in the role of alcohol in precipitating seizures.
- Educate the patient and his family about prognosis, activity, and job precautions; teach airway protection by positioning and caution against the insertion of a tongue blade into the mouth.
- Elicit and discuss all patient questions and apprehensions thoroughly; discourage unnecessary restriction of activity.

ANNOTATED BIBLIOGRAPHY

Annegers JF, Brabow JD et al: Seizures after head trauma: A population study. Neurology 30:683, 1980 (*Emphasizes that a remote history of head trauma is often not a sufficient explanation for new onset seizures.*)

Delgado-Escueta AV, Treiman DM, Walsh GO: The treatable epilepsies. N Engl J Med 308:1508, 1576, 1983 (*An extensive review including the classification, natural history, and clinical presentation of epilepsies; includes a thoughtful discussion of the trade-off between freedom from seizures and drug toxicity.*)

Drugs for epilepsy. Med Lett 25:81, 1983 (*Best recent summary.*)

Engel J, Troupin AS, Crandall PH et al: Recent developments in the diagnosis and therapy of epilepsy. Ann Intern Med 97:584, 1982

(*Reviews clinical and electroencephalographic classification of seizure disorders, advances in diagnosis, and new therapeutic drugs and alternative approaches.*)

Hauser WA, Kurland LT: The epidemiology of epilepsy in Rochester, Minnesota, 1935 through 1967. Epilepsia 16:1, 1975 (*Thorough review of epilepsy in patients of all ages including incidence, types, etiology, and prognosis. 10-year follow-up.*)

Hauser WA, Anderson E, Loewenson RB et al: Seizure recurrence after a first unprovoked seizure. N Engl J Med 307:522, 1982 (*May temper the use of long-term anticonvulsants for the patient with none of the risk factors for recurrent seizures.*)

Ramirez-Lassepas M: The value of computed tomographic scanning in the evaluation of adult patients after their first seizure. Ann Neurol 15:536, 1984 (*Emphasizes that, though the yield is not high, this procedure should be offered to all patients with a first seizure.*)

Reynolds EH: Chronic antiepileptic toxicity: A review. Epilepsia 16: 319, 1975 (*Very thorough.*)

Russ LS: The diagnostic assessment of single seizures. Arch Neurol 40:744, 1983 (*Excellent discussion in the context of readily available CT scanning.*)

Schomer DL: Partial epilepsy. N Engl J Med 309:536, 1983 (*A brief but useful review of clinical manifestations, workup and management.*)

Slater E, Beard AW: The interictal behavior syndrome of temporal lobe epilepsy. Br J Psychiatry 109:95, 1963 (*55 pages of detailed psychiatric and neurologic study. There are more recent studies, but this is excellent.*)

Troupin AS: The measurement of anticonvulsant agent levels. Ann Intern Med 100:854, 1984 (*Reviews the reliability and clinical uses for anticonvulsant drug levels.*)

Wolf SM: Controversies in the treatment of febrile convulsions. Neurology 29:287, 1979 (*A rational approach to a fairly common problem—summarizes all the previous literature.*)

Woodbury DM et al: Antiepileptic Drugs. New York: Raven Press, 1972 (*Detailed review of pharmacology.*)

Woodcock S, Cosgrove SBR: Epilepsy after the age of 50: A 5-year follow-up study. Neurology 14:34, 1964 (*Montreal study of 80 patients older than 50. Suffers from lack of CT scanner at the time [PEG used] so results are not entirely applicable now. Definition of cerebrovascular disease is also rather vague.*)

165

Approach to the Patient With Transient Ischemic Attacks

AMY A. PRUITT, M.D.

Transient ischemic attacks (TIAs) are episodes of temporary, focal cerebral dysfunction due to vascular disease. Onset is rapid (often less than 1 minute) and, strictly defined, the symptom may last up to 24 hours; however, the vast majority of TIAs last only a few minutes. Clearing is as rapid as onset, and the attack leaves no neurologic deficits.

Recognition of TIAs and differentiation from similar nonvascular events are of critical importance. The symptom may be the initial clue to the presence of significant cerebrovascular disease. Although figures vary, it appears that about one-third of patients with TIAs progress to a completed stroke within 5 years. Unfortunately, clinical criteria that identify patients at greatest risk are not well established. Furthermore, the precise benefit of anticoagulation or endarterectomy in reducing stroke risk is not known. However, the primary physician should be able to recognize the occurrence of a TIA and should keep abreast of the extensive and evolving literature on the subject. In this chapter, the available data are discussed in the context of the practical problem of recognizing patients who require urgent evaluation for potentially operable vascular lesions or anticoagulation therapy.

PATHOPHYSIOLOGY AND CLINICAL PRESENTATION

Investigators have long disagreed about pathogenesis of TIAs. Some suggest that transient lowering of blood pressure in the presence of hemodynamically significant stenosis leads to symptoms, while the majority believe that emboli of platelets and fibrin or of atheromatous material break off from a vessel wall (usually the carotid) and transiently occlude branches of cerebral vessels. TIAs are known to occur on the side of a totally occluded vessel. In this case, small clots are presumed to form on the distal end of the thrombus and then dislodge.

On rare occasions, focal symptoms are caused by cardiac arrhythmias; but, recent studies indicate that blood pressure reduction alone rarely results in focal symptoms unless a stenotic lesion is already present.

In certain rare instances, TIAs may be attributable to steal phenomena (such as subclavian steal) or to hyperviscosity states such as polycythemia. Far more commonly (and more importantly for differential diagnosis) emboli from heart valves with rheumatic disease, mitral valve prolapse, or endocarditis, may produce recurrent focal neurologic deficits.

TIAs can be divided into those that indicate disease in the carotid circulation and those that point to disease in the vertebrobasilar territory. Symptoms of *carotid disease* include transient paresis (usually in the face and/or arm), paresthesias, dysphasia, or amaurosis fugax (transient monocular blindness). The last symptom is due to occlusion of the ophthalmic artery or branches ipsilateral to the carotid stenosis and classically is described by the patient as a "shade" or "curtain" that descends over the affected eye.

Symptoms of *vertebrobasilar disease* include binocular visual disturbance, vertigo, paresthesias, diplopia, ataxia, dysarthria, light-headedness, generalized weakness, loss of consciousness, and transient global amnesia. Any of these may be an isolated symptom of posterior circulation disease.

One particularly troublesome problem is that of the patient who presents with isolated vertigo. As a symptom of vertebrobasilar insufficiency, this complaint is rather uncommon and more often is attributable to labyrinthine pathology (see Chapter 160). Dizziness in vertebrobasilar disease is usually not true vertigo and usually is accompanied by other brain stem signs.

Certain clinical features are likely to be associated with carotid or vertebrobasilar disease, but no single feature is a consistently reliable sign. In one series, 95 patients with carotid territory TIAs were evaluated by arteriography. These patients had either tight carotid stenosis (defined as a residual vessel lumen of less than 2 mm), carotid occlusion, or normal vessels. Fifty-two patients had transient hemispheric attacks, 33 had amaurosis fugax, and 10 had both. Sixty-seven had recurrent episodes of the same general type. Two clinical features were correlated with the arteriographic state of the artery. First, duration of hemispheric attacks over 60 minutes, whether single or multiple, was significantly associated with a normal carotid (and presumably attacks were due to emboli from the heart). Second, the nonsimultaneous occurrence of both transient hemispheric episodes and transient monocular blindness was correlated with an 80 percent incidence of carotid disease. No difference between normal and diseased carotid groups was found when the cumulative number of attacks per patient was considered. Similarly, division according to pure ocular or pure hemispheric symptoms did not distinguish the two groups. Future similar studies may reveal other diagnostic and prognostic features of the clinical presentation.

DIFFERENTIAL DIAGNOSIS

Transient focal motor or sensory dysfunction does not have to be of vascular origin. Focal seizures (see Chapter 164) can produce a similar picture, as can the focal aura of migraine, which is not always followed by the diagnostic headache (see Chapter 166). Hyperventilation can produce distal tingling and numbness. Cervical discs can also produce transient focal motor or sensory disturbance, sometimes precipitated by manipulation of the head or neck (see Chapter 161). Carpal tunnel syndrome may present with intermittent (often nocturnal) paresthesias in a median nerve distribution. Meniere's disease presents with episodic vertigo and hearing loss, but without signs and symptoms of brain stem dysfunction (see Chapter 160).

The age group affected by TIAs of vascular origin is similar to that affected by cardiovascular disease, and the risk factors for cerebrovascular disease are similar. In general, the other disorders mentioned above do not usually present a practical problem in differential diagnosis (see Chapter 161).

WORKUP

The goals in evaluating a TIA are to establish the risk for significant vascular disease, to identify those patients whose symptoms dictate intervention, and to provide an adequate explanation for the event, should cerebrovascular disease prove not to be the etiology.

History. Questioning should first confirm that the transient episode is indeed a TIA. There ought to be the rapid onset of temporary focal cerebral dysfunction and equally rapid resolution with complete clearing. Duration of symptoms beyond 24 hours rules out TIA. The onset of headache during resolution of the neurologic deficit is more suggestive of a migrainous episode (see Chapter 166). Careful description of symptoms is needed to distinguish vertebrobasilar involvement from carotid disease. In addition, the frequency of episodes, date of first onset, and presence of hypertension and cardiac disease are important to ascertain. These items of the history may help predict clinical course. Patients with carotid symptoms are more likely to develop a disabling stroke than are those with vertebrobasilar dysfunction; the patient is at greatest risk for stroke in the first few months after onset of TIAs. The presence of hypertension, cardiac disease, or advanced age (greater than 65) increases the risk of subsequent stroke.

Physical Examination should be directed to the nervous system and vascular structures. Hypertension, atrial fibrillation, and cardiac murmurs should be noted. Ocular examination involves a search for visible atheromatous plaques in retinal artery branches. Neurologic examination, provided the patient has not had a previous completed stroke, is likely to be normal.

Carotid arteries should be palpated for upstroke and volume and should be auscultated for bruits. The presence of a bruit does not invariably herald significant stenosis (a bruit can be present with hemodynamically insignificant lesions or with complete occlusion), but in as many as 70% to 80% of cases, the bruit does identify ipsilateral carotid disease. Palpation of facial and superficial temporal pulses with simultaneous assessment of supratrochlear and supraorbital pulses may confirm collateral flow to the latter two vessels by way of the external carotid artery and suggest occlusion of the internal carotid artery. Unfortunately, the vertebrobasilar circulation is not accessible to accurate physical examination.

Laboratory Studies. At present, there is no entirely reliable noninvasive test for carotid or vertebrobasilar disease. *Doppler ultrasonography, thermography, carotid ultrasound,* and *phonangiography* are helpful in diagnosing hemodynamically significant carotid lesions. The combination of Doppler and B-mode ultrasound allows determination of lumen size and visualization of the arterial lesion. However, in some instances, one cannot tell if the carotid artery is completely occluded or only tightly stenosed. *Digital subtraction angiography* with injection of contrast intravenously instead of intra-arterially can give excellent views of the carotids, but is not always satisfactory for the vertebrobasilar circulation, cannot always exclude complete carotid occlusion, and is risky for diabetic patients and for those with angina. Thus *arteriography* remains the definitive diagnostic procedure. Many neuroradiologists advise using the above listed noninvasive tests only in the atypical case to "rule in" doing an arteriogram when symptoms are equivocal, but not to "rule out" doing an arteriogram in an otherwise suspicious case. However, arteriography should be performed only if the physician would proceed to endarterectomy in the case

of carotid disease or to anticoagulation in the case of vertebrobasilar disease; that is, the procedure should lead to a critical management decision.

PRINCIPLES OF MANAGEMENT

The literature of therapeutic options is complex and often confusing. Many studies are not well controlled, and, frequently, study populations are not well defined or well characterized. In a large multicenter controlled study done in Canada, *aspirin* was found to reduce risk of stroke by 31% and TIA occurrence by 19%; both effects were seen only in men. Other antiplatelet drugs do not seem to enhance the protective effect of aspirin. Aspirin and *warfarin* have not been compared in a well-controlled study, and no study of *warfarin* is as well designed as the recent Canadian trial on efficacy of aspirin in TIAs. Similarly, aspirin, warfarin, and surgery have never been directly compared in a thoroughly evaluated, prospectively randomized series. However, surgical morbidity from endarterectomy has been greatly reduced, and it appears that surgery may be the best treatment for tightly stenotic, symptomatic carotid lesion in a patient who has no contraindication to an operative procedure.

Bearing in mind that optimal therapy for TIAs is not yet clearly defined and the new information will be forthcoming, the following guidelines for management are recommended at the present time:

1. Those under 65 years of age who are good surgical risks and have recurrent TIAs, or TIAs within 2 months of examination, require prompt attention. If adequate radiologic support is available, these patients should have arteriography as soon as possible. Some physicians directly admit such patients to the hospital and immediately place them on intravenous heparin until arteriography can be performed if there is an unavoidable delay. Patients with residual carotid lumens of less than 2 mm or with ulcerated plaques should undergo endarterectomy. The physician should refer surgical candidates to a center where many endarterectomies are done.

2. Those with normal carotid vessels should have thorough cardiac evaluation to rule out an embolic source from the heart. In the absence of atrial fibrillation, valvular heart disease, or carotid disease, the proper treatment (anticoagulation with warfarin or aspirin or other therapy) is not known. While natural history studies suggest that these patients are at risk for future stroke, efficacy of available treatment is unclear. After the results of the American and Canadian aspirin studies became known, it became common to place such patients on aspirin prophylactically. While there is some evidence to recommend this practice, it should be clear that these studies did not address the question of TIA or stroke from noncarotid sources.

3. A sense of urgency is equally appropriate in the evaluation of patients with progressing neurologic deficit or with fixed, mild deficit and continuing TIAs. They, too, may benefit from anticoagulation and endarterectomy.

4. Patients over 65, patients with a single remote event, and patients seen in settings where angiographic and surgical services are unavailable may benefit from prophylactic administration of aspirin, although the proper dose is presently in question (doses in studies range from 60 mg to 1.2 g/day; most evidence favors doses at the lower end of the range). Hypertension and other risk factors should be eliminated. Other antiplatelet agents are being studied (no form of antiplatelet therapy yet has been shown to be effective in women).

The Asymptomatic Carotid Bruit

The incidental discovery on physical examination of an asymptomatic bruit is often a source of concern. Epidemiologic studies indicate the finding is associated with an increased risk of stroke, coronary disease, and death, but interestingly, not necessarily with increased risk of stroke on the side of the bruit. Moreover, risk of stroke is actually quite low, especially in patients without severe stenosis. In a large prospective study of 500 patients with asymptomatic bruits followed for an average of 2 years by clinical and Doppler examinations, the overall risk of stroke in patients who remained asymptomatic was 1% at 1 year, and 1.7% if those who developed TIAs were included. A major predictor of stroke was the severity of carotid stenosis (greater than 75% stenosis was a significant predictor of enhanced risk). Other predictors of stroke were preexisting heart disease and progression of the stenosis on repeat Doppler study. Most authors report that an initial warning TIA occurs in up to 70% of patients who eventually suffer a completed thrombotic carotid stroke.

Thus, the detection of a carotid bruit in an asymptomatic patient need not be considered a necessarily worrisome development. The patient should have a noninvasive carotid evaluation to confirm the carotid origin of the bruit and to determine severity of stenosis. Emphasis is placed on recognition and prompt reporting of any TIA-like symptoms and modification of cardiovascular risk factors such as smoking, hypertension, and hypercholesterolemia. Those with severe stenosis (greater than 75%) who experience a TIA are at markedly enhanced risk of stroke and should be referred to the neurologist for consideration of treatment. Carotid endarterectomy may be the best therapy for such patients, but prospective, randomized studies on its efficacy are lacking. Moreover, there is little controlled data on the relative merits of aspirin, warfarin, and other forms of medical therapy. Methods of effective stroke prophylaxis remain to be defined. The literature should be followed closely for future randomized prospective studies of therapy.

ANNOTATED BIBLIOGRAPHY

Ackerman RH: The relative effectiveness of six noninvasive tests for carotid disease. Neurology 26:379, 1976 (*Concise summary of a new and important area of diagnosis.*)

Brust JCM: Transient ischemic attacks: natural history and anticoagulation. Neurology 27:701, 1977 (*Excellent review of all previously published studies with critical analysis of their conflicting results.*)

Canadian cooperative stroke study group: A randomized trial of aspirin and sulfinpyrazone in threatened stroke. N Engl J Med 299: 53, 1978 (*Our best available evidence on the subject.*)

Caplan LR: Carotid-artery disease. N Engl J Med 315:886, 1986 (*An editorial suggesting that patients with asymptomatic bruits be studied noninvasively, educated about the symptoms of a TIA, and followed expectantly, reserving surgery for those who develop TIAs and have severe stenosis.*)

Cebul RD, Ginsberg MD: Noninvasive neurovascular test for carotid artery disease. Ann Intern Med 97:867, 1982 (*Reviews the use of phonoangiography, ultrasonic scanning, Doppler imaging, digital subtraction angiography, ophthalmodynamometry, and oculoplethysmography; clinical indications and combined use of tests are discussed.*)

Chambers BR, Norris JW: Outcome in patients with asymptomatic neck bruits. N Engl J Med 315:860, 1986 (*An important natural history study; risk of stroke greatest in those with severe stenosis.*)

Duncan GW et al: Concomitants of atherosclerotic carotid artery stenosis. Stroke 8(6):665, 1977 (*Shows carotid disease following same risk factors as Framingham study established for cardiac disease.*)

Fields WS: Aspirin for prevention of stroke. Am J Med 84:61A, 1983 (*A useful discussion and review of the issue.*)

Genton EG et al: Cerebral ischema: The role of thrombosis and of antithromobtic therapy. Stroke 8(1):150, 1977 (*A critical overview.*)

Heyman A: Risk of stroke in asymptomatic persons with cervical arterial bruits: A population study in Evans, County, Georgia, N Engl J Med 302:838, 1980 (*The risk of stroke ipsilateral to the auscultated bruit was very low, and the authors suggest that aggressive diagnostic studies are not appropriate unless symptoms have occurred.*)

Kistler JP, Lees RS, Miller A et al: Correlation of spectral phonoangiography and carotid angiography with gross pathology and carotid stenosis. N Engl J Med 305:417, 1981 (*Demonstrates the value of this noninvasive method in estimating residual lumen diameter among patients with carotid stenosis.*)

Kistler JP, Ropper AH, Heros RC: Therapy of cerebral vascular disease due to atherothrombosis. N Engl J Med 311:27, 100, 1984 (*Comprehensive discussion of evaluation and therapy; 175 references.*)

Levine M, Hirsh J: Hemorrhagic complications of long-term anticoagulant therapy for ischemic cerebral vascular disease. Stroke 17:111, 1986 (*A critical review of the utility and safety of anticoagulant therapy.*)

Pessin MS et al: Clinical and angiographic features of carotid transient ischemic attacks. N Engl J Med 296:358, 1977 (*Discussed in this chapter in detail. Provides useful clinical guidelines for evaluation.*)

Sandok BA: Guidelines for the management of transient ischemic attacks. Mayo Clin Proc 53:605, 1978 (*A reasonable compromise.*)

166
Management of Migraine and Other Vascular Headaches

Migraine

Migraine afflicts about 5% to 10% of the adult population and causes considerable misery. There is no cure for migraine, but medical therapy can reduce the frequency and severity of attacks. The primary physician should be able to offer relief to the patient with migraine through the design of a program that is safe and effective for both prophylaxis and treatment of attacks.

CLINICAL PRESENTATION AND COURSE

There are several forms of migraine. *Classic migraine* accounts for 10 to 15 per cent of cases. It is characterized by a prodrome of transient visual, motor, or sensory disturbances (*e.g.,* scintillating scotomata, zig-zag patterns, hemianopsia, paresthesias, hemiparesis, difficulty speaking) followed by onset of a hemicranial throbbing headache, nausea, photophobia, and sensitivity to noise. Typically the aura resolves as the headache begins. *Common migraine* occurs in 80% of patients with migraine. It differs from the classic variety in that there is no prodrome; sometimes the headache is bilateral or shifts sides. Nausea, photophobia, and related symptoms usually accompany the headache. Classic migraine may produce a prodrome without headache; this can lead to considerable diagnostic confusion, for there may be only a transient sensory or motor deficit. Since migraine is generally a self-limited disorder, neurologic dysfunction that lasts longer than 24 to 36 hours should suggest another diagnosis (see Chapter 159).

The list of reported precipitants of migraine includes fatigue, hunger, changes in the weather, menstrual period, emotional stress, alcohol, oral contraceptives, and certain foods. Cheese, nuts, avocados, ripe cheeses, and chocolate have been known to cause attacks in certain patients. Food cured with nitrates or flavored with monosodium glutamate has also brought on attacks. In over 50% of cases, there is a family history. Many patients were troubled by motion sickness or cyclic vomiting during childhood. All age groups are affected, but attacks usually begin before the third decade and subside by the fifth. Migraine occurs in women about four times as often as in men and may begin or terminate during menopause. It often subsides during pregnancy, but occasionally it may actually worsen during this time.

PRINCIPLES OF MANAGEMENT

There is no cure for migraine, but prophylaxis and symptomatic treatment are reasonably effective. Although the disease is self-limited, attacks may continue for decades, and chronic exposure to some of the drugs used in prophylaxis and treatment may be damaging or addicting. Consequently, design of a long-term management program requires attention to safety as well as efficacy.

Prophylaxis. Prevention of attacks involves *nonpharmacologic measures* as well as drug treatment. Since migraine may be precipitated by emotional stress or psychologic conflict, it is important to investigate family and social circumstances in designing a program of prevention. Regular exercise (*e.g.,* jogging) or *relaxation techniques* (see Chapter 222) may significantly decrease the frequency and severity of headaches. These activities help reduce the impact of stress. Many patients prefer to try them before attempting other forms of therapy.

Some patients bothered by migraine are overly competitive, very aggressive, and feel considerable need to succeed. They often harbor repressed hostility toward parents or other loved ones. An analysis of the circumstances associated with attacks may provide a clue to the presence of these factors. Therapy for such patients should include helping them to express their feelings and deal with these issues. Although extensive psychotherapy may not reduce attacks, it is worth trying to determine areas of stress and search with the patient for ways to resolve them. Recommending rest or a vacation might not suffice; in fact, flare-ups are common during vacations and weekends.

Biofeedback methods are of unproven benefit and probably no better than relaxation exercises and other nonpharmacologic methods. Lack of adequately designed studies limits conclusions regarding biofeedback.

Drug therapy should be added when nonpharmacologic measures do not suffice. *Beta-adrenergic blocking agents* (*e.g.,* propranolol, timolol, and others) have been shown to reduce the frequency and severity of attacks in double-blind crossover studies and are FDA-approved for prevention of common migraine attacks. In studies with propranolol, about two thirds of patients benefit from therapy; one third achieve a 50% or greater reduction in number of attacks; one third report no benefit or an increase in severity. Initial propranolol dose is 80 mg per day, increasing to as much as 160 to 240 mg per day. Beta blockade does not need to be achieved in order to attain a prophylactic effect. Asthma, heart failure, and heart block are the major contraindications (see Chapter 25). Tolerance has not been reported in trials lasting as long as 6 months.

Methysergide, a serotonin antagonist, has been relegated to a second-line position in migraine prophylaxis because of its association with retroperitoneal, pleuropulmonary, and valvular fibrosis when used for prolonged, uninterrupted periods. In view of its potentially serious side-effects, methysergide should be prescribed under close supervision and only after simpler measures have proven inadequate. However, the drug is effective; 60% to 80% of patients who take methysergide achieve at least a 50% or greater reduction in frequency of headaches. An initial dose of 1 mg should be given; the dose is then gradually increased over a 2-week period to a maximum of 6 mg per day. After a reduction in episodes of migraine has been achieved, the daily amount should be tapered to the minimum effective dose. Methysergide should be withheld for 1 month after every 6-month course of treatment to reduce the likelihood of fibrotic complications, which may develop silently. If therapy is uninterrupted, a yearly intravenous pyelogram should be obtained to detect any early signs of ureteral obstruction from retroperitoneal fibrosis. Upon initial administration, about 30% of patients experience nausea, vomiting, indigestion, myalgias, insomnia, restlessness, or feelings of depersonalization; about 10% cannot tolerate the drug for these reasons. Because the drug produces vasoconstriction, methysergide is relatively contraindicated in patients with peripheral vascular disease, coronary artery disease, and severe hypertension. Its concurrent use with ergotamine may increase the risk of severe vasospasm and occlusion. Active peptic ulcer disease, arteritis, liver or renal failure, and pregnancy are other relative contraindications.

Calcium channel blockers have emerged as a potentially useful new class of agents for prophylaxis of migraine. Although most drugs in this class have provided some benefit, *verapamil* and *nimodipine* (currently under investigation) appear to work best for prophylaxis of migraine. Nimodipine demonstrates the greatest affinity for cranial vessels and may prove to be the calcium channel blocker of choice for migraine. Both prodromal and headache symptoms are prevented. This class of drugs works best in patients with classic migraine (response rates of 80% to 90%), though a substantial fraction (50% to 60%) of patients with common migraine also report complete cessation or reduction in frequency and severity of attacks. Prophylactic effect does not begin to occur until 10 to 14 days into therapy, with a full response taking as long as 2 to 4 weeks. Cardiovascular side effects are greatest with use of verapamil and nifedipine (see Chapter 25), and relatively minimal with nimodipine.

Tricyclic antidepressants have been found capable of reducing the frequency of migrainous attacks, especially when depression is a prominent problem, but also when there are few depressive symptoms reported. *Antianxiety agents* may contribute to the prophylactic effort when acute situational stress and marked anxiety appear to be responsible for episodes. The efficacy of the popular combination drug *Fiorinal* is probably due to its barbiturate component, because it additionally contains only aspirin and caffeine. Clonidine, aspirin, and dipyridamole have all been tried with variable results; none approach the prophylactic efficacy of beta-blockers.

Treatment of an Acute Attack. Some patients with migraine find that attacks can be relieved by simple *physical measures* such as hot or cold packs or temporal massage. Dimming the lights and lying down in a quiet room also help to lessen the discomfort. Biofeedback techniques are under study.

Ergotamine tartrate is the drug most effective for relief of acute attacks. It has been found to constrict the arteries of the scalp, and it is therefore believed to counteract the vasodilatation phase of the migraine headache. Complete or partial relief from the headache occurs in about 70% of patients. To be effective, ergotamine must be taken at the first sign of an attack, such as during the prodromal phase of classic migraine. The lack of a prodrome in common migraine means there is often little advance warning, and this may limit ergotamine's usefulness.

The initial dose of ergotamine is 2 mg sublingually. There is some evidence to suggest that the sublingual form is faster acting and more effective than the oral route. An inhaled form is also rapid in onset of action. *Caffeine* potentiates ergotamine by increasing its absorption; as a result, some patients note even better results when using an ergot–caffeine preparation. Because of nausea and vomiting, some patients prefer to use a rectal suppository preparation of ergotamine. The ergotamine should be repeated every hour if there is no relief, until a maximum 24-hour dose of 6 to 8 mg is taken. Further doses are generally not helpful and may lead to toxicity.

Ergotamine is reasonably safe when used properly. Serious reactions occur in only 0.1% of patients. Adverse effects include nausea, vomiting, myalgias, paresthesias, chest discomfort, peripheral ischemia, angina, rebound headache, and dependency. Dependency and rebound headaches are managed by discontinuing the drug and controlling the headache with other medications.

Ergotamine is contraindicated in patients with vascular disease such as Raynaud's syndrome, coronary artery disease, thromboangiitis obliterans, thrombophlebitis, and severe atherosclerosis. The drug should not be taken during pregnancy because it causes uterine contractions as well as vasoconstriction.

Analgesics are required when the headache is well established and unresponsive to ergotamine. Control of mild headache may be obtained with 600 mg of *aspirin* or *acetaminophen* every 4 hours. The combination preparation Midrin, containing acetaminophen 325 mg, dichloralphenazone 100 mg, and the vasoconstrictor isometheptene mucate 65 mg, has been found, in controlled studies, to be superior to acetaminophen alone. The dose of this preparation is 2 capsules at the onset of the headache, followed by 1 capsule every hour until relief occurs, up to 5 capsules per 12 hours. Adverse reactions are chiefly transient dizziness and skin rash. *Narcotics* may be needed for very severe headaches but should be used sparingly. Codeine sulfate, 30 to 60 mg every 4 to 6 hours, usually will suffice.

Fiorinal is a very popular drug for migraine; it is an aspirin–caffeine preparation combined with a small dose of barbiturate (butalbital). Long-term use of Fiorinal exposes the patient to the risk of barbiturate dependence. Fiorinal previously contained phenacetin, which in large cumulative doses causes interstitial nephritis (see Chapter 139). Since migraine is a chronic, recurrent problem, the drug should be prescribed with caution if used at all on a chronic basis.

Photophobia responds to treatment of the headache, but nausea may persist, requiring separate antiemetic therapy. *Prochlorperazine,* 10 mg orally every 6 hours or 25 mg rectally every 12 hours, is indicated if incapacitating nausea and vomiting are present. At times, the nausea may be worsened by ergotamine intake; if ergotamine has been effective and its continued use is desired, addition of prochlorperazine may be helpful. *Metoclopramide* taken before ergot can prevent some of the nausea ergot induces.

PATIENT EDUCATION

The importance of careful instruction in the use of medications for prophylaxis and treatment of migraine cannot be overemphasized, because efficacy and safety depend on correct usage. Migraine is a problem that may last for decades, and it is essential to establish good habits related to drug use early on so that complications due to chronic misuse can be avoided. For example, the patient on methysergide must be informed of the need to cease the drug for a full month after every 6 consecutive months of use in order to avoid fibrotic complications. Ergotamine is not likely to be effective unless taken at the first sign of migraine. Patients should be advised that Fiorinal is not to be used continuously because of the risk of barbiturate dependence.

THERAPEUTIC RECOMMENDATIONS

Prophylaxis

- Identify any precipitating factors such as situational stress or psychologic conflict and attend to them directly (see Chapter 222). Relaxation techniques and regular exercise may help reduce the impact of stress.
- Begin a beta-blocker (*e.g.,* propranolol, 80 mg per day) if attacks are frequent and severe enough to interfere with the patient's normal activities. Increase the daily dose until a reduction in severity or number of episodes is noted or a dose of 240 mg per day is reached.

- If propranolol is effective, continue therapy on a daily basis for 6 months, then taper and watch for recurrence.
- If propranolol is ineffective and prophylaxis is definitely needed, begin *methysergide,* 2 mg daily, and increase dose to 6 mg per day over the next 2 weeks. If there is no improvement, stop the drug. If improvement is apparent, taper to the minimum effective dose. Do not use methysergide for more than 4 to 6 months. There must be a medication-free interval of 4 weeks after every 6-month course of treatment to prevent fibrotic complications.
- As an alternative to methysergide, consider a calcium channel blocker (*e.g.,* verapamil or nimodipine).
- Consider a tricyclic antidepressant (see Chapter 223) for prophylaxis if depression is accompanied by migraine, or if other agents fail to achieve reduction in frequency or severity of attacks.

Treatment of Acute Attacks

- Begin ergotamine tartrate, 2 mg sublingually, at the first sign of migraine. A caffeine-containing preparation may help speed onset of action.
- Repeat every hour until relief is obtained or a maximum of 6 to 8 mg has been taken in 24 hours.
- If the headache is severe, well-established, and unresponsive to ergotamine, treat the attack with codeine sulfate, 30 to 60 mg every 4 hours.
- If the headache is mild, aspirin, 600 mg every 4 hours, or acetaminophen, 600 mg every 4 hours, should suffice.
- Avoid chronic use of barbiturate-containing compounds (*e.g.,* Fiorinal).
- Treat incapacitating nausea and vomiting with prochlorperazine suppositories, 25 mg rectally every 12 hours or 10 mg tablets orally every 6 hours.
- Consider use of metoclopramide (10 mg before use of ergot) if ergot-induced nausea is troublesome.

Cluster Headaches

Cluster headaches are a form of vascular headache, but lack the vasoconstrictive component characteristic of migraine. They cause a sharp, steady (rather than pounding) type of headache (see Chapter 159). Episodes typically occur every night for several weeks or months, then resolve spontaneously, only to recur years later. In about 10% of patients, the attacks persist. Propranolol, tricyclic antidepressants, lithium, prednisone, ergotamine, and methysergide have been tried with variable results. *Calcium channel-blocking agents* offer new hope for these patients. Very encouraging results have been obtained using nimodipine, verapamil, and nifedipine. Prophylactic efficacy is reported in up to 80% of patients, with most noting partial or complete relief of headache attacks.

A.H.G.

ANNOTATED BIBLIOGRAPHY

Diamond S et al: Propranolol in prophylaxis of migraine headache. Headache 22:268, 1982 (*A single-blind study showing a response rate of 70%; no tolerance developed after 6 months of continued use.*)

Elkind AH et al: Silent retroperitoneal fibrosis associated with methysergide therapy. JAMA 206:5, 1968 (*Documents this important complication of long-term methysergide therapy.*)

Feuerstein M, Adams H: Cephalic vasomotor feedback in modification of migraine headache. Biofeedback Self Regul 2:241, 1977 (*Describes some of the biofeedback techniques for control of migraine.*)

Graham JR: Methysergide for prevention of headache. N Engl J Med 270:67, 1964 (*Classic paper on the effectiveness of the drug for prophylaxis.*)

Health and Public Policy Committee, American College of Physicians: Biofeedback for headaches. Ann Intern Med 102:128, 1985 (*Concludes that there is insufficient data to recommend biofeedback for migraine, and that there is no evidence suggesting it is any better than relaxation techniques.*)

Linet MS, Stewart WF: Migraine headache: Epidemiologic perspectives. Epidemiol Rev 6:107, 1984 (*Exhaustive review detailing descriptive epidemiology of migraine, genetic and physiologic predisposing factors, and factors associated with onset and frequency of attacks.*)

Meyer JS: Calcium channel blockers in the prophylactic treatment of vascular headache. Ann Intern Med 102:395, 1985 (*Reviews evidence for their use and argues they are likely to play a major role in prophylaxis of migraine and cluster headache.*)

Stellar S, Ahrens SP, Meibohm AR et al: Migraine prevention with timolol. JAMA 252:2576, 1984 (*Sixty-five percent with timolol had a favorable response compared to 40% with placebo in this randomized trial.*)

Solomon GE, Steel JG, Spaccavento LJ: Verapamil prophylaxis of migraine. JAMA 250:2500, 1983 (*A small double-blind crossover study in which 10 of 12 patients had fewer migraines during verapamil therapy.*)

Waters WE: Controlled clinical trial of ergotamine tartrate. Br Med J 1:325, 1970 (*Casts some doubt on the efficacy of oral administration of ergot and argues for sublingual or rectal route.*)

Wideroe TE, Vigander R: Propranolol in the treatment of migraine. Br Med J 2:699, 1974 (*A double-blind crossover trial using 30 patients demonstrated significant reduction in mean frequency of migraine attacks when propranolol was used prophylactically.*)

167
Management of Parkinson's Disease

AMY A. PRUITT, M.D.

The development of improved drug therapy for Parkinson's disease has brought new hope and relief to thousands suffering from this immobilizing condition. Proper treatment requires careful timing and skillful utilization of drugs, because there are important difficulties associated with pharmacologic therapy. The agents used for Parkinson's disease often cause *drug–drug* interactions and produce substantial side effects (including some that resemble symptoms of the disease). Moreover, drug efficacy declines over time, and therapeutic response may be blunted by improper timing or inappropriate selection of antiparkinsonian agents.

The frequency of Parkinson's disease, its ability to interfere with daily activity and independent functioning, and the availability of drug therapy make it important for the primary physician to know the details of management.

CLINICAL PRESENTATION AND COURSE

Tremor is the most obvious initial finding, but it is absent in 20% of patients. Parkinson's disease may begin insidiously with vague, aching pain in the limbs, neck, or back and with decreased axial dexterity before tremor is noted. Other early subtle symptoms are decreases in the caliber of handwriting and the volume of the voice; both reflect disturbances in extrapyramidal motor function. More disabling are rigidity and bradykinesia, which can interfere with daily activity. Distressing episodes of frozen rigidity, sudden loss of postural control, and immobile facies that may be mistaken for depression can result.

Before the introduction of levodopa (L-dopa), the disease had a fairly predictable course. At 5 years from onset, 60% of patients were severely disabled, and at 10 years, nearly 80% were. The rate of progression varied widely. Mortality was three times that of an age-matched population. Death rarely was a direct result of parkinsonism; rather, it was a consequence of immobility (aspiration pneumonia, urinary tract infections) or of trauma. Trauma has actually become more frequent as patients gain mobility but continue to have poor postural control.

L-dopa produces a marked improvement in functional capacity, although treatment does not alter the underlying pathologic process. However, by preventing complications that result from immobility, levodopa does extend the life span of severely affected patients. Over a period of 5 years of therapy, one-third of the 85% of patients who initially respond to treatment retain their benefit, one-third lose some of the response, and one-third lose all initial benefit and are considerably worse than they were when treatment began.

PRINCIPLES OF MANAGEMENT

Dopamine and acetylcholine are neurotransmitters. The normally high concentration of dopamine in the basal ganglia has been found to be depleted in parkinsonian patients. Clinically, these patients appear to have excessive cholinergic activity. These findings have led to the notion of treating Parkinson's disease by either dopaminergic repletion or cholinergic antagonism.

Anticholinergic agents were the mainstay of parkinsonian therapy for more than a century, and they have remained important even with the introduction of levodopa because more than half of the patients who have benefited from levodopa note additional improvement when anticholinergic agents are added. Moreover, levodopa response decreases after the first few years of therapy (regardless of the extent of initial improvement or the severity of the disease), making it necessary to employ a second drug.

One commonly used anticholinergic is trihexyphenidyl (Artane), which resembles the belladonna alkaloids. Adverse effects include blurred vision, urinary retention, and drying of mucous membranes. Similar agents are benztropine (Cogentin) and some antihistamines with weak anticholinergic effect, such as diphenhydramine (Benadryl).

Amantadine, initially used for prophylaxis of influenza A, is believed to act by releasing dopamine from nigrostriatal terminals that are still intact. Amantadine acts maximally within a few days but loses efficacy within 6 to 8 weeks of continuous treatment. Side effects are minimal, although macular degeneration and livido reticularis of the legs have appeared infrequently.

Levodopa has been in common use for a full decade and is now available by itself or in combination with the dopa-decarboxylase inhibitor carbidopa. L-dopa is rapidly absorbed after oral administration, reaches peak effect at 30 minutes to 2 hours, and has a half-life of 1 to 3 hours. The rate of absorption is decreased by eating a protein-rich meal. When used alone, only 1% of an L-dopa dose eventually reaches the brain, but the addition of a peripheral dopa-decarboxylase inhibitor ensures greater delivery to the central nervous system.

Therapeutic efficacy is impressive. Over three-quarters of patients show some response to levodopa. All symptoms diminish, but bradykinesia and rigidity improve more than does tremor.

Adverse reactions are many. Nausea, vomiting, anorexia, hypotension, dyskinesias, and hallucinations can be quite disturbing. Recently defined problems include declining efficacy, a distressing "on–off" phenomenon with sudden fluctuations in disability, and deterioration of intellectual function. Decarboxylase inhibitors have decreased the early gastrointestinal side effects but have led to increased incidence of dyskinetic and psychiatric reactions.

Regardless of duration of disease, the best results with levodopa are obtained in the first 3 years after initiation of therapy. With time there is a declining threshold for the development of adverse central side effects; this may necessitate a decrease in daily dose. The phenomenon has been explained as a kind of denervation hypersensitivity of dopamine-depleted terminals. On the other hand, an increasing dose of medication is required over time to forestall the inevitable disappearance of responsiveness. Decline in effect is believed related to a reduction in dopaminergic receptor sites or to the depletion of the dopa-converting enzyme that is required to form the active metabolite when levodopa is administered orally. A progressive dementia has been noted in rare cases in patients on prolonged levodopa therapy. Although this symptom has come to be recognized as part of the disease process itself, levodopa clearly has played a direct causative role in some reported cases. Other psychiatric symptoms, including nightmares, hallucinations, and increased sexual drive, are being seen more frequently because higher doses of levodopa are delivered centrally by the combination preparations. The disturbing "on–off" phenomenon, which has been linked to impaired absorption and transport of L-dopa, may limit therapy in young patients with otherwise good response to levodopa. Paradoxically, increased mobility has in some instances led to increased disability as a result of sudden falls by previously rigid patients.

The physician is able to offer the parkinsonian patient much benefit, but one is still quite limited by the toxicity of treatments. The goal of therapy is to maintain the patient at a maximal or at least tolerable level of function with minimal medication. Initiation of L-dopa therapy should be delayed as long as possible, because *regardless of the initial severity of the disease or the initial benefit from the drug, levodopa's efficacy decreases with time.* The patient and physician must tolerate many of the early signs of parkinsonism, which are sufficient to prompt medical consultation, but, aside from provoking psychologic discomfort, are not threatening. Clearly, this philosophy must be individualized; the violinist with a tremor is much more drastically disabled by his symptoms than is a retired businessman.

Attempts to abolish all evidence of parkinsonism often necessitate use of doses of levodopa that produce intolerable side effects. The appearance of dyskinesias may require a decrease in dose and a compromise between parkinsonism and dyskinesia, allowing some signs of the original disease to re-emerge. For practical purposes, the target symptom of most importance is rigidity. A reasonable therapeutic end point is mobilization of the patient; complete abolition of all parkinsonian symptoms may not be feasible.

Several suggested means of dealing with the disadvantages of levodopa therapy have been proposed; results are variable. Temporary withdrawal of levodopa therapy neither enhances the efficacy nor prevents complications of long-term use, although it may transiently relieve drug-related problems. Untested is the suggestion that protein intake be spread out and medication be taken on an empty stomach to counter the "on–off" phenomenon.

Initiating Therapy. Each newly diagnosed patient should be evaluated for extent of disability at home and at work, including the effect of the illness on social interactions. Mild tremor that is well tolerated need not be treated; follow-up visits at regular intervals will suffice. If symptoms are more disturbing, one can prescribe an anticholinergic agent such as trihexyphenidyl (Artane), beginning with 2 mg once or twice a day; an alternative is to start amantadine, at 200 mg per day.

Finally, L-dopa, the most potent currently available treatment, should be started when patients need immediate symptom relief or are quite advanced at the time of presentation. If early minor signs are treated with levodopa, maximal benefit at a later, more symptomatic time may be impaired. During the initial "induction" phase, treatment is started at a subtherapeutic level with, usually, one of the combination dopa-decarboxylase-levodopa preparations. Treatment may be started with 1 tablet containing 25 mg carbidopa/250 mg levodopa (Sinemet) three times a day after meals; 1 tablet may be added every 2 to 4 days. The daily dose is increased gradually to minimize gastrointestinal side effects. Patients who have been taking large doses of levodopa may be switched to Sinemet by decreasing the total daily levodopa dose by about 50% to 75% and using the large size combination tablet (25 mg carbidopa/250 mg levodopa).

Several practical concerns inevitably arise. A protein meal, while decreasing gastrointestinal toxicity, also decreases absorption. Nevertheless, it is reasonable to give the medication with meals to minimize GI upset. Pyridoxine enhances activation of dopa-decarboxylase, and, in the amounts present in many common multivitamin preparations, may decrease the therapeutic effect of levodopa, although not that of the combination preparations. Phenothiazines and haloperidol worsen parkinsonism, and monoamine oxidase (MAO) inhibitors may interact with levodopa to cause a dangerous elevation of blood pressure.

Direct dopamine agonists such as *bromocriptine* have been used for patients who have become refractory to the Sinemet combinations. Unfortunately, many of the same psychiatric and "on–off" side-effects are at least as great with these medicines. Constant infusion of L-dopa has been tried recently and helpful experimentally in reducing the incidence of fluctuations in mobility in advanced Parkinsonism. This remains an experimental procedure at present.

Maintenance. A maintenance phase follows the establishment of a therapeutic dose schedule. Day-to-day and even hour-to-hour fluctuations in clinical status should not be surprising. The clinical situation may not stabilize for at least 2 months from onset of therapy. The physician commonly receives frequent calls from the patient. The occurrence of gastrointestinal side effects from use of L-dopa often necessitates adjustment in the program; if L-dopa is being used alone, switching to a combination agent may allow for a lowering of the L-dopa intake without a loss of therapeutic effect. If bradykinesia and rigidity appear late in the afternoon, it may be worthwhile to add a 25-mg carbidopa–250-mg levodopa combination tablet at 4 PM. It is sometimes necessary to decrease the evening dose of L-dopa at the expense of some stiffness during the late evening hours in order to minimize the occurrence of vivid nightmares, frequently experienced by some patients.

PATIENT EDUCATION

Patient and family education is essential to the success of therapy. The patient and family should receive careful explanation of the side effects and potential benefits of drugs. The need for trial and error to obtain maximal benefit with minimal side effects must be explained. Therapy can be proposed optimistically. The diminishing efficacy of the drug must be anticipated, but the development of newer agents, such as direct dopaminergic agonists, is in progress and may obviate the problem of decreased sensitivity to levodopa.

THERAPEUTIC RECOMMENDATIONS

- Mild tremors that do not interfere with activity or bother the patient do not require treatment. Those that do can be managed by starting an anticholinergic agent such as trihexyphenidyl 2 mg once or twice daily; levodopa should not be introduced unless the anticholinergic agent does not suffice or is poorly tolerated.
- Amantadine (200 mg per day) is immediately effective and may be added early in the course of Parkinson's disease to control both bradykinesia and tremor. Its efficacy is lost over time; thus it should not be used as the sole agent.
- Levodopa should be introduced when symptoms interfere significantly with the patient's life *and* other agents have not provided adequate relief. L-dopa treatment should be initiated utilizing the combination preparation containing 25 mg carbidopa and 250 mg levodopa. The starting dose is 1 tablet after each meal, increasing the dose by 1 tablet every 2 to 4 days. This schedule will help to minimize gastrointestinal side effects and the cumulative dose of levodopa.
- The development of the disabling side effects of L-dopa usually responds to reduction in dose, but the appearance of uncontrollable dyskinesias or the "on–off" phenomenon requires consultation with an experienced neurologist.

ANNOTATED BIBLIOGRAPHY

Bianchine JR: Drug therapy of parkinsonism. N Engl J Med 295: 814, 1976 (*Good, brief review.*)

Boshes B: Sinemet and the treatment of parkinsonism. Ann Intern Med 94:364, 1981 (*Good review for the generalist.*)

Calne DB: Progress in Parkinson's disease. N Engl J Med 310:523, 1984 (*An editorial discussing advances in pathophysiology and treatment.*)

Fahn S, Calne BB: Considerations in the management of parkinsonism. Neurology 28:5, 1978 (*A sober note of caution about initial treatment with levodopa.*)

Lieberman A et al: Treatment of Parkinson's disease with bromocriptine. N Engl J Med 295:1400, 1976 (*Encouraging reports of improvement in patients who are levodopa nonresponders.*)

Marsden CD, Parles JD: Success and problems of long-term levodopa therapy in Parkinson's disease. Lancet 1:345, 1977 (*Reviews reasons for failure of levodopa therapy against the background of the natural history of Parkinson's disease.*)

Mayeux R, Stern Y, Mulvey K, et al: Reappraisal of temporary levodopa withdrawal ("drug holiday") in Parkinson's disease. N Engl J Med 313:724, 1985 (*Temporary withdrawal was not helpful.*)

Nutt JG, Woodward WR, Hammerstad JP, et al: The "on–off" phenomenon in Parkinson's disease. N Engl J Med 310:483, 1984 (*Provides data suggesting interference by food and amino acids with the absorption and transport of L-dopa.*)

Sweet RD, McDowell FH: Five years of treatment of Parkinson's disease with L-dopa. Ann Intern Med 83:456, 1975 (*A large case series with lucid discussion of the state of the art.*)

Vance ML, Evans WS, Thorner MB: Bromocriptine. Ann Intern Med 100:78, 1984 (*Comprehensive review of the drug; 134 references.*)

Weiner WT, Bergen D: Prevention and management of the side effects of levodopa. *In* Klawans HL (ed): Clinical Neuropharmacology, vol. 2, p 1–23. New York, Raven Press, 1977 (*A detailed, rather biochemical explanation of side-effects with some practical management suggestions.*)

168

Management of Alzheimer's Disease

MICHAEL A. JENIKE, M.D.

It is estimated that between 2 and 4 million Americans currently suffer from senile dementia of the Alzheimer's type (SDAT). As more individuals survive into old age, the prevalence of this disorder will increase. About 5% to 7% of those over age 65 and as many as 20% of those over age 80 will develop Alzheimer's disease. Almost half of all nursing home patients have progressive dementing illnesses. The primary care physician who is going to manage such patients must be familiar with the course of the illness, the treatment of its psychiatric concomitants (psychosis, anxiety, depression, behavioral disturbances), the types of social services available, and approaches to family counselling.

CLINICAL PRESENTATION AND COURSE

During the earliest stages, most patients seem *mildly forgetful* and complain of such memory deficits as forgetting names or where they placed household items. The patient may seem concerned but has no social or employment problems and shows no evidence of memory deficit during a clinical interview.

The next stage of mild cognitive decline is characterized by decreased performance in demanding work or social situations. Patients complain of *poor concentration* and difficulty finding words and names, and may report that co-workers have noticed their relatively poor performance. Some patients present initially with *visuospatial deficits,* while others may have difficulty with *speech* early in the course of the illness. Later, patients may get lost when traveling to an unfamiliar location. Anxiety and depression are common, and many patients begin to deny symptoms.

As the illness progresses, patients become unable to travel alone and are unable to handle their personal finances. *Memory* for *recent events* will be drastically impaired, and patients display decreased knowledge of current events. Complex tasks are impossible, but patients remain well-oriented to time and person and can travel to very familiar places, like the corner drugstore. Many patients are aware of their deficits and are capable of understanding what is happening to them. Patients instinctively withdraw from previously challenging situations. *Denial* may become pronounced.

During the next phase, patients can no longer survive without some assistance. They are unable to recall major relevant aspects of their current lives or even the names of close friends and family members. *Delusions* are common. For example, the spouse is accused of being an imposter or the patient talks to imaginary persons or to his own reflection in the mirror. *Depression, agitation,* and violent behavior may occur. Frequently patients are disoriented to time or place. However, they generally remain able to eat and use the toilet without assistance, but may have difficulty properly choosing and putting on clothing.

In the last stages of the disease, patients become totally *incapacitated* and *disoriented.* They eventually forget their own name and may not recognize their spouse. *Incontinence* is common. *Personality* and *emotional changes* become very pronounced, though these occasionally occur even in the earliest stages. Eventually all verbal abilities are lost, motor skills deteriorate, and patients require total care. Generalized cortical and focal neurologic signs and symptoms are frequently present. Death usually occurs from total debilitation or infection.

The course of Alzheimer's disease varies from 2 to as long as 20 years from onset to death. The average is around 6 to 8 years. Typically, the illness progresses at a fairly constant rate. If it has rapidly developed over the past year, it is likely to continue at that rate. A slowly progressive illness over the past 5 to 10 years suggests that the patient may survive for a number of years.

PRINCIPLES OF MANAGEMENT

Once treatable causes for dementia have been ruled out (see Chapter 163), the physician faces the challenge of a chronic, progressive illness. Management involves the skillful interplay of care by family members (who often choose to maintain the patient at home), psychopharmacologic therapy, and the help of community agencies.

Drugs for Memory Enhancement. A wide variety of pharmacologic agents have been investigated for the treatment of cognitive decline in Alzheimer's disease; therapies have reflected ongoing hypotheses about the disease's cause. Evidence has been accumulating which suggests defects in acetylcholine synthesis and metabolism. These findings have stimulated trials of medications and dietary supplements (*e.g., lecithin*) to bolster the failing acetylcholine system. To date, none has proven effective.

Another group of drugs classified loosely as "metabolic enhancers" has been tried. *Ergoloid mesylate* (*Hydergine*) remains the most commonly prescribed drug for SDAT patients, and a number of controlled studies have shown minimal cognitive improvement with Hydergine. Individual effects are generally small; the most significant change is in depression. Even though study results are weak, experienced clinicians occasionally report an individual patient with a good response to a 3- to 6-month trial of this agent. If there is no improvement after 6 months, it should be discontinued.

Even though the body of basic information about SDAT has increased dramatically in the last few years, the pharmacologic treatment remains in its infancy. Research has thus far produced no consistently effective agents that the primary care physician can use to treat SDAT patients. It is likely, however, that breakthroughs will occur in the next decade. All patients with mild or moderate SDAT should be referred to research centers for experimental protocols when this is feasible.

Drugs to Control Psychiatric Symptoms. Many SDAT victims will experience concomitant depression, anxiety, behavioral abnormalities, or psychosis. Selective use of psychopharmacologic therapy can be helpful. *Depression* often responds to a tricyclic agent or a monoamine oxidase inhibitor (see Chapter 223). The condition is not an irreversible or inevitable consequence of Alzheimer's disease; in fact, most patients do not experience it. However, it is treatable and should be sought and treated vigorously. Cautious use of anxiolytic agents (see Chapter 222) can help with bouts of excessive *anxiety* (see below). Behavioral disturbances and psychoses also may respond to psychopharmacologic intervention, utilizing neuroleptics and sedative–hypnotic drugs (see below). The safe and effective use of psychotropic medication in Alzheimer patients necessitates adjustments in drug selection, dose, and frequency to accommodate the alterations in drug uptake and metabolism that occur in the elderly. Such adjustments are particularly important when using neuroleptics and sedative–hypnotics (see Appendix).

Management of Behavioral Disorders. Certain behaviors are particularly troublesome to family members. Among those cited most frequently are catastrophic reactions (including violent behavior), wakefulness, suspiciousness, and incontinence.

Catastrophic reactions are massive emotional overresponses typically precipitated by task failure or minor stress. Hitting and violent resistance to care are extreme forms of such reactions. Most excessive emotional responses can be minimized by teaching the family to avoid or remove the precipitating task or stress, to remain quiet and calm, and to gently change the focus of attention. Neuroleptic drugs (*e.g.,* haloperidol 0.5 mg qd or bid) are sometimes helpful in difficult cases, but only as an adjunct to behavioral techniques.

Wakefulness and *night walking* often deprive the caregiver of much-needed rest. Helpful environmental interventions include placing locks on each door so that the patient will not wander out of the house at night, keeping the patient physically active during the day, and not allowing a nap. Sedative–hypnotics, such as a short-acting benzodiazepine (*e.g.,* lorazepam 1.0 mg qhs) or chloral hydrate, may be helpful (see Chapter 228). Occasionally, low doses of a neuroleptic may be needed (see Appendix).

Suspiciousness and accusatory behaviors are believed to result from the brain-injured person's efforts to explain misplaced possessions or misinterpreted events. If the family understands this, their frustration, hurt, and anger may be reduced. Simple interventions, such as keeping an orderly house or making a sign pointing to where an object is kept, may help (see below). Neuroleptics may be used as a last resort.

Incontinence is typically a late manifestation of SDAT, and when present early, it warrants a careful search for other causes, such as urinary tract infection (see Chapter 133).

SDAT patients may decompensate cognitively and behaviorally when they experience a *superimposed illness.* Coexistent medical problems, such as asthma, diabetes, and congestive heart failure, should be carefully controlled. Even a minor upper respiratory tract or urinary tract infection can worsen behavior. Patients are susceptible to *medication-induced delirium;* close supervision of drug regimens is imperative.

Family members can be assured that *inappropriate sexual behavior* is very uncommon. In the rare instances where it occurs, self-stimulation is the usual form; Alzheimer's patients are not child molesters.

The Home Environment. As mentioned earlier, families need to be encouraged to maintain a *structured,* predictable environment for the patient. Any change can be devastating and stressful to a demented patient and may produce a massive emotional overresponse. A schedule in which activities such as arising, eating, taking medication, and exercise occur at the same time each day maximizes the patient's familiarity with his personal environment. At times, use of an *orientation center* in the home with pertinent information such as the date, time, schedule of household events, and pictures of relevant people is very helpful.

Not infrequently patients will want to drive when it is clear that they are no longer safe on the roads. If possible, it is best to avoid direct confrontation. Simple techniques such as hiding the keys, disconnecting distributor wires, or giving the patient a nonfunctional set of keys have usually been successful in discouraging patients from driving.

Firearms should not be kept in the home for obvious reasons. In addition, smoking and cooking become potentially dangerous activities. Environmental modifications, such as removing stove knobs, having a stove cut-off switch placed in an inconspicuous place, locking rooms or closets, or locking up matches, are important for safety.

Management of the Family. Some family members may well react with dread and depression to the fact that their relative has Alzheimer's disease. Those members who have a preexisting psychiatric illness may decompensate. Others will have suspected the diagnosis and are relieved to have an understanding physician who will be available and helpful over the course of the illness. Family members who are initially stunned and ask few questions should not have information forced upon them. Careful explanation about any further evaluative tests should be given and a follow-up appointment within a week arranged. Common questions include: How long will the patient live? How rapidly will he deteriorate? What are the chances of other family members developing the disease—is it hereditary? Is there a treatment?

Within the first few weeks of making the diagnosis, family members should see a *social worker* who is aware of community resources such as visiting nurse services, meals-on-wheels, financial aid, and nursing homes. For the very early Alzheimer's patient, this may seem premature, but family members will be reassured by the knowledge that help will be available when needed in the future. Most families read about the illness and become acutely aware of the devastating course of the illness.

Guilt, unrealistic expectations, and assumption of excessive responsibility are common responses of families. In discussing these and similar issues, the physician should focus both on physical realities and on the family's emotional responses to the patient. One frequently encountered source of difficulty is the reversal of parent/child roles that the care of an elderly person often represents. There is no one way to handle this issue; however, in the overwhelming majority of such cases, just allowing family members to discuss these and other issues will be therapeutic in and of itself.

Family members report that *lack of time for themselves* and sleep disturbances in patients are the least tolerable aspects of home care. Families do best when relatives and friends visit frequently and when provisions are made for the primary caregiver to have breaks in his or her responsibilities. Visiting nurses or day-care centers can be invaluable. Family support is the major variable in keeping the cognitively impaired elderly at home.

Even with a compassionate and empathetic physician, many families feel alone with this illness and are unable to find friends who understand. Embarrassment may make them withdraw from previous social contacts. To meet the need for communication and information, families in many areas have established *volunteer organizations* that are involved in helping each other, sharing solutions to management problems, exchanging information, supporting needed legislation and research, and educating the community. These organizations welcome members who are concerned about all of the dementing illnesses, of which Alzheimer's disease is the most common. The number of such support groups is growing rapidly, and families consistently report how helpful they are.

These local volunteer organizations have established a national organization, the *Alzheimer's Disease and Related Disorders Association* (ADRDA), whose goals are family support, education, advocacy, and encouraging research. The address of ADRDA is 70 E. Lake St., Chicago, IL 60601. The national organization will give family members the addresses of local groups.

Each family member should be encouraged to read one of the available lay books on Alzheimer's disease. *The 36-Hour Day* is required reading for anyone (including the physician) who is dealing with an individual with a progressive dementing illness.

THERAPEUTIC RECOMMENDATIONS

- Once a patient has been diagnosed as having a progressive dementing illness, the primary care physician will become the main coordinator of the patient's care and advisor to the family. The physician should consciously decide whether to take on this responsibility or to refer the patient and family for care by a group specializing in the management of such patients.

- Family members should be apprised of the patient's diagnosis and an open discussion should be part of the initial management.
- Early in the course of the illness, a social worker should meet with the family to help plan for care and provide support.
- A predictable, well-structured home environment should be established.
- When patients develop a concomitant psychiatric problem, such as depression, anxiety, behavioral disorder, or psychosis, psychopharmacologic intervention can be helpful. For depression, begin a low dose of a well-tolerated tricyclic agent (*e.g.,* 25 mg of desipramine qhs; see Chapter 223); for anxiety or sleep consider a low dose of a short-acting benzodiazepine (*e.g.,* 1.0 mg of lorazepam; see Chapter 222); for psychotic behavior or catastrophic reactions a low dose of a neuroleptic may prove useful (*e.g.,* 0.5 mg haloperidol qhs or bid; see Appendix). Drug treatment should be brief (except in depression) and with the smallest dose possible.
- A number of drugs are available to treat cognitive impairment. None is consistently effective and results are modest at best. There is no evidence that vitamin or dietary supplements (*e.g.,* lecithin) have any effect.
- Family members should be advised to join the local chapter of ADRDA and to become knowledgeable about the disease and its course by reading one of the currently available books (*The 36-Hour Day*) is an excellent resource.)

ANNOTATED BIBLIOGRAPHY

Albert M: Assessment of cognitive functioning in the elderly. Psychosomatics 25:310, 1984 (*Discusses the cognitive changes associated with both normal aging and dementing illness.*)

Bartus RT, Dean RL, Beer B et al: The cholinergic hypothesis of geriatric memory dysfunction. Science 217:408, 1982 (*An excellent review of the basis for using cholinergic agents in an attempt to improve cognitive function.*)

Crook T, Gershon S: Strategies for the Development of an Effective Treatment for Senile Dementia. New Canaan, CT, Mark Powley Associates, 1981 (*An excellent review by experts of various research approaches to the treatment of senile dementia.*)

Ferris SH (ed): Psychopharmacology in the elderly. *In* Psychopharmacology Bulletin. Public Health Service. Washington. Vol. 19, 1983 (*Excellent, but often technical, review.*)

Jenike MA: Handbook of Geriatric Psychopharmacology. Littleton, MA, PSG Publishing, 1985 (*Covers drug treatment of depression, psychosis, anxiety, and insomnia as well as a chapter on Alzheimer's disease.*)

Katzman R: Alzheimer's disease. N Engl J Med 314:964, 1986 (*A concise update with an emphasis on pathophysiology, but also discussions on diagnosis and management.*)

Kosick KH, Growdon JH: Aging, memory loss, and dementia. Psychosomatics 23:1982 (*A concise review of the major elements of the evaluation and pharmacotherapies for Alzheimer's disease.*)

Mace NL, Rabins PV: The 36-Hour Day. Baltimore, The Johns Hopkins University Press, 1981 (*Required reading for all who care for patients with dementing illnesses. Excellent for family members.*)

Rabins PV, Mace NL, Lucas MJ: The impact of dementia on the family. JAMA 248:333, 1982 (*Interview reports from primary caregivers of 55 patients suffering from irreversible dementia. Excellent perspective on the social impact and likely problems to be encountered with dementia.*)

Appendix: Use of Psychotropic Drugs in the Elderly

Pharmacokinetic Changes Associated With Aging. With aging, clinically important changes in drug absorption, distribution, protein binding, hepatic metabolism, and renal excretion ensue. Gastric *p*H increases and splanchnic blood flow decreases, altering drug solubility and absorption. Total body fat rises from 10% of body weight at age 20 to 24% at age 60, increasing the volume of distribution for lipid-soluble drugs, such as diazepam and its metabolites, and greatly prolonging drug half-life. In addition, total body water may decrease from 25% to 18% in the same period, causing water-soluble drugs, such as ethanol, to have higher concentrations due to decreased reservoir size. Serum albumin levels decline by 10% to 15%, decreasing protein-binding sites and liberating more free active drug into the circulation, thus raising the risk of toxicity. Drug metabolism slows; the activity of hepatic cytochrome P-450 decreases, as does demethylation. The result is higher levels of unmetabolized drug.

After age 40, there is a progressive decline in glomerular filtration rate and renal plasma flow. By age 70, the reduction is about 50%, prolonging drug action and increasing the likelihood of toxicity if dosage is not adjusted downward.

In addition to these pharmacokinetic changes, decreased CNS dopamine and acetylcholine levels, respectively, can lead to increased sensitivity to extrapyramidal and anticholinergic side-effects. An increased tendency to CNS disinhibition in the elderly increases the likelihood of drug-associated confusion, sedation, and paradoxical reactions.

Neuroleptics. Violence, rage, and psychosis are common problems in patients with Alzheimer's disease. The drugs most commonly used to treat these problems are the neuroleptics. All of the neuroleptics are equally effective in treating the above symptoms. Choice of a particular drug is based on its side-effects and toxicity. The main side-effects of the neuroleptics are sedation, orthostatic hypotension, extrapyramidal symptoms, and anticholinergic symptoms. There is a fairly consistent relationship between potency of the neuroleptic and side-effects: as the milligram potency of a neuroleptic increases, the frequency and severity of sedation, or-

Table 168-1. Neuroleptics

NAME (TRADE NAME)	APPROXIMATELY EQUIVALENT DAILY DOSE (MG)
High-Potency Agents	
haloperidol (Haldol)	2
thiothixene (Navane)	5
trifluoperazine (Stelazine)	5
fluphenazine (Prolixin)	2
Low-Potency Agents	
chlorpromazine (Thorazine)	100
thioridazine (Mellaril)	95
Medium-Potency Agents	
perphenazine (Trilafon)	10
loxapane (Loxitane)	15
molindone (Moban)	10

thostatic hypotension, and anticholinergic symptoms decrease and extrapyramidal symptoms increase (see Table 168-1).

Side-effects can be used therapeutically. The patient who has trouble falling asleep will find sedating neuroleptics to be of more use than nonsedating agents. Sedating neuroleptics may also be used to calm an agitated patient during the day. More commonly, however, sedation is an unwanted side-effect. Daytime sedation may cause or aggravate nighttime insomnia, and sedation may also increase confusion and disorientation in the demented patient. As disorientation and confusion increase, the patient typically becomes more agitated.

One of the most severe dangers when using neuroleptics is the possibility of inducing *orthostatic hypotension,* which can lead to falls and fractures, stroke, or even heart attack.

Hypotensive episodes are especially apt to occur at night when the elderly patient awakens and gets up to urinate.

High-potency neuroleptics, such as *haloperidol, thiothixene,* and *fluphenazine,* are generally safe to use in the elderly, but should be started at very low doses, such as 0.5 mg of haloperidol once or twice daily. Although generally safe, these drugs are more likely than low-potency agents (such as chlorpromazine or thioridazine) to produce extrapyramidal symptoms in the elderly. As many as 50% of all patients between 60 and 80 years who receive neuroleptics develop extrapyramidal symptoms, and those with brain damage, dementia, or Parkinson's disease are much more sensitive to these effects. The most troubling extrapyramidal symptoms are akathisia, parkinsonism, and akinesia (see Table 168-2).

Akathisia is a feeling of motor restlessness associated with a subjective sensation of discomfort, often described as anxiety. Sleep is usually disturbed because the individual is unable to find a comfortable, motionless position. Sometimes this restlessness is misinterpreted as an increase in psychotic symptoms and is treated with an increase in neuroleptic dosage. A most effective treatment for akathisia is lowering the dose. Other treatments include anticholinergic agents, benzodiazepines, amantadine, and propranolol.

Neuroleptic-induced *parkinsonism* appears identical to the postencephalitic or idiopathic forms. An occasional patient will be exquisitely sensitive to this side-effect and as little as one dose of a high-potency agent may precipitate the syndrome. Parkinsonism can usually be treated effectively with small doses of anticholinergic agents or with the addition of amantadine in dosages of 100–200 mg/day (see Chapter 167).

One of the unfortunately common and severe side-effects of any neuroleptic agent is the development of *tardive dys-*

Table 168-2. Extrapyramidal Reactions to Major Tranquilizers

REACTION	TIME INTERVAL AFTER DRUG	CHARACTERISTICS	TREATMENT
Acute dystonia	1–5 days	Spasm of muscles of neck, tongue, face, back; occasionally trismus (lockjaw)	Benzotropine 1–2 mg/day IM or Diphenhydramine 25–50 mg/day IM
Akathisia	5–60 days	Motor restlessness, jitteriness, constant pacing	Propranolol 30–80 mg/day PO or Benztropine 1–8 mg/day PO or Trihexyphenidyl 2–10 mg/day PO or Amantadine 100–200 mg/day PO
Parkinsonism	5–30 days	Bradykinesia, cogwheel rigidity, tremor	Benztropine 1–8 mg/day PO or Trihexyphenidyl 2–10 mg/day PO or Amantadine 100–200 mg/day PO
Tardive dyskinesia	Late	Involuntary, repetitive movement of face and tongue	Often irreversible, no drugs consistently effective

kinesia, manifested by a wide variety of movements, including lip-smacking, sucking, jaw movements, writhing tongue movements, chorea, athetosis, dystonia, tics, and facial grimacing. In severe cases, speech, eating, walking, and even breathing can be seriously impaired. Onset is gradual, usually after long-term, high-dose administration, but on rare occasions it can occur with short-term or low-dose use. Advancing age correlates not only with increased prevalence, but also with severity. Once tardive dyskinesia has developed, it is much less likely to reverse in an elderly patient than it is in a younger one.

The best way to *prevent* tardive dyskinesia is to avoid the use of neuroleptics. Obviously, these drugs are sometimes required, but they should not be used when indications are unclear or when less potentially toxic drugs may be as efficacious. Neuroleptics should never be used for simple anxiety, uncomplicated depression, or for long periods in patients who were suffering from an *acute* psychotic episode. It is important to make a baseline examination prior to starting neuroleptics and to note any early signs of tardive dyskinesia, such as fine vermicular movements or restlessness of the tongue, mild choreiform finger or toe movements, and facial tics or frequent eye blinks. The patient should be monitored for the development of early tardive dyskinesia at least every 3 months. Currently, there are no consistently effective agents that are useful in the treatment of tardive dyskinesia. In view of the significant risk to the elderly patient and the ineffective treatment options, physicians should avoid the use of neuroleptic drugs in elderly patients whenever possible.

Antidepressants. See Chapter 223.

Anxiolytics. See Chapter 222.

Hypnotics. See Chapter 228.

ANNOTATED BIBLIOGRAPHY

Ferris SH (ed): Psychopharmacology in the elderly. Psychopharmacol Bull 19(2):1983 (*Excellent review.*)

Jenike MA: Tardive dyskinesia: Special risk in the elderly. J Am Geriatr Soc 31:71, 1983 (*A detailed discussion of this important complication.*)

169
Management of Bell's Palsy
AMY A. PRUITT, M.D.

Bell's palsy is an idiopathic paralysis of the facial muscles innervated by the seventh cranial nerve. The condition encompasses 80% of all facial palsies. Satisfactory explanations for the condition are lacking, although viral infection and ischemia with subsequent edema of the facial nerve and adjacent structures have been invoked. Other causes of facial paralysis involve injury to the facial nerve and include bacterial infection (from a source in the ear), herpes zoster, diabetes mellitus, sarcoidosis, Guillain-Barré syndrome, tumor (acoustic neuroma, pontine glioma, neurofibroma, cholesteatoma), and trauma (fracture of the temporal bone).

The primary physician should be able to distinguish Bell's palsy from other, more ominous causes of facial palsy and temper therapeutic intervention by knowledge of the disease's self-limited course and good prognosis.

CLINICAL PRESENTATION AND COURSE

The distinction between Bell's palsy and other facial paralyses is usually not difficult. The onset of Bell's palsy is acute, involving the peripheral seventh nerve. There are no rashes, signs of trauma or sarcoidosis, history of diabetes, or evidence of ear infection. The patient appears with drooping face and mouth and occasionally with drooling. Maximal deficit develops over a few hours. The condition is almost always unilateral and in two thirds of the cases may be accompanied by pain in or behind the ear. Fever, tinnitus, and mild hearing diminution may be present during the first few hours.

Voluntary and involuntary motor responses are lost. Upper and lower parts of the face are affected, distinguishing this peripheral facial nerve lesion from a central supranuclear one, in which only lower facial muscles are affected. The palpebral fissure appears widened and the forehead smooth. Bell's phenomenon (the normal upward deviation of the eye with lid closure) is prominent because of orbicularis oculi weakness. The corneal reflex may be decreased on the involved side. Lacrimation is only rarely defective and, depending on the level of the injury, loss or perversion of taste on the anterior two thirds of the tongue or hyperacusis may be noted.

Seventy-five percent to 90% of cases recover to a cosmetically acceptable level without treatment. Recovery is best in children; poor prognosis has been associated with increasing age, hyperacusis, diminished taste, and severity of the initial motor deficit. Prognosis can be predicted by electromyographic (EMG) testing of the involved muscles at 14 to 18 days from onset. If EMG shows no signs of nerve degeneration by this time, there is usually notable clinical improvement, and recovery is almost uniformly complete. If, however, there is EMG evidence of degeneration, recovery may require several months and be less than total. It should be remembered that even though nerve conduction may remain abnormal in up to 20% of cases, the resulting motor function is usually satisfactory from the patient's point of view. The upper face, involved earliest as the disease develops, is the first to recover.

Complications of Bell's palsy result from abnormal regeneration of damaged nerve fibers. Lacrimation with eating or "crocodile tears" result when autonomic fibers regrow and connect with salivary glands instead of lacrimal ducts. Abnormal movements may occur if regenerating motor fibers innervate inappropriate muscles. Contracture of the involved site may be noted during voluntary movement. Seven percent of patients experience recurrent facial paralysis.

PRINCIPLES OF MANAGEMENT

Of greatest practical importance during the acute stage of the illness is the prevention of injury to the cornea, which is left exposed by weakness of the orbicularis muscle. When the lid is weak, methylcellulose drops should be prescribed for used twice a day and at bedtime; in addition, the lid may need to be taped shut at night.

The prognosis for most cases of Bell's palsy is good. Often little or no treatment is necessary. However, if paralysis is severe and the patient is seen within a few days of onset, a short course of corticosteroid therapy will increase the chances for maximal recovery. One study reported full facial recovery in 88% of the group treated with prednisone and in 64% of the untreated control group. Another study found a decrease in the frequency of chronic autonomic dysfunction (from 10% to 1%) when prednisone was used early in the course of illness. Associated ear pain diminished more quickly when steroids were used. Nevertheless, the benefits from use of steroids are often difficult to demonstrate, because the disease has such a good prognosis. Steroid therapy seems to make a difference only in cases with poor prognostic signs.

Other treatments have been used. Based on the theory that nerve swelling contributes to the deficit, surgical decompression has been tried, but without much success. Some patients have been followed with EMG stimulation of the muscles to hasten particularly stubborn paralyses. The possible role of EMG stimulation in management is unclear; it has not been subjected to controlled study.

THERAPEUTIC RECOMMENDATIONS AND INDICATIONS FOR REFERRAL

- Ascertain that the condition is indeed Bell's palsy. Check for involvement of other cranial nerves and ear infection. Examine for zosteriform lesions on the tympanic membrane, in the external auditory canal, and behind the ear.
- Explain the benign nature and good prognosis of the condition and caution the patient about corneal abrasion. Prescribe use of methylcellulose eyedrops twice a day and at sleep, with taping of the especially weak lid. Tarsorrhaphy may be considered when severe lid weakness exists.
- If the palsy is complete, the patient is seen within 3 or 4 days of onset, and there is no important contraindication to corticosteroid use, a short course of prednisone may be prescribed on the following schedule: 60 mg for 10 days, 40 mg for 2 days, 30 mg for 2 days, 10 mg for 1 day, and 5 mg for 2 days. If postauricular pain recurs when the dose is tapered, the immediately preceding dose may be reinstituted.
- In the 10% of patients who do not achieve acceptable recovery, autografting with a portion of the greater auricular nerve may provide reasonable cosmetic results and afford lasting protection of the eye. Patients in this category should be referred to an otolaryngologist or to a neurosurgeon.

ANNOTATED BIBLIOGRAPHY

Adour KK: Diagnosis and management of facial paralysis. N Engl J Med 307:348, 1982 (*A superb succinct clinical review not only of Bell's palsy but also of facial paralysis due to herpes zoster, trauma, otitis media, neoplasms, and other causes.*)

Adour KK et al: Prednisone treatment for idiopathic facial paralysis (Bell's palsy). N Engl J Med 287:1268, 1972 (*Controlled part of this study stopped when authors felt pain relief and recovery were clearly aided by prednisone. However, the results for both groups were very good.*)

Hauser WD et al: Incidence and prognosis of Bell's palsy in the population of Rochester, Minnesota. Mayo Clin Proc 46:258, 1971 (*Gives natural history and establishes excellent prognosis.*)

Wolf SH et al: Treatment of Bell's palsy with prednisone. A prospective, randomized study. Neurology 28:158, 1978 (*There was incomplete recovery in 16% [mild in 14%]. No diabetics were included.*)

170

Management of Tic Douloureux (Trigeminal Neuralgia)

Tic douloureux is among the most excruciating of pain syndromes seen in office practice. There are 15,000 new cases annually in the United States; most patients are middle-aged or elderly. Some have found the pain so intolerable that they consider suicide. The primary physician needs to know how to use available medical therapies and when to send the patient for neurosurgical consultation.

CLINICAL PRESENTATION AND NATURAL HISTORY

The illness is characterized by paroxysms of unilateral lancinating facial pain involving the jaw, gums, lips, or maxillary region (areas corresponding to branches of the trigeminal nerve). Attacks are often precipitated by minor, repeated contact with a trigger zone, setting off brief but fierce pain that usually lasts up to a few minutes. Repeated paroxysms may continue day and night, for several weeks. The disease is unilateral and unaccompanied by demonstrable sensory or motor deficits, which distinguishes it from other causes of trigeminal pain, such as tumor.

The condition can be chronic, although spontaneous remissions are not uncommon. Women are more often affected than men, and the incidence rises with age. The etiology of the condition remains unknown. Despite much speculation, no definitive evidence links it to herpes simplex virus. The pathologic lesion found in some electron micrographs appears to be a breakdown of myelin.

PRINCIPLES OF MANAGEMENT

Treatment is symptomatic. Because the condition may be self-limited and agents that give temporary relief are available, drug therapy should be tried before surgery is contemplated. *Carbamazepine* (Tegretol) is the drug of choice; it was initially tried because anticonvulsants were believed to be helpful in causalgic pain. Studies have shown impressive short-term effects; most patients report marked pain relief within 24 to 72 hours on 400 mg to 600 mg per day. The maintenance dosage ranges from 400 mg to 800 mg per day.

Unfortunately, by 3 years, 30% no longer obtain relief from carbamazepine; alternative therapy is needed. Moreover, the incidence of serious side-effects (bone marrow suppression, rash, liver injury) is high (5%–19%), requiring cessation of therapy. Fortunately, marrow suppression is often reversible if the drug is stopped early. Skin rash often precedes other serious side-effects; it may be erythematous and pruritic.

The onset of a skin rash is an early indication to halt therapy. Annoying side-effects include nausea, diarrhea, ataxia, dizziness, and confusion. Neurologic reactions are reported most commonly and affect about 15% of patients. Starting carbamazepine at 200 mg daily helps to avoid many of the annoying minor side-effects. During the first 3 months of therapy, complete blood and platelet counts should be obtained weekly; later, the frequency of monitoring can be about once a month. It is advisable to attempt reduction or cessation of carbamazepine therapy at least once every 2 to 3 months.

If carbamazepine alone begins to lose its effectiveness, *phenytoin* can be added. Before carbamazepine was available, phenytoin was used alone with some success. Regarded by many as a second-line agent, it is still preferred by others, since it may be better tolerated and requires less frequent hematologic monitoring (see Chapter 164).

Baclofen, an agent capable of inhibiting synaptic transmission, has been used with success in some cases. Treatment is initiated at dosages of 10 mg bid and increased slowly. Abrupt cessation of therapy can lead to hallucinations and seizures, so discontinuation must be gradual.

When drug therapy proves inadequate, *surgical approaches* can be considered. The procedure producing the least deficit with the greatest relief of symptoms is percutaneous electrocoagulation of the preganglionic rootlets that feed the trigger zone. The poorly myelinated pain fibers are destroyed, while the more heavily myelinated touch fibers that supply the relevant zone are spared. The procedure has produced lasting relief in 90% of those treated once; only 5% have experienced undesirable loss of sensation. The late recurrence rate is 10%, and a repeat procedure achieves pain relief in these patients; few need further treatment.

Formerly used treatment methods include alcohol injection or partial section of the sensory root of the fifth nerve. These techniques provided pain relief, but often only for 1 to 2 years, and at the price of unacceptable permanent sensory deficits. Total tooth extraction is an ineffective and erroneous treatment method.

PATIENT EDUCATION

The patient needs to be told that the condition can be controlled and is often self-limited. This knowledge can prevent a distraught sufferer from attempting suicide. The physician must keep in mind the anguish these patients may experience; they require close support. Obvious hints, such as avoiding repetitive contacts with the trigger zone, have usually been discovered by the patient, but can be helpful and are worth mentioning. Patients treated with carbamazepine must be taught to recognize the early symptoms and signs of marrow suppression (fever, sore throat, mouth ulcers, petechiae, easy bruising) and instructed to discontinue the drug and report to the physician immediately if these occur.

THERAPEUTIC RECOMMENDATIONS AND INDICATIONS FOR REFERRAL

- Teach the patient to avoid repetitive contact with the trigger zone.
- Begin drug therapy for disabling and frequent episodes of pain, starting with 100 mg (half a tablet) of carbamazepine twice daily, and increase the dosage by 200 mg per day until control of symptoms is achieved or a dosage of 800 mg per day is reached.
- During the first 3 months of carbamazepine therapy, monitor complete blood count and platelet count weekly; thereafter, monthly checks will suffice.
- Stop drug therapy immediately if any significant fall in count occurs or if skin rash, easy bruising, fever, mouth sores, or petechiae develop.
- If carbamazepine alone is not sufficient to control symptoms, add phenytoin at a dosage of 300 mg per day.

- In refractory cases, begin a trial of baclofen, 10 mg bid. Increase the dosage by 10 mg every 3 days until a response or a maximum of 60 mg is reached. Discontinue the medication gradually; do not withdraw it abruptly.
- Avoid use of narcotics, because they are unlikely to be of help for long-term control of pain and may only lead to drug dependency.
- Refer the patient who cannot be managed by pharmacologic measures to a neurosurgeon skilled in selective percutaneous electrocoagulation of the preganglionic rootlets.

A.H.G.

ANNOTATED BIBLIOGRAPHY

Crill WE: Carbamazepine. Ann Intern Med 79:844, 1975 (*A review of the pharmacology and use of this agent. Argues for its use as the first line of therapy in tic douloureux.*)

Hershey R: Baclofen for neuralgia. Ann Intern Med 100:905, 1984 (*An editorial note discussing its use in patients with neuralgic pain.*)

Lunsford LD: Treatment of tic douloureux by percutaneous retrogasserian glycerol injection. JAMA 248:449, 1982 (*After this treatment, 23 of 30 patients remained pain-free for 5 to 12 months.*)

Sweet WH: The treatment of trigeminal neuralgia (tic douloureux). N Engl J Med 315:174, 1986 (*A concise and authoritative review of both medical and surgical approaches to treatment by a pioneer in surgical therapy for this condition.*)

12

Dermatologic Problems

171
Screening for Skin Cancers
ARTHUR J. SOBER, M.D.

Neoplasms of the skin are among the most common cancers in humans. It has been estimated that more than 400,000 new tumors occur annually in the United States. The majority are basal cell carcinomas, relatively benign, locally mutilating tumors associated with few deaths. Squamous cell carcinoma, the second most common cutaneous malignancy, causes approximately 1500 deaths annually. Malignant melanoma, of which there are more than 20,000 cases annually, is responsible for approximately 7500 deaths annually. The first two types of tumor derive from the epidermal keratinocytes; the latter develops from the melanocytes along the basal layer of the epidermis.

Screening for these tumors is important because they are relatively easy to diagnose in early stages when cure is possible by simple measures. This is particularly true for malignant melanoma, because we are in the midst of a striking, unexplained increase in melanoma incidence. In the past decade, the incidence of melanoma in the United States has approximately doubled. Since 1960, mortality resulting from melanoma has increased more rapidly than any other cancer mortality except for that of lung cancer among women.

EPIDEMIOLOGY AND RISK FACTORS

Basal cell carcinomas are probably the most common malignancy in man. They are distinctly solar-related. In one study of over 800 tumors, approximately 90% of the lesions occurred on the head and neck. The frequency of these lesions is increased in people who work out-of-doors, such as farmers and sailors. Etiologic factors other than solar exposure are responsible for some basal cell carcinomas. For example, the basal cell nevus syndrome is a genetically transmitted autosomal-dominant disorder in which multiple basal cell carcinomas occur in relatively young individuals in association with palmer pits, bone cysts, and frontal bossing. Basal cell lesions can develop in persons exposed to arsenic. Scars from radiation dermatitis and from thermal burns can also provide sites favorable to development of basal cell tumors. Previously identified disease is also a risk factor. Once a single basal cell carcinoma has developed, there is a 20% chance that a second one will ensue within 1 year; after two have developed, there is a 40% likelihood that a third or more will occur within 1 year.

Squamous cell carcinomas may develop from actinic keratoses and may also occur following arsenic ingestion or in areas of scarring from radiodermatitis or thermal burns. Two thirds of these tumors occur on sun-exposed surfaces. Those arising in sun-damaged skin usually behave biologically in a less aggressive fashion than those that occur on surfaces not exposed to the sun. It is the latter group that apparently metastasize more frequently.

Malignant melanoma, while far less common than basal cell and squamous cell cancers, accounts for 70% of the deaths caused by tumors of the skin. The incidence of malignant melanoma has been increasing rapidly over the past decade, and in certain areas, such as Canada, its rate of increased incidence is exceeded only by that of carcinoma of the lung. The current annual incidence exceeds those of Hodgkin's disease, carcinoma of the thyroid, and carcinoma of the pharynx and larynx. The sex ratio for melanoma in the United States is approximately 1:1. A second primary develops in about 2% of patients; 6% to 10% have affected relatives.

Giant hairy nevus is a form of congenital nevus that has been associated with malignant degeneration in 2% to 40% of cases. Recent studies estimate the overall risk of malignancy to be about 6%. Melanomas may arise in these lesions anytime throughout life, but they usually do so by age 10. Smaller *pigmented congenital nevi* occur in about 1% of the population. Malignant melanoma occasionally arises in these nevi, but the frequency is unknown.

The risk of developing skin cancer is not equal in all persons. Individuals with fair skin who burn easily on exposure to sun and who tan poorly are especially at risk. Conversely, blacks and dark-skinned whites have a much lower risk. This observation appears to be valid for malignant melanoma, but the association is less convincing than with other forms of skin cancer.

Because of the rapid rise in melanoma incidence, attention has focused on melanoma precursors and risk factors. Precursor lesions include *congenital nevi* and *dysplastic nevi.* While congenital nevi occur in approximately 1% of all newborns, most of these are small (less than 1.5 cm in diameter). Melanoma risk has been most clearly associated with medium (1.5 cm–20 cm) and large (greater than 20 cm) nevi; lifetime melanoma risk for persons with large congenital nevi has been estimated between 5% and 20%.

Dysplastic nevi occur in between 2% and 8% of people. They usually develop early in adolescence. Among those with dysplastic nevi, the lifetime risk of melanoma has been estimated at 10%, or 15 times that of all whites in the United States. The 8- to 12-fold risk of melanoma among first-degree relatives of persons with melanoma may be partly explained by the fact that predisposition to dysplastic nevi is inherited.

Sun exposure is a critical risk factor for both nonmelanoma and melanoma skin cancers. It has been suggested that total accumulated sun exposure is associated with risk of basal cell and squamous cell carcinoma. Melanoma, however, is more likely to result from episodic, intense sun exposure.

NATURAL HISTORY OF SKIN CANCERS AND EFFECTIVENESS OF THERAPY

Basal cell carcinomas rarely metastasize, but they can be locally invasive and disfiguring; few deaths result. Only about 400 basal cell carcinomas have been reported to have metastasized. This extremely infrequent event usually occurs in patients who have delayed therapy for many years and who have large, locally invasive, eroded lesions.

Several effective forms of therapy exist, all yielding a cure rate of approximately 95%: surgical excision, radiation therapy, dessication and curettage, and cryotherapy with liquid nitrogen applied by special spray apparatus. Treatment of the 5% of basal cell carcinomas that recur presents a greater challenge. The cure rate of a recurrent basal cell carcinoma is about 66%. In the most difficult recurrent and infiltrative basal cell carcinoma, a special form of surgery called Mohs chemosurgery has been developed. In this technique, the tissue is fixed with zinc chloride paste and is examined directly under the microscope to determine whether the tumor has been completely removed. Additional sections of skin are removed until all the borders are histopathologically clear of tumor. With the Mohs technique, cure rates of recurrent tumors exceed 90%. A recent modification of the Mohs technique allows for microscopically controlled surgery without the need for zinc chloride fixation. The use of 5-fluorouracil has been advocated by some physicians for the treatment of superficial basal cell carcinoma. Experience has not been sufficient to be able to place this modality in relationship to the other forms of therapy that have a clearly established track record, but it may have some role in patients with multiple lesions in whom other techniques cannot be employed.

Squamous cell carcinomas may begin as actinic keratoses, of which perhaps 1 in 1000 eventually undergoes malignant change. There are several effective therapeutic modalities for actinic keratoses. Application of 5-fluorouracil cream or solution twice daily for 2 to 3 weeks will usually result in the destruction of these lesions. Some clinically inapparent lesions will also be destroyed by this therapy. The patient must be warned about the impressive inflammation that occurs when 5-fluorouracil is used. The inflammation can be decreased by the concomitant use of a topical steroid cream. Because 5-fluorouracil is also a photosensitizing agent, treatment in late fall or winter, when solar exposure is diminished, is preferred. Other effective modalities include cryotherapy with liquid nitrogen and light dessication. If a cutaneous horn is present, biopsy of the lesion is warranted to rule out the presence of a squamous cell carcinoma. Actinic keratoses are extremely common and usually present no great threat to life. Treatment is often of cosmetic consequence only.

Bowen's disease or squamous cell carcinoma *in situ* is substantially less common than actinic keratoses. It represents the next grade of neoplasia in the keratinocytic line. Surgical removal of Bowen's disease lesions is probably the most effective treatment. Alternatively, this tumor can be treated satisfactorily by cryotherapy with liquid nitrogen. Five percent 5-fluorouracil solution, applied two to three times daily and covered by a plastic occlusive dressing for 6 weeks, may also be employed for treatment of Bowen's disease.

Effective treatment of squamous cell carcinomas includes surgical excision and radiation; the latter is reserved for people over 60 years of age.

There are four primary types of *malignant melanomas:* superficial spreading, nodular, lentigo maligna melanoma, and acral lentigenous. The *superficial spreading type* is the most common in the United States and represents 70% of all malignant melanomas diagnosed. The early lesion exists 1 to 7 years before a nodule develops, indicating that deep penetration has occurred. During this 1 to 7 years, the lesion grows superficially; removal during this time is associated with a 5-year survival rate approaching 100%.

Nodular melanoma has a poorer prognosis. It may arise *de novo* or within a nevus as an invasive tumor from onset. Even with early recognition, metastasis will already have occurred in a certain percentage of patients. This type of tumor can occur on any cutaneous surface, as can the superficial spreading melanoma. Nodular melanoma represents about 15% of all melanomas.

Lentigo maligna melanoma, the third type, represents about 5% of malignant melanomas and occurs on sun-damaged skin of elderly patients. It is the least aggressive of the melanomas and may be present for 5 to 50 years before an invasive nodule develops. Prior to nodule formation, the lesion is termed lentigo maligna. Local excision is satisfactory in the treatment of lentigo maligna; in lentigo maligna melanoma, excision with at least a 1-cm margin is advocated. Surgical outcome in this type of tumor is almost uniformly favorable, although recurrence is sometimes seen. Nonetheless, it is unusual for a patient to die from disseminated lentigo maligna melanoma.

Acral lentigenous melanoma occurs on palms, soles, subungual areas, and mucous membranes. This is the most common type to affect blacks and Orientals, but it may also occur in Caucasians. The lesion begins as a flat pigmented lesion that may be irregular in its border and pigment pattern. Early biopsy is essential to achieve cure before metastasis has occurred.

Systems for determining prognosis now exist so that the extent of surgery can be matched to the degree of severity of the lesion. The earliest widely used system was that of Clark, in which the anatomic level of invasion of the primary tumor is determined. Four levels of invasion are employed: Level II penetrating into the papillary dermis, Level III filling the papillary dermis, Level IV penetrating into reticular dermis, Level V penetrating into the subcutaneous fat. Five-year survival rates at Massachusetts General Hospital for clinical stage I patients (those with localized disease only on clinical grounds) are as follows: Level II, 99%; Level III, 95%; Level IV, 75%; Level V, 39%. Spread to the lymph nodes greatly worsens the prognosis, in that the overall 5-year survival rate varies from 18% to 42%, depending on whether nodal involvement is gross or microscopic.

Measurement of the thickness of the primary tumor is a sound system for determination of prognosis and has become the most widely utilized prognostic technique; tumor thickness is measured with an ocular micrometer on a standard microscope from the granular cell layer down to the deepest tumor cell. This system, along with the anatomic leveling system, has been useful in further refining the prognosis within groups of patients. Lesions thinner than 0.85 mm have a uniformly favorable prognosis, while those greater than 3.00 mm have a fairly poor prognosis (<0.85, 99% survival; 0.85–1.69 mm, 94%; 1.70–3.64 mm, 78%; >3.65 mm, 42%).

At present, wide local excision is the treatment recommended for primary melanoma. The width of excision in our institution is based on primary tumor thickness. For tumors <0.85 mm thick, 1.5 cm margins are recommended; 3 cm margins are recommended for tumors thicker than 0.85 mm. As mentioned earlier, 1-cm margins are considered adequate for lentigo maligna melanoma regardless of thickness. The usefulness of elective lymph node dissection is still being debated; current evidence suggests that this procedure has no benefit over delaying removal until the nodes become clinically involved. Nodal dissection is still useful as a staging procedure to identify high-risk patients, enabling meaningful stratification for adjuvant therapy studies.

The treatment of *disseminated melanoma* is at present a difficult and unrewarding problem. The most effective and widely used drug, dimethyl triazenoimidazole carboxamide, has a response rate of approximately 20%. The nitrosoureas such as methyl CCNU are also utilized, and have approximately the same response rate. Even patients who respond usually relapse and die after a few months. Combinations of chemotherapy are currently being evaluated.

Since the prognosis in disseminated melanoma is so poor, attempts are being made to use adjuvant therapy postoperatively in patients who are at high risk for recurrence. At present, none have proved beneficial.

Early surgical removal of *giant hairy nevus* (Fig. 171-1) is necessary to prevent development of malignancy. Our current recommendation for treatment of congenital raised, pigmented *melanocytic nevi* is to consider prophylactic removal. This view is not universally accepted; some advocate a wait-and-see approach.

SCREENING AND DIAGNOSTIC TESTS

Skin cancers are unique in their accessibility and the frequency with which a tissue diagnosis can be made. In the case of *basal cell carcinomas,* the lesion may take several forms. The typical appearance is that of a translucent papule with telangiectasias over the surface (Fig. 171-2) that slowly

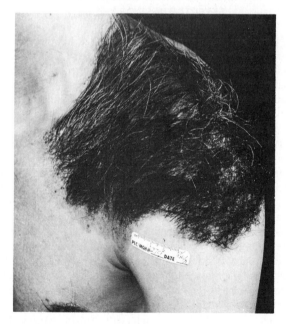

Figure 171-1.   Giant hairy melanocytic nevus.

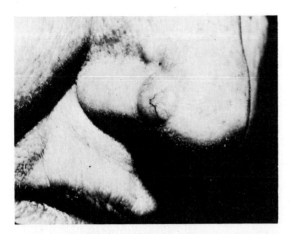

Figure 171-2. Nodular basal cell carcinoma. Note telangiectasia.

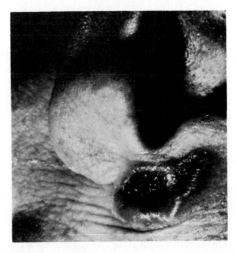

Figure 171-3. Basal cell carcinoma—"rodent ulcer."

enlarges and subsequently develops a central ulceration (Fig. 171-3). This lesion has been termed the "rodent ulcer." Basal cell carcinoma may also become pigmented in darker-skinned individuals and be confused with malignant melanoma of the nodular or superficial spreading type. Superficial forms of basal cell carcinoma exist, most commonly on the back, and have the appearance of an erythematous plaque. Usually some papular elements will be present at the border to assist in diagnosis. In a sclerotic form of basal cell carcinoma called the "morphealike" basal cell, nests of tumor cells are interspersed with thick fibrotic bundles. This tumor is more resistant to treatment.

Differential diagnosis of basal cell carcinoma includes dermal nevi and other appendage tumors such as trichoepithelioma. Trichoepithelioma may be clinically indistinguishable from basal cell carcinoma. On histopathologic examination of a basal cell carcinoma, proliferation of ba-

sophilic staining cells is seen, usually in nests surrounded by discrete lacunae located in the upper dermis. This tumor is relatively easy for the pathologist to diagnose microscopically. Because basal cell carcinomas are more common in those who have already had one, patients should be followed on an annual basis for early detection of new lesions.

Clinically, *actinic keratoses* appear as flat to slightly raised, scaly erythematous patches, which may be single or multiple and occur predominantly in sun-exposed areas (Fig. 171-4). Often, this lesion is more easily felt (sandpapery) than observed. It appears to go through cycles from macular erythematous lesions through raised scaly lesions. In the later stages a crusted surface, and sometimes even a horn of keratin, develops. Histopathologic examination of these lesions reveals atypical keratinocytes in the basal cell layer of the epidermis.

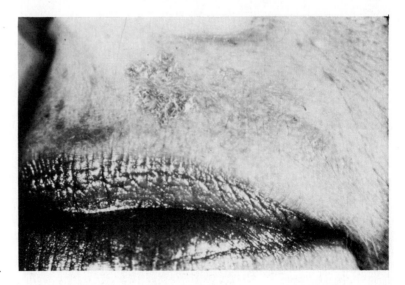

Figure 171-4. Actinic keratosis on the upper lip.

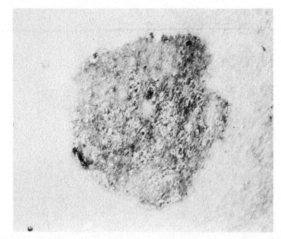

Figure 171-5. Bowen's disease—squamous cell carcinoma *in situ.*

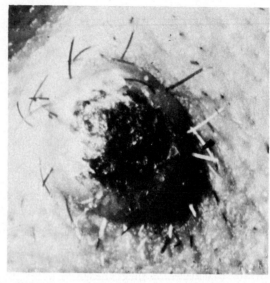

Figure 171-7. Keratoacanthoma. Note the central keratotic plug.

Bowen's disease usually presents as a chronic, asymptomatic, nonhealing, slowly enlarging erythematous patch usually having a sharp but irregular outline. It may resemble eczematous dermatitis but does not respond to topical steroid therapy (Fig. 171-5). Within the patch, there are generally

areas of crusting. The sharp borders, chronicity, and lack of symptoms are clues that suggest the necessity of performing a biopsy. In dark-skinned people, such as some of Mediter-

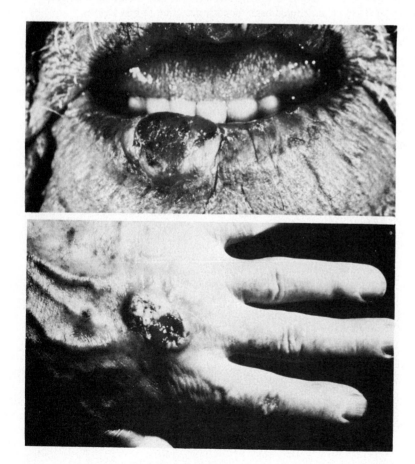

Figure 171-6. Squamous cell carcinoma in typical locations.

ranean descent, these lesions may have a brown to blue-gray coloration. Bowen's disease can occur on any part of the skin and on mucocutaneous sites such as the vulva. In the vulvar area, differential diagnosis includes lichen sclerosis et atrophicus, lichen simplex chronicus, squamous cell carcinoma, and, when pigmented, malignant melanoma. On histopathologic examination, atypical keratinocytes are noted throughout the epidermis. There is no invasion of keratinocytes into the dermis.

In the case of *squamous cell carcinoma,* the lesion begins as a flesh-colored, asymptomatic nodule, which enlarges and often undergoes ulceration and crusting (Fig. 171-6). The lesion may become quite keratotic and have a thickened surface. A cutaneous horn may result. Excisional biopsy with close margins is the procedure of choice for the diagnosis of this lesion. Squamous cell carcinoma may sometimes be confused with a benign keratinocytic lesion, which is dome-shaped and exhibits a prominent central plug called a kera-

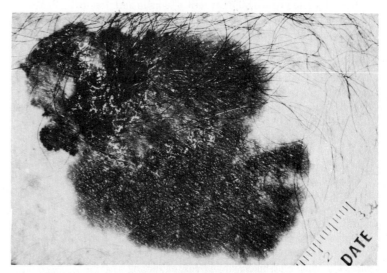

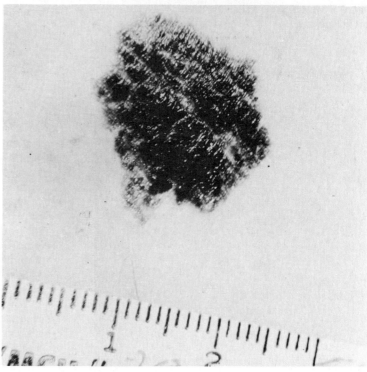

Figure 171-8. Malignant melanoma of the superficial spreading type. Note the irregularity of the border and prominent notch.

toacanthoma (Fig. 171-7). The keratoacanthoma usually exhibits more rapid growth and often regresses spontaneously.

Under the microscope, the squamous cell carcinoma has fingers of atypical keratinocytic cells infiltrating into the dermis. The nuclei are clearly atypical; mitoses are frequently found.

Melanomas have some common characteristics. Hallmarks for clinical recognition of the majority of melanomas include the following features: (1) irregularity of the border (sometimes a notch is present; Fig. 171-8) and (2) variegation in the color and pigmentation pattern. Colors in addition to brown and tan, such as red, white, blue, and their admixtures, grays, pinks, and purples, are of great use in distinguishing the overwhelming number of benign pigmented lesions from those that are melanomas. The preceding characteristics are sometimes found in pigmented basal cell carcinoma and pigmented Bowen's disease. In addition, odd dermal or compound nevi, irritated seborrheic keratoses, and occasionally vascular lesions will be clinically confused with melanoma. The benign blue nevus also shares similar clinical features. Biopsy and histopathologic evaluation by the pathologist are warranted if a lesion meets the criteria previously noted.

Each of the different types of melanoma has distinguishing features. *Superficial spreading melanomas* have some irregularity in the border and some alteration in the regularity of pigment pattern and coloration (see Fig. 171-8). *Nodular melanoma,* which arises *de novo* or within nevi as an invasive tumor from the onset, has no radial growth component. It exists as a blue, blue-black, gray nodule of varying size (Fig. 171-9). Most of these lesions are deeply invasive at the time of diagnosis.

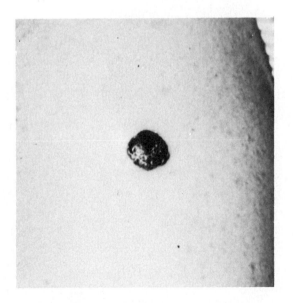

Figure 171-9.   Malignant melanoma, nodular type.

The *lentigo maligna* begins as a frecklelike lesion that slowly expands. It has a markedly irregular pigmentation pattern and usually an extremely irregular border. Spontaneous regression may occur; the border may advance on one side while regressing on another, so that the lesion may appear to march across the skin surface. Since about 2% of patients with melanoma develop a second primary tumor, it is worthwhile to examine the entire skin surface to look for the development of a second tumor upon each encounter. In familial melanoma as many as 30% of patients with melanoma may develop a second primary tumor. Because a trait favoring the development of melanoma appears to occur in families, family members of patients who have had melanoma should be examined.

Distribution of malignant melanoma across the body surface is not uniform. In both males and females, there is an aggregation on the back, head, and neck. In the female, the lower extremity is heavily affected, but is spared in males, in whom the anterior torso is more likely to be involved. The bra and swim trunk areas are spared in the female, and the swim trunk area and thighs are spared in the male.

CONCLUSIONS AND RECOMMENDATIONS

Screening for skin cancer represents one of the best examples of detection leading to effective treatment. For example, the current 5-year survival rate for clinical stage I malignant melanoma is 85%. It is estimated that by educating patients and physicians about signs of disease and the importance of early diagnosis, the 5-year survival rate for malignant melanoma could approach 85% to 90%.

Every primary physician should be able to recognize the common skin cancers, and his patients should be taught to avoid risk factors and report suspicious lesions. In particular, the following precautions should be observed:

- All fair-skinned persons who sunburn easily, and those in whom evidence of solar damage or skin cancer has already developed, should be warned about the hazards of continued high-intensity solar exposure. Rather than suggesting nocturnal activities, it is sufficient to advise that exposure be avoided between 11:00 A.M. and 2:30 P.M.; 70% of the harmful ultraviolet radiation can thus be avoided. The use of sunscreens containing PABA will also serve to decrease the amount of damaging ultraviolet radiation penetrating the skin. A high solar protection factor (SPF) sunscreen should be recommended.

- Patients with a history of exposure to arsenic or previous x-ray therapy with radiation dermatitis should be watched closely for the development of cancer.

- In nonmelanomatous skin cancer, the patient is asked to report any new, slowly growing, nodular or papular lesions that are flesh-colored or translucent. The patient should see a physician if bleeding, ulceration, or horn formation occurs. Areas of maximum solar exposure are at greatest risk.

- In malignant melanoma, the patient is asked to see the physician about any pigmented lesion that has an irregular border or a variation in color, especially blue, gray, or black. Any growth in a pigmented lesion should also arouse suspicion.

If any doubt exists, the physician's obligation is either to biopsy the lesion or to refer the patient to an experienced specialist for an opinion. If patients and physicians work together, the incidence of skin cancer and the deaths associated with it can be greatly reduced.

ANNOTATED BIBLIOGRAPHY

Andrade R, Gumport SL, Popkin G et al (eds): Cancer of the Skin. Philadelphia, WB Saunders, 1976 (*Recent two-volume compendium on all aspects of skin cancer.*)

Clark WH (ed): Human cutaneous malignant melanomas. Semin Oncol 2:81, 1975 (*Entire issue devoted to melanoma. Covers developmental biology, clinical diagnosis, epidemiology, immunology, surgery, and chemotherapy.*)

Epstein EH, Levin DL, Croft JD et al: Mycosis fungoides: Survival, prognostic features, response to therapy, and autopsy findings. Medicine 51:61, 1972 (*Comprehensive description of a rare problem.*)

Fitzpatrick TB, Sober AJ: Sunlight and skin cancer. N Engl J Med 313:818, 1985 (*Editorial accompanying a case-control study finding association between skin exposure and ocular melanoma. Reviews the evidence for sun exposure, particularly episodic intense exposure in the case of melanoma, as the principal risk factor for skin cancer.*)

Greene MH, Clark WH, Tucker MA et al: Acquired precursors of malignant melanoma. N Engl J Med 312:91, 1985 (*An important description of the natural history of both common and dysplastic nevi, including a color atlas. An accompanying editorial provides a prospective on melanoma risk associated with dysplastic nevi.*)

Haynes HA: Primary cancer of skin. In Petersdorf RG, Adams RD, Braunwald E et al (eds): Harrison's Principles of Internal Medicine, 10th ed, pp 835–836. New York, McGraw-Hill, 1983 (*Brief discussion of basal cell carcinoma, squamous cell carcinoma, and mycosis fungoides [lymphoma].*)

Kopf AW et al: Malignant melanoma: A review. J Dermatol Surg Oncol 3:41, 1977 (*Recent comprehensive review.*)

Lee JAH: Melanoma and exposure to sunlight. Epidemiol Rev 4:110, 1982 (*An exhaustive review of melanoma epidemiology and the evidence supporting a causal association between sunlight and melanoma.*)

Lever WF, Schaumburg-Lever G: Tumors and cysts of the epidermis (Chapter 26), and Tumors of the epidermal appendages (Chapter 27). In Histopathology of the Skin, ed Philadelphia, JB Lippincott, 1983 (*Clinical and histopathologic description of cutaneous malignancies.*)

Mihm MC, Fitzpatrick TB, Lane-Brown MM et al: Early detection of primary cutaneous malignant melanoma: A color atlas. N Engl J Med 289:989, 1973 (*Eighteen color plates illustrating typical malignant melanomas.*)

National Institute of Health Consensus Development Panel: Precursors to malignant melanoma. JAMA 251:1864, 1984 (*Consensus statement including descriptions, evidence regarding risk of melanoma, and management recommendations for both dysplastic and congenital nevi.*)

Sober AJ: Immunology and cutaneous malignant melanoma. Int J Dermatol 15:1, 1976 (*Review for the general physician of the immunology and immunotherapy of malignant melanoma.*)

Sober AJ, Fitzpatrick TB, Mihm MC et al: Early recognition of cutaneous melanoma. JAMA 242:2795, 1979 (*Self-assessment approach to the recognition of early lesions in this color atlas.*)

Trozak D, Rowland WD, Hu F et al: Metastatic malignant melanoma in prepubertal children. Pediatrics for the Clinician, February 1975 (*Grave indictment of metastatic potential of giant congenital melanocytic nevi.*)

172
Evaluation of Pruritus

Pruritus is an unpleasant sensation that provokes the urge to scratch. It may be a clinical presentation of underlying disease or even a prognostic variable. The clinical challenge for the primary physician is to identify any underlying disease and to provide symptomatic relief.

PATHOPHYSIOLOGY AND CLINICAL PRESENTATION

Itching is a cutaneous sensation that arises from sensory unmyelinated nerve endings located between cells of the epidermis, with higher concentrations in the flexor aspects of the wrist and ankles. The itching sensation is carried by pain fibers in the spinothalamic tracts and is integrated in the thalamus.

Various external stimuli decrease the threshold to itching. These include inflammation, dry skin, and vasodilation. Many chemical mediators of itching have been suggested, including histamine, serotonin, kinins, and prostaglandins. Persons vary in their response to itching. There is a psychological influence on the perception of itching, which explains why a physician may experience itching after attending a patient with scabies or pediculosis.

DIFFERENTIAL DIAGNOSIS

The many conditions that cause itching may be dermatologic, environmental, systemic, or psychological. Dermatologic entities associated with itch include infestation such as pediculosis and scabies, contact dermatitis, urticaria, neurodermatitis, psoriasis, lichen planus, and dermatitis herpetiformis. The most common cause of itching is xerosis. Environmental factors that cause itching include sunburn, cats, fiberglass, prickly heat, and overdrying of the skin.

Systemic diseases associated with itching include the endocrine disorders of diabetes mellitus, carcinoid syndrome, hypercalcemia, and hypo- or hyperthyroidism. Generalized itching is said to occur in between 4% and 11% of patients with Graves' disease, usually when the disease is long-standing. Increased kinin activity and slightly elevated skin temperatures are suggested mechanisms. Liver disease, particularly obstructive cholestatic jaundice—most notably primary biliary cirrhosis—produces itching. It has been estimated that 20% to 25% of patients with jaundice are plagued with itching, though it is rare in the absence of cholestasis. Pruritus occurs in oral contraceptive users after the first cycle in 50% and within the first six cycles in 90% of affected women. Pruritus of cholestasis is related to the accumulation of bile salts, although it may not be a direct effect but rather may occur as a result of proteases being liberated in the skin by the bile salts.

Hematologic disorders cause itching, including lymphoma, mycosis fungoides, systemic mastocytosis, polycythemia, and iron-deficiency anemia. The itching of polycythemia vera affects 30% to 50% of patients and is usually exacerbated by a hot shower or bath. In Hodgkin's disease, mycosis fungoides pruritus has been suggested as an adverse prognostic factor. Histamine released by an increased number of circulating basophiles is a suggested pathophysiologic mechanism. Chronic renal failure is an important cause of itching, particularly with the increasing number of patients undergoing hemodialysis. Secondary hyperparathyroidism, which results in elevated histamine levels, is the probable mechanism. Other investigations have implicated endopeptidases or kinins as substances that may accumulate in uremia. Peripheral neuropathy may contribute to itching. Itching during the last trimester of pregnancy has been reported in up to 1% to 3% of expectant women. Allergies to drugs, malignant neoplasms, neurologic syndromes, opiate ingestion, and venous stasis all may be implicated. Bites and parasitic infections may cause itching. There are a group of patients who suffer from psychogenic itching. This condition occurs more often at night when other stimuli are lacking, and may be associated with excoriations from intense efforts to remove the itching stimulant, causing a pseudoparasitic infestation.

WORKUP

History should focus on trying to determine how severe and widespread the itching is and any symptoms that point to a specific underlying diagnosis. The physician should ask if itching disturbs sleep, if it occurs primarily at night, and if it interferes with daytime activities. If itching does interfere with sleep or activity, treatment is much more imperative. Symptoms should be reviewed for the possibility of associated diseases such as hyperthyroidism, renal failure, liver disease or for the use of drugs.

Physical Examination begins with a careful and complete inspection of the skin for evidence of scratching marks, excoriations, or lichenification. The skin should be examined for evidence of inflammation, lice, the interdigital lesions of scabies, or rash suggestive of specific dermatologic diagnosis. The skin, particularly on the legs, should be examined for scaling and dryness. Lymph nodes should be palpated for enlargement.

Laboratory Examination reveals relatively common and treatable conditions. A complete blood count, urinalysis, and blood urea nitrogen test (BUN) constitute adequate initial screening. If there is no environmental stress, such as winter dryness or obvious skin rash, determinating thyroxine (T_4), calcium, and bilirubin levels and obtaining a chest radiograph are justified.

SYMPTOMATIC THERAPY

The patient with itching should be reassured when there is no underlying systemic disease. Many patients may be managed with a conservative therapeutic trial directed at relieving xerosis. Topical approaches include sponging the skin with cool water, substitution of superfatted soaps, humidification of the internal environment, and lubrication before bedtime. The patient should avoid lotions and creams unless they are recommended by the physician. The most effective topical agents available include camphor and phenol, which have an anesthetic quality; menthol, which substitutes a cool sensation for the itch; and hydrocortisone cream or lotion. Calamine lotion is adequate but drying and, therefore, should be limited to use on weeping lesions. A menthol-phenol combination is useful, but corticosteroid creams or sprays are more effective. Pramoxine with or without hydrocortisone is an effective nonsensitizing topical antipruritic. Recently it has been combined with menthol in a moisture-retaining base marketed as an over-the-counter preparation called Pramegel. If environmental manipulation and topical agents are not effective, then systemic medication must be considered.

The systemic medications that are most used are antihistamines, sedatives, and aspirin. *Antihistamines* are believed to work by occupying the histamine receptors, but they are specific only for allergically mediated itch. Studies have shown that in most cases antihistamines are no more effective than aspirin. Antihistamines have a sedative quality and can be an effective bedtime medication in patients who have sleep difficulties. The choice of an ideal agent is by found trial and error on the basis of the placebo, sedative, and anticholinergic effects of the drug. A good choice is *hydroxyzine,* an antihistamine with minimal soporific effects, or *cyproheptadine,* which is effective but more expensive. *Terfenadine,* a peripherally acting antihistamine, can be effective without causing sedation. *Sedatives,* most commonly *diazepam* or *chlordiazepoxide,* are useful for patients who have difficulty sleeping because of the itching. *Aspirin,* with its low cost and relatively low toxicity, may reduce itching through an anti-inflammatory, antikinin, or prostaglandin-inhibitor effect. *Cimetidine* is particularly useful in treating itching associated with polycythemia or uremia. *Pimozide,* a neuroleptic, is effective for treating delusions of parasitosis. Dermatologic conditions require specific therapy. Systemic steroids suppress itching but should not be used for symptomatic relief.

The chelating agent *cholestyramine* is good for cholestatic itching. Ultraviolet radiation and intravenous xylocaine have been reported successful in treating uremic pruritus. Photochemotherapy, activated charcoal, exchange transfusion, and parathyroidectomy have all been used for recalcitrant uremic pruritus. The opiate antagonist naloxone has been shown in some studies to improve pruritus, and in others it appeared to worsen it.

PATIENT EDUCATION

All patients with itching can be helped with relatively little risk by several changes in their behavior. They should be told to trim their fingernails and keep them clean to prevent excoriation or infection. It should be noted if vasodilating drugs or foods such as coffee, spices, or alcohol precipitate itching, and these should be avoided. Frequent bathing should be avoided because it eliminates the normal oil protection, contributing to dryness. Patients should shower for a short time. The physician should warn against applying lotions or cream except on his recommendation. A simple lubricant can be useful (refer to Chapter 184 for details). Static electricity is known to precipitate itching; therefore, it is sometimes helpful to change one sheet at a time to reduce static electricity. It can also be useful to add Alpha Keri or other lubricating agents to the rinse cycle when sheets are washed. The physician should advise patients to substitute superfatted soaps for regular soap. They should avoid rough clothing, particularly wool, and use cotton clothing that has been dou-

bly rinsed of detergents. Indoor moisture can be maintained during the winter with humidifiers or by placing bowls of water near radiators. These measures can be helpful to itching of any etiology and will often reduce or eliminate itching without the need to resort to pharmacologic therapy. In the absence of a proven etiology, empiric trials of modalities with low toxicity are recommended.

L.A.M.

ANNOTATED BIBLIOGRAPHY

Bernstein JE, Swift R: Relief of intractable pruritus with naloxone. Arch Dermatol 115:1366, 1979 (*Another option in difficult cases.*)

Denman ST: A review of pruritus. J Am Acad Dermatol 14:375, 1986 (*A superb current review emphasizing pathophysiology workup and treatment; 142 references are included.*)

Feiner AS et al: Prognostic importance of pruritus in Hodgkin's disease. JAMA 240:2738, 1978 (*A bad sign.*)

Garden JM, Ostrow JD, Roenigle HH: Pruritus in hepatic cholestasis: pathogenesis and therapy. Arch Dermatol 121:1415, 1985 (*An excellent review.*)

Gilchrest BA: Pruritus pathogenesis, therapy, and significance in systemic disease states. Arch Intern Med 142:101, 1982 (*A superb review, with a great bibliography.*)

Kligman AM: Water-induced itching without cutaneous sign. Arch Dermatol 122:183, 1986 (*A well-characterized subset of elderly patients in which age, dry skin, and seasonal weather conditions define patients who respond well to local measures.*)

Pederson JA, Matter BJ, Czerisinski AD: Relief of idiopathic generalized pruritus in dialysis patients treated with activated oral charcoal. Ann Intern Med 93:446, 1980 (*A safe therapy.*)

Shelley WB, Arthur RP: The neurohistology and neurophysiology of the itch sensation in man. Arch Dermatol 76:296, 1957 (*A classic paper on the pathophysiology of itch.*)

Weick JK, Donavan PB, Najean Y: The use of cimetidine for the treatment of pruritus in polycythemia-vera. Arch Intern Med 142: 241, 1982 (*Another anectodal option in a specific disease causing itching.*)

Winkelmann RK: Pharmacologic control of pruritus. Med Clin North Am 66:1119, 1982 (*A review of therapeutic alternatives.*)

Winkelmann RK, Muller SA: Pruritus. Annu Rev Med 15:53, 1964 (*A scholarly review of the literature, emphasizing the prevalence of itching in systemic diseases.*)

173
Evaluation of Urticaria
WILLIAM V. R. SHELLOW, M.D.

Urticaria is a usually pruritic eruption of circumscribed wheals on an erythematous base. It is estimated that 10% to 20% of the population experience it at some time. Individual lesions are usually short-lived, but successive eruptions may occur. Chronic urticaria is defined by persistence of more than 6 to 8 weeks. The primary physician must be capable of evaluating the cause of an urticarial eruption and providing symptomatic treatment. Finding the cause of urticaria may be elusive and frustrating to both the patient and the doctor.

PATHOPHYSIOLOGY

Urticaria is a vascular reaction pattern that leads to extravasation of protein-rich fluid from small blood vessels whose permeability has increased. Localized accumulation of fluid produces the characteristic clinical lesions of erythematous papules, which are pruritic and blanch on pressure. When extravasation occurs in deep layers of the skin, the cutaneous manifestation is less well circumscribed and is known as "angioedema."

The pathogenesis of urticaria is incompletely understood. It may be precipitated by immunologic or nonimmunologic stimuli, but the cutaneous eruption results from activation of a final common pathway. Mediators, such as histamine, are released from tissue mast cells or circulating basophils, producing a vascular reaction pattern. Histamine may be released by an innocent-bystander reaction or by activation of the complement enzyme system, which may produce holes in the mast cell membrane allowing histamine to escape. The reaction pattern can be activated by drugs, infection, food allergy, or physical agents such as cold, heat, or light. A second pathogenetic mechanism is cutaneous hyperreactivity to acetylcholine, which may be due to inadequate production of cholinesterase. This condition is known as "cholinergic urticaria." In time, better definition of the precipitants of histamine release and probably other mediators of the urticarial reaction will be demonstrated.

DIFFERENTIAL DIAGNOSIS

Urticaria may be due to exogenous factors such as inhalants, ingestants, and physical agents, or endogenous sources such as bacterial, fungal, amebic, or parasitic infection. Urticaria is associated with systemic diseases and psychological stresses.

Inhalants that produce urticaria include mold, dust, and pollens. *Candida albicans,* which is resident in the gastrointestinal (GI) tract, may have a contributory effect. Aerosols and animal and plant substances are etiologic considerations. Ingestants may cause both acute and chronic urticaria. Food, particularly nuts, chocolate, shellfish, cheese, milk, eggs, corn, soybean, and, rarely, wheat may cause urticaria. Drugs and chemicals may be ingested with foods in the form of artificial colors, preservatives, or antioxidants. Penicillin in milk, tartrazine dye in pills, fluoride in drinking water, and even menthol cigarettes have been reported as causes of chronic urticaria. Drugs, including penicillin, aspirin, or barbiturates, may cause urticaria on an allergic basis. Histamine releasers, such as morphine, codeine, thiamine, and pilocarpine, may be urticariagenic agents on a nonallergic basis. It is important to remember that precipitating agents may be absorbed through the conjunctival, gastrointestinal, vaginal, rectal, or oral mucosa.

Physical agents cause urticaria. Heat causes cholinergic urticaria, while light or cold may produce noncholinergic urticaria. Cold urticaria may be related to cryoglobulinemia, or it may be essential, either familial or acquired. Mechanical stimulation of the skin may give rise to dermographic urticaria.

Endogenous causes of urticaria are predominantly infectious. Infections such as dental abscesses, sinusitis, cholecystitis, or prostatitis can cause urticaria. Viral infection, particularly mononucleosis, is part of the differential diagnosis. Dermatophytosis and candidiasis are frequent causes of urticaria. *Entamoeba histolytica, Giardia lamblia,* and *Trichomonas vaginalis* may be responsible for urticaria. Parasitic infestations associated with urticaria include strongyloidiasis, ascariasis, uncinariasis, and trichuriasis. Marked eosinophilia may be indicative of parasitosis. Malaria, schistosomiasis, and filariasis may also manifest with chronic urticaria. Systemic diseases that have been associated with urticaria include renal disease, hepatitis, neoplasia, collagen vascular disease, and thyroid disorders. Urticaria associated with collagen disease has a burning quality, persists for more than 24 hours, and leaves residual hyperpigmentation. Psychogenic urticaria resulting from emotional stress must be considered. It should also be noted that two agents may combine to create a urticarial eruption. Hereditary angioedema is a distinct clinical entity with a strong family history and associated GI symptoms.

WORKUP

History. The emphasis of the workup is the history. An exhaustive list of questions may help determine the proximate cause of the urticarial reaction. Recent illness, drug use, foods, and inhalants that have been associated with urticaria should be ascertained. Patients should be encouraged to keep a diary of foods eaten. Screen items of daily use, such as toothpaste, cosmetics, food additives, or birth control pills. Ask about milk products or beer because penicillin in dairy products or yeast in beer may precipitate urticaria. Associated parasympathetic symptoms such as cramps, diarrhea, headache, salivation, or diaphoresis may point to cholinergic urticaria. It should be determined if heat, cold, or light precipitates lesions. A travel history may identify amebic or parasitic infection.

Physical Examination is important in evaluating the extent and, occasionally, the etiology of urticaria. Some dermatologists suggest that the clinical appearance is helpful. Bizarre, gyrate hives have been associated with internal malignancy. Lesions without pseudopods suggest allergy. Small lesions with erythematous flares are typical of cholinergic urticaria. The physician should evaluate the extent of urticaria, looking for periorbital or labial swelling and excoriations on the body. He should examine the patient's teeth for tenderness to percussion and palpate for sinus tenderness. He should also palpate for adenopathy, seeking evidence of lymphomas, and examine joints for signs that suggest collagen vascular disease.

Laboratory Examination can be selective or exhaustive. It is usually unproductive to seek possible etiologies through laboratory examination without corroborating historical or examination points. Therefore, a complete blood count, eosinophil count, sedimentation rate, and urinalysis should suffice. When a collagen disease is suspected, obtain an ANA, C_3, C_4, and CH_{50}. The physician should avoid expensive laboratory or radiographic determinations until the clinical evidence points to an underlying etiology.

Several provocative tests can help ascertain the etiology. An ice cube on the skin may induce cold urticaria, and stroking may result in dermographic urticaria. Cholinergic urticaria may be revealed by an intradermal injection of methecholine, 0.1 cc of a 1:500 dilution. Extensive skin testings for molds, dusts, pollens, or food allergies are difficult to interpret and rarely indicated. The current popularity of cytotoxic food allergy testing has no scientific validity and should be firmly discouraged.

It is sometimes difficult to separate workup from treatment, but a number of therapeutic trials are worth trying in order to identify an etiology. An elimination diet that consists of lamb, rice, string beans, fresh peas, tea, sugar, salt, and rye crackers excludes most common food allergens. A more limited approach is to eliminate dairy products, beer, nuts, shellfish, berries, and food additives. It may be useful to stop all drugs or change preparations or brands to eliminate tartrazine dyes or peculiarities of certain brand-name toothpastes or cosmetics.

The diagnosis of chronic urticaria can be a significant challenge to the physician in terms of both patient and disease management. Some clinicians admit patients for control of diet and long periods of observation. This expensive procedure is notoriously unrewarding because of its expense and the high percentage of patients who remain undiagnosed. A small percentage of patients with chronic urticaria are later found to have an underlying neoplasm or a serious systemic disease, but that is not a universal justification for an extensive workup.

SYMPTOMATIC MANAGEMENT

Antihistamines are the drugs of choice. The most effective agent is hydroxyzine in doses of 10 to 100 mg, four times a day; cyproheptadine, 12 to 20 mg per day in divided doses, is effective and may be particularly good for treating cold urticaria. Chlorpheniramine, because of low cost and over-the-counter availability, might be tried in dosage of 12 to 24 mg per day. *Cimetidine* in combination with antihistamine has been demonstrated effective in some refractory cases. *Doxepin* in low doses three times a day has been shown to be more effective than antihistamine in one controlled study. Subcutaneous aqueous epinephrine ameliorates acute attacks, but it is not helpful for chronic urticaria. Acute urticaria may be aborted by parenteral corticosteroids, but in chronic urticaria, corticosteroids that may suppress the eruption are not worth the risks.

Occasionally, therapeutic trials to eliminate common causes of urticaria are worthwhile. Nystatin, 500,000 units, three times a day, or *ketoconazole,* 200 mg daily, may improve the clinical picture by eliminating *Candida.* The association of urticaria with chronic bacterial infection has led to successful resolution with a broad-spectrum antibiotic given for 7 to 10 days. Urticaria patients with asymptomatic trichomonas vaginitis may attain relief with a course of metronidazole (see Chapter 115). Occasionally treatment of tinea pedis is helpful.

PATIENT EDUCATION

It is important to educate the patient in advance of the workup that an etiology is often not found. Emphasize the variable natural history of hives and the probability that the lesions will disappear spontaneously. Prepare the patient for the likelihood that urticaria will recur. Reassure the patient that the medical workup will exclude serious and or treatable diseases and that many options are available to shorten the process and alleviate symptoms.

ANNOTATED BIBLIOGRAPHY

Akers WA: Chronic urticaria: Seek at least two causes. Cutis 10:591, 1972 (*An effective demonstration of the multifactorial etiology of chronic urticaria.*)

Beakey JF: An allergist looks at urticaria. Cutis 18:247, 1976 (*A succinct review, emphasizing the need for careful instruction in elimination diets.*)

Beall GN: Urticarias: A review of clinical and laboratory observations. Medicine 43:131, 1964 (*Excellent review, although somewhat dated pathophysiology explanations.*)

Berman BA, Ross RN: Hereditary angioedema. Cutis 31:124, 1983 (*A succinct article discussing the pathophysiology of HAE.*)

Buckley RH, Matthews KP: Common allergic skin diseases. JAMA 248:2611, 1982 (*Extensive review of atopic dermatitis, allergic contact dermatitis, and urticaria.*)

Champion RW et al: Urticaria and angioedema—A review of 554 patients. Br J Dermatol 81:588, 1969 (*Seventy-nine percent unknown etiology; atopic history not more frequent; 21% exacerbated by aspirin.*)

Green SL, Reed CE, Schroeter AL: Double blind crossover study comparing doxepin with diphenhydramine for treatment of chronic urticaria. J Am Acad Dermatol 12:669, 1985 (*Doxepin at low doses, 10 mg tid, is statistically more effective than diphenhydramine, 25 mg tid, in the treatment of chronic idiopathic urticaria.*)

Harvey RP et al: A controlled trial at therapy in chronic urticaria. J Allergy Clin Immunol 68:262, 1981 (*A small controlled trial demonstrating the superiority of a combination of hydroxyzine plus cimetidine in treating chronic urticaria.*)

Jorizzo, JL, Smith EB: The physical urticarias: An update and review. Arch Dermatol 118:194, 1982 (*Review article of the less common forms of urticaria; 84 references are included.*)

Lockshin NA, Hurley H: Urticaria as a sign of viral hepatitis. Arch Dermatol 105:571, 1972 (*An important article that reports the association of urticaria and antigen-antibody reactions in hepatitis.*)

Matthews KP: Urticaria and angiodema. J Allergy Clin Immunol 72:1, 1983 (*A practical discussion of the various types of urticaria including diagnostic procedures and treatment recommendations; 62 references are included.*)

Neittaanmaki H: Cold urticaria. J Am Acad Dermatol 13:636, 1985 (*A current review.*)

Ramsay CA: Solar urticaria. Int J Dermatol 19:233, 1980 (*Review of the topic.*)

Zamm AV: Chronic urticaria: A practical approach. Cutis 9:27, 1972 (*A superb classification of the types of urticaria, with outlines for the workup of chronic urticaria.*)

174
Evaluation of Hyperhidrosis
WILLIAM V. R. SHELLOW, M.D.

Excessive sweating is not an uncommon complaint, but it rarely signifies underlying pathology. Medical consultation may be sought because of abnormal wetness, a change in the pattern or amount of sweating, sweaty palms, stained clothing, or offensive odor. There is much variation in the amount people sweat in response to the physiologic stimuli of heat, emotion, or eating. The interaction of the person, the environment, and his emotions influences the amount of sweating. The primary physician must offer scientific explanation and symptomatic management to the person who complains of excessive sweating.

PATHOPHYSIOLOGY AND CLINICAL PRESENTATION

Sweating helps maintain temperature and fluid and electrolyte homeostasis, particularly under the environmental stresses of heat. There are two kinds of sweat glands, eccrine and apocrine. Cooling results from evaporation of eccrine sweat. Eccrine glands are concentrated on the palms and soles and are present on the face, axillae, and, to a lesser extent, the back and chest. Heat causes sweating on the face, upper chest, and back. Sweating of the palms and soles is a characteristic response to stress. Gustatory sweating occurs on the face, particularly the upper lip, and following ingestion of spiced foods. The eccrine glands have no anatomic relationship to other cutaneous appendages.

Sebaceous and apocrine glands are intimately associated with hair follicles. The apocrine glands are concentrated in the axillae, areolae, groin, and perineum. Apocrine secretion consists of minuscule drops, viscid and milky, that produce odor after bacteria act on it.

Eccrine sweating is controlled by neural factors or a reflex. Thermal sweating is governed by the hypothalamus, and emotional sweating by the cerebral cortex. The innervation of eccrine glands is anatomically sympathetic, but for unexplained reasons the sweat glands are under cholinergic control. Excess sweating may be induced by abnormalities of the autonomic nervous system. Autonomic overactivity of the sweat glands may occur without identifiable cause. Sweating is associated with medical diseases that increase metabolic activity, causing the need for dissipation of heat. Though the eccrine glands are under cholinergic control, epinephrine stimulates excessive sweating.

DIFFERENTIAL DIAGNOSIS

Most cases of excess sweating are due to exaggerated physiologic responses or functional variations of no pathologic consequence. Hyperhidrosis most commonly involves the palms, soles, or axillae. This may be a result of an increase in impulses from the central nervous system (CNS), or it may reflect underlying problems with the sweat glands. There is often a relationship to emotional stress, and the problem is disabling when it interferes with work or social interactions. Axillary hyperhidrosis is less common than palmar or plantar, producing the need for frequent clothing changes. The most common pathologic cause of hyperhidrosis is fever. It is well known that during defervescence sweating occurs, particularly at night. Night sweats indicate the possibility of underlying infectious disease (see Chapter 6). Central neurologic injury from stroke or tumor may produce hyperhidrosis. Peripheral neuropathy associated with the autonomic nerves may produce excess sweating. Medical conditions associated with abnormal sweating include menopause (see Chapter 117), thyrotoxicosis (see Chapter 101), and, uncommonly, pheochromocytoma. Parkinson's disease may cause increased sweating and sebaceous activity. Various drugs, such as antipyretics, insulin, meperidine, emetics, alcohol, and pilocarpine, may induce sweating. Gustatory sweating, though uncommon, may be due to compensatory diabetic neuropathy, damage to the seventh nerve during parotid surgery, the rare Frey syndrome, or injury to the sympathetic trunk following surgery. Excess sweating because of anxiety or the perception of excess sweating resulting from functional disorder must always be considered.

WORKUP

History. The workup should identify whether excess sweating is restricted to the axillae, affects the palms and soles, or is more generalized. In patients with axillary hyperhidrosis, the physician should inquire about family history because there is a familial form of this disorder. The physician should determine if sweating occurs primarily at night and, if so, whether or not fever, fatigue, or any other symptom of a subacute infectious or malignant process is present. He should inquire about symptoms of thyroid overactivity, and note if the patient has recently entered menopause. A careful drug history is needed, emphasizing agents that are known to cause excess sweating. The physician should ask whether excess sweating began relatively recently and can be correlated with stress.

Physical Examination can identify objective evidence of excess sweating. The patient should be examined for signs of hyperthyroidism. Blood pressure determination is important because, if paroxysmal hypertension, flushing, and sweating are present, pheochromocytoma should be considered. The cranial nerves and retina should be examined because of the possibility of CNS disease. There are no mandatory laboratory investigations, but a thyroxine (T_4), blood sugar, or urine vanillylmandelic acid (VMA) should be ordered if there is a clinical indication.

SYMPTOMATIC MANAGEMENT

The primary etiology of excess sweating is usually unknown, and its significance is restricted to the extent of interference with employment or cosmesis. Many therapies have been used. Topical therapies include 10% formalin compresses, which can induce allergic sensitization. Buffered glutaraldehyde is effective but stains the skin. Scopolamine and other anticholinergics have been effective, but they may precipitate glaucoma or obstruction from prostatic hypertrophy.

The following steps can be used in symptomatic management:

- Reassure the patient that excess sweating is not due to a pathologic condition.
- For axillary sweating, recommend frequent washing and changes of clothing.
- For excess sweating of the palms or the axillae, the most effective agent currently available is a 20% alcoholic solution of aluminum chloride hexahydrate (Drysol). A 6.25% aluminum tetrachloride (Xerac) is an effective alternative. It should be applied at bedtime and covered with a plastic wrap or polyethylene gloves. In the morning, it should be washed with soap and water. Clinical improvement in axillary hyperhidrosis may be seen after one to three consecutive treatments per week.
- Electrical current may be used to temporarily block sweat glands. The device (Drionic), used daily for 1 week, may relieve sweating for up to 1 month.
- If topical therapy and reassurance fail, surgery may be considered if hyperhidrosis significantly interferes with occupational or social life. Axillary hyperhidrosis may be cured with surgical extirpation of the eccrine glands in the axillae. Palmar sweating may respond to sympathectomy.

PATIENT EDUCATION

Patient education is crucial to the treatment of excess sweating. Providing the patient with a scientific explanation and firm understanding of sweating is helpful in relieving anxiety. Patients with night sweats should record their temperature so that any significant febrile illness can be identified. The application of topical agents should be well explained and carefully used by patients. Surgical intervention for a problem as minor as hyperhidrosis requires the patient's understanding of the risks and benefits of such a procedure and the active involvement of the primary physician in helping the patient reach a decision.

ANNOTATED BIBLIOGRAPHY

Adar R, Kurchin A, Zweig A: Palmar hyperhidrosis and its surgical treatment. A report of 100 cases. Ann Surg 186:34, 1977 (*A report of an 89% success rate in 93 patients who underwent bilateral upper dorsal sympathectomy for palmar hyperhidrosis; a good review of surgical approaches; 40 references are included.*)

Bloor K: Gustatory sweating and other responses after cervicothoracic sympathectomy. Brain 92:137, 1969 (*Incidence as high as 36%. This study showed 29 of 146 patients.*)

Chalmers JM, Keele CA: The nervous and chemical control of sweating. Br J Dermatol 64:43, 1952 (*Definitive review of the pathophysiology of eccrine sweat production.*)

Cunliffe WJ, Tan SG: Hyperhidrosis and hypohidrosis. Practitioner 216:149, 1976 (*A good review of differential diagnosis and treatment.*)

Hurley HJ, Shelley WB: Axillary hyperhidrosis. Clinical features and local surgical management. Br J Dermatol 78:127, 1966 (*The surgical technique of removing eccrine sweat glands from the axilla.*)

Hurley HJ, Shelley WB: A simple surgical approach to the management of axillary hyperhidrosis. JAMA 186:109, 1963 (*Surgical excision of the eccrine glands in the axilla can be used in refractory hyperhidrosis.*)

Levit F: Treatment of hyperhidrosis by tap water iontophoresis. Cutis 26:193, 1980 (*Use of galvanic generator to control palmar and plantar hyperhidrosis.*)

Shelley WB, Hurley HJ: Studies on axillary antiperspirants. Acta Derm Venereol (Stockh) 55:241, 1975

175
Evaluation of Purpura

Purpura represents bleeding into the skin. In the office setting, it may be encountered as a complaint related to easy or spontaneous bruising or to a rash. *Petechiae* (red macules that measure less than 3 mm in diameter) usually reflect a defect in platelets or vessel walls. *Ecchymoses* are larger than 3 mm in diameter and appear with disorders of the clotting system as well as with vascular and platelet problems. Many cases of purpura are caused by unappreciated trauma. Patients who complain of easy or spontaneous bruising need to be evaluated for a bleeding diathesis. In those with petechial rashes, consideration of vasculitis and bacteremia, as well as disorders of platelets and connective tissue, is required.

PATHOPHYSIOLOGY AND CLINICAL PRESENTATION

Purpura results from a break in small dermal blood vessels and occurs in perfectly normal people in response to significant trauma. The appearance of purpura in multiple sites simultaneously or in areas where trauma was trivial or absent suggests a problem in the hemostatic mechanism. The integrity of vessels is maintained by quantitatively and qualitatively adequate platelets and healthy connective tissue. A break in a vessel triggers formation of platelet plug followed by a fibrin clot. Disturbances of platelets present in the skin as petechial lesions, usually in dependent areas. Damage to the capillary endothelium produces a similar clinical picture. Coagulation defects cause delayed but more prolonged blood loss, during which continuous oozing due to inadequate fibrin clot formation results in ecchymoses rather than petechiae.

Platelet disorders are among the most common causes of purpura. *Thrombocytopenic purpura* is not encountered until the platelet count falls below 50,000. The onset and severity of purpura is highly variable; no difficulty may be noted until the platelet count drops well below 10,000, perhaps reflecting the continued integrity of the blood vessel wall in the presence of even a scant population of platelets. Bleeding from other sites may ensue before purpura appears (see Chapter 80).

Defective platelet function is often related to drugs that inhibit adenosine diphosphate (ADP) release, though hereditary thrombocytopathies sometimes account for easy bruising. Aspirin, indomethacin, phenylbutazone, and other nonsteroidal anti-inflammatory agents block ADP release. The effect can be induced by as little as 600 mg of aspirin and persists for the life span of the platelets made during the time aspirin is present. Significant bleeding rarely results solely from use of platelet-active drugs, but an underlying bleeding diathesis may be aggravated and hemorrhage precipitated. Platelet function is also impaired in patients with cirrhosis or uremia. Generalized oozing from many sites is sometimes a serious problem in renal failure; the platelet defect can be reversed by dialysis. Platelet function in dysproteinemias may become a problem because of coating with abnormal globulins. *Excess platelets*—as in polycythemia vera—may not function normally, and lead to bleeding (see Chapter 80).

Vascular and *connective tissue defects* compromise vessel walls and supportive extravascular structures, leading to easy bruising. Purpura may be caused by pressure applied by clothing or, in elderly patients and those taking corticosteroids, result from trivial trauma. The presentation is usually in the face, neck, dorsum of the hands, forearms, and legs; degeneration of dermal collagen is the presumed cause. A variant is the production of stasis or orthostatic purpura, usually occurring in the lower extremities of an elderly patient following a prolonged period of standing. Stasis dermatitis also causes petechial lesions in the legs resulting from a capillaritis. Scurvy compromises the vascular endothelium, and perifollicular purpura develops because of increased capillary fragility. In amyloidosis, deposition of amyloid in the skin and subcutaneous tissue causes fragile vessels with ecchymoses forming when the skin is pinched.

Small vessel vasculitis represents immunologically mediated inflammation and necrosis of arterioles and capillaries. The skin, mucous membranes, brain, lung, heart, kidneys, muscle, and gastrointestinal tract may be affected. Precipitants include drug hypersensitivity reactions (sulfonamides, penicillin, tetracycline, quinidine, guanethidine, phenacetin, phenothiazines, propylthiouracil) and connective tissue diseases such as rheumatoid arthritis, systemic lupus erythematosus, and cryoglobulinemia. Petechial papules (palpable purpura) that do not blanch are characteristic of vasculitis and appear in symmetric fashion; they predominate in dependent areas. Urticaria, vesicles and necrotic ulcerations may also develop. Fever, arthralgias, myalgias, arthritis, pulmonary infiltrates, effusions, pericarditis, peripheral neuropathy, abdominal pain, bleeding, and encephalopathy can occur along with the petechial rash. The skin commonly itches, stings, or burns. Hematuria and proteinuria are often detected.

Infections that enter the bloodstream may lead to vascular injury and formation of petechiae, which sometimes are palpable. Petechial lesions associated with subacute bacterial endocarditis are flat, do not blanch, and appear on the upper chest, neck, and extremities in addition to the mucous membranes. In gonococcal and meningococcal septicemias, petechiae develop early, become pustular, and then turn hemorrhagic and necrotic. The lower extremities are a common site for the gonococcal lesions, which resolve within 5 to 7 days. The rash of Rocky Mountain spotted fever begins as pink macules on the wrists, soles, ankles, and palms, spreads centripetally, and by the fourth day becomes petechial and papular. Hemorrhagic, ulcerated lesions may follow.

Anticoagulant use, unless excessive, and mild hepatocellular failure do not cause spontaneous bleeding into the skin. Easy bruising following trivial trauma, with formation of ecchymoses, occurs when anticoagulant levels are far beyond therapeutic range or from severe hepatocellular failure. The bleeding is typically oozing and slow to stop. Abuse of these agents is seen in health care personnel. *Coumadin necrosis* is an idiosyncratic hemorrhagic necrosis of unknown etiology that occurs in patients who are in therapeutic range (see Chapter 85).

Autoerythrocyte sensitization is a puzzling form of purpura characterized by spontaneous, painful ecchymosis surrounded by erythema and edema. Headache, nausea, and vomiting sometimes accompany the purpura. Intradermal injection of autologous red cells can reproduce the clinical picture. Many patients with this condition have pronounced psychoneurotic complaints.

Purpura simplex is a designation for idiopathic disease. The patient is typically a woman who is otherwise in good health.

DIFFERENTIAL DIAGNOSIS

Purpura can be conveniently divided into thrombocytopenic and nonthrombocytopenic categories (see Chapter 80). Nonthrombocytopenic purpuras are classified according to whether platelet function is defective, abnormalities exist in connective tissue, or vascular integrity has been compromised by degeneration or inflammation. The most common causes of purpura are trauma, benign purpura simplex, senile purpura, and drug-induced impairment of platelet function. The extensive list of disorders that must be considered in the patient presenting with petechial or purpuric lesions is presented in Table 175-1.

WORKUP

The workup of the patient complaining of purpuric lesions must emphasize history and physical examination to avoid costly and nonproductive laboratory evaluations. A careful characterization of the site, size, and duration of the lesions is essential. Lesions smaller than 6 cm localized to areas in which trauma is common, such as the thighs, are less likely to be of pathologic significance.

Table 175-1. Important Causes of Purpura

Thrombocytopenic (see Chapter 80)

Nonthrombocytopenic
Platelet defects
    Nonsteroidal anti-inflammatory agents
    Uremia
    Thrombocytopathies (hereditary)
    Dysproteinemias
    Thrombocythemia (polycythemia vera)

Vascular defects
    Trauma
    Venous stasis
    Vasculitis (drugs, connecctive tissue disease, infection)
    Amyloidosis
    Scurvy
    Hereditary hemorrhagic telangiectasia

Extravascular support defects
    Age
    Cushing's syndrome or corticosteroid use

Coagulation defects
    Excessive anticoagulant use
    Hereditary conditions
    Hepatocellular failure

Idiopathic
    Purpura simplex
    Erythrocyte autosensitization (psychogenic purpura)
    Coumarin necrosis

History. A carefully taken history should include inquiry into blood loss from other sites, easy bruisability, and prolonged, heavy bleeding with menstruation, surgery, or dental work. The family history is important because there are numerous hereditary familial purpuric syndromes and a variety of thrombocytopathies, particularly the autosomal-dominant von Willebrand's disease. The drug history is essential, focusing on anticoagulants and antiplatelet agents (*e.g.,* aspirin, dipyridamole, phenylbutazone, sulfinpyrazone, indomethacin, and the other nonsteroidal anti-inflammatory agents [NSAID] such as ibuprofen, tolectin, and naproxen). Drugs that cause hypersensitivity reactions (antibiotics, quinidine, phenothiazines) may cause purpura.

Associated symptoms—such as fever, itching, pleuritic chest pain, abdominal pain, vaginal or penile discharge, myalgias, arthralgias, arthritis, morning stiffness, numbness, paresthesias—provide important diagnostic information. Symptoms of renal disease or hepatocellular failure should be noted.

Physical Examination begins with inspection of the skin lesions. Petechiae do not blanch when a glass slide is pressed over them; many nonpurpuric erythematous lesions do. Blanching lesions must not be dismissed too hastily, because telangiectasias and spider angiomas are signs of conditions predisposing to purpura. The size, number, and location of purpuric lesions should be recorded, and note made of whether they are palpable or macular, petechial or ecchymotic. Tenderness suggests psychogenic purpura. It is sometimes helpful to circle ecchymoses so that extension or regression may be followed objectively.

A general physical examination is performed, looking for temperature elevation, cushingoid appearance, jaundice, mucosal petechiae, adenopathy, pleural effusion, heart murmur, rub, hepatomegaly, ascites, splenomegaly, purulent vaginal or urethral discharge, joint inflammation, edema, and nuchal rigidity; excessively neurotic behavior may be noted.

The tourniquet test has been used to assess capillary fragility. The test can be performed in the office by inflating the blood pressure cuff to a point halfway between systolic and diastolic blood pressure, maintaining it for 5 minutes, and then releasing it. A positive tourniquet test is demonstrated by 15 or more petechiae in an area the size of a nickel. This test is diagnostic not of thrombocytopenia, but rather of increased capillary fragility. False positives sometimes occur; petechiae have been demonstrated in 8% of normal individuals.

Laboratory Studies. A few tests usually suffice (see also Chapter 80). The *peripheral blood smear* is studied for presence of platelets. If they are present, significant thrombocytopenia is unlikely. A platelet count can be used to confirm the impression obtained from peripheral smear and to detect any thrombocytosis. A count greater than 800,000 identifies

thrombocythemia. A *bleeding time* is the best screening test for platelet function. The Ivy method is widely used and best performed with a template to ensure an incision 1 mm deep and 1 cm long. The cut is made in an avascular area of the forearm while venous return is obstructed with a blood pressure cuff inflated to 40 mm Hg. Blotting paper is applied to the edge of the incision. A normal result is cessation of blotter-detected oozing by 9 minutes.

Ecchymotic lesions should be evaluated with *prothrombin* (PT) and *partial thromboplastin times* (PTT) to be sure there are no defects in the extrinsic or intrinsic coagulation pathways. Patients on oral anticoagulants and those with hepatobiliary disease are also candidates for a PT and PTT.

When palpable purpura is noted, a *skin biopsy* is needed to confirm vasculitis; it should also be cultured and Gram stained for organisms. If fever is present in conjunction with petechiae, blood cultures must be obtained. An ANA and rheumatoid factor may be of help, as well.

A *stool guaiac* test and *urinalysis* are performed for detection of occult blood loss; in addition, protein and casts are looked for in the urine. In the elderly patient who is at risk for dysproteinemia, a *sedimentation rate* and serum globin level can be used for screening, and immunoelectrophoresis obtained if these determinations are elevated.

SYMPTOMATIC MANAGEMENT AND PATIENT EDUCATION

Detailed reassurance needs to be given to the patient with no hematologic or systemic abnormality, but only *after* thorough evaluation has been completed. In the elderly patient, supportive explanation that this is a normal concomitant of aging is often helpful. Cessation of drugs that impair platelet function, such as aspirin, indomethacin, phenylbutazone, or newer nonsteroidal anti-inflammatory agents, is advisable but not mandatory. Patients who need these drugs for the treatment of a chronic disease may learn to accept the cosmetic unpleasantness of ecchymoses. Occasionally, otherwise healthy patients buy and take large doses of vitamins C and K in hopes of lessening easy bruisability. Such self-treatment is without any proven efficacy and adds an unnecessary expense. However, the patient with hepatocellular failure may show mild improvement with parenteral vitamin K, provided some synthetic function remains. Patients with thrombocytopenia must pay careful attention to avoiding trauma (see Chapter 80).

INDICATIONS FOR ADMISSION

Any patient with fever and purpura requires prompt hospital admission, since vasculitis and septicemia are possible. The person who gives evidence of bleeding from multiple sites is best hospitalized. Absence of platelets on smear and a very prolonged bleeding time are more safely evaluated in the inpatient setting.

L.A.M.
A.H.G.

ANNOTATED BIBLIOGRAPHY

Goldenberg LA, Altman A: Benign skin changes associated with chronic sunlight exposure. Cutis 34:33, 1984 (*Sun exposure contributes to senile purpura.*)

Kramer J: Capillary resistance and its relation to bleeding. In Johnson SA, Monto RW, Rebuck JW, et al (eds): Blood Platelets. Boston, Little, Brown, 1961 (*A good description of capillary fragility testing showing that at least 8% of normal individuals have increased capillary fragility.*)

Nalbandian RM, Mader IJ, Barre HJL et al: Petechiae, ecchymosis,

and necrosis of skin induced by coumarin congeners. JAMA 192: 603, 1965 (*Description of this unusual complication.*)

Ratnoff OD, Agle DP: Psychogenic purpura: A re-evaluation of the syndrome of autoerythrocyte sensitization. Medicine 47:476, 1968 (*A careful analysis of this syndrome of painful ecchymoses and a characteristic personality profile.*)

Tattersall RN, Seville R: Senile purpura. QJ Med 19:151, 1951 (*Good epidemiologic data.*)

Wallerstein RO, Wallerstein RO Jr: Scurvy. Semin Hematol 13:211, 1976 (*A review of this uncommon deficiency state showing that hemorrhage may be deep as well as superficial.*)

Zucker S, Mielke CH, Durocher JR et al: Oozing and bruising due to abnormal platelet function (thrombocytopathia). Ann Intern Med 76:725, 1972 (*A good article showing minor platelet dysfunction in patients complaining of purpura.*)

(See also Bibliography for Chapter 80.)

176

Evaluation of Disturbances in Pigmentation

WILLIAM V. R. SHELLOW, M.D.

Disturbances in pigmentation are conspicuous and common. Patients complain about general darkening, brown spots, or depigmented areas. Pigmentary alterations may be manifestations of a genetic, endocrine, metabolic, nutritional, infectious, or neoplastic problem. Physical and chemical factors also can be important.

PATHOPHYSIOLOGY AND CLINICAL PRESENTATION

Pigmentary changes are caused by melanin being absent, increased, decreased, abnormally placed, or distributed. Hyperpigmentation may result from an increased rate of melanosome production, an increased number of melanosomes transferred to keratinocytes, or a greater size and melanization of the melanosome. Hyperpigmentation is perceived as blue when melanin is located deeply, because of the Tyndall phenomenon. The pathophysiologic mechanisms that produce hyperpigmentation through the melanocyte system include elevated adrenocorticotropic hormone (ACTH), which has a melanocyte-stimulating action, ultraviolet radiation, and certain drugs.

Hypomelanosis, or depigmentation, may result from genetic loss of melanocytes or destruction by inflammation. Inflammation may be secondary to infection or burns or associated with a variety of immunologically mediated diseases.

DIFFERENTIAL DIAGNOSIS

Hyperpigmentation

The differential diagnosis of hyperpigmentation is organized on the basis of whether the hyperpigmentation is circumscribed or diffuse.

Circumscribed Hyperpigmentation includes freckles (ephelides), lentigines, and melasma. *Freckles* are small macular lesions seen on areas exposed to the sun. Freckles may become less dark in adults, but they darken after exposure to long-wave ultraviolet radiation.

Lentigines are macular, and are larger and darker than freckles. Histologically, the two are easily distinguishable. Senile lentigines appear on sun-exposed areas in older patients. They are termed "liver spots" by patients.

Melasma or *chloasma* is a blotchy hyperpigmentation that occurs on the forehead, cheeks, and upper lip, usually in women. Pregnancy, oral contraceptives, and other hormones contribute to their appearance, but exposure to sunlight appears to perpetuate the condition. During pregnancy, a physiologic darkening of the linea alba, pigmented nevi, nipples, and genitalia occurs as a result of melanocyte-stimulating hormone (MSH) and increased estrogen and progesterone.

Diffuse Hyperpigmentation results from increased amounts of melanin in the epidermis. The color may be accentuated in sun-exposed areas, over pressure points or body folds, or in areas of trauma such as new scars. Increased pigmentation occurs in *Addison's disease* as a result of increased amounts of MSH and ACTH from the pituitary because of decreased cortisol levels.

Metabolic disease such as Wilson's disease, von Gierke's hemochromatosis, biliary cirrhosis, and porphyria cutanea tarda may be accompanied by diffuse melanosis. On occasion, rheumatoid arthritis, Still's disease, and scleroderma have been associated with hyperpigmentation.

Drugs such as busulfan and cyclophosphamide may produce diffuse melanosis, as can topical nitrogen mustard. Chronic inorganic arsenic poisoning causes diffuse hyperpigmentation with normal or lighter skin areas scattered throughout, colorfully called "rain drops in the dust." Chlorpromazine and antimalarials tend to produce a bluish gray hyperpigmentation. Silver (argyria) and gold (chrysiasis) may accumulate in the skin, leading to hyperpigmentation depending on the dosage given.

Diffuse melanosis may be seen during *starvation,* with *hepatic insufficiency, malabsorption syndromes,* and *lymphomas and other malignancies.* Also included in the differential diagnosis are *deficiencies* of vitamins A, C, and B_{12}, niacin, and folic acid.

Postinflammatory hyperpigmentation may occur secondary to a number of precipitants. For example, phytophotodermatitis occurs after contact with photosensitizing agents present in meadow grass, citrus fruits, and edible plants that cause an exaggerated sunburn. Hyperpigmentation follows the acute phase. Skin contact with organic dyes and aromatic compounds may lead to photosensitization followed by hyperpigmentation. Tar, pitch, and oils may induce similar changes.

Physical trauma, friction, and heat may also lead to postinflammatory pigmentary changes, as may inflammatory dermatoses that stimulate melanin formation.

Hypopigmentation

Hypopigmentation may be hereditary or acquired. A hereditary disorder may be associated with a lack or deficiency of melanin. Melanocytes that are deficient or lacking occur in the depigmented areas of partial albinism (piebaldism). A white forelock may be present. In oculocutaneous albinism, melanocytes are normal in number but unable to produce melanin secondary to defective or absent tyrosinase.

Diseases involving abnormal amino acid metabolism, such as phenylketonuria and homocystinuria, have associated hypopigmentation of skin and hair. In tuberous sclerosis, elongated hypopigmented patches are seen. Certain cutaneous diseases lead to loss of melanin into the dermis, lending a gray appearance to the skin.

Vitiligo is a common, acquired disorder of hypopigmentation that may become progressive. Any area of the skin,

usually in early adult life, may be the first affected. Lesions may be symmetrical, primarily on exposed skin, on intertriginous areas, over bony prominences, or around orifices. In involved areas, the hair may be white. The border may be sharp and hyperpigmented. Occasionally, vitiligo assumes a segmental or zosteriform pattern. Halo nevi, centrifugal areas of depigmentation that surround a pigmented nevus, accompany one third of the cases of vitiligo. Premature graying of the hair occurs in 35% of vitiligo patients.

Partial repigmentation of vitiligo may occur in sun-exposed areas, but vitiliginous patches may burn because of the lack of protective pigmentation. Vitiligo has been associated with autoimmune diseases such as pernicious anemia, collagen diseases, and hypo- and hyperthyroidism. Diabetes mellitus, alopecia areata, male hypogonadism, hypopituitarism, and Cushing's syndrome have been associated with diffuse hypopigmentation.

Depigmentation may be caused by a variety of chemical agents, rubber, antioxidants, germicides, and, most notably, phenolic compounds that interfere with tyrosinase activity. Dermatitis may precede the loss of pigment, and areas remote from the inflamed sites may also lose pigment.

Dermatoses and infections may result in localized areas of pigment loss. Such areas may be more noticeable in dark-skinned persons. Small hypopigmented areas occur on women's legs and may be related to the trauma of shaving. Tinea versicolor, pityriasis alba, and various eczematous conditions may present as areas of hypopigmentation.

WORKUP

Hyperpigmentation

Evaluation of the patient with localized hyperpigmentation requires inspection of the lesions and inquiry about previous dermatoses and the use of oral contraceptives that may produce melasma. The majority of localized hyperpigmented areas are postinflammatory and of only cosmetic concern. Diffuse hyperpigmentation necessitates a careful history that specifies the time of onset and possible sun exposure. A drug history that emphasizes agents known to produce pigmentary changes should be pursued. There should be general review of systems, noting weakness associated with Addison's disease; itching and hepatic dysfunction associated with biliary cirrhosis. The physician should consider the possibility of severe vitamin deficiency or malnutrition. The history should be followed by a physical examination that notes hyperpigmentation in creases and scars, as are characteristic of Addison's disease, and clues to obvious underlying pathology, as may occur with malignancy, hepatic insufficiency, or malabsorption. Laboratory investigation must be based on clinical signs of underlying disease. Biopsy may be indicated when heavy metal deposition or hemosiderosis is a diagnostic consideration.

Hypopigmentation

Hypopigmentation requires a careful history of approximate time of onset and possible exposure to bleaching agents, most notably phenol-containing products. Hypopigmented areas should be scraped, and a KOH wet mount examined microscopically to diagnose tinea versicolor. The total depigmentation of vitiligo should be differentiated from partial postinflammatory hypopigmentation. Patients with vitiligo should undergo a careful general review of systems and a physical examination that seeks to identify diseases such as pernicious anemia, thyroid disease, diabetes, or collagen vascular disease known to be associated with the condition. Ophthalmoscopic examination should be performed to detect retinal pigmentary changes.

SYMPTOMATIC THERAPY

Hyperpigmentation

In treating hyperpigmented areas, the chief symptomatic advice is strict avoidance of sunlight. Topical bleaching with hydroquinone cream may be effective. Strong topical corticosteroid preparations have a pigment-lightening effect, as does retinoic acid. A bleaching solution of retinoic acid 0.1%, hydroquinone 5%, and dexamethasone 0.1% in a hydrophilic ointment or alcohol is quite effective.

Hypopigmentation

Hypopigmented areas can usually be masked by appropriate cosmetics, by bleaching normal skin, or by repigmentation with psoralens and ultraviolet radiation. Hundreds of treatments may be required. The primary physician must assess the desire for treatment and inform the patient of the alternatives. Age, sex, or duration of vitiligo does not affect the response. Lesions on the face and abdomen tend to repigment more rapidly than those on the hands, feet, and bony prominences. Treatment should probably be supervised by a dermatologist experienced in using these agents to achieve optimal cosmetic results.

It is important to reassure the patient that there is no systemic disease and that the condition is not contagious. The primary physician should advise the patient about cosmetic alternatives and help the patient decide on an appropriate course of treatment.

ANNOTATED BIBLIOGRAPHY

Albert DM, Nordlund JJ, Lerner AA: Ocular abnormalities occurring with vitiligo. Ophthalmology 86:1145, 1979 (*One third of 112 vitiligo patients had lesion of the retinal pigment epithelium or choroid.*)

Bleehen SS, Pathak MA, Hori Y et al: Depigmentation of skin with 4-isopropylacatechol, mercaptoamines and other compounds. J Invest Dermatol 50:103, 1968 (*An investigative screening of 33 compounds to assess depigmenting ability.*)

Cunliffe WJ et al: Vitiligo, thyroid diseases and autoimmunity. Br J Dermatol 80:135, 1968 (*Confirms the association of vitiligo with thyroid disease, pernicious anemia, alopecia areata, and diabetes mellitus.*)

El Mofty AM, El Mofty M: Vitiligo: A symptom complex. Int J Dermatol 19:237, 1980 (*Discussion of vitiligo and its association with systemic disease.*)

Fulk CS: Primary disorders of hyperpigmentation. J Am Acad Dermatol 10:1, 1984 (*A review article that contains 135 references.*)

Kahn G: Depigmentation caused by phenolic detergent germicides. Arch Dermatol 102:177, 1970 (*Brings attention for the first time to the depigmenting properties of disinfectants used by hospital workers.*)

Kenney JA, Grimes PE: How we treat vitiligo. Cutis 32:347, 1983 (*Practical approaches for treating vitiligo from the Vitiligo Research Center.*)

Kumari J: Vitiligo treated with Topical Clobetasol Propionate. Arch Dermatol 120:631, 1984 (*Clobetasol produced repigmentation of 90% to 100% in more than 80% of the patients with facial lesions and more than 40% of patients on other parts of the body.*)

Lerner AB, Nordlund JJ: Vitiligo! What is it? Is it important? JAMA 239:1138, 1978 (*A comprehensive review.*)

Pathak MA, Daniels F Jr, Fitzpatrick TB: The presently known distribution of furocoumarins (psoralens) in plants. J Invest Dermatol 39:225, 1962 (*A scholarly article that lists all plants that elicit phytophotodermatitis.*)

Resnick S: Melasma induced by oral contraceptive drugs. JAMA 199:601, 1967 (*An important article on a major side-effect of oral contraceptive agents—29% of 212 patients developed melasma.*)

Tsuji T, Hemada T: Topically administered fluorouracil in vitiligo. Arch Dermatol 119:722, 1983 (*Abrasion plus 5-FU produced partial or complete repigmentation in 18 of 28 patients.*)

177
Evaluation of Alopecia
WILLIAM V. R. SHELLOW, M.D.

Alopecia may be described as the lack of hair in areas where it normally grows. The most noticeable area for alopecia is the scalp, but loss of body hair may also occur. Patients may seek medical care for what is perceived as excessive hair loss even when there is no alopecia. Whether the problem is genetically induced male pattern baldness or alopecia as a result of systemic illness, the primary care physician may be the first to whom the problem is presented and must offer the patient a rational approach to diagnosis and treatment.

PATHOPHYSIOLOGY

Hair is a product of keratinocytes in the hair bulb. The hair shaft is made of hard keratin. Synthesis results from mitoses of cells within the hair matrix. The growth of hair is cyclical, with the length of the cycle varying with the location. Scalp hair grows from 3 to 10 years, involutes over 3 months, and rests for another 3 months. In healthy young persons, about 90% of all scalp hairs are in anagen, actively growing. Telogen, or resting hair, accounts for most of the remainder.

Hairs that grow for long periods and rest briefly are most susceptible to interruption of the growth cycle, and variations in the growing-to-resting ratio are most noticeable. The longer the growing period, the longer the hair. Scalp hair grows at the rate of approximately 0.35 mm per day, but there are factors that may affect the rate.

Hair loss must be distinguished from hair breakage, which results from physical or chemical stress to the shaft. The term proximal trichorrhexis is sometimes used to describe hair breakage that occurs within the first centimeter from the scalp, while distal trichorrhexis is that which occurs beyond this point. Hair straightening may give rise to proximal trichorrhexis. Patients often recognize distal breakage as splint ends, which may be accelerated by sunshine or swimming in chlorinated pools.

The primary pathogenic mechanisms of hair loss are destruction of the hair matrix by physical agents and infectious or immunologically mediated inflammation. Hair loss may occur secondary to a slowing of hair growth from metabolic diseases, antimetabolites, or other drugs. Physiologic alterations may also produce hair loss by altering the relationship of the growing and resting phases of hair follicles. During pregnancy, fewer hairs are shed, producing fewer telogen hairs. After parturition, the percentage of telogen hairs increases, and there is loss of hair. The process is diffuse and short-lived. This alteration in the relationship of resting hairs to the total may also develop secondary to pharmacologic changes induced by oral contraceptives. Destructive pathogenic mechanisms often produce scarring alopecia, whereas systemic illnesses and drugs usually result in nonscarring alopecia.

DIFFERENTIAL DIAGNOSIS

The standard classification of alopecia is scarring (or cicatricial) and nonscarring (noncicatricial). In the latter, the hair follicles are retained and the process is potentially reversible. In the scarring type, follicles are destroyed and hair never regrows. A few conditions that begin as nonscarring may later scar as a result of chronicity.

SCARRING ALOPECIA generally involves significant *inflammation*. Physical trauma such as burns, radiation, injuries, and chronic traction are often implicated. Traction alopecia usually results from braiding or tight hair rollers. The pattern of hair loss is dependent on the styling. The process is initially reversible but progresses to a scarring phase with chronicity. Hot combs in combination with petrolatum used to straighten hair may result in inflammation with consequent fibrosis and hair loss. *Infections*—whether they be bacterial, resulting in deep cellulitis, fungal with *Trichophyton schoenleini,* or viral, such as recurrent herpes simplex or herpes zoster—produce inflammatory change and alopecia. *Dermatologic processes* such as discoid lupus erythematosus, scleroderma, lichen planus, cutaneous neoplasms, or granulomas may produce scarring alopecia. Factitial causes and neurotic excoriations must also be considered.

NONSCARRING ALOPECIA. Alopecia is most often nonscarring, with the most common cause being male and female pattern baldness. *Male pattern baldness* (androgenetic alopecia) is symmetrical, usually beginning in the frontoparietal scalp. The development of male baldness is related to age, genetic predisposition, and the presence of androgenic hormones. The inheritance is probably dominant, with incomplete penetrance. The process is permanent with pigmented scalp hairs replaced by fine unpigmented vellus hairs. *Female pattern baldness,* also androgenetic alopecia, is more diffuse, usually in the central and frontal areas without complete baldness. Age, family tendency, and androgenic hormones are important factors. The presence of a male pattern hair loss in a female should provoke concern about androgen excess.

Nonscarring alopecia often involves systemic disease, medication, or metabolic abnormality. *Alopecia areata,* a condition of unknown etiology in which hair is rapidly lost, usually in circular patterns, is probably the second most common cause of nonscarring alopecia. *Alopecia totalis* is loss of all the scalp hair, and alopecia universalis includes loss of facial and body hair as well. The course of alopecia areata is unpredictable. Some persons have one episode with one or several bald spots and spontaneous regrowth. Others may develop new areas of baldness and become totally bald. Onset before puberty is associated with a poorer prognosis. Many authors believe that there is an autoimmune mechanism and an association with other autoimmune diseases.

Alopecia may follow *infectious diseases* with high persistent fevers such as typhoid or pneumonia. Secondary syphilis, superficial folliculitis, and tinea capitis may produce nonscarring alopecia. *Medication,* notably antineoplastic agents such as 5-fluorouracil, cyclophosphamide, or methotrexate, produce hair loss. Other drugs such as heparin, allopurinol, thiouracil, and quinine and hypervitaminosis A have been associated with alopecia.

Oral contraceptives, hyperandrogenism, and pregnancy are known to interfere with the relationship of resting and growing hairs and to produce hair loss. Diffuse hair thinning may occur with *thyroid disease* and *iron deficiency.* Less commonly, hypopituitarism and parathyroid disease produce hair loss. Alopecia is a manifestation of collagen vascular diseases, notably systemic lupus erythematosus and dermatomyositis. Occasional patients have self-induced hair loss, a condition known as *trichotillomania.* These patients may not be aware that they are plucking hairs, and the condition may indicate significant psychiatric disturbance.

WORKUP

History should identify the date of onset and determine whether the patient is troubled by a specific area of hair loss or by the perception of excessive loss. The history may reveal specific physical causes. The physician should ask about the use of curlers, rollers, bleaching, permanent waves, hair straightening, or hot combs, which may produce traction or physical destruction. Febrile illness within the last 6 to 12 weeks may be important. Drug history, noting particularly antimetabolites, colchicine, estrogens, androgens, antithyroid drugs, anticoagulants, or vitamin A, should be pursued. Less common causes that may be revealed by the history include delivery of a baby 3 months before, or recent severe dieting. A family history may suggest probable male or female pattern baldness.

Physical Examination is essential to distinguish scarring from nonscarring alopecia. The physician should observe whether the pattern is localized or diffuse and whether the hair loss reveals a genetic pattern or suggests a mechanical cause. The physician should note hirsutism and masculinizing signs in women with baldness.

The scalp should be examined carefully for areas of reduced hair growth, actual areas of alopecia, and scarring. When the circular areas characteristic of alopecia areata are seen, light traction on the hairs at the edge of the bald area will indicate if the disease is active at that location. If hairs come out with ease, then extension of the alopecic area is to be expected. The physician should examine the area surrounding the hair loss for evidence of inflammation, cellulitis, folliculitis, or fungal infection. Also, the physician should note the presence of short broken hairs, which suggests pulling of the hair. It is useful to examine the nails; the presence of Beau's lines may correlate with a systemic process affecting both nail and hair growth.

The "pluck" or "pull" test may be helpful. A dozen or so hairs are grasped between the thumb and index finger, and moderate traction is applied. Three areas should be tested in this fashion: the vertex, the occiput and the parietal scalp. Extraction of two or fewer hairs per area indicates that hair loss is probably not excessive. In instances of telogen effluvium and in active androgenetic alopecia, more than six hairs will be removed. The interpretation of finding between two and six hairs is less precise, and additional studies, sometimes including scalp biopsy, are indicated.

It is often helpful to collect objective evidence of hair loss to distinguish perceived from genuine problems of hair loss. The patient can collect the hairs that he loses daily, count them, place them in an envelope, and note the daily total. It may be found that 100 hairs a day are being lost, and that is within normal limits. Examination of an area of alopecia with a Wood's light may reveal fluorescent fungal infection. The physician should always scrape for microscopic examination and culture any areas of inflammation. Some dermatologists perform telogen counts by removing 100 hairs and counting how many are in the telogen phase. Telogen hair is identified by the presence of a terminal club on the hair shaft. This procedure can separate conditions resulting from telogen excess from those resulting from broken hairs, but it may be too time-consuming to be useful to the primary physician.

Laboratory Studies. A biopsy may be helpful, particularly in cases of scarring alopecia, both to add histologic evidence to diagnose according to etiology and also to determine areas of activity that might respond to anti-inflammatory therapy. Performance of laboratory tests for systemic disease, such as blood count, serum iron, thyroxine, antinuclear antibody, and others, depends on the history and physical evidence.

SYMPTOMATIC MANAGEMENT

The primary physician can provide the patient with reassurance, advice, and, occasionally, specific therapy. The treatment of alopecia depends on identification of a probable etiology. Patients with the perception of excessive hair loss that is not substantiated by the presence of alopecia and furthermore with a normal hair loss count should be reassured. Patients with hair loss following pregnancy should be reassured with a careful explanation of why it is occurring. Drugs associated with hair loss should be discontinued. Infection, either bacterial or fungal, should be specifically treated. Underlying diseases such as hypo- or hyperthyroidism should be treated, and hair loss will often resolve.

Alopecia areata may respond to specific medical therapy, which should be undertaken by a dermatologist or physician skilled in the technique. A traditional treatment for stimulating new hair growth has been irritation with phenol or ultraviolet light. Topical fluorinated corticosteroids under occlusion may be helpful, and this may be tried by the primary physician. It is often necessary to inject a dilute steroid solution into the scalp, preferably triamcinolone, which appears to be less likely to cause atrophy than other steroids. Small volumes are used, and several injections may be necessary to cover a large area. Systemic corticosteroids have, on occasion, been helpful, but their effectiveness is often lost when the drugs are discontinued, and the risks of chronic therapy (see Chapter 103) outweigh the benefits. They should be used only under exceptional circumstances and only by a dermatologist experienced in treating patients with hair problems. In young women with androgenic alopecia, spironolactone improved the condition in one study, but more data are necessary before recommending this approach.

A number of newer approaches are under investigation. Dinitrochlorobenzene (DNCB), has been shown to induce sufficient hypersensitivity to produce erythema and scaling with regrowth of hair in approximately 70% of patients. The treatment often needs to be repeated and DNCB has the cloud of a positive Ames test showing mutagenicity. Squaric acid dibutylester is another control-sensitizing chemical that has been used to treat alopecia areata. It has not been shown to be mutagenic in the Ames assay. Anthralin, used in the management of psoriasis, has been used to stimulate hair growth but it must be applied nightly and removed in the morning. Psoralen and ultraviolet A light (PUVA) therapy has also been used with some success. Hair growth takes as long as 6 months and almost always take more than 6 weeks before any improvement is noted. Cooling the scalp helps prevent hair loss induced by chemotherapy.

One of the most promising approaches is the use of the antihypertensive *minoxidil* in the topical form. Trials are in progress for the treatment of both alopecia areata and male pattern baldness. The drug's long-term efficacy and safety remain to be determined. Until the data are available, topical minoxidil should be considered investigational.

Despite the substantial interest and literature extolling various therapies, no approach can be judged effective enough to recommend. Many experienced clinicians believe that treatment accelerates resolution in approximately 50% of alopecia areata sufferers, who would spontaneously regrow hair. Some argue that, outside of a study situation, expectant treatment is medically correct and cost-effective.

PATIENT EDUCATION

Patient education can be the most important part of the primary physician's management of the patient with alopecia. Once diagnosis is established or serious diseases are excluded, the patient should be reassured. Patients are often concerned that the hair loss will progress, and the most useful information that can be given is the likelihood of continued or total hair loss. Men with genetic baldness are often reassured to know that there is no systemic disease. Women may be helped by advice on how to restyle hair. Patients are often well aware of the option of wigs and ask the physician about such issues as having their hair woven or having hair transplants. Weaving is a relatively safe procedure performed by nonphysicians. It is successful but must be repeated periodically and thereby becomes expensive and a nuisance. Hair transplants are expensive. The procedure is painful and is usually not covered by insurance. Patients with coarse dark hair are the best candidates for hair transplants. The use of artificial hair implants should be discouraged because they usually fall out or elicit a chronic foreign body reaction. Patients seek advice about shampooing and the treatment of hair. They should be told to avoid alkaline pH shampoo and excessive toweling after washing their hair and that a conditioner may be helpful. It is useful to advise patients that combing is less injurious to hair than brushing and that if one must brush, to gently disentangle the hair from the brush. It is safest to use a natural bristle brush or a nylon brush with rounded edges. Patients should avoid bleaching, permanent waving, straightening, use of hot combs, or excessive exposure to the sun. Success in the management of the patient with alopecia is often dependent on the physician's ability to teach the patient to accept the reality of hair loss.

ANNOTATED BIBLIOGRAPHY

Case PC, Mitchell AJ, Swanson NA: Topical therapy of alopecia areata with squaric acid dibutylester. J Am Acad Dermatol 10: 447, 1984 (*Eleven of 26 patients treated with this contact sensitizer had excellent regrowth of hair.*)

Claudy AL, Gagnaira D: PUVA treatment of alopecia areata. Arch Dermatol 119:975, 1983 (*This method is successful in about half of those treated.*)

Fiedler-Weiss VC, West DP, Buys CM: Topical minoxidil dose-response effect in alopecia areata. Arch Dermatol 122:180, 1986 (*Topical 5% minoxidil produced terminal hair regrowth in 40 of 47 patients (85%) after 48 to 60 weeks of therapy. Regrowth was* generally not cosmetically acceptable, but higher dosing produced better results without toxicity.)

Groverman HD, Ganiats T, Klauber MR: Lack of efficacy of polysorbate 60 in the treatment of male pattern baldness. Arch Intern Med 145:1454, 1985 (*A scientific dismissal of an anecdotally tested baldness cure.*)

Hanke CW, Bergfeld WF: Fiber implantation for pattern baldness. JAMA 241:146, 1979 (*Describes the serious deficiencies associated with this procedure, which is probably an unacceptable alternative to baldness.*)

Happle R, Cebulla K, Echternacht-Happle K: Dinitrochlorobenzene therapy for alopecia areata. Arch Dermatol 114:1629, 1978 (*Eighty-nine percent of patients treated with DNCB regrew hair.*)

Kasick JM, Berfeld WF, Steck WD et al: Adrenal androgenic female-pattern alopecia: Sex hormones and the balding woman. Cleve Clin 50:111, 1983 (*A discussion of endocrinologic abnormalities in women with balding. Discusses spironolactone therapy; 52 references are included.*)

Mitchell AJ, Krull EA: Alopecia areata. Pathogenesis and treatment. J Am Acad Dermatol 11:763, 1984 (*The current use of immunotherapy, including systemic agents; 158 references are included.*)

Muller SA, Winkelmann RV: Alopecia areata: An evaluation of 736 patients. Arch Dermatol 88:290, 1963 (*A review emphasizing natural history.*)

Satterwhite B, Zimm S: The use of scalp hypothermia in the prevention of doxorubicin hair loss. Cancer 54:34, 1984 (*A chemocap with cryogel reduced hair loss in 9 of 12, to the point that a wig was not required.*)

Weiss VC, West DP, Fu TS et al: Alopecia areata treated with topical minoxidil. Arch Dermatol 120:457, 1983 (*Using a 1% topical solution, 25 of 48 patients showed some regrowth, but in only 11 was it cosmetically acceptable.*)

178

Management of Acne

RONALD M. REISNER, M.D.

Acne, the most common of all skin disease, is a polygenic, multifactorial disease that, depending on the strictness of its definition, afflicts between 50% and 100% of adolescents in the United States. It ranges in severity from a few scattered whiteheads and blackheads to disfiguring, painful, deep-seated, pus-filled, and bleeding nodulocystic lesions. About 15% of surveyed patients with acne seek medical care. The primary care physician is in a unique position to identify and treat a high proportion of acne sufferers. Properly managing acne requires a thorough understanding of the development of acne in all its phases so that therapy appropriate to the circumstances can be selected from the available modalities. Early effective treatment will minimize the physical scarring of the disease and prevent or reduce equally important psychic trauma.

PATHOPHYSIOLOGY AND CLINICAL PRESENTATION

The pathogenesis of acne is proving to be increasingly complex. It involves the interaction of enzymatic, immunologic, and chemotactic effects of normal cutaneous microflora; hormonal influences; abnormal keratinization of the sebaceous follicular duct wall; follicular fragility and host responsiveness.

Acne is a disease of the sebaceous follicles. There are approximately 5000 sebaceous follicles scattered predominantly on the face and central upper back and chest. The initial event in the pathogenesis of acne is conversion of the loose, easily shed, horny layer of the epithelium lining the follicular duct wall to a self-adhering mass that gradually obstructs the (follicular) duct. This has been called "retention hyperkeratosis." It takes 1 to 2 months for the accumulated mass of keratin, sebum, and bacteria to reach visible size as a closed comedone or whitehead. Whiteheads may expand the duct ("pore") opening to communicate freely with the outside. The compact, melanin-rich tip then gives the appearance and name "blackhead."

Chemotactic agents produced within the duct attract leukocytes, and in ensuing events follicular duct walls may rupture, releasing their contents into the surrounding dermis. This provokes a profound inflammatory response, leading to the development of papules, pustules, nodules, and suppurative nodules that are commonly, but mistakenly, termed "cysts." These inflammatory lesions may lead to permanent scarring.

Acne may most conveniently be divided into two categories, obstructive and inflammatory. The former, resulting from the impaction of horny material, bacteria, and sebum in the dilated follicular duct wall, is characterized by closed comedones (whiteheads) and open comedones (blackheads). Leakage of intrafollicular contents from comedones produces an inflammatory response. Depending on the level of leakage into the dermis and the amount of material released, lesions vary from small, erythematous papules and superficial pustules to deeper pustules and larger, persistent, or suppurative nodules. Genetic immunologic factors contribute to an exaggerated inflammation response and more severe cystic forms of acne.

PRINCIPLES OF THERAPY

The goals of therapy are removal of existing lesions and prevention of new ones. The modalities employed depend on the kind of lesion.

The first principle of therapy is to remove acnegenic agents. Some cosmetics, oils, and creams may be capable of producing comedones, and their use should be stopped. Women should cease taking oral contraceptives with androgenic progestational components such as norethindrone and norgestrel. The physician should advise against using acnegenic drugs such as androgens, steroids, iodides, and bromides. Consider an underlying endocrinopathy in the evaluation of an adult with acne of recent onset.

OBSTRUCTIVE ACNE should be approached by removing closed comedones. Removal is accomplished by atraumatically nicking the covering epidermis with a No. 11 blade or blood lancet and extracting the contents with a comedone extractor. The expression of open comedones has little influence on future inflammatory lesions but does improve appearance. After removing existing comedones, the physician should prescribe a comedolytic agent. The two most effective agents available are *retinoic acid* and *benzoyl peroxide*. The frequency of application should be adjusted to produce minimally visible erythema and desquamation. Initial therapy may be 5% benzoyl peroxide gel, once or twice daily, followed after several weeks by the addition of 0.05% retinoic acid of application or use of a more concentrated solution or gel is indicated by the patient's response. The order of therapy may be reversed with retinoic acid started first and benzoyl peroxide added after 3 to 6 weeks.

The combination of agents loosens existing comedones, making extraction easier, and helps prevent formation of new lesions. Retinoic acid thins the outer, horny layer of the epidermis; therefore, the patient should discontinue other topical medications, avoid excessive cleansing, and minimize sun exposure. Patients should be warned of a possible transient pustular flare when therapy is initiated. Topical agents may be used concomitantly with tetracycline (see below). Benzoyl peroxide, which oxidizes bacteria, and retinoic acid, which diminishes hyperkeratosis, have largely replaced compounds that contain sulfur, salicylic acid, and resorcinol.

Patients with acne may have oily skin, but *cleansing measures* to remove excess oil do not affect the course of acne. Cleansing may improve an undesirable oily appearance, and gentle cleansing methods such as use of mild soap and water are tolerated. Astringents, generally mixtures of alcohol or acetone and water, are a convenient means of removing excessive oil.

INFLAMMATORY ACNE. Mild inflammatory acne may be treated with topical agents used for obstructive lesions. *Benzoyl peroxide* increases the rate of resorption of small erythematous papules and thin-roofed pustules. Ultraviolet light produces erythema and desquamation-enhancing inflammatory lesions, but sunlamps should not be recommended.

Severe inflammatory acne—characterized by large, deep papules and pustules and the destructive suppurating, nodular lesions—requires long-term *systemic antibiotics. Tetracycline* is used if an intensive topical regimen fails. Alternatively, *erythromycin* is effective. Systemic antibiotics suppress the organism *Propionibacterium acnes,* a normal inhabitant of the follicular canal in humans. This organism may participate in the initiation and aggravation of inflammatory lesions by elaborating enzymes, including lipases, that act on sebum to release potentially irritating free fatty acids. Hyaluronidase increases permeability of the follicular duct wall, and protease damages the follicular duct wall, causing leakage of materials into the surrounding dermis. *P. acnes* produces chemotactic substances that contribute to the initiation and evolution of inflammatory lesion. Tetracycline, though it diminishes bacteria, may actually work most effectively by reducing chemotactic substances.

Antibiotics prevent the development of new lesions but do not affect existing ones. *Topical antibiotics* such as *erythromycin* and *clindamycin* (clindamycin should not be used systemically) are used before systemic drugs in milder inflammatory acne. Topical clindamycin is less oily but more expensive than erythromycin. Clinical results are not ordinarily seen before 4 to 6 weeks of therapy, at which time the formation of new lesions should decrease. Existing papulopustular lesions may persist for 7 to 10 days and deep, nodulocystic lesions may remain for months.

Two decades of experience with antibiotic therapy, including a detailed review of indications and hazards of such therapy by an *ad hoc* committee of the American Academy of Dermatology, has established it as rational, effective, and remarkably safe. The usual oral regimen is to initiate therapy with tetracycline, 250 mg four times a day, for 2 to 4 weeks, gradually reducing the dosage according to the response. In some patients, 250 mg of tetracycline every other day suppresses new eruptions. Generic tetracycline is cheapest, but doxycycline allows twice-daily dosage with less uncertainty about absorption and fewer GI side-effects. Minocycline is frequently used, but its superiority has not been established. Therapy should be stopped periodically to determine whether or not continued antibiotics are necessary. Flares occur between 2 and 4 weeks after the antibiotics are discontinued. Contraindications to tetracycline are known hypersensitivity, pregnancy, and age under 12.

Benzoyl peroxide and *retinoic acid* appear to be synergistic with antibiotic therapy, possibly increasing the concentration of tetracycline in the follicular duct. Tetracycline should be given at least 1 hour before or 2 hours after meals, and absorption or patient compliance can be evaluated by examining either the oral mucosa with a Wood's light for greenish yellow fluorescence or the large pores of the nose, which lose their coral red fluorescence as the *P. acnes* population is reduced. An occasional complication of systemic antibiotic therapy is the development of a gram-negative folliculitis with pustules around the nose and mouth and spreading onto the cheeks. Culture of the lesions, with identification of the organisms—usually *Klebsiella* or *Enterobacter*—is indicated. It usually responds within 2 or 3 days to trimethoprim–sulfa. More recently, 13-cis-retinoic acid has proved useful for gram-negative folliculitis.

Intralesional corticosteroids may hasten involution of nodulocystic lesions, reducing the risk of permanent scarring. *Triamcinolone acetonide* 2.0 mg or 2.5 mg/cc in saline injected with a 30-gauge needle directly into specific lesions, is often remarkably effective. Pseudoatrophy is a danger. The physician should avoid dosages in excess of 20 mg per week, which may suppress the pituitary–adrenal axis. Some dermatologists prefer to use cryotherapy with liquid nitrogen. This requires experience to avoid excessive freezing and tissue destruction.

There is no evidence that *diet* has a significant effect on acne. Diuretics, vitamin A, and vaccines, which have been advocated, do not appear to have demonstrable therapeutic value. Radiation therapy is rarely if ever indicated.

Cyclic estrogen–progestin therapy may be considered in highly selected situations with full awareness of and careful monitoring for side-effects. Sulfones are reserved for the most severe inflammatory acne and have been supplanted by 13-cis-retinoic acid.

Systemic *13-cis-retinoic acid* has given us a powerful new agent for the treatment of acne. The recommended dosage for severe acne is 60 to 80 mg a day; however, dosages of 10 to 40 mg daily produce fewer side-effects and are effective in controlling less severe forms of acne, but are less likely to induce permanent remission. The drug has some severe effects, including teratogenesis. The FDA approval is reserved for severe nodulocystic acne, which is unresponsive to conventional therapy. To prevent birth defects and spontaneous abortion in women receiving 13-cis-retinoic acid during pregnancy, treatment should be preceded by a pregnancy test, which is repeated at monthly intervals during therapy. Hypertriglyceridemia, pseudotumor cerebri, idiopathic skeletal hyperostosis, cheilitis, nasal mucosal dryness, nosebleeds, conjunctivitis, skin fragility, arthralgia, headaches, and transaminase elevations all occur, but most of these effects are reversible. Despite these problems, it is a remarkable medication for the treatment of nodular cystic acne. One or two 15- to 20-week courses often bring severe acne under complete control, with little or no further therapy.

THERAPEUTIC RECOMMENDATIONS

- Explanation to the patient is an essential part of treating acne, so that understanding and cooperation can be enlisted.
- Eliminate acnegenic drugs, such as steroids or androgens, exposure to oils, and habits such as rubbing the face.
- For obstructive acne, use retinoic acid 0.05% to a point just short of clinically visible erythema. A topical antibiotic or benzoyl peroxide may be used if papules are present concurrently.
- In inflammatory acne, prescribe an antibiotic, usually tetracycline, 250 mg, reducing the dosage once control is achieved.
- In acne characterized by large nodules, intralesional steroids or, in the hands of experts, liquid nitrogen may be tried.
- For severe nodulocystic acne, resistant to conventional therapy, 13-cis-retinoic acid should be considered with full awareness of its risks and appropriate monitoring of the blood.
- For people with acne scars, dermabrasion should be considered, in consultation with a dermatologist highly experienced in the procedure.

PATIENT EDUCATION

Treatment of acne falls within the domain of the primary physician. The dermatologist should be consulted if basic topical and antibiotic therapy fail and in cases of severe disfiguring lesions that require techniques such as intralesional steroids or acne surgery. Patient education and cooperation are crucial to the success of therapy. Patients must understand the chronic nature of the process and not be discouraged when lesions continue to appear. Patients who unrealistically expect cure may become discouraged, uncooperative, and finally angry.

A vast mythology about acne has developed. The patient should be assured that acne has no relationship to diet, masturbation, sexual activity or inactivity, constipation, dirt, or angry feelings. The patient should be helped to gain perspective and discouraged from self-examination in brightly lit mirrors, which often produce a distorted self-image. The patient begins to perceive himself as "acne with a person attached," rather than a person with acne. Describing this process to the patient often brings an answering smile of recognition and is reassuring. Instructions for the use of topical and systemic agents must be precise and carefully followed. The patient should be reminded that therapeutic results are not achieved immediately, and treatment must be continued for 6 to 8 weeks before a response is seen.

ANNOTATED BIBLIOGRAPHY

Ad Hoc Committee on Antibiotic Treatment of Acne: Systemic antibiotics for treatment of acne vulgaris—efficacy and safety. Arch Dermatol 111:630, 1975 (*This authorative report concludes that systemic antibiotics, particularly tetracycline, are safe.*)

Bernstein JE, Shalita AR: Topically applied erythromycin in inflammatory acne vulgaris. J Am Acad Dermatol 2:318, 1980 (*Two percent erythromycin evaluated, compared with vehicle control in 349 patients.*)

Chalker DK, Shalita A, Smith JC: A double-blind study of the effectiveness of a 3% erythromycin and 5% benzoyl peroxide combination in the treatment of acne vulgaris. J Am Acad Dermatol 9:433, 1983 (*The combination was successful presumably because benzoyl peroxide transcends the stratum corneum to allow better penetration of the erythromycin.*)

Dicken CH: Retinoids: A review. J Am Acad Dermatol 11:541, 1984 (*The state of the art in using retinoids.*)

Fulton JE Jr, Pay SA, Fulton JE III: Comedogenicity of current therapeutic products, cosmetics and ingredients in the rabbit ear. J Am Acad Dermatol 10:96, 1984 (*The scientific basis for decisions about cosmetics.*)

Fulton JE, Plewig G, Kligman AM: Effect of chocolate on acne vulgaris. JAMA 210:2071, 1979 (*Debunking another myth, concluding that chocolate has no impact.*)

Gammon WR, Meyer C, Lantiss: Comparative efficacy of oral erythromycin versus oral tetracycline in the treatment of acne vulgaris. J Am Acad Dermatol 114:183, 1986 (*Two hundred patients with moderate to moderately severe acne; 77% of erythromycin-treated patients, and 88% of tetracycline patients were markedly improved by week 12.*)

Hubbell CG, Hobbs ER, Rist T et al: Efficacy of minocycline compared with tetracycline in treatment of acne vulgaris. Arch Dermatol 118:989, 1982 (*Both are effective. Improvement is seen more quickly in minocycline-treated patients.*)

Levine RM, Rasmussen JE: Intralesional corticosteroids in the treatment of nodule cystic acne. Arch Dermatol 119:486, 1983 (*Guidance for this form of acne surgery.*)

Marynick SP, Chakmakjian ZH, McCaffree DL et al: Androgen excess in cystic acne. N Engl J Med 308:981, 1983 (*Documents high dehydroepiandrosterone sulfate levels in both men and women with long-standing cystic acne resistant to conventional therapy; symptoms improved when levels were reduced by dexamethasone in men and dexamethasone and/or the oral contraceptive demulen in women.*)

Melski JW, Arndt KA: Topical therapy for acne. N Engl J Med 302:503, 1980 (*This concise review of topical therapy can help the primary care physician avoid the toxic effects of systemic approaches.*)

Mills OH, Kligman AM: Acne detergicans. Arch Dermatol 111:65, 1975 (*A description suggesting that obsessive washing may actually produce comedones.*)

Peck GL et al: Prolonged remissions of cystic and conglobate acne with 13-cis-retinoic acid. N Engl J Med 300:329, 1979 (*A seminal article establishing the efficacy of this important drug.*)

Pochi PE: Hormonal therapy of acne. Dermatol Clin 1:377, 1983 (*An up-to-date review of the therapeutic option of hormones in acne.*)

Reisner RM: Antibiotic and anti-inflammatory therapy of acne. Dermatol Clin 1:385, 1983 (*A comprehensive discussion of topical and systemic antibiotics, including mechanisms of action and complications.*)

Shalita AR, Smith EB, Auer E: Topical erythromycin versus clindamycin therapy for acne, a multicenter double-blind comparison. Arch Dermatol 120:351, 1984 (*Comparable efficacy with reduction of inflammatory lesions by 62% and 59%; 73% of the erythromycin patients and 62% of the clindamycin had excellent to good responses.*)

179

Management of Acne Rosacea and Other Variants

WILLIAM V. R. SHELLOW, M.D.

Acnelike eruptions occur in adults but are often ignored. Middle-aged women and men may be affected by acne rosacea, younger women by perioral dermatitis, and older people by periorbital comedones. These conditions occasionally cause a patient to seek medical attention, but more often are noted incidentally by an examining physician seeing a patient for another reason. The primary care practitioner's responsibility involves identification of the patient with acne variants and institution of effective therapy.

PATHOPHYSIOLOGY AND CLINICAL PRESENTATION

ACNE ROSACEA is a chronic condition involving the blush area of the face. Persistent erythema is a prominent component and may coexist with telangiectasia. Papules and pustules recur periodically. The condition occurs more commonly in women, but when it occurs in men it tends to be more severe. Presentation may include flushing, telangiectasia, papules, pustules, or nodules. Comedones are rarely seen. Rhinophyma, a thick and lobulated overgrowth of connective tissue and sebaceous glands of the nose, may be an associated feature. Ocular complications commonly include blepharitis, conjunctivitis, and episcleritis, and infrequently include iritis and keratitis.

PERIORAL DERMATITIS, a papular erythema around the mouth, chin, upper lip, and nasolabial folds, is seen primarily in young women. Eruption is usually bilateral and symmetrical; occasionally, papulopustular lesions are widespread.

PERIORBITAL COMEDONES are most frequently seen in older people. The condition is related to senile loss of elasticity of the skin; opened pores favor the accumulation of keratin and sebaceous materials. Senile comedones recur less rapidly than comedones associated with acne vulgaris.

The pathophysiology of all these conditions is incompletely understood. Hot liquids such as coffee and tea, alcohol, and spicy foods aggravate rosacea. It is also exacerbated by menopause and periods of emotional unrest. The follicle mite, *Demodex folliculorum,* is found in the pilosebaceous follicles of patients with rosacea, but its causative role is questionable.

The cause of perioral dermatitis is unknown, but it may be due to hormonal factors or the use of oily cosmetics. The condition can be replicated by chronic use of fluorinated corticosteroid creams or ointments. An association with the use or discontinuance of oral contraceptives has been noted.

PRINCIPLES OF THERAPY

The principles of therapy involve removal of exacerbating conditions and the use of systemic antibiotics. In rosacea, conditions that lead to flushing or vasodilation should be minimized. Exposure to sunlight, extreme heat or cold, and ingestion of hot foods known to exacerbate the condition should be interdicted. Agents containing sorbic acid or benzoic acid may increase flushing, erythema, and edema. Topical therapy can be similar to that for acne vulgaris, utilizing agents that enhance the turnover of skin and the restoration of normal skin. Topical agents such as *benzoyl peroxide* or *retinoic acid* may be used. The most effective therapy is systemic *tetracycline,* which may be required for prolonged periods of time. It is most important to caution against use of fluorinated corticosteroids, which produce an initial response only to result in atrophy of skin and development of permanent telangiectasia.

Perioral dermatitis should be approached by interdicting greasy cosmetics and cold creams. Topical acne preparations that increase turnover of skin have been useful. Fluorinated steroid creams should not be used, but hydrocortisone 1% may provide more rapid resolution of the dermatitis. Topical antibiotic preparations of erythromcyin or clindamycin in an oil-free vehicle are being used instead of systemic antibiotics.

Periorbital comedones may be treated by expression of the blackheads. Redevelopment of blackheads is relatively slow, so that periodic expression at 3- or 4-month intervals is adequate. Retinoic acid applied judiciously is effective in resolving the condition, but compliance may be difficult to obtain in the older population.

THERAPEUTIC RECOMMENDATIONS

Acne Rosacea

- Tetracycline, 250 mg four times a day, continued for a period of time with gradual reduction in dosage down to 250 mg every other day before it is stopped. Prolonged low-dose treatment may be necessary.
- Sunlight, fluorinated steroids, fluoridated toothpaste, and foods known to exacerbate the condition should be interdicted.
- A surgical approach possibly with lasers is necessary to improve rhinophyma.

Perioral Dermatitis

- Treatment should begin with tetracycline, 250 mg three times a day, gradually reduced over a period of weeks once resolution has occurred.
- Greasy creams and cosmetics should be scrupulously avoided.
- Hydrocortisone cream with a topical erythromycin lotion may be tried before systemic antibiotics are used.

Periorbital Dermatitis

- Periodically express the blackheads.
- Retin-A may be useful in patients who are concerned about their appearance and capable of compliance.

PATIENT EDUCATION

The major element of patient education is to explain that these conditions are common and treatable. Many patients are bothered by a single pimple, while others can sustain the disfigurement of acne rosacea without complaint.

ANNOTATED BIBLIOGRAPHY

Bartholomew RS, Reid BS, Cheesbrough MJ: Oxytetracycline in the treatment of ocular rosacea, a double-blind trial. Br J Ophthalmol 66:386, 1982 (*Tetracycline is the treatment of choice for ocular rosacea.*)

Bikowski JB: Topical therapy for perioral dermatitis. Cutis 31:678, 1983 (*Erythromycin topical solution plus hydrocortisone valerate are effective for this condition.*)

Epstein S: Perioral dermatitis. Cutis 10:317, 1972 (*Excellent clinical description with treatment recommendation.*)

Kligman AM, Mill OH Jr: Acne cosmetica. Arch Dermatol 106:843, 1972 (*A common acne variant seen in adult women is attributable to the long-term use of facial cosmetics.*)

MacDonald A, Felwel M: Perioral dermatitis: Aetiology and treatment with tetracycline. Br J Dermatol 87:315, 1972 (*A good description of the problem and its treatment.*)

Milhan R, Ayres S Jr: Perioral dermatitis. Arch Dermatol 89:803, 1964 (*Original description of this condition.*)

Mullanax MG, Kierland RR: Granulomatous rosacea. Arch Dermatol 101:206, 1970 (*Separates this condition from cutaneous tuberculosis.*)

Wilkins JK: Rosacea. Int J Dermatol 22:393, 1981 (*A good review.*)

180
Management of Psoriasis
NICHOLAS J. LOWE, M.D.

Psoriasis is a chronic skin disease characterized by discrete erythematous papules and plaques covered by a silvery white scale. Patients with psoriasis are concerned with cosmetic disfigurement that their disease causes, and there may also be associated itching and sometimes pain resulting from fissuring of the lesions.

The onset is frequently in early adult life, but the disease may be seen first in childhood or old age. Between 1.5% and 2% of the population of the United States is affected. Psoriasis may be inherited as a simple autosomal dominant with incomplete penetrance, or as a polygenic trait. Affected individuals have an increased incidence of HLA-13 and HLA-17 antigens. HLA-Cw6 and HLA-DRw7 have recently also been linked with psoriasis vulgaris. An increased incidence of HLA-27 is found in patients with psoriatic arthritis. The arthritis associated with psoriasis is often polyarticular, but may be monoarticular. A characteristic type is arthritis of the distal interphalangeal joints with juxta-articular destruction of bone. Arthritis is seen in 5% to 10% of patients with psoriasis.

The primary physician should be able to treat mild to moderate cases of psoriasis. An understanding of the pathophysiology of the disease and knowledge of the different treatment modalities available will facilitate collaboration with a dermatologist for those patients with severe disease.

PATHOPHYSIOLOGY AND CLINICAL PRESENTATION

The epidermal turnover time for a cell to travel from the basal cell layer of the epidermis to the granular layer is normally 14 days; in psoriatic skin, it is a brief 2 days. Normal cell maturation cannot take place in this short time, and subsequent keratinization is faulty. Clinically, this is seen as scaling. Histologically, the epidermis is thickened, and immature nucleated cells are seen in the horny layer. An accompanying dilatation of the subepidermal blood vessels and infiltration with mononuclear cells accounts for erythema. Neutrophils are often seen within the stratum corneum, forming characteristic micropustules.

Epidermal proliferation in psoriatic skin has been studied using radioactive tracers and precursors of nucleic acids. There are numerous explanations for the increased cell turnover. There may be a loss of the normal control mechanisms for epidermal cell production, which then leads to hyperproliferation, impaired maturation, and abnormal keratinization. Active research attempting to determine the etiology of pso-

riasis is extensive, but to date, the exact causes of abnormal cellular proliferation remain unknown.

Clinically, psoriasis presents with well-marginated erythematous elevated papules or plaques, which, if not previously treated by the patient, also show thick, silvery scaling. Removal of this scale reveals punctate bleeding points known as Auspitz's sign. Nails often show punctate pitting and a characteristic discoloration of the surface of the nail that resembles an oil spot. Subungual collections of keratotic material are also common. Mucous membranes are rarely involved.

Other clinical types include guttate psoriasis, which presents with small, discrete, erythematous papular lesions. An exfoliative or erythrodermic form of psoriasis shows generalized erythema without any characteristic lesions. Localized pustular psoriasis of the palms and soles may also be seen without characteristic lesions of psoriasis elsewhere. An uncommon but serious variation is that of generalized pustules, often accompanied by systemic symptoms. Patients with this type of psoriasis usually require hospitalization and intensive treatment. At times, generalized pustular psoriasis is life-threatening.

PRINCIPLES OF MANAGEMENT

Topical Therapy

Topical Steroids. Topical corticosteroids are widely used, especially for ambulatory patients, because they are relatively easy to apply. The ability of topical steroids to produce vasoconstriction, with resultant pallor of the skin, has been used to rank them for anti-inflammatory potency. In most psoriatics, the more potent steroids are usually required to produce a good response. They are sometimes effective in clearing psoriasis and may be used in certain situations—for example, for exposed and unsightly areas of psoriasis and flexural psoriasis; however, caution is needed in their use.

Side-effects seen with potent topical steroids include skin atrophy, rebound worsening of psoriasis after discontinuing use, a tendency to convert "stable" psoriasis to "unstable" (erythrodermic or pustular types), significant skin absorption and systemic steroid effect in patients with extensive psoriasis, and the possibility of a rosacealike syndrome after long-term use of potent topical steroids on the face.

Coal Tar Preparations. Goeckerman described the combination of ultraviolet (UV) light and coal tar, in 1925. Numerous modifications of this treatment have been proposed. Crude coal tar application may be no more effective than petrolatum when combined with aggressive erythemogenic UVB (290–320 nm) therapy for psoriasis. However, suberythemogenic UVB and 1% crude coal tar or a coal tar extract in oil have proven more effective than suberythemogenic UVB and petrolatum. Thus, coal tars themselves are probably therapeutic and enhance the effects of suberythemogenic UVB. The long-term safety of erythemogenic UVB without tar compared with suberythemogenic UVB with tar remains to be determined.

Anthralin is trihydroxy-anthracene, an aromatic compound with three benzene rings, used topically for psoriasis since the 19th century. It is available commercially in creams and ointments. Use of concentrations of 0.1% to 1% anthralin for at least 8 hours daily improves psoriasis. The relapse rate is increased by the addition of topical corticosteroids to the regimen. Interestingly, the application of much higher concentrations (1% and above) of anthralin, which are then washed off after 10 to 30 minutes improves psoriasis and makes outpatient psoriasis treatment with anthralin practical. Caution is needed to avoid skin irritation. Anthralin may also stain adjacent skin reddish brown.

Systemic Treatment of Psoriasis

Systemic treatment is indicated only for severe or incapacitating psoriasis. This indication includes generalized pustular psoriasis, generalized exfoliative psoriasis, severe psoriatic arthropathy, severe uncontrolled psoriasis, and socially incapacitating psoriasis.

Systemic Corticosteroids, particularly triamcinolone acetonide and prednisone, are occasionally used in the treatment of psoriasis. These drugs are to be avoided unless the patient has been treated previously with a systemic steroid and has become "steroid dependent."

Systemic steroids used for stable psoriasis vulgaris may have led to some cases of severe generalized psoriasis. Occasionally one has to use systemic steroids in the acute disease when other forms of systemic treatment are contraindicated. Withdrawal of systemic steroid treatment may lead to a worsening of the psoriasis. Some physicians use short courses of systemic steroids given by oral or intramuscular routes for the treatment of acute guttate psoriasis. Rebound worsening of the psoriasis may follow such treatment.

Systemic Antimitotic Drugs. In psoriasis there is an increased mitotic rate and DNA synthesis in the epidermis. Systemic antimitotic agents can be used in the control of this disease, but it must be emphasized that this group of drugs carries a significant number of potential side-effects.

The most widely used of the antimitotic agents in the United States is *methotrexate,* usually given orally, though it may be given by intramuscular or intravenous routes. Some recommend that pretreatment liver biopsies be taken to be sure there is no evidence of hepatic fibrosis (a significant potential side-effect of methotrexate). Adequate blood cell counts (including platelets) and hepatic and renal function must be confirmed before treatment is given. Methotrexate should be reserved for chronic unresponsive psoriasis in patients past the reproductive age. The patient must be willing to have initially weekly, then monthly, blood samples taken to monitor side-effects.

Oral regimens may be either three doses per week, spaced at 12-hour intervals, or one dose weekly by mouth. If there is significant nausea from oral use, then the intramuscular route can be used. Usually a test dose of 5 mg to 7.5 mg is given, and the patient response is observed over the next 5 to 7 days. Increased dosage is then given until good clinical response is seen. A complete blood count should be done at each visit, and biochemical studies checked regularly.

Bone marrow suppression may occur, but other side-effects such as renal, bowel, and lung toxicity are not expected in dosages used for psoriasis therapy.

Photochemotherapy of Psoriasis. Another effective treatment for recalcitrant, severe psoriasis is psoralen photochemotherapy (PUVA). This treatment involves the use of the photosensitizing drug *psoralen (P)* and long-wave-length (320–400 nm) *ultraviolet light (UVA).* It has proven very effective, but there is concern about its side-effects. It is not known to what extent delayed side-effects such as premature skin aging and carcinogenesis will be seen as a result of this treatment. Long-term (10- to 15-year) follow-up data are needed. PUVA treatment appears to be carcinogenic for the skin in susceptible individuals. Patients most at risk for skin cancer following PUVA are those with lighter skin who sunburn readily and those who have received previous x-ray therapy to their skin. They should not receive PUVA therapy. Early and usually mild transient side-effects include pruritus and phototoxic erythema. Occasionally nausea is a problem.

At present, PUVA should be reserved for severe or recalcitrant psoriasis resistant to topical therapy. It may help some patients with generalized pustular or exfoliative psoriasis, but great care is needed to avoid worsening the condition.

Synthetic Retinoids such as the aromatic retinoid *etretinate* (Tegisone) have significantly improved some psoriatics in clinical trials. The oral dosage has to be monitored closely to control side-effects (including cheilitis, itching, fragile skin, thirst, sore mouth, and peeling of the palms and soles). In 60% to 70% of patients, good responses are achieved, and the benefits of treatment outweigh the side-effects. An unresolved problem with the systemic synthetic retinoids is abnormalities of serum lipids in some patients. The significance of this finding remains unknown.

Oral 13-cis-*retinoic acid* (isotretinoin) was approved by the FDA in 1982 for treatment of severe pustulocystic acne.

Some psoriasis patients have been treated with combinations of 13-cis-retinoic acid alone and also with anthralin or UVB phototherapy. The drug is not effective for plaque-stage psoriasis but is useful to control generalized pustular psoriasis.

THERAPEUTIC RECOMMENDATIONS

- The primary physician should be able to treat mild to moderate cases of psoriasis. More chronic or extensive cases require care by a dermatologist.
- Sunlight exposure, taken cautiously, helps many patients, but the patient must avoid sunburning.
- Psoriasis is a chronic and relapsing disease; hence, constant patient reassurance is important.
- No permanent cure is available, but it is possible to achieve complete clearance for a time in many patients.
- Complications such as generalized erythroderma and pustulation are best treated in a hospital.
- The use of cytotoxic or phototoxic (PUVA) therapy for the severe, intractable, or potentially lethal forms of psoriasis requires careful supervision.
- Topical steroid treatment used sparingly and locally is sometimes effective under plastic wrap occulsion, but remission times are often relatively short. Occasionally, sudden withdrawal of topical steroid makes the disease "unstable."
- Systemic use of steroids in the past frequently led to a severe relapse upon withdrawal. This therapy is now rarely indicated.
- Newer systemic agents such as synthetic retinoids are becoming available for the therapy of psoriasis, resistant to either topical therapy or ultraviolet phototherapy.

ANNOTATED BIBLIOGRAPHY

Ellis CN, Goldfarb MT, Roenigle H: Effects of oral meclofenamate therapy in psoriasis. J Am Acad Dermatol 14:49, 1986 (*One hundred and three patients studied revealed no improvement in the group taking meclofenamate, but there was also no worsening, making it a reasonable consideration for the treatment for psoriatic arthritis.*)

Ellis CN, Kary S, Grekin RC: Etretinate therapy for psoriasis. Arch Dermatol 121:877, 1985 (*Reduction of cell-mediated antibody-dependent cytotoxicity of polys as a mechanism of the success of oral retinoid in treating psoriasis.*)

Goeckerman WH: The treatment of psoriasis. NW Med 24:229, 1925 (*Describes the combination of coal tars and ultraviolet radiation for treatment of psoriasis.*)

Kaplan R, Russell DH, Lowe NJ: Etretinate therapy for psoriasis. J Am Acad Dermatol 8:95, 1983 (*Describes the use of synthetic retinoid etretinate in psoriasis.*)

Levine MJ, White HAD, Parrish JA: Components of the Goeckerman regimen. J Int Dermatol 10:455, 1979 (*Evaluation of the different components of this therapy. With erythemogenic ultraviolet treatment, emollient ointments are as effective as coal tars.*)

Lowe NJ: Psoriasis therapy: A current perspective. West J Med 139: 184, 1983 (*A review of current therapeutic alternatives.*)

Lowe NJ, Ashton RE, Koudsi H et al: Anthralin for psoriasis. J Am Acad Dermatol 9:69, 1984 (*Short contact therapy compared with topical steroid and conventional anthralin.*)

Lowe NJ, Wortzman MS, Breeding J et al: Coal tar phototherapy for psoriasis reevaluated. J Am Acad Dermatol 9:781, 1983 (*Coal tars are a superior vehicle when using suberythemogenic ultraviolet therapy. Tars also have mild antipsoriatic properties when used alone.*)

Momtax TK, Parish JA: Combination of psoralen and ultraviolet A and ultraviolet B in the treatment of psoriasis vulgaris: A bilateral comparison study. J Am Acad Dermatol 10:481, 1984 (*Good clearing of psoriasis was obtained by combining PUVA and UVB therapies.*)

Muller SA, Perry HO: The Goeckerman treatment in psoriasis: Six decades of experience at the Mayo Clinic. Cutis 34:265, 1984 (*The standard [2% crude coal tar in petrolatum with 1% polysorbate 80] applied to the skin followed by ultraviolet radiation still gives excellent results.*)

Parrish JH, Fitzpatrick T, Tanenbaum I: Photochemotherapy of psoriasis with oral methoxsalen and long-wave ultraviolet light. N Engl J Med 291:1207, 1974 (*Early description of use of PUVA in psoriasis.*)

Roegnigk H, Averback R, Maibach HI: Methotrexate guidelines revised. J Am Acad Dermatol 2:145, 1982 (*Guidelines for using methotrexate in severe psoriasis.*)

Stern RS, Laird N, Melski J et al: Cutaneous squamous cell carcinoma in patient treated with PUVA. N Engl J Med 310:1156, 1984 (*The relative risk of squamous cell carcinoma among patients exposed to high dose as opposed to low dose PUVA was 13. The authors counsel careful follow up of patients treated with PUVA.*)

Weinstein GD, Van Scott EJ: Autoradiographic studies of normal and psoriatic epidermis. J Invest Dermatol 45:257, 1965 (*This shows the hyperplastic nature of psoriatic epidermis using radio-labeled precursors of nucleic acids.*)

181
Management of Contact Dermatitis
MARVIN J. RAPAPORT, M.D.

Contact dermatitis is an inflammatory reaction of the skin that is subdivided into two types: primary irritant dermatitis and allergic contact dermatitis. The irritant type accounts for 75% of cases. Very strong chemicals that irritate the skin of most people include lye, paint removers, solvents, and acids. Milder irritants such as soaps, mineral oils, polishes, and bleaches affect fewer people and less often. Allergic contact dermatitis is limited to individuals who were previously sensitized to a chemical. Rubber, nickel, formaldehyde, chromates, botanical plants, acrylics, cosmetic preservatives, and topical medicaments such as antibiotics are examples of allergens. Uncommonly, sensitization is caused by a chemical allergen plus the ultraviolet portion of sunlight. The primary physician should be able to treat the active dermatitis, and to attempt to identify and remove the eliciting agent.

PATHOPHYSIOLOGY AND CLINICAL PRESENTATION

The common denominator of contact dermatitis is cutaneous inflammation produced by exogenous agents. Irritating chemicals produce a direct toxic effect on the epidermis. Allergic contact dermatitis results from a delayed type of hypersensitivity reaction. It is a cutaneous expression of an immunologic reaction to an allergen. This allergen, called a hapten, combines with a carrier protein in the skin. The hapten-carrier protein complex is processed by epidermal macrophages (Langerhan cells) and then presented to T lymphocytes where sensitization occurs. The process takes place in regional lymph nodes, after which effector lymphocytes return to the skin and initiate the clinical reaction seen as dermatitis. The initial sensitization takes 1 to 3 weeks, but reexposure produces a reaction within days. It is known that the amnestic cells have a finitie life span, so that the hypersensitivity reaction to a specific allergen may decrease or disappear with time.

The severity of the clinical reaction depends on the potency of the provocative agent, its concentration, and the duration of exposure. Factors that contribute to the development and severity of contact dermatitis include friction, pressure, occlusion, sweating, previous maceration, extremes of temperature, and coexistent dermatologic disease. Areas of the skin that are more readily sensitized include the eyelids, (flexural) neck, and genital areas, whereas the scalp, palms, and soles are relatively resistant.

Mild irritation produces erythema, microvesiculation, and oozing. Stronger reactions cause blistering, bullae, erosions, and ulcers. Repeated exposures will result in a chronic dermatitis consisting of dryness, thickening, and lichenification. At times, contact dermatitis can result in an urticarial response when the chemical touches the skin. Foodstuffs and some oxidizing agents may produce this type of reaction.

WORKUP

One attempts to confirm that the dermatitis is caused by a contactant. Exposure may occur at home or at work, or it may be related to a hobby. Ask about new exposure to medications, insecticides, cosmetics, or clothing as well as gardening and travel experiences. Referring to a list of agents known to produce contact dermatitis may help. Corroboration of the suspected allergenic agents can be achieved by patch testing. Standard antigens are available for such testing, and suspected contactants from the patient's environment should also be used.

Standard *patch test* trays often contain mixtures of chemicals. When a positive patch test is obtained, then the patient is tested to the individual components of the mixture. Some of the ingredients in a standard tray are the following:

- Fragrance mixture—These ingredients help to identify patients who are sensitive to perfumes and fragrances. Cross-reactions of food, dentifrice, and medication flavorings may elicit a positive patch test to this mixture.
- Paraphenylenediamine—PPDA is present in permanent hair dyes. Patients may show cross-reaction with semipermanent hair dyes, PABA sunscreens, "caine" anesthetics, and sulfonamide drugs.
- Mercaptobenzothiazole—MBT is a rubber accelerator found in rubber boots and gloves, as well as in elastics and rubber adhesives.
- Neomycin sulfate—Neomycin may show cross-reactions with gentamicin, streptomycin, and kanamycin.
- Paraben mix—The parabens are used as preservatives in many cosmetics as well as in topical creams, ointments, and lotions, including corticosteroid preparations.

- Epoxy resins—These adhesives are widely used and there are many opportunities at work and in the home to become sensitized to them.
- "Caine" mix—This contains the topical anesthetics commonly found in over-the-counter products that many patients use for itching or irritation.
- Ethylenediamine—This is the stabilizer found in Mycolog cream (but not in the ointment). It may cross-react with many antihistamines related to ethylenediamine and also to aminophylline.
- Potassium dichromate—The dichromates are very common industrial sensitizers.
- Formaldehyde—Patients encounter this chemical in paper, cosmetics, and wash-and-wear clothing. It is also found widely in industry.
- Nickel sulfate—This is the most common contact allergen in the United States, along with the Rhus family of plants (poison ivy, oak, and sumac). Many women become sensitized to nickel when their ears are pierced. Many products in the home and in industry contain nickel, and subsequent dermatitis results from these contacts.

Other allergens not included in the standard tray include the following:

- Balsam of Peru—This is found in many medications and in perfumes. Some sources of exposure include lip preparations, flavorings, insect repellents, cough syrups, suppositories, shampoos, and other hair products.
- Turpentine—This is a paint solvent that is also found in polishes, cleaning agents, medications, and adhesives. Cross-reactions may occur in patients sensitive to ragweed and pyrethrum.

The basic patch test screening tray, which is not difficult to use, may be ordered from the American Academy of Dermatology, Inc. (1567 Maple Avenue Evanston, IL 60201).

PRINCIPLES OF MANAGEMENT

If the causative agent has been identified by patch testing, then specific advice on avoiding this agent (and others that may cause cross-reactions) should be given. In the absence of a specific allergen or an identifiable irritant, patients should decrease exposure to potential irritants within the home, such as abrasive soaps, detergents, solvents, bleaches, and moist vegetables. It may be helpful to use rubber or plastic gloves (preferably those with cotton liners that absorb sweat and prevent maceration) and wash thoroughly after exposure to any irritants or potential allergens. Barrier creams containing silicones may be worthwhile in preventing hand dermatitis. Only hypoallergic cosmetics should be used.

Vesicular or exudative lesions of acute contact dermatitis should be dried using compresses of *Burow's solution* in a 1:20 dilution (one package or tablet in 8 oz of water). The water used should be cool, and ice cubes can be added to make the compresses even more soothing. Clean cotton torn from old bedsheets, pillowcases, T-shirts, or pajamas makes excellent cloth for a compress. Wet dressings should be applied for 20 to 40 minutes two to four times daily. As the cloth dries out, it must be remoistened in the solution. In more generalized exudative eruptions, *colloidal oatmeal baths* will produce a soothing and drying effect. Oral antipruritics can be prescribed if itching is severe.

Inflammation should be treated with *topical corticosteroids,* usually a fluorinated cream preparation for acute, oozing conditions, but an ointment is better for more chronic and lichenified eruptions. When the dermatitis is bullous, or when large areas of skin are involved, a short course of *systemic corticosteroids* is indicated. Oral prednisone, 40 to 60 mg daily for 5 to 7 days is used, with tapering to discontinuation over a 10- to 14-day period. Alternatively, intramuscular triamcinolone in a dosage of 40 mg can be given. Subacute dermatitis is treated with topical agents alone. In chronic contact dermatitis, hydrophobic emollients (*e.g.,* Aquaphor) are used to rehydrate the skin, and the use of topical corticosteroids under occlusion or Cordran tape may lessen lichenification and itching.

THERAPEUTIC RECOMMENDATIONS

- Help the patient identify and avoid irritant or allergenic contactants; interdict all home remedies.
- Advise the patient to use barrier creams or gloves even if the irritant has not been identified.
- Advise the patient to wash thoroughly after exposure to potential irritants or allergens.
- Treat acute exudative lesions with cold compresses of Burow's solution; in more generalized dermatitis, colloidal oatmeal baths can be used.
- Apply fluorinated corticosteroid creams for acute dermatitis. Use a preparation that is paraben-free. A corticosteroid ointment is used to treat chronic contact dermatitis.
- In bullous or extensive acute contact dermatitis, oral predisone, begun at 40 to 60 mg per day and rapidly tapered, may be indicated. Intramuscular triamcinolone acetonide can be given in lieu of oral medication.
- Itching may be reduced with oral antipruritic agents such as hydroxyzine, 40 to 200 mg per day.

The crucial element in managing patients with contact dermatitis is the identification of the contactant. The experienced dermatologist is aware of many environmental contactants and possibilities of exposure. If the contact dermatitis recurs after successful treatment, referral to a dermatologist for additional workup is indicated. Patients can assist their physician by helping to identify irritants or allergens in their work or home environment and by maintaining diaries. Limitation of exposure to contactants by the patient is essential to long-term control of the dermatitis. Patch testing with standard patch test allergens and other suspected environmental agents can often establish the etiologic agent.

ANNOTATED BIBLIOGRAPHY

Adams RM: Patch testing—a recapitulation. J Am Acad Dermatol 5:629, 1981 (*A review of the patch test and its role in identifying the cause of allergic contact dermatitis.*)

Buckley RH, Matthews KP: Common allergic skin diseases. JAMA 248:2611, 1982 (*Extensive review for the generalist of atopic dermatitis and allergic contact dermatitis.*)

Eiermann H, Larsen W, Taylor J: Prospective study of cosmetic reactions: 1977–1980. J Am Acad Dermatol 6:1, 1982 (*Four-hundred and eighty-seven cases of cosmetic-induced dermatitis were analyzed. The most common sensitizers are discussed.*)

Fisher AA: Allergic reactions to topical corticosteroids or their vehicles. Cutis 32:122, 1983 (*A discussion of the likely sensitizers in topical steroid preparations. Sometimes it is the steroid itself!*)

Fisher AA: The chromates: Prime causes of industrial allergic contact dermatitis. Cutis 32:34, 1983 (*Contains a list of occupations exposed to chromates.*)

Guin JD: Contact sensitivity to topical corticosteroids. J Am Acad Dermatol 10:773, 1984 (*Five cases of contact sensitivity to topical corticosteroids are described, and the literature is reviewed.*)

Larsen WG: Perfume dermatitis. J Am Acad Dermatol L2:1, 1985 (*Discusses allergic contact dermatitis to fragrances and includes a complete list of ingredients and how to patch test.*)

Stoner J, Rasmussen J: Plant dermatitis. J Am Acad Dermatol 9:1, 1983 (*An excellent review of seven major categories of dermatitis caused by plants, with a discussion of the chemical constituents responsible for the dermatitis.*)

182

Management of Eczematous Dermatitis

WILLIAM V. R. SHELLOW, M.D.

Acute and chronic dermatitis constitutes a major portion of cutaneous disease. Eczema is defined clinically by the observable changes in the skin, which reflect a common cutaneous reaction to a variety of pathologic processes.

Acute eczematous dermatitis is characterized by erythema, edema, vesiculation, oozing, crusting, or scaling; the chronic stage is characterized by excoriation, thickening, hyperpigmentation, and often lichenification. Eczematous dermatitis is common, demanding that the primary care physician render basic therapy. Treatment is often frustrating, and consultation with a dermatologist is frequently required.

PATHOPHYSIOLOGY AND CLINICAL PRESENTATION

Histopathologically, acute dermatitis is characterized by inter- and intracellular edema, with intraepidermal vesicles. In the dermis there is edema, vascular dilatation, and perivascular inflammatory cell infiltration. Chronicity causes thickening of the epidermis (acanthosis), capillary proliferation, and cellular infiltration with lymphocytes, histiocytes, and fibroblasts. The inflammation may be secondary to a variety of pathogenic mechanisms, the most common being contact with an allergic or irritant agent and atopic dermatitis. Eczematous dermatitis of the hands may be due to fungal infection with "id" reaction, contact, household irritants, or the poorly understood abnormal sweating condition referred to as dyshidrosis. Nummular eczema is a morphologically distinct process with coin-shaped lesions. Chronic eczematous change may lead to lichen simplex chronicus. Dermatologic syndromes such as seborrheic or stasis dermatitis may produce eczematous change.

Atopic dermatitis is characterized by intense itching leading to scratching, eczematous change, and lichenification. Two thirds of atopic patients have family members with asthma, hay fever, or atopic dermatitis. In adults, the lesions characteristically involve the neck, wrists, the area behind the ears, and the antecubital and popliteal flexural areas. Certain fabrics, notably wool, may induce itching. Lesions are exacerbated by extremes of temperature and humidity. Psychological stress may induce flares.

Nummular eczema is a variant recognized by distinctive round lesions located on the external aspects of the extremities, buttocks, and posterior aspect of the trunk. The lesions are pruritic; they ooze, crust, and may become purulent. The course varies; there may be a few constant lesions or a gradual increase in the number of lesions. The prognosis is good, with eventual clearing, although it may take years.

Chronic dermatitis of the hands or feet may be irritant in nature, like "housewives' hands," pustular (chronic pustular eruption), or vesicular (pompholyx or dyshidrosis). These conditions may be acute or chronic. Chronic eczema of the hands presents a diagnostic and therapeutic challenge that may tax the most experienced dermatologist.

Lichen simplex chronicus is a localized neurodermatitis consisting of a circumscribed plaque, thickened skin with increased markings, some scaling, and papulation. The occipital region is a common site. Lesions may also be seen on the wrists, thighs, or lower aspects of the legs. Women are more frequently affected. The prognosis is variable but when scratching is stopped, lesions regress.

PRINCIPLES OF THERAPY

The management of eczema embodies the fundamental principles of dermatologic therapy: precipitants should be eliminated, wet lesions dried, dry lesions hydrated, and inflammation treated with steroids. Frustration should be anticipated, and if basic management fails, referral to an experienced dermatologist should be prompt. Acute dermatitis should be treated with drying measures such as *Burow's compresses.* A search for precipitating factors is mandatory. *Topical corticosteroids* are always required. Systemic corticosteroids are sometimes used on a short-term basis for generalized or incapacitating dermatitis. Secondary bacterial infection may require systemic antibiotics.

Topical Steroids. Understanding the principles of topical corticosteroid therapy is essential. Steroids exert anti-inflammatory, antipruritic, and antiproliferative effects. There is a wide variation in the potency of steroids as measured by vasoconstriction assays (see Table 182-1). The strongest steroid is 500 times more effective in blanching the skin than is the weakest. The vehicle affects potency with ointment formulations more potent than creams. Nongreasy cream bases are cosmetically more acceptable. Greasy ointments are often

Table 182-1.   Selected Topical Steroids
in Various Categories*

Highest Potency
Betamethasone dipropionate (Diprolene)
Clobetasol propionate (Temovate)

High Potency
Amcinonide (Cyclocort)
Betamethasone dipropionate (Diprosone)
Desoximethasone (Topicort)
Fluocinonide (Lidex)
Halcinonide (Halog)
Diflorasone (Maxiflor)

Medium Potency
Betamethasone valerate (Valisone)
Fluocinolone (Synalar, Synemol, Fluonid)
Hydrocortisone valerate (Westcort)
Triamcinolone acetonide (Aristocort, Kenalog)

Low Potency
Hydrocortisone butyrate 1% (Lodoid)
Desonide (Tridesilon)
Hydrocortisone 1% and 2.5% (Hytone, Synacort)
Dexamethasone (Decadron)
Clocortolone (Cloderm)

* The primary care physician should chose one agent from each group based on cost, cosmetic acceptability, and efficacy and become familiar with its use.

reserved for thick, scaling lesions. Gels can be used in hairy areas as well as on glabrous skin, though gels are somewhat drying when used on nonhairy skin. Lotions may be creamy or alcohol-based, but in either case they are more drying than creams. Specialized formulations include aerosol sprays, which are used in the scalp or to cover large areas of skin in acute dermatitis.

Occluding the skin enhances penetration, with up to 100 times more blanching observed in vasoconstriction tests when polyethylene film is used over a given formulation than is seen without occlusion. Steroid-impregnated tape (Cordran) provides its own occlusion but may not justify the additional expense. Ointments are generally not occluded because folliculitis may develop.

The potent halogenated corticosteroids are the most likely to cause atrophy, telangiectasia, purpura, striae, and an acneiform eruption. Suppression of the pituitary–adrenal axis as measured by plasma cortisol levels may be demonstrable, but is rarely clinically significant. Thin-skinned areas are especially susceptible to development of atrophy; less potent formulations should also be used on areas such as the face, dorsum of the hands, and the scrotum. Fluorinated steroids may cause rosacea when used on the face. Only low-potency ophthalmic preparations should be used around the eye. Low-potency products should be used in the groin and axilla because striae may occur. Purpura is seen on the dorsal aspect of the forearms and hands after long-term use of potent topicals.

A basic principle is to use a potent formulation initially to improve the condition and then to reduce the potency if maintenance therapy is indicated. Over-the-counter topical steroids cannot exceed ½% hydrocortisone, compared to 1% or 2½% in prescription products. Lower concentrations of hydrocortisone may be effective for mild dermatitis, but the patient often selects the wrong vehicle—for example, an ointment when a lotion or cream would be better. It is axiomatic that patients for whom the OTC preparation are effective will not visit a physician.

Topicals are normally applied two to four times daily, but the reservoir effect of retention of steroid in the stratum corneum makes one or two applications per day probably as effective as more frequent applications.

In chronic eczema, identification of irritants is necessary. Mild irritants include detergents, gasoline, polishes, and other occupational and household products. Frequent baths or showers, hot water, and drying "soaps" should be interdicted. Systemic steroids are contraindicated in chronic eczema. Potent topical agents sometimes used with occlusive dressing may be helpful in chronic eczema. In prescribing a topical agent, it is helpful to estimate the quantity of topical medication that will be required. A 10-day to 2-week course of therapy applied two to three times daily requires 30 g for the face, 45 g for feet or hands, 60 g for arms or legs, 60 to 90 g for the trunk and 120 to 150 g for the whole body.

THERAPEUTIC RECOMMENDATIONS

- Identify and remove potential contacts, allergens and irritants. Use of rubber gloves with cotton linings may be beneficial.
- Oozing lesions should be dried with Burow's solution compresses applied three to four times a day; colloidal oatmeal baths are indicated for more generalized lesions.
- Patients with dry skin should be managed as described in Chapter 184.
- Fluorinated corticosteroid creams can be used for acute dermatitis. Chronic, lichenified eruptions should be treated with ointments or, if unresponsive, steroid cream under occlusion. In refractory cases, intralesional injection or a diluted triamcinolone solution (2.0 or 2.5 mg/cc) given by an experienced physician may be effective.
- Reduce the potency of the steroid as soon as the acute inflammation has been controlled.
- Pruritus should be suppressed, if possible, with aspirin or an antihistamine.
- Patient education about the need for chronic therapy cannot be overemphasized. Simple measures such as clipping fingernails or wearing cotton gloves can reduce secondary excoriation. Early identification of eczematous exacerbations helps facilitate treatment.

ANNOTATED BIBLIOGRAPHY

Clobetasol—A potent new topical corticosteroid. Med Lett 28:57, 1986 (*Up-to-date data on generic availability and cost of most topical steroids.*)

Dobson RL: Diagnosis and treatment of eczema. JAMA 235:2228, 1976 (*A succinct review of classification and principles of treatment.*)

Epstein E: Hand dermatitis: Practical management and current concepts. J Am Acad Dermatol 10:395, 1984 (*A review article describing the causes and various methods of treatment of this clinical condition.*)

Fusaro RM, Kingsley DN: Topical glucocorticoids. How they are used and misused. Postgrad Med 79:283, 1986 (*An excellent summary of therapeutic considerations and a good bibliography.*)

Glickman FS, Silvers SH: Hand eczema and atopy in housewives. Arch Dermatol 95:487, 1967 (*Eighty-two percent of 50 patients with hand eczema had an atopic history.*)

Hanifin JM: Atopic dermatitis. J Am Acad Dermatol 6:1, 1982 (*A comprehensive review emphasizing pathogenesis, with 134 references.*)

Lynfield YL, Schechter S: Choosing and using a vehicle. J Am Acad Dermatol 10:56, 1984 (*An evaluation of the average amount of cream, ointment, and liquid needed to thinly cover the skin of adults when self-applied.*)

Roth HL, Kierland RD: The natural history of atopic dermatitis. Arch Dermatol 89:209, 1964 (*Case record review of 492 patients seen at the Mayo Clinic 20 years earlier, with follow-up questionnaire.*)

Tan PL, Barnett GL, Flowers FP: Current topical corticosteroid preparations. J Am Acad Dermatol 114:79, 1986 (*A compilation of available preparations including manufactured dosage form, available size, and vehicles.*)

Weidman AI, Sawicty HH: Nummular eczema. Review of the literature: Survey of 516 case records and follow-up of 125 patients. Arch Dermatol 73:58, 1956 (*Review of the literature; 516 cases with 125 follow-ups.*)

Wright S, Burton JL: Oral evening primrose-feed oil improves atopic eczema. Ti. 1120, 1983 (*An intriguing treatment for a difficult problem.*)

183

Management of Seborrheic Dermatitis

WILLIAM V. R. SHELLOW, M.D.

Seborrheic dermatitis is a chronic inflammatory disease that is constitutionally determined but without known cause. Seborrheic dermatitis affects particular areas of the skin, making the condition quite distinctive. It is a benign disorder, but its high prevalence and incurability render it a therapeutic challenge. The primary physician must be capable of treating seborrheic dermatitis and educating the patient about chronicity and the need for continued management.

PATHOPHYSIOLOGY AND CLINICAL PRESENTATION

Seborrheic dermatitis presents scaly patches that are occasionally slightly papular, surrounded by minimal to moderate erythema. The borders of the lesions are not well demarcated. The scales may be greasy and appear yellow. The lesion is usually asymptomatic, but pruritus may occur. The scalp is most commonly involved and is distinguished from common dandruff by its association with erythema. More extensive disease involves the forehead at the margin of the hair, eyebrows, nasal folds, and the retroauricular and presternal area. In more severe cases, intertriginous areas, the external ear canal, and the umbilicus are involved. In these areas, there are erythema and exudation, progressing to chronic dermatitis with scaling.

A number of neurologic conditions, notably Parkinson's

disease, are associated with oily skin and seborrheic dermatitis. Obesity and endocrinopathies may also be present. Cutaneous diseases such as acne vulgaris, rosacea, or psoriasis may be associated with seborrhea.

The pathogenesis of seborrheic dermatitis is unknown. Organisms such as *Pityrosporon ovale,* once thought to be saprophytic, may explain why seborrhea occurs in AIDS. The anatomic localization correlates with areas of sebaceous gland concentration, although a direct relationship with sebaceous activity has not been established. Empiric data on the bacteriology of people with seborrheic dermatitis have failed to reveal a pathogenic microbiologic mechanism. Seborrheic dermatitis appears to be a constitutional diathesis that may be exacerbated by emotional stress and tension. The mechanism for these exacerbating phenomena is not understood.

PRINCIPLES OF THERAPY

The first principle is to explain that seborrhea is not contagious or curable. It can be controlled with chronic treatment. The treatment to suppress the lesions must be effective, convenient, and respectful of cost.

Therapy should remove scaling, reduce oiliness, eliminate redness, and control itching when it is present. Therapy should be guided by the severity, anatomic location, and relative degree of scale, erythema, and oiliness. For most patients, the regular use of an over-the-counter dandruff or antiseborrheic shampoo is usually sufficient. The ingredients in the over-the-counter preparations include sulfur, which is a drying agent; resorcinol, which is anti-inflammatory; salicylic acid or tar, which are keratolytic; and zinc pyrithione or selenium, which decreases the turnover of skin cells. Most preparations contain multiple agents but have one predominant active ingredient. Sebulex, Ionil, and Vanseb contain sulfur and salicylic acid. Zinc pyrithione is found in Head and Shoulders and Zincon. Tar, the prominent ingredient in Sebutone, Pentrax, T-Gel, and Zetar, should be used cautiously, if at all, in blond or light gray-haired people because it may change the color of the hair. The patient should use a list of seborrheic agents as a guide to try to find one suitable to his preference for lather, odor, and efficacy. Many patients find that a shampoo works for a period of time then becomes less effective and that a new product must be chosen.

Patients with particularly oily seborrhea may have to shampoo daily. If over-the-counter shampoos have failed, and frequently patients have tried many before reaching the physician, then a 2.5% selenium sulfide shampoo should be prescribed. Capitrol, a recently developed prescription-alternative drug that contains chloroxine, is effective and may be tried for refractory seborrhea.

The keratolytic component of the over-the-counter preparations removes most scales, but patients with heavy crusting should rub warm mineral oil into the scalp 30 minutes before shampooing. Occasionally, a patient may need to apply a more potent 3% salicylic acid, 3% sulfur, and 4% tar cream, known as Pragmatar, to remove heavy crust. Antiseborrheic scalp preparations that contain salicylic acid and an antibacterial agent may occasionally be useful, but are not necessary to the effective treatment of seborrhea.

The presence of significant erythema requires use of a corticosteroid preparation. In hairy areas, a lotion, spray, or gel may be applied two to four times daily. Creams should be avoided because they cause hair to become matted. Ointments are satisfactory to use at night, but they make the hair greasy, necessitating shampooing again in the morning. On the scalp a fluorinated steroid lotion is acceptable. Mild erythema on glabrous skin should be treated by washing with a mild soap twice a day, followed by application of hydrocortisone cream, 0.5% to 1.0%. Hydrocortisone is relatively inexpensive and has considerably less risk of causing telangiectasia and atrophy; a 1% concentration may be used for erythematous or papular lesions. After initial success, there may be a period of tachyphylaxis, requiring increased concentrations of cream or potent fluorinated steroids. There is considerable danger of telangiectasia with the long-term use of these products, and they should be avoided on the face. Intertriginous seborrheic dermatitis may require Burow's solution compresses for exudative lesions, followed by a fluorinated steroid lotion. Superinfection that requires antimicrobial agents may occur in intertriginous areas.

In selected cases, alleviation of stress with the use of minor tranquilizers may be considered.

THERAPEUTIC RECOMMENDATIONS

- Provide the patient with a list of over-the-counter shampoos to meet personal preferences. For oily hair, advise shampooing daily for the first week, decreasing to two to three times a week for maintenance.
- Remove heavy crusts by softening in mineral oil, or use a keratolytic agent before shampooing.
- When erythema is present, prescribe a corticosteroid preparation, a fluorinated lotion for the scalp, and hydrocortisone for the face.
- Blepharitis may be treated hygienically, gently rubbing the eyelashes with a coarse washcloth. Occasionally, a steroid-containing eye ointment, such as Metimyd or Blephamide solution, may be used, cautiously, because of the hazard of steroid in the eye.
- Treat exudative intertriginous lesions with drying and a fluorinated topical steroid.
- Patient education is essential. The patient should be taught about the chronic noncurable nature of the disease, its relation to stress, and the need not to become discouraged. The patient should be cautioned about the deleterious effects of overusing topical steroids. The goal is to suppress inflammation by regular use of an appropriately effective antiseborrheic agent, while remaining cognizant of the chronic nature of the disease.

ANNOTATED BIBLIOGRAPHY

Ingram JT: The seborrheic diathesis. Arch Dermatol 76:157, 1967 (*Philosophically discusses the various factors that influence seborrheic dermatitis.*)

Mathes BM, Douglass NC: Seborrheic dermatitis in patients with acquired immuno-deficiency syndrome. J Am Acad Dermatol 13:947, 1985 (*A high prevalence of seborrheic dermatitis occurs in AIDS; 83% in comparison to 3% of historic controls. The severity of seborrheic dermatitis is greater than usual, and it is associated with a poor prognosis in AIDS.*)

Parrish JS, Arndt KA: Seborrheic dermatitis of the beard. Br J Dermatol 87:241, 1972 (*Facial hirsutism may be accompanied by seborrheic dermatitis. Shaving is not necessary to control the problem.*)

Pinkus H, Mehregan AH: The primary histologic lesion of seborrheic dermatitis and psoriasis. J Invest Dermatol 46:109, 1966 (*Leukocytes and serum are discharged from engorged capillaries in both diseases.*)

Shuster S: The aetiology of dandruff and the mode of action of therapeutic agents. Br J Dermatol 3:236, 1984 (*An essential review.*)

Skinner RB, Noah PW, Tayler RM: Double-blind treatment of seborrheic dermatitis with 2% ketoconazole cream. J Am Acad Dermatol 12:852, 1985 (*The possibility of a microbial etiology is raised by response to a topical antifungal.*)

184
Management of Dry Skin
WILLIAM V. R. SHELLOW, M.D.

Dry skin, or xerosis, commonly seen during the winter months, occurs more often in the elderly. The most common clinical presentation is mild to moderate itching (see Chapter 172). Severe chronically dry skin can become eczematous and may be referred to as "asteatotic eczema." The primary physician must recognize dry skin and use simple measures and effective patient education to relieve the symptom.

PATHOPHYSIOLOGY AND CLINICAL PRESENTATION

Skin is dry because it lacks water. A pathophysiology of cutaneous desiccation may be excessive water loss through the stratum corneum. The lipids that aid retention of water within the stratum corneum diminish with age. Xerosis in the elderly reflects a decrease in both the number and activity of sebaceous glands and a slower rate of perspiration. Excessive use of soap, detergent, or disinfectants damages the stratum corneum and increases water loss up to 50 times the normal rate. Environmental factors such as low humidity, forced air heat, or cold winter winds contribute to dryness. There is an unexplained familial tendency toward the development of dry skin. There are a variety of hygroscopic water-soluble chemicals, which include lactic acid, urea, and sodium pyrrolidine carboxylic acid. Collectively these substances are referred to as natural moisturizing factor.

Dry skin is characterized by scaling and loss of suppleness and elasticity. The clinical appearance is fine scaling of the lower portions of the legs. In severe xerosis, loss of elasticity leads to cracking and fissuring, producing a superficial appearance of "cracked porcelain," referred to as "erythema craquelé." Itching is a common concomitant and may lead to scratching and excoriation. Occasionally, dry skin is associated with systemic diseases such as hypovitaminosis A, drug reactions, hypothyroidism, or ichthyosis.

PRINCIPLES OF THERAPY

The primary principle of therapy is to restore water. The modalities available include environmental manipulations, modifications in habits, and the judicious use of agents that hold water in the skin. It is important to humidify the external environment, particularly during the winter months. In cold climates, humidification can be economically achieved by leaving pails of water near radiators, but, if necessary, humidifiers may be installed into forced-air heating systems.

Avoid soaps or detergents and frequent bathing, which dry the skin. A bath is more drying than a brief shower, and many toilet bars that are essentially detergents are extremely dehydrating. The principles to follow are to reduce the frequency of bathing to less than once a day; if baths are taken, add a bath oil; avoid detergent soaps, and substitute a well-oilated soap. It is also wise to avoid exposure to mild irritants such as solvents and wool clothing.

The treatment of preexisting dryness requires the addition of water and the application of hydrophobic agents. The physician should instruct patients to soak affected areas several minutes and apply a hydrophobic substance. A variety of agents are available; plain petrolatum is inexpensive and effective, but it is not as pleasant to use as many proprietary preparations. The patient should avoid lanolin-based emollients if he is allergic to wool. Lubriderm and Keri lotions are light, easily applied, but less occlusive than the lanolin substances. Aquaphor and Eucerin are greasier than the above-mentioned lotions and creams. Crisco may be the most economical emollient. To avoid the greasiness felt with petrolatum-based preparations, newer formulations such as Moisturel use esterified alcohols as emollients. The plethora of expensive skin creams do little to retain moisture in the skin. Hygroscopic agents such as urea, alpha hydroxy acids, sorbitol, and glycerol extract atmospheric moisture and are thought to hold it in the skin. The apparent benefit may be due as much to their ability to plasticize the stratum corneum as to any real increase in moisture. In severe cases or in order to achieve immediate results, topical corticosteroids, often with occlusive dressing, produce effective and rapid results. Occasionally, oral antipruritic agents such as the antihistamines may be required for severe itching. The physician should emphasize patient education to prevent recurrence.

THERAPEUTIC RECOMMENDATIONS

- Instruct the patient on environmental modifications to increase ambient humidity. Keep room temperature as low as is compatible with comfort.
- Caution the patient to avoid dehydrating soaps, solvents, or disinfectants. Do not scrub the skin.
- Encourage the use of bath oils and well-oilated soaps. The patient should soak in the tub for 1 to 10 minutes before the bath oil is added. Warn the patient about the potential for bath oil to cause slipping.
- Emollients should be used after showering or bathing. Try a variety of agents beginning with the cheapest to find one that is acceptable. The newer emollients utilizing esterified alcohols or emulsifiers are the most cosmetically acceptable and costly.
- Lotions or creams that contain from 2% to 20% urea or 12% lactate help hold water in the stratum corneum and may increase the plasticity of the skin.

- In the presence of eczematous change or for a patient who insists on rapid resolution, topical corticosteroid ointments with or without occlusion may be used.
- The most important aspect of management is patient education. The physician should reinforce the adjustments that prevent the development of dryness.

ANNOTATED BIBLIOGRAPHY

Blank IH: Action of emollient creams and their additives. JAMA 164:412, 1959 (*Emollients help to retain water—rather than aiding as "lubricants."*)

Middleton JO: The effects of temperature on extensibility of isolated corneum and to relation to skin chapping. Br J Dermatol 81:717, 1969 (*The suppleness of stratum corneum is reduced easily when the temperature is lowered, perhaps a mechanism in chapping.*)

Steigleder R, Raab WP: Skin protection afforded by ointments. J Invest Dermatol 38:129, 1962 (*Various ointments were compared for their barrier ability; white petrolatum proved to be the best.*)

Van Scott ES, Yu RS: Hyperkeratinization, corneocyte adhesion and alpha hydroxy acids. J Am Acad Dermatol 11:867, 1984 (*Humectants such as lactic acid, malic acid, and glycolic acid maintain the thickness of the stratum corneum.*)

Wehr R, Krochmel L, Bagatell F: A controlled two center study of lactate 12% lotion and a petrolatum based creme in patients with xerosis. Cutis 37:205, 1986 (*Lactate 12%, available by prescription, was significantly superior.*)

185

Management of Intertrigo and Intertriginous Dermatoses

WILLIAM V. R. SHELLOW, M.D.

Intertrigo is a dermatitis that affects the body folds. It is more common in obese people and is exacerbated by warm weather. The areas of involvement are the axillary, inguinal, and inframammary folds. The primary physician should be capable of distinguishing intertrigo from other body-fold eruptions such as erythrasma, seborrheic dermatitis, psoriasis, and dermatophyte infections, as well as rendering appropriate treatment.

PATHOPHYSIOLOGY AND CLINICAL PRESENTATION

Intertrigo presents as erythematous exudative inflammation in the body folds. Patients may complain of soreness and itching, and with secondary invasion, overt purulence may occur. The pathogenic mechanism is mechanical. Heat, moisture, and the retention of sweat produce maceration and irritation, an environment that promotes bacterial infection.

Early intertrigo is characterized by slight maceration and erythema. The moisture initially comes from eccrine sweat that cannot evaporate in the intertriginous areas. With time, redness becomes more intense, and the epidermis becomes eroded or even denuded. Subsequent inflammation causes exudation of serous fluid. Increased moisture may lead to bacterial colonization, which accounts for the odor that may be associated with intertrigo. The groin and intergluteal areas may be colonized by gram-negative organisms. Incontinence of urine or feces may add to the maceration.

Intertrigo in the groin must be distinguished from tinea cruris and moniliasis. Tinea cruris is a fungal infection characterized by small, red, scaly patches. The lesions form circinate plaques with scaly or vesicular borders and central clearing. The diagnosis can be confirmed by scraping scales, adding 20% potassium hydroxide solution, and finding hyphae under low microscopic power. Moniliasis produces deep, beefy-red lesions with characteristic satellite vesicopustules outside the border of the primary lesion. Involvement of the scrotum is common, unlike tinea, which usually spares the scrotum.

The groin may be affected by sexually transmitted diseases such as condylomata, herpes, scabies, or pediculosis. These will cause an erythematous and pruritic eruption with characteristics that point to the underlying diagnosis. Severe forms of intertrigo, such as lichen sclerosus et atrophicus and lichen simplex chronicus, must be considered.

Eruptions in the axilla may be caused by intertrigo as well as *Candida,* tinea, erythrasma, or contact dermatitis. *Candida* presents with an erythematous eruption, tinea corporis in the axilla demonstrates an active border with scale, erythrasma has a reddish brown discoloration, and contact dermatitis usually spares the axillary vault. A condition known as benign familial pemphigus (Hailey–Hailey disease) should also be considered. When an axillary lesion is nodular or raised, Fox–Fordyce disease and hidroadenitis suppurativa enter the differential. In the intertriginous area below the breast, intertrigo, with or without candidal infection, predominates.

PRINCIPLES OF THERAPY

The primary principle of therapy is to alter the conditions that cause maceration and irritation when skin is in close apposition. The goal is to promote drying. This can be accomplished by exposing the intertriginous areas to air, possibly adding a fan or electric bulb to promote drying. Addition of a nonmedicated absorbing powder is helpful. Encourage the patient to wear dry, cotton, loose-fitting clothing. Women should wear bras that provide good support. The patient should avoid hot, humid environments and clothing made of wool, nylon, or synthetic fibers. Men with groin involvement should be encouraged to wear boxer shorts rather than briefs, and women cotton panties rather than nylon. The physician should forbid ointments and greasy preparations that retain moisture and exacerbate the condition.

There is no evidence that antibacterial soaps are more effective than ordinary toilet soaps. Medicated powders should be banned, but Zeasorb made from corn cobs is useful. Exudative lesions should be treated by the application of Burow's compresses in 1:20 or 1:40 dilutions.

Secondary bacterial infection should be treated. Pustules or scales should be examined microscopically and cultured for evidence of bacteria, *Candida,* or dermatophytes. Therapy with the appropriate antimicrobial agents should be instituted. In uninfected intertrigo, corticosteroids may be added to reduce inflammation. Lotions with an alcohol base are quite drying and may sting. Fluorinated steroids should not be used for prolonged periods because intertriginous striae and

atrophy are common complications. Popular preparations such as Vioform-Hydrocortisone are effective, but they stain clothing yellow. Mycolog has antibacterial, antimonilial, and anti-inflammatory activity, but the preservative ethylenediamine is a sensitizing agent. Hydrocortisone cream is an effective, safe, and cost-saving approach. Lotrisone, which combines medium-potency beclomethasone with clotrimazole, is useful as initial therapy in quite erythematous and pruritic eruptions. Topical medication should be used sparingly to avoid retention of moisture. Concurrent medical conditions such as diabetes or obesity should be treated.

THERAPEUTIC RECOMMENDATIONS

- It is essential in therapy of intertrigo to eliminate precipitating conditions. Carefully dry the area that separates folds with absorbent material, dust with drying powders, and wear loose, absorbent clothing. In exudative lesions, a drying agent such as Burow's solution should be used to compress.
- Treat secondary bacterial or fungal infection with appropriate antibiotics.
- Identify potential contactants in axillary eruptions and interdict their use.
- Treat inflammatory areas with topical hydrocortisone and if necessary, with fluorinated steroids for short periods of time.
- The patient must understand the mechanical effects of skin occluding skin and be encouraged to use support bras, cotton clothing, or sandals to ensure adequate aeration. The patient should inspect intertriginous zones to detect the development of erythema and maceration so that effective therapy can be instituted early. In elderly immobile patients, the physician should educate the family or a friend to inspect intertriginous areas to prevent maceration and secondary infection.

ANNOTATED BIBLIOGRAPHY

Brophy MC, Dunagin WG: Intertriginous dermatoses. Postgrad Med 78:105, 1985 (*An excellent review of differential considerations.*)

Epstein NN, Epstein WL, Epstein JH: Atrophic striae in patients with intertrigo. Arch Dermatol 87:450, 1963 (*Covers hazards of treating intertrigo with potent topical corticosteroids.*)

Sarkany I, Taplen D, Blank H: The etiology and treatment of erythrasma. J Invest Dermatol 37:283, 1961 (*Excellent bacteriologic study of the disease.*)

Sarkany I, Taplin D, Blank H: Incidence and bacteriology of erythrasma. Arch Dermatol 85:578, 1962 (*Concise discussion of the disease and its etiology.*)

Smith MA, Waterworth PM: The bacteriology of some cases of intertrigo. Br J Dermatol 74:323, 1962 (*Brief discussion of the bacterial flora found in intertriginous areas.*)

186

Management of Corns and Calluses

WILLIAM V. R. SHELLOW, M.D.

Corns and calluses are common and vexing lesions. They may not be a presenting complaint, but the primary care physicians will frequently be asked about them. Calluses can be confused with plantar warts but may be distinguished by the maintenance of normal skin markings, in contrast to verrucae in which these markings are interrupted. The primary physician can provide diagnosis, simple therapy, advice on prevention, and referral to a dermatologist or podiatrist when indicated.

PATHOPHYSIOLOGY AND CLINICAL PRESENTATION

Corns (helomas or clavi) and calluses (tylomas or tyloses) have a common pathology. Friction and pressure on the skin overlying bony prominences lead to hyperemia, hypertrophy of dermal papillae, and proliferation of keratin. Corns often have a central hard core that is painful when the lesion is pressed. The pressure of shoes on the corn may cause pain with walking. Corns may develop at any joint, but the most common site is over the dorsum of the proximal interphalangeal joint. Hard corns show a translucent avascular core with interruption of normal skin markings. Soft corns appear macerated, resemble dermatophytosis, and are painful. The first and fourth web spaces are favored sites. Persons who do not wear shoes may develop calluses but usually do not develop corns. Calluses do not contain a central core, preserve normal skin markings, and occur preferentially across the metatarsal head area.

PRINCIPLES OF THERAPY

The primary physician's major contribution to therapy is to encourage prevention. The elimination of friction and pressure is the *sine qua non* of prevention. Shoes must fit correctly, and pressure over the toes must be evenly distributed. Softer shoe materials and sandals are often helpful. Stockings must fit properly and should cushion the foot. Keeping the feet dry with powder and by changing shoes daily also reduces friction.

Symptomatic relief of calluses can be achieved by paring hyperkeratotic lesions with a No. 10 or No. 15 scalpel. Keratin should be shaved off with the blade held parallel to the skin. Repeated strokes of the blade should be made in a direction least likely to cause penetration, should the patient move suddenly. Movement from proximal to distal is best. Once a callus is removed, it is essential that previous weightbearing not be continued, or the callus will return.

Patients can treat corns and calluses themselves with intermittent debridement, using keratolytic agents. Salicylic and lactic acid combinations and 40% salicylic acid plasters are used to reduce the thickness of tissue. The patient should cut a piece of 40% salicylic acid plaster smaller than the lesion and apply it to the skin. It may be left overnight or for as long as several days. The dressing should be removed and the foot soaked. The softened and macerated skin is removed with a Buf-Ped or pumice stone. The plaster may be carefully reapplied as often as is necessary, to keep the lesions flat and asymptomatic.

A technique recently advocated is the injection of silicone under corns to cushion the skin from underlying bone. This technique has been reported as successful, but removal from the market of medical-grade silicone fluid makes this technique impractical. The principles of treating soft corns involve reducing excess perspiration. Use of absorbent lamb's wool, soaking the foot in potassium permanganate, 1:4,000 solution, or silver nitrate cauterization have all been successful.

Referral to a podiatrist or orthopedic surgeon is indicated when simple measures and advice fail to reduce symptoms or recurrences. Intrinsic bony problems subject the foot to uneven pressure. Pronation, flat feet, and medial and lateral imbalances should be treated. Padding of lesions with felt moleskin or lamb's wool may prevent uneven external pressure. Foam rubber surrounding the lesion will distribute pressure around the lesion rather than directly on it. Latex, plastic, or silicone molds may be individually adapted to prevent localized pressure from producing corns or calluses. Shoes may be constructed by a podiatrist to redistribute weight and pressure. Occasionally, surgical removal of a subjacent bony prominence eliminates the source of abnormal pressure on the skin.

THERAPEUTIC RECOMMENDATIONS

- Shoes must fit. The physician should advise the patient to avoid tight, pointed-toed shoes, and shoes should be changed frequently. Socks should cushion the sensitive area.
- Corns and calluses may be treated by the patient with proprietary plasters. The physician or patient can apply 40% salicylic acid plaster to the lesion for several days. The lesion may then be pared down by the patient or physician. The physician should instruct the patient never to pull loose skin. Moleskin may be used to protect the tender area after paring. Once the lesions have been removed, the physician

should ensure that the foot is not subjected to the same pressures that originally produced the corns or calluses. The physician should care for diabetics and others with impaired vascular systems.

• In many cases, patient education and simple office techniques are successful. Refractory or unusual lesions should be referred to a podiatrist or orthopedist for definitive treatment of structural problems. Careful explanation of the objectives is essential to ensuring patient compliance.

ANNOTATED BIBLIOGRAPHY

Balkin SW: Treatment of corns by injectable silicone. Arch Dermatol 111:1143, 1975 (*The use of silicone as a cushion to prevent hyperkeratoses.*)

Gibbs RC: Calluses, corns, warts. Am Fam Physician 3:92, 1971 (*Succinct and practical treatment of the subject for the primary practitioner.*)

Mann RA, Duvales HL: Intractable plantar keratosis. Orthop Clin North Am 4:67, 1973 (*Describes surgical techniques for this condition.*)

Montgomery RM: Differential diagnoses of plantar hyperkeratoses. Cutis 1:74, 1965 (*A practical discussion of keratotic lesions of the foot.*)

Montgomery RM: Relieving painful feet. Geriatrics 29:137, 1974 (*Practical tips useful in the office.*)

Schwartz N: Callus formation. J Am Podiatry Assoc 65:666, 1975 (*A brief discussion of some of the causes of plantar keratoma.*)

187

Management of Stasis Dermatitis, Stasis Ulcers, and Decubitus Ulcers

Skin ulceration can be an extremely troublesome and potentially dangerous skin problem. It is most prevalent among the elderly because of vascular insufficiency and immobility. The primary physician who recognizes the early skin changes can prevent many of the debilitating consequences.

PATHOPHYSIOLOGY AND CLINICAL PRESENTATION

The major mechanisms of skin ulceration are venous and arterial insufficiency and prolonged pressure.

Venous Insufficiency. The initial manifestation of venous insufficiency is edema, usually absent upon arising and severe at the end of the day. The pathophysiology is faulty venous valves caused by age, thrombophlebitis, or the hereditary tendency to develop venous varicosities. All three mechanisms cause abnormally high venous pressure during ambulation. Protein-rich fluid from the vein accumulating in the intravascular space produces congestion and edema. The exchange of oxygen and metabolites is impaired, with the development of pigmentation, induration, dermatitis, and finally ulceration. The rupture of delicate venules releases hemoglobin, which changes to hemosiderin, and produces pigmentation.

Scaling and oozing develop when the skin is scratched. Vesicles may indicate a contact dermatitis resulting from a topical medication. Secondary bacterial invasion occurs and may lead to cellulitis.

Stasis ulcerations then develop within the areas of dermatitis or indurated cellulitis. They occur most frequently above the medial malleolus because of its poor vascular supply and sparse subcutaneous tissue. Minor trauma may precipitate ulceration. The size of stasis ulcers varies from small erosions to a size that encircles the ankle. They may or may not be painful; if they are painful, elevation of the leg helps to relieve the discomfort. The base of the ulcer is usually moist with exuberant granulation tissue. Purulence occurs secondary to infection.

Arterial Insufficiency. The leg is cool and appears pale or cyanotic, and peripheral pulses are lost or reduced (see Chapter 17). Ulcers resulting from ischemia are initially small and superficial but, with worsening ischemia, become larger and deeper. Ischemic ulcers affect the sides of the feet, the heels, the toes, and the nailbeds. Arteriography can delineate whether or not the vessels can be repaired surgically (see Chapter 29).

Hypertensive ulcers are characteristically seen over the lateral malleoli. They begin as painful, blue-red plaques, which soon become ulcers. A purpuric halo may surround the ulceration. Vasculitis, as palpable purpuric lesions or hemorrhagic vesicles, may eventuate in ulcerations. The underlying cause may be systemic disease such as SLE or rheumatoid arthritis or drug sensitivity.

Hematologic causes of leg ulcers include sickle cell disease, hereditary spherocytosis, thalassemia, polycythemia vera, leukemia, and dysproteinemias.

Infrequent causes of leg ulcers are deep fungal infections such as histoplasmosis, cryptococcosis, blastomycosis, and coccidioidomycosis. Mycobacterial or spirochetal infections are rare causes of leg ulcers. Kaposi's sarcoma has become more important with the recent AIDS epidemic. Biopsy is indicated when ulcers are suspected to be squamous cell carcinoma, malignant melanoma, basal cell carcinoma, histio-cytic lymphoma, or Kaposi's sarcoma.

Decubitus Ulcer. The pressure sore or decubitus ulcer is common in bed-ridden or semiambulatory patients. Factors contributing to the development of pressure sores include shearing forces, friction, and moisture. Decubiti usually occur over bony prominences. The pressure gradient occludes lymphatic vessels and overloads the microvascular system, leading to the accumulation of waste products and ultimately to necrosis. The lower part of the body and sacrococcygeal area are the predominate sites, with the hip, malleolus, and heel being the other important areas. Pressure sores can lead to cellulitis, bacteremia, osteomyelitis, and even meningitis.

PRINCIPLES OF THERAPY

The principles of ulcer care are essentially the same, independent of etiology or location. The four principles of management are to *remove pressure, debride necrotic tissue, keep* the ulcer *clean,* and *prevent further injury.* External compressive bandages or stockings may be used to reduce venous pressure in the lower extremities. Graduated *compressive surgical stockings* are expensive but can be helpful (see Chapter 30). The patient should apply the compression in the morning before getting out of bed. Prolonged standing should be interdicted, weight loss emphasized, and periods of leg elevation encouraged.

Leg Ulcers. The skin of the leg and ankle should be washed with a mild soap and emollients used to prevent xerosis. *Stasis dermatitis* is treated with *topical corticosteroid* creams or ointments. Oozing dermatitis requires wet-to-dry compresses and bed rest. Scratching, use of over-the-counter medications, and adhesive tape on the dermatitic areas should be discouraged. *Secondarily infected* dermatitis should be treated with systemic *oral antibiotics* such as dicloxacillin, amoxicillin/clavulanate (Augmentin), or erythromycin. Topical antibiotic preparations may be used, but neomycin should be avoided because of its tendency to induce contact sensitization and dermatitis.

If the ulcer has a clean base, the application of an *Unna paste boot* will often encourage healing and reepithelization. An Unna boot is a flesh-colored roll bandage impregnated with zinc oxide, calamine, glycerin, and gelatin. Topical enzymes and hydrophilic beads are sometimes useful adjunctive agents. Hydrocolloid occlusive dressings have been used to treat leg ulcers. Although the healing time may not decrease, they are convenient and relieve pain. Available dressings include polyurethane films (Opsite, Tegaderm), polyethylene oxide hydrogel with polyethylene film backing (Vigilon), and a combination hydrocolloid of gelatin-pectin (DuoDerm). The patient must be warned to expect an unpleasant odor caused by a buildup of fluid when the dressing is removed 2 to 3 weeks after the exudative phase has ended.

Decubitus Ulcers. Nutritional repletion to reverse catabolism and to correct all factors that affect the oxygenation of tissue such as anemia, edema, and vascular problems is important. Reducing pressure on the affected area is critical. The basic principle of *debridement* is to use *wet-to-dry dressings.* A variety of biochemical agents that dissolve debris are purported to promote healing, though double-blind evidence for their efficacy is generally lacking. Occasionally grafts are required to close the ulceration.

The microbiology of decubiti is polymicrobial, and the organisms that cause the most problems, including life-threatening bacteremias, are group A *Streptococci, Staphylococcus aureus, E. coli,* and *B. fragilis.* If fever occurs, hospitalization and intravenous therapy should be instituted with an aminoglycoside plus clindamycin or a third-generation cephalosporin such as ceftazidime. Decubiti are associated with extremely high mortality when associated with anemia and hypoalbuminemia. A shallow ulcer may hide a deep infective sinus or a tunnel to an osteomyelitis.

Future therapy includes use of laser sterilization and vascular grafts. The best treatment remains primary prevention.

PATIENT EDUCATION

In most ulcers, prevention is the key. Patients and family must be educated to look for the preulcerative changes in stasis dermatitis and to use compensatory measures at that time before ulceration occurs. In patients with chronic vascular disease, strict advise about nail cutting, treating sores early, and seeking medical care at the first sign of a break in skin is important. For people confined to beds or chairs, it is important to educate the family to prevent prolonged pressure on a bony prominence. The primary care physician can reduce ulceration by identifying patients at risk with stasis dermatitis, vascular insufficiency, vasculitic disease, or immobility that leads to decubiti.

THERAPEUTIC RECOMMENDATIONS

- In all patients with stasis changes, edema should be controlled by avoidance of dependency, rest and elevation, and external compression with stockings or bandages.
- Nutritional deficiency, hypertension, diabetes, congestive heart failure, and edema should be treated.
- Pruritus should be treated with low- or midrange-potency topical corticosteroids. Ointments are indicated if the area is dry and scaly, and creams should be used if the area is moist.
- Acute exudative dermatitis should be treated with cool Burow's compresses (1:40 dilution) two to three times daily for 30 to 60 minutes.
- Neomycin-containing topical antibiotics should be avoided.
- Scratching and use of over-the-counter medicants should be discouraged.

Adjunctive measures for stasis ulceration:
- Wet-to-dry compresses should be used, followed by cleaning and gentle debridement with gauze sponges several times daily. Dilute hydrogen peroxide can be used to clean the ulcerated area.
- Topical steroids can be applied to the dermatitic areas surrounding the ulcer.
- Secondary infection is treated with systemic oral broad-spectrum antibiotics such as dicloxacillin or erythromycin.
- Aerobic and anaerobic bacterial culture should be performed.
- Persistent ulcers of long duration require x-rays of the area to rule out underlying osteomyelitis.
- Failure of ulcers to heal after good management with a compliant patient indicates the need for surgical consultation. Surgical debridement and split-thickness or full-thickness skin grafting may be necessary.
- Occlusive dressings are worth a trial because they may ease pain, debride ulcers, and lead to healing without need for surgical intervention.

L.A.M.

ANNOTATED BIBLIOGRAPHY

Alper JC, Welch EA, Maguire P: Use of the vapor permeable membrane for cutaneous ulcers: Detail of application and side effects. J Am Acad Dermatol 11:858, 1984 (*The authors report good success utilizing their technique employing vapor permeable membrane dressings and 10% benzoyl peroxide lotion.*)

Andersen KE, Jensen O, Kuorning SA et al: Prevention of pressure sores by identifying patients at risk. Br Med J 284:1370, 1982 (*Coma, dehydration, and paralysis are major risk factors, while age greater than 70, restricted mobility, incontinence, emaciation, and redness over bony prominences are additional risk factors.*)

Falanga V, Eaglscein WH: A therapeutic approach to venous ulcers. J Am Acad Dermatol 14:777, 1986 (*The systematic approach to the treatment of venous ulcers, emphasizing the usefulness of newer and more effective occlusive dressings.*)

Friedman SJ, Su D: Management of leg ulcers with hydrocolloid occlusive dressing. Arch Dermatol 120:1329, 1984 (*Twenty-two patients with 31 leg ulcers of various causes were treated with different regimens, including oxygen impermeable hydrocolloid dressings. Convenience of management and relief of pain were major advantages.*)

Hendricks WM, Swallow RT: Management of stasis leg ulcers with Unna's boots versus elastic support stockings. J Am Acad Dermatol 12:90, 1985 (*The healing time of patients with leg ulcers due to stasis was greatly decreased by the use of Unna boots.*)

Kidawa AS, Lemont H: Vascular diseases of the lower extremities. Clin Dermatol 1:67, 1983 (*An in-depth discussion of many vascular diseases of the legs including venous insufficiency.*)

Reuler JB, Cooney TG: The pressure sore: Pathophysiological principles of management. Ann Intern Med 94:661, 1981 (*A complete review.*)

188
Management of Cellulitis
ELLIE J. C. GOLDSTEIN, M.D.

Cellulitis represents infection of the skin involving the deeper subcutaneous layers. In an outpatient practice, older patients commonly present with redness and swelling of the lower extremities, and cellulitis from changes due to vascular insufficiency needs to be differentiated from that due to phlebitis. Once cellulitis is identified, the primary physician has to decide who can be managed at home on oral antibiotics and who requires hospitalization.

PATHOPHYSIOLOGY AND CLINICAL PRESENTATION

Any process that causes a break in the integrity of the skin will allow normal skin flora to gain access to the underlying subcutaneous tissue and initiate an inflammatory response; trauma, stasis ulceration, ischemia, and most causes of chronic edema are common precipitants. Contiguous or hematogenous spread from other sites is uncommon but does occur.

Any condition that impairs host response may predispose to cellulitis caused by opportunistic organisms such as gram-negative bacteria. The organisms producing cellulitis are often the normal inhabitants of the skin: the streptococci and, less frequently, *Staphylococcus aureus*. Cellulitis in the perineum may be caused by enteric aerobic and anaerobic bacteria. Injury to mucosal surfaces predisposes to infection with unusual organisms. Once the connective tissue is involved, the infection spread occurs along fascial planes. Staphylococci produce disease through their ability to multiply and through the production of extracellular enzymes, including alpha- and beta-hemolysin, leukocidin, coagulase, hyaluronidase, and lipases. Streptococci also produce more than 20 extracellular enzymes. Recent studies have emphasized the role of anaerobes in diabetic foot ulcers, abscesses, and traumatic wounds.

Cellulitis, in certain settings, may be caused by unusual organisms. In individuals who handle fish, poultry, or meat, cellulitic infection with *Erysipelothrix rhusiopathiae* may occur. In cases of water-related injury and sometimes in immunosuppressed patients, *Aeromonas hydrophila* may produce cellulitis. Animal bites or scratches, especially from cats, may produce a cellulitis caused by a *Pasteurella multocida* organism. *Vibrio* species have been implicated in salt-water-related injuries. Gram-negative organisms including *E. coli, Pseudomonas,* and *Klebisella* may occur in immunosuppressed patients, diabetics, or alcoholics.

Recurrent cellulitis has been described in the saphenous venectomy limbs of patients who have undergone coronary artery bypass. The pathophysiologic mechanisms in understanding these cases may include tinea infection, which allows entry of bacteria, or may occur as a result of hypersensitivity to streptococcal exotoxins.

Anaerobic infection should be suspected in crush injuries and when disproportionate pain occurs without discharge. The mechanism is mixed aerobic and anaerobic strep, producing a fasciitis and cellulitis. Bites are ports of entry for conventional strep or staph cellulitis, but one must also consider the unusual spreading cellulitic infections of a recluse spider or a fire ant. Unusual cause of cellulitis simulating a septic thrombophlebitis may occur from *Campylobacter* infection, often with concurrent diarrheal illness.

Cellulitis presents with local redness, heat, swelling, and tenderness coming on over a few days. Fever, chills, or rigors are manifestations of potential bacteremia. The clinical presentation does not allow delineation of the specific microbial etiology. Red streaks extending proximally in conjunction with tender lymph nodes indicate an associated lymphangitis. Crepitus indicates gas production and suggests anaerobic involvement.

WORKUP

Cellulitis first needs to be distinguished from other causes of focal erythema, swelling, and tenderness. Superficial thrombophlebitis may present very similarly, but the inflammatory response is usually centered in the involved vein, which is tender and palpable. The dependent rubor of arterial insufficiency is generalized, nontender, and associated with diminished or absent pulses and a cold extremity. Erythema nodosum differs clinically from cellulitis in that the lesions are typically multiple, exquisitely tender, and often pretibial in location. It should be remembered that cellulitis may occur concurrently with phlebitis or arterial insufficiency.

History. Once it is established that cellulitis is present, predisposing factors should be identified. Inquiry into history of diabetes, congestive failure, recent trauma, leg edema, claudication, previous infection, and loss of sensation is helpful. Ask about intravenous drug use, occupational exposure, or recent bites. A history of fever with rigors suggests bacteremia.

Physical Examination should include a careful check for elevated temperature, lymphangitic streaking, proximal lymphadenopathy, heart murmur, peripheral edema, diminished peripheral pulses, skin atrophy or ulceration, and loss of sensation. Marking the borders of the lesion with an in-

delible pen allows assessment of progression. The presence of a discharge, crepitus, or foul odor is important; the latter are suggestive of anaerobic infection. Palpate for fluctuance and inspect the vitality of surrounding tissue. Identify factors that may have predisposed to cellulitis, such as tinea, dermatitis, venous insufficiency, or previous injury.

Laboratory Studies begin with a complete blood count and differential. When rigors, fever, heart murmur, or lymphangitic spread is present, two blood cultures should be obtained. Most cellulitis is due to streptococci or staphylococci and, therefore, culture of the cellulitis area is not routinely performed. Moreover, it is difficult to culture the offending organism from unbroken skin, and there is no evidence that aspiration from the advancing margin is superior to aspiration from any other part of the skin. Culture is indicated in patients who have open, weeping wounds or infection in unusual areas such as the perineum; in such cases, anaerobic and aerobic cultures should be planted. Blood cultures are positive in 5% to 10% of cellulitis cases, and should be obtained in toxic or immunocompromised patients. If crepitus, fluctuance, or devitalization is present, obtain an x-ray film to look for gas. In diabetic or immunocompromised patients, or in situations of previous injury, an x-ray is important to be sure osteomyelitis does not underly the cellulitis.

PRINCIPLES OF MANAGEMENT

The need for hospital admission must be considered. Hospitalization is required in patients who are compromised hosts or in whom cellulitis is rapidly progressive or recurrent. Cellulitis of the orbit, face, or perineum, or elsewhere, when accompanied by fever and lymphangitis, is most safely treated in an inpatient setting. When the patient appears unreliable and unable to care for himself at home, admission is indicated.

The majority of patients, however, may be treated as outpatients with oral antibiotics and supportive measures. Patients who are afebrile and in whom adenopathy and lymphangitis are absent may not even require antibiotics, but cellulitis is usually treated with antibiotics. The drugs of choice are either penicillin or a penicillinase-resistant semisynthetic penicillin preparation. There is little definitive evidence on which to base antibiotic selection. The high prevalence of streptococci, the sensitivity of some community-acquired staphylococci to penicillin, and the low cost of penicillin suggest that a reasonable approach is to start patients on penicillin and monitor them carefully. If after 48 hours the patient is still febrile or not improving, a penicillinase-resistant preparation can be substituted. Antibiotic therapy should continue for 7 to 14 days, depending on rate of clinical resolution. Infections of the perineum, face, or hands and those in a compromised host should be treated in consultation with an infectious disease specialist.

In patients with open wounds, the risk of tetanus should be considered. If a booster has not been obtained within 5 years, it should be given. Patients who have not had an initial tetanus series should receive both tetanus toxoid and tetanus immune globulin (see Chapter 4).

Supportive measures, in addition to antibiotics, can be important. These include elevation of the affected part and scrupulous prevention of new trauma. The addition of heat may help in resolution of cellulitis by promoting blood flow to the area. In patients with underlying conditions such as congestive failure, stasis dermatitis, or vascular insufficiency, control of edema and maintenance of skin moisturization may be necessary for prevention of recurrent episodes.

THERAPEUTIC RECOMMENDATIONS AND INDICATIONS FOR ADMISSION

- Hospitalize the patient unable to care for himself at home reliably, as well as anyone with high fever, rigors, lymphangitis, rapid progression, compromised host defenses, or involvement of the face, orbit, or perineum. Consultation with an infectious disease specialist is advisable.
- If the uncomplicated, mildly ill patient can be followed closely on an ambulatory basis, begin oral therapy with phenoxymethyl penicillin, 500 mg every 6 hours, and monitor over the next 48 hours. If close contact with the patient is not possible or if inflammation and fever do not resolve within 48 hours, a penicillinase-resistant penicillin, such as dicloxacillin, 500 mg every 6 hours, should be substituted. In patients allergic to penicillin, erythromycin, 500 mg every 6 hours, is the drug of choice.
- All patients should receive supportive care, including the application of heat, elevation of the affected part, and strict avoidance of trauma.
- Patients without a recent tetanus booster and with an open wound should be given 0.5 cc of tetanus toxoid intramuscularly.

PATIENT EDUCATION

The patient should be instructed to remain in bed most of the time, but may have bathroom privileges. If there is leg edema, he should be encouraged to keep the swollen foot elevated and do foot exercises to reduce the possibility of thrombophlebitis. It is crucial to protect the affected area and to insist that the patient not scratch. The importance of taking antibiotic therapy as instructed should be reinforced, as well as the need to take penicillin on an empty stomach. The patient should be asked to record progression and temperature on a daily basis and to call if there is persistent elevation or a failure of resolution of the cellulitic area. The patient needs to know that cellulitis usually resolves within 5 to 7 days and that he should return promptly for follow-up if improvement is not evident.

ANNOTATED BIBLIOGRAPHY

Baddour LM, Bisro AL: Recurrent cellulitis after coronary bypass surgery. JAMA 251:1049, 1984 (*Nine patients with recurrent cellulitis were studied, seven of whom had tinea pedis.*)

Ginsberg MB: Cellulitis: Analysis of 101 cases and review of the literature. South Med J 74:530, 1981 (*A good review.*)

Louie TM, Bartlett JG, Tally FP et al: Aerobic and anaerobic bacteria in diabetic foot ulcers. Ann Intern Med 85:461, 1976 (*Twenty diabetic patients were studied showing both aerobic and anaerobic bacteria, which should be considered in the selection of antimicrobial therapy.*)

Meislin HW, Lerner SA, Graves MH et al: Cutaneous abscesses: Anaerobic and aerobic bacteriology and outpatient management. Ann Intern Med 87:145, 1977 (*One-hundred and thirty-five patients were studied, and the microbiologic finding are discussed. Primary therapy was felt to be incision and drainage. Antibiotics were considered adjunctive.*)

Wannamaker LW: Differences between streptococcal infections of the throat and of the skin. N Engl J Med 282:23, 1970 (*A discussion of nephrogenic serotypes and site of antecedent infection.*)

189

Management of Pyodermas

WILLIAM V. R. SHELLOW, M.D.

Primary cutaneous bacterial infections are usually initiated by a single organism such as coagulase-positive staphylococci or beta-hemolytic streptococci. Primary infection develops on normal skin whereas secondary infection is defined as a bacterial component superimposed on diseased skin. Cutaneous bacterial infections may be classified according to the depth of the infection and the propensity for scarring. Infection demands prompt recognition by the primary physician and effective antibiotic treatment.

PATHOPHYSIOLOGY AND CLINICAL PRESENTATION

The pathogenic mechanism of pyodermas is infection. The clinical expression of the infection reflects the organism, environmental factors, skin appendages, and host resistance. The common pyodermas include impetigo, ecthyma, folliculitis, furunculosis, and erysipelas.

Impetigo is a common lesion caused by staphylococci or beta-hemolytic streptococci. Some observers believe that intense erythema at the base of a pustule suggests streptococcal causation. Impetigo is seen most frequently in children, but it also occurs in adults. Poor hygiene may predispose persons to the development of infection. Impetigo is less highly contagious in adults than among infants.

Impetigo begins as a small erythematous macular lesion that evolves into a vesicle. Vesicles are located beneath the stratum corneum, and the thin-roofed collection of fluid ruptures easily, leaving denuded, oozing areas. The fluid dries and builds up to form a honey-colored crust. New lesions appear in the same location, and they coalesce. When the honey-colored crusts are removed, the skin appears raw. Individual lesions usually do not exceed 2 cm in size. The face is the most common site of involvement. Ordinary lesions do not produce scarring but may leave erythematous marks for a time. Untreated infections may last for weeks.

Ecthyma, usually caused by streptococci, is a deeper version of impetigo. Ecthyma may be a sign of gram-negative or fungal sepsis. Erosion of the epidermis creates ulcerative, crusted lesions. The heaped-up crust conceals the underlying erosion. Healing is accompanied by some scarring because of the depth of the lesions. The legs are commonly involved, and children are more susceptible than adults. Antecedent conditions include eczema, scabies, arthropod bites, trauma, and hot, humid climates. The brown recluse spider bite, characterized by necrotizing ulcer and spreading ecthyma, is important to recognize because it requires specific therapy with dapsone.

Folliculitis is infection of the hair follicles, usually caused by coagulase-positive staphylococci, and may be divided into superficial and deep types. Superficial folliculitis consists of a small pustule pierced by the hair shaft. It may be seen on the scalp or other hairy portions of the body. Occupational exposure to cutting oils, coal tar products, or topical corticosteroids under occlusion may precipitate folliculitis. Rarely, small pustules with surrounding erythema caused by *Propionibacterium acnes* may develop around the occiput in males. *Pseudomonas folliculitis* has been described in association with hot tubs.

Furuncles or *boils* may develop from a preceding folliculitis. They are not seen where there is no hair. The erythematous and tender lesion usually becomes fluctuant after 4 days. A yellowish, pointed area may be seen on the surface, and if the lesion ruptures spontaneously, pus and necrotic tissue are extruded. The buttocks, axillae, neck, face, and waist areas are common sites of involvement. Systemic factors such as diabetes, malnutrition, obesity, and hematologic disorders predispose persons to furunculosis. Carbuncles are a coalescence of deep furuncles with multiple points of drainage.

Erysipelas, caused by beta-hemolytic streptococci, is characterized by a peripherally spreading, infiltrated, erythematous, sharply circumscribed plaque. The lesion is warm to touch. The face, scalp, hands, and genitals are frequently involved. Rapid evolution of the lesions is seen, and some patients have constitutional symptoms such as fever and malaise. Poor hygiene and lowered resistance promote infection. Trauma may elicit infection, and recurrent erysipelas may lead to brawny edema. Less common cutaneous infections include staphylococcal scalded-skin syndrome, toxic shock, scarlatina, and erythema marginatum associated with rheumatic fever.

PRINCIPLES OF THERAPY

The principles of therapy are the use of physical measures to enhance resolution and make the skin surface less amenable to colonization by bacteria and to treat infecting agents with antimicrobial drugs. The physical measures employed differ with the pyoderma being treated. Impetigo must be debrided to remove the crust in order to expose the surface where bacteria are present. Furuncles and carbuncles are treated with hot compresses to enhance drainage. Fluctuant lesions may require incision. Exudative lesions require drying compresses to remove detritus and desiccate the lesion. Saline, tap water, or Burow's solution may be applied for 10 to 20 minutes, three to four times a day. Dehydration improves the appearance of the skin and destroys many organisms.

The principle of reducing colonization is particularly important in the treatment of recurrent furunculosis. Frequent cleansing with soap, particularly chlorhexidene, is useful. Nails should be clipped and vigorously scrubbed. Antibiotic cream should be instilled into the anterior nares. Before shaving, the beard should be soaked with hot water for 5 minutes, and blades should be discarded after each use. The razor should be soaked in alcohol. Separate towels, sheets, and clothing should be used, and everything should be laundered and changed frequently. If vigorous reduction of colonization is unsuccessful, consideration should be given for replacement of the pathogenic staphylococcal flora with a less pathogenic strain.

Antibiotics are essential in treating infections. Lesions may be treated on clinical appearance, but microscopic examination of Gram-stained material is a quick and inexpensive way to confirm a diagnosis. Culture and sensitivity are usually not necessary for superficial infections, but are for more destructive lesions or if the patient is not improving. Topical therapy is usually sufficient for impetigo and folliculitis, particularly when it is combined with cleansing and debridement. Most pyodermas are caused by gram-positive organisms and respond to erythromycin or bacitracin. Neomycin is effective, but it should be used sparingly because of potential allergic sensitization. Systemic antibiotic therapy is indicated when there are constitutional symptoms or if the patient is uncooperative.

Glomerulonephritis is an uncommon complication secondary to cutaneous streptococcal infection. There is not evidence that antibiotics prevent postimpetigo glomerulonephritis. When systemic antibiotics are required for streptococcal infections, penicillin is adequate. Erythromycin is effective against both staphylococci and streptococci. Resistant staphylococci must be treated with semisynthetic penicillins.

THERAPEUTIC RECOMMENDATIONS

- Impetigo should be treated with Burow's compresses for 20 minutes, two to four times daily, followed by gentle debridement using a washcloth and cleansing with a chlorhexidene-containing agent. A topical antibiotic such as erythromycin or a bacitracin-polymyxin combination should be applied lightly to the area after drying. Ointments may be used at night. The lesions should not be covered, and the family should be instructed to avoid using the same towel or washcloth and to keep children away from the patient with impetigo.
- Folliculitis should be treated with debridement and topical antibiotics. Furuncles and carbuncles should be treated with hot compresses until the lesions are fluctuant and spontaneous drainage occurs. Larger lesions may require removal of the core with a 4-mm biopsy punch to facilitate drainage. Furuncles or carbuncles associated with cellulitis, fever, or located on the face must be treated with systemic antibiotics such as erythromycin, 1 g a day for 10 days, or a semisynthetic penicillin. Recurrent furunculosis requires a 10- to 14-day course of a systemic antibiotic, combined with removal of bacteria from potential sources such as the skin, nares, nails, razor, or other fomites. Aggressive hygienic measures and occasionally replacement with nonpathogenic *Staphylococcus* can resolve recurrent furunculosis. Erysipelas should be treated with cool compresses and penicillin G.
- The nasal carrier state of staph must be eradicated. Dicloxacillin, given orally in combination with topical antibiotics, is usually effective. The addition of rifampin should be considered in recalcitrant cases.
- A primary consideration in the therapy of all pyodermas is patient education. Aggressive and regular use of cleansing and debridement are essential to the successful resolution of the infection.

ANNOTATED BIBLIOGRAPHY

Bisno AL: Cutaneous infections: Microbiologic and epidemiologic considerations. Am J Med 76:172, 1984 (*Important review.*)

Dillon HC Jr: Impetigo contagiosa: Suppurative and nonsuppurative complications. Am J Dis Child 115:530, 1968 (*Excellent discussion of clinical epidemiologic and bacteriologic characteristics of impetigo in 497 children.*)

Dillon HC Jr: The treatment of streptococcal skin infections. J Pediat 76:676, 1970 (*Intramuscular benzathine penicillin G was the drug of choice for these pyodermas.*)

Dillon HC Jr et al: Epidemiology of impetigo and acute glomerulonephritis. Results of serologic typing of group A streptococci. Am J Epidemiol 86:710, 1967 (*Certain strains of streptococci causing impetigo are nephritogenic.*)

Duncan WC, Dodge BG, Knox JM: Prevention of superficial pyogenic skin infections. Arch Dermatol 99:465, 1969 (*The regular use of an antibacterial soap reduced the incidence of superficial bacterial infections.*)

McNally TP: Antimicrobial agents. Chemotherapy 25:422, 1984 (*Rifampin was the most effective approach to eradicating nasal carriage of staph.*)

Steele RW: Recurrent staphylococcal infection in families. Arch Dermatol 116:189, 1980 (*Controlled study that showed 83% retention of inoculated* S. aureus *organisms after 6 months.*)

Storrs FJ: Treatment of nonbullous impetigo. Cutis 16:886, 1975 (*Brief discussion of the various topical and systemic methods of treating impetigo.*)

Zayhoun ST, Uwayda MM, Kurban AC: Topical antibiotics in pyoderma. Br J Dermatol 90:331, 1974 (*Patients treated with topical gentamicin did no better than those on a placebo cream. Antibacterial soap was used and crusts were removed.*)

190
Management of Superficial Fungal Infections
WILLIAM V. R. SHELLOW, M.D.

Superficial fungal infections are prevalent and easily diagnosed. It is paradoxical that such infections are undiagnosed, or nonfungal dermatoses are incorrectly treated, as fungal infections. The primary physician must be familiar with definitive methods of diagnosis and cost-effective therapy. It is essential that the physician diagnose superficial fungal infection precisely to treat it specifically. Though neither dangerous nor life-threatening, fungal infections can be irritating and recurrent. The primary physician must educate patients to reduce recurrence.

PATHOPHYSIOLOGY AND CLINICAL PRESENTATION

A pathophysiologic consideration that is still incompletely understood is why most people resist these ubiquitous pathogens while others seem unable to rid themselves of infections. Systemic diseases such as diabetes increase susceptibility to *Candida* infection. Studies suggest that hereditary factors may be involved, but an important factor may be local susceptibility caused by maceration of the skin.

Fungal infection occurs when one of these ubiquitous organisms invades the superficial layers of the skin. Dermatophytes do not invade below the level of keratin because a potent antifungal factor prevents deeper infection. Candidal infection produces inflammatory change through elaboration of an endotoxinlike substance.

Tinea versicolor is characterized by brown, scaly patches that occur on the chest, back, and shoulders. Tinea versicolor, particularly during the summer, may present as hypopigmented areas, often erroneously interpreted as vitiligo. The organism appears to prevent pigment transfer from melanocytes to epidermal cells. The diagnosis can be suspected if scratching a macular area raises a fine and branny scale. Examination of the skin with a Wood's light reveals gold or orange-brown fluorescence. The infection is diagnosed by scraping a scaly lesion and examining it with a drop of 20% potassium hydroxide for characteristic short hyphae and spores, sometimes referred to as "spaghetti and meatballs."

Dermatophytic and candidal infections are scaly, mildly erythematous, with defined margins occurring in characteristic areas of the body that promote the growth of fungi.

Dermatophyte infections are defined by the area of the body they affect. The most common are tinea cruris, which involves the groin, inner thigh, and sometimes the abdomen and buttocks, and tinea pedis, characterized by blisters and inflammation on the soles and interdigital areas of the feet. Tinea corporis affects the nonhairy portion of the skin, particularly the face, arms, and shoulders. Tinea capitis, or scalp ringworm, occurs almost exclusively in children. Tinea barbae has become relatively uncommon. Onychomycosis is characterized by the accumulation of subungual keratin, which produces a thickened, distorted, and crumbly nail.

Diagnosis requires microscopic examination for hyphae and spores in a potassium hydroxide wet-mount. Occasionally, a scraping will have to be planted on Sabouraud agar to culture the fungus.

Candida infections of the skin occur principally in intertriginous locations such as the axillae, groin, intergluteal folds, inframammary area, or interdigital web spaces. Crusted involvement of the labial commissures, known as perlèche, and involvement of the glans penis also occur. Lesions are pustular, thin-walled, on a red base, often producing burning and itching. Candidiasis may be clinically suspected as a result of the presence of characteristic satellite pustules outside of the margin of the primary lesion. Diagnosis requires microscopic demonstration of budding spores and pseudohyphae.

PRINCIPLES OF MANAGEMENT

Fungal infections require management of the conditions that predispose to infection and use of specific antifungal agents. The elimination of moisture reduces the likelihood of fungal infection. Inflammatory or weeping lesions should be dried with the application of a desiccating agent such as aluminum acetate, available as Burow's solution. Once predisposing factors have been reduced and the lesions dried, specific antifungal medication is appropriate. There are a host of effective agents available; the physician should prescribe the least expensive effective agent that produces the fewest annoying side-effects. The physician must instruct the patient on how to keep the skin dry and on the proper use of the topical antifungal agents, including manner of application, duration of application, and treatment course.

It may be worthwhile to investigate host factors that predispose to fungal infection, such as corticosteroids or coexistent disease, such as diabetes.

MANAGEMENT RECOMMENDATIONS

Tinea Versicolor. The etiologic agent of tinea versicolor, *Malassezia furfur,* can be treated effectively with selenium sulfide, sodium thiosulfate, zinc pyrithione, sulfa-salicylic acid combinations, or with one of the antifungal agents miconazole, clotrimazole, econazole, ketoconazole, or ciclopirox. For effectiveness, convenience, and least expense, a 2.5% suspension of selenium sulfide or a 1% (zincon) or 2% (sebulon) zinc pyrithione shampoo can be applied with a rough washcloth. It should be allowed to remain on the affected areas for 10 minutes and then rinsed off. Daily application for 1 week is recommended. In refractory cases, selenium sulfide suspension can be left on the skin overnight. Sodium thiosulfate 25% (Tinver) is malodorous and rarely used. The topical antifungal agents are much more expensive but useful in recalcitrant involvement of small areas. Systemic ketoconazole, 200 mg daily, is effective for extensive involvement.

Other Diffuse Tineas. In tineas other than versicolor, *Trichophyton rubrum, Trichophyton mentagrophytes,* and *Epidermophyton floccosum* are the most common infecting organisms. The actual agent is less important than establishment of a fungal etiology. Treatment is independent of location; the lesion should be kept dry and an effective topical agent applied. The patient should dry oozing lesions by applying compresses soaked in Burow's solution from 30 to 60 minutes one to three times daily. A nonmedicated or antifungal powder may be used to absorb moisture. Topical treatment suffices for involvement of glabrous skin, but systemic drugs should be considered when hair sheaths are involved, widespread involvement exists, or associated folliculitis occurs.

A number of effective topical antifungal agents are available. Tolnaftate (Tinactin, Aftate) and miconazole (MicaTin) are available over the counter, and if these are effective the patient will not visit the physician. Clotrimazole (Lotrimin, Mycelex), econazole (Spectazole), ciclopirox (Loprox), and ketoconazole (Nizoral) are all quite effective.

There are no firm guidelines to choosing topical antifungals, but some observations may be helpful. The imidazoles, such as clotrimazole, are the least irritating. Spectazole tends to burn in intertriginous areas, and ciclopirox penetrates the nail plate. Topical lotions are more drying and can be applied in the morning and upon return from work; a cream should be used at night. In erythematous pruritic lesions therapy may be initiated with an antifungal in combination with a steroid such as Lotrisone (clotrimazole and beclomethasone). Refractory cases may be managed by using a combination of agents, one during the day and a different preparation at night. If lesions persist, it may be necessary to prescribe systemic antifungal therapy, such as ketoconazole, 200 mg daily. However, the cost and risk of hepatotoxicity may outweigh the benefit of treating this relatively minor condition.

Tinea Pedis is common and sometimes difficult to treat. The patient must be instructed to wear nonocclusive leather footwear or sandals and absorbent cotton socks, and to dry the feet frequently without rubbing, such as by using a hair dryer. Topical antifungals alone often suffice, but when widespread scaling with hyperkeratosis occurs, so-called moccasin foot keralytic agents are required. The nightly application of Keralyt Gel under occlusion with antifungal creams used two or three times daily may successfully treat this difficult problem.

Onychomycosis is extremely refractory but may respond to *griseofulvin*. A polyethylene glycol vehicle preparation may facilitate absorption; 250 mg two to four times daily, depending on the response, must be taken for as long as it takes the infected portion of the nail to grow out. Monthly blood counts are advised because leukopenia has been observed. It may be necessary to remove the affected nail. Even when a cure is obtained, reinfection is common. Men should be counseled to live with their toenail infections. Women have the option of using nail polish to cover cosmetic unsightliness. Reducing the hyperkeratotic nail with filing will help the appearance. Fingernail infections usually respond better than toenail infections. Topical *ciclopirox* (Loprox) may penetrate the nail plate and might be tried with nightly applications under occlusion.

Candidiasis. Treatment requires meticulous drying of the area, adequate exposure to air, and specific therapy. Gentian violet or Castellani's paint are time-proven but quite messy and have largely been abandoned. Imidazole creams or lotions should be used two or three times daily, but ointments should be avoided because they maintain a moist local environment. In highly inflamed infections, initiating therapy with a topical corticosteroid cream in combination with clotrimazole (Lotrisone) applied lightly is useful. Oral ketoconazole is rec-

ommended for difficult candidal infections. Predisposing factors such as use of systemic corticosteroids, birth control pills, tetracycline, or other antibiotics should be considered. Pregnancy, diabetes, Cushing's syndrome and acquired immunodeficiency also predispose the patient to candidiasis.

Candidal paronychia are difficult to treat. Therapy consists of avoiding exposure to water, and rubber gloves with cotton lining should be worn whenever contact is unavoidable. Nystatin or amphotericin B (Fungizone) lotion should be applied two to four times daily to the affected area. In highly inflamed conditions, nystatin or clotrimazole with steroids may be applied overnight under a fingercot. Nails grow out normally after the paronychia has healed. Ketoconazole should be given orally if local therapy fails.

Referral should be made to a dermatologist when a fungal infection proves refractory to conventional treatment. The primary physician should evaluate patients with recurring infection for predisposing factors and immunocompetence.

PATIENT EDUCATION

At the time of the first incident, patients with fungal infection should be instructed in appropriate measures to prevent recurrence. Dryness is the essential condition that the patient should maintain. This is particularly important in tinea pedis, tinea cruris, and candidal infections. Preventive measures should be taken in areas that have shown a tendency to become infected.

Additionally, the patient should be told to apply powder liberally to naturally moist areas of the body and to wear cotton clothing and loose-fitting underwear. Also, patients with tinea pedis should always wear socks and avoid sneakers and rubber-soled shoes, and the physician should encourage exposure of feet to the air as frequently as possible. Last, people who sweat profusely should change clothing more frequently, shower, and apply nonmedicated talcum powder.

It is important for the physician to instruct the patient carefully in appropriate therapy and length of treatment. Prophylactic measures may reduce recurrences. After treatment for fungal infections, patients do not usually need to return to the physician. Patients with tinea versicolor should be examined, for continued scaling is evidence of persistent activity. The patient should be advised that depigmentation may persist though the infection has been adequately treated. Patients should be instructed to call at the first sign of recurrence and to institute appropriate drying measures and specific therapy after physician consultation.

ANNOTATED BIBLIOGRAPHY

DeVillez RL, Lewis CW: Candidiasis seminar. Cutis 19:69, 1977 (*A good review of the epidemiologic, diagnostic, and therapeutic considerations in treating Candida.*)

Griffith ML, Flowers FP, Araujo OE: Superficial mycoses. Therapeutic agents and clinical application. Postgrad Med 79:151, 1986 (*A timely review.*)

Jones HE, Reinhardt JH, Rinaldi MG: A clinical, mycological and immunological survey of dermatophytosis. Arch Dermatol 108: 61, 1973 (*An in-depth scientific discussion of the pathophysiology of dermatophyte infections.*)

Kligman AM, Bogaert H, Cordero C: Evaluation of ciclopirox olamine cream for the treatment of tinea pedis: Multicenter, double-blind comparative studies. Clin Ther 7:409, 1985 (*The 1% ciclopirox cream [Loprox] proved superior to 1% clotrimazole for treating tinea pedis.*)

Leyden JJ, Kligman AM: Interdigital athlete's foot: New concepts in pathogenesis. Postgrad Med 61:113, 1977 (*A review of the role of bacteria and fungi as well as how to prevent this common disease.*)

Lyddon FE, Coundersen K, Maibach HI: Short-chain fatty acids in the treatment of dermatophytoses. Int J Dermatol 19:24, 1980 (*Reviews topical antifungal therapy with emphasis on undecylenic acid.*)

Maibach HI: Iodochlorhydroxyquin-hydrocortisone treatment of fungal infections. Arch Dermatol 114:1773, 1978 (*Double-blind investigation proved that the combination was effective in the treatment of cutaneous fungal infections.*)

Maibach HI, Kligman AM: The biology of experimental human cutaneous moniliasis (*Candida ablicans*). Arch Dermatol 85:233, 1962 (*The definitive monograph on the nature of disease produced by* Candida albicans.)

Quiñones CA: Tinea versicolor: New topical treatments. Cutis 25: 386, 1980 (*Use of various imidazole antifungal creams.*)

Rudolph AH: The diagnosis and treatment of tinea capitis due to *Trichophyton tonsurans.* Int J Dermatol 24:426, 1985 (*A discussion of Trichophyton tonsurans as the predominant agent causing tinea capitis today.*)

Sanchez JL, Torres VM: Double-blind efficacy study of selenium sulfide in tinea versicolor. J Am Acad Dermatol 11:235, 1984 (*Daily, 10-minute, application of 2.5% selenium sulfide for 1 week proved an effective, convenient treatment, with 87% success at the end of 4 weeks.*)

Savin RC: Systemic ketoconazole in tinea versicolor: A double-blind evaluation and one (1) year follow up. J Am Acad Dermatol 101: 824, 1984 (*A daily dose of 200 mg for weeks produced a 97% cure—33 of 34 patients—but after 1 year, only 21 [64%] were still clear.*)

Zaias N: Onychomycosis. Arch Dermatol 105:263, 1972 (*A lucid discussion of fungal infections of the nails.*)

191
Management of Cutaneous and Genital Herpes Simplex

JEFFREY E. GALPIN, M.D.

Herpes simplex virus (HSV) is a ubiquitous virus that clinically affects man. HSV type I is the prototype for cutaneous disease of the upper body; HSV type II generally produces genital and lower body infections. The viruses share 50% common genetic material and may be interchangeable clinically. They differ in sensitivity to viral drugs and in their ability to cause specific disease in other organs.

Many patients seek help to confirm the herpes infection they suspect, or because they have frequent recurrent rashes and symptoms. The primary care physician must seek a prompt diagnosis, know how to utilize the approaches to treatment, and address the concerns and negative social stigmata that often accompany genital infection.

PATHOPHYSIOLOGY AND CLINICAL PRESENTATION

Primary HSV I infection may go unnoticed, but usually presents as severe exudative pharyngitis or gingivostomatitis, with high fevers and tender lymphadenopathy. The illness often is mistaken for streptococcal disease or other bacterial infections of the oropharynx.

Primary HSV II infection also may be missed or misdiagnosed. In its most overt form, an exudative painful vulvovaginitis is seen in the female and penile ulceration with tender inguinal nodes in the male. Although suppurative lymphadenopathy is not seen as a result of HSV infections, superimposed bacterial infections can occur, which do produce this finding. Primary genital infection usually occurs at adolescence, although infection may take place at the time of birth.

In a comprehensive review of 268 patients, genital lesions were described as painful by 95% of men and 99% of women. Local symptoms increased over the first 6 to 7 days of illness and peaked between days 8 and 10, then gradually decreasing over the next week. Lymph nodes enlarged and were firm and tender, but suppurative lymphadenopathy was not seen. Systemic symptoms of fever and malaise occurred in 67%, dysuria in 63%, and tender adenopathy in 80% of patients. Complications of primary infections included aseptic meningitis in 8%, sacral autonomic nerve dysfunction in 2%, extragenital lesions in 20%, and secondary yeast infections in 11%.

An unusual form of primary infection results from implantation of virus into broken skin, producing a *herpetic whitlow* characterized by pain, swelling, and erythema of the fingers with pronounced adenopathy. Wrestlers may develop *herpes gladiatorum,* a primary herpes infection on exposed parts of the body that are inoculated during the rough activity of wrestling.

The most common presentation is *recurrent herpes labialis* or *genitalis.* The virus, which resides in the associated dorsal root ganglion, circulates along the endoneural sheath to the skin if there is a breakdown in host defenses. Loss of cytotoxic killer cell activity, a decrease in local secretory IgA, or local skin damage permits reactivation, causing a localized, self-limited form of illness. It may begin with a prodrome of tingling or discomfort, as well as more generalized symptoms such as nausea, fatigue, or even fever. Some patients develop pain without rash, but most experience the typical maculopapular to vesicular eruption. The lesions become turbid as interferon is produced in the vesicles and as lymphocytes stimulated by interleukin-2 begin controlling the infection. During the initial 3 to 4 days, some patients autoinoculate themselves in other areas, but secondary infections are usually brief, mild, self-limited, and incapable of establishing disease in new regions. Recurrent infections can occur in different distributions along the same ganglia, and there is heterogeneity in the illness.

Eventually, there is reepithelialization of the skin, usually without scarring. Secondary bacterial infections caused by streptococci or staphylococci can lead to cellulitis and lymphangitis; these must be watched for. The risk of transmission is greatest in the first 96 hours after the appearance of the rash. Even without evidence of disease, silent shedding occurs in 2% to 5% of patients, particularly those with recurrent genital disease.

Complications of local recurrent infections are few. Sacral or perirectal disease can lead to proctitis or colitis. Sacral disease is also associated with risk of recurrent aseptic meningitis. Recurrent disease sometimes takes the form of erythema multiforme without evidence of vesicles. In atopic individuals, HSV can produce a devastating generalized eczema herpeticum.

DIAGNOSIS

The diagnosis of herpes simplex infection is important, especially identifying type II disease, because of its social and psychological significance. Approximately 50% of ulcerative lesions in the genital area are herpetic. Herpes infection, however, may overlap with a diagnosis of syphilis or chancroid caused by *Hemophilus ducreyi* (see Chapter 138). Ulcerations may also occur from noninfectious causes such as Behcet's syndrome, inflammatory bowel disease, or simply as a result of excoriations and secondary bacterial infections caused by vigorous sexual activity. Syphilis serology should always be performed when genital HSV is suspected (see Chapter 123).

The most specific diagnostic method is *viral culture.* Cytologic (Tzanck preparation) and *antigen detection techniques* are less sensitive. DNA probes may provide a more sensitive,

specific, and much more rapid approach to viral isolation. Promising monoclonal and oligoclonal detection methods are under development. *Serology* can confirm type and whether herpes infection has been present before; but it is less useful in documentating the herpetic origin of a recurrent infection, because titers often do not rise sufficiently and there is cross-reactivity between HSV I and II. Serology also has the disadvantage of not producing data within the period that the patient is clinically affected, and patients, once exposed, carry titers forever whether or not they ever reactivate. High IgE levels seem to occur during active recurrences.

PRINCIPLES OF THERAPY

Herpes infection is self-limited. The goals of therapy are to increase the speed of healing and reduce the length of symptoms, the frequency and severity of recurrences, and the risk of complications.

The mainstay of treatment is *oral acyclovir,* which is a purine analogue substrate for viral thymidine kinase. The kinase is uniquely activated in cells that are infected with HSV. Acyclovir is effective against both types of HSV, although HSV I is more sensitive than HSV II. Oral acyclovir shortens viral shedding and reduces the time to healing and crusting of lesions. Continuous use of acyclovir in patients with frequent recurrences reduces the number and severity of repeat episodes. Unfortunately, once the drug is discontinued, its effect on recurrences ceases. Long-term use is associated with slow adaptation of the virus to the drug, but clinically important resistance does not emerge. Cessation of use results in reversion to original sensitivity.

Intravenous acyclovir produces higher, more consistent blood levels; only 15% of oral acyclovir is absorbed. The oral vehicle is acceptable for mucocutaneous manifestations in immunocompetent hosts. Intravenous administration is indicated in *immunocompromised hosts* and in disseminated disease such as meningoencephalitis.

There is little place for *topical acyclovir,* although it has limited efficacy in primary infection. Topical acyclovir is also of little use in keratoconjunctivitis. In this dangerous illness, trifluorothymidine ointment plus oral or intravenous acyclovir should be used.

Adjuncts to acyclovir treatment of HSV include good local care and the use of drying agents to speed the transition from active vesicle to crusting. Topical surfactants such as ether or chloroform seem to give some additional relief. Some have advocated, with little evidence, the associated use of cimetidine because of research evidence suggesting that histamine-2 antagonists have antiherpes activity. Vidarabine, ribavirin, and bromodeoxyuridine, as well as DHPG, have some promise of antiviral activity.

Some clinicians use topical corticosteroids to abort progression of herpetic lesions. This empiric approach often works, though it lacks scientific evidence; it raises a theoretical concern about spread, though no evidence has been published to document this danger. Over-the-counter preparations such as Blistex, Campho-Phenique, or Anbesol may provide some minimal symptomatic relief, but do not affect the course of the eruption. Considering the long history of ineffective therapy, physicians should remain skeptical about new remedies offered.

There is growing evidence that long-term modulation of the immune system by *vaccines* is capable of maintaining benign latency. The *in vivo* stimulation of natural killer cells, interferon, interleukin-2, and other lymphokines by several vaccines is being studied in this country and in Europe. Initial results have been encouraging.

PATIENT EDUCATION

Reassurance of the frightened genital herpes patient is critical. Herpes has acquired an unjustifiably vicious reputation in the media. The only substantial danger is during childbirth, which can be addressed simply by frequent culture and the use of C-section if there is a question of active lesions or culturable infection. There is a small and probably real danger of herpes infection contributing to the development of cervical cancer, but this is a screenable disease and only requires greater diligence on the part of physician and patient (see Chapter 105). The stigma associated with this disease must be reduced. The patient must be made to understand that herpes infection is common and is not a badge of disgrace, nor is the patient a constant threat for transmission to other people. Guilt should be assuaged, and the patient should be educated to know the probable signs of disease and to recognize that asymptomatic recurrence does occur and that is occasionally difficult to prevent recurrences. Condom use can be of some help. By confirming the presence of antibody in a sexual partner, anxiety surrounding sexual relations can be eliminated.

Pamphlets about the disease are available through the Centers of Disease Control, the National Institutes of Health, and the American Social Health Association. These are superior sources to many of the lay-initiated hotlines, which may overplay the emotional problems of the disease. It should be emphasized that recurrent infections are far less likely to produce discomfort or pain than primary infection.

THERAPEUTIC RECOMMENDATIONS

- Symptomatic lesions should be treated with oral acyclovir, 200 mg five times a day. The earlier the treatment is instituted the better. Patients should be given enough medication to restart therapy at the first suspicion of reactivation. Patients with prodromal signs have an advantage.
- Patients who have frequent recurrences of more than six to eight times a year may benefit from chronic use of acy-

clovir with the dose titrated to the lowest level possible without reactivation. Treatment should be limited to 6 to 12 months at a time.
- Educate patients about transmissibility. It is important they know when the illness spreads most easily. The concept of silent spreading must also be appreciated by the patient. Transmission is less likely with the use of condoms, but is still possible.
- Care of skin lesions is important in the immunocompromised or eczematous host in whom dissemination and autoinoculation can lead to serious consequences. Keratoconjunctivitis should be treated with trifluorothymidine along with acyclovir. In all cases of the illness, secondary infection with bacteria must be watched for.
- It is most important to follow genital infections during pregnancy; recurrences at the time of delivery can lead to neonatal disseminated herpes. A C-section is advocated in these cases. Genital herpes is also a major cause of type 2 and 3 Pap smear abnormalities and should be routinely sought when these changes are seen.

ANNOTATED BIBLIOGRAPHY

Barringer JR: Recovery of herpes simplex virus from human sacral ganglion. N Engl J Med 291:828, 1974 (*Gives evidence for residence of the latent type II HSV within human sacral sensory ganglia.*)

Bierman SM: Recurrent genital herpes simplex infection. A trivial disorder. Arch Dermatol 121:173, 1985 (*A good normative statement placing this illness in perspective.*)

Corey L, Spear PG: Infection with herpes simplex viruses. N Engl J Med 314:686, 749, 1986 (*A two-part state of the art review.*)

DiGiovanna JJ, Blank H: Failure of lysine in frequently recurring herpes simplex infections. Arch Dermatol 120:48, 1984 (*Double-blind placebo-controlled study failed to show any benefit for lysine.*)

Douglas JM, Critchlow C, Benedetti J et al: A double-blind study of oral acyclovir for suppression of recurrences of genital herpes simplex virus infection. N Engl J Med 310:1551, 1984 (*Oral acyclovir given for 4 months markedly reduced, but did not eliminate, recurrences. The natural history of recurrences was not affected.*)

Luby ED, Klinge V: Genital herpes: A pervasive psychosocial disorder. Arch Dermatol 121:494, 1985 (*An article emphasizing the adverse effect of herpes on intimate sexual relationships.*)

Marlowe SI: Medical management of genital herpes. Arch Dermatol 121:467, 1985 (*A good summary of the state of the art.*)

Mertz GJ, Critchlow CW, Benedetti J et al: Double-blind placebo controlled trial of oral acyclovir in first-episode genital herpes simplex virus infection. JAMA 252:1147, 1984 (*Acyclovir treatment shortened the duration of viral shedding, symptoms, and lesions, but did not reduce subsequent recurrences.*)

Reichman RC, Badger GJ, Mertz GJ et al: Treatment of recurrent genital herpes with acyclovir, a controlled trial. JAMA 251:2103, 1984 (*Oral acyclovir shortened viral shedding and, when patient-initiated, shortened the course of clinical recurrences. The best effects were achieved when therapy was patient initiated.*)

Sabin AB: Misery of recurrent herpes: What to do. N Engl J Med 293:986, 1975 (*Recommendation of topical ether therapy.*)

Solomon A, Rasmussen JE, Varani J: The tzanck smear in the diagnosis of cutaneous herpes simplex. JAMA 251:633, 1984 (*Viral culture was superior to tzanck prep, but still a useful, cost-effective aid in early diagnosis.*)

Spruance SL, Overall JC, Kern ER et al: The natural history of re-current herpes simplex labialis: Implications for antiviral therapy. N Engl J Med 297:69, 1977 (*Recent observations on untreated herpetic lesions of the lip, and the difficulties in studying antiviral medications.*)

Straus SE, Rooney JF, Sever SL et al: NIH conference. Herpes simplex virus infection: Biology, treatment and prevention. Ann Intern Med 103:404, 1985 (*A superb review.*)

192

Management of Herpes Zoster

JEFFREY E. GALPIN, M.D.

Herpes zoster (shingles) is a common viral cutaneous eruption estimated to affect 300,000 persons a year in the United States. The infection presents with radicular pain followed by the appearance of grouped vesicles on an erythematous base in a dermatomal distribution. The incidence increases with age. A Mayo Clinic community-based study noted 100 cases per 100,000 person years between the age of 15 to 35 rising with each decade to reach 450 cases per 100,000 by age 75. The seasonal variation seen with varicella does not occur with zoster. Shingles may present as a pain syndrome without vesicles and pose a diagnostic problem. Shingles is rarely an epidemic illness; most cases represent reactivation of the varicella-zoster virus. The primary physician must recognize zoster, make the patient comfortable, and prevent complications.

PATHOPHYSIOLOGY AND CLINICAL PRESENTATION

Varicella, the chickenpox virus, usually affects people early in life and then lies dormant in a nerve ganglion in a genomic state until reactivation occurs. A decrease in cellular immunity may provide the trigger that allows the latent virus to reactivate and spread along the nerve resulting in clinical zoster. Helper T-cells and several lymphokines produced by other T-cell subsets usually protect the host from reactivation. The disorder occurs with increased frequency among immunocompromised patients and the elderly, probably as a consequence of defects in cellular immunity. Humoral immunity does not appear to be an important factor; even severely infected patients show significantly elevated antibody titers to zoster. It has been suggested that every person who has had chickenpox harbors latent virus, that 50% of all people who live to the age of 85 will have an attack of zoster, and that approximately 10% will have at least two attacks.

There is no evidence of an increased risk of latent cancer in those with herpes zoster. In a large study of 590 patients followed for 9389 person years, the relative cancer risk was only 1.1 times that of the general population. There is a ten-uous suggestion of a somewhat higher than average risk of colon cancer.

The risk of transmission is low despite the fact that zoster contains large amounts of virus transmitted to normal hosts. Immunosuppressed patients and those who have never had chickenpox are at risk from patients with zoster. In a New York study, only 4.5% of persons born in the United States did not possess varicella antibody. Recent reports have demonstrated reactivation on exposure to zoster in a few patients with a previous history of chickenpox.

Typically, zoster presents with *dermatomal pain,* itch, or tenderness that precedes the cutaneous lesion by 1 to 7 days. Patients may describe burning, tingling, itching, sharp knife-like pricking, or deep boring discomfort. The nerve root changes consist of necrotization and sometimes cyst formation. The Mayo Clinic study showed that more than half of the patients have unilateral involvement of one or more of the thoracic dermatomes. The cranial dermatomes account for approximately 15%, while cervical and lumbar dermatomes each accounts for approximately 10% of the cases.

The cutaneous eruption is characterized by *tense vesicles* that arise on an *erythematous base* distributed along a *dermatome.* They become pustular within a few days followed by crusting and healing over 14 to 21 days. The crust is often dark, almost black. Depending on the depth of the lesion, scarring and atrophy may occur. Malaise, low-grade fever, and adenopathy may accompany the eruption. The total course is related to the time of new vesicle development; several days of vesicle development usually leads to a 2½-week course, whereas vesicles that persist over a week predict a longer course.

In the Mayo Clinic study, 12% experienced at least one complication. Major complications include postherpetic neuralgia, uveitis, motor deficits, infection, systemic involvement such as meningoencephalitis, pneumonia, deafness, or dissemination. Vesicles on the tip of the nose were thought to indicate nasociliary involvement, but a recent review of ophthalmic zoster does not confirm the validity of this clinical pearl. *Postherpetic neuralgia* occurs most frequently in patients over 50 years of age. The pain of postherpetic neuralgia is often excruciating and does not respond well to conventional methods of pain reduction. The presence of more than 10 lesions outside a single dermatome of distribution is early evidence of dissemination.

AIDS patients may have varicella-zoster virus (VZV) infections as part of the AIDS-related complex (ARC). In most cases it presents as typical dermatomal illness; occasionally it is disseminated and can be complicated by hepatitis, pneumonia, meningitis, or proctitis. In immunocompromised hosts, VZV and herpes simplex infections may present in similar and atypical fashion, sometimes without vesicles, at others in unusual distributions.

DIAGNOSIS

The diagnosis of herpes zoster is generally not difficult when pain and the typical dermatomal rash is present. The most serious diagnostic problem occurs during the prodromal days when patients present with a pain syndrome. Periorbital headache, unexplained back pain, or chest wall pain may represent the prodromal period of herpes zoster. Prodromal zoster pain has been mistaken for myocardial infarction, cholecystitis, and appendicitis. The characteristic eruption may not appear until 2 to 5 days later. In patients with the characteristic rash, a positive *Tzanck preparation* demonstrating *multinucleated giant* cells is supportive evidence of zoster. *Culture,* though slow to report, provides confirmation. The diagnosis may be confirmed by demonstrating *rising antibody titer,* which requires two separate determinations, or by immunofluorescence.

PRINCIPLES OF THERAPY

The goals of therapy are to dry the vesicles, relieve pain, and prevent secondary infection and complications. Lesions are kept clean and dry by the application of a wet-to-dry compress soaked with Burow's solution three to four times a day. If purulence or erythema develops, suggesting secondary infection, antibiotics are indicated. There are no data to support the use of prophylactic antibiotics.

Relief of pain and itching is important. Pain relief can usually be achieved with a mild analgesic such as aspirin or acetaminophen, but one should not hesitate to use *codeine* if need be. The pain of thoracic zoster may be reduced by splinting the affected area with a *tight wrap.* Lesions are covered with a nonadherent dressing and then the area wrapped with an elastic bandage. Malaise reflects viremia and should be treated with rest. Severe local pain can be ameliorated with *intralesional injections* of *triamcinolone,* 2 mg/cc in lidocaine. There is little evidence to suggest that pain or the rate of healing can be ameliorated by use of *systemic corti-*

costeroids; however, such treatment may reduce the incidence of postherpetic neuralgia. Steroids should be used only in patients over 50 (they are at increased risk for postherpetic neuralgia) who have no contraindications to steroid use. Itching may be relieved by oral *antihistamines* (see Chapter 172) or *calamine lotion,* which both reduces itching and dries the rash.

Acyclovir, given orally or intravenously, has been shown to improve and shorten the course of VZV infections, if therapy is begun early in the syndrome. VZV is much more resistant to acyclovir than herpes simplex virus (HSV); double-dose therapy is required. Oral acyclovir should be administered at a dosage of 400 mg five times a day for 5 to 7 days. Intravenous acyclovir should be given at 15 mg/kg three times daily for the same time interval. There is growing acceptance of acyclovir treatment in adults who develop zoster. Limited evidence suggests that early therapy can decrease the likelihood of complications and may reduce the occurrence of postherpetic neuralgia. A 6-deoxy prodrug of acyclovir (BW ASISU) is under development and may prove more efficacious.

A varicella *vaccine* is completing trials and should soon be available for administration. This attenuated vaccine may benefit adults who have not had chickenpox and some adults at risk for reactivation. It is hoped that the vaccine will stimulate T-cell subsets and make reactivation less likely.

The use of *lymphokine therapy* with or without hyperimmune globulin to VZV may have an adjunctive effect on the immunocompromised host in whom zoster develops and then disemminates. In investigational trials, *vidarabine* accelerated cutaneous healing and decreased dissemination and visceral complications if given within 72 hours of onset of the rash in immunosuppressed patients. Side-effects include nervousness, hallucinations, nausea, vomiting, and diarrhea.

Treatment of *complications* is difficult. Ophthalmologic consultation is indicated if there is any suggestion of *intraocular involvement.* Antivirals should be prescribed in all cases of zoster ophthalmicus. *Post-herpetic neuralgia* is sometimes avoided with early steroid therapy in high-risk patients, but can be one of the most disabling and frustrating consequences of zoster. Nonnarcotic methods such as antidepressants, transcutaneous nerve stimulation, and the anticonvulsive drug carbamazepine have been used with some efficacy. Success has been reported with the use of repeated triamcinolone injections into symptomatic areas or as a sympathetic ganglion block. Other clinicians have found that chlorprothixene (Taractan) in doses of 25 to 50 mg or Triavil, three to four times daily, reduces pain. Recent work has suggested roles for L-dopa and Tagamet in the management of postherpetic neuralgia. Adenosine monophosphate injections into the area of pain has been dramatic in one study. The severity of postherpetic neuralgia pain and its refractoriness to treatment has provided some of the stimulus for early use of steroids in patients over 50 to reduce the risk of complication.

ANNOTATED BIBLIOGRAPHY

Balfour HH Jr: Acyclovir therapy for herpes zoster: Advantages and adverse effects. JAMA 255:387, 1986 (*An editorial position on using acyclovir for zoster.*)

Burgoon CF, Burgoon JS: The natural history of herpes zoster. JAMA 164:265, 1957 (*Discussion of the course of herpes zoster in 206 unselected cases. Complications developed in 16.9%; about half of these were cases of postherpetic neuralgia.*)

Eaglestein WH, Katz R, Brown JS: The effects of early corticosteroid therapy on the skin eruption and pain of herpes zoster. JAMA 211:1681, 1970 (*The duration of postherpetic neuralgia was decreased by oral triamcinolone therapy begun early in the disease course.*)

Hirsch MS, Swartz MN: Antiviral agents. N Engl J Med 302:903, 949, 1980 (*A review of the chemoprophylactic and therapeutic uses of amantadine, vidarabine, interferon, and acyclovir.*)

Liesegang TJ: The varicella-zoster virus: Systemic and ocular features. J Am Acad Dermatol 11:165, 1984 (*A superb review with emphasis on ophthalmic zoster; includes 135 references.*)

McKendrick MW, Care C, Burke C et al: Oral acyclovir in herpes zoster. J Antimicrob Chemother 14:661, 1984 (*Uncertain benefits for oral acyclovir in zoster.*)

Palmer SR, Caul ED, Donald DE: An outbreak of shingles? Lancet 2:1108, 1985 (*Suggests that shingles can be provoked by reexposure to varicella-zoster virus.*)

Ragozzino MW, Melton LJ, Kurland LT et al: Risk of cancer after herpes zoster. N Engl J Med 307:393, 1982 (*A retrospective cohort study that found no increased risk of cancer among patients with herpes zoster.*)

Sklar SH, Blue WH, Alexander EJ et al.: Herpes-zoster. The treatment and prevention of neuralgia with adenosine monophosphate. JAMA 253:1427, 1985 (*A remarkably effective treatment for both acute zoster, and postherpetic neuralgia.*)

Solomon AR, Rasmussen JE, Weiss JS: A comparison of the tzanck smear and viral isolation in varicella-herpes zoster. Arch Dermatol 122:282, 1986 (*Tzanck prep was superior to viral isolations in obtaining positive results in early lesion.*)

Taub A: Relief of postherpetic neuralgia with psychotropic drugs. J Neurosurg 39:235, 1973 (*Guidance for treatment of the difficult problem.*)

Weller TH: Varicella and herpes zoster. N Engl J Med 309:1362, 1434, 1983 (*An extensive review of the epidemiology, natural history, prevention, and therapy of infections due to this ubiquitous virus.*)

193
Management of Warts
WILLIAM V. R. SHELLOW, M.D.

In the past several years it has been recognized that each type of wart is associated with a separate class of DNA human papilloma virus (HPV). Warts may be transmitted by direct contact with a wart or by autoinoculation. The papilloma virus is epithelotropic and causes tumors of the epidermis. Warts are seen frequently in young people, as well as in adults; they may heal spontaneously, presumably through immunologic mechanisms. Approximately two thirds of warts disappear spontaneously within 2 years of their appearance; however, if left untreated, additional warts may develop from the original one. The primary care physician should be able to distinguish warts from other skin tumors and to treat them.

PATHOPHYSIOLOGY, CLINICAL PRESENTATION, AND COURSE

The pathophysiology of warts is infection by a DNA virus. Almost 30 different types of HPV have been identified. Typing is accomplished by serologic analysis of virion proteins and by molecular hybridization of viral DNA. Five types of HPV have been shown to be oncogenic. Two types have been implicated in cervical carcinoma and three in squamous cell carcinoma.

The clinical presentation of warts varies. The *common wart, verruca vulgaris* (associated with HPV2 and HPV4), is a flesh-colored or grayish white lesion with a hyperkeratotic surface that appears "warty." It may be seen anywhere but commonly affects the elbows, knees, fingers, and palms. Filiform warts are more delicate and threadlike. *Flat warts, verruca plana* (associated with HPV3), are smaller than common warts, and their surface is smoother. They may be present in great numbers on the hand, on the beard area in men, and on the shaved legs in adult women. The *plantar wart, or verruca plantaris* (associated with HPV1 and HPV4) derives its name from the location where it is found, and appears as grayish or yellow interruptions in the skin lines on the bottom of the foot. This wart is less elevated because the weight of the patient presses it inward. These may be solitary, multiple, or confluent, in which instance the term "mosaic wart" is used. Superficial thrombosed capillaries appear as black dots on the surface of plantar warts and also on common warts. *Anogenital warts, condylomata acuminata* (associated with HPV6 and HPV16), grow on mucous membranes and are most often sexually transmitted. They may become very large and cauliflowerlike. It is interesting to note that, according to CDC figures for 1981, office visits for *condylomata acuminata* were more than three times those for genital herpes

(946,000 versus 295,000). The physician should always look for internal warts and coexistent venereal disease.

Warts are usually asymptomatic, although plantar warts may be painful when one is walking because they act like a foreign body. Anogenital warts may become friable, bleed, and cause discomfort. Periungual lesions may become fissured.

DIFFERENTIAL DIAGNOSIS

Although warts are usually easy to diagnose, a differential diagnosis may be indicated. Verrucae vulgaris should be differentiated from squamous cell carcinoma and also from a cutaneous horn arising from an actinic keratosis. Multiple verrucae planae on the face should be differentiated from trichoepitheliomas, syringomas, or the cutaneous lesions of sarcoidosis. Anogenital warts must be differentiated from condylomata lata or squamous cell carcinomas. Bowenoid papulosis (associated with HPV16) appears as wartlike lesions on the male and female genitals. Histopathologically these lesions show cellular atypia characteristic of carcinoma *in situ,* but they have little biologic tendency to become malignant. With condylomata acuminata, a serologic test for syphilis should be done, and in the female, cervical biopsy is needed because of increased risk of cervical carcinoma (see Chapter 105).

PRINCIPLES OF THERAPY

Once a firm diagnosis has been made, the physician must decide if and how the warts should be treated. Warts disappear spontaneously, and because therapy may cause scarring, the patient and the physician may occasionally decide not to treat. The location of the wart and the treatment modalities available to the practitioner often influence the decision. Larger warts of long duration, and plantar, perianal, or periungual areas are the most difficult to treat. The patient's occupation, skin pigmentation, and body area should be considered when designing therapy. The goal is to destroy the epidermal tumor while minimizing damage to the underlying dermis. The greater the dermal injury, the greater is the risk of scar formation. Only minimal scarring should be expected or considered acceptable.

Liquid nitrogen applied with a cotton-tipped applicator causes the wart to separate from the underlying dermis. After freezing, the wart usually falls off within 2 weeks. Before freezing, the thickened keratin should be pared off. It is best to freeze a few millimeters of the surrounding normal tissue. The patient should be warned that the area may hurt for several hours following treatment and occasionally hemorrhagic bullae develop. If not completely gone, the wart can be retreated within 2 to 3 weeks. Liquid nitrogen has the advantage of being quick, bloodless, and not too painful, but the liquefied gas evaporates quickly and requires storage in special containers. Commercial kits generating sticks of "dry ice" from compressed carbon dioxide gas are available, but because the sticks are not as cold as liquid nitrogen, they require more pressure and a longer duration of application. They are less effective.

Light *electrodesiccation* and *chemical cautery* with nitric acid or mono-, bi-, or trichloroacetic acid are alternatives. Curettage with or without electrodesiccation is effective but time-consuming, and scarring can result if treatment is too vigorous. Plantar warts are usually treated by nonsurgical methods because scarring in this location can cause permanent discomfort. The lesion should be pared and application of 40% *salicylic acid plasters* taped in place for 1 to 3 days, followed by scraping off of the macerated skin. This procedure is used for 2 to 3 weeks. Liquid nitrogen can be used on plantar warts in non-weight-bearing areas. Daily 10% formalin or 25% glutaraldehyde compresses are sometimes used for mosaic plantar warts. Cantharidin, which causes an acantholytic blister, is another option, but is rarely used. Topical *5-fluorouracil* cream or solution or *retinoic acid* cream or gel is effective for flat warts, especially those on the face.

Twenty percent to 40% *podophyllum* in compound tincture of benzoid is used to treat *moist anogenital warts.* It must be applied sparingly, only to the wart, and allowed to dry thoroughly before the patient dresses. The medication is washed off by the patient 1 to 4 hours after application. Repeat treatment is the rule. Podophyllum is contraindicated in pregnancy. Evaluation for concurrent veneral disease is mandatory in patients presenting with genital warts.

Dinitrochlorobenzene (DNCB) sensitization followed by repeated applications of diluted DNCB has been used to treat resistant warts. This form of immunotherapy is sometimes effective, but DNCB has been shown to be a potential carcinogen in some studies. The intralesional injection of *bleomycin* has also been used to treat warts. Although is said to be safe, it must be considered adventuresome therapy. There is no evidence that autogenous wart *vaccines* are more effective than placebos.

THERAPEUTIC RECOMMENDATIONS

The primary care physician should observe the basic principle that warts are benign tumors, which often regress spontaneously. Treatment should not be so aggressive as to produce permanent scarring. Simple and safe treatments should be employed. Repeated failure of modalities necessitates referral to a dermatologist.

- Liquid nitrogen is good therapy for many types of warts.
- Moist anogenital warts can be treated with podophyllum; the patient should be reminded to remove the medication within a few hours.
- Flat warts can be treated with 5-fluorouracil, retinoic acid, or Keralyt, a 6% salicylic acid gel.
- Plantar warts are shaved down with a scalpel and a piece

of 40% salicylic acid plaster is cut to the shape, but slightly smaller than the wart. It is covered with occlusive adhesive tape and left in place for 24 to 72 hours. The patient may continue this treatment at home and can pare away the macerated wart and then reapply the salicylic acid plasters. The physician should check on progress every few weeks.

• When topical treatment proves ineffective, *electrocoagulation* or *surgical excision* is indicated. Excision with histologic confirmation is indicated to rule out malignancy in large venereal warts that do not respond to podophyllum.

PATIENT EDUCATION

Prevention of warts entails avoiding others with warts and removing warts from the patient so that the viral reservoir is reduced. Although warts may have initially come from contact with others, biting and picking warts by the patient may result in additional lesions.

Treatment of warts by any method may be both time-consuming and expensive for the patient. Recurrences of warts are seen around one third of the time. The patient must be made to understand that warts are caused by a virus, and physicians are unable to eliminate the virus. The length of treatment, cost, discomfort, and possible failure of therapy should be candidly discussed before treatment is initiated. In most instances the patient's immune system will eventually prevent the HPV virus from causing the clinical lesion, the wart, although the virus is still present.

Finally, although over-the-counter preparations containing salicylic acid and lactic acid (Compound W) may be effective in removing some lesions, the physician will most likely be seeing a self-selected group of patients for whom these remedies have failed.

ANNOTATED BIBLIOGRAPHY

Adler MW: ABC of sexually transmitted diseases: Genital warts and molluscum contagiosum. Br Med J 288:213, 1984 (*Succinct review.*)

Bender ME, Ostrow RS, Watts S et al: Immunology of human papilloma virus: Warts. Pediatr Dermatol 1:121, 1983 (*A discussion of the techniques used for identifying HPV in clinical conditions, and the immune responses produced by these viruses.*)

Crum CP et al: Human papilloma virus type 16 and early cervical neoplasia. N Engl J Med 310:880, 1984 (*Association of type 16 subtype of papilloma virus with cervical neoplasia.*)

Daling JR, Sherman KS, Weiss NS: Risk factors for condyloma acuminatum in women. Sex Transm Dis 13:16, 18, 1986 (*Long-term cigarette smoking and/or oral contraceptive use dramatically increased the risk of genital warts.*)

Litt JZ: Don't excise—exorcise: Treatment for subungual and periungal warts. Cutis 22:673, 1978 (*Describes the use of phenol and nitric acid, plus the powerful effect of suggestion in treating warts.*)

Madison MD, Morris R, Jones LW: Autogenous vaccine therapy for condyloma acuminatum: A double-blind controlled study. Br J Vener Dis 58:62, 1982 (*In a double-blind cross-over study in 34 patients, an autogenous wart vaccine was not significantly more effective than a placebo.*)

Massing AM, Epstein WL: Natural history of warts. Arch Dermatol 87:306, 1963 (*One thousand children with warts were observed for 2 years. Without treatment there was an increase in the total number of verrucae.*)

Sanders BB, Stretcher GS: Warts: Diagnosis and treatment. JAMA 235:2859, 1976 (*A review emphasizing the design of a treatment regimen based on the type of wart being treated.*)

194
Management of Scabies and Pediculosis
WILLIAM V. R. SHELLOW, M.D.

Scabies has been pandemic in the United States over the past two decades. Pediculosis capitis is a serious problem in primary schools. Although less common, pediculosis pubis is embarrassing and may be associated with other sexually transmitted diseases. The primary physician, therefore, must be able to properly diagnose and treat these ectoparasitic infestations.

PATHOPHYSIOLOGY AND CLINICAL PRESENTATION

Scabies is a worldwide disease that occurs in cycles. It is due to an infestation with *Sarcoptes scabei var. hominis,* which is transmitted by close personal contact with infested individuals. It may affect patients of any socioeconomic level. Once contracted, scabies usually persists until the diagnosis is made and specific therapy is prescribed.

The scabies mite is $1/60$ inch. The adult female attaches to skin and digs into the horny layer where it is thin. Copulation with a wandering male has rendered the female fertile for life. Once in the skin, she remains there for the rest of her life, which may be more than a month. She remains within her burrow, laying two or three eggs a day. These eggs hatch within 3 to 4 days. Mature adults develop over the next 10 to 14 days. While in her burrow, the female chews on epidermal cells and feeds on liquid oozing from them. The average number of female mites on the body is 11. Eighty-five percent of infested individuals have burrows on the hands and wrists. Other common sites of mite recovery are extensor aspect of elbows (40%), feet and ankles (37%), penis and scrotum (36%), buttocks (16%), and axillae (15%). The rash seen in patients with scabies reflects sensitization to the organism, and it does not correspond to places where the mite is found. In patients who have never been infested, the pruritic rash takes several (2–4) weeks to develop.

Nocturnal itching is the cardinal symptom, although patients with scabies also itch when they remove their clothing or become overheated. The scabetic rash may become eczematous, crusted, excoriated, and secondarily infected. The diagnosis is made by finding topical grayish white *burrows,* a millimeter or 2 long, perhaps with a black speck (the mite) at the end. Burrows should be looked for in hand, wrist, ankle, and genital areas, where the recovery rate is highest. The roof of the burrow is shaved off with a scalpel and the base is scraped. The material is placed on a microscope slide and a drop of light mineral oil and a cover slip are added. In mineral oil, but not in potassium hydroxide, movement of the mite is seen. The lowest power objective should be used. The presence of adult mites, immature mites, ova, or fecal pellets (tan-brown in color) confirms the diagnosis. Presumptive diagnosis can also be made based on the symptoms, the appearance of the rash, and the history of contacts who are also itching.

Pediculosis. Head and body lice represent two forms of the organism *Pediculus humanus.* They are elongated insects that are transmitted by contact with infested clothing, combs, or bedding. Body lice are seen most commonly in people with poor personal hygiene, more often in indigent populations. The adult louse lives and lays eggs in clothing, often in the seams, and travels onto the skin for a blood meal. *Vertical excoriations* on the trunk are the cardinal sign. The head louse typically infests the occipital portion of the scalp and sometimes the postauricular region. Although there are few adults, there are many oval eggs (nits) cemented to the hair. The diagnosis is made by plucking a hair and identifying the full or empty egg case under the microscope. Head lice have been a substantial public health problem among school children. Pyoderma of the nape or the occiput requires that pediculosis capitis be ruled out.

Pediculosis pubis is usually a sexually transmitted infestation caused by *Phthirus pubis,* the crab louse. This organism has a more rounded body, and the second and third pair of legs are claws that clasp hairs tightly. The eyelashes, axillary, chest, and thigh hairs can be involved. Itching is the cardinal symptom, caused by the lice injecting saliva, digestive juices, and feces into the skin. Although only a few adult lice may be found at the base of the hair, numerous nits are usually seen. Often the patient's underwear is speckled with blood. Characteristic asymptomatic macular blue discolorations,

called *maculae caeruleae* are sometimes seen on the trunk and thighs.

PRINCIPLES OF THERAPY

Killing of the mites or lice and prevention of infestation among close contacts are the aims of treatment. Secondary bacterial infection should be treated with systemic antibiotics.

Scabies. Both mites and ova are killed by 1% lindane (gamma benzene hexachloride [GBH]). This must be applied to the entire body from the neck down, with special attention to the folds and creases. Close contacts must also be treated. Lindane must be used with caution in infants, and never in pregnancy, because overzealous application has resulted in neurotoxicity. Topical steroids and systemic antihistamines help control the rash and pruritus. Occasionally systemic steroids are indicated. Persistent postscabetic papules may be treated by the intralesional injection of corticosteroids.

Pediculosis. In pediculosis corporis, the lice living in clothing can be killed by boiling, laundering, dry cleaning, or ironing. Proper hygiene, bathing, and a change of underclothing and bedding usually suffice.

In pediculosis capitis, lindane shampoo is effective. Malathion lotion 0.5% has been used recently. Synergized pyrethins are effective for ridding fomites of infestation. Nits remaining on the hair must be removed with a fine-toothed comb. Pyoderma should be treated with antibiotics as necessary.

Pubic lice are treated with lindane cream or lotion. Lindane shampoo may also be used. As with pediculosis capitis, nits must be removed by mechanical means.

Phthirus pubis palpebrum may be treated with nonirritating, nontoxic petrolatum. The lice either suffocate or slip off the greased hairs.

THERAPEUTIC RECOMMENDATIONS

- The treatment of choice for scabies is 1% lindane cream or lotion (Kwell, Scabene) applied to the entire body below the neck, and left on for 6 hours, then washed off. About 30 ml is sufficient for the average adult. Underwear and bed linen must be changed. Only one prescription should be given, to prevent overuse.
- Crotamiton 10% (Eurax cream or lotion) is a satisfactory scabicide with some inherent antipruritic properties. It should be applied from the neck downward nightly for two nights. Twenty-four hours after the second application, the medication is washed off. Intimate apparel and bed linen must be changed, laundered, or dry cleaned after treatment.
- Only if reinfestation has occurred should a second course of treatment be necessary.
- Pruritus is usually controlled by topical corticosteroids and oral antihistamines. Residual irritation may be controlled by a mild corticosteroid cream or lotion.

- Pediculosis capitis is treated with lindane shampoo left on the scalp for 4 minutes. Nits are removed with a fine-toothed comb. Malathion lotion 0.5% (Prioderm) is applied to the hair, let dry for 8 to 12 hours, then shampooed out. Synergized pythretins are available as over-the-counter preparations. Combs and brushes should be soaked in rubbing alcohol.
- Pediculosis pubis is treated by applying lindane shampoo and lathering well, then leaving it on for 4 minutes. A thin layer of lindane lotion can be applied and left on for 12 hours and then washed off. If new eggs appear, or itching recurs, reapplication in a week is indicated.
- Eyelash infestation is treated by twice-daily thick applications of petrolatum for 8 days, followed by mechanical removal of nits. Physostigmine ointment is a reasonable second choice.
- In all infestations, the patient should be given written instructions on how the medication is to be used. Treatment failure is usually the result of poor patient compliance.

ANNOTATED BIBLIOGRAPHY

Burkhart CG: Scabies: An epidemiologic reassessment. Ann Intern Med 98:498, 1983 (*Reviews the epidemiology, clinical manifestations, treatment, and prevention of scabies infection.*)

Couch JM, Green WR, Hirst LW: Diagnosing and treating phthirus pubis palpebrarum. Surv Ophthalmol 26:219, 1982 (*Petrolatum is the treatment of choice for lice in eyelashes.*)

Kramer MS: Operational criteria for adverse drug reactions. An updated evaluation of 1% gamma benzene hexachloride. Drug Int Bull 82:140, 1982 (*The appropriate warnings for the use of Kwell.*)

Meinking TL, Taplin D, Kalter DC: Comparative efficacy of treatment for pediculosis capitis infection. 122:267, 1986 (*Also editorial in the same issue* [259, 1986], *questions whether Kwell is the best treatment, and argues for vigorous mechanical removal of nits.*)

Richey HK, Fenskey NA, Cohen LE: Scabies: Diagnosis and management. Hosp Pract 21:124A, 1986 (*A comprehensive review.*)

Taplin D, Castillero PM, Spiegel J: Malathion for treatment of pediculosis humanus var capitis infestation. JAMA 247:3103, 1982 (*A 98.4% cure rate 1 week after a 12-hour application of malathion 5% lotion.*)

195

Management of Animal and Human Bites

ELLIE J. C. GOLDSTEIN, M.D.

Animal bites are common, and patients frequently present to the primary physician for information and therapy. Human bites are less common but potentially more serious. Clenched-fist injuries result from striking the mouth. Patients may appear shortly after injury concerned about rabies, tetanus, or repair of a disfiguring tear. They may delay seeking medical care only to present later with infection. The primary physician must provide first aid and tetanus prophylaxis, decide when antibiotics are necessary, and be able to estimate the risk of rabies.

PATHOPHYSIOLOGY AND CLINICAL PRESENTATIONS

Bite wounds produce a break in the skin, allowing inoculation by bacteria that normally inhabit the skin and oral cavity. Once the protective barrier of the skin is compromised, conditions favoring infection have been established. The risk of infection increases the longer the wound is left unattended. The infecting organisms are usually the normal flora of the oral mucosa. *Pasteurella multocida* is a frequent etiologic agent, present in 50% of animal oral cavities and in 20% of animal bite wounds. Bites from animals who ingest feces may become infected with enteric organisms. In humans, the mouth flora is more abundant than in most animals and includes *Streptococcus viridans*, *Eikenella corrodens*, *Bac-*

teroides species, anaerobic diphtheroids, vibrios, fusobacteria, and spirochetes. Wounds may also be infected by skin flora such as a streptococcus or staphylococcus. Human bites are responsible for most severe bite wound infections because of the heavy inoculum of bacteria received.

Bites initially thought to be trivial may become infected hours or days later. Cat bites occasionally lead to severe cellulitis, and an occasional patient presents with cat scratch fever. Lymphadenopathy is the usual presentation of cat scratch fever.

The most serious bite wounds are caused by clenched-fist injuries. Damage occurs when the tendons and other tissues of the exterior area of the finger are stretched to full length, the skin is broken, and the tendon and possibly the joint are exposed. As the fingers are straightened, the damaged parts relax, and infecting organisms are carried into the tissues, producing infection in wounds that initially appear minor. If the joint capsule is penetrated, the risk of osteomyelitis is increased.

PRINCIPLES OF THERAPY

Principles of therapy include characterization of the injury, vigorous cleansing, tetanus prophylaxis, and appropriate antibiotics. It is important to elicit a history of the circumstances surrounding the injury. If an animal bite occurred, the type of animal and the animal's behavior need to be detailed, as well as whether the animal has been vaccinated and whether the attack was provoked or unprovoked.

Since 1967, there have been only one or two cases of rabies in man each year in the United States. There have been no cases of rabies in man in New York or Los Angeles for many years. In 1981, 7211 animals in the United States were reported to have rabies—195 foxes, 216 dogs, 285 cats, 465 cattle, 481 racoons, 858 bats, and 4,480 skunks. Rabies is a concern if the attack is unprovoked, occurs in a rural setting, or involves a bat, a skunk, or an animal that is behaving in a peculiar manner. The local health department provides data regarding the local incidence of rabies and should be notified for follow-up and statistical reasons. It is unlikely that the patient will need treatment for rabies. When rabies is a possibility, *duck embryo vaccine* should be given along with *rabies immune globulin* without delay. When a person is bitten by a pet, the animal should be watched at home by the owner for 2 weeks and reported to the local health department.

It is important to determine if the patient has had an initial series of tetanus shots and a booster within the past 5 years. Those who have not had an initial series should be given both *tetanus toxoid* and *tetanus immune globulin* (see Chapter 4). In those who have had the initial series but no recent booster, 0.5 cc of *tetanus toxoid* intramuscularly should be administered. Most minor puncture wounds from animal bites may be cleansed with soap and water and treated expectantly without antibiotics. Copious *irrigation* of wounds with normal saline or hydrogen peroxide is an important therapeutic adjunct.

Therapy of tear wounds is problematic. There have been no controlled trials of closure nonclosure, with or without antibiotics. The principles of therapy are to trim loose edges and cleanse and debride the wound. After the wound is left open for 24 to 48 hours, the edges can be approximated with Steri-strips or sutured, and phenoxymethyl penicillin, 250 to 500 mg four times a day, can be given for 3 to 5 days. Secondary closures may be done when it is apparent that no infection is present. Facial wounds should be closed and antibiotics given. It may be useful to refer these patients to a plastic surgeon.

Patients may present after 24 hours with infection. Principles of treatment include debridement, drainage, cleansing, delayed closure of the wound, and institution of appropriate antibiotic therapy. Penicillin is the drug of choice because it is effective against *P. multocida,* some staphylococci, streptococci, anaerobes, and *E. corrodens.* In penicillin-allergic patients tetracycline is preferred because *P. multocida* is often resistant to erythromycin. Amoxicillin plus clavulanate (Augmentin) is considered an acceptable alternative, but probably should be reserved for nonmammal bites involving gram-negative organisms. It is not an adequate antistaph agent.

Human bites are usually located on an extremity; wounds of the hand are more serious than those located elsewhere. The same principles of cleansing, drainage, and debridement apply. Human bites should not be closed primarily, though edges may be approximated if the tear is severe. Antibiotics should be instituted as soon as wound cultures are taken. Penicillin and penicillinase-resistant penicillin should be administered pending culture results to cover oral anaerobes and gram-positive cocci, particularly *S. aureus.* In one series, 44% of wounds grew *S. aureus.* Infrequently, a penicillin-resistant gram-negative organism may be present, necessitating a change in antibiotic regimen. Tetanus toxoid 0.5 cc should be administered to all those previously immunized who have not had a booster in the previous 5 years. Follow-up is essential, because of the potential delayed presentation of serious infection.

Clenched-fist injuries usually require specialized care. Radiographs should be taken to rule out fractures and to provide a baseline for future assessment of osteomyelitis. Extension and flexion of digits should be carefully checked and sensation tested. The third metacarpophalangeal joint is most frequently affected. The integrity of the joint capsule needs to be determined; this should be done by an experienced surgeon. If the capsule is intact, the hand is cleaned, debrided, immobilized, and elevated. Penicillin and a penicillinase-resistant penicillin are started and tetanus toxoid administered. Patients seen within 8 hours of injury with intact joint capsules may be managed as outpatients with careful follow-up. Those with torn capsules need to be admitted for surgery and treatment with intravenous antibiotics. Patients who present after 8 hours should be admitted for observation whether the capsule is intact or interrupted.

THERAPEUTIC RECOMMENDATIONS AND PATIENT EDUCATION

- Clean all wounds vigorously with soap and water. Copious irrigation with normal saline or dilute hydrogen peroxide is advisable.
- Immunize against tetanus with 0.5 cc of tetanus toxoid intramuscularly in those who have previously been immunized but have not had a booster in the past 5 years.
- Animal puncture wounds that are small and clean require no other treatment.
- Treat fresh, uninfected tear wounds with cleansing, debridement, and phenoxymethyl penicillin (250 mg four times a day), followed by secondary closure in 24 to 48 hours if there are no signs of infection.
- Treat infected animal bite wounds with debridement, drainage, and cleansing. Culture the wound, delay wound closure until infection subsides, and begin penicillin, 500 mg four times daily. Dicloxacillin, 500 mg four times a day, should be used when erythema appears to be spreading or when *S. aureus* is suspected. Treat for 7 to 10 days, pending culture results. If the patient is allergic to penicillin, use

tetracycline, 500 mg four times a day, for initial antibiotic therapy.

- Treat *all* human bites initially with *both* penicillin and a penicillinase-resistant agent. Delay closure of the wound.
- Elevate affected limbs for 3 to 5 days.
- Clenched fist injuries should be immobilized, usually in a plaster splint. Inspect the injury in 24 hours. The expertise of a hand surgeon is often needed.
- Instruct the patient to watch the wound for signs of infection, such as redness, warmth, swelling, or purulent exudate.

ANNOTATED BIBLIOGRAPHY

Baile WE, Stowe EC, Schmitt AM: Aerobic bacterial flora of oral and nasal fluids of canines with reference to bacteria associated with bite. J Clin Microbiol 7:223, 1978 (*Aerobic oral and nasal flora of 50 dogs was determined. P. multocida, II-j, EF-4, and S. aureus were all recovered, with high incidence. No anaerobic work was done.*)

Callahorn ML: Dog bite wounds. JAMA 244:2327, 1980 (*A reasonable review of the topic, except we disagree with the use of a penicillinase-resistant penicillin or cephalexin as the "drug of choice."*)

Callahorn ML: Treatment of common dog bites: Infection risk factors. J Am Coll Emerg Physicians 7:83, 1978 (*A retrospective study of 106 patients demonstrated an increased risk of infection in patients older than 50 who delayed seeking treatment and had puncture wounds located on the upper extremities.*)

Chuinard RG, D'Ambrosia RD: Human bite infections of the hand. J Bone Joint Surg 59:416, 1977 (*Forty-two patients were studied retrospectively, and another 59 prospectively. Recommends early and aggressive surgical management and stresses the need for determination of capsule integrity.*)

Ellenbaas RM, McNabuey WK, Robinson WA: Prophylactic oxacillin of dog bite wounds. Ann Emerg Rev 11:248, 1982 (*A prospective study of 63 patients treated with placebo versus oxacillin. The findings that the placebo group did as well as the oxacillin group is at variance with most other studies. No microbiological data are given.*)

Francis DP, Holmes MA, Brandon G: *Pasteurella multocida* infection after domestic animal bites and scratches. JAMA 233:42, 1975 (*A retrospective study attempting to define the role of P. multocida.*)

Goldstein EJC, Citron DM, Miller TA et al: Infections following clenched fist injury: A new perspective. J Hand Surg 3:455, 1978 (*Uses optimal microbiologic methods. Notes significant number of anaerobes [9/16] and Eikenella corrodens [5/15] isolated in wounds. Both penicillin and a penicillinase-resistant penicillin are recommended as initial empiric therapy.*)

Goldstein EJC, Citron DM, Wield B et al: Bacteriology of human and animal bite wounds. J Clin Microbiol 8:667, 1978 (*Stresses the range of organisms, both aerobic and anaerobic, found in bite wounds, and the need for complete microbiology.*)

Mann RJ, Hoffeld TA, Farmer CB: Human bites of the hand: Twenty years of experience. J Hand Surg 2:97, 1977 (*One hundred and thirty-six patients over 20 years were studied retrospectively and another 38 patients were studied prospectively. S. viridans was the most common aerobic pathogen; 44% of wounds had S. aureus. The use of penicillinase-resistant penicillin is recommended.*)

Taylor GA: Management of human bite injuries of the hand. Can Med Assoc J 133:191, 1985 (*A well-conceived approach.*)

196
Management of Minor Burns

Accidental minor burns are common; the majority of the estimated 2 million burn victims can be treated as outpatients. The primary physician will frequently be asked to give advice about immediate care and should render definitive treatment for localized partial thickness burns.

PATHOPHYSIOLOGY AND CLINICAL PRESENTATION

Burns represent direct thermal injury to the cells of the skin and underlying structures. The clinical presentation is dependent on the degree of damage, which is a direct function of the intensity and duration of exposure to heat. The skin in *first-degree burns* is painful, red, and swollen; it blanches with pressure and shows little or no edema. Ultraviolet radiation, scalding, low-intensity exposure to steam, or contact with a hot object are common causes. Complete recovery usually occurs within a week, often with peeling and sometimes with postinflammatory hyperpigmentation. *Second-degree burns* present as painful red blisters or broken epidermis exposing a weeping edematous surface. They are most often caused by scalds or brief exposure to a flame. Recovery requires 2 to 3 weeks; sometimes scarring occurs. *Third-degree burns* usually result from prolonged contact with steam, hot objects, or flames. They present with ulceration, tissue necrosis, and are painless because nerve tissue in the area has been destroyed.

Sunburn is one of the most common types of burns presenting to the office-based physician. It has two phases: an immediate, initial, erythematous phase, which generally fades within 30 minutes after exposure, and a delayed response—what patients call sunburn—occurs 3 to 6 hours after the exposure to the sun and peaks in 12 to 24 hours. Sunburn is characterized by erythema, pruritus, and tenderness, but may proceed to edema, vesiculation, and even blistering.

Sun-related eruptions may also occur as a result of photosensitizing medications. The primary culprits are thiazide diuretics, sulfa-containing agents, tetracyclines (particularly demeclocycline), griseofulvin, phenothiazines, and nalidixic acid. Topical substances, particularly furocoumarins, found in parsley, celery, carrots, certain perfumes, and aftershave lotions, are also photosensitizing.

PRINCIPLES OF THERAPY

The first task is to document the depth of injury and ascertain the area involved. Outpatient management should be limited to patients with partial thickness burns that involve less than 5% to 10% of the body and spare the face, perineum, hands, and feet. Feasibility of outpatient management is determined by the extent of the burn, the patient's reliability, and the support available at home.

The goals of therapy are to reduce inflammation, prevent infection, relieve pain, and promote healing. *First aid* to minor burns involves immediate application of *ice packs* or *cold compresses* of water, milk, or oatmeal. Cold reduces discomfort, edema, and hyperemia and may diminish the extent of injury. The application of cold should continue until the burn is pain-free. Superficial burns require no medication or dressing.

Chemical burns should be placed under *running water* for at least 15 to 30 minutes before cleansing or debridement is started. Patients complaining of pain or displaying anxiety should be given an analgesic or a sedative prior to manipulation of the injured area.

If the skin is broken by a *second-degree burn,* it is important to protect the wound so that healing may occur without infection. This involves gently washing the area of the burn with water and a *mild antiseptic soap,* such as one containing chlorhexidine. Washing is followed by gentle *irrigation* with *sterile isotonic saline* and application of a *sterile occlusive dressing.* Dressings are prepared by applying a nonadherent fine mesh gauze soaked in sterile saline to the burn, and covering this with a bulky dressing that allows drainage into but not through, it. The patient should be examined in 2 days for pain, adenopathy, or fever, and the dressing should be checked. If no evidence of infection is noted, the dressing may remain for 5 to 7 days when the area is reexamined to determine the need for a dressing change.

Controversy exists over the prophylactic use of topical antibiotics in minor burns. The evidence from the literature suggests that they have little or no effect. Topical anesthetics provide symptomatic relief but should be avoided because of the risk of sensitization.

Tetanus prophylaxis includes administering tetanus toxoid booster to previously immunized patients. Pain can usually be relieved with aspirin or acetaminophen. Aspirin has the advantage of suppressing inflammation and is particularly helpful in sunburn. In cases of extensive sunburn, a topical corticosteroid lotion or spray may provide symptomatic relief. Systemic corticosteroids do not reduce the edema associated with sunburn and are not indicated.

THERAPEUTIC RECOMMENDATIONS AND INDICATIONS FOR ADMISSION

- For first-degree burns, immediately apply cold and maintain it until the area is free of pain even after the cold is withdrawn.
- If the skin is broken, cleanse with a mild soap and water before applying cold water or ice.
- No dressing or emollient or antibiotic is needed for first-degree burns. Topical corticosteroid lotion may provide symptomatic relief of extensive sunburn. Aspirin, 600 mg every 4 hours, will provide some analgesia and help limit inflammation. Occasionally systemic steroids are needed for extensive sunburn.
- Second-degree burns with broken skin should be covered by nonadherent gauze impregnated with sterile petrolatum. Wrap the area with several layers of gauze for protection.
- The topical antibiotic silvadene may be used to prevent infection in high-risk second-degree burns.
- Systemic antibiotics, usually dicloxacillin, should be used to treat secondary cellulitis. Prophylactic antibiotic should not be used for fear of selecting out gram-negative organisms.

PATIENT EDUCATION

Patient education is extremely important to the successful resolution of a burn. The patient should be carefully instructed to keep the wound clean and watch for signs of infection. Following healing of the burn, the new epithelial layer may tend to dry and crack; this problem can be reduced by applying lanolin-containing creams for 4 to 8 weeks following healing. Patients with a healed burn should avoid prolonged exposure to direct sunlight for at least 6 months, as well as constricting clothing and strong soaps. The need to tan gradually should be stressed, and the patient should be encouraged to use a sunscreen containing para-aminobenzoic acid to prevent sunburn in the future.

L.A.M.

ANNOTATED BIBLIOGRAPHY

Moncrief JA: Burns. I. Assessment. II. Initial treatment. JAMA 242: 72, 1979 (*A review focusing on emergency management.*)

Nance FC, Lewis VL Jr, Hines JL et al: Aggressive outpatient care of burns. J Trauma 12:144, 1972 (*An approach for the emergency physician.*)

Pathak MA: Sunscreens: Topical and systemic approaches for protection of human skin against the harmful effects of solar radiation. J Am Acad Dermatol 7:285, 1982 (*An excellent review of how to prevent burns and the malignant sequelae of solar radiation.*)

Shuck JM: Outpatient management of the burned patient. Surg Clin North Am 58:1107, 1978 (*A practical and well-reasoned approach to treating burns.*)

Sorenson B: First aid in burn injuries: Treatment at home with cold water. Mod Treat 4:1199, 1967 (*The rationale behind using cold water as an initial treatment.*)

197
Minor Surgical Office Procedures for Skin Problems

ERIC KORTZ, M.D.
CHARLES J. McCABE, M.D.

SIMPLE LACERATIONS

Treatment of simple lacerations is one of the most commonly performed outpatient surgical procedures. All lacerations should be evaluated for the extent of injury to surrounding structures, particularly nerves. This is most important with lacerations of the face, hand, and wrist. All injuries involving peripheral nerves should be referred to an emergency room; digital nerve branches can be approximated with excellent long-term benefit. All tendon injuries should receive the attention of a hand surgeon. Those lacerations complicated by bone fracture should be treated by an orthopedic surgeon.

In uncomplicated wounds, foreign material around and within the wound, including devitalized tissue, should be removed prior to definitive closure.

The following materials are used to treat simple lacerations:

Anesthetic

1. 1% or 2% Xylocaine without epinephrine
2. 5-cc to 10-cc syringes
3. 19-G to 22-G needles

Prep Solution

1. Gentle soap solution
2. Betadine
3. Normal saline

Drapes

1. Three or four sterile towels

Instruments

1. Adson forceps
2. Needle holders (plastic)
3. Hemostat
4. Irrigation bulb syringe
5. Suture scissors
6. Suture material (see Table 197-1)
7. 6 to 12 sterile gauze pads
8. Sterile gloves

Dressings

1. Xeroform gauze
2. Two gauze pads
3. Tape or gauze roll

Anesthesia

- Infiltration of the wound edges may either precede or follow wound cleansing and debridement, depending on the patient and the wound.
- The path of the injecting needle should proceed from clean, prepped areas to deeper tissue levels. The interior of the wound should be avoided.
- Aspiration should precede infiltration of anesthetic to prevent intravascular injection.

Skin-Wound Preparation and Draping

- Copiously irrigate the wound with normal saline under moderate pressure. Foreign material and devitalized tissue are removed at this time. The wound and surrounding skin is then cleansed with a gentle detergent, followed by an antiseptic such as Betadine applied to the surrounding skin only.
- Sterile drapes are placed to isolate the wound completely including enough surrounding skin to allow easy approach and a working surface area.

Wound Closure

- Hemostasis is obtained. Bleeding is usually minimal. Closure proceeds in one or several layers, depending on the depth of the wound. Subcutaneous sutures are of the absorbable type, either 3-0 or 4-0 Dexon or chromic. These sutures should be simple interrupted stitches secured with minimal tension.
- Skin closure for minor lacerations is best achieved with a nonabsorbable, monofilament suture. Nylon is an inexpensive and excellent choice. The suture placement technique should be simple, interrupted, and allow for approximation of the wound edges without inducing ischemia. As Figure 197-1 demonstrates, the curved needle should enter the skin at an acute angle (Fig. 197-1). Advancement is

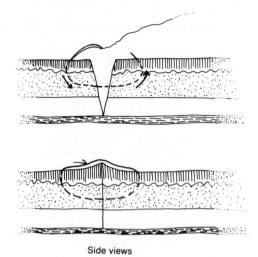

Side views

Figure 197-1. Simple interrupted stitch for skin closure. Notice the path of the needle; the needle enters and leaves the skin at acute angles, which allows eversion of the skin edges. (Grossman JA: Minor Injuries and Disorders: Surgical and Medical Care, p 52. Philadelphia, JB Lippincott, 1984)

then with the natural curve of the needle and includes all layers (epidermis, dermis, and the upper subcutaneous tissue). Care should be taken to maintain equal depth and width from the wound edge with each stitch. A good technique is to sequentially divide the wound in half. The first stitch is placed directly in the center of the laceration. Subsequent sutures subdivide the remaining open surface. Corresponding parts of an irregular wound should be approximated first.

Dressings

- Once the entire wound is closed, normal saline or a gauze sponge can be used to clean the skin of dried blood and Betadine.
- The wound is then covered with a strip of xeroform gauze and dry sterile dressing.
- Lacerations involving the fingers, palm, or wrist should be immobilized.
- Follow-up for patients with minor lacerations can be done at the time of suture removal. A convenient schedule for suture removal is presented in Table 197-1.

SIMPLE PARONYCHIA

Paronychia (Fig. 197-2) represents a soft tissue infection and abscess formation along the nail border. The patient usually complains of pain, and the area surrounding the nail base is red, swollen, and tender.

The following materials are used to treat simple paronychia:

Table 197-1. Suture Selection and Removal Time

LOCATION	SUTURES	REMOVAL TIME (DAYS)
Scalp	3-0	10–14
Face	5-0, 6-0	4–5
Neck	3-0, 4-0	7–10
Trunk	3-0	7–10
Extremities	3-0	8–12
Hands	4-0, 5-0	8–12
Feet	3-0, 4-0	8–12
Oral mucosa	4-0, 3-0 chromic	10–14

Anesthetic

1. 1% or 2% Xylocaine without epinephrine
2. 5-cc to 10-cc syringes
3. 19-G to 22-G needles

Prep Solution

1. Gentle soap solution
2. Betadine or alcohol
3. Normal saline

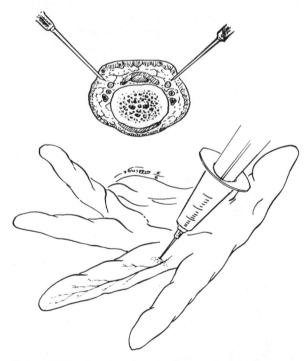

Figure 197-2. Metacarpal block. Entrance of needle is at the palmar base of finger, medial and lateral. The needle path is then toward the palmar metacarpal head. (Van Way CW III, Buerk CA (eds): Surgical Skills in Patient Care, p 55. St Louis, CV Mosby, 1978)

Drapes

1. Three or four sterile towels

Instruments

1. Adson forceps
2. Pediatric suture scissors
3. Kelly clamps
4. No. 15 scalpel blade
5. Scalpel handle
6. Sterile gloves

Dressings

1. Nu-Gauze ¼ inch
2. Two gauze pads
3. Tape or gauze roll

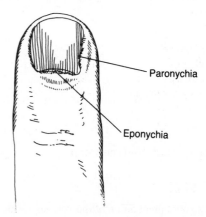

Figure 197-3. Simple paronychia. (Grossman JA: Minor Injuries and Disorders: Surgical and Medical Care, p 253. Philadelphia, JB Lippincott, 1984)

Anesthesia

Complete anesthesia of the finger may be accomplished with a metacarpal block (see Fig. 197-2). After alcohol preparation of the skin over the metacarpophalangeal joint is performed, points for needle entrance are selected on the medial and lateral palmar surface of the metacarpal head. Care is taken to aspirate each time prior to the infiltration of 1 cc to 2 cc of Xylocaine.

Preparation of Skin

The entire digit, including the metacarpal head, may be washed with a gentle soap solution, followed by application of a uniform layer of Betadine.

Draping

Placement of sterile towels must achieve isolation of the digit involved and exposure of the metacarpal area. (Additional anesthesia is sometimes necessary.)

Incision and Drainage

Treatment of the laterally based infection (Fig. 197-3) involves incising the skin along the lateral edge of the nail; a small incision is made directly over the swollen fluctuant area. After drainage of purulent material, a wick is used to prevent premature wound closure. The wick is removed after 24° to 36° and soaking of the digit is begun on a twice-daily schedule.

Occasionally, a portion of the nail must be removed to establish adequate drainage, particularly if the infection has established penetration of the subungual space. A small scissors is used to separate the nail from the underlying matrix. This dissection is carried out from the tip of the nail to the base in a vertical strip involving ¹/₆ inch to ¼ inch of the nail

surface. The nail is then incised with a No. 15 blade or a scissors along this vertical line. A Kelly clamp is then used to grasp the portion of nail to be removed and tease the nail from beneath the eponychium.

Dressing

Xeroform or Vaseline gauze is placed within the wound created by nail removal, taking care to place a layer between the matrix and the eponychium to ensure that nail growth can occur in the area of resection. A gauze pad covers this dressing, which is secured in place. Routine administration of antibiotics is unnecessary; however, those patients with diabetes should be placed on antistreptococcal and antistaphylococcal coverage for 7 days.

ABSCESS

A subcutaneous abscess is seen frequently. The patient will usually complain of pain and swelling. Abscesses commonly occur in the perianal region. If fluctuance is present, incision and drainage should be performed.

The following materials are used to treat abscesses:

Anesthetics

1. 1% to 2% Xylocaine without epinephrine
2. 5-cc to 10-cc syringes
3. 19-G to 22-G needles

Prep Solution

1. Betadine

Drapes

1. Three or four sterile towels

Instruments

1. No. 11 or 15 scalpel blade
2. Scalpel handle
3. Kelly clamps
4. Adson forceps
5. Five or six gauze pads
6. Sterile gloves

Dressing

1. ¼-inch to ½-inch Nu-Gauze strip

Anesthesia

After alcohol preparation of the skin, superficial skin infiltration is carried out in a linear course across the abscess. A second linear course is then traversed directly perpendicular to the first. Care is taken to remain superficial to the abscess cavity.

Skin Preparation

A single layer of Betadine is applied to the abscess and sufficient surrounding skin for adequate exposure.

Drapes

Placement of drapes ensures isolation of the abscess and the prepared surrounding skin.

Incision and Drainage

A linear incision is made through the skin, entering the abscess cavity. The cavity is opened widely across the entire abscess dimension. If more drainage is desired, a second incision is made perpendicular to the first, forming a cruciate design.

Dressing

After complete drainage of the cavity, placement of strip gauze within the wound is necessary to maintain drainage and ensure secondary healing of the wound. Although antibiotics are not necessary for most, those patients with diabetes or accompanying cellulitis may benefit from 24 to 48 hours of gram-positive coverage. Continued packing of the wound should proceed with daily changes until healthy closure of the defect occurs.

BURNS

Burns of the skin can result from many sources: flame, steam, scald, electrical, and chemical. These agents cause variable cellular damage to the layers of epidermis, dermis, and subcutaneous fat, depending on the depth. Classification,

and therefore treatment, of burn wounds is based on the depth and surface area of skin involved. *First-degree burns* are those that involve just the superficial layers of the epidermis (Fig. 197-4). *Second-degree burns* involve the epidermis and dermis; a broad distinction is made between superficial and deep burns, based on the amount of dermis involved. Deep second-degree burns involve the entire papillary dermis, with penetration to some or all of the reticular dermis. *Third-degree burns* involve all layers of the epidermis and dermis, with penetration into underlying fat and muscle.

The surface area of burns has traditionally been based on the rule of nines. Each arm is considered 9% of the body surface area, each leg is 18%, the anterior and the posterior trunk are each 18%, the head is 9%, and perineum/genitalia is 1%.

Using these classifications, the treatment of burns can proceed in an organized fashion. All second-degree burns greater than 20%, all third-degree burns, any burns associated with electrical current, and all burns of the ears, eyes, face, hands, feet, and perineum should be immediately referred to a major hospital familiar with burn care. The remaining first-degree burns and second-degree burns less than 10% to 15% can be cared for on an outpatient basis with adequate wound care and follow-up.

The following materials are used to treat burns:

Prep Solution

1. pHisoHex, gentle soap
2. Normal saline

Drapes

1. Three or four sterile drapes

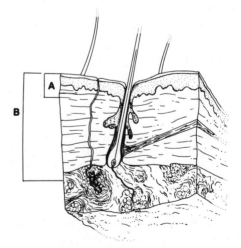

Figure 197-4. Anatomy of the skin demonstrating (*A*) epidermis, (*B*) epidermis and dermis (*i.e.,* full thickness). (Grossman JA: Minor Injuries and Disorders: Surgical and Medical Care, p 71. Philadelphia, JB Lippincott, 1984)

Instruments

1. Adson forceps
2. Suture scissors
3. Silvadene cream
4. Sterile gloves

Dressings

1. Sterile gauze pads
2. Roll gauze

Skin Preparation

Chemical burns should first receive generous lavage with normal saline to dilute the irritant. First- and second-degree burns should be washed with a gentle soap solution. For second-degree burns with ruptured bullae, all free skin should be debrided.

Draping

The cleansed, debrided area of a burn is isolated on a sterile field.

Dressing

Silvadene cream is applied to the surface of the burn in a thin, even layer. Application with a tongue depressor works nicely. Silvadene is subsequently covered with dry gauze pads, which are secured with rolled gauze. Complete dressing change should then be done twice daily, with complete cleansing of the wound before a new dressing is applied. Healing for first-degree burns can be expected in 3 to 4 days; second-degree burns will require 10 to 20 days. Although controversial, treatment with oral penicillin at moderate dosages, 250 mg four times a day for 3 days, may help to prevent deepening of the burn wound secondary to strep infection.

SKIN BIOPSY

The following materials are used in skin biopsies:

Anesthesia

1. 1% or 2% Xylocaine without epinephrine
2. a 5-cc syringe
3. a 22-G needle

Prep Solutions

1. Gentle soap solution
2. Betadine

Drapes

1. Three or four drapes

Instruments

1. No. 15 scalpel blade and handle
2. Sterile skin biopsy punch

3. Adson forceps
4. Suture scissors
5. Needle holders
6. Nylon suture
9. Five or six sterile gauze pads
10. Pathology specimen container
11. Sterile gloves

Dressings

1. Xeroform gauze
2. Gauze pad
3. Tape or gauze roll

Anesthesia

After alcohol preparation of the skin is done, complete superficial skin infiltration is accomplished, including the lesion of interest.

Skin Preparation

After the area is cleansed with a gentle soap, a single layer of Betadine is applied.

Draping

The entire prepared area is isolated from surrounding skin and environment.

Biopsy

If a scalpel blade is to be used, an ellipse, surrounding the lesion in question, is created. The entire depth of the epidermis and dermis should be penetrated. Care is taken in the creation of the ellipse to ensure sufficient local skin mobility to allow edge approximation after skin excision has been done. Skin excision is accomplished by elevating one of the corners and sharply separating it from underlying subcutaneous tissue with sharp scissors. Hemostasis is easily obtained by gentle pressure for 1 to 2 minutes. Wound closure then follows, as described for lacerations.

Alternatively, skin biopsy can be performed by using a skin punch. After anesthesia and skin preparation, the circular punch is pressed against the skin, and cutting is achieved with a gentle twisting motion. Once the entire depth of skin has been traversed, it is separated from underlying subcutaneous tissue with sharp scissors. Wound closure is accomplished with several simple sutures. The specimen is then placed in the proper pathology container and solution.

Dressing

The sutured wound should be covered with a strip of Vaseline-impregnated gauze. A dry sterile gauze pad is placed and held securely with tape or gauze roll.

13

Ophthalmologic Problems

198
Screening for Glaucoma
CLAUDIA U. RICHTER, M.D.

Glaucoma affects more than 1 million Americans and is the cause of 12% of the cases of blindness in the United States. The disease is characterized by damage to the optic nerve caused primarily by abnormally high intraocular pressure. Strictly speaking, the disease process is neither preventable nor curable, but clinicians agree that visual loss can be prevented or minimized if the patient is identified early and the intraocular pressure is controlled.

Secondary glaucoma is associated with ocular inflammation, trauma, systemic disease, or neoplasm and often occurs in patients already under the care of an ophthalmologist. Angle-closure glaucoma is a symptomatic disease: patients present with eye pain or headache associated with decreased visual acuity during an attack. Primary open-angle glaucoma, by far the most prevalent type, is an insidious cause of blindness. Detection of the asymptomatic patient who may be developing irreversible loss of vision depends on routine glaucoma screening by the primary care provider.

EPIDEMIOLOGY AND RISK FACTORS

The prevalence of glaucoma in populations of adults over age 40 is about 2%. Prevalence increases with age and may be greater in nonwhite populations. Rates as high as 6.4% have been reported in medical clinics.

Elevated intraocular pressure is the principal risk factor for glaucomatous visual loss. Although the mean level of intraocular pressure in adult populations is 15 mmHg, both the mean and the standard deviation increase with age.

There is a genetic predisposition to the development of primary open-angle glaucoma: the prevalence among first-degree relatives is approximately 10%. Other risk factors include increasing age, being male, and being black. Diabetes and arterial disease, including vascular hypertension, atherosclerotic heart disease, and cerebrovascular disease, are risk factors.

NATURAL HISTORY AND EFFECTIVENESS OF EARLY THERAPY

The pathophysiology of visual loss in glaucoma is not completely understood and represents a combination of factors. Increased intraocular pressure increases vascular resistance, causing decreased vascular perfusion of the optic nerve and ischemia; it interferes with axoplasmic flow in the ganglion cell axons, causing cell dysfunction and death; and it compresses the lamina cribrosa, the sievelike structure through which axons pass when leaving the eye. The altered supporting struture may then interfere with axonal function. These mechanisms vary in importance in different patients, but the end result is that elevated intraocular pressure causes optic nerve damage and loss of vision.

The relationship between intraocular pressure and glaucomatous field defects is highly variable among individuals. The mean duration of high intraocular pressure before development of field defects has been estimated to be 18 years. The incidence of glaucomatous field defects among patients with ocular hypertension has been shown to be about 1% per year of follow-up.

Visual field loss due to glaucoma is irreversible. The disease process cannot be arrested in an absolute sense, regardless of the stage at which therapy is instituted. Glaucoma is controlled by lowering intraocular pressure by medical, laser, or surgical therapy. Early diagnosis and treatment are important because the clinical consensus is that the optic nerve is more vulnerable to any increase in intraocular pressure once damage has occurred and lower pressure must be maintained to prevent progression in more advanced cases. Several studies support this impression, but it has never been tested with controlled investigation.

SCREENING METHODS

Tonometry. For the primary physician who is not an ophthalmologist, Schiotz tonometry is the most feasible method for measuring intraocular pressure. Applanation tonometry is generally agreed to be both more accurate and more precise, but the equipment is expensive and the technique demands considerable skill. Newer tonometers using an air jet to measure pressure are not available to most primary physicians, but hand-held applanation devices may be.

While measurement error using the Schiotz tonometer can be significant, particularly in myopic patients, the uncertain relationship between intraocular pressure and glaucomatous visual loss is a more important problem in tonometric screening. Within limits, the physician chooses the sensitivity and specificity of tonometric screening by his choice of the level of intraocular pressure used as an indication for referral. Referring patients with modestly elevated pressures will result in a fairly sensitive but nonspecific screen. One study found a sensitivity of about 70% and a specificity of 80% for a referral level of 21.9 mmHg. Raising the referral level to 25.8 mmHg increased specificity to 95%, but at a cost of reducing sensitivity to 50%.

Ophthalmoscopy. Changes in the contour of the optic cup provide the first definitive evidence of glaucoma damage. The optic cup is the depressed area in the center of the optic disc. The usual cup has a round, regular contour; the cup in early glaucoma becomes notched on the superotemporal or inferotemporal rim. Later changes include an increase in the depth and width of the physiologic cup, nasal displacement of the central retinal vessels, and progressive pallor of the optic nerve head. Other disc changes associated with glaucoma are asymmetric discs and disc hemorrhages.

There is disagreement about the value of ophthalmoscopy in detecting early glaucoma; while some authors feel that it is equal to tonometry in detecting definite glaucoma, at least one study has demonstrated unacceptably low sensitivity and specificity. Nevertheless, ophthalmoscopy should be viewed as an important, inexpensive, and convenient screening adjunct, because characteristic glaucomatous disc changes have been well described, and few subjects are found to have both abnormal intraocular pressure and disc abnormalities on screening. Many nonophthalmic physicians are reluctant to perform tonometry, yet routinely perform ophthalmoscopy.

Visual Field Testing. Traditional manual visual field testing is inadequate for mass glaucoma screening because of the time and technical difficulty in performing an adequate examination. The development of automated perimetry has, however, stimulated interest in screening by visual field examination. One study suggested that automated perimetry is a more effective screening method than tonometry or ophthalmoscopy: automated perimetry demonstrated 92% sensitivity and 46% specificity; ophthalmoscopy, 72% sensitivity and 64% specificity; and tonometry, 72% sensitivity and 60% specificity. Automated perimetry is still being investigated as a screening tool and several important guidelines have been found: the screening examination should take 60 to 90 seconds per eye, with a total time of less than 5 minutes per person. The visual field screening device should cost no more than $1000 to $1500 and be extremely simple to operate, and the results should be reported as normal or abnormal.

CONCLUSIONS AND RECOMMENDATIONS

- Glaucoma is highly prevalent in the adult population. It is a major cause of blindness.
- Risk factors for primary open-angle glaucoma include age, sex (males greater than females), race (blacks greater than whites), family history, diabetes mellitus, and vascular disease including vascular hypertension, atherosclerotic heart disease, and cerebrovascular disease.
- Clinical consensus holds that treatment early in the course of the disease is more effective and more likely to prevent visual loss. Such early treatment depends on detection of the asymptomatic patient.
- Schiotz tonometry should be performed on all individuals over 40 years of age. Individuals with elevated levels (>21.9 mm Hg torr) and asymmetry >4 mmHg should be referred for examination by an ophthalmologist.
- Fundoscopic examination is an important screening adjunct and should be used by all primary care physicians.
- Automated perimetry has potential for being an important screening adjunct in the future.
- There are little data on which to base recommendations regarding the frequency of tonometric screening. The apparently long duration of elevated intraocular pressure before development of visual field deficits indicates that pressure measurement every 3 to 5 years is sufficient after a stable baseline is established for the individual patient.

ANNOTATED BIBLIOGRAPHY

Anderson DR: The management of elevated intraocular pressure with normal optic discs and visual fields. I. Therapeutic approach based on high-risk factors. Surv Ophthalmol 21:479, 1977 (*Excellent review of relationship between ocular hypertension and glaucoma.*)

Eddy DM, Sanders LE, Eddy JF: The value of screening for glaucoma with tonometry. Surv Ophthalmol 28:194, 1983 (*A structured review of the test, the effectiveness if therapy and costs—concludes that screening with tonometry is not warranted.*).

Gottlieb LK, Schwartz B, Pauker SG: Glaucoma screening. A cost-effectiveness analysis. Surv Ophthalmol 28:206, 1983 (*A more inclusive analysis than Eddy et al; makes the interesting point that tonometry, ophthalmoscopy, and perimetry have different relative values in different age groups.*)

Keltner JL, Johnson CA: Screening for visual field abnormalities with automated perimetry. Surv Ophthalmol 28:175, 1983 (*Review of studies indicating that automated perimetry can be an effective screening method.*)

Kirsch RE, Anderson DR: Clinical recognition of glaucomatous cupping. Am J Ophthalmol 75:442, 1973 (*Study that defines the characteristic changes of glaucomatous discs.*)

Kitazawa Y et al: Untreated ocular hypertension. Arch Ophthalmol 95:1180, 1977 (*Seven of 75 ocular hypertensives followed a minimum of 9 years developed typical glaucomatous visual field defects. Early clinical findings were not helpful in predicting course.*)

Levi L, Schwartz B: Glaucoma screening in the health care setting. Surv Ophthalmol 28:164, 1983 (*Review of screening surveys and results of a study showing that health care studies had a higher percentage of referrals and that physicians should use ophthalmoscopy in screening.*)

Packer, H et al: Efficiency of screening tests for glaucoma. JAMA 192:693, 1965 (*Provides estimates of sensitivity and specificity for tonometric screening over a range of possible cutoff points.*)

Perkins ES: The Bedford glaucoma survey. I. Long-term follow-up of borderline cases. Br J Ophthalmol 57:179, 1973 (*Four percent of 141 patients followed for 5 to 7 years because of ocular hypertension, suspicious discs, or a positive family history developed glaucoma.*)

Pollack IR: The challenge of glaucoma screening. Surv Ophthalmol 13:4, 1968 (*An extensive review recognizing problems with available screening methods. Recommends age-specific screening levels: age 20 to 39, 21 mmHg; 40 to 59, 22 mmHg; 60 to 79, 24 mmHg.*)

Schwartz JT: Influence of small systematic errors on the results of tonometric screening. Am J Ophthalmol 60:409, 1965 (*Points out that a consistent measurement error of 2 mmHg can increase or decrease the number of patients referred by 60%.*)

199
Evaluation of the Red Eye
ROGER F. STEINERT, M.D.

The red eye is the most common eye problem encountered by the primary care physician. Most cases represent benign self-limited disorders that can be expeditiously diagnosed and treated by the primary physician; however, because redness of the eye may signal serious disease that threatens vision, the physician must be aware of the differential diagnosis and able to conduct a proper initial evaluation.

PATHOPHYSIOLOGY AND CLINICAL PRESENTATION

Redness of the eye and the periocular tissues reflects inflammation and/or hemorrhage. Causes of inflammation include bacterial, viral, chlamydial, and fungal infections, allergic responses, immune disorders, elevated intraocular pressure, environmental and pharmacologic irritants, foreign bodies, and trauma. Hemorrhage may be due to laceration, contusion, coagulopathy, or concomitant infection.

The pattern of conjunctival injection provides important clues in differential diagnosis. Corneal or intraocular inflammation produces "ciliary flush," dilatation of the fine capillaries around the corneal border producing a red-violet halo. Larger, deep episcleral vessels may also be engorged. Primary conjunctivitis induces diffuse vessel engorgement on the palpebral as well as bulbar conjunctiva, without a ciliary flush. The clinical presentations of various causes of red eye are quite distinctive (see Table 199-1).

A red eye may be due to pathology in the conjunctiva, cornea, uveal tract, eyelids, or orbit.

Conjunctival Pathology

CONJUNCTIVITIS is the most common cause of a red eye. Discharge, conjunctival erythema (especially of the peripheral bulbar segment), normal vision, lids stuck together in the morning, and absence of photophobia are the major manifestations. The etiology may be infectious, allergic, or chemical.

BACTERIAL CONJUNCTIVITIS is characterized by a mucopurulent discharge and usually occurs unilaterally without preauricular adenopathy. The eyelids have a thick crust on them after a night's sleep. *Pneumococcus* is most commonly the infectious agent in temperate zones, and *Hemophilus aegyptius* in tropical climates. Grossly purulent conjunctivitis suggests *Neisseria infection,* which may scar or perforate the cornea or lead to systemic dissemination. Chronic conjunctivitis is often due to *S. aureus* or *Moraxella lacunata.* Concomitant sterile marginal corneal ulcers are common with chronic staph infection.

CHLAMYDIAL CONJUNCTIVITIS, transmitted from the genitourinary tract, occurs as bilateral "inclusion conjunctivitis" in sexually active young adults. Exudate is profuse, and preauricular adenopathy is common.

TRACHOMA is the leading cause of blindness worldwide

Table 199-1.   The Red Eye

	CONJUNCTIVITIS			CORNEAL INJURY OR INFECTION	IRITIS	ACUTE GLAUCOMA
	Bacterial	*Viral*	*Allergic*			
Vision	−	−	−	↓ or ↓↓	↓	↓↓
Pain	−	−	−	+	+	+++
Photophobia	−	±	−	+	++	−
Foreign body sensation	−	±	±	+	−	−
Itch	±	±	++	−	−	−
Tearing	+	++	+	++	+	−
Discharge	Mucopurulent	Mucoid	−	−	−	−
Preauricular adenopathy	−	+	−	*	−	−
Pupils	−	−	−	NL or small†	Small	Mid-dilated and fixed
Conjunctival hyperemia	Diffuse	Diffuse	Diffuse	Diffuse and ciliary flush	Ciliary flush	Diffuse and ciliary flush
Cornea	Clear	Sometimes faint punctate staining or infiltrates	Clear	Depends on disorder	Clear or lightly cloudy	Cloudy
Intraocular pressure	NL	NL	NL	NL‡	↓, NL or ↑	↑↑

* In herpes keratitis.

† Indicates secondary iritis.

‡ Very low in perforating trauma.

but is rare in the United States except among American Indians in the Southwest. However, the rapidly increasing rate of chlamydial cervicitis (see Chapter 115) among young women raises the risk of trachoma in a much wider population of newborns.

VIRAL CONJUNCTIVITIS is characterized by watery, sometimes mucoid discharge, often beginning in one eye but spreading to the other eye several days later. Preauricular adenopathy is common. It may be associated with fever and pharyngitis (pharyngoconjunctival fever), particularly in children. Epidemic keratoconjunctivitis (EKC) is a highly contagious adenoviral infection that may be accompanied by corneal epithelial defects in the first week and subepithelial infiltrates in the second week, with some diminution of vision. Pseudomembranes or scarring of the conjunctiva may occur and sometimes are painful.

Bilateral itching and clear tears characterize *allergic conjunctivitis,* which may be associated with seasonal allergies and atopic dermatitis. Vernal keratoconjunctivitis is a chronic recurrent hypersensitivity reaction that may lead to the formation of corneal ulcers. Bilateral *sterile conjunctival inflammation* occurs in acne rosacea, Reiter's syndrome, and Stevens-Johnson syndrome.

HYPERSENSITIVITY to eye medications may cause erythema of the external lids, especially at the lateral canthus. *Angioneurotic edema* of the lids may occur bilaterally as an allergic response to a systemic allergen, often food, or unilaterally secondary to exposure to local allergens such as topical chemicals, poison ivy, and insect bites; it develops rapidly and resolves in 1 to 2 days. Edema without erythema suggests allergy.

PINGUECULA is a yellow harmless nodule of the scleral conjunctiva, usually found on the nasal side, causing only mild discoloration. However, a related disorder, *pterygium,* is vascularized. It causes redness and encroaches on the cornea. The condition is most common in patients heavily exposed to strong sunlight.

SUBCONJUNCTIVAL HEMORRHAGE is distinctive in appearance. In most cases the bleeding occurs secondary to trauma. The patient may be unaware of the minor trauma involved. In patients receiving anticoagulant medications, spontaneous subconjunctival hemorrhage may be a sign of overdosage. Massive subconjunctival hemorrhage accompanied by proptosis and limited extraocular movements, usually after trauma, signals orbital hemorrhage, which may compromise the optic nerve and retinal circulation.

FOREIGN BODY on the bulbar conjunctiva or under either the upper or lower lid may result in copious tearing, conjunctival injection, and a sensation that something has gotten "into" the eye. On occasion, the foreign body may be well tolerated, with the eye remaining white and quiet.

EPISCLERITIS is usually a benign inflammation of superficial episcleral vessels. The conjunctiva manifests areas of circumscribed nodular inflammation, seen in association with collagen disease, gout, allergic conditions, and such skin diseases as psoriasis. The patient complains of tender irritated eyes; vision and lids are normal; the cornea is clear; the conjunctiva shows local raised areas of redness.

SCLERITIS, often associated with rheumatoid arthritis and other immune disorders, is a potentially destructive inflammation of the collagen in the deep episcleral vessels and the sclera itself. The eye is sometimes painful. Fortunately, scleritis is rare. An experienced observer is required to make the diagnosis.

Corneal Disease

KERATITIS presents with a perilimbal ciliary flush, accompanied by clear tears and photophobia. Corneal ulcers detected by fluorescein staining may be sterile or caused by bacteria, viruses, or fungi. Particularly distinctive is the "dendritic" figure of herpes simplex keratitis, in which the epithelium stains in a fine, branching pattern. Herpes simplex and zoster may also cause broader, "geographic" defects. *S. aureus* may cause a sterile infiltrate in the corneal limbus.

CORNEAL ABRASIONS stain with fluorescein but have no infiltrate unless they are untreated for several days. *Hyphema* (blood layering in the anterior chamber) indicates severe trauma and requires ophthalmologic consultation. *Recurrent erosion* presents as an epithelial defect at the site of an abrasion that occurred months or years before and was often caused by organic material (*e.g.,* tree branch, fingernail). It may also occur in corneal dystrophies. In both instances, it is due to a defect in epithelial adherence to the underlying stroma. A *corneal foreign body* may cause tearing and hyperemia with little sensation of a foreign body. This is particularly true of rust rings left by ferrous foreign bodies. Dry eyes can cause intense reactions secondary to superficial keratitis, as does overwearing of contact lenses (corneal hypoxia) and ultraviolet keratitis. *Corneal laceration* with perforation is suggested by a shallow or absent anterior chamber, markedly decreased intraocular pressure, and eccentric pupil with iris prolapse into the wound.

CHEMICAL KERATOCONJUNCTIVITIS is a common industrial injury due to a splash of an irritant solution. The conjunctiva is uniformly red, the pupil constricted, vision decreased, the cornea hazy, and the eye painful because of spasm of the iris.

Uveal Tract Disease

UVEITIS refers to inflammation of the uveal tract, including the iris, ciliary body, and choroid. The diagnosis is suggested by pain, photophobia, redness, and ciliary flush. Iritis presents with eye pain, photophobia, redness, and pupillary contraction. It may be unilateral or bilateral; if uni-

lateral, the pupil is smaller than that of the other eye because of spasm. Flashlight examination shows a slightly cloudy anterior chamber. Slit lamp examination discloses cells in the anterior chamber and "flare," representing increased aqueous humor protein. Inflammatory cells, called "keratic precipitates," may collect in clusters on the posterior cornea.

Iritis and uveitis are usually idiopathic, but may be associated with a large number of systemic and ocular diseases. Ankylosing spondylitis, sprue, granulomatous colitis, tuberculosis, sarcoidosis, and juvenile rheumatoid arthritis are sometimes associated with uveitis. The HLA-B27 tissue antigen is strongly associated with iritis, often accompanied by ankylosing spondylitis or Behçet's disease. Secondary iritis occurs in response to blunt trauma or corneal inflammation.

Eyelid and Orbital Disease

BLEPHARITIS connotes inflammation involving the structures of the lid margin with redness, scaling, and crusting. Examination of the lid margin may reveal inspissated sebaceous material. Staphylococcal blepharitis causes dry scales, lash loss, and sometimes conjunctivitis and corneal limbal infiltrates. Seborrheic blepharitis is associated with greasy scales and less redness. Blepharitis tends to be chronic with acute flare-ups, and is more common in fair-skinned people.

HORDEOLUM is an acute staphylococcal infection of the meibomian glands (internal hordeolum) or of the glands of Zeis or Moll around the lashes (external hordeolum or sty). It may present as diffuse redness, tenderness, and edema, localized only by an inspissated meibomian gland. An internal hordeolum may point either to the skin or conjunctival side of the lid, while an external hordeolum always points to the skin. Hordeolum may produce a diffuse superficial lid infection known as "preseptal cellulitis."

CHALAZION is a sterile granulomatous inflammation of the meibomian gland, which may be tender and mildly inflammed or a quiet, discrete mass.

ACUTE DACRYOCYSTITIS is a tender, warm, localized infection of the tear ducts over the lateral nose; purulent material may be expressed from the tear duct upon the application of pressure.

HEMORRHAGE in the lids or forehead, either spontaneous or traumatic, may rapidly dissect along the tissue planes of the lids and cause an impressive generalized ecchymosis, greatly alarming the patient.

ORBITAL CELLULITIS is usually caused by gram-positive organisms that enter the orbit either directly from the sinuses or through venous channels. It presents as swollen, red eyelids with chemosis, exophthalmos, pain, fever, and leukocytosis. If it progresses, it may lead to paresis of the third, fourth, and sixth cranial nerves, or the ophthalmic division of the fifth, signs of the very serious complication *cavernous sinus thrombosis.*

Intraocular Disease

ACUTE GLAUCOMA is an ocular emergency that presents as a painful, red eye with prominent ciliary flush. The pupil is middilated and fixed, and the cornea is cloudy secondary to edema. Intraocular pressure is above 40 and may reach 70 to 80. The patient reports cloudy vision, colored rings around lights (due to corneal edema), and unilateral headache, often accompanied by nausea and vomiting, occasionally leading the physician to consider an acute abdomen. Acute glaucoma is usually due to closure in eyes with narrow angles, but may be due to inflammatory cells or red blood cells in the anterior chamber, neovascularization of the iris (rubeosis iridis), or peripheral anterior synechiae.

DIFFERENTIAL DIAGNOSIS

The causes of red eye can be divided anatomically into the categories of conjunctival, corneal, uveal, eyelid–orbital, and intraocular disease (see Table 199-2). Differentiation can usually be made on clinical grounds (see Table 199-1).

WORKUP

History is directed toward ascertaining the duration of redness, rapidity of onset, the patient's activity at the time,

Table 199-2. Some Important Causes of Red Eye

Conjunctival Disease
Infection (bacterial, viral, chlamydial)
Allergy
Foreign body
Subconjunctival hemorrhage
Pinguecula
Pterygium
Episcleritis
Scleritis
Abrasion

Corneal Disease
Herpes simplex
Adenovirus
Herpes zoster
Keratoconjunctivitis sicca
Exposure keratopathy
Chemical trauma
Corneal ulceration (with or without concomitant infection)

Uveal Tract Disease
Primary iritis and choroiditis
Secondary iritis (infection, trauma)
Systemic diseases (collagen vascular)

Diseases of the Eye and Orbit
Blepharitis
Chalazion
Hordeolum
Dacryocystitis
Cellulitis
Hemorrhage

Intraocular Disease
Acute glaucoma

and the degree and quality of symptoms. Ophthalmologic history and medications should be noted. Key symptoms include visual changes, pain, itching, crusting in the morning, tearing, mucoid or purulent discharge, photophobia, and foreign body sensation. While usually helpful, the history can be misleading, as viral conjunctivitis may be accompanied by itching or a foreign body sensation, or the patient may ascribe the symptoms of herpes simplex keratitis to a "chemical in the eye" because she first noted the symptoms after a home hair permanent.

Examination. Accurate measurement of visual acuity, preferably at a distance, is essential. If it is abnormal, it is important to check for uncorrected optical abnormality by use of a pinhole. Any patient with reduced vision not readily explained by a preexisting or obviously harmless condition needs immediate referral to an ophthalmologist. Mucus and tearing may reduce vision one or two lines at most. Corneal lesions may further reduce vision, with only partial improvement on pinhole testing; a central epithelial abrasion typically maintains vision at about 20/100 or better. Preauricular nodes should be palpated. A complete examination of the eye and fundus is important. The lid margins should be inspected for crusting, ulceration, inspissations, and masses, and the conjunctiva for distribution of redness, ciliary flush, foreign bodies (including lid eversion) and, if a slit lamp is available, follicles and papillae. Corneal clarity is noted with a flashlight, and a direct ophthalmoscope set at about +15 diopters can be used to magnify corneal details.

If fluorescein stain is available it can be used in conjunction with a blue filter to visualize the cornea for infection and other injury. However, if there is any suspicion of corneal injury, referral is needed quickly for slit lamp examination.

Intraocular pressure should be determined if glaucoma is suspected. Depth of the anterior chamber of the other eye can be assessed by a flashlight shined parallel to the iris (coronal plane) from the temporal side. A shallow anterior chamber is usually convex and will cast a shadow on the nasal iris.

Laboratory Studies are usually the responsibility of an ophthalmologist. The primary practitioner may attempt conjunctival smears, which show polymorphonuclear leukocytes in acute bacterial conjunctivitis, lymphocytes in viral or late bacterial conjunctivitis, and eosinophils in allergic reactions. This is time-consuming and generally not necessary. Purulent discharges should be cultured on blood agar and, if *Neisseria* is suspected, chocolate agar; Gram stain may reveal gram-negative diplococci in such cases. Scrapings for inclusion bodies in suspected chlamydial or viral disease are usually unrewarding, and scraping and culture of an infected corneal ulcer requires an ophthalmologist.

White blood cell and differential counts are indicated, as are blood cultures, in suspected cellulitis. Clotting studies for subconjunctival hemorrhage are not indicated unless other evidence of coagulopathy is present or the patient is being treated with anticoagulants (see Chapter 85).

PRINCIPLES OF MANAGEMENT AND INDICATIONS FOR REFERRAL

Red eye problems associated with eye pain, visual disturbance, or corneal damage require immediate referral, as does acute glaucoma. In most other situations, the primary physician can provide symptomatic relief or at least first aid.

Blepharitis usually responds to lid hygiene measures and topical antibiotics. One can instruct the patient to dilute Johnson's baby shampoo 50:50 with water and use a cotton ball to scrub the lids well with the eyes closed. After rinsing with water, a hot compress is applied to the closed lids for 5 to 10 minutes, and then erythromycin or bacitracin ophthalmic ointment is instilled in the inferior fornix. Carrying out this procedure three to four times daily will improve most cases. Normal lids can be maintained by nightly lid hygiene and warm compresses. A *hordeolum* may respond to this treatment or, like *chalazia,* may require incision and curettage by an ophthalmologist.

Minor *cellulitis* of the lid margin (preseptal cellulitis) responds to topical treatment plus oral antibiotics. Dicloxacillin (250 mg qid) is a good first choice. Erythromycin, 250 to 500 mg PO tid, is an effective alternative for patients who are penicillin allergic. Warm compresses and oral antibiotics are also indicated for *acute dacryocystitis,* but persistent localized abscess requires incision and drainage by an ophthalmologist. Orbital cellulitis and cavernous sinus thrombosis are medical emergencies that require immediate hospitalization for intravenous therapy.

Mild hypersensitivity reactions of the lids respond rapidly to discontinuation of the offending agent and application of cool compresses. Systemic antihistamines are useful in moderate reactions, and steroids in severe reactions.

Cool compresses and ice packs applied early can minimize *lid ecchymoses* from trauma; later, warm compresses speed resolution.

Conjunctivitis, in which there is no photophobia, no eye pain, and no change in visual acuity, can be treated by the primary physician. Erythromycin ophthalmic ointment, four times daily, is usually an effective antimicrobial treatment for *bacterial conjunctivitis.* Bacitracin ophthalmic ointment and sodium sulfacetamide are alternative medications. Neomycin causes allergic keratitis in 5% of patients treated topically and should be avoided if possible. *Neisseria* requires systemic penicillin therapy. Bacterial conjunctivitis improves in several days; viral conjunctivitis may take several weeks. Viral conjunctivitis is quite contagious, and live virus is shed in the tears for up to 2 weeks. The patient should be instructed to refrain from rubbing the eye and transmitting infection to

the other eye or to another person. Cases that fail to respond should be reevaluated by an ophthalmologist. A nonophthalmologist should never prescribe topical steroid or steroid–antibiotic combination drops, as infection may worsen and a corneal ulcer may rapidly form and cause perforation.

Allergic conjunctivitis in seasonal allergies is relieved by cool compresses and decongestant–antihistamine drops (Vasocon-A, Albalon-A) four times a day, as well as oral antihistamines. Long-term use of these drops is not recommended, because marked rebound vasodilation may develop. Severe allergic conditions may require topical steroid therapy instituted by an ophthalmologist. Cromolyn 4% ophthalmic solution has recently emerged as an alternative to steroids. However, its onset of action is slow, taking up to a week to show an effect.

Subconjunctival hemorrhage usually requires only reassurance; compresses (initially cool, then warm) and erythromycin ophthalmic ointment or a lubricating ointment may reduce discomfort in cases with marked swelling.

Conjunctival foreign bodies are usually easily removed with a cotton swab or fine forceps; erythromycin ointment tid for 2 days is adequate for healing.

Corneal ulcers require intensive emergency evaluation and treatment by an ophthalmologist. Patients with typical herpes simplex dendritic keratitis may be started on idoxuridine or vidarabine ointment five times daily and erythromycin ointment twice daily if an ophthalmologist is not available. *Corneal abrasions* heal rapidly with erythromycin ointment and a tight sterile patch that prevents lid motion for 24 to 48 hours. If the initial abrasion was sizable (roughly 25% of the cornea or more), healing should be checked after removal of the patch. Lesions of this size also require cycloplegia for relief of painful secondary iritis during healing (see iritis treatment). After reepithelialization occurs, ointment applied three times daily for 4 days helps complete the healing process. Cases involving *foreign bodies* and rust rings are treated like abrasions once the body has been removed. Foreign bodies may be irrigated and then removed with a cotton swab, a sterile "golf stick," or an 18-gauge needle with a syringe as a handle. Rust on the surface is easily debrided, but scraping is prohibited as it will damage Bowman's membrane and cause permanent scarring. Left untreated, rust may be irritating, but will surface and slough in 1 or 2 weeks. *Contact lens overwear* and *ultraviolet keratitis* respond to brief cycloplegia, erythromycin ointment, and sterile pressure patching for 24 hours. The associated pain often requires codeine.

Suspected *corneal laceration* and *perforation* is an ophthalmic emergency. A protective metal shield ("Fox shield") should be placed over the eye; no medication should be instilled.

An ophthalmologist must evaluate and treat *primary iritis,* but initial cycloplegia by tropicamide 1% qid or cyclopentolate 1% qid will prevent posterior synechia formation and relieve pain. *Iritis* secondary to corneal abrasion may be treated with these medications or, in an eye that will be patched for 1 or 2 days, several drops of scopolamine 0.25% will provide longer cycloplegia. The nonophthalmologist should avoid atropine, as its effects persist for 1 to 2 weeks.

Acute glaucoma should be treated by immediate administration of acetazolamide, 500 mg IV, and glycerol, 120 cc orally in orange juice. Pilocarpine 2% should be begun with instillation as frequently as every 15 minutes to break the attack. Immediate attention by an ophthalmologist is necessary, because the only definitive treatment is laser or surgical iridotomy.

ANNOTATED BIBLIOGRAPHY

Baum JL: Ocular infections. N Engl J Med 299:28, 1978 (*Succinct overview.*)

Cromolyn sodium for allergic conjunctivitis. Med Let 27:7, 1985 (*Brief review of its efficacy.*)

Drugs for bacterial conjunctivitis. Med Lett 18:70, 1976 (*A succinct, critical review of topical agents; external infections with gonococci. C. trachomatis, and Pseudomonas require systemic as well as topical treatment. Caution is suggested in the use of topical corticosteroids. A table of suggested treatments for the major organisms involved in bacterial conjunctivitis is presented.*)

Hazelman BL: Ocular manifestations of rheumatoid diseases. Practitioner 217:83, 1978 (*Details of the many findings.*)

Jones ELR: The red eye. Practitioner 219:59, 1977 (*An excellent review that divides the red eye into those in which vision is affected, watery eyes in which vision is not affected, and red sticky eyes in which vision is not affected. A flowchart is presented.*)

Leibowitz HM, Pratt MV, Flagstad IJ et al: Human conjunctivitis: Diagnostic evaluation. Arch Ophthalmol 94:1747, 1976 (*A diagnostic approach is presented showing little correlation between clinical signs and ultimate etiologic diagnosis.*)

Perkins RE, Kundsin RB, Pratt MV et al: Bacteriology of normal and infected conjunctiva. J Clin Microbiol 1:147, 1975 (*A careful bacteriologic study that shows that anaerobic organisms may be responsible for many cases of chronic conjunctivitis.*)

Smolen G, Okumoto M: Staphylococcal blepharitis. Arch Ophthalmol 95:812, 1977 (*A review of this very common cause of red eye, emphasizing detailed treatment.*)

Thoft RA: Corneal disease. N Engl J Med 298:1239, 1978 (*A short review for the generalist.*)

Vaughan D, Asbury T: General Ophthalmology. Ed 8. Los Altos-Lange, 1977 (*A practical and inexpensive reference with photographs and details.*)

200
Evaluation of Impaired Vision
CLAUDIA U. RICHTER, M.D.

Patients with decreasing or blurred vision often refer themselves directly to an eye specialist, but at times they first present to their primary physician. Sudden visual loss is a medical emergency. Gradual diminution of sight raises the specter of eventual blindness and inability to function independently. Paradoxically, some elderly patients may not volunteer that their vision is decreasing because they consider it a natural part of aging. Consequently, the primary physician needs to screen elderly patients for treatable causes of decreased vision. In addition, one should be capable of distinguishing between visual impairment due to refractive error, cataracts, glaucoma, retinal disease, and trauma to provide proper initial care and appropriate referral.

PATHOPHYSIOLOGY AND CLINICAL PRESENTATION

Vision is impaired when there is a change in the refracting surfaces of the eye, opacification of the transparent ocular media, damage to the photoreceptor cells of the retina, or a lesion of the optic nerve, its radiations, or the visual cortex. Anatomic orientation provides a framework for considering the pathophysiology of visual difficulties, beginning with the cornea and working inward.

Refractive error remains the most common cause of decreased visual acuity. It results from the inability of the eye to focus light precisely on the retina and may be due to an abnormality in the cornea, lens, or size of the globe. Myopic patients commonly present during their teens and early 20s. Patients in their 40s may report decreased visual acuity but, in fact, simply cannot accommodate to near distances and require reading glasses. Early cataracts can increase myopia before they opacify and block transmission of light. Uncontrolled diabetes mellitus produces swelling of the lens and myopia, which resolves with control of the blood sugar. Sulfonamides, thiazides, and anticholinergic agents, may cause blurred vision.

Occasionally, sudden visual loss results from *eyelids* being closed by *swelling* due to trauma, insect bites, cellulitis, or angioneurotic edema. Acute *blepharospasm* secondary to ocular surface pain may be described as inability to see.

The *cornea* is the major refracting surface of the eye, and any change in it can lead to visual disturbances. A *corneal abrasion,* herpes simplex virus keratitis, or ulcer causes irregularity of the corneal epithelium and opacity of the normally clear cornea. *Acute glaucoma* causes sudden visual loss by producing corneal edema. Corneal dystrophies or degenerations result in a more gradual reduction in visual acuity, often progressing over a period of years.

The *anterior chamber* may be opacified by inflammatory cells resulting from iritis or red blood cells resulting from a *hyphema.*

Cataracts, opacifications of the lens, are a leading cause of gradual vision loss in older patients. The usual history is one of a painless, slow deterioration of eyesight. However, a traumatic cataract may develop over a period of hours to days.

Vitreous opacification occurs most often from *hemorrhage,* less commonly from inflammation or infection. Proliferative diabetic retinopathy, a retinal hole or detachment, trauma, sickle cell retinopathy, hypertension, and clotting abnormalities may cause vitreous hemorrhage. A vitreous *floater* may transiently blur vision or be called a blind spot.

Glaucoma may damage nerve fibers at the optic disk and cause visual field defects. Four types of visual field defects occur: paracentral scotomas occurring along the distribution of the arcuate nerve fiber bundle, arcuate scotomata, sector-shaped defects, and nasal steps. As the disease progresses, these visual field defects enlarge. Central vision remains intact until late in the disease, but even this may be lost. Acute angle-closure glaucoma produces a red eye, fixed pupil, hazy cornea, eye pain, and acute impairment of vision. Acute angle-closure glaucoma accounts for less than 5% of all glaucoma cases. Most visual loss due to glaucoma is gradual and progressive (see Chapter 206).

The *retina* may be compromised by degeneration, inflammation, trauma, detachment, or ischemia. *Senile macular degeneration* occurs in patients over age 55 and is a leading cause of legal blindness. Central vision is impaired while peripheral vision remains intact. Fundoscopic examination may show loss of the foveal reflex, macular drusen, atrophy of the retinal pigment epithelium with prominent choroidal vessels, subretinal edema or hemorrhage, or a central fibrous scar. Some 15% patients with senile macular degeneration have treatable disease, presenting with early visual symptoms and a subretinal neovascular net that can be obliterated with laser photocoagulation. They need to be seen promptly to maximize their chances of effective treatment. Those at particular risk of developing exudative senile macular degeneration have drusen or a disciform scar in one macula; they should screen their central vision daily with an Amsler grid.

A host of other retinal problems may lead to loss of vision. *Central serous retinopathy* is an idiopathic, spontaneous *detachment* of the retina in the macular area. Patients range in age from 20 to 50 years. Central vision is reduced, but recovery is usually spontaneous within a few months. *Inflammation* of the retina and choroid, such as histoplasmosis,

toxoplasmosis, cytomegalovirus, or herpes virus infections, can involve the macula or produce a vitritis, decreasing vision. *Trauma* may cause retinal edema and decreased visual acuity when it occurs in the macular region. This edema resolves within a few days.

Retinal detachment may be extensive and cause decreased visual acuity or be small and noted as a minor field defect. Flashing lights and a *shower of vitreous floaters* may presage a retinal detachment. As a detachment extends, the patient may note that the visual field defect progresses like a shade being drawn. A detached retina appears ballooned forward with undulating folds.

The *vasculature* of the *retina* or *optic nerve* may be compromised, leading to sudden visual loss. The vascular diseases involving the arteries include central retinal artery occlusion, giant-cell arteritis, and anterior ischemic optic neuropathy. In *central retinal artery occlusion,* there is sudden, painless loss of ability to perceive light or hand movements. The patient may have had previous episodes of amaurosis fugax with fleeting blindness lasting 10 to 15 minutes. Ophthalmoscopy reveals a pale optic disc, attenuated arterioles, "boxcar" veins, hazy edematous retina, and a *cherry-red spot* in the macula. Occasionally, an *embolus* may be seen at a bifurcation of a retinal arteriole. The most common embolic source is an atheromatous plaque in the ipsilateral carotid artery.

Giant-cell or *temporal arteritis,* a granulomatous inflammation of the medium and large arteries in elderly people, may cause sudden visual loss (see Chapter 156). These patients may have premonitory visual symptoms similar to amaurosis fugax and may have symptoms of polymyalgia rheumatica. The fundus examination may reveal a swollen optic disc, a normal optic disc, or a central retinal artery occlusion.

Anterior ischemic optic neuropathy is produced by ischemia to the anterior portion of the optic nerve. The patient notes decreased visual acuity and/or a visual field defect, usually involving the superior or inferior visual field and the macula. The optic disc initially appears edematous, sometimes in just one portion, with a few flame-shaped hemorrhages. Optic atrophy follows the disc edema. The most common etiology is *thrombosis* of an arteriosclerotic vessel. The patients tend to be younger than those affected by giant-cell arteritis and have hypertension or diabetes mellitus.

Central or branch *retinal vein occlusions* cause a sudden painless decrease in visual acuity. In central retinal vein occlusion, the *fundus* has a classic *"blood and thunder"* appearance: the veins are tortuous and dilated and the retina is edematous and covered with flame-shaped hemorrhages. The optic disc margin is blurred. The fundus changes in branch retinal vein occlusion are similar, but limited to the distribution of the involved vein. Decreased visual acuity is due to macular edema and ischemia. In central retinal vein occlusion, 20% of patients have preexisting chronic open-angle glaucoma, and 50% of men have preexisting hypertension. In branch retinal vein occlusion, 75% have preexisting hypertension.

Optic neuritis, inflammation of the optic nerve, presents with a relatively acute impairment of vision. It is usually idiopathic but can be associated with multiple sclerosis. Clinically, there is progressive loss of vision over hours to days, typically unilateral, with pain on eye motion and improved visual function in the second to third week. Examination reveals an afferent pupillary defect, globe tenderness, visual field defects, and impairment of color vision.

Infiltrative or compressive lesions of the optic nerve, such as pituitary adenomas, meningiomas, gliomas, or internal carotid artery aneurysms, cause gradual visual field loss. It is unusual for lesions posterior to the optic chiasm to present with decreased visual acuity because of the decussation of fibers in the optic chiasm. Unilateral lesions, such as a tumor or a cerebrovascular accident, cause a homonymous hemianopsia or related visual field defect. Bilateral central nervous system lesions may cause profound visual loss.

Many patients complain of blurred vision at night. Rarely, these patients may be found to have true *night blindness* caused by retinitis pigmentosa or vitamin A deficiency. More commonly, no etiology is found; a slight decrease in visual acuity at night is common and normal.

Systemic diseases may involve the retina and cause decreased vision. Hypertension, diabetes mellitus, anemia, leukemia, Waldenstrom's macroglobulinemia, and systemic lupus erythematosus are examples. Also, hysterical patients and malingerers may present with complaints of visual loss.

DIFFERENTIAL DIAGNOSIS

The causes of visual impairment can be logically considered in terms of anatomic site affected (Table 200-1).

WORKUP

History is most important in evaluating a complaint of visual loss. It is necessary to determine the length and pattern of visual loss, whether the loss is bilateral or unilateral, and if pain is present. The presence of premonitory symptoms is helpful. Acute loss is suggestive of a vascular event or retinal detachment. Preceding episodes of amaurosis fugax indicate central retinal artery occlusion or giant-cell arteritis. A sudden flurry of flashes of light and vitreous floaters may herald a retinal detachment. Progressive visual loss points to a chronic disturbance, such as cataract, macular degeneration, or glaucoma. Previous episodes of decreased visual acuity with halos around lights and pain indicate angle-closure glaucoma. A foreign body sensation indicates a corneal abrasion, foreign body, or herpes simplex keratitis. The presence of other diseases such as diabetes mellitus, hypertension, heart disease, or sickle cell anemia may be contributory. A history of trauma is important to note.

Table 200-1. Causes of Impaired Vision

Eyelids
  Edema
  Blepharospasm

Cornea
  Abrasion
  Edema
  Degeneration

Anterior chamber
  Inflammatory cells (from iritis)
  Hyphema

Lens
  Cataract
  Swelling (as in poorly controlled diabetes)

Vitreous
  Hemorrhage
  Floaters

Retina
  Senile macular degeneration
  Central serous retinopathy
  Inflammation
  Trauma
  Detachment
  Diabetes
  Hypertension

Vasculature
  Central retinal artery occlusion
  Giant-cell (cranial or temporal) arteritis
  Anterior ischemic optic neuropathy
  Retinal vein occlusion

Optic nerve
  Compression (glaucoma, tumor)

Psychiatric
  Hysteria
  Malingering

Refractive error

Physical Examination and Laboratory Studies. Vision should be *tested* one eye at a time. If the patient complains of pain, a topical anesthetic such as proparacaine should be used to allow examination. If the lids are tightly swollen, it may be necessary to pry them apart forcibly. The patient should wear his glasses. A Snellen eye chart with its standardized letter sizes is most convenient, but if one is not available any printed material can be used. One notes the size of the smallest print the patient can read and the distance at which he can read it. If letters cannot be read, the distance at which the patient can accurately count fingers or identify hand motions is noted. If targets cannot be seen, it is important to determine whether or not the eye can perceive light. Vision is rechecked with the patient looking through a pinhole to eliminate any residual refractive error.

The *pupils* should be examined carefully, noting size, direct and consensual reactions to light, and presence of any afferent pupillary defect. An afferent pupillary defect may be found in optic neuritis, central retinal artery occlusion, giant-cell arteritis, and extensive retinal diseases. A fixed pupil in conjunction with a red eye is indicative of acute angle-closure glaucoma.

The *conjunctiva* is examined to determine whether the eye is red and inflamed or white and quiet. With the exception of trauma, acute glaucoma, and infection, the diseases that cause sudden visual loss do not cause a red eye (see Chapter 199). The *cornea* normally is clear with a crisp light reflex and no fluorescein stain. If a tonometer is available, the *intraocular pressure* should be measured.

Ophthalmoscopy is important; it should first be noted whether the *fundus* can be visualized or if a dense cataract or vitreous opacity is present. If the fundus can be visualized, the optic disk is examined for papilledema or atrophy. The *macula* is examined, looking for a cherry-red spot, hemorrhages, and scars. The *vessels* are examined, with attention paid to the caliber and the presence of visible emboli. Patients over age 50 with sudden visual loss should have an *erythrocyte sedimentation rate* to check for temporal arteritis (see Chapter 156).

If a patient is a malingerer or hysterical, the examination of the eye will be normal. It may be necessary to trick the patient to make a diagnosis of hysterical blindness. An easy way is to test *opticokinetic responses,* one eye at a time: to have normal opticokinetic responses, the eye must be able to fixate on the test object. Passing a newspaper front page before the eyes of the patient is a useful test: normal opticokinetic responses with headlines correlate with 20/200 vision. Stereoscopic vision remains normal. Finally, *visual field* testing at different distances is helpful. If one doubles the distance between the patient and the testing screen, the size of the visual field should double. For most hysterical and malingering patients, the size of the visual field remains unchanged.

SYMPTOMATIC MANAGEMENT AND INDICATIONS FOR REFERRAL

Patients with sudden visual loss need immediate ophthalmologic consultation. If an ophthalmologist is not immediately available, there are appropriate emergency measures that should be taken.

If a *central retinal artery occlusion* exists that is less than 24 hours old, it is reasonable to attempt heroic measures to salvage vision. The goal is to encourage the embolus to break apart or at least to move distally. First, one can gently *massage the globe* with the fingers to attempt to dislodge the embolus. Next, have the patient *breathe a mixture* of *5% CO_2 and 95% O_2*; this will cause the retinal vessels to vasodilate and allow delivery of a high pO_2 to any viable retinal cells. If this mixture is not available, have the patient *breathe into a paper bag.* Next, give the patient *500 mg intravenous acetazolamide* to decrease the production of aqueous humor and lower intraocular pressure.

If the physician suspects *giant-cell arteritis,* the patient should be started at once on *60 mg* of *prednisone* a day. Some vision may be salvaged in the affected eye, and the other eye is protected (see Chapter 156).

Acute angle-closure glaucoma should be treated at once with *topical pilocarpine 2%* in both eyes and *acetazolamide 500 mg intravenously.* The pilocarpine acts therapeutically in the involved eye and prophylactically in the uninvolved eye. Pain medication and antiemetics are appropriate. If available, osmotic agents such as intravenous *mannitol* or oral *glycerol* should be used. All patients with acute angle-closure glaucoma need a laser iridotomy or peripheral iridectomy to prevent further attacks.

INDICATIONS FOR REFERRAL

All patients with acute loss of vision should be seen immediately by an ophthalmologist. Individuals suspected of having glaucoma, macular degeneration, or retinal vein occlusion, as well as those in whom the cause of impaired vision is unclear, should have early ophthalmologic consultation. Referral for cataracts can wait until some functional impairment is noted by the patient.

ANNOTATED BIBLIOGRAPHY

Chisolm IA: Gradual visual loss. Practitioner 219:64, 1977 (*A good review with clear branching logic.*)

Cullen JF, Coleiro JA: Ophthalmic complications of giant cell arteritis. Surv Ophthalmol 20:247, 1976 (*An excellent review of temporal arteritis and its visual manifestations.*)

Gass JDR: Drusen and disciform macular detachment and degeneration. Arch Ophthalmol 90:206, 1973 (*A follow-up study of 200 patients with macular drusen to determine the cause of central visual loss.*)

Hayreh SS: Central retinal vein occlusion: Differential diagnosis and management. Trans Am Acad Ophthalmol Otolaryngol 83: OP379, 1977 (*An excellent discussion of the different clinical presentations and of the inadequacy of therapy.*)

Kornzweig AL: Visual loss in the elderly. Hosp Pract 12:51, 1977 (*A paper on ocular and systemic causes of visual loss.*)

Lessel S: Optic neuropathies. N Engl J Med 299:533, 1978 (*A superb review of the characteristics and differentiation of ischemic, compressive, and inflammatory optic nerve disorders.*)

Macular Photocoagulation Study Group: Argon laser photocoagulation for senile macular degeneration: Results of a randomized clinical trial. Arch Ophthalmol 100:912, 1982 (*Evidence that laser photocoagulation decreases visual loss in a subgroup of patients with senile macular degeneration.*)

Repka MX, Savino PJ, Schatz NJ et al: Clinical profile and long-term implications of anterior ischemic optic neuropathy. Am J Ophthalmol 96:478, 1983 (*Younger patients with anterior ischemic optic neuropathy have a higher incidence of hypertension and diabetes mellitus.*)

Sanders MO: Sudden visual loss. Practioner 219:43, 1977 (*A straightforward review emphasizing differential diagnosis.*)

201

Evaluation of Eye Pain

ROGER F. STEINERT, M.D.

Pain in the eye is most often produced by conditions that do not threaten vision. However, at times the discomfort may result from corneal or intraocular pathology that is capable of compromising eyesight. The first responsibility of the primary physician is to promptly determine if there is an immediate threat to vision that requires urgent therapy or quick referral to the ophthalmologist; minor problems can be treated symptomatically in the office.

Ocular pain is usually not the only presentation of injury or disease. Several distinct pain categories can be identified that, when combined with assessment of inflammation (see Chapter 199) and vision (see Chapter 200), allow the primary physician to categorize the nature of the problem and make appropriate disposition.

PATHOPHYSIOLOGY AND CLINICAL PRESENTATION

The external ocular surfaces (lid, conjunctiva, and cornea) and the uveal tract are richly innervated to detect pain. Localization within these structures is relatively less precise. The orbit and sinuses may give rise to pain localized to the eye. Pathology confined to the vitreous, retina, or optic nerve is rarely a source of pain.

Eyelids. Inflammation of the eyelid causes tenderness and foreign body sensation. Common causes are hordeolum (stye), trichiasis (inturned lashes), and tarsal foreign bodies. Redness and edema may accompany the pain.

Conjunctiva. Viral and bacterial conjunctivitis cause mild burning and foreign body sensation, whereas allergic conjunctivitis primarily elicits itching (see Chapter 199). Toxic, chemical, and mechanical injuries are commonly responsible for unilateral disease.

Cornea. The cornea is densely innervated by pain fibers, so that even a minor injury may result in considerable discomfort. Pain arises from exposure of nerve endings in the epithelium; the patient complains of a burning or foreign body sensation. Reflex photophobic lacrimation may accompany the discomfort. Blinking exacerbates the pain, which is generally relieved by a pressure patch holding the lid shut. *Keratitis* (inflammation of the cornea) occurs with trauma, infection, exposure, vascular disease, or decreased lacrimation. Cellular infiltration and loss of corneal luster ensue. If blood vessels invade the normally avascular corneal stroma, vision may become cloudy. Severe pain is a prominent

symptom; movement of the lid typically exacerbates symptoms. Fluorescein stain reveals the epithelial defects quite well and allows identification with a penlight.

Sclera. Compared to disease of the eyelids, scleral problems are more likely to cause dull, deep pain. If the condition involves the anterior sclera, it may be readily visible as an area of redness. The blood supply to the sclera is not extensive and its metabolism is relatively inactive; consequently, inflammatory conditions of the sclera tend to be rather torpid; many are associated with connective tissue disease.

Uveal Tract. Anterior uveitis or iritis is accompanied by a dull ache and photophobia due to the irritative spasm of the pupillary sphincter. Posterior uveitis without anterior involvement may be painless or cause deep-seated aching. Profound ocular and orbital pain radiating to the frontal and temporal regions accompanies sudden elevation of pressure, as in acute angle-closure glaucoma. Vagal stimulation with high pressure may result in nausea and vomiting. Often the patient gives a history of mild intermittent episodes of blurred vision preceding the onset of an attack of throbbing pain, nausea, vomiting, and decreased visual acuity; halos about lights are sometimes noted. A fixed, midposition pupil, redness, and a hazy cornea may be present (see Chapter 206).

Orbit. Inflammation and rapidly expanding mass lesions may cause deep pain. Displacement of the globe and diplopia may ensue. In optic neuritis, eye movement may cause sharp pain due to meningeal inflammation; the extraocular rectus muscles insert along the dura of the nerve sheath at the orbital apex. Most cases are idiopathic, but 10% to 15% are associated with multiple sclerosis. Symptoms include pain on eye movement, abnormal color vision, and some loss of central vision. In most instances, the optic disk appears normal, but occasionally there is edema. A central scotoma may be found. Sinusitis may also cause secondary orbital inflammation and tenderness on extremes of eye movement. In orbital cellulitis there is proptosis, limitation of extraocular movement, injection, and diminished vision.

Other Sources. Mild headache referred to the orbit is associated with refractive error, ocular muscle imbalance, sinusitis (see Chapter 217), and other causes of nonocular headache, such as tension headache, temporal arteritis, and the prodromal phase of herpes zoster (see Chapter 192). Severe aches in the eye cannot be attributed to refractive error, nor can aches about the eye that are noted on awakening in the morning.

DIFFERENTIAL DIAGNOSIS

Extraocular causes of eye pain include diseases of the lid, conjunctiva, cornea, and sclera. Common lid conditions are hordeolum (a small abscess of the lid), acute dacryocystitis, cellulitis, and chalazion. Incipient herpes zoster involving the ophthalmic branch of the fifth nerve may cause eye pain. Conjunctival irritation related to prolonged sun exposure, pollution, occupational irritants, aerosol propellants, wind, dust, or lack of sleep, as well as that due to viral or bacterial infection, is an important source of eye discomfort. Episcleritis and scleritis can present with severe pain. The most common causes of corneal pain are abrasions, foreign bodies, ulcers, ingrown lashes, contact lens abuse, excessive exposure to sun or other forms of ultraviolet radiation, and viral or bacterial infection.

The important intraocular conditions that produce eye pain may compromise vision and include acute angle-closure glaucoma, acute anterior uveitis, and retrobulbar optic neuritis. The list of conditions associated with anterior uveitis includes the collagen diseases, sarcoidosis, and inflammatory bowel disease; however, most cases are idiopathic. Any orbital tumor or inflammatory process may cause eye pain.

Pain may be referred to the eye from the sinuses, teeth, or other cranial structures.

WORKUP

The initial task is to be sure that there is no threat to vision. Most intraocular conditions that cause eye pain may compromise vision and should be carefully checked for, as should corneal injuries.

History. The quality of the pain needs to be considered. Deep pain is suggestive of an intraocular problem; a foreign body sensation makes it likely that the problem is on the surface of the eye. The patient should be asked about any change in visual acuity or color vision, because any report of deteriorating vision requires urgent ophthalmologic consultation. A history of diplopia and displacement of the eye raises the possibility of an orbital problem. Ascertaining the aggravating and alleviating factors can aid diagnosis. Pain exacerbated by lid movement and relieved by cessation of lid motion is very suggestive of a foreign body or corneal lesion. Pain worsened by eye motion may be due to retrobulbar optic neuritis, especially if accompanied by loss of central vision and a normal appearing optic disc. Photophobia is often prominent in acute anterior uveitis. Localization of a extraocular lesion by history is often difficult, because most of the time the foreign body sensation is felt in the outer portion of the upper lid, regardless of the lesion's location.

In considering causes of conjunctival irritation, it is important to ask about occupational exposures, trauma, sun, sun lamp, and other forms of ultraviolet radiation (*e.g.,* arc welding), as well as foreign body contact. History of sinusitis and headaches should be noted.

Physical Examination. An ophthalmoscope, penlight, ability to perform lid eversion, and use of fluorescein stain can be very helpful for assessment. First, visual acuity, color vision, and extraocular movements should be tested and recorded. The eye, lid, and conjunctiva are inspected for masses and redness, the pupil for reactivity, the cornea for clarity, and the fundus for any abnormalities of the disc. A cloudy cornea in conjunction with a fixed, midposition pupil is consistent with acute glaucoma; the eye may be red. A constricted pupil in the presence of an eye that is tearing excessively suggests anterior uveitis; in severe cases, the eye also may be reddened and the anterior chamber hazy. Finding a central scotoma should raise suspicion of retrobulbar neuritis; a normal appearing disc supports the diagnosis. The upper lid should be inverted with a Q-tip to check for a foreign body or chalazion. The penlight can then be used to survey the cornea for gross injury; examination is facilitated by use of a small hand lens. The iris ought to be examined for evidence of dilated vessels around the limbus; this ciliary flush is characteristic of intraocular inflammation and occurs in anterior uveitis. Often the flush cannot be seen without the aid of a slit lamp.

All but very small corneal epithelial lesions can be detected without the use of a slit lamp if *fluorescein* and a cobalt blue filtered light are employed in the eye examination. Because of the ease of *Pseudomonas* contamination of the fluorescein, it must be instilled by means of either a single-dose container or sterile fluorescein strips wetted with sterile saline. The strip is touched to the inferior cul de sac while the patient looks upward; the patient is then asked to blink once. The fluorescein stains into denuded areas of corneal epithelium, producing a bright green color when viewed by normal light. The intensity of staining is enhanced if the eye is illuminated with a cobalt blue light. Among the lesions that can be identified by fluorescein staining are the dendritic ulcers of herpes keratitis, abrasions, small foreign bodies, and punctate defects caused by irradiation.

If pain is not clearly related to the external eye or adnexa, the intraocular pressure should be measured (see Chapter 198) to rule out glaucoma, provided there is no infection and the globe is intact without external or penetrating foreign bodies.

INDICATIONS FOR REFERRAL

Significant loss of vision always requires prompt ophthalmic evaluation. Progressive pain, redness, or discharge that fails to respond to conservative treatment must be evaluated. Care must be taken not to mistake penetrating trauma for a simple abrasion. An eccentric pupil or shallow chamber may indicate loss of aqueous humor. Never instill antibiotic ointment if there is a possibility of a perforation; simply patch the eye with a metal or plastic shield, which protects the eye, and arrange referral; do not place any pressure on the globe.

SYMPTOMATIC MANAGEMENT

Foreign Bodies. Irrigation with normal saline from a squirt bottle, syringe without a needle, or intravenous tubing may flush out foreign material. Use of cotton-tip applicators and needles for foreign body removal, especially from the cornea, requires topical anesthesia, good visualization, and experience. If irrigation fails, no further attempt should be made by the nonophthalmologist to remove the foreign body if it is firmly embedded in the cornea; use of a dry cotton-tipped applicator will only remove much normal corneal epithelium.

Abrasions. Superficial epithelial abrasions usually heal well with prophylactic antibiotic medication (*e.g.,* erythromycin ointment) and a tight pressure patch for 24 to 48 hours.

For discussions of *conjunctivitis* and *glaucoma* (see Chapters 199 and 206, respectively).

ANNOTATED BIBLIOGRAPHY

Paton D, Goldberg MF: Management of Ocular Injuries. Philadelphia, WB Saunders, 1976 (*A concise text intended for ophthalmologists but readable and helpful in many aspects of primary trauma care. Includes instructions on foreign body removal and patching.*)

Records RE: Primary care of ocular emergencies: Traumatic injuries. Postgrad Med 65:143, 1979 (*Well-illustrated guide to common injuries.*)

202

Evaluation of Dry Eyes

DAVID A. GREENBERG, O.D., M.P.H.

The normal tear film provides important protection to the eye. Defects in tear production are uncommon, but often occur in conjunction with systemic disease. The primary physician must decide if systemic disease does exist, provide symptomatic relief, and know when referral is needed.

PATHOPHYSIOLOGY AND CLINICAL PRESENTATION

The ocular tear film performs a host of functions, including maintenance of the corneal and conjunctival epithelium, lubrication of lid motion, delivery of oxygen and uptake of CO_2 from the cornea, carriage of antimicrobial defenses, clearance of foreign matter and tissue debris, and smoothing of the anterior ocular surface for clear vision. The tear film is inherently unstable, depending on the interaction of its three components for stability.

The outermost layer of the tear film is lipid, excreted by the lid meibomian glands. This layer retards evaporation and counters gravitational forces on the aqueous layer. The middle layer is aqueous, secreted by the main and accessory lacrimal glands. The innermost layer is mucinous, primarily secreted by conjunctival goblet cells and attaching to the corneal epithelium; this converts the corneal surface from a hydrophobic to a hydrophilic one. Each blink redistributes and replenishes the tear film. Dry eyes ensue from a defect in maintenance of the tear film.

Aqueous Deficiency. Approximately 90% of the tear film is aqueous in composition. A defect in production of the aqueous phase causes dry eyes or *keratoconjunctivitis sicca.* The condition most often occurs as a physiologic consequence of *aging,* but may develop in the setting of connective tissue (*e.g.,* rheumatoid-associated Sjögren's syndrome), drug use, or neurologic disease. In *Sjögren's syndrome,* the triad of dry eyes, dry mouth, and arthritis characterize the clinical presentation. Facial telangiectasias, parotid enlargement, Raynaud's phenomenon, and dental caries complete the list of findings associated with the condition. Patients complain first of burning and a sandy, gritty, foreign body sensation, particularly later in the day. Increased eye debris and mucus are noted. Secondary bacterial infection develops in severe cases. Occasionally, dry eyes present paradoxically as watery eyes, when the ocular irritation stimulates excess reflex tearing.

Systemic *medications* with *anticholinergic* properties can reduce aqueous production. These include phenothiazines, atropinic agents, and antihistamines.

Mucin Deficiency. Reduction in mucin production may occur from primary goblet cell deficiency resulting from *vitamin A deficiency;* when this is combined with protein deficiency (as occurs in underdeveloped parts of the world), keratomalacia results. Secondary loss of goblet cells and mucin deficiency follows chemical *burns,* benign ocular *pemphigoid,* and *trachoma.* With loss of main and accessory lacrimal production, a combined mucin-aqueous deficiency ensues. Dry eyes linked to problems in mucin production have been noted in patients using the antiacne preparation isotretinoin (Accutane).

Lipid Abnormalities. Chronic *blepharitis* and *meibomitis* (see Chapter 199) lead to a qualitative change in sebaceous secretions, with release of free fatty acids and focal drying of the corneal epithelium.

Eyelid Defects. Compromised lid function may affect the entire tear film, because of impaired rewetting. Incomplete blinking, 5th or 7th cranial nerve palsy, exophthalmos, and exposure during sleep are among the conditions that result in drying of the inferior interpalpebral cornea. Lid movement may also be hindered by scar formation.

Patients with dry eye will rarely present with that complaint. The clinical presentation that suggests dry eye is grittiness, itching, burning, soreness, difficulty in moving the eyelids, or the sensation of a foreign body in the eye. Ironically, a number of patients with dry eye seek treatment for excessive tearing. Rarely, patients present with corneal ulcers and a red eye.

DIFFERENTIAL DIAGNOSIS

The most common cause of keratoconjunctivitis sicca is the generalized diminution of lacrimal secretion associated with old age. This physiologic alteration is often exacerbated by the desiccating effect of dry environmental conditions, which probably accounts for the majority of dry eye complaints. Systemic diseases associated with keratoconjunctivitis sicca include Sjögren's syndrome, rheumatoid arthritis, sarcoidosis, Hodgkin's disease, systemic lupus erythematosus, scleroderma, and Mikulicz's syndrome of dacryoadenitis and parotitis. It is also seen as a side effect of anticholinergic drugs such as atropine and antihistamines. It may also result from neurogenic hyposecretion, associated with such uncommon conditions as basal skull fracture or the Ramsay-Hunt syndrome. Dry eye secondary to mucin or lipid abnormalities is somewhat less common. The causes include trachoma of the upper lid, erythema multiforme of the lower lid, Reiter's syndrome, benign mucosal pemphigoid, chemical irritation, dermatitis herpetiformis, and hypovitaminosis A. Mechanical causes of dry eye include exposure keratitis, which causes aqueous layer evaporation, possibly due to exophthalmos, deficient lid closure, ectropion, or absence of blinking.

WORKUP

History. The workup should begin by noting the duration and frequency of symptoms and particularly if onset is related to dry environmental conditions. Symptoms of keratoconjunctivitis sicca are usually more pronounced as the day progresses and are frequently exacerbated by tobacco smoke. The physician should ask if tears are produced with crying and if the patient finds himself removing strands of mucus from the inner canthi upon awakening (a very suggestive symptom). It is important to note any associated dry mouth,

joint pains, prior ocular disease, infection, or surgery. A drug history is helpful.

Physical Examination. The physician should observe the patient without the patient's awareness. Attention is paid to frequency and completeness of blinking and note taken of any lid pathology. Blepharitis and meibomitis are evident as lid margin crusting and engorgement of the meibomian glands, respectively. Other physical findings may include thick yellow mucous strands in the lower fornix, hyperemic and edematous bulbar conjunctiva, and corneal dullness. Abnormal corneal sensitivity reflex may indicate a neuroparalytic keratitis or facial nerve palsy. It is mandatory to check for completeness of lid closure as well as position of eyelashes. The skin and joints should be examined as indicated.

Studies. The *Schirmer test* diagnoses aqueous deficiency by measuring wetting of a filter paper strip (Whatman No. 41 filter paper, 5 mm by 35 mm). A folded end is hooked over the lower lid nasally and the patient is instructed to keep the eyes lightly closed during the test. In the Schirmer I test, wetting is measured after 5 minutes; less than 5 mm is usually abnormal. A basal Schirmer test using topical anesthetic to prevent reflex tearing caused by the paper strip is sometimes performed; its need is debated.

SYMPTOMATIC MANAGEMENT AND INDICATIONS FOR REFERRAL

As long as there are no signs of ocular disease, the primary physician may attempt symptomatic relief. The first attempt should be to reduce the environmental dryness that exacerbates the aqueous deficiency of aging. Often this can be accomplished by use of a room humidifier. A 2-week trial of one of the many commercially available *artificial tear substitutes* is recommended. Methylcellulose (Visulose, 0.5% or 1%), polyvinyl alcohol (Liquifilm Tears, 1.4%, or Liquifilm Forte, 3%), and hydroxypropyl methylcellulose, 1% (Ultra Tears, Tears Naturale and Adsorbotear) have all been used successfully.

These nonprescription drops are soothing and, through a variety of formulations, provide aqueous replacement and sometimes mucomimetic substances. Believed to be harmless, drops may be instilled as often as desired; mild cases are usually treated at least four times a day. Each drop probably persists ½ hour at best. Topical application of 1 or 2 drops, four times a day, is a useful starting dosage. The patient may increase the frequency of application to as often as hourly to achieve comfort; a bland ointment can be used at night. Toxicity is uncommon, but topical sensitivity or corneal epithelial damage may occur. Topical steroids or antibiotics should not be used unless they are specifically indicated. More severe cases may warrant a trial of slow-release methylcellulose inserts (Lacrisert); acceptance of these has been limited.

The patient should be instructed to seek immediate

ophthalmologic attention in the event of a red eye, visual disturbance, or eye pain. An eye specialist should be consulted when simple symptomatic treatment does not give rapid relief.

PATIENT EDUCATION

It is critical for the primary physician to be certain that the patient knows how to instill the drops into his eye. Instructions should include the careful instillation of the drop into the lower fornix without contact occurring between the dropper and the eye and the utilization of digital pressure in the punctal or inner region of the lower lid to reduce drainage and prolong contact. The patient should also be educated that the instillation of more than one drop at a time exceeds the physical capacity of the inferior fornix and is wasteful.

ANNOTATED BIBLIOGRAPHY

Barsam PC et al: Treatment of the dry eye and related problems. Ann Ophthalmol 4:122, 1972 (*A series demonstrating subjective relief of symptoms in patients with idiopathic ocular discomfort and dry eye using an artificial tear substitute.*)

Baum JL: Keratoconjunctivitis sicca. Trans Am Acad Ophthalmol Otolaryngol 81:519, 1976 (*A scholarly review of the current understanding of the dry eye syndrome.*)

Holly FJ, Lemp MA: Tear physiology and dry eyes. Surv Ophthalmol 22:69, 1977 (*Still the best review.*)

Jones DB: Prospects in the management of tear deficiency states. Trans Am Acad Ophthalmol Otolaryngol 83:OP692, 1977 (*A superb review with a comprehensive table listing the causes by mechanism.*)

Moutsopoulos HM et al: Differences in the clinical manifestations of sicca syndrome in the presence and absence of rheumatoid arthritis. Am J Med 66:733, 1979 (*An article suggesting that the sicca syndrome in the absence of rheumatologic disease may represent a distinct pathology with specific systemic effects.*)

Moutsopoulos HM et al: Sjogren's syndrome (sicca syndrome): Current issues. Ann Intern Med 92:212, 1980 (*A comprehensive update.*)

Sjögren H, Block KJ: Keratoconjunctivitis sicca and Sjögren's syndrome. Surv Ophthalmol 16:143, 1971 (*A comprehensive review of the ocular consequences of Sjögren's syndrome.*)

Wright P: The dry eye. Practitioner 214:631, 1975 (*A terse review focusing on the components of the ideal tear replacement drop.*)

203
Evaluation of Excessive Tearing
ROGER F. STEINERT, M.D.

The presence of watery eyes reflects an increased production of tears or a decreased ability to drain them. Patients complain of watery eyes or may actually describe tears overflowing and running down their cheeks, a condition called epiphora. The primary physician must decide if structural pathology exists or if reassurance is the appropriate treatment.

PATHOPHYSIOLOGY AND CLINICAL PRESENTATION

Tears are produced by the main and accessory lacrimal glands. They flow out through upper and lower puncta, which open into canaliculi. These, in turn, drain into the lacrimal sac and then into the nasolacrimal duct, which opens under the inferior turbinate in the nose.

In the presence of a normal lacrimal drainage system, epiphora most often results from hypersecretion. Common stimulants are blepharitis and keratitis of any etiology (*e.g.,* infectious, foreign body), atopy, and sinusitis. Pseudoepiphora is reflex tearing in the presence of dry eyes (see Chapter 202). Aberrant regeneration of the seventh nerve may result in gustatory lacrimation ("crocodile tears").

Many abnormalities are capable of interfering with lacrimal drainage. Tear film movement may be obstructed by eyelid margin lesions or conjunctival redundancy or folds.

Tears do not flow down the drainage system merely by gravity, but rather are pumped by lid motion. This pump may be impaired by seventh nerve palsy or conditions stiffening the lids, such as scars or scleroderma. The puncta must be properly positioned; ectropion prevents tears from gaining access to the canaliculus. This condition is common in the elderly and is characterized by a sagging lower lid. The punctum itself or the canaliculus may be occluded congenitally, by chemical or thermal injury, or by neoplasms. In addition, canalicular infections may cause occlusion. The most common of these are *Actinomyces israeli* (*Streptothrix*) and *Candida*. Finally, obstruction of the lacrimal sac and nasolacrimal duct may be idiopathic, congenital, or caused by neoplasms, ethmoiditis, and turbinate disease.

The more distal the obstruction, the more likely that the epiphora will be accompanied by purulent discharge or dacryocystitis, as the stagnant tears become infected. Digital pressure may express purulent material from the puncta.

DIFFERENTIAL DIAGNOSIS

The most common causes of watery eye are senile ectropion and increased physiologic tearing. These problems are more common in the elderly. Excessive moisture may be the complaint in a patient who has an inflammatory process such as keratitis, blepharitis, or conjunctivitis.

Obstruction in the drainage system most commonly results from dacryocystitis. The puncta may be obstructed by a myriad of causes: tumors, burns, erythema multiforme, or redundant skin. The lacrimal passage may be obstructed by a stone, laceration, burn, surgery, senile atresia, or infection of the lacrimal duct. The puncta may be rendered ineffective by ectropion, sagging of the lower lid. Excessive tearing accompanies facial palsies but is rarely the primary complaint.

WORKUP

History. The physician should determine if tears actually run down the cheek and, if so, how frequently. Overflowing tears in the absence of environmental irritants suggests structural pathology. Watery eyes noted upon exposure to cold, air conditioning, or a dry environment may be due to an exaggerated perception of physiologic tearing.

Inquiry into whether the problem is unilateral or bilateral can be helpful. Unilateral tearing is more often obstructive, but stenosis can be bilateral; environmental irritants should cause bilateral epiphora. Any sinus disease, facial fractures, infections, and surgery should be noted as possible etiologic factors, as should symptoms suggestive of sicca syndrome (see Chapter 144).

Physical Examination. Lid structure and motion should be observed. Patency of the puncta is visualized under low magnification. Gentle pressure is applied over the lacrimal sac on the side of the nose and over the canaliculi to attempt to express purulent material for examination and culture. Examination for signs of dry eye (see Chapter 202) is needed to rule out paradoxical tearing, which requires an entirely different therapeutic approach.

Studies. The ophthalmologist may also evaluate the lacrimal drainage system in several ways. Fluorescein dye instilled in the conjunctival sac should make its way to the nose (Jones test). Saline irrigation and probing may prove patency or localize an obstruction. Dacryocystography (radiocontrast dye injection) may dramatically outline the obstruction and the proximal lacrimal system. Dacryoscintigraphy, in which aqueous radioactive tracer is introduced into the tear film and followed during blinking, may demonstrate functional impairment (pump failure).

SYMPTOMATIC MANAGEMENT AND INDICATIONS FOR REFERRAL

Irritants must be eliminated. Sicca is treated with appropriate lubricants (see Chapter 202). Dacryocystitis is treated with hot compresses at least four times a day and systemic antibiotics (usually erythromycin 250 mg qid or dicloxicillin 250 mg qid directed against staphylococcal species). Patients without infection can be reassured the condition is not harmful.

Unresponsive patients are properly referred to an ophthalmologist for further evaluation and treatment. In symptomatic cases, lid surgery to correct malposition, or dacryocystorhinostomy to relieve nasolacrimal obstruction may be indicated.

ANNOTATED BIBLIOGRAPHY

Jones LT, Linn ML: The diagnosis of the causes of epiphora. Am J Ophthalmol 67:751, 1969 (*Still the classic presentation on the workup of epiphora.*)

Victor WH: Watery eye. Western J Med 144:759, 1986 (*A review written for the primary care physician; emphasizes a practical approach.*)

204

Evaluation of Common Visual Disturbances: Flashing Lights, Floaters, and Other Transient Phenomena

CLAUDIA U. RICHTER, M.D.

Patients often come to their primary physician with reports of transient visual disturbances, including flashes of light, specks, halos, and discolorations. Flashes of light (photopsia) and dark moving lines and specks (floaters) are particularly common, usually benign occurrences, but on occasion, they herald a retinal detachment or tear. Other short-lived disturbances accompany such diverse conditions as migraine, digitalis toxicity, and acute glaucoma. The primary physician needs to know when these visual phenomena are likely to be harmless and when they presage a serious ophthalmologic or systemic event that requires prompt attention.

PATHOPHYSIOLOGY AND CLINICAL PRESENTATION

Floaters are vitreous opacities that cast a shadow on the retina. They can be single or multiple, characteristically moving across the visual field and transiently blurring if they cross the macula. They are most notable when gazing at a clear blue sky or a blank white wall. Floaters usually form from condensation of vitreous sheets or glial tissue on the posterior vitreous surface; under these circumstances, they are a harmless development that increases with age. Floaters may also represent minute remnants of the hyaloid vascular system, inflammatory cells, red cells, cholesterol crystals, mineral crystals, tumor cells, or retinal fragments. When occurring as a consequence of *aging,* they increase imperceptibly over time; however, when they are due to *chronic intraocular inflammation,* their number increases slowly but noticeably. When they are caused by *acute retinitis,* the increase is still more rapid; a *vitreous detachment* or *retinal tear* can cause a sudden shower of them.

Flashes (photopsia) refers to the perception of bright, small flickering lights. The retina responds to any type of stimulation by reporting the sensation of "light." Consequently, when a light is shined on the eye or when the retina is subjected to mechanical stimulation by rubbing or trauma, the sensation of light is experienced (*e.g.,* "seeing stars" when struck in the head or coughing hard). Photopsia can result from traction on the retina, as well as from irritation of the retina, optic nerve, or geniculocalcarine pathway in the brain.

The clinical circumstances under which these and related visual phenomena occur range from the harmless to the worrisome, including vitreous detachment, retinal tear and detachment, classic migraine, and visual hallucinations.

Vitreous detachment is a consequence of aging. The vitreous gel liquefies with age, and its fibrous matrix contracts, causing it to pull away from the retina. Because the vitreous is attached to the retina at several sites (including the optic nerve), the traction can cause photopsia. If the vitreoretinal traction tears superficial retinal vessels, vitreous bleeding may ensue and present as an acute shower of floaters. Vitreoretinal traction may lead to a *retinal tear,* allowing vitreous to flow behind the retina and cause *retinal detachment,* marked by a new visual field defect. The patient may complain of a curtain or shadow coming over the visual field; if the macular area is reached, central vision deteriorates. Fundoscopic examination may reveal a retinal tear, though usually this occurs too peripherally to be seen with a hand-held ophthalmoscope. One might, however, note a ballooning white area of retina where it has detached.

Classic migraine headache also can present with flashing lights as part of a complex set of visual prodromal phenomena (see Chapter 166). The photopsia in this setting tends to be more complex and includes flashes of light with associated transient blind spots (*scintillating scotomata*); there may also be rhythmically flashing zig-zag lines (*fortification phenomena*). With onset of the headache, these resolve and leave no residual deficit. Some patients with migraine will experience the visual prodrome without developing the headache.

A host of other conditions can cause transient visual phenomena. *Digitalis toxicity* (see Chapter 25) represents another etiology of lightning flashes; the condition also tends to cause yellow discoloration or the appearance of frost over objects. Often, *acute glaucoma* (see Chapter 206) produces colored halos around lights, not lightning flashes. *Visual hallucinations* caused by *seizure* activity in the occipital cortex and the adjacent association area produce static light and stars; hallucinations from the parastriate area 18 cause luminous sensations or colored flashes and rings. These hallucinations are usually perceived bilaterally.

DIFFERENTIAL DIAGNOSIS

Although most cases of floaters and photopsia are harmless, the occurrence of an acute shower of floaters and flashes of light can be a sign of important ocular or central nervous system pathology. Causes of these phenomena can be listed according to clinical presentation (see Table 204-1).

WORKUP

History. A complete and detailed description of the patient's symptoms uninfluenced by leading questions is the most important part of the history, followed by information regarding their onset, course, and presence of any associated symptoms (*e.g.,* headache, compromise in vision). The sudden onset of a shower of flashing lights and floaters is highly suggestive of vitreoretinal traction, possibly in association with a posterior vitreous detachment, retinal tear, or retinal detachment. New floaters may also be due to acute retinitis, although onset in this condition is less dramatic. Flashes of light upon waking and rubbing the eyes are usually harmless, as are floaters that have been present for an extended time

Table 204-1.   Causes of Floaters and Flashing Lights

Acute Shower of Floaters
Vitreous detachment
Retinal tear
Retinal detachment

Chronic Floaters
Normal occurrence (if no increase over time)
Chronic intraocular inflammation (gradual increase)
Acute retinitis (more rapid increase)

Flashing Lights
Classic migraine (with scotomata)
Retinal detachment or tear
Vitreous detachment or traction
Minor mechanical stimulation (cough, rubbing the eyes, hear trauma)
Seizure activity in the visual cortex (static light, colored flashes)

without marked increase in number. Patients who complain of halos deserve consideration for glaucoma; the patient on digitalis who experiences visual disturbances needs to be checked for drug toxicity.

Physical Examination should include visual acuity testing and careful ophthalmoscopy, looking for a ballooning white area suggestive of a retinal detachment. Confrontation field testing may indicate an area of loss coinciding with a retinal detachment. The failure to find a detachment does not rule out the condition, for it may be too peripheral to be seen with the hand-held ophthalmoscope. Only by careful examination of the peripheral retinal can a retinal tear or detachment by discovered before it becomes extensive. Patients with migraine will have a perfectly normal physical examination, unless they have other prodromal phenomena such as hemiplegia or hemianopia (see Chapter 166).

Studies. The most important study in patients with new onset of a shower of flashes and floaters is indirect ophthalmoscopy and scleral depression done by the opthalmologist. The patient with halos needs to be checked for glaucoma (see Chapter 198); the person on a digitalis preparation who experiences visual disturbances should have a drug serum level obtained (see Chapter 25).

PATIENT EDUCATION AND INDICATIONS FOR REFERRAL

There is no symptomatic therapy for flashes or floaters. Flashes that occur in a situation easily attributed to minor mechanical stimulation require only reassurance and explanation. Light flashes in association with migraine headaches or temporal or occipital lobe disease should be explained as part of the underlying pathologic process.

A sudden shower of new floaters with or without flashes requires urgent referral to an ophthalmologist. If a field loss is detected by the patient or examiner, referral is even more urgent. Patients with chronic flashes and floaters should have a complete ophthalmologic examination, including indirect ophthalmoscopy, but it is not urgent. All patients with flashes and floaters need to be warned that a sudden shower of new floaters or the appearance of a peripheral visual field defect may represent a retinal hole or detachment and that they should see an ophthalmologist promptly.

ANNOTATED BIBLIOGRAPHY

Aring CD: The scintillating scotoma. JAMA 220:519, 1972 (*A review of flashing lights in migraine syndrome.*)

Boldrey EE: Risk of retinal tears in patients with vitreous floaters. Am J Ophthalmol 96:783, 1983 (*A series of 589 patients: visual symptoms of diffuse dots, many vitreous cells, and grossly visible vitreous or preretinal blood had the strongest association with retinal tears.*)

Jaffe NS: Complications of acute posterior vitreous detachment. Arch Ophthalmol 79:568, 1968 (*Flashes of light are associated with acute posterior vitreous detachment.*)

Moore F: Subjective "lightning flashes." Am J Ophthalmol 23:1255, 1940 (*A classic article.*)

Morris PH, Scheie HG, Aminlari A: Light flashes as a clue to retinal disease. Arch Ophthalmol 91:179, 1974 (*One hundred patients complaining of light flashes were studied: 23% had demonstrable vitreoretinal disease; of these, 16% had retinal breaks.*)

Murakami K, Jalkh A, Avila MP et al: Vitreous floaters. Ophthalmology 90:1271, 1983 (*The vitreous changes in 148 eyes with sudden onset of vitreous floaters were evaluated by slit-lamp examination and documented photographically.*)

205
Evaluation of Exophthalmos
CLAUDIA U. RICHTER, M.D.

Exophthalmos is defined as protrusion of the eye. It may be a variation of normal physiognomy or a sign of systemic or orbital disease. The primary physician must be able to recognize it and evaluate the patient for a possible endocrinologic, neoplastic, or vascular cause and decide on the need for further study or referral.

PATHOPHYSIOLOGY AND CLINICAL PRESENTATION

Pathologic forms of exophthalmos may result from inflammation, infiltration, a mass lesion, or a vascular abnormality. The ophthalmopathy of *Graves' disease* occurs as a consequence of an inflammatory infiltrative process affecting the soft tissues of the orbit. In its mildest form, there is minor lid retraction, stare, lid lag, and mild protrusion of the eye (proptosis). The severe form, "malignant" exophthalmos, causes edema of the lids and conjunctiva, marked proptosis, limitation of extraocular movements, and optic nerve compression. Although it is usually a bilateral disease, it may present unilaterally or asymmetrically. Pathologically, there is an inflammatory infiltrate of lymphocytes, mucopolysaccharides, and edema. Later, fibrosis of the extraocular muscles may develop. The condition does not parallel the degree of hyperthyroidism and, in fact, may worsen with treatment of thyrotoxicosis. Its precise mechanism remains unclear (see Chapter 101).

Neoplasms of the orbit, such as gliomas, produce exophthalmos by mass effect. Some vascular lesions, such as a *hemangioma,* produces only a mass effect, whereas a *carotid-cavernous sinus fistula* may present with a diffusely congested orbit with exophthalmos, prominent episcleral vessels, and elevated intraocular pressure. Neoplasms and vascular abnormalities are unilateral diseases. Clinical presentations are varied. When ocular mobility is impaired, the initial complaint may be one of diplopia. Inability to close the eye leads to exposure keratitis. Stretching or compression of the optic nerve impairs visual acuity.

Orbital cellulitis and *cavernous sinus thrombosis* are extremely serious, though rare, causes of proptosis. Because the orbit is bordered on three sides by paranasal sinuses, orbital infection can result from sinusitis caused by direct extension of infection through the lamina papyracea. Lid edema, ptosis, proptosis, chemosis, and diminished ocular movements make for a dramatic clinical presentation. Retrograde extension can lead to thrombosis of the cavernous sinus (see Chapter 217).

DIFFERENTIAL DIAGNOSIS

Bilateral exophthalmos is usually caused by Graves' disease, but occasionally it occurs with Cushing's syndrome, acromegaly, or lithium ingestion. Unilateral disease is most often due to tumor; occasionally the cause is an inflammatory or infectious condition. In a combined series of 668 patients with unilateral exophthalmos, 54% had tumor, predominantly hemangioma, meningioma, or optic nerve glioma; 15% had thyroid disease; 8% had carotid-cavernous sinus fistula. Primary orbital tumors may arise from any tissue in the orbit. Orbital pseudotumor mimics a mass lesion. Tumors extending into the orbit include those originating in the eye, lids, and paranasal sinuses. Among inflammatory etiologies are sarcoidosis, orbital cellulitis, foreign body, orbital thrombophlebitis, and ruptured dermoid cyst. Hemangioma, aneurysm, varices, carotid-cavernous sinus fistula, and cavernous sinus thrombosis constitute the important vascular etiologies.

Skeletal abnormalities (*e.g.,* Paget's disease) may produce exophthalmos. Asymmetry of the orbits, severe unilateral myopia, facial nerve paresis, and congenital glaucoma may give the appearance of exophthalmos. Ptosis or enophthalmos of the opposite eye can mimic exophthalmos.

WORKUP

The finding that directs the workup is the presence of either bilateral or unilateral orbital involvement. The differential diagnosis of bilateral involvement is so often thyroid disease that few patients require workup other than thyroid function tests and eye examination. Unilateral orbital involvement has a much longer differential diagnosis that requires evaluation. The physician should search for systemic disease and the ocular complications associated with exophthalmos.

History should include inquiry into the time course of the exophthalmos and the presence of associated symptoms, whether they are of an underlying etiology or a complication of the proptosis. Old photographs are helpful in determining if the problem is new in onset or simply a long-standing anatomic variant. Change in visual acuity, diplopia, pain, excessive lacrimation, photophobia, and foreign body sensation are indications of adverse effects from the exophthalmos. A history of trauma to the orbit, severe sinus infection, worsening headache, or use of lithium may have etiologic significance. Any symptoms of hyperthyroidism (see Chapter 101) ought to be noted, as should a history of goiter.

Physical Examination begins with documenting the degree of exophthalmos. The distance to be measured is from the lateral orbital wall to the apex of the cornea. The normal range is 18 mm to 24 mm; a difference between both eyes of 2 mm is considered significant. Visual acuity, intraocular pressure, and ocular motility should be tested. Ophthalmoscopic examination might demonstrate a pale or swollen optic nerve head. The globe and orbit need to be auscultated for bruits and pulsation suggestive of vascular fistula; the sinuses are checked for tenderness and discharge. A complete physical examination should include a search for associated signs of Graves' disease, such as pretibial edema.

Laboratory Studies. Thyroid function tests are useful, but normal levels of free T_4 and total T_3 do not rule out the diagnosis of Graves' ophthalmopathy (see Chapter 101). All patients with unilateral exophthalmos should have orbital radiographs. Ultrasonography has proven very useful for evaluation of suspected orbital masses; computed tomography may follow or precede in selected cases. If there is facial asymmetry, marked sinus tenderness, and purulent discharge, sinus films are indicated. Specialized tests that are the provence of the ophthalmologist include orbitography and vascular studies. Some patients require surgical exploration for definitive diagnosis and histologic confirmation.

SYMPTOMATIC MANAGEMENT AND INDICATIONS FOR REFERRAL

The primary physician must be cognizant of potential ocular complications and give advice for relief of minor symptoms. Periorbital and lid edema may be reduced by elevating the head of the bed at night. Exposure keratopathy causes a foreign body sensation, which can be relieved with use of 1% methylcellulose drops, occasionally as often as hourly while the patient is awake, and taping the eyelids closed at night. If such simple measures are inadequate, referral to the ophthalmologist for consideration of tarsorrhaphy or section of Muller's muscle may be necessary. Sunglasses help improve a patient's cosmetic appearance and reduce photophobia and tearing. Underlying hyperthyroidism should be treated carefully, avoiding precipitous hypothyroidism, which may exacerbate Graves' ophthalmopathy.

Emergency admission is needed if orbital cellulitis is suspected. Ophthalmologic consultation should be obtained early in unilateral, severe, or unexplained exophthalmos. Eye changes from Graves' disease may require systemic steroids, radiation therapy, or even orbital decompression when corneal integrity or optic nerve function is endangered; consultation is indicated. Exophthalmos due to neoplasm may require surgery, radiation therapy, or chemotherapy. Carotid-cavernous sinus fistulas need careful vascular surgery. It is judicious to discontinue lithium in patients with exophthalmos.

Patient education is important because evaluation, treatment, and the underlying disease process itself may be lengthy. The primary physician should explain that the eye findings may represent an underlying disease and that the evaluation needs to be methodical and thorough. The need for the patient to recognize symptoms of ocular compromise necessitates a review of important symptoms to watch for (diplopia, excessive tearing, change in vision, etc.). Patients with Graves' disease ought to understand that, while it is possible to reverse the hyperthyroidism, the eye changes are likely to persist, although probably not worsen substantially as long as a precipitous decline in thyroid function is not induced.

ANNOTATED BIBLIOGRAPHY

Chard H, Norman D: The use of computer tomography and ultrasonography in the evaluation of orbital masses. Surv Ophthalmol 27:49, 1982 (*A review of the characteristics and techniques of computed tomography and ultrasonography in the evaluation of orbital masses. The advantages and limitations of each modality are discussed.*)

Gamblin GT, Harper DG, Galentine P et al: Prevalence of increased intraocular pressure in Graves' disease—evidence of frequent subclinical ophthalmopathy. N Engl J Med 308:420, 1983 (*Patients with Graves' disease but no exophthalmos may have increased intraocular pressure on upgaze, indicating the presence of subclinical ophthalmopathy.*)

Gorman C: Ophthalmopathy of Graves' disease. N Engl J Med 308: 453, 1983 (*Excellent update on the problem.*)

Grove AS: Evaluation of exophthalmos. N Engl J Med 292:1005, 1975 (*A comprehensive review detailing the various radiographic techniques used in diagnosis of exophthalmos.*)

Hamburger JI, Sugar HS: What the internist should know about the ophthalmopathy of Graves' disease. Arch Intern Med 129:131, 1972 (*A great review focusing on physical findings in exophthalmos.*)

Moss HM: Expanding lesions of the orbit: A clinical study of 230 consecutive cases. Am J Ophthalmol 54:761, 1962 (*A classic series.*)

Segal RL, Rosenblatt S, Eliasoph I: Endocrine exophthalmos during lithium therapy of manic-depressive disease. N Engl J Med 289: 136, 1974 (*Five of 44 patients [11%] started on lithium developed exophthalmos.*)

Smigiel MR, MacCarty CS: Exophthalmos: The more commonly encountered neurosurgical lesions. Mayo Clin Proc 50:345, 1975 (*A good review making the point that 54% of unilateral exophthalmos is caused by tumor.*)

Solomon DH: Identification of subgroups: Euthyroid Graves' ophthalmopathy. N Engl J Med 296:181, 1977 (*A subset of patients with clinically classic Graves' ophthalmopathy but no abnormality in thyroid function.*)

Werner SC, Coleman J, Franzen LA: Ultrasonographic evidence of a consistent orbital involvement in Graves' disease. N Engl J Med 290:1447, 1974 (*Consistent involvement in Graves' disease was demonstrated on ultrasonography in 44 out of 77 cases.*)

206
Management of Glaucoma
CLAUDIA U. RICHTER, M.D.

Glaucoma is a disease of elevated intraocular pressure leading to optic nerve cupping and visual field loss. Elevated intraocular pressure is statistically defined as a pressure greater than 21 mm Hg and may occur in as much as 15% of the elderly population. Glaucoma is difficult to define and diagnose precisely because modestly elevated pressures may never cause glaucomatous damage in some patients while statistically normal intraocular pressure causes damage in others. Although the primary physician is not responsible for the diagnosis or treatment of glaucoma, he needs to screen patients for ocular hypertension (see Chapter 198) and recognize early stages of optic nerve change that might ensue from such hypertension. One must also be able to recognize

acute angle-closure glaucoma to institute proper initial therapy or at least to arrange prompt referral. In addition, many patients with glaucoma have multiple medical problems, necessitating an understanding of the medical therapy for glaucoma and how it might be affected by or affect treatment of other medical conditions.

PATHOPHYSIOLOGY AND CLINICAL PRESENTATION

The essential pathophysiologic feature of glaucoma is an intraocular pressure that is too high for the optic nerve. The exact mechanism of optic nerve damage has not been established and is probably a combination of factors. Increased intraocular pressure increases vascular resistance, causing decreased vascular perfusion of the optic nerve and ischemia. The increased pressure can interfere with axoplasmic flow in the ganglion cell axons, causing cell dysfunction and death; and it can compress the lamina cribrosa, the sievelike structure through which axons pass when leaving the eye. The altered supporting structure may then interfere with axonal function. These different mechanisms of axonal damage are of variable importance in different patients, but the final result is loss of ganglion cells and their axons, increased optic nerve cupping, and visual field loss.

The *pathophysiology* of increased intraocular pressure can best be understood in terms of the anatomy and physiology of aqueous flow. The iris divides the front of the eye into anterior and posterior chambers that communicate through the pupil. Aqueous humor is produced by the ciliary body, fills the posterior chamber, flows through the pupil into the anterior chamber, and leaves the eye through the trabecular meshwork, a connective tissue filter at the angle between the iris and the cornea. The aqueous passes through the trabecular meshwork into Schlemm's canal and into the episcleral venous system.

The pressure in the eye is maintained by the dynamic equilibrium of aqueous production and outflow. An increase in production or an obstruction to outflow will cause elevated intraocular pressure. In primary open-angle glaucoma, the obstruction exists at a microscopic level in the trabecular meshwork. In angle-closure glaucoma, the iris obstructs the trabecular meshwork. Secondary causes of glaucoma include inflammation, trauma, neoplasm, neovascularization, and corticosteroid therapy.

The most common presentation of *open-angle glaucoma,* accounting for more than 90% of glaucoma cases, is detection of *asymptomatic* elevated intraocular pressure by a primary physician, an optometrist, or an ophthalmologist. It is frequently called the "silent blinder," because extensive damage may occur before the patient is aware of visual field loss. The patient is usually over 40. Glaucomatous *cupping* of the optic nerve may be noted on routine ophthalmoscopy.

Acute *angle-closure glaucoma* presents with a *painful red eye.* The physical findings include decreased visual acuity, redness, fixed and unreactive pupil in middilation, and corneal haziness. Occasionally, the principal symptoms are nausea and vomiting and the patient may be thought to have abdominal or coronary disease. Patients with acute angle-closure glaucoma require emergency treatment. Patients susceptible to angle-closure can be identified by shining a light parallel to the iris plane from the temporal side of the globe: eyes with narrow angles will have a shadow fall on the nasal iris. This screening is particularly important in patients with a positive family history, episodes of halos, or of painful, blurred vision.

PRINCIPLES OF THERAPY

Chronic Open-Angle Glaucoma. The objective of treatment is stabilization of the intraocular pressure in a range that will prevent optic nerve damage and visual field loss. Therapy involves medications that reduce aqueous production or facilitate outflow. Topical medications include cholinergic agents, anticholinesterases, sympathomimetics, and topical beta-adrenergic antagonists. *Pilocarpine,* the most frequently used parasympathomimetic, acts by contracting the ciliary body, which opens the trabecula to facilitate aqueous outflow. Ocular side-effects include headache with initial administration, a miotic pupil with dimming of vision, fluctuating myopia, conjunctival hyperemia, and retinal detachment. Systemic side-effects include diaphoresis, diarrhea, and leukocytosis.

Anticholinesterases act to increase endogenous cholinergic effects and are used to treat patients in whom pilocarpine is unsuccessful or who prefer the less frequent dosage. The most commonly used anticholinesterase is *echothiophate iodide* (Phospholine Iodide). The ocular side-effects are similar to those of pilocarpine, but also include cataract formation. A patient on an anticholinesterase who is unknowingly treated with succinylcholine may have appreciably prolonged respiratory depression.

Epinephrine is a sympathomimetic drug that decreases aqueous production and may increase aqueous outflow. It is additive in effect to pilocarpine and may be used in combination. The ocular side-effects of epinephrine include a burning sensation, conjunctival pigmentation, conjunctival hyperemia, and allergic reactions. Many topical side-effects may be reduced by using *dipivefrin* hydrochloride (Propine), an epinephrine prodrug that is converted to epinephrine intraocularly. Systemic effects including tachycardia, palpitations, and hypertension may occur with either agent.

Beta-adrenergic antagonists decrease aqueous humor production when applied topically and, because they have fewer ocular side-effects than pilocarpine and need only twice-daily administration, they have become important first-line topical agents for treatment of glaucoma. *Timolol,* the prototype drug in this class for ophthalmic use, is a nonselective beta-blocker; although extremely well tolerated, beta-blockers are absorbed into the systemic circulation and can precipitate heart block, heart failure, and exacerbation of asthma in patients who are predisposed to these conditions. *Betaxolol,* a newer, more selective $beta_1$-blocker is probably less likely at low dosages to trigger an attack of asthma, but may also be slightly less efficacious in controling glaucoma.

Carbonic anhydrase inhibitors, such as *acetazolamide,* reduce aqueous production and are used when topical medications do not adequately lower intraocular pressure. They are usually used in combination with and are additive in effect to the topical medications discussed earlier. They have a variety of systemic effects, including mild metabolic acidosis, paresthesias of the face and extremities, metallic taste, anorexia, nausea, vomiting, diarrhea, and renal stones.

Most patients are treated first with topical timolol, then with epinephrine, pilocarpine, anticholinesterases, and finally carbonic anhydrase inhibitors. (The primary physician should take note of his patient's ocular medications and be familiar with their side-effects.) When medical therapy is inadequate or not tolerated, laser trabeculoplasty and then surgery are indicated.

Laser trabeculoplasty effectively lowers intraocular pressure in many patients inadequately controlled by medical therapy. The argon laser is used to place approximately 100 50-μm spots circumferentially on the trabecular meshwork. Its effectiveness appears to be due to a "tightening" of the untreated trabecular meshwork and improved aqueous outflow. Approximately 75% of treated patients have an adequate decrease in intraocular pressure to avoid glaucoma surgery. The major complication is a postlaser elevation of intraocular pressure, which can be largely avoided by performing the laser trabeculoplasty in two sessions.

Surgical intervention should be considered when maximal medical therapy and laser trabeculoplasty do not lower the intraocular pressure to a level protective to the optic disc and visual field. The usual surgical procedure is to create a filtering or drainage route from the anterior chamber to the subconjunctival space. If filtering surgery fails or cannot be performed, a cyclodialysis, separating the ciliary body from the sclera, or cryotherapy to the ciliary body, may be performed to decrease aqueous production.

Acute Angle-Closure Glaucoma. This requires prompt recognition and treatment with a miotic agent such as pilocarpine, followed by urgent referral to the ophthalmologist. *Pilocarpine* is given as 1 drop of the 4% solution in the involved eye every 20 minutes. Then *acetazolamide,* 250 mg, is given by mouth or 500 mg intravenously, and the patient is taken to the ophthalmologist. Laser iridotomy or a surgical peripheral iridectomy is necessary to prevent recurrent attacks. A laser program is preferred to spare the patient intraocular surgery. The iridectomy provides communication between the posterior and anterior chambers for the aqueous humor and prevents the iris from being forced anteriorly against the trabecular meshwork. A prophylactic laser iridotomy is indicated in the unaffected eye.

THERAPEUTIC RECOMMENDATIONS

Drugs that increase intraocular pressure should be used cautiously. These include systemic and topical steroids, particularly when applied to the eye. Drugs with anticholinergic effects may precipitate angle-closure glaucoma in patients with narrow angles. Reports of hypotensive optic neuropathy following precipitous lowering of blood pressure suggest that a gradual reduction in blood pressure done in consultation with an ophthalmologist is preferable in patients with coincident systemic and ocular hypertension.

Most patients are treated first with topical beta-adrenergic antagonists, then with epinephrine, pilocarpine, an anticholinesterase, and finally a carbonic anhydrase inhibitor. The primary physician should know his patients' ocular medications and their systemic side-effects. If medical therapy proves inadequate or intolerable, then laser trabeculoplasty and surgery deserve consideration.

PATIENT EDUCATION

A chief responsibility of the primary physician is to educate the patient about the meaning of elevated intraocular pressure and the need to screen for it (see Chapter 198). Patients may be told that they are "glaucoma suspects," should their intraocular pressures reach the middle 20s. When their optic nerves are healthy, these patients can be safely followed without treatment. Patients may call their primary physician for reassurance about the side-effects of drugs, and the physician should provide an explanation and facilitate consultation with the ophthalmologist. For patients diagnosed with glaucoma and on medication, the importance of careful follow-up examinations and compliance with medication regimens to prevent visual loss needs to be emphasized.

ANNOTATED BIBLIOGRAPHY

Bulpitt CJ, Hodes C, Everett MG: Intraocular pressure and systemic blood pressure in the elderly. Br J Ophthalmol 59:717, 1975 (*Reviews some of the data about precipitous changes in systemic blood pressure exacerbating glaucoma.*)

Hayreh S: Optic disc changes in glaucoma. Br J Ophthalmol 56:175, 1975 (*An excellent review of the optic disc changes one should detect as a sign of glaucoma.*)

Kini MM, Leibowitz HM, Colton T et al: Prevalence of senile cataract, diabetic retinopathy, senile macular degeneration, open angle glaucoma in the Framingham eye study. Am J Ophthalmol 85:28, 1978 (*An important landmark in epidemiology of eye disease, including presentation of important data on glaucoma.*)

Leier CV, Baker ND, Weber PA: Cardiovascular effects of ophthalmic timolol. Ann Intern Med 104:197, 1986 (*Documents substantial cardiovascular effects in a normal population.*)

Leske MC, Rosenthal J: Epidemiologic aspects of open-angle glaucoma. Am J Epidemiol 109:250, 1979 (*A consummate review; 105 references are included.*)

Quigley HA: Long-term follow-up of laser iridotomy. Ophthalmology 88:218, 1981 (*One hundred and forty eyes were treated with laser iridotomy; complications were limited to cataract progression similar to age-matched controls treated with surgical iridectomy.*)

Schwartz B: Current concepts in ophthalmology: The glaucomas. N Engl J Med 299:182, 1978 (*A superb, succinct review.*)

Two new beta-blockers for glaucoma. Med Lett 28:45, 1986 (*Reviews betaxolol and levobunolol and compares them to timolol.*)

Wise JB: Long-term control of adult open angle glaucoma by argon laser treatment. Ophthalmology 88:197, 1981 (*Report of excellent results of argon laser trabeculoplasty.*)

Zimmerman TJ, Kass MA, Yablonski ME et al: Timolol maleate: Efficacy and safety. Arch Ophthalmol 97:656, 1979 (*A randomized double-blind trial of various concentrations of timolol solution revealed it to be a safe and effective ocular hypotensive agent.*)

207
Management of Cataracts
ROGER F. STEINERT, M.D.

Cataracts are opacifications of the crystalline lens of the eye. They are unusual in young patients, but the incidence rises sharply in later years, such that virtually all elderly patients have some degree of cataract. Because of the implications of this diagnosis, the term "cataract" is best reserved for opacities resulting in functional impairment. The primary care physician should be able to detect cataract formation, monitor its progression, advise the patient on when to seek ophthalmologic consultation, help the ophthalmologist assess medical candidacy for surgery, and support the patient in the perioperative and rehabilitation phases.

PATHOPHYSIOLOGY AND CLINICAL PRESENTATION

Cataracts may arise from a variety of causes. Occasionally, they are *congenital;* a few develop during the early years of life, usually in association with specific diseases such as diabetes, Wilson's disease, Down's syndrome, and other metabolic diseases. The majority of cataracts occur in the elderly and reflect senescent change occasionally associated with systemic diseases. Trauma is another important precipitant.

Presenile and Senile Cataract. Age-related lens opacity results from protein denaturation and hydration. Sodium and calcium concentrations increase, potassium and ascorbate diminish, and glutathione disappears. The underlying metabolic changes leading to senile cataract are unknown. In diabetes mellitus, excess sugar is diverted to the sorbitol pathway. An insoluble alcohol accumulates, and this osmotic load causes the protein to hydrate. Clinical trials are now beginning to assess the ability of medication to interrupt this pathway.

As the human lens ages, the nucleus hardens (nuclear sclerosis). The first visual event may be a shift toward nearsightedness because of the increased refractive index of the sclerotic nucleus. As a result, the patient may temporarily experience enhanced reading vision without glasses ("second-sight"), and a change in spectacles may be the only treatment. Eventually the nucleus acquires a yellow-brown coloration ("brunescent cataract") and becomes progressively more opaque. Only a few patients are aware of the gradual spectral change, with a yellow cast to the visual world; they usually acknowledge it only after the cataract is removed. Visual impairment initially is more marked at distance than near, and a patient may fail a driver's license exam and still be able to read a newspaper. Loss of contrast sensitivity may cause a functional impairment out of proportion to the results of a standard visual acuity test.

Posterior subcapsular cataracts form at the back of the lens, usually centrally. This type of cataract is often responsible for the "presenile" cataract in the 40- to 50-year-old age group. It may be spontaneous but is often associated with prolonged use of topical or systemic steroids or with diabetes mellitus. The central location of the opacity causes the vision to worsen when the pupil becomes small, as in reading or on bright days. The refractile nature of the opacity commonly causes severe difficulty with glare, such as driving at night. Pupillary dilatation from mydriatic or cycloplegic drops or use of subdued light improves vision in such cases, as more light is allowed to enter the eye.

Presenile and senile cataract formation is painless and generally progresses over months or years.

Traumatic Cataract. These most commonly result from intraocular foreign bodies that perforate the lens capsule, allowing the lens protein to hydrate and thereby denature and opacify. Occasionally a lens will opacify after severe, blunt nonpenetrating trauma. Electric shock and high-dose ionizing radiation may lead to protein denaturation and lens opacification. Traumatic cataracts are frequently associated with intraocular inflammation and glaucoma.

WORKUP

Initial evaluation by the primary physician includes *visual acuity* determination at a distance and near. The lenticular opacity can be appreciated with the *direct ophthalmoscope* while attempting to visualize the fundus. If the angle is not shallow, dilation with one drop of 2.5% phenylephrine or 1% tropicamide is helpful. With the ophthalmoscope lens set at zero and standing about 12 inches from the patient, a bright red reflex is seen in the normal eye. Cataract formation is clearly seen by the disruption of the red reflex. Plus power (black numbers) in the ophthalmoscope of about 15 or 20 diopters will then put the lens of the eye in focus as the physician approaches the eye. The fundus should be examined for retinal abnormalities, particularly macular degeneration (manifested by hemorrhage, scarring, and drusen), which will cause loss of vision symptomatically similar to that from cataract. In all cases of visual impairment, an ophthalmic consultation is indicated.

PRINCIPLES OF MANAGEMENT

At present, the only established treatment for cataract is *surgery.* Surgery is urgent in some congenital and juvenile cataracts because of the threat of amblyopia. Traumatic cataracts and very advanced senile cataracts may cause inflammation and glaucoma, for which emergency surgery is mandatory. However, most cataract surgery is elective. The patient should understand that a cataract is not a tumor or a "growth" and that the cataract will not harm the eye.

In early nuclear sclerosis, modification of the patient's spectacles may improve vision adequately to defer surgery. Sometimes chronic pupillary dilation will suffice for a patient with posterior subcapsular cataract. When, despite these measures, the patient feels that visual function is intolerably impaired, cataract surgery can be discussed as a treatment option.

Cataract surgery is often performed under local anesthesia with mild sedation and monitoring by qualified anesthesia personnel. Patient movement during surgery may be disastrous, however, and the primary physician can assist the ophthalmologist in assessing whether or not age, mental status, and medical condition make general anesthesia appropriate.

There are several options for cataract surgery. These are *intracapsular extraction,* in which the entire lens is removed in one piece, and *extracapsular extraction,* in which the lens capsule is opened and the contents removed, leaving the posterior capsule of the lens. A variant of extracapsular extraction is called "phaco-emulsification," which uses ultrasonic energy to break up the hard nucleus and aspirate it through a small opening. Adherence of the youthful vitreous to the lens capsule makes extracapsular extraction mandatory under the age of about 40. For older patients, extracapsular extraction has become the most common surgical approach. The patient is best served by referral to a skilled and caring ophthalmologist and avoiding inappropriate emphasis on particular surgical techniques.

Postoperatively, the surgeon will prescribe topical medications and restrict activity to some extent. Modern microsurgical wound closure allows earlier rehabilitation than in the past, but cataract wounds generally require 6 to 8 weeks to achieve full strength, and the surgeon may prohibit vigorous exertion during this period. Final visual correction will also await this 2-month healing period.

Three methods of *visual rehabilitation* are available: eyeglasses, contact lenses, and lens implants. *Cataract spectacles* must be powerful to correct for the absence of the crystalline lens. In addition to thickness and weight, these spectacles magnify approximately 25%. This magnification prohibits the use of a cataract lens for only one eye, because a double image would result.

The spectacle thickness also severely limits side vision, with a midperipheral blind spot. These problems make adjustment to cataract glasses difficult at best, and some patients find ambulation nearly impossible with these spectacles.

Contact lenses are optically superior to spectacles. Because the lens power is so much closer to the eye, magnification is only 5 to 7%, and most patients will not perceive diplopia with a contact lens, although stereoscopic acuity will be reduced. Peripheral vision will be normal. Many elderly patients have difficulty handling contact lenses; extended wear lenses (usually soft) may be tolerated for weeks to months between removals for cleaning. Use of these lenses is not without difficulty, however. Lens deposits, damage, and loss may result in frequent visits to the ophthalmologist, with high cost and time lost.

Intraocular lens implantation has been refined to the point that it is standard practice where not specifically contraindicated. At the time of cataract extraction (and occasionally as a secondary procedure in cases of spectacle and contact lens intolerance) the surgeon implants a delicate plastic device with optical power to replace the cataractous lens. In 1984, over 70% of cataract patients had primary implantation of an intraocular lens. The implant is permanent, requires no care, and restores normal optics without magnification. Although once controversial, with advances in manufacturing and surgical technique there is minimal extra risk to the implant. The implant is contraindicated in some conditions, such as chronic uveitis, which is assessed by the ophthalmologist preoperatively.

For a limited number of patients with contraindications to the above techniques, optical rehabilitation may be provided by means of a corneal refractive surgical procedure.

PATIENT EDUCATION

The primary physician should help the patient understand that although surgical correction is highly successful, it is not risk free; occasionally, complications do occur. When vision is good in one eye and there are no particular social or economic constraints, it may be preferable to defer surgery; careful refraction may improve vision sufficiently. The primary physician should not advise cataract surgery in patients who have a limited life expectancy. Following surgery, it may take several months for the patient to adjust to the aphakia unless he has had an intraocular lens implant. Some patients adapt rapidly and other never do.

ANNOTATED BIBLIOGRAPHY

Abrahamson IA: Cataract update. Am Fam Phys 24:111, 1981 (*A thoughtful and well-illustrated discussion of cataract diagnosis and therapy.*)

Chylack LT Jr, Kinoshita JH: A biochemical evaluation of a cataract induced in a high glucose medium. Exp Eye Res 8:401, 1969 (*A landmark study, providing the foundation for research and clinical trials of medical treatment for diabetic cataract.*)

Jaffe NS: Current concepts in ophthalmology: Cataract surgery—a modern attitude toward a technological explosion. N Engl J Med 299:235, 1978 (*Although already technologically dated, the basic wisdom of preoperative evaluation remains valid.*)

Kahn HA, Leibowitz HM, Ganley JP *et al*: The Framingham eye study outline and major prevalence findings. Am J Epidemiol 106:17, 1977 (*Documents incidence and prevalence of cataract diagnosis and therapy.*)

208

Management of Diabetic Retinopathy

CLAUDIA U. RICHTER, M.D.

Diabetic retinopathy is a leading cause of blindness in the United States; its incidence has increased with the increase in long-term survival of diabetics. The prevalence increases with age and duration of disease; women slightly outnumber men. Promising treatment for prevention of some of retinopathy's most serious complications now exists, making it most important that the primary physician routinely check for early signs of retinopathy and know when referral is appropriate. Diabetes can also cause refractive changes, cataracts (see Chapter 207), glaucoma (see Chapter 206) and reversible cranial nerve palsies, all of which the primary physician needs to be aware of in providing comprehensive care for the diabetic (see Chapter 100).

PATHOPHYSIOLOGY AND CLINICAL PRESENTATION

Diabetic retinopathy is of two types, background and proliferative, and is diagnosed by ophthalmoscopic examination. *Background retinopathy* occurs in the posterior pole of the retina. The early structural changes include a breakdown of the blood–retinal barrier with loss of intramural pericytes and thickening of the capillary basement membrane resulting from the deposition of extra basement membrane material, fibrin, erythrocytes, and platelets. Despite the multiple layers of basement membrane, the capillaries become permeable to water and large molecules, allowing exudate and edema to form in the retina. The characteristic findings of background diabetic retinopathy include microaneurysms, venous dilation, exudates, hemorrhages, and retinal edema. *Microaneurysms* are dilatations of capillaries in which intramural pericytes are absent. "*Hard*" *exudates* are sharply defined, yellow, irregular, and consist of lipid. Occasionally the lipid accumulates in a ring around leaking microaneurysms, forming a circinate pattern. *Retinal edema* occurs from serum leakage through retinal blood vessels and may not be detectable by direct ophthalmoscopy even while causing decreased visual acuity. *Hemorrhages* are circular when they result from bleeding in the deeper retinal layers, or flame-shaped when located in the ganglion cell layer. Background diabetic retinopathy is often asymptomatic, but may cause decreased visual acuity when exudates or edema occur in the macula.

Proliferative retinopathy has a much graver prognosis and is caused by retinal hypoxia. The pathogenesis of capillary occlusion causing the retinal hypoxia is unknown. The presence of retinal hypoxia is noted by the appearance of "*soft*" or "*cotton-wool exudates,*" which are nerve-fiber-layer infarcts caused by occlusion of precapillary arterioles, venous beading, and intraretinal microvascular abnormalities. Proliferative retinopathy occurs after capillary occlusion and dropout have occurred. *Neovascularization* represents proliferation of a delicate network of new vessels that form in response to the hypoxia. The neovascularization may be on the optic disc or elsewhere in the retina. The proliferative vessels usually arise from veins, beginning as a collection of fine, naked vessels, proliferate further with connective tissue formation, and frequently grow toward areas of retinal ischemia. The vessels commonly grow onto the posterior vitreal surface. Movement of the vitreous (as with abrupt head movement, mild trauma, or shrinkage) pulls on the network of fragile vessels, causing *vitreous hemorrhage,* retinal breaks, and *retinal detachment,* all of which may seriously compromise visual acuity. Neovascular *glaucoma* is another complication of retinal hypoxia and proliferative retinopathy. It may be heralded by neovascularization of the iris.

Proliferative retinopathy usually presents as a physical finding, but minor bleeding into the vitreous may produce specks or cobwebs. An occasional patient will present with the flashing lights and visual loss because of vitreal bleeding or retinal detachment.

The incidence of diabetic retinopathy increases with the duration of the disease. Juveniles with insulin-dependent diabetes of less than 5 years' duration usually do not have retinopathy. Those patients who have had diabetes for 5 to 10 years have a 27% incidence of retinopathy, while those with diabetes for greater than 10 years have a 71% incidence.

WORKUP

Because some of the complications of diabetic retinopathy may now be prevented, it is important that the primary physician carefully examine the eyes of the diabetic every 6 to 12 months. An ophthalmoscopic assessment through dilated pupils can detect important retinopathic changes before they become symptomatic and compromise vision. Of particular importance are signs of proliferative retinopathy (*e.g.*, neovascular proliferation) and retinal ischemia (cotton-wool spots). Any suggestion of proliferative or ischemic change necessitates referral to the ophthalmologist for more detailed examination.

PRINCIPLES OF MANAGEMENT

Although the means to prevent retinopathy are still not at hand—strict control of hyperglycemia has not proven capable of preventing or controlling retinopathic changes (see Chapter 100)—effective treatment to limit proliferative retinopathy is now available.

The major therapeutic modality is *panretinal photocoagulation.* The energy of a well-focused, intense light (either xenon arc, ruby laser, or, most commonly, the argon laser) is absorbed by the retinal pigment epithelial cells and converted to heat; this coagulates the adjacent retinal cells. By ablating large portions of the retina, the neovascularization stimulus is reduced and neovascularization may regress or at least not progress. In a 2-year follow-up of a multicenter trial, 61% fewer eyes became blind in the group treated with photocoagulation. The potential complications are loss of peripheral visual field, reduction in visual acuity, inadvertent burn of the fovea, hemorrhage, and angle-closure glaucoma. Focal laser photocoagulation to areas of capillary leakage and clinically significant macular edema has been shown to substantially reduce the risk of visual loss.

Other medical approaches to managing diabetic retinopathy have been tried: clofibrate has been used to reduce lipid exudates, but the studies were not well controlled; *aspirin* is being evaluated because of its antiplatelet activity. A retrospective study has shown less retinopathy in nonsmoking diabetics. Any concurrent hypertension should be treated diligently, because it can exacerbate retinopathy.

A number of surgical approaches have been undertaken. *Vitrectomy* is a surgical procedure for evacuating hemorrhagic or fibrous tissue in the vitreous that has not spontaneously resorbed. The timing of vitrectomy following vitreous hemorrhage is still being evaluated. The Diabetic Retinopathy Vitrectomy Study Research Group found that early vitrectomy in patients with type I diabetes resulted in better final visual acuity than vitrectomy done after 1 year. Early vitrectomy did not result in better visual acuity than late vitrectomy in patients with type II diabetes.

The fortuitous discovery that *hypophysectomy* arrested the development of retinopathy led to its brief use. However, hypophysectomy is not currently the treatment of choice be-

cause of the difficulty of endocrine management of these patients and the success of panretinal photocoagulation.

Refractive changes occur because of osmotic swelling of the lens when a patient's blood glucose is uncontrolled. The induced myopia resolves when the blood glucose is controlled. *Diplopia* may ensue if third, fourth, and sixth cranial nerve palsies develop in patients with diabetes, possibly because of localized demyelinization of the nerve secondary to focal ischemia. Extraocular muscle function usually recovers within 1 to 3 months. Cataracts may also form. Considerable progress has been made in their management (see Chapter 207).

INDICATIONS FOR REFERRAL

The decision about whether and how to treat diabetic retinopathy should be made by an ophthalmologist. The timing of referral is the responsibility of the primary physician. Referral should be made to an ophthalmologist in the following instances:

- When a diabetic patient reports a change in vision or the appearance of floaters.
- When the physician observes background or proliferative retinopathy.
- When neovascularization is found, be it on the fundus or even on the iris.
- When the physician is unable to examine the fundus clearly.
- When the patient reports eye pain.

PATIENT EDUCATION

Patient education about the nature and prognosis of diabetic retinopathy and continued support by the primary physician are important in management. The physician should explain that most diabetic patients do not lose their vision but that regular examinations and prompt reporting of decreased vision or symptoms such as spots, cobwebs, or flashing lights are essential. Cigarette smoking will accelerate retinopathy and should be interdicted.

ANNOTATED BIBLIOGRAPHY

The Diabetic Retinopathy Study Research Group: Photocoagulation treatment of proliferative diabetic retinopathy: The second report of Diabetic Retinopathy Study findings. Ophthalmology 85:82, 1978 (*The report that demonstrates the important role of photocoagulation in proliferative diabetic retinopathy.*)

The Diabetic Retinopathy Vitrectomy Study Research Group: Early vitrectomy for severe vitreous hemorrhage in diabetic retinopathy. Arch Ophthalmol 103:1644, 1985 (*Early vitrectomy helps achieve better final visual acuity in type I diabetics.*)

Early Treatment Diabetic Retinopathy Study Research Group: Photocoagulation for diabetic macular edema. Arch Ophthalmol 103:1796, 1985 (*Focal photocoagulation of "clinically significant" diabetic macular edema substantially reduces the risk of visual loss.*)

Klein R, Klein BEK, Moss SE et al: The Wisconsin epidemiologic study of diabetic retinopathy. II. Prevalence and risk of diabetic retinopathy when age at diagnosis is less than 30 years. Arch Ophthalmol 102:520, 1984 (*The frequency and severity of retinopathy is associated with the duration of diabetes.*)

Klein R, Klein BEK, Moss SE et al: The Wisconsin epidemiologic study of diabetic retinopathy. III. Prevalence and risk of diabetic retinopathy when age at diagnosis is 30 or more years. Arch Ophthalmol 102:527, 1984 (*The severity of retinopathy is correlated with longer duration of diabetes, younger age at diagnosis,* *higher glycosylated hemoglobin levels, higher systolic blood pressure, use of insulin, presence of proteinuria, and small body mass.*)

Knowler WC, Bennett PH, Ballantine EJ: Increased incidence of retinopathy in diabetics with elevated blood pressure. N Engl J Med 302:645, 1980 (*Twice the number of exudates in diabetics with systolic blood pressures greater than 145.*)

Paetkau MD, Boyd TAS, Winship B et al: Cigarette smoking and diabetic retinopathy. Diabetes 26:46, 1977 (*A sample of 181 diabetics was analyzed, showing that proliferative retinopathy rose with increasing tobacco consumption.*)

14

Ear, Nose, and Throat Problems

209
Screening for Oral Cancer
JOHN P. KELLY, D.M.D., M.D.

Cancer arising in the oral cavity will affect nearly 30,000 new patients this year in the United States, representing 4% of new cancer cases in males and 2% in females. Over 9,000 deaths result from oral cancer yearly, the death rates for both men and women being unchanged over the past 25 years. Despite the ready accessibility of the oral cavity to inspection by physicians, dentists, and patients themselves, 50% of total cancers already have metastasized at the time of diagnosis.

Pain is the most common symptom which leads the patient to seek medical attention, but the early stages of oral carcinoma are notoriously painless. Hence, careful examination on a routine basis will enable more patients to be diagnosed in the early stages of their disease when treatment can be most effective.

EPIDEMIOLOGY AND RISK FACTORS

The peak incidence of oral carcinoma is in the sixth decade for women and is equally frequent in each decade after the age of 50 for men. However, the appearance of the disease in the third and fourth decades is not rare, and must not be overlooked.

Exposure to tobacco in all its forms is highly correlated with the risk of development of oral cancers. Unlike cancers of the lung and larynx, which are related to cigarette smoking, malignancies of the mouth are associated with use of cigars, pipes, and chewing tobacco as well as cigarettes. Among non-smokers, cancers of the tongue and buccal mucosa are seen more frequently than are lesions of the floor of the mouth or other oral sites.

The most common form of oral cancer is that of the lower lip. Chronic exposure to the ultraviolet rays of the sun appears to play a significant causal role. Squamous cell or epidermoid carcinoma of the lower lip has high incidence among fair-skinned people residing in sunny climates and in those whose occupations subject them to prolonged exposure to the sun. On the other hand, such cancers are rare among blacks, probably because of pigmentary protection against actinic radiation.

An epidemiologic association between alcohol consumption and oral carcinoma has long been recognized. However, no direct correlation can be made, because most heavy users of alcohol are also users of tobacco products. It has been suggested that alcohol may chronically irritate the oral tissues, facilitating the carcinogenic properties of tobacco products, or that the nutritional deficiencies associated with alcoholism predispose the oral mucosa to malignant change.

Cancer of the tongue is highly correlated with the atrophic glossitis seen with tertiary syphilis. Mucosal atrophy from other causes is also associated with an increased incidence of oral cancers. Most notably, chronic iron deficiency leading to Plummer–Vinson syndrome is known to alter mucosal tissues and this change may be related to the increased incidence of oral carcinoma.

Chronic irritation of the oral mucosa by ill-fitting dentures, poorly restored teeth, or particularly spicy diets has often been mentioned as contributing to the development of oral carcinoma. However, there are no epidemiologic data to support this view.

The precise etiology of oral cancer is unknown. The etiology factors mentioned above probably act as cocarcinogens, effecting malignant change in concert with some primary agent not yet elucidated.

NATURAL HISTORY

The 5-year survival rate for localized oral cancer is over 67%, but only 30% of patients with metastatic disease survive for 5 years. When untreated, oral carcinoma metastasizes to the regional lymph nodes of the neck, ultimately leading to respiratory embarrassment or involvement of the great vessels.

Ipsilateral node involvement is most common, but metastasis to the contralateral side—especially from primary lesions of the tongue or floor of the mouth—occurs with such frequency that treatment for control of metastasic disease is very difficult. Hence, early diagnosis and control of the primary site is essential. The lungs are the most frequently involved sites of extranodal metastasis.

Local recurrence is seen, although many such recurrences may, in fact, be new primary sites of disease. The appearance of multiple separate cancers within the oral cavity has led to use of the term "field cancerization" to characterize the susceptibility of the entire oral mucosa to malignant change in affected patients. As many as one patient in five may be expected to develop a second primary oropharyngeal cancer, with smokers who do not quit incurring the greatest risk.

SCREENING AND DIAGNOSTIC TESTS

The challenge to primary care health providers is to recognize malignancies of the oral cavity in their earliest stages. Lesions that show deep ulceration and fungating borders are easily recognized and the patient can readily be referred for treatment, but the greatest hope for control of the disease exists prior to the appearance of the grossly invasive lesion.

Thorough examination of the tissues of the oral cavity, both by inspection and by palpation, must be included in the routine evaluation of the patient. Recognition of the normal appearance of the mucosa in contrast with either atrophic or hyperplastic tissue serves as a baseline. Similarly, familiarity with normal anatomic structures, such as the circumvallate papillae of the tongue and the lingual tonsils, is necessary in order to differentiate such structures from neoplasms.

For many years, the term *leukoplakia* was used as a clinicopathologic term signifying a premalignant or frankly carcinomatous lesion. More appropriately, however, the term is now employed to indicate the development of a "white patch" on the oral mucosa. Such lesions include hyperkeratosis of various etiologies, ectopic sebaceous glands in the buccal mucosa, leukoedema, chemical burns (most commonly, from aspirin), lichen planus, candidiasis, and pemphigus vulgaris, as well as malignancies. Approximately 6% of leukoplakic lesions eventually show malignant histology.

Recently, the diagnostic significance of *erythroplasia* has been stressed. The appearance of a red, hyperplastic area of mucosa is highly suggestive of an early carcinoma. While most cancer screening protocols have emphasized a search for white lesions, the predominant color in premalignant or early lesions is red, not white. In fact, while some white lesions may only be "premalignant," the red lesions must be considered to be true malignancies unless proven otherwise by biopsy.

The oral mucosa may show pigmented lesions of black, blue, or brown color. Benign conditions such as vascular malformations, heavy metal ingestion, amalgam tattooing, pigmented nevi and the pigmentations associated with such systemic conditions as neurofibromatosis, intestinal polyposis, and Addison's disease, must be differented from the blue-black lesion of malignant melanoma. Biopsy is essential if this diagnosis is suggested by the appearance of the lesion.

Initial evaluation of a suspicious lesion begins with eliciting appropriate historical data in order to eliminate such relatively harmless lesions as the acute aspirin burn. Irritative lesions can be identified by removing or repairing jagged teeth and poorly fitting or protruding dental prostheses and following the clinical healing of the mucosal wound. In any patient with a suspicious lesion, use of a noxious agent such as tobacco must be eliminated at the outset.

Any red or white lesion which persists for 2 weeks after initial recognition and elimination of irritating agents demands further investigation. Many authors have suggested the use of exfoliative cytology or in vivo staining with toluidine blue for screening purposes, but neither of these procedures yields unequivocal results and, even if they are positive, biopsy will be necessary for confirmation of the diagnosis. Hence, referral of the patient to an oral and maxillofacial surgeon for biopsy is preferable as the definitive diagnostic maneuver. High-risk patients, specifically those with histories of smoking and drinking, should be referred for biopsy promptly, as should any patient with a deeply ulcerative or fungating lesion.

Any swelling beneath a normal-appearing oral mucosa must be evaluated by an appropriate specialist for diagnosis or treatment. Such lesions are commonly benign and are the result of infection, bony exostosis, or mucous retention phenomena, but they may represent neoplasms of the minor salivary glands or other submucosal structures.

RECOMMENDATIONS

- A thorough visual and manual examination of the oral cavity should be a part of every patient's evaluation; red or white mucosal patches are sought.
- A high index of suspicion must be maintained for patients with a history of smoking, drinking, and heavy exposure to sunlight.
- Atrophic or hyperplastic areas of the oral mucosa must be viewed with suspicion, particularly if they are red or white (erythroplasia or leukoplakia) and last more than 2 weeks after cessation of smoking, drinking and exposure to irritants.
- Referral for definitive biopsy is indicated for persistent lesions.

ANNOTATED BIBLIOGRAPHY

Baker HW, Rickles NH et al: Oral Cancer. New York, American Cancer Society, 1973 (*A well-illustrated booklet on the diagnosis, treatment, and rehabilitation of the oral cancer patient.*)

Ballard BR, Suess GR et al: Squamous cell carcinoma of the floor of the mouth. Oral Surg 45:568, 1978 (*A good review of the epidemiology, clinical staging, and prognosis of 100 recently treated patients.*)

Connolly GN, Winn DL, Hecht SS et al: The re-emergence of smokeless tobacco. N Engl J Med 314:1020, 1986 (*An extensive review documents health risks and points out alarming rise in popularity. An editorial by the Surgeon General reinforces the message.*)

Decker J, Goldstein JC: Risk factors in head and neck cancer. N Engl J Med 306:1151, 1982 (*Reviews the epidemiology of oral malignancy emphasizing the importance of smoking, alcohol, and poor oral hygeine.*)

Mashberg A: Erythroplasia: The earliest sign of asymptomatic oral cancer. J Am Dent Assoc 96:615, 1978 (*A significant recent contribution to the literature with good illustration and description of the early malignant lesion.*)

Nash DB: National implications of smokeless tobacco: A National Institutes of Health Consensus Development Conference. Ann Int Med 104:436, 1986 (*Reviews findings of NIH symposium and condemns use of smokeless tobacco.*)

Silverman S et al: Tobacco usage in patients with head and neck carcinomas. JAMA 106:33, 1983 (*A study of the risk of tobacco usage both before and after the development of an oropharyngeal carcinoma.*)

210
Evaluation of Impaired Hearing

AINA J. GULYA, M.D.

It is estimated that approximately 10% of the population of the United States has a hearing problem. People with seriously impaired hearing often become withdrawn or appear confused. Subtle hearing loss may go unrecognized. Patients with hearing loss can often be greatly helped, particularly if the loss is due to a conductive problem. The primary physician has the responsibility to detect hearing loss, to search for an etiology, and to decide when referral to an otolaryngologist is indicated.

PATHOPHYSIOLOGY AND CLINICAL PRESENTATION

Impaired hearing may result from an interference with the conduction of sound, its conversion to electrical impulses, or its transmission through the nervous system. Hearing involves an acoustic stage during which sound waves cause the tympanic membrane to vibrate. Ossicles amplify the sound, and the oscillation of the footplate of the stapes in the oval window transmits the sound waves to the perilymph of the inner ear. The endolymph of the scala media (or cochlear duct) is wedged between the perilymph of the scala vestibuli and scala tympani. Displacement of the basilar membrane stimulates the hair cells, converting sound waves to neural impulses, which are conveyed to the temporal lobes. Interference with mechanical reception or amplification of sound, as occurs with disease of the auditory canal, tympanic membrane, or ossicles, creates conductive hearing loss. Degeneration or destruction of hair cells or the acoustic nerve produces sensorineural hearing loss.

Conductive Hearing Loss presents with diminution of volume, particularly for low tones and vowels. There is often a history of previous ear disease. In the Weber test, the tuning fork is perceived more loudly in the conductively deaf ear. The Rinne test shows that bone conduction is better than air conduction. The physical examination may reveal a specific etiology, such as obstruction of the auditory canal by impacted cerumen, a foreign body, or exostoses, scarring or perforation of the drum due to chronic otitis, external otitis, or ongoing serous otitis media with effusion.

Exostoses are bony excrescences of the external auditory canal. They are characteristically located in the anterior, posterior, and superior quadrants of the canal. Nearly always bilaterally symmetric, their occurrence seems to be related to repetitive exposure to cold water, for example, as in ocean swimming. They cause symptoms by blockage of the external auditory canal, resulting in conductive hearing loss, or by sequestration of debris with subsequent infection.

Otosclerosis, a surgically remediable cause of conductive hearing loss, is a disorder affecting the architecture of the bony labyrinth which may fix the footplate of the stapes in the oval window. In a white population, evidence of otosclerosis upon histopathologic examination is found in roughly one out of ten cases; however, clinical otosclerosis, that is, that associated with a hearing loss, is seen in only approximately one out of 100 patients. The incidence in the black population is approximately one tenth of that in the white population. Approximately 65% of the patients with clinical otosclerosis are females; there also appears to be an association between pregnancy and hearing loss in otosclerosis. The condition is inherited in an autosomal dominant fashion, with varying clinical expressivity. It generally presents in the second or third decade of life.

External otitis (swimmer's ear) is a painful inflammation of the external auditory canal; because the inflammation causes edematous or purulent obstruction of the canal, there is an associated conductive hearing loss.

Developmental defects, such as failure of canalization of the external auditory canal (canal atresia) or ossicular malformations or both, may underlie conductive hearing loss. There may or may not be an associated abnormality of the pinna.

Chronic otitis media, in conjunction with tympanic membrane perforation and scarring, may also cause ossicular erosion, disrupting the ossicular chain, or tympanosclerotic fixation, both of which are attended by conductive hearing loss.

Glomus tumors, or nonchromaffin paragangliomas, are benign, highly vascular tumors derived from normally occurring glomus formations of the middle ear and jugular bulb. Presenting symptoms include conductive hearing loss (from middle ear mass effect), spontaneous hemorrhage from the canal, and paralysis of cranial nerves IX, X, and XI (the jugular foramen syndrome). With progression, they may involve the intracranial space or cause bony destruction of the base of the skull.

Sensorineural Hearing Loss characteristically produces impairment of high tone perception. Patients may complain that they can hear people speaking but have difficulty deciphering words because discrimination is poor. Shouting may only exacerbate the problem. The patient with high frequency loss may have difficulty hearing doorbells, telephones, or a ticking watch. More difficulty may be noticed in hearing the higher-pitched female voice. Recruitment, an abnormally rapid increase in perceived loudness with increased sound intensity, may be present and indicates cochlear dysfunction. Air conduction is reported better than bone conduction. Tinnitus is often a concomitant complaint.

Presbycusis is hearing loss associated with aging and is the most common cause of diminished hearing in the elderly. There are four types of presbycusis, distinguished according to the correlated pathologic changes in the cochlea. Hair cell loss and cochlear neuron degeneration are the most widely recognized changes related to presbycusis. Characteristically, the hearing loss is bilaterally symmetric and gradual in onset. The majority of cases begin with a loss of the high frequencies with slow progression. Eventually, middle and low frequency sounds also become difficult to perceive (see Appendix, Figs. 210-4 and 210-5). Clear enunciation, not merely elevated volume of speech, along with directly facing the presbycusic patient while engaged in conversation, optimizes verbal communication.

Noise-induced hearing loss is of major epidemiologic and economic significance. Chronic exposure to sound levels in excess of 85 to 90 dB causes hearing loss, particularly in the frequency range around 4000 c/s. The patient may be unaware of the problem because the speech frequencies (50, 1000, and 2000 c/s) are initially unaffected. The first stage

of noise-induced hearing loss is referred to as temporary threshold shift, in which there is a reversible rise in threshold for sound perception. The ear may feel full, or the patient may complain of a sense of pressure. If exposure to loud noise ceases at this stage, hearing returns to its previous level. If exposure persists, however, a permanent threshold shift ensues. The term "acoustic trauma" more specifically relates to a particular, single noise event, for example, a shotgun blast, which induces an immediate hearing loss.

Drug-induced hearing impairment has become more frequent due to the increased use of agents which are ototoxic. The aminoglycoside antibiotics are the most potent of the common offending agents; ethacrynic acid, quinidine, furosemide, and salicylates are of lesser importance. The daily dose of acetylsalicylic acid that has been found to cause toxicity averages between 6 to 8 g/day; fortunately, salicylate toxicity is completely reversible. Among the aminoglycosides, dihydrostreptomycin, neomycin, and kanamycin are the most ototoxic. The first sign of gentamicin ototoxicity is disequilibrium; monitoring blood levels is the best way to avoid such problems with toxicity.

Meniere's disease produces a fluctuating, unilateral, low-frequency impairment, usually associated with tinnitus, a sensation of fullness in the ear, and intermittent episodes of vertigo. The vertiginous attacks may be the presenting symptom of Meniere's disease, with later onset of fluctuating hearing loss. With time, progression of hearing loss may occur, with loss eventually encompassing the higher frequencies as well.

Acoustic neuromas, benign tumors of the eighth cranial nerve, comprise a rare but important cause of hearing loss; there may be an associated disequilibrium (see Chapter 160). The patient's speech discrimination is much worse than predicted by the deficit in pure tone perception. Unlike Meniere's disease, the symptoms related to the acoustic neuroma are in general more relentless, not fluctuating.

Sensorineural deafness, generally bilaterally symmetric, may be genetically determined. Many syndromes have been identified in which hereditary hearing loss is associated with anomalies in other organ systems. Congenital malformations of the inner ear, not necessarily hereditary, may also underlie sensorineural hearing loss.

Sudden deafness of the sensorineural variety can be due to head trauma or can appear without obvious cause or warning. In idiopathic sudden sensorineural deafness, recovery appears to be predicted by the pattern of hearing loss sustained, age (greater or less than 40); presence or absence of vertigo, and electronystagmogram pattern. The etiology of the idiopathic variant is still a matter of debate, but viral infection seems to be the most likely precipitant. Uncommonly, an acoustic neuroma may present with sudden hearing loss. Sudden hearing loss demands expeditious referral to an otolaryngologist for further evaluation and possible therapy.

Injury to the inner ear or eighth nerve will produce asymmetric sensorineural loss of hearing. Skull fracture, meningitis, otitis media, scarlet fever, and mumps are major etiologic factors. Trauma may also cause conductive hearing loss, for example, hemotympanum, tympanic membrane perforation, or ossicular dislocation.

Congenital syphilis may produce sensorineural hearing loss with onset in adult life. One or both ears may be affected; the course can be variable, with remissions and exacerbations. Vertigo is sometimes present as well.

DIFFERENTIAL DIAGNOSIS

The causes of hearing loss can be grouped according to whether the problem is conductive or sensorineural in etiology (Table 210-1). The categorization is of practical use because the conductive defects lend themselves to correction in many instances.

WORKUP

History. Evaluation of the patient with hearing loss should focus on detection of a correctable lesion; this search is aided by identifying whether the impairment is conductive or sensorineural. History is of some help. Conductive disease often results in loss of low-frequency hearing, while sensorineural problems cause high-frequency hearing loss. It is worth trying to find out the sounds or situations in which the patient has most trouble hearing. Difficulty deciphering spoken words suggests sensorineural disease. Inquiry into drug use is essential, focusing on aminoglycosides, quinine derivatives, salicylates, and the diuretics—furosemide and ethacrynic acid. A history of otitis or head trauma should be noted.

Table 210-1.   Common and Important Causes
of Impaired Hearing

CONDUCTIVE	SENSORINEURAL
Impacted cerumen	Presbycusis
Foreign body	Noise-induced deafness
Occlusive edema of auditory canal	Drugs (aminoglycosides, loop diuretics, quinidine, aspirin)
Perforation of tympanic membrane	Meniere's disease
	Acoustic neuroma
Chronic otitis media	Hypothyroidism (mild loss)
Serous otitis media	Idiopathic sudden deafness
External otitis	Congenital syphilis
Otosclerosis	Diabetes
Exostoses	
Developmental defects	
Glomus tumors	

Inquiry into acoustic trauma is important, especially the details of occupational exposure. Family history is no less important, particularly in the consideration of such entities as otosclerosis or acoustic neuromas (associated with von Recklinghausen's disease).

Physical Examination. The *Rinne* and *Weber tests* will separate most sensorineural cases from those due to a conductive problem. A tuning fork which vibrates at a frequency of 512 c/s is adequate; the 128-c/s tuning fork used for testing vibratory sensation is not. Testing should be done near the threshold of perception. A common technique is to test by a gentle rap of the fork on the knee to produce sufficient but not excessive intensity. The maximum output of a tuning fork is in the vicinity of 60 dB.

The normal response to a vibrating fork placed midline on the skull (the *Weber test*) is equal loudness in both ears. The sound will be heard more clearly in the ear with a conductive defect. If there is a sensorineural loss in one ear, sound will be better perceived in the other.

When the vibrating fork is placed on the mastoid process (the *Rinne test*), it is heard for a period of time and then dies away; it is heard again if the same fork is promptly moved without any reactivation to the external auditory meatus. Normal persons will hear sound conducted by air for about twice as long as a sound conducted by bone, because of the greater sound transmission efficiency of the middle ear apparatus. In the Rinne test, sound by air conduction is normally heard for twice as long as sound by bone conduction. With a marked conductive loss, the reverse is found. With lesser degrees of conductive impairment, the ratio is closer to 1:1. The normal ratio is preserved in patients with sensorineural loss, but hearing via both bone and air conduction is reduced.

In the *Schwabach test,* the examiner's hearing by bone conduction is compared with the patient's. The vibrating tuning fork is alternately placed on the mastoid process of examiner and patient. If the examiner's hearing is normal, he will perceive the sound for a longer time than the patient with a sensorineural deficit and for a shorter time than the patient with a conductive problem.

Other simple hearing tests can be performed in the office and are of qualitative use. The *watch tick* is an easy, although crude, method of detecting high-frequency impairment. *Whispering* from 2 feet after full exhalation is another rough means of gauging capacity to hear. The best words to use are familiar bisyllabic ones in which one syllable is clearly accented over the other (*e.g.,* pancake, hotdog). Patients with sensorineural loss hear a spoken voice much better than a whisper, even if the whisper is loud, because they have impairment of high-frequency hearing.

Physical examination of the ear includes inspection of the external auditory canal for obstruction by impacted cerumen, a foreign body, external otitis, or exostoses. Removal of the foreign body and retesting will identify its contribution to the hearing loss. Otoscopic examination of the tympanic membrane should include a check for inflammation, perforation, and scarring. One should check for the presence of fluid in the middle ear. A reddish mass visible through the intact tympanic membrane may indicate a high-riding jugular bulb, an aberrant internal carotid artery, or a glomus tumor. Pneumatic otoscopy assesses tympanic membrane mobility, which, if reduced, will impair hearing.

Cranial nerve examination is essential, especially if vertigo is an associated symptom (see Chapter 160). A glomus tumor may present with a jugular foramen syndrome (dysfunction of cranial nerves IX through XI). Nasopharyngeal examination is indicated in patients with persisting serous otitis media, particularly if it is unilateral.

Laboratory Studies. An *audiogram* is an essential component of the workup of impaired hearing. The pattern of hearing loss has considerable diagnostic and therapeutic importance, helping to establish the type of hearing loss and localize the site of pathology. Interpretation usually requires the joint efforts of otolaryngologist and audiologist, but a few common patterns are useful for the primary physician to recognize (see Appendix). Ordering the study before referral is of help to the otolaryngologist.

CT scanning has assumed an important role in the radiologic evaluation of the patient with a suspected acoustic neuroma or glomus tumor. This study must be performed with contrast (for acoustic tumors, air contrast may suffice). For those patients with iodine allergy, a nuclear magnetic resonance (NMR) study may become the procedure of choice. *Brainstem-evoked response audiometry* has also been found useful in the site-of-lesion testing of hearing loss, as has *electronystagmography* (see Chapter 160). Both tests require expert performance and interpretation and should be ordered only in consultation with consultants experienced in their use and interpretation.

SYMPTOMATIC MANAGEMENT AND INDICATIONS FOR REFERRAL

The primary physician's role in the treatment of hearing loss is relatively limited. Maneuvers that are available include removal of impacted cerumen, cessation of ototoxic drugs, treatment of otitis media (see Chapter 216), advising patients exposed to occupational noise to use earplugs and avoid further acoustic trauma, and identification and correction of metabolic abnormalities.

Cerumen removal may be accomplished by gentle, bodytemperature water irrigation using a syringe or an irrigation jet. Removal of wax, as well as some foreign bodies, may be performed using a cerumen spoon or forceps under direct visualization provided by headlight and speculum. Harder objects may be "hooked" out using a blunt-tipped right angle pick. Insects are better exterminated by instillation of mineral oil into the canal before removal is attempted.

Referral to an otolaryngologist for further evaluation and treatment is indicated when a conductive etiology or acoustic neuroma is suspected, or when simple symptomatic measures do not suffice and the hearing impairment is disabling. The otolaryngologist needs to determine whether or not the patient is a candidate for medical or surgical therapy and whether a hearing aid is appropriate. There is a great variety of *hearing aids* available on the market. Patients with sensorineural hearing losses—especially those with a flat threshold and good discrimination—benefit from amplification and deserve as much consideration as those patients with conductive hearing losses. Even those patients with steeply sloping, high-frequency sensorineural hearing loss with poor discrimination may find amplification useful. Only after an adequate trial, after careful otolaryngologic evaluation and competent hearing aid fitting, can one finally make a decision regarding the helpfulness of amplification.

A true sudden hearing loss demands immediate otolaryngologic referral.

ANNOTATED BIBLIOGRAPHY

Glasscock ME, Jackson CG, Josey AF: Brain Stem Electric Response Audiometry. New York, Thieme-Stratton, Inc., 1981 (*A basic guide to the principles and use of electric response audiometry.*)

Heffler AJ: Hearing loss due to noise exposure. Otolaryngol Clin N Am 11:723, 1978 (*A good review of this increasingly important cause of hearing loss.*)

Laird N, Wilson WR: Predicting recovery from idiopathic sudden hearing loss. Am J Otolaryngol 4:161, 1983 (*This paper presents the logic and computation of the likelihood of recovery from idiopathic sudden hearing loss.*)

Meyerhoff WL, Paparella MM: Diagnosing the cause of hearing loss. Geriatrics 33(2):95, 1978 (*Provides a practical approach to the assessment of hearing loss in adults, with emphasis on problems seen in the elderly.*)

Quick CA: Chemical and drug effects on the inner ear. *In* Paparella MM, Shumrick DA (eds): Otolaryngology: Ear, Vol 2, p 391. Philadelphia, WB Saunders, 1973 (*An excellent discussion of ototoxic agents.*)

Schuknecht HF: Pathology of the Ear, pp 388–403. Cambridge, Massachusetts, Harvard University Press, 1974 (*The classic in pathology of the ear; these pages give an in-depth discussion of presbycusis.*)

Wilson WR, Nadol JB, Jr: Quick Reference to Ear, Nose, and Throat Disorders. Philadelphia, JB Lippincott, 1983 (*A concise, easy-to-read, and up-to-date reference to otolaryngological diseases, specifically written for the generalist.*)

Zwislocki JJ: Middle ear, cochlea, and Tondorff. Am J Otolaryngol 2:240, 1981. (*A review of the development of knowledge concerning sound transmission mechanisms of the middle ear.*)

Appendix: Laboratory Studies for Evaluation of Impaired Hearing

AUDIOMETRY

Audiometry helps to classify a hearing loss as conductive or sensorineural. The basic audiogram consists of pure tone air and bone conduction testing with evaluation of speech reception threshold and speech discrimination. The *pure tone air thresholds* are obtained by stimulating each ear individually with a standard spectrum of sound frequencies (pitch) from 250 c/s (low tones) to 8000 c/s (high tones). The minimal intensity (decibel) at which the patient perceives each tone is charted at the threshold for that frequency. The responses are recorded as indicated in Figures 210-1 and 210-2. The pure tone air threshold curve measures both the conductive and sensorineural components of hearing. In order to appreciate a conductive component to a hearing loss, bone conduction thresholds are obtained.

In *bone conduction testing,* the mastoid process of each ear is directly stimulated with an oscillator or vibrator over a similar frequency spectrum and results are graphically recorded (see Fig. 210-3). The bone conduction audiogram by-

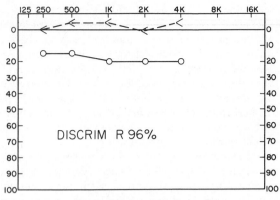

Figure 210-3. Air–bone gap.

passes the ossicular chain, tympanic membrane, and canal by directly vibrating the skull, thus measuring cochlear/eighth nerve capacity. With standardization the bone thresholds approximate those obtained by air. A discrepancy between air-

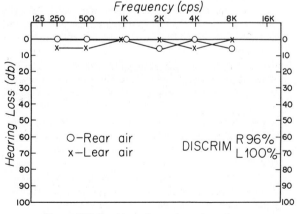

Figure 210-4. Presbycusis due to hair cell loss. Note good hearing thresholds at the speech frequencies 250 to 2000 c/s.

Figure 210-1. Symbol key.

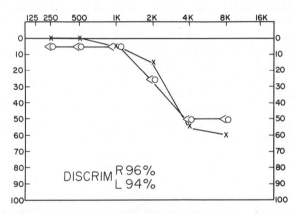

Figure 210-5. Presbycusis due to loss of cochlear neurons. Note poor discrimination.

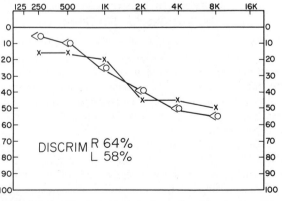

Figure 210-2. Normal pure tone air audiogram.

conducted sound waves and those conducted by the skull (see Fig. 210-5), or a so-called air–bone gap, is indicative of impaired sound conduction, be it ossicular or more laterally located, involving a perforated tympanic membrane or a blocked ear canal.

Because of the capacity of the bones of the skull to conduct airborne sound waves striking it at an intensity greater than 40 dB, masking (the presentation of broad-band white noise in the ear not undergoing testing) is necessary to ensure that sounds are perceived by the tested ear.

Additional testing includes *speech reception threshold* (SRT) and speech discrimination testing. The SRT is defined as the lowest intensity at which the patient can correctly identify 50% of presented words. The SRT should match, within a few decibels, the average of the pure tone thresholds at 500, 1000, and 2000 c/s; this checks the validity of the hearing test. The SRT also determines the intensity at which speech discrimination testing is to be performed.

Discrimination testing evaluates the comprehension of speech, and as such is an extremely important measure of useful hearing. The test is conducted at a loudness 40 dB above the determined SRT for each ear. Speech discrimination, for example, the understanding of words, that is markedly diminished in proportion to the recorded hearing loss is indicative of auditory nerve pathology; in fact, this is a useful diagnostic clue to acoustic neuroma, when the speech discrimination is poor and the pure tone thresholds are relatively good. Ordinarily, patients with good pure tone hearing should hear speech (words) well also.

BRAINSTEM-EVOKED RESPONSE AUDIOMETRY AND ELECTRONYSTAGMOGRAPHY

Brainstem-evoked response audiometry (BSERA) uses computer averaging techniques to record responses of the auditory pathways to a presented sound stimulus (click or tone burst). Five waves of response are recognized, sequentially associated with the cochlear nerve action potential, the cochlear nucleus, the superior olive, the lateral lemniscus, and the inferior colliculus. Conduction delays or aberrancies of waveform are indicative of pathology; the site of the abnormality gives a clue to the site of the lesion of the sound conduction pathway (so-called site-of-lesion testing). BSERA also is useful for obtaining "hearing" thresholds in infants or other difficult-to-test patients, such as retarded, unconscious, or malingering patients. The quality of the tracing obtained is highly operator-dependent, and appropriate interpretation by a skilled audiologist is mandatory for maximal usefulness of the study.

The *electronystagmogram* (ENG) provides a permanent recording on ECG-like paper of nystagmus at rest and in response to vestibular stimulation, be it positional changes or calorics (warm and cold water irrigation of the ear canals). ENG patterns are recognized which may suggest peripheral vestibular system disorder (*e.g.,* the semicircular canals or the vestibular component of the eighth cranial nerve) or a more central basis (brain stem or cerebellum) for dizziness and disequilibrium. This test requires careful interpretation by an otolaryngologist, an otoneurologist, or a neurologist.

211
Approach to Epistaxis
WILLIAM R. WILSON, M.D.

Most spontaneous nosebleeds are self-limited. Patients present for medical care when the bleeding becomes unusually brisk, will not stop, or episodes become frequent. Severe or recurrent bleeding necessitates evaluation for nasal pathology and, less commonly, an underlying generalized disorder. The immediate therapeutic objective is control of bleeding.

PATHOPHYSIOLOGY AND CLINICAL PRESENTATION

Etiologies. The primary mechanism of epistaxis is disruption of the nasal mucosa, primarily caused by *trauma.* In patients with deviated septum or septal spurs in the anterior portion of the nose, trauma occurs easily, either from the drying effects of poorly humidified air or secondary to probing in or bumps on the nose. Picking, rubbing, or forceful blowing

may also trigger bleeding when the nasal mucosa is inflamed from a viral, bacterial, or allergic cause.

Ulcerations, which tend to form over septal deviations and spurs, bleed easily. Repeated mucosal exposure to cocaine leads to anoxic tissue necrosis from drug-induced intense vasospasm; perforation may result and cause chronic crusting and bleeding. Collagen diseases such as lupus are occasionally responsible for ulceration.

Bleeding diatheses sometimes present as epistaxis (see Chapter 80). For example, patients with Osler-Weber-Rendu syndrome manifest a positive family history, telangiectasia, and onset of repeated bleeding episodes in midlife. Adolescent boys with a nasopharyngeal angiofibroma experience brisk posterior epistaxis.

Wegener's granulomatosis, midline granuloma, and *nasal malignancy* share a presentation of epistaxis, unremitting sinus infection, and opacified sinuses on x-ray. Posterior epistaxis is commonly attributed to hypertension, but epidemiologic studies show that few hypertensives experience nosebleeds.

Site of Bleeding. Regardless of etiology, the site of bleeding has distinguishing clinical characteristics. Active *anterior epistaxis* usually presents as unilateral, continuous, moderate bleeding from the septum. Recurrent episodes of bleeding, lasting a few minutes to half an hour over the preceding few days and controlled by pinching the anterior nose are characteristic. The majority of adult cases and almost all spontaneous nasal hemorrhage in children occur on the anterior aspect of the nasal septum. Most are venous, but an arterial source becomes more common with advancing age and mucosal and vascular atrophy.

Posterior epistaxis is associated with intermittent, very brisk arterial bleeding, with blood flowing into the pharynx unless the patient is leaning forward. When the patient is leaning forward, the blood may run from one or both sides of the nose. Spontaneous posterior hemorrhage is more common in the older age groups and following severe facial trauma. The vessel rupture is usually just superior or inferior to the posterior tip of the inferior turbinate on the lateral nasal wall.

DIFFERENTIAL DIAGNOSIS

The differential diagnosis of nosebleeds can be divided into local and systemic disorders. The local causes are most commonly inflammatory or traumatic. The most notable inflammatory lesions are upper respiratory infections, allergies, and chronic sinusitis. Trauma may be induced by habitual picking, constant rubbing, or forceful blowing of the nose. Chronic occupational exposure to volatile chemical irritants and repeated nasal use of cocaine are becoming increasingly frequent. Local vascular lesions include angiomas and hereditary hemorrhagic telangiectasia. More than 90% of bleeds are related to local irritation; most occur in the absence of a specific underlying anatomic lesion.

Nosebleeds occasionally occur during the course of certain infectious diseases such as chickenpox and influenza. Granulomatous disease (Wegener's midline granuloma, sarcoidosis) may lead to nasal bleeding. The patient with an underlying hematologic disease, a clotting problem, or a disorder of platelet function may present with bleeding from the nose (see Chapter 80). A rare hypertensive patient with severe pressure elevation may experience epistaxis.

WORKUP

History should begin with inquiry into the amount of bleeding, its duration, and frequency. After the bleeding is under control, the patient can be questioned about easy bruising, hematuria, melena, heavy periods, family history of bleeding disorders, the use of oral anticoagulants or drugs with antiplatelet effects (aspirin, etc.), occupational exposure to irritating chemicals or dust, dry home, chronic cocaine use, and repeated noseblowing or picking.

Physical Examination should be performed with the patient sitting and leaning forward so that the blood flows from the nose. This allows the physician to assess the rate and site of bleeding, as well as to prevent the swallowing of blood, which will quickly lead to emesis. The pulse and blood pressure should be taken and the skin and conjunctiva checked for rash, pallor, purpura, petechiae, and telangiectasias. Lymph nodes should be examined for enlargement, suggesting sarcoidosis, tuberculosis, or malignancy. The sinuses are percussed for evidence of sinusitis, which would make Wegener's, midline granuloma, and nasal tumor considerations.

Laboratory Studies are best ordered on the basis of findings from the history and physical examination. The patients suspected of a bleeding diathesis should have a bleeding time, PT, PTT, and blood smear or platelet count obtained (see Chapter 80). Sinus films are appropriate to evaluate the patient with recurrent bouts of sinus pain, tenderness, and bleeding.

PRINCIPLES OF MANAGEMENT

The first objective is to stop the bleeding. The approach depends upon whether the source is anterior or posterior.

Anterior Septal Bleeding. A few simple first-aid measures suffice for the vast majority of cases. The patient should *sit up* (this reduces venous pressure) and *lean forward* (which prevents the swallowing of blood if the bleeding is anterior). A small piece of cotton or cotton balls soaked in 1:1000 epinephrine or a vasoconstricting nosedrop such as *phenylephrine* (Neo-Synephrine) or *oxymetazoline* (Afrin) is placed in the vestibule of the nose and pressed against the bleeding site for 5 to 10 minutes. It is then removed to observe for rebleeding. This will stop almost all venous types of anterior nosebleeds. Humidification and a lubricant such as petrolatum ointment help promote healing.

If these remedies fail, the mucous membrane can be anesthetized by applying cotton soaked with 4% cocaine or 4% lidocaine for 5 minutes. A *silver nitrate stick* can then be applied to the bleeding site and to any prominent vessels.

Occasionally, a small artery in the septal mucous membrane will either fail to stop bleeding or rebleed a short time later. These episodes can usually be controlled by anesthetizing and recauterizing the area. This is followed by placing a small amount of *oxidized regenerated cellulose* (Surgigel) against the bleeding artery, or a small *packing of petroleum gauze* strip in the nasal vestibule for 24 hours.

Patients with bleeding disorders require especially careful treatment to prevent abrading the mucous membrane. Therapy involves use of humidity, copious lubricants, and soft cotton tamponades wetted with long-acting vasoconstricting drops (oxymetazoline 0.1%; Afrin nasal solution). Packing should be avoided at all costs, but if unavoidable can be accomplished with a piece of oxidized cellulose which does not require removal. Further treatment is best directed at the underlying bleeding disorder.

Posterior Epistaxis constitutes an inherently more serious problem, because of the relative rapidity of blood loss and the relatively inaccessible and poorly visualized bleeding site in the posterior nose. Initial efforts should be made to bring the bleeding under control while awaiting an otolaryngologic consult. Hematocrit, blood pressure, and pulse should be immediately obtained, and if necessary, a sample sent for type and crossmatch. The patient should be instructed to *sit up* and *lean forward,* and if there has been a temporary interruption in the bleeding, no treatment other than *spraying* the nose with a topical anesthetic and vasoconstricting substance, such as *4% cocaine,* should be attempted. The nose should be suctioned or blown clear only when the medical personnel present are prepared to deal with brisk epistaxis. If the patient's blood pressure permits, a parenteral analgesic such as Demerol 50 or 100 mg intramuscularly should be given prior to the surgeon's *electrocautery* of the posterior nose, or the placement of *compressing* balloons, packs, or tampons.

PATIENT EDUCATION

Prevention. Once septal bleeding is controlled in the office or emergency ward, measures to prevent recurrence should be instituted. The patient should keep the septum well coated with petrolatum-based ointment such as zinc oxide, A and D ointment, or an antibiotic ointment until healed, usually in 3 to 5 days. The fingernails of children should be trimmed short. Minor recurrent bleeding can be controlled by the patient's use of cotton pledgets soaked in vasoconstricting solutions and pressed against the bleeding site. Instruct the patient on the need to avoid traumatizing the mucosa. Specifically, warn against habitual nose picking, constant rubbing with a handkerchief, and excessively forceful blowing. Explain the importance of humidifying the home environment. This may be done by keeping a few windows partially open, by placing containers of water near radiators or stoves, or by installing a humidifier. Occasionally, patients may benefit from use of a water-based lubricant applied to the rims of the nostrils in order to maintain mucosal moisture; however, this does involve a very small risk of lipoid pneumonia, and should be avoided in children and the elderly.

First-Aid. Few patients understand the proper treatment for care of minor nosebleeds at home; simple telephone instruction may obviate the need for an office or emergency room visit. The patient should be instructed to *sit up* and remain calm, *lean forward* and *press the ala* of the vestibule against the septum on the side than is bleeding in order to tamponade the flow. The nose can then be sprayed with any of the over-the-counter nasal sprays that contain *phenylephrine* (e.g., Neo-Synephrine) or oxymetazoline (Afrin). A small *pledget of cotton* is then lightly soaked with the spray and pressed against the bleeding portion of the septum. After 10 minutes, most nosebleeds will have stopped. A *petrolatum-based ointment,* such as zinc oxide or Bacitracin, can be applied to the septum to prevent further drying and abrasion of the septum. It is left in for a few days and the patient instructed to limit heavy lifting, other forms of straining, bending over, intake of spicy or hot foods, hot showers, and medications which might impair hemostasis (see Chapter 80).

Reassure the patient when the nosebleed is purely a local phenomenon; many people attribute nosebleeds to hypertension and fear cerebral hemorrhage.

INDICATIONS FOR REFERRAL AND ADMISSION

Patients with active posterior bleeding should be admitted to the hospital immediately for emergency treatment to control the bleeding. Posterior packing can cause airway obstruction, particularly in elderly patients, due to downward displacement of the soft palate and subsequent palatal edema and swelling or slipped packing. All patients with nasal packing should be closely observed for signs of hypoxia and hypercarbia. Unfortunately, packs must be left in place for a minimum of 5 days to be effective. Posterior packing is associated with a great deal of discomfort; the patients generally require intravenous hydration because of poor oral intake due to painful swallowing, antibiotics to prevent sinusitis, pain medications, and careful observation by the nursing staff for impending airway obstruction.

ANNOTATED BIBLIOGRAPHY

Hallberg OE: Severe nosebleed and its treatment. JAMA 148:355, 1952 (*A classic article that is still very useful.*)

Kirchner JA: Epistaxis. N Engl J Med 307:1126, 1982 (*A review of anatomy, etiology, and therapy of epistaxis.*)

Lingeman RA: Epistaxis. Am J Fam Phys 14(6):78, 1976 (*A brief, practical article that clearly illustrates methods for nasal packing.*)

Wilson WR, Nadol JB Jr: Quick Reference to Ear, Nose, and Throat Disorders. Chapter 8, Nasal and Facial Emergencies, p 145. Philadelphia, JB Lippincott, 1983 (*A discussion of emergency measures.*)

212
Evaluation of Facial Pain and Swelling
JOHN P. KELLY, D.M.D., M.D.

The primary care physician often encounters patients whose presenting complaint of facial pain or swelling is related to the masticatory apparatus (teeth, gums, jaws, muscles) or salivary glands. Dental decay is the most prevalent disease in the United States and a major cause of conditions leading to facial pain and swelling. Because symptoms may be referred to nondental structures and because an odontogenic infection may involve areas of the head and neck seemingly unrelated to the teeth, the patient may first seek the advice of a physician rather than of a dentist. Prompt recognition and effective initial treatment may well prevent development of a serious complication such as abscess formation.

PATHOPHYSIOLOGY AND CLINICAL PRESENTATION

Odontogenic Infection. Dental decay is a multifactorial disease that encompasses dietary factors (most notably, refined carbohydrates), environmental factors (such as availability of fluoride ion during the production of the enamel of the teeth) and various host factors (not the least of which is the patient's oral hygiene habits). Oral bacteria utilize dietary carbohydrates to form plaque on the enamel of the teeth; susceptible enamel is then decalcified, resulting in a "cavity" or carious lesion.

In its initial stages, *decay* is asymptomatic. However, when the dentin beneath the enamel is exposed, the patient may complain of aching pain when the affected tooth comes into contact with hot, cold, or sweet substances. The frequent finding of referred pain may make localization of the offending tooth difficult and is one reason why a patient may first consult his physician rather than his dentist.

Progressive decay of the tooth will result in *inflammation of the pulp* (pulpitis); the symptoms will be unchanged until the dental pulp becomes necrotic and, eventually, suppurative. The cardinal symptom then is deep, throbbing pain on exposure to hot foods or drinks; the pain is abruptly relieved by ice or cold water. This symptom complex is quite distinct from the paroxysmal, lancinating pain of trigeminal neuralgia, which has no relationship to extremes of temperature, but which may be related to eating because of the presence of trigger zones in the oral cavity (see Chapter 170).

Simple dental decay, pulpitis, and pulpal necrosis all are recognized by pain and by clinical and radiographic examination. They are not associated with fever, swelling, or leu-

kocytosis. However, when the infection of the pulp spreads beyond the confines of the tooth to involve the periodontal ligament and the adjacent alveolar bone, an acute *alveolar abscess* may ensue. In this condition, the affected tooth is tender to percussion or to masticatory forces and is mobile. The adjacent soft tissues begin to show the classic signs of acute inflammation: edema, erythema, heat, and tenderness. The location of the involved tooth will determine the location of the swelling. Abscessed maxillary teeth will produce labial or infraorbital edema; an infected mandibular tooth will produce submandibular edema. Lymphadenopathy of the cervical chain can be seen in either maxillary or mandibular infection. Fever, leukocytosis, and dehydration are frequent concomitants of the acute alveolar abscess with facial cellulitis.

Spread of the infection along the fascial planes of the head and neck can result in life-threatening complications, such as cavernous sinus thrombosis, meningitis, or mediastinitis. Such devastating complications were once quite common; they are still seen today, even with the availability of antibiotics.

A typical history obtained from a patient with a *facial cellulitis* reveals a previous episode of toothache with pain suggestive of pulpitis, which may regress spontaneously. An asymptomatic period, corresponding to pulpal necrosis, then precedes the onset of swelling and pain when the necrotic pulp becomes infected and the process spreads to adjacent anatomic structures.

Periodontal Infection. Acute bacterial infection of the periodontal tissues is most often localized to the gingiva or mucosa adjacent to the involved tooth. The typical patient will complain of a "gum boil," and examination will reveal a discrete, fluctuant swelling which may drain easily on manual palpation.

In the late adolescent years, infection of the soft tissue surrounding erupting third molars or wisdom teeth (pericoronitis) is common. Low-grade, chronic infection may be accompanied by symptoms described as "teething"; acute infection will result in pain, swelling and difficulty in opening the mouth (trismus) as the adjacent masticator space becomes involved.

Salivary Gland Swelling. Acute infection of the major salivary glands (parotid, submandibular, and sublingual) may be either viral or bacterial. *Viral parotitis* (mumps) is a disease well known to family practitioners, occurring most frequently in school-age children and appearing either unilaterally or bilaterally. The efficacy of immunization programs should make this disease a relative rarity in the future. Viral lymphadenopathy in the preauricular area, such as that seen in infectious mononucleosis and in cat-scratch disease, may masquerade as parotid swelling and must be considered.

Sialadenitis, bacterial infection of the salivary glands, commonly affects a single gland. The infection is generally an ascending infection in which bacteria gain access to a gland made susceptible to infection by stasis of saliva. Obstruction of the salivary duct by a stone or mucinous plug is the usual inciting event, but any low-flow state can lead to sialadenitis. The condition is frequently seen in elderly, debilitated or postoperative patients, in whom dehydration may lead to decreased salivary flow and consequent infection. The parotid gland is the usual target organ for this infectious process and involvement is more often unilateral than bilateral. Purulent drainage can be obtained from the duct orifice. Previous episodes of parotitis or congenital abnormality of the acinar structure of the parotid gland may produce sialoangiectasis, which facilitates pooling and stasis of saliva within the gland and increases the patient's susceptibility to episodes of acute infection.

Noninfectious salivary swelling is a component of a number of *systemic conditions,* including diabetes mellitus, uremia, Laennec's cirrhosis, chronic alcoholism, and malnutrition. A toxic reaction to a variety of drugs, such as iodine, mercury, and guanethidine, causes a painless bilateral parotid gland swelling. A specific triad of keratoconjunctivitis sicca, salivary gland swelling, and rheumatoid arthritis is known as *Sjögren's syndrome.* Since its original description with rheumatoid arthritis, the syndrome has also been related to other chronic autoimmune connective tissue disorders, such as systemic lupus erythematosus (SLE), and polyarteritis nodosa. The diagnosis of Sjögren's syndrome may be made initially without apparent systemic disease and may be the stimulus for further workup to detect the presence of rheumatoid disease. Development of lymphoma in a patient with longstanding Sjögren's syndrome has been recently recognized and must be considered.

Infiltration of both major and minor salivary glands by lymphoproliferative processes is an important consideration in the differential diagnosis of salivary swelling. Lymphomas, tuberculosis, and sarcoidosis (uveoparotid fever) have all been first diagnosed from salivary gland enlargement.

DIFFERENTIAL DIAGNOSIS

The causes of facial pain or swelling can be divided into odontogenic, nonodontogenic, and salivary gland etiologies (Table 212-1).

WORKUP

History. Evaluation of facial pain and swelling requires thorough consideration of the pain's onset, severity, quality, location, radiation, aggravating or ameliorating factors, and duration. The various stages of dental infection can be characterized by specific pain histories. For example, pain brought on by contact with hot, cold, or sweet substances is indicative of dental caries, whereas aggravation by heat and relief by cold suggests a periapical abscess. If fever and swelling ensue, an alveolar abscess must be considered. Lancinating pain precipitated by contact with a trigger zone is typical of trigeminal neuralgia; it can be distinguished by history from abscess formation because symptoms are unrelated to the temperature of the contacting substance, and swelling is absent.

In the patient who complains of salivary gland enlargement, it is important to inquire about site(s) of involvement, presence of fever or tenderness, history of chronic illness, malignancy, toxin or drug exposure, and symptoms of rheumatologic disease or sicca syndrome (dry eyes, dry mouth). Unilateral painful swelling of acute onset suggests sialadenitis, especially when seen in an elderly, debilitated, or postoperative patient. A unilaterally enlarged, painless parotid may be due to tumor, particularly if there is a history of progressive increase in size and extension beyond the gland. Bilateral involvement requires consideration of lymphoma and sarcoidosis as well as Sjögren's syndrome (which is bilateral in about half of cases).

It is important to keep in mind that episodic jaw pain may be due to angina (see Chapter 14).

Physical Examination. A semisitting position will usually allow both patient comfort and examiner access. While a flashlight can be used, a lighting fixture that can illuminate the oral cavity and leave the examiner with both hands free is preferable.

Inspection of the mouth for fractured, decayed, or heavily restored teeth and for heavy deposits of debris and calculus ("tartar") on the teeth and gingiva requires little experience and will direct the examiner's attention to odontogenic disease as a likely source of the pain or swelling. A dental mirror or a short-handled laryngoscopy mirror serves as a better retractor than does a wooden tongue blade. Palpation of the teeth to determine tenderness or mobility will help to identify an abscessed tooth. The soft tissues should be palpated to detect the presence of indurated or fluctuant swelling adjacent to a suspicious tooth. Tenderness to percussion of a tooth, using a short, sharp tap with the dental mirror handle, is diagnostic of an abscessed tooth. The salivary glands are palpated bimanually intraorally and extraorally; the salivary duct orifices should be observed for salivary flow or purulent drainage during palpation of the individual glands. Cervical lymph nodes should be checked for enlargement and tenderness.

Table 212-1.   Important Causes of Facial Pain or Swelling

CAUSE OF PAIN	SYMPTOMS
Odontogenic pain	
Caries	Hot, cold, or sweet sensitive; brief
Pulpitis	Hot and cold aggravate; prolonged; more severe; radiation of pain
Periapical abscess	Heat aggravates, cold relieves; sensitivity to percussion; mobility of tooth
Alveolar abscess	Swelling, malaise
Nonodontogenic pain	
Neuralgia	Lancinating pain; trigger zone
Myalgia	Trismus or pain on opening; deviation of jaw to affected side; tender muscle
Referred	Angina
Salivary Pain and Swelling	
Viral infection (mumps)	
Bacterial infection	
Obstructed flow	
Chemical, metabolic agents	
Lymphoproliferative diseases	
Autoimmune diseases (Sjögren's syndrome)	
Tumors	
Lymphadenopathy	
Masseter hypertrophy	

Laboratory Studies. Suspicion of dental caries can be confirmed by x-ray, as can abscess formation. Most other conditions produce few radiologic changes. White blood count in the potentially toxic patient or blood sugar in the diabetic patient may aid in subsequent management. Suspicion of Sjögren's syndrome can be confirmed by lip biopsy. It is important to obtain any purulent drainage for Gram stain, culture, and sensitivity testing.

INDICATIONS FOR REFERRAL

Early recognition of dental decay and gingival inflammation with consequent referral to a general dentist for complete evaluation and treatment is the most effective means of preventing infection. In the patient with valvular heart disease, full dental evaluation on a periodic basis is mandatory and is particularly indicated prior to consideration of a valvular prosthesis so that potential sources of dental sepsis may be eliminated. Adequate antibiotic prophylaxis for subacute bacterial endocarditis must be provided for such patients at the time dental procedures are performed (see Chapter 11).

When physical examination indicates no other source of facial pain, referral for dental evaluation is indicated. Abscess formation necessitates prompt referral for definitive drainage.

When the patient's clinical appearance demonstrates involvement of deep fascial spaces, as evidenced by fever, trismus, elevation of the tongue, ophthalmoplegia, and so forth, referral to an oral surgeon and admission to the hospital for parenteral antibiotics are urgent.

The patient with acute salivary swelling should be seen by an oral surgeon for radiographic examination, by which sialoliths causing obstruction are sought. Gentle dilatation of the duct may help to relieve the obstruction; in some cases, surgery is necessary to remove the stone. Sialography, or examination of the salivary system with radiographic contrast injections, is contraindicated in the acute period of infection.

When salivary swelling is chronic in nature, no antibiotics are indicated. Sialography is highly diagnostic in this group of patients. If the differential diagnosis includes Sjögren's syndrome, sarcoidosis, or lymphoma, a biopsy of one of the minor salivary glands of the lower lip will usually confirm the diagnosis, without necessitating a more complex parotid biopsy.

SYMPTOMATIC MANAGEMENT

While awaiting dental evaluation, the very uncomfortable patient may require strong analgesia (*e.g.,* codeine sulfate,

30 mg every 4 to 6 hours). Penicillin remains the primary antibiotic of choice in treatment of odontogenic infection and for patients with valvular heart disease who need prophylaxis for dental work. Initiation of an oral penicillin-VK regimen of 250 mg every 6 hours is appropriate at the first recognition of swelling associated with an infected tooth or periodontal tissue. A 2.0 g oral dose 1 hour before dental work and a 1.0 g oral dose 6 hours later is sufficient for endocarditis prophylaxis. Antibiotics are not indicated in the absence of swelling. Erythromycin is the preferred drug for the patient allergic to penicillin. Referral of the patient to an oral surgeon for definitive drainage of the infection at the earliest opportunity is indicated and should be made simultaneously with the prescribing of antibiotics.

Acute swelling of a salivary gland, accompanied by purulent or inspissated saliva from the involved duct, requires antibiotic treatment. Stimulation of salivary flow with sour candies and warm compresses is a helpful local measure. The submandibular gland tends to be infected with the same flora as is found in odontogenic infections. Hence, penicillin is the drug of choice for submandibular sialadenitis. Acute bacterial parotitis, on the other hand, is associated with staphylococcal species, and one of the penicillinase-resistant antibiotics, such as dicloxacillin, is preferred. Antibiotic treatment for other infections which may have preceded the onset of the salivary infection can alter the oral flora and produce infection of the salivary system by unusual organisms, such as *E. coli*. Thus, culturing of the purulent saliva is suggested.

ANNOTATED BIBLIOGRAPHY

Chow AW, Roser SM, Brady FA: Orofacial odontogenic infections. Ann Intern Med 88:392, 1978 (*A comprehensive review of pertinent oral microbiology, surgical anatomy of the spread of infection, and the signs and symptoms of patients with odontogenic infection.*)

Guralnick WC, Dinoff RB, Galbadini J: Tender parotid swelling in a dehydrated patient, J Oral Surg 26:669, 1968 (*A good differential diagnosis of salivary gland swelling.*)

Kaye D: Prophylaxis for infective endocarditis: An update. Ann Intern Med 104:419, 1986 (*A review of the latest recommendations.*)

213

Approach to the Patient with Hoarseness

WILLIAM R. WILSON, M.D.

Hoarseness is a symptom of laryngeal disease. The majority of acute episodes are self-limited and due to viral upper respiratory tract infection or voice abuse. However, the patient bothered by persistent hoarseness requires careful assessment, because carcinoma of the larynx, tumor-associated damage to the recurrent laryngeal nerve, and other serious conditions may be responsible. Prompt evaluation maximizes the chances of detecting an early lesion and achieving a cure.

PATHOPHYSIOLOGY AND CLINICAL PRESENTATION

Vocal quality is determined by complex factors, including the distance between vocal cords, tenseness of the cords, and the rapidity of vibration. Hoarseness results from interference with normal apposition of the cords. Inflammatory, traumatic, and neoplastic lesions cause hoarseness by altering cord structure and function.

Often the quality of the voice disturbance reflects the underlying pathophysiology. A "breathy" voice occurs when the vocal cords do not approximate completely, allowing air to escape during vocalization. The cords may be kept apart by tumor, polyps, or nodules. A similar presentation occurs when the cords fail to approximate due to unilateral or bi-lateral cord paralysis. Patients with hysterical aphonia purposefully hold the cords apart while speaking.

A "raspy" or harsh voice ensues from cord thickening due to edema or inflammation. This is the voice quality characteristic of many heavy smokers. The voice is of lowered pitch and poor clarity. Associated inspiratory or expiratory cervical stridor results from laryngeal obstruction.

A high, "shaky" voice or a low, soft vocalization are consequences of decreased respiratory force (phonasthenia). These voices characterize elderly or debilitated patients, who may complain of additional voice difficulties, such as change in voice pitch or poor vocal projection.

The presentations of a number of etiologies are best considered in terms of whether they are acute or chronic.

Acute Hoarseness

Acute laryngitis leads to vocal cord edema and erythema. Viral infection, vocal abuse, sudden excessive smoking, inhalation of irritant gases, aspiration, and occasionally allergy (hay fever) constitute the list of important precipitants. *Vocal cord nodules* may develop when edematous cords are used excessively. Fibrous tissue begins to collect at the junction of the anterior one-third and the posterior two-thirds of the cord. This results in a lowered breathy voice which can harm a singing or speaking career.

Acute laryngeal edema may present as part of a generalized edematous allergic response involving the lips, tongue, and other hypopharyngeal tissues. *Foods* are important precipitants, especially seafoods and nuts; medications can have a similar effect. Edema can develop from hereditary deficiency of C-1-esterase inhibitor (*hereditary angioneurotic edema*). Swelling forms in response to mechanical trauma, such as dental surgery or intubation for general anesthesia. In the pediatric population, subglottic edema from viral laryngotracheal bronchitis (*croup*) can obstruct the airway. In adults, *acute epiglottitis* has been noted with increasing frequency. It is associated with risk of airway obstruction, especially in the setting of *H. influenzae* infection. Symptoms include severe sore throat, dyspnea, and hoarseness.

Chronic Hoarseness

Chronic laryngitis causes a low, raspy voice, a nonproductive cough, and a "dry throat" sensation. There is little or no pain. The voice waxes and wanes, becoming worse as the day progresses. The typical patient is a heavy smoker who continually talks, subjecting himself to a combination of chemical irritation and vocal abuse. In rare instances, an infectious or chronic inflammatory condition (*e.g.,* tuberculosis or sarcoidosis) may produce a similar picture. Chronic laryngeal edema with development of *dependent polyps* represents another form of chronic laryngitis; it may arise in the setting of hypothyroidism, radiation therapy to the neck, or chronic sinusitis with persistent drainage and cough. Patients with this condition speak in a lowered, gravelly voice with short phonation time.

Leukoplakia, another form of chronic laryngitis, is the term for the white, scalelike appearance of hyperkeratotic changes involving the vocal cords. It occurs secondary to chemical irritation, especially from *tobacco* smoke and *alcohol.* Symptoms include hoarseness but no pain. Leukoplakia, which may be a premalignant state, cannot be distinguished visually from squamous cell carcinoma in situ, or early invasive cancer.

Contact ulcers of the larynx occur on the posterior third of the vocal cords where the arytenoid cartilage is covered only by a thin layer of mucosa. Once this mucosa is abraded, an ulcer often forms. Symptoms are painful phonation and a weakened, "breathy" voice. Chronic ulcerations may in time develop into granulations that hold the cords apart, and at times these may become large enough to cause some respiratory obstruction. The ulcerations result most commonly from acute or chronic laryngeal *intubation* but classically are the result of *vocal abuse* by orators who misuse their larynx attempting to lower the pitch of their voices when speaking forcefully.

Vocal cord paralysis occurs with nerve injury; usually just one cord is paralyzed (except in patients with severe CNS

disease) giving a weak, breathy voice. The position of the cord is affected by the amount of time that has elapsed since injury, as paralyzed cords tend to move toward the midline. The degree of paralysis and the clinical presentation depend on where the neural injury is located. Injury to a vagus nerve results in the loss of all ipsilateral laryngeal muscle function and sensation, leading to aspiration and a weak, breathy voice. A more peripheral injury of the recurrent laryngeal nerve leads to little if any aspiration and a voice that is hoarse and somewhat weak, but less breathy. Viral neuritis is the most common cause; function usually returns in 6 to 9 months.

Laryngeal carcinoma usually occurs in patients with a history of smoking and drinking. If the vocal cords are involved, progressive hoarseness is an early sign, but if the tumor arises on the epiglottis, hypopharynx, or false cords, hoarseness may be a late development. Pain secondary to ulceration is also a late symptom and is often perceived as referred otologic pain, especially when swallowing. These patients may have a mildly fetid breath. Patients with a hypopharyngeal or laryngeal cancer can present with an unexplained lymph node in the neck.

DIFFERENTIAL DIAGNOSIS

The causes of hoarseness are best considered in terms of acute and chronic etiologies (see Table 213-1).

Table 213-1.   Important Causes of Hoarseness

ACUTE HOARSENESS	CHRONIC HOARSENESS
Acute laryngitis	Chronic laryngitis
Viral infection	Chronic or recurrent vocal
Vocal abuse	abuse
Toxic fumes	Smoking
Allergy (seasonal)	Allergy
	Persistent irritant exposure
Acute laryngeal edema	
Angioneurotic edema	Carcinoma of larynx
Infection	Intrinsic to vocal cords
Direct injury	Extrinsic to vocal cords
Nephritis	
	Vocal cord lesions
Acute epiglottitis	Polyps
	Leukoplakia
	Contact ulcer and granuloma
	Vocal nodule (see vocal abuse)
	Benign tumors
	Vocal cord paralysis
	Laryngeal nerve injury (tumor,
	neck surgery, aortic
	aneurysm)
	Brain stem lesion
	Vocal cord trauma
	Chronic intubation
	Systemic disorders
	Hypothyroidism
	Rheumatoid arthritis
	Virilization
	Psychogenic

WORKUP

History. The evaluation of hoarseness depends on the chronicity of the condition. One needs to determine whether the onset was sudden or gradual and the course self-limited or progressive. Difficulty in breathing or stridor suggests obstruction and is an indication for emergency hospital admission. It is helpful to find out if hoarseness is exacerbated by talking; also whether the voice completely disappeared and, if so, for how long. Any recent upper respiratory tract infection, sore throat, fever, chills, sputum or myalgias should be noted, as well as excessive voice use. Exposure to dust, fire, smoke, or irritant fumes should be documented, as should tobacco and alcohol intake. A history of neck mass, neck surgery, intubation, or lung tumor may provide important clues to etiology. Symptoms of hypothyroidism (see Chapter 102) are worth checking for when the etiology is not readily evident.

Physical Examination. There are two rules of thumb regarding patients with hoarseness: first, hoarseness of more than 2 to 3 weeks' duration requires an examination of the larynx, and second, this examination will provide, in the majority of cases, an immediate diagnosis.

A good view of the hypopharynx and larynx is somewhat difficult to obtain, but the primary physician is encouraged to try, and with practice can master the technique. *Indirect laryngoscopy* with a head light and warmed laryngeal mirror is a time-honored method and still provides the best and most rapidly obtained view of the area. For the gagging patient, premedication with 10 mg of diazepam orally and an analgesic throat spray (Cetacaine, xylocaine 1% spray) are of benefit. For patients with uncontrollable gag reflexes, referral for examination with a fiberoptic laryngoscope will be necessary. As this instrument is introduced through the nose, the nasal passages are vasoconstricted and anesthetized (cocaine 4% solution is ideal). It is rare when a good laryngeal view cannot be obtained in this manner.

Even if laryngoscopy cannot be carried out, some clues as to etiology can be gleaned by a careful physical examination and noting voice quality. One needs to examine the oropharynx and carefully palpate the thyroid and cervical lymph nodes. The hoarse patient with an unexplained neck mass or lymph node requires a thorough check of the nose, paranasal sinuses, and nasopharynx. A breathy voice suggests poor cord apposition, which may be due to tumor, polyp, or nodule. A raspy voice is indicative of cord thickening due to edema or inflammation, as with chemical irritation, vocal abuse, and infection. The patient with a high, shaky voice or a very soft one is having trouble mounting adequate respiratory force. Dyspnea is an indication for laryngoscopy.

Laboratory Studies. In most instances, the selection of studies depends upon the findings at laryngoscopy and should be done in conjunction with the otolaryngologist. The patient with unilateral paresis of the right vocal cord may have a recurrent laryngeal nerve syndrome secondary to a Pancoast tumor, necessitating radiologic evaluation of the right lung apex. If the cords appear chronically edematous and there is clinical suspicion of hypothyroidism, a check of a serum TSH is in order (see Chapter 102). Patients with a suspected carcinoma involving the larynx or with an unexplained neck node and hoarseness need a thorough evaluation of the aerodigestive tract prior to biopsy. Open biopsy of neck nodes done without definitive surgery will reduce chances for survival in patients with carcinoma of the aerodigestive tract. Small needle biopsies have circumvented the need for some open biopsies. The patient with recurrent edematous episodes and a positive family history might have angioneurotic edema; a check of the C-1-esterase inhibitor level is indicated. Soft tissue films may be of use in the dyspneic patient.

PRINCIPLES OF THERAPY AND MANAGEMENT RECOMMENDATIONS

Regardless of causes, all patients with hoarseness should be strongly advised to *quit smoking* immediately (see Chapter 49). It is often in the setting of an associated medical problem that a smoker will finally decide to quit. Other measures are a function of the underlying etiology.

Acute Laryngitis. The best treatment is *voice rest;* when it is necessary to speak, the patient should use a moderate voice and not whisper. Warm *sialogogues,* such as hot tea with sugar and lemon, may be helpful. Antibiotics are not indicated unless there is documented bacterial infection. *Cough suppressants,* particularly with mucolytic agents, may be helpful. Also, *humidity* is of benefit; inhalation of steam in a hot shower or breathing through a moist, hot towel will provide immediate partial relief. When hay fever is the cause, a topical steroid spray such as dexamethasone or flunisolide helps provide symptomatic relief, but steroids should not be used unless there is an allergic etiology.

Patients who are professional singers or speakers should be advised to rest their voice when they become hoarse (especially during upper respiratory infections), in order to prevent permanent injury to the vocal cords. A vasoconstricting spray and analgesics are used by professionals when use of their voice is absolutely necessary. Occasionally, professional singers may be given a short course of topical steroids to get through a singing commitment, but further cord injury may ensue.

Acute laryngeal edema represents a medical emergency; hospitalization is urgent. Treatment is based on the degree of swelling and subsequent airway compromise. An *emergency airway* is established if necessary; 0.3 ml of *adrenalin* 1 to 1000 is administered subcutaneously, and steroids such as *dexamethasone* (Decadron 12 mg) may be given intravenously.

Vocal cord nodules should be treated early because often they respond to voice rest and vocal therapy. Nodules that do not respond to conservative therapy can be removed; use of an atraumatic technique (microlaryngeal surgery, carbon dioxide laser) is mandatory.

Angioneurotic edema does not respond to adrenalin or steroids. In an acute situation, intubation or tracheotomy may be required to maintain an airway. Treatment is prophylactic: namely, avoidance of trauma and stress. Prophylaxis prior to mandatory surgery may include fresh plasma transfusions or the short-term use (because of fear of phlebitis) of epsilon aminocaproic acid prior to and after surgery. The androgens danazol and tranexamic acid have been used in clinical trials for prophylactic treatment. Work is progressing on the synthesis of C-1-esterase inhibitor.

Persistent vocal cord paralysis can be treated symptomatically by the injection of Teflon paste into the musculature of the paralyzed cord, moving it to the midline. This permits the functioning cord to better approximate, thereby improving vocal quality.

Carcinoma of the larynx can be cured, if detected in its early stages (T1N0); surgery, laser treatment, and radiation are all capable of achieving a 90% cure rate. Selection of modality depends on the type of expertise available locally and the location of the lesion. A better voice is usually obtained with laser or irradiation. Metastases and a poor prognosis usually do not occur until the vocal cord cancer becomes larger (T3 to T4) and extends beyond the true cords. Early supraglottic carcinomas arising above the true cords can be cured in about 75% of patients with radiation therapy, partial laryngectomy, or a combination of the two. Larger lesions require total laryngectomy and irradiation, with a cure rate of 40%. Induction chemotherapy is utilized for advanced stages of disease. Prevention remains the best treatment; all smokers must be told to quit.

Leukoplakia is treated by vocal cord stripping under microscopic control. Regular follow-up examinations of the larynx are necessary; repeated vocal cord stripping may be needed once or twice a year, particularly if the patient fails to limit use of irritants.

Dependent polyps are removed by microsurgery.

INDICATIONS FOR REFERRAL AND ADMISSION

If the primary care physician does not feel competent to visualize the vocal cords, a decision must be made about whether to refer the patient to an otolaryngologist. Hoarseness of greater than 3 weeks duration, particularly when there has not been a history of an acute infectious process, requires referral; any patient with concurrent dyspnea should be immediately hospitalized. In those who have a resolving process and are at low risk for malignancy (young, nonsmoker, nondrinker), a complete otolaryngologic examination may be deferred pending full resolution.

Among patients who do undergo indirect laryngoscopy by the primary care physician, any with a cord nodule, thickening, or paralysis by indirect laryngoscopy requires referral, as does the patient with persistent unexplained hoarseness of more than 2 to 3 weeks' duration and inability to tolerate indirect laryngoscopy.

Referral for voice therapy can help foster healthful vocal habits and is indicated for patients who experience repeated vocal trauma or who have organic disease and are in need of voice rehabilitation.

ANNOTATED BIBLIOGRAPHY

Decker J, Goldstein JC: Risk factors in head and neck cancer. N Engl J Med 306:1151, 1983 (*A good segment in this review on laryngeal cancer.*)

Vaughan CW: Diagnosis and treatment of organic voice disorders. N Engl J Med 307:863, 1983 (*A terse review for the general reader.*)

214
Evaluation of Smell and Taste Disturbances

Impairment of taste and smell, in addition to being intrinsically unpleasant, is annoying because it interferes with the ability to derive pleasure from food. Moreover, a diminished ability to detect noxious agents in the environment leaves the patient vulnerable to them. Patients may complain of total loss, attenuation, or perversion of these senses. Problems of smell are often reported as alterations of taste because much of the awareness of taste is olfactory. The primary physician should be capable of recognizing taste and smell disturbances that are manifestations of serious illness requiring detailed evaluation, as well as simple forms in which symptomatic relief will suffice.

PATHOPHYSIOLOGY AND CLINICAL PRESENTATION

Smell. The olfactory area is located high in the nasal vault above the superior turbinate. The neurons of the first cranial nerve penetrate the cribriform plate and travel to the cortex at the base of the frontal lobe on top of the cribriform plate. The most common mechanism of anosmia or hyposmia is *nasal obstruction* that prevents air from reaching olfactory areas high in the nose. Food is tasteless while the problem persists. In most instances, such as those related to the common cold or allergic rhinitis, the process is fully reversible, but sometimes more lasting damage is done. *Chronic infection* may lead to partial replacement of olfactory mucosa with respiratory epithelium. *Influenza* is known for its ability to cause permanent destruction of the nasal receptors; the onset is often acute. Another mechanism of acute anosmia is *head trauma,* in which the nerve filaments coming through the cribriform plate are damaged.

More gradual onset of reduced smell is typical of an expanding *mass lesion* at the base of the frontal lobe; meningiomas and aneurysms of the anterior cerebral circulation are the most importance sources of this problem. Upward extension of mass lesion into the frontal lobe is manifested by lack of initiative, personality change, and forgetfulness; posterior extension may involve the optic chiasm.

Perversion of smell (parosmia) can result from local nasal pathology such as *empyema* of the nasal sinuses, or *ozena,* a chronic rhinitis of unknown etiology causing thick greenish discharge and crusting (see Chapter 217); *Klebsiella* and *Pseudomonas* are often cultured from the discharge. *Olfactory hallucinations* are central in origin and may present as the aura of a seizure; the responsible lesion is typically found in the area of the uncus. *Olfactory delusions* are reported by schizophrenic patients while their sense of smell remains intact.

Many disorders of smell are of unknown cause. The mechanisms of reduced smell associated with *hypothyroidism, hypogonadism,* and *hepatitis* are not understood. A recent subject of speculation has been the influence of various trace metals, particularly copper and zinc, on the production and treatment of smell disorders.

Taste. The tongue, seventh and ninth cranial nerves, and the hippocampal region of the cerebral cortex make up the taste apparatus. The front of the tongue detects sweet and salty tastes, the sides sense sour tastes, and the large papillae in the back detect bitter tastes. The pharynx also has the ability to sense taste. The taste buds are concentrated in the anterior two thirds of the tongue, which is innervated by the chorda tympani branch of the seventh cranial nerve. The posterior third of the tongue and palate are supplied by the glossopharyngeal nerve.

The most frequent source of diminished fine taste is *impairment of smell.* In addition, the taste buds may be directly injured by *alcohol* and *smoking.* The common observation that food tastes better after these habits are terminated is due to improvement in both the olfactory receptors and the taste buds. *Age* is associated with a decrease in taste buds. Diseases and drugs that dry the mouth, for example, *Sjögren's syndrome* and *tricyclic antidepressants,* reduce the threshold for taste. Chorda tympani and seventh nerve lesions are rarely

bilateral and therefore do not produce a complete loss of taste. Cerebral mass lesions usually do not involve the hippocampal gyrus. Depression, endocrinopathies, and a host of drugs are associated with complaints of altered taste. The mechanisms are unknown, but in many instances the primary disturbance seems to be in part an alteration of smell.

DIFFERENTIAL DIAGNOSIS

Most of the conditions which disrupt taste are annoying but not life-threatening (Table 214-1). However, a disturbance in the sense of smell may be a sign of more serious illness (Table 214-2).

WORKUP

Smell

History. A primary objective is to distinguish local nasal pathology from a central or cranial nerve lesion. History of

Table 214-1. Some Important Causes of Impaired Taste

A. Disturbances in smell
B. Injury to taste buds
  1. Age
  2. Smoking
  3. Hot liquids
  4. Dental disease
  5. Sjögren's syndrome
  6. Idiopathic conditions
C. Cranial nerve lesions (seventh or ninth, partial loss only)
  1. Ear Surgery
  2. Bell's palsy
  3. Ramsay-Hunt syndrome (herpes zoster infection of the geniculate ganglion)
  4. Cholesteatoma
  5. Cerebellopontine angle tumors (advanced disease)
D. Central lesions
  1. Head trauma
  2. Tumors (very rare)
E. Psychiatric disorders
  1. Depression
F. Drugs
  1. Captopril
  2. Imipramine (and other tricyclic agents)
  3. Clofibrate
  4. Lithium
  5. L-dopa
  6. Acetazolamide
  7. Metronidazole
  8. Glipizide
  9. Iron
  10. Tetracycline
  11. Allopurinol
G. Metabolic–endocrine conditions
  1. Hypogonadism
  2. Uremia
  3. Hypothyroidism
  4. Hepatitis
  5. Pregnancy

Table 214-2.   Causes of Disturbances in Smell

A. Nasal
  1. Upper respiratory tract infection
  2. Polyps
  3. Ozena
  4. Chronic sinusitis
  5. Allergic rhinitis
  6. Influenza and other virus
  7. Chemical injury (*e.g.,* tar, formaldehyde)
B. Cranial nerve
  1. Trauma
  2. Meningioma
  3. Cerebral aneurysm
C. Cerebral cortex
  1. Seizure disorder
  2. Meningioma
  3. Aneurysm
  4. Schizophrenia
D. Metabolic–endocrine
  1. Hypothyroidism
  2. Hypogonadism
  3. Liver disease

head trauma, worsening headaches, olfactory hallucinations, change in personality, unexplained forgetfulness, visual disturbances, gradual onset or steady progression of symptoms suggests disease beyond the nasal cavity. History of head congestion, nasal discharge, allergies, sinus problems, influenza, chemical exposure, or a recent cold suggests the nose as the source of difficulty. Inquiry into symptoms of hepatitis (see Chapter 70) and hypothyroidism (see Chapter 102) may uncover an endocrine-metabolic etiology. A careful psychiatric history is needed when there is description of abnormal smells in the absence of any other pathology.

Physical Examination. One can document the disorder by challenging each nostril with a representative sample of each primary odor: pungent, floral, mint, and putrid. Smell is most accurately assessed by the use of chemicals, such as pyridine, garlic-like odor, nitrobenzene, bitter almond, thiophene, and burnt rubber odor. Kits are available which contain these substances. Ammonia, which will produce a response by irritation even in the absence of olfactory powers, should be avoided.

On physical examination, the head is assessed for trauma and the nares are inspected for polyps, deviated septum, mucosal inflammation, and discharge. The sinuses are transilluminated to look for evidence of sinusitis. Fundi are checked for blurring of the disc margins, and the visual fields are tested by confrontation for evidence of optic chiasm compression. The skin, thyroid, and ankle jerks are examined for signs of hypothyroidism (see Chapter 102), and the hair, voice, muscles, and testes for hypogonadism. Any jaundice, hepatomegaly, ascites, or asterixis should be noted.

Laboratory Studies. Sinus films should be reserved for patients with clinical evidence of sinusitis. Routine skull x-rays are of low yield; only if there is a history of recent head

trauma or there are signs on physical examination of a cerebral mass is a skull film worthwhile, in which case fracture or shift of pineal to one side is sought. Far more sensitive for detection of an intracranial mass lesion is computed tomography (CT). CT will be needed if the presence of an intracranial lesion is strongly suspected. Liver, thyroid function, and gonadotropin tests are useful only when there are relevant findings on history and physical examination, not in otherwise asymptomatic individuals with impaired smell.

Taste

History. The initial objective of the evaluation is to localize the problem. Intracranial disease is distinctly rare, so assessment can be concentrated on disease in the mouth, in the area of chorda tympani, and seventh nerve. Alcohol abuse, smoking, dental disease, and severe mouth dryness suggest a buccal cavity source. Facial palsy, herpes zoster rash about the ear, recent ear surgery, hearing problems, vertigo, and tinnitus are clues to diseases which may injure the seventh nerve. Drug use and concurrent metabolic or endocrinologic problems (see Table 214 and above) deserve exploration. Isolated reduction in taste requires inquiry into smell impairment and concurrent depression. Dry eyes in conjunction with dry mouth suggest Sjögren's syndrome, especially if rheumatoid arthritis is present.

Physical Examination. Careful examination of the nose, ears, oral cavity, tongue, and teeth is essential. The condition of the gums and teeth is worth noting. Taste should be assessed by challenging the withdrawn tongue with sweet, salty, bitter, and sour stimuli on each side and asking the patient to indicate what he tastes. Lateralizing the defect suggests a lesion of the seventh nerve. Examination of the cranial nerves needs to concentrate on testing of olfaction, hearing and facial motor functions.

Laboratory Studies. If history or physical examination suggests hypothyroidism, a TSH level should be obtained; likewise a BUN and creatinine if renal disease is suspected. Sjögren's syndrome can be confirmed by lip biopsy. Suspicion of a cerebellopontine angle tumor is an indication for CT scan.

SYMPTOMATIC MANAGEMENT

Smell. Local nasal pathology is often self-limited, but when chronic sinusitis or allergic rhinitis persists, definitive therapy is indicated (see Chapters 217 and 220). Avoidance of toxic fumes (*e.g.,* formaldehyde) and removal of nasal polyps should also help. When influenza has caused sudden, complete, and permanent loss of smell, little can be done. Ozena sometimes requires local or even systemic antibiotic therapy; saline irrigations to remove obstructing crusts are helpful (see Chapter 220). Correction of hypothyroidism improves smell. A literature has developed suggesting that zinc salts will restore normal olfaction and taste, although a recent double-blind controlled trial showed zinc to be no better than placebo.

Taste. Regardless of the cause of reduced taste, the patient should be encouraged to stop smoking and reduce alcohol consumption; often the development of a disability such as altered taste is sufficient motivation to get the patient to stop (see Chapter 49). If possible, medications which may impair taste should be stopped or reduced to determine what contribution, if any, they make to the taste disturbance. Any dental disease of consequence should be corrected. The same pertains to hypothyroidism (see Chapter 102). Concurrent depression may respond to a tricyclic antidepressant, but the drug may impair taste by causing a dry mouth (see Chapter 223); forewarning the patient can prevent side-effects from becoming an unpleasant surprise. Disease related to the brainstem, chorda tympani, and inner ear requires referral for treatment.

INDICATIONS FOR REFERRAL

Olfactory hallucinations, change in personality, visual field defects, and impairment of memory in conjunction with disorders of smell, and multiple cranial nerve defects, vertigo, and tinnitus in conjunction with altered taste, are indications for neurologic consultation. Patients with ozena, nasal polyps, deviated nasal septum, refractory sinusitis, or a chorda tympani lesion may benefit from evaluation by the otolaryngologist.

A.H.G.

ANNOTATED BIBLIOGRAPHY

Henkin RI et al: The molecular basis of taste and its disorders. Ann Intern Med 71:791, 1969 (*A comprehensive review of the pathophysiology of taste disorders.*)

Henkin RI et al: Idiopathic hypogeusia with dysgeusia, hyposmia and dysosmia: A new syndrome. JAMA 217:434, 1971 (*A report of 35 patients presenting with an apparently new syndrome. Pathologic changes in taste buds were observed on electromicroscopy.*)

Henkin RI et al: Abnormalities of taste and smell in Sjögren's syndrome. Ann Intern Med 76:375, 1972 (*An important cause to consider.*)

Henkin RI et al: A double-blind study of the effects of sulfate on taste and smell dysfunction. Am J Med Sci 272, 1976 (*Zinc and placebo were equally effective.*)

McConnell RJ et al: Defects of taste and smell in patients with hypothyroidism. Am J Med 59:254, 1975 (*A study of 18 unselected patients, 9 who were aware of alteration in taste, and 7 of alteration in sense of smell.*)

Rollin H: Drug-related gustatory disorders. Ann Otol Rhinol Laryngol 87:1, 1978 (*A review of drugs that alter taste.*)

Schecter PJ et al: Abnormalities of taste and smell after head trauma. J Neurol Neurosurg Psychiatry 37:802, 1974 (*Decreased taste and smell acuity were studied in 29 patients after head trauma.*)

Schiffman SS: Taste and smell in disease. N Engl J Med 308:1275, 1983 (*Comprehensive review.*)

Smith FR, Dell RB et al: Disordered gustatory function in liver disease. Gastroenterology 70:568, 1976 (*A common complication and probably a contributor to anorexia.*)

215

Evaluation of Tinnitus
AINA J. GULYA, M.D.

Tinnitus is an important but nonspecific symptom of otologic disease. "Ringing," "buzzing," or "roaring" are terms used to describe the sensation, which can be annoying and a source of concern. The occurrence of tinnitus requires assessment for a serious or treatable otologic problem. In the absence of a specifically treatable etiology, it is still important to provide the patient with some symptomatic relief, especially at night.

PATHOPHYSIOLOGY AND CLINICAL PRESENTATION

The pathophysiology of tinnitus remains very poorly understood. Research on the problem is often limited to studies of therapeutic responses to empirical treatments. The most that can be said with certainty is that tinnitus is usually a nonspecific manifestation of disease in the ear, eighth nerve, or central auditory apparatus; it is often accompanied by hearing loss. Tinnitus may be subjective (head noise) or objective. In the latter case, the examiner may also hear the tinnitus by means of a Toynbee tube. It may be pulsatile or nonpulsatile (see below).

External and Middle Ear Conditions. Tinnitus due to such problems as impacted cerumen, perforation of the tympanic membrane, and fluid in the middle ear is commonly described as low-pitched, intermittent, and accompanied by muffled hearing and a change in the sound of one's own voice. In otosclerosis, tinnitus is constant but may disappear as the disease progresses. Acute otitis media (see Chapter 216) sometimes produces a pulsating type of tinnitus that resolves as inflammation subsides. Pulsatile tinnitus is also associated with glomus tumors and posttraumatic arteriovenous fistulae.

Inner Ear and Eighth Nerve Disease. Presbycusis and acoustic trauma can give rise to a high-pitched tinnitus that is near the frequency of greatest hearing loss. Transient tinnitus that follows acute noise exposure is a forerunner of hearing loss and a warning sign to avoid repeated exposure. Ototoxic drugs, such as the aminoglycoside antibiotics, may produce high-pitched tinnitus and hearing loss that often persist after cessation of drug use. Salicylates are frequently responsible for reversible, dose-related tinnitus. Meniere's disease results in transient, low-pitched tinnitus that varies with the intensity of the condition's other symptoms, often worsening when vertigo and hearing loss are imminent. Acoustic neuroma produces a similar set of symptoms but usually the clinical course is progressive, with tinnitus frequently preceding other symptoms, such as vertigo (see Chapter 160).

Other Sources. Tinnitus cerebri is described as a roaring in the head and is believed to be vascular or neurologic in origin. A vascular aneurysm with an audible bruit, a jugular megabulb anomaly, palatal myoclonus with audible muscle contraction, and an unusually patent eustachian tube that transmits respiratory sounds are examples of "objective" tinnitus in which the sounds can be heard by the examiner. When ambient noise is reduced, most people will notice some head sounds. These may be due to the rushing of blood (severest in aortic insufficiency) or contraction of auditory muscles. Loss of hearing due to conductive defects accentuates the problem. Tinnitus may also be associated with temporomandibular joint dysfunction (Costen's syndrome). Depressed and neurotic individuals have less tolerance for these normal head sounds and complain of them when in quiet settings. The ability to withstand tinnitus is also subject to much individual variation; tolerance is lessened by fatigue and emotional stress.

DIFFERENTIAL DIAGNOSIS

Most tinnitus results from the same conditions that cause hearing loss, whether conductive or sensorineural, peripheral or central (see Chapter 210). Subjective complaints of ear or head noise in the absence of otologic pathology may be a concomitant of psychogenic disease. Objective tinnitus suggests cerebrovascular pathology, palatal myoclonus, or a patulous eustachian tube.

There are few data on the frequency of the various conditions responsible for tinnitus. Of interest is the fact that reports from otologic practice list as many as 50% of cases being of unknown etiology.

WORKUP

The diagnostic assessment of tinnitus follows the same pattern as that for hearing loss (see Chapter 210).

History. The pitch of the tinnitus is unfortunately of limited use in diagnosis, although some conditions are more likely than others to be associated with tinnitus of a certain pitch. Distinguishing pulsatile, nonpulsatile, subjective, and objective tinnitus may be more helpful. Any association of the sound with respiration, drug use, vertigo, noise trauma, or ear infection should be checked. A history of head trauma should be sought, as it may be associated with an arteriovenous fistula, or an aneurysm of the intrapetrous portion of the internal carotid artery. When the problem is present only at night, it suggests increased awareness of normal head sounds. Most patients with tinnitus of otologic origin have an associated hearing defect or soon develop one, whereas those without other signs of ear disease may have a vascular lesion or an accentuated awareness of normal head noises.

Physical Examination. One ought to conduct an inspection of the external ear and tympanic membrane for cerumen impaction, foreign bodies, perforation, signs of otitis media (see Chapter 216), and abnormal middle ear masses. Weber and Rinne testing should be performed to determine if there is sensorineural or conductive hearing loss (see Chapter 210). The cranial nerves are examined for evidence of brainstem damage, a sign of an advanced acoustic neuroma, or a glomus tumor. Testing for nystagmus (see Chapter 160) is worthwhile if vertigo is reported. The skull should be auscultated for a bruit if the origin of the problem remains obscure. Compression of the ipsilateral jugular vein will abolish the objective tinnitus associated with the jugular megabulb anomaly.

Laboratory Studies. An *audiogram* can help to identify and localize an otologic lesion. If acoustic neuroma is suspected because of progressive worsening of hearing loss, vertigo, and tinnitus, an audiogram can provide suggestive evidence for the condition. Further workup by the otolaryngologist (see Chapter 210) includes brainstem-evoked response audiometry, and CT scanning with and without contrast. Definitive diagnosis sometimes requires posterior fossa myelography. Temporal bone polytomography will reveal destructive vascular lesions of the petrous pyramid, as well as an enlarged jugular bulb.

INDICATIONS FOR REFERRAL

Referral is essential when a conductive hearing loss is discovered, because many of these lesions are correctable. Suspicion of an acoustic neuroma, glomus tumor, or cerebrovascular abnormality is also an indication for consultation, especially before embarking on an expensive workup. Referral to the otolaryngologist may be necessary to satisfy the anxious patient that everything has been explored and that there is no serious or correctable underlying condition.

SYMPTOMATIC MANAGEMENT AND PATIENT EDUCATION

The patient with a lesion that cannot be cured will still want relief from the annoyance of the tinnitus. Drugs of all types have been tried, including nicotinic acid, vasodilators, and tranquilizers. None has proven superior to placebo. The symptom is most troublesome at night and in quiet rooms. Nighttime use of a clock radio that shuts off after a half hour of playing background music often allows the patient to fall asleep. Keeping a radio on during the day when the patient has to work in a quiet room is also helpful. Many devices are promoted that one wears like a hearing aid (tinnitus maskers) to help mask tinnitus; they are of questionable value. Biofeedback may help in certain cases in which the tinnitus is related to stress.

ANNOTATED BIBLIOGRAPHY

Fowler EP: Head noises in normal and disordered ears. Arch Otolaryngol 39:498, 1944 (*A classic article on the causes of tinnitus.*)

House JW: Treatment of severe tinnitus with biofeedback training. Laryngoscope 88:406, 1978 (*A discussion of the use of biofeedback in tinnitus.*)

Meyerhoff WL, Cooper JC: Chapter 39, Tinnitus. *In* Paparella MM, Shumrick DA (eds): Otolaryngology. Philadelphia, WB Saunders, 1980, pp 1861–1870 (*A thorough review of the subject.*)

Michel RG et al: A practical approach to the treatment of subjective tinnitus. Eye, Ear, Nose, Throat Monthly 55:96, 1976 (*A paper that describes supportive therapy and the use of masking devices.*)

Myers E, Berstein J: Salicylate ototoxicity. Arch Otolaryngol 82:483, 1965 (*A clinical and experimental study documenting reversibility of aspirin ototoxicity.*)

Pulec JL, Hodell SF, Anthony PF: Tinnitus: Diagnosis and treatment. Ann Otolaryngol 87:821, 1978 (*A study of 64 patients from an otologic practice, with emphasis on use of hearing aids and/or tinnitus maskers to relieve the symptoms.*)

Vernon J: Attempts to relieve tinnitus. J Am Audiol Soc 2:124, 1977 (*An extensive and excellent review of measures that have been employed to treat tinnitus.*)

216
Approach to the Patient with Otitis

AINA J. GULYA, M.D.

Not infrequently a patient presents complaining of ear pain or purulent discharge. Inspection of the ear often reveals signs of otitis media or external otitis. The primary care provider should know how to recognize and treat these common conditions so that only refractory or complicated cases need to be referred.

PATHOPHYSIOLOGY AND CLINICAL PRESENTATION

Acute Otitis Media is an extremely common problem in early childhood; its incidence declines with increasing age, and it is an uncommon infection in adults. Purulent otitis media results when bacteria ascend from the nasopharynx to the normally sterile middle ear. Abnormal eustachian tube reflux or obstruction caused by viral nasopharyngitis are considered important in the pathogenesis of acute otitis media. Pain, fever, and hearing loss are the classic presenting complaints. Tympanic membrane perforation and otorrhea may occur.

The most common cause of otitis media is the *Pneumococcus*. While *H. influenzae* was once considered important only in young children, a recent study identified these organisms in 36% of patients with otitis media between 5 and 9 years of age. Other organisms implicated in some patients include streptococci, *Neisseria catarrhalis,* and *Staph. epidermidis.* Gram-negative bacilli and *Staph. aureus* can cause acute otitis in neonates. Viruses and Mycoplasma are not etiologically important. Anaerobic bacteria have recently been implicated in some cases.

The prognosis for acute otitis media is excellent. Chronic serous otitis, hearing loss, and recurrent purulent otitis are the most common difficulties encountered in the antibiotic era. In the past, acute suppurative mastoiditis was the most common sequela of acute otitis, and purulent labyrinthitis, meningitis, lateral sinus thrombosis, and brain abscess were disastrous, if less common, complications.

Serous Otitis Media is a noninfectious variant of otitis media in which fever and pain are absent. Clear fluid is present in the middle ear, the tympanic membrane remains retracted, and bony landmarks are intact. It often follows eustachian tube obstruction, which may result from viral upper respiratory tract infection in adults.

Chronic Otitis Media is seen in all age groups and results from neglected or recurrent acute otitis media. Pain and fever are usually absent, but can occur during sporadic flare-ups in activity. Diminished hearing and foul otorrhea are the major symptoms. Physical examination discloses perforation of the tympanic membrane. Central perforations of the pars tensa are associated with benign disease, but marginal or peripheral perforations may be associated with invasive cholesteatomas. X-rays may reveal sclerosis of the mastoid air cells and bone destruction. A great variety of organisms can be cultured from the drainage in cases of chronic otitis media, including staphylococci, streptococci, *Pseudomonas aeruginosa,* and enteric gram-negative bacilli.

External Otitis is a common, generally benign inflammatory condition usually precipitated by excessive moisture in or trauma to the external auditory canal. Patients complain of pruritus or pain, which may be severe. Crusting, inflammation, and discharge in the canal are typical findings. The pain, which results from movements of the external ear, helps distinguish otitis externa from otitis media. A broad range of organisms including gram-positive cocci, gram-negative bacilli, and fungi can cause otitis externa.

DIAGNOSIS

The cornerstone of the clinical diagnosis of acute purulent otitis media is the finding of a bulging tympanic membrane with impaired mobility and obscuration of the bony landmarks. The other diagnostic possibility is a serous otitis media, in which fever and pain are absent and, although fluid is present in the middle ear, the tympanic membrane is usually retracted and the bony landmarks are preserved. Cultures of the nasopharynx are not helpful in defining the etiology of acute otitis media. Needle aspiration of the middle ear can be used to confirm the diagnosis and to identify the causative organism; however, this is rarely necessary in clinical practice because the bacteriology of acute otitis media is relatively well defined and the response to antibiotics is easy to monitor.

In chronic otitis media, a perforated drum and discharge strongly support the diagnosis. Pain, erythema, and discharge in the external auditory canal are diagnostic of otitis externa.

PRINCIPLES OF MANAGEMENT AND THERAPEUTIC RECOMMENDATIONS

Acute Otitis Media therapy includes use of analgesics, decongestants, and antibiotics. *Amoxicillin* (or ampicillin) is generally the drug of choice in the pediatric age group, while *penicillin* (*e.g.,* Pen-Vee-K 250 mg qid for 7–10 days) usually suffices in adults. Unfortunately, ampicillin-resistant strains of *H. influenzae* have now been implicated in 2.4% to 8% of all cases of otitis media. When such organisms have been isolated or when patients fail to respond to amoxicillin or are penicillin-allergic, combinations of erythromycin and sulfisoxazole or *trimethoprim–sulfamethoxazole* (one double-strength tablet bid) have proved excellent alternatives. (Sulfisoxazole has been useful in the chemoprophylaxis of recurrent otitis in children.) A *sympathomimetic decongestant* may help when the otitis occurs in the setting of an upper respiratory tract infection and eustachian tube obstruction. However, routine use of a decongestant–antihistamine preparation is ineffective. Myringotomy does not hasten recovery but is indicated in patients with intractable pain, progressive deafness, or early mastoiditis, and in those who have had a poor response to medical therapy.

Serous Otitis Media secondary to eustachian tube obstruction from allergy or upper respiratory infection may im-

prove with use of *sympathomimetic decongestants* (see Chapter 220). When allergic in origin, an antihistamine might be utilized to obtain relief, although definitive evidence for efficacy is lacking and antihistamines tend to thicken and dry secretions, impeding clearance.

Chronic Otitis. Antibiotics are generally of little benefit and surgery is required in advanced cases. Without therapy, chronic otitis media can cause the same intracranial suppurative complication as acute otitis media. Topical otic drops are used prior to surgery. Cortisporin otic suspension and ophthalmic antibiotic eye drops tend to be less irritating. Irrigation of the ear with a solution of half vinegar and half sterile water helps to cleanse the ear and to restore its normal *p*H. Without therapy, chronic otitis media can cause the same intracranial suppurative complications as acute otitis media.

Otitis Externa is treated topically; eardrops containing polymyxin and neomycin produce excellent results. Two drops are applied three times daily for a week, in combination with elimination of water contact (a cotton ball coated with petrolatum ointment usually suffices). The neomycin-containing ear drops, such as Cortisporin, can cause allergic reactions; a simple band-aid patch test will diagnose such a potential problem. More severe cases of external otitis, in which the canal is obstructed by edema or purulent debris or both, require careful suction removal of debris, and insertion of a 2 × 2 gauze sponge to act as a wick for the antibiotic drops. Referral to an otolaryngologist is appropriate in such instances.

True Cellulitis of the external ear requiring systemic antibiotics may develop in some patients. *Malignant otitis externa* is a rare but life-threatening infection in diabetics caused by *Pseudomonas aeruginosa;* prompt hospitalization and parenteral antibiotics are required.

INDICATIONS FOR REFERRAL

An otolaryngologist should be consulted if acute otitis media fails to respond to medical therapy or if complications such as tympanic membrane perforation, recurrent acute otitis, serous otitis, or chronic otitis media develop.

PATIENT EDUCATION

The pain of acute otitis media almost always impels the patient to seek prompt medical attention, so little education or encouragement is required. Patients with recurrent external otitis can learn to recognize symptoms and treat themselves. Patients who have active external otitis or chronic otitis media with perforation of the eardrum should be instructed to avoid swimming and water entering the ear. Ear plugs usually do not suffice to keep out water, but, as already noted, a cotton ball coated with petrolatum ointment provides a simple yet effective water barrier.

Patients with otitis media who must fly should use oral or intranasal decongestants (see Chapter 220), especially in anticipation of descent when the risk of barotrauma is greatest. Self-inflation of the eustachian tubes can provide symptomatic relief in serous otitis. The patient is instructed to pinch the nose shut, take a deep breath, close the mouth, and try to blow the nose while keeping it pinched shut.

ANNOTATED BIBLIOGRAPHY

Bluestone CD: Otitis media in children: to treat or not to treat. N Engl J Med 306:1399, 1982 (*An excellent review of the pathogenesis, diagnosis, and management of otitis media.*)

Brook I, Anthony BF, Finegold SM: Aerobic and anaerobic bacteriology of acute otitis media in children. J Pediatr 92:13, 1978 (*A bacteriologic study of 62 children with acute otitis media. Pneumococci and H. influenzae were isolated from 57%; a wide group of organisms occurred in the remainder of cases.*)

Cantekin EI et al: Lack of efficacy of a decongestant–antihistamine combination for otitis media with effusion ("secretory" otitis media) in children. N Engl J Med 308:297, 1983 (*A double-blind randomized study of 553 infants and children, which shows that the traditional use of decongestant–antihistamine therapy is of no benefit.*)

Doroghazi RM et al: Invasive external otitis. Am J Med 71:603, 1981 (*A study of 21 patients with this devastating Pseudomonas infection; occurs almost exclusively in diabetics.*)

Henderson FW et al: A longitudinal study of respiratory viruses and bacteria in the etiology of acute otitis media with effusion. N Engl J Med 306:1377, 1982 (*Viral upper respiratory tract infections were important precursors of otitis media in this 14-year longitudinal study.*)

Schwartz RH et al: Trimethoprim–sulfamethoxazole in the treatment of otitis media caused by ampicillin-resistant strains of H. influenzae. Rev Inf Dis 4:514, 1982 (*The drug proved beneficial in 14 of 15 patients who failed to respond to ampicillin because of drug resistance.*)

Schwartz RH et al: Acute purulent otitis media in children older than 5 years. JAMA 238:1032, 1977 (*H. influenzae was identified as the cause of acute otitis media in 36% of 58 children with otitis between the ages of 5 and 9.*)

Schwartz RH et al: The increasing incidence of ampicillin-resistant Hemophilus influenzae. JAMA 239:320, 1978 (*A study of 625 children with otitis. Overall, 8% of those infections were caused by ampicillin-resistant strains of H. influenzae.*)

217

Approach to the Patient with Sinusitis

HARVEY B. SIMON, M.D.

While infections of the paranasal sinuses are common, they tend to be overdiagnosed by patient and physician alike. Often a frontal headache or congested sensation is attributed to "sinus trouble" and self-medicated with over-the-counter decongestants. Individuals with allergic or vasomotor rhinitis may present seeking treatment for their "sinus condition." The primary physician should be able to distinguish true sinusitis from other causes of nasal congestion, treat uncomplicated cases, and recognize complications.

PATHOPHYSIOLOGY AND CLINICAL PRESENTATION

True sinusitis may be acute or chronic. *Acute purulent sinusitis* is characterized by nasal congestion, purulent nasal discharge, facial pain (that typically increases when the patient stoops forward), and, often, fever and other constitutional symptoms. Viral, allergic, or vasomotor rhinitis are frequent antecedent events. The presence of nasal polyps or deviation of the nasal septum may also predispose the patient to purulent sinusitis by obstructing sinus drainage. Other contributing factors may include rapid changes in altitude, trauma, intranasal foreign bodies or tumors, and, occasionally a systemic process such as cystic fibrosis or Kartagener's syndrome (situs inversus, bronchiectasis, and sinusitis).

The sinuses may be involved singly or, more often, in combination. Maxillary and frontal sinusitis are common in adults; ethmoiditis is more common in children. The signs and symptoms of sinusitis depend upon which sinuses are involved. *Frontal sinusitis* produces pain and tenderness over the lower forehead and purulent drainage from the middle meatus of the nasal turbinates. *Maxillary sinusitis* produces pain and tenderness over the cheeks; in addition, pain is often referred to the teeth, and the hard palate may be edematous in severe cases. Purulent drainage is present in the middle meatus. Patients with *ethmoid sinusitis* complain of retro-orbital pain, and may have tenderness and even erythema over the upper lateral aspect of the nose. Drainage from the anterior ethmoid cells occurs through the middle meatus, while drainage from the posterior cells is through the superior meatus. Isolated *sphenoid sinusitis* is uncommon, but can present as retro-orbital, frontal, or facial pain, with purulent drainage from the superior meatus.

Symptoms of *chronic sinusitis* include nasal congestion and discharge, but pain and headache are usually mild or absent, and fever is uncommon.

Because of technical difficulties in obtaining valid cultures, the *bacteriology* of sinusitis has been incompletely defined. The most common pathogens in acute sinusitis are pneumococci, streptococci, and *Hemophilus influenzae.* Although some studies report the isolation of *Staphylococcus aureus* from significant numbers of patients with acute sinusitis, these studies have been based on nasal cultures and probably reflect nasal contamination rather than a true etiology. In contrast, small numbers of *S. aureus* were recovered in one study from operative cultures in 18% of patients with chronic sinusitis. In the same study, heavy growths of anaerobic organisms were isolated in 28% of patients with chronic sinusitis; anaerobic streptococci and *Bacteroides* species predominated. The importance of anaerobes in chronic sinusitis is reflected by the predominace of anaerobes in brain abscesses of sinus origin. Viruses have been considered rare causes of sinusitis but may be etiologically important in some patients. Rarely, fungi such as *mucor, Rhizopus,* and *Aspergillus* species can produce invasive sinusitis in poorly controlled diabetics or leukemics. Gram-negative bacilli may cause sinusitis in hospitalized patients who are nasotracheally intubated or immunocompromised.

Complications of sinusitis have become uncommon in the antibiotic era but can be life-threatening. Frontal sinusitis can lead to osteomyelitis of the frontal bones, especially in children. Patients present with headache, fever, and a characteristic doughy edema over the involved bone, which is termed "Pott's puffy tumor." The organisms involved are the same as those responsible for the underlying sinusitis except that *S. aureus* is more common. Osteomyelitis of the maxilla is an infrequent complication of maxillary sinusitis.

Because the orbit is surrounded on three sides by paranasal sinuses, orbital infection can result from sinusitis. This is most frequently a complication of ethmoid sinusitis due to direct extension of infection through the lamina papyracea. *Orbital cellulitis* usually begins with edema of the eyelids and rapidly progresses to ptosis, proptosis, chemosis, and diminished extraocular movements. Patients are usually febrile and acutely ill. Pressure on the optic nerve can lead to visual loss which can be permanent, and retrograde spread of infection can lead to intracranial infection.

Retrograde extension of infection along venous channels from the orbit, ethmoid or frontal sinuses, or nose can produce septic *cavernous sinus thrombophlebitis.* These patients are highly febrile and appear "toxic." Lid edema, proptosis, and chemosis are present, but unlike uncomplicated orbital cellulitis, third, fourth, and sixth cranial nerve palsies are prominent, the pupil may be fixed and dilated, and fundoscopic examination may reveal venous engorgement and papilledema. Although the process is usually unilateral at first, spread across the anterior and posterior intercavernous sinuses results in bilateral involvement. Patients may exhibit alterations of consciousness.

Finally, sinusitis can lead to intracranial suppuration either by direct spread through bone or via venous channels. A great variety of syndromes can result, including epidural abscess, subdural empyema, meningitis, and brain abscess. Clinical findings vary greatly, ranging from subtle personality changes with frontal lobe abscesses to headache, symptoms of elevated intracranial pressure, alterations of consciousness, visual symptoms, focal neurologic deficits, seizures, and ultimately, coma and death.

DIFFERENTIAL DIAGNOSIS

The common cold and allergic or vasomotor rhinitis (see Chapter 220) are by far the most common causes of "sinus" symptoms, but polyps, tumors, cysts, foreign bodies, and vasculitides such as Wegener's granulomatosis occasionally produce symptoms resembling sinusitis.

WORKUP

History is checked for presence of a purulent nasal discharge and frontal, maxillary, retro-orbital, or vertex pain which worsens on bending forward. Risk factors such as nasal polyps, deviated nasal septum, trauma, foreign bodies and rapid changes in altitude are inquired about. Special attention is paid to toxic symptoms of high fever and rigors in association with complaints suggestive of extension of infection, such as edema of the eyelids and diplopia.

Physical Examination may reveal a purulent discharge draining from one of the turbinates. The diagnosis of sinusitis can be confirmed by the finding of opacity on transillumination of the frontal or maxillary sinuses and tenderness to percussion.

Laboratory Studies. Confirmation of the diagnosis can also be achieved by radiographic findings of mucosal thickening, sinus opacification, or air–fluid levels. Bone erosion can be present in chronic sinusitis. Nasal cultures correlate poorly with actual sinus fluid and cannot be relied upon. Tomograms and CT scans provide precise definition of sinusitis in complicated cases but are not indicated in patients with routine sinus infection.

PRINCIPLES OF MANAGEMENT AND THERAPEUTIC RECOMMENDATIONS

The patient with acute sinusitis can be made more comfortable by employing local application of heat. Decongestants are of paramount importance. *Pseudoephedrine* can be administered by mouth and by nasal spray. The danger of "rebound" following short-term use of nasal spray has probably been exaggerated. Patients should be instructed to spray each nostril once, and then wait a minute to allow the anterior nasal mucosa to shrink; a repeat spray will then reach the upper and posterior mucosa including the nasal turbinates and sinus ostea. This procedure can be repeated every 4 hours for several days if needed. *Antihistamines* may provide additional decongestion if there is an allergic component to the problem, but because they can thicken secretions, they should not be used unless allergy is present. Steroids are not necessary in most patients and may be harmful.

Most patients with acute sinusitis respond well to decongestants and analgesics without the use of *antibiotics.* There is little controlled data to support the use of antibiotics in acute sinusitis, much less to dictate the choice of drugs. Nevertheless, many physicians administer *ampicillin, penicillin, trimethoprim–sulfa, erythromycin,* or a *cephalosporin* in conjunction with decongestants. Antibiotics should be used in "toxic" patients, in those who fail to respond to decongestants, and in those with complications. Surgical intervention should be avoided in acute sinusitis unless patients fail to respond to medical therapy and complications are present. Sinus irrigation or surgical drainage may be necessary in chronic sinusitis.

INDICATIONS FOR ADMISSION AND REFERRAL

Any patient who appears toxic or has clinical evidence suggestive of extension to the orbit, bone, brain, or cavernous sinus requires urgent admission for emergency assessment and high-dose intravenous antibiotics. Warning symptoms include high fever, rigors, lid edema, diplopia, pupillary abnormalities, ptosis, and palsies of extraocular movements. The patient should be seen by both an otolaryngologist and infectious disease consultant. Antibiotic coverage is directed against both staphylococci and gram-negative rods. Surgical drainage may be urgently needed.

PATIENT EDUCATION

Patients should understand that nasal congestion and frontal headaches are much more commonly caused by viral upper respiratory infections and allergic or vasomotor rhinitis than by true sinusitis. Nevertheless, decongestants are indicated in all of these conditions to promote sinus drainage and prevent purulent sinusitis. The patient with recurrent symptoms should learn to recognize them and begin decongestant therapy, but the decision to begin antibiotics should be reserved by the physician.

ANNOTATED BIBLIOGRAPHY

Axelson A, Brorson JE: The correlation between bacteriological findings in the nose and maxillary sinus in acute maxillary sinusitis. Laryngoscope 83:2003, 1973 (*A Swedish study which shows that nasal cultures correlate poorly with cultures obtained by sinus puncture. Staphylococci were common nasal contaminants but were rarely recovered from the sinus tap. Pneumococci and H. influenzae were the most common causes of sinusitis.*)

Berlinger NT: Sinusitis in immunodeficient and immunosuppressed patients. Laryngoscope 95:29, 1985 (*A broad range of bacterial and fungal pathogens can cause severe necrotizing sinusitis in the impaired host.*)

Evans FW et al: Sinusitis of the maxillary antrum. N Engl J Med 293:735, 1975 (*An intensive study of 24 patients with maxillary sinusitis. Opacity on transillumination and marked mucosal edema on x-ray were suggestive of purulent sinusitis.*)

Frederick J, Braude AI: Anaerobic infection of the paranasal sinuses. N Engl J Med 290:290, 1974 (*A heavy growth of anaerobic bacteria in pure culture was obtained in 23 of 83 surgical specimens from patients with chronic sinusitis.*)

Lew D et al: Sphenoid sinusitis: A review of 30 cases. N Engl J Med 309:1149, 1983 (*A detailed study of the varied presentations of this uncommon but potentially serious type of sinusitis.*)

Price CD, Hameroff SB, Richards RD: Cavernous sinus thrombosis and orbital cellulitis. Southern Med J 64:1243, 1971 (*A study of nine patients with orbital cellulitis and four with cavernous sinus thrombosis, showing clinical differentiation of these two serious complications of sinusitis.*)

218
Approach to the Patient with Pharyngitis
HARVEY B. SIMON, M.D.

A wide variety of organisms may be responsible for pharyngitis, but the differential diagnosis usually comes down to determining whether the cause is viral or streptococcal. The differentiation is important because acute rheumatic fever is a preventable complication of *Streptococcus pyogenes* infec-

tion. Unfortunately, in most cases clinical features are not distinctive enough to separate viral from streptococcal pharyngitis.

The objectives of management should be to maximize the chances that a patient with streptococcal infection will be identified and treated and to minimize unnecessary use of antibiotics, delay of therapy, inconvenience, and expense. The strategy for achieving these goals has been the subject of recent study and much unresolved debate. Determining the best approach to the sore throat remains a surprisingly complex problem; the primary physician needs to know the advantages and shortcomings of available alternatives.

PATHOPHYSIOLOGY AND CLINICAL PRESENTATION

Respiratory viruses and group A beta-hemolytic streptococci account for the majority of sore throats in adults. A host of other bacteria, viruses, fungi, and spirochetes have also been identified as etiologic agents. Trauma, inhalation of irritant gases, and dehydration are among the noninfectious causes of sore throat.

Streptococcal Pharyngitis accounts for about 10 to 15% of sore throats in adults who are subjected to throat culture. The onset of discomfort is typically acute, with difficulty swallowing often noted. Pharyngeal erythema, exudate, cervical adenopathy, and fever greater than 101°F (38.3°C) are common but by no means pathognomonic. Children with "strep throat" exhibit exudate and high fever with greater frequency than do adults with the same disease. Cough, rhinorrhea, and other symptoms of upper respiratory infection are reported in less than 25%. About one quarter of adult patients give a history of recent exposure to streptococcal infection. The pharyngitis is self-limited; symptoms usually resolve within 7 to 10 days.

Peritonsillar cellulitis and *abscess formation* are important suppurative complications of streptococcal pharyngitis. The peritonsillar tissue and then the tonsils become edematous and inflamed; abscess formation may ensue unless antibiotic therapy is instituted. One or both tonsils may be involved. A grayish-white exudate forms on the tonsils; high fever, rigors, and leukocytosis are associated symptoms. Other suppurative complications include retropharyngeal and parapharyngeal space infections. Scarlet fever is a rare complication in adults, due to infection with a toxigenic strain of *S. pyogenes*.

Acute rheumatic fever is the most important nonsuppurative complication of group A beta-hemolytic streptococcal infection. However, its incidence has declined dramatically over the past 30 years. It appears most frequently among children aged 5 to 15, but about 15% of hospitalized patients with rheumatic fever are over the age of 18. The chances of developing rheumatic fever increase with length of time that the organism persists in the pharynx and with the intensity of the immunologic response. *Acute glomerulonephritis* is another nonsuppurative complication. Unlike rheumatic fever, it does not seem to be preventable by means of antibiotic therapy.

OTHER STREPTOCOCCI. Groups C and G streptococci can cause pharyngitis, but with far less frequency than group A organisms. Suppurative complications are rare and rheumatic fever and glomerulonephritis never follow.

Viruses. Respiratory viruses are the most common causes of sore throat. Pharyngitis can be the only manifestation of illness or may be accompanied by conjunctivitis, cough, sputum production, rhinitis, and systemic symptoms. Pharyngeal erythema, exudates, tonsillar enlargement, and cervical adenopathy are often present, but with less frequency than in streptococcal disease.

Epstein–Barr virus is the agent responsible for *infectious mononucleosis* and, as such, is sometimes a cause of sore throat. Prodromal symptoms of mononucleosis include malaise, headache, and fatigue followed by fever, sore throat, and cervical lymphadenopathy. Sore throat is the most common feature; the pharynx shows hyperplasia of lymphoid tissue, erythema, and edema. About half of patients develop tonsillar exudates. Petechiae at the junction of the hard and soft palate occur in about a third of patients and are highly suggestive of the diagnosis of mononucleosis. Both anterior and posterior cervical adenopathy may develop; generalized lymphadenopathy often follows. Splenomegaly is noted in about half of cases, and hepatomegaly and tenderness are present in about 10%; clinical hepatitis sometimes ensues. A faint, maculopapular rash and transient supraorbital edema occasionally appear. IgM antibody is the first to appear.

Other causes of pharyngitis include *herpes simplex* and *Coxsackie A* virus. Herpes infection is typically in the form of a stomatitis that involves the buccal mucosa and tongue as well as the pharynx; vesicles and small ulcers develop. Coxsackie A infection is characterized by vesicles and ulcers on the tonsillar pillars and soft palate.

Other Organisms. In patients engaging in orogenital sexual activity, *gonococci* can lead to sore throat, pharyngeal exudate, and lymphadenopathy, or just asymptomatic colonization of the pharynx. In rare instances, bacteremia may result. *Hemophilus influenzae* is a rare cause of pharyngitis in adults, but the infection can be extremely painful; epiglottitis with airway obstruction is a life-threatening complication. Serologic evidence of infection with *Chlamydia trachomatis* or *Mycoplasma pneumoniae* has been obtained in a surprising percentage of patients presenting with pharyngitis. The significance of this finding remains unclear. Outbreaks of diphtheria, which is caused by *Corynebacterium diphtheriae,* have taken place in unimmunized populations. The infection is characterized by development of an adherent whitish-blue pharyngeal exudate ("pseudomembrane") that covers the pharynx and causes bleeding if removal is attempted.

About 5% to 15% of healthy people harbor *meningococci* in the pharynx. Although sore throat may be a prodromal symptom of meningococcemia, isolated pharyngitis due to meningococcal infection is very rare; most instances of meningococcal recovery from the pharynx represent asymptomatic colonization.

Although numerous other bacterial species can be cultured from the pharynx in both symptomatic and asymptomatic individuals, they do not cause pharyngitis except under most unusual circumstances. In particular, it should be emphasized that while pneumococci and staphylococci commonly reside in the nasopharynx and can cause severe disease in other parts of the respiratory tract, they do not cause pharyngitis. However, mixed infections with normal mouth flora do occur in debilitated patients.

Fusobacteria and *spirochetes* can cause gingivitis ("trenchmouth") or necrotic tonsillar ulcers ("Vincent's angina"). Patients present with foul breath, pain, pharyngeal exudate, and a dirty gray membranous inflammation which bleeds easily. A similar combination of bacteria and spirochetes can produce an extremely serious invasive gangrene of the mouth known as cancrum oris; this process occurs only in malnourished infants or patients with advanced malignancy and immunosuppression, and is fortunately rare. *Treponema pallidum* can cause pharyngitis as part of primary or secondary syphilis. The diagnosis requires a high index of suspicion and serologic confirmation.

Among other organisms that can cause pharyngitis, *M. tuberculosis* is very rare. While most forms of fungal pharyngitis are also rare, *Candida albicans,* present in the normal mouth flora, can produce pharyngitis if antibiotics, immunosuppressive agents, or debilitating illnesses upset microbial interactions or host defenses. Oropharyngeal moniliasis (thrush) can be painful and is characterized by a cheesy, white exudate which can be scraped off to demonstrate yeast forms by smear and culture. As noted above, the significance of positive serology for *Mycoplasma pneumoniae* in patients with isolated pharyngitis remains unclear; diagnosis is rarely made clinically in the absence of pneumonitis.

WORKUP

History. As with many other upper respiratory tract infections, the signs and symptoms of pharyngitis do not usually enable the physician to establish an etiologic diagnosis. However, questions concerning family members with documented strep throats, orogenital sexual contact, concurrent steroid or immunosuppressive therapy, and previous history of rheumatic fever are appropriate. Any dyspnea must be noted.

Physical Examination of the pharynx is useful for identifying a less common cause of pharyngitis such as thrush, characterized by its white cheesy exudate; gingivitis or necrotic tonsillar ulcers suggest fusobacteria and spirochetes. Associated physical findings, such as a viral exanthem, conjunctivitis, petechiae, generalized lymphadenopathy, splenomeg-

aly, or hepatic tenderness, may provide important clues to etiology. The dyspneic patient needs laryngoscopy.

Laboratory Studies. While *throat culture* remains the most reliable and practical means of diagnosing streptococcal pharyngitis, the test is not needed in every case of sore throat. Patients at very high risk of rheumatic fever (*i.e.,* those with a history of rheumatic fever and those in a closed population that is currently experiencing an epidemic of streptococcal pharyngitis) can be managed without dependence on culture results. In other circumstances, the need for a throat culture is more pressing because the clinical assessment of the likelihood of strep infection is very crude; most clinical data are, at best, only suggestive. But, those with recent household exposure, fever greater than 101°F, pharyngeal exudate, cervical adenopathy, and absence of cough probably could forego culturing and be treated directly. Culturing and treating in a few days if the culture is positive is quite safe. Because delay of a day or two in initiating therapy does not increase the risk of rheumatic fever, antibiotics can be withheld until culture results are ready. Available techniques for office plating and culturing of pharyngeal specimens are inexpensive and reliable when performed correctly. Proper technique for culturing the throat includes swabbing the tonsils and posterior pharynx. Patients with no clinical evidence of streptococcal infection, and with typical symptoms and signs of viral upper respiratory infection, do not need a throat culture; the incidence of streptococcal infection in this group has been found to be less than 5%.

Although the throat culture remains the standard for identification of streptococcal pharyngitis, it has some shortcomings. Not all patients with positive cultures have infection; it has been estimated that the carrier rate is as high as 20% to 30%. This represents colonization rather than true infection. There is some evidence to suggest that patients with cultures showing less than ten colonies per plate are either colonized or have very mild infection that is not likely to lead to serious sequelae. Definitive identification of significant infection with risk of rheumatic fever necessitates serologic testing for an antibody response. Such testing is of little practical use because results do not become available in time to be of help.

Rapid office diagnosis of group A streptococci in the pharynx is becoming possible with the development of *latex agglutination* and *ELISA techniques* for immunologically identifying streptococcal antigens on pharyngeal throat swabs. The sensitivity of these methods ranges from 77% to 95%, with specificity of 86% to 100% making them acceptable for clinical use. Issues of cost–benefit remain to be determined; the time it takes office staff to perform the test (15 to 20 minutes) may prove too long to be acceptable in some office practices unless one does the test in batches.

In sum, despite the frequency of sore throat and the risk

of resultant rheumatic fever, no firm guidelines are available for selection of patients in whom throat cultures are indicated. Even when the culture is positive for group A strep, there is at present no clinically proven method to distinguish between the carrier state and active infection without waiting for the results of serologic tests.

Viral pharyngitis due to respiratory pathogens is essentially a clinical diagnosis and requires no laboratory investigation. On the other hand, the patient with sore throat and diffuse lymphadenopathy, splenomegaly, or pharyngeal petechiae deserves evaluation for infectious mononucleosis. A *heterophile* is a useful test, provided there is no prior history of infectious mononucleosis. It may take as long as 3 weeks for the heterophile to become positive, necessitating a repeat test in a few weeks if it is initially negative. Alternatively, one can check serology for antibodies to Epstein-Barr virus. IgM antibodies can be demonstrated during the second week of illness, replaced later by IgG antibodies. Heterophile-negative mononucleosis may be due to CMV infection.

The patient with a history of orogenital contact should be cultured for gonococcal infection (see Chapter 116). Some cultures for gonococci will grow out meningococci, which in most instances represents a carrier state. Suspected candidal infection can be confirmed by scraping off the exudate and examining a wet prep.

PRINCIPLES OF MANAGEMENT AND THERAPEUTIC RECOMMENDATIONS

Suspected Group A Streptococcal Infection

The rationale for treating group A streptococcal infection is to prevent rheumatic fever, suppurative complications such as peritonsillar or retropharyngeal abscess, and the spread of streptococcal infection. Treatment does not shorten the course of the pharyngitis.

Rheumatic fever can be prevented by prompt eradication of *S. pyogenes* from the throat. The attack rate for rheumatic fever is reduced by over 90% if antibiotic therapy is instituted within a week of the onset of sore throat. However, the efficacy of prophylactic therapy is substantially reduced if there is a marked delay in initiating treatment. Starting antibiotics 2 weeks after sore throat is first noted is associated with a reduction in attack rate of only 67%, and delaying treatment until 3 weeks into the illness provides no more than a 40% reduction in attack rate.

Treatment Strategies. There are several approaches to treatment of pharyngitis that can be employed; the choice depends on the probability of strep infection, the likelihood of patient compliance, the chance of an adverse reaction to antibiotics, and the benefits of treating immediately versus waiting for culture results. Patients who are symptomatic and have a household member with a documented group A beta-streptococcal infection should receive treatment without need for culture. Patients with a classic presentation of exudative

pharyngitis, fever, and bilateral cervical adenopathy also can be started on treatment immediately, since they have at least a 30% chance of having streptococcal infection. Some argue that it is unnecessary to culture such people since the likelihood of strep infection is already quite high.

In the majority of pharyngitis patients with a less distinctive presentation, the choice is between starting therapy at the time a culture is obtained or waiting until the results are available before prescribing antibiotics. In favor of the first approach is more rapid relief of symptoms; antibiotic therapy has now been shown to speed resolution of symptoms. Against is the unavoidable treatment of patients who will prove not to have strep infection, subjecting them to the risk of unnecessary antibiotic exposure. Awaiting culture results before initiating treatment minimizes unnecessary antibiotic exposure but requires good patient compliance to check back with the physician for results and instructions. Regardless of which approach is taken, one should not order a culture unless committed to stopping antibiotics if the culture is negative.

To be effective, antibiotic therapy must completely eradicate the streptococcus from the pharynx. This can be achieved by a single intramuscular injection of 1.2 million units of benzathine penicillin or a 10-day course of oral penicillin V, 250 mg four times per day. The advantages of the intramuscular route are the certainty of full treatment and convenience; its major disadvantage is a five- to tenfold increase in the incidence of serious allergic reactions to penicillin. In the patient allergic to penicillin, oral erythromycin, 250 mg four times daily for 10 days, is an effective alternate. Treatment of asymptomatic individuals who have small numbers of group A streptococci on throat culture is probably unnecessary, except in very high-risk patients who have a prior history of rheumatic fever; however, most of these patients should already be on prophylactic therapy (see Chapter 12).

Other Types of Pharyngitis

The *meningococcal carrier state* sometimes presents a therapeutic dilemma, in terms of both selecting patients who actually need treatment and choosing antibiotics. Carriers should be treated only when there is evidence of active meningococcal disease in household or dormitory contacts. Penicillin will not eradicate the meningococcal carrier state, and since many strains are now sulfonamide-resistant, rifampin should be used.

In *gonococcal pharyngitis,* the usual penicillin and tetracycline regimens are effective (see Chapter 116), but spectinomycin is not. In the case of *diphtheria,* antitoxin is necessary to prevent myocarditis and peripheral neuritis and is the mainstay of therapy. Both erythromycin and penicillin can eliminate the organism from the upper respiratory tract. In *epiglottitis,* hospitalization is needed.

Necrotizing pharyngitis due to fusobacterial infection responds to penicillin and good nutrition. *Candida* infections require gargling with oral nystatin suspension; the frequent administration of large doses may be necessary. *Viral sore throats* are treated symptomatically. Voice rest, humidification, and lozenges or hard candy provide some relief; saline gargling and aspirin or acetaminophen also help.

PATIENT EDUCATION

Many patients insist on antibiotic therapy for a sore throat, often because they think they will obtain symptomatic relief more rapidly from such treatment. Much of the unnecessary antibiotic exposure associated with management of pharyngitis is probably due as much to patient insistence as to the physician's desire to do something. When the etiology is viral, patients ought to be informed that antibiotics are not indicated. On the other hand, the patient who proves to have group A streptococcal infection should be carefully instructed on the importance of completing a full 10-day course of antibiotic therapy; otherwise, many patients will stop taking the medication when symptoms resolve.

ANNOTATED BIBLIOGRAPHY

Bisno AL: Diagnosis of streptococcal pharyngitis. Ann Intern Med 90:426, 1979 (*An editorial reviewing the difficulties of diagnosing the cause of sore throat, with particular critique of the use of the Gram stain.*)

Brook I: The role of beta lactamase-producing bacteria in the persistence of streptococcal tonsillar infection. Rev Infect Dis 6:601, 1984 (*Beta lactamase produced by Bacteroides species and S. aureus may account for persistence of streptococci following penicillin therapy in some patients.*)

Glezen WP et al: Group A streptococci, mycoplasmas, and viruses associated with acute pharyngitis. JAMA 202:119, 1967 (*A clinical study of the various etiologies of acute pharyngitis.*)

Holmberg SD, Faich GA: Streptococcal pharyngitis and acute rheumatic fever in Rhode Island. JAMA 250:2307, 1983 (*The incidence of acute rheumatic fever was only 0.2 per 100,000, yet more than 157,000 throat cultures were performed in a year among a population of about 900,000; throat cultures were often misused, judging by the fact that 40% of physicians continued antibiotics regardless of culture results.*)

Komaroff AL, Aronson MD, Pass TM et al: Serologic evidence of chlamydial and mycoplasmal pharyngitis in adults. Science 222:927, 1983 (*Serologic evidence of C. trachomatis infection was found in 20% and of Mycoplasma in 10% of 763 adults presenting with sore throat.*)

Krober MS, Bass JW, Michels GN: Streptococcal pharyngitis; clinical response to penicillin therapy. JAMA 253:1271, 1985 (*Early penicillin therapy did significantly ameliorate symptoms.*)

Markowitz M: The decline of rheumatic fever: The role of medical intervention. J Pediatr 106:545, 1985 (*A review of progress since 1950, when penicillin was first used.*)

MayoSmith MF, Hirsch PJ, Wodzinski SF et al: Acute epiglottitis in adults. N Engl J Med 314:1133, 1986 (*A potentially dangerous, not well-appreciated condition.*)

Paradise JL et al: Efficacy of tonsillectomy in recurrent throat infection in severely affected children. N Engl J Med 310:674, 1984 (*Although children who undergo tonsillectomy do experience significantly decreased infection rates during the first 2 postoperative years, medically treated children also do well.*)

Peter G, Smith AL: Group A streptococcal infections of the skin and pharynx. N Engl J Med 297:311, 1977 (*An authoritative review of the biology of the group A streptococcus with an up-to-date discussion of streptococcal pharyngitis.*)

Rapid office diagnostic tests for streptococcal pharyngitis. Med Let 27:49, 1985 (*A good review of available office tests for rapid diagnosis.*)

Tompkins RK, Burnes DC, Cable WE: An analysis of the cost-effectiveness of pharyngitis management and acute rheumatic fever prevention. Ann Intern Med 86:481, 1977 (*An examination of various strategies for workup and treatment of sore throat.*)

Walsh BT, Bookheim WW, Johnson RC, Tompkins RK: Recognition of streptococcal pharyngitis in adults. Arch Intern Med 135:1493, 1975 (*Attempts to identify a cluster of clinical findings that suggest an increased likelihood of streptococcal infection.*)

Wannamaker LW: Perplexity and precision in the diagnosis of streptococcal pharyngitis. Am J Dis Child 124:352, 1972 (*A forthright account of the surprising number of uncertainties and controversies surrounding this common problem.*)

Weisner PJ, Tronen E, Bonin P et al: Clinical spectrum of pharyngeal gonococcal infection. N Engl J Med 288:181, 1973 (*A comprehensive study of patients in a venereal disease clinic, describing the incidence, clinical features, and therapy of gonococcal pharyngitis.*)

219
Approach to Hiccup

Hiccup is usually a transient, innocuous symptom, but when persistent it may become an exhausting and disabling problem. Intractable hiccup has been attributed to a host of metabolic, peridiaphragmatic, neurologic, and psychogenic conditions, but many cases are of unknown etiology. The primary physician should be able to offer the exasperated patient symptomatic relief while conducting a judicious evaluation to determine the source of difficulty.

PATHOPHYSIOLOGY AND CLINICAL PRESENTATIONS

No useful function has been found for the hiccup, which occurs as a result of synchronous clonic spasm of intercostal muscles and diaphragm that causes sudden inspiration followed by prompt closure of the glottis and inhibition of respiratory activity. It is believed to be a reflex. There is debate about whether it is centrally mediated. The afferent pathway is from T10 to T12, and the efferent limb is along the phrenic nerve. During the hiccup, the glottis is closed. Some investigators believe the hiccup is related more to gastrointestinal than to respiratory function. Current understanding of pathophysiology does not yet permit an explanation of how the presumptive etiologies operate to produce the hiccup, though the classic explanation is that it is due to stimulation of the phrenic nerve.

It is often unclear whether the reported causes of hiccup are etiologies or only associations. In a series of 220 cases seen at the Mayo Clinic men outnumbered women by 5 to 1, and most were in their 60s. Over 90% of the women had no concurrent illness other than an emotional problem, whereas only 7% of men were labeled as having a psychogenic disorder. About 20% of men who experienced hiccup did so after undergoing intra-abdominal, intrathoracic, or neurologic surgery. About 25% had a diaphragmatic hernia, another 20% had cerebrovascular disease or another CNS problem, 5% had a metabolic illness, and in 10% no associated disease or psychiatric problem was identified.

DIFFERENTIAL DIAGNOSIS

The causes of persistent hiccup typically listed are clinical associations and cannot be considered proven etiologies (Table 219-1).

WORKUP

Persistent hiccup that proves refractory to simple measures is an indication for further investigation. Extensive workup is usually not very productive, but a check for a previously unsuspected metabolic or subdiaphragmatic process is sometimes rewarding.

History. Questioning should include inquiry into recent abdominal, thoracic, or neurologic surgery, abdominal pain (especially that which radiates to the tip of the shoulder or is worsened by respiration), prior renal disease, excess consumption of alcohol, fever, cough, diabetes, and emotional problems. Also of help is reviewing the various methods that the patient has tried for relief of symptoms. Any neurologic complaints should be noted.

Physical Examination should include a temperature determination, a check of the tympanic membranes, percussion of the lungs for evidence of reduced diaphragmatic excursion, and auscultation for signs of an infiltrate, effusion, or pleuritis. The abdomen is examined for distention, organomegaly, upper abdominal tenderness, and signs of peri-

Table 219-1. Conditions Associated with Persistent Hiccup*

A. Diaphragmatic Irritation/Gastrointestinal Disease/Head and Neck Disease
  1. Pericarditis
  2. Tumor
  3. Subdiaphragmatic abscess
  4. Pneumonia
  5. Pleuritis
  6. Myocardial infarction
  7. Hiatus hernia
  8. Peritonitis
  9. Gastric dilatation
  10. Pancreatitis
  11. Biliary tract disease
  12. Tympanic membrane irritation
B. Metabolic Disturbances
  1. Uremia
  2. Diabetes
  3. Alcoholism
C. CNS Disease
  1. Tumor
  2. Infection
  3. Surgery
D. Psychogenic Disease
  1. Hysteria
  2. Anorexia nervosa
  3. Anxiety

* These are not proven etiologies.

tonitis. A careful neurologic examination is needed if there is a history of neurologic difficulties.

Laboratory Studies. Patients with an acute bout of hiccups need no laboratory studies, but those with *refractory hiccups* that persist for days need to be evaluated for a pharyngeal, thoracic, diaphragmatic, intra-abdominal, CNS, or metabolic/pharmacologic etiology. If a careful physical examination that includes a check of the tympanic membranes, pharynx, chest, heart, abdomen, and CNS is unrevealing, one ought to obtain a chest x-ray, serum sodium, creatinine, and BUN determinations, and consider a CT scan of the abdomen, concentrating on the subdiaphragmatic region. If central nervous system disease is suspected by history or physical examination, a CT or magnetic resonance scan may help detect the lesion. Treatment of the underlying etiology is the best means of curing refractory hiccups.

SYMPTOMATIC THERAPY AND INDICATION FOR REFERRAL

For patients with *self-limited* causes of hiccuping, several home remedies are capable of interrupting the reflex arc; others simply suppress it temporarily. *Breath holding* and breathing into a *paper bag* will decrease the frequency of hiccups, but if the underlying stimulus has not disappeared, they usually return after these maneuvers are terminated.

Swallowing a teaspoonful of *granulated sugar* works by irritating the pharynx sufficiently to inhibit further hiccuping. A more noxious maneuver is to have the patient put his finger into the back of his pharynx and *stimulate the gag reflex.* Drinking from the wrong side of the glass is another gag reflex stimulant. Rubbing the nasopharynx with a cotton swab is sometimes effective. Passage of a *nasogastric tube* causing hypopharyngeal stimulation will usually work if other methods have failed.

When symptoms are *persistent* and the cause remains undiagnosed or untreatable, symptomatic relief becomes an important goal. *Chlorpromazine* in doses of 25 to 50 mg intravenously will often terminate refractory hiccups and can be followed by oral maintenance therapy of 25 mg qid. *Metoclopramide* given intravenously, followed by oral therapy (10 mg tid), has also proven effective. Atropine and quinidine have been used, but with less success. *Phenytoin* and *carbamazepine* are helpful in patients with a CNS etiology.

When all other measures have failed, and the hiccups remain disabling, consideration of surgical *infiltration of the phrenic nerve* is appropriate. Fluoroscopy is needed to see if one leaf of the diaphragm is responsible and can be singled out for treatment. In addition, one needs to be sure one leaf is not already paralyzed, a circumstance which would rule out this therapeutic option. The phrenic nerve serving the offending diaphragm is infiltrated with a long-acting anesthetic; if it works, but the hiccups return, reinfiltration with alcohol or *crushing* may be necessary. If both leaves of the diaphragm are involved, one phrenic nerve is treated.

In most instances, hiccups will resolve spontaneously or respond at least partially to one of these therapeutic maneuvers.

L.A.M. and A.H.G.

ANNOTATED BIBLIOGRAPHY

Editorial: Hiccup. Br Med J 1:235, 1971 (*A terse review of pathophysiology and the significance of the hiccup.*)

Engleman EG, Lankton J, Leakton B: Granulated sugar as treatment for hiccups in conscious patients. N Engl J Med 285:1489, 1971 (*A letter reported successful relief of hiccups in 19/20 patients following swallowing a teaspoon of ordinary dry white sugar.*)

Salem MR et al: Treatment of hiccups by pharyngeal stimulation in anesthetized and conscious subjects. JAMA 202:321, 1967 (*Therapeutic success in 84/86 patients by introduction of a catheter through the nose and stimulating the pharynx at the level of C2–3.*)

Samuels L: Hiccup: A ten-year review of anatomy, etiology, and treatment. Can Med Assoc J 67:315, 1952 (*The classic hiccup paper with differential diagnosis.*)

Souadjian JV et al: Intractable hiccup: Etiologic factors in 220 patients. Postgrad Med 43:72, 1968 (*A review of 220 patients from the Mayo Clinic presenting probable causes and arguing for a psychogenic etiology in 92% of females in the series.*)

Williamson BWA, MacIntyre JMC: Management of intractable hiccup. Br Med J 2:501, 1977 (*A succinct review of therapeutic approaches, finding chlorpromazine and metoclopramide the most effective drugs; 39 refs.*)

220

Approach to the Patient with Chronic Nasal Congestion and Discharge

It is estimated that 15% to 20% of the population suffer from recurrent or chronic nasal problems. Allergic rhinitis accounts for many such cases, but vasomotor rhinitis, mechanical obstruction, certain drugs, and abuse of decongestants are also responsible for symptoms in many people. These conditions cause a great deal of discomfort and absenteeism, and result in the expenditure of many millions of dollars for therapy. The primary physician needs to be able to distinguish an allergic etiology from one due to obstruction, inflammation, or vasomotor instability. Moreover, one must know the proper uses of antihistamines, decongestants, and topical corticosteroids as well as the indications for skin testing and referral to the allergist or ENT specialist.

PATHOPHYSIOLOGY AND CLINICAL PRESENTATION

Allergic Rhinitis is due to IgE-mediated release of histamine, slow-reacting substance, bradykinin, and other mediators from mast cells in the nasal mucosa, resulting in nasal congestion and rhinitis. The reaction develops in response to inhalation of allergen that forms antigen-IgE complexes on receptors in the nasal mucosa. The condition is *seasonal* when the antigen is a pollen ("hay fever") and *perennial* when the allergens are dusts, molds, or animal danders. Patients living in the northern half of the United States who are sensitive to tree pollen will become symptomatic in late March and early April; those sensitive to grasses, in mid-May to late

June. Patients affected by ragweed and other summer weeds experience difficulty in late August until the first frost. Patients with seasonal allergic rhinitis outnumber those with perennial complaints by a ratio of about 10 to 1. It is not unusual for an individual to be allergic to a number of antigens and to show increased sensitivity to chemical irritants as well. The incidence of allergy among patients with nonallergic parents is about 10%; incidence rises to 25% if one parent is allergic, and to 60% if both are. Antigen-specific responses are controlled by regulatory genes.

In some instances, the patient has all the earmarks of perennial allergic rhinitis but no evidence of IgE mediation, and skin tests for inhaled allergens are negative. Such patients have been designated as having *nonallergic rhinitis,* even though their nasal secretions often contain large numbers of eosinophils and they respond to corticosteroids.

Onset of allergic rhinitis is usually during childhood, but may occur at any age; childhood cases frequently continue into adulthood. Some patients have asthma, but there is no evidence that allergic rhinitis predisposes to development of asthma. However, there is an increased incidence of recurrent upper respiratory infections and sinusitis. The condition often improves with time.

Nasal congestion, sneezing, and profuse watery discharge dominate the initial clinical presentation. Itching of the nose, throat, and eyes is common, as is postnasal drip and tearing. Often the nasal mucosa appears pale and edematous. Symptoms typically vary over the course of the day; they are most severe in the morning, lessen in the afternoon, and worsen again by evening.

Vasomotor Rhinitis may mimic perennial allergic rhinitis and is believed by some clinicians to be a diagnosis of exclusion when no allergen is identified. Others consider the condition a readily distinguishable entity characterized by a normal-appearing nasal mucosa and persistent nasal stuffiness without itching, that is worsened by changes in ambient temperature and humidity. Although congestion is the most prominent symptom, a discharge may also be present. Sneezing is relatively absent. The pathophysiology is poorly understood but believed to involve abnormal autonomic responsiveness and vascular dilatation of the submucosal vessels. IgE levels are normal and the number of eosinophils in nasal secretions is usually, but not always, normal. Abnormal autonomic reactivity is felt to account for the nasal stuffiness or rhinorrhea sometimes occurring with *emotional upset* and *sexual arousal.*

Drugs. Overuse of topical alpha-adrenergic *nasal decongestants* (rhinitis medicamentosa) can result in a worsening of symptoms. Response to these agents becomes blunted (tachyphylaxis), leading to increased use, often on an hourly basis. As soon as the vasoconstrictor effect subsides, nasal stuffiness returns worse than ever, presumably due to marked reflex vasodilatation. The nasal mucosa appears erythematous. The problem resolves in 2 to 3 weeks if topical decongestants are stopped. Agents with adrenergic blocking activity can aggravate pre-existing rhinitis and cause mild nasal congestion in normal patients. *Reserpine* and *guanethidine* are the major offenders. *Cocaine abuse* is also a cause.

Hormonal Etiologies. *Hypothyroidism* and *pregnancy* may cause the turbinates to become pale and edematous, leading to nasal congestion. Hypothyroidism may otherwise be subclinical save for the chronic nasal obstruction. Symptoms resolve with correction of the hypothyroidism or with delivery.

Mechanical Obstruction. Unilateral congestion and discharge are characteristic of mechanical obstruction due to tumor, polyp, or deviated septum. *Neoplasm* is rare but is suggested by a blood-tinged discharge. *Polyps* occur in association with allergic and vasomotor rhinitis, chronic sinusitis, aspirin-induced asthma, cystic fibrosis, and reserpine use. The mechanism of formation is unknown. Polyps move freely since they are pedunculated and nontender, and appear as soft, pale gray, smooth structures. Patients with asthma and nasal polyps are often hypersensitive to aspirin. Polyps do not regress spontaneously and may become large or multiple, causing considerable obstruction. A *deviated septum* is sometimes the source of obstructive symptoms. Most are not traumatic in origin and develop during growth. Associated sinus occlusion is rare.

Obstruction due to crusting is seen with *atrophic rhinitis.* The condition is of unknown etiology, appears mostly in women, and is characterized by dry atrophic nasal turbinates, mucosal crusts, and a foul or fetid greenish discharge referred to as ozena. The purulent discharge is believed due to secondary infection.

Chronic Inflammatory Disease. A number of serious chronic inflammatory conditions may cause obstruction. *Midline granuloma* is an uncommon illness of unknown etiology that causes ulcerative destruction of upper respiratory tract structures. It often presents as nasal stuffiness, crusting, and granulations, but progresses steadily as ulcerations form in the nasal septum and elsewhere. The majority of patients are over 50 and many have histories of allergic rhinitis. *Wegener's granulomatosis* may have a similar insidious presentation with nasal obstruction, rhinorrhea, or chronic sinusitis. Necrotizing granulomatous lesions and vasculitis are found in the upper and lower airway. Middle-aged men and women are equally affected. *Sarcoidosis* may present as bilateral nasal obstruction.

DIFFERENTIAL DIAGNOSIS

The causes of nasal congestion and discharge can be organized pathophysiologically and are listed in Table 220-1.

Table 220-1. Important Causes of Chronic or Recurrent Nasal Congestion

A. Allergic
  1. Seasonal allergic rhinitis (pollens)
  2. Perennial allergic rhinitis (dusts, molds)
B. Vasomotor
  1. Idiopathic (vasomotor rhinitis)
  2. Abuse of nose drops
  3. Drugs (reserpine, guanethidine, prazosin, cocaine abuse)
  4. Psychologic stimulation (anger, sexual arousal)
C. Mechanical
  1. Polyps
  2. Tumor
  3. Deviated septum
  4. Crusting (as in atrophic rhinitis)
  5. Hypertrophied turbinates (chronic vasomotor rhinitis)
  6. Foreign body (usually in children)
D. Chronic Inflammatory
  1. Sarcoidosis
  2. Wegener's granulomatosis
  3. Midline granuloma
E. Infectious
  1. Atrophic rhinitis (secondary infection)
F. Hormonal
  1. Pregnancy
  2. Hypothyroidism

WORKUP

Although it is important to rule out mechanical obstruction, chronic inflammatory disease, and drug-induced illness, the usual diagnostic task is to distinguish between allergic and vasomotor disease.

History should focus on timing of symptoms and aggravating and alleviating factors. Nasal congestion that coincides with periods of pollenation is virtually diagnostic of seasonal allergic rhinitis. Continuous waxing and waning of symptoms throughout the year, with exacerbations during the hay fever season, suggests a combination of perennial and seasonal allergic disease.

When symptoms occur chronically without respect to seasons, one may be dealing with vasomotor rhinitis, perennial allergy, mechanical obstruction, or a chronic inflammatory condition. Perennial rhinitis is a possibility when the patient reports frequent "colds."

Patients bothered by dusts are generally atopic, whereas those whose symptoms are aggravated by quick changes in temperature, emotion, or drugs fall into the vasomotor category. Use of antihypertensive agents and topical nasal decongestants needs to be explored, as does exposure to fur-bearing animals, feathers, other possible sources of animal danders, or chemical irritants. Pollutants are often more irritating to allergic patients, but may also cause symptoms in nonatopic people.

Symptoms accompanying nasal congestion sometimes provide useful diagnostic clues. Fever and a purulent nasal discharge are evidence of an infectious etiology. A cold is the most likely cause of acute discharge, but chronic discharge that is fetid, foul-smelling, and accompanied by crusting indicates secondary infection as in atrophic rhinitis, Wegener's granulomatosis, and midline granuloma. Bloody discharge and unilateral obstruction suggest tumor. Mechanical obstructions are often unilateral as well. The presence of asthma or aspirin sensitivity increases the likelihood of nasal polyps. Sneezing, postnasal drip, and itching are nonspecific and of little help in distinguishing among etiologies. When the cause is obscure, exploration for cocaine abuse, hypothyroidism, or possible pregnancy may provide explanations.

Epidemiologic data need to be considered. Onset in childhood is typical of allergic disease, but onset of symptoms during adulthood does not rule out atopy. When chronic progressive nasal congestion develops in a middle-aged patient, particularly a woman, one must consider atrophic rhinitis or one of the necrotizing inflammatory diseases. The allergy histories of the patient's parents should be ascertained.

Physical Examination includes inspection of the nasal mucous membranes for color, atrophy, edema, crusting, and discharge; the presence of polyps, erosions, and septal perforations or deviations should be noted. A nasal speculum markedly improves visualization of the nasal cavity and ought to be used in every examination. Some findings are nonspecific. For example, a pale boggy appearance to the mucosa is allegedly a classic sign of allergic disease, but erythema sometimes occurs in allergy and its presence certainly does not rule it out. Transillumination and percussion of the sinuses, pharyngeal examination for erythema and discharge, a look in the ears for evidence of otitis, cervical node examination for adenopathy, and auscultation of the chest for wheezes complete the physical examination.

Laboratory Studies. When the differentiation between allergic and nonallergic disease is difficult to make on the basis of clinical findings, *skin testing* might prove helpful. Preparations of commonly inhaled allergens (dusts, molds, animal danders, and local pollens) are injected into the skin to see if there is an immediate wheal and flare reaction. A positive skin test only indicates atopy. Correlation with history and physical examination is needed to establish an etiologic role for the antigen. Antihistamines must be omitted for 12 to 24 hours before testing to avoid a false-negative result. A common cause of false-positive testing is the presence of dermographism; because 15% to 20% of the population exhibits dermographism, a saline control injection should be given along with injections of allergens.

Other studies are available for detection of an allergic etiology, but are not as inexpensive, easily performed, or necessarily more sensitive than skin testing; moreover, results of some tests take over a week to become available. *Radioallergosorbent testing (RAST)* involves adding the patient's serum to a purified allergen absorbed to an inert particle. If the serum contains high concentrations of specific IgE antibodies to the allergen, it will give a positive test. The shortcomings of RAST testing are its expense and only modest sensitivity. The test is best used in conjunction with skin testing rather than instead of it. Determination of *total IgE* is helpful if the level is markedly elevated, but some cases of allergic rhinitis are not associated with high serum concentrations. Thus a normal result is not useful for diagnosis. The same is true for the *total eosinophil count.* A count at the time of an exacerbation that is in excess of 500 cells per mm³ is suggestive of an allergic etiology. The absence of peripheral eosinophilia does not rule out allergic rhinitis. Smears of nasal secretions for eosinophils should be done but are of limited specificity, because eosinophils may be present in substantial numbers in both vasomotor and allergic rhinitis. The smears can be of use when infection is in question, because neutrophils should be present in abundance.

Purulent discharges not associated with an obvious cold are worth culturing. Sinus films should be obtained if fever, facial asymmetry, opacification, or tenderness suggests an accompanying sinusitis (see Chapter 216).

PRINCIPLES OF MANAGEMENT AND PATIENT EDUCATION

Allergic Rhinitis

Avoidance Measures. The basic approach to relief of symptoms begins with avoidance of known allergens. Patients with allergic seasonal rhinitis can be advised to avoid long walks in the woods during the pollenation period and to stay indoors with the windows closed when symptoms are severe and the pollen count is high (*e.g.,* hot windy sunny days). Some patients find air conditioners helpful, but the machine's filter does little to remove pollen from the air. The air conditioner simply makes it more tolerable to stay indoors with the windows closed on a hot day. The hot air vent on the air conditioner should be kept closed to avoid the intake of pollenated air. If ragweed is a problem, daisies, dahlias and chrysanthemums should not be kept indoors. Preventing accumulation of excess dust in the bedroom and avoiding irritants such as tobacco smoke, chemical vapors, and strong perfumes lessen symptoms.

Control of perennial allergic rhinitis requires particular attention to allergens in the home, but recommendations should be practical. Cleaning the house and especially the bedroom with a damp mop two to three times a week will reduce dust. Feather pillows should be replaced by Dacron or polyester ones, and mattresses should be covered with an elastic fabric casing. Areas where mold can collect, such as piles of old newspapers or furniture in a damp basement, should be cleaned up. A dehumidifier may prevent mold growth. Throwing out carpets and draperies is excessive, but

new furnishings made of synthetic fabrics are preferable to cotton and wool to minimize dust collection. Humidification of air in winter also helps keep down dusts. Patients allergic to molds should avoid having African violets and geraniums in the home. No new fur-bearing pets should be obtained; most pets usually have to be removed from the home entirely if symptoms are disabling. Simply keeping the pet out of the bedroom does not help sufficiently, because the dander circulates in the air throughout the house.

When history provides ready identification of allergens, there is little need for skin testing, but if drastic environmental measures are being contemplated, documentation of the specific allergens is worthwhile.

Pharmacotherapy is indicated in patients who find allergen avoidance impractical or ineffective. The commonly utilized agents include antihistamines, which block the effects of histamine on end organs; beta-adrenergic agents, which block degranulation of mast cells and basophils; corticosteroids, which act on degranulation, late phase reactions, and end-organ response; and alpha-adrenergic agents, which decongest by means of vasoconstriction.

ANTIHISTAMINES. The problem with antihistamines has been their sedating effect, which has made daytime use difficult. The development of antihistamines that do not cross the blood–brain barrier represents an important improvement in symptomatic treatment of allergic rhinitis. The H₁-receptor antagonist *terfenadine* is the first of such agents, being no more sedating in double-blind controlled studies than placebo. Clinical trials have shown it to be equal in efficacy to the widely used antihistamine chlorpheniramine, with control of symptoms in about 60% of cases. Terfenadine is rapidly absorbed after oral intake; onset of action begins within 1 to 2 hours and lasts for up to 12 hours. Terfenadine appears effective in perennial as well as seasonal allergic rhinitis. The dose is 60 mg bid. Cost is approximately seven times that for chlorpheniramine, making it a very expensive choice that is best reserved for daytime use when sedation is unacceptable. At night, an equally effective, more sedating antihistamine will suffice and hold down costs. Adverse effects are few; anticholinergic side-effects are similar to those of other antihistamines.

SYMPATHOMIMETICS. Adrenergic stimulation has long been used in combination with antihistamines, in part to counter the latter's sedative effects as much as for their decongestant properties. Phenylpropanolamine, ephedrine, and pseudoephedrine are widely used and available in over-the-counter formulations, often in combination with antihistamines such as chlorpheniramine. *Phenylpropanolamine* is essentially an alpha-adrenergic agent; *ephedrine* and *pseudoephedrine* have a combination of alpha and beta effects. All are effective decongestants, but those with beta properties are preferred by some when drowsiness is a problem. A typical regimen is use of pseudoephedrine, 60 mg/every 4 to 6 hours;

lower doses may suffice in mild cases. Sympathomimetics can produce nervousness, increased heart rate, and elevation in blood pressure. Their prolonged use in patients with hypertension or coronary artery disease is inadvisable. Empirical trials of various antihistamines and decongestants are often necessary to select the best agent(s) and dose(s). Combination preparations are convenient if the fixed doses match the doses needed; these preparations should not be used as initial therapy.

Topical decongestant sprays have a limited role because of the risks of tachyphylaxis and rebound nasal congestion. They are best used for keeping the eustachian tubes patent in patients who ride in airplanes (see Chapter 216). An application of *phenylephrine* (Neo-Synephrine) or *oxymetazoline* (Afrin) every 3 to 4 hours while the patient is airborne should suffice, especially when preceded by an oral decongestant an hour before flight time. Rebound congestion occurs if sprays are used repeatedly for more than 4 or 5 days in a row.

INTRANASAL TOPICAL CORTICOSTEROIDS are safe and effective for symptomatic relief of both seasonal and perrenial allergic rhinitis. They also enhance responsiveness to antihistamines, making combined use quite effective. Recommended preparations for intranasal use are beclomethasone and flunisolide, which have supplanted dexamethasone because of their superior topical activity and fewer systemic effects. *Beclomethasone dipropionate* is supplied as a freon-propelled aerosol that delivers 50 μg of the drug in a fine powder with each spray. Sometimes, it provides relief within hours, especially in cases of seasonal rhinitis (hay fever), but regular use for as long as 1 to 2 weeks may be necessary before benefit is noted. The most convenient dose is two inhalations in each nostril bid. *Flunisolide* comes in an aqueous suspension delivered as a metered spray of 25 μg by a hand-activated pump. Dosage is two inhalations in each nostril bid; 200 μg of flunisolide is as effective as 400 μg of beclomethasone.

Each preparation is packaged in a container providing a 25-day supply; they cost about the same. Patients with copious nasal secretions and marked congestion may need preliminary adrenergic or even systemic steroid therapy to permit the topical preparation to reach the nasal mucosa. Patients with dryness and crusting of the nasal mucosa may prefer flunisolide because it is a liquid. Topical inhalation therapy does not benefit allergic conjunctivitis.

At recommended doses and frequencies, adrenal suppression does not occur with these topical corticosteroids, even when used chronically. However, suppression can occur with excessive dosage or increased frequency. Other adverse effects include increased mucosal friability leading to an occasional nosebleed. Mucosal ulceration is rare. Application of the spray can cause transient burning and sneezing. Atrophic rhinitis is a risk of chronic use. Colonization of the nose with *Candida* has been reported. Topical steroid therapy should be considered when antihistamines and sympathomimetic agents either do not adequately control symptoms or the patient cannot tolerate their side-effects.

Cromolyn sodium (see Chapter 45) has been found moderately effective in double-blind crossover studies of some patients with allergic rhinitis. The agent is administered either as an inhaled powder or as a dissolved liquid. Cromolyn works by preventing degranulation of mast cells and is used prophylactically. Patients with very high IgE levels are most responsive; many others are not.

IMMUNOTHERAPY (hyposensitization) is indicated as a last resort in patients who remain incapacititated despite a full pharmacotherapy program and face prolonged (more than 6 weeks) exposure to a known allergen. Hyposensitization reduces IgE production and stimulates synthesis of IgG blocking antibody; it may also induce IgE suppressor lymphocyte activity or reduce mast cell and basophil responsiveness. Prevention of local reaction to pollens, cat dander, and dust mites has been demonstrated in patients with allergic rhinitis. Hyposensitization involves cutaneous administration of incremental doses of allergen extract, initially at intervals of 1 to 2 weeks, progressing to intervals of 3 to 6 weeks after several months of treatment.

This form of therapy should be considered an adjunct to medication; most responses are not dramatic. Skin testing and frequent visits over a prolonged period mean patient inconvenience and high cost. Assessment of response to immunotherapy (improvement in symptoms, reduction in medication requirements) should be made every 6 months and therapy discontinued if substantial benefit is not evident after 12 to 18 months.

For the patient with allergic rhinitis whose condition is inadequately controlled on a well-designed medical regimen, referral to an allergist for skin testing and consideration of immunotherapy is a reasonable step.

Vasomotor Rhinitis

Vasomotor rhinitis is difficult to treat. Avoidance of tobacco smoke, rapid changes in temperature or humidity, and irritant chemical vapors is helpful. Humidification of the home in winter is also worthwhile. Cessation of nasal spray use is essential; altering antihypertensive medications may be needed. A mild adrenergic agent with some alpha activity (*e.g.,* pseudoephedrine) sometimes provides partial improvement. Addition of an antihistamine for its nonspecific drying effect may give some extra relief but is ineffective by itself.

Immunotherapy and steroids are of no proven benefit. Patients bothered severely by nasal obstruction may benefit from cryosurgical treatment of the inferior and middle turbinates. Profuse rhinorrhea is occasionally treated by sectioning the parasympathetic nerve supply to the nose. Consideration of surgical approaches should be reserved for patients seriously impaired by the condition.

INDICATIONS FOR REFERRAL

The patient should be referred to an otolaryngologist for removal of polyps or foreign bodies, for management of a suspected tumor, necrotizing inflammatory condition, or atrophic rhinitis, and for correction of deviated septa. An allergist can be of help when an allergic etiology cannot be distinguished from vasomotor rhinitis, when the antigen(s) must be identified for management purposes, and when immunotherapy is contemplated.

A.H.G.

ANNOTATED BIBLIOGRAPHY

Broder I et al: Epidemiology of asthma and allergic rhinitis in a total community. Tecumseh, Michigan. IV. Natural history. J Allergy Clin Immunol 54:100, 1974. (*Demonstrates that asthma is neither a common accompaniment nor a consequence of allergic rhinitis; also showed that the remission rate for perennial allergic rhinitis was 5 to 10% over 4 years of follow-up.*)

Intranasal corticosteroid aerosols for noninfectious rhinitis. Medical Letter 23:101, 1981 (*A review of the evidence for their use; concludes they are safe and effective.*)

Matthews KP: Respiratory atopic disease. JAMA 248:2587, 1982 (*One of a primer on allergic and immunologic diseases; provides an exhaustive review of allergic rhinitis and bronchial asthma.*)

Naclerio RM, Proud D, Togias AG et al: Inflammatory mediators in late antigen-induced rhinitis. N Engl J Med 313:65, 1985 (*An important study delineating the mediators of allergic rhinitis; basophils seem to play a major role.*)

Racklin RE: Clinical and immunologic aspects of allergen-specific immunotherapy in patients with seasonal allergic rhinitis and/or allergic asthma. J Allergy Clin Immunol 72:323, 1983 (*A review of immunotherapy, its procedures, and its efficacy.*)

Seebohm PM: Allergic and nonallergic rhinitis. In Middleton E, Ellis E (eds): Allergy: Principles and Practice, p 868. St. Louis, CV Mosby, 1978 (*An excellent critical summary of these conditions, with emphasis on clinically relevant data.*)

Slavin RG: Diagnostic tests in clinical allergy. Postgrad Med 67(3): 72, 1980 (*Critical review of skin testing and other techniques used to detect allergic rhinitis.*)

Terfenadine—A nonsedating antihistamine. Medical Letter 27:65, 1985 (*The manufacturer's claims that this new histamine$_1$-receptor antagonist is as effective and much less sedating than other antihistamines appear to be valid.*)

221
Management of Aphthous Stomatitis

Aphthous stomatitis (canker sores) is a common recurrent condition involving painful ulcers of the oral mucosa. About 20% of the population is affected at one time or other; prevalence is high among upper middle class individuals; women are more commonly affected than men. The lesions can be very painful, and the primary physician should be capable of providing symptomatic relief.

PATHOPHYSIOLOGY, CLINICAL PRESENTATION, AND COURSE

The etiology of aphthous stomatitis has not been established, although there is some evidence for an immunologic pathogenesis. For example, aphthous stomatitis is associated with diseases presumed to be caused by immune mechanisms, such as Crohn's disease and chronic ulcerative colitis. Moreover, exposure to oral epithelial antigens or cross-reacting microbial antigens leads to elevated levels of IgA and production of hemagglutinating antibodies to oral mucosa. Lymphocytes from affected patients cause cytotoxic changes in tissue cultures of oral epithelium. Low titers of antimucosal antibodies have been found in the sera of patients with aphthous stomatitis.

Although the condition seems to involve injury, other factors may be important. For example, an association of aphthous stomatitis with nutritional deficiencies of iron, folate, and B$_{12}$ has also been found; lesions clear with correction of the deficiency. Infection seems to play a contributing role; after mucosal breakdown has occurred, the lesions are invaded by mouth flora and become secondarily infected. Emotional stress can precipitate an attack.

Aphthous stomatitis develops in four clinical stages.

1. *Premonitory*—tingling, burning, or hyperesthetic sensation, lasting up to 24 hours
2. *Preulcerative*—lasting from 18 hours to 3 days, characterized by moderately painful erythematous macules or papules with erythematous halos
3. *Ulcerative*—lasting 1 to 16 days, characterized by painful discrete ulcers covered by gray-yellow membrane with a dusky erythematous halo. Pain ceases during this stage
4. *Healing*—usually without scarring, averages 2 weeks (range ½ to 5 weeks).

Aphthous ulcers are classified according to size. The majority are "minor," that is, are less than 1 cm in diameter and appear in crops of four or five. "Major" lesions are greater than 1 cm, solitary, indolent, and heal with scarring. Minor lesions heal without scarring within 7 to 10 days. Lesions are painful and may occur anywhere within the oral cavity. In two-thirds of patients, recurrent lesions do not develop, but in one-third, recurrences continue for up to 40 years.

PRINCIPLES OF THERAPY

Aphthous stomatitis is a difficult problem to treat. The goals of therapy are to provide acute relief and prevent recurrence. *Tetracycline liquid* used as a mouthwash several times a day has been the most effective symptomatic therapy. *Carbamide peroxide gel* is an oxidizing agent which releases oxygen on contact with the oral mucosa. It has some bactericidal effect against many mouth organisms and is a mild debriding agent. In the presence of extremely painful lesions, use of *topical anesthetic agents* (*e.g.,* viscous lidocaine) before meals may allow the patient to eat. Avoidance of abrasive foods also helps.

Immunologically targeted therapies have been tried. *Corticosteroids* should be helpful, but the physical environment within the oral cavity makes topical use difficult. One approach to overcome this problem is to instruct the patient to take a 5-mg hydrocortisone tablet and to keep it on or near the ulcer so that it dissolves into and around the lesion. Vehicles that help the steroid component cling to the mucous membrane (*e.g.,* Orabase) slow the release of the active ingredient. In cases associated with severe pain, intralesional corticosteroids may be tried by a clinician experienced in their use. *Levamisole,* which stimulates immune response, has been reported efficacious in about two-thirds of cases, but the unknown long-term safety of this antihelmintic agent limits its use.

Women with a definite premenstrual flare may be helped by estrogen-dominated oral contraceptives. Identification and correction of an existing deficiency of folate, B_{12}, or iron may cure aphthous stomatitis. For lesions precipitated by emotional stress, judicious use of tranquilizers is reasonable. Chemical cauterization by means of silver nitrate sticks ($AgNO_3$) is used by some practitioners to treat acute lesions, but this involves the distinct possibility of destroying normal tissue and should not be used by inexperienced physicians. Avoidance of local trauma to the oral mucosa and maintenance of good oral hygiene and nutrition are important supplements to therapy.

THERAPEUTIC RECOMMENDATIONS AND PATIENT EDUCATION

- Any deficiency of iron, B_{12}, or folate should be identified and corrected.
- Tetracycline, 250-mg capsules, dissolved in a teaspoonful of warm water can be used as a mouthwash three or four times a day. The solution should be expectorated.
- Oxygen-liberating agents such as carbamide peroxide gel have a temporary soothing effect and may supplement tetracycline.
- Viscous lidocaine, 1 teaspoonful, retained in the mouth for several minutes and then expectorated, may allow patients with intense pain to eat.
- Patients whose conditions are refractory to other topical therapies can be given a trial of dissolving a 5-mg hydrocortisone tablet over the ulcer once a day; the hydrocortisone is expectorated after the tablet has fully dissolved.
- Patients should avoid stressful situations as much as possible, and diazepam may be taken before bedtime for a brief period (see Chapter 222).
- Patient education ought to stress good mouth hygiene. The use of a fluoride toothpaste sometimes helps. Patients can be advised to avoid food with sharp surfaces, salt, and talking while chewing and to use a soft-bristled toothbrush. It may be comforting for the patient to know that the condition is self-limited, though the possibility of recurrence should also be explained.

L.A.M. and A.H.G.

ANNOTATED BIBLIOGRAPHY

Cooke BED: Recurrent oral ulceration. Br J Dermatol 81:159, 1969 (*Classification of the various types of recurrent aphthous lesions.*)

Lehner T: Immunologic aspects of recurrent oral ulcers. Oral Surg 33:80, 1972 (*Discusses the various immunologic changes which have been described in recurrent aphthous stomatitis.*)

Olson JA, Nelms C, Silverman S et al: Levamisole, a new treatment for recurrent aphthous stomatitis. Oral Surg 41:588, 1976 (*The use of levamisole in the treatment of this condition. Open trial in 50 patients: 6% remission, 56% improvement, 38% no change.*)

Sircus W, Church R, Kelleher J: Recurrent aphthous ulceration of the mouth. A study of the natural history, aetiology, and treatment. Q J Med 26:235, 1957 (*An investigation of the natural history and factors which affect course.*)

Stanely HR: Aphthous lesions. Oral Surg 33:407, 1972 (*Description of the various stages of aphthous lesions and their duration.*)

15

Psychiatric and Behavioral Problems

222
Approach to the Patient with Anxiety

JERROLD F. ROSENBAUM, M.D.

Patients with anxiety pose an ongoing challenge to the primary care physician, presenting with feelings of distress and concern about disease in the absence of objective evidence for a medical problem. Suffering no less from the subjective nature of the ailment, such patients fear something is amiss with their bodies and persistently seek an acceptable explanation and relief. Anxiety disorders are prevalent, with an estimated 5% of the general population affected. Given the array of associated somatic symptoms, anxiety is a frequent precipitant of visits to the nonpsychiatric physician.

Anxiousness is a normal human affect; distinguishing it from pathologic anxiety and anxiety disorders often requires systematic evaluation and a thorough understanding of the individual patient's physical and psychologic status. Since the autonomic arousal accompanying anxiety may affect many organ systems, anxiety can be a great imitator of physical disease. Moreover, anxiety and anxietylike symptoms may be consequent to a variety of medical ailments and their treatments. Unrecognized and untreated, anxiety disorders render the patient vulnerable to further morbidity, including demoralization, hypochondriasis, depression, and varying degrees of disability.

A comprehensive and empathetic assessment of anxious patients permits a reasoned and often therapeutically effective approach to the difficult problems they pose.

PATHOPHYSIOLOGY AND CLINICAL PRESENTATION

Anxiety is the distressing experience of dread, foreboding, or panic, accompanied by a variety of autonomic—primarily sympathetic—bodily symptoms. The distress, therefore, is both psychic and physical. As with pain, patients vary considerably in their ability to tolerate anxiety.

Most patients in the primary physician's office present with some combination of motor tension (restlessness, edginess, jitteriness), apprehension, vigilance (including distractibility, trouble concentrating, and insomnia), and autonomic hyperactivity. The latter may be manifested by diaphoresis, cardiac symptoms (palpitations, chest tightness, tachycardia), gastrointestinal complaints (stomach distress, diarrhea), urinary frequency, neurologic difficulties (dizziness, paresthesias), or respiratory symptoms (dyspnea, increased respiratory rate).

Generalized anxiety disorder is diagnosed when these symptoms have persisted, often with low-grade intensity, for greater than 4 weeks. In most cases, however, the patient identifies the problem as being present for years with periods of improvement or exacerbation. Frequently, this persistent anxiousness will be associated with intermittent acute spells or attacks of anxiety. When these spells are sudden and severe with prominent symptoms of sudden sympathetic arousal (tachycardia, trembling, hyperventilation, dyspnea), they may be attended with a fear of dying, a feeling of panic, and/or a need to flee from the setting where they have occurred. Such spells are now termed "panic attacks."

Panic attacks. Many patients suffer from occasional panic attacks and from the persistent generalized form of anxiety in the interval between attacks. Some have attacks only at the onset of their chronic smoldering symptoms. Others experience persistent symptoms with no history of acute spells, while still others report intermittent panic attacks separated by relatively asymptomatic periods.

Recurrent panic attacks, or "*panic disorder,*" may become disabling to the patient, who frequently views these spells as indicative of a serious underlying physical disorder. Phobic avoidance of places with restricted escape (crowds, theaters, tunnels, elevators) may follow as the patient fears being trapped during an attack. Some become homebound, afraid to leave places of safety or to be left alone (agoraphobia).

The paroxysmal nature of the panic attacks and the prominence of autonomic symptoms often suggest cardiac or neurologic events. The patients become focused on their bodies, vigilant to premonitory symptoms of the next attack.

Whether generalized anxiety without panic is related to panic anxiety or is a distinct syndrome remains unresolved. Those with panic attacks, however, are more often female, have a family history of the disorder, have had an onset in early adult life (often following the loss of a loved one or after a physical injury or illness), have a childhood history of separation difficulty (as in school phobia), and manifest some phobic avoidance. One series reports a higher than expected rate of premature mortality from cardiovascular illness in males with panic disorder.

Given the exceptional distress of the symptoms, these patients will persist in seeking a physical explanation, will "doctor shop" if necessary, and ultimately become demoralized and depressed. Since benzodiazepine drugs such as diazepam offer partial relief, they may be overused in the patient's effort to gain relief.

Generalized anxiety and panic disorder, with or without agoraphobia, usually will appear to be autonomous; that is, the reasons for the suffering or the causes of specific attacks are obscure, as if the syndrome has a course of its own. These autonomous disorders will tend to be the more perplexing to the physician and most often confused with other medical illnesses.

Situational anxiety. Other presentations of anxiety in the medical setting will be more consistent with "normal" anxiety. The patient will suffer symptoms similar to generalized anxiety, but in a time-limited way, and evidently related to a physical or emotional precipitant or a specific setting. Such "situational" anxiety typically coincides with an identifiable interpersonal or social upheaval. One familiar example of situational anxiety is some patients' response to the office visit itself.

"*Social*" *phobia* is a form of situational anxiety that continually recurs in settings where the patient feels scrutinized by others. *Posttraumatic stress disorder* is an anxiety state that follows upon serious physical trauma or a life-threatening event. *Performance anxiety,* or stagefright, is a brief but at times severe anxiety state precipitated by exposure to an audience. A variety of specific *phobias* may generate severe but circumscribed symptoms, as with fear of flying. Anxiety symptoms, including panic attacks, may also accompany a major *depression* (see Chapter 223).

The *mitral valve prolapse* syndrome (MVP) is associated with anxietylike symptoms. Twenty to fifty percent of patients with panic disorder are discovered to have MVP. MVP is more common in women and predisposes to arrhythmias (see Chapter 20). They appear no different from those with panic attacks alone in terms of course, the anxiety illness, family history, and response to treatment.

As illustrated by the case of MVP, the presence of a physical finding does not exclude the diagnosis of an anxiety disorder; there may be interactions, with one condition exacerbating the other in a repetitive cycle of anxiety, increased physical symptoms, and more anxiety.

DIFFERENTIAL DIAGNOSIS

The medical differential diagnosis of the symptoms associated with anxiety is extensive (see Table 222-1). Some reports suggest that undiagnosed medical ailments are responsible for a significant number of psychiatric referrals for

Table 222-1.   Medical Causes of Anxiousness

TYPE OF CAUSE	SPECIFIC CAUSE
Cardiovascular	Angina pectoris, arrhythmias, congestive heart failure, hypertension, hypovolemia, myocardial infarction, syncope (of multiple causes), valvular disease, vascular collapse (shock)
Dietary	Caffeinism, monosodium glutamate (Chinese-restaurant syndrome), vitamin-deficiency diseases
Drug-related	Akathisia (secondary to antipsychotic drugs), anticholinergic toxicity, digitalis toxicity, hallucinogens, hypotensive agents, stimulants (amphetamines, cocaine, and related drugs), withdrawal syndromes (alcohol or sedative-hypnotics)
Hematologic	Anemias
Immunologic	Anaphylaxis, systemic lupus erythematosus
Metabolic	Hyperadrenalism (Cushing's disease), hyperkalemia, hyperthermia, hyperthyroidism, hypocalcemia, hypoglycemia, hyponatremia, hypothyroidism, menopause, porphyria (acute intermittent)
Neurologic	Encephalopathies (infectious, metabolic, and toxic), essential tremor, intracranial mass lesions, postconcussion syndrome, seizure disorders (especially of the temporal lobe), vertigo
Respiratory	Asthma, chronic obstructive pulmonary disease, pneumonia, pneumothorax, pulmonary edema, pulmonary embolism
Secreting tumors	Carcinoid, insulinoma, pheochromocytoma

"anxiety." Unrecognized arrhythmias, thyroid disease, insulin reactions, and drugs (*e.g.,* caffeine, stimulants, alcohol and sedative-hypnotic withdrawal) are important precipitants.

Besides physical illness, *other psychiatric disorders* are included in the differential diagnosis of anxiety. Most critical to recognize is *depression;* besides anxiousness, the patient manifests impaired mood, sleep, appetite, sex drive, energy, and concentration (see Chapter 223).

Most other psychiatric syndromes, including *psychosis, dementias,* alcohol withdrawal, and drug-related disorders, may present with anxiousness as a component.

WORKUP

The medical differential diagnosis of the symptoms associated with anxiety is too extensive to permit exhaustive medical evaluation of every patient. A reasonable approach to the evaluation of anxiety in the medical patient is to begin by considering the possible role of the illness(es) for which the patient is already under treatment, including symptoms of the illness, patient fears, and therapies. Next, a detailed review of the patient's symptoms is in order with special focus on those conditions most commonly linked to anxiety (*e.g.,* dysrhythmias, hyperthyroidism, severe hypoglycemia, drugs).

If the patient has a single prominent symptom, such as dizziness or chest discomfort, further evaluation should focus on that symptom. When symptoms are paroxysmal, the patient may be suffering the "spells" of panic attacks, which at times may occur without the usual accompaniment of a psychic panic state. In this case, reviewing the features of panic attacks may help identify this "masked" panic: female predominance, onset in early adult life, phobic avoidance and the urge to flee, homeboundedness, family history of similar symptoms, childhood history of school phobia, and partial relief with benzodiazepines. At times, one feature of a panic attack predominates, such as hyperventilation or tachycardia. While hyperventilation, for example, may generate further symptoms such as paresthesias secondary to hypercarbia, its recognition is not tantamount to diagnosis.

The interview of the anxious patient includes a compassionate inquiry into recent life events. Furthermore, the physician should recall that anxiety symptoms are typically manifested in three dimensions: psychologic (worry, dread, fear, terror); bodily (autonomic symptoms, usually cardiac, neurologic, or gastrointestinal); and behavioral (avoidance behavior). A thorough physical examination is essential, checking for signs of illnesses that may present as anxiety (see Table 222-1).

Since there are effective treatments for severe anxiety, a diagnostic trial of antianxiety or antipanic intervention can help resolve difficult diagnostic questions. However, simple suppression of symptoms does not rule out a medical disorder.

PRINCIPLES OF MANAGEMENT

The treatment strategies for anxiety include pharmacologic, psychotherapeutic, and behavioral interventions. For many patients, all three are used in treatment.

Psychotherapy

For those with reactive or situational anxiety, compassionate inquiry that helps guide the patient to an understanding of the association between circumstance, emotion, and symptoms may be an adequate intervention. Constraints of time may necessitate referral for more frequent or in-depth psychotherapeutic work. The reactive and time-limited nature of the symptoms are underscored. Many situationally anxious patients have been through this pattern of response before, and past recovery, after adequate coping with stressors, may be recalled. When symptomatic suffering impairs daily function, temporary introduction of low doses of benzodiazepine drugs may be offered to diminish, but rarely to eradicate, symptoms (see below).

Reassurance in the form of "all is well," even if given in a sympathetic, nonpatronizing manner, will be demoralizing and disappointing. Such perfunctory reassurance is greatly overvalued in responding to the anxious patient who is worried by the physical symptoms. While a negative finding may reassure some patients, the panic disorder patient, in particular, is not relieved because he is experiencing distinctive, intrusive, and distressing symptoms, as if a bolus of epinephrine had been administered blindly.

Reassurance serves to heal only when the patient understands what is wrong and when a course of action is initiated to offer relief. Effective reassurance stems from a systematic physical and psychiatric evaluation and a responsible formulation derived from this clinical data. If "situational" anxiety is implicated as the source of a patient's distress, the physician should have discovered the acute pathogenic setting or event, in addition to recognizing characteristic symptoms. Then a clinical hypothesis is evident that can be tested by response to treatment.

If an autonomous disorder such as panic attacks is diagnosed, the patient is first helped by an explanation that emphasizes the syndromic nature of the illness, the benign but typically alarming quality of the symptoms, and the role of both physical predisposing as well as stress-related factors. Then a treatment strategy can be outlined.

Behavioral Therapy

For those patients whose symptoms are phobic in nature or when avoidance behavior predominates, behavioral therapies offer a direct and effective intervention. Such techniques as "in vivo exposure," desensitization, and general relaxation-response training (see Appendix) will prove adequate treatment for some patients and a useful adjunct to pharmacotherapy for others. Rebreathing training is a popular self-help measure often taught to patients; although useful in mild situational stresses, it will rarely suffice when panic attacks are the trigger of hyperventilation.

Pharmacotherapy

For generalized anxiety symptoms, whether chronic or situational, the benzodiazepines (BZD) are generally considered the drugs of choice. BZDs are more selectively anxiolytic, offering less sedation and diminished morbidity and mortality in overdose and acute withdrawal than barbiturates and nonbarbiturate sedative agents such as meprobamate, ethchlorvynol, glutethimide, and others. Beta-adrenergic blocking agents are useful for performance anxiety and bothersome catechol-induced symptoms.

Benzodiazepines. While there is a small number of patients for whom maintenance treatment with BZDs offers substantial if not complete relief, the usual goal of treatment with BZDs is a diminution of symptomatology and improvement in a patient's ability to perform tasks that had been impaired by anxiety symptoms.

There is wide *individual variation* in clinical response to BZDs and in plasma level and dosage requirements. While the occasional patient will show dramatic and persistently beneficial effect over time, more typically these drugs have only an adjunctive role to play in managing patient distress. Patients should be told to expect that treatment will be of limited duration and will diminish their disorder but not eradicate it. Overuse of medication and drug-seeking from multiple sources does occur in a small percentage of patients using BZDs, although rarely with the intensity and risks associated with opiates, barbiturates, and other sedatives. Nevertheless, the physician should know the patient well before prescribing, be alert for alcohol or drug dependence, evaluate the efficacy of treatment with follow-up visits, avoid prescribing by telephone, and calculate the precise quantity of the drug required for the interval between visits.

Since prescribing a BZD represents a clinical decision to offer symptomatic relief, the critical assessment is to evaluate the patient's response. The patient's coping should be enhanced and avoidance behavior diminished to justify continued treatment.

SELECTION OF AGENT. The available BZDs appear equally effective for the management of generalized anxiety symptoms. The essential differences between agents are pharmacokinetic. Much has been made by drug manufacturers of the various pharmacokinetic differences among these agents. The relevance of pharmacokinetic data to drug selection depends primarily on whether the drug is to be used in acute or intermittent (single-dose) fashion as opposed to a maintenance or multidose manner.

When selecting an agent for occasional or *single-dose use,* the important pharmacokinetic issues are *rate of absorption* and *extent of distribution.* The rate of absorption of a drug will determine the rapidity of the onset of its clinical effect. The degree to which a BZD is lipophilic will determine how rapidly it is distributed into lipid stores and determine the offset of clinical effect after a single dose. Diazepam, despite its long half-life, has its single-dose action terminated by being rapidly redistributed into lipid stores. Thus, despite its rather long half-life, as a single-dose agent diazepam has a rapid and potent onset of clinical effect and a quick offset. Short half-life, therefore, is not a relevant criterion on which to base the selection of a drug for single dosing.

When one considers placing a patient on *maintenance treatment* involving multiple or daily doses, *half-life* becomes more relevant. The longer half-life agents will be more likely to accumulate, but shorter half-life drugs do not accumulate. Except for older male patients and patients with hepatic disease, accumulation does not appear to be a major clinical concern. One reason for this is the development of tolerance to the sedative effects of these drugs with increasing plasma level. Drug selection is best based on pharmacokinetic considerations to achieve the onset and offset desired, with or without systemic accumulation (see Table 222-2).

DETERMINATION OF DOSAGE. The only reasonable guideline to selecting dosage is to begin with low doses and titrate up as necessary, expecting that most nonpanic patients rarely achieve additional benefit above a daily dose of 30 mg of diazepam or its equivalent. Starting doses in the elderly should be no more than 50% of those for younger patients, and maximum doses the equivalent of 10 mg of diazepam (see below).

SIDE-EFFECTS AND DEPENDENCE. Side-effects with BZDs include drowsiness—especially in combination with alcohol—impaired memory acquisition, and occasionally a paradoxical reaction of increased hostility and aggression. Daily use of BZDs over a period of months can lead to psychologic and physical *dependence. Withdrawal* is usually accompanied by only mild symptoms; those distinct from anxiety include tinnitus, involuntary movements, and perceptual changes. Severe withdrawal symptoms are unlikely unless high doses of a potent preparation (especially a short-acting one) have been used daily for a prolonged period of time and therapy is halted abruptly. A delirium tremens-like syndrome may occur with abrupt cessation. Seizures have been reported upon sudden halting of alprazolam after as short a time as 1 to 2 months of daily therapy. For less potent, long-acting BZDs, the risk of an abstinence syndrome is less, allowing daily use of usual doses for up to 4 months, provided the patient has no prior history of sedative use or abuse.

Chronic daily treatment is best discontinued by tapering doses over a several week period. Benzodiazepine dependence is uncommon, but can be a serious problem, often precipi-

Table 222-2. Pharmacokinetic Properties
of Commonly Used Benzodiazepines

DRUG	APPROXIMATE DOSE EQUIVALENCE (MG)	RELATIVE RAPIDITY OF EFFECT	HALF-LIFE (H)
Alprazolam (Xanax)	0.5	Fast–intermediate	6–20
Chlordiazepoxide (Librium)	10	Intermediate	5–30
Clorazepate (Tranxene)	7.5	Fast	30–200
Diazepam (Valium)	5	Fastest	20–100
Lorazepam (Ativan)	1	Intermediate	10–20
Oxazepam (Serax)	15	Slower	5–15
Prazepam (Centrax)	10	Slowest	30–200

tated by careless prescribing and inadequate patient education about proper drug use. Once it develops, it can be hard to treat and is best accomplished by referral to one who is experienced in managing this difficult problem.

Other drug discontinuation syndromes include *recurrence* (return of the original symptoms) and *rebound* (a worsening of the original symptoms). Again, preparations with a short half-life are more likely to trigger such developments.

Beta-Adrenergic Blocking Agents blunt the peripheral catecholamine-mediated manifestations of anxiety and, as such, are very useful when used on an as-needed basis for performance anxiety and stagefright. For generally anxious patients with prominent somatic adrenergic symptoms (diaphoresis, tremulousness, palpitation), beta blockers have offered control when used alone and in combination with BZDs. They should be used with caution if at all in patients with asthma, heart failure, and heart block (see Chapter 25); moreover, they may worsen symptoms if the cause of the anxiety is an underlying depression.

Treatment of Panic Attacks

Most BZDs are inadequate or only partially effective in blocking panic attacks. However, with the advent of the potent agent *alprazolam* (Xanax), a triazolobenzodiazepine, panic attacks can now be more readily controlled than was possible with previously utilized medications. However, large doses are commonly necessary. While treatment with alprazolam may begin with standard daily doses (1 to 3 mg in divided doses), antipanic efficacy is often not evident until higher dosages (4 to 6 mg/day) are reached. Typically, 4 to 8 months of continuous therapy for panic attacks are nec-

essary before withdrawal of medication can be attempted. The result is a potential for developing alprazolam dependence and its attendant risk of withdrawal symptoms in patients with panic attack disorders. In patients with an otherwise disabling panic attack disorder unresponsive to other forms of medication, the risk of dependency may be acceptable. As with any BZD, alprazolam therapy should be carried out with the patient fully understanding the potential risk of dependence.

Among the antipanic agents with minimal potential for habituation, certain *tricyclic antidepressants* (*e.g.,* imipramine) and *monoamine oxidase inhibitors* (MAOI) (*e.g.,* phenelzine) have proven clinically and experimentally capable of preventing attacks. Accumulating data suggest that other tricyclics may be similarly effective. Typically, the response to treatment with a tricyclic agent proceeds in two stages. Initially many of these patients will tolerate only low doses or will transiently experience increased symptomatology potentially leading to premature abandonment of treatment. The patient should be encouraged to remain with the treatment and given very low initial doses which are increased over several days to more typical antidepressant levels; at this point many patients will experience a dramatic improvement. The MAOIs in some cases appear to have an advantage by being better tolerated and possibly more effective. Often the secondary behavioral disability, such as agoraphobia, will spontaneously remit when panic attacks have been effectively controlled.

Regardless of which agent is used, the goal of treatment is prevention of panic spells. Following relief of attacks, periodic efforts at gradual withdrawal may be attempted after 4 to 8 months of well-being.

Sometimes physicians will prescribe therapies designed to treat specific peripheral symptoms (*e.g.,* beta-blocking drugs for tachycardia). Such an approach leaves other components of the syndrome unchecked.

Use of Antianxiety Agents in the Elderly

In the elderly, the *benzodiazepines* are the safest, most effective sedative-hypnotics available. They are less addicting than earlier sedatives (*e.g.,* phenobarbital, meprobamate) and are unlikely to cause lethal overdosage when taken alone. Most fatalities associated with benzodiazepine use have occurred when other respiratory depressants such as alcohol were also ingested.

The antianxiety effects of these drugs are usually manifested at dosages that do not cause sedation. Although there are many similarities among the benzodiazepines, interdrug differences exist that are clinically significant in elderly patients. *Short-acting drugs* are conjugated to glucuronide in the liver and then eliminated in the urine, metabolic activities that do not decline markedly with age. *Lorazepam* and *oxazepam,* two such short-acting drugs, are often recommended for use in the elderly because they have no active metabolites and their metabolism is affected only slightly if at all by the physiologic changes that accompany aging. The main disadvantages of these drugs include need for frequent doses, daytime anxiety if used only qhs, and rebound insomnia if abruptly stopped after prolonged use. Initial dosage should be 10 mg of oxazepam or 0.5 mg of lorazepam 2 to 3 times daily. Intake should be limited to short (5- to 10-day) courses or to occasional prn use.

The long-acting agents such as *diazepam, chlordiazepoxide, clorazepate,* and *prazepam* have active metabolites and are slowly eliminated from the body. Their metabolism is more affected by the physiologic concomitants of aging. For example, a half-life of diazepam of 20 hours at age 20 may increase to as much as 90 hours by age 80. The long half-lives of these drugs in the elderly can lead to accumulation and an increase in side-effects in some patients, including diminished alertness that may be mistaken for senility or dementia. Their main advantage is that they can be given once a day or even every other day. Initial dosages of these drugs should be in the range of 2 to 5 mg/day of diazepam or its equivalent. Dosage should be increased cautiously, because it may take more than a week for steady-state levels to be reached with the longer-acting agents.

Agitation in the elderly (a state of motor drivenness distinct from anxiety) occasionally requires low doses of a high-potency *neuroleptic* such as haloperidol, thiothixene, and fluphenazine. Low-potency neuroleptics such as chlorpromazine and thioridazine have more associated hypotensive, cardiovascular, and anticholinergic side effects (see Chapter 168). Neuroleptics are often useful in agitated elderly patients with organic brain disease. Patients may feel much better and exhibit less agitation, paranoia, antisocial behavior, and insomnia with doses as low as 0.5 mg of *haloperidol* or 1 mg of *thiothixene* twice daily. To minimize risk of adverse effects to which the elderly are particularly susceptible (extrapyramidal symptoms, hypotension), use should be limited to short courses of therapy at low doses (see Chapter 168).

Beta-adrenergic blocking agents such as *propranolol* (40 to 80 mg/day) can be useful for control of adrenergic symptoms, but must be used with considerable care in the elderly due to their ability to trigger or worsen congestive heart failure, heart block, and bronchospasm (see Chapters 25 and 44). In large doses, nightmares and depression may occur. Other antianxiety drugs also can aggravate depression.

THERAPEUTIC RECOMMENDATIONS AND INDICATIONS FOR REFERRAL

Situational Anxiety

- Reassurance occurs in the context of identification of specific provocative stressors and their association with the onset of symptoms.
- If the distress represents one of many such episodes in a pattern of emotional upheaval, psychotherapy referral is indicated.
- When distress from anxiety symptoms impairs daily function, benzodiazepine drugs (BZDs) may be used for transient reduction of symptom intensity, avoiding maintenance treatment for acute problems.
- If symptoms endure beyond the presumed stressful period or worsen despite treatment, referral to a psychiatrist is in order.

Panic Attacks and Agoraphobia

- Effective control of panic attacks is critical to avoid phobic avoidance, demoralization, depression, and disability.
- When depressive symptoms are present a tricyclic antidepressant (TCA) (*e.g.,* imipramine) or a monoamine oxidase inhibitor (MAOI) (*e.g.,* phenelzine) is indicated.
- TCA treatment begins with low, "test" doses (*e.g.,* imipramine 10 to 25 mg hs) and proceeds when tolerated to full antidepressant levels (*e.g.,* imipramine 100 to 200 mg hs).
- MAOIs are most effective; their use requires familiarity with the drug and a tyramine-restricted diet. A dose of 1 mg/kg is the average required. Referral for this treatment may be necessary.
- Alprazolam (beginning with 1 to 3 mg/day in divided doses) may be an alternative for panic attack control. Caution is necessary in initiating chronic therapy because dependency can develop after as little as 6 to 8 weeks of daily use.
- Prominent phobic avoidance without panic spells or despite pharmacologic control of panic indicates a need for behavioral therapies and psychiatric referral.

Generalized Anxiety

- A short course of benzodiazepine therapy may be useful for periods of exacerbation; patients with disabling chronic anxiety need psychiatric referral.
- Avoid chronic BZD therapy due to risk of dependency. If the patient is coming off long-term therapy, taper over several weeks according to the patient's ability to tolerate decreases. Monitor for any withdrawal symptoms (*e.g.*, tinnitus, perceptual changes, involuntary movements).
- Psychotherapy or counselling may help diminish the role of psychosocial stressors in the disorder.
- A history of associated panic attacks or depression suggests a role for TCAs or MAOIs.

ANNOTATED BIBLIOGRAPHY

Baldessarini RJ: Drugs and the treatment of psychiatric disorders. In Gilman AG, Goodman LS, Gilman A (eds): Goodman and Gilman's The Pharmacological Basis of Therapeutics, 6th ed, pp 391–447. New York, Macmillan, 1980 (*An excellent review of preclinical pharmacology of anxiolytic drugs.*)

Brown JT, Mulrow CD, Stoudemire GA: The anxiety disorders. Ann Intern Med 100:558, 1984 (*Reviews diagnostic criteria and therapy as well as theories of anxiety.*)

Busto U, Sellers EM, Naranjo CA et al: Withdrawal reaction after long-term therapeutic use of benzodiazepines. N Engl J Med 315: 854, 1986 (*A controlled study describing a mild, but clinically important withdrawal syndrome. The results suggest that gradual reduction is the preferred technique for cessation of therapy.*)

Gorman JM, Fyer AF, Gliklich J et al: Effect of imipramine on prolapsed mitral valves of patients with panic disorder. Am J Psychiatry 138:977, 1981 (*MVP and panic attacks.*)

Greenblatt DJ, Shader RI, Abernethy DR: Current status of benzodiazepines (second of two parts). N Engl J Med 309:354, 410, 1983 (*State-of-the-art review of clinical pharmacology of BZDs.*)

Jenike MA: Treating anxiety in elderly patients. Geriatrics 38:115, 1983 (*A practical review.*)

Klein DF, Rabkin JG (eds): Anxiety: New Research and Changing Concepts. New York, Raven Press, 1981 (*Compilation of several papers dealing with diagnosis, phenomenology, and treatment of panic attacks and agoraphobia.*)

Matuzas W, Glass RM: Treatment of agoraphobia and panic attacks. Arch Gen Psychiatry 40:220, 1983 (*Reasoned discussion of the role of drugs and behavioral therapy, particularly "in vivo exposure" treatment.*)

Mavissakalian M: Pharmacologic treatment of anxiety disorders. J Clin Psychiatry 43:487, 1982 (*Straightforward review of standard therapeutic options.*)

Mellinger GD, Balter MB, Uhlenhuth EH: Prevalence and correlates of the long term regular use of anxiolytics. JAMA 251:375, 1984 (*A nationally representative survey indicating that less than 2% of adults between ages 18 and 79 are long-term anxiolytic users.*)

Noyes R, Clancey J, Coryell WH: A withdrawal syndrome after abrupt withdrawal of alprazolam. Am J Psychiatry 142:114, 1985 (*Sei-*

zures and other serious withdrawal symptoms within 3 days of ceasing therapy.)

Rosenbaum JF: Current concepts in psychiatry: The drug treatment of anxiety. N Engl J Med 306:401, 1982 (*Guidelines for the general physician on the rationale and approach to prescribing BZDs.*)

Schuckit MA: Anxiety related to medical disease. J Clin Psychiatry 44:11(sec 2):31, 1983 (*A discussion of anxiety as a reaction to illness, symptom of a physical disorder, and part of a chronic disease. This issue of the journal contains other relevant articles.*)

Sheehan DV: Panic attacks and phobias. N Engl J Med 307:156, 1982 (*Reviews the natural history, diagnosis, and epidemiologic aspects as well as psychological, behavioral, and pharmacological therapy.*)

Sheehan DV, Ballenger J, Jacobsen G: Treatment of endogenous anxiety with phobic, hysterical, and hypochondriacal symptoms. Arch Gen Psychiatry 37:51, 1980 (*New classic paper demonstrating the efficacy of TCAs and MAOIs in panic disorder and agoraphobia; finds MAOIs tend to be most effective.*)

Zitrin CM, Klein DF, Woerner MG: Behavior therapy, supportive psychotherapy, imipramine, and phobias. Arch Gen Psychiatry 35:307, 1978 (*Report illustrating the role of TCAs combined with behavioral treatments and support.*)

Appendix: Strategies for Stress Management
WILLIAM E. MINICHIELLO, Ed.D.

Stress itself is not harmful when managed effectively. With the increased awareness of the impact of stress on the body has come a variety of stress-reducing techniques derived from behavior therapy. Stress management training enables the patient to condition his body to cope more adaptively with stress or anxiety. As part of a comprehensive treatment program, the primary care physician may choose to train the patient in one or more of the self-regulatory procedures. Relaxation training is by far the most effective of the procedures.

Before proceeding to train the patient in relaxation as a self-control procedure, the physician should advise reduction or elimination of caffeine from the patient's diet, since relaxation training is aimed at lowering the patient's autonomic arousal level and caffeine augments arousal.

Progressive deep muscle relaxation, autogenic training, and diaphragmatic breathing represent the major techniques practical for use in the primary care setting.

Progressive Deep Muscle Relaxation

Progressive deep muscle relaxation is probably the most extensively used and most effective relaxation technique today for the treatment of anxiety and stress-related problems. A brief, modified version can be taught to the patient in one session. The rationale for the technique is the view that anxiety and relaxation are mutually exclusive; that is, anxiety cannot be experienced when the muscles are relaxed.

Progressive deep muscle relaxation is a simple procedure

contrasting tension with relaxation. Since a person generally has very little awareness of the sensation of relaxation, he is asked first to tense a set of muscles as hard as he can until he can feel tension in the muscles. Then he allows those muscles to relax and tries to become aware of ("to feel internally") the difference between tension and relaxation.

This relaxation technique entails the systematic focus of attention on specific gross muscle groups throughout the body. The patient is instructed to actively tense each muscle group for 10 to 15 seconds, after which he is told to let go of the tension in the muscles, observe the difference, and relax the muscles. The sequence of tensing the muscles, letting go of the tension, and noting the difference between tension and relaxation is systematically applied to the following muscle groups: forehead and scalp, eyes, nose, face, tongue, jaws, lips, neck, right fist and forearm, left fist and forearm, right leg, left leg, back, chest, stomach, buttocks, thighs, calves, ankles, toes. (see Fig. 222-1)

Autogenic Training

Autogenic training is a relaxation technique composed of a set of exercises that are intended to induce heaviness and warmth in the muscles through mental imagery.

Progressive Deep Muscle Relaxation

Practice is to be done while sitting in a chair with your back straight, head on a line with your back, both feet on the floor and hands resting on your lap. Each muscle is to be tightened, held in tightened position for 15–20 seconds, and then slowly let go while studying the difference between tension and relaxation.

Forehead. Wrinkle up your forehead by arching your eyebrows and creasing your forehead, hold the tension, and then slowly let go of the tension.

Eyes. Squeeze your eyes together tightly, hold the tension, and then slowly let go of the tension.

Nose. Wrinkle up your nose and spread your nostrils, hold the tension, and then slowly let go of the tension.

Face. Put a forced smile on your face and spread your face, hold the tension, and then slowly let go of the tension.

Tongue. Push your tongue hard against the roof of your mouth, hold the tension, and then slowly let go of the tension.

Jaws. Clench your jaws together tightly, hold the tension, and then slowly let go of the tension.

Lips. Pucker up your lips and spread them, hold the tension, and then slowly let go of the tension.

Neck. Tighten the muscles of your neck by pulling your chin in and shrugging up your shoulders, hold the tension, and then slowly let go of the tension.

Right Arm. Tense your right arm and hand by stretching it out in front of you and clenching your fist tightly, hold the tension, and then slowly let go of the tension.

Left Arm. Tense your left arm and hand by stretching it out in front of you, and then slowly let go of the tension.

Right Leg. Extend your right leg in front of you (at the height of the chair seat), tense your thigh and leg by pointing your toes inward toward your face, hold the tension, and then slowly let go of the tension.

Left Leg. Extend your left leg in front of you, tense your thigh and leg by pointing your toes inward toward your face, hold the tension, and then slowly let go of the tension.

Upper Back. Tense your back muscles by sitting slightly forward in the chair, bending your elbows and trying to get them to touch each other behind your back, hold the tension, and then slowly let go of the tension.

Chest. Tense your chest muscles by pulling your stomach in and thrusting your chest upward and outward, hold the tension, and then slowly let go of the tension.

Stomach. Tense your stomach muscles, making them hard by pushing your stomach out, hold the tension, and then slowly let go of the tension.

Buttocks and Thighs. Tense your buttocks and thighs by placing your feet squarely on the floor, pointing your toes into the floor and forcing your heels to remain on the floor while pushing forward, hold the tension, and then slowly let go of the tension.

Practice should be engaged in twice daily for a period of 12–15 minutes. Mastery of the technique is after 2–4 weeks of twice daily practice.

Figure 222-1. Instructions to patients.

Autogenic training typically involves the patient sitting comfortably in an armchair in a quiet room with his eyes closed. Verbal formulae are introduced (*e.g.,* "my arm is heavy"), and the patient is instructed to visualize and feel the relaxation of the muscle being focused on while silently repeating and passively concentrating on that formula. The formulae, which consist of verbal somatic suggestions, are intended to facilitate concentration and "mental contact" with the parts of the body indicated by the formula.

Training consists of six psycho-physiologic exercises which are practiced several times a day. The training begins with the theme of heaviness (*e.g.,* "my arm feels heavy and relaxed"). The second group of formulae involve warmth (*e.g.,* "my arm feels warm and relaxed"). Following warmth training, the patient continues with passive concentration on cardiac activity (*e.g.,* "my heartbeat feels calm and regular"). The fourth exercise focuses on breathing and respiration. In the next exercise the patient focuses on warmth in the chest and abdomen, and in the last exercise the focus is passive concentration on cooling of the forehead. In modern practice, the time and the six standard exercises have been condensed so that a whole round can be practiced in a very brief period of between 5 and 10 minutes. In this condensed version the autogenic training phrases are focused primarily on the physiologic aspect used in the training, interspersed with general suggestions for relaxation. Each phrase is said slowly, allowing time for the patient to begin to feel some awareness of the effect of the suggestion (see Fig. 222-2).

Diaphragmatic Breathing

The quickest and simplest method of relaxation is to breathe slowly and deeply from the belly. Diaphragmatic breathing is an effective means of coping with and reducing stress.

For centuries, students of yoga and zen have been aware that a mastery of breathing could slow heart rate, lower blood pressure, and calm the body. Diaphragmatic breathing involves parasympathetic nervous system stimulation. Diaphragmatic breathing prevents the possibility of hyperventilation and, after 50 to 60 seconds of such breathing, brings a feeling of quiescence to the body and reduction in bodily symptoms of stress.

Training in diaphragmatic breathing can be done either sitting or lying down. In either position a pillow should be placed at the small of the back to force the belly out. Breathing should begin by pushing the stomach out as inhalation takes place slowly and deeply. Care should be taken to minimize the movement of the chest with each inhalation. The word "relax" should be said silently prior to exhaling and the stomach should fall with exhalation. While breathing *in,* the stomach should be pushed *out;* while breathing *out,* the stomach should come *in* (see Fig. 222-3).

Autogenic Training

Practice is to be done while sitting in a soft, comfortable chair with your eyes closed. As attention is called to specific groups of muscles, try to *visualize* and *feel* the relaxation of those muscles. Try to let *happen* what is being suggested. Repeat each formula 2–3 times.

My forehead and scalp feel heavy, limp, loose, and relaxed.

My eyes and nose feel heavy, limp, loose, and relaxed.

My face and jaws feel heavy, limp, loose, and relaxed.

My neck, shoulders, and back feel heavy, limp, loose, and relaxed.

My arms and hands feel heavy, limp, loose, and relaxed.

My chest, solar plexus, and the central part of my body feel quiet, calm, comfortable, and relaxed.

My stomach feels heavy, limp, loose, and relaxed.

My buttocks, thighs, calves, ankles, and toes feel quiet, heavy, limp, loose, and relaxed.

My whole body feels quiet, heavy, limp, and relaxed.

Practice should be engaged in twice daily for a period of 6–8 minutes. Mastery of the technique is after 1–3 weeks of twice daily practice.

Figure 222-2. Instructions to patients.

Diaphragmatic Breathing

While sitting or lying down with a pillow at the small of your back

1. Breathe in slowly and deeply by pushing your stomach out.
2. Say the word "relax" silently to yourself prior to exhaling.
3. Exhale slowly, letting your stomach come in.
4. Repeat entire procedure 10 times consecutively, with emphasis on slow, deep breaths.

Practice should take place 5 times per day, 10 consecutive diaphragmatic breaths each sitting. Time for mastery is after 1–2 weeks of daily practice.

Figure 222-3. Instructions to patients.

223
Approach to the Patient with Depression

STEVEN E. HYMAN, M.D.
MICHAEL A. JENIKE, M.D.

The vast majority of patients with depression present to primary care physicians, often complaining of somatic symptoms. The frequency, treatability, and potentially serious consequences of depression make its diagnosis and management high priorities for the primary care physician. Unfortunately, the diagnosis is not always evident because the symptoms may masquerade as a variety of psychiatric or somatic conditions.

CLINICAL PRESENTATION

"*Depressed mood*" is usually the major symptom, though some clinicians prefer to use the term "*dysphoric mood*" because patients often complain of feeling irritable, worried, discouraged, or frustrated rather than sad or despondent (see Table 223-1). Some depressed patients focus on disturbances in behavior or thought such as memory loss, inability to concentrate, lack of self-confidence, or poor self-esteem. Others are troubled by low energy, poor sleep, or a variety of somatic

Table 223-1.   Clinical Presentation
of Depressive Syndromes

Psychologic Symptoms and Signs
Mood sad, blue, "down in the dumps"
Depressed affect
Poor self-esteem
Anxiety
Irritability or anger
Loss of interest in environment
Anhedonia (lack of pleasure)
Social withdrawal
Guilt (may be delusional)
Feelings of helplessness or hopelessness
Multiple physical complaints or hypochondriacal fears
Rumination, obsessive thoughts
Poor concentration
Decreased libido
Recurrent thoughts of death or suicide
Psychotic symptoms may occur (*e.g.*, delusions)

Vegetative Symptoms
Decreased energy
Sleep disturbance (most commonly early morning awakening)
Appetite disturbance (usually loss of interest in food; anorexia)
Diurnal variation in mood (usually worse in the morning)
Psychomotor retardation or agitation

pains and concerns. Disordered sleep, poor appetite, lack of energy, and a diurnal variation in mood (independent of the day's events), are referred to as *neurovegetative symptoms,* or melancholia; they suggest the presence of a drug-responsive disorder (see below).

Abnormal affect (a disturbance in the patient's predominant emotional state) is the sign of depression that corresponds to the patient's subjective feeling of dysphoria. Although sadness is the most common presentation, irritability, anger, or apathy may predominate. Depressed affect can be subtle, at times only noticed when sadness ensues from talking with the patient. As depression worsens, psychomotor abnormalities may occur. Most common is *psychomotor retardation,* with slow movements, slow speech, and a long latency before the patient answers questions. Conversely (especially in the elderly), some patients may manifest *agitation* with motor restlessness and rapid speech. These patients are often anxious and irritable rather than sad.

No diagnostic classification of depressions has met with universal approval. Nonetheless, the current standard of diagnosis, the American Psychiatric Association's *Diagnostic and Statistical Manual,* Third Edition (DSM III), provides an adequate schema for characterization of depression, one which can be used to guide treatment (see Table 223-2).

Major Depression is the DSM III term for serious *episodic* depression that is accompanied by *neurovegetative symptoms.* Prior terms for this disorder were *endogenous depression* and *unipolar depression.* Dysphoric mood typically dominates the clinical picture and is relatively persistent. In addition, the patient must have at least four of the following eight symptoms for at least 2 weeks: appetite disturbance, sleep disturbance, psychomotor retardation or agitation, anhedonia (lack of pleasure in any activities), loss of energy, feelings of worthlessness or guilt, decreased cognitive functioning, or suicidal thoughts.

When the symptoms and signs of major depression are present, the history or absence of a precipitating event is not critical to the diagnosis. Onset is variable. Although symptoms usually develop over weeks to months, they may develop suddenly. At least half of all patients have recurrent episodes. Major depression is more common in women than in men.

Delusions, hallucinations, or bizarre behavior (depression with psychotic features) may occur. Such psychotic symptoms

Table 223-2. Classification of Depressive Syndromes

Major Affective Disorders

Major depression (severe and episodic, including
  neurovegetative symptoms; previously called unipolar or
  endogenous depression)
  Treatment: an antidepressant

Bipolar disorder (severe and episodic, with a history of a manic
  episode)
  Treatment: lithium (plus an antidepressant in depressed
  phase)

Other Specific Affective Disorders

Dysthymic disorder (less severe, chronic; may represent residual
  major depression or characterological depression)
  Treatment: Trial of antidepressant if vegetative symptoms
  present; psychotherapy

Cyclothymic disorder (less severe, chronic mood swings)
  Treatment: lithium

Atypical Affective Disorders

Atypical depression (some presentations include
  pseudodementia, chronic pain syndromes, some
  hypochondrias, some phobic and anxiety states, some
  paranoid states, and catatonia)
  Treatment: an antidepressant

Organic Brain Syndromes

Organic affective disorder (depression or mania due to an
  organic cause)
  Treatment: treatment of underlying medical problem; trial of
  antidepressant if necessary

Other Conditions

Adjustment disorders with depressed mood (reactive depression)
  Treatment: psychotherapy; antidepressant if some vegetative
  symptoms present and troublesome

are not pathognomonic of schizophrenia; in fact, they are usually congruent with the patient's mood (*e.g.,* delusions of guilt or of physical decay), though other psychotic symptoms may occur (*e.g.,* paranoid ideas). In the elderly, depression can mimic dementia. The patient may appear withdrawn, unkempt, inattentive, and even confused. This state may be due to depression alone (pseudodementia) or to a combination of depression and dementia.

A family history of a major affective disorder (major depression or dipolar disorder) is common, as is one of alcoholism, though the relationship between alcoholism and depression remains controversial (see below).

Bipolar Disorder, Depressed Phase. The presentation of depression in the bipolar (manic-depressive) patient is identical to that of major depression. The crucial difference is a history of prior *manic* or *hypomanic episodes* (periods of elation or expansive mood, increased energy, decreased need for sleep, inflated self-esteem, and overinvolvement in activities, with a decreased concern for their consequences). If the patient has only had hypomania, depression may be difficult to recognize.

Dysthymic Disorder (Chronic Low-grade Depression). Some patients complain of life-long feelings of depression.

Symptoms are less severe than those of major depression, and the neurovegetative symptoms are minor or absent. These patients seem to have depression as an essential part of their character (hence the older term of *characterologic depression*). Often, they are frustrating to treat because of chronic dysphoria, self-pity, and development of irrational patterns of negative thinking (*i.e.,* that things always go wrong for them). The physician feels helpless and may unconsciously communicate a wish that the patient would go away.

Not all dysthymic patients have the same underlying disorder. Typically, those with a truly characterologic depression have onset in adolescence or early adult life and manifest other symptoms of a personality disorder, such as a history of difficulty with interpersonal relationships, manipulativeness, and predominant feelings of emptiness and lack of an identity. They are unlikely to respond to pharmacologic interventions and often respond poorly to psychotherapy as well.

Some patients with chronic depression have either *residual symptoms* of a major affective disorder or an *attenuated chronic form of major depression*. There is either a prior history of a major depressive episode without a full recovery or the presence of at least some neurovegetative symptoms. These patients usually have onset later in life after a period of good functioning.

Cyclothymic Disorder. This disorder resembles bipolar disease, but the mood swings are less severe. These patients have a chronic mood disturbance characterized by periods of depression and periods of elevated mood, but not of sufficient severity or duration to meet the criteria for major depressed or manic episodes. Interspersed may be periods of normal mood lasting as long as several months. There is often a family history of major affective disorders.

Adjustment Disorder With Depressed Mood (Reactive Depression). Probably the most common type of depression is a *reactive* or situational depression. By definition this occurs following a *significant life stress*. Patients usually present with depressed mood associated with feelings of hopelessness, helplessness, worthlessness, and anxiety. Thoughts are often dominated by the problems that precipitated the episode. Sleep and appetite disturbance are common, but are less severe and less persistent than in major depression. Any patient with symptoms severe enough to meet the criteria for major depression (described above) should receive that diagnosis regardless of the history of a precipitant. Reactive depression is usually *self-limited* and improves when the stress is removed or the individual finds a better coping mechanism.

DIFFERENTIAL DIAGNOSIS

It is important to rule out possible organic causes of depression and other psychiatric disorders that can masquerade as depression.

Organic Affective Syndromes. The clinical presentation may be identical to that of a functional depression (see Table 223-3). Even psychotic symptoms may occur. Confusion or alterations in level of consciousness (which strongly suggest organicity) are often not present. In some medical illnesses, for example, *pancreatic cancer* (see Chapter 73) depression may even dominate the early clinical picture. Probably the most common medical cause of depression is use of medications. In drug-induced illness, onset is temporally related to medication use. Depression due to *reserpine* has decreased in frequency as better antihypertensives have replaced it, but *alpha methyldopa* and *beta blockers* remain potential precipitants (see Chapter 21). In the elderly, use of *sedative-hypnotics* can produce a picture of depression or dementia. When depression is due to an endocrine disorder, other symptoms are usually present, although they may be subtle as in *apathetic hyperthyroidism* of the elderly (see Chapter 101) or early Cushing's syndrome.

Alcoholism and Drug Dependence. Many alcoholic patients appear depressed, but it is not possible to sort out which symptoms are due to alcohol and which, if any, might be due to a primary affective disorder until the patient has been fully detoxified. Other substance abuse disorders may mimic depression, especially abuse of *sedative-hypnotics* (including *benzodiazepines*). *Withdrawal* from *cocaine* and *amphetamines* can lead to depression.

Uncomplicated Bereavement. Symptoms may be identical to those of depression. The question of a superimposed depression should be raised if mourning continues for more than 6 months, if neurovegetative symptoms are particularly severe, or if there is severe impairment in the patient's ability to function.

Personality Disorders. This group of patients frequently complains of depressive symptoms, with periods of severe dysphoria, but their affective symptoms often fluctuate markedly with environmental changes (especially with changes in interpersonal relationships). Poor impulse control, histories of unstable relationships, and a striking quality of manipulativeness are other characteristics.

WORKUP

History. The possibility of depression should always be raised by the presence of neurovegetative symptoms such as poor energy, poor sleep (especially with early morning awakening), loss of interest in food and sex, and diurnal variation in mood. Multiple bodily complaints out of proportion to physical findings represents another important clue. Depression should always be considered when patients express feelings of hopelessness or poor self-esteem. The onset of depressive symptoms and signs in patients with chronic debilitating disorders or chronic pain can be slow and subtle and should not be overlooked.

When depression is suspected, further inquiry is needed. Since many patients, especially those with somatic complaints, might deny psychologic difficulties, it is often less threatening to ask first about sleep, appetite, and energy. Then one can inquire about mood and any loss of interest in sex, family, job, and other sources of interest or pleasure. In addition, the patient should be queried about his self-opinion and any self-critical feelings. With every depressed patient, it is most important to ask about suicidal thoughts (see below).

Family history can provide important information, but may be difficult to elicit because of shame about any family history of mental illness. It helps to explain that depression often runs in families perhaps because of a biochemical imbalance. A family history of major depression, bipolar disorder, or suicide helps confirm a diagnosis of depression in the patient. A family history of schizophrenia is not necessarily evidence against an affective disorder, because mania was frequently misdiagnosed as schizophrenia in the past. It is sometimes worth reviewing the family member's symptoms and attempting a tentative rediagnosis.

Discussion of the *home environment* can provide important information. Does the patient live alone? If not, is the

---

Table 223-3. Organic Etiologies of Depression

1. *Drug induced:* reserpine, beta blockers, alpha-methyldopa, levodopa, estrogens, corticosteroids, cholinergic drugs, benzodiazepines, barbiturates, and similarly acting drugs
2. *Related to drug abuse:* alcohol abuse, sedative-hypnotic abuse, cocaine and other psychostimulant withdrawal
3. *Toxic-metabolic disorders:* hyperthyroidism (especially in the elderly), hypothyroidism, Cushing's syndrome, hypercalcemia, hyponatremia, diabetes mellitus
4. *Neurologic disorders:* stroke, subdural hematoma, multiple sclerosis, brain tumors (especially frontal), Parkinson's disease, Huntington's disease, uncontrolled epilepsy, syphilis, dementias
5. *Nutritional disorders:* vitamin B_{12} deficiency, pellagra
6. *Other:* pancreatic carcinoma; viral infections (especially mononucleosis and influenzae)

family environment accepting and supportive or, conversely, contributing to the patient's discomfort? The availability of responsible family members to observe and supervise the patient might mean the difference between outpatient treatment and hospitalization if the patient is very depressed or debilitated.

Examination. While obtaining the history, the physician should also note the patient's *mental status.* Is there psychomotor retardation or agitation? The form of the patient's speech should be observed. Does the patient offer anything spontaneously or is there a long period of hesitation before answering? Is the speech slow? Is normal inflection present? The patient's *affect* should be observed. Sadness, tearfulness, despondency, irritability, anxiety, or anger suggest depression.

It should be noted whether the patient is able to maintain attention or is distractable. Inattention may occur in depression, delirium, dementia, or severe anxiety, and will interfere with the patient's overall cognitive performance. Any inattention is worth documenting by testing ability to recall a series of random numbers (digit span). Patients should be able to repeat a series of at least 5 to 7 numbers without error.

One notes both the form and the content of the patient's thought. Is the patient's thought clear and coherent or perhaps tangential, circumstantial, or nonsensical? Are there ideas of worthlessness, helplessness, hopelessness, guilt, suicidal thoughts, and homicidality? It should be noted whether the patient appears guarded or expresses paranoid or other delusions. Inquiry into any unusual experiences such as hearing voices or seeing things that other people could not see is important. If appropriate, tests of memory, calculation, and other higher cortical functions should be made.

Even if the history, mental status, and family history suggest depression, it is still necessary to obtain a full medical history and review of systems and to perform a physical examination. Depression may be the first symptom of a metabolic, infectious, neoplastic, or neurologic disorder. It is especially important to obtain a detailed drug history, of both prescription and other.

Laboratory Studies. Unfortunately, there are *no* useful chemical tests to confirm a diagnosis of depression. It was thought that measurement of urinary metabolites of catecholamine metabolism (*e.g.,* MHPG) or an overnight *dexamethasone suppression test* (DST) might be diagnostic of major depression or predictive of tricyclic responsiveness, but these tests have proven too inaccurate for routine clinical use. While approximately half of the patients with major depression have abnormalities of the hypothalamic–pituitary–adrenal axis as measured by the DST (4 PM cortisol above 5 μg/dl on the day after an 11 PM oral dose of 1 mg of dexamethasone), the test has proven unacceptably insensitive and nonspecific. Thus, depression remains very much a clinical diagnosis. However, medical causes of fatigue may mimic depression and need to be tested for (see Chapter 5).

Evaluation for Suicide Risk. The assessment of suicide risk stands out as one of the most critical tasks in evaluation of the depressed patient, and is especially important because suicide is often preventable. Depression is responsible for more than half of all suicides. Conversely, about 15% of all patients with major affective disorders take their own lives. Other conditions precipitating suicide include chronic alcoholism, personality disorders, and both functional and drug-induced psychoses, in which delusional beliefs or hallucinations may lead to self-destruction.

With proper intervention, most suicidal patients change their minds about wanting to die. Unfortunately, the task of predicting a suicide attempt is difficult even among patients who complain of suicidal thoughts. Adequate assessment requires careful, empathetic history-taking that allows the patient an opportunity to express his feelings. A common pitfall is to prematurely interrupt the patient who mentions suicide in order to talk him out of it or to send him immediately to an emergency room.

The physician must take any mention of suicide seriously and ask every depressed patient about suicide. Suicide is an extremely personal issue that necessitates a circumspect, calm approach without any implied criticism of the patient. The question might be broached by first eliciting the patient's feelings of hopelessness or suffering and then asking, "Are you feeling so badly that sometimes you would prefer not to go on living?" This query can be followed with a more direct question about self-destructive thoughts. Asking patients about suicide does not put the idea into their heads. It is an error to avoid the subject for fear of doing so. Truly suicidal patients may even be relieved to be asked about it.

Assessing risk of suicide requires attention to the patient's *thoughts* (ideas, wishes, motives), *intent* (the degree to which the patient intends to act on the thoughts), and *plans.* A well worked out, realistic, and potentially lethal plan suggests great risk, as does the act of putting one's affairs in order. Mental status, especially the patient's ability to resist suicidal thoughts, is important to consider. An extremely impulsive, psychotic, or intoxicated patient has no meaningful internal controls and will need hospitalization. Demographic factors associated with an increased risk, such as living alone and being unemployed (see Table 223-4), deserve review.

There is no simple formula for assessing suicide risk; it requires careful clinical judgment. If the patient is severely depressed and, on the basis of the evaluation, appears to be a significant suicide risk (*e.g.,* lacking reliable internal resources to resist suicidal impulses), emergency psychiatric consultation should be arranged. Such patients should be closely supervised and not allowed to transport themselves. Patients with severe or worsening depression who are judged to be at lesser risk should be given a prompt, confirmed appointment with a psychiatrist. Low-risk patients who seem trustworthy and have external social supports can be treated by the primary physician, so long as frequent visits can be

Table 223-4. Demographic Risk Factors for Suicide

1. History of prior attempts
2. Depression
3. Alcoholism
4. Positive family history of suicide
5. Living alone
6. Age: in males risk increases with age, peaking at 75; in females the peak for successful suicide is between 55 and 65
7. Sex: females attempt suicide 3–4 times more often than men, but men are successful 2–3 times more often than women
8. Marital status: those who have never married are at greatest risk, followed by widowed, then separated or divorced, then married without children, then married with children
9. Employment: the unemployed and unskilled are at greater risk than the employed and skilled
10. Physical illness; half of all patients who attempt suicide have a physical illness; those at highest risk are patients with chronic pain, a chronic disease, recent surgery, or a terminal illness

arranged and the depression responds to treatment. Patients with suicide potential should never be given more than 1 g or a week's supply of a tricyclic antidepressant (see below).

PRINCIPLES OF MANAGEMENT

Successful management of depression depends on good rapport with the patient as well as a proper diagnosis. Management has two facets, psychologic and medical. The availability of effective medical treatments (antidepressant medications and electroconvulsive therapy) has dramatically improved prognosis. The choice of treatments (psychotherapy, medication, or a combination of the two) depends on the nature of the depression and the wishes of the patient. There are currently ideologic splits among psychiatrists as to whether psychologic and somatic treatments are compatible; the best evidence suggests that the benefits may be complementary. If there is an organic cause (secondary depression), one treats the causative medical illness and discontinues any potentially offending medications. If the medical condition responds slowly or is untreatable, trials of an antidepressant or supportive psychotherapy might prove useful.

The cornerstone of treatment for *major depression* (unipolar or endogenous depression) is *antidepressant medication.* Psychotherapy can be helpful in sorting out feelings and in dealing with both intrapsychic and interpersonal problems, but alone, does not appear to be curative in serious depressions. If the patient has *bipolar disease, lithium* will be needed in addition to an antidepressant, and treatment is best undertaken by a psychiatrist. *Reactive depression* (DSM III adjustment disorder with depressed mood) may be treated by the primary care physician with *supportive psychotherapy.* If moderate sleep and appetite disturbances are present (as they

may be even in reactive depressions), a tricyclic antidepressant can provide relief.

Psychologic Management (Supportive Psychotherapy). All patients suffering from depression, regardless of diagnostic type, require careful psychologic management. A clear, empathetic, and hopeful manner facilitates treatment. A detailed explanation of the diagnosis combined with reassurance that it is eminently treatable can do much to calm a fearful patient. When patients feel hopeless or undeserving, it is useful to point out that these are symptoms of depression and will gradually improve.

While conveying hope and optimsm, the physician must take care not to dismiss as insignificant the patient's fears, pains, and negative feelings. Many feel overwhelmed by life stresses. It is important to identify these stresses; empathetic listening and thoughtful comment can help the patient devise strategies for coping.

At the outset of treatment one should see the patient every week or two for a half hour. Appointments can then be spaced out according to the patient's needs. If a patient becomes severely depressed, agitated, or psychotic (it becomes impossible to have a conversation with him), emergency psychiatric referral should be made. When the acute depressive episode has resolved, the patient should be informed that depressions can recur, and that it is important to contact the physician should symptoms return.

Social and Environmental Interventions. A caring family willing to monitor the severely depressed patient may make the difference between outpatient treatment and hospitalization. Family members can ensure proper use of medication and keeping of follow-up appointments. Exploring with the family stressful elements in the patient's environment might serve as a first step toward modifying them. Involvement of the family serves to decrease social isolation, which both results from and exacerbates depression. Patients worried about taking time off from work should be advised that depression is a real medical illness and assured that the physician is willing to contact the patient's employer to help arrange a reduced schedule or a short absence if indicated.

Antidepressant Medication is the treatment of choice for major depression (endogenous depression) and is effective in other subtypes of depression when neurovegetative symptoms are present (regardless of whether or not an environmental precipitant can be identified). Antidepressants are usually not helpful in characterologic depressions but may be useful in chronic depressions due to other etiologies. The tricyclic compounds and related newer drugs serve as first-line antidepressants. The monoamine oxidase inhibitors and lithium are reserved for special situations.

TRICYCLICS. There are currently a large number of tricyclic and other heterocyclic antidepressants available. Used in the proper dosages, all are effective, although onset of improvement might not be noted until 2 to 4 weeks into therapy. The major differences are in the degree of anticholinergic and sedative side-effects. Drug choice for a given patient can be made according to the side-effect profile (see Table 223-5). The primary care physician should become comfortable with the use of two or three of these drugs, including at least one sedating and one nonsedating compound. In general, it is best to avoid drugs with the high levels of anticholinergic activity in order to maximize patient comfort and compliance.

Selection of agent. Patients with severe *insomnia* might do best with a strongly sedating drug, such as *doxepin* (Adapin or Sinequan) given at bedtime. The very sedating drug *amitriptyline* (Elavil) has long been popular with physicians, but because of its strong anticholinergic side-effects, it is probably not an optimal first-choice agent. Patients without insomnia, especially if elderly or with prostatic hypertrophy, should receive one of the nonsedating tricyclics that has relatively mild anticholinergic activity (*e.g.,* desipramine [Norpramin] or nortriptyline [Aventyl or Pamelor]). Nortriptyline has the advantage among tricyclics of causing the least postural hypotension. *Imipramine* (Tofranil) is moderately sedating and moderately anticholinergic, but is the least costly.

The prescribing of *fixed combination drugs* containing a tricyclic and a neuroleptic (*e.g.,* Triavil) or a tricyclic and a benzodiazepine (*e.g.,* Limbitrol) is irrational and should be avoided. Combinations make it difficult to achieve therapeutic levels of the tricyclic without administering too much of the other compound. Indeed, except for the depressed patient with delusions, *neuroleptics* (which carry a risk of causing tardive dyskinesia) have no place in the treatment of depression.

Adverse effects. The most significant danger with use of tricyclics is their *lethal potential* when taken in overdose. One should never prescribe more than 1 gm of a tricyclic to a potentially suicidal patient or a patient whom one does not know well. The most common serious side-effect of the tricyclic drugs is *postural hypotension.* Especially in the elderly, this can lead to falls and other complications. If postural hypotension is a problem, nortriptyline should be used; if the hypotension is always worse in the morning, it may be useful to give the nortriptyline in three divided doses. Patients should be instructed to be careful when rising from recumbency or sitting.

Many patients complain of *dry mouth, lassitude, constipation,* and *mild mental clouding* and assume that these conditions are drug-related. Depressed patients frequently have low tolerance for any somatic discomfort, and these may be symptoms of depression as well as possible anticholinergic drug side-effects. Such symptoms present no reason in themselves to discontinue medication or decrease dosage. The patient should be reassured that these symptoms usually lessen with time.

Rarely, more severe dose-related anticholinergic symptoms occur, especially in the elderly. These include *tachyarrhythmias, ileus, urinary retention,* and, very rarely, a full anticholinergic syndrome with agitation or delirium and fever in addition to other anticholinergic signs. The most common reason for the emergence of this syndrome is the simultaneous use of more than one anticholinergic drug. Most often implicated along with the tricyclic antidepressants (especially amitriptyline) are thioridazine (Mellaril), anticholinergic antiparkinsonian drugs, antihistamines, antispasmodics, and over-the-counter sleep medications containing antihista-

Table 223-5.   Antidepressants

GENERIC NAME	TRADE NAME	RELATIVE ANTICHOLINERGIC EFFECT	SEDATIVE EFFECT	USUAL DOSE AND RANGE (MG/DAY)*	THERAPEUTIC SERUM LEVEL (NG/ML)
Tricyclic Tertiary Amines					
Amitriptyline	Elavil and others	8	High	150 (50–300)	—†
Imipramine	Tofranil and others	2	Moderate	150 (50–300)	>225‡
Doxepin	Sinequan, Adapin	2	High	150 (50–300)	—†
Tricyclic Secondary Amines					
Desipramine	Norpramin, Pertofrane	1	Low	150 (50–300)	>125
Protriptyline	Vivactil, Triptil	4	Low	30 (15–60)	—†
Nortriptyline	Aventyl, Pamelor	2	Low	75 (25–150)	50–150
Others					
Amoxapine	Ascendin	2	Low	150 (75–300)	—†
Maprotiline	Ludiomil	2	Moderate	150 (75–200)	—†
Trazodone	Desyrel	0	High	200 (150–600)	—†

* Dose is reduced by half for use in the elderly.

† Relation between serum level and therapeutic efficacy remains to be established.

‡ Sum of parent drug plus N-desmethyl metabolite.

mines. The number of anticholinergic compounds should be closely monitored, especially in the elderly.

In all patients over 40, it is good practice to obtain a baseline electrocardiogram prior to starting a tricyclic. At therapeutic levels, tricyclics have anticholinergic effects on the heart, which could cause a *rise in heart rate,* and effects similar to those of quinidine and may *delay conduction.* In patients without underlying conduction system disease, tricyclics rarely cause problems. In patients with bundle branch block, atrioventricular block, or sinus node disease, there is an increased risk of higher degrees of heart block. A rule of thumb is that if a patient has a conduction disorder that would contraindicate the use of quinidine for ventricular ectopy, it would also relatively contraindicate the use of tricyclics for depression. There appears to be no extra safety with newer tetracyclic drugs. If the depression is very severe, the best alternative to tricyclics might be electroconvulsive therapy. If the depression is mild, alprazolam might be effective since it is free of cardiac toxicity (see below).

Dosage. Tricyclics are started at a low dose with gradual increases until the therapeutic dose range is achieved. Finding the right tricyclic dose for a patient often involves a process of trial and error. The most common error leading to treatment failure is inadequate dosage. In healthy adults, a typical *starting dose* is the equivalent of 50 mg of desipramine. (Nortriptyline has twice the milligram potency of most tricyclics; thus its starting dose is 25 mg.) The daily dose is best prescribed to be taken at bedtime to facilitate compliance. Dosage can be increased by 50 mg every 3 to 4 days to a dose of 150 to 200 mg at bedtime. Elderly patients should receive one-third to one-half the usual adult dose (see below). The final dosage chosen is one that provides a therapeutic response without intolerable side-effects. The usual *maximum dosage* is 300 mg of desipramine or the equivalent (150 mg for nortriptyline).

If a patient has no response after 4 weeks on a full dosage with documented therapeutic blood levels, then the drug trial should be considered a failure. If the depression successfully remits, the tricyclic is maintained for at least 6 months. At that time the dosage can be slowly tapered over a period of 4 weeks while watching for the re-emergence of depressive symptoms. Should symptoms recur, the dosage is returned to its prior level and maintained for at least another 3 months. A small number of patients will require long-term maintenance treatment with a tricyclic.

Tricyclic *blood levels* are helpful to document a therapeutic dosage in patients who initially do not respond or who have severe side-effects on relatively low oral doses. Blood levels have been found to vary widely among patients for any given oral dose due to differences in drug absorption and metabolism. Those drugs whose blood levels are best studied and most likely to be clinically meaningful are imipramine, desipramine, amitriptyline, and nortriptyline. The only real usefulness of blood levels for other drugs is to monitor com-

pliance. Many clinical laboratories are unreliable in measuring these compounds. It is worth establishing which local laboratory is best at detecting tricyclics before levels are sent.

OTHER ANTIDEPRESSANTS. Depressed patients who fail to respond to therapeutic levels of a tricyclic or who are unable to tolerate a tricyclic because of a cardiac conduction disturbance or problems with side effects should be referred to a skilled psychopharmacologist. (It is important in establishing referral patterns to find out which psychiatrists specialize in this area.) The *monoamine oxidase inhibitors* (MAOI) and *lithium* have antidepressant efficacy. Lithium is best prescribed initially by physicians familiar with its use because of its potential toxicity. MAOIs are quite useful in treating the elderly (see below).

Trazodone represents one of the nontricyclic antidepressants now in common use. It offers some advantages over earlier drugs, such as a very low incidence of anticholinergic side-effects, although some patients complain of dry mouth. The lack of anticholinergic side-effects is probably responsible for the low incidence of therapy dropouts in comparative studies with tricyclics and other agents. The elderly seem to tolerate trazodone very well, although postural hypotension can be a problem (see below). Clinically, trazodone is very sedating and particularly helpful for depressed patients who cannot sleep. Other common side-effects include indigestion, nausea, and headaches. Priapism has been reported. Trazodone appears to have fewer cardiac side-effects than the tricyclics, but caution is still recommended in using trazodone in patients with pre-existing cardiac disease. The drug is less dangerous than tricyclics when taken in overdosage; there have been no reported life-threatening complications. Trazodone is about half as potent as imipramine, and has a wide dosage range of 150 to 600 mg/day. Since trazodone has a short half-life, it should be administered in divided doses; however, with the major portion can be given at night to minimize daytime drowsiness.

Other nontricyclics also have little anticholinergic activity or hypotensive effect; however, such adverse reactions as seizures (*maprotiline*) and tardive dyskinesias (*amoxapine*) limit their safety and usefulness, especially in the elderly. The benzodiazepine *alprazolam* (Xanax) has excellent antianxiety effects and mild antidepressant action. However, prolonged use is associated with significant risk of dependency.

Treatment of Depression in the Elderly

Loss, sadness, and grief are common experiences of old age. Depression may affect nearly a million older Americans and is by far the most common psychiatric disorder of the elderly. Primary treatment modalities include electroconvulsive therapy (reserved for very severe, refractory, or life-threatening cases) and drugs, such as tricyclic antidepressants, monoamine oxidase inhibitors, stimulants, and newer nontricyclic agents such as trazodone and maprotiline.

Although *tricyclics* are considered the drug of choice for depression, the elderly are particularly susceptible to some of their adverse effects, such as *orthostatic hypotension,* which can lead to falls and debilitating fractures. Amitriptyline and imipramine are among the agents most likely to cause such hypotension. In addition, these tertiary amines, doxepin, and trazodone tend to produce more *sedation,* presumably by preferentially blocking synaptic serotonin re-uptake and affecting histamine receptors.

The elderly are particularly vulnerable to *anticholinergic side-effects,* such as tachycardia, dry mouth, urinary retention, and confusion. If desipramine is designated an anticholinergic potency of 1, amitriptyline would be 8 times more anticholinergic. The other tricyclics lie somewhere in between, with a relative potency of about 2. The combination of pronounced anticholinergic activity and danger of orthostatic hypotension makes amitriptyline the least desirable of all the available tricyclics for use in the elderly.

Prior to starting tricyclic antidepressant medication in the elderly patient, postural signs and an electrocardiogram should be performed. One starts with a very low dose of medication—a maximum of 25 mg for most patients (except 5 mg for protriptyline and 50 mg for trazodone). The dosage can be raised slowly every few days, while monitoring subjective response and heart rate and watching for anticholinergic, cardiovascular, and CNS side-effects. One slows the increase in dose if tachycardia, excessive sedation, or orthostatic hypotension develops. Often the patient is the last to know that he is getting better and family members commonly report that the patient is sleeping and eating better before the dysphoria resolves. An adequate trial may take twice as long in the elderly as in younger patients.

If there is little improvement after a reasonable trial at presumably therapeutic doses, a blood level should be obtained to assess compliance and attainment of a therapeutic serum level. When the level is not in the appropriate range, dosage should be adjusted. If this does not produce clinical improvement, a trial of a monoamine oxidase inhibitor or electroconvulsive therapy should be considered.

Monoamine oxidase inhibitors (*MAOIs*) have been used sparingly in the treatment of elderly patients because of fears of adverse reactions. It is now known that these fears are largely unfounded, and that these agents can be used safely in the elderly. Many older patients who do not respond to tricyclics or some of the other antidepressants will improve with MAOIs. The enzyme, monoamine oxidase, increases in the brain with increasing age. Its primary function is to decrease brain catecholamines. Catechol reductions are believed to account for at least some depressions in elderly and demented patients.

MAOIs have essentially no anticholinergic effects and are useful in patients who are sensitive to such side-effects. The elderly patient who has urinary retention with as little as 10 mg of desipramine may do very well on an MAOI. The pri-

mary side-effects are *hypotension* and *insomnia.* Hypotension is not dose-dependent and may occur up to a month after starting the drug. Hypotension will rarely necessitate stopping the drug. Insomnia can be minimized by giving the last daily dose no later than 4 PM.

Dietary and drug precautions must be given to all patients taking MAOIs. Patients generally comply very well with these restrictions and rarely complain about them. A *low-tyramine diet* is required, necessitating avoidance of foods such as fermented cheese, large amounts of yogurt, excessive caffeine and chocolate, beer, and red wine. Patients can, however, drink white wine, vodka, gin, and whiskey, and a blanket instruction to avoid all alcohol is not only unwarranted but also may decrease compliance dramatically. Combination cold tablets, nasal decongestants, appetite suppressants, and amphetamines must be avoided; however, pure antihistamines and plain expectorants can be used.

Ingestion of a large amount of tyramine can produce a hypertensive crisis. Treatment involves immediately discontinuing the monoamine oxidase inhibitor and instituting antihypertensive therapy. Phentolamine, 5 mg given slowly intravenously, is recommended. Fever should be managed by means of external cooling.

Tranylcypromine is the preferred MAOI in the elderly because when discontinued, its effects usually reverse within 24 hours. In contradistinction, *phenelzine's* effects may persist for over a week after discontinuation. Tranylcypromine should be started at a dose of 10 mg twice daily and gradually increased as needed over a few weeks. Usually 20 to 30 mg daily will suffice, but occasional patients require as much as 60 mg per day.

Patients who are refractory to drug therapy and incapacitated by their depression should be referred for consideration of other therapeutic modalities, such as electroconvulsive treatment.

INDICATIONS FOR REFERRAL AND ADMISSION

The vast majority of depressed patients can be treated as outpatients by their primary care physician; however, some should be referred for psychiartric evaluation. These include bipolar patients, psychotic patients, patients at risk for suicide, those with very severe depression, and those with a history of treatment-resistant depression. In addition, those patients who appear to be treatment failures after 1 to 2 months of appropriate treatment should have a psychiatric consultation. Many of these patients can be referred back to their primary physician for follow-up after one or two psychiatric appointments. Under some circumstances, psychiatric hospitalization is indicated. These include a high risk of suicide, lack of reliable social supports (if the depression is very severe), history of previously poor response to treatment, and symptoms that are so severe that the patient requires constant observation and nursing care.

PATIENT EDUCATION

The patient should be told that depression is a real medical illness, the treatment of which includes medication. If the patient comes from a background that stigmatizes mental illness or opposes psychotropic medication, he should be counselled that there is no blame in having a depression and that compliance with the prescribed regimen is medically important. Compliance with prescribed tricyclics can be difficult for patients because of side-effects, but also because patients may attribute their own depressive symptomatology to the drugs. Some stop their medication after only a few days because they do not notice an immediate improvement. Prior to initiating therapy, one should note that tricyclic drugs often take weeks to work, that some mild physical symptoms may occur, and that the drugs do not work if taken only on a prn basis. The importance of prolonged, regular use must be emphasized. If the patient already has a tendency toward constipation, the prescription of a stool softener may make the tricyclic more acceptable. Patients should be instructed to report side-effects rather than stopping the medication on their own, and to call if suicidal thoughts develop or if the depression markedly worsens.

Both the patient and the family should be educated about the symptoms of depression and attempts should be made to decrease stresses at home. With elderly or severely depressed patients, the family should be taught about the proper use of tricyclics and asked to monitor compliance.

THERAPEUTIC RECOMMENDATIONS

- If a depressive syndrome is identified, try to make a specific diagnosis.
- With all depressed patients make an assessment of suicide risk.
- If the patient appears to be at risk for suicide, has psychotic symptoms, is severely depressed with no social supports, or is unable to care for himself, arrange prompt psychiatric consultation with a view to possible hospitalization.
- For other patients, begin supportive therapy and make any social and environmental interventions that may help. Especially with elderly or severely depressed patients, involve the family in the treatment.
- For patients who have major depression (or patients with other subtypes who have neurovegetative symptoms) begin a tricyclic. If insomnia is severe choose a more sedating drug (doxepin or imipramine). Otherwise choose a drug that minimizes anticholinergic effects (desipramine or nortriptyline). If postural hypotension is a problem, switch to nortriptyline. All patients over 40 should have a baseline electrocardiogram to rule out conduction system disease.
- Start tricyclics at a dose of 50 mg qhs and increase by 50 mg every 3 to 4 days until 150 to 200 mg/day is reached. If no benefit occurs after 2 weeks slowly increase (up to a

maximum of 300 mg). Nortriptyline is twice as potent as the others, so its doses should be halved. In the elderly use one half to one third the normal adult dose of the chosen tricyclic.

- If high doses produce no benefit or low doses seem to produce excessive side-effects, check a blood level and adjust accordingly. The goal is a dosage that yields a good response without intolerable side-effects.
- Psychiatric consultation should be obtained if there is no benefit after a 4-week trial at a therapeutic dosage or if the patient is bipolar and therefore requires lithium.
- If the patient responds to the tricyclic, it should be continued for at least 6 months and then slowly tapered.
- Never prescribe more than a week's supply or a total of 1 gm of a tricyclic if there is suicidal risk.
- Explain to patients that tricyclics must be taken regularly; that they may take weeks to work; and that there may be mild side effects which do not warrant discontinuation of the drug.

ANNOTATED BIBLIOGRAPHY

Akiskal HS: Dysthymic Disorder: Psychopathology of proposed chronic depressive subtypes. Am J Psychiatry 140:11, 1983 (*Although somewhat complex, this is an excellent review of chronically depressed patients, with an attempt to divide them into treatment groups.*)

American Psychiatric Association Task Force on Nomenclature and Statistics: Diagnostic and Statistical Manual of Mental Disorders, 3rd ed. Washington DC: American Psychiatric Association, 1980 (*The current standard diagnostic classification. The primary care physician should have at least some familiarity with it.*)

Barreira P: Depression. In Hyman SE (ed): Manual of Psychiatric Emergencies. Boston, Little, Brown, 1984 (*A practical review of emergency diagnosis and management.*)

Brown JT, Stoudemirer GA: Normal and pathological grief. JAMA 250:378, 1983 (*A succinct description of three faces of the normal grief process and guidelines for physician recognition and management of pathologic reactions.*)

Crowe RR: Electroconvulsive therapy. N Engl J Med 311:163, 1984 (*Reviews the indications and effectiveness as well as adverse effects of electroconvulsive therapy.*)

Glassman AH, Bigger JT: Cardiovascular effects of therapeutic doses of tricyclic antidepressants. Arch Gen Psychiatry 38:815, 1981 (*A good review pointing out the relative safety of tricyclics.*)

Glassman AH, Roose SP: Tricyclic drugs in the treatment of depression. Med Clin N Am 66:1037, 1982 (*A good review for the nonpsychiatrist which reviews side effects and use of blood levels.*)

Hirschfeld RMA, Koslow SH, Kupfer DJ: The clinical utility of the dexamethasone suppression test in psychiatry. JAMA 250:2172, 1983 (*The summary of the National Institute of Mental Health Workshop concluding that there is no indication for routine use of this test in diagnosis or clinical management of depression.*)

Hyman SE: Suicide. In Hyman SE (ed): Manual of Psychiatric Emergencies. Boston, Little, Brown, 1984 (*A guide to the estimation of suicide risk and subsequent management.*)

Jenike MA: Handbook of Geriatric Psychopharmacology, chapter 4, Affective Illness. Littleton, Mass., PSG Publishing, 1986 (*A good review on treatment of the elderly patient.*)

Keller MB, Klerman GL, Lavori PW et al: Long term outcome of episodes of major depression. JAMA 252:788, 1984 (*Long-term followup of 97 patients with major depressive disorder, indicating that recovery is more likely early and that more than 20% remained ill for more than 2 years.*)

Keller MB, Lavore PW, Lewis CE et al: Predictors of relapes in major depressive disorder. JAMA 250:3299, 1983 (*The probability of relapse into a major depressive disorder was highest in the months immediately after recovery; prior episodes of depression and older age made relapse more likely.*)

Klerman GL: Psychotherapies and somatic therapies in affective disorders. Psychiatr Clin N Am 6:85, 1983 (*Demonstrates the benefits of combining somatic and psychologic treatments.*)

Klerman GL: Affective disorders. In Nicholi AM (ed): The Harvard Guide to Modern Psychiatry. Cambridge, Harvard University Press, 1978 (*A clearly written comprehensive overview of the topic.*)

Veith RC, Raskind MA, Caldwell JH et al: Cardiovascular effects of tricyclic antidepressants in depressed patients with chronic heart disease. N Engl J Med 306:954, 1982 (*There was no effect noted on left ventricular function nor any significant adverse effect on ventricular irritability; suggests depressed patients with heart disease can be treated with tricyclic therapy.*)

224
Approach to the Patient with Excessive Alcohol Consumption
ELEANOR Z. HANNA, Ph.D.

Alcohol abuse is a complex problem, with elements of a medical illness, a dependency syndrome, and a learned behavioral disorder. Its societal and personal costs are staggering; the annual economic impact approaches 45 billion dollars, with 12.5 billion for medical care alone. It is estimated that 9 to 10 million adults and 3.3 million youths in the United States have drinking or alcohol-related problems. Nevertheless, most problem drinkers are employed, employable, or in families, indicating that the scope of the problem extends far beyond the skid row stereotype drinker, who accounts for only 5% of patients.

The medical consequences include a mortality rate 2.3 times that of aged-matched persons, with 56% of deaths directly related to alcohol. In terms of violence and traumatic death, alcohol is a factor in 30% of traffic injuries, 50% of automobile deaths, nearly 50% of industrial accidents and fatalities, 50% of homicides, 80% of fire burns, 70% of drownings, and 40% of child abuse cases.

The primary care physician is in the unique position to detect and treat an alcohol problem in its very early phases long before it becomes disabling and more difficult to manage. Given the extent to which alcohol abuse contributes to morbidity and mortality, assessment of alcohol use should be a routine part of every medical evaluation. One seeks to help the patient accept his problem, understand its consequences, and recognize the need for treatment. The objective then shifts to negotiating and carrying out an acceptable treatment plan, one that is personalized and multifaceted.

CAUSES OF ALCOHOL ABUSE

Our understanding of the causes of alcohol abuse remains incomplete. Biologic, sociocultural, psychologic, and psy-chologic–behavioral factors have been elucidated. Their precise contributions are often unclear, but models based on them are useful to researchers and may be utilized by clinicians to guide assessment and treatment. No single model is sufficient to account for all clinical presentations.

Biologic Model. The development of alcoholism is attributed to predisposing *biogenetic defects.* The view is based on studies demonstrating that genetic factors influence the metabolism of alcohol and the effects of alcohol on neurotransmitters, receptors, and the structure and composition of cell membranes. Such factors may account for the differences that alcohol has on behavior and on the development of medical sequelae among patients with and without a family history of alcohol abuse.

Sociocultural Model. In this model, external factors such as *poverty, socialization patterns,* and *cultural differences* in the rules governing alcohol use are emphasized. In addition, attention is directed toward *parental* and *peer values,* attitudes, and behaviors regarding alcohol. This model explains the increased use of alcohol among women and younger people.

Psychologic–Psychodynamic Model. Underlying *psychopathology* (*e.g.,* dependency conflict, depression, excessive need for power or sensation seeking, gender identification problems) is viewed as predisposing a person to drink in an abusive or alcoholic fashion to either mask or solve a psychologic problem; drinking is seen as merely a symptom. The emphasis in this model is not on the drinking but rather on intrapsychic restructuring, without which there can be no symptom removal.

Psychologic–Learning Theory/Behavioral Model. Alcoholism is seen as a *learned behavior* that is reversible, time-limited, on a continuum with normal drinking behavior, and established by a series of learning and *reinforcement experiences.* Certain precipitants and consequents (or maintainers) become associated with drinking and later with problem drinking. These precipitants can be:

1. Social (modeling the behavior of others, social interactions, and situations)
2. Emotional (anxiety, depression, or any unpleasant or unmanageable affect aroused in the setting of a particular event, situation, or person)
3. Cognitive (negative, retaliatory, and guilty thoughts)
4. Physiologic (reduction in pain, allowance of sleep, prevention of withdrawal)

Any of these precipitants coupled with learned expectations about the effects of alcohol and deficits in social skills will initiate and maintain drinking behavior leading to alcohol abuse.

Debate continues about which of these models best explains alcohol abuse. Alcoholism is a multivariate problem and the diagnoses and treatment of any given patient should reflect that complexity.

CLINICAL PRESENTATION AND COURSE

Alcohol abuse has a continuum of presentations ranging from the social drinker with a tendency to occasionally use alcohol in excess when under stress to the constantly intoxicated vagrant. The most commonly encountered presentations include:

- The *normal social drinker* is one who varies consumption and beverage according to internal cues and external circumstances. If he chooses to drink, he does so in drinking-appropriate circumstances and will rarely exceed the one-to two-drink limit that is seen as an accepted social lubricant. He is not likely to drive if under the influence (he might have his drink on arrival at a party and switch to something nonalcoholic later), nor is he likely to drink in order to deal with problems, escape, or get drunk. However, he may have a propensity to overindulge occasionally or to use alcohol in order to help cope with internal (*e.g.,* anxiety, depression) or external (*e.g.,* loss of a loved one, shift in employment status) stress. A serious problem with alcohol can develop from what appear to be relatively innocuous beginnings.
- The *heavy social drinker* is one who continues to drink in socially appropriate circumstances; however, he either seeks out or lives a life in which occasions for drinking are omnipresent. This patient will exist in a drinking context (*e.g.,* part of his job, social life, eating) and will have more than two drinks every day. He will eventually seek out more situations in which to drink and may often overconsume,

even though he matches the consumption of his peers. It is from this population that problem drinkers are drawn, for although he may never appear drunk or seem affected in his social and work routine, as his drinking continues and escalates it becomes increasingly related to both the physical and psychologic relief or escape. However, neither the person nor others in his life would suspect a potential problem with misuse of alcohol.

- The *problem drinker* is one who meets the criteria for heavy drinking, gets drunk on occasion, and who has also exhibited some medical, legal, social, or psychologic problem as a direct consequence of his alcohol consumption. In addition, he may have made or thought of making attempts at cutting down or refraining completely from alcohol consumption. Functioning may vary from seemingly intact behavior to an inability to cope. The patient may still try to deny he has a problem with drinking and attribute blame to external events or persons. Denial is common even among those with multiple arrests for drunk driving.
- The *alcohol-dependent patient* will consume the same amount of alcohol regardless of factors such as mood and situation. His pattern may change only if external circumstances constrain his drinking for a time. These people are not necessarily "skid row bums"; in fact, they are in the work force, often fairly high up. Alcohol is given top priority in all situations (the patient goes to a party to drink and not to socialize). Tolerance develops, and he notices that he consumes without effect more than the ordinary person. He will experience repeated withdrawal symptoms of mood disturbance, tremor, nausea, and sweats during the workday when his blood alcohol level drops and drink to relieve these symptoms at lunch and cocktail hour when his tasks are completed. He is aware of his compulsion to drink. Even this person will be difficult to reach unless his family or employer notes a problem or there are very serious medical complications involved.
- The *severely deteriorated patient* maintains a constant state of intoxication, having no care for his person or anything around him. He undergoes hospitalizations for detoxification and for medical care necessary after alcohol-related trauma or organ damage. These patients are most likely to present in the emergency room or inpatient setting with such medical complications as Wernicke's encephalopathy, Korsakoff's dementia, alcoholic dementia, cerebral atrophy, withdrawal phase disorder, tuberculosis, cirrhosis, alcoholic hepatitis, fatty liver, gastritis, oral cancers, esophagitis, pancreatitis, cardiac arrhythmias, or cardiac myopathy. While they do represent the worst possible case of what could happen to anyone who uses alcohol improperly and is allowed to do so without restraint, their state is not the necessary end point for all who drink.

Some medical sequelae of alcohol abuse, such as impotence and fetal alcohol syndrome, may appear in earlier phases of disease. *Impotence* and *loss of libido* may result from impaired testosterone synthesis, enhanced hepatic metabolism, and inhibition of gonadotropin release and often predate end stage disease. At times the cause is underlying depression, but a hypogonadal state is not uncommon. A *fetal alcohol syndrome* occurs in infants born to mothers who drink heavily during pregnancy. Features include permanently stunted growth, mental retardation (IQ in the 50 to 75 range), microcephaly, short palpebral fissures, musculoskeletal abnormalities, fine tremor, poor coordination, and cardiac malformations. The incidence and severity of the syndrome appear related, at least in crude fashion, to the degree and duration of alcohol intake during pregnancy. Incidence approaches 33% among pregnant women who drink more than 150 g of alcohol per day. Another third of children born to such women will have mental retardation, though they may be spared the full syndrome. There are no data available on when and how much alcohol can be taken safely during pregnancy.

Several groups of patients who used to be considered at low risk for development of alcoholism are demonstrating such increases in frequency of alcohol-related problems that they are now being labelled as *high risk.* These groups include professionals, executives, young people, women, and the elderly. *Executives* and *professionals* may be expected to drink and have the opportunity to do so during work functions. They may be able to hide the consequences of their drinking for extended periods before functioning becomes so disturbed as to emerge from efforts to conceal it. As many as 30% to 40% of *young people* (under age 25) report alcohol-related problems. Even as drug use declines, alcohol abuse continues to rise at alarming rates in this age group. *Women,* as a result of social change, are consulting alcohol clinics at double the former rates. *Elderly* patients may begin to use alcohol for stress, especially in reaction to loss of a loved one or because of difficulty with sleep. The older person who has always drunk may develop a problem from increasing his intake because the effects of alcohol are blunted with advancing age or because of tolerance. A peak period for onset of alcohol-related problems is 65 to 74 years of age.

Clinical Course

There is considerable variation in onset and progression. Onset ranges from an initial phase of social drinking to immediate heavy drinking starting as early as age 10 (as noted in some inner city neighborhoods). Most alcoholics report starting with heavy drinking in their late teens. The prognosis remains relatively favorable until dependence sets in. Once alcohol abuse is an ingrained habit and the addiction is psychologic or physiologic, it is difficult to break and the clinical course is often progressive. At the point of addiction, one can expect no more than long periods of abstinence or controlled drinking, punctuated by episodic drinking or pro-

longed relapses and further progression, especially if there is no expert intervention.

There is major controversy regarding whether or not total abstinence is required to halt progression. Once school of thought disputes the notion of inevitable progression and argues that some patients can learn to modify their drinking behavior and reduce their risk of progression without total abstinence. A contrary view states that alcoholics are addiction-prone patients who can never truly attain a controlled-drinking state. Prospective, controlled, randomized studies will be needed to resolve the issue.

As regards the medical sequelae, the risk of organ damage is related in part to the dose and duration of alcohol exposure, with some conditions (*e.g.,* alcoholic cardiomyopathy) manifesting reversibility with abstinence, while others (*e.g.,* cirrhosis) seeming to progress inexorably once severe hepatocellular damage is done. Risk appears to be a function of a genetic predisposition as well as alcohol dosage and chronicity of exposure.

DIAGNOSIS AND STAGING

The *differential diagnosis* of alcohol abuse includes abuse of other substances. The patient who is acutely intoxicated, in withdrawal, or comatose may be under the influence of any one of a host of CNS *depressants,* alone or very commonly in combination with alcohol. Clinical *withdrawal* from alcohol is similar to that from *sedatives, hypnotics,* and *tranquilizers;* in addition, cross-tolerance and cross-dependence exist between alcohol and other CNS depressants. Alcoholics can present with any *psychiatric disorder* as an antecedent or consequence of alcoholism. Depressed patients are particularly prone to heavy drinking, but there is no such entity as an "alcoholic personality."

There are several major *classification systems* for the diagnosis and staging of alcoholism (see Table 224-1). They differ in their views of etiology and natural history and thus in their diagnostic criteria.

The *Jellinek system* describes four stages: psychologic dependence without loss of control, physiologic complications, physiologic tolerance with psychologic dependence, and total inability to abstain. This is the oldest and most widely accepted system; it is based on observation and retrospective histories of alcoholics in treatment. It implies a relentless progression with continued drinking and suggests that total abstinence is necessary to halt the risk of progression.

The National Council on Alcoholism Criteria. This complex system lists 43 criteria detailing expected behaviors, attitudes, and clinical syndromes encompassing four stages of disease: pre-alcoholic, prodromal, crucial, and chronic. It too implies progression from pre-alcoholism to chronic disease with continued drinking. Diagnosis is achieved under this system by finding evidence of psychologic, physiologic, behavioral, and attitudinal manifestations. The system is useful

Table 224-1. Systems for Diagnosis and Staging

Jellinek System Criteria

STAGE	CHARACTERISTICS
α	Alcohol abuse without loss of control
β	Physiologic complications resulting from alcohol use/abuse without either psychologic or physiologic dependence on the substance
Γ	Physiologic tolerance together with psychologic dependence and loss of control once one begins to drink
Δ	Psychologic and physiologic dependence with an inability to abstain plus all factors that obtain for the Γ alcoholic

The National Council on Alcoholism Criteria

STAGE	CRITERIA (SAMPLE LIST)
Pre-alcoholic	Very heavy drinking for personal effects or relief of stress
Prodromal	Blackouts, surreptitious drinking, guilt
Crucial	Loss of control, remorse, morning drinking, medical problems
Chronic	"Benders," cognitive impairment, obsession with alcohol, downward social drift

DSM III Criteria

Alcohol abuse: Necessary daily use of alcohol to function; an inability to decrease or stop alcohol intake; repeated efforts to control alcohol use; blackouts; occasional consumption of a fifth or more of alcohol; and continued drinking, despite a health problem that is caused or exacerbated by alcohol use. Some impairment in social or occupational functioning as a consequence of alcohol use; disturbance must be of at least 1 month's duration. Pattern of abuse must be distinguished from nonpathological use of alcohol, which may include episodes of intoxification without pathological use.

Alcohol dependence: Pathological use of alcohol, with impairment of functioning in the social and economic spheres; plus, either tolerance or withdrawal. Tolerance is either a need for increased amounts of alcohol to achieve the desired effects or markedly diminished effect with regular use of the same amount. Withdrawal is development, within several hours of stopping or reducing drinking, of a coarse tremor of the hands, tongue, and eyelids and at least one of the following: Nausea and vomiting, malaise or weakness, autonomic hyperactivity, anxiety, depression or irritability, orthostatic hypotension. Must be certain withdrawal symptoms attributable to cessation of alcohol and not to any other physical or mental disorder.

Johns Hopkins Criteria

Consequences of abuse: "benders," blackouts, impotence, medical complications

Signs of addictive drinking: loss of control, attempts to limit time and places of drinking, drinks on awakening, drinks nonbeverage alcohol

Social problems: family members, friends, and acquaintances object to the patient's drinking; patient thinks he drinks too much and feels guilty about drinking; loses friends

---

as a reference to the many possible presentations of alcohol abuse, though there is somewhat excessive emphasis on late-stage manifestations.

DSM III, the diagnostic manual of the American Psychiatric Association, distinguishes between alcohol abuse and alcohol dependence. It differs from the other systems in that it requires application of a time limit and distinguishes between abuse and dependence. A problem need not be seen as either progressing to a disastrous end point or requiring a single solution at all stages.

The Johns Hopkins system is a useful tool for the measurement of problem drinking and alcoholism, especially in allowing for an earlier diagnosis of problem drinking. It focuses on the consequences of abuse, the signs of addictive drinking, and social problems.

One can use these diagnostic and staging systems as guides for the recognition of an alcohol problem, eclectically taking from each that which seems most useful. Early detection remains the major diagnostic challenge (*e.g.,* evaluating the

steady two to three drink per day individual who may exhibit seemingly innocuous early signs of an alcohol problem).

WORKUP

No patient, whether a colleague, a successful executive or professional, a seemingly intelligent, articulate, intact person whose drinking pattern seems acceptable, a bright college or high school athlete, or a sweet old lady, should be exempt from an alcohol-use history as a routine part of every medical checkup or evaluation. Primary physicians are often the first to see the patient with an alcohol problem who might complain of anxiety, sleep disorder, inability to fight infection, or present with an alcohol-related illness in its earliest stages. It is with these patients in particular that care must be taken in eliciting the alcohol history so that early or incipient alcohol problems can be dealt with before they become insoluble.

In addition to those who present with the predictable and obvious medical sequelae (see above) or telltale signs (see below), one should be alert to alcoholism when there is evidence of child abuse, in patients with multiple psychosomatic problems, in patients who make multiple requests and switch symptoms frequently, in those who are anxious, suicidal, or depressed and are unable to articulate their feelings, and in patients who have interpersonal, occupational, financial, or legal problems.

Taking an Alcohol History. For the patient in whom there is no clinical evidence or suspicion of alcohol abuse, a series of screening questions (the CAGE Questions; see Fig. 224-1) has proven useful. A self-administered questionnaire (the MAST test; see Fig. 224-2) is another convenient means of early detection.

For the patient with a drinking problem, usually the situation must be overwhelming before he will volunteer that he has a drinking problem and wants help. Consequently, the onus of early detection falls on the primary physician. In the patient with a suspected but unadmitted problem, one has to use an interview technique that is kind and supportive, yet firm and even confrontative when there are substantial clinical findings and concerns about ability to function. Involving family members, friends, and even the employer may facilitate both history-taking and therapy.

A detailed drinking history is in order for all patients suspected of having an alcohol problem on the basis of:
* Symptomatology; family complaint
* A daily drinking pattern of two to three drinks accompanied by seemingly innocuous complaints that might be related to drinking
* A life-style that will perpetuate increased, prolonged drinking
* The occurrence of intrapsychic or interpersonal problems, or actual changes in life events
* Suggestive manifestations on physical examination, such as alcohol on the breath, spider angiomata, plethoric facies, tremor, multiple bruises, other signs of hepatocellular failure (see Chapter 71)
* Abnormal liver function tests; macrocytic anemia

The Drinking Profile. In taking a drinking history, it is critical that one go beyond issues of quantity, frequency, and development of tolerance. One must determine the rate at which a patient drinks, exactly what meaning alcohol (drink-

ing) holds, and something about the nature of the patient's social life as it pertains to alcohol. It is also useful to determine whether other drugs are used. With women and the elderly, especially, this would include an emphasis on prescription drugs. A profile of the patient's drinking behavior over a given time period will prove most useful. The drinking profile should include attention to:
* Setting: time, place, and occasion for drinking
* Social network: the people involved with the drinking and their relationship to the patient
* Consumption: quantity, frequency, and rate of consumption as it relates to that of others in the drinking context and as it relates to the patient's expected consumption
* Pressures (internal or external) to drink
* Other activities related to drinking

In short, the physician should suspect *anyone who drinks* and is in a *drinking context on a regular basis*—that means most patients who present for treatment. Not only will a drinking profile help characterize an alcohol abuser or alcoholic, it will also identify those not suspected of having a problem. The profile is an effective tool for confronting the resistant patient, treating a willing patient, and educating a person with a potential problem. This technique fits the notion of drinking as a learned behavior which, because it is learned and reinforced, can be reshaped or extinguished if the relevant dimensions are known.

Causes for Missing the Diagnosis. The diagnosis of alcohol abuse may be overlooked for several reasons: subtlety of presentation; definitions of alcoholism that do not encompass its early manifestations (see above); the view that the patient is normal so long as he can perform his daily activities; societal acceptance of dangerous levels of alcohol intake; and general expectations of alcohol consumption at most social occasions. There may be unintentional collusion with the patient in denying the problem, especially if the patient is of similar or higher social status, has similar habits and lifestyle, or is attractive, verbal, and intelligent.

PRINCIPLES OF MANAGEMENT

Management is most successful when it is multifaceted, personalized, and long-term. For many alcoholics, the primary care physician remains the one constant medical figure

---

Have you ever felt the need to **C**ut down on drinking?
Have you ever felt **A**nnoyed by criticism of drinking?
Have you ever had **G**uilty feelings about drinking?
Have you ever taken a morning **E**ye opener?

Figure 224-1.   The CAGE test. (Mayfield D, McLead G, Hall P: The CAGE questionnaire. Am J Psychiatry 131:1121, 1974)

1. Do you feel you are a normal drinker?	(No 2)	Yes
2. Have you ever awakened in the morning after some drinking the night before and found that you could not remember part of the evening?	(Yes 2)	No
3. Does your wife (or husband or parents) ever worry or complain about your drinking?	(Yes 1)	No
4. Can you stop drinking without a struggle after one or two drinks?	(No 2)	Yes
5. Do you ever feel badly about your drinking?	(Yes 2)	No
6. Do you ever try to limit your drinking to certain times of day or to certain places?	(Yes 0)	No
7. Do your friends or relatives think that you are a normal drinker?	(No 2)	Yes
8. Are you always able to stop when you want to?	(No 2)	Yes
9. Have you ever attended a meeting of Alcoholics Anonymous?	(Yes 5)	No
10. Have you gotten into fights when drinking?	(Yes 1)	No
11. Has drinking ever created problems with you and your wife (husband)?	(Yes 2)	No
12. Has your wife (husband or other family member) ever gone to anyone for help about your drinking?	(Yes 2)	No
13. Have you ever lost friends or girlfriends/boyfriends because of drinking?	(Yes 2)	No
14. Have you ever gotten into trouble at work because of drinking?	(Yes 2)	No
15. Have you ever lost a job because of drinking?	(Yes 2)	No
16. Have you ever neglected your obligations, your family or your work for two days or more in a row because of drinking?	(Yes 2)	No
17. Do you ever drink before noon?	(Yes 1)	No
18. Have you ever been told you have liver trouble?	(Yes 2)	No
19. Have you ever had DTs (delerium tremens), severe shaking, heard voices or seen things that weren't there after heavy drinking?	(Yes 2)	No
20. Have you ever gone to anyone for help about your drinking?	(Yes 5)	No
21. Have you ever been in a hospital because of drinking?	(Yes 5)	No
22. Have you ever been a patient in a psychiatric hospital or on a psychiatric ward of a general hospital where drinking was part of the problem?	(Yes 2)	No
23. Have you ever been seen at a psychiatric or mental health clinic, or gone to a doctor or clergyman for help with an emotional problem in which drinking has played a part?	(Yes 2)	No
24. Have you ever been arrested, even for a few hours, because of drunken behavior?	(Yes 2)	No
25. Have you ever been arrested for drunk driving or driving after drinking?	(Yes 2)	No

A score of three points or less is considered nonalcoholic; a score of four points is suggestive, and a score of five points or more indicates alcoholism.

Figure 224-2.   The Michigan Alcoholism Screening Test (MAST). (Selzer ML: The Michigan Alcoholism Screening Test. Am J Psychiatry 127:1653, 1971)

in the patient's life and the person he probably trusts most. Whether one intends to personally care for the alcoholic patient or refer him to a specialist in alcohol problems, the primary physician has the important initial task of assisting the patient in acknowledging his drinking problem and accepting a treatment program.

Dealing with Denial. When the patient denies that there is a problem, one should first listen carefully to how he explains the findings. If it seems that he accepts the situation

internally but feels the need to protect himself publicly, it is worth trying to present the case over time in a manner that shows interest in helping him discover the problem for himself. One might ask the patient to keep a journal or weekly log of drinking events and then review it, taking care to note and explore links between drinking and particular environmental, interpersonal, and psychologic factors. This will provide an opportunity to determine exactly how much the patient drinks without confronting him directly in the absence of actual evidence.

This same technique, with some additions, can be used for the patient who is hiding the problem from himself. In such a case, one would do best to detail all the positive findings and present evidence on how alcohol is directly involved in the patient's health problem. Alcoholism screening tests, such as the Michigan Alcohol Screening Test (MAST) or CAGE (see Fig. 224-1) might be used, or the clinical impression presented in terms of a specific diagnostic classification system. If the patient continues to resist, then one can bring in family, friends, or employer to present the patient with their evidence of how destructive his drinking is to himself and them. Again, these sessions should be factual, nonjudgmental discussions of the relationship of alcohol to the patient's health and behavior, and its impact on those important to him.

Dealing with Resistence to Treatment. The patient who agrees he has a problem yet continues to refuse help or to relinquish alcohol should be handled similarly, but with more focus on his fears and his resistance. The hostile or belligerent patient should be dealt with firmly, but in a manner which enhances his ability to objectify and control his anger; the physician helps him to identify the sources of anger and lets him know he will not give up on him because of his behavior.

It is pointless to force the patient into treatment when no medical emergency exists. It is better to present the options available, continue exploring the issue, and provide health education while treating the patient's medical problems, until he is willing to acknowledge the alcohol problem and seek help on the basis of the physician's recommendations.

Often those who resist treatment must first fear the loss of something very important (*e.g.,* spouse, job) before seeking help. Unfortunately, once out of imminent danger, such patients often return to old habits, unless they are worked with over a lifetime. The doctor–patient relationship can be used to change life-style, identify and restructure destructive patterns, and learn new coping skills. It is simply not enough to medically detoxify a patient, prescribe Antabuse, and send him to AA. Effective care requires being available on a regular basis to provide the monitoring, instruction, and support needed by any patient with a chronic disease. If such support is beyond the scope of the individual primary physician, he should at least ensure a proper and smooth referral for specialized care.

Patient Selection for Management by the Primary Physician. Long-term management by the primary care physician is best indicated for those patients:

• whose medical complications are the foremost concern
• who have a strong personal tie to the primary physician
• who are socially stable
• who demonstrate only minor psychopathology
• who are intelligent and pragmatic
• who put great faith in physicians
• who have an intact and supportive social network

It is important to remember that the treatment will be long and arduous. If and when the physician should find himself unable to cope, the patient should be referred to a specialist with the primary physician remaining as the coordinator of care.

Determinants of Successful Treatment. *Early detection* and *treatment* are essential to success. Major studies cite success rates of 50% to 90% in patients who were drinking without impairment, who are of a higher socioeconomic status, and who were not yet diagnosable as alcoholics per se. Success rates also depend on the length of time a person stays in treatment, his involvement in goal setting and treatment planning, and his continued attachment to family or an integrated social network.

It is best to involve *family members* or significant others in the confrontation and treatment, as they are crucial in assisting and supporting the life-style changes which must be made if the destructive drinking pattern is to be arrested. This is especially true for women and younger problem drinkers. Their families often have a hard time providing support and structure because of their shock in discovering that a problem exists.

However, despite the importance of patient factors in eventual treatment success, the major problem remains getting the patient to accept and then stay in treatment. The onus here falls on the primary physician, who must recognize that the majority of patients go untreated because their problem is undetected and undiagnosed until it is very advanced. The patient may be lost between the referral source and the treatment person if active coordination does not take place, especially if the referring physician has not worked with the patient long enough to determine what the best treatment would be and to enlist the patient's own cooperation in decision making. The best way to ensure that the patient keeps an appointment is to engage the family, make both the family and patient full participants, keep the waiting period brief, and remind him a day or two ahead.

Once in treatment, a variety of methods appropriate to the multifaceted nature of the disorder/illness must be used (see below). The treatment plan should be gone over in depth and continually re-evaluated, with the patient taking an active part lest there be a wide discrepancy between doctor and patient expectations. Past treatment failures and/or early dropout should be explored. Efforts to give immediate relief when satisfying dependency needs, providing medications when necessary, and increasing social stability by coordinating arrangements for housing or employment are also helpful.

As noted earlier, the therapist must recognize that the patient's behavior is sick and often will be directed at him in either a covert or overtly hostile manner. One must keep in mind that the ultimate goal is to help the patient gain self-control, regulation, and a sense of responsibility. One must not counterattack.

Treatment Modalities

Therapies can be classified as biological, psychological, behavioral, or sociocultural. Selection is best done on an individualized basis to meet the patient's specific needs. The biologic approaches include use of drugs to decrease alcohol consumption and inpatient programs to achieve detoxification and freedom from physiologic dependence.

Drugs to Decrease Alcohol Consumption. Despite little evidence supporting their efficacy, drugs are reported to be used by over 90% of physicians in private practice for the treatment of alcoholism. Pharmacologic agents are prescribed to reduce the urge to drink, to blunt withdrawal symptoms, and to treat underlying psychiatric problems that may be contributing to alcohol abuse.

DISULFIRAM (Antabuse) is an aversive therapy that sensitizes the patient to the effects of alcohol by inhibiting hepatic aldehyde-NAD oxidoreductase. Within minutes of taking of as little as 1 ounce of alcohol, the patient experiences an increase in serum acetaldehyde concentration that leads to palpitations, flushing, tachypnea, tachycardia, and shortness of breath. Nausea, vomiting, and headache develop if a greater amount of alcohol is taken. Symptoms last about 90 minutes and usually are self-limited; occasionally marked hypotension or a cardiac arrhythmia may occur. Fatalities from myocardial infarction and stroke have been reported. Controlled studies demonstrate no more than short-term improvement in alcohol consumption and underscore the greater importance of nonpharmacologic factors in determining outcome. Side-effects include drowsiness and lethargy, which are countered by administering the drug before bed. The standard dose is 250 mg at bedtime. The agent can worsen depression and schizophrenia.

Important drug–drug interactions occur with antihypertensive agents (potentiation of hypotensive effect with intake of alcohol), benzodiazepines (reduced intensity of the disulfiram reaction), tricyclic antidepressants and phenothiazines (potentiation of CNS effects), and drugs metabolized by hepatic microsomes (prolongation of their half-lives).

Candidates for disulfiram therapy require careful medical and psychiatric evaluation prior to initiating therapy. Patients best suited for this therapy are those who seek total abstinence, request the drug, have no underlying cardiovascular, depressive, or schizophrenic disease, and are willing to return monthly for evaluation of therapy. The goal is to provide the patient time to organize the supports necessary for achievement of long-term abstinence. Disulfiram should not be considered an option for chronic use. Duration of therapy is individualized. Treatment ought to be terminated if the patient fails to keep appointments, resumes drinking, becomes pregnant or depressed, or develops abnormalities in liver function tests or cardiovascular status.

PSYCHOACTIVE DRUGS. Pharmacologic treatment of underlying psychopathology has been proposed as a means of cutting down on drinking. Anxiolytic agents such as the *benzodiazepines* (BZDs) have been used with a modicum of success in patients who drink because of an *anxiety disorder.* There is no evidence for long-term efficacy in reduction of alcohol use, but some data suggest a short-term reduction in anxiety that could enable a patient to engage in more comprehensive forms of therapy. BZDs have also been proposed as a means of reducing the desire to drink that might emanate from a postulated chronic withdrawal syndrome. Supporting data for both the syndrome and the efficacy of long-term drug treatment are minimal. *Tricyclic antidepressants* may be effective when there is an underlying *depression,* especially when it is accompanied by neurovegetative symptoms (see Chapter 223). There is preliminary evidence for reduced alcohol consumption with use of *lithium* in patients with *bipolar disease.*

In sum, drug therapy plays only a supportive role in the outpatient care of the alcoholic patient, mainly providing a brief respite from alcohol consumption to enable the patient to engage in a more comprehensive and durable treatment program.

Drugs for Withdrawal. Manifestations of the *acute withdrawal* syndrome (tachycardia, elevation in blood pressure, tremor, hyperreflexia, increased irritability) can be blunted by the use of *beta-blockers* or *benzodiazepines,* and progression of seizures, hallucinations, and delirium tremens usually prevented. In a randomized, double-blind study in a community hospital setting, atenolol (50 to 100 mg per day) proved effective in treating the acute withdrawal syndrome, reduced the requirement for benzodiazepine therapy, and shortened the length of hospital stay. The efficacy of drug therapy for treatment of the postulated *chronic withdrawal* syndrome awaits clarification of the syndrome and its symptoms.

Alcohol Inpatient Programs. These treatment programs attempt to achieve detoxification and total abstinence using drug therapy and a variety of psychological and social manipulations. They typically involve a minimum stay of 28 days. The programs use educational and confrontative techniques, and attempt to teach social skills. There is little free time or individualized care. Alcoholics Anonymous (AA) meetings are an integral part of most programs and patients are often expected to follow a life-regimen planned and monitored at the conclusion of the hospitalization. This program is suited to people who can afford to be taken out of their social and work environments for prolonged periods, with whom all other forms of treatment have failed, and who will not deal with the problems so long as they are in environments that maintain destructive drinking. It is a costly approach and should be used as a last recourse.

Outpatient Psychotherapy places emphasis on psychic restructuring and removal of the presumed underlying psychopathology. The modalities used include the various individual and group psychotherapies such as transactional analysis, Gestalt, and Reality as well as psychoanalysis. This treatment may be suitable for a person whose interpersonal or psychologic problems outweigh his alcohol abuse, which takes the form of spree, binge, or controlled drinking. In addition, the patient should be socially intact, sophisticated, intellectually curious, and eager to be involved in the process. However, people with alcohol problems have special needs that are not always met in traditional psychotherapy settings. The therapist should not leave the alcohol problem undiscussed but must be active, provide structure, guidance, support, nurturance, and instruction in helping the patient control drinking while working on other issues. Because of this, the therapist to whom the patient is referred should either be a staff member of a specialized alcohol treatment program or have demonstrated interest and experience with this problem.

Behavioral–Cognitive Therapies are based on the notion of alcoholism as a learned behavior that can be extinguished and reshaped, with controlled drinking a possible outcome. Behavioral modalities include *aversive* conditioning to either eliminate alcohol use or train patients to drink no more than what would bring them to a safe blood alcohol level (usually 0.05%). Alternative behaviors are taught via operant conditioning. These are suitable for patients who are rigid, repressed, and resistant to anything that does not have a defined, tangible end point. In addition, they are helpful in dealing with problems involving role changes and behaviors in specific situations.

Cognitive therapy takes this one step further and is often a useful adjunct to any treatment. Its focus is on pathologic drinking being on a continuum with normal drinking, and it forces the patient and therapist to deal with the observables of the drinking behavior:

1. Frequency, duration, derivation, and quantity
2. Time, place, activity
3. Age-, sex-, role-appropriate drinking behavior
4. Problems associated with excessive use, identifying the precipitants to abuse and the factors that maintain and perpetuate it

Sociocultural treatment emphasizes altering external factors; it includes *residential care, halfway houses,* and direct social manipulation, such as *finding jobs,* helping with *shelter* and *money,* and removing a person from his family. This is a treatment appropriate for homeless, jobless, unstable persons whose social functioning is impaired, for repeated treatment failures, for young people, and for others with severe family problems.

Community Services

Alcoholics Anonymous combines most other forms of treatment, but usually in only a very superficial way, except in the cases of those who commit themselves to the total program as a way of life. It does provide social support, caring, and structure, but is usually not effective except as an adjunct to other treatment. However, the person willing to dedicate himself to a lifetime of sobriety can achieve the goal in this carefully delineated manner.

Alanon and *Alateen* assist family members of the alcoholic. Various social service and guidance centers can deal with marital and family problems. *Employee assistance programs* are usually available in most large companies and their counselors can work in tandem with physicians. Specific legal, occupational, social, and financial programs are usually available through state or federal agencies or organizations such as the YMCA. Coordination with clergy is important with a religious patient.

PATIENT EDUCATION AND ALCOHOLISM PREVENTION

It is insufficient to simply prohibit the use of alcohol, nor is it enough to warn people of the chronic and acute hazard to their physical and mental health which results from alcohol use. As noted earlier, primary care physicians are the ideal persons to begin the preventive and educational process. They can provide important information on alcohol and its effects on health in the context of a general medical evaluation. By taking a drinking history, one can educate the patient and provide suitable guidelines for drinking behavior as one would regarding smoking, exercise, stress, or wearing seat belts; it is an important part of the patient's yearly checkup.

People who choose not to drink need support to know their decision is right for them; they need not feel odd and succumb to social pressure. People who do drink need to know how alcohol can affect them, how to behave responsibly when drinking, and how to drink to prevent drunkenness (see Tables 224-2 and 224-3). Individuals should know that their attitudes and behaviors will affect how their children/ spouses drink. All should be cautioned that drinking is a dangerous solution for insomnia and emotional problems.

This instruction can be complemented by waiting room literature, a direct talk with the patient after the examination, and hospital or community health education programs. National campaigns are focusing on alcohol-related accidents and crimes with their resultant loss of life or permanent disability. Advertisements which point to the family and work problems of the alcoholic are now frequently shown on television. In addition, there is a much more positive approach to dealing with the subject in all the media.

These are all attempts to help the individual modify his life-style. The goal is to eventually change the cultural significance of drinking, much in the same way that has been the case with regard to smoking, exercise, and diet.

Table 224-2. Blood Alcohol Level* and Behavior

TIME ELAPSED SINCE FIRST DRINK (IN HOURS)	NUMBER OF DRINKS†									
	1	**2**	**3**	**4**	**5**	**6**	**7**	**8**	**9**	**10**
1	0.01	0.03	0.05	0.08	0.10	0.13	0.15	0.17	0.20	0.22
2	0.00	0.02	0.04	0.06	0.09	0.11	0.14	0.16	0.19	0.21
3	0.00	0.005	0.02	0.05	0.07	0.10	0.12	0.14	0.17	0.19
4	0.00	0.00	0.01	0.03	0.06	0.08	0.11	0.13	0.15	0.18
5	0.00	0.00	0.00	0.02	0.04	0.07	0.09	0.11	0.14	0.16

* Determined by the number of drinks consumed in a circumscribed time period by a presumably normal 150-pound male. Females, because they are affected more quickly, require less alcohol to achieve these levels.

† Blood alcohol levels as a function of weight, time, and number of drinks consumed:
One drink = 1.5 oz 80-proof spirits (40% alcohol)
          3.0 oz fortified wine (20% alcohol)
          5.0 oz table wine (12% alcohol)
          12.0 oz beer (4.5% alcohol)

INDICATIONS FOR ADMISSION AND REFERRAL

Acute hospitalization is indicated for the following complications of alcohol abuse:

1. Respiratory depression
2. Ventricular irritability and other major dysrhythmias
3. Gastrointestinal bleeding
4. Lactic acidosis
5. Marked hypoglycemia
6. Severe hypokalemia
7. Severe hepatocellular failure

Hospital admission also is indicated for withdrawal from alcohol in the high-risk patient (prior history of severe withdrawal, concurrent medical or psychiatric illness, chronic and severe alcohol-related illness) and in the patient complaining of tremor, agitation, hallucinations, or seizures. A free-standing detoxification center may suffice for the otherwise uncomplicated patient, who because he is alone or unreliable, could benefit from the nursing care and supervision.

Patients with major psychopathology, poor ties to the physician, or a disintegrated social network have serious drawbacks to successful treatment by even the most willing primary care physician. Such patients should be referred in a coordinated way for specialized care, ensuring continuity

as well as a personalized treatment program. The primary physician can perform a major service for these patients by understanding available specialized referral resources in one's community and matching them to the patient's needs.

MANAGEMENT RECOMMENDATIONS

Some basic guides to follow regardless of which treatment is offered:
- First establish rapport. Let the patient know you accept and understand him by approaching the problem in a way that is comfortable for him.
- Offer appropriate and sufficient instruction and explanation as you go along, always engaging the patient in establishing realistic goals and not pushing him beyond his limits.
- Maintain a proper balance of support, caring, and limit-setting; remain flexible and adaptable to the patient's needs.
- Think of treatment as a series of short-term programs in order to develop and increase the patient's sense of mastery.
- Never insist on immediate abstinence. This is a goal to be negotiated. Only if all else fails should there be confrontation and control in this area, unless, of course, serious health problems will result from any alcohol intake.

Table 224-3. Behavior Expected at Various Blood Alcohol Levels (BAL)

BAL	BEHAVIORAL EFFECTS
0.05	Relaxation; possibility of thought, judgment, and self-control being affected
0.10	Obvious impairment of voluntary motor action; legally drunk in most states
0.20	Considerable motor impairment and loss of emotional control; definite intoxication
0.40–0.50	Unconsciousness and probable death resulting from respiratory failure

- If a patient comes to a session drunk, kindly and calmly explain why it would be pointless to have a session and reschedule the appointment. If this behavior continues, the treatment agreement should be renegotiated to include rules about it.
- Keep motivation high, not only by utilizing the patient's fear of losing something or someone very important, but by getting him to seek and define his own reinforcers.
- Teach the patient to identify, objectify and deal with anger, depression, anxiety, guilt, mistrust, etc., so that self-control in the emotional area is also enhanced.
- When the patient is ready, help him pinpoint the actual behaviors to be changed and work on them progressively. One may need to provide information, modeling, practice, feedback, and homework as the patient learns to handle feelings and to develop new social skills, the tools necessary to assess and modify his behavior.
- Encourage self-monitoring of drinking behavior via logs, teaching the patient to detect causes, consequences, and maintaining factors, and thus helping him learn alternate ways of coping with the people, places, situations, and feelings associated with heavy drinking.
- Select those components of available specialized treatment programs (see below) that are most appropriate for the individual patient; that is, personalize the treatment program to match to the patient's needs, wants, and ability to cope. The standard formula of detoxification—disulfiram and AA—is no longer either the recommended or the most acceptable treatment for alcoholism.
- For patients whose interpersonal or psychologic problems are predominant, who exhibit binges, sprees, or controlled drinking, and who are socially intact, intellectually curious, and psychologically minded, consider outpatient psychotherapy. There should be a willingness to engage in a therapeutic program that may take as long as 2 years.
- For patients strongly motivated to attain total abstinence and specifically requesting disulfiram therapy, begin 250 mg qhs and renew on a monthly basis, re-evaluating the need for continued drug therapy while working on psychosocial interventions that will sustain long-term abstinence. Treatment is contraindicated in those with underlying psychiatric illness or cardiovascular disease.
- For patients who are rigid, repressed, and resistant to open-ended therapies, consider behavioral–cognitive methods.
- For patients willing to dedicate themselves to a lifetime of sobriety or who will benefit from peer counselling, consider AA, especially if there is a religious interest.
- For patients who are homeless, jobless, or have other serious social problems, refer to a community social service agency for direct aid.
- For patients who have failed outpatient treatments, can afford the time, and need to be taken out of their environment to cease drinking, consider an inpatient alcohol program.

- Patients who are reliable, have a supportive family who can provide supervision, and have no underlying medical illnesses or a prior history of severe withdrawal symptoms can be withdrawn from alcohol on an outpatient basis. Prescribe 50 mg of atenolol per day if the resting heart rate is less than 80 beats per minute and 100 mg per day if greater than 80. Treat for 1 week and hospitalize promptly should any significant withdrawal symptoms develop (*e.g.*, tachycardia, tremor, hallucinations, increased irritability).

ANNOTATED BIBLIOGRAPHY

Criteria Committee: National Council on Alcoholism Criteria for the Diagnosis of Alcoholism. Am J Psychiatry 129:127, 1972 (*Clinical criteria necessary to definition and diagnosis of problem in various phases.*)

Donovan J, Jessor R, Jessor L: Problem drinking in adolescence and young adulthood: A follow-up study. J Stud Alcohol 44:109, 1983 (*Updates a survey of drinking patterns and correlates to problem drinking in high school students.*)

DSM III Diagnostic and Statistical Manual of Mental Disorders (3rd ed) Washington, DC: American Psychiatric Association, 1980 (*Latest diagnostic system of the American Psychiatric Association.*)

Edwards G: Alcohol dependence: Provisional description of a clinical syndrome. Br Med J 1:1058, 1976 (*An attempt to move from the disease theory to alcohol dependence as a result of normal drinking behavior.*)

Gerstel EK, Harford TC: Age-related patterns of daily alcohol consumption in metropolitan Boston. J Stud Alcohol 42:1062, 1981 (*A breakdown of how, when, and where people drink, and of changes with age.*)

Geuien J, Rosenberg C, Manohar V: Disulfiram maintenance in outpatient treatment of alcoholism. Arch Gen Psychiatry 28:798, 1973 (*Details of disulfiram treatment and its utility in alcoholism treatment.*)

Hanna E: Attitudes toward problem drinkers: A critical factor in treatment recommendations. J Stud Alcohol 39:98, 1978 (*A review of relevant literature and study of disposition of patients presenting to a walk-in psychiatric clinic who self-label as alcoholics.*)

Institute of Medicine: Alcoholism, Alcohol Abuse, and Related Problems: Opportunities for Research. Washington, DC: National Academy Press, 1981 (*Summary of the state of the art in alcoholism and recommendations for the future by a panel of experts.*)

Jellinek E: The Disease Concept of Alcoholism. New Jersey, Hillhouse Press, 1960 (*The classic attempt at understanding alcoholism which remains as the basis for much current thought.*)

Knight R: The dynamics and treatment of chronic alcohol addiction. Bull Menninger Clin 1:233, 1937 (*Classic psychoanalytic approach to alcoholism and the "alcoholic personality."*)

Kraus ML, Gottlieb LD, Horwitz RI et al: Randomized clinical trial of atenolol in patients with alcohol withdrawal. N Engl J Med 313:905, 1985 (*Atenolol proved effective in this double-blind study of treatment for acute withdrawal in the community hospital setting.*)

Lerner WD, Fallon HJ: The alcohol withdrawal syndrome. N Engl J Med 313:951, 1985 (*Summarizes developments in pathogenesis and treatment.*)

Lundberg GD: Ethyl alcohol—ancient plague and modern poison. JAMA 252:1911, 1984 (*An editorial introducing and discussing eight articles about alcohol abuse and its effects appearing in this theme issue of HAMA. It includes ten provocative proposals for changes in society's approach to alcohol and its use.*)

Mendelson J, Mello N: Biological concomitants of alcoholism. N Engl J Med 303: 1979 (*An excellent and comprehensive review with extensive bibliography of the most recent advances in behavioral and biological studies of alcoholism. If you were to read only one paper, this should be it!*)

Mendelson J, Babor T, Mello N et al: Alcoholism and prevalence of medical and psychiatric disorders. J Stud Alcohol 47:361, 1986 (*A study of admissions for alcoholism treatment indicates a high prevalence of significant medical problems; treatment in hospitals with medical expertise, and resources for early detection would lead to reduced mortality and morbidity from alcoholism and its concomitant medical disorders.*)

Miller W, Munoz R: How to Control Your Drinking. New Jersey, Englewood Cliffs, Prentice Hall, 1976 (*A practical approach to behavioral modification of drinking; could be used as a self-help manual or in instructing patients to understand and control their drinking.*)

Nace EP: The role of craving in the treatment of alcoholism. National Assoc Prev Pub Health J 13:27, 1982 (*A guide to mastery over and understanding of wish/need to drink, leading to greater self control.*)

Parker E, Noble E: Alcohol consumption and cognitive functioning in social drinkers. J Stud Alcohol 38:1224, 1977 (*Details the effects of light, moderate, and heavy drinking on abstracting and adaptive abilities of social drinkers.*)

Patterson E, Kaufman E: Encyclopedic Handbook of Alcoholism. New York, Gardner Press, 1982 (*Covers the entire field. A good handbook for reference.*)

Pollick J, Armor D, Braiker H: The Course of Alcoholism: Four Years After Treatment. Santa Monica, Rand Corporation, 1980 (*Evaluation of treatment effectiveness based on a national survey. Compares patient and treatment types and contains much practical information necessary to understanding alcoholism and its treatment.*)

Rosett H: A clinical perspective of the fetal alcoholism syndrome. Alcoholism: Clinical and Experimental Research 4:119, 1980 (*Effects of drinking during pregnancy on mental and motor development of the child.*)

Sellars EM, Maranjo CA, Peachey JE: Drugs to decrease alcohol consumption. N Engl J Med 305:1255, 1981 (*Reviews various pharmacotherapies for alcoholism and concludes that they can only serve as adjuncts to other therapies.*)

Shuckit MA: Genetics and the risk for alcoholism. JAMA 254:2614, 1985 (*This article reflects the current state of biogenetic research in alcohol, an area that should be followed as it is most relevant to prevention and treatment of people with family histories positive for alcoholism.*)

Skinner HA, Holt S et al: Identification of alcohol abuse using laboratory tests and a history of trauma. Ann Intern Med 101:847, 1984 (*A brief trauma history was more sensitive than laboratory tests in detecting problem drinking.*)

Streissguth A, Barr H, Martin D et al: Effects of alcohol, nicotine, and caffeine use during pregnancy on infants' mental and motor development at eight months. Alcoholism: Clinical and Experimental Research 4:152, 1980 (*Points to risk of drinking 4 oz or more of alcohol daily during pregnancy even in a low-risk sample.*)

Tournier R: Alcoholics Anonymous as treatment and ideology. J Stud Alcohol 40:230, 1979 (*Author proposes argument that Alcoholics Anonymous has fettered innovation, precluded early intervention, and limited treatment in the alcoholism field. Comments on above, Ibid 318–338, by various authorities in agreement and opposed to position taken.*)

Wechsler H, Levine S, Idelson R et al: The physician's role in health promotion—A survey of primary care practicioners. N Engl J Med 308:97, 1983 (*Importance of physicians in promoting healthy behavior is supported by practicioners who engage in and are interested in expanding their skills in this area.*)

Weissman M, Myers J: Clinical depression in alcoholism. Am J Psychiatry 137:372, 1980 (*Epidemiologic survey using research diagnostic criteria reports the incidence of coexisting depression and alcoholism and the rates of secondary and primary depression when the disorders coexist.*)

Resource Materials

National Clearinghouse for Alcohol Information
P.O. Box 2345
Rockville, MD 20852

Addiction Research Foundation
33 Russell Street
Toronto, Ontario, Canada
M5S 2SI

National Council on Alcoholism, Inc.
733 Third Avenue
New York, NY 10017

Local state alcoholism agency

Local Alcoholics Anonymous chapter

225
Approach to the Patient with Sexual Dysfunction

LINDA C. SHAFER, M.D.

There is an important relationship between one's sexual life and emotional and physical well-being. It has been estimated that approximately 15% of medical outpatients come to primary care physicians with complaints that are primarily or secondarily sexual in nature. The incidence of sexual problems in any medical practice is a function of the frequency with which physicians take a sexual history. The primary care physician needs to know how to take a sexual history and carry out basic types of sexual counselling and supportive therapy.

DEFINITIONS

Disorders are classified as "*primary*" when there has never been a period of satisfactory functioning, and "*secondary*" when the difficulty occurs after adequate functioning had been obtained.

Male Disorders

Impotence (erectile dysfunction) is defined as the inability of a male to maintain an erection sufficient to engage in intercourse and is considered a problem if it occurs in over 25% of attempts. *Premature ejaculation* is the loss of voluntary control of the ejaculatory reflex. Masters and Johnson have defined the condition in terms of the inability to satisfy the female partner at least 50% of the time. However, this presupposes that the female has no problem with orgasm. Premature ejaculation is most often defined as ejaculation that occurs in less than 2 minutes after penetration or upon fewer than 10 thrusts. *Retarded ejaculation* is the inhibition of the ejaculatory reflex. There is a persistent failure to ejaculate in the presence of a satisfactory erection. *Retrograde ejaculation* is a physical impairment of internal vesical sphincter activity.

Female Disorders

Frigidity is a term applied to a wide variety of conditions in the female, from complete lack of any sexual response to various inadequacies in orgasmic response. As it is nonspecific and has a derogatory connotation, the term has been eliminated from most recent classifications. *Generally unresponsive female* (excitement phase dysfunction) is defined as the in-

ability to respond to sexual stimulation with lubrication and genital vasocongestion. *Orgasmic dysfunction* refers to the inability to release the orgastic reflex and have an orgasm, despite ability to enjoy sexual intercourse and have normal sexual desire. There is no distinction between "healthy" vaginal and "infantile" clitoral orgasm. Some women who can have orgasm with direct clitoral stimulation find it impossible to reach orgasm during intercourse. This is a normal variant of sensitivity requiring the pairing of direct clitoral contact with intercourse. *Vaginismus* is an involuntary spasm of the musculature of the outer third of the vagina, making penile penetration impossible.

Both Sexes

Dyspareunia is a condition defined as painful intercourse in both sexes leading to avoidance of sexual contact. *Low libido* is defined as a lack of desire to engage in sexual activity for both males and females.

PSYCHOLOGIC MECHANISMS AND CLINICAL PRESENTATIONS

While organic conditions should never be overlooked (see Chapters 113 and 131), the vast majority of sexual problems in both sexes are at least partially psychologic in origin. There are usually complex and multiple causes. Although there are no rigid correlations between certain background factors and dysfunctional syndromes, sexual disorders can be related to prior experiences. Early sexual attitudes may be negatively shaped by parental communication that sex is bad, dirty, or sinful, by inadequate information about sex, or by myths and misconceptions such as the ever-ready penis or mutual climax. Other negative experiences include previous unpleasant sexual encounters and rape. Intrapsychic conflicts ranging from fear of sexual failure to concerns about sexual identity and profound depression may be responsible. Interpersonal issues of a sexual as well as nonsexual nature sometimes interfere with sexual functioning, especially in the setting of inadequate communication and lack of cooperation between partners. Sexual problems may develop from such nonsexual factors as situational stress and financial pressures. Lastly, sexual difficulty may occur in the context of the anxiety generated by an organic illness, such as fear of death after a heart attack. Once a sexual problem ensues, regardless of the cause, a vicious cycle of fear of failure, anxiety, and guilt is likely to ensue and remain self-perpetuating.

Just as the causes of sexual problems are multiple, the clinical presentations of these disorders may also be complex. The real nature of the problem can be uncovered as gradual trust between the patient and the clinician develops. Common somatic presentations which have no apparent medical cause include headaches, low back pain, generalized pelvic pain, and vulvar pruritus.

Presentation

Impotence. Most normal men experience an occasional erectile failure due to fatigue, too much alcohol, or any number of transient unfavorable circumstances. The diagnosis of impotence should not be made until there is a failure at intercourse in 25% of attempts. The incidence ranges from 1% of men under 35, to 25% of men over age 70. Although statistics show an increase in the problem with aging, they also indicate that a large number of men can continue normal sexual lives with advanced age.

The prognosis for the condition is directly related to the length of time that the symptom has been present. Prolonged impotence and primary impotence are much more likely to be associated with medical disorders (see Chapter 131) or more serious psychologic issues, such as fears of intimacy, feelings of intense hostility toward women, and gender identity questions.

Premature Ejaculation is the most common male sexual disorder and its increasing incidence is linked with women wanting more sexual satisfaction, particularly orgasm. If the premature ejaculation occurs over a long period of time and remains untreated, secondary impotence may result. It is often easily treated in the context of a good relationship. The prognosis is very good. Of course, physical factors must be ruled out (see Chapter 131).

The psychologic causes of the disorder range from early conditioning to ambivalence and hostility toward women. Once premature ejaculation occurs, it can easily be reinforced by the negative attitudes expressed by the partner. In addition, prolonged periods of no sexual experience seem to make the premature ejaculation worse.

Retarded Ejaculation occurs in 0.3% of males, most often younger and more sexually inexperienced. In its milder form, which is often related to anxiety-provoked situations, the prognosis is excellent. However, the long-standing condition often signifies deeper-seated psychopathology. The men have significant fears of rejection involved with letting go. Issues of control and commitment are important as well as unconscious conflicts regarding female genitals or pregnancy. Physical causes are rare but must be considered (see Chapter 131).

Generally Unresponsive Women (excitement phase dysfunction) often present with a complete avoidance of sexual activity or an aversion of sex, which is stoically endured. There is often a deep-seated conflict about sexuality which makes the outcome less favorable. There may be concomitant depression and interpersonal problems as well as a history of medications and pelvic pathology (see Chapter 113).

Orgasmic Dysfunction is the most frequent female sexual complaint and occurs more often during the early years of sexual activity. The capacity for orgasm appears to increase with sexual experience and that includes the aging female. Again, the psychologic factors involved are variable and the prognosis for the condition is a function of which factors are responsible. These range from fears of loss of control and unrealistic expectations about sexual performance to poor partner communication. Depression must not be overlooked. Organic factors, although unlikely, should also be considered (see Chapter 113).

Vaginismus is associated with a high incidence of pelvic pathology (see Chapter 113). A careful gynecologic examination is always warranted and, in fact, is the only definitive way to make a diagnosis. Vaginismus is one cause of *dyspareunia*. When related to psychologic factors, vaginismus can be considered a conditioned response and treatment must be approached behaviorally. There is often confusion about sexual anatomy and physiology leading to fears of penetration and concerns about femininity. If the condition is longstanding, partners of these women can become seriously affected, developing secondary impotence. This disorder has been at the center of many cases of unconsummated marriages of long duration.

WORKUP

The Sexual History. A brief screening sexual history should be taken as part of every routine medical evaluation. It is most easily done in conjunction with the gynecologic and menstrual review of systems in women and the genitourinary review in men. In this way, sexual concerns can be comfortably elicited in the context of routine history-taking, especially if the physician displays an open, nonjudgmental, unembarrassed, and accepting attitude. One needs to take into account differences in social values, class, and age. Helpful screening questions include: "Does your present sexual functioning meet your expectations?" "Has there been a change in your sexual functioning?" "Would you like to change anything about your sexual functioning?"

If a sexual problem is uncovered, the chief complaint should be explored in detail. Ask the patient to describe the problem in his own words, noting its duration, the circumstances under which it occurs, possible precipitating and alleviating factors, and severity. A thorough description sometimes helps to distinguish an organic from a functional etiology. For example, preservation of erectile function during masturbation or upon awakening in the impotent patient suggests a psychologic cause.

Also try to elicit what type of treatment is viewed as potentially helpful, be it medicine, information, or support. Anything that tends to alleviate the problem, even if only temporarily, should be sought, as should any psychosocial precipitants. While a detailed description of past sexual activity and experiences may be indicated in some cases, the collection of such data is usually deferred until a more intensive psychologic evaluation is undertaken and can be obtained in that context.

Physical Examination And Laboratory Studies. After a clear description of the presenting sexual problem is obtained, a careful physical examination is conducted to search for evidence of a medical etiology; selected laboratory studies may also be indicated (see Chapters 113 and 131). Although most sexual problems are psychogenic in origin, many may have an organic basis or an organic component; this necessitates a thorough medical workup in every case.

PRINCIPLES OF TREATMENT

The primary care physician is often the first person consulted by a patient with a sexual problem. Even the physician without formal training in sex therapy can help many patients deal effectively with their sexual difficulties. When the problem stems from guilt and misinformation, the physician can use his position as an authority figure to give *permission* and *reassurance,* relabelling as "neutral" or "positive" sexual activities that the patient might fear are "bad" or "sinful." *Educating* patients and correcting misinformation is a function that should not be overlooked or underestimated. Giving permission or providing information may be all that is necessary to help many patients.

When the problem goes beyond misinformation, a trial of *behavioral methods* with specific suggestions to patient and partner (see below) can be helpful and is an appropriate next step. The objectives are to increase communication between partners, decrease performance anxiety and "spectatoring," change the goal of sexual activity towards feeling good and away from emphasis on erection or orgasm, and relieve the pressure to perform at each sexual encounter. A trial of such therapy is reasonable when there is no evidence of important underlying psychopathology or organic illness. Behavioral therapy will often lead to improved sexual function without the need for referral; however, couples who fail such therapy might benefit from consultation with a mental health professional trained in dealing with sexual problems.

BEHAVIORAL TECHNIQUES

For Impotence

1. First educate the patient as to his ability to satisfy his partner without having penile vaginal intercourse.
2. Then begin "sensate focus" exercises, which start with

nongenital massage and progress to genital massage. There should be a prohibition against intercourse, even if erections occur.
3. After erection is obtained by genital massage, progress to attempting intercourse. In the female-superior position, the female may manually stimulate the penis, and if erection is obtained, she may insert it into her vagina in a slow, nondemanding fashion, relieving the male of any responsibility for insertion. This may also be done with a partial erection. Gradual movement is begun. There is an emphasis on the pleasures of vaginal containment.

For Premature Ejaculation

1. Educate the patient that his condition has little to do with the sensitivity of the penis but is usually the result of previous conditioning and anxiety.
2. Suggest an increase in the frequency of sexual activity.
3. Teach the Masters and Johnson "squeeze" technique. In this technique, the female manually stimulates the penis. When ejaculation is approaching the point of inevitability, as indicated by the male, the female squeezes the penis with her thumb on the frenulum, her index finger placed above, and her middle finger below the coronal ridge on the dorsal side of the penis. The pressure is applied until the male no longer feels the urgency to ejaculate (15 to 60 seconds). The "squeeze" technique should be repeated two or three times before ejaculation is allowed to occur.
4. Once there are good results with the squeeze technique, the couple can try intercourse. In the female-superior position, the female remains motionless to accustom the male to vaginal containment. Gradual thrusting begins using the "squeeze" technique as excitement intensifies.
5. An alternative to the "squeeze" technique is the "stop–start" method. The female stimulates the male to the point of ejaculation, at which time she stops the stimulation. The erection may or may not subside. She then resumes stimulating the penis. After several stop-start procedures, the male may ejaculate.

For Retarded Ejaculation (During Intercourse)

1. The female stimulates the penis, asking for directions (verbal and physical) to enhance the feeling.
2. Extravaginal ejaculation is obtained by continued stimulation. In the male's mind, the female should become associated with ejaculatory release.
3. The female stimulates the penis manually until orgasm becomes inevitable. The penis is then inserted and the female thrusts demandingly. Manual stimulation is repeated if there is no successful ejaculation.

For Generally Unresponsive Female (Excitement Phase Disorder)

This disorder often results from more severe psychopathology and usually requires referral for treatment. However, on the practical side, suggestions regarding the supplemental use of lubrication such as saliva or KY jelly should be made.

For Orgasmic Dysfunction

1. Change the goal of sexual activity away from orgasm toward enjoyment of the experience.
2. Give permission to the female to express sexual feelings.
3. Begin sensate focus exercises, nongenital massage to genital massage. Use the back-protected position (male in a seated position with female between his legs with her back against his chest) with female in control to alleviate self-consciousness or spectatoring.
4. Instruct the male in stimulative technique: he should not force responsivity but rather seek to accommodate desires; he should not approach the clitoris directly because of sensitivity.
5. After success in manual genital stimulation, controlled intercourse in the female-superior position with the male making no demands comes next. This is followed by a lateral position which allows for mutual freedom of pelvic movement.
6. For women who have never experienced orgasm, suggestions regarding self-stimulation are appropriate. The use of fantasy material is most helpful.
7. For women who do have orgasms with masturbation but not intercourse, the "bridge technique" may be useful. After insertion of the penis, the male can stimulate the female (clitorally) manually or with a vibrator. This pairing can be helpful in achieving orgasm, and often after the female experiences orgasm in this way, the need for supplementary stimulation disappears.

For Vaginismus

1. Explain to the patient and her partner that this condition is involuntary and not willfully caused. Physical demonstration of the involuntary vaginal spasm may be done by inserting a gloved finger into the vaginal entrance.
2. The couple is asked to refrain from intercourse during the early treatment.
3. In a stepwise, gradual fashion, the woman is encouraged to accept larger and larger objects into the vagina. This may be accomplished with the use of graduated Hegar dilators to be used in the office and at home, or the woman may begin by using her fingers, first one, then several approximately the size of the penis. She may use her partner's fingers. Syringe containers of different sizes make good dilators.
4. In the female-superior position, the woman gradually inserts the penis.

INDICATIONS FOR REFERRAL

After trying these techniques, the patient's condition may still not be improved. This is often a sign that a referral to a psychiatrist who specializes in the area is indicated, and that the patient needs more intensive therapy. Often, direct referral to the specialist is indicated for patients with chronic psychopathology, such as those with "primary" sexual dysfunctions, gender identity questions or homosexual conflicts, marked personality disorders or significant past psychiatric history (especially of psychosis), or overt evidence of a clinical depression underlying the sexual complaint. Moreover, chronic severe problems in the relationship with one's partner signal the need for a referral.

PATIENT EDUCATION

Early in one's practice, it becomes clear that patients have many sexual questions and concerns. Inadequate or inaccurate information about sexual anatomy, physiology, and practices is the basis for many sexual problems. Therefore, sex education should not be overlooked. Patients can sometimes obtain supplemental information from suggested reading material. Several books which might be helpful to the patients include *For Yourself: The Fulfillment of Female Sexuality* by Lonnie Garfield Barbach, New York, Doubleday, 1975; *Male Sexuality* by Bernie Zilbergeld, Boston, Little, Brown, 1978; and *The Joy of Sex,* edited by Alex Comfort, New York, Simon and Schuster, 1972. Of course it is helpful to be available to answer questions which come up in the context of reading. As noted above, an accepting, nonjudgmental, and open approach is essential to helping patients through their sexual difficulties.

ANNOTATED BIBLIOGRAPHY

Croft HA: Managing common sexual problems. Postgrad Med 60(3): 200; 60(4):193; 60(5):186; 60(6):164, 1976 (*Excellent series of articles geared for use by primary care physicians treating sexual problems.*)

Ende J et al: The sexual history in general medical practice. Arch Intern Med 144:558, 1984 (*Recent study looking at aspects of taking the sexual history by the primary care specialist.*)

Kaplan HS: The New Sex Therapy. New York, Brunner/Mazel, 1974 (*Excellent general reference for all aspects of sexuality.*)

Levine SB: Marital sexual dysfunction: Erectile dysfunction. Ann Intern Med 85:342, 1976 (*Good review with many references. Emphasis on definitions of sexual dysfunction.*)

Levine SB, Rosenthal M: Marital sexual dysfunction: Female dysfunctions. Ann Intern Med 86:588, 1977 (*Second part of this general review, with many references.*)

Masters W, Johnson V: Human Sexual Inadequacy. Boston, Little, Brown, 1970 (*Revolutionized the treatment of sexual disorders by proposing a behavioral framework for treatment.*)

Nadelson C: Sexual dysfunction, and treatment of sexual dysfunction. In Lazare A (ed): Outpatient Psychiatry, Chapter 24, p 307 and Chapter 39, p 526, Baltimore, Williams & Wilkins, 1979 (*Good summary of subject with especially detailed and easy to follow considerations of treatment techniques.*)

226

Approach to the Somatizing Patient

ARTHUR J. BARSKY, III, M.D.

The somatizing patient presents with bodily complaints or disability out of proportion to any demonstrable organic pathology. Included in this category are anxious and depressed patients, hypochondriacs, chronic pain patients, and malingerers. These people are among the most frustrating and troublesome encountered in office practice, but they can be evaluated and managed successfully. Attention to the causative psychologic disorder helps to render symptoms understandable, enables the physician to distinguish them from those due to organic pathology, and facilitates management.

PSYCHOLOGIC MECHANISMS AND CLINICAL PRESENTATIONS

Anxiety (see Chapter 222). Individuals suffering from *chronic anxiety* focus on and become alarmed by normal bodily sensations. They report headache, gastrointestinal disturbance, or musculoskeletal pain. *Acute anxiety* can have somatic manifestations; individuals complain of palpitations, chest pain, tachycardia, dyspnea, choking sensations, diarrhea, cramps, dizziness, and fainting.

Depression (see Chapter 223). Depression's neurovegetative symptoms may overshadow the characteristic affective, cognitive, and behavioral changes. As many as one half of somatizing ambulatory medical patients over age 40 are depressed. The chief complaint may be headache, constipation, weakness, fatigue, abdominal pain, insomnia, anorexia, or weight loss. Depressed patients worry about and focus attention upon their bodies; a positive review of systems, chronic pain, or complaints involving multiple organ systems typify the clinical presentation, and symptoms recur with the periodicity characteristic of depressions.

Personality Disturbances exist in a considerable number of somatizers. The terms *crock, hypochondriac,* and *chronic complainer* refer to patients whose symptoms, illness, role as patient, and pursuit of medical care have become a way of life. For them, illness and medical treatment provide a vocabulary for interacting with other people, a way of responding to stress, and a means for expressing psychologic needs and conflicts. Their somatic symptoms are disproportionate to demonstrable structural pathology. They are preoccupied with their bodies and their health, convinced that they have some occult serious medical disease; at the same time, they

fear disease intensely. Their symptoms shift and fluctuate over time, being nonspecific, diffuse, and similar to the transient sensations felt by healthy individuals. Worry about being ill is remarkably persistent, and it is not assuaged by reassurance after thorough medical evaluation. At times, they may have genuine medical problems, but their suffering, disability, and medical care needs are typically in excess of any objective pathology. By their reports, medical care has been disappointing, failing to provide a cure or even relief of symptoms.

When interviewed, they talk mainly about their illnesses and medical care; one hears little about friends, work, or hobbies. They often seem more concerned with establishing the authenticity of their complaints than with obtaining relief. They adamantly refuse to consider the possibility of an emotional cause for their symptoms (in contrast to many patients with demonstrable physical disease, who are willing to consider the possibility).

In attempting to understand these patients, some authorities have emphasized the unconscious meaning and gratification of pain and discomfort. Bodily complaints may be amplified by the deprived and needy person who has only experienced caring and attention when sick or in pain. Suffering and illness can thus become ways to express and gratify yearnings for contact, comfort, and support. Other hypochondriacal individuals are angry and hostile, feeling rejected or wronged in some way. For them, physical symptoms offer a nonverbal way of expressing their anger, recrimination and blame, by reproaching and belaboring others with their suffering. Finally, symptoms and illness can unconsciously serve to distract these individuals from an even more painful sense of themselves as fundamentally worthless and defective as people. They can thus attribute their failures, disappointments, and rejections to a physical incapacity rather than to any personal inadequacy.

Chronic complainers gain self-esteem and a sense of identity from their ability to endure suffering, survive misfortune, and tolerate discomfort. Their requests for relief and cure can be understood as attempts to be respected for their ability to endure and survive rather than as a true desire to end discomfort.

Postconcussion Syndrome is a self-limited condition that follows mild to moderate head trauma. A variety of somatic symptoms (headache, dizziness) accompany emotional ones (depression, sleeplessness, irritability).

Hysterical Conversion Reactions are acute physical disabilities that suggest medical disorder but which are actually the expression of a psychologic need or conflict. The emotional distress is thought of as being "converted" into, or expressed as, physical distress. Symptoms are either sensory or neuromuscular (*e.g.,* weakness, paralysis, ataxia, blindness, aphasia, deafness, anesthesia, paresthesias, or seizures). Conversion symptoms are generally of short duration. The process is unconscious and not objectively provable, but there is often a prior history of similar reactions, major emotional stress prior to onset, apparent symbolic meaning to the symptom (*e.g.,* "heartache" following the loss of a loved one; blindness after viewing a horrifying event), inappropriate lack of concern about the symptom ("la belle indifférence"), major secondary gain, and the presence of other significant psychopathology.

Compensation (or Accident) Neurosis is marked by a wide range of somatic symptoms of undetermined cause that follow an accident in which there is litigation pending. The patient is not consciously aware of any relationship between the symptoms and the legal proceedings, yet the condition subsides when the litigation is concluded.

Somatic Delusions are seen in schizophrenia, severe affective disorders, and organic brain syndromes. These are false, fixed ideas that are often vivid, bizarre, or extraordinary. Unlike hypochondriacal concerns, they do not fluctuate. The individual may believe some extraordinary change has occurred in his body, for example, that his organs are shriveling up, that body parts are deformed or missing, or that foreign objects are inside an orifice or organ.

Malingering is relatively rare outside situations in which illness confers some obvious benefit, as in prisons, among drug addicts, or in individuals under some legal threat. Symptoms are exaggerated, and the subject's description of them may vary with each interview. When the patient is unaware that he is being observed, he may relax the simulation and thus betray himself. Such individuals are frequently sociopaths or drug addicts; some may have worked in a medically related field.

DIFFERENTIAL DIAGNOSIS

The differential diagnosis of somatizing includes anxiety, depression, postconcussion syndrome, conversion reaction, compensation neurosis, hypochondriacal personality disturbance, schizophrenia, and malingering. Multiple sclerosis (see Chapter 161) and polymyalgia rheumatica (see Chapter 156) are among the medical conditions sometimes mistaken for somatization.

WORKUP

Differentiating psychologically induced symptoms from those of organic disease is not always easy (see Chapters 222 and 223), but the quality, timing, and precipitants of symptoms, as well as the patient's response to illness, attitude, and choice of words can be of considerable help (see below). Once a psychogenic etiology is suspected on the basis of the clinical presentation, evaluation should proceed to better define the underlying psychopathology.

Attention is first directed to the symptoms. A complaint whose characteristics are anatomically and physiologically nonsensical is very likely to be psychogenic in origin. For example, psychogenic sensory complaints often cross the midline or involve a combination of sensory modalities that is neurologically impossible (see Chapter 161). Multiple complaints involving many organ systems and many parts of the body suggest depression (see Chapter 223). Hysterical seizures do not involve incontinence or tongue-biting, and the hysterically blind exhibit a withdrawal or startle reflex when a hand is flashed before the face. Psychogenic aphonia may be differentiated from true aphasia in that the ability to read and write is unimpaired in the former. With hysterical paralysis of the upper extremity, the patient's arm avoids the face after being held above it and released. In hysterical paralysis of one lower extremity, attempts to move the afflicted leg do not invoke contraction of the other leg, as is the case in neurologic disease.

Psychogenic pain is typically unaffected by activity or by the passage of time, and the patient often seems more concerned with the physician's accepting the authenticity of his pain than with relieving it. The presence of a significant psychogenic component to a symptom can be suspected when it is exactly like a symptom that afflicted someone important to the patient.

The patient's description may provide important evidence of a psychological cause. Excessively vague, diffuse, and inconsistent descriptions as well as overly detailed, vivid, and elaborate ones are very suggestive. Psychologic factors may be revealed in the choice of words (*e.g.,* "pain in the neck," or "not having a leg to stand on").

Timing and relation to prior events may be helpful clues. Although both physical and psychologic illness can be precipitated by stress, the onset of psychogenic complaints is often closely associated with significant emotional stress, such as the loss of a loved one, or the onset of a major interpersonal conflict or sexual problem. Functional complaints are also prone to occur on the anniversary of a psychologically meaningful event, such as the death of a loved one.

The attitude of the patient toward the symptom should be noted. When the patient is unconcerned, inappropriately calm, or more concerned with establishing the authenticity of his symptoms than with obtaining relief, one should suspect a strong emotional component. Patients with psychogenic complaints who unconsciously derive considerable gain from their illness are often reluctant to consider an emotional cause for their symptoms.

History. The workup of the somatizing patient needs to include inquiry into possible precipitants and response to illness. History is searched for ongoing psychological stress, pending litigation, prior medical complaints without a demonstrable physical cause, depression, anxiety, prior psychosis, and recent head trauma. Details of previous medical care experiences can be revealing. A history of consulting many physicians for the same complaints, or of the immediate replacement of a treated symptom with a new one, help in the diagnosis of psychogenic illness.

It is important to determine if illness, discomfort, and disability have become important parts of the patient's personality and to what extent they are used to deal with emotional discomfort, interpersonal difficulties, and environmental stress. Does the patient see himself as the suffering unfortunate one whose life is filled with disappointment, "bad luck," and defeat, as well as with illness? Expressions of anger and hostility may be indirect, as in cynicism, sarcasm, and uncooperativeness. The individual feels deprived and put upon and is likely to recriminate, accuse and blame. Finally, excessive dependence upon others may be a feature of his personality. One senses an overpowering desire for care, attention, sympathy, and human contact. The patient's attitude toward the physician may have a clinging and hungry quality.

In addition to information about the patient's personality, other psychologically relevant data are helpful for diagnosis and sound management. What personal significance does he attach to his symptoms or to the suspected illness? Are there possible secondary gains, such as (1) receiving sympathy, attention, and support (including financial support) from family and friends, (2) being excused from duties, challenges, and responsibilities (*e.g.,* competing for a promotion at work, having to care for children), and (3) acquiring the power to influence and manipulate others because he is sick.

Physical Examination and Laboratory Studies. A thorough physical examination and a careful mental status examination are essential; not only may unexpected evidence of organic illness turn up, but a normal examination is a prerequisite for effective reassurance and the avoidance of unnecessary laboratory testing. Unless there is evidence that is strongly suggestive of organic pathology, elaborate and, particularly, invasive studies should be avoided. Performing a noninvasive test to help provide reassurance can be constructive, but radiologic and biochemical hunting expeditions may only add to confusion and expense. The likelihood of a false-positive result is high (see Chapter 2).

PRINCIPLES OF MANAGEMENT

Support. Management must be directed at the underlying psychopathology as well as at the presenting bodily com-

plaints. The first step is to put the complaint in perspective, while recognizing that the patient has come because of physical symptoms. When the results of the workup are presented, the reality of the symptoms should not be denied, nor should it be implied that they are imaginary. The patient can be told that serious, damaging organic disease has been ruled out and that stress can amplify real bodily sensations and disrupt normal function. It is important to avoid making the patient feel foolish because there is "nothing wrong." The presence of symptoms is an indication of considerable distress, which the patient should be encouraged to discuss. The patient needs to know that the relationship with his physician will not terminate because the medical workup is negative. Additional visits should be scheduled to provide time to further discuss personal and situational problems on a regular basis. By offering the patient a long-term relationship that is not contingent upon organic symptoms, one may remove a major stimulus for their development. Refractory cases may benefit from referral to a psychiatrist.

Drug Therapy. Nonspecific attempts to suppress somatization pharmacologically should be avoided. All too often, patients are told that their symptoms are due to their "nerves" and sent away with a prescription for a minor tranquilizer. Such an approach to therapy usually fails, and it often alienates the patient. It is especially important to recognize depression because of its high prevalence, subtle manifestations, and good response to therapy. The neurovegetative symptoms of depression respond well to antidepressant medication (see Chapter 223). Anxiety disorder may be helped by the use of a benzodiazepine (see Chapter 222); schizophrenia, by a phenothiazine. The postconcussion syndrome is self-limited, resolving within 6 to 24 months.

Personality Disorders. The primary care physician can manage the majority of somatizing patients having personality disturbances, because the best treatment is supportive. Medical intervention should be minimized whenever possible; in particular, major diagnostic workups involving expensive and invasive tests, especially for equivocal or questionable findings, should be avoided, as should pain medication and tranquilizers. Even though medication is often requested, these patients generally do not respond to it and tend to be especially prone to development of troublesome side effects and adverse reactions.

The patient's need to remain disabled, distressed, and symptomatic must be recognized. The physician must not expect cure, because the patient loses no time in reporting that he is no better, and perhaps is worse. To avoid struggles, the patient, especially if hostile and angry, should be involved as much as possible in therapeutic and diagnostic decisions. The physician ought to make it clear that his role is to help the patient tolerate discomfort rather than to eliminate it. Therapeutic suggestions should be made with the implication that although they may be of some palliative value, they will probably not help dramatically.

The patient's self-esteem needs bolstering. Acknowledging his strength to endure suffering, tolerate discomfort, and survive hardship and misfortune is particularly gratifying to him. These qualities are the ones the patient values most in himself and are the source of what little self-esteem he has.

Conversion Reactions. There are two aspects to the treatment of hysterical conversion reactions: symptom removal and management of the internal conflict to avoid the development of bodily complaints. The first is done through the use of suggestion—hysterical patients are exceptionally suggestive—and education. The patient should be assured that the disorder is self-limited and that the symptoms will gradually improve and finally vanish. Conversion symptoms are likely to recur, however, unless psychotherapy is arranged to alter the psychologic forces at work.

Compensation Neurosis. The best treatment for compensation neurosis is settlement of litigation. Interim therapy includes encouraging the patient not to stop work, minimizing medical treatment of the injury, and stressing its favorable prognosis. Litigation should be completed as soon as possible.

Malingering. Malingering is generally resistant to treatment. Diagnostic and therapeutic procedures should be avoided whenever possible because they reinforce pathologic behavior. Any abnormal laboratory tests or physical findings are suspect.

INDICATIONS FOR REFERRAL

Most somatizing patients can be well managed by the primary physician. Referral is indicated when a patient has accepted a psychologic explanation of his symptoms and wants to see a psychiatrist; when a conversion reaction, serious anxiety disorder, or psychosis is present; or when the primary physician has such a negative reaction to the patient with a personality disorder that he cannot serve him well.

TREATMENT RECOMMENDATIONS

- Explain the results of the medical workup without denying the reality of the patient's discomfort.
- Encourage discussion of psychosocial problems and set up a regular schedule of appointments for further elaboration and supportive therapy. Make it clear to the patient that he need not have physical symptoms to see the doctor. Avoid prn appointments.

- Treat the underlying psychological problem specifically; do not attempt the nonspecific suppression of symptoms with tranquilizers.
- Do not try to remove or cure symptoms in the patient with a somatizing personality disorder. Acknowledge the suffering and provide support. Avoid the use of medication and the extensive workup of vague symptoms. Make adaptation to chronic discomfort the goal of care.

ANNOTATED BIBLIOGRAPHY

Adler G: The physician and the hypochondriacal patient. N Engl J Med 304:1394, 1981 (*A brief review.*)

Barsky AJ: Patients who amplify bodily sensations. Ann Intern Med 91:63, 1979 (*The presence or absence of medical disease is not crucial in managing somatizing patients.*)

Barsky AJ, Klerman GL: Overview: hypochondriasis, bodily complaints, and somatic styles. Am J Psychiatry 140:273, 1983 (*Review of the different conceptualizations that have been advanced to understand hypochondriasis.*)

Brown HN, Vaillant GE: Hypochondriasis. Arch Intern Med 141:723, 1981 (*Clear, explicit, and practical discussion of the role of hostility, aggression, and anger.*)

Drossman DA: The problem patient. Ann Intern Med 88:366, 1978 (*Presents an approach that is useful clinically.*)

Engel GL: "Psychogenic" pain and the pain-prone patient. Am J Med 26:899, 1959 (*This classic article makes the psychology of many types of somatizing comprehensible.*)

Lazare A: Conversion symptoms. N Engl J Med 305:745, 1981 (*Reviews the incidence, etiology, diagnosis, prognosis and treatment of conversion symptoms.*)

Lipsitt DR: Medical and psychological characteristics of "crocks." Psychiatry Med 1:15, 1970 (*How to understand and manage the chronic somatizer.*)

Monson RA, Smith GR, Jr: Somatization disorder in primary care. N Engl J Med 308:1464, 1983 (*A brief review stressing the importance of a long-term physician/patient relationship, recognition that these patients' lives revolve around physical distress, and the importance of regularly scheduled visits.*)

Rosen G, Kleinman A, Katon W: Somatization in family practice: a biopsychosocial approach. J Fam Pract 14:493, 1982 (*Emphasizes the role of the family and sociocultural forces.*)

Smith GR, Monson RA, Ray DC: Patients with multiple unexplained symptoms. Arch Intern Med 146:69, 1986 (*A concise review.*)

Smith GR, Monson RA, Ray DC: Psychiatric consultation in somatization disorder. N Engl J Med 314:1407, 1986 (*A controlled randomized study showing that consultation reduced health care utilization but did not improve health status or satisfaction with care.*)

227
Approach to the Angry Patient
ARTHUR J. BARSKY, III, M.D.

Patients often become angry in response to the suffering and disability caused by disease, adverse life events, or the psychologic threats intrinsic to being a patient. When faced with an angry patient, the primary physician needs to be able to recognize the source of the patient's anger, prevent it from interfering with therapeutic efforts, and help the patient to cope.

PSYCHOLOGIC MECHANISMS

People become angry when they feel threatened or when their wishes and aims are frustrated. Illness often leads to anger since it presents the threat of disfigurement, pain, lost opportunity, abandonment, and even death. Some patients are particularly enraged by the helplessness, lack of control, and enforced passivity that disease confers.

Other patients are uncomfortable in the doctor–patient relationship because it represents the threat of dependence upon the physician—of allowing someone powerful to take control of, take care of, and be responsible for them. They use anger to defend themselves against the intimacy, closeness, and warmth that develop with the doctor in the course of receiving medical care. Anger, then, can be an attempt to drive the physician away and allay the threat of dependency or intimacy which is inherent in the doctor–patient relationship.

Patients commonly express to their clinicians anger derived from threats and stresses they have encountered elsewhere in their lives. In such instances, the animosity and hostility seem inappropriate to the situation and out of proportion to any provocation the doctor can think of. This usually occurs when patients are in conflict with people important to them to whom they cannot express their anger, such as an employer or a spouse.

Other patients appear to have a personality and life-style permeated by a quick temper, chronic resentments, and dissatisfactions. The physician is little more than a screen onto which they project hostility garnered elsewhere. Globally angry patients may have a borderline personality organization. Both in their relationships to the physician and in the other aspects of their lives, they seem to be generally abusive, uncooperative, and ungrateful people. These patients have long histories of relating to physicians and others in a dependent and demanding fashion, exhibiting hostility toward and devaluation of the very people upon whom they depend so desperately. Their anger expresses their sense that people are

menacing and unsympathetic; it also reflects their disappointment at having been let down and not having received the help they feel they need and deserve.

RECOGNIZING THE ANGRY PATIENT

Anger may be expressed verbally in direct statements that convey demands, annoyance, and resentment, as well as in personal histories of temper outbursts and undirected violence (*e.g.,* slamming doors). It may be expressed more obliquely through cynicism, sarcasm, negativism, and behavior which, while superficially compliant, innocent, and cooperative, is actually obstructive. Anger may be evidenced by behavior as well as words, for example, failure to adhere to a medical regimen, keep appointments, or quit self-destructive health habits. Helpful nonverbal clues may be observed during the interview. The angry patient clenches his fists and jaws or knits his forehead in a frown. The palpebral fissures are narrowed, lips compressed, and nostrils widened. Gestures and gait may be explosive. Finally, the interviewer's own subjective, emotional response to the patient during the interview may convey important diagnostic information. Whenever the interviewer is aware of being irritated or bored with the patient, he should question himself as to whether these feelings are an unconscious response to anger and hostility.

It is important not only to recognize that the patient is angry but also to learn what he is angry about. During the interview, the physician should note the subject matter that brings out irritation, annoyance, or hostility. The themes which seem to evoke anger are obvious and important clues to issues that are troubling the patient.

The globally angry patient with a borderline personality organization can be recognized by a few clinical characteristics: (1) interpersonal relationships are either superficial or very dependent and manipulative; (2) emotions are intense and labile, and extreme emptiness and anger predominate; (3) social and intellectual skills may be well developed, but the patient's life is marked by lack of fulfillment and frequent failures; (4) impulsive, manipulative, and self-destructive behavior is present; and (5) past history may include brief psychotic episodes.

PRINCIPLES OF MANAGEMENT

Once the physician has recognized that the patient is angry and has defined any specific threats or frustrations that are fueling the anger, he can proceed to acknowledge the patient's feelings and reassure him that they will not destroy their relationship. This often helps bring about a more open give-and-take discussion between doctor and patient. The physician need not agree that the patient's feeling is justified, but he should acknowledge its existence by explicitly presenting the patient with his observations and the reasons for concluding that the patient is angry. Such discussion can introduce an atmosphere of frankness, honesty, and sensitivity into the therapeutic relationship. The physician conveys the sense that he is not afraid of the patient's feelings and that he will respond not by rejecting but by helping the patient.

If the patient's hostility interferes with communication, the therapeutic regimen, or optimal coping with illness, the doctor should point this out. The physician needs to indicate that while he recognizes the patient's anger and his right to have it, it nonetheless represents a problem because it is self-destructive, interfering with therapy and recovery. One need not be bullied by the globally angry patient; it is possible and necessary to set limits on the patient's behavior while making it clear that there will be no counterattack in retribution.

By defining the specific frustrations and threats, the physician should be able to approach the patient more effectively. For the patient who is angry about being ill, detailed investigation of exact fears and sources of despair is helpful. For the patient who is angry about having to be a patient, the doctor may be able to structure their relationship so as to minimize those aspects which most threaten the patient. If the patient most fears dependency, the physician should assume a somewhat cool, reserved, and proper stance, while still conveying his support and sympathy. Finally, if the anger seems to be displaced upon the physician from some other situation or relationship, this may be pointed out, without specifically encouraging the direct and immediate venting of the hostility upon its actual source.

The physician should take care that he does not react with his own hostility to the angry and provocative patient. Maintaining an objective perspective on the situation will help the physician to recognize when anger is not a criticism of him but rather is a response to the inner torment of threats and frustrated wishes. By doing so, one is in a good position to work with the angry patient, to preserve the therapeutic relationship, to help the patient, and to get on with the business of optimal medical care.

ANNOTATED BIBLIOGRAPHY

Adler G: Valuing and devaluing in the psychotherapeutic process. Arch Gen Psychiatry 22:454, 1970 (*Psychiatric patients express hostility toward their psychiatrists as protection against wishes for nurturance, against envy, against low self-esteem, and as a focal point for rage coming from elsewhere in their lives.*)

Crutcher JE, Bass MJ: The difficult patient and the troubled physician. J Fam Pract 11:933, 1980 (*Empirical research on the types of patients and patient problems that irritate and dismay physicians.*)

Groves JE: Taking care of the hateful patient. N Engl J Med 298: 883, 1978 (*Discussion includes the physician's own emotional responses to patients, and the ways to use these responses constructively.*)

Gunderson J, Singer M: Defining borderline patients. Am J Psychol 132:1, 1975 (*An excellent review identifying basic characteristics of such patients, including intense, often hostile, affect; 87 refs.*)

Kahana RJ, Bibring GL: Personality types in medical management. *In* Zinberg N (ed): Psychiatry and Medical Practice in a General Hospital. New York, International University Press, 1965 (*Though not dealing specifically with the angry patient, this is an excellent discussion of the emotional meaning that illness holds for particular personality types.*)

228

Approach to the Patient with Insomnia

JEFFREY B. WEILBURG, M.D.

Occasional difficulty falling asleep or staying asleep is a universal and normal human experience. Insomnia, defined as persistent difficulty falling or staying asleep that compromises daytime functioning, is also a common problem, with a prevalence of 15% to 20%. Insomnia affects patients of all ages and is particularly troublesome in the elderly.

Most patients with insomnia try a host of techniques, home remedies, and nonprescription drugs before seeking medical help. They frequently come to the primary physician requesting more potent sleep medication. The primary care doctor needs to be skilled in the assessment and therapy of insomnia, not only because the problem is extremely common and a cause of considerable misery but also because it is an important precipitant of excessive drug use and habituation. Almost a billion dollars are spent each year in the United States on medication for sleep.

PHYSIOLOGY AND CLINICAL PRESENTATION

There are various pathophysiologic processes that can cause a patient to experience difficulty falling asleep or staying asleep. These processes have been categorized as the *Disorders of the Initiation and Maintenance of Sleep* (DIMS). In this schema, the term *insomnia* designates the end product (*i.e.,* the symptom) of a DIMS and is formally defined as the complaint of long-standing (more than 2 weeks) trouble falling or staying asleep that is associated with compromised daytime functioning.

By using the polysomnogram (a continuous, all-night recording of a patient's respirations, eye movements, electroencephalogram (EEG), muscle tone, blood oxygen saturation and electrocardiogram), *normal sleep* can be divided into two basic phases: *REM,* or *rapid eye movement sleep,* and *nonREM (NREM).* REM is a state of mental and physical activation. Pulse and respiration are increased but muscle tone is diminished, so little body movement occurs. The brain is active, and the EEG shows a pattern similar to that seen during waking. Most dreaming occurs during REM. In contrast, NREM is a time of deep rest. Pulse, respiration, and EEG all slow, and the patient goes from light sleep, called stages 1 and 2, to deep or delta sleep, called stages 3 and 4. REM and NREM normally cycle in a reciprocal pattern, giving a typical "architecture" to the polysomnogram. The entire cycle lasts about 90 minutes, and is repeated smoothly four or five times during the night.

There is no polysomnographic pattern pathognomonic of insomnia. Some insomniacs have slightly shorter than normal sleep times, some have less stages 3 and 4 sleep, but most have normal-appearing polysomnograms. Recent data suggest that slight disruptions of the normal smooth cycling caused by frequent brief arousals may be related to subjectively unsatisfying sleep. Other data indicate that psychologic variables strongly influence an insomniac's perceptions of the time spent in bed and its influence on satisfaction during the day.

Psychiatric disorders are believed by most experts to be the underlying cause of DIMS in about half of all insomnia cases. Among the psychiatric etiologies, the affective disorders—major depression and dysthymic disorder (mild depression, or the old "neurotic" depression)—account for approximately 50% of the cases. Patients suffering from *dysthymic disorder* typically complain of feeling tired (see Chapter 223). They often feel irritable, have difficulty falling asleep, and report that they cannot get enough sleep to feel rested. Sometimes they deny feeling sad or depressed and focus only on their physical complaints. Indeed, insomnia may be the major presenting complaint in many of these patients.

Patients with *major depression* complain of either difficulty falling asleep or of waking in the early morning and being unable to return to sleep. Diurnal variation of mood is often noted. Severe depression with agitation may lead to markedly diminished total sleep and overall exhaustion (see Chapter 223).

Patients in the *manic phase* of affective disorder have diminished total sleep time but do not report feeling tired during waking times.

Character disorders make up about 40% of the other psychiatrically based DIMS. Patients with anxiety and obsessive disorders frequently have great difficulty falling asleep because they lie in bed and ruminate. Patients with narcissistic or borderline character disorders characteristically feel angry or entitled and may have difficulty falling asleep because they focus on their lack of sleep as the source of all their troubles. They lie in bed, furiously trying to make themselves sleep. Such patients may use their insomnia as a justification for their inability to function or to improve their lives; indeed, some even use it as a rationale for their inability to comply with the treatment of the insomnia itself.

Active psychosis of any type (*e.g.,* schizophrenia) produces disturbed sleep and accounts for the other 10% of psychiatric insomnia. The other signs and symptoms of psychotic illness appear along with the insomnia, facilitating recognition of this problem.

The remaining 50% of DIMS are nonpsychiatrically based. Drug and alcohol abuse are responsible for about 10 to 15% of this group. *Alcohol* induces sedation, but the resulting sleep is often shallow, fragmented, and not restorative. Alcoholics can have prematurely "aged" sleep (*i.e.,* shallow and short) during and for months after cessation of drinking. *Sedatives,* such as most benzodiazepines and especially barbiturates, when used on a regular, long-term basis lead to shallow, fragmented sleep. *Rebound insomnia* and rebound anxiety prompt reuse, and tolerance leads to dose escalation, so patients get caught in a vicious cycle. Sedatives and alcohol depress respiratory function, which can lead to very poor quality sleep in patients with sleep apnea (see below). *Stimulant drugs* such as amphetamine or methylphenidate, activating antidepressants such as phenelzine or protriptyline, and the phenylpropanolamine found in many over-the-counter decongestant, cold, and diet remedies can induce significant difficulty falling asleep. Terbutaline, aminophylline, and other antiasthmatics can produce insomnia. The caffeine and stimulant xanthines found in tea, coffee, cola drinks, and chocolate may produce difficulty falling asleep in most people if used in large enough quantities, and if used at all in some who are sensitive. Finally, the nicotine and other substances found in cigarette smoke have been shown to disrupt sleep induction and continuity.

Medical problems of all types can cause insomnia, and make up approximately 10% of all the DIMS. Pain, of whatever source, is a frequent cause of insomnia in the elderly. Delerium is another frequent cause of insomnia in the elderly. Dementia, unrecognized infection, and even medication toxicity (sometimes secondary to the anticholinergic agents used to induce drowsiness in over-the-counter sleep remedies) are common sources of delerium. Cardiovasacular dysfunction leading to orthopnea, paroxysmal nocturnal dyspnea, or nocturnal angina; chronic obstructive pulmonary disease; hyperthyroidism, and urinary frequency also can produce insomnia.

Primary sleep disorders make up approximately 10% to

20% of all DIMS. *Sleep apnea* is a disorder characterized by repeated, prolonged cessation of respiration, due to transient airway collapse, failure of inspiratory effort, or both. In severe cases, behavioral changes, pulmonary hypertension, cardiac arrhythmias, and death can occur. Patients are often unaware of how disrupted their sleep is and complain only of "insomnia"—that is, they feel exhausted during the day so that they believe they need more or better sleep. As noted above, sedating these patients can be dangerous, as it worsens the apnea. *Nocturnal myoclonus,* characterized by repetitive twitching of the legs, which is also unrecognized by the patient, can produce poor quality sleep and lead to the complaint of "insomnia." *Phase shifts,* which are disruptions in the normal 24-hour wake and sleep cycle, can result from alternating shift work or jet travel across time zones, and can cause patients to be unable to fall asleep at a given clock time, prompting them to complain of insomnia. Endogenous disruptions of the brain's internal circadian rhythm-setter can produce a similar picture.

The remaining 10% to 15% of DIMS include (1) the *primary,* or *idiopathic insomnias,* in which patients have objectively verified difficulty initiating or maintaining sleep in the absence of any identifiable underlying pathology. Some recent studies suggest that these patients may need more, rather than less, sensory input to fall asleep, rather like hyperactive children who require stimulants to control their activity. (2) *Conditioned,* or *"psychophysiologic" insomnia.* These patients have learned to associate bedtime with frustration, anxiety, and sleep-preventing behaviors. They typically sleep very well while away from their usual bedroom, for example, while on vacation or on the living room couch. (3) Persistent complaint of insomnia without objective evidence. These patients persistently complain of insomnia but have objectively normal polysomnograms and no other DIMS. (4) DIMS produced by rare, poorly understood polysomnographic aberrations, such as the intrusion of alpha EEG into delta sleep.

DIFFERENTIAL DIAGNOSIS

Clarification of the patients' complaint is the first step in the differential diagnosis of insomnia (see Table 228-1). Those patients who have excessive daytime somnolence (*e.g.,* they actually fall asleep during the day against their will) do not have "insomnia." Those who are natural "short sleepers" (regularly have less than 7 hours of well-maintained sleep and have no problems other than too much time on their hands at night) likewise do not have insomnia. Those who have a brief, time-limited disturbance of sleep related to stressful events in their lives also do not have "insomnia." The same pertains to the normal elderly patients who experience the decline in total sleep time, depth, and continuity which is a natural part of the aging process.

Table 228-1.   Disorders in the Initiation and Maintenance of Sleep (DIMS)

1. Psychiatric Disorders—50%
   A. Affective disorders: major depression, dysthymic disorder, manic depressive disorder
   B. Character disorders: Anxiety, obsessive-compulsive, borderline, narcissistic character disorders
   C. Psychosis: schizophrenia, other
2. Drug and Alcohol Abuse—10% to 15%
   A. Sedatives: alcohol, benzodiazepines, barbiturates, narcotics
   B. Stimulants: amphetamines, methylphenidate, pemoline, stimulating antidepressants (phenelzine, protriptyline), caffeine and stimulant xanthines in coffee, tea, cola, and chocolate
   C. Antiasthmatics, decongestants: terbutaline, aminophylline, phenylpropanolamine
   D. Cigarettes
3. Medical/Surgical Problems—10%
   A. Cardiovascular: nocturnal angina, orthopnea, PND
   B. Respiratory: COPD
   C. Renal: UTI, urinary frequency
   D. Endocrine: hyperthyroidism and hypothyroidism
   E. Pain of any source
   F. Delirium: dementia, infection, metabolic derangement, medication toxicity (*e.g.,* anticholinergic delirium secondary to OTC sleep aids)
4. Primary Sleep Disorder—10% to 20%
   A. Sleep apnea
   B. Nocturnal myoclonus
   C. Phase shift
5. Other—10%
   A. Idiopathic insomnia
   B. Psychophysiologic, or conditioned, insomnia
   C. Persistent complaint without objective evidence
   D. Unusual polysomnographic patterns: alpha–delta sleep

WORKUP

A careful clinical history, which systematically addresses the host of possible etiologies of DIMS, is the key to the workup of insomnia. Close attention must be given to medication, drug, and food intake, current mental and physical status, past and family medical and psychiatric history, as well as occupational and travel patterns. Physical examination, including laboratory tests (such as urine toxic screens), should be conducted when indicated. Whenever possible, interviewing the spouse, bed partner, or family member is of great value. Finally, the use of a *sleep log,* or diary, which includes time in bed, estimate of time asleep, any awakenings, time of morning arousal, estimate of sleep quality, and comments on unusual events, recorded by the patient directly upon getting up each morning, should be standard procedure in every insomnia workup.

Referral to the sleep laboratory is indicated only if a primary sleep disorder, such as sleep apnea or nocturnal myoclonus, is suspected, or if careful workup fails to reveal the source of the DIMS. Psychiatric consultation is indicated or when character problems interfere with diagnosis or ma

agement, or if the nature of a suspected mental or emotional problem is obscure.

PRINCIPLES OF MANAGEMENT

Precise elucidation of the particular DIMS causing the patient's complaint allows for effective management.

For Depression-Related DIMS. If an affective disorder is present, treatment with a *sedating tricyclic antidepressant* is indicated (see Chapter 223). Patients with dysthymic disorder, and many patients with anxiety disorders, can often benefit from even low doses of sedating tricyclics (such as 25 to 50 mg of amitriptyline or doxepin) taken an hour before bedtime, for a month or more.

For Anxiety-Related DIMS. Most authorities believe that *benzodiazepines* (*BZDs*) can be used safely and effectively in the management of DIMS due to anxiety and other character disorders. However, controversy remains as to the proper frequency and duration of therapy when insomnia is a long-standing problem. Most believe it is best to treat insomnia with a short (1-week) course of BZD therapy, which often helps to reestablish a more normal sleep pattern. Occasional patients require a program of BZD use two to three times per week over longer periods. Before initiating therapy, one should check for such contraindications to treatment as sleep apnea and substance abuse. Alcohol and other sedatives should not be used concurrently because of the risk of oversedation. For patients requiring prolonged therapy, careful monitoring is essential to ascertain efficacy, check for adverse effects, and assure proper dosage and frequency. Drug holidays and attempts at alternative treatment are important components of any therapeutic program that involves prolonged BZD intake. Withdrawal symptoms may develop within 3 to 20 days after cessation of chronic BZD use, especially if abrupt. It is best to taper therapy slowly over several weeks in patients with a history of prolonged intake (see Chapter 222).

Debate also continues on *choice of BZD preparation.* In most instances, the optimal BZD for treatment of anxiety-related DIMS is one with rapid onset of action. Whether one chooses a short-acting or long-acting agent depends upon how much daytime sedation is desired (see Chapter 222). *Flurazepam* (Dalmane) is a widely prescribed, effective agent that induces sleep quickly. Its effects may persist for many hours, making the drug useful for patients in whom daytime anxiety adds to the insomnia problem. Caution must be taken, especially in the elderly, to see that drug accumulation and compromise of daytime function do not appear. Two dosage sizes are available; the 15 mg tablet may be as effective as the 30 mg one and should be tried first. *Diazepam* (Valium) is clinically similar to flurazepam in onset and duration of

effect. Its wider range of available dosage sizes affords more opportunity to identify the smallest effective dose. Tolerance to hypnotic effects and propensity for abuse limit the utility of diazepam. *Temazepam* (Restoril) is effective, but onset of action can be slow, necessitating intake an hour or more before bedtime, which potentially limits its usefulness in patients whose primary problem is difficulty in falling asleep. Rebound insomnia and agitation have been reported. *Triazolam* (Halcion) is a very potent, short-acting BZD, with rapid onset of action. Because of its potency, the potential for adverse reactions is high, especially in the elderly. Care must be taken to use triazolam at the lowest possible dosage (no more than 0.125 mg per day in the elderly).

Chloral hydrate has an unpleasant smell but can be effective in patients for whom benzodiazepines are not indicated. *Antihistamines* such as diphenhydramine can be used for some patients in whom the small but measurable decrement in respiratory drive produced by other sedatives is a problem; however, anticholinergic side-effects can be troublesome.

In the elderly, sedatives should be used in reduced dose and with caution, if at all (see Chapter 222). Explanation of how the normal aging process affects sleep, emphasis on sleep hygiene (see below), and empathetic support are often the best course for many patients. *Barbiturates, meprobamate,* and *over-the-counter drugs* should not be used.

Psychotherapy, often in conjunction with medication, can be useful for patients with affective or character problems. *Antipsychotic agents* can relieve insomnia and agitation in psychotic or delirious patients. Treatment of pain or underlying medical problems, proper withdrawal and then abstinence from drugs or alcohol, and attention to any primary sleep disorder are effective when these DIMS are present.

PATIENT EDUCATION

The overall promotion of good "*sleep hygiene*" is useful for many patients. Establishing a regular bed and wake time, avoiding any and all naps, having regular exercise (although not at night), using bed only for sleeping or lovemaking (rather than reading or watching TV), and getting in bed only when ready for sleep (leaving bed if sleep is not forthcoming) are useful suggestions. Avoidance of caffeinated foods, stimulants, cigarettes, and alcohol are necessary for some sensitive patients.

Instructing patients about these basic rules of sleep hygiene, and helping them to avoid trying too hard to fall asleep, is often useful. Disabusing patients of the myth that everyone must have 8 hours of sleep every night makes many people feel relieved. Also, informing patients that much of the time they spend in bed believing they are "only drowsy" is time

spent actually in the lighter stages of sleep can ameliorate some patients' frustration.

THERAPEUTIC RECOMMENDATIONS

- If the DIMS is related to affective disorder, begin a sedating tricylic antidepressant, such as amitriptyline 25 mg or doxepin 25 mg, to be taken an hour before bedtime every night for at least a month. Increase the dose as needed.
- If the DIMS is related to anxiety or other personality disorder, offer psychiatric consultation and treatment, require close adherence to good sleep hygiene. If the insomnia persists and daytime anxiety is also a problem, begin therapy with a before-bed dose of flurazepam (15 mg). If daytime sedation is not desired, treat with triazolam (0.125 mg qhs).
- If the DIMS is related to drug, alcohol, or other substance use, clearly inform the patient that improvement is based on proper substance withdrawal and the maintenance of abstinence. Supervise withdrawal; support the patient's efforts at maintaining abstinence. Try to avoid treating "dry" alcoholics with sedatives, as this may rekindle their drinking.
- Treat any underlying medical DIMS; a brief course of benzodiazepine therapy after treatment can re-establish the sleep pattern and boost patient confidence.
- Use reduced dose and caution when prescribing sedatives for the elderly.
- Withdraw benzodiazepine therapy slowly in tapering fashion over 1 to 2 weeks to avoid rebound insomnia if drug therapy has been used daily for more than 6 to 8 weeks.
- Refer patients with primary sleep disorders, or those who are refractory to all efforts, for evaluation by a sleep laboratory.

ANNOTATED BIBLIOGRAPHY

Association of Sleep Disorders Centers: Diagnostic Classification of Sleep and Arousal Disorders (1st ed). Prepared by the Sleep Disorders Classification Committee, Roffwarg HP, Chairman. Sleep 2(1):21, 1979 (*Outline of the current classification of all the sleep disorders, with description of each disorder.*)

Choice of benzodiazepines. Medical Letter 23:41, 1981 (*Authoritative discussion of criteria for drug selection, with reference to speed of onset and duration of action as important properties to consider in selection.*)

Coleman RM et al: Sleep–wake disorders based on a polysomnographic diagnosis. JAMA 247:997, 1982 (*More technical discussion of the various sleep disorders based on the PSG.*)

Consensus Conference: Drugs and insomnia. The use of medications to promote sleep. JAMA 1251:2410, 1984 (*Good discussion of hypnotics, in terms of efficacy and side effects.*)

Kales A, Caldwell AB, Soldatos CR et al: Biopsychosocial correlates of insomnia. II. Patterns specifity and consistency with the Minnesota Multiphasic Personality Inventory. Psychosom Med 45: 341, 1983 (*One of an excellent, long-running series of articles on insomnia. Good bibliography.*)

Kales A, Kales J: Sleep disorders. N Engl J Med 290:487, 1974 (*A classic article nicely outlining the sleep disorders and their treatment.*)

Kales A, Soldatos CR, Bixler EO, Kales JD: Rebound insomnia and rebound anxiety: A review. Pharmacology 26:121, 1983 (*Supplements above article; good clinical focus.*)

Triazolam—a new benzodiazepine for insomnia. Medical Letter 25: 32, 1983 (*Concludes it is an effective short-acting, rapid-onset agent useful for short-term treatment of insomnia, with little production of residual drowsiness.*)

229
Approach to the Patient with Obesity
CAROLYN J. CRIMMINS, M.P.H., R.D.

Obesity is a major public health problem. Eighty million Americans are considered overweight and 40 million are clinically obese. Thirty percent of men and 40% of women between the ages of 40 and 49 are at least 20% above the "ideal" weight as defined by insurance company studies. The prevalence of obesity is higher with advancing age and with decreasing socioeconomic status. Recent statistics indicate that the weight of the general U.S. population, particularly that of men of the same height, has been increasing over the last few decades.

Obesity costs billions of dollars annually when medical complications, lost wages, and expenditures for weight reduction efforts are taken into account. Obese persons may or may not be fat for psychologic reasons, but their obesity can be the cause of untold psychic pain and physical discomfort. Morbid obesity (>100% or >100 pounds overweight) is a health hazard with 12-fold increase in mortality for persons aged 25 to 34. The earlier (ages 20 to 29) the onset of overweight in adult life the more pronounced an effect it has on mortality later in life. The most important medical complication of obesity is an increase in mortality from coronary artery disease, due to the development or exacerbation of such cardiac risk factors as adult-onset diabetes, hypertension, and hyperlipidemia. The Framingham heart study illustrated that obesity is a significant *independent* predictor of cardiovascular disease. Obesity is also associated with increased incidence of impaired pulmonary function, surgical risk, osteoarthritis, gallbladder disease, and cancer mortality.

Weight loss is not a cure for obesity. It has been reported that 95% of people who lose weight regain lost pounds and often some more, within the first year. To properly manage the obese patient the primary physician must understand and identify the factors contributing to obesity as well as demonstrate sensitivity to its social and psychologic hazards (see below).

One must be able to put dieting in perspective and recommend the most comprehensive, safe, and effective weight reduction program for each patient. Utilizing a registered dietitian can facilitate the effort. Therapy focuses on physical activity, behavior modification, and, in moderately and morbidly obese persons, more aggressive methods for promoting weight loss. Patients frequently go from one fad diet to another, sometimes jeopardizing their health in the process. Consequently, the components and health consequences of popular diets and nonprescription drugs must be understood, as well as the methods and efficacy of the various self-help weight loss group programs available in the community.

PATHOPHYSIOLOGY AND CLINICAL PRESENTATION

In the simplest sense, obesity results when intake of food exceeds caloric needs. Why this happens is usually far from clear, inasmuch as the mechanisms responsible for alteration of appetite and caloric needs and stimulation of excessive food intake are still not well understood. The hypothalamus plays a role in the regulation of appetite. Destructive lesions of the ventromedial nucleus lead to appetite arousal, including hyperphagia. A lateral but less well-defined region of the hypothalamus seems to be responsible for integration of food-selecting behavior: injury to this region can result in aphagia and inactivity in other spheres.

A small fraction of obese patients have an identifiable genetic, neurologic, or endocrinologic disorder. More often, psychologic, developmental, dietary, exertional, socio-occupational, and pharmacologic factors operate and interact in a complex fashion to precipitate weight gain. Contrary to popular belief, there is no definitive evidence that obese people utilize food more efficiently than slender people. However, some obese patients have demonstrated a physiologic resistance to slimming, and some slender normal volunteers have shown a resistance to experimental fattening.

Psychologic Factors. Emotional problems frequently contribute to the onset and perpetuation of obesity. In many, obesity results from overeating as a pattern of coping with emotional turmoil during important events. *Loss* often prompts overeating, be it loss of a significant person, body part, or function. Sometimes it is not the loss itself that causes the problem but merely the threat of separation or rejection. Another major setting for "compensatory" eating is *frustration,* such as that due to anger at a spouse in the context of a dependent-hostile relationship. In either loss or frustration, eating becomes a *defense* to ward off the pangs of anxiety, depression, or even self-destruction. Other people lose their appetite when they are angry, tense, or "blue." There is no known explanation of why some people develop reactive hyperphagia while others react to stress with anorexia. Indeed, considerable research has been unable to determine any particular personality organization or cluster of psychologic defense mechanisms clearly linked to obesity.

Developmental obesity refers to excessive weight gain that begins in childhood as a result of prenatal influences, constitutional and environmental factors, and, probably most important, rearing practices. The prognosis for reversal of childhood onset obesity is generally poor. Eighty percent of overweight children become overweight adults. There is a 70% to 75% likelihood of becoming obese if both parents are obese; a 40% chance of obesity if one parent is obese and the other lean; and if both parents are lean there is a 10% chance of obesity. Although fat children can in themselves pose many problems for their parents, most often it is the parents who have deep-seated psychologic conflicts long antedating the child's overeating and overweight. Obesity that begins in early childhood is associated with changes in fat cell numbers and composition, body image distortion, and refractoriness to later weight reduction (often because of a striking depression that accompanies weight loss).

Despite the negative medical and societal responses to obesity and the poor self-image associated with it, many obese people have *difficulty keeping weight off.* Often this is because of emotional problems that arise during such efforts. Weight reduction can *precipitate severe depression* or even psychosis, especially in people with a history of childhood-onset obesity or weight loss-induced depression. Those with the *night-eating syndrome,* characterized by insomnia, massive late evening "refrigerator raids," and morning anorexia also experience particular emotional distress when trying to reform their eating behavior. Usually there are coinciding social stresses as well. Indeed, because of the rigors of weight reduction, people undergoing considerable situational distress should be advised to defer weight reduction programs until the psychosocial situation has stabilized.

Having survived the pitfalls and potential *complications* of weight reduction, the formerly obese person faces new problems. Many now find that previously unsatisfactory, though stable, relationships begin to fall apart when their morbid image is shed. Moreover, *new sexual demands* may be encountered by people who previously had avoided such demands by remaining fat and physically unattractive. Some obese women have prominent fantasies of promiscuity and fear they would "act out" sexually should they lose weight and become physically attractive. In sum, loss of obesity poses new psychologic and interpersonal challenges which may be resisted and compromise efforts for change.

Biologic Factors. Theories continue to emerge on the biologic factors which contribute to development of obesity. Problems with thermogenesis, numbers of fat cells, and biologic set point have been postulated. Animal experiments examining *thermogenesis* by brown fat suggest that this tissue might serve as an energy buffer. Brown adipose tissue dissipates substantial amounts of energy in the form of heat during eating and during exposure to cold. It is hypothesized that obese people might be more susceptible to weight gain because they have a *disturbance* in the mechanism of normal *energy release* which should occur at time of food intake. Too little energy dissipation would result in greater preservation of calories and, eventually, in obesity, even under conditions of modest food intake which might not lead to obesity in a person with normal brown fat thermogenesis. To date, studies have been limited to animals, but the findings are intriguing and might help to at least partially explain why some people eat unrestrictedly and never gain weight while others become obese in spite of strenuous efforts to limit intake.

The *fat cell theory* holds that hyperplastically obese people (a small subset of the total obese population) are likely to be very heavy because of their large number of fat cells and very efficient lipoprotein lipase, which facilitates accumulation of energy and results in a lower caloric requirement for weight maintenance and gain.

The *set point theory* views each person as having an ideal biologic weight that is maintained by internal physiologic and psychologic signals. The body resists being displaced from this set point weight by adjusting rates of energy expenditure. After weight loss, the number of calories needed for weight maintenance is reduced because of this marked decrease in the rate of energy expenditure. The set point is defended by control of both the ingestion of food and its rate of energy expenditure. Exercise, not dieting, lowers the set point.

Neurochemical research has provided new insights into appetite regulation. The neurotransmitter *serotonin* may influence regulation of food choice, specifically the ability to choose a desired proportion of carbohydrates in the diet. Common abnormalities in eating behavior, such as *carbohydrate craving,* may be related to disturbances in serotonin-mediated neurotransmission.

Some patients seem to have an unwise preference for foods high in fat and calories. It has been shown that these people may have a *biologic predisposition* to consume foods high in energy density. In our society this problem is more pronounced because these "fattening" foods are not only readily available but their consumption is often encouraged. Another factor in dietary obesity involves the *timing of food intake.* There is some evidence that those who eat once daily,

particularly before going to bed, may be prone to accumulate adipose tissue.

The contribution of *decreased physical activity* to the initiation, propagation, and maintenance of obesity is unclear, but available evidence suggests a role. It has been noted that obese people exercise and move about less than nonobese people. The question of whether inactivity precedes or follows obesity is unanswered. The athlete who stops running a mile a day and does not reduce his caloric intake can gain 11 to 22 pounds a year.

Pharmacologic agents have been shown in many instances to stimulate food intake, especially of carbohydrate-rich products. For example, amitriptyline (Elavil), the *tricyclic antidepressant,* often produces the "blind munchies" several weeks to months after the patient has begun to recover from depression. *Antipsychotic agents* such as chlorpromazine, thioridazine, trifluoperazine, and haloperidol also have been associated with considerable appetite stimulation and weight gain. Among the *antipruritic agents,* cyproheptadine (Periactin) has produced significant increases in appetite and weight gain; the same occurs when a patient is initially placed on *corticosteroids.*

Endocrine disturbances are more often the result rather than the cause of excess weight. However, *hypothyroidism* has been found to account for up to 5% of cases in some series (see Chapter 102). *Cushing's syndrome* is a rare cause and is usually accompanied by characteristic features of truncal obesity and peripheral muscle wasting. *Stein–Leventhal syndrome*—polycystic ovaries, absent menses, and moderate hirsutism (see Chapter 109)—often goes unrecognized as an endocrinologic form of obesity; the precise mechanism of the obesity is unknown. *Eunichism* and *hyperinsulin states* may also be associated with obesity.

Neurologic causes of obesity are usually not cryptic; they mostly result from *hypothalamic injury,* as occurs with craniopharyngiomas, encephalitis, or trauma. Visual field defects or headaches are usually present. Two rare types of neurologic disease without obvious CNS symptoms have been described. Kleine–Levin syndrome consists of periodic hyperphagia and hypersomnia. A second syndrome is characterized by preoccupation with food and accompanying electroencephalographic abnormalities that respond to phenytoin.

The importance of *genetic influences* in determining human fatness was underscored in a large-scale Danish study of adopted subjects. There was a strong relation between weight class of adoptees and their biologic parents, but none between adoptees and their adopted parents. A large American twin study reaffirmed the premise that obesity is under substantial genetic control.

Socio-occupational obesity is commonplace. Excess weight occurs far more frequently among people in lower socioeconomic classes (1 in 3) than among those in upper socioeconomic classes (1 in 20). Whether this difference represents dietary preference, socially motivated behavior, or interactional factors is unclear. In certain occupations, such as wrestling, obesity is a help, not a hindrance. In former times, corpulence was a sign of prosperity and cultivated by bankers and businessmen.

WORKUP

Determination of Obesity. Obesity is a pathologic condition characterized by an accumulation of fat much in excess of that necessary for optimal body function. To establish whether an individual is obese requires first a measurement of body fat. It is then necessary to relate body fatness to some standard or range of acceptable degrees of fat for the particular population under study.

The *"eyeball test"* for obesity still holds true: if a person looks fat, he is fat. However, the most widely used quantitative indices used to identify obesity are the *anthropometric measurements* such as height, weight, and skinfold thickness. These measurements correlate well with the more sophisticated methods for determining obesity, such as total body radioactive potassium-40 densitometry, that are for research purposes only and impractical in clinical practice.

The best single simple determinations of adiposity are measurements of *skinfold thickness.* Use of suitable skinfold calipers on triceps and subscapular skinfolds provides a reasonable index of an individual's fatness. However, reliability can be a problem when using skinfolds as a measure of fatness, because body fat increases with age, grossly obese patients are difficult to measure, and results vary among providers using the calipers.

The chief advantage of utilizing *height* and *weight tables* to assess overweight is the simplicity with which measurements can be made. There are serious limitations, however, to the use of these tables as yardsticks of overnutrition. Standard charts often list "ideal" or desired weights that are based on actuarial data indicating weights associated with lowest mortality or greatest longevity, yet it is not necessarily the weight per se that minimizes morbidity or incidence of disease. The person having a significant percentage of lean body mass, such as a physical laborer, may well exceed "ideal" body weight yet not be obese. On the other hand, some individuals may be within the ideal range but have noninsulin-dependent diabetes mellitus, mild hypertension, or other conditions that would benefit from modest weight reduction.

The Metropolitan Life Insurance Company has published revised reference weights in an attempt to isolate the effect of weight alone on longevity; individuals with major diseases, such as cancer, diabetes, or heart disease were omitted from the study (see Table 229-1). However, the consensus of the American Heart Association and the National Institutes of Health is to recommend continued use of 1959 tables, arguing that basing tables only on mortality ignores possible nonfatal risks of increased weight.

Table 229-1.   Optimal Weights,* in Pounds, for Adults Aged 25 and Over (Light Clothing)

HEIGHT (IN SHOES)	SMALL FRAME	MEDIUM FRAME	LARGE FRAME
Men			
5 ft 2 in	112–120	118–129	126–141
5 3	115–123	121–133	129–144
5 4	118–126	124–136	132–148
5 5	121–129	127–139	135–152
5 6	124–133	130–143	138–156
5 7	128–137	134–147	142–161
5 8	132–141	138–152	147–166
5 9	136–145	142–156	151–170
5 10	140–150	146–160	155–174
5 11	144–154	150–165	159–179
6 0	148–158	154–170	164–184
6 1	152–162	158–175	168–189
6 2	156–167	162–180	173–194
6 3	160–171	167–185	178–199
6 4	164–175	172–190	182–204
Women			
4 10	92–98	96–107	104–119
4 11	94–101	98–110	106–122
5 0	96–104	101–113	109–125
5 1	99–107	104–116	112–128
5 2	102–110	107–119	115–131
5 3	105–113	110–122	118–134
5 4	108–116	113–126	121–138
5 5	111–119	116–130	125–142
5 6	114–123	120–135	129–146
5 7	118–127	124–139	133–150
5 8	122–131	128–143	137–154
5 9	126–135	132–147	141–158
5 10	130–140	136–151	145–163
5 11	134–144	140–155	149–168
6 0	138–148	144–159	153–173

* Weights associated with the lowest mortality rates (derived from actuarial data, Metropolitan Life Insurance Company).

Body Mass Index (BMI = [body weight in kilograms] divided by [height in meters]^2) based on the 1959 tables shows a direct and continuous relationship to morbidity and mortality in studies of large populations. The National Institutes of Health Consensus Development Conference on the Health Implications of Obesity recommended that health professionals adopt this as an index for evaluating obesity (see Fig. 229-1).

A *height/weight formula* provides a quick and easy way for determining a patient's ideal body weight as well as estimating the degree of overweight.

Female: allow 100 lb for first 5 feet of height plus 5 lb for each additional inch.
Male: allow 106 lb for first 5 feet of height plus 6 lb for each additional inch.

Appropriate weight goals for patients can be determined only by a thorough analysis of the medical history and physical findings, supplemented by appropriate laboratory evaluation.

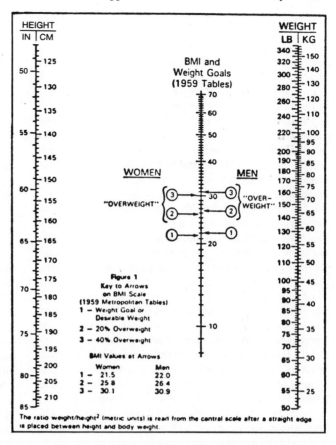

Figure 229-1. Nomogram for body mass index (kg/m²). Weights and heights are without clothing. With clothes, add 5 lb (2.3 kg) for men and 3 lb (1.4 kg) for women and 1 in. (2.5 cm) in height for shoes. (J Am Diet Assoc 85:1119, 1985. New weight standards for men and women. Stat Bull Metrop Life Ins Co 40:1, 1959)

Weight and Diet History. An extensive weight history should include age of onset of obesity, identifiable circumstances associated with the onset of obesity, and highest and lowest adult weight. The patient's past dieting attempts, duration of the effort, and the weight loss attained and maintained should be noted, as well as physical activity patterns. This information can be used to arrive at some mutually agreed upon short-term and long-term goals. A careful review of ongoing psychologic and situational stress is also essential.

Workup for Underlying Medical Etiology. Brief workup for an underlying endocrinologic or neurologic cause should be carried out because of its implications for treatment. *History* should include questions about cold intolerance, hoarseness, change in skin and hair texture, amenorrhea, hirsutism, easy bruising, weakness, drug use, visual disturbances, and headaches. In the *physical examination,* it is important to check for moon facies, hirsutism, dry, thickened skin, coarse hair, truncal obesity, pigmented striae, goiter, adnexal masses, lack of secondary sex characteristics, delayed relaxation of ankle jerks, and visual field deficits. Evaluation should include assessment for consequences of obesity, such as symptoms and signs of hypertension (see Chapter 13), diabetes (see Chapter 100), and osteoarthritis (see Chapter 144).

Laboratory testing is probably more productive for de-

tecting the metabolic consequences of obesity than for revealing etiology. Two-hour postprandial glucose, cholesterol, fasting triglyceride, and uric acid tests are sufficient to detect common metabolic abnormalities resulting from excess weight. Thyroid-stimulating hormone (TSH) is the most sensitive indicator of primary hypothyroidism and worth ordering if there is a clinical suspicion based on history of physical examination. Laboratory testing for Cushing's syndrome is of low yield unless symptoms or signs are suggestive. An overnight 1 mg dexamethasone suppression test is a reasonable screening procedure. When a mass lesion in the region of the sella turcica is suspected, computed tomography is much more sensitive than simple skull films for detection of sellar enlargement.

PRINCIPLES OF MANAGEMENT

Treatment of any underlying medical etiology takes priority over other forms of therapy and may in itself suffice. For the vast majority of obese patients without a definite medical cause there are guidelines for selection of a treatment modality.

In our society there is enormous pressure to be thin. Overweight persons tend to be preoccupied with their weight and have a persistent concern with dieting. Recognition that obesity is a physiologic process rather than simply a problem of deficient will power must be considered; this recognition aids in understanding why it is difficult for some patients to lose weight and keep it off once lost. Stunkard states, "Much of a physician's job is to help patients to exercise cognitive controls over powerful biological systems, in effect, learning to live in a semistarved manner."

Weight loss should not be the only attainable goal for patients embarking on a weight reduction program; careful attention must be focused on treatment of weight obsessions such as poor self- and body-image, disordered eating patterns created by dieting, disordered life-style marked by inadequate exercise, and metabolic depression produced by dieting.

The physician can help select the appropriate weight reduction method by having a knowledge of available treatment programs, community resources, and the patient's preferences. No one program has been shown to be effective for all obese persons. A key factor is motivating patients to alter their current life-style habits.

Patients seeing the physician for the first time about obesity, whether it is of recent onset or long-standing, often respond to dietary and exercise counselling. The decision to lose weight may be part of a complex decision to improve the conduct of one's life; consequently, the physician should be aware that by the visit the patient may be asking for permission to make environmental or life-style changes, or to resolve some nagging conflicts in a close relationship.

The conventional treatments of obesity include diet, self-help groups, fasting, drug therapy, and surgery. Promising approaches to weight reduction involve concentration on dietary counselling, exercise, behavior modification, and very low calorie diets that produce rapid weight loss.

Diet. A Public Health Service report stated that at any given time at least 20% of the population—40 million people—are on some kind of weight loss diet (see Appendix). The word "diet" has a negative connotation implying that going on a diet is followed by going off a diet, with resumption of old eating patterns. *The most effective diet is not a diet at all but rather a gradual change in eating habits and exercise that can be followed for a lifetime.* Any weight reduction diet should be nutritionally adequate except for calories and include a variety of foods. Most fad diets are neither nutritionally sound nor based on proven scientific evidence (see Appendix).

A direct approach to weight reduction has been one of prescribing a diet specifically reduced in calories. The central concept is that when intake exceeds expenditure any food will be stored in the body as fat. A deficit of 500 kcal per day can bring about a loss of 1 lb per week (3500 calories deficit = 1 pound weight loss).

One crude formula used to determine the number of calories necessary to maintain an obese person's weight, based on activity levels is:

- Obese female: 8 to 10 calories × present weight in pounds
- Obese male: 10 to 12 calories × present weight in pounds (sedentary female patients allow 8 kcal per pound, active male patients allow 12 calories per pound)

When following a prescribed dietary regimen, the patient must realize that initial rapid weight loss may occur because of a negative fluid balance. After 2 to 3 weeks the rate of weight loss slows down. Most subsequent loss reflects the catabolism of fat. Loss of fat is directly proportional to the size and duration of the energy deficit. Patients often become discouraged when they enter the slower phase. Some individuals tend to adjust to caloric restriction by unknowingly diminishing their energy expenditures. Some form of physical activity is essential to any weight reduction program.

Self-Help Groups. Self-help group programs offer available, cost-effective services for the obese and others who seek the benefit of group support (see Appendix). Weight control programs into which behavioral self-management techniques are incorporated have been shown to be an effective treatment for mildly to moderately overweight patients.

Diet Workshop and *Weight Watchers* are examples of group programs with a nutrition component. Cookbook approaches to dieting are offered, (*e.g.,* preprinted calorie-restricted balanced diets). The background qualifications and experience of instructors vary widely. A registered dietitian usually serves as a consultant or is on staff at headquarters. Members attend at least one meeting a week, at which they are weighed. Tips on coping, low-calorie recipes, and other strategies for dealing with weight control are discussed.

Overeaters Anonymous (OA) is a self-help group modeled after alcoholics anonymous, having 12 steps, 12 "traditions," and a view that overeating is an addiction that can be controlled but not cured. It appeals to those who see themselves as "compulsive eaters." The program's primary emphasis is on controlling the addictive behavior. Members are encouraged to follow any diet that works for them; some use the available deficit-calorie diet plans. The support system is extended beyond the meetings by pairing new members with more experienced members, who act as advisors. Before eating in the morning new members phone in their meal plan for the day. This serves as a commitment and a daily food record, in addition to providing a daily contact for motivation.

Pharmacologic Treatment. Pharmacologic treatment is commonly requested by patients who have trouble controlling their food intake. *Amphetamines* and amphetaminelike drugs have been the most widely used agents for appetite suppression, but they can produce bothersome side-effects such as *sleep disturbances,* nervousness, and diarrhea, not to mention their serious potential for addiction and development of tolerance. Weight loss is at best temporary, even with continued use, since eating habits are usually not altered. Prolonged use may lead to fatigue and depression. The role of amphetamines and amphetaminelike agents in weight reduction is debatable;

if used at all, these agents should be prescribed for a brief period to supplement other efforts.

Over-the-counter diet pills usually contain phenylpropanolamine and/or benzocaine, often in combination with vitamins or caffeine. There is no available evidence proving their efficacy for weight control, and they can be dangerous, especially those containing phenylpropanolamine. They have received much attention in the lay press because some published reports show small degrees of weight loss with their use. *Phenylpropanolamine* is a sympathomimetic substance used as a nasal decongestant and promoted as an active weight-reducing agent. It is found in many over-the-counter appetite suppressants (*e.g.,* Dexatrim, Appedrine, Dietac, Dex-a-Diet, Prolamine). Phenylpropanolamine is contraindicated for patients with heart disease, hypertension, diabetes, or hyperthyroidism. Reported adverse reactions include acute psychotic episodes, hypertension, hypertensive crisis, renal failure, cardiac arrhythmias, and death. *Benzocaine,* a topical anesthetic, is sold in candy and gum to dieters. Use of such nonprescription agents should be strongly discouraged.

When drugs with appetite-stimulating effects are being used in treatment of a severe psychiatric disorder, such as schizophrenia or endogeous depression, the substitution of *molindone* for other neuroleptics and of *desipramine* or protriptyline for amitriptyline can lessen drug-initiated excessive eating.

In the rare instance of abnormal food preoccupation and binge eating in association with electroencephalographic abnormalities, *phenytoin* may alleviate the problem. More commonly, binge eaters have primitive, impulsive characters often diagnosed as borderline states. With successful psychotherapy, these regressive episodes tend to disappear as more healthy defenses and a less chaotic life-style emerge.

Dietary Counselling. Dietary counselling is an ongoing process provided by registered dietitians. Registered dietitians (RD) are skilled professionals whose education and training are specifically directed to translating the science of nutrition and food and the art of food preparation to the provision of nutritional assessment and dietary counselling services. In individual or group counselling, the RD attempts to help people assess and change their attitudes toward food and what are usually lifelong problem eating habits, to provide people with sufficient knowledge to make appropriate decisions in a multitude of eating-related situations faced every day, and to encourage people to increase their daily activity. An assessment is made integrating medical concerns with the individual and/or family life-style, economic status, learning ability, and psychologic needs. The RD uses a multi-intervention approach, individualized for the patient. Nutrition counselling offers distinct promise for increasing patient adherence to a dietary regimen which maximizes optimal care.

Exercise. An exercise or physical fitness component should be included in any weight loss program. Most obese persons are less active than lean people, but it is not known whether this is a cause or consequence of obesity. Energy expenditure and basal metabolic rate decrease with weight loss on calorically restricted diets. Exercise, in conjunction with a low-calorie diet, increases the metabolic rate. Thermogenesis produced by eating is enhanced and the metabolic rate has been shown to increase for a number of hours after the exercise is completed.

Increased physical activity for many obese people can promote weight loss and decrease body fat. Lean body mass is preserved when exercise and diet are combined. Obese individuals use more energy and burn more body fat for the same amount of activity than normal-weight individuals because the energy cost of most exercise is proportional to body weight. The amount of exercise needed to decrease body fat is related to duration and intensity of the exercise.

Exercise may also benefit the dieter by increasing feelings of self-control, reducing stress, improving appearance and alleviating depression.

A critical element in any exercise prescription is to be able to provide specific guidelines for an obese person ready to begin an exercise program (see Chapter 10). To tell a patient to "get more exercise" is not enough to mobilize a sedentary obese person. Adherence to exercise programs has a poor track record. Thirty percent or more of obese patients have been found to drop out of physical training programs— swimming or jogging—and one study reported that only 32% of obese women completed a 1-year exercise program requiring just walking.

General guidelines which may aid in implementing a realistic exercise plan with the patient include:

1. Begin at the patient's level of current activity (see Chapter 10). Walking for 10 minutes a day may be a lot for a sedentary individual. Encourage routine activity (*e.g.,* park some distance from destination, use stairs instead of the elevators).
2. Encourage a specific time of the day to exercise regularly (early morning, lunch hour, after work).
3. Exercise needs to be done consistently (like brushing the teeth every morning). Patients should work toward a 30-minute session four or five times a week.
4. Encourage use of a diary to chart progress. Self-monitoring reinforces effort.
5. Encourage activity with a friend, co-worker, or family member. Referral to a credible group-exercise facility may be indicated.
6. When an activity other than walking is undertaken it must be easily accessible and fit the patient's life-style. Swimming is not a reasonable activity for a patient who does not live near a pool (or who cannot swim.)

In order to keep weight off once lost, exercise must become a permanent component of an individual's life-style.

Behavior Modification

Behavior modification has come into prominence as a method of weight reduction since the best results ever recorded in outpatient treatment of obesity were published in 1967. Behavioral treatment is directed toward the mildly to moderately obese. Operant conditioning techniques appear to be somewhat more effective than aversive techniques, in which a noxious stimulus is paired with food. Experimental data have shown that obese patients are more prone to respond to external cues than are control subjects of normal weight. Each individual has a pattern of eating behavior; the stimuli that trigger a complex system of response chains may be situational, physiologic, or emotional. The aim of the behavioral approach is to substitute an alternative eating behavior that is practical and leads to decreased caloric intake.

Four general principles are utilized:

1. Description of the behavior to be controlled (*e.g.,* patients are instructed to keep records of all eating behaviors, including daily weight, time and place of eating, stimuli preceding eating that the individual is aware of, and description of surroundings)
2. Modification and control of stimuli
3. Development of techniques to control the act of eating (*e.g.,* decreasing speed of eating by counting mouthfuls)
4. Prompt reinforcement of behaviors that delay and control eating

Patients are advised to eat only in one room (cue elimination), to have company while eating (cue supervision), to develop methods of making diet food attractive (cue strengthening), to arrange for deviations from the diet, and to arrange for positive feedback if they comply with exercise and diet programs. Distracting activities such as watching television or reading while eating are discouraged. Eating behavior is made to be associated with highly specific stimuli.

Group programs utilizing behavioral techniques have been developed. Studies have shown that members of behavior modification groups achieve greater weight reductions than individuals treated with traditional methods, including supportive psychotherapy, instruction in nutrition and dieting, and use of appetite suppressants upon demand. The results are encouraging, but few carefully controlled studies are available. Long-term follow-up studies may suggest that the really significant role of behavior modification is in helping people maintain weight loss regardless of how it was achieved.

Extreme Measures

Very Low Calorie Diets. Very low calorie diets (VLCD) are defined as less than 500 kcal per day. They are potentially dangerous, require close medical supervision, and inappropriate as a "do-it-yourself" regimen. They were introduced in the late 1960s and early 1970s to achieve the more rapid and sustained rate of weight reduction associated with complete starvation while avoiding the inherent risks of starvation.

Protein-sparing modified fasts (PSMF) and liquid protein regimens are two examples of VLCDs. PSMFs provide high-quality protein and essential amino acids as opposed to liquid protein diets, which contain low-quality protein and are deficient in essential amino acids.

The *protein-sparing modified fast* should be restricted to patients more than 30 to 40% above ideal weight; it requires medical supervision. Included in this supervision should be an initial cardiac evaluation and ongoing surveillance. Goals in PSMFs are optimal nitrogen balance and muscle tissue sparing. The PSMF consists of 1.5 g protein/kg ideal body weight per day in the form of lean meat, fish, or fowl; noncaloric beverages; a multivitamin and mineral supplement containing folic acid; 1500 cc fluid/day; 25 mEq potassium, and calcium supplement. The combination of PSMF and behavior modification appears promising. Average weight losses on the diet are 45 lb in fasting periods that last approximately 12 weeks: The PSMF is not recommended for those who are moderately overweight or for children, adolescents, pregnant or lactating women, or the elderly. Also, it should be avoided by those suffering from cardiovascular disease, essential hypertension, insulin-dependent diabetes mellitus, and severe renal or hepatic impairment. Follow-up studies do not exist on this approach. However, comprehensive programs combining very low-calorie diet (to achieve a large initial weight loss) with dietary counselling, exercise training, and behavior modification may offer a solution to the problem of sustained weight loss and maintenance, the limiting factor in long-term success.

Liquid protein diets contain protein of low quality (typically hydrolyzed gelatin or collagen) and should be avoided. They have been associated with *cardiac arrhythmias* and some *fatalities.* Collagen and gelatin are proteins of low biologic value; liquid protein preparations are deficient in potassium, magnesium, phosphorus, and trace elements. Cardiac arrhythmias have been suggested as the major cause of sudden death among patients on liquid protein diets.

Surgical Treatment. Over 25 years ago, surgical interventions were initiated for control of morbid obesity. The morbid form of severe obesity has been defined as "100 lb overweight" or over 200% of desirable weight as defined by the Metropolitan Life Insurance Company tables. The prevalence of severe obesity is only 0.5% of the obese population, yet physicians often encounter these people in clinical practice; morbidity and mortality accelerates rapidly among men and women as their overweight becomes increasingly severe. Medical treatments for the severely obese have been ineffective; surgical methods have been devised.

The choice for surgical intervention should be undertaken only after careful consideration of the risks and benefits with the patient. Selection should be limited to highly motivated morbidly obese patients without serious medical or psychosocial problems who have failed to achieve and maintain significant weight loss with suitable nonsurgical treatments, that is, calorie restriction and behavioral therapy. Specific criteria include absence of untreated psychoses, severe depression, or alcoholism; lack of masochistic or other type of severe characterologic pathology; absence of progressive myocardial, liver, or kidney disease; and availability of adequate financial support should repeated hospitalizations be needed. Patients who are over age 50 may be a greater risk due to their difficulties in adjusting to the potential complications of these surgical procedures. If the Pickwickian syndrome is present, the patient should first go on an inhospital fast until the P_{CO_2} comes back to normal.

The *jejunoileal bypass* was one of the first surgical treatments used, in which the absorptive surface of the intestine was decreased to 18 inches in order to decrease the area available for absorption of fat and other nutrients. Inevitable side effects and severe complications have been associated with this procedure. Side-effects include *severe diarrhea, hypokalemia,* and *hypocalcemia.* The complications include a high incidence of oxalate-containing *kidney stones,* excessive flatulence, arthritis, *liver failure* and development of various nutritional deficiencies, including *protein malnutrition.*

Gastric reduction operations, involving construction of a small 15- to 50-ml pouch connected through a small stoma to an outflow tract, are the current surgical procedures of choice for morbid obesity. Food passes first into the pouch and then into the jejunum in the *gastric bypass type* of reduction procedure, and into the distal stomach and duodenum in the *gastroplasty type.* Gastric bypass appears more effective in promoting weight loss, but gastroplasty is associated with fewer complications. Surgical mortality ranges from 0% to 4%. After surgery, patients must be instructed to *eat small amounts,* eat slowly, chew carefully, avoid eating when not hungry, and take no liquids with meals. Results are impressive, with an average of 50% of excess weight lost in the first 12 months, although it is not clear whether the cause is early satiety or aversive conditioning due to epigastric pain and vomiting with eating too much at one time.

Compared to those associated with intestinal bypass surgery, complications are much less severe and less frequent. They include *outlet obstruction,* deficiencies in thiamine, B_{12}, and folate, and some temporary hair loss believed due to inadequate protein intake. Most of the serious complications of intestinal bypass surgery do not occur, but an increased incidence of *gallstones* has been reported.

Benefits of this procedure include improvement in glucose intolerance, reduction in blood pressure for hypertensive patients, reversal of cardiorespiratory impairment, and reduction of serum cholesterol. Psychosocial benefits are dependent on the degree of weight loss and independent of side effects and complications. The patient with significant weight loss has shown improvement in employability, sex life, physical activity, and self-esteem, and a more gregarious outlook on life.

Suction lipectomy, a cosmetic procedure for removal of localized fat accumulations, has given variable results. Success depends on elastic properties of the overlying skin. Temporary loss of skin sensation, wavy contour, and blood loss are adverse effects.

Total Fasting. Total fasting has been *abandoned* as a drastic form of treatment for obesity due to physical danger to patients and poor maintenance of weight losses. In the 1970s deaths related to fasting were reported.

PATIENT EDUCATION

Motivation is a key factor for successful weight control. The patient must be committed to altering his exercise and eating patterns and must understand that shedding unwanted pounds permanently is not easy. Quick weight loss attempts are popular, but the long-term success rate is discouraging. Patients need to have a realistic attitude about goals and expectations. Support and encouragement are important. Obstacles that may inhibit a patient's progress in a weight reduction program include poor self image and body image, erratic eating patterns, inadequate exercise, and psychologic barriers such as feelings of loneliness, boredom, anger, and depression. Patients need to be informed of the inadequacy of fad diets (see Appendix).

Components of any weight loss program should include:

1. *Nutrition Education.* Knowledge must be provided about basic nutrition principles, such as caloric value of foods and practical methods for changing eating habits. A weight control plan must be individualized to each patient's needs and food preferences. Dietary changes must be gradually implemented to ensure lifelong positive eating habits.
2. *Behavior Modification.* These techniques are effective in promoting weight loss and maintenance:

- Recording of food intake
- Cue elimination (eating only in one place, using smaller plate, no other activity while eating, keeping food out of sight)
- Planning meals (shop from a list, have low-calorie foods available, brown bag lunch, plan strategy before eating out, at parties positioning away from the food table)
- Substituting an alternate activity for eating
- Increased physical activity

INDICATIONS FOR REFERRAL

A weight control plan that includes a well-balanced diet moderately reduced in calories and regular aerobic exercise can be successful for a patient with only a few pounds to lose. When special help is needed for education and guidance the primary physician should recommend an available weight reduction program that is under the direction of a registered dietitian. When emotional problems are too great for primary physician and registered dietitian to handle, patients should be referred to a psychiatrist. Surgical referral is indicated only when nonsurgical approaches have failed and the risks associated with the surgery are less than those of remaining morbidly obese.

MANAGEMENT RECOMMENDATIONS

- A comprehensive approach to weight reduction must be undertaken for successful weight loss and maintenance. Key components include a balanced deficit-calorie diet in conjunction with dietary counseling, behavior modification, and increased physical activity.
- Changes in eating and exercise patterns should be individualized and made gradually in order to maximize the potential for long-term compliance.
- Self-help group programs offer available, cost-effective services for the obese and others who seek the benefit of group support.
- Diets based on unsubstantiated medical claims have popular appeal but are ineffective for long-term weight control. Patients who chronically go from one fad diet to another would benefit from an RD-supervised weight management program.
- Protein-sparing modified fast should be restricted to patients more than 30% to 40% above ideal weight; it requires medical supervision.

Appendix: Popular Dietary Programs for Weight Reduction

According to a 1978 Nielson survey, 45% of all U.S. households have somebody dieting during the course of a year. Fifty-six percent of women aged 25 to 34 said they were dieting. It is rare when a popular diet is not ranked highly on bestseller book lists. People become desperate to lose weight fast and will search vainly for that magic combination of foods that results in loss of excess pounds. Most fad diets capture the attention of dieters by their offer of hope and provision of strict dietary regimens that people believe in.

Popular diets can be categorized into several groups: high protein, ketogenic diets; specific food diets; and calorie-conscious commercial programs. The primary physician must be familiar with the rationale, efficacy, side effects, and complications of the more popular diets and commercial diet programs in order to advise the patient adequately and help in the choice of a safe and practical program for weight loss.

High-Protein, Ketogenic Diets

These diets are very popular in the lay press. They appeal to dieters because there is an initial rapid weight loss. Unlimited amounts of high-protein foods are allowed but with few or no carbohydrates. Low-carbohydrate diets induce fluid loss due to diuresis caused by ketosis. Also, by excluding whole categories of food, there is simply a reduction in the total amount of calories consumed. These diets can be boring

but often attract those people who do not want to make decisions about food.

However, these diets are nutritionally unbalanced. Accumulation of ketones from fat metabolism causes nausea, dizziness, fatigue, and apathy. Excess protein stresses kidneys. High saturated fat intake increases risk of coronary heart disease. Lack of fiber results in constipation. Vitamin and mineral deficiencies are also potential problems. Postural hypotension is not uncommon in the minimally obese subject. No attention is given to the potential for acute gouty attacks resulting from competition of ketoacids and uric acid for renal tubular excretion (see Chapter 155). Examples are:

1. *Atkins Diets.* Unsubstantiated claim that high-protein, high-fat diet triggers secretion of "fat-mobilizing hormone" (FMH) that promotes utilization of fat stores. Claims unused calories are lost via urinary ketones and acetone excretion through expiration. No data exist to support this claim.

   Dietary regimen: Rigid carbohydrate restriction.

   Special conditions: Check ketones daily. Initially permitted to ingest unlimited amounts of certain foods in a fat-to-protein ratio of 40:60% of total calories.

2. *Cambridge Diet (The University Diet).* Very low calorie diet in powdered form. Rapid weight loss with goal of protein-sparing. The FDA has received reports of several cases associated with this diet in which acute illness required hospitalization.

   Dietary regimen: Liquid formula composed of 44 g carbohydrate, 33 g protein and 3 g fat, total 330 calories. Two hundred percent of the United States Recommended Daily Allowance for all vitamins and minerals are included. The FDA has required product labels warning of possible illness or death from such low-calorie formulas.

   Special conditions: Sold directly to the public via ads and door-to-door as part of a pyramid system.

3. *Herbalife Diet Plan.* Similar to Cambridge Diet.

4. *Stillman Quick Weight Loss Diet (Water diet).* Unsubstantiated claim that a food's specific dynamic action (SDA) provides a calorie deficit (*i.e.,* calories are wasted as heat rather than preserved in the form of ATP.) Protein supposedly causes the "system to burn more calories daily." The SDA for protein is approximately 20% of the energy value of food ingested; for carbohydrate the figure is 6%, for fat 4%.

   Dietary regimen: Unlimited quantities of lean meat, poultry, lean fish, eggs, low fat cheese.

   Special conditions: Drink 6-8 glasses of noncaloric fluids a day.

5. *The Complete Scarsdale Medical Diet.* Devised by a famous doctor in Scarsdale, NY, it makes the unsubstantiated claim that "combination of foods can increase fat burning process in the human system." High-protein, low-

carbohydrate diet targeted to busy executive who does not have time to make food decisions.

Dietary regimen: Strict regimen with specific menus.

Special conditions: Stay on diet 2 weeks, no substitutions permitted. After 2-week maintenance program diet resumed for further weight loss.

Specific Food Diets

Emphasis is often on the combination of foods and its effect on metabolism. The diets are monotonous yet require no calorie counting. Unrealistic eating habits are promoted. Serious vitamin and mineral deficiencies could result if these are followed for more than a few days. Examples are:

1. *Beverly Hills Diet.* Unsubstantiated claim that protein and carbohydrate digestive enzymes cannot work together. "Conscious combining" recommended, which involves consuming protein with other proteins, fats, and carbohydrates only with other carbohydrates and fats, and fruits alone.

Dietary regimen: Low-calorie fruit diet.

Special conditions: Combining theory as described above.

2. *High-Carbohydrate Diets* (*e.g.,* Jane Fonda, Pritikin, Bloomingdale's, "Eat to Succeed"). Their premise is that eating high-carbohydrate, high-fiber foods aids weight loss through better satiation on fewer calories. Some are nutritionally balanced, others are not.

3. *Mayo Diet or Grapefruit Diet* (No connection to Mayo Clinic.) Makes unsubstantiated claim that grapefruit contains enzymes that somehow subtract calories by increasing the fat-burning process.

Dietary regimen: Unlimited quantities of meat, fish, bacon, eggs. Limiting sugar and starches.

Special conditions: Eat grapefruit before each meal.

4. *Dr. Berger's Immune Power Diet.* States food allergies responsible for obesity (an unsubstantiated claim) and uses nutritional supplements, which Dr. Berger sells.

Calorie-Conscious Commercial Programs

These programs offer group support and motivation for the dieter. The printed diet plans between 800 and 1500 calories a day. Participants are encouraged to eat a wide variety of foods. Most of these diets can be followed indefinitely, except for those with strict caloric restrictions. These programs should not be recommended without medical supervision and adequate financial resources. (Participation often requires $500 to $2500.)

1. *Weight Loss Clinic.* Promotes eclectic program and quick weight loss.

Dietary regimen: 500 calories a day. Food sources lean animal protein, fruit, and vegetables (45 to 70 g protein, 15 to 25 g fat, 15 to 30 g carbohydrate).

Special conditions: Participants are required to make daily visits to check weight, food records, blood pressure, and urinary ketones; high fees.

ANNOTATED BIBLIOGRAPHY

Anderson T, Backer OG, Stokholm KH et al: Randomized trial of diet and gastroplasty compared with diet alone in morbid obesity. N Engl J Med 310:352, 1984 (*While there was no difference in maximum weight loss, surgical patients sustained their lower weight and had a more favorable outcome at 2 years.*)

Atkinson RL, Russ CS, Ciavarella PA et al: A comprehensive approach to outpatient obesity management. J Am Diet Assoc 84: 439, 1984 (*Successful long-term treatment programs for obesity are nonexistent. An optimistic model for treatment of this chronic disease is outlined.*)

Brownell KD: The psychology and physiology of obesity: Implications for screening and treatment. J Am Diet Assoc 84:406, 1984 (*A review of the psychologic and physiologic causes and consequences of obesity. Current screening and treatment modalities are outlined. Motivation is critical as well as social support, behavior modification, physical activity.*)

Buckwald H: True informed consent in surgical treatment of morbid obesity: The current case for both jejunoilelal and gastric bypass. Am J Clin Nutr 33:482, 1980 (*The risks/benefits of obesity surgery reviewed.*)

Burros M: Diet game, where chances of winning are slim. NY Times Wednesday July 16, 1986 p C1 (*An excellent review of fad diets; for the layman.*)

Callaway CW: Weight standards: Their clinical significance. Ann Intern Med 100:196, 1984 (*Discussion of setting realistic weight goals for patients.*)

Carney RM, Goldberg AP: Weight gain after cessation of cigarette smoking. A possible role for adipose tissue lipoprotein lipase. N Engl J Med 310:616, 1984 (*Interesting finding correlating lipoprotein lipase activity in adipose tissue and the rate at which smokers gain weight after smoking cessation. Authors suggest measurement of enzyme activity may be a useful clinical tool for predicting potential for weight gain for exsmokers.*)

Felig P: Very low calorie protein diets. N Engl J Med 310:589, 1984 (*Editorial providing insight regarding the appropriate clinical use of very low calorie diets.*)

Gastric operations for obesity. Medical Letter 26:113, 1984 (*Concludes these can result in marked weight loss in the massively obese. Fewer short-term complications and so far fewer serious long-term ones compared to ileal bypass.*)

Himms-Hagen J: Thermogenesis in brown adipose tissue as an energy buffer. N Engl J Med 311:1549, 1984 (*An intriguing theory of energy regulation and its implications for obesity and weight control.*)

Hocking MP, Duerson MC, O'Leary P et al: Jejunoileal bypass for morbid obesity. N Engl J Med 308:995, 1983 (*Documents a high rate of continuing side-effects and complications of this procedure.*)

Hubert HB, Feinleib M, McNamara PM et al: Obesity as an independent risk factor for cardiovascular disease: A 26-year follow-up of participants in the Framingham heart study. Circulation 67:968, 1983 (*Significant findings illustrate the independent influence of obesity on cardiovascular disease. These data show the benefits of weight reduction in obesity as well as the harmful effects of weight gain.*)

Leibel RL, Hirsch J: Diminished energy requirements in reduced-obese patients. Metabolism 33:164, 1984 (*Findings in this study show that obese patients who have reduced have an approximately 25% lowered caloric requirement for weight maintenance. Confirms major problem of long-term maintenance of weight losses.*)

Mason AE, Printen KJ, Blommers TJ et al: Gastric bypass in morbid obesity. Am J Clin Nutr 33:395, 1980 (*History and current techniques used in gastric surgery described. Gastric surgery for morbid obesity has become the preferred surgical treatment for weight reduction because of less complicated long-term care required after the gastric procedures.*)

National Institutes of Health Consensus Development Conference: Health implications of obesity. Ann Intern Med 103:977, 1985 (*A definitive review of the issue; finds obesity is a major contributor to morbidity and mortality; essential reading for all primary physicians.*)

Phenylpropanolamine for weight reduction. Medical Letter 26:55, 1984 (*Concludes that effectiveness is limited and risks considerable.*)

Simopoulos AP, Van Itallie TB: Body weight, health and longevity. Ann Intern Med 100:285, 1984 (*Review of epidemiologic studies suggesting that duration of obesity is an independent risk factor for cardiovascular disease and reduced life expectancy. Recommendations for a reference data table that relates body weight to health and longevity are outlined.*)

Suction lipectomy. Medical Letter 26:95, 1984 (*Finds the cosmetic procedure of limited usefulness.*)

Stunkard AJ, Sorensen TIA, Hanis C et al: An adoption study of human obesity. N Engl J Med 314:193, 1986 (*Strong relationship between weight class of adoptees and their biologic parents, but not between them and their adoptive parents.*)

Stunkard AJ, Stellar E (eds) Eating and Its Disorders. Research Publications: Association for Research in Nervous and Mental Disease. Vol 62. New York, Raven Press, 1984 (*Excellent review and comprehensive text on obesity research. Several theoretical models provide insight for the clinical management of the obese patient.*)

Thompson WR, Amaral JI, Caldwell MD et al: Complications and weight loss in 150 consecutive gastric exclusion patients. Am J Surg 146:603, 1983 (*Effectiveness of procedure for weight loss illustrated by these patients followed for 6 years. Complications were mainly postsurgical biliary disease and ventral hernias.*)

Van Itallie TB: Bad news and good news about obesity. N Engl J Med 314:239, 1986 (*An editorial exploring the "nature vs. nurture" issue.*)

Wadden TA, Stunkard AJ, Brownell KD: Very low calorie diets: their efficacy, safety, and future. Ann Intern Med 99:675, 1983 (*Extensive review, composition, dietary treatment, and medical benefits discussed. Short-term use of these diets promote rapid weight loss.*)

Weigley ES: Average? Ideal? Desirable? A brief overview of height–weight tables in the United States. J Am Diet Assoc 84:417, 1984 (*Historical overview of the "reference weight for height" tables. Height–weight tables reflect that stated weights of policyholders aged 25 to 59 at which mortality is lowest. Important to be aware of their derivation if used in clinical setting.*)

230
Approach to Eating Disorders
NANCY A. RIGOTTI, M.D.

Anorexia nervosa and bulimia (the binge–purge syndrome) are psychiatric disorders of disturbed eating behavior that can have serious medical consequences. Over the past decade, they appear to have increased in incidence. Both are more common in women and usually develop during adolescence or early adulthood. The prevalence of anorexia approaches 1 in 200 adolescent females in Western countries, while bulimia may exist in up to 15% of college women. Primary care physicians should recognize these syndromes, be able to evaluate patients for medical complications, assist in ambulatory management, and determine when a patient requires hospitalization.

PSYCHOPATHOLOGY, PATHOPHYSIOLOGY, AND CLINICAL PRESENTATION

Anorexia nervosa is a syndrome of severe weight loss due to inadequate food intake by individuals with no medical reason to lose weight (Table 230-1). Instead, an intense fear of fatness leads to a relentless pursuit of an unreasonable and unhealthy thinness. Weight is lost in two ways. Restrictive anorectics essentially starve themselves. A second group, with coexistent bulimia, loses weight by purging after eating, usually by vomiting or taking laxatives. Bulimic anorectics have a graver prognosis and more medical problems.

Table 230-1.   Diagnostic Criteria for Anorexia Nervosa and Bulimia*

Anorexia Nervosa
1. Refusal to maintain body weight over a minimal normal weight for age and height; weight loss leading to maintenance of body weight 15% below expected.
2. Intense fear of becoming obese, even when underweight.
3. Disturbance in the way in which one's body weight, size, or shape is experienced.
4. In females, absence of at least three consecutive menstrual cycles when otherwise expected to occur (primary or secondary amenorrhea)
5. Absence of any physical illness to account for weight loss.

Bulimia
1. Recurrent episodes of binge eating (rapid consumption of a large amount of food in a discrete period of time).
2. During the eating binges there is fear of not being able to stop.
3. The individual regularly engages in either self-induced vomiting, use of laxatives, or rigorous dieting, exercise, or fasting in order to counteract the effects of the binge eating.
4. A minimum average of two binge-eating episodes per week for at least 3 months.

* Adapted from Diagnostic and Statistical Manual of Mental Disorders, 3rd ed (revised). American Psychiatric Association, 1986.

Anorexia often begins as a diet that gets out of control. The onset frequently coincides with a time of separation from home or the loss of a loved one by illness, death, or divorce. Originally more prevalent in high socioeconomic groups, it is now becoming more evenly distributed among social classes. Psychologic studies portray patients as bright, compulsive, and perfectionistic individuals who perform well at school or work.

Bulimia is characterized by repeated episodes of binge eating, during which individuals rapidly consume large amounts of high-calorie foods, usually in secrecy. The binge is followed by self-deprecating thoughts and, to prevent weight gain, purging. Most bulimics purge by inducing vomiting or using laxatives, but some use diuretics or exercise excessively. Bulimic patients fear losing control of their eating behavior and are ashamed when it happens. Binges may be repeated several times daily. At other times, bulimics may diet rigorously or use diet pills. In severe cases, there may be no regular eating pattern. The result of this behavior is frequent weight fluctuations but not severe weight loss.

Anorectic and bulimic patients differ. Anorectics deny that they are ill, but their emaciation attracts attention. In contrast, bulimics are aware that their behavior is abnormal but often conceal the illness because of embarrassment. The bulimic's near-normal weight permits the illness to be hidden. Detection of surreptitious vomiting or laxative abuse is a challenge for the primary care physician.

Etiologic Factors. The etiology of anorexia nervosa and bulimia is unknown. Anorectics have well-documented neu-roendocrine abnormalities, but these appear to be the consequence, not the cause, of their starvation. Some attribute anorexia and bulimia to problems in emotional development or disturbed family interactions. Others view eating disorders as variants of depression. Anorectics and bulimics share clinical features with depressed patients and may respond to antidepressants. Bulimics have a high prevalence of alcohol and drug abuse, leading some to postulate that bulimia is part of an impulse control disorder.

Cultural pressure to be thin probably contributes to the apparently increasing prevalence of both disorders. Both anorectics and bulimics commonly report that a diet preceded their disease. Bingeing has been observed when experimentally starved normal individuals resume eating, leading to speculation that strict dieting contributes to bulimia.

Clinical Manifestations and their Pathophysiology

Anorexia Nervosa. As noted above, the presentation of the patient with anorexia nervosa is remarkable for the lack of complaints. The anorectic often claims to *feel well* and appears unconcerned about her emaciation, in contrast to patients losing weight because of medical illness, who express concern about their weight loss. Hunger is not a complaint, but patients may report *difficulty sleeping,* abdominal discomfort and *bloating* after eating, *constipation, cold intolerance,* and *polyuria. Amenorrhea* is uniformly present in females. Unlike other starving individuals, anorectics are not fatigued until malnutrition is very severe. Listlessness is an ominous sign. Most are restless and physically active, and some exercise to excess.

Physical examination reveals an *emaciated* patient bundled in clothing. Skin is dry and may be pale (due to anemia) or yellow-tinged (due to carotenemia). Hands and feet are cold and blue. *Fine downy hair,* termed lanugo, may cover face and arms. In women, the female pattern of fat distribution disappears, but axillary and pubic hair are preserved. *Bradycardia, hypotension,* and *hypothermia* are common. The presentation may suggest hypothyroidism or panhypopituitarism.

Restrictive anorexia nervosa is similar to starvation. Diets are deficient in carbohydrates and total calories, but protein and vitamin intake is relatively preserved. Consequently, vitamin deficiencies are unusual. Inadequate nutrient intake results in a loss of weight, fat stores, and muscle mass. Cardiac muscle atrophies, with reduction in left ventricular wall thickness and cardiac output, but congestive failure does not occur. *Arrhythmias* and electrocardiographic changes, primarily low-voltage ST segment depression and T-wave flattening, have been documented. Prolonged QT intervals have been reported shortly before death in three patients. Autopsies of some patients dying suddenly have showed degeneration of myocardial cells, which may predispose to arrhythmias.

Weight loss is also accompanied by a compensatory slowing of metabolism, which reduces energy expenditure and conserves body mass. This is achieved by an *alteration* in *thyroid hormone metabolism.* In starvation, thyroxine is preferentially converted to the inactive reverse-T_3 rather than to the more potent triiodothyronine, as normally occurs. Levels of thyroxine are in the low-normal range, but triiodothyronine levels are reduced, and anorectics have clinical features suggesting hypothyroidism, such as bradycardia, hyopthermia, dry skin, cold intolerance, and constipation. However, there is no compensatory rise in TSH to suggest thyroid gland failure.

The metabolic slowing is accompanied by characteristic clinical and laboratory features. There is a reversible bone marrow depression. Although *mild anemia* is common, it is rarely due to iron, folate, or B_{12} deficiency. Despite *leukopenia,* there is no increased susceptibility to infection. Thrombocytopenia is unusual. *Increased cholesterol* and carotene levels occur in some patients, probably due to an acquired defect in lipoprotein metabolism rather than excess dietary intake of yellow vegetables or cholesterol-rich foods. Blood levels of glucose, protein, amino acids, and insulin are normal or mildly reduced. Severe hypoglycemia and coma have been reported when starvation is very advanced. *Delayed gastric emptying* occurs and explains some of the symptoms of abdominal bloating. The combination of slowed peristalsis and the meager dietary intake results in constipation.

Another consequence of starvation is reversible *dysfunction* of the *hypothalamic–pituitary axis,* which explains the amenorrhea, cold intolerance, and polyuria of anorectics. *Amenorrhea* is accompanied by estrogen deficiency and reduced gonadotropin secretion. A critical amount of body fat must be present to initiate the cyclic gonadotropin release necessary for ovulation. However, weight loss does not entirely explain the amenorrhea, because up to 25% of anorectics lose menses before weight loss is significant, and amenorrhea may persist after weight is regained.

Reduced vasopressin secretion from the posterior pituitary accounts for polyuria. The anorectic's hypothalamus defends core temperature poorly in the face of changes in environmental temperature, resulting in *hypothermia.* Many anorectics have *elevated plasma cortisol* levels that do not respond to an overnight dexamethasone suppression test. However, there are no clinical signs of Cushing's syndrome. Anorectic women have *reduced skeletal mass.* Those with long-standing weight loss may develop *osteoporosis* and vertebral fractures.

Refeeding the anorectic frequently leads to *fluid retention,* which complicates the interpretation of weight changes and frightens the patient. This is a greater problem in the anorectic who purges and is volume-depleted. If fluid retention is severe, congestive heart failure may develop as the increased intravascular volume exceeds the capacity of the weakened heart. Refeeding can also be followed by gastric dilatation, ileus, and transient elevations of liver function tests due to fatty liver. Rehydration may unmask anemia.

Bulimia. The medical consequences of bulimia depend on the specific behaviors present. *Bingeing* has few complications, although *abdominal pain* due to distention is common. Acute gastric dilatation and rupture are rare.

Chronic vomiting has more serious consequences. Repeated regurgitation of stomach contents produces *volume depletion* and a *hypochloremic metabolic alkalosis.* Dizziness, syncope, thirst, orthostatic changes in vital signs, and an elevated BUN occur in the volume-depleted patient. Renal compensation for the alkalosis and volume depletion causes *potassium depletion* and *hypokalemia,* which may predispose to cardiac arrhythmias. Serum and urine chloride are low. Symptoms of hypokalemia are nonspecific: muscle cramps and weakness, paresthesias, polyuria, constipation. T-wave flattening and U waves are seen on the electrocardiogram.

Reversible painless *swelling* of the *parotid glands* can occur with chronic vomiting and is often accompanied by *hyperamylasemia.* Irreversible dental problems also occur. Repeated exposure of the teeth to stomach acid causes *enamel decalcification* and *erosion.* Teeth diminish in size and become discolored and sensitive to temperature changes. Many vomiters have symptoms of *reflux esophagitis.* Sore throat due to mucosal trauma from inducing vomiting is common but hematemesis is unusual. Some patients use *emetine* (ipecac) to induce vomiting. Its chronic use has been reported to cause a reversible proximal *myopathy* and a potentially fatal cardiomyopathy.

The abuse of *laxatives* is a common and potentially dangerous form of purging. It may begin as a response to constipation and continue because of the temporary weight loss it causes. Weight loss is secondary to fluid depletion rather than to a reduced absorption of calories. Stimulant laxatives are used most often. They increase colonic motility, producing *abdominal cramps* and loss of electrolytes in a *watery diarrhea.* Volume depletion, hyponatremia, hypokalemia, and either *metabolic acidosis* or *alkalosis* may result. Calcium and magnesium depletion have also been reported. Irritation of intestinal mucosa or hemorrhoids from rapid fecal transit may cause *rectal bleeding,* and rectal *prolapse* can occur. When laxative abuse stops, transient fluid retention, edema, and constipation are common.

Patients use *diuretics* more often to prevent fluid retention than to induce weight loss. They contribute to a *hypochloremic metabolic alkalosis, hypokalemia,* and *volume depletion.* Dilutional hyponatremia may also occur. In contrast to vomiters and laxative abusers, diuretic users do not have low urine sodium and chloride. Fluid retention and edema occur when diuretics are stopped.

NATURAL HISTORY

About 5% of patients with anorexia nervosa die. Most deaths are sudden, apparently due to cardiac arrhythmias. Fatal hypoglycemic coma has also been reported. The risk of death appears to be higher in patients whose weight loss exceeds 40% of premorbid weight (or 30% if it has occurred within 3 months). Bulimic anorectics with metabolic abnormalities are probably at higher risk.

In follow-up studies, over 75% of anorectics regain weight to near-normal levels, and the majority resume menstruation, but abnormal eating habits and psychosocial problems often persist. Some become bulimic. About 15% of anorectics develop a chronic syndrome, and 5% become obese. Bulimic symptoms, lower weight, and older age at presentation are associated with poor outcome. Little is known about the mortality and natural history of bulimia, but the behaviors can persist for decades.

WORKUP

Anorexia Nervosa

History. Anorexia nervosa should be suspected in patients with unexplained weight loss (see Chapter 7). A careful history can strongly suggest the diagnosis. The history should explore the patient's attitude toward the weight loss, desired weight, and eating habits. A 24-hour dietary recall is more revealing than asking general questions about diet. Detailed weight and menstrual histories should be obtained, including the date and circumstances at the onset of weight loss, minimum and maximum weights, and recent weight changes. Ask all patients about bingeing, vomiting, laxatives, diuretics, diet pills, and emetics, and quantify daily exercise. Patients should be asked about symptoms of malnutrition (fatigue, skin or hair changes), dehydration (lightheadedness, syncope, thirst), hypokalemia (cramps, weakness, paresthesias, polyuria, palpitations), and other symptoms common in purgers (heartburn, abdominal pain, rectal bleeding).

Physical Examination, supplemented by laboratory studies, excludes other etiologies of weight loss and quantifies the severity of malnutrition and dehydration. Height and weight should be measured without street clothing, and orthostatic vital signs and temperature recorded. A careful physical examination is performed, taking particular note of the skin, lungs, heart, abdomen, and extremities.

Laboratory investigation should include a complete blood count, serum electrolytes, BUN, creatinine, liver function tests, glucose, thyroid function tests, and an electrocardiogram. If unusual abdominal pain or diarrhea is present, consider barium studies and stool examination to exclude occult bowel disease. Patients with neurologic signs or symptoms warrant consideration of computed tomography and electroencephalography to exclude tumors and seizure disorders.

Extensive evaluation of symptoms or laboratory abnormalities common to anorexia is not necessary, but if the clinical picture is atypical, the physician must consider other etiologies for weight loss, including malignancy, chronic in-

fection, intestinal disorders (malabsorption, inflammatory bowel disease, or hepatitis), and endocrinopathies (hyperthyroidism, panhypopituitarism, adrenal insufficiency, diabetes mellitus). Tumors of the central nervous system mimic anorexia nervosa in rare cases. Psychiatric illness that can be confused with anorexia include depression, schizophrenia, and obsessive-compulsive neurosis.

Bulimia

History. Making the diagnosis of bulimia requires maintaining a high index of suspicion, because bingeing and purging may be concealed and there are no characteristic physical signs. Clues include a preoccupation with weight and food, a history of frequent weight fluctuations, and complaints common to patients who purge and become dehydrated (dizziness, thirst, syncope) or hypokalemic (muscle cramps or weakness, paresthesias, polyuria). Vomiters may also have hematemesis or heartburn, while laxative abusers may complain of constipation, rectal bleeding, and fluid retention. When the diagnosis is suspected, the physician should ask directly about bingeing and purging and should order serum electrolytes. A direct inquiry may elicit the history from a patient seeking help but ashamed to volunteer the information.

Physical Examination should include a check of postural signs for evidence of volume depletion and a noting of any salivary gland enlargement or scars on the dorsum of the hand suggestive of chronic self-induced vomiting. The teeth are examined for erosion and discoloration. A careful neurologic examination is also indicated to rule out any focal abnormalities indicative of a CNS tumor or seizure disorder which, in rare instances, can mimic bulimia.

Laboratory Studies. Most useful are serum and urine electrolytes, BUN, creatinine, and electrocardiogram. Calcium and magnesium should be measured in laxative abusers. The pattern of serum and urine electrolytes helps to determine the mode of purging.

Any suspicion of CNS disease may be excluded with an electroencephalogram and computed tomography. Some patients who vomit deny that it is voluntary. Organic causes of chronic vomiting should be excluded in these cases with barium studies and liver function tests. The combination of unexplained hypochloremic alkalosis, concern about weight gain, and absence of other pathology strongly suggests bulimia.

PRINCIPLES OF MANAGEMENT AND PATIENT EDUCATION

There is *no single treatment of choice* for anorexia or bulimia. A number of therapies produce short-term weight gain in anorectics, but relapse is common. There is little evaluation of treatments for bulimia. Consequently, most treatment is *multidisciplinary,* combining medical, nutritional, psychologic, and pharmacologic approaches. *Psychologic treatments* include individual or group psychotherapy, behavior modification, and family therapy. Antipsychotics, antidepressants, anticonvulsants, and appetite stimulants have been tried for anorectic and bulimic patients, but few carefully controlled studies have been done. *Antidepressants* have received the most attention and widest use. Both tricyclics and monoamine oxidase inhibitors (see Chapter 223) can decrease the frequency of binge eating in bulimia, even in patients without coexistent depression. Antidepressants are less effective in anorectic patients.

Treatment of the patient with an eating disorder requires attention to both medical and psychosocial problems. In most cases, the primary care physician works with a psychiatrist or psychologist to develop a *coordinated treatment plan* in which the physician assumes responsibility for the patient's physical care while the psychiatrist coordinates psychosocial treatment. The team approach eases the physician's burden when treating a patient who may deny the seriousness of the illness, can be deceptive, manipulative, and angry, and has difficulty trusting the physician. All caretakers must agree on overall goals and stay in contact during treatment. The patient should understand that anorexia is a life-threatening illness and that the first priority is to protect life so that psychiatric treatment can proceed.

The physician should *inform the patient* of the nature of the illness, its seriousness, and potential complications. For anorectics, the necessity of weight gain must be emphasized. Patients who purge should be educated about the consequences of their behavior. The ineffectiveness of laxative or diuretic use for real weight loss should be explained. The connection between the eating disorder and any symptoms or laboratory abnormalities present should be pointed out.

The physician should set guidelines for outpatient management. For anorectics, these should include a *weight goal* and a minimum acceptable weight, below which hospitalization will be required. The minimum weight is usually set at a 40% weight loss from premorbid or ideal body weight. The weight goal is more difficult to determine and is often a point of disagreement between physician and patient. An estimate of desirable weight for height can be derived from standard tables. The weight goal should be at least 85% of this chart weight and, for females, be a weight at which the patient has menstruated. Unless the patient had been obese, it is usually close to the patient's premorbid weight. The patient and all caregivers should know of and agree to these weight guidelines.

One monitors the *weight* and *vital signs* regularly. Weight should be regained slowly, at a rate of 1 to 2 pounds per week, to avoid the risk of congestive heart failure. A dietitian can help formulate an eating plan. *Nutritional supplements* should be added if the patient is unable to gain weight at an acceptable rate. Patients with severe postprandial *bloating* due to poor gastric emptying may benefit from *metoclopramide* (5 to 10 mg orally before meals and at bedtime).

In bulimics or anorectics who purge, *serum potassium* and *orthostatic vital signs* must be monitored, and the patient instructed to eat potassium-rich foods. Maintaining normal electrolytes should be a condition of continued outpatient treatment. If the potassium level falls below normal despite dietary measures, *supplemental potassium* is indicated. This must be given as potassium chloride to correct the metabolic alkalosis that maintains the hypokalemia. Patients should be instructed to take the supplement at a time when purging will not occur; often this is at bedtime. Patients not able to maintain a normal potassium level with supplements require hospitalization.

Complications of refeeding and rehydration should be anticipated and explained. Patients with *pedal edema* can be aided by *support stockings, leg elevation,* mild *salt restriction,* and reassurance that the condition is temporary. Congestive heart failure is treated in the conventional way.

Patients who vomit should be referred for dental evaluation and the irreversibility of enamel loss pointed out. Those using laxatives should be informed of the ineffectiveness of these agents for real weight loss and urged to stop, either abruptly or by gradual tapering. To prevent constipation, patients should increase *dietary fiber,* and may benefit from fiber supplements or stool softeners. A re-equilibration period of several weeks may occur with temporary constipation, fluid retention, and weight gain. For bulimic patients who do not respond rapidly, a trial of *tricyclic antidepressants* should be considered (see Chapter 223). Physicians caring for bulimics should be alert to the possibility of drug and alcohol abuse, which are more common in these patients.

INDICATIONS FOR ADMISSION AND REFERRAL

The primary care physician should assess, then monitor, the patient's physical state to determine whether hospitalization is necessary. It is indicated for severe weight loss, dehydration, and metabolic derangements. Medical criteria for hospitalization include: (1) weight loss of >40% of premorbid or ideal weight (>30% if within 3 months), (2) rapidly progressing weight loss, (3) cardiac arrhythmias, (4) persistent hypokalemia unresponsive to outpatient treatment, and (5) symptoms of inadequate cerebral perfusion or mentation (syncope, severe dizziness, listlessness).

In addition, psychiatric hospitalization may be required for behavior beyond the patient's control or for incapacitating depression.

TREATMENT GUIDELINES

1. Assist in diagnosis by excluding other etiologies for weight loss (see Chapter 7) or purging.

2. Assess the degree of malnutrition, dehydration, and electrolyte disturbance.
3. Educate the patient about the medical complications of the illness.
4. Set guidelines for outpatient management:
   Minimum acceptable weight
   Weight goal
   Weight gain of 1 to 2 lb per week for underweight patients
   Maintenance of normal electrolytes
5. Treat hypokalemia with potassium chloride.
6. Monitor weight, vital signs, and electrolytes during treatment.
7. Consider referral to psychiatrist and nutritionist to aid in management.
8. Criteria for hospitalization are:
   >40% loss of weight (>30% if weight loss occurred within 3 months)
   Rapidly progressing weight loss
   Cardiac arrhythmias
   Persistent hypokalemia unresponsive to outpatient treatment
   Symptoms of inadequate cerebral perfusion or mentation (syncope, severe dizziness, listlessness)
   Severe depression

ANNOTATED BIBLIOGRAPHY

Adler AG, Walinksy P, Krall RA et al: Death resulting from ipecac syrup poisoning. JAMA 243:1927, 1980 (*Repeated use of ipecac to induce vomiting may lead to fatal cardiomyopathy.*)

Bo-Linn GW, SantaAna CA, Morawski SG et al: Purging and calorie absorption in bulimic patients and normal women. Ann Intern Med 99:14, 1983 (*Laxative use does not reduce the proportion of calories absorbed after a standard meal; the weight loss that occurs is by fluid loss from the colon.*)

Harris RT: Bulimarexia and related serious eating disorders with medical complications. Ann Intern Med 99:800, 1983 (*Reviews the medical complications of weight loss and the binge-purge syndrome.*)

Herzog DB, Copeland PM: Eating disorders. N Engl J Med 313:295, 1985 (*An update on diagnosis, pathogenesis, natural history, physical manifestations, and treatment of anorexia nervosa and bulimia.*)

Isner JM, Roberts WC, Heymsfield SB et al: Anorexia nervosa and sudden death. Ann Intern Med 102:49, 1985 (*QT intervals were prolonged on premortem ECGs in three patients who died, with ventricular tachyarrhythmias as the terminal rhythm.*)

Oster JR, Materson BJ, Rogers AI: Laxative abuse syndrome. Am J Gastroenterol 74:451, 1980 (*Reviews medical complications of chronic laxative use, with particular attention to the pathophysiology of electrolyte disturbances.*)

Palmer EP, Guay AT: Reversible myopathy secondary to abuse of ipecac in patients with major eating disorders. N Engl J Med 313:1457, 1985 (*Two patients who chronically used ipecac developed a diffuse myopathy, characterized by proximal muscle weakness and electrocardiographic abnormalities. Myopathy gradually resolved when ipecac was stopped.*)

Pyle RL, Mitchell JE, Eckert ED: Bulimia: A report of 34 cases. J Clin Psychiatry 42:60, 1981 (*An early description of the binge-purge syndrome in normal-weight women.*)

Ratcliffe PJ, Bevan JSL: Severe hypoglycemia and sudden death in anorexia nervosa. Psychol Med 15:679, 1985 (*Report of two patients with anorexia who developed hypoglycemic coma; one died.*)

Rigotti NA, Nussbaum SR, Herzog DB et al: Osteoporosis in women with anorexia nervosa. N Engl J Med 311:1601, 1984 (*Anorectic women have a lower critical bone density than normal controls, and vertebral fractures may occur.*)

Schwabe AD, Lippe BM, Chang RJ et al: Anorexia nervosa. Ann Intern Med 94:371, 1981 (*Review of the clinical, nutritional, and endocrine features of the disease.*)

Schwartz DM, Thompson MG: Do anorectics get well? Current research and future needs. Am J Psychiatry 138:319, 1981 (*Most anorectics regain weight to within 15% of normal, but disordered attitudes toward food and psychiatric symptoms persist in over half. Mortality rate is 6%.*)

Yates A, Leehey K, Shisslak CM: Running—An analogue of anorexia? N Engl J Med 308:251, 1983 (*Speculative article pointing out similar features of anorectics and compulsive runners.*)

Index

Page numbers followed by a *t* indicate tabular material. Page numbers followed by an *f* indicate illustrations.

ISBN 0-397-50717-8

90000

9 780397 507177